COLD SPRING HARBOR SYMPOSIA ON QUANTITATIVE BIOLOGY

VOLUME LII

COLD SPRING HARBOR SYMPOSIA ON QUANTITATIVE BIOLOGY

VOLUME LII

Evolution of Catalytic Function

COLD SPRING HARBOR LABORATORY
1987

COLD SPRING HARBOR SYMPOSIA ON QUANTITATIVE BIOLOGY
VOLUME LII

© 1987 by The Cold Spring Harbor Laboratory
International Standard Book Number 0-87969-054-2
International Standard Serial Number 0091-7451
Library of Congress Catalog Card Number 34-8174

COLD SPRING HARBOR SYMPOSIA ON QUANTITATIVE BIOLOGY

Founded in 1933 by
REGINALD G. HARRIS
Director of the Biological Laboratory 1924 to 1936

Previous Symposia Volumes

I (1933) Surface Phenomena
II (1934) Aspects of Growth
III (1935) Photochemical Reactions
IV (1936) Excitation Phenomena
V (1937) Internal Secretions
VI (1938) Protein Chemistry
VII (1939) Biological Oxidations
VIII (1940) Permeability and the Nature of Cell Membranes
IX (1941) Genes and Chromosomes: Structure and Organization.
X (1942) The Relation of Hormones to Development
XI (1946) Heredity and Variation in Microorganisms
XII (1947) Nucleic Acids and Nucleoproteins
XIII (1948) Biological Applications of Tracer Elements
XIV (1949) Amino Acids and Proteins
XV (1950) Origin and Evolution of Man
XVI (1951) Genes and Mutations
XVII (1952) The Neuron
XVIII (1953) Viruses
XIX (1954) The Mammalian Fetus: Physiological Aspects of Development
XX (1955) Population Genetics: The Nature and Causes of Genetic Variability in Population
XXI (1956) Genetic Mechanisms: Structure and Function
XXII (1957) Population Studies: Animal Ecology and Demography
XXIII (1958) Exchange of Genetic Material: Mechanism and Consequences
XXIV (1959) Genetics and Twentieth Century Darwinism

XXV (1960) Biological Clocks
XXVI (1961) Cellular Regulatory Mechanisms
XXVII (1962) Basic Mechanisms in Animal Virus Biology
XXVIII (1963) Synthesis and Structure of Macromolecules
XXIX (1964) Human Genetics
XXX (1965) Sensory Receptors
XXXI (1966) The Genetic Code
XXXII (1967) Antibodies
XXXIII (1968) Replication of DNA in Microorganisms
XXXIV (1969) The Mechanism of Protein Synthesis
XXXV (1970) Transcription of Genetic Material
XXXVI (1971) Structure and Function of Proteins at the Three-dimensional Level
XXXVII (1972) The Mechanism of Muscle Contraction
XXXVIII (1973) Chromosome Structure and Function
XXXIX (1974) Tumor Viruses
XL (1975) The Synapse
XLI (1976) Origins of Lymphocyte Diversity
XLII (1977) Chromatin
XLIII (1978) DNA: Replication and Recombination
XLIV (1979) Viral Oncogenes
XLV (1980) Movable Genetic Elements
XLVI (1981) Organization of the Cytoplasm
XLVII (1982) Structures of DNA
XLVIII (1983) Molecular Neurobiology
XLIX (1984) Recombination at the DNA Level
L (1985) Molecular Biology of Development
LI (1986) Molecular Biology of *Homo sapiens*

All Cold Spring Harbor Laboratory publications may be ordered directly from Cold Spring Harbor Laboratory, Box 100, Cold Spring Harbor, New York 11724. Phone: 1-800-843-4388. In New York, (516)367-8423.

Symposium Participants

ALTMAN, SIDNEY, Dept. of Biology, Yale University, New Haven, Connecticut

ARMSTRONG, JOHN, Dept. of Drug Metabolism, Smith, Kline & French Research Ltd., Welwyn Herts, England

BAKER, MICHAEL, University of California, San Diego, La Jolla

BALDWIN, ANNE, Dept. of Biochemistry, Stanford University Medical Center, California

BALDWIN, ROBERT, Dept. of Biochemistry, Stanford University Medical Center, California

BALL, ANDREW L., Dept. of Microbiology, University of Alabama, Birmingham

BARTLETT, PAUL, Dept. of Chemistry, University of California, Berkeley

BASHFORD, DONALD, Dept. of Chemistry, Harvard University, Cambridge, Massachusetts

BELFORD, MARLENE, Wadsworth Laboratories, New York State Dept. of Health, Albany

BENKOVIC, STEPHEN, Dept. of Chemistry, Pennsylvania State University, University Park

BENNER, STEVEN, Laboratory for Organic Chemistry, Swiss Federal Institute of Technology, Zurich

BERG, JEREMY, Dept. of Chemistry, Johns Hopkins University, Baltimore, Maryland

BIEBRICHER, CHRISTOF, Dept. of Biochemical Kinetics, Max-Planck Institut, Gottingen, Federal Republic of Germany

BLAKE, COLIN C.F., Laboratory of Molecular Biophysics, University of Oxford, England

BOSWELL, ROSS, Dept. of Haematological Medicine, University of Cambridge Clinical School, England

BOUBLIK, MILOSLAV, Dept. of Biochemistry, Roche Institute of Molecular Biology, Nutley, New Jersey

BRÄNDÉN, CARL, Dept. of Chemistry and Molecular Biology, Uppsala Biomedical Center, Sweden

BRESLOW, RONALD, Dept. of Chemistry, Columbia University, New York, New York

BRUICE, THOMAS, Dept. of Chemistry, University of California, Santa Barbara

BURKE, JOHN, Dept. of Chemistry, Williams College, Williamstown, Massachusetts

CARRELL, ROBIN, Dept. of Haematology, University of Cambridge, England

CARTER, PAUL, Genentech, South San Francisco, California

CAVALIER-SMITH, THOMAS, Dept. of Biophysics, Cell and Molecular Biology, Kings College, London, England

CECH, THOMAS, Dept. of Chemistry and Biochemistry, University of Colorado, Boulder

CEDERGREN, ROBERT, Dept. of Biochemistry, University of Montreal, Canada

CHOTHIA, CYRUS, MRC Laboratory of Molecular Biology, Cambridge, England

CRAIK, CHARLES, Dept. of Pharmaceutical Chemistry, University of California, San Francisco

CREIGHTON, THOMAS, MRC Laboratory of Molecular Biology, Cambridge, England

DARNELL, JAMES, Rockefeller University, New York, New York

DAUTER, ZBIGNIEW, European Molecular Biology Laboratory, Hamburg, Federal Republic of Germany

DAVIES, WAYNE, Allelix, Inc., Mississauga, Ontario, Canada

DEGRADO, WILLIAM, E.I. du Pont de Nemours and Company, Wilmington, Delaware

DOMANICO, PAUL, E.I. du Pont de Nemours and Company, Wilmington, Delaware

DOOLITTLE, RUSSELL, Dept. of Chemistry, University of California, San Diego, La Jolla

DOOLITTLE, W. FORD, Dept. of Biochemistry, Dalhousie University, Halifax, Nova Scotia, Canada

DORIT, ROBERT, Dept. of Cellular and Developmental Biology, Harvard University, Cambridge, Massachusetts

DOUDNA, JENNIFER, Dept. of Molecular Biology, Massachusetts General Hospital, Boston.

EIGEN, MANFRED, Dept. of Biophysikalische Chemie, Max-Planck Institute, Gottingen, Federal Republic of Germany

EISENBERG, DAVID, Dept. of Chemistry, University of California, Los Angeles

EISENSTEIN, EDWARD, Dept. of Molecular Biology and Virus Laboratory, University of California, Berkeley

EPSTEIN, LLOYD, Dept. of Biological Science, Florida State University, Tallahassee

ERIKSSON, ELISABETH, Dept. of Molecular Biology, Uppsala University, Sweden

FERRIS, JAMES, Dept. of Chemistry, Rensselaer Polytechnic Institute, Troy, New York

FITCH, WALTER, Dept. of Biological Sciences, University of Southern California, Los Angeles

FREY, PERRY, Enzyme Institute, University of Wisconsin, Madison

GARDELL, STEPHEN, Dept. of Biological Chemistry, Merck, Sharpe & Dohme Research Laboratories, West Point, Pennsylvania

GERBI, SUSAN, Division of Biology and Medicine, Brown University, Providence, Rhode Island

GILBERT, WALTER, Dept. of Cellular and Developmental Biology, Harvard University, Cambridge, Massachusetts

Gō, Mitiko, Dept. of Biology, Kyushu University, Higashi-ku Fukuoka-shi, Japan

Goodman, Morris, Anatomy Department, Wayne State University School of Medicine, Detroit, Michigan

Grabowski, Paula, Center for Cancer Research, Massachusetts Institute of Technology, Cambridge

Gregory, Steven, Dept. of Experimental Biology, Roswell Park Memorial Institute, Buffalo, New York

Gumport, Richard, Dept. of Biochemistry, University of Illinois, Urbana

Hackert, Marvin, Dept. of Chemistry, University of Texas, Austin

Hall, Timothy, Dept. of Biology, Texas A&M University, College Station

Harayama, Shigeaki, Dept. of Medical Biochemistry, University of Geneva, Switzerland

Hilvert, Donald, Dept. of Molecular Biology, Scripps Clinic and Research Foundation, La Jolla, California

Hingorani, Vijay, Dept. of Biological Chemistry, University of Illinois, Chicago

Humphreys, John, Dept. of Biotechnology, Miles Laboratories, Inc., Elkhart, Indiana

Inoue, Tan, The Salk Institute, La Jolla, California

Jencks, William, Dept. of Biochemistry, Brandeis University, Waltham, Massachusetts

Jones, Alwyn, Dept. of Molecular Biology, University of Uppsala, Sweden

Joyce, Gerald, The Salk Institute For Biological Studies, San Diego, California

Jukes, Thomas, Space Sciences Laboratory, University of California, Berkeley

Jurka, Jerzy, Dept. of Biostatistics, Dana Farber Cancer Institute, Boston, Massachusetts

Karplus, Martin, Dept. of Biophysics, Harvard University, Cambridge, Massachusetts

Keller, Walter, Dept. of Cell and Molecular Biology, German Cancer Research Center, Heidelberg, Federal Republic of Germany

Kendall, Debra, Dept. of Bioorganic Chemistry and Biochemistry, Rockefeller University, New York, New York

Kim, Byung-Dong, Dept. of Plant Science, University of Rhode Island, Kingston

Klar, Amar, Cold Spring Harbor Laboratory, New York

Klug, Aaron, MRC Laboratory of Molecular Biology, Cambridge, England

Knowles, Jeremy, Dept. of Chemistry, Harvard University, Cambridge, Massachusetts

Kolakofsky, Daniel, Dept. of Microbiology, University of Geneva Medical School, Switzerland

Komives, Elizabeth, Dept. of Chemistry, Harvard University, Cambridge, Massachusetts

Korant, Bruce, Dept. of Central Research and Development, E.I. du Pont de Nemours & Company, Wilmington, Delaware

Koshland, Daniel, Dept. of Biochemistry, University of California, Berkeley

Koster, Hubert, MilliGen-Division of Millipore, Bedford, Massachusetts

Kremsky, Jonathan, Genetics Institute, Cambridge, Massachusetts

Krenitsky, Thomas, Dept. of Experimental Therapy, Wellcome Research Laboratories, Research Triangle Park, North Carolina

Kretsinger, Robert, Dept. of Biology, University of Virginia, Charlottesville

Krug, Robert, Dept. of Molecular Biology and Virology, Memorial Sloan-Kettering Cancer Center, New York, New York

Kurkinen, Markku, UMDNJ-Robert Wood-Johnson Medical School, Piscataway, New Jersey

Lai, Michael, Dept. of Microbiology, University of Southern California School of Medicine, Los Angeles

Lake, Jim, Dept. of Biology, University of Southern California, Los Angeles

Laskowski, Michael, Jr., Dept. of Chemistry, Purdue University, West Lafayette, Indiana

Lerner, Richard, Dept. of Molecular Biology, The Research Institute of Scripps Clinic, La Jolla, California

Levitt, Michael, Dept. of Chemistry, Weizmann Institute, Rehovot, Israel

Li, Wen-Hsiung, Dept. of Demographic and Population Genetics, University of Texas Health Science Center, Houston

Mandecki, Wlodek, Abbott Laboratories, Abbott Park, Illinois

Mandiyan, Valsan, Dept. of Biochemistry, Roche Institute of Molecular Biology, Nutley, New Jersey

Marsh, Loren, Dept. of Biology, Texas A&M University, College Station

Massey, Richard, IGEN Inc., Rockville, Maryland

Matthews, Charles, Dept. of Chemistry, Pennsylvania State University, University Park

McLachlan, Andrew, MRC Laboratory of Molecular Biology, Cambridge, England

Mertz, Ronald, Max-Planck-Institut für Biochemie, Martinsried, Federal Republic of Germany

Michel, François, Centre de Genetique Moleculaire du CNRS, Gif-sur-Yvette, France

Milkman, Roger, Dept. of Biology, University of Iowa, Iowa City

Miller, Stanley, Dept. of Chemistry, University of California, San Diego, La Jolla

Mills, Donald, Dept. of Genetics and Development, Columbia University College of Physicians, Surgeons, New York, New York

Miyata, Takashi, Dept. of Biology, Kyushu University, Fukuoka, Japan

MOORE, PETER, Dept. of Chemistry, Yale University, New Haven, Connecticut

MORAS, DINO, Institute de Biologie Moleculaire and Cellulaire, Strasbourg, France

MOWBRAY, SHERRY, Dept. of Biochemistry, University of California, Berkeley

NIERHAUS, KNUD, Max-Planck-Institut für Molekulare Genetik, Berlin, Federal Republic of Germany

NINIO, JACQUES, Institut Jacques Monod, Paris, France

NOLLER, HARRY, University of California, Santa Cruz

NOMURA, MASAYASU, Dept. of Biochemistry, University of California, Irvine

NORTH, GEOFFREY, *Nature,* London, England

OLSEN, GARY, Dept. of Biology and Institute of Molecular and Cellular Biology, Indiana University, Bloomington

ORGEL, LESLIE, Chemical Evolution Laboratory, Salk Institute for Biological Studies, San Diego, California

OSAWA, SYOZO, Biology Laboratory of Molecular Genetics, Nagoya University, Japan

OZEKI, HARUO, Dept. of Biophysics, Kyoto University, Japan

PACE, NICK, Dept. of Biochemistry, Texas A&M University, College Station

PACE, NORMAN, Dept. of Biology, Indiana University, Bloomington

PEEBLES, CRAIG, Dept. of Biological Science, University of Pittsburgh, Pennsylvania

PENNY, DAVID, DEPT. of Botany and Zoology, Massey University, Palmerston North, New Zealand

PERUTZ, MAX, MRC Laboratory of Molecular Biology, Cambridge, England

PETSKO, GREGORY, Dept. of Chemistry, Massachusetts Institute of Technology, Cambridge

PETTER, RUSSELL, Dept. of Chemistry, University of Pittsburgh, Pennsylvania

PICCIRILLI, JOE, Laboratorium für Organische Chemie, ETH Zentrum, Zurich, Switzerland

PILKIS, SIMON, Dept. of Physiology and Biophysics, State University New York, Stony Brook

PLUCKTHUN, ANDREAAS, Dept. of Molecular Biology, Ludwig-Maximilians-Universitat, Martinsried, Federal Republic of Germany

POWELL, MICHAEL, IGEN Inc., Rockville, Maryland

QUIOCHO, FLORANTE, Baylor College of Medicine, Houston, Texas

RAJAVASHISTH, TRIPATHI, School of Medicine, University of California, Los Angeles

RAO, NAGIARAJA, Molecular Genetics Research, Lilly Corporate Center, Indianapolis, Indiana

REANNEY, DARRYL, Science Focus, East Hawthorn, Victoria, Australia

REYNOLDS, FREDERICK, Oncogene Science Inc., Mineola, New York

RHEINBERGER, HANS-JORG, Max-Planck-Institut für Molekulare Genetik, Berlin, Federal Republic of Germany

RICHARDS, FREDERIC, Dept. of Molecular Biophysics and Biochemistry, Yale University, New Haven, Connecticut

ROBERTUS, JON, Dept. of Chemistry, University of Texas, Austin

SAAVEDRA, RAUL, Dept. of Biology, California Institute of Technology, Pasadena

SANTER, MELVIN, Dept. of Biology, Haverford College, Pennsylvania

SCHEINMAN, ANDREW, Dept. of Molecular Biology, University of California, Los Angeles

SCHULTZ, PETER, Dept. of Chemistry, University of California, Berkeley

SCHULZ, GEORG, Institut für Organische Chemie und Biochemie, Universitat Freiburg, Federal Republic of Germany

SCHWARTZ, ALAN, Dept. of Exobiology, University of Nijmegen, The Netherlands

SHARP, PHILLIP, Center for Cancer Research, Massachusetts Institute of Technology, Cambridge

SHUB, DAVID, Dept. of Biological Sciences, State University of New York, Albany

SIGLER, PAUL, Dept. of Biochemistry and Molecular Biology, University of Chicago, Illinois

STACY, DAVID, St. Joseph's Hospital, Atlanta, Georgia

STEITZ, THOMAS, Dept. of Molecular Biophysics and Biochemistry, Yale University, New Haven, Connecticut

STEWART, CARO-BETH, Dept. of Biochemistry and Biophysics, University of California, San Francisco

STOLZFUS, ARLIN, Dept. of Biology, University of Iowa, Iowa City

STUBBE, JOANNE, Dept. of Biochemistry, University of Wisconsin, Madison

SUGIMOTO, NAOKI, Dept. of Chemistry, University of Rochester, New York

SYMONS, ROBERT, Dept. of Biochemistry, University of Adelaide, Australia

TABAK, HENK, Dept. of Molecular Biology, University of Amsterdam, The Netherlands

TAKAHASHI, TADASHI, Biotechnology Developing Center, Olympus Corporation, Lake Success, New York

THILLET, JOELLE, Institut Jacques Monod, Paris, France

THOMPSON, BOB, Dept. of Biology, University of Colorado, Boulder

THORSNESS, PETER, Dept. of Biochemistry, University of California, Berkeley

TINOCO, IGNACIO, JR., Dept. of Chemistry, University of California, Berkeley

TOMITA, FUSAO, Kato Memorial Bioscience Laboratries, Kyowa Hakko Kogyo Co. Ltd., Tokyo, Japan

TURNER, DOUGLAS, Dept. of Chemistry, University of Rochester, New York

UHLENBECK, OLKE, Dept. of Chemistry and Biochemistry, University of Colorado, Boulder

VYAS, NAND, Howard Hughes Medical Institute,

Structural Biology Laboratory, University of Texas, Houston

WATSON, JAMES, Cold Spring Harbor Laboratory, New York

WEINER, ALAN, Dept. of Molecular Biophysics and Biochemistry, Yale University School of Medicine, New Haven, Connecticut

WEISS, ROBERT, Howard Hughes Medical Institute, University of Utah, Salt Lake City

WELLS, JAMES, Dept. of Biocatalysis, Genentech, South San Francisco, California

WERTZ, GAIL, Dept. of Microbiology, University of Alabama, Birmingham

WESTHEIMER, FRANK, Dept. of Chemistry, Harvard University, Cambridge, Massachusetts

WILLS, PETER, Dept. of Physics, University of Auckland, New Zealand

Wimmer, Eckard, Dept. of Microbiology, State University New York, Stony Brook

YANAGAWA, HIROSHI, Mitsubishi-Kasei Institute of Life Sciences, Tokyo, Japan

YONATH, ADA, Dept. of Structural Chemistry, Weizmann Institute, Rehovot, Israel

ZARLING, DAVID, Dept. of Molecular Biology, SRI International, Menlo Park, California

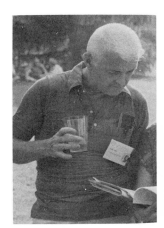
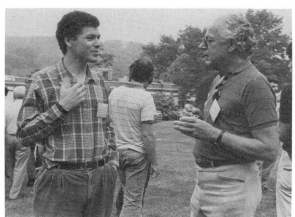
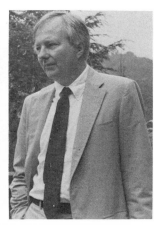
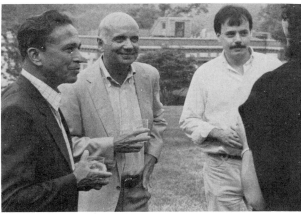
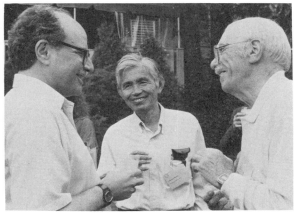
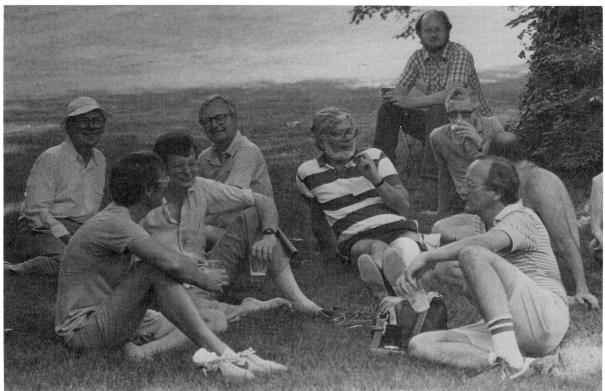

First row: W. Fitch; J. Berg, T. Bruice; J. Darnell
Second row: S. Deodhar, G.M. Browne, J. Maroney; W. Gilbert, M. Nomura, T. Jukes
Third row: Picnic

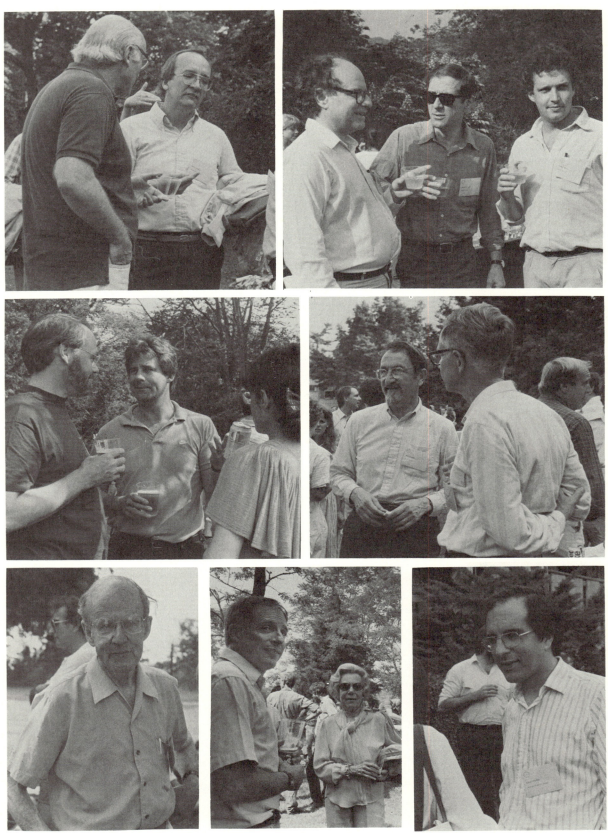

First row: P. Sigler, M. Hackert; W. Gilbert, J. Knowles, R. Dorit
Second row: P. Sharp, J. Hicks, T. Grodzicker; M. Karplus, R. Baldwin
Third row: M. Perutz; D. Eisenberg, L.A. Hazen; C. Chothia

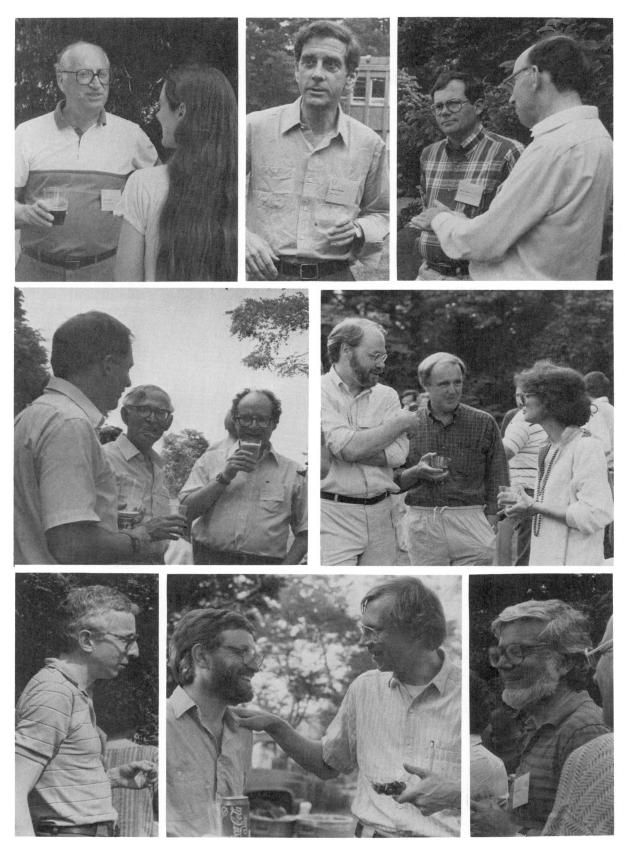

First row: D.E. Koshland, S. Mowbray; J. Knowles; G. Petsko, A. McLachlan
Second row: D. Eisenberg, A. Klug, W. Gilbert; P. Sharp, R. Lerner, E. Watson
Third row: S. Benkovic; M. Mathews, T. Cech; T. Steitz

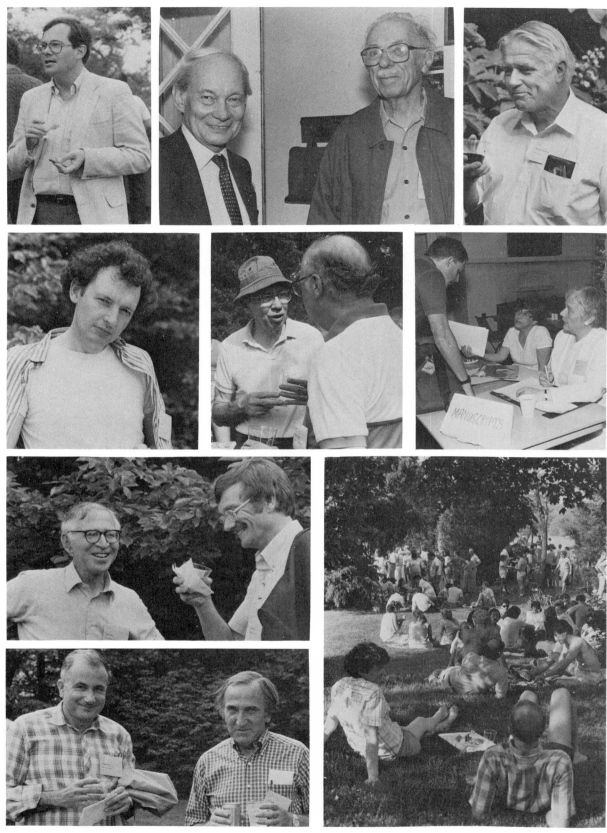

First row: G. Petsko; M. Eigen, T. Jukes; F. Richards
Second row: T.A. Jones; R. Doolittle, D. Koshland; D. Eisenberg, M. Cozza, J. Ebert
Third row: A. Klug, J. Robertus; Picnic
Fourth row: J. Ninio, L. Orgel

Foreword

For all too long, RNA never had the essential simplicity we wanted from it. Unlike DNA, the closer we got to it, the more complex it seemed. Initially, we focused on its informational properties, postulating that it carried the genetic information from DNA to the cytoplasmic sites of protein synthesis. It then seemed natural to believe that the main RNA molecules within ribosomes were the templates for the ordering of amino acids during protein synthesis. Quickly, however, this idea was overturned with the discovery first of transfer RNA and then of the true templates, messenger RNA itself. These seminal discoveries had the positive impact of permitting the basic outlines of protein synthesis to be established, as well as permitting the elucidation of the genetic code. At the same time, the dilemma arose of why RNA played so many different roles. In some profound way, the explanation had to lie in the molecular events that gave rise to the origin of life.

Rationally thinking about events so distant in the past, however, was then and still is a major intellectual challenge. Francis Crick rose to the occasion by postulating that RNA had to have an enzymatic role, as well as template and structural roles, functioning during the early stages of life as the enzyme for its own self-replication. Under this scheme, the first genetic molecule was RNA, with DNA coming later, after the essential outlines of the genetic code were established. But logical as this idea was, it had little impact, and for almost 20 years, thinking about the origin of life was regarded at best as a safe haven for minds unable to keep up with the extraordinary rush of a recombinant-DNA-driven assault on the nature of life as it exists today.

Then in 1982, the discovery of the first example RNA self-splicing suddenly led to the realization that RNA molecules do have the capability to act as catalysts. Over the past several years, many more examples of self-splicing have been found, and the fact that the catalytic activity of RNase P resides in its RNA component has been demonstrated. With Crick's conjecture now a fact and with the recent rapid progress in understanding today's enzymes and ribosomes, the time had thus arrived to bring together a diverse collection of pure chemists, biochemists, molecular biologists, and evolutionary biologists to discuss the evolutionary events that may have given rise to the living organisms that now exist on earth. As a title, we chose the Evolution of Catalytic Function to help assure that this Symposium would bring together minds that think in terms of chemistry, as well as about genetic information.

The first plans for this our 52nd Symposium arose at a meeting at Harvard in August 1986 between Walter Gilbert, Jeremy Knowles, and myself. Subsequently, I greatly benefited from suggestions given by Leslie Orgel, Daniel Koshland, Russell Doolittle, Tom Cech, and Jim Darnell. The final program comprised 110 speakers, each speaking some 30 minutes. These presentations led to one of our intellectually most demanding meetings, since the talks were arranged to be longer than customary in view of the very diverse nature of the audience, which this year consisted of some 167 scientists. The majority of this year's attendees presented papers, resembling the situation in the very first Symposia. At its start, I worried that our program might be too wide-ranging for true intellectual exchanges. But by the end, I was more than pleased by the high spirits expressed by virtually all participants, who felt that this was a truly historic gathering in which the need to think evolutionary had at last become an accepted way of thinking for molecular biologists. Helping assure this success were the wide-ranging opening talks by Daniel Koshland, Leslie Orgel, and Manfred Eigen as well as the gracefully lucid summary by Alan Weiner.

The bringing together of so many speakers required many sources of financial backing. In addition to our long-time Symposium supporters, the National Cancer Institute/ National Institutes of Health, the National Science Foundation, and the Department of Energy, we are greatly indebted to special help provided by the Sloan Foundation and the Lucille P. Markey Charitable Trust. Essential funds were also provided by our Corporate Sponsor Program, which provides core support for the Cold Spring Harbor Meetings Programs: Abbott Laboratories; American Cyanamid Company; Amersham International plc; AMGen; Becton Dickinson and Company; Boehringer Mannheim GmbH; Bristol-Myers Company; Cetus Corporation; Ciba-Geigy Corporation; Diagnostic Products Corporation; E.I. du Pont de Nemours & Company; Eastman Kodak Company; Genentech, Inc.; Genetics Institute; Hoffman-La Roche Inc.; Johnson & Johnson; Eli Lilly and Company; Millipore Corporation; Monsanto Company; Oncogene Science, Inc.; Pall Corporation; Pfizer Inc.; The Procter & Gamble Company; Schering-Plough Corporation; Smith Kline & French Laboratories; Tambrands Inc.; The Upjohn Company; The Wellcome Research Laboratories; Burrough Wellcome Co.; and Wyeth Laboratories.

Our Meetings Office staff, Maureen Berejka, Karen Otto, Diane Tighe, Michela McBride, and Barbara Ward, again performed at a high level, looking after the registration and housing of Symposium participants and making each of our participants feel thoroughly wanted. The audiovisual setups were again ably provided by Herb Parsons, and the massive correspondence and telephoning needed to put together a Symposium was cheerfully performed by Andrea Stephenson. As in the past several years, our Publications Department has worked hard to ensure the publication of these books by the end of the year, and for their efforts we are indebted to Nancy Ford, Managing Director of Publications, and editors Patricia Barker and Dorothy Brown, ably assisted by Joan Ebert and Mary Cozza.

James D. Watson, Director
October 19, 1987

Contents

Templates

Putting a Protein Together

CONTENTS

Proteins

Structure

Cofactors

Function

Exons and Introns

Summary

COLD SPRING HARBOR SYMPOSIA ON QUANTITATIVE BIOLOGY

VOLUME LII

Evolution of Catalytic Function

D.E. KOSHLAND, JR.

University of California at Berkeley, Berkeley, California 94720

To lead off a volume on the evolution of catalytic function is a major challenge, especially since reconstructing evolution from the organisms that exist today is a little like deducing the nature of communications between prehistoric cavemen by examining in excruciating detail the workings of the Bell Telephone System. It is extrapolation fraught with peril, but it is, fortunately, unlikely to be falsified by replication.

The job is made even more difficult by recent discoveries that convincingly demonstrate that RNA has catalytic powers (Cech 1986). Evolution of catalytic function was, until recently, the exclusive domain of protein chemists. Unfortunately, a group of nucleic acid chemists developed suggestions of an "RNA world" (Cech 1986; Gilbert 1986) that cannot be ignored in the evolution of catalytic function. Since that is even more speculative than protein evolution, I first examine the evolution of catalytic function in proteins and then attempt to extend those principles to a few aspects of the RNA world.

One of Darwin's fundamental conclusions with regard to the evolution of species was gradualism. This appears to be eminently applicable to the evolution of catalytic function. There is, of course, a possibility that evolution proceeds by discontinuous jumps; e.g., a million polymers are made in order to have one or two appear as superb catalysts. That kind of stochastic approach to evolution, although not mathematically impossible, seems unlikely. Rather, we expect a gradual evolution from an inefficient primordial catalyst to the highly efficient enzymes of today. This, in turn, suggests structures that are also modified gradually, and the first postulate would therefore be that enzymes became large molecules at some fairly early stage. Anyone who has tried to construct oriented catalytic groups on a small framework, such as a steroid, learns quickly

that even minor changes in side chains result in major orientation differences among catalytic groups. On the other hand, a large protein can be modified by amino acid substitution far from the active site in ways that cause small changes in the active site itself. Thus, it is not surprising that enzymes are large and appear to change by incremental amino acid modification.

If the catalytic function is to change incrementally, then it would be desirable to have a number of different catalytic devices and to have ways of optimizing each of them by structural changes that improve the catalyst. Table 1 presents the sources of catalysis that we recognize in the protein catalysts of today (Koshland and Neet 1968; Westley 1969; Cunningham 1977; Walsh 1977). They clearly provide just the features we want. First of all, there are a number of different contributors to catalysis, which means that a catalyst that functions using one property can be further improved by adding a second and third type of catalysis. Moreover, the nature of each of these properties is such that they can be improved incrementally.

To illustrate this, Figure 1 shows a hypothetical active site containing two substrates and two catalytic groups. It is quite apparent that a four-body collision in solution is unlikely. But constructing an enzyme (utilizing the energy of the sun) to bring two catalytic groups

Table 1. Contributions to Catalysis of Proteins

Proximity: Juxtaposition of reactive groups and catalytic groups

Orientation: Precise orientation of the catalytic and reactive groups

Microenvironment: Ability of the heterogeneous protein surface to juxtapose polar and nonpolar components

Polarizing groups: Lewis acids, Lewis bases, nucleophiles, etc.

Structural complementarity: Special affinity for transition complex

Covalent catalysis: Groups on enzyme that attack, form covalent bond, and leave so rapidly that they serve as catalysts

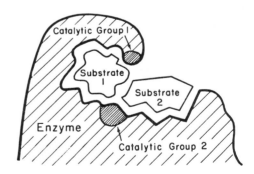

$$\text{Proximity Effect} = \frac{(E_t)(55)(55)(55)}{(S_1)(S_2)(C_1)(C_2)}$$

$$= \frac{(10^{-6})(55)^3}{(10^{-5})^4} = 2 \times 10^{19}$$

Figure 1. A typical enzyme surface with two substrates held in orientation and proximity by noncovalent attractions and two catalytic groups held in place because of their covalent attachments in the sequence of the protein. The low probability of a four-body collision in solution is obviated by the design of the enzyme active site achieved ultimately through the energy of the sun channeled into the protein structure.

to the right location and to provide binding sites for the two substrates can change the four-body collision to a situation with high probability. The first calculation of proximity to explain such a phenomenon used 55 M for the effective concentration of a juxtaposed neighbor (Koshland 1962), and as shown in Figure 1, this will give an overall enzymatic enhancement factor of 10^{12}, assuming four molecules (two substrates and two catalysts) at 10^{-5} M for the collision reaction and an enzyme at a concentration of 10^{-6} M for the enzymatic reaction. This figure is actually a minimum, since orientation was later shown to make an additional large contribution (Storm and Koshland 1970; Dafforn and Koshland 1971, 1973). The factors of orientation and proximity can be calculated in a variety of ways (Bruice and Pandit 1960; Westheimer 1962; Page and Jencks 1971). Other types of catalysis shown in Table 1 can be added, and each of these factors can be improved incrementally by improving the binding groups and the organization of the binding groups.

The enzyme surface can provide further forms of catalysis by utilizing amino acid side chains, as acids or basis, or by attracting cofactors and metal ions that can generate polarizations that catalyze decarboxylations, condensations, oxidation reductions, etc. A further catalytic power of enzymes is achieved by the microheterogeneity of the surface. In solution, reactions occur in a bulk dielectric of a single type. Some reactions are aided by a low and others by a high dielectric constant. However, many times one part of a reaction would improve in a high dielectric and another part would improve in a low one. An active site of an enzyme embeds the substrate in groups that can alternate between hydrophobic and charged side chains. In effect, these provide adjacent microscopic high-dielectric and low-dielectric regions. Since charged acids are known to be very strong in low-dielectric solvent, the pushing of water out of an active site by the binding power of the substrate can create a situation in which a charged group is essentially surrounded by hydrophobic residues, thus making it a much stronger Lewis acid. This type of "microenvironment effect," sometimes called electrostatic catalysis (Pocker and Ellsworth 1977), is a special feature of enzymes as they are known today. Covalent catalysis, in which an enzyme intermediate is formed and speeds up the reaction, can provide another type of catalysis and can provide other functions such as stereochemistry and preservation of high-energy intermediates.

The final, and certainly not the least important, type of catalysis is the stabilization of the transition state, the concept initially promulgated by Linus Pauling (1946) which suggests that the enzyme is designed to interact specifically with the transition state in order to lower the activation energy and accelerate the appearance of products. Here, the catalytic groups are those that bind, provide the microenvironment, orientation, etc., to stabilize the transition state in preference to the enzyme-substrate ground state.

Since each of these types of catalysis has been dis-

cussed elsewhere, I will only comment that each of them can be gradually optimized by changes in the quality of the catalytic groups and by improvements in the orientation and juxtaposition of these groups in the final catalyst. The preparation of mutants with lower activity indicates that amino acid changes can improve the catalytic function incrementally. It would be presumptuous to say that we can detail the exact reasons for the structure of any one protein catalyst today, but certainly we know most of the ingredients of that catalyst and can ascribe rough factors that come close to explaining the enormous catalytic power of current enzymes.

From the point of view of protein chemistry, therefore, it is not difficult to imagine some polymers existing in the primordial soup that was imagined by Oparin (1957), which contained one or two catalytic groups to provide crude catalysis. Polyhistidine, for example, is known to catalyze esterase reactions. Reactions might have had half-lives of days or months in the prebiotic soup, which would be refined through evolutionary selection to the millisecond half-lives of the superb catalysts we have today. Thus, incremental changes in structure would improve the polarizing effectiveness, the stabilization of protein intermediates, and transition state complexes. By changing amino acids outside the active site, small perturbations in the active site would be engineered and the efficiency of each component of catalysis could be optimized.

Protein Flexibility

Would the evolution of a protein catalyst have developed monotonically along the lines of ever-increasing catalytic power, as described above? The answer would appear to be "no." An extremely important feature of the catalytic power of enzymes is their specificity. A template-type structure, into which some substrates would fit and others would not, must have evolved gradually at early stages. As these more specific catalysts arose, the ubiquity of oxygen and water would mean that the hydroxylic compounds certainly were utilized early in evolution. As a result, specificity in the modification of hydroxyl groups of substrates would of necessity require discrimination against water in many cases. To do this, flexible enzymes of the induced-fit category (Koshland 1958, 1963, 1964, 1973) would be needed, as illustrated in Figure 2. The induced-fit property would serve not only to exclude water, but to exclude other small molecules as well, to enhance the specificity of a protein.

In recent times, some investigators have derived mathematical models that appear to imply that induced fit cannot produce specificity (Fersht 1985). This conclusion is peculiar, since induced fit was designed to explain specificity and led to predictions of conformational changes in enzymes that have been extensively verified (Yankeelov and Koshland 1965; delaFuente et al. 1970; Anderson and Steitz 1975; Lipscomb 1983). These conclusions against specificity almost invariably

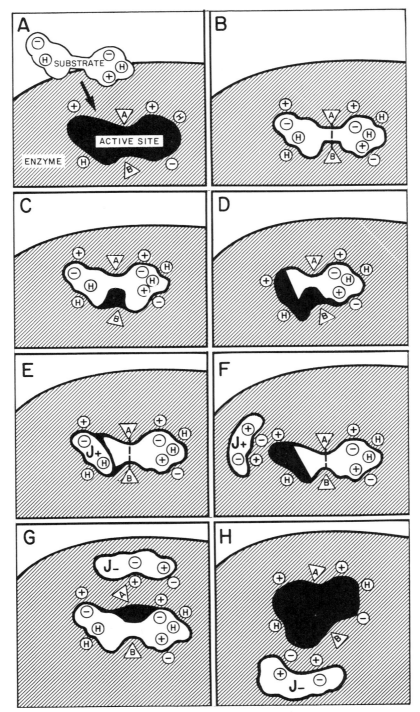

Figure 2. Illustration of induced conformational changes. (*A*) Substrate approaches active site. (*B*) Substrate binds and induces conformational change to provide correct alignments in the transition state. (*C,D*) Too-large and too-small substrate analogs bind but fail to induce the proper protein conformation. (*E,F*) Added effectors (J⁺) activate the enzyme for a too-small substrate analog by providing the needed conformational change immediately adjacent to the substrate or at a more distant site. (*G*) Inhibitor (J⁻) distorts the protein so a bad substrate does not react. (*H*) Inhibitor (J⁻) distorts the enzyme so substrate does not bind.

3

involve mistaken assumptions, e.g., that the poor substrate and the good substrate have the same protein transition state, a self-fulfilling prophecy inconsistent with the induced-fit hypothesis. An even more peculiar criticism is the argument that induced fit would be unlikely because it is wasteful to invest some of the binding energy of the substrate to induce the proper conformation of the enzymatic transition state. Induced conformational changes can be extremely fast, and binding energy far higher than needed, for catalysis can be devised by addition of binding groups. Enzymes are probably selected for intermediate levels of K_m (10^{-5} M) because products, which are usually structurally similar to the substrates, must leave the protein surface or dissociation will be rate-limiting. Antibodies that have routinely lower K_D values than enzymes indicate that it is quite possible to select protein sites for lower K_D values (higher affinity) if needed. Moreover, as discussed below, it is not necessary that all enzymes operate at diffusion velocity speeds. In many cases, the sacrifice of a little catalytic power to achieve specificity is well worth the price for an evolving cellular system.

The fact that a part of a substrate molecule that was not part of the catalytic reaction itself, e.g., the nonpolar side chain in the elastase reaction, could influence the structure of a protein meant that other nonreacting structures, not even part of the substrate molecule, could also influence that reactivity. Thus, the induced-fit prediction that xylose could increase the ATPase activity of hexokinase, shown schematically in Figure 2, was proven to be correct (delaFuente and Sols 1970; delaFuente et al. 1970). The development of this type of specificity and the regulation through allosteric sites led to the feedback regulation needed for a complex cell.

An example (Byers and Koshland 1975) of induced-fit specificity that is relevant to evolution is the effect of NAD on the reactivity of various groups in the glyceraldehyde-3-phosphate dehydrogenase enzyme. One of these studies involves the influence of NAD on the reactivity of an SH group with iodoacetic acid and iodoacetamide. There is no physiological function for iodoacetic acid acting on glyceraldehyde-3-phosphate dehydrogenase. However, the fact that the nonreactant molecule NAD can change the structure of the protein around the SH group is illustrative of the way bound cofactors and covalent modification can alter the reactivity of adjacent or even distant residues in a protein molecule. A physiologically important application of this principle from the same study is seen in Table 2, where the effect of NAD on the relative rates of phosphorylation and hydrolysis of acyl intermediates is documented. In this case, the binding of NAD to the protein surface enormously increases the rate of phosphorylation (by 10^5) relative to the rate of hydrolysis. This is an example of an induced-fit effect to improve specificity and an effective evolutionary outcome (cf. Fig. 2 for schematic illustration). If hydrolysis produces a wasteful loss of an intermediate in the glycolytic pathway, the NAD changes the protein structure to

Table 2. Effect of NAD on Reactions of Cysteine-149 Residue of Yeast Glyceraldehyde-3-Phosphate

	$k_{(+NAD)}/k_{(-NAD)}$
Hydrolysis of phosphoglyceryl enzyme	60
Phospholysis of phosphoglyceryl enzyme	$>4 \times 10^6$
ICH_2CONH_2 alkylation	0.1
ICH_2COO alkylation	15.8

favor phosphorolysis and decreases hydrolysis. This is a simple case in which a nonparticipant in the direct catalytic process can enormously change the specificity, and clearly, a similar protuberance in the substrate or an allosteric effector can do the same thing.

The existence of the flexible enzyme provided the basis for a further sophistication of enzymatic power: the ability to be regulated by molecules that do not look like the substrate at all. Once a functioning cell had evolved, it would have been important to modify enzymatic velocity, depending on the needs of the cell and the environment. Having all enzymes operating at full speed all the time could not produce an adapting biological organism. Feedback and control were therefore essential and are aided enormously by enzyme flexibility (Gerhart and Pardee 1962; Monod et al. 1963). Covalent modification of a protein is analogous to binding at a distant regulatory site as it induces conformational changes that travel through the protein to the active site.

The regulatory aspects of enzymes undoubtedly came later than the need for flexibility; but once pathways had developed, the need for feedback was clear.

Multisubunit Effects

The initial formation of multisubunit protein and the need for maintenance of these proteins when there is no cooperativity are still a mystery, although various suggestions have been made (Koshland 1976a). However, once such multisubunit proteins existed, cooperativity became possible. Since the structure of one subunit, altered under the induced fit, could be transmitted to neighboring subunits, binding curves appreciably steeper or appreciably shallower than the classical Michaelis-Menten hyperbola could be generated. These cooperative properties are an important feature of the fine tuning of enzymes and are observed extensively in species today. Cooperativity could come later in evolution than feedback, since it involves a refinement of control.

There is an advantage of multiple subunits beyond cooperativity as illustrated in Figure 3. In addition to the changes in the steepness of curves, their midpoints change simply because of changes in the subunit interactions. It is an extremely important feature of enzymatic power that its effective K_m be appropriate to the physiological concentration of its substrate or allosteric effector. If the substrate in a cell is 10^{-8} M, an enzyme with a midpoint of 10^{-3} M would be ineffective.

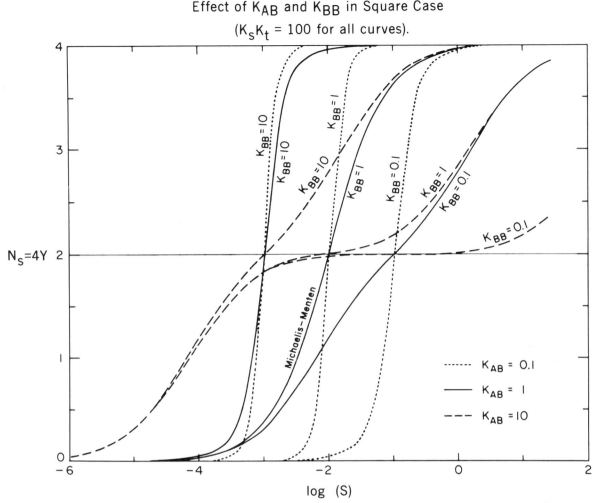

Figure 3. Binding curves for a tetrameric protein in which only subunit interactions are changed. Both steepness of curves and midpoints shift even though active sites remain the same.

The evolution of a new species might mean that the concentration of its particular substrate in the cellular milieu would be changed because the species had moved from the sea to land. Instead of having to redesign the active site (a finely tuned delicate structure) the new protein could simply change its subunit interactions. The active site would remain the same, but the subunit interaction would produce a K_m appropriate to the new species.

A similar logic explains the need for calmodulin (Keller et al. 1982) as the subunit in a number of proteins or for the GTP-binding protein and many similar peptide subunits. One might ask why it would not be simpler to design a calcium-binding site on the new protein, rather than devise a subunit-binding site for the calmodulin protein. The answer would seem to be that designing a site that binds calcium usually at concentrations in the range of 10^{-8} to 10^{-7} M, which can discriminate against magnesium (a very similarly structured ion) usually present in cells in the millimolar range, is a difficult and demanding task. Once such a

binding site has been obtained, it is a lot easier to devise subunit-binding sites on the periphery of the calmodulin molecule than to redesign the specific calcium-binding site for each protein.

Enzymatic Perfection and Imperfection

It is important at this stage to consider what we are selecting for. In some cases, we are selecting for very fast enzymes. As defined by J. Knowles, enzymatic perfection occurs when an enzyme has a turnover number equal to the diffusion velocity of the substrate (Albery and Knowles 1976). An enzyme cannot perform more effectively than that, and certain enzymes have achieved that excellence. It would be a mistake, however, to believe that all enzymes are selected for speed. Since covalent regulatory control has been found to be an important regulator of enzyme function, many futile cycles of phosphorylation-dephosphorylation are set up to maintain a steady state of phosphorylation. The higher the turnover rate of such proteins, the greater the waste of ATP energy. Would it not be desirable to make them very slow to save ATP? The answer is "yes and no" (Koshland 1984). These regulatory enzymes exist to respond to environmental signals. If that signal occurs in a neuron, the need for change may be in milliseconds. If it occurs in a muscle cell, the need for change may require response in fractions of minutes. If it occurs in developmental cells, the need may require days or weeks. In such cases, the optimum would be as slow as possible to save energy and as fast as needed for the physiological response. Thus, it should not surprise protein chemists who are working with localized mutagenesis to find that some enzymes will be improved by modification, since not all enzymes are at their optimum catalytic potential. One example of such selection is isocitric dehydrogenase in microorganisms. In this case, an experiment has been done in which growth on acetate cannot occur if an optimized highly catalytic isocitric dehydrogenase is present in the system (LaPorte et al. 1985). A selection process shows growth can occur if a less catalytically effective enzyme is obtained (LaPorte et al. 1985).

Framework and Modular Structure

The next question that arises is how such enzymes are selected. Do we always start de novo? Do we always start from the same primordial enzyme? Can we shuttle parts of proteins back and forth? Do introns and extrons provide the answer? The answer to these questions is again "yes and no."

The developing understanding of evolutionary sequences and protein structure indicates that various permutations of the above exist. Domain swapping does occur in certain cases. On the other hand, there is convergent evolution in other cases. In some cases, introns clearly mark the end of the domain and in other cases they do not. Domain swapping occurs in some bacterial proteins where introns do not exist. Furthermore, it has been suggested that introns in the middle of a domain can provide a mechanism of accelerated mutagenesis, which would provide more rapid selection for function. These subjects are discussed at length in this volume.

There is good evidence that the concept of frameworks (Schulz and Schirmer 1979; Pain 1982; Bajaj and Blundell 1984) that can be made by many different amino acid sequences is utilized in evolution. It has been shown that many proteins of very different specificities and functions have basic modular structure (Richardson 1981; Rossmann and Argos 1981; C.-I. Bränden, pers. comm.). In fact, a further generalization can be made that the specific functional features are frequently (but not always) located in the loops between α helixes on β barrels. The example of a hydrophobic core turns up in most proteins. But very few of them are identical (Brown 1987), suggesting that the principle of a hydrophobic center was used in early enzymes and then fine-tuned by minor changes to improve the catalytic power of the particular reaction. The same is true of more closely related sequences

such as trypsin and chemotrypsin, derived from common ancestors. These proteins have 30% homology (Neurath 1985), which means that 70% of the amino acids have changed and not just in the active site, where the specificity changes are obvious. Thus, fine tuning of active sites or hydrophobic cores for new purposes occurs extensively. It seems clear that exchanges of portions of DNA occur through recombination, virus infection, gene conversion, and other methods to produce modular-type switches in proteins which are then fine-tuned for specific functions.

The RNA World

What do these lessons in regard to catalytic functions of protein allow us to say about catalytic function of RNA? The case for the evoluntionary significance of RNA catalysts has been made elegantly by Cech and other investigators (Cech 1986; Gilbert 1986; Guerrier-Takada et al. 1983). There are important similarities and some important differences between RNA and modern enzymes. First, the process of base pairing makes the development of specificity for replication simpler than designing the active site of an enzyme. High specificity could be obtained with a few bases, depending of course on how many similar bases existed in the primordial soup. Nucleic acids could have many different types of side chains for catalysis, some of which probably exist today in tRNAs and some of which may have been erased over evolutionary time. Such molecules would be more suitable for replicating themselves than modern proteins. Moreover, they might have obtained some structural organization by binding proteins to themselves to form some larger complexes. One could imagine a complex gradually becoming more sophisticated and including more reactions until ultimately proteins that would have more flexibility would take over the catalytic function and leave the hereditary function to nucleic acids.

The properties of flexibility and microheterogeneity might be more difficult for a nucleic acid to solve, possibly because the double-stranded version would be more one dimensional than proteins. Designing small incremental changes or optimizing the orientation of catalytic groups would seem to be more difficult with such molecules. Thus, although there seems to be no bar on the design of catalytic molecules on RNA, and there is of course excellent evidence that a limited range of catalytic reactions are currently carried out by RNA in today's cellular environment (Cech 1986), it would seem likely that at some stage in evolution, the more complex alternatives offered by large proteins would begin to cause a shift to proteins as the optimal catalysts. If that occurred, one might erase most of the evidence for the early vestigial ribonucleic acid catalysts, leaving today, as suggested by Cech, those catalysts that are specifically designed for RNA functions. The finding by S. Altman (Guerrier-Takada et al. 1983) of the RNA-protein complex, which has catalytic power, further advances the idea that there was an intermediate world in which RNA and protein acted together, and some of that world is still evident in today's cells.

The Cell

It would seem that the membrane surrounding a cell of organized pathways had to come at a moderately advanced stage in evolution. The problems of transport in and out of a cell are formidable and need a complex organization. Thus, one might expect early systems to be aggregates held together by noncovalent association with rather porous shells. As the shells become more like the membranes we know today, the pathways would, of necessity, have to be sophisticated for control, ingress of nutrients, and egress of waste products.

CONCLUSION

Dhobzansky (1973) said, "Nothing makes sense except in the light of evolution." Darwin pointed out the survival of the fittest. Perhaps the enormous extrapolations required to understand evolution select for the fittest investigators. It seems to me that's why Jim Watson brought us together: to test our survival.

ACKNOWLEDGMENT

The author gratefully acknowledges support for this work from the National Institutes of Health and the National Science Foundation.

REFERENCES

Albery, W.J. and J.R. Knowles. 1976. Evolution of enzyme function and development of catalytic efficiency. *Biochemistry* **15:** 5632.

Anderson, W.F. and T.A. Steitz. 1975. Structure of yeast hexokinase: Low resolution structure of enzyme-substrate complexes revealing negative cooperativity and allosteric interactions. *J. Mol. Biol.* **92:** 279.

Bajaj, M. and T.L. Blundell. 1984. Evolution and the tertiary structure of proteins. *Annu. Rev. Biophys. Bioeng.* **13:** 453.

Brown, A.L. 1987. Positively Darwinian molecules. *Nature* **326:** 12.

Bruice, T.C. and U.K. Pandit. 1960. The effect of geminal substitution ring size and rotamer distribution on the intramolecular nucleophilic catalysis of the hydrolysis of monophenyl esters of dibasic acids. *J. Am. Chem. Soc.* **82:** 5858.

Byers, L.D. and D.E. Koshland, Jr. 1975. The specificity of induced conformational change in yeast glyceraldehyde-3-phosphate dehydrogenase. *Biochemistry* **14:** 3661.

Cech, T. 1986. A model for the RNA-catalyzed replication of RNA. *Proc. Natl. Acad. Sci.* **83:** 4360.

Cunningham, E.B. 1977. *Biochemistry: Mechanisms of metabolism.* McGraw-Hill, New York.

Dafforn, A. and D.E. Koshland, Jr. 1971. Theoretical aspects of orbital steering. *Proc. Natl. Acad. Sci.* **68:** 2463.

———. 1973. Proximity, entropy and orbital steering. *Biochem. Biophys. Res. Commun.* **52:** 779.

delaFuente, G. and A. Sols. 1970. The kinetics of yeast hexokinase in the light of the induced fit involved in the binding of its sugar substrate. *Eur. J. Biochem.* **16:** 234.

delaFuente, G., R. Lagunas, and A. Sols. 1970. Induced fit in yeast hexokinase. *Eur. J. Biochem.* **16:** 226.

Dobzansky, T.H. 1973. Nothing in biology makes sense except in the light of evolution. *Am. Biol. Teach.* **35:** 125.

Fersht, A. 1985. *Enzyme structure and mechanism.* W.H. Freeman, New York.

Gerhart, J. and A.B. Pardee. 1962. The enzymology of control by feedback inhibition. *J. Biol. Chem.* **237:** 891.

Gilbert, W. 1986. The RNA world. *Nature* **319:** 618.

Guerrier-Takada, C., K. Gardiner, T. Marsh, N. Pace, and S. Altman. 1983. The RNA subunit of ribonuclease P is the catalytic subunit of the enzyme. *Cell* **35:** 849.

Keller, C.H., B.B. Olwin, W. Heidman, and D.R. Storm. 1982. Energetics and chemistry for interactions between calmodulin and calmodulin-binding proteins. *Calcium Cell Funct.* **3:** 103.

Koshland, D.E., Jr. 1958. Mechanism of transfer enzymes. In *The enzymes*, revised edition (ed. P. Boyer et al.), p. 305. Academic Press, New York.

———. 1962. The comparison of non-enzymic and enzymic reaction velocities. *J. Theor. Biol.* **2:** 75.

———. 1963. Correlation of structure and function in enzyme action. *Science* **142:** 1533.

———. 1964. The role of flexibility in enzyme action. *Cold Spring Harbor Symp. Quant. Biol.* **28:** 473.

———. 1973. Protein shape and biological control. *Sci. Am.* **229:** 52.

———. 1976a. The evolution of function in enzymes. *Fed. Proc.* **35:** 2104.

———. 1976b. Role of flexibility in the specificity, control and evolution of enzymes. *FEBS Lett.* **62:** E47.

———. 1984. Control of enzyme activity and metabolic pathways. *Trends Biochem. Sci.* **9:** 155.

Koshland, D.E., Jr. and K.E. Neet. 1968. The catalytic and regulatory properties of enzymes. *Annu. Rev. Biochem.* **37:** 359.

LaPorte, D.C., P.E. Thorsness, and D.E. Koshland, Jr. 1985. Compensatory phosphorylation of isocitrate dehydrogenase: A mechanism for adaptation to the intracellular environment. *J. Biol. Chem.* **260:** 10563.

Lipscomb, W.N. 1983. Structure and catalysis of enzymes. *Annu. Rev. Biochem.* **52:** 17.

Monod, J., J.P. Changeux, and F. Jacob. 1963. Allosteric proteins and cellular control mechanisms. *J. Mol. Biol.* **6:** 306.

Neurath, H. 1985. Proteolytic enzymes, past and present. *Fed. Proc.* **44:** 2907.

Oparin, A.I. 1957. *The Origin of Life on Earth.* Academic Press, New York.

Page, M.I. and W.P. Jencks. 1971. Entropic contributions to rate accelerations in enzymic and intramolecular reactions and the chelate effect. *Proc. Natl. Acad. Sci.* **68:** 1678.

Pain, R.H. 1982. The evolution of enzyme activity. *Nature* **299:** 486.

Pauling, L. 1946. Molecular architecture and biological reactions. *Chem. Eng. News* **24:** 1375.

Pocker, Y. and D.L. Ellsworth. 1977. Electrostatic catalysis by ionic aggregates. *J. Am. Chem. Soc.* **99:** 2276.

Richardson, J.S. 1981. Anatomy and taxonomy of protein structure. *Adv. Protein Chem.* **34:** 167.

Rossmann, M.G. and P. Argos. 1981. Protein folding. *Annu. Rev. Biochem.* **50:** 497.

Schulz, G.E. and R.H. Schirmer. 1979. *Principles of protein structure.* Springer, New York.

Storm, D.R. and D.E. Koshland, Jr. 1970. A source for the special catalytic power of enzymes: Orbital steering. *Proc. Natl. Acad. Sci.* **66:** 445.

Walsh, C. 1977. *Enzymatic reaction mechanisms.* W.H. Freeman, San Francisco.

Westheimer, F.H. 1962. Mechanisms related to enzymic catalysis. *Adv. Enzymol.* **24:** 456.

Westley, J. 1969. *Enzymic catalysis.* Harper and Row, New York.

Yankeelov, J.A. and D.E. Koshland, Jr. 1965. Evidence for conformation changes induced by substrates of phosphoglucomutase. *J. Biol. Chem.* **240:** 1593.

Evolution of the Genetic Apparatus: A Review

L.E. ORGEL

Chemical Evolution Laboratory, The Salk Institute for Biological Studies, San Diego, California 92138

Compelling fossil evidence shows that cells with morphologies similar to those of modern blue-green algae were already abundant 3.5 billion years ago, i.e., within at most a billion years of the formation of the earth. It seems safe to infer that evolution based on a conventional system of nucleic acids and proteins has led from these or similar simple cells to the diversity of living organisms.

I review here the largely speculative literature on the earlier period of evolution—that preceding the fixation of the nucleic acid/protein system in its contemporary form. A period of speculative fever in this field arose in the late 1960s and early 1970s (Woese 1967; Crick 1968; Orgel 1968; Sulston and Orgel 1971a,b). Most of the ideas discussed here, including the hypothesis of a protein-free, catalytic-RNA-dependent organism, were put forward at that time. Often, the same idea occurred independently to several researchers, whereas a single author may have waxed and waned in his or her enthusiasm for a particular strand in the argument. The situation is not dissimilar today: The new wave of speculation is inspired by the remarkable experimental discoveries of introns and catalytic RNAs. However, it may be useful to remember the words of a distinguished molecular biologist, "An honest man, armed with all the knowledge available to us now, could only state that in some sense, the origin of life appears at the moment to be almost a miracle, so many are the conditions which would have had to have been satisfied to get it going" (Crick 1981).[1] I fear that he may still be right.

The problem that concerns us is the evolution of a genetic system based on nucleic acids and proteins from a prebiotic soup containing organic molecules that accreted with the earth or were formed in its oceans and atmosphere. The ease with which amino acids and the organic components of nucleic acids are formed from simple molecules such as ammonia, formaldehyde, and hydrogen cyanide justifies the belief that these molecules were present in the prebiotic soup (Miller and Orgel 1974). Whether they were sufficiently abundant relative to potential inhibitors of the earliest "genetic chemistry" is an important question, to which we will return.

The first appearance of a mechanism of molecular memory based on replication was a crucial event in the origins of life. Any macromolecule, however remarkable its properties, must ultimately have decomposed. Without a memory mechanism, it could have had no

long-term effect on the chemistry of its environment. Only macromolecules that operated on their environment to produce further copies of themselves had an evolutionary future. This seems to be generally accepted. Everything about the nature of the first replicating molecules on the primitive earth remains controversial.

Two fundamentally different replication paradigms have been suggested. The more popular is based on the known enzymatic mechanisms of DNA and RNA synthesis. It proposes residue-by-residue replication, in which each subunit of a copolymer directs an identical or complementary subunit into a growing chain. The "replicating-clay" hypothesis (Cairns-Smith 1982) is a two-dimensional variant of this paradigm. An alternative view suggests that the first replicating systems consisted of cycles of catalysts (usually polypeptides), each of which facilitated the synthesis of one or more different members of the cycle (Kauffman 1986).

In my opinion, cyclic systems of polypeptide catalysts seem implausible if one considers realistically the minimum length needed to obtain specific catalysis with a polypeptide. If a cyclic system was composed of five 20 mers, for example, it would be necessary to synthesize 95 peptide bonds, which is an average of 19 bonds for each catalyst. Clearly, a 20 mer could not catalyze 19 different specific reactions. No completely convincing escape from this dilemma has been suggested.

If we accept residue-by-residue replication as the more probable mechanism, we must next consider the chemical nature of the first replicating entity. The following possibilities are among the most popular:

1. Early functional proteins replicated directly. They "invented" nucleic acids and were ultimately enslaved by them.
2. Early nucleic acids or related molecules replicated directly. They "invented" protein synthesis. Uncoded polypeptides may or may not have been involved in the earliest precoding replication mechanism.
3. Nucleic acid replication and genetic coding of proteins coevolved.
4. The first form of life on the earth was based on some inorganic or organic system unrelated to proteins or nucleic acids. It has been suggested, for example, that it consisted of a family of self-replicating clay particles (Cairns-Smith 1982). The early system "invented" the nucleic acid/protein system, or a precursor of it.

Possibilities 2 and 3 have always appealed to molecular biologists. The recent discovery that certain RNA

---

[1]The author qualifies this statement to make it clear that he does not believe that the origin of life was a miracle.

molecules, in the total absence of protein, can catalyze highly sequence-specific hydrolytic and transesterification reactions of polynucleotides (Kruger et al. 1982; Guerrier-Takada et al. 1983) has greatly increased popular support for possibility 2. I examine this view in detail and suggest that it needs to be modified in certain important details. Many of the topics touched on here have been discussed in greater detail in an earlier publication (Orgel 1986).

What Can RNA Do without the Help of Enzymes?

Template-directed reactions. The group of non-biological reactions that have been studied most intensively are called template-directed condensations. They correspond to the biological reactions carried out by DNA or RNA polymerases and DNA ligases. The first of these reactions was reported by Naylor and Gilham (1966), who showed that a poly(A) template would facilitate the synthesis of $(pT)_{12}$ from $(pT)_6$. Subsequently, a large number of related reactions were described.

The way in which a template facilitates the synthesis of complementary oligomers is illustrated in Figure 1. A complex between the template and the substrate is formed that brings together the activated 5′-phosphate of one substrate molecule and the 2′(3′)-hydroxyl of another. This may facilitate the formation of an internucleotide bond. Clearly, there are two requirements for effective template-directed synthesis. First, the experiment must be carried out at a temperature below the melting point of the helical complex. Second, the

detailed stereochemistry of the complex must bring the template-bound substrates together in an orientation that favors reaction.

Template-directed reactions of mononucleotides are limited to systems in which polymer-monomer complexes are stable (Ts'o 1974). No reactions of monomeric U derivatives on poly(A) are possible, since poly(A)·mono(U) complexes are never stable. No reactions of monomeric C derivatives on poly(G) are possible for a different reason: Helical self-complexes of oligo(G) are so stable that, under normal conditions, oligo(G):mono(C) complexes do not form. 2 Poly-(U)·mono(A) complexes are usually stable between 0°C and 25°C, and poly(C)·mono(G) complexes are stable up to somewhat higher temperatures. Homopolymer:monomer reactions are thus restricted to polypyrimidine:monopurine systems.

The most striking fact about template-directed reactions is that, with ribonucleotide substrates, they almost always work, more or less, provided the substrate is appropriately activated and the template-substrate complex is stable at the temperature of the experiment (Orgel and Lohrmann 1974). Condensation reactions with deoxynucleotide substrates or with derivatives of pentose sugars other than ribose are much less efficient (Lohrmann and Orgel 1977).

When the reactions are studied in detail, a wide range of efficiency and regiospecificity can be seen. Activated derivatives of A, such as adenosine 5′-phosphorimidazolide (ImpA) (Fig. 2), form triple-helical complexes with poly(U). The self-condensation of ImpA in such a helix leads to the formation of oligo(A)s up to about eight residues long with high efficiency. However, the polymers are almost entirely 2′,5′-linked. The condensation of ImpG on poly(C) takes place in a double helix at pH values above 7.5. It is somewhat more efficient than the corresponding reaction of ImpU on poly(A) and gives products containing 2′,5′ and 3′,5′ phosphodiester bonds in roughly equal abundance (Orgel and Lohrmann 1974).

Metal ions have a profound influence on almost all of these reactions. The Pb^{++} ion catalyzes an extremely efficient polymerization of ImpG on poly(C), which yields long, all 2′,5′-linked products (Lohrmann and Orgel 1980). Under the same conditions, the Zn^{++} ion also catalyzes the efficient synthesis of long oligo(G)s, but with almost exclusively the natural 3′,5′ linkage (Bridson and Orgel 1980).

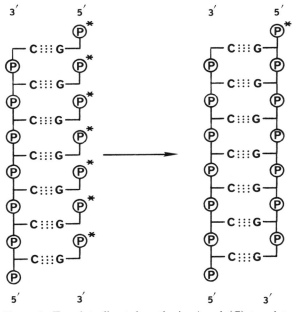

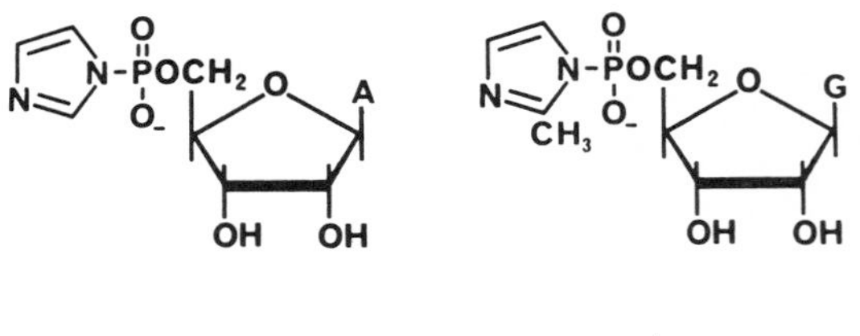

Figure 1. Template-directed synthesis. A poly(C) template forms a double-helical complex with an activated derivative of guanosine-5′-phosphate. The orientation must be such as to facilitate the formation of phosphodiester bonds. For simplicity, the double-helical structure is shown diagrammatically as though it were unwound.

Figure 2. Structure of nucleoside-5′-phosphorimidazolides. (*a*) ImpA; (*b*) 2-MeImpG.

We have studied one particular set of reactions—the condensation of guanosine 5′-phosphoro-2-methyl-imidazolide (2-MeImpG) and related activated nucleotides (Fig. 2)—in great detail, as a model of an RNA polymerase. The condensation of 2-MeImpG on poly(C) is a very efficient, regiospecific reaction that yields long, all 3′,5′-linked oligo(G)s (Fig. 3a–d). The condensation proceeds in a Watson-Crick double helix by extension of oligo(G)s in the 5′ → 3′ direction. The fidelity of the reaction is high. If poly(C) is incubated with equal amounts of the four nucleoside phosphoro-2-methylimidazolides, bases other than G are discriminated against by factors in the range of 100–500 (Inoue and Orgel 1982). Short oligonucleotides such as C_5 (or dC_5) are also efficient templates, but sometimes yield rather complex mixtures of isomeric products (Chen et al. 1985).

Random copolymer templates direct the oligomerization of substrate nucleotides that are complementary to the bases of the template: Poly(CU), for example, directs the co-oligomerization of 2-MeImpG and 2-MeImpA (Inoue and Orgel 1983). The reactions are sequence-specific, since the short template CCGCC facilitates the synthesis of the complementary sequence GGCGG (Inoue et al. 1984). Many similar reactions have been examined, and accurate complementary synthesis on templates as long as d(CCCGCCCGCC-CGCC) has been reported (Haertle and Orgel 1986; Acevedo and Orgel 1987).

Although "transcription" of a number of sequences has been achieved, the model lacks the generality of the enzymatic process. Synthesis occurs only on templates containing an excess of C residues and is inhibited if the template can form an intramolecular base-paired self-structure. The reaction stops once the template is filled by complementary products. In many cases, initiation occurs at internal positions on the template strand.

The template-directed reactions of short oligomeric substrates have been studied much less completely (Ninio and Orgel 1978). However, it is clear that they proceed in much the same way as the reaction of monomers and that they display a comparably wide range of efficiencies and regiospecificities. In one special case, autocatalytic synthesis of a hexadeoxynucleotide derivative from two trinucleotide derivatives has been demonstrated (von Kiedrowski 1986). A large number of template-derived ligation reactions of longer oligonucleotides have been studied by Shabarova and her colleagues. They have shown that ligation is a useful procedure, particularly for the synthesis of oligonucleotides containing unusual linkages (e.g., phosphoramidate linkages) in their backbones (Shabarova 1984).

A second group of template-directed reactions, al-

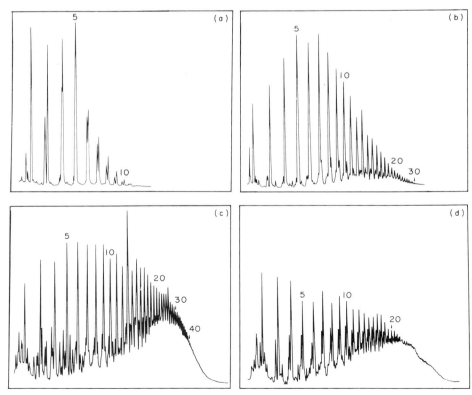

Figure 3. HPLC elution profiles of self-condensation of 2-MeImpG on poly(C) at various pH values. Reaction conditions: 0°C for 14 days; 0.4 M 2,6-lutidine · HCl buffer, 0.1 M 2-MeImpG, 0.1 M poly(C), 1.2 M NaCl, 0.2 M $MgCl_2$; (a) pH 7.0; (b) pH 7.7; (c) pH 8.2; (d) pH 9.0. Numbers above selected peaks are the lengths of the corresponding oligomers. Conditions for HPLC: elution with a linear $NaClO_4$ gradient (pH 12, 0 to 0.06 M, 90 min). UV absorption monitored at 262 nm.

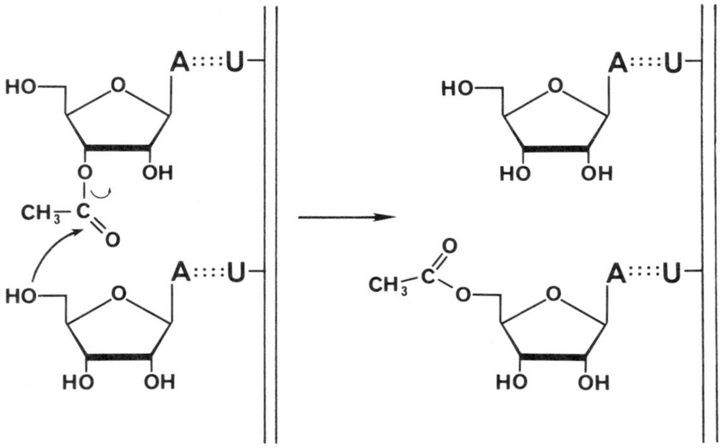

Figure 4. Intermolecular transfer of an acetyl group between 3′-acetyl adenosine and the 5′-OH group of adenosine is catalyzed by a poly(U) template.

though studied less intensively, is particularly relevant to RNA catalysis. The transfer of reactive groups from one nucleotide to another, and reactions between reactive groups attached to nucleotides, can be facilitated by their alignment on a complementary template (Fig. 4). Acetyl groups, for example, are transferred in an intermolecular template-directed reaction between the 3′ and 5′ positions of adjacent adenine nucleosides and nucleotides on a poly(U) template (Chung et al. 1971). Poly(U) has a catalytic effect on the synthesis of glycylglycine from the glycylester of pA (Weber and Orgel 1980). The possibility that template-directed reactions of this kind contributed to preenzymatic "biosynthesis" must be taken seriously.

Nonenzymatic template-directed polymerization and ligation reactions of the kind that are needed to permit molecular replication are well established. However, there are still many obstacles facing any attempt to develop a general, efficient transcription reaction that depends on plausibly prebiotic, activated mononucleotides as substrates. It is also difficult to formulate a mechanism by means of which strands could be separated and prevented from reannealing under prebiotic conditions. Could RNA catalysis help overcome some of these difficulties? Before trying to answer this question, it is necessary to summarize what is already known about RNA-catalyzed reactions.

Reactions catalyzed by ribozymes. A number of specific aspects of ribozyme catalysis are discussed further in other chapters in this volume. General reviews of the subject are readily available (Cech 1987). Consequently, I present only a minimal discussion of the salient features of the best-known reactions.

The simplest reactions known to be catalyzed by ribozymes are hydrolyses of specific phosphodiester bonds in RNA. The RNA component of ribonuclease P from *Escherichia coli*, for example, cleaves a precursor of tRNA at one particular phosphodiester bond to yield the mature tRNA. A ribozyme derived from the intron of the pre-rRNA of *Tetrahymena thermophila* will hydrolyze a variety of RNA substrates, including the

pre-rRNA itself. These reactions are remarkable in that they generate a terminal nucleoside 5′-phosphate and a terminal 3′-OH group. The spontaneous hydrolysis of RNA always yields a 2′(3′) phosphate and a free 5′-OH group.

In another set of related reactions, spontaneous sequence-specific hydrolysis of viroid and related RNAs occurs via the normal intermediate, the 2′,3′-cyclic phosphate (Buzayan et al. 1986; Prody et al. 1986). An interesting analog of this mode of hydrolysis in which a short oligonucleotide acts as catalyst for the hydrolysis of viroid RNA has been described by F.X. Sullivan and O.C. Uhlenbeck (pers. comm. and Uhlenbeck 1987). This group of reactions is perhaps less surprising than those that are involved in self-splicing, since hydrolysis via a cyclic phosphate intermediate proceeds spontaneously under mildly alkaline conditions and, in tRNA, is catalyzed in a sequence-specific manner by the Pb^{++} ion. Usher has shown that poly(U) is an excellent catalyst for the hydrolysis, via a 2′,3′-cyclic phosphate, of 2′,5′-linked phosphodiester bonds between A residues (Usher and McHale 1976). This system could be considered as the first ribozyme model.

A second well-established group of ribozyme-catalyzed reactions involves transesterification. Such residues are involved in the self-splicing of certain group I and group II introns. The biologically relevant reactions all display considerable site specificity, but a ribozyme derived from the intervening sequence of *Tetrahymena* pre-rRNA will catalyze transesterifications between dinucleotide substrates (Kay and Inoue 1987)

$$CpU + pGpN \rightleftharpoons CpUpN = pG \ (N = U, C, A, \text{ or } G)$$

In the context of the origins of life, ribozyme-catalyzed transesterification reactions of the type

$$C_n + C_n \rightleftharpoons C_{n+1} + C_{n-1} \ (n \geqslant 3)$$

have received much attention (Zaug and Cech 1986), since they seem to provide a mechanism for building longer oligonucleotides from shorter ones. The scope and limitations of such reactions as models for RNA replication and transcription are discussed further below.

The report of a ribozyme only 31 bases long that brings about the branching of a long-chain polyglucan is particularly exciting (Shvedova et al. 1987). If confirmed, it will demonstrate for the first time that ribozymes can act on substrates that do not contain nucleoside bases or similar planar, hydrogen-bonding groups.

Hypothetical ribozymes: RNA polymerases. The discovery of ribozymes has opened the gates to a flood of speculation. What should one believe? The most conservative attitude is to refuse to think about RNA-catalyzed reactions that have not been demonstrated experimentally. The least critical attitude is to suppose that there was a ribozyme wherever there is now an enzyme and that once upon a time bacteria lived happily without the help of proteins. It is hard to be sure which is the more appropriate point of view, and so I discuss here some of the possibilities and some of the difficulties.

Many investigators have realized that a ribozyme for RNA replication is an attractive candidate for the role of an ancestral catalyst (Woese 1967; Crick 1968; Orgel 1968). Furthermore, it has been suggested that the known ribozyme-catalyzed transesterification reactions could be prototypes of RNA replication (Pace and Marsh 1985; Sharp 1985; Cech 1986). First, we must examine this claim.

The dismutation reaction of C_5 described by Zaug and Cech (1986) differs from the reactions carried out by RNA polymerases in two important respects. First, it leads to the formation of an "equilibrium" mixture of oligomers, some smaller than the pentamer and some longer; no new phosphodiester bonds are formed. Second, the experimentally demonstrated reaction depends on a particular internal template and not on an arbitrary external template; in some ways, it is more closely related to the oligomerization of CDP by polynucleotide phosphorylase than to transcription or RNA replication.

It must be recognized that the equilibrium mixture of products formed by the oligomerization even of a "high-energy" compound such as ATP would include few very long molecules. The formation of long polymers by RNA or DNA polymerase is made possible by the kinetic properties of the enzymes. Clearly, if the formation of a dinucleotide from a pair of monomers was as rapid as the extension of a preformed oligomer chain, dimers and short oligomers would predominate in the reaction product. The essential requirement for the formation of long oligomers is that the initiation of new oligomer chains from monomers should be much slower than the extension of an oligomer chain once it is formed. One way of meeting this requirement is to make the catalyst highly processive, although this is not the only way.

We can thus see that the dismutation reaction (Zaug and Cech 1986) is not competent to produce long product molecules from short substrates. However, if we are prepared to speculate that a similar but much more processive reaction is possible, it might be able to produce high-molecular-weight products from C_2, for example. Since the reaction

$$C_2 + C_n \rightleftharpoons C + C_{n+1}$$

is essentially "energy-neutral," a smaller proportion of the substrate could be converted to long oligomers than is possible with CTP as substrate.

The claim that the C_5 dismutation reaction provides evidence for the possibility of ribozyme-catalyzed replication of RNA involves an important assumption. The ribozyme involved would need to recognize the growing end of the replication complex, without the help of the groups on the substrates that normally participate in Watson-Crick base pairing. It is not yet clear that ribozymes can operate on a wide range of substrates other than nucleotides and oligonucleotides. However, since a ribozyme that catalyzes the branching of a polyglucan has been reported (Shvedova et al. 1987), we think it plausible that other RNA-catalyzed transformations of this type, including RNA replication, are possible.

If we consider reactions only slightly more distant from the presently known transesterification reactions, we arrive at a more plausible class of replication models. We assume that an activated mononucleotide (e.g., a 5'-triphosphate) can transfer the mononucleotide moiety to the end of a growing chain, under the influence of a ribozyme. This is just another way of describing the ribozyme equivalents of an RNA polymerase. However, the proposed reaction is also an analog of the transesterification (and transphosphorylation) reaction brought about by ribozymes. Since uncatalyzed nucleotide transfers from many kinds of activated nucleotides are much easier reactions than the nucleotide transfers involved in transesterification, I believe that activated mononucleotides are the most attractive substrates for a hypothetical ribozymic RNA polymerase.

Hypothetical ribozymes: Metabolism. The appearance of RNA catalysts for the copying of RNA strands may have been crucial in the evolution of systems of replicating and competing RNA molecules. However, a primitive, protein-free RNA analog of a modern organism would also have required some form of RNA-catalyzed metabolism. How likely is this?

There is only one relevant experimental publication (Shvedova et al. 1987). These authors claim that a specific RNA molecule containing many modified bases is the catalytic component of a polyglucan branching enzyme. If the unmodified RNA has similar activity, it will provide a foundation for theories of RNA-based metabolism.

Many investigators have suggested that there is evidence in biochemistry that RNA once played a role as a catalyst in many reactions that now depend on proteins (Woese 1967; Crick 1968; Orgel 1968). It was noted that many of the most important coenzymes involve an organic catalyst bound via a pyrophosphate link to a nucleotide (Woese 1967; Orgel 1968). Are these molecules chemical fossils of a period when, for example, DPN oxidized UDP glucose, while both were attached by hydrogen bonds to an RNA catalyst? Is imidazole glycerol phosphate the fossil of a "catalytic nucleotide"? Many similar questions can be asked, but as yet none can be answered.

It is by no means established that a primitive form of life evolved prior to the invention of protein synthesis. However, in the light of recent work on ribozymes, this seems to me to be a possibility worth considering. I next explore some of the questions raised by the hypothesis that, before the evolution of the genetic code, there was a period in evolution when RNA replication was efficient and RNA catalysts supported at least a primitive metabolism.

What Preceded RNA?

If it turns out that RNA-based life once existed on the primitive earth (Cech 1986; Darnell and Doolittle 1986; Gilbert 1986; Westheimer 1986), it will not be the final solution to the "origins of life" problem. One will have to ask: Where did the mononucleotide substrates of RNA replication come from?

The origin of the nucleotides is particularly hard to understand (Miller and Orgel 1974). There is only one plausible prebiotic synthesis of ribose, the polymerization of formaldehyde. Ribose is formed as one of a large number of sugars and never as a major product. Similarly, the condensation of adenine or guanine with ribose leads to complex isomeric mixtures containing a relatively small amount of the natural nucleoside. The prebiotic synthesis of pyrimidine nucleosides is even more difficult. The possibility that the accurate replication of an oligoribonucleotide could occur directly in an unfractionated, racemic, prebiotic soup seems remote (Joyce et al. 1987). We must conclude that RNA is an evolutionarily advanced molecule that was preceded by one or more simpler genetic polymers.

Of course, once ribozymes (or enzymes) were available, the catalyzed synthesis of ribose might have been possible, and similarly for the subsequent steps in nucleotide synthesis. But what happened before that? We seem to face a new problem as serious as the one that ribozymes are alleged to solve. The most primitive organized system must have evolved in a milieu that originally included organic molecules in their "natural" abundance, i.e., in the relative proportions obtained without the intervention of ribozymes or enzymes. Various concentration and separation mechanisms could have simplified the prebiotic soup to a great extent, but it is still hard to believe that a series of well-defined $3',5'$-linked oligo-β-D-ribonucleotides could have formed de novo. It seems more likely that different types of monomers and short oligomers would have copolymerized and that the predominant monomers would have been simpler than ribonucleotides. Obviously, I do not know the identity of those simpler RNA analogs. However, the idea that some flexible backbone (Fig. 5), like the glycerol-phosphate backbone of teichoic acids, preceded the nucleic acid backbone seems very plausible (Schwartz and Orgel 1985; Joyce et al. 1987).

The nature of the original "bases" is also a subject for speculation. A replicating system that employed only two bases, A and I, might be possible (Crick 1968). Alternatively, some of the "bases" may not have been purines or pyrimidines. Perhaps, as we learn more about earlier phases in the evolution of life, we will come to recognize that the earliest genetic polymer was very different from DNA. The principle of structural complementarity between monomeric subunits may be all that has been conserved. Guessing the nature of the "ur RNA," the very first self-replicating genetic polymer, is likely to become a growth industry.

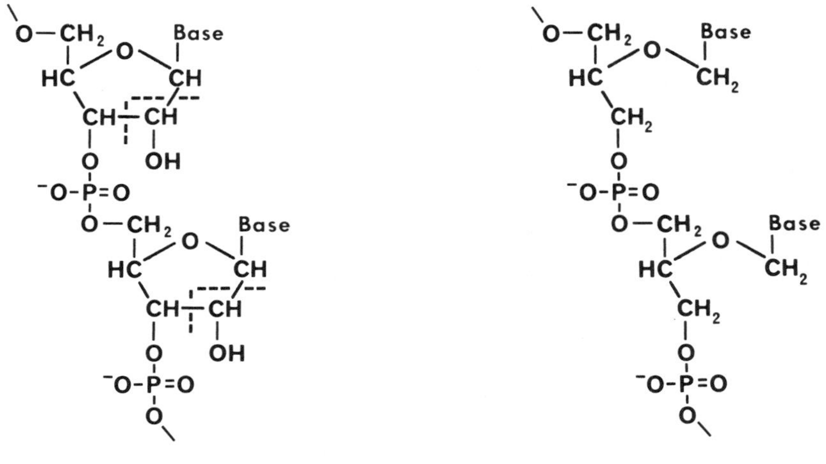

Figure 5. Comparison of the structures of RNA and of a much simpler polymer derived from glycerol.

At present, the central unsolved problem of chemical evolution seems to me to be the identification of the first informational molecules and the reconstruction of the path from them to DNA, RNA, and proteins. There are a number of constraints that must be satisfied by any acceptable theory:

1. The very first informational system must have had some capacity for self-replication in the absence of information-rich catalysts. Its monomeric subunits must have been abundant components of a prebiotic mixture of inorganic and organic compounds, and the chemistry involved in their polymerization must have proceeded easily in the appropriate prebiotic environment.

2. The "evolved" informational macromolecules at each stage must have had two properties. First, they must have functioned within the scope of their own system to improve the efficiency and accuracy of replication. Second, they must have facilitated the transition from their own system to the next more-advanced system. Thus, if glycerol derivatives were involved in place of ribose in a proto-nucleic acid, it must have been possible to build protoribozymes with glycerol derivatives that catalyzed the replication of poly (glycerol-nucleotide) oligomers and other glycerol-based catalysts that led to the synthesis or preferential utilization of ribonucleotides.

3. The transition to more modern biochemistry required the invention of genetic coding. This could, in principle, have occurred at any stage, either before or after the transition from proto-nucleic acids to nucleic acids.

The Evolution of Protein Synthesis

It is clear that in the course of recent eukaryotic evolution, introns have in some way facilitated the shuffling of the domains of proteins to produce molecules with new and useful properties (Gilbert 1985). At the present time, it also seems likely, but perhaps not certain, that introns were already present in proteins before the divergence of the eukaryotes from the bacteria (Gilbert et al. 1986). The evidence for these claims is discussed in this volume. What impact, if any, have these discoveries had on our ideas about the origins of protein synthesis?

Work on the positions of introns in the genes for universal enzymes, for example, the enzymes of glycolysis, may allow us to penetrate further back into the history of protein synthesis than ever before. There is some evidence supporting the suggestion that early enzymes were assembled from modules consisting of a short α-helix followed by a turn and then a short β-strand (Gilbert et al. 1986). Modules consisting of pairs of antiparallel β strands joined through a β-turn are also likely to have been important (Orgel 1977). Whether modules were at first joined together covalently, or whether they at first aggregated noncovalently in aqueous solution, is obscure.

These new discoveries somewhat simplify the problem of the evolution of the genetic code. They suggest that something useful could be achieved by coding for polypeptides as short as 12–30 amino acids in length. However, it does not seem to me that the new work provides insights into earlier stages in the evolution of the genetic code. In this area, only speculation is possible.

Contemporary protein synthesis is a complex process that involves many families of proteins, e.g., ribosomal proteins, activating enzymes, initiation factors, elongation factors, and termination factors. The first form of polynucleotide-directed polypeptide synthesis must have been much simpler. One appealing idea is that an early version of the genetic code involved a small number of amino acids. Alternatively, a few classes of amino acids rather than individual amino acids may have been assigned to codons (Woese 1967). Even with this simplification, the problems of controlling initiation and termination and of preventing a growing peptide chain from migrating during the course of synthesis seem to me insuperable in any but a highly evolved system.

An escape from this dilemma that I have proposed earlier (Orgel 1972, 1977; Brack and Orgel 1975) is to demand less of early protein synthesis. Perhaps the earliest coded polypeptides acted only as a porous membrane or a glue to hold together the polynucleotides that had guided their synthesis. Then, a simple error-resistant code that mapped polynucleotides with alternating purine-pyrimidine sequences onto peptides with alternating hydrophobic-hydrophilic sequences could have got the system started.

The origin of catalytic activity in peptides takes on a new look if we suppose that ribozymes preceded catalytic polypeptides. Then it seems reasonable to suppose that polypeptides first acted to make ribozymes more efficient. Ultimately, the polypeptides usurped the functions of the polynucleotides and became independent of them. Ribonuclease P can be thought of as a catalyst that has not progressed past the earlier stages in the sequence (see Westheimer 1986).

The ultimate origin of the genetic code remains a mystery. Some of the outstanding and as yet unanswerable questions are (1) Was there a stage in evolution when the attachment of amino acids to oligonucleotides (or their precursors) conferred selective advantage through a function other than peptide-bond formation? (2) Was there a stage in evolution when oligonucleotides (or their precursors) facilitated peptide-bond formation independently of any code or message? (3) Are the assignments in the genetic code a frozen accident or do they depend on specific interactions involving the codons (or anticodons) and the corresponding amino acids?

These are difficult questions, and it is not possible to suggest approaches that are likely to answer them soon. In the past, major contributions to our understanding of prebiotic chemistry and chemical evolution have come from unexpected discoveries in other disciplines. One can only hope that more such surprises are in store.

ACKNOWLEDGMENTS

I am grateful to Francis Crick and Jerry Joyce for their helpful comments, Sylvia Bailey for manuscript preparation, and Aubrey Hill, Jr., for drafting the figures. Some sections of this paper are adapted from a previous publication (Orgel 1986). This work was supported by grants from the National Institutes of Health and the National Aeronautics and Space Administration.

REFERENCES

Acevedo, O. and L.E. Orgel. 1987. Non-enzymatic transcription of an oligodeoxynucleotide 14 residues long. *J. Mol. Biol.* **197:** 187.

Brack, A. and L.E. Orgel. 1975. β structures of alternating polypeptides and their possible prebiotic significance. *Nature* **256:** 383.

Bridson, P.K. and L.E. Orgel. 1980. Catalysis of accurate poly(C)-directed synthesis of 3'-5'-linked oligoguanylates by Zn^{2+}. *J. Mol. Biol.* **144:** 567.

Buzayan, J.M., W.L. Gerlach, and G. Bruening. 1986. Non-enzymatic cleavage and ligation of RNAs complementary to a plant virus satellite RNA. *Nature* **323:** 349.

Cairns-Smith, A.G. 1982. *Genetic takeover and the mineral origins of life.* Cambridge University Press, Cambridge, Great Britain.

Cech, T.R. 1986. A model for the RNA-catalyzed replication of RNA. *Proc. Natl. Acad. Sci.* **83:** 4360.

———. 1987. The chemistry of self-splicing RNA and RNA enzymes. *Science* **236:** 1532.

Chen, C.B., T. Inoue, and L.E. Orgel. 1985. Template-directed synthesis on oligodeoxycytidylate and polydeoxycytidylate templates. *J. Mol. Biol.* **181:** 271.

Chung, N.M., R. Lohrmann, and L.E. Orgel. 1971. Template catalysis of acetyl transfer reactions. *Biochim. Biophys. Acta* **228:** 536.

Crick, F.H.C. 1968. The origin of the genetic code. *J. Mol. Biol.* **38:** 367.

———. 1981. *Life itself; Its origin and nature.* p. 88. Simon and Schuster, New York.

Darnell, J.E. and W.F. Doolittle. 1986. Speculations on the early course of evolution. *Proc. Natl. Acad. Sci.* **83:** 1271.

Gilbert, W. 1985. Genes-in-pieces revisited. *Science* **228:** 823.

———. 1986. The RNA world. *Nature* **319:** 618.

Gilbert, W., M. Marchionni, and G. McKnight. 1986. On the antiquity of introns. *Cell* **46:** 151.

Guerrier-Takada, C., K. Gardiner, T. Marsh, N. Pace, and S. Altman. 1983. The RNA moiety of ribonuclease P is the catalytic subunit of the enzyme. *Cell* **35:** 849.

Haertle, T. and L.E. Orgel. 1986. The template properties of some oligodeoxynucleotides containing cytidine and guanosine. *J. Mol. Evol.* **23:** 108.

Inoue, T. and L.E. Orgel. 1982. Oligomerization of (guanosine 5'-phosphor)-2-methylimidazolide on poly(C): An RNA polymerase model. *J. Mol. Biol.* **162:** 201.

———. 1983. A nonenzymatic RNA polymerase model. *Science* **219:** 859.

Inoue, T., G.F. Joyce, K. Grzeskowiak, L.E. Orgel, J.M. Brown, and C.B. Reese. 1984. Template-directed synthesis on the pentanucleotide CpCpGpCpC. *J. Mol. Biol.* **178:** 669.

Joyce, G.F., A.W. Schwartz, S.L. Miller, and L.E. Orgel. 1987. The case for an ancestral genetic system involving simple analogues of the nucleotides. *Proc. Natl. Acad. Sci.* **84:** 4398.

Kauffman, S.A. 1986. Autocatalytic sets of proteins. *J. Theor. Biol.* **119:** 1.

Kay, P.S. and T. Inoue. 1987. Catalysis of splicing-related reactions between dinucleotides by a ribozyme. *Nature* **317:** 343.

Kruger, K., P.J. Grabowski, A.J. Zaug, J. Sands, D.E. Gottschling, and T.R. Cech. 1982. Self-splicing RNA: Autoexcision and autocyclization of the ribosomal RNA intervening sequences of *Tetrahymena. Cell* **31:** 147.

Lohrmann, R. and L.E. Orgel. 1977. Reactions of adenosine 5'-phosphorimidazolide with adenosine analogs on a polyuridylic acid template. The uniqueness of the 2'-3'-unsubstituted β-ribosyl system. *J. Mol. Biol.* **113:** 193.

———. 1980. Efficient catalysis of polycytidylic formation by Pb^{2+}. *J. Mol. Biol.* **142:** 555.

Miller, S.L. and L.E. Orgel. 1974. *The origins of life on the earth.* Prentice Hall, Englewood Cliffs, New Jersey.

Naylor, R. and P.T. Gilham. 1966. Studies on some interactions and reactions of oligonucleotides in aqueous solution. *Biochemistry* **5:** 2722.

Ninio, J. and L.E. Orgel. 1978. Heteropolynucleotides as templates for non-enzymatic polymerizations. *J. Mol. Evol.* **12:** 91.

Orgel, L.E. 1968. Evolution of the genetic apparatus. *J. Mol. Biol.* **38:** 381.

———. 1972. A possible step in the origin of the genetic code. *Isr. J. Chem.* **10:** 287.

———. 1977. β-turns and the evolution of protein synthesis. In *The organization and expression of the eukaryotic genome. Proceedings of the International Symposium, May 3–6, 1976, Tehran* (ed. E.M. Bradbury and K. Javaherian), p. 499. Academic Press, London.

———. 1986. RNA catalysis and the origins of life. *J. Theor. Biol.* **123:** 127.

Orgel, L.E. and R. Lohrmann. 1974. Prebiotic chemistry and nucleic acid replication. *Acc. Chem. Res.* **7:** 368.

Pace, N.R. and T.L. Marsh. 1985. RNA catalysis and the origin of life. *Origins Life* **16:** 97.

Prody, G.A., J.T. Bakos, J.M. Buzayan, I.R. Schneider, and G. Bruening. 1986. Autolytic processing of dimeric plant virus satellite RNA. *Science* **231:** 1577.

Schwartz, A.W. and L.E. Orgel. 1985. Template-directed synthesis of novel, nucleic acid-like structures. *Science* **228:** 585.

Shabarova, Z.A. 1984. Chemical ligation—An alternative method for assembly of natural and modified DNA duplexes. *Sov. Sci. Rev. Sect. D Biol. Rev.* **5:** 1.

Sharp, P.A. 1985. On the origin of RNA splicing and introns. Minireview. *Cell* **42:** 397.

Shvedova, T.A., G.A. Korneeva, V.A. Otroshchenko, and T.V. Venkstern. 1987. Catalytic activity of the nucleic acid component of the 1,4-α-glucan branching enzyme from rabbit muscles. *Nucleic Acids Res.* **15:** 1745.

Sulston, J.E. and L.E. Orgel. 1971a. Polynucleotides and the origin of life. In *De la physique théorique à la biologie* (ed. M. Marois), p. 109. Editions du Centre National de la Recherche Scientifique, Paris.

———. 1971b. Polynucleotide replication and the origin of life. In *Prebiotic and biochemical evolution* (ed. A.P. Kimball and J. Oro), p. 89. Elsevier/North-Holland, Amsterdam.

Ts'o, P.O. 1974. *Basic principles in nucleic acid chemistry,* vol. I. Academic Press, New York.

Uhlenbeck, O.C. 1987. A small catalytic oligoribonucleotide. *Nature* **328:** 596.

Usher, D.A. and A.H. McHale. 1976. Hydrolytic stability of helical RNA: A selective advantage for the natural 3',5'-bond. *Proc. Natl. Acad. Sci.* **73:** 1149.

von Kiedrowski, G. 1986. A self-replicating hexadeoxynucleotide. *Angew. Chem. Int. Ed. Engl.* **25:** 932.

Weber, A.L. and L.E. Orgel. 1980. Poly(U)-directed peptide-bond formation from the 2'(3')-glycyl esters of adenosine derivatives. *J. Mol. Evol.* **16:** 1.

Westheimer, F.H. 1986. Polyribonucleic acids as enzymes. *Nature* **319:** 534.

Woese, C.R. 1967. *The genetic code: The molecular basis for genetic expression.* Harper and Row, New York.

Zaug, A.J. and T.R. Cech. 1986. The intervening sequence RNA of *Tetrahymena* is an enzyme. *Science* **231:** 470.

Which Organic Compounds Could Have Occurred on the Prebiotic Earth?

S.L. MILLER

Department of Chemistry, B-017, University of California, San Diego, La Jolla, California 90293

In the past three decades, a wide variety of experiments have been designed to simulate conditions on the primitive earth and to demonstrate how organic compounds that made up the first living organisms were synthesized. This paper reviews this work and indicates the status of such syntheses. There is too much material to review in detail, and the reader is directed to a number of more complete discussions (Miller and Orgel 1974; Kenyon and Steinman 1969; Lemmon 1970).

Composition of the Primitive Atmosphere

There is no agreement on the constituents of the primitive atmosphere. It is to be noted that there is no geological evidence concerning the conditions on the earth from 4.5×10^9 to 3.8×10^9 years, since no rocks older than 3.8×10^9 years are known. Even the 3.8×10^9-year-old Isua Rocks in Greenland are not sufficiently well preserved to infer details of the atmosphere at that time. Proposed atmospheres and the reasons given to favor them are not discussed here. As described below, the more reducing atmospheres favor the synthesis of organic compounds in terms of both yields and the variety of compounds obtained. Some of the organic chemistry can give explicit predictions about atmospheric constituents. Such considerations cannot prove that the earth had a certain primitive atmosphere, but the prebiotic synthesis constraints should be a major consideration.

Energy Sources

A wide variety of energy sources have been utilized with various gas mixtures since the first experiments using electric discharges. The importance of a given energy source is determined by the product of the energy available and its efficiency for organic compound synthesis. Even though both factors cannot be evaluated with precision, a qualitative assessment of the energy sources can be made. It should be emphasized that a single source of energy or a single process is unlikely to account for all the organic compounds on the primitive earth (Miller et al. 1976). An estimate of the sources of energy on the earth at the present time is given in Table 1.

The energy from the decay of radioactive elements was probably not an important energy source for the synthesis of organic compounds on the primitive earth, since most of the ionization would have taken place in

silicate rocks, rather than in the reducing atmosphere. The shock-wave energy from the impact of meteorites on the earth's atmosphere and surface and the larger amount of shock waves generated in lightning bolts have been proposed as energy sources for primitive earth organic synthesis. Very high yields of amino acids have been reported in some experiments (Bar-Nun et al. 1970), but it is doubtful whether such yields would be obtained in natural shock waves. Cosmic rays are a minor source of energy on the earth at present, and it seems unlikely that any increase in the past could have been so great as to make them a major source of energy.

The energy in the lava emitted at the present time is a significant, but not a major, source of energy. It is generally supposed that there was a much greater amount of volcanic activity on the primitive earth, but there is no evidence to support this. Even if the volcanic activity was a factor of 10 greater than at present, it would not have been the dominant energy source. Nevertheless, molten lava may have been important in the pyrolytic synthesis of some organic compounds.

UV light was probably the largest source of energy on the primitive earth. The wavelengths absorbed by the atmospheric constituents are all below 2000 Å, except for ammonia (< 2300 Å and $H_2S < 2600$ Å). Whether it was the most effective source of organic compounds is not clear. Most of the photochemical reactions would occur in the upper atmosphere, and the products formed would, for the most part, absorb the

Table 1. Present Sources of Energy Averaged Over the Earth

Source	Energy	
	(cal/cm^2/yr)	(J/cm^2/yr)
Total radiation from sun	260 000	1 090 000
Ultraviolet light		
<3000 Å	3 400	14 000
<2500 Å	563	2 360
<2000 Å	41	170
<1500 Å	1.7	7
Electric discharges	4[a]	17
Cosmic rays	0.0015	0.006
Radioactivity		
(to 1.0 km depth)	0.8	3.0
Volcanoes	0.13	0.5
Shock waves	1.1[b]	4.6

[a] 3 cal/cm^2/yr of corona discharge +1 cal/cm^2/yr of lightning.
[b] 1 cal/cm^2 yr of this is in the shock wave of lightning bolts and is also included under electric discharges.

longer wavelengths, and so be decomposed before they reached the protection of the oceans. The yield of amino acids from the photolysis of CH_4, NH_3, and H_2O at wavelengths of 1470 and 1294 Å is quite low (Groth and von Weyssenhoff 1960), probably due to the low yields of hydrogen cyanide. The synthesis of amino acids by the photolysis of CH_4, C_2H_6, NH_3, H_2O, and H_2S mixtures by UV light of wavelengths greater than 2000 Å (Khare and Sagan 1971; Sagan and Khare 1971) is also a low-yield synthesis, but the amount of energy is much greater in this region of the sun's spectrum. Only H_2S absorbs the UV light, but the photodissociation of H_2S results in a hydrogen atom having a high kinetic energy, which activates or dissociates methane, ammonia, and water. This appears to be a very attractive prebiotic synthesis. However, it is not clear whether a sufficient partial pressure of H_2S could be maintained in the atmosphere, since H_2S is photolyzed rapidly to elemental sulfur and hydrogen. The same applies to other molecules that might generate hot hydrogen atoms.

A photochemical source of HCN using the very short wavelengths of the Lyman continuum (796–912 Å) has been proposed by Zahnle (1986). The N atoms produced diffuse lower into the atmosphere and react with CH_2 and CH_3, producing HCN. The process depends on N atoms reacting with nothing else before the CH_2 and CH_3. Whether this is valid remains to be determined.

The most widely used sources of energy for laboratory syntheses of prebiotic compounds are electric discharges. These include sparks, semicorona, arc, and silent discharges, with the spark being the most frequently used type. The ease of handling and high efficiency of electric discharges are factors favoring their use, but the most important reason is that electric discharges are very efficient in synthesizing hydrogen cyanide, whereas UV light is not. Hydrogen cyanide is a central intermediate in prebiotic synthesis, being needed for amino acid synthesis from the Strecker reaction, or by self-polymerization to amino acids, and most importantly for the prebiotic synthesis of adenine and guanine.

An important feature of all these energy sources is the activation of molecules in a local area, followed by quenching off this activated mixture, and then protecting the organic compounds from further influence of the energy source. The quenching and protective steps are critical because the organic compounds will be destroyed if subjected continuously to the energy source.

Prebiotic Synthesis of Amino Acids

Mixtures of CH_4, NH_3, and H_2O with or without added H_2 are considered strongly reducing atmospheres. The atmosphere of Jupiter contains these species, with H_2 in large excess over CH_4. The first successful prebiotic amino acid synthesis was carried out using an electric discharge as an energy source (Miller 1953, 1955). The result was a large yield of amino acids (the yield of glycine alone was 2.1% based on the carbon), together with hydroxy acids, short aliphatic acids, and urea. One of the surprising results of this experiment was that the products were not a random mixture of organic compounds, but rather a relatively small number of compounds produced in substantial yield. In addition, the compounds were, with a few exceptions, of biological importance.

The mechanism of synthesis of the amino and hydroxy acids was investigated (Miller 1957, 1959). It was shown that the amino acids were not formed directly in the electric discharge but were the result of solution reactions of smaller molecules produced in the discharge, in particular hydrogen cyanide and aldehydes. These rections are presented in Scheme 1.

$$RCHO + HCN + NH_3 \rightleftharpoons RCH(NH_2)CN \xrightarrow{H_2O} RCH(NH_2)\overset{O}{\overset{\|}{C}}-NH_2 \xrightarrow{H_2O} RCH(NH_2)COOH$$

$$RCHO + HCN \rightleftharpoons RCH(OH)CN \xrightarrow{H_2O} RCH(OH)C-NH_2 \xrightarrow{H_2O} RCH(OH)COOH$$

The reactions were subsequently studied in detail, and the equilibrium and rate constants of these reactions were measured (Miller and Van Trump 1981). These results show that amino and hydroxy acids can be synthesized at high dilutions of HCN and aldehydes in a primitive ocean. It is also to be noted that the rates of these reactions were rather rapid. The half-lives for the hydrolysis of the amino and hydroxy nitriles are less than 10^3 years at 0°C.

This synthesis of amino acids, called the Strecker synthesis, requires the presence of NH_4^+ (and NH_3) in

Table 2. Yields from Sparking a Mixture CH_4, NH_3, H_2O, and H_2.

Compound	Yield	
	μmoles	%
Glycine	630	2.1
Glycolic acid	560	1.9
Sarcosine	50	0.25
Alanine	340	1.7
Lactic acid	310	1.6
N-Methylalanine	10	0.07
α-Amino-n-butyric acid	50	0.34
α-Aminoisobutyric acid	1	0.007
α-Hydroxybutyric acid	50	0.34
β-Alanine	150	0.76
Succinic acid	40	0.27
Aspartic acid	4	0.024
Glutamic acid	6	0.051
Iminodiacetic acid	55	0.37
Iminoacetic-propionic acid	15	0.13
Formic acid	2330	4.0
Acetic acid	150	0.51
Propionic acid	130	0.66
Urea	20	0.034
N-Methyl urea	15	0.051
Total		15.2

The present yields are based on carbon; 59 mmoles (712 mg) of carbon was added as CH_4.

the primitive ocean. On the basis of the experimental equilibrium and rate constants, it can be shown (Miller and Van Trump 1981) that equal amounts of amino and hydroxy acids are obtained when the NH_4^+ concentration is about 0.01 M at pH 8 and 25°C, with this NH_4^+ concentration being insensitive to temperature and pH. This translates into a pNH_3 in the atmosphere of 2×10^{-7} atm at 0°C and 4×10^{-6} atm at 25°C. This is a low partial pressure, but it would seem to be necessary for amino acid synthesis. A similar estimate of the NH_4^+ concentration in the primitive ocean can be obtained from the equilibrium decomposition of aspartic acid (Bada and Miller 1968). Ammonia is decomposed by UV light, but mechanisms for resynthesis are available. The details of the ammonia balance on the primitive earth remain to be worked out.

In a typical electric-discharge experiment, the partial pressure of CH_4 is 0.1–0.2 atm. This pressure is used for convenience, and it is likely, but never demonstrated, that organic compound synthesis would work at much lower partial pressures of methane. There are no estimates available for pCH_4 on the primitive earth, but 10^{-5} to 10^{-3} atm seems plausible. Higher pressures are not reasonable because the sources of energy would convert the CH_4 to organic compounds in the oceans too rapidly for higher pressures of CH_4 to build up.

UV light acting on this mixture of gases is not effective in producing amino acids except at very short wavelengths (< 1500 Å), and even then the yields are very low (Groth and von Weyssenhoff 1960). The low yields are probably due to the low yields of HCN produced by UV light. If the gas mixture is modified by adding gases such as H_2S or formaldehyde, then reasonable yields of amino acids can be obtained at relatively long wavelengths (< 2500 Å), where considerable energies from the sun are available (Khare and Sagan 1971; Sagan and Khare 1971). It is possible, but not demonstrated, that HCN and other molecules are produced, which then form amino acids in the aqueous part of the system.

Pyrolysis of CH_4 and NH_3 gives very low yields of amino acids. The pyrolysis conditions are from 800°C to 1200°C, with contact times of 1 second or less (Lawless and Boynton 1973). However, the pyrolysis of CH_4 and other hydrocarbons gives good yields of benzene, phenylacetylene, and many other hydrocarbons. It can be shown that phenylacetylene would be converted to phenylalanine and tyrosine in the primitive ocean (Friedmann and Miller 1969). Pyrolysis of the hydrocarbons in the presence of NH_3 gives substantial yields of indole, which can be converted to tryptophan in the primitive ocean (Friedmann et al. 1971).

A mixture of CH_4, N_2, and traces of NH_3, and H_2O is a more realistic atmosphere for the primitive earth because large amounts of NH_3 would not have accumulated in the atmosphere since NH_3 would dissolve in the ocean. It is still, however, a strongly reducing atmosphere. This mixture of gases is quite effective with an electric discharge in producing amino acids (Ring et al. 1972; Wolman et al. 1972). The yields are somewhat

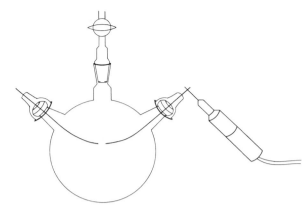

Figure 1. Spark-discharge apparatus. The 3-liter flask is shown with the two tungsten electrodes and a spark generator. The second electrode is usually not grounded. In the experiments described in Table 3, the flask contained 100 ml of 0.05 M NH_4Cl brought to pH 8.7 giving pNH_3 of 0.2 torr. The pCH_4 was 200 torr and pN_2 was 80 torr. Since the temperature was about 30°C during the sparking, pH_2O was 32 torr.

Table 3. Yields from Sparking CH_4 (336 mmoles), N_2, and H_2O with Traces of NH_3

	μmoles
Glycine	440
Alanine	790
α-Amino-n-butyric acid	270
α-Aminoisobutyric acid	~30
Valine	19.5
Norvaline	61
Isovaline	~5
Leucine	11.3
Isoleucine	4.8
Alloisoleucine	5.1
Norleucine	6.0
tert-Leucine	<0.02
Proline	1.5
Aspartic acid	34
Glutamic acid	7.7
Serine	5.0
Threonine	~0.8
Allothreonine	~0.8
α,γ-Diaminobutyric acid	33
α-Hydroxy-γ-aminobutyric acid	74
α,β-Diaminopropionic	6.4
Isoserine	5.5
Sarcosine	55
N-Ethylglycine	30
N-Propylglycine	~2
N-Isopropylglycine	~2
N-Methylalanine	~15
N-Ethylalanine	<0.2
β-Alanine	18.8
β-Amino-n-butyric acid	~0.3
β-Amino-isobutyric acid	~0.3
γ-Aminobutyric acid	2.4
N-Methyl-β-alanine	~5
N-Ethyl-β-alanine	~2
Pipecolic acid	0.05

Yield based on the carbon added as CH_4. Glycine = 0.26%, Alanine = 0.71%, total yield of amino acids in the table = 1.90%.

lower than with higher partial pressures of NH_3, but the products are more diverse. Hydroxy acids, short aliphatic acids, and dicarboxylic acids are produced along with the amino acids (Peltzer and Bada 1978; Peltzer et al. 1984). Of the 20 amino acids that occur on proteins, 10 are produced directly in this experiment. Counting asparagine and glutamine, which are formed but hydrolyzed before analysis, and methionine, which is formed when H_2S is added (Miller and Van Trump 1972), one can say that 13 of the 20 amino acids in proteins can be formed in this single experiment. Cysteine was found in the photolysis of CH_4, NH_3, H_2O, and H_2S (Khare and Sagan 1971). The pyrolysis of hydrocarbons, as discussed above, leads to phenylalanine, tyrosine, and tryptophan. This leaves only the basic amino acids: lysine, arginine, and histidine. There are so far no established prebiotic syntheses of these amino acids. There is no fundamental reason the basic amino acids cannot be synthesized, and this problem may be solved before too long.

Mildly Reducing and Nonreducing Atmospheres

There has been less experimental work with gas mixtures containing CO and CO_2 as carbon sources instead of CH_4. Spark discharges have been the source of energy most extensively investigated (Abelson 1965; Schlesinger and Miller 1983a,b; Stribling and Miller 1987). Figure 2 compares amino acid yields using CH_4, CO, and CO_2 as carbon sources with various amounts of H_2. Separate experiments were performed with and without added NH_3. In the case of CH_4 without added NH_3, the yield of amino acids is 4.7% at $H_2/CH_4 = 0$ and drops to 1.4% at $H_2/CH_4 = 4$. With CO and no added NH_3, the amino acid yield is 0.05% at $H_2/CO = 0$ and rises to a maximum of 2.7% at $H_2/CO = 3$. With

CO_2 and no added NH_3, the amino acid yield is 7×10^{-4} at $H_2/CO_2 = 0$. This is close to the level of reagent contamination and is so low that this could not be considered as a significant source of amino acids on the primitive earth. At higher H_2/CO_2 ratios, however, the yield is about 2%. With both CO and CO_2, the presence of added NH_3 increases the yield of amino acids by a factor of approximately 10 at low H_2/CO and H_2/CO_2 ratios. The amino acids produced in the CH_4 experiments were similar to those shown in Table 3. With CO and CO_2, glycine was the predominant amino acid, with little else besides an alanine being produced (Table 4).

A mixture of $CO + H_2$ is used in the Fischer-Tropsch reaction to make hydrocarbons in high yields. The reaction requires a catalyst, usually Fe or Ni supported on silica, a temperature of 200–400°C, and a short contact time. Depending on the conditions, aliphatic hydrocarbons, aromatic hydrocarbons, alcohols, and acids can be produced. If NH_3 is added to the $CO + H_2$, then amino acids, purines, and pyrimidines can be formed (Hayatsu and Anders 1981). The intermediates in these reactions are not known, but it is likely that HCN is involved, together with some of the intermediates postulated for the electric discharge processes.

A mixture of $CO + H_2O$ with electric discharges is not particularly effective in organic compound synthesis, but UV light that is absorbed by water ($<$1849 Å) results in the production of formaldehyde and other aldehydes, alcohols, and acids in fair yields (Bar-Nun and Hartman 1978; Bar-Nun and Chang 1983). The mechanism seems to involve splitting H_2O to H + OH, with OH converting CO to CO_2 and H reducing another molecule of CO.

Electric discharges and UV light do not give substan-

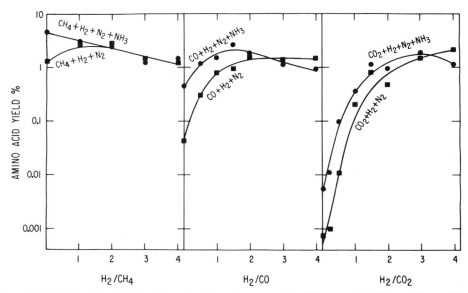

Figure 2. Amino acid yields based on initial carbon. In all experiments, $pN_2 = 100$ torr, and pCH_4, pCO, or $pCO_2 = 100$ torr and 100 ml H_2O. The flask was kept at room temperature, and the spark generator was operated continuously for 48 hr.

Table 4. Mole Ratio of Amino Acids Relative to Glycine = 100

Amino acid	$H_2/CH_4 = 3.0$	$H_2/CO = 3.0$	$H_2/CO_2 = 0.5$	$H_2/CO_2 = 3.0$
Glycine	100 (0.40)	100 (1.42)	100 (0.01)	100 (1.53)
Alanine	101	2.4	7.0	0.87
α-Amino butyric	30	0.04	<0.001	0.09
Valine	1.2	0.005	<0.001	<0.001
Norvaline	1.3	0.01	<0.001	<0.001
Aspartic acid	1.6	0.09	0.22	0.14
Glutamic acid	1.5	0.01	0.06	<0.001
Serine	3.1	0.15	0.40	0.23

The percent yield of glycine based on carbon is given in parentheses. Adapted from Schlesinger and Miller (1983a).

tial amounts of organic compounds with a mixture of $CO_2 + H_2O$. Ionizing radiation (e.g., 40 MEV helium ions) gives small yields of formic acid and formaldehyde (Garrison et al. 1951). Calculations using one-dimensional photochemical models of $CO_2 + H_2O$ atmospheres show that substantial amounts of H_2CO can be produced in these atmospheres by solar UV light (Pinto et al. 1980; Kasting et al. 1984).

The action of γ-rays on an aqueous solution of CO_2 and ferrous iron gives fair yields of formic acid, oxalic acid, and other simple products (Getoff 1962). UV light gives similar results. In these reactions, the Fe^{++} is a stoichiometric reducing agent rather than a catalyst. Nitrogen in the form of N_2 does not react, and experiments with NH_3 have not been tried.

The implications of these results in considering the composition of the primitive earth is that CH_4 is the best carbon source for prebiotic synthesis, especially for amino acid synthesis. Although glycine was essentially the only amino acid synthesized in the spark discharge experiments with CO and CO_2, other amino acids (e.g., serine, aspartic acid, and alanine) would probably have been formed from this glycine, H_2CO, and HCN as the primitive ocean matured. Since we do not know which amino acids made up the first organism, we can only say that CO and CO_2 are less favorable than CH_4 for amino acid synthesis; however, these amino acids may have been adequate. The synthesis of purine and sugars described below would not be greatly different with CH_4, CO, or CO_2 with adequate H_2. Although the spark discharge yields of amino acids, HCN, and H_2CO are about the same with CH_4 and with $H_2/CO > 1$ and $H_2/CO_2 > 2$, it is not clear how such high H_2/carbon ratios could have been maintained in the primitive atmosphere, since H_2 escapes from the earth's atmosphere into outer space. These problems are poorly understood and beyond the scope of this paper.

Purine and Pyrimidine Synthesis

Hydrogen cyanide is used in the synthesis of purines as well as amino acids. This is illustrated in a remarkable synthesis of adenine. If concentrated solutions of ammonium cyanide are refluxed for a few days,

adenine is obtained in up to 0.5% yield, along with 4-aminoimidazole-5-carboxamide and the usual cyanide polymer (Oro and Kimball 1961, 1962). The probable mechanism of adenine synthesis under these concentrated conditions in these experiments is probably via the HCN tetramer and formamidine.

The difficult step in the synthesis of adenine just described is the reaction of tetramer with formamidine. This step may be bypassed by the photochemical rearrangement of tetramer to aminoimidazole carbonitrile, a reaction that proceeds readily in contemporary sunlight (see Scheme 3) (Ferris and Orgel 1966; Sanchez et al. 1967, 1968).

A further possibility is that tetramer formation may have occurred in an eutectic solution. High yield of tetramer (>10%) can be obtained by cooling dilute cyanide solutions to between $-10°C$ and $-30°C$ for a few months (Sanchez et al. 1966a). The cyanide polymerization reaction to adenine is even more complex than indicated here, with the synthesis proceeding through 8-cyanoadenine and 2-cyanoadenine under some conditions (Voet and Schwartz 1983).

Guanine, hypoxanthine, xanthine, and diaminopurine would have been synthesized by variations of the adenine synthesis, as shown in Scheme 4, using aminoimidazole carbonitrile and aminoimidazole carboxamide.

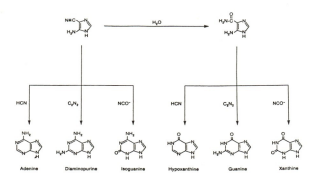

The prebiotic synthesis of the pyrimidine cytosine involves cyanoacetylene, which is synthesized in good yield by sparking mixtures of $CH_4 + N_2$. Cyanoacetylene reacts with cyanate to give cytosine (Sanchez et al. 1966b; Ferris et al. 1968), and the cytosine can be converted to uracil (see Scheme 5).

Cyanate can come from cyanogen or by decomposition of urea. A related synthesis starts with cyanoacetaldehyde, from the hydration of cyanoacetylene, which reacts with guanidine to give diaminopyrimidine. This is then hydrolyzed to cytosine and uracil (see Scheme 6) (Ferris et al. 1974).

Another prebiotic synthesis of uracil starts from β-alanine and cyanate and UV light (see Scheme 7) (Schwartz and Chittenden 1977).

Sugars

The synthesis of reducing sugars from formaldehyde under alkaline conditions was discovered by Butlerow (1861). However, the Butlerow or formose reaction is very complex and incompletely understood. It depends on the presence of a suitable catalyst, with calcium hydroxide and calcium carbonate being the most popular heterogeneous catalysts. In the absence of catalysts, little or no sugar is obtained. At 100°C, clays such as kaolin serve to catalyze formation of monosaccharides, including ribose, in significant yield from dilute (0.01 M) solutions of formaldehyde (Gabel and Ponnamperuma 1967; Reid and Orgel 1970).

The reaction is autocatalytic and proceeds in stages through glycolaldehyde, glyceraldehyde, and dihydroxyacetone, tetroses, and pentoses to give finally hexoses, including glucose and fructose. One proposed reaction sequence is depicted in Scheme 8.

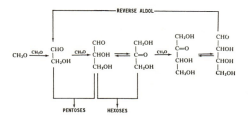

There are two problems with the formose reaction as a source of sugars on the primitive earth. The first is the stability of sugars. They decompose in a few hundred years at most at 25°C. There are a number of possible ways to stabilize sugars, the most interesting being to convert the sugar to a glycoside of a purine or pyrimidine. The second problem is that the formose reaction gives a wide variety of sugars, both straight chain and branched. Over 40 sugars have been separated from one reaction mixture (Decker et al. 1982). Ribose is in this mixture, but is not particularly abundant. It is difficult to envision how the relative yield of ribose could be greatly increased in this reaction or how any prebiotic reaction of sugars could give mostly ribose. It has therefore become apparent that ribonucleotides could not have been the first components of the prebiotic nucleic acids. A number of alternatives to the ribonucleoside (I) have been proposed (Joyce et al. 1987), which include the compounds (II, III, IV) shown in Scheme 9.

There are many other possibilities, but the ones shown are attractive because they are open chain, flexible, and prochiral. The prebiotic synthesis of these compounds has not yet been demonstrated.

Other Prebiotic Compounds

There are a number of compounds that have been synthesized under primitive earth conditions, but space does not permit an adequate discussion. These include dicarboxylic acids, tricarboxylic acids, fatty acids C_2-C_{10} (branched and straight), fatty alcohols (straight chain via Fischer-Tropsch reaction), porphin, nicotinonitrile and nicotinamide, triazines, and imidazoles. Other prebiotic compounds that may have been involved in polymerization reactions include cyanate [NCO^-], cyanamide [H_2NCN], cyanamide dimer [$H_2NC(NH)NH-CN$], dicyanamide [$NC-NH-CN$], cyanogen [$NC-CN$], HCN tetramer, diimino succinonitrile, acylthioesters, and phosphate polymers.

Compounds That Have Not Been Synthesized Prebiotically

It is a matter of opinion as to what constitutes a prebiotic synthesis. In some cases, the conditions are so forced (e.g., the use of anhydrous solvents) or the concentrations are so high (e.g., 10 M formaldehyde) that such conditions could not have occurred extensively on the primitive earth. Reactions under these and other extreme conditions cannot be considered prebiotic.

There have been many claimed prebiotic syntheses in which the compound has not been properly identified. The best method for unequivocal identification these days is gas chromatography–mass spectrometry of a suitable derivative, although melting points and mixed melting points can sometimes be used. The amino acid analyzer alone or chromatography in multiple solvent systems does not prove the identification of a compound.

Some of the compounds that do not yet have adequate prebiotic syntheses are arginine, lysine, histidine, straight chain fatty acids, porphyrins, pyridoxal, thiamine, riboflavin, folic acid, lipoic acid, and biotin. It is probable that prebiotic syntheses will be available before too long for some of these compounds. In other cases, the compounds may not have been synthesized prebiotically, so their occurrence in living systems is a result of early metabolic syntheses.

Organic Compounds in Carbonaceous Chondrites

On September 28, 1969, a type II carbonaceous chondrite fell in Murchison, Australia. Surprisingly, large amounts of amino acids were found by Kvenvolden et al. (1970, 1971) and Oro et al. (1971). The first report identified seven amino acids (glycine, alanine, valine, proline, glutamic acid, sarcosine, and α-aminoisobutyric acid), of which all but valine and proline had been found in the original electric discharge experiments (Miller 1953, 1955, 1957). The most striking are sarcosine and α-aminoisobutyric acid. The second report identified 18 amino acids, of which 9 had previously been identified in the original electric discharge experiments, but the remaining 9 had not.

At that time, we had identified the hydrophobic amino acids from the low-temperature electric discharge experiments described above, and therefore we examined the products for the nonprotein amino acids found in Murchison. We were able to find all of them (Ring et al. 1972; Wolman et al. 1972).

There is a striking similarity between the products and relative abundances of the amino acids produced by electric discharge and the meteorite amino acids. Table 5 compares the results. The most notable difference between the meteorite and the electric discharge amino acids is pipecolic acid, the yield being extremely low in the electric discharge. Proline is also present in relatively low yield from the electric discharge. The amount of α-aminoisobutyric acid is greater than α-

Table 5. Relative Abundances of Amino Acids in the Murchison Meteorite and in an Electric-discharge Synthesis

Amino acid	Murchison meteorite	Electric discharge
Glycine	****	****
Alanine	****	****
α-Amino-n-butyric acid	***	****
α-Aminoisobutyric acid	****	**
Valine	***	**
Norvaline	***	***
Isovaline	**	**
Proline	***	*
Pipecolic acid	*	<*
Aspartic acid	***	***
Glutamic acid	***	**
β-Alanine	**	**
β-Amino-n-butyric acid	*	*
β-Aminoisobutyric acid	*	*
γ-Aminobutyric acid	*	**
Sarcosine	**	***
N-Ethylglycine	**	***
N-Methylalanine	**	**

Mole ratio to glycine (=100): * 0.05–0.5; ** 0.5–5; *** 5–50; **** <50.

amino-n-butyric acid in the meteorite, but the reverse is the case in the electric discharge. Reasonable differences in ratios of amino acids do not detract from the overall picture. Indeed, the ratio of α-aminoisobutyric acid to glycine is quite different in two meteorites of the same type, being 0.4 in Murchison and 3.8 in Murray (Cronin and Moore 1971). A similar comparison has been made between the dicarboxylic acids in Murchison (Lawless et al. 1974) and those produced by an electric discharge (Zeitman et al. 1974), and the product ratios are quite similar.

The close correspondence between the amino acids found in the Murchison meteorite and those produced by electric discharge synthesis, both as to the amino acids produced and as to their relative ratios, suggests that the amino acids in the meteorite were synthesized on the parent body by means of an electric discharge or analogous processes. A quantitative comparison of the amino acid and hydroxy acid abundances (Peltzer and Bada 1978) shows that these compounds can be accounted for by a Strecker-Cyanohydrin synthesis on the parent body (Peltzer et al. 1984). Electric discharges appear to be the most favored source of energy, but sufficient data are not available to make realistic comparisons with other energy sources.

Our ideas on the prebiotic synthesis of organic compounds are based largely on the results of experiments in model systems. It is extremely gratifying to see that such synthesis really did take place on the parent body of the meteorite, and so it becomes plausible but not proved that they took place on the primitive earth.

Interstellar Molecules

In the past 10 years, a large number of organic molecules have been found in interstellar dust clouds mostly by emission lines in the microwave region of the spectrum (for a summary, see Mann and Williams 1980). The concentration of these molecules is very low (a few molecules per cm^3 at the most), but the total amount in a dust cloud is high. The molecules found include formaldehyde, hydrogen cyanide, acetaldehyde, and cyanoacetylene. These are important prebiotic molecules, and this immediately raises the question of whether the interstellar molecules played a role in the origin of life on the earth. For this to have taken place, it would have been necessary for the molecules to have been greatly concentrated in the solar nebula and to have arrived on the earth without being destroyed by UV light or pyrolysis. This appears to be difficult to do. In addition, it is necessary for some molecules to be continuously synthesized (unless life started very quickly) because of their instability, and an interstellar source could not be responsible for these.

For these reasons, it is generally felt that the interstellar molecules played at most a minor role in the origin of life. However, the presence of so many molecules of prebiotic importance in interstellar space, combined with the fact that their synthesis must differ from that on the primitive earth where conditions were very different, indicates that some molecules are particularly easily synthesized when radicals and ions recombine. In other words, there appears to be a universal organic chemistry, which shows up in interstellar space, in the atmospheres of the major planets, and in the reducing atmosphere of the primitive earth.

Production Rates and Concentrations of Hydrogen Cyanide, Formaldehyde, and Amino Acids in the Primitive Ocean

The number of quantitative data available for the synthesis of HCN and H_2CO by various energy sources is limited, but a preliminary calculation of production rates can be made (Stribling and Miller 1987).

Figure 3 shows the corona discharge synthesis of HCN and H_2CO at various H_2/CH_4, H_2/CO, and H_2/CO_2 ratios (Stribling and Miller 1987). For CH_4 atmospheres, the energy yield is about 5 nmoles/J. Taking the corona discharge energy as 12.6 J/cm^2/yr gives about 60 nmoles/cm^2/yr. The calculated lightning yields in $CH_4 + N_2$ atmospheres are about 500 nmoles/J (Chameides and Walker 1981), but preliminary experiments indicate that much lower yields of about 30 nmoles/J are obtained. The calculated yields are very low for CO and CO_2 atmospheres.

A photochemical source of HCN has been proposed by Zahnle (1986) as discussed earlier. The yields of HCN range between a maximum of 520 nmoles/cm^2/yr when the production of N atoms is limiting, and 5–50 nmoles/cm^2/yr at lower CH_4 fluxes. We will assume a combined production rate of HCN of 100 nmoles/cm/yr for a CH_4 atmosphere. The production rates would not be much lower in CO and CO_2 atmospheres if the Zahnle N atom process were important. In the absence of this mechanism, the HCN production rates would be one or two orders of magnitude lower.

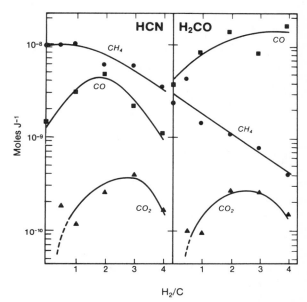

Figure 3. Energy yields for the synthesis of HCN and H_2CO by a spark discharge with H_2/CH_4, H_2/CO, and H_2/CO_2 ratios of 0 to 4.

The production rates of H_2CO from corona discharge are also shown in Figure 3. This is an effective energy source, especially with a CO-containing atmosphere. There are also photochemical experiments of about 3 nmoles/J from $CH_4 + H_2O$ (Ferris and Chen 1975) and about 8 nmoles/J from $CO + H_2O$ (Bar-Nun and Hartman 1978; Bar-Nun and Chang 1983).

The production rate of H_2CO in a model CO_2 atmosphere has been calculated by Pinto et al. (1980). The rain-out rate is about 15 nmoles/cm^2/yr. The assumed atmosphere is relatively reducing, since $H_2/CO_2 = 3$. Another calculation by Kasting et al. (1984) gives 1.6–45 nmoles/cm^2/yr. An important part of these calculations is the rain-out rate of the H_2CO, since H_2CO absorbs UV at 3200 Å. It is not clear whether this factor has been adequately treated. As in the case with HCN, the H_2CO production rates from the various sources, including the results of our experiment, are generally comparable.

These production rates of HCN allow a calculation of the steady-state concentration in the primitive ocean. We assume that all the HCN produced in the atmosphere enters the ocean and remains there and that the only pathway for the loss of HCN is hydrolysis to formamide and then to formic acid. At steady state, the production rate (S_{HCN} in moles/cm^2/yr) equals the rate of hydrolysis

$$S_{HCN} = \frac{d(HCN)}{dt} V_o$$

where (HCN) is the molar concentration, and V_o is the volume of the ocean in liters/cm^2 (now 300 liters/cm^2). Writing the hydrolysis rate of HCN as a pseudo first-order reaction

$$-\frac{d(\text{HCN})}{dt} = k_1(\Sigma\text{HCN})$$

where k_1 is the pseudo first-order rate constant in yr^{-1} and depends on temperature and pH, and $\Sigma\,\text{HCN} = \text{HCN} + \text{CN}^-$.

The hydrolysis of HCN is both acid- and base-catalyzed (for discussion, see Stribling and Miller 1987). The results for several pH values and temperatures are given in Table 6. The concentrations of HCN are proportional to the production rate, the H^+ concentration, and inversely proportional to the volume of the ocean.

The results of Table 6 make it clear that low temperatures and pH favor higher concentrations of HCN, but even at pH 7 and 0°C, a concentration of 3.5×10^{-5} M is much lower than the usual prebiotic experiment. Concentrations of HCN of 10^{-6} M are sufficient to make amino acids by the Strecker synthesis (Miller and Van Trump 1981), but adenine synthesis would require a concentration mechanism, with freezing being the most likely (Sanchez et al. 1967).

The spark discharge synthesis of HCN would have been only 1 nmole/cm^2/yr for $\text{H}_2/\text{CO}_2 = 1$ and 4 nmoles/cm^2/yr for H_2/CO_2, which is considerably lower than the 100 nmoles/cm^2/yr assumed in this calculation. This would lead to HCN concentrations 25–100 times lower than those given in Table 6, which might raise problems for amino acid and purine synthesis. If the Zahnle N atom synthesis were as efficient on the primitive earth as calculated, then this problem would not arise.

Concentration of Amino Acids in the Primitive Ocean

The production rates of HCN and H_2CO estimated above permit us to calculate the rate of buildup of amino acids in the primitive ocean and their steady-state concentration. Provided the concentrations of HCN and aldehydes do not drop too low, the Strecker synthesis will be effective in the primitive ocean (Miller and Van Trump 1981). We will assume an amino acid yield of 10% based on the HCN production. This is the approximate yield reported with CH_4, CO, and CO_2 atmospheres (Schlesinger and Miller 1983a,b). The yield is much higher ($\sim 90\%$) with the Strecker synthesis, whereas the cyanide polymerization gives only about 1% (Lowe et al. 1963; Ferris et al. 1978).

Taking a combined HCN production rate of 100 nmoles/cm^2/yr, the steady-state amino acid production rate would then have been 10 nmoles/cm^2/yr. Taking the volume of the ocean as 300 liters/cm^2, the increase in amino acid concentration would have been 3.3×10^{-11} moles/yr. Assuming no losses, this gives 3.3×10^{-4} M in 10 million years. In a low-temperature ocean, the losses from thermal decomposition should be low for amino acids such as glycine and alanine, but considerably greater for less stable amino acids such as serine. The losses from adsorption on clays, ionizing radiation, and UV light are much more difficult to estimate. The most important loss mechanism was probably the submarine vents, in which sea water is heated to at least 350°C, thereby decomposing all the amino acids. Since the entire ocean on the average passes through the vents in 10 million years (Edmond et al. 1982), the amino acid concentration could not have risen higher than 3×10^{-4} M with the above assumptions. Increasing the production rate of HCN or decreasing the size of the ocean would increase proportionally the steady-state concentration of amino acids.

It is more difficult to estimate the concentration of adenine and other purines because the details of the different pathways from HCN are not known. In the Murchison meteorite, the purines are about one-twentieth of the amino acids. A figure for the primitive ocean of 1% of the amino acid concentration (within an order of magnitude) is in accord with general experience in prebiotic chemistry. An adenine concentration of 3×10^{-5} M seems low, and a means to concentrate it may have been needed.

As discussed for the HCN production, CO_2 atmospheres give considerably lower HCN yields from spark discharges. Without the HCN production from the Zahnle N atom mechanism, the amino acid concentrations would be 25–100 times lower than the 3×10^{-4} M. There is no way at the present time to estimate the amino acid and purine concentrations needed for life to arise. A detailed mechanism of the process leading to the origin of life is needed to place constraints on the amino acid concentrations as well as the atmosphere conditions and composition required for the synthesis of necessary amino acids and purines.

ACKNOWLEDGMENT

This work was supported by NASA grant NAGW-20.

Table 6. Half-lives for Hydrolysis of HCN and the HCN Concentrations in the Primitive Ocean

	0°C	25°C	50°C
$t_{1/2}$ (yr) pH 8	7,000	40	0.5
$t_{1/2}$ (yr) pH 7	70,000	400	5
M_{HCN} pH 8	4×10^{-6}	2×10^{-8}	3×10^{-10}
M_{HCN} pH 7	4×10^{-5}	2×10^{-7}	3×10^{-9}

These figures are based on a HCN production rate of 100 nmoles/cm^2/yr and an ocean of 300 liters/cm^2.

REFERENCES

Abelson, P.H. 1965. A biogenic synthesis in the Martian environment. *Proc. Natl. Acad. Sci.* **54**: 1490.

Bada, J.L. and S.L. Miller. 1968. Ammonium ion concentration in the primitive ocean. *Science* **159**: 423.

Bar-Nun, A. and S. Chang. 1983. Photochemical reactions of water and carbon monoxide in earth's primitive atmosphere. *J. Geophys. Res.* **88**: 6662.

Bar-Nun, A. and H. Hartman. 1978. Synthesis of organic compounds from carbon monoxide and water by UV photolysis. *Origins Life* **9**: 93.

Bar-Nun, A., N. Bar-Nun, S.H. Bauer, and C. Sagan. 1970. Shock synthesis of amino acids in simulated primitive environments. *Science* **168:** 470.

Butlerow, A. 1861. Formation synthetique d'une substance sucree. *C.R. Acad. Sci.* **53:** 145.

Chameides, W.L. and J.C.G. Walker. 1981. Rates of fixation by lightning of carbon and nitrogen in possible primitive atmospheres. *Origins Life* **11:** 291.

Cronin, J.R. and C.B. Moore. 1971. Amino acid analyses of the Murchison, Murray, and Allende carbonaceous chondrites. *Science* **172:** 1327.

Decker, P., H. Schweer, and R. Pohlmann. 1982. Identification of formose sugars, presumable prebiotic metabolites, using capillary gas chromatography/gas chromatography-mass spectrometry of *n*-butoxime trifluoroacetates on OV-225. *J. Chromatogr.* **225:** 281.

Edmond, J.M., K.L. Von Damm, R.E. McDuff, and C.I. Measures. 1982. Chemistry of hot springs on the east Pacific Rise and their effluent dispersal. *Nature* **297:** 187.

Ferris, J.P. and C.T. Chen. 1975. Chemical evolution. XXVI. Photochemistry of methane, nitrogen, and water mixtures as a model for the atmosphere of the primitive earth. *J. Am. Chem. Soc.* **97:** 2962.

Ferris, J.P. and L.E. Orgel. 1966. An unusual photochemical rearrangement in the synthesis of adenine from hydrogen cyanide. *J. Am. Chem. Soc.* **88:** 1074.

Ferris, J.P., R.A. Sanchez, and L.E. Orgel. 1968. Studies in prebiotic synthesis. III. Synthesis of pyrimidines from cyanoacetylene and cyanate. *J. Mol. Biol.* **33:** 693.

Ferris, J.P., P.C. Joshi, E.H. Edelson, and J.G. Lawless. 1978. HCN: A plausible source of purines, pyrimidines and amino acids on the primitive earth. *J. Mol. Evol.* **11:** 293.

Ferris, J.P., O.S. Zamek, A.M. Altbuch, and H. Frieman. 1974. Chemical evolution. XVIII. Synthesis of pyrimidines from guanidine and cyanoacetaldehyde. *J. Mol. Evol.* **3:** 301.

Friedmann, N. and S.L. Miller. 1969. Phenylalanine and tyrosine synthesis under primitive earth conditions. *Science* **166:** 766.

Friedmann, N., W.J. Haverland, and S.L. Miller. 1971. Prebiotic synthesis of the aromatic and other amino acids. In *Chemical evolution and the origin of life* (ed. R. Buret and C. Ponnamperuma), p. 123. North-Holland, Amsterdam.

Gabel, N.W. and C. Ponnamperuma. 1967. Model for origin of monosaccharides. *Nature* **216:** 453.

Garrison, W.M., D.C. Morrison, J.G. Hamilton, A.A. Benson, and M. Calvin. 1951. Reduction of carbon dioxide in aqueous solutions by ionizing radiation. *Science* **114:** 416.

Getoff, N. 1962. Über die Bildung organischer Substanzen aus Kohlensäure in wasseriger Lösung mittels ^{60}CO-Gamma-Strahlung. *Z. Naturforsch.* **17b:** 751.

Groth, W. and H. von Weyssenhoff. 1960. Photochemical formation of organic compounds for mixtures of simple gases. *Planet. Space Sci.* **2:** 79.

Hayatsu, R. and E. Anders. 1981. Organic compounds in meteorites and their origins. *Top. Curr. Chem.* **99:** 1.

Joyce, G.F., A.W. Schwartz, S.L. Miller, and L.E. Orgel. 1987. The case for an ancestral genetic system involving simple analogues of the nucleotides. *Proc. Natl. Acad. Sci.* **84:** 4398.

Kasting, J.F., J.B. Pollack, and D. Crisp. 1984. Effects of high CO_2 levels on surface temperature and atmospheric oxidation state of the early earth. *J. Atm. Chem.* **1:** 403.

Kenyon, D.H. and G. Steinman. 1969. *Biochemical predestination.* McGraw-Hill, New York.

Khare, B.N. and C. Sagan. 1971. Synthesis of cystine in simulated primitive conditions. *Nature* **232:** 577.

Kvenvolden, K.A., J.G. Lawless, and C. Ponnamperuma. 1971. Nonprotein amino acids in the Murchison meteorite. *Proc. Natl. Acad. Sci.* **68:** 486.

Kvenvolden, K., J.G. Lawless, K. Pering, E. Peterson, J. Flores, C. Ponnamperuma, I.R. Kaplan, and C. Moore.

1970. Evidence for extraterrestrial amino-acids and hydrocarbons in the Murchison meteorite. *Nature* **228:** 923.

Lawless, J.G. and C.G. Boynton. 1973. Thermal synthesis of amino acids from a simulated primitive atmosphere. *Nature* **243:** 405.

Lawless, J.G., B. Zeitman, W.E. Pereira, R.E. Summons, and A.M. Duffield. 1974. Dicarboxylic acids in the Murchison meteorite. *Nature* **251:** 40.

Lemmon, R.M. 1970. Chemical evolution. *Chem. Rev.* **70:** 95.

Lowe, C.U., M.W. Rees, and R.M. Markham. 1963. Synthesis of complex organic compounds from simple precursors: Formation of amino acids, amino-acid polymers, fatty acids and purines from ammonium cyanide. *Nature* **199:** 219.

Mann, A.P.C. and D.A. Williams. 1980. A list of interstellar molecules. *Nature* **283:** 721.

Miller, S.L. 1953. Production of amino acids under possible primitive earth conditions. *Science* **117:** 528.

———. 1955. Production of some organic compounds under possible primitive earth conditions. *J. Am. Chem. Soc.* **77:** 2351.

———. 1957. The formation of organic compounds on the primitive earth. *Ann. N.Y. Sci.* **69:** 260. In *The origin of life on the earth* (ed. A. Oparin), p. 123. Pergamon Press, Oxford.

Miller, S.L. and L.E. Orgel. 1974. *The origins of life on the earth.* Prentice Hall, Englewood Cliffs, New Jersey.

Miller, S.L. and J.E. Van Trump. 1972. Prebiotic synthesis of methionine. *Science* **178:** 859.

———. 1981. The Strecker synthesis in the primitive ocean. In *Origin of life* (ed. Y. Wolman), p. 135. Reidel, Dordrecht, Holland.

Miller, S.L., H.C. Urey, and J. Oro. 1976. Origin of organic compounds on the primitive earth and in meteorites. *J. Mol. Evol.* **9:** 59.

Oro, J. and A.P. Kimball. 1961. Synthesis of purines under primitive earth conditions. I. Adenine from hydrogen cyanide. *Arch. Biochem. Biophys.* **94:** 221.

———. 1962. Synthesis of purines under possible primitive earth conditions. II. Purine intermediates from hydrogen cyanide. *Arch. Biochem. Biophys.* **96:** 293.

Oro, J., S. Nakaparksin, H. Lichtenstein, and E. Gil-Av. 1971. Configuration of amino acids in carbonaceous chondrites and a Precambrian chert. *Nature* **230:** 107.

Peltzer, E.T. and J.L. Bada. 1978. α-Hydroxy carboxylic acids in the Murchison meteorite. *Nature* **272:** 443.

Peltzer, E.T., J.L. Bada, G. Schlesinger, and S.L. Miller. 1984. The chemical conditions on the parent body of the Murchison meteorite: Some conclusions based on amino, hydroxy and dicarboxylic acids. *Adv. Space Res.* **4(12):** 69.

Pinto, J.P., C.R. Gladstone, and Y.L. Yung. 1980. Photochemical production of formaldehyde in the earth's primitive atmosphere. *Science* **210:** 183.

Reid, C. and L.E. Orgel. 1970. Synthesis of sugar in potentially prebiotic conditions. *Nature* **228:** 923.

Ring, D., Y. Wolman, N. Friedmann, and S.L. Miller. 1972. Prebiotic synthesis of hydrophobic and protein amino acids. *Proc. Natl. Acad. Sci.* **69:** 765.

Sagan, C. and B.N. Khare. 1971. Long-wavelength ultraviolet photoproduction of amino acids on the primitive earth. *Science* **173:** 417.

Sanchez, R.A., J.P. Ferris, and L.E. Orgel. 1966a. Conditions for purine synthesis: Did prebiotic synthesis occur at low temperatures? *Science* **153:** 72.

———. 1966b. Cyanoacetylene in prebiotic synthesis. *Science* **154:** 784.

———. 1967. Studies in prebiotic synthesis. II. Synthesis of purine precursors and amino acids from aqueous hydrogen cyanide. *J. Mol. Biol.* **30:** 223.

———. 1968. Studies in prebiotic synthesis. IV. The conversion of 4-aminoimidazole-5-carbonitrile derivatives to purines. *J. Mol. Biol.* **38:** 121.

Schlesinger, G. and S.L. Miller 1983a. Prebiotic synthesis in atmospheres containing CH_4, CO, and CO_2. I. Amino acids. *J. Mol. Evol.* **19**: 376.

———. 1983b. Prebiotic synthesis in atmospheres containing CH_4, CO, and CO_2 II. Hydrogen cyanide, formaldehyde and ammonia. *J. Mol. Evol.* **19**: 383.

Schwartz, A.W. and G.J.F. Chittenden. 1977. Synthesis of uracil and thymine under simulated prebiotic conditions. Biosystems. **9**: 87.

Stribling, R. and S.L. Miller. 1987. Energy yields for hydrogen cyanide and formaldehyde syntheses: The HCN and amino acid concentrations in the primitive ocean. *Origins Life* **17**: 261.

Voet, A.B. and A.W. Schwartz. 1983. Prebiotic adenine synthesis from HCN—Evidence for a newly discovered major pathway. *Bioinorg. Chem.* **12**: 8.

Wolman, Y., W.J. Haverland, and S.L. Miller. 1972. Nonprotein amino acids form spark discharges and their comparison with the Murchison meteorite amino acids. *Proc. Natl. Acad. Sci.* **69**: 809.

Zahnle, K.J. 1986. The photochemistry of hydrocyanic acids (HCN) in the earth's early atmosphere. *J. Geophys. Res.* **91**: 1819.

Zeitman, B., S. Chang, and J.G. Lawless. 1974. Dicarboxylic acids from electric discharge. *Nature* **251**: 42.

Prebiotic Synthesis: Problems and Challenges

J.P. FERRIS

Department of Chemistry, Rensselaer Polytechnic Institute, Troy, New York 12180

The spontaneous synthesis of amino acids in electric discharge experiments, the direct formation of purines form HCN, and the synthesis of oligonucleotides by the template-directed condensation of activated nucleotides are selected experiments which suggest that the field of chemical evolution is making rapid progress in its search for an understanding of the chemical processes leading to the origins of life. But it is quite apparent to most of us working in this field that many important questions must be answered before we can claim that a complete picture of even the early stages of chemical evolution has emerged. Some gaps in our understanding of prebiotic reaction pathways are reviewed in this paper, and an alternative approach to the experimental study of these and other problems in chemical evolution is outlined.

Amino Acids and Peptides

A diverse array of amino acids and carboxylic acids have been identified as products of the action of an electric discharge on methane, water, nitrogen, and ammonia mixtures. Ten of the protein amino acids (Table 1) (Ring et al. 1972) are formed together with 23 nonprotein amino acids (Table 2) (Wolman et al. 1977). Carboxylic acids and other products are also formed (Fig. 6) (Miller 1957; Yuen et al. 1981). Basic and aromatic amino acids are not formed and histidine is conspicuous by its absence. The formation of histidine may have proceeded by a route that did not involve the direct action of an electric discharge such as the reaction of ammonia with sugars (Shen et al. 1986).

Several questions need to be answered if it is assumed that the array of amino acids formed in a discharge was the reservoir from which the first polypeptides were formed. How were the ten coded amino acids selected from this mixture? How was it possible to differentiate between the amino acids with primary amino groups and those with secondary amino groups? How were the α amino acids selected from the β and γ amino acids? How were polypeptides formed from the α amino acids in the presence of these other amino acids and carboxylic acids? It would be expected that nonprotein amino acids and carboxylic acids would have been chemically activated to react in the same way that the α amino acids were activated to form polypeptides. Some of these points have been discussed from a theoretical point of view (Weber and Miller 1981), but there have been virtually no experiments dealing with these questions (Brack 1986).

These problems are partially solved if carbon monoxide or carbon dioxide (with hydrogen) is used in place of methane as the carbon source in the discharge studies (Table 1) (Schlesinger and Miller 1983). A much smaller array of amino acids is obtained, with the amount of glycine being 10–100-fold greater than that of any other amino acids (Table 2). It does not appear likely that the polypeptides formed from this much smaller ensemble of amino acids would possess useful catalytic properties.

Table 1. Protein Amino Acids from the Miller-Urey Experiment

Amino acid	$CH_4/N_2/NH_4Cl^a$ (1:1:0.05 M)	$CO/N_2/H_2^b$ (1:1:3)	$CO_2/H_2/N_2^b$ (1:3:1)
Glycine	100	100	100
Alanine	180	2.4	0.87
Valine	4.4	0.005	<0.001
Leucine	2.6	—	—
Isoleucine	1.1	—	—
Proline	0.3	—	—
Aspartic	7.7	0.09	0.14
Glutamic	1.7	0.01	<0.001
Serine	1.1	0.15	0.23
Threonine	0.2	—	—

Mole ratios normalized to glycine as 100.
[a]Data from Ring et al. (1972).
[b]Data from Schlesinger and Miller (1983).

Table 2. Nonprotein Amino Acids from the Miller-Urey Experiment

Amino acid	$CH_4/N_2/NH_4Cl$
Sarcosine	12.5
N-Ethylglycine	6.8
N-Propylglycine	0.5
N-Isopropylglycine	0.5
N-Methylalanine	3.4
N-Ethylalanine	trace
β-Alanine	4.3
α-Amino-*n*-butyric	61
α-Aminoisobutyric	7
β-Amino-*n*-butyric	0.1
β-Aminoisobutyric	0.1
γ-Aminobutyric	0.5
N-Methyl-β-alanine	1.0
N-Ethyl-β-alanine	0.5
Pipecolic	0.01
α-Hydroxy-γ-aminobutyric	17
α,β-Diaminobutyric	7.6
α,β-Diaminopropionic	1.5
Isoserine	1.2
Norvaline	14
Isovaline	1
Norleucine	1.4
Allothreonine	0.2

Mole ratios normalized to glycine at 100. Data from Wolman et al. (1972) and Ring et al. (1972).

Table 3. Amino Acids from Aqueous HCN

Protein amino acids	
glycine	0.6%
alanine	+
aspartic	+
glutamic	±
Nonprotein amino acids	
diaminosuccinic	0.1%
guanidinoacetic	0.03%
β-alanine	+
α-aminoisobutyric	+

Yields based on starting HCN (Ferris et al. 1978).

An alternative route to amino acids is by the hydrolysis of the oligomers formed by the self-condensation of HCN in aqueous solution (Ferris and Hagan 1984). Four of the coded amino acids have been identified as the products of this reaction mixture, along with appreciable amounts of the diastereomeric forms of diaminosuccinic acid and smaller amounts of other substances (Table 3) (Ferris et al. 1978). The relative amounts and composition of the protein amino acid mixture are comparable to those obtained in electric discharge experiments using carbon monoxide or carbon dioxide as the carbon source (Table 2).

Polypeptides

The prebiotic synthesis of polypeptides has been investigated using purified samples of amino acids. Thermal condensation reactions were performed under anhydrous conditions at temperatures of 120–200°C (Fig. 1) (Fox and Dose 1977). These condensation reactions proceed most efficiently to form polymers with an average molecular weight of 4500 when either lysine, aspartic, or glutamic acid is present in tenfold excess. Since it has not been possible to detect lysine in primitive earth simulation experiments, its use in large excess does not appear to constitute a valid prebiotic model. The use of aspartic and glutamic acids in excess assumes the selective concentration of these amino acids in the mixture that was heated on the primitive

ASPARTIC ACID	42%
GLUTAMIC ACID	38%
15 OTHER AMINO ACIDS	1.25% each

120°C
Anhydrous
7 Days

OLIGOMER

1. MEAN MOLECULAR WEIGHT 4500
2. SLOW AND INCOMPLETE ENZYMIC HYDROLYSIS OF PEPTIDE BONDS
3. β-ASPARTYL AND γ-GLUTAMYL BONDS

Figure 1. Polypeptide synthesis by thermal fusion of amino acids (Fox and Dose 1977).

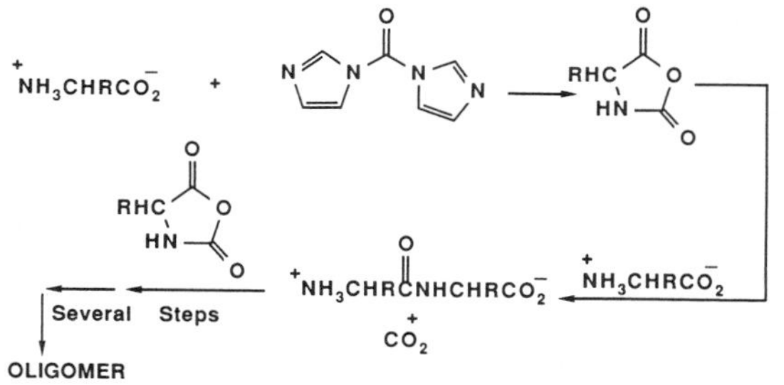

1. MAXIMUM MOLECULAR WEIGHT 800-1000
2. ASPARTIC AND GLUTAMIC DO NOT REACT VIA Beta-or Gamma-CARBOXYL GROUPS.
3. Gamma-AMINO ACIDS AND Alpha-SUBSTITUTED AMINO ACIDS 5-10 FOLD LESS REACTIVE THAN Alpha-AMINO ACIDS.

Figure 2. Peptide formation using aqueous diimidazole carbonyl (Brack 1986).

earth, but it is not clear how this may have taken place. The presence of excess glutamic and aspartic acids in the reaction mixture results in the formation of oligomers with β-aspartyl and γ-glutamyl groupings (Fox and Dose 1977). There have been no studies of the effect of other components of the mixtures formed in the prebiotic synthesis of amino acids (e.g., fatty acids and β and γ amino acids) on the composition or molecular weight of the oligomers formed by thermal synthesis.

An alternative approach to the prebiotic synthesis of polypeptides involves the polymerization of N-carboxyanhydrides in aqueous solution (Fig. 2) (Brack 1986). The advantage of this proposed synthesis is that the N-carboxyanhydride of α amino acids condenses somewhat more rapidly than the corresponding anhydride formed from γ amino acids. In addition, α-aminoisobutyric acid, an amino acid that is produced in most of the prebiotic syntheses of amino acids, is incorporated into the polypeptide less efficiently under these reaction conditions. Thus, this procedure results in the preferential selection of protein amino acids from the other amino acids formed in the electric discharge. A major disadvantage of this approach is that the elongation of the polypeptide chain stops after incorporation of six to ten amino acid residues when the oligomer precipitates from solution. In addition, it is unlikely that the condensing agent used in these studies, diimidazole carbonyl, was present on the primitive earth.

Ribonucleic Acids

It is hoped that the discovery of the catalytic properties of RNA (Cech 1986) will provide an escape from the problems of prebiotic peptide synthesis, as well as the apparent inability of protein to store genetic information. A biopolymer like RNA with the ability to both catalyze reactions and store information is exactly what was needed for the first living system. It is not difficult to imagine the evolution to protein and DNA once the first replicating RNA polymers were in place.

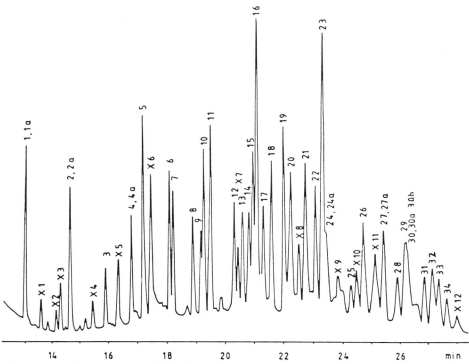

Figure 3. Gas chromatographic separation of the trifluoroacetyl *n*-butoxime derivatives of the sugars formed by the formose reaction. The syn and anti isomers of the oxime derivative result in two peaks for each sugar. The isomeric ribose derivatives are peaks 8 and 14. (Reprinted, with permission, from Decker et al. 1982.)

However, many sticky problems remained to be solved concerning the prebiotic synthesis of RNA; the difficulties are comparable to those outlined for the prebiotic formation of polypeptides.

It is generally agreed that the purine bases of RNA could have formed from HCN as described by Ferris and Hagan (1984). This reaction proceeds in 0.1–0.01 M HCN solution. Smaller yields of pyrimidines are also obtained via HCN oligomerization, and reactions of cyanoacetylene provide additional routes to pyrimidine bases (Ferris et al. 1974).

A more difficult problem is the prebiotic formation of ribose and nucleosides by the reaction of ribose and bases. It was first pointed out by Reid and Orgel (1967) that there are many problems with the proposed prebiotic synthesis of ribose by the self-condensation of formaldehyde in mildly basic solution. Complex mixtures of pentoses, hexoses, and other sugars are obtained, and the small yield of ribose slowly decomposes under the reaction conditions. An example of the complexity of the reaction mixture is shown in Figure 3 (Decker et al. 1982). It is not completely certain that ribose would not be produced in significant amounts by this route because the amount of material with the same high-performance liquid chromatography (HPLC) retention time as ribose increases as the reaction time increases (Harsch et al. 1983). Ribose is described as a "...stable minor product..." in this study, although the problem of its further conversion to acidic compounds (Socha et al. 1981) may have been a

problem on the primitive earth. There have been no suggestions about how ribose was separated on the primitive earth from the other sugars, all of which have virtually identical chemical and physical properties.

The inefficient formation of nucleosides by condensation of purine bases with ribose and the lack of reaction between ribose and pyrimidines are major barriers in the proposed prebiotic synthesis of RNA (Fuller et al. 1972a,b). The reaction of purines with ribose proceeds in low yield when purine bases, ribose, and calcium chloride or magnesium chloride are heated in the dry phase at 100°C for 2 hours to give mixtures of the α- and β-isomers of the ribofuranosides (Fig. 4) (Fuller et al. 1972b). No pyrimidine nucleosides are formed under these reaction conditions. No other pre-

$$\text{PURINE + RIBOSE + SEA WATER}^* \xrightarrow[\text{DRY}]{\text{100°C, 4h}} \text{NUCLEOSIDE}$$

$$^*\text{Na}^+, \text{Mg}^{+2}, \text{Ca}^{+2}, \text{Cl}^-, \text{SO}_4^=$$

	α – NUCLEOSIDE	β – NUCLEOSIDE
	(%)	
ADENOSINE	1-2	2.3
GUANOSINE	-	5
XANTHOSINE	-	2.1
INOSINE	3	8

Figure 4. Nucleoside formation (Fuller et al. 1972b).

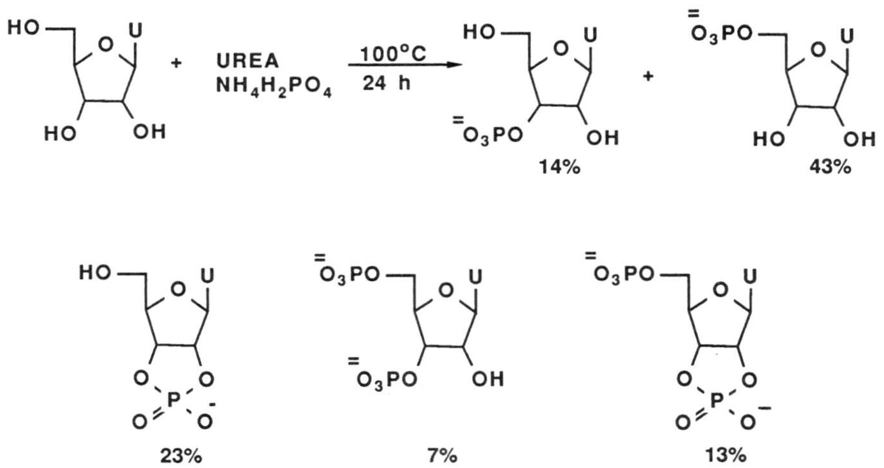

Figure 5. Nucleotide synthesis (Osterberg et al. 1973).

biotically plausible routes to nucleosides have been reported.

The phosphorylation of nucleosides to nucleotides is a dry-phase reaction that proceeds in good yield (Fig. 5) (Osterberg et al. 1973). Mixtures of isomers and different levels of phosphorylation are observed; however, their fractionation or selective reaction under prebiotic conditions has not been investigated. The activation and further condensation of nucleotides are discussed in subsequent papers in this volume.

Lipids

If the problems associated with the synthesis of RNA polymers are overcome, it is still not clear how it was possible to maintain a primitive earth environment where these RNA species replicated and catalyzed chemical processes. One proposal is that the system may have been anchored to a mineral in a gradient of organic or inorganic nutrients such as those observed in hydrothermal vents today. There have been no experimental studies of this model. Another proposal is that it may have been packaged in a container that was located in a relatively stable environmental niche on the primitive earth. It is not surprising that phospholipid vesicles have been considered as possible containers for the first life forms, and some studies of the prebiotic synthesis of phospholipids have been undertaken. The main difficulty is the lack of formation of long-chain linear fatty acids under primitive earth reaction conditions (Fig. 6) (Yuen et al. 1981; Allen and Ponnamperuma 1967). Branched-chain fatty acids and hydrocarbons are formed in electric discharge reactions. These branched-chain acids have carbon numbers as high as C_{12} after 4 days of reaction (Allen and Ponnamperuma 1967). It is likely that these high-molecular-weight acids are formed as a result of the multiple excitation of the smaller acids that are produced initially, since C_6 is the highest carbon number of the hydrocarbons formed on one pass of methane through a discharge (Goto et al. 1986). Whether a

multiple excitation of water-soluble acids would have taken place on the primitive earth is open to question. A C_{10}–C_{12} linear fatty acid is the minimum size required to form a bilayer membrane (Deamer 1986), and it is not clear that the branched C_{10}–C_{12} acids produced in the discharge would form a stable bilayer. The Fischer-Tropsch synthesis yields long-chain (C_6–C_{18}) linear fatty acids, but the reaction conditions required (400°C, high pressure, and Fe catalyst) are not likely to have been prevalent on the primitive earth (Leach et al. 1978). Such fatty acids may have been formed in the higher-temperature processes that occurred during the formation of the earth from an interstellar dust cloud, a suggestion that receives some support from the observation that lipid-like material can be extracted from the Murchison meteorite (Deamer 1986). The condensation of fatty acids, glycerol, and phosphate under primitive earth conditions appears to be a feasible prebiotic process (Eichberg et al. 1977; Epps et al. 1978). If it were possible to synthesize linear fatty acids of sufficient chain length, then the problem of the selection of long-chain linear fatty acids from the shorter-chain fatty acids could have been based on

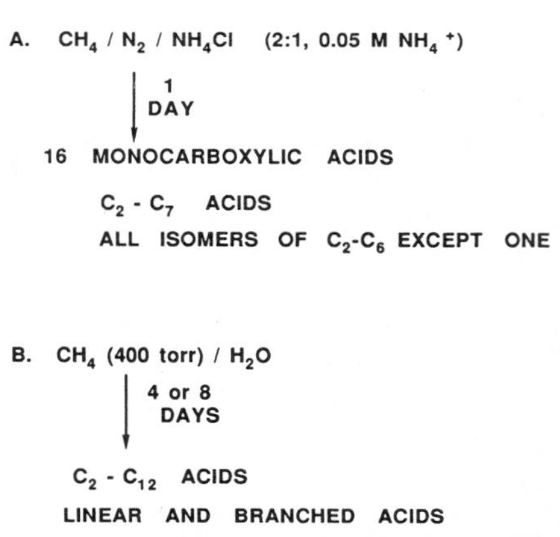

Figure 6. Carboxylic acid synthesis in an electric discharge (*A*, Yuen et al. 1981; *B*, Allen and Ponnamperuma 1967).

greater stability of the membranes formed from the longer-chain fatty acids.

The peptide oligomers formed by the dry-phase heating of amino acids has also been suggested as a source of membranes. Saturated solutions of these oligomers form microspheres that appear to have an outer membrane boundary when observed under a microscope (Fox and Dose 1977). This boundary material does not appear to have the properties needed for a suitable container for a primitive living system. It is permeable to most water-soluble substances and it dissolves when the concentration of oligomers drops below that of a saturated solution.

One of the first proposals for a primitive cell was the coacervate hypothesis of Oparin (1957). It was proposed that these coacervates originated from organic material that formed an insoluble phase in an aqueous environment on the primitive earth. It was proposed that this insoluble phase extracted organic compounds from the aqueous phase and provided a more hospitable environment for organic and biochemical processes to proceed. A problem with this hypothesis is that the stability of this organic phase is governed solely by solubility factors, and there is no barrier to diffusion between the organic and the aqueous phases.

Chirality

The problem of enantiomeric selectivity has not been addressed in the chemical processes outlined above. There are many theories for the origins of chirality, but none of them has a firm experimental base. Polymers composed of building blocks with mixed chirality will have different properties from those composed of building blocks with the same chirality. Some experiments have been performed which suggest that the chirality of the monomers in a polymer chain will have a major influence on the chirality of the next building block to be added to the chain (Goldberg et al. 1986). In more sophisticated template-directed polymerizations, incorporation of the opposite enantiomer in the growing polymer chain results in the termination of the polymerization process (Joyce et al. 1984). There has been extensive investigation of possible processes by which chiral forces on the primitive earth may have led to the excess of one enantiomer over another (Tokay et al. 1986; Keszthelyi 1987), but to date there have been no studies that provide any clue to how chiral selection occurred. The experimental studies are difficult because the extents of chiral enrichments are small, and as a consequence, different results are obtained when different scientists try to reproduce the same experiment. The use of achiral monomers that form chiral polymers may provide a solution to this problem (Spach 1984; Schwartz and Orgel 1985).

Mineral Catalysis

Why, more than 35 years after the Miller-Urey experiment, are there so many gaps in schemes designed to understand chemical events on the primitive earth? It certainly is due in large part to our lack of knowledge of reaction conditions on the primitive earth and the timing for the origins of life. This ignorance results in an insufficient number of constraints on possible primitive earth scenarios, so that it is difficult to select among the possible reaction conditions. I believe that the success of the early experimental studies in generating biological molecules also contributed to the gaps in our understanding. Early on, there was a general feeling that the reaction pathways would become apparent if one did enough electric discharge, thermal, or irradiation experiments on the proper mix of chemicals. Few experimentalists carried out more insightful experimental studies of the problem. For example, although it was recognized by Bernal (1949) before the Miller-Urey study that mineral catalysis must have played a central role in the formation of biological polymers, there have been few rigorous experimental studies of the possible role of mineral catalysis in the origin of life. Since life today is impossible without enzymes, it is very likely that catalysis had an important role in the origin of life.

We have demonstrated in a simple model system how clay mineral catalysis facilitates the formation of the phosphodiester bond in aqueous solution using a derivative of HCN as the condensing agent (Ferris et al. 1984). HCN spontaneously reacts in aqueous solution to form a tetramer, diaminomaleonitrile (DAMN), a compound that is oxidized by Fe^{+3} and other oxidizing agents to diiminosuccinonitrile (DISN), the condensing agent in our system. DISN reacts readily with phosphate compounds, but it is also hydrolyzed with water. Mixtures of DISN and 3'-AMP yield 2',3'-cAMP, presumably via a type of mixed anhydride (Fig. 7). This reaction does not proceed efficiently unless there is an

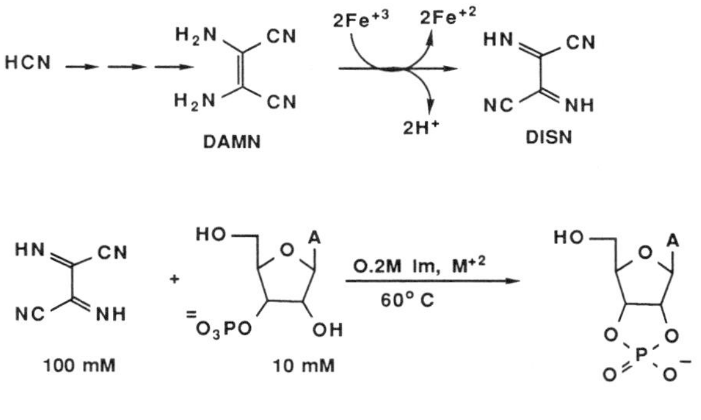

M^{+2} (10 mM)	YIELD (%)
--	9.0
Ca^{+2}	8.5
Mn^{+2}	31.5
Fe^{+3}	6.1
Zn^{+2}	14.4

Figure 7. Model system for phosphate ester bond formation (Ferris et al. 1984; Ferris and Hagan 1986).

appreciable excess of DISN because of its destruction by hydrolysis. The formation of 2',3'-cAMP proceeds more efficiently if it is performed in the presence of montmorillonite clay and the DISN is generated in situ from DAMN (Ferris and Hagan 1986; Ferris et al. 1986). In this process (Fig. 8), the 3'-AMP binds to the clay surface, the Fe^{+3} in the clay lattice oxidizes the DAMN to DISN on the surface of the clay in the presence of the adsorbed 3'-AMP, and the clay catalyzes the reaction between DISN and 3'-AMP to form 2',3'-cAMP. The 2',3'-cAMP is released from the clay surface because it binds much less strongly than does 3'-AMP. This is not a complete catalytic cycle because there is no oxidation of the Fe^{++} in the clay lattice back to Fe^{+3}. This oxidation reaction could have occurred on the primitive earth either by direct photolysis or by reaction with oxidants that are generated photochemically. This simple model system demonstrates the potential of mineral catalysis for the formation of the phosphate ester bond. Additional studies using 5'-AMP have shown that in the presence of montmorillonite, dimers and trimers that contain the phosphodiester bond are formed, whereas in the absence of montmorillonite, pyrophosphate bond formation is the principal reaction pathway (J.P. Ferris, unpubl.).

This example of montmorillonite catalysis provides a hopeful ending to what would otherwise be a litany of problems in the field of chemical evolution. It suggests that a detailed study of the mechanism of mineral catalysis is likely to provide new insights into reaction pathways that may have been important on the primitive earth. These catalysts need not be limited to clays. Iron oxides, metal sulfides and phosphates, and silicates are but a few of the mineral types that can be investigated. These studies will take time because one must first investigate how each of these minerals interacts with organic compounds before meaningful studies of their possible role as catalysts can be carried out. However, I am optimistic that a study of the mineral-catalyzed formation of biopolymers will lead to an understanding of the chemical processes that led to the origins of life.

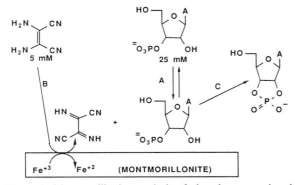

Figure 8. Montmorillonite catalysis of phosphate ester bond formation (Ferris et al. 1986; Ferris and Hagan 1986).

ACKNOWLEDGMENT

This research was supported by National Science Foundation grant CHE-8606377.

REFERENCES

Allen, W.V. and C. Ponnamperuma. 1967. A possible prebiotic synthesis of monocarboxylic acids. *Curr. Mod. Biol.* **1:** 24.

Bernal, J.D. 1949. The physical basis of life. *Proc. R. Soc. Lond.* A **62A:** 537.

Brack, A. 1986. Emergence and survival of protein-like peptides in water. *Origins Life* **16:** 486.

Cech, T.R. 1986. RNA as an enzyme. *Sci. Am.* **235(5):** 64.

Deamer, D.W. 1986. Role of amphiphilic compounds on the evolution of membrane structure on the early earth. *Origins Life* **17:** 3.

Decker, P., H. Schweer, and R. Pohlmann. 1982. Identification of formose sugars, presumably prebiotic metabolites, using capillary gas chromatography/gas chromatography-mass spectrometry on *n*-butoxime trifluoroacetate on OV25. *J. Chromatogr.* **244:** 281.

Eichberg, J., E. Sherwood, D.E. Epps, and J. Oro. 1977. Cyanamide mediated synthesis under plausible primitive earth conditions. IV. The synthesis of acylglycerols. *J. Mol. Evol.* **10:** 221.

Epps, D.E., E. Sherwood, J. Eichberg, and J. Oro. 1978. Cyanamide mediated synthesis under plausible primitive earth conditions. V. The synthesis of phosphatidic acids. *J. Mol. Evol.* **11:** 279.

Ferris, J.P. and W.J. Hagan, Jr. 1984. HCN and chemical evolution: The possible role of cyano compounds in prebiotic synthesis. *Tetrahedron* **40:** 1093.

———. 1986. The adsorption and reaction of adenine nucleotides on montmorillonite. *Origins Life* **17:** 273.

Ferris, J.P., C.-H. Huang, and W.J. Hagan. 1986. Clays as prototypical enzymes for the prebiological formation of phosphate esters. *Origins Life* **16:** 473.

Ferris, J.P., P.C. Joshi, E.H. Edelson, and J.G. Lawless. 1978. HCN: A plausible source of purines, pyrimidines and amino acids on the primitive earth. *J. Mol. Evol.* **11:** 293.

Ferris, J.P., O.S. Zamek, A.M. Altbuch, and H. Freeman. 1974. Chemical evolution. XVIII. Synthesis of pyrimidines from guanidine and cyanoacetaldehyde. *J. Mol. Evol.* **3:** 301.

Ferris, J.P., H. Yanagawa, P.A. Dudgeon, W.J. Hagan, Jr., and T.E. Mallare. 1984. The investigation of the HCN derivative diiminosuccinonitrile as a prebiotic condensing agent. The formation of phosphate esters. *Origins Life* **15:** 29.

Fox, S.W. and K. Dose. 1977. *Molecular evolution and the origin of life.* Marcel Dekker, New York.

Fuller, W.D., R.A. Sanchez, and L.E. Orgel. 1972a. Studies in prebiotic synthesis. VII. Solid-state synthesis of purine nucleosides. *J. Mol. Evol.* **1:** 249.

———. 1972b. Studies in prebiotic synthesis. VI. Synthesis of purine nucleosides. *J. Mol. Biol.* **67:** 25.

Goldberg, S.I., J.M. Crosby, N.D. Iusem, and U.E. Younes. 1986. Racemic origins of the stereochemical homogeneity of the biosphere. Isotactic biasing in the formation of oligomeric peptides. *Origins Life* **16:** 475.

Goto, K., M. Kinjo, K. Hashimoto, and M. Ishigami. 1986. Synthesis of hydrocarbons under presumed prebiotic conditions using high-frequency discharge. *J. Mol. Evol.* **23:** 113.

Harsch, G., M. Harsch, H. Bauer, and W. Voelter. 1983. Produktverteilung und Mechanismus der Gesamtreaktion der Formose-Reaktion. *Z. Naturforsch.* **38b:** 1269.

Joyce, G.F., G.M. Visser, C.A.A. van Boeckel, J.H. van Boom, L.E. Orgel, and J. van Westrennen. 1984. Chiral selection in poly(C)-directed synthesis of oligo(G). *Nature* **310**: 602.

Keszthelyi, L. 1987. Asymmetries of nature and origin of biomolecular handedness. *Biosystems* **20**: 15.

Leach, W.W., D.W. Nooner, and J. Oro. 1978. A biotic synthesis of fatty acids. In *Origins of Life: Proceedings of the 2nd ISSOL meeting, 5th ICOL meeting* (ed. H. Noda), p. 113. Center for Academic Publications, Japan; Japan Scientific Societies Press, Tokyo.

Miller, S.L. 1957. The mechanism of synthesis of amino acids by electric discharges. *Biochim. Biophys. Acta* **23**: 480.

Oparin, A.I. 1957. *The origins of life on earth.* Oliver and Boyd, Edinburgh.

Osterberg, R., L.E. Orgel, and R. Lohrman. 1973. Further studies of urea-catalyzed phosphorylation reactions. *J. Mol. Evol.* **2**: 231.

Reid, C. and L.E. Orgel. 1967. Synthesis of sugars in potentially prebiotic conditions. *Nature* **216**: 455.

Ring, D., Y. Wolman, N. Friedmann, and S.L. Miller. 1972. Prebiotic synthesis of hydrophobic and protein amino acids. *Proc. Natl. Acad. Sci.* **69**: 765.

Schlesinger, G. and S.L. Miller. 1983. Prebiotic synthesis in atmospheres containing CH_4, CO and CO_2. *J. Mol. Evol.* **19**: 376.

Schwartz, A.W. and L.E. Orgel. 1985. Template-directed synthesis of novel nucleic acid-like structures. *Science* **228**: 585.

Shen, C., L. Yang, S. Miller, and J. Oro. 1986. Prebiotic synthesis of imidazole-4-acetaldehyde, imidazole-4-glycol and imidazole-4-ethanol. *Origins Life* **16**: 275.

Socha, R.F., A.H. Weiss, and M.M. Sakharov. 1981. Homogeneously catalyzed condensation of formaldehyde to carbohydrates. VII. An overall formose reaction model. *J. Catal.* **67**: 207.

Spach, G. 1984. Chiral versus chemical evolutions and the appearance of life. *Origins Life* **14**: 433.

Tokay, R.K., B. Norden, and J.-O. Liljenzin. 1986. Has nuclear chirality been a prebiotic source of optical purity of living systems? The quantum yields of gamma- and beta-decarboxylation of $1\text{-}^{14}C$-labelled D- and L-leucine in the solid state can indicate considerable selectivity. *Origins Life* **16**: 421.

Weber, A.L. and S.L. Miller. 1981. Reasons for the occurrence of the twenty coded amino acids. *J. Mol. Evol.* **17**: 273.

Wolman, Y., W.J. Haverland, and S.L. Miller. 1972. Nonprotein amino acids from spark discharges and their comparison with Murchison meteorite amino acids. *Proc. Natl. Acad. Sci.* **69**: 809.

Yuen, G.U., J.G. Lawless, and E.H. Edelson. 1981. Quantification of monocarboxylic acids from a spark discharge synthesis. *J. Mol. Evol.* **17**: 43.

In Search of RNA Ancestors

A.W. Schwartz, J. Visscher, R. Van der Woerd, and C.G. Bakker
Laboratory of Exobiology, Faculty of Science, University of Nijmegen,
Toernooiveld, 6525 ED, Nijmegen, The Netherlands

The recent discoveries of catalytically active RNA species have reinforced the view that a key step in the emergence of life on earth may have been the development of self-replicating RNA molecules. Although much progress has been made in recent years toward the development of an experimental model of RNA replication, there remain many problems that have yet to be overcome (Joyce et al. 1984a; Joyce and Orgel 1986). Perhaps the most serious difficulty is that of understanding the prebiotic synthesis of the nucleosides and of the specifically phosphorylated and activated derivatives required for template-directed reactions. The major obstacle in the formation of the nucleosides is not the synthesis of purines and pyrimidines, for which quite reasonable pathways are available (at least for adenine and uracil), rather, it is the question of the source of ribose and deoxyribose that has remained troublesome over the years. Although the "formose" reaction is often cited in this connection, a very serious complication is the large number of isomeric carbohydrates that are formed, even under carefully controlled conditions. A gas-chromatographic analysis, for example, reveals nearly 50 individual carbohydrate species, not including stereoisomers, of which ribose is only a minor member (Decker et al. 1982).

The data of Joyce et al. (1984b) demonstrate that, even in the unlikely circumstance that a suitably activated mononucleotide could somehow be formed, as a result of yet unsuspected selection mechanisms involving preferential formation of ribose and its fortuitous condensation with a purine under appropriate conditions (including the selection of the correct anomeric configuration), enantiomeric cross-inhibition would interfere with template-directed oligomerization. Considerations of this sort have led some authors to dispair of finding a rational explanation for the origins of prebiotic polynucleotide replication (Shapiro 1986). There is, however, quite a different conclusion possible. These technical difficulties make it seem likely that some more readily available class of prebiotic molecules played a transitional role in the evolutionary steps leading up to autocatalytic RNA.

Recent results suggest the possibility that nucleic acid analogs that are capable of maintaining Watson-Crick base-pairing but have novel "backbone" anatomy could have performed just this function. A number of examples are known of template-directed oligomerizations that are catalyzed by "conventional" polynucleotides but produce unusual backbones. One of the earliest reported of these was the 2'-5' phosphodiester-linked oligoguanylic acids produced under the influence of Pb^{++} catalysis (Lorhmann et al. 1980). These products, although linked via phosphodiester bonds, are based on a seven-atom repeating structural unit, rather than the usual six. It is known that such structures can have a biological function (Kerr and Brown 1978). The oligomerization of 3'-amino-3'-deoxynucleoside-5'-phosphoimidazolides produces 3'-5'-linked phosphoramidates (Zielinski and Orgel 1985). Pyrophosphate-linked products have been synthesized by the oligomerization of deoxynucleoside-3',5'-diphosphates (see Schwartz and Orgel 1985). The syntheses of these structures, based on an eight-atom average repeating group, are catalyzed by complementary templates, but they also proceed more slowly in the absence of a template (Schwartz et al. 1987). Significantly, the acyclic analog 9-(1,3-dihydroxy-2-propoxy)methylguanine, $\tilde{G}$, was also shown to undergo a template-directed oligomerization (of the diphosphoimidazolide) in the presence of poly(C) (Schwartz and Orgel 1985). This compound (Fig. 2), which is formally derivable from guanine, formaldehyde, and glycerol, represents the first example of a possible prochiral precursor of contemporary polynucleotides. Such precursors could have circumvented the problem of enantiomeric cross-inhibition (Joyce et al. 1987).

As a first step toward testing the hypothesis that structurally simpler analogs might have served as the basis for a primitive information-transfer system, we have developed a synthetic strategy for the preparation of pyrophosphate-linked deoxynucleoside oligomers of defined sequence. Here, we report some initial results of a study on the oligomerization of one such dimer.

METHODS

The syntheses of diimidazolides of monomers such as pdAp and pdGp (Schwartz et al. 1987), p$\tilde{G}$p (Schwartz and Orgel 1985), and pd(3')Ap (Visscher and Schwartz 1987) have been described. Pyrophosphate-linked dimers of pdAp were synthesized following the procedure (see Fig. 1) of Van der Woerd et al. (1987). Oligomerizations were carried out in the presence of the water-soluble condensing agent 1-ethyl-3-(dimethyl-aminopropyl)-carbodiimide hydrochloride (EDAC). To ensure nearly quantitative conversion of the terminal phosphate groups to phosphoimidazolides, the following procedure was applied. To 37.5 μl of a solution 2 M in EDAC and 2 M in imidazole (pH 6.5), 18.5 μl of 0.15 M dimer was added at 0°C. After 2 hours at 0°C,

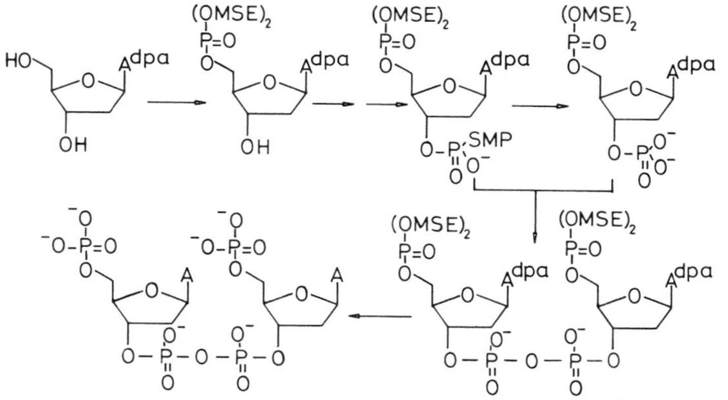

Figure 1. Scheme for the synthesis of the 3'-3' pyrophosphate-linked dimer of pdAp. The 5'-5'- and 3'-5'-linked isomers were synthesized by analogous procedures (for conditions, see van der Woerd et al. 1987).

conversion to diphosphoimidazolide was at least 90% complete, as determined by high-performance liquid chromatography (HPLC) and ^{32}P-NMR. Aliquots (2.5 μl) of this solution were then added to tubes containing 7.5 μl H$_2$O, 2 μmoles MgCl$_2$, 1 μmole NaCl, and, when required, 0.5 μmole poly(U) (monomer-equivalent). Final concentrations were therefore 0.0125 M dimer-diphosphoimidazolide, 0.2 M MgCl$_2$, 0.1 M NaCl, and, if added, 0.05 M poly(U) (monomer-equivalent). Reactions were carried out in a volume of 10 μl in Pyrex tubes, at 4°C for 2 weeks. At the conclusion of the reaction, 2.5 μl of KEDTA (1 M, pH 9.0) and 7.5 μl of K$_4$P$_2$O$_7$ (1 M, pH 9.0) were added, and the reaction mixture was stored at −25°C. Prior to analysis, poly(U) was destroyed by digestion with pancreatic ribonuclease (1 μl of hydrolyzed reaction mixture was added to 100 μl of Tris-HCl [0.05 M, pH 7.6] containing 10 units of enzyme; incubation was carried out for 12 hr at 37°C). When necessary, surviving imidazolides were destroyed by hydrolysis at pH 4.0 (1 μl of reaction mixture was added to 100 μl of 0.1 M sodium acetate, pH 4.0, and heated at 50°C for 4 hr). Analysis was by HPLC on RPC-5 in 0.02 M NaOH, with a linear gradient of NaClO$_4$ (0–0.04 M over 60 min) at a flow rate of 1.0 ml/min. Peak detection was by absorbance monitoring at 254 nm.

RESULTS AND DISCUSSION

In addition to the template-directed and spontaneous oligomerizations of the diimidazolides of pdAp and pdGp reported previously (Schwartz et al. 1987), we have recently observed similar reactions with a related compound, 3'-deoxyadenosine-2',5'-diphosphoimidazolide (Fig. 2). Oligomerizations of this compound are extremely efficient, due to the inability of the activated phosphate groups to cyclize (Visscher and Schwartz 1987). Such cyclization is a major competing reaction in the oligomerization of the analogous 2'-deoxynucleoside diphosphoimidazolides. More importantly, these

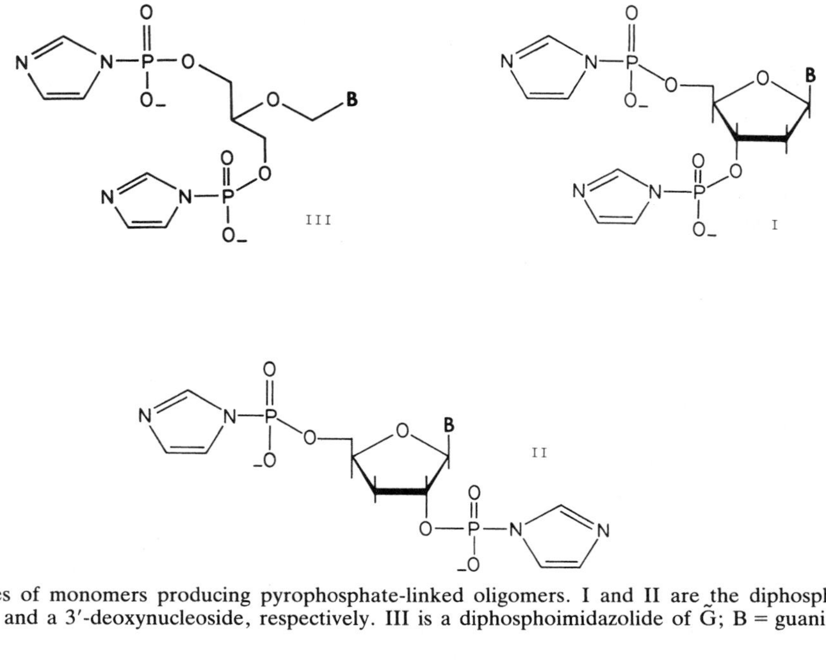

Figure 2. Structures of monomers producing pyrophosphate-linked oligomers. I and II are the diphosphoimidazolides of a 2'-deoxynucleoside and a 3'-deoxynucleoside, respectively. III is a diphosphoimidazolide of G̃; B = guanine.

oligomers represent an additional class of analog, since the average structural unit of the backbone is a nine-atom repeating group.

Results of the oligomerization of the 3'-5' pyrophosphate-linked dimer of pdAp are illustrated in Figure 3. It is clear that the presence of a poly(U) template increases the proportion of longer oligomers formed, as well as increasing the total yield of all oligomeric products (under these conditions, from 21% to 77%). Preliminary results obtained with the 3'-3'- and 5'-5'-linked dimers suggest that the influence of the template on these oligomerizations is much less pronounced.

Several reaction systems have now been described in which the oligomerization of nucleotide analogs is catalyzed by polynucleotide templates. In all such catalyzed oligomerizations, it is a reasonable presumption that the formation of a hybrid double or triple helix occurs between the template and the complementary product oligomers. This suggests the possibility that information transfer in a totally analog system might be possible. New lines of evidence now support this possibility. The recent demonstration that a phosphoramidate-linked dimer containing cytosine and guanine can be oligomerized to produce long, self-complementary chains in a yield in excess of 70% (Zielinski and Orgel 1987) suggests that the products may be acting as self-templates. All 3'-3'-, 5'-5'-, 3'-5'-, and 5'-3'-linked isomers of dimers of pdAp and pTp will soon be available, enabling us to test for similar effects in the pyrophosphate-linked system.

ACKNOWLEDGMENTS

We thank René Tros for technical assistance. This research has been supported by U.S. National Aeronautics and Space Administration grant NGR-05067.

REFERENCES

Decker, P., H. Schweer, and R. Pohlmann. 1982. Bioids. X. Identification of formose sugars, presumable prebiotic metabolites, using capillary gas chromatography/gas chromatography-mass spectrometry of n-butoxime trifluoroacetates on OV-225. *J. Chromatogr.* **244:** 281.

Joyce, G.F. and L.E. Orgel. 1986. Non-enzymatic template-directed synthesis on RNA random copolymers. Poly-(C,G) templates. *J. Mol. Biol.* **188:** 433.

Joyce, G.F., T. Inoue, and L.S. Orgel. 1984a. Non-enzymatic template-directed synthesis on RNA random copolymers. Poly(C,U) templates. *J. Mol. Biol.* **176:** 279.

Joyce, G.F., A.W. Schwartz, S.L. Miller, and L.E. Orgel. 1987. The case for an ancestral genetic system involving simple analogues of the nucleotides. *Proc. Natl. Acad. Sci.* **84:** 4398.

Joyce, G.F., G.M. Visser, A.A. van Boeckel, J.H. van Boom, L.E. Orgel, and J. van Westrenen. 1984b. Chiral selection in poly-(C)-directed synthesis of oligo(G). *Nature* **310:** 602.

Kerr, I.M. and R.E. Brown. 1978. pppA2'p5'A2'p5'A: An inhibitor of protein synthesis synthesized with an enzyme fraction from interferon-treated cells. *Proc. Natl. Acad. Sci.* **75:** 256.

Lohrmann, R., P.K. Bridson, and L.E. Orgel. 1980. Efficient metal-ion catalyzed template-directed oligonucleotide synthesis. *Science* **208:** 1464.

Schwartz, A.W. and L.E. Orgel. 1985. Template-directed synthesis of novel, nucleic acid-like structures. *Science* **228:** 585.

Schwartz, A.W., J. Visscher, C.G. Bakker, and J. Niessen. 1987. Nucleic acid-like structures. II. Polynucleotide analogues as possible primitive precursors of nucleic acids. *Origins Life* **17:** 351.

Shapiro, R. 1986. *Origins—A skeptics guide to the creation of life on earth.* Summit Books, New York.

Van der Woerd, R., C.G. Bakker, and A.W. Schwartz. 1987. Synthesis of P1,P2-dinucleotide pyrophosphates. *Tetrahedron Lett.* **28:** 2763.

Visscher, J. and A.W. Schwartz. 1987. Nucleic acid-like structures. III. Oligomerization of 3'-deoxyadenosine-2',5'-diphosphate. *J. Mol. Evol.* (in press).

Zielinski, W.S. and L.E. Orgel. 1985. Oligomerization of activated derivatives of 3'-amino-3'-deoxy-guanosine on poly(C) and poly(dC) templates. *Nucleic Acids Res.* **13:** 2469.

———. 1987. Oligoaminonucleoside phosphoramidates. Oligomerization of dimers of 3'-amino-3'-deoxynucleotides (GC and CG) in aqueous solution. *Nucleic Acids Res.* **15:** 1699.

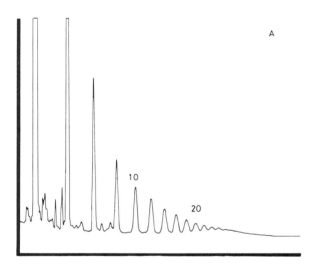

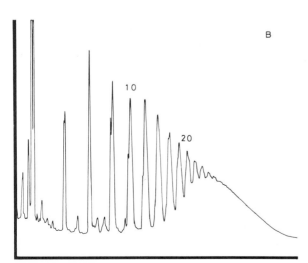

Figure 3. HPLC analyses of reaction products obtained from the oligomerization of the 3'-5' pyrophosphate-linked dimer of pdAp in the absence of a poly(U) template (*A*) and in the presence of template (*B*). For conditions, see text.

Nonenzymatic Template-directed Synthesis of Informational Macromolecules

G.F. JOYCE
The Salk Institute for Biological Studies, San Diego, California 92138

Biological evolution is a remarkably effective mechanism for the generation of catalytically active materials. A compendium of the known biological enzymes includes a large and functionally diverse array of proteins (Webb 1984) and a small but growing number of catalytic RNAs (for review, see Cech 1987). The key to evolution's effectiveness is its use of a few basic structural units (the 20 amino acids or the 4 ribonucleotides), which are assembled into functional macromolecules according to historically validated genetic information. All biological catalysts are informational catalysts in that their structure and function derive from choices that were made during the course of their evolutionary development. These choices are linked to the survival of the organism and result in a particular ordering of monomeric subunits within the structure of the polymeric catalyst.

Two informational processes are fundamental to the operation of an evolving system. First, the genetic information must be replicated in order to compensate for the inevitable loss of individual copies due to chemical degradation. Second, the genetic information must be expressed as a behavioral phenotype so that its usefulness can be assessed by natural selection. In biology, both of these processes rely on the use of a polymerase enzyme. Following the central dogma, replication utilizes a DNA-dependent DNA polymerase to produce additional copies of itself, whereas expression utilizes a DNA-dependent RNA polymerase to produce mRNA, which is then translated to protein. A modern extension of the central dogma would include RNA viral genomes that can be replicated by an RNA-dependent RNA polymerase and RNA enzymes that are transcribed directly from DNA.

In trying to capture the ability to evolve catalytic materials in the laboratory, we ask, What are the minimum requirements for the construction of a chemical evolving system? The basic requirement is for an informational macromolecule that can be replicated irrespective of its primary sequence and can be expressed as a behavioral phenotype in a way that is sequence-dependent. If the system is to be self-sustaining, then it is also required that the ability to carry out replication and expression be part of the expressed phenotype. Taking a cue from biology, the most attractive candidates for the role of informational macromolecule are those compounds that have inherent template properties. Templating greatly simplifies the task of information transfer during the replication process. The ideal candidate would be a polymer that acts as a template to direct the synthesis of additional copies of itself. Biology has settled on a slightly more complicated solution by relying on the reciprocal synthesis of complementary templates.

The problem of phenotypic expression can be reduced to a question regarding the range of behaviors that are available to the genetic material itself. If these behaviors include a replicase function, then the minimum requirements for an evolving system can be met without resorting to the introduction of a transcription/translation apparatus. However, as we shall see, chemical attributes that allow a compound to express a range of interesting phenotypes often make it difficult for that compound to serve as a good substrate for replication. Biology has found it advantageous to separate genotype and phenotype into specialized macromolecules. Whether or not this separation has been in effect since the time of life's origins is open to speculation (Woese 1967; Crick 1968; Orgel 1968; Eigen and Schuster 1978). In the laboratory, rather than face the enormous task of trying to design a transcription/translation apparatus, we instead focus on the problem of replication and on trying to copy genetic information without the aid of an external catalyst.

In the discussion that follows, I review the progress that has been made in the area of nonenzymatic template-directed RNA synthesis. This work, most of which has been carried out by Leslie Orgel and his co-workers, has led to the development of chemical systems for macromolecular information transfer. It is possible to transfer sequence information from RNA to RNA and from DNA to RNA, in analogy to the behavior of an RNA-dependent or DNA-dependent RNA polymerase (for review, see Orgel 1986). These reactions are not general with respect to template sequence, and thus do not easily lend themselves to the construction of a self-replicating system. Self-replication has been demonstrated in a very limited sense using chemically modified RNA substrates and a well-chosen self-complementary template (von Kiedrowski 1986; Zielinski and Orgel 1987). However, until systems of this kind can be expanded to include a variety of template sequences, there is no way to conduct an evolutionary search for alternative sequences that are associated with novel behavioral phenotypes.

From Monomer to Polymer

Attempts to construct a self-replicating system should be distinguished from attempts to model self-replicating systems that existed during the earliest stages of life on earth. In the former, we are less concerned with restrictions that result from a consideration of plausible prebiotic conditions and more concerned with pragmatic issues, such as the availability of suitable starting materials and the applicability of established analytic techniques. From the point of view of prebiotic chemistry, RNA appears to be an unlikely candidate for the role of the first genetic material (Shapiro 1986; Joyce et al. 1987). But from the point of view of the modern laboratory, it offers a number of practical advantages.

As discussed above, one of the most appealing properties of RNA (and other RNA-like materials) is its inherent template ability. There is preferential interaction between complementary nucleotides based on the specificity of Watson-Crick pairing. This property can be exploited in order to bind monomers at complementary sites along a preformed template. Then, with the help of a suitable condensing agent, the adjacent template-bound monomers can be joined to form oligomeric products. The main difficulty in implementing a reaction system of this kind is that although each of the nucleotide bases must be sufficiently dissimilar so as to maintain the specificity of complementary pairing, the dissimilarity results in other sequence-dependent properties that tend to limit the generality of the reaction.

We begin with a consideration of template-directed synthesis on homopolymer RNA templates. Poly(C) and pG form helical complexes that are stable at 0°C (Howard et al. 1964). The stoichiometry of these complexes is critically dependent on pH. Below pH 7, a poly(C)·pG·poly(CH$^+$) protonated triple helix is formed, whereas above pH 8, a poly(C)·pG Watson-Crick double helix is obtained (Howard et al. 1964; Davies and Davidson 1971). Poly(U) and pA form a 2 poly(U)·pA triple helix that is stable at 0°C over a wide range of pH values (Howard et al. 1966; Huang and Ts'o 1966). Poly(G) and pC are unable to form a helical complex because of the strong tendency of poly(G) to self-associate, and poly(A)·pU complexes are unstable because of the poor base-stacking interaction between adjacent uridine residues (Ts'o 1974). Thus, template-directed reactions involving homopolymer templates and complementary monomers are limited to the synthesis of oligopurines.

Two different methods have been employed in order to facilitate the condensation of template-bound monomers. The first involves the use of a water-soluble carbodiimide that can combine with a mononucleotide to produce an activated intermediate. The second involves the use of a preactivated nucleotide derivative, such as a nucleoside 5'-phosphorimidazolide (Fig. 1). Using either method, it is possible to synthesize short oligo(G)s or oligo(A)s in the presence of a complementary template (Sulston et al. 1968, 1969; Weimann et al. 1968; Lohrman and Orgel 1978a). The major condensation products are dimers and trimers, although a small amount of longer oligomers are also produced. The products contain predominantly 2'-5' phosphodiester linkages, reflecting the intrinsically greater reactivity of the nucleotide 2'-OH (Lohrman and Orgel 1978b). It would be preferable, of course, if they contained only 3'-5' linkages, thus maintaining the backbone structure that is present in the template. It is difficult enough to cooptimize the oligomerization reaction for the various nucleotide bases without introducing the added complication of linkage isomerism. Furthermore, as a purely practical consideration, most of the enzymatic techniques that are available for the analysis of RNA base composition and sequence can only be applied to 3'-5'-linked oligomers.

Both the efficiency and regiospecificity of the oligomerization reaction are highly sensitive to the precise stereochemical orientation of adjacent template-bound reactants. For example, in the absence of a template, adenosine 5'-phosphorimidazolide (ImpA) undergoes an inefficient dimerization reaction that yields 2'-5'- and 3'-5'-linked isomers in a ratio of about 6:1. With the addition of a poly(U) template, the overall yield increases more than fivefold and the 2'-5':3'-5' ratio rises to about 18:1 (Lohrmann and Orgel 1978b). Comparing the poly(U):ImpA reaction to a similar reaction

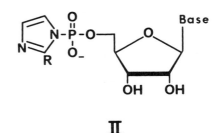

Figure 1. Structure of activated mononucleotides used in template-directed condensation reactions. (I) Activated intermediate formed by the addition of a water-soluble carbodiimide to the 5'-phosphate of a nucleotide; typically, R=(CH$_2$)$_3$N(CH$_3$)$_2$ and R'=C$_2$H$_5$. (II) Activated phosphorimidazole derivative of a nucleoside; R=H, nucleoside 5'-phosphorimidazole; R=CH$_3$, nucleoside 5'-phospho-2-methylimidazolide.

involving poly(C) and ImpG, the overall yields are roughly the same, but for poly(C):ImpG, the isomer ratio is reversed, favoring 3'-5' linkages by about 2:1 (Ninio and Orgel 1978). These results suggest that factors which alter the relative orientation of template-bound reactants may also influence the efficiency and regiospecificity of the oligomerization reaction.

Enhancement of the Oligomerization Reaction

The addition of divalent metal cations was found to have a profound effect on template-directed reactions involving ImpA or ImpG. In particular, the addition of 1–10 mM Pb^{++} to a reaction mixture containing 100 mM poly(U) and 50 mM ImpA results in a fourfold increase in the yield of oligomeric products of pentamer length and longer. In sharp contrast to the reaction in the absence of Pb^{++}, the Pb^{++}-catalyzed products contain predominantly 3'-5' phosphodiester linkages (Sleeper and Orgel 1979). Pb^{++} is also an effective catalyst for the condensation of ImpG on a poly(C) template, enhancing the yield of oligomeric products by a factor of 5. In this case, however, the products remain almost entirely 2'-5'-linked (Lohrmann and Orgel 1980). If 10–100 mM Zn^{++} is used in place of Pb^{++} in the poly(C):ImpG reaction, the yield of oligo(G)s is still enhanced and the regiospecificity is reversed to favor 3'-5' linkages almost exclusively (Bridson and Orgel 1980). Thus, in both the poly(U):ImpA and poly-(C):ImpG reactions, it is possible to obtain 3'-5'-linked oligomers in good yield simply by adding the appropriate metal ion.

The mechanism by which Pb^{++} and Zn^{++} catalyze the template-directed synthesis of 3'-5'-linked oligomers is not known. It is assumed that they alter the relative orientation of donor and acceptor molecules such that the activated phosphate of the donor is brought into position to react with the 3'-OH of the acceptor. In an attempt to achieve this same stereochemical effect without the addition of a metal ion, a large number of modified guanosine 5'-phosphorimidazolides were tested in the poly(C):ImpG reaction. It was found that guanosine 5'-phospho-2-methylimidazolide (2-MeImpG; see Fig. 1) is oligomerized with high efficiency, even higher than the efficiency of ImpG oligomerization in the presence of Zn^{++}. The products of 2-MeImpG oligomerization are almost exclusively 3'-5'-linked (Inoue and Orgel 1981). In a typical reaction mixture, containing 0.1 M poly(C), 0.1 M 2-MeImpG, 0.2 M $MgCl_2$, and 1 M NaCl, incubated at pH 8 and 0°C, the yield of oligomeric products of tetramer length and longer after 7 days is about 85% (Inoue and Orgel 1982). The product distribution can be characterized in detail using high-pressure liquid chromatography (HPLC) on an RPC-5 column. Oligomers are separated on the basis of chain length and phosphodiester-linkage isomerism (Fig. 2). The major peaks in the HPLC profile correspond to all

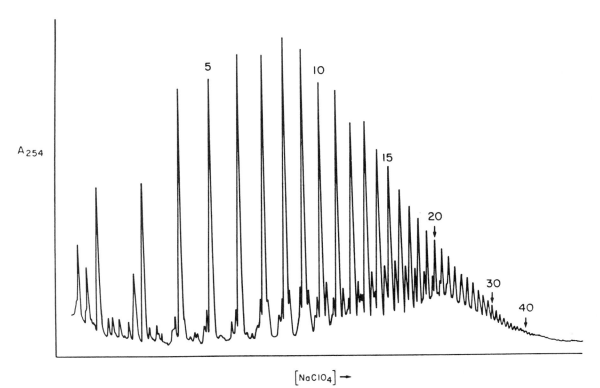

Figure 2. HPLC elution profile of 2-MeImpG condensation on a poly(C) template. The numbers above the peaks are the lengths of the corresponding 3'-5'-linked oligo(G)s. The materials were eluted from an RPC-5 column using a linear $NaClO_4$ gradient (pH 12, 0–60 mM, 90 min), and UV absorption was monitored at 254 nm.

3'-5'-linked oligo(G)s of successive lengths. The cluster of very small peaks preceding each of the major peaks corresponds to oligo(G)s that contain one or more 2'-5' linkages.

The poly(C)-directed oligomerization of 2-MeImpG is a very robust reaction, as long as a few simple requirements are met (Inoue and Orgel 1982). There is an absolute requirement for divalent cation in order to ensure the stability of the poly(C) · oligo(G) helical complex. For the same reason, the reaction temperature must be below about 37°C, although typically a temperature of 0°C is used. The preferred pH is in the range of 7.6–9.0. Below pH 7.6, a poly(C) · 2-MeImpG · poly(CH$^+$) triple helix begins to form (Miles and Frazier 1982), whereas above pH 9.0, guanine begins to lose a proton at N-1. Either of these changes is likely to alter the orientation of template-bound reactants and thus disturb the already optimized oligomerization reaction. Finally, the concentration of 2-MeImpG and

the concentration of 2-MeImpG relative to that of poly(C) must be sufficient to allow monomer-monomer interaction in free solution and monomer-oligomer interaction along the template.

The interaction of monomers in free solution results in the formation of dimers, which are subsequently bound to the template and elongated (Fakhrai et al. 1984). Elongation proceeds in the 5' → 3' direction and involves the addition of a template-bound monomer to the 3' terminus of an adjacent oligo(G) (Inoue and Orgel 1982). The relative rates of initiation and elongation, which are dependent on duplex stability and the concentration of both monomer and template, determine the overall yield and the distribution of products in the oligomerization reaction. The faster the rate of elongation relative to initiation, the greater the yield of oligomers (beyond the dimer) and the longer the chain length of the average oligomer.

Although the 2-methylimidazole derivative of guano-

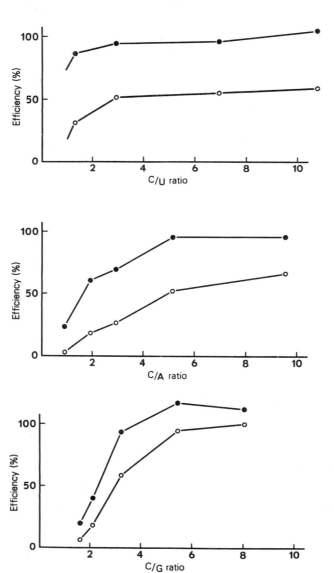

Figure 3. Efficiency of monomer incorporation in self-condensation of 2-MeImpG and 2-MeImp$X$ on poly-(C,X') as a function of the base composition of the template. (*Top*) Poly(C,U) templates; (*middle*) poly(C,A) templates; (*bottom*) poly(C,G) templates; (●) efficiency of G incorporation; (○) efficiency of X incorporation (X=A, U, or C). Efficiency measures the yield of oligomeric products of tetramer length and longer, multiplied by a factor m/t, where m is the initial concentration of monomer and t is the concentration of complementary sites on the copolymer template.

sine 5'-phosphate undergoes efficient condensation in the presence of poly(C), the corresponding derivative of adenosine 5'-phosphate does not oligomerize in the presence of poly(U). However, when a poly-(C,U) random copolymer template is used, 2-MeImpG and 2-MeImpA are co-oligomerized to yield a variety of oligo(G,A)s. More generally, any random, mixed polymer template that contains a substantial excess of cytosine residues can be used to direct the synthesis of oligomers whose base composition is complementary to that of the template. Monomers are incorporated into newly synthesized oligomers if and only if their complement is present in the template (Inoue and Orgel 1983). This remarkable result demonstrates that the specificity of Watson-Crick pairing is sufficient to provide the basis for information transfer in template-directed oligomerization reactions. It is, of course, inappropriate to discuss information transfer in the context of a random, mixed polymer template. However, studies involving templates of defined sequence (as will be described below) have shown that sequence information is transferred from template to product.

The major limitation of the poly(C,N)-directed reactions is the requirement that the template contain a substantial excess of cytosine residues. This is necessary in order to maintain the favorable structure of the poly(C):2-MeImpG duplex. If the ratio of cytosine to noncytosine in the template is decreased, the template begins to take on a different character, and the efficiency of the reaction drops sharply (Fig. 3). This is a severe obstacle to chemical self-replication, because it means that any cytosine-rich polynucleotide that can serve as a good template will produce a cytosine-poor complementary strand that is unable to direct further rounds of synthesis. It is conceivable that there is some other reaction system that can accommodate templates that do not have an abundance of cytosine residues. After all, the polymerase enzymes manage to operate on templates that contain only about 25% cytosine residues. In a nonenzymatic system, however, nucleotide polymerization should be regarded as consisting of 16 different reactions, involving the addition of any one of the four activated monomers to an oligomer terminated by any one of the four nucleotides. It will not be easy to find a reaction system that allows all 16 of these reactions to proceed at an acceptable rate.

Information Transfer

An ideal reaction system would allow sequence information to be transferred from template to product with high fidelity and would be able to copy a very large number of possible sequences with comparable efficiency. The fidelity of template-directed synthesis, as determined by the selectivity of complementary base pairing, sets a limit on the length of a sequence that can be maintained against its distribution of error copies (Eigen 1971). In the template-directed reactions described above, the fidelity of complementary synthesis appears to be quite high. When poly(C) is incubated with an equimolar mixture of the four nucleoside 5'-phospho-2-methylimidazolides, 2-MeImpG is incorporated preferentially into oligomeric products with a discrimination factor of up to 500 (Inoue and Orgel 1982). The transfer of information from U to A, from G to C, and especially from A to U is likely to be somewhat less accurate, but in general, the fidelity of complementary synthesis is not a limiting factor in the transfer of information from template to product. The main limitation stems from the fact that only cytosine-rich template sequences can be copied. The average information content of a template message is given by $\Sigma p_i \log p_i$, where p_i is the probability of occurrence of a particular message x_i. Therefore, the smaller the set of sequences that can be copied, and the greater the disparity in the efficiency with which individual sequences are copied, the lower the information content of the average message.

In an attempt to expand the message set and to smooth the differences in the efficiency of copying, we studied the poly(C,N)-directed reactions in some detail. The poly(C,U)-directed synthesis of oligo(G,A)s was found to be constrained by the relatively poor incorporation of adenine, which is particularly a problem on templates that are rich in uracil. The incorporation of adenine is limited by an intrinsically less-efficient condensation reaction when adenine is stacked on the 3' end of a growing chain and by the masking of uracil sites as a result of $G \cdot U$ noncomplementary (wobble) pairing (Joyce et al. 1984). Adenine incorporation can be improved simply by increasing the concentration of 2-MeImpA relative to 2-MeImpG. This allows adenine to compete effectively at wobble sites and does not disrupt the incorporation of guanine at complementary sites.

The poly(C,A)-directed synthesis of oligo(G,U)s is the least efficient of the three poly(C,N) copolymer template reactions. In this case, the problem is the poor stacking interaction of adjacent uracil residues, which makes it very difficult to copy a template sequence that contains two or more consecutive adenine residues. The efficiency of the reaction can be improved marginally by increasing the concentration of 2-MeImpU and by choosing reaction conditions that maximize duplex stability (G.F. Joyce and L.E. Orgel, unpubl.). However, it appears that messages that contain a run of consecutive adenines will always be poorly suited as templates in a nonenzymatic reaction system.

The poly(C,G)-directed synthesis of oligo(G,C)s is a very interesting reaction, since templates containing roughly equal amounts of cytosine and guanine would direct the synthesis of complementary strands with base composition similar to that of the template. In reactions involving cytosine-rich poly(C,G) templates, cytosine is incorporated readily into oligomeric products due to the intrinsically efficient condensation reaction between 2-MeImpC and an adjacent template-bound oligomer. The poor stacking ability of cytosine is compensated in part by the strength of $G \cdot C$ complementary pairing and can be further offset by increasing the concentration of 2-MeImpC in the reaction mixture (Joyce and Orgel 1986). The problem with poly(C,G) templates that do not contain an excess of cytosine is that the template has a tendency to form inter- and intramolecular duplex structures. Template-directed synthesis is then limited to regions of the template that are not involved in self-structure.

Overcoming template self-structure is a very difficult problem, since it calls for conditions in which short duplex regions are favored in order to allow template-directed synthesis to occur, whereas long duplex regions are disfavored in order to permit access to the entire template sequence. Intermolecular self-structure could, at least in principle, be overcome by decreasing the concentration of poly(C,G) or by segregating individual template molecules along a surface. Intramolecular self-structure is a more difficult problem because there is no possibility of isolating complementary regions that lie close together within a single molecule. It would be possible to lessen the degree of self-complementarity by introducing occasional adenine and uracil residues into the template sequence. However, by changing to a four-base system, one is faced with a complex set of coconstraints related to the efficient incorporation of each of the activated monomers.

Reactions Involving Defined-sequence Templates

The first unambiguous demonstration of information transfer in a nonenzymatic template-directed reaction system used the defined-sequence template CCGCC to direct the condensation of 2-MeImpG and 2-MeImpC (Inoue et al. 1984). The 3'-5'-linked GGCGG is substantially the most abundant pentameric product formed in the reaction (Fig. 4). The yield of GGCGG is never large (<20% compared to the amount of template), presumably because off-template reactions consume a sizable portion of the partial template-directed products. The elongation of GG to GGC, in particular, appears to be the bottleneck in the reaction. This step is quite slow, allowing the misdirected conversion of GG to GGG to occur. However, once GGC is formed, it is converted efficiently to GGCG and GGCGG.

It is clear that small differences in template size and sequence can make a considerable difference in the efficiency of the template-directed reaction. For example, whereas CCGCC is a reasonably good template, CGC is completely inert (Inoue et al. 1984). To investigate systematically the effect of template size and sequence on the efficiency of the reaction, one would like to examine a large number of closely related templates. Unfortunately, the chemical synthesis of

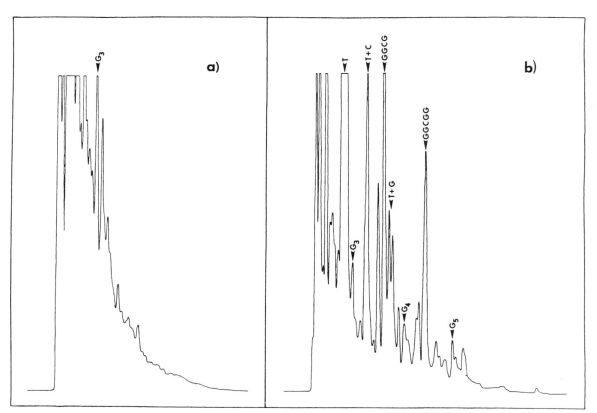

Figure 4. HPLC elution profiles of 2-MeImpG and 2-MeImpC condensation in the absence of template (*a*) and in the presence of the template CCGCC (*b*). (T) Template; (T + C) C adducts to the template; (T + G) G adducts to the template; (G_3, G_4, and G_5) oligo(G)s from trimer to pentamer; (GGCG and GGCGG) complementary products of template-directed synthesis.

RNA oligomers is a time-consuming and expensive process. Recently, a new enzymatic technique has become available allowing RNA to be synthesized from a complementary single-stranded DNA template (Lowary et al. 1986). An even simpler solution would be to use DNA oligomers themselves in the template-directed condensation reaction. This is not an unreasonable idea considering the fact that both RNA · RNA duplexes and DNA · RNA hybrids preferentially exist in the A form of the double helix (Milman et al. 1967; Zimmerman and Pheiffer 1981). In fact, it has been shown that the template-directed oligomerization of 2-MeImpG occurs with comparable efficiency and regiospecificity in the presence of either poly(C) or poly-(dC) (Chen et al. 1985).

A series of experiments were carried out using oligo(dC) templates of length 3 through 7. The oligomerization of 2-MeImpG in the presence of dC_3 is no more efficient than the reaction in template-free controls. dC_4 has a slight influence on the synthesis of oligo(G)s, whereas dC_5, dC_6, and dC_7 result in a very efficient reaction (Chen et al. 1985). At early times in these reactions, the major products contain all 3′-5′ linkages. As the reactions proceed, oligomers containing a single 2′-5′ linkage tend to accumulate. The 2′-5′ linkage is usually found at the 2′(3′) end of the growing chain and is most likely to occur in oligomers whose length is close to that of the template.

The obvious interpretation of these findings is that the regiospecificity of the reaction is lower when synthesis occurs near the 5′ end of the template. Once a 2′-5′ linkage is formed, it tends to distort the 2′(3′) terminus of the oligomer, thus acting as a chain terminator. Interestingly, as long as monomers are joined to the growing chain by a 3′-5′ linkage, elongation can continue, yielding oligomers whose length may even exceed the length of the template (Chen et al. 1985). This is possible on a homooligomer template because of the phenomenon of "chain sliding." Chain sliding is thought to involve the formation of a "bulge" loop at one end of the helix, diffusion of the loop along the helix, and resolution of the loop defect at the opposite end (Pörschke 1974). As a result, the complementary strand is able to move relative to the template, exposing previously occupied template sites that can then be used to direct further elongation. The complementary strand may slide partway off one template and take up a position spanning two template molecules, permitting synthesis to continue up to the length of the second template.

On mixed oligomer templates, sliding is less important because the reading frame soon becomes fixed by complementary pairing. The cocondensation of 2-MeImpG and 2-MeImpC on a $d(C_7GC_7)$ template yields oligomeric products of the form $(pG)_i pC(pG)_j$; the oligomers with $i = 6$ or 7 are the most abundant (Haertle and Orgel 1986a). The reaction begins with the synthesis of oligo(G) along the heptacytidine portions of the template. Oligo(G) is able to slide and elongate until a cytosine residue is added, at which

point the reading frame is fixed. Further elongation then occurs by the addition of guanosine residues downstream from cytosine. The template $d(5′-GC_7-3′)$ yields the same products as dC_7, whereas the template $d(5′-C_7G-3′)$ yields oligomers of the form pG_i and $pG_i pC$ ($i = 1,7$) (Haertle and Orgel 1986b). These results emphasize that initiation occurs mainly at oligocytidine sites on the template and suggest that in order to fix complementary synthesis to an unambiguous reading frame, one should employ a single initiator site, preferably at the 3′ end of the template.

The longest defined-sequence template used to direct the synthesis of its complement from activated monomers is the 15-mer $d(C_3GC_3GC_3GC_3)$ (Acevedo and Orgel 1987). The major products are the 3′-5′-linked oligomers of the form GGGC... and GGC... (Fig. 5a). Somewhat surprisingly, products of the form GGC... are the most abundant, suggesting that GG is converted more rapidly to GGC than to GGG. When the 14-mer template $d(5′-C_3GC_3GC_3GC_2-3′)$ is used, the major products up to the 12-mer are oligomers of the form GGGC... and GGC..., but the major products of length 12 and longer are all of the form GGC... (Fig. 5b). This reflects the fact that to produce an oligomer of length 12 or longer, initiation must occur opposite the sequence CC at the 3′ end of the template.

On the basis of the results of experiments involving templates of defined sequence, it appears that a large number of messages can be transferred from the template to the complementary product with good fidelity. This number is only a small fraction of the total number of possible template messages, since several restrictions must be applied. First, the template must have an oligocytidine (preferably dicytidine) initiator sequence at its 3′ end. Second, the template must not contain a region of stable self-structure that cannot be overcome by the competing oligomerization reaction. Third, the template must not contain long runs of any one of the four nucleotide bases. Long runs of cytosine would provide alternative initiation sites and prevent the entire template sequence from being copied. Long runs of any one of the other bases, particularly adenine, would be difficult to copy with reasonable efficiency. One is left with a family of cytosine-rich sequences, containing a scattering of uracil and guanine residues and a lesser amount of adenine. The crucial question is whether any of these RNA sequences are associated with an interesting behavioral phenotype. Specifically, do any of these sequences have the ability to catalyze their own synthesis?

Self-replication of Oligonucleotide Analogs

The question of catalytic behavior can be addressed in the context of self-replication. Given a population of self-replicating RNA molecules competing for a limited supply of activated monomers, those individuals that are best able to direct the incorporation of monomers into additional copies of themselves will eventually grow to dominate the population. Since self-replication

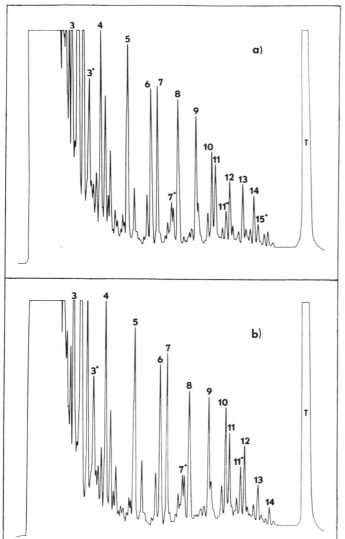

Figure 5. HPLC elution profiles of 2-MeImpG and 2-MeImpC condensation in the presence of the 15-mer template d($C_3GC_3GC_3GC_3$) (*a*) and the 14-mer template d($5'$-$C_3GC_3GC_3GC_2$-$3'$) (*b*). The numbers above the peaks are the lengths of the corresponding $3'$-$5'$-linked complementary oligomers. (T) Template. The profiles contain two series of peaks, corresponding to oligomers of the form GGGC... and oligomers of the form GGC.... The two peaks are coincident at any oligomer length for which the base composition of GGGC... and GGC... are identical. At the 3-mer, 7-mer, and 11-mer, the two peaks are resolved; those that correspond to oligomers of the form GGGC... are indicated by an asterisk.

proceeds with less than perfect fidelity, mutant copies of the dominant individuals are often generated. If a mutant has an even better ability to direct its own production compared to the dominant individuals in the population, it may grow to supplant those individuals and become the new dominant species. This is an expression of evolutionary behavior (Eigen 1971). The suggestion is that by repeating the process of mutation and selection, it may be possible to develop RNA catalysts from a population of self-replicating RNA molecules. The most natural product of such an evolving system would be an RNA molecule that has primitive replicase activity. It is not known whether a replicase function is within the realm of potential phenotypes for RNA. More to the point, it is not known whether a replicase function can be evolved in the laboratory starting from the restricted population of molecules that can be replicated by template-directed synthesis alone.

At the present time, there are two examples of self-replication in a template-directed reaction system, both of which involve chemically modified nucleotide substrates and a self-complementary (palindromic) template. The first utilizes two trideoxynucleotide substrates, d($5'$-Me-CCGp-$3'$) and d($5'$-CGGp-*o*-PhCl-$3'$), and a hexadeoxynucleotide template, d($5'$-Me-CCGCGGp-*o*-PhCl-$3'$) (von Kiedrowski 1986). The two substrates are bound to the template by complementary pairing and, in the presence of water-soluble carbodiimide, undergo condensation to form a new template molecule (Fig. 6a). The template-template complex can dissociate to yield two free template molecules, each of which is then able to bind additional substrate and begin a new round of synthesis. On the basis of this reaction scheme, it is predicted that the initial rate of template formation will follow an equation of the form: $(d[T]/dt)_{init} = K_a + K_b[T]^{1/2}$, where [T] is the template concentration and K_a and K_b are

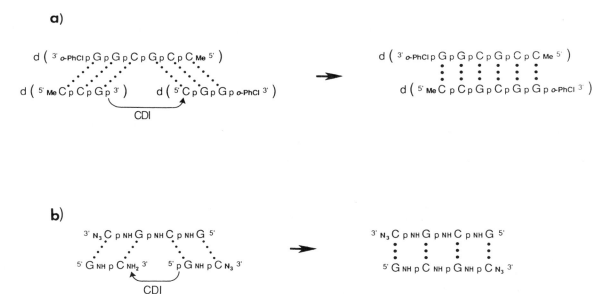

Figure 6. Mechanism of two self-replication reactions involving palindromic oligonucleotide-analog templates. (*a*) The 3'-terminal phosphate of CCG is activated by water-soluble carbodiimide (CDI), and in the presence of a template, it reacts with the 5'-terminal hydroxyl of CGG to produce 5'-CCGCGG-3'. (*b*) The 5'-terminal phosphate of GC is activated by CDI, and in the presence of a template, it reacts with the 3'-terminal amine of GC to produce 5'-GCGC-3'.

constants. Kinetic data are in close agreement with this prediction, consistent with the autocatalytic nature of the reaction (von Kiedrowski 1986).

The other example of self-replication involves the use of nucleotide analogs in which the 3'-OH of ribose has been replaced by a 3'-amine. The purpose of this modification is to enhance the nucleophilicity of the 3' terminus of a growing chain, thereby decreasing the sensitivity of the oligomerization reaction to the precise stereochemical orientation of template-bound reactants. For example, compared to 2-MeImpG, ImpG undergoes rather inefficient oligomerization in the presence of poly(C) or poly(dC). The 3'-deoxy-3'-amino derivative of ImpG, however, condenses with high efficiency and regiospecificity (Zielinski and Orgel 1985). The resulting oligomers contain 3'-5' phosphoramidate linkages, rather than the conventional 3'-5' phosphodiester linkages.

In the self-replication reaction, a tetranucleoside triphosphoramidate template, 5'-GNHpCNHpGNHpCN$_3$-3', was used to direct the condensation of two dinucleoside phosphoramidate substrates, 5'-GNHpCNH$_2$-3' and 5'-pGNHpCN$_3$-3' (Zielinski and Orgel 1987). The reaction scheme is similar to that described above, except that a 5'-phosphate rather than a 3'-phosphate is activated by water-soluble carbodiimide (Fig. 6b). Again, the kinetic data show a roughly square-root dependence of the initial reaction rate on the concentration of template, consistent with autocatalytic synthesis (Zielinski and Orgel 1987).

Neither of the two self-replication reactions described here involves information transfer, since in each case there is only one possible product. Without information transfer, the system has no capacity to evolve. Current studies involve the use of more complicated mixtures of chemically modified nucleotide substrates in an attempt to expand the set of messages that can be replicated. As a matter of practicality, it appears to be advantageous to work with the 3'-deoxy-3'-amino nucleotide analogs since they can be oligomerized on templates that do not support oligomerization of the nucleoside 5'-phospho-2-methylimidazolides (Tohidi et al. 1987). The problem of specifying a single initiation site at the 3' end of the template and the problem of avoiding stable template self-structure have yet to be overcome.

Several authors have suggested that there may be another route to the development of an RNA molecule with replicase activity; it may be possible to construct a replicase by modifying the core structure of a modern ribozyme (Sharp 1985; Pace and Marsh 1985; Cech 1986a; Szostak 1986). With such a molecule in hand, one could explore the landscape of potential RNA phenotypes by launching "evolutionary probes" into different regions of RNA sequence space. The problem with this scenario is that, based on our current understanding of modern ribozymes, it is likely to be extremely difficult (if not impossible) to transform a molecule that has been designed to catalyze sequence-specific transesterification into a molecule that catalyzes template-directed polymerization.

The *Tetrahymena* ribozyme, derived from a group I intron of pre-rRNA in *Tetrahymena thermophila*, is the most extensively studied catalytic RNA (for review, see Cech 1986b). This molecule is able to catalyze a dismutation reaction of the form: $C_i + C_j \rightleftharpoons C_{i+1} + C_{j-1}$, where $i \geq 3$ and $j \geq 4$, utilizing an internal template to bind the oligo(C) substrates (Zaug and Cech 1986). By altering the sequence of the internal template, it is possible to alter the substrate specificity of the reaction (Zaug et al. 1986). However, to convert this reaction to a polymerization reaction that operates on an external template of arbitrary sequence, three obstacles must be overcome. First, the kinetic barrier to the formation of long oligomers must be surmounted if template-directed dismutation is to result in the synthesis of a complete product. Templates at least as long as the catalyst, which contains about 100–300 nucleotides, must be copied in their entirety. Second, the template must be able to move through the active site of the catalyst in a processive manner, making its entire sequence available for complementary synthesis. Third, the secondary structure of both template and partially synthesized product must not interfere with the ongoing dismutation reaction.

These requirements are certainly a tall order for an RNA enzyme, particularly one that has already evolved to perform a specific task in biology. At the present time, it is difficult to say whether the "top-down" approach, beginning with an evolved ribozyme, or the "ground-up" approach, beginning with short oligomers that replicate by template-directed synthesis, will provide the best route to the development of an RNA replicase. Perhaps a combination of the two approaches, using template-directed synthesis to produce oligonucleotide subunits that can be ligated to form an RNA molecule with cleavage/ligation activity, will prove most fruitful.

ACKNOWLEDGMENTS

I am grateful to Dr. Leslie Orgel for many helpful discussions. This work was supported by NASA grant NGR-05067001. The author is a Merck fellow of the Life Sciences Research Foundation.

REFERENCES

Acevedo, O.L. and L.E. Orgel. 1987. Non-enzymatic transcription of an oligodeoxynucleotide 14 residues long. *J. Mol. Biol.* (in press).

Bridson, P.K. and L.E. Orgel. 1980. Catalysis of accurate poly(C)-directed synthesis of 3'-5'-linked oligoguanylates by Zn^{2+}. *J. Mol. Biol.* **144:** 567.

Cech, T.R. 1986a. A model for the RNA-catalyzed replication of RNA. *Proc. Natl. Acad. Sci.* **83:** 4360.

———. 1986b. Catalytic RNA. *Sci. Am.* **255:** 64.

———. 1987. The chemistry of self-splicing RNA and RNA enzymes. *Science* **236:** 1532.

Chen, C.B., T. Inoue, and L.E. Orgel. 1985. Template-directed synthesis on oligodeoxycytidylate and polydeoxycytidylate templates. *J. Mol. Biol.* **181:** 271.

Crick, F.H.C. 1968. The origin of the genetic code. *J. Mol. Biol.* **38:** 367.

Davies, R.J.H. and N. Davidson. 1971. Base pairing equilibria between polynucleotides and complementary monomers. *Biopolymers* **10:** 1455.

Eigen, M. 1971. Self-organization of matter and the evolution of biological macromolecules. *Naturwissenschaften* **58:** 465.

Eigen, M. and P. Schuster. 1978. The hypercycle: A principle of natural self-organization, part C: The realistic hypercycle. *Naturwissenschaften* **65:** 341.

Fakhrai, H., T. Inoue, and L.E. Orgel. 1984. Temperature-dependence of the template-directed synthesis of oligoguanylates. *Tetrahedron* **40:** 39.

Haertle, T. and L.E. Orgel. 1986a. Template-directed synthesis on the oligonucleotide d(C_7-G-C_7). *J. Mol. Biol.* **188:** 77.

———. 1986b. The template properties of some oligodeoxynucleotides containing cytidine and guanosine. *J. Mol. Evol.* **23:** 108.

Howard, F.B., J. Frazier, M.N. Lipsett, and H.T. Miles. 1964. Infrared demonstration of two- and three-strand helix formation between poly C and guanosine mononucleotides and oligonucleotides. *Biochem. Biophys. Res. Commun.* **17:** 93.

Howard, F.B., J. Frazier, M.F. Singer, and H.T. Miles. 1966. Helix formation between polyribonucleotides and purines, purine nucleosides, and nucleotides. *J. Mol. Biol.* **16:** 415.

Huang, W.M. and P.O.P. Ts'o. 1966. Physiochemical basis of the recognition process in nucleic acid interactions. I. Interactions of polyuridylic acid and nucleosides. *J. Mol. Biol.* **16:** 523.

Inoue, T. and L.E. Orgel. 1981. Substituent control of the poly(C)-directed oligomerization of guanosine 5'-phosphorimidazolide. *J. Am. Chem. Soc.* **103:** 7666.

———. 1982. Oligomerization of (guanosine 5'-phosphor)-2-methylimidazolide on poly(C): An RNA polymerase model. *J. Mol. Biol.* **162:** 201.

———. 1983. A nonenzymatic RNA polymerase model. *Science* **219:** 859.

Inoue, T., G.F. Joyce, K. Grzeskowiak, L.E. Orgel, J.M. Brown, and C.B. Reese. 1984. Template-directed synthesis on the pentanucleotide CpCpGpCpC. *J. Mol. Biol.* **178:** 669.

Joyce, G.F. and L.E. Orgel. 1986. Non-enzymatic template-directed synthesis on RNA random copolymers: Poly-(C,G) templates. *J. Mol. Biol.* **188:** 433.

Joyce, G.F., T. Inoue, and L.E. Orgel. 1984. Non-enzymatic template-directed synthesis on RNA random copolymers: Poly(C,U) templates. *J. Mol. Biol.* **176:** 279.

Joyce, G.F., A.W. Schwartz, S.L. Miller, and L.E. Orgel. 1987. The case for an ancestral genetic system involving simple analogues of the nucleotides. *Proc. Natl. Acad. Sci.* **84:** 4398.

Lohrmann, R. and L.E. Orgel. 1978a. Template-directed polynucleotide condensation as a model for RNA replication. In *Origins of life: Proceedings of the 2nd ISSOL meeting, 5th ICOL meeting* (ed. H. Noda), p. 235. Center for Academic Publications, Japan; Japan Scientific Societies Press, Tokyo.

———. 1978b. Preferential formation of (2'-5')-linked internucleotide bonds in non-enzymatic reactions. *Tetrahedron* **34:** 853.

———. 1980. Efficient catalysis of polycytidylic acid-directed oligoguanylate formation by Pb^{2+}. *J. Mol. Biol.* **142:** 555.

Lowary, P., J. Sampson, J. Milligan, D. Groebe, and O.C. Uhlenbeck. 1986. A better way to make RNA for physical studies. In *Structure and dynamics of RNA* (ed. P.H. van Knippenberg and C.W. Hilbers), p. 69. Plenum Press, New York.

Miles, H.T. and J. Frazier. 1982. Infrared study of G·C complex formation in template-dependent oligo(G) synthesis. *J. Mol. Biol.* **162:** 219.

Milman, G., R. Langridge, and M.J. Chamberlin. 1967. The structure of a DNA-RNA hybrid. *Proc. Natl. Acad. Sci.* **57:** 1804.

Ninio, J. and L.E. Orgel. 1978. Heteropolynucleotides as templates for non-enzymatic polymerizations. *J. Mol. Evol.* **12:** 91.

Orgel, L.E. 1968. Evolution of the genetic apparatus. *J. Mol. Biol.* **38:** 381.

————. 1986. Molecular replication and the origins of life. In *The lesson of quantum theory* (ed. J. de Boer et al.), p. 283. Elsevier Science Publishers, Amsterdam.

Pace, N.R. and T.L. Marsh. 1985. RNA catalysis and the origin of life. *Origins Life* **16:** 97.

Pörschke, D. 1974. Model calculations on the kinetics of oligonucleotide double helix coil transitions. Evidence for a fast chain sliding reaction. *Biophys. Chem.* **2:** 83.

Shapiro, R. 1986. *Origins — A skeptic's guide to the creation of life on earth*. Summit Books, New York.

Sharp, P.A. 1985. On the origin of RNA splicing and introns. *Cell* **42:** 397.

Sleeper, H.L. and L.E. Orgel. 1979. The catalysis of nucleotide polymerization by compounds of divalent lead. *J. Mol. Evol.* **12:** 357.

Sulston, J., R. Lohrmann, L.E. Orgel, and H.T. Miles. 1968. Nonenzymatic synthesis of oligoadenylates on a polyuridylic acid template. *Proc. Natl. Acad. Sci.* **59:** 726.

Sulston, J., R. Lohrmann, L.E. Orgel, H. Schneider-Bernloehr, B.J. Weimann, and H.T. Miles. 1969. Nonenzymatic oligonucleotide synthesis on a polycytidylate template. *J. Mol. Biol.* **40:** 227.

Szostak, J.W. 1986. Enzymatic activity of the conserved core of a group I self-splicing intron. *Nature* **322:** 83.

Tohidi, M., W.S. Zielinski, C.B. Chen, and L.E. Orgel. 1987. Oligomerization of 3'-amino-3'-deoxyguanosine-5'-phosphorimidazolidate on a d(CpCpCpC) template. *J. Mol. Evol.* **25:** 97.

Ts'o, P.O.P. 1974. *Basic principles in nucleic acid chemistry*, p. 453. Academic Press, New York.

von Kiedrowski, G. 1986. A self-replicating hexadeoxynucleotide. *Angew. Chem. Int. Ed. Engl.* **25:** 932.

Webb, E.C. 1984. *Enzyme nomenclature 1984.* (Recommendations of the nomenclature committee of the International Union of Biochemistry on the nomenclature and classification of enzyme-catalysed reactions.) Academic Press, Orlando, Florida.

Weimann, B.J., R. Lohrmann, L.E. Orgel, H. Schneider-Bernloehr, and J.E. Sulston. 1968. Template-directed synthesis with adenosine-5'-phosphorimidazolide. *Science* **161:** 387.

Woese, C. 1967. *The genetic code*, p. 186. Harper and Row, New York.

Zaug, A.J. and T.R. Cech. 1986. The intervening sequence RNA of *Tetrahymena* is an enzyme. *Science* **231:** 470.

Zaug, A.J., M.D. Been, and T.R. Cech. 1986. The *Tetrahymena* ribozyme acts like an RNA restriction endonuclease. *Nature* **324:** 429.

Zielinski, W.S. and L.E. Orgel. 1985. Oligomerization of activated derivatives of 3'-amino-3'-deoxyguanosine on poly(C) and poly(dC) templates. *Nucleic Acids Res.* **13:** 2469.

————. 1987. Autocatalytic synthesis of a tetranucleotide analogue. *Nature* **327:** 346.

Zimmerman, S.B. and B.H. Pheiffer. 1981. A RNA·DNA hybrid that can adopt two conformations: An x-ray diffraction study of poly(rA)·poly(dT) in concentrated solution or in fibers. *Proc. Natl. Acad. Sci.* **78:** 78.

Natural Selection, Protein Engineering, and the Last Riboorganism: Rational Model Building in Biochemistry

S.A. BENNER, R.K. ALLEMANN, A.D. ELLINGTON, L. GE, A. GLASFELD, G.F. LEANZ,
T. KRAUCH, L.J. MACPHERSON, S. MORONEY, J.A. PICCIRILLI, AND E. WEINHOLD
Laboratory for Organic Chemistry, Swiss Federal Institute of Technology, CH-8092 Zurich, Switzerland

The behavior of biological macromolecules can be interpreted both functionally and historically (Benner et al. 1985). Functional interpretations presume natural selection and require a distinction between macromolecular behaviors that are the products of selection and those that reflect neutral drift. Historical interpretations require distinctions between "primitive traits" present in a common ancestor and "derived" traits that arose more recently.

These distinctions are extremely difficult to make. Therefore, appropriate research strategy involves construction of formal models that can be set in opposition to each other and experimentally tested. The building and testing of historical and functional models are described in this paper. We hope to illustrate how rigorous model building can (1) help distinguish between selected and nonselected behaviors in proteins, (2) permit the engineering of the catalytic properties of enzymes, and (3) define the role of RNA in early catalysis.

To show how model building can help distinguish between selected and nonselected behaviors in proteins, let us consider a single trait, stereospecificity, of a single class of enzymes, alcohol dehydrogenases dependent on nicotinamide cofactors (NAD^+ and $NADP^+$). NADH bears two hydrogens (Fig. 1) at the 4-position, labeled R and S. The hydrogens are different, and individual dehydrogenases catalyze the transfer of only

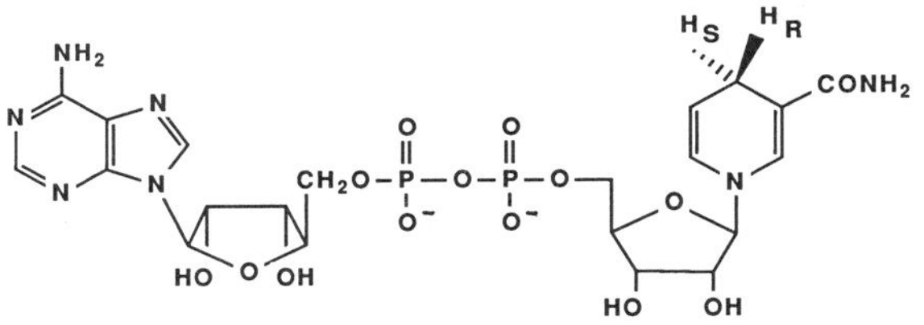

Figure 1. Two hydrogens at the 4-position of reduced nicotinamide cofactors are different and are designated R and S. Dehydrogenases selectively transfer only one of these hydrogens (Table 1).

one of them. This is a trait that displays diversity; about half of the dehydrogenases examined transfer H_R and half transfer H_S.

When dehydrogenases are organized by their Enzyme Commission catalog number, stereospecificity appears to be random (see Table 1), consistent with the hypothesis that the trait is not selected. Either stereospecificity is drifting or it is a randomly fixed historical accident that has been conserved for unspecified reasons. Data exist that rule out the possibility that stereospecificity is drifting (You 1985). For example, all lactate dehydrogenases, including enzymes from bacteria, plants, and animals, transfer H_R, inconsistent with the notion that this trait is drifting. Rather, a historical model must make two assumptions: (1) All lactate dehydrogenases are descendants of a single

Table 1. Stereospecificity of Dehydrogenases Organized by Enzyme Commission Catalog Number

E.C. no.	Enzyme	Stereospecificity
1.1.1.1	ethanol dehydrogenase	R
1.1.1.3	homoserine dehydrogenase	S
1.1.1.6	glycerol dehydrogenase	R
1.1.1.8	glycerol-3-phosphate dehydrogenase	S
1.1.1.26	glyoxylate reductase	R
1.1.1.27	L-lactate dehydrogenase	R
1.1.1.28	D-lactate dehydrogenase	R
1.1.1.30	3-hydroxybutyrate dehydrogenase	S
1.1.1.35	3-hydroxyacyl-CoA dehydrogenase	S
1.1.1.37	malate dehydrogenase	R
1.1.1.38	malic enzyme	R
1.1.1.50	3-hydroxysteroid dehydrogenase	S
1.1.1.60	tartronate semialdehyde reductase	R
1.1.1.62	estradiol dehydrogenase	S
1.1.1.100	3-oxoacyl ACP Reductase	S
1.1.1.108	carnitine dehydrogenase	S

ancestral lactate dehydrogenase that transferred H_R (for no functional reason) and (2) stereospecificity is rigorously conserved during the divergence of plants, animals, bacteria, and mycoplasma (e.g., *Acholeplasma laidlawaii*).

Alternatively, a functional model might argue that the uniform stereospecificity displayed by lactate dehydrogenases reflects either convergent evolution of stereospecificity or a functional constraint on the drift of stereospecificity during the divergent evolution of lactate dehydrogenases. In both cases, the transfer of H_R is assumed to confer a selective advantage on the host organism.

In the two decades preceding 1980, the historical explanation came to be accepted as the only explanation for the origin of this particular trait (You 1985). This was largely due to the absence of an alternative, mechanistically reasonable functional model. One such model was recently proposed (Benner et al. 1985) on the basis of three hypotheses: (1) Which hydrogen is transferred is controlled by the conformation of bound NADH and is determined in part by stereoelectronic considerations, (2) different conformers of NADH have different redox potentials, and (3) functionally optimal enzymes match the redox potential of bound NADH to the redox potential of the natural substrate of the dehydrogenase.

A model based on these assumptions makes a simple prediction: Enzymes that have evolved to reduce unstable carbonyl substrates should have evolved to transfer H_R, whereas enzymes that have evolved to reduce stable carbonyl substrates should have evolved to transfer H_S. As shown in Table 2, this prediction is, in general, confirmed by experiment.

The ability of a functional model to create order in the distribution of an apparently random macromolecular behavior itself strongly supports the model, at least as a working hypothesis. However, the correlation in Table 2 is also consistent with a modified historical model that assumes that (1) there existed *two* ancestral dehydrogenases, one transferring (randomly) H_R and the other transferring (randomly) H_S; (2) the ancestral enzyme transferring H_R had a preference for unstable carbonyl substrates, whereas the enzyme transferring H_S must have had a preference for stable carbonyl substrates; and (3) both stereospecificity *and* substrate type were rigorously conserved during divergent evolution.

Implicit in the functional model and in the correlation shown in Table 2 is the statement that stereospecificity is not strongly selected in those enzymes acting on substrates with intermediate stabilities. A simple interpretation of the functional model suggests that if stereochemical diversity is to be observed in analogous enzymes from different organisms, it will be observed in enzymes acting on substrates such as ethanol or glycerol-3-phosphate, where the equilibrium constant of the overall reaction is approximately 10^{-11} M. The historical model predicts that such enzymes will have the same stereospecificity. This then might provide some grounds for distinguishing between the two models.

We have examined several enzymes that catalyze the reduction of substrates with the general structure R-CH_2CHO. The equilibrium constants for the redox reactions of these substrates are at the "break" in the correlation in Table 2. Thus, one naively expects that enzymes from different organisms acting on these substrates might have different stereospecificities. This is in fact the case. Ethanol dehydrogenases (e.g., from *Drosophila* and yeast) and hydroxymethyl glutaryl–coenzyme A (HMG-CoA) reductases (e.g., from *Acholeplasma* and mammal) both display stereochemical heterogeneity and act on substrates with redox potentials such that the functional model predicts that either particular stereospecificity would not be strongly selected.

Of course, these data do not by themselves rule

Table 2. Stereospecificity of Dehydrogenases Organized by Redox Potential of Presumed Natural Substrate

log K_{eq}	Enzyme	Stereospecificity
−17.5	glyoxylate reductase	R
−13.5	tartronate semialdehyde reductase	R
−12.8	glycerate dehydrogenase	R
−12.1	malate dehydrogenase	R
−12.1	malic enzyme	R
−11.6	L-lactate dehydrogenase	R
−11.6	D-lactate dehydrogenase	R
−11.2	ethanol dehydrogenase	R
−11.1	glycerol-3-phosphate dehydrogenase	S
−10.9	homoserine dehydrogenase	S
−10.9	carnitine dehydrogenase	S
−10.5	3-hydroxyacyl-CoA dehydrogenase	S
−8.9	3-hydroxybutyrate dehydrogenase	S
−7.7	estradiol 17-dehydrogenase	S
−7.6	3-oxoacyl ACP Reductase	S
−7.6	3-hydroxysteroid dehydrogenase	S

Of the 130 dehydrogenases studied to date, about 120 fit the correlation, perhaps 10 do not. For discussion, see Benner et al. (1985) and Oppenheimer (1984).

out all historical models. Perhaps all enzymes from organisms such as *Drosophila* are stereochemically "unusual," or perhaps enzymes acting on substrates with redox potentials far from the break also display stereochemical diversity. We have looked for evidence to support either argument, but have found none. For example, the functional model predicts that malate dehydrogenases from all organisms should transfer H_R. The enzymes from mammals, birds, fish, insects (e.g., *Drosophila*), fungi, eubacteria (e.g., *Clostridium acidiurici*), plants, and archaebacteria (e.g., *Halobacter halobium*) in fact all transfer H_R.

To explain the facts, the historical model must now assume two ancestral dehydrogenases for both ethanol and HMG-CoA as substrates (but not for malate and lactate as substrates), or postulate that stereospecificity can drift in ethanol dehydrogenases or HMG-CoA reductases (but not lactate dehydrogenases or malate dehydrogenases). These modifications, although possible, are ad hoc. Furthermore, in the absence of explanations as to why some enzymes have multiple ancestors or why stereospecificity can diverge in some enzymes and not in others, historical models with such ad hoc modifications are not predictive.

An independent argument suggests that stereospecificity may not be absolutely conserved within a group of homologous enzymes. We recently showed that the ethanol dehydrogenase from *Drosophila* transfers H_S, in contrast to the ethanol dehydrogenase from yeast, which transfers H_R (Benner et al. 1985). Earlier, Jornvall et al. (1981) noted sequence similarities in the dinucleotide-binding domain of these two proteins and suggested that these two enzymes might therefore be homologous. If their suggestion is correct, stereospecificity with respect to cofactor is not the same in at least some homologous dehydrogenases.

Historical models consistent with these data are too ad hoc to permit direct experimental test. Reasonable criteria for separating dehydrogenases into separate lineages, including sequence analysis, metal ion requirements, and substrate specificity, all fail to predict stereospecificity in any but the most trivial examples. In contrast, the functional model, although controversial (Oppenheimer 1984), remains a subject for intensive experimental investigation and has proved to be remarkably successful in anticipating experimental and

theoretical results on enzymatic and model systems related to dehydrogenases. Several of these are listed in Table 3.

On the basis of similar models, well-studied macromolecular behaviors can be divided into two groups (Table 4). In one, working functional models exist that are predictively satisfactory, whereas in the other group, historical models are proving to be more satisfactory.

Even a limited distinction between functional and nonfunctional behavior in proteins can be valuable. For example, it can assist those attempting to engineer the behavior of proteins via molecular biological tools that allow the biochemist to alter the structure of catalytic proteins. Although "engineered enzymes" are widely recognized as desirable entities, there is at present no good theory to suggest which residues to change to achieve a desired perturbation in behavior. Therefore, residues generally are changed in the active sites of proteins and are chosen by inspection of a crystal structure. Not surprisingly, many of these changes have enormous (and often undesirable) impact on the behavior of the enzyme. Loss of a factor of 10^5 in catalytic activity is not uncommon (Cronin et al. 1987).

Alterations in structure at a distance from the active site offer the prospect of engineering more delicate changes; this strategy is more consistent with that followed by Nature as she engineers the behavior of proteins. However, the biochemist has difficulty with this strategy because of the number of mutations that are possible in residues remote from the active site.

We have argued for some time (Nambiar et al. 1986) that if we can distinguish in a general way between the results of selection and drift in macromolecular structure, an alternative rationale can be implemented for engineering of the behaviors of proteins by deliberate alteration of amino acid residues remote from the active site. In a strategy termed "evolutionary guidance," comparison of the structure and behavior of homologous enzymes, tempered by available understanding of selection and drift in proteins, provides guidance for changing the structure of a particular protein to yield new proteins with properties that are not simply the average of the properties of modern homologous proteins.

Consider, for example, a simply stated problem in

Table 3. Recent Results Consistent with the Functional Model

Computational verification of stereoselectivity based on conformation in reduced nicotinamide cofactors (Wu and Houk 1987)

Correlation between stereoselectivity and redox potential in nicotinamide model systems (Ohno et al. 1986)

Experimental and theoretical confirmation of arguments regarding adjustment of internal equilibrium constants in certain enzymes (Ellington and Benner 1987)

Convergent stereospecificity of nonhomologous dihydrofolate reductases (Matthews et al. 1986)

Stereospecificity of $NAD^+/NADP^+$ transhydrogenases (Kaplan 1967)

Table 4.   Candidates for Selectable Macromolecular Traits

Stereoselection between diastereomeric transition states
   NADH-dependent redox reactions
   phosphoryl transfer reactions
Internal equilibrium constants
Kinetic parameters ±10%
Stability/instability
Substrate specificity against compounds present physiologically
Candidates for neutral macromolecular traits
Stereoselection between enantiomeric transition states
   decarboxylation of beta-keto acids
   pyridoxal-dependent decarboxylation of amino acids
Nonequilibrium dynamic motion of proteins (Stackhouse et al. 1985)
Substrate specificity against compounds not present physiologically

protein engineering: How can we make yeast alcohol dehydrogenase, an enzyme that reduces acetaldehyde to ethanol, reduce acetaldehyde faster? The task is especially difficult for two reasons. ADH from yeast is already an exceptionally fast enzyme. Furthermore, a crystal structure for the enzyme from yeast is not available. The closest structure is for the alcohol dehydrogenase from horse liver, an enzyme sharing only 35% sequence identity with the enzyme from yeast. However, a simple rationale exists for designing a faster enzyme. The rate-limiting step in the reduction reaction is not the hydride transfer, but the release of NAD^+. Therefore, a mutant form of the enzyme, where the free energies of all bound species are raised together (Fig. 2), might well be faster. Such a "uniform binding change" (Albery and Knowles 1976) can be effected by weakening the interaction between the enzyme and the adenine portion of the cofactor somewhat, but not by too much.

A comparison of the sequences of homologous dehydrogenases (Fig. 3) in a region near the adenine-binding site identified residue 211 as a position where variation in amino acid substitution might alter the binding of cofactor uniformly. The residue was changed from arginine to threonine. Representative kinetic constants of the resulting mutant enzyme are shown in Table 5. The results are notable in several respects. First, the increased dissociation constants of NAD^+ and NADH in the mutant dehydrogenase were as predicted. Second, the residue that was changed was remote from the active site. It would not have been targeted by a rationale based on simple inspection of a crystal structure. Third, the mutant enzyme had kinetic properties that were not the average properties of the enzymes found in nature. Indeed, mutant R211T appears to be a faster "acetaldehyde reductase" than any natural enzyme studied so far. "Evolutionary guidance" as a strategy for deliberately engineering the behavior of proteins must still be explored. However, it has passed an important test.

How can this approach be used to address questions regarding RNA catalysis and the origin of life? Here again, the interesting questions revolve around an analysis of contrasting functional and historical models, proposals that distinguish between primitive and derived traits, and distinctions between selection and drift

as mechanisms for evolving observed behaviors. Here again, there is a virtue to rigorous model building.

A simple model for the involvement of RNA molecules as early catalysts is based on three assumptions: (1) The first life form consisted of an RNA-directed RNA polymerase that itself was an RNA

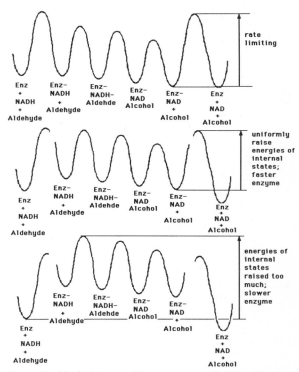

Figure 2. (*Top*) Abstract "free-energy profile" for the reaction catalyzed by yeast alcohol dehydrogenase. As evidenced by the small primary deuterium isotope effect ($V_H/V_D=1.4$), the rate-limiting step is not the transfer of hydrogen, but rather the release of NAD^+ cofactor. Therefore, moving the free energies of all internal states up by a modest amount (*middle*) is expected to increase the rate of the reaction. However, a uniform loosening of the binding of all internal states can easily be overdone (*bottom*), leading to a slower enzyme with another rate-limiting step. Thus, mutations at the active site are likely to be insufficiently delicate to produce the change desired to the extent desired. We have used "evolutionary guidance," based on an analysis of different sequences and behaviors of a set of homologous proteins, to identify residues remote from the active site that, when altered, will produce mutants with the desired kinetic properties.

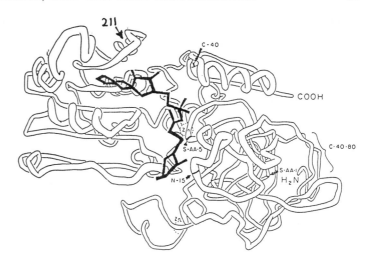

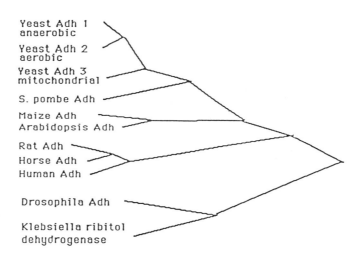

Figure 3. Analysis of the sequences and behaviors of a set of homologous proteins connected by the tree shown above identifies a region above the adenine-binding site where mutations might influence uniformly the binding of NAD$^+$ and NADH. Residues here, remote from the active site, would not be the targets of site-directed mutagenesis experiments had simple inspection of a crystal structure been the sole basis for the mutagenesis rationale. However, alterations here produce the desired change in binding and a faster enzyme (Table 7).

molecule; (2) the first synthesis of proteins was done by RNA catalysts; and (3) at some point, proteins took over most of the catalytic tasks previously performed by RNA catalysts.

Although a rudimentary form of this model was proposed by Woese, Crick, and Orgel in the late 1960s (Woese 1967; Crick 1968; Orgel 1968), the development of the model in the 1970s should not be overlooked. For example, in 1976, Usher and his co-workers discovered what we believe to be the first clear example of catalytic RNA (Usher and McHale 1976). Furthermore, the significance of the structure of many "ribo-cofactors," mentioned by Orgel (1968), was explored by White in 1976. Finally, in what might be

regarded as the apogee of theoretical development of this model to date, Visser and Kellogg (1978) were able to correlate the model, the structure of ribo-cofactors, and their chemical reactivities.

The model, especially as developed in the 1970s, solves four specific problems presented by the biochemistry of modern organisms: (1) the "chicken or egg" problem, originating in the simultaneous need for DNA to make proteins and proteins to make DNA, (2) the intermediacy of mRNA between DNA and proteins, (3) the presence of rRNA as the prinicipal component of ribosomes, and (4) the fact that many cofactors contain RNA-like moieties that do not participate in the chemical reaction and that can be removed with no ill effect on catalysis. The last point may be the most important (Fig. 4). Ribo-cofactors are distributed in nature in a pattern that suggests that these structures are primitive. The RNA parts of the cofactors almost certainly have no intrinsic function. Analogous molecules with similar reactivities that perform identical biological functions are known that lack any RNA component (Fig. 4). Without the historical model out-

Table 5. Kinetic Properties of Native and Mutant Alcohol Dehydrogenases

Protein	NAD$^+$ (K_D)	NADH (K_D)	V_H/V_D	Red (V_{max}; relative)
ADH 1	1.2 mM	0.075 mM	1.4	100
R211T	1.6 mM	0.185 mM	1.8	141

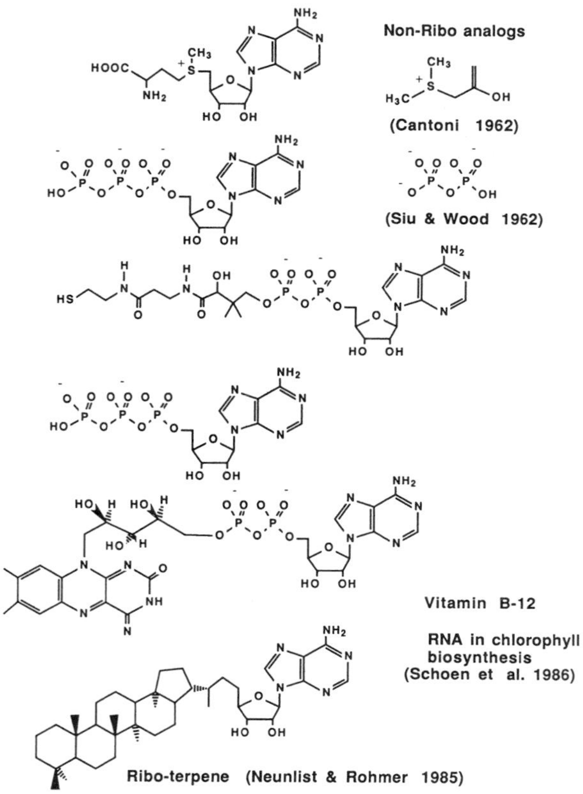

Figure 4. Many cofactors contain fragments of RNA that serve no apparent role in catalysis. Although arguments occasionally are made that these fragments serve some function (Fierke and Jencks 1986), their presence cannot reflect intrinsic function, as simpler variants of several of these cofactors (right-hand column) are chemically similar in other enzymatic systems. The wide distribution in nature of this apparently nonfunctional trait strongly suggests that ribo-cofactors are primitive structures. A model that presumes a *complex* ribometabolism based nearly exclusively on RNA as a catalyst offers a simple explanation for these structures. Models that presume a *primitive* ribometabolism preceding the advent of translation are logically inadequate to provide an analogous explanation. Finally, cofactors that arose during a period when proteins and RNA molecules both served as catalysts (a period that apparently extends from the time of the breakthrough organism to the present day) are expected to contain chemically nonessential fragments that include protein-like moieties. Acyl-carrier protein may well be an example of such a cofactor.

enigmatic structures are explained as vestiges of an ancient metabolism based on RNA catalysts.

In more recent discussions of the "ribo-world" (Table 6) (Sharp 1985; Darnell and Doolittle 1986; Gilbert 1986; Westheimer 1986), the model has lost some of its logical force for three reasons.

1. The revised model has focused almost exclusively on RNA-catalyzed intron splicing and RNA processing, beginning with an assumption that these traits, and the related genetic structure of various species, are primitive vestiges of an earlier world.
2. The revised model views the geological time during which RNA served as catalyst as short.
3. The revised model focuses on the development of translation machinery as the first step in the evolution of a primitive riboorganism.

Each of these assumptions is problematical. Introns and their self-catalyzed splicing are not "obviously primitive traits" either chemically or by their distribution in nature. Transesterification reactions of phosphodiesters are readily catalyzed (see below); introns, self-splicing, and protein-catalyzed splicing display peculiar distribution in the modern world, and the diversity of splicing mechanisms is perplexing a priori. Modern examples of RNA catalysis can presently be explained equally well as vestiges of an ancient state or as a trait derived recently as an inexpensive way to remove introns that serve roles that are either regulatory (as perhaps is the case in T4 phage) (Ehrenman et al. 1986) or unknown. In the context of the historical model outlined above, RNA-catalyzed splicing may be viewed as confirming the historical model based on other grounds. However, it is a poor foundation for a historical model and does not make a convincing case if forced to stand alone. Furthermore, a model based on the notion that translation evolved before complex metabolism is not logically equipped to explain the data it is intended to explain. If the model is intended to explain the structure of NAD^+ as a vestige of a riboorganism, it must assume that the *breakthrough riboorganism*, the first organism to synthesize proteins by translation, had ribozymes catalyzing redox reactions using NAD^+. In fact, the model must assume that the breakthrough organism had several ribodehydrogenases; otherwise, it cannot easily explain why the ribocofactor structure was conserved across the breakthrough. This is also true for *S*-adenosylmethionine (implying that the breakthrough organism had ribo-

lined above, the repeated occurrence of nonfunctional RNA in cofactors whose structures are almost certainly primitive represents a problem. With the model, these

Table 6. Some Representative Comments Concerning the Plausibility of a Complex Metabolism in Riboorganisms

Lehninger (1972): "It is quite plausible that a primitive nucleotide-based life could have existed in the absence of proteins. But it is quite clear that not much evolutionary progress could have been made without proteins."

Visser (1984): "The catalytic capabilities of RNA molecules suggest that a short but decisive evolution towards primitive metabolism was possible even before the origin of the genetic code."

Orgel (1986): "The transition to a more modern biochemistry required the invention of genetic coding."

transmethylases), flavin adenine dinucleotide (ribo-oxidases), adenosine triphosphate (ribophosphate metabolism), riboterpenoids (ribozyme-based isoprenoid chemistry), CoA (ribozyme-catalyzed Claisen condensations), and other ribo-cofactors (Fig. 4).

This is simply not a description of an organism with a primitive metabolism. Rather, for the model to explain the vestigal RNA structures that are distributed in catalytic roles throughout the biological world, it must assume that the breakthrough organism had a fully developed metabolism.

One cannot dilute this picture without damaging the explanatory coherence of the model. For example, many current models attempt to introduce protein participation in the RNA world as early as possible to assist RNA as a catalyst. This attempt is apparently based on the assumption that RNA molecules "need" proteins, without which they are ineffective catalysts. Although this view can be questioned on chemical grounds (see below), explanations based on this modified model are necessarily weakened. To the extent that models assume the involvement of proteins in the world where ribo-cofactors evolved (which must also be the world where metabolism dependent on ribo-cofactors evolved), the model cannot explain why the nonfunctional fragments of cofactors are RNA and not (for example) proteinaceous. In the context of a logically explanatory model, acyl carrier protein is a cofactor that evolved in a ribonucleic acid–protein world; nicotinamide adenine dinucleotide is not. In the context of the model, the modern world is the world where proteins doubled with RNA as catalysts, not the ancient world.

To provide a logically coherent solution to the four problems mentioned above, the model must postulate a breakthrough riboorganism with complex metabolism. With an eye toward the chemistry of modern metabolic processes, one might inspect modern metabolic pathways to generate a model for the metabolism of this breakthrough organism. Although the details of the model vary depending on the rules one uses to construct the model, one plausible metabolism is shown in Table 7.

Table 8 illustrates how modern bioorganic data can be used to address a single question arising in the model: Was the breakthrough organism photosynthetic? Here again, the value of the discussion is not that it resolves this issue, but that it is a rich source of suggestions for future experimental work. The question is especially intriguing for another reason. The participation of RNA in the biosynthesis of chlorophyll in the modern world (Schoen et al. 1986) is consistent with the possibility that the breakthrough organism was photosynthetic (Table 8). The origin of photosynthesis can be approximately dated by the appearance of oxidized sediments in datable geological strata (Strother and Barghoorn 1980). Fossils of organisms are known preceding this time. Thus, if the metabolism outlined in Table 7 is correct, these fossils are fossils of riboorganisms.

The assumption that complex metabolism arose before ribosome-based translation has advantages in addition to its making the model explanatory. Translation is among the most complex biological processes known. It requires many chemical transformations, including the charging of tRNA molecules with appropriate amino acids, the translation step itself, and the modification of RNA bases. In chemical terms, it is more complex than many pathways. It is unreasonable on chemical grounds to argue that translation emerged before complex metabolism. Furthermore, many of the most perplexing problems discussed regarding the origin of translations are perplexing because it is assumed that translation arose in a metabolically primitive organism. These problems are lessened (but not solved) by models that presume a metabolically complex breakthrough organism.

Could RNA catalyze the chemical reactions that the historical model must presume are part of the breakthrough metabolism? Many have doubted this possibility (Table 6), although recent dramatic discoveries by Cech (Bass and Cech 1984), Altman (Guerrier-Takada and Altman 1983), Szostak (1986), and their co-workers have removed some of these doubts. However, accounting for catalysis by RNA molecules is not difficult in many cases, and catalysis by RNA in general is not a priori more problematic than catalysis by proteins. For example, in accounting for the transesterification reactions catalyzed by self-splicing RNA molecules, hydrophobic interactions have been largely overlooked (Fig. 5). Binding a phosphate in a hydrophobic region of RNA will raise the pK_a of the phos-

---

Table 7. One Model for the Breakthrough Organism

Reactions Part of the Breakthrough Organism's Metabolism
  Oxidation/reduction reactions, aldol condensations, Claisen
    condensations, transmethylations
  Lived in an aerobic environment, were photosynthetic
  Degraded fatty acids, synthesized terpenes
  Used DNA to store information
  Energy metabolism based on ATP
  Modified RNA bases

Reactions Not Part of the Breakthrough Organism's Metabolism
  Biotin-dependent carboxylations
  Fatty acid synthesis
  Pyridoxal chemistry, transaminations

Table 8. Was the Breakthrough Organism Photosynthetic?

YES: The first step in the "C_5" pathway for the biosynthesis of chlorophyll involves RNA intimately in the catalytic step (Schoen et al. 1986).

NO: The C_5 pathway is not distributed in modern organisms as one would expect for a primitive trait. Plants have it. But both mammals and bacteria on opposite sides of the tree have an alternative pathway.

YES: But this distribution merely suggests that the enzymes catalyzing the first step of the alternative pathway in bacteria and mammals are not homologous. Bio-organic data suggest that this may be true. The enzyme from *Rhodopseudomonas spheroides* has a lysine in the active site, whereas the corresponding enzyme from rat may have an active-site cysteine (Nandi 1978).

AMBIGUITIES:
1. Arguments for an active-site cysteine in the mammalian enzyme are not strong.
2. At least some bacterial enzymes appear homologous by sequence to mammalian enzymes. However, a cysteine is highly conserved, not a lysine.
3. Some organisms have both pathways.

The area is rich with suggestions for new experiments.

phodiester from 2 to well above 10. Favorable binding interactions between the substrate and the RNA catalyst can compensate for the unfavorable energy of interaction between the catalyst and the phosphate group. The "unhappy" phosphate monoanion will pick up a proton from solvent; the protonated phosphate is 10^6 times more reactive toward transesterification than the diester monoanion. Proper orientation of the attacking nucleophile is worth an additional two to three orders of magnitude in rate enhancement. Although this mechanism postulates the involvement of a proton from solvent in the reaction, it does not require a general acid or general base attached to the catalyst itself. The proposed mechanism illustrates that hydrophobicity in an active site, if used judiciously, can, in

principle, account for the majority of the catalysis observed in self-splicing.

For more complicated reactions implicit in the ribometabolism listed in Table 7, catalysis by RNA need not be viewed as more problematic than catalysis of similar reactions by proteins. Although it appears to be a widespread belief that catalysis by proteins is easier to account for than catalysis by RNA because proteins have more functional groups than RNA, this view of the catalytic power of RNA molecules, especially in a metabolically sophisticated breakthrough organism, is not supported by chemical considerations.

Table 9 lists functional groups known to occur in RNA and protein molecules. In terms of available

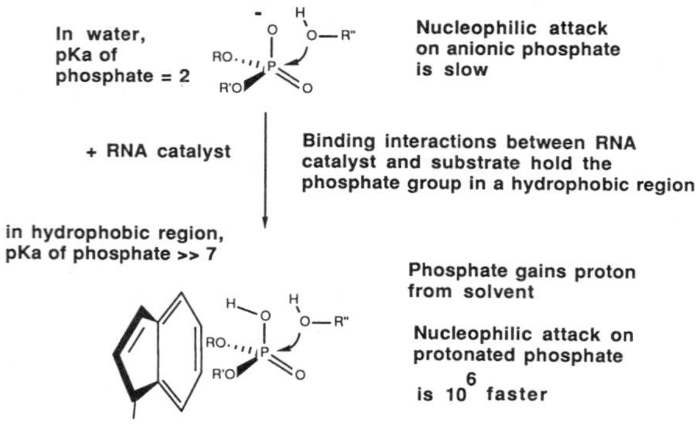

Figure 5. Mechanism for RNA-catalyzed transesterifications. Binding a phosphodiester (via favorable interactions between the RNA molecule and other portions of the diester) between two bases in an RNA catalyst brings the diester into a region with an effective dielectric of approximately 12. This will raise the pK_a of the phosphate from 2 to well above 10. The bound phosphate monoanion will therefore gain a proton from solvent. The protonated phosphate is 10^6 times more reactive toward transesterification than the diester monoanion. Proper orientation of the attacking nucleophile should provide an additional two to three orders of magnitude in rate enhancement. Thus, hydrophobic regions and "proximity" together can account for most of the rate acceleration observed in RNA self-splicing and processing reactions.

Table 9. Functional Groups in RNA and Protein Molecules

On Building Blocks	
Hydrogen bonding	Hydrogen bonding
Hydrophobic groups	Hydrophobic groups
Phosphates	
Sugars	
	Aliphatic amines
	Carboxylates
	Sulfur
	Hydroxyl groups
	Imidazole
Posttranscriptional (Translational) Modification	
Aliphatic amines	
Carboxylates	
Sulfur	
Hydroxyl groups	
	Phosphates
	Sugars
Ketones	Ketones
Selenium	Selenium
Available on Cofactors	
Nicotinamide	Nicotinamide
R-SH	
Flavin	Flavin
Sulfonium ions	Sulfonium ions
Acyl anions	Acyl anions
Metals	Metals

Data from Adams et al. (1976).

functional groups, RNA and protein catalysts are not very different. Both biopolymers have certain functional groups built into the building blocks. Both lack other functional groups, but obtain these by post-transcriptional (translational) modification and from cofactors. This fact presents an interesting puzzle. The fact that most modern catalysts are *not* RNA molecules suggests, in the context of this model, that proteins are superior to RNA molecules as catalysts. What is the chemical basis for this superiority? There are two interesting possibilities. There may be some special features of a polypeptide backbone (e.g., lack of charge) that make proteins better suited as catalysts. Alternatively, a higher fraction of the functional groups found in RNA molecules are obtained by posttranscriptional modification. Posttranscriptional modification requires information, which is undoubtedly costly. This may represent a disadvantage for an organism that uses RNA as its principal catalyst.

The latter problem reflects a shortage of building blocks for RNA molecules, which, in turn, reflects the fact that RNA molecules exploit only two of eight possible hydrogen-bond-pairing schemes theoretically available for a "pyrimidine-purine-like" base pair (Fig. 6). The two that are exploited (uracil and cytosine as the "pyrimidine"; see Fig. 6) are the only two where the "pyrimidine-like" base is joined to the ribose by a carbon-heteroatom bond. To construct base pairs using other hydrogen-bonding schemes, pyrimidine analogs must be joined to a ribose via a *carbon-carbon* bond. These constructions are difficult to envision as products of prebiotic chemistry. This may be why these other hydrogen-bonding schemes are not used in RNA.

As organic chemists, we are not constrained by prebiotic chemistry. We have synthesized a new base pair, where a new hydrogen-bonding pattern is exploited using pyrimidine analogs joined to ribose via a carbon-carbon bond. An outline of the synthetic scheme is shown in Figure 6. Thus, we have expanded the number of "letters" in the RNA "alphabet," offering the potential of increasing the number of functional groups that can be introduced into RNA directly, diminishing the number that must be introduced posttranscriptionally, and improving the intrinsic power of RNA as a catalyst.

This advance comes 2 billion years too late to help those organisms that tried to use only RNA catalysis to compete with the breakthrough organism. However, pseudouridine, a naturally occurring nucleoside formed posttranscriptionally with a base joined to a ribose by a carbon-carbon bond, may reflect an effort by a breakthrough organism to do by chance billions of years ago what we have done in the last year using organic synthesis.

An important final comment about the origin of life also follows from the historical model. The traits of a primitive organism can be guessed only by comparison of the traits of many of its descendants. We cannot infer the structure of a primitive organism by examining a single descendant simply because we cannot distinguish traits in the descendant that are primitive from those that are derived.

A metabolically complex breakthrough organism living in an ecologically diverse world does not resemble the first organism. Furthermore, evidence suggests that only a single breakthrough organism existed (Lake 1985). This implies that competing rriboorganisms (those that did not participate in the breakthrough) became extinct (Fig. 7). Therefore, even if we were to deduce a complete and accurate model of the breakthrough organism, we could not extrapolate past the evolutionary bottleneck back to the properties of more primitive organisms. Our view to primeval times is necessarily obscured. Examining the modern world for clues to the origin of life is futile.

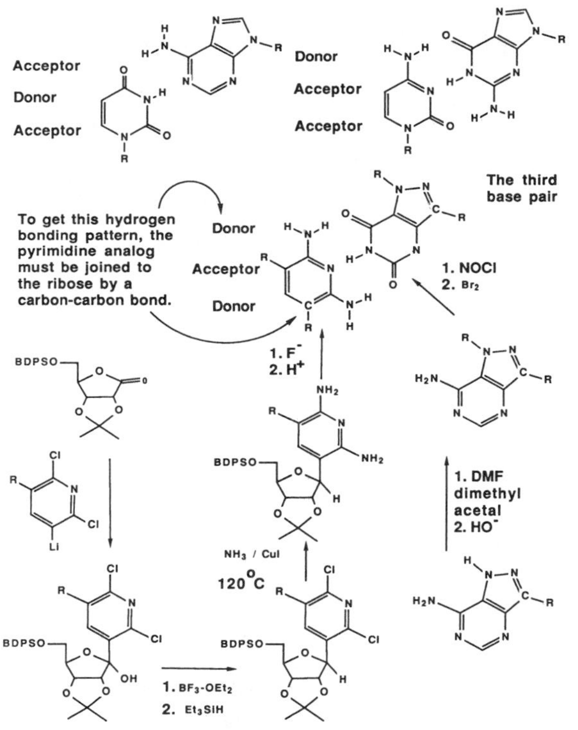

Figure 6. Only two of the eight possible "standard" Watson-Crick hydrogen-bonding schemes available to RNA are used in modern biochemistry. Those involving U and C as the pyrimidine-like unit are the only ones where the pyrimidine base is attached to the sugar by a carbon-nitrogen bond. To achieve other base-pairing schemes (*center*), the pyrimidine-like unit must be attached to the sugar by a carbon-carbon bond. Such molecules are almost certainly not found in prebiotic soups, and their absence in modern biochemistry may reflect a constraint imposed upon the evolution of nucleic acids by prebiotic chemistry. However, the presence of pseudouridine in modern RNA may reflect an ancestral effort by rriboorganisms to relax this constraint. Organic chemists are not constrained by prebiotic chemistry. We have synthesized the molecules necessary to construct the "third base pair" (*bottom*). This is the first step toward the development of RNA molecules built from eight or more building blocks, capable of bearing a more diverse set of functional groups, and (presumably) inherently better catalysts.

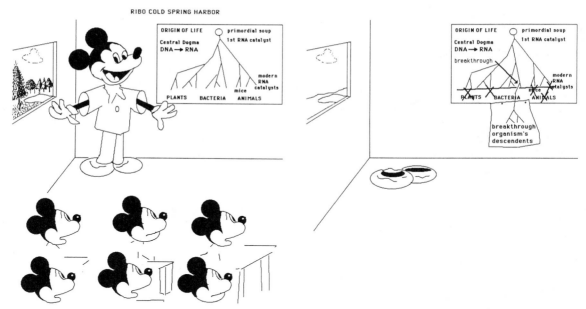

Figure 7. Ribo-Mickey is shown delivering a seminar on the origin of life at a Ribo-Cold Spring Harbor Symposium at the time of the breakthrough some 2 billion years ago. The metabolic diversity required in the breakthrough organism implies ecological diversity as well, as metabolically complex organisms based on RNA catalysis would be expected to have the same pressures to diversify in order to occupy specialized ecological niches that apply to modern organisms based on protein catalysis. Because the ribo-descendants of the primitive organism are all around him, and can be studied directly, Ribo-Mickey can examine many descendants of the primeval organism to infer which traits are primitive and construct a model for the very first form of life. However, the breakthrough organism, the first to invent the synthesis of proteins by translation (most likely not a ribo-mouse), most likely caused a general extinction of competing ribo-organisms. Therefore, at a Cold Spring Harbor Symposium today, modern organisms are all descendants from a single breakthrough organism. Data from these modern organisms can be used to infer the structure of the breakthrough organism, but no further. Ribo-Mickey, and all of his ribohomologs, have become extinct, taking with them the information that is necessary to extrapolate back to the properties of the primeval organism. Thus, if the model developed in this paper is correct, arguments that attempt to extrapolate from modern biochemistry back to the origin of life are futile. However, understanding the breakthrough organism itself has some rewards. For example, some models of the breakthrough organism raise the possibility that fossils of rioorgansims are already known.

SUMMARY

A detailed study of the chemical behavior of modern catalysts (here, exemplified by dehydrogenases dependent on NAD^+) allows us to construct models that distinguish between selected and drifting behaviors in biological macromolecules. These models enable us to manipulate rationally the properties of enzymes, here to design an "acetaldehyde reductase" dependent on NAD^+ that is faster than any given us by nature.

When applied to the origin of protein catalysis, models that explain the structures of ribo-cofactors (e.g., NAD^+) must postulate a metabolically complex breakthrough organism. This means that: (1) The view from the present day back to the truly primeval organism is obscured; it is futile to try to deduce the detailed structure of the first life by examining the behaviors of modern organisms. (2) Riboorganisms dominated life on earth for a long time before translation evolved; indeed, fossils of riboorganisms might already be known. (3) Using organic synthesis, we have expanded the number of bases available for making RNA and making accessible RNA molecules that are likely to be intrinsically better catalysts.

REFERENCES

Adams, R.L.P., R.H. Burdon, A.M. Campbell, and R.M.S. Smellie. 1976. *The biochemistry of nucleic acids*, 8th edition. Chapman and Hall, London.

Albery, W.J., and J.R. Knowles. 1976. Evolution of enzyme function and the development of catalytic efficiency. *Biochemistry* **15**: 5631.

Bass, B.L. and T.R. Cech. 1984. Specific interaction between the self-splicing RNA of tetrahymena and its guanosine substrate: Implications for biological catalysis by RNA. *Nature* **308**: 820.

Benner, S.A., K.P. Nambiar, and G.K. Chambers. 1985. A stereochemical imperative in dehydrogenases: New data and criteria for evaluating function-based theories in bioorganic chemistry. *J. Am. Chem. Soc.* **107**: 5513.

Cantoni, G.L. 1962. Dimethylthetin-homocysteine methylpherase. *Methods Enzymol.* **5**: 743.

Crick, F. 1968. The origin of the genetic code. *J. Mol. Biol.* **38**: 367.

Cronin, C.N., B.A. Malcolm, and J.R. Kirsch. 1987. Reversal of substrate charge specificity by site-directed mutagenesis of aspartate aminotransferase. *J. Am. Chem. Soc.* **109**: 2222.

Darnell, J.E. and W.F. Doolittle. 1986. Speculations on the early course of evolution. *Proc. Natl. Acad. Sci.* **83**: 1271.

Ehrenman, K., J. Pedersen-Lane, D. West, R. Herman, F. Maley, and M. Belfort. 1986. Processing of phage T4 td-encoded RNA is analogous to the eukaryotic group I splicing pathway. *Proc. Natl. Acad. Sci.* **83**: 5875.

Ellington, A. and S.A. Benner. 1987. Free energy differences between enzyme bound states. *J. Theor. Biol.* (in press).

Fierke, C.A. and W.P. Jencks. 1986. Two functional domains of coenzyme A activate catalysis by coenzyme A transferase. *J. Biol. Chem.* **261**: 7603.

Gilbert, W. 1986. The RNA world. *Nature* **319**: 818.

Guerrier-Takada, C. and S. Altman. 1983. Catalytic activity of an RNA molecule prepared by transcription in vitro. *Science* **223**: 285.

Jornvall, H., M. Persson, and J. Jeffrey. 1981. Alcohol and polyol dehydrogenases are both divided into two protein types, and structural properties cross-relate the different enzyme activities within each type. *Proc. Natl. Acad. Sci.* **78**: 4226.

Kaplan, N.O. 1967. Beef heart TPNH-DPN pyridine nucleotide transhydrogenases. *Methods Enzymol.* **10**: 317.

Lake, J.A. 1985. Evolving ribosome structure: Domains in archaebacteria, eocytes, and eukaryotes. *Annu. Rev. Biochem.* **54**: 507.

Lehninger, A. 1972. *Biochemistry.* Worth, New York.

Matthews, D.A., S.L. Smith, D.P. Baccanari, J.J. Burchall, S.M. Oatley, and J. Kraut. 1986. Crystal structure of a novel trimethoprim-resistant dihydrofolate reductase specified in *Escherichia coli* by R-plasmid R67. *Biochemistry* **25**: 4194.

Nambiar, K.P., J. Stackhouse, S.R. Presnell, and S.A. Benner. 1986. Evolutionary guidance and the engineering of enzymes. In *Enzymes as catalysts in organic synthesis* (ed. M. Schneider), p. 325. D. Reidel, New York.

Nandi, D.L. 1978. Delta-aminolevulinic acid synthase of *Rhodopseudomonas spheroides.* *Arch. Biochem. Biophys.* **188**: 266.

Neunlist, S. and M. Rohmer. 1985. A novel hopanoid, 30-(5'-adenosyl)hopane, from the purple non-sulphur bacterium *Rhodopseudomonas acidophila*, with possible DNA interactions. *Biochem. J.* **228**: 769.

Ohno, A., M. Ohara, and S. Oka. 1986. NAD(P)⁺-NAD(P)H models. 61. An interconversion between central and axial chiralities as an evidence for a functional model of chemical evolution of an enzyme. *J. Am. Chem. Soc.* **108**: 6438.

Oppenheimer, N.J. 1984. Stereoselectivity of enzymic transfer of hydrogen from nicotinamide coenzymes: A stereochemical imperative? *J. Am. Chem. Soc.* **106**: 3032.

Orgel, L.E. 1968. Evolution of the genetic apparatus. *J. Mol. Biol.* **38**: 381.

———. 1986. RNA catalysis and the origins of life. *J. Theor. Biol.* **123**: 127.

Schoen, A., G. Krupp, S. Gough, S. Berry-Lowe, C.G. Kannangara, and D. Soell. 1986. The RNA required in the first step of chlorophyll biosynthesis is a chloroplast glutamate tRNA. *Nature* **322**: 281.

Sharp, P.A. 1985. On the origin of RNA splicing and introns. *Cell* **42**: 397.

Siu, P.M.L. and H.G. Wood. 1962. Phosphoenolpyruvic carboxytransphosphorylase, a CO_2 fixation enzyme from propionic acid bacteria. *J. Biol. Chem.* **237**: 3044.

Stackhouse, J., K.P. Nambiar, J.J. Burbaum, D.M. Stauffer, and S.A. Benner. 1985. Dynamic transduction of energy and internal equilibria in enzymes: A reexamination of pyruvate kinase. *J. Am. Chem. Soc.* **107**: 2757.

Strother, P.K. and E.S.H Barghoorn. 1980. *Origins of life and evolution* (ed. H.O. Halvorsen and K.E. van Holde), p. 14. A.R. Liss, New York.

Szostak, J.W. 1986. Enzymatic activity of the conserved core of a group I self-splicing intron. *Nature* **322**: 83.

Usher, D.A. and A.H. McHale. 1976. Hydrolytic stability of helical RNA: A selective advantage for the natural 3', 5'-bond. *Proc. Natl. Acad. Sci.* **73**: 1149.

Visser, C.M. 1984. Evolution of biocatalysis. *Origins Life* **14**: 291.

Visser, C.M. and R.M. Kellogg. 1978. Biotin. Its place in evolution. *J. Mol. Evol.* **11**: 171.

Westheimer, F.H. 1986. Polyribonucleic acids as enzymes. *Nature* **319**: 534.

White, H.B. III. 1976. Coenzymes as fossils of an earlier metabolic state. *J. Mol. Evol.* **7**: 101.

Woese, C.R. 1967. *The origins of the genetic code.* Harper and Row, New York.

Wu, Y.-D. and K.N. Houk. 1987. Theoretical transition structures for hydride transfer to methyleniminium ion from methylamine and dihydropyridine. On the nonlinearity of hydride transfers. *J. Am. Chem. Soc.* **109**: 2226.

You, K.-S. 1985. Stereospecificity for nicotinamide nucleotides in enzymatic and chemical hydride transfer reactions. *CRC Crit. Rev. Biochem.* **17**: 313.

Economics of Enzyme Catalysis

W.P. JENCKS

Graduate Department of Biochemistry, Brandeis University, Waltham, Massachusetts 02254

ECONOMICS OF ENZYME CATALYSIS

What Do Enzymes Do?

One of the revolutions of this century is the development of our knowledge of catalysis by enzymes to the point where it can be examined in ordinary chemical terms. There is optimism that chemistry can explain enzymatic catalysis without requiring vitalistic or mystical hypotheses. Nevertheless, it is clear that we are far from being able to provide such a chemical explanation today and that very little is known quantitatively about the enormous rate accelerations brought about by enzymes for reactions of their specific substrates. With few exceptions, chemical catalysts do not begin to approach the catalytic efficiency or specificity of enzymes.

The most obvious and important difference between enzymes and most chemical catalysts is the availability of noncovalent binding interactions between an enzyme and its specific substrates. Synthetic catalysts can provide chemical catalysis through one or several groups, X'Y' in Figure 1, that accelerate the reaction of XY groups on a substrate. An enzyme that utilizes these same groups for chemical catalysis can also utilize the energy from noncovalent binding interactions between the enzyme and a specific substrate to accelerate the reaction. This acceleration can be very large. The initial half-reaction catalyzed by coenzyme A (CoA) transferase involves the transfer of CoA from succinyl CoA to a COO^- group on the enzyme to form a new thiol ester with the enzyme. The transfer of CoA from this specific substrate is 10^{12} faster than the transfer of a short-chain thiol with the same pK, methyl mercaptopropionate, from the corresponding thiol ester, which has the same chemical reactivity as the thiol ester of CoA (Eq. 1).

$$ECOO^- + \text{succinyl-SCoA} \rightarrow ECSCoA + \text{succinate}$$
$$\left.\begin{array}{l} \\ \\ \end{array}\right\} > 10^{12} \quad (1)$$
$$ECOO^- + \text{succinyl-SR} \rightarrow ECSR + \text{succinate}$$

Thus, the noncovalent binding interactions of the side chain of CoA with the enzyme are directly responsible for a rate increase of 10^{12}. This rate increase is within a factor of 10 of the overall rate acceleration brought about by this enzyme (Moore and Jencks 1982b).

Comparable rate accelerations are brought about in phosphoglucomutase by the sugar ring and phosphate of the specific substrate, glucose-1-phosphate, compared with H_2O (Ray and Long 1976; Ray et al. 1976). Similar, if less dramatic, examples are known for many

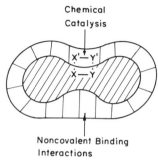

Figure 1. A chemical catalyst and an enzyme can use catalytic groups, X' and Y', to accelerate a reaction, but an enzyme can also use noncovalent binding interactions with its specific substrates for catalysis.

enzymes (Jencks 1975). The problem is to understand the source of these rate increases; in general, it is not known. However, some of the factors responsible for the rate increase of CoA transferase can be roughly identified (Table 1) (Moore and Jencks 1982b): (1) The observed binding of CoA substrates is 10^3 stronger than that of nonspecific substrates. (2) The side chain of CoA causes an increase of 10^2–10^3 in the nonspecific chemical reactivity of the enzyme-CoA intermediate toward reagents that do not resemble the normal substrates, such as H_2O, BH_4^-, and RS^-. This may be regarded as a destabilization of the thiol ester relative to the transition states for its reactions with nucleophiles, which is brought about by the side chain of CoA. (3) The advantage from exact positioning of the bound substrate at the active site is not known, but it certainly is significant. Advantages from intramolecularity by factors of 10^4–10^5 compared with 1 M reactants in solution are well documented for several enzymes (Thompson 1974; Jencks 1975, 1981; Bode 1979; Nakamura and Abeles 1985). Finally, there is evidence for a conformational change induced by CoA that appears to be unfavorable by a factor of $\sim10^4$ in the absence of CoA; however, this factor may overlap one or more of the other factors.

The principal conclusion is that it is very likely that the acceleration brought about by CoA involves several modest contributions rather than a single large effect.

Table 1. CoA Transferase Interactions with CoA

Observed binding	10^3
Activation: H_2O, RS^-, BH_4^-	10^2–10^3
Intramolecularity	10^5?
Conformational change	10^4

This is likely to be the case for most such substrate-induced rate increases (Jencks 1975; Ray and Long 1976). How should we think about the mechanisms for such rate accelerations? Three topics that are important for enzyme catalysis, but are often confusing, are briefly reviewed below.

Are Strain and Destabilization Important?

Comparisons of the second-order rate constants for the reaction of the substrate with a group at the active site of an enzyme and with the same group in a nonenzymatic reaction provide a measure of the catalytic effectiveness of the enzyme. It has been pointed out that strain and destabilization of a bound substrate do not increase the second-order rate constant for an enzymatic reaction, k_{cat}/K_m (Fersht 1974). This is apparent in Figure 2: Destabilization of the enzyme-substrate (ES) complex has no effect on the difference in energy between $E + S$ and the transition state, $ES^{\ddagger}$, which corresponds to k_{cat}/K_m. It might therefore be concluded that strain and destabilization are not important for enzyme catalysis.

Nothing could be further from the truth. Destabilization of the ES complex is absolutely essential for enzymatic catalysis. It is true that *small* changes in this destabilization have no effect on k_{cat}/K_m (Fig. 2), but destabilization is essential for the *large* increase in rate that enzymes bring about (see Fig. 3) (Jencks 1975).

It is well known that enzymatic catalysis involves stabilization by the enzyme of the transition state for the catalyzed reaction. (There have been several reports supporting the "hypothesis" that enzymes catalyze reactions by stabilizing the transition state, but such stabilization is required by the definitions of catalysis and of the transition state.) Figure 3a shows the barrier for a nonenzymatic reaction, and Figure 3b shows the

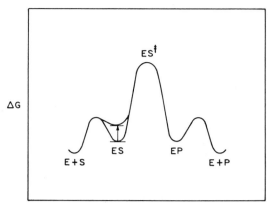

Figure 2. Strain or destabilization of the ES complex has no effect on the barrier for reaction of $E + S$ or on k_{cat}/K_m.

barrier for the same reaction mechanism catalyzed by an enzyme, in which the enzyme has stabilized both the transition state and the ES and enzyme-product (EP) complexes by a large amount. This produces a totally useless enzyme, because the barrier for reaction of the S of the ES complex is exactly the same as the barrier for the reaction of free S. The barrier for reaction of $E + S$ is small, but the concentration of free E at any useful concentration of S is so small that no significant catalysis will be observed. Thus, stabilization of the transition state is *necessary*, but it is not *sufficient* to give catalysis.

To obtain catalysis, the Gibbs free energy of the ES and EP complex *must* be increased so that the transition state can be reached easily from ES and EP. This represents destabilization of the ES complex, ΔG_D, which can occur by physical strain, desolvation, and other mechanisms. This destabilization must be relieved in the transition state. The Gibbs energy of the ES complex is also increased by loss of entropy when

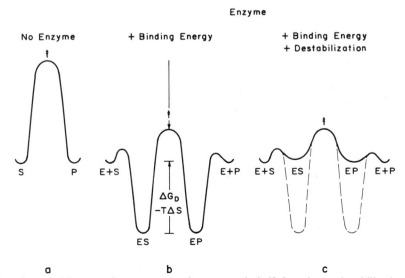

Figure 3. Stabilization of a transition state by an enzyme gives no catalysis if there is equal stabilization of the ES complex. Catalysis requires that ΔG of the ES complex must be increased, so that the transition state can be reached easily.

the reacting groups in the ES complex are held in precisely the correct position for reaction, which involves a decrease in entropy, $-T\Delta S$. The resulting active enzyme is shown in Figure 3c.

The economics of this system are unpleasant but important—you must pay for what you get. The enzyme must use up, or *utilize*, the specific binding energy made available upon the binding of substrate in order to overcome the strain, destabilization, and entropy loss (which might be thought of as "entropic strain") (Jencks 1966). The observed binding of a substrate to the enzyme represents the difference between the intrinsic binding energy that is available from binding forces and the destabilization and loss of entropy that must be overcome when binding occurs. The essential point—that there must be an imbalance between the binding and stabilization of the transition state and of the ES complex—was made clearly and concisely by Pauling (1946). This point is illustrated for CoA transferase in Figure 4, which is an energy bar graph that describes the thermodynamic box of Equation 2.

$$
\begin{array}{ccc}
S^{\neq} & \overset{\Delta G_2}{\rightleftharpoons} & ES^{\neq} \\
\Delta G_1 \Big\updownarrow & & \Delta G_3 \Big\updownarrow \\
S & \overset{\Delta G_4}{\rightleftharpoons} & ES
\end{array}
\qquad (2)
$$

The Gibbs energy of activation for the nonenzymatic reaction is approximately 30 kcal/mole and that of the ES complex is 15 kcal/mole. The enzyme stabilizes the substrate by 4 kcal/mole upon forming the ES complex. Completion of the diagram shows that the enzyme stabilizes the transition state by 19 kcal/mole. Much of this stabilization represents expression of the binding

energy of the CoA moiety of the substrate, which gives a rate increase of 10^{12} (16 kcal/mole). But this stabilization is not sufficient to give catalysis. If the ES complex were equally stabilized (it has essentially the same groups to bind to the enzyme), the barrier for the reaction of the ES complex would also be 30 kcal/mole, as shown by the dashed lines in Figure 4. This would be a useless enzyme.

For the enzyme to work, the Gibbs energy of the ES complex must be increased so that the transition state can be reached easily. In fact, it is increased by 15 kcal/mole. This is an *interaction energy;* it represents the amount by which the energy changes differ on any two opposite sides of the thermodynamic box. The interaction energy is a simple, poorly appreciated, but extraordinarily important quantity; in fact, I will assert that almost anything interesting that happens in biology involves an interaction energy. For enzymes, the interaction energy reflects the amount of strain, destabilization, and entropy loss that prevents strong binding of the substrate to the enzyme in the ES complex. It is the difference between the observed expression of binding energy in the ES complex and in the transition state (the interaction energy can be so large that parts of the substrate may not fit into the active site at all in the ES complex). Understanding catalysis by CoA transferase, then, involves evaluation and characterization of this interaction energy. Fierke approached this problem by examining the activity of fragments of the CoA molecule to determine the roles of the different parts of the molecule in catalysis (Fierke and Jencks 1986).

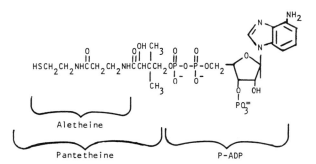

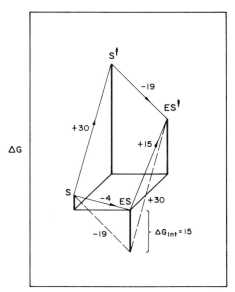

Figure 4. Bar graph of Gibbs free energy for the reaction catalyzed by CoA transferase in the presence and absence of the enzyme.

Acetoacetyl pantetheine is a very poor substrate for CoA transferase. For years it was thought to be completely inactive; later, it was found to be 10^6 less reactive than acetoacetyl CoA. Therefore, we concluded that the 3'-ADP moiety of CoA is essential for catalysis and thought that it provided the activation of the physiological substrate.

Fierke, however, chose to examine the role of pantetheine more thoroughly by following the reaction in the reverse direction. She spent a long time attempting to prepare the enzyme-pantetheine thiol ester intermediate in order to examine its reaction with acetoacetate, but she failed to isolate it. It finally turned out that it could not be isolated because it undergoes hydrolysis in less than 1 minute, 100 times faster than the covalent intermediate of the enzyme and coenzyme A, E-CoA.

She was able to prepare it in solution and to measure its reactivity with acetoacetate and succinate by a competition technique. To our astonishment, its reactivity with specific substrates was found to be very similar to that of E-CoA, only about 10 times slower. The data are summarized in Table 2. Removal of the pantoic acid moiety of pantetheine, to give the alatheine derivative, results in loss of this activation.

The results (Table 2) showed that the hypothesis that the pantetheine moiety does not provide activation for catalysis is wrong. The pantetheine group has a reactivity very similar to that of CoA once it is held in the active site; it is only the free substrate that has a low activity. This curious situation shows that the binding and the activation brought about by CoA reside in different parts of the molecule: The pantetheine moiety provides the activation but does not have enough binding energy to pull acetoacetyl pantetheine into the active site. The 3'-ADP moiety provides little activation but has enough binding energy to pull the pantetheine moiety of a CoA substrate into the active site, kicking and screaming, where it is destabilized and activated to react (Fig. 5).

This example illustrates the economics of binding and destabilization energy nicely, because they are located in different parts of the CoA molecule. In particular, it shows how binding energy can be expressed in the transition state and give catalysis even if it is not at the site of the chemical reaction. This may be a general (although not universal) principle; there are numerous examples of specificity for catalysis (not binding) that involve parts of the molecule that are some distance from the site of reaction. We can speculate that the cleavage of sugars by glycosidases, for example, involves desolvation of the COO^- group at the active site upon binding of the sugar, which is made possible by the binding energy of the nonreacting part of the substrate (Fig. 6). This destabilization is relieved in the carbocation-like transition state, so that the binding energy is fully expressed in the transition state. There is little or no stabilization that arises from interaction of the COO^- with the developing carbocation in the transition state (sodium chloride does not form stable ion pairs in water); instead, there is relief of the destabilization that allows expression of the intrinsic binding energy of other parts of the substrate (Vernon 1967; Jencks 1983).

This pattern, however, is certainly not universal. With phosphoglucomutase, addition of the separated portions of the complete glucose-1-phosphate molecule causes progressive increases in activity, which finally

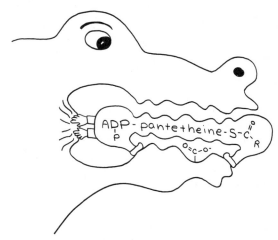

Figure 5. The phospho-ADP moiety of acetoacetyl CoA provides binding energy to pull the pantetheine moiety of the substrate into the active site, where it is activated for reaction.

reaches a level close to that of the intact substrate even when the portions are not connected by covalent bonds (Ray and Long 1976; Ray et al. 1976).

The difference in binding energy for the substrate and the transition state, and the nature of the interaction energy (Fig. 3 and 4), can be characterized by examination of transition state analogs in order to obtain information about mechanisms of activation and catalysis. The tight binding of Analog 1 (see below) to proline racemase, for example, suggests that the enzyme stabilizes a planar transition state more than the tetrahedral substrate (Cardinale and Abeles 1968).

However, there are only a few enzymes for which there is evidence for catalysis by strain, distortion, or compression, presumably because enzymes cannot provide the large force constants that are required for small distortions that require large energies. Large differences in energy can be obtained by stabilization and destabilization of charges, and the tight binding of Analog 2 to isopentenyl pyrophosphate isomerase is consistent with much tighter binding of a carbocation-like transition state than of the uncharged substrate to this enzyme, for example (Reardon and Abeles 1985).

Acceleration of the decarboxylation of the pyruvate-thiamine adduct by pyruvate decarboxylase provides an

Table 2. CoA Transferase

	Rate constants in both directions		
	k, M^{-1} min^{-1}		
	CoA	pantetheine	alatheine
E + AcAc-SR	4×10^8	220	3×10^{-3}
E-SR + AcAc	3×10^7	3×10^6	2×10^{-1}
E-SR + H_2O (min^{-1})	0.014	2.0	2×10^{-4}

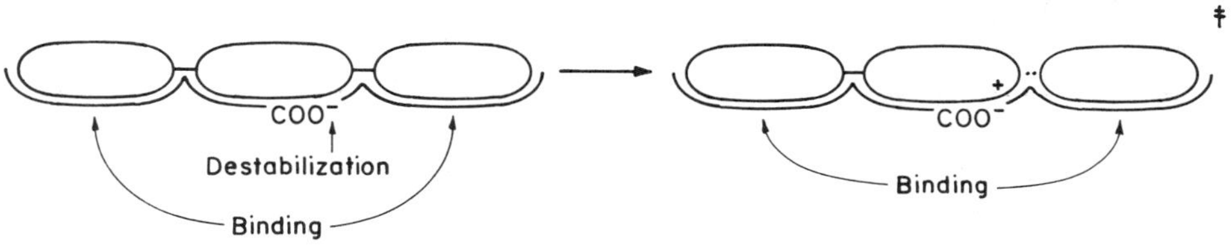

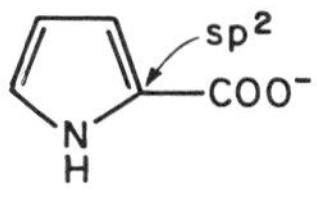

Figure 6. Sugar residues in a polysaccharide may provide binding energy to overcome destabilization from desolvation of a carboxylate group. If this destabilization is relieved in the transition state, the binding energy will be expressed and result in a net stabilization of the transition state.

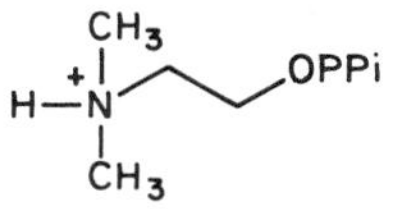

excellent example of the utilization of binding energy for substrate destabilization and catalysis. Decarboxylation of an analog of this adduct (Analog 3) is accelerated by factors of 10^5 or more in nonaqueous solvents that destabilize the reactant relative to the transition state by providing poor solvation for the $-COO^-$ group (Crosby et al. 1970).

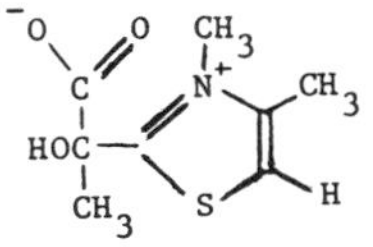

Other decarboxylation reactions show rate increases of up to 10^8 in nonhydroxylic solvents (Kemp and Paul 1975). There is evidence that the active site of the enzyme is hydrophobic and an uncharged transition state analog, thiamine thiazolone pyrophosphate (Analog 4), binds to the enzyme irreversibly with an apparent K_i of $\leq 5 \times 10^{-10}$ M, which is much smaller than $K_d = 10^{-5}$ M for thiamine pyrophosphate (Gutowski and Lienhard 1976).

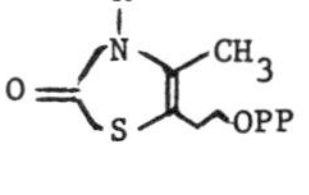

Thiamine and, presumably, the pyruvate-thiamine adduct bind to the enzyme relatively weakly because much of the intrinsic binding energy is used up to pay for the loss of solvation when the COO^- and N^+ groups are pulled into the active site.

Is Entropy a Dirty Word?

No one likes entropy—we spend our lives trying to avoid disorder, confusion, uncertainty, and messiness. Schrödinger's description of living systems as highly improbable states of high information content and negative entropy is better (Schrödinger 1967), but it is still a double negative. What is still worse is that negative entropy is hard to come by; it has to be paid for by a large input of useful energy, with little to show for it in the end. It is no wonder that enough new words to fill a dictionary have been coined to describe the advantages of induced intramolecularity in enzyme catalysis without using the term entropy.

One of the most confusing aspects of the advantage from binding of a substrate to an active site is that it appears in two places—in the observed binding of the substrate and in precise binding once binding has occurred. Furthermore, the fact that entropy loss has to be paid for with binding energy means that tight binding is weak, whereas loose binding is strong. Is this Orwellian double speak?

Consider the advantage of intramolecularity in a model reaction for CoA transferase. There is evidence that the transfer of CoA from succinyl CoA to the enzyme COO^- group proceeds through an anhydride intermediate (White and Jencks 1976; Pickart and Jencks 1979). The nonenzymatic formation of an anhydride from thiol esters of succinate is 6×10^5 faster than the reaction of 1 M acetate with the same thiol ester of acetate (Eq. 3) (Moore and Jencks 1982a). This means that if the enzyme can hold its COO^- group next to the carbonyl group of bound succinyl CoA as accurately as the carboxylate group of the succinate thiol ester is positioned relative to the carbonyl group of the ester in the intramolecular reaction, it will produce an advantage of 5×10^5 M, compared with the bimolecular reaction from this factor alone.

(reaction scheme, Eq. 3: top $0.0012 \text{ M}^{-1}\text{min}^{-1}$; bottom 760 min^{-1}; $+ \ ^-\text{SPhNO}_2$ $\quad 6 \times 10^5$ M) (3)

The maximum advantage is $\sim 10^3$ higher than this if the rotations of succinate are frozen into the correct position for reaction, and rate increases of 10^8 M have been observed for a number of other intramolecular chemical reactions in the absence of strain.

The overall advantage that can be gained from induced intramolecularity may be described by comparisons of enzymatic and nonenzymatic reactions as shown in Equations 4 and 5. Equation 4 divides the nonenzymatic reaction into positioning the reactants in the correct position to react, with the dissociation constant K_N, and reaction within this complex, with the rate constant k_N. The advantage from intramolecularity (Eq. 3) shows that K_N is, at least, 6×10^5 M and could be 10^8 M. If the enzyme brings the reactants into the same position when they bind and the rate constant for the bound reactants is the same as in the nonenzymatic reaction, so that $k_E = k_N$, the total advantage from induced intramolecularity in the enzymatic reaction is 2×10^8 (Eq. 5).

(reaction scheme, Eq. 4): $\text{RCOO}^- + \text{CH}_3\text{CSR} \underset{K_N}{\rightleftharpoons} \text{CH}_3\text{CSR} \xrightarrow{k_N} \text{CH}_3\text{C} \cdots \text{O} + \ ^-\text{SR}$ (4)

(reaction scheme): $\text{ECOO}^- + \text{CH}_3\text{CSR} \underset{K_E}{\rightleftharpoons} \text{CH}_3\text{CSR} \xrightarrow{k_E} \text{CH}_3\text{C} \ ^-\text{SR}$

$$\frac{V_E}{V_N} = \frac{k_E K_E}{k_N / K_N} = \frac{6 \times 10^5 \text{ M}}{3 \times 10^{-3} \text{ M}} = 2 \times 10^8$$

$$\text{or} \qquad \frac{10^8 \text{ M}}{3 \times 10^{-3} \text{ M}} = 3 \times 10^{10}$$

(5)

This example shows how the advantage from induced intramolecularity arises partly from the observed binding ($K_E = 3 \times 10^{-3}$ M) and partly from the advantage from intramolecularity once binding has occurred ($K_N = 6 \times 10^5$ M). If this advantage is 10^8 M, the total advantage is a factor of 3×10^{10} (Eq. 5).

The very exact binding required for these large rate accelerations does not come easily. It is improbable; it involves a large loss of entropy. This is paid for by the intrinsic binding energy of the substrate (Figs. 2 and 3). A loss of entropy, $-T\Delta S$, corresponds to a positive ΔG; the binding energy offsets, or pays for, the loss of entropy. This is why tight, exact binding will have a relatively small observed association constant; it will be weak. Less exact binding can have a larger association constant and be stronger. Suppose a molecule can bind in any of 1000 almost identical positions with the same binding energy. This would result in an observed binding that is 1000 times stronger than it would be if the molecule were restricted to only one of these positions. However, the molecule will be up to 1000 times more likely to form a new covalent bond if it is held in the one correct position to form that bond.

An essential problem in enzymology is the determination of how large this rate acceleration from induced intramolecularity actually is in particular enzymes. The nonphysiological reaction of free CoA with an inactive thiol ester at the active site, E-SR, to form E-SCoA with CoA transferase is 10^5 faster than the corresponding nonenzymatic reaction. At least part of this advantage reflects the noncovalent binding of CoA in the correct position to react intramolecularly.

Better estimations of this advantage can be obtained from comparisons of the binding to an enzyme of two molecules, A and B, with the binding of a single molecule, A-B, that contains the elements of A and B. The difference between the binding energy of A-B and A gives an estimate of the binding energy of B, with relatively little or no loss of translational and rotational entropy; this is a limiting value for the intrinsic binding energy of B. The difference between this binding and the observed binding of B gives the advantage from intramolecularity, or the "effective molarity," of B. Although other explanations are possible in special cases, the most probable interpretation of this effective molarity is that it represents a measure of the advantage from intramolecularity that results from the reduced requirement for loss of entropy in the binding of A-B (Jencks 1981).

There are now enough examples of induced intramolecularity in enzymatic reactions to give a firm conclusion that advantages of 10^4–10^5 M can be obtained; it is not unlikely that larger values will be found.

(structures of Compactin (A-B), B, and A)

Compactin
A-B   B   A
K 2×10^{-10} M $\gt 5 \times 10^{-4}$ M   0.02 M

The inhibitor compactin (A-B) binds to β-hydroxy-β-methylglutaryl CoA reductase with $K_d = 2 \times 10^{-10}$ M, whereas 3,5-dihydroxyvaleric acid (A) binds with $K_d = 0.02$ M. The absence of detectable binding of the other portion of compactin sets a limit of $K_d \geqslant 5 \times 10^{-4}$ M for the binding of B. The difference gives a value of $\geqslant 5 \times 10^4$ M for the effective molarity of B in compactin (Nakamura and Abeles 1985).

The strong binding of peptide aldehyde inhibitors to proteolytic enzymes arises largely from induced intramolecularity. The probability of hemiacetal formation from reaction of the carbonyl group with the active-site nucleophile is greatly increased because of its high effective molarity when the peptide chain has bound in the active site. For elastase, this advantage is approximately 10^5 M (Thompson 1974; Jencks 1975). An effective molarity of 4×10^4 M for amino-terminal isoleucylvaline compared to the free dipeptide has been observed for the conversion of trypsinogen to an active form (Bode 1979).

Large differences in binding with very small changes in structure provide another means for probing the importance of exact fit in enzymes. Exact positioning requires that bound groups be held firmly to within a fraction of an angstrom of their position in the transition state, so that molecules of only slightly different size should show large differences in binding. The low reactivity of proteolytic enzymes following interchange of S and O in the active sites of cysteine proteases may represent such behavior, although differences in hydrogen bonding and other chemical properties may also be involved (Clark and Lowe 1978).

The activity of phosphono and arsono analogs of 3-phosphoglycerate as substrates for phosphoglycerate kinase provides a striking example of a large difference in activity that arises from a small difference in substrate structure. The 3-phosphono analog shows only a 30% decrease in k_{cat} and a threefold increase in K_m, compared with 3-phosphoglycerate (Orr and Knowles 1974); however, Dixon and co-workers have found that the arsono analog (Analog 5) shows a 1300-fold decrease in k_{cat} with a 5-fold increase in K_m (Adams et al. 1983).

$$\begin{array}{cc} = \text{O} & \text{OH} \\ | & | \\ \text{O}{=}\text{AsCH}_2\text{CH}_2\text{CHCOO}^- \\ | \\ \text{O} \end{array}$$

$\underset{\sim}{5}$

The difference in the size of these analogs is very small, with bond lengths of 0.167 nm for As-O and 0.150 nm for P-O in the monoanions of the arsono and phosphono analogs, respectively (Kamiya et al. 1983). Such a large change in activity with a small change in the size of a substituent at the opposite end of the molecule from the site of phosphorylation suggests that the enzyme is capable of recognizing extremely small differences in the position of the bound substrate in the transition state. This means that exact positioning is very important for catalysis.

The requirement for a large advantage from induced intramolecularity is that the reactants must be held very firmly indeed; "freezing" is not enough. Entropies of fusion are small, so that a solid is not much better than a liquid for holding reacting groups together. Formation of a covalent bond, or reaching the transition state for the formation of a covalent bond, requires a much larger loss of entropy than the formation of a crystalline solid (Jencks 1975). The large effective molarities that have been observed for enzymatic reactions show that enzymes are capable of bringing about such tight fixation. This requires considerable restriction of motion and may involve compression of reacting groups. However, the large effective molarities for nonenzymatic reactions of succinate derivatives show that some motions are allowed. What are not allowed are low-frequency vibrations and motions, such as those found for a particle rattling about in a solvent cavity. Simply bringing molecules next to each other in solution causes very little loss of entropy (Jencks 1975).

One of the greatest difficulties with entropies (or enthalpies) is that it is difficult or impossible to evaluate their contribution to the advantage from intramolecularity, strain, or other aspects of catalysis by measuring thermodynamic parameters for reaction or activation. The reason is that almost anything that occurs in aqueous solution gives rise to large, compensating, solvent-derived changes in entropy and enthalpy that obscure the contributions from intramolecularity and binding interactions derived from dispersion interactions (Evans and Polanyi 1936; Lumry and Rajender 1970; Bolton and Hepler 1971; Jencks 1975). It has been known for a long time that observed values of ΔG are often a better measure of potential energy changes than observed enthalpy changes (Hammett 1940). Changes in "water structure" are a major cause of this problem. Because the solvent is at equilibrium, with a mixture of structures at a minimal ΔG, any small perturbation of this equilibrium will have a small ΔG, although it may involve large, compensating changes in ΔH and $T\Delta S$ (Grunwald 1984).

To Move or Not to Move?

Conformational changes in enzymes are popular; they convey a sense of movement, freedom, liberty, and action. Experiments and calculations have shown that proteins move, shake, and flop; motion pictures of these movements convey a sense of great activity. At the extreme, proteins have been compared to liquids.

How can these motions be reconciled with the requirements for rigidity, severe limitation to movement, and absence of low-frequency vibrations that are inferred from the large effective molarities that have been observed with enzymes? It is clear that however much enzymes flutter and shake, they are still able to guide one reacting group toward another with extraordinary precision. If an enzyme can change into 1000 different conformations and only one of these is the active conformation, its activity will be reduced by a factor of 1000. Clearly, it is desirable to limit the freedom of an enzyme to explore inactive conformations.

There are several reasons why enzymes must undergo conformational change. Many active sites are in crevices, holes, or junctions between domains and some have flaps that close over the bound substrates, so that a conformational change is required for binding. This makes possible a firm, exact positioning of the reactants with respect to each other and to catalytic groups. It can also provide additional intrinsic binding energy from interaction with portions of the enzyme that cover the bound substrates (Wolfenden 1976). Conformational changes also provide a mechanism for allosteric control of enzyme activity. However, the usefulness of conformational changes is not as large as is sometimes believed. Under most circumstances a conformational change from an inactive to an active form that is brought about by a bound substrate, as in "induced fit," does not increase the specificity of the enzyme toward the substrate unless it provides additional intrinsic binding energy to stabilize the transition state; it only decreases k_{cat}/K_m relative to that for an enzyme that always remains in the active form. This decrease is the same for both specific and nonspecific substrates, because it requires overcoming the unfavorable energy of the change in conformation to the active form (Fersht 1974; Herschlag 1987). Nevertheless, there are special circumstances, some of which may be of physiological significance, in which induced fit can increase specificity (Herschlag 1987).

The resolution of the dichotomy must reside in the structure of proteins, particularly the fact that they are held together by the covalent bonds of the peptide chain. Cross-links can provide additional restrictions. Furthermore, proteins are close-packed. Their fraction of occupied volume is 0.75, which is the same as that for close-packed spheres, much larger than the values for organic liquids (0.44 for carbon tetrachloride), and still larger compared with the value of 0.36 for water (Klapper 1971; Richards 1974); it is responsible for the fact that proteins have a high density and can be sedimented in the ultracentrifuge. These structural characteristics provide severe restrictions to motion of parts of the protein. Most internal rotations are forbidden, or decreased to such a small angle that they involve a small entropy change. Again, the high reactivity of succinate derivatives shows that even large rotational motions are compatible with high effective molarities if other low-frequency motions are restricted by a covalent backbone.

The close packing of proteins means that many motions are not possible unless other groups move out of the way to make the movement possible (Richards 1974). This correlation between movements or "correlated fluctuations" (Careri 1974; McCammon et al. 1977) further decreases entropy. High density and restricted motion also play an important role in providing a large intrinsic binding energy, from dispersion interactions and other forces, to bring about catalysis of the reactions of specific substrates. Motions of domains

relative to each other can be important in fixing a bound substrate firmly in the active site. It involves only a small loss of entropy if the number of possible states is small. Thus, the important property of a protein, with respect to enzyme catalysis, is that it does *not* resemble a fluid. Enzymes can undergo structural changes that are needed for activity and regulation, but at the same time they preserve a highly ordered structure that is responsible for a large fraction of the remarkable catalytic activity that enzymes exhibit toward their specific substrates. The recent reports of catalytic activity of nucleic acids show that other polymers can have comparable activities (Cech et al. 1981; Guerrier-Takada and Altman 1984).

REFERENCES

Adams, S.R., M.J. Sparkes, and H.B.F. Dixon. 1983. The arsonomethyl analogue of 3-phosphoglycerate. *Biochem. J.* **213**: 211.

Bode, W. 1979. The transition of bovine trypsinogen to a trypsin-like state upon strong ligand binding. II. The binding of the pancreatic trypsin inhibitor and of isoleucine-valine and of sequentially related peptides to trypsinogen and to p-guanidinobenzoate-trypsinogen. *J. Mol. Biol.* **127**: 357.

Bolton, P.D. and L.G. Hepler. 1971. Polar substituent effects and the ionization of acids. *Q. Rev. Chem. Soc.* **25**: 521.

Cardinale, G.J. and R.H. Abeles. 1968. Purification and mechanism of action of proline racemase. *Biochemistry* **7**: 3970.

Careri, G. 1974. The fluctuating enzyme. In *Quantum statistical mechanics in the natural sciences* (ed. B. Kursunoglu et al.), p. 15. Plenum Press, New York.

Cech, T.R., A.J. Zaug, and P.J. Grabowski. 1981. In vitro splicing of the ribosomal RNA precursor of tetrahymena: Involvement of a guanosine nucleotide in the excision of the intervening sequence. *Cell* **27**: 487.

Clark, P.I. and G. Lowe. 1978. Conversion of the active-site cysteine residue of papain into a dehydro-serine, a serine and a glycine residue. *Eur. J. Biochem.* **84**: 293.

Crosby, J., R. Stone, and G.E. Lienhard. 1970. Mechanisms of thiamine-catalyzed reactions. Decarboxylation of 2-(1-carboxy-1-hydroxyethyl)-3,4-dimethylthiazolium chloride. *J. Am. Chem. Soc.* **92**: 2891.

Evans, M.G. and M. Polanyi. 1936. Further considerations on the thermodynamics of chemical equilibria and reaction rates. *Trans. Soc. Faraday* **32**: 1333.

Fersht, A.R. 1974. Catalysis, binding and enzyme-substrate complementarity. *Proc. R. Soc. Lond. B.* **187**: 397.

Fierke, C.A. and W.P. Jencks. 1986. Two functional domains of coenzyme A activate catalysis by CoA transferase: Pantetheine and adenosine 3' phosphate 5' diphosphate. Communication. *J. Biol. Chem.* **261**: 7603.

Grunwald, E. 1984. Thermodynamic properties, propensity laws, and solvent models in solutions in self-associating solvents. Application to aqueous alcohol solutions. *J. Am. Chem. Soc.* **106**: 5414.

Guerrier-Takada, C. and S. Altman. 1984. Catalytic activity of an RNA molecule prepared by transcription in vitro. *Science* **223**: 285.

Gutowski, J.A. and G.E. Lienhard. 1976. Transition state analogs for thiamin pyrophosphate-dependent enzymes. Communication. *J. Biol. Chem.* **251**: 2863.

Hammett, L.P. 1940. *Physical organic chemistry*, p. 120. McGraw-Hill, New York.

Herschlag, D. 1987. The role of induced fit and conformational changes of enzymes for specificity and catalysis. *Bioorg. Chem.* (in press).

Jencks, W.P. 1966. Strain and conformation change in enzymic catalysis. In *Current aspects of biochemical energetics* (ed. N.O. Kaplan and E.P. Kennedy), p. 273. Academic Press, New York.

———. 1975. Binding energy, specificity and enzymic catalysis: The Circe effect. *Adv. Enzymol.* **43:** 219.

———. 1981. On the attribution and additivity of binding energies. *Proc. Natl. Acad. Sci.* **78:** 4046.

———. 1983. On the economics of binding energies: Design and synthesis of organic molecules based on molecular recognition. In *Proceedings of the 18th Solvay Conference on Chemistry,* Brussels, Belgium. (ed. G. Van Binst), p. 59. Springer-Verlag, Berlin.

Kamiya, K., W.B.T. Cruse, and O. Kennard. 1983. The arsonomethyl group as an analogue of phosphate. An X-ray investigation. *Biochem. J.* **213:** 217.

Kemp, D.S. and K. Paul. 1975. The physical-organic chemistry of benzisoxazoles. III. The mechanisms and the effects of solvents on the rates of decarboxylation of benzisoxazole-3-carboxylic acids. *J. Am. Chem. Soc.* **97:** 7305.

Klapper, M.H. 1971. On the nature of the protein interior. *Biochim. Biophys. Acta.* **229:** 557.

Lumry, R. and S. Rajender. 1970. Enthalpy-entropy compensation phenomena in water solutions of proteins and small molecules: A ubiquitous property of water. *Biopolymers* **9:** 1125.

McCammon, J.A., B.R. Gelin, and M. Karplus. 1977. Dynamics of folded proteins. *Nature* **267:** 585.

Moore, S.A. and W.P. Jencks. 1982a. Model reactions for CoA transferase involving thiol transfer: Anhydride formation from thiol esters and carboxylic acids. *J. Biol. Chem.* **257:** 10882.

———. 1982b. Formation of active site thiol esters of CoA transferase and the dependence of catalysis on specific binding interactions. *J. Biol. Chem.* **257:** 10893.

Nakamura, C.E. and R.H. Abeles. 1985. Mode of interaction of β-hydroxy-β-methylglutaryl coenzyme A reductase with strong binding inhibitors: Compactin and related compounds. *Biochemistry* **24:** 1364.

Orr, G.A. and J.R. Knowles. 1974. The interaction of the phosphonate analogue of 3-phospho-D-glycerate with phosphoglycerate kinase. *Biochem. J.* **141:** 721.

Pauling, L. 1946. Molecular architecture and biological reactions. *Chem. Eng. News* **24:** 1375.

Pickart, C.M. and W.P. Jencks. 1979. Formation of stable anhydrides from CoA transferase and hydroxamic acids. *J. Biol. Chem.* **254:** 9120.

Ray, W.J., Jr., and J.W. Long. 1976. Thermodynamics and mechanism of the PO_3 transfer process in the phosphoglucomutase reaction. *Biochemistry* **15:** 3993.

Ray, W.J., Jr., J.W. Long, and J.D. Owens. 1976. An analysis of the substrate-induced rate effect in the phosphoglucomutase system. *Biochemistry* **15:** 4006.

Reardon, J.E. and R.H. Abeles. 1985. Time-dependent inhibition of isopentenyl pyrophosphate isomerase by 2-(dimethylamino)ethyl pyrophosphate. *J. Am. Chem. Soc.* **107:** 4078.

Richards, F.M. 1974. The interpretation of protein structures: Total volume, group volume distributions and packing density. *J. Mol. Biol.* **82:** 1.

Schrödinger, E. 1967. *What is life? The physical aspect of the living cell.* Cambridge University Press, Cambridge, England.

Thompson, R.C. 1974. Binding of peptides to elastase: Implications for the mechanism of substrate hydrolysis. *Biochemistry* **13:** 5495.

Vernon, C.A. 1967. The mechanisms of hydrolysis of glycosides and their relevance to enzyme-catalysed reactions. *Proc. R. Soc. Lond. B.* **167:** 389.

White, H. and W.P. Jencks. 1976. Mechanism and specificity of succinyl-CoA: 3-ketoacid coenzyme A transferase. *J. Biol. Chem.* **251:** 1688.

Wolfenden, R. 1976. Transition state analog inhibitors and enzyme catalysis *Annu. Rev. Biophys. Bioeng.* **5:** 271.

Artificial Enzymes

R. BRESLOW

Department of Chemistry, Columbia University, New York, New York 10027

There are two general purposes to the study of artificial enzymes and enzyme mimics. One purpose is to furnish additional understanding of natural enzymes themselves. We tend to "understand" things by relating them to other simpler things that we already believe we understand. Thus, in the case of enzymes, it is common to try to explain their extraordinary rates and stabilities in terms of the properties of simpler chemical model systems. One of the important functions of the creation of artificial enzymes and enzyme mimics is to produce such model systems. Their behavior is a test of our understanding and also furnishes additional relevant chemistry that can be used to interpret enzymatic processes. In this kind of enzyme model, chemistry serves as an assistant to biochemistry; i.e., the chemistry is done in order to help with the understanding of the biochemical reactions.

There is another very important function of enzyme models in which the roles are reversed: The properties and structures of enzymes help to inspire the construction of novel chemical catalysts. The aim is to produce new catalytic systems that might have some of the same high selectivities and high rates characteristic of enzyme processes but that might have special advantages over natural enzymes. Such catalysts need not be proteins; so they could have improved stabilities. In addition, such catalysts could be prepared to perform reactions for which no natural enzymes occur. Many of the most important chemical processes of interest to us in chemical manufacturing, for instance, are not processes that are also performed enzymatically in nature. However, appropriately developed artificial enzymes could in principle perform these useful chemical reactions with an enzymatic style and with the resultant advantages of selectivity and rate characteristic of this style.

We have been active in this field for approximately 30 years and have coined the term "Biomimetic Chemistry" to describe it (Breslow 1972). We have also reported the first synthesis of a catalyst described as an "artificial enzyme" (Breslow and Overman 1970). Since this work has involved a very large effort and has been reviewed elsewhere (Breslow 1986), the present paper will be somewhat selective. I describe here some of the more interesting systems that we have prepared and also indicate the most recent developments of these types of systems.

Enzymes operate by binding a substrate and then performing a selective catalyzed reaction within the enzyme-substrate complex. The geometry of the complex and the geometric placement of various catalytic functional groups within the complex help determine both the rates and the specificities of the reactions. In our earliest work, we examined the use of metal binding as a way to link catalysts and substrates (Breslow and Chipman 1965), and to some extent, we still pursue this kind of approach. However, the most useful general kind of binding seems to be hydrophobic inclusion inside a cavity. This process permits the binding of many organic molecules or groups that do not have the ability to coordinate to metal ions. In fact, in some early work (Breslow and Overman 1970), we showed how hydrophobic binding in a cavity could be used to bring a simple organic compound close enough to a metal to permit metal-catalyzed reactions, even though the substrate itself is not a normal metal ligand. Some related studies are described toward the end of this paper.

The cyclodextrins (Bender and Komiyama 1977; Tabushi 1982) are cyclic molecules with a relatively hydrophobic interior and hydroxyl groups that make them water soluble. In addition to cyclodextrins, a number of totally synthetic molecules with hydrophobic cavities have been made. In our laboratory, we have pursued such examples (O'Krongly et al. 1985), and many other laboratories around the world are also focused on the construction of synthetic hydrophobic cavities that can be used in the construction of enzyme mimics. However, the ready availability of cyclodextrins made them attractive in the first constructions of artificial enzymes. With these molecules already at hand, we could focus on attaching functional groups and studying the reactions that occur within hydrophobic complexes. Many other investigators around the world have also used cyclodextrins for this purpose (Tabushi 1982), and indeed we were not the first (Heinrich and Cramer 1965).

Catalysis by Cyclodextrins

A very simple illustration of the power of such complexing is seen in studies on the selective chlorination of anisole induced by binding into a cyclodextrin cavity (Breslow and Campbell 1969, 1971). We found that a chlorination reaction that would ordinarily be relatively random, directed to both the ortho and para positions, became completely selective for the para position in the presence of cyclodextrins, particularly α-cyclodextrin (with six glucose members in a ring). This molecule binds anisole fairly tightly into the cavity, and then a chlorine is delivered specifically to the para position of the anisole by one of the hydroxyl groups of the cyclodextrin molecule (Fig. 1). This mechanism has been

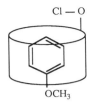

Figure 1. Anisole binds into the cavity of a cyclodextrin and is selectively chlorinated at the para position.

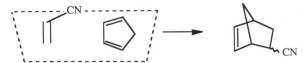

Figure 2. Diels-Alder addition of acrylonitrile to 1,3-cyclopentadiene is catalyzed by mutual binding into a cyclodextrin cavity.

rather well established by detailed studies. In later work, it was possible to turn this into a relatively practical process by converting the cyclodextrin into a polymer (Breslow et al. 1976), in which case this chlorination process could be run with continual reuse of the catalyst.

Although the enzyme chlorinase will chlorinate anisole, it does so relatively randomly (Brown and Hager 1967). Thus, this represents a simple illustration of the fact that selective chemical processes of interest to chemists may well be performed better by even simple enzyme mimics, rather than by enzymes, when nature has not produced selective enzymes for the particular process of interest. Recently, this type of study has been extended in a number of directions by other workers. Quite a few selective synthetic chemical reactions, especially substitution reactions, have been performed inside cyclodextrin cavities by using more or less the scheme we devised.

In the example just described, the cyclodextrin performed several functions. It bound a substrate into the cavity in an oriented fashion, used that orientation to select a particular reactive position on the substrate, and then performed the substitution with the catalytic assistance of the hydroxyl groups of the cyclodextrin molecule; i.e., it held a chlorine atom and an aromatic ring together in a specific way. Another very simple version of an artificial enzyme involves the use of cyclodextrin cavities to hold two different reacting species together *within* the cavity, promoting a bimolecular process.

A striking example of a class of chemical reactions of great interest to organic and manufacturing chemists and for which there are no available enzyme catalysts are Diels-Alder reactions. A diene and a dienophile react together in a process called a cycloaddition. During this process, no protons have to move nor are any large charges developed. Thus, the opportunity for catalyzing such a process with normal catalytic functional groups is relatively limited. However, the reaction should of course be catalyzed by any system that holds the two components together to promote their reaction.

Molecular model building made it clear that certain typical Diels-Alder reactions could occur inside the cavity of β-cyclodextrin (the molecule with seven glucose residues in a ring). A simple diene such as cyclopentadiene could fit into the cavity, but there was still enough room for a dienophile such as acrylonitrile to fit in as well (Fig. 2). Furthermore, the two would be

held next to each other in the geometry required for reaction, and both the transition state for the reaction and the final product looked as if they could also fit nicely into the cavity. Accordingly, we examined the possibility that β-cyclodextrin would indeed catalyze such Diels-Alder reactions. The findings (Rideout and Breslow 1980) were just as predicted from the models. Dienes and dienophiles that could both occupy the same β-cyclodextrin cavity reacted with each other with significant rate increases, but it was also possible to inhibit these reactions. If the smaller α-cyclodextrin was used, it could bind one of the components but not both, and it slowed the reaction. Furthermore, if β-cyclodextrin was used with larger dienes and dienophiles, it also acted as an inhibitor, not a catalyst, since it bound one of the components but not both of them. Thus, simple cyclodextrin molecules proved to be catalytic for reactions of interest for which no natural enzyme catalysts exist.

In the course of this work, a very striking finding emerged that helped to clarify some other aspects of reaction in solution. The Diels-Alder reactions in cyclodextrin cavities were much faster than comparable reactions in typical organic solvents, in which they are normally performed. However, the Diels-Alder reaction in water alone also proved to be accelerated, although not by as much as in the cyclodextrin cavities. In this case, the water alone was able to promote association of the diene and the dienophile because of the hydrophobic effect; i.e., the two components of the reaction were forced together in water solution by the same kind of force that normally forces organic substrates to enter the cyclodextrin cavity.

Evidence for this was clearly furnished by the effects of dissolved salts on the reaction rate (Rideout and Breslow 1980) and the reaction selectivity (Breslow et al. 1983a; Breslow and Maitra 1984). The addition of lithium chloride is known to increase hydrophobic effects in water (von Hippel and Schleich 1969), and it increased the rate of the Diels-Alder reaction as well and its selectivity for formation of the more compact product isomer. The addition of guanidinium chloride to the water is known to decrease hydrophobic effects (von Hippel and Schleich 1969), and it decreased the reaction rate and selectivity of the Diels-Alder reaction in water solution. Thus, in this case, water alone can do a pretty good job of promoting the association needed for Diels-Alder reaction, but of course, it does not have the size selectivity described above for the reactions catalyzed by cyclodextrins with well-defined cavity dimensions. In recent work, we and other investigators have been exploring other reactions promoted by water, as well as bimolecular reactions occurring in cyclodextrin cavities and in other synthetic cavities.

One of the most striking studies on cyclodextrin-promoted reactions was the early work by Bender (Bender and Komiyama 1977) on acylation reactions of phenyl esters bound into cyclodextrin cavities. He showed that one could achieve about a 10^2 acceleration of the deacylation of some nitrophenyl esters as the result of binding of the substrate into the cavity followed by acyl transfer to a cyclodextrin hydroxyl. Of course, such accelerations are relatively modest in enzymatic terms. We examined these systems in models and concluded that they were not optimal. Although the substrate fits the cavity nicely, the transition state for reaction is extensively pulled out of the binding site. For rapid reactions, it is important that the *transition state* be bound, not simply (and perhaps not even necessarily) the substrate.

We devised a new group of nitrophenyl esters based on ferrocene derivatives (Trainor and Breslow 1981; Breslow et al. 1983b; Le Noble et al. 1983). In these substrates, it looked as if the transition state, or at least the tetrahedral intermediate, would bind about as well as the substrate did. We found that in these cases, very large accelerations were observed, i.e., as much as 10^8 acceleration of deacylation. Even though this was a relatively simple system, with no catalytic functional groups except for the hydroxyl groups of cyclodextrin, the acylation of a cyclodextrin hydroxyl group (Fig. 3) was accelerated to a greater extent than is the acylation of chymotrypsin by nitrophenyl esters such as *p*-nitrophenyl acetate. From this work, it was clear that with appropriate molecular design and geometry, very large accelerations of individual steps were possible.

Of course, the acylation of the hydroxyl group is not a catalytic reaction, and for that matter, the cleavage of nitrophenyl esters is not of great interest. Systems have been examined in other laboratories to turn such acyl transfer reactions of *p*-nitrophenyl esters into overall catalytic processes. However, we have focused instead on trying to develop systems that would perform the catalytic hydrolysis of more normal but difficult substrates, such as amides.

Peptide Cleavage

The ability of carboxypeptidase to hydrolyze a bound peptide in 10 msec or so under very mild conditions is a great challenge to artificial enzyme chemistry, a challenge that has not yet been met. We have approached this problem by studying the mechanism of action of the enzyme carboxypeptidase itself (Breslow and Wernick 1976, 1977; Breslow et al. 1983c), and we have come up with fairly good evidence for a particular mechanism of action of this enzyme (Breslow and Schepartz 1987; Schepartz and Breslow 1987) on the basis of work from our laboratory and the work of many others in the field. We have also studied a simple model for this very effective peptidase enzyme. We see rather rapid cleavage of a bound peptide under bifunctional catalysis by a metal and a carboxyl group (Breslow and Schepartz 1987; Schepartz and Breslow 1987), as occurs in the enzyme itself. Efforts in our laboratory are now directed at turning such a model system into a true catalytic system. There are currently many enzyme models and mimics, including antibodies, that will cleave nitrophenyl esters with pretty good rates. The much more difficult problem of hydrolyzing relatively stable structures such as peptide bonds still remains to be solved in this field.

The cyclodextrin nucleus is a very attractive framework on which to mount catalytic groups. Indeed, many years ago, we produced the first molecule described as an artificial enzyme by attaching a metal-binding group to a cyclodextrin so as to permit metal-catalyzed reaction of ligands that are principally bound by the cyclodextrin cavity (Breslow and Overman 1970). Typical enzymes utilize at least two functional groups, so we set out some years ago to produce a cyclodextrin-based artificial enzyme carrying more than one catalytic functionality.

Ribonuclease Mimics

For a variety of reasons, we were attracted to ribonuclease as our target for inspiration. Many hydrolytic enzymes perform their cleavage reactions in two steps, in which an intermediate is formed with a covalent bond to the enzyme. Thus, for enzymatic turnover, it is necessary in such cases that a second reaction also be catalyzed, in which this covalent bond is broken. For instance, in the work described above on acylation reactions, our early studies did not address this problem, and thus we were not dealing with true catalytic turnover. However, the enzyme ribonuclease cleaves RNA in a two-step sequence in which the intermediate is *not* covalently attached to the enzyme. Instead, a covalent intermediate is formed by the nucleophilic attack of a hydroxyl group from the substrate; in the second step, the resulting cyclic phosphate ester is hydrolyzed with enzyme catalysis. If we could induce an

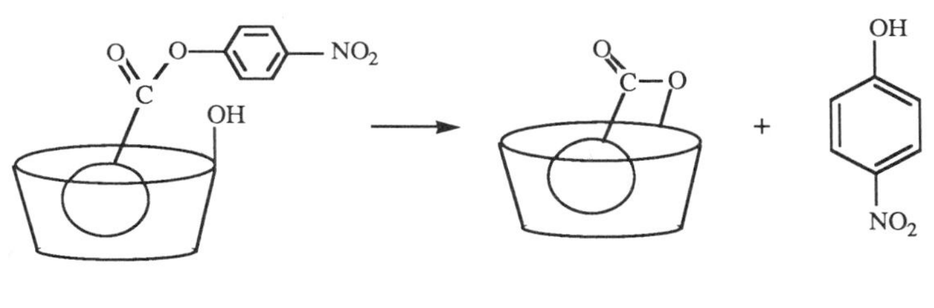

Figure 3. Very rapid acylation of cyclodextrin by a bound nitrophenyl ester occurs if the geometry of the complex is correct.

artificial enzyme to mimic either the first or the second step, it should thus perform the process with turnover catalysis. We were able to make such a system, and it was indeed a turnover catalyst.

The simplest version of this involved attaching two imidazole groups to cyclodextrin. Tabushi (1982) discovered a simple way to functionalize two of the positions in the cyclodextrin nucleus. Although his procedure was not completely selective for the relative positions of these two new groups, we were both (Breslow et al. 1980a; Tabushi 1982) able to develop methods that were selective. Using such compounds, we were able to attach two imidazole rings to the cyclodextrin nucleus, and thus cyclodextrin bisimidazole was our simple artificial enzyme (Breslow et al. 1978).

It would have been interesting to use this material to cleave RNA itself or the corresponding cyclic phosphate. Unfortunately, the geometry of binding of RNA groups into a cyclodextrin cavity was inappropriate to hold the system in the correct position for catalytic reaction (Lipsey 1980). However, we were able to construct a cyclic phosphate ester substrate that would bind to the cyclodextrin cavity and that could be hydrolyzed under the bifunctional influence of these two catalytic imidazole rings (Breslow et al. 1978).

It is perhaps not surprising that an artificial enzyme may well require an artificial substrate as well if its geometry is not optimal for natural substrates. With the artificial enzyme cyclodextrin derivative, the cyclic phosphate substrate was rapidly hydrolyzed, and the pH rate profile was bell-shaped. This indicated that the mechanism was indeed bifunctional, with cooperative catalysis by both the basic imidazole and the acidic imidazolium groups. This is, of course, the mechanism generally postulated for the enzyme as well. Furthermore, the cleavage of this substrate was quite selective. The product obtained was that expected from the geometric control exerted by this catalyst in the enzyme-substrate complex (Fig. 4). In contrast, in a different catalyst in which the functional groups were differently attached (Breslow et al. 1980a), the selectivity was changed. This also made sense in terms of the preferred geometry in the latter system.

Our bifunctional catalyst showed good turnover, although the product was an inhibitor, as also occurs in many enzymatic reactions. The fact that our catalyst was not able to cleave RNA is an indication of the substrate selectivity seen in the system; for that matter,

we found that the enzyme ribonuclease is not able to hydrolyze our artificial substrate (Lipsey 1980). However, it is clearly desirable to develop artificial catalysts that can cleave RNA.

As an initial study in this direction, we developed a good kinetic method to follow the cleavage of RNA by enzymatic or nonenzymatic means (Corcoran et al. 1985) and used it to study the ability of imidazole to catalyze this cleavage. Imidazole rings are, of course, the catalytic groups in the enzyme itself, as well as being the catalytic groups in the artificial enzyme we have just described. In a detailed kinetic study (Breslow and Labelle 1986), we found that catalysis of RNA cleavage does indeed occur with imidazole buffer. The process shows a bell-shaped pH-rate profile as in the enzyme and in our artificial enzyme, but the other kinetic information about this simple system indicated that it does not involve concerted bifunctional catalysis. Instead, the data are consistent with a *sequential* mechanism in which the basic imidazole ring does not simply remove a proton, but instead removes it and transfers it to a phosphate oxygen. The imidazolium ring then catalyzes cleavage of the five-coordinate intermediate produced. This mechanism had not been previously considered for the enzyme. However, it is consistent with everything known about the enzyme, and it is the mechanism apparently preferred in this simple model system. Possibly, this model has given us some new insights into the enzymatic process.

We have prepared a variety of polyimidazole compounds with binding groups attached to see if we could get improved rates of catalysis of RNA cleavage. Unfortunately, these more sophisticated attempted mimics of the enzyme ribonuclease have so far been no more effective than simple imidazole itself. Some metal-based catalysts that can cleave molecules related to RNA are described later in this paper.

Enzyme-Coenzyme Mimics

Not all enzymes catalyze reactions using only functional groups supplied by the side chains of amino acids. Instead, coenzymes may be required to perform the sort of special chemistry not possible with simple acids, bases, or nucleophiles as catalysts. A good example of this is the elaborate chemistry involved in amino acid metabolism, performed by enzymes that use pyridoxal phosphate and pyridoxamine phosphate as

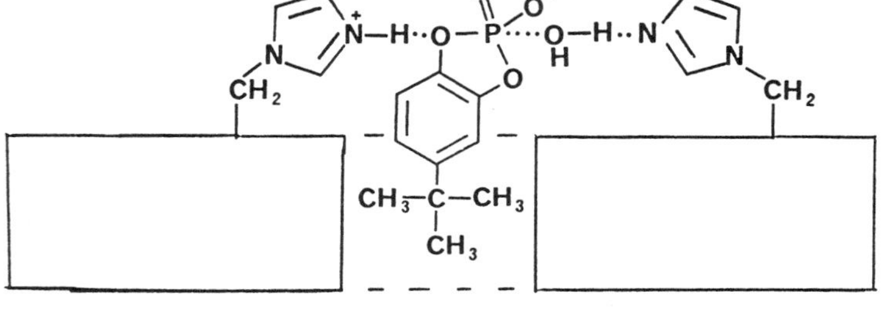

Figure 4. A cyclodextrin bis-imidazole catalyzes the selective hydrolysis of a bound phosphate substrate using a bifunctional mechanism like that used by the enzyme ribonuclease.

coenzymes. We decided to try to incorporate such systems into artificial enzymes. We hoped to combine a binding group and a coenzyme and a basic group to perform certain proton transfers involved in the typical catalyzed reactions.

In our first study (Breslow et al. 1980b), we attached pyridoxamine to the primary side of β-cyclodextrin and produced a catalyst combining a coenzyme with a binding group. This material was indeed able to perform the reductive amination of keto acids, just as pyridoxamine itself can (Fig. 5). However, in contrast to pyridoxamine, this compound showed a preference for keto acids that could also bind into the cyclodextrin cavity. Thus, in competitive experiments, phenylpyruvic acid was converted to phenylalanine and indolepyruvic acid was converted to tryptophan more rapidly than simple pyruvic acid was converted into alanine. In our earliest estimates, the rate advantage was rather high, but some of that advantage came from the fact that the slower processes were accompanied by more decomposition of the catalytic material. More recently, we estimated that the rate advantage in such systems (Breslow et al. 1986) ranges from 15 to 50.

We also were able to attach pyridoxamine to the secondary face of β-cyclodextrin (Breslow and Czarnik 1983). In this compound, we saw a similar preference for substrates that could also bind into the cavity. Finally, we also attached pyridoxamine to a totally synthetic artificial cavity unrelated to the cyclodextrins, and in this compound as well, we saw a preference for substrates that could bind (Winkler et al. 1983).

The reactions that occurred with the cyclodextrin-derived materials produced the amino acids in an optically active preferred form. This of course does not happen with simple pyridoxamine itself without an enzyme, but in our case, the complex that is bound into the cavity is in an asymmetric environment. In one interesting series, the stereochemical preference was reversed on going from the derivative attached to the cyclodextrin to the other derivative attached to the secondary side. However, such accidents in the asymmetric environment are obviously not the best way to achieve stereospecific production of amino acids.

As a second approach, we set out to establish that basic groups attached to pyridoxamine would catalyze the proton transfers that are part of every one of these biochemical transformations. In particular, we wanted to see if a single basic group would remove the proton from the methylene group of pyridoxamine and transfer it, in the covalent intermediate, to the carbon that picks up a proton in the conversion of a keto acid to an amino acid. If this 1,3-proton transfer could be demonstrated, in particular if the proton on the amino acid carbon is delivered by the basic group, then one could hope that asymmetric placement of this group would lead to the production of optically active amino acids.

In our first study (Zimmerman et al. 1983), we demonstrated that attached basic groups would indeed accelerate the amination reaction performed by pyridoxamine. In particular, the relationship between rate and structure established that the best catalytic groups were long enough to reach not only the carbon that must give up a proton, but also the more distant carbon that must accept a proton in the production of the amino acid. This strongly suggested that an asymmetric placement of such a basic group would successfully lead to the production of optically active amino acids.

Another study (Weiner et al. 1985) addressed a different kind of transformation, one catalyzed by pyridoxamine and in which proton removal (and not proton transfer) was involved. In this case, there was a preference for shorter base groups that could reach the nearby methylene carbon of pyridoxamine, since no distant proton transfer was required. This confirmed our interpretation that the previous preference for longer base groups in transamination did indicate that they were involved in proton delivery, not just in proton removal.

Armed with this information, we set out to make a pyridoxamine derivative (Fig. 6) in which a basic group is attached on one side of the pyridine plane, so that any proton transfers it performed would automatically put the new hydrogen atom in an asymmetric position on the newly developed amino acid. With a somewhat lengthy synthesis, a compound was prepared in which an extra ring was fused to the pyridoxamine so that a group coming off this ring would have to be on either the front or the back face of the system (Zimmerman and Breslow 1984). The optically resolved compound was indeed able to produce optically active amino acids with rather good asymmetric preferences, better than 10:1 and approaching 20:1. The catalytic groups used were not, in fact, the best catalysts we have developed for such reactions; so one might expect even better optical preferences with better proton transfer catalysts.

Finally, this work has resulted in the preparation of a single material that can do everything that is required. This material has a cyclodextrin-binding group, a pyridoxamine, and an asymmetrically mounted basic

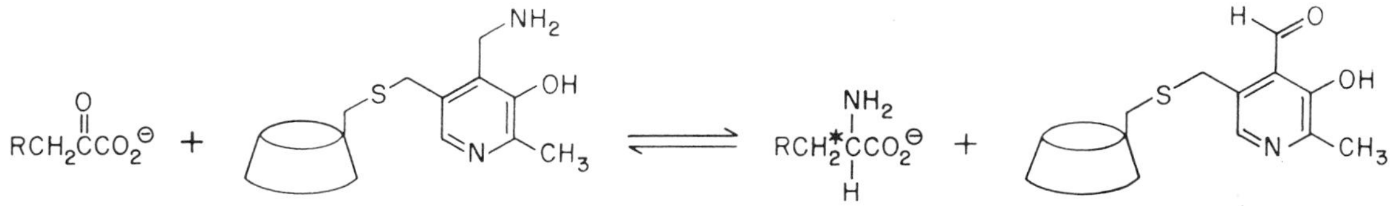

Figure 5. Attachment of pyridoxamine to cyclodextrin produces an artificial enzyme that can reductively aminate keto acids with substrate selectivity and some stereoselectivity in the product amino acids.

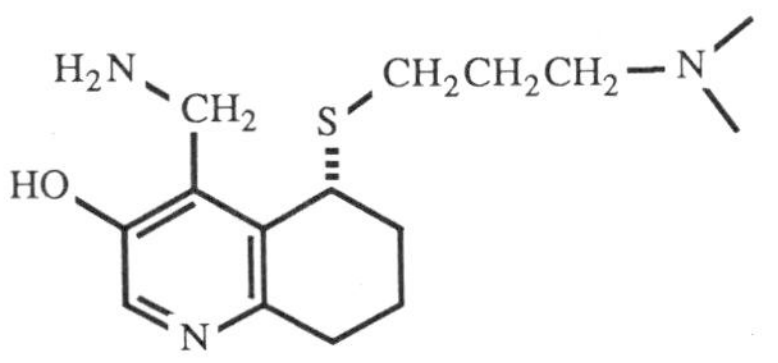

Figure 6. A basic group constrained to one face of a pyridox-amine catalyzes transaminations of keto acids with high stereoselectivity.

group in a position to catalyze the proton transfers and produce an optically active amino acid. Actually, two such approaches have been followed. One of them was an international cooperation largely carried out in Japan by the research group of Tabushi, in collaboration with us (Tabushi et al. 1985). In this approach, pyridoxamine was attached to a cyclodextrin, and a base group was attached to a different sugar residue of cyclodextrin. The isomers were then separated so that two different catalysts were on hand, one going from the pyridoxamine to the base in a clockwise direction and the other in a counterclockwise direction. As hoped, these two different catalysts were quite selective in the production of optically active amino acids, with close to a 50:1 preference in some cases.

In our research group, a different approach has been under study for some time, and it is essentially complete (R. Mehra et al., unpubl.). We attach a cy-clodextrin to a pyridoxamine compound that carries the base group mounted asymmetrically (Fig. 7). In the earliest versions of this approach, we also obtained production of optically active amino acids, although the preference ($\sim$6.7:1) was not as high as we would have liked. However, the proton-transfer catalyst groups in this case are not yet optimal; it remains to be seen whether this proves to be as good an approach to the general problem.

Closely related to this approach are studies in which other coenzyme groups are attached to binding groups. We have attached thiamine-like species to cyclodextrin (Hilvert and Breslow 1984), and more recently, Diederich has prepared a thiamine-like compound attached to a synthetic binding cavity (Lutter and Diederich 1986). Both of these systems show interesting substrate selectivities, performing thiamine-cata-

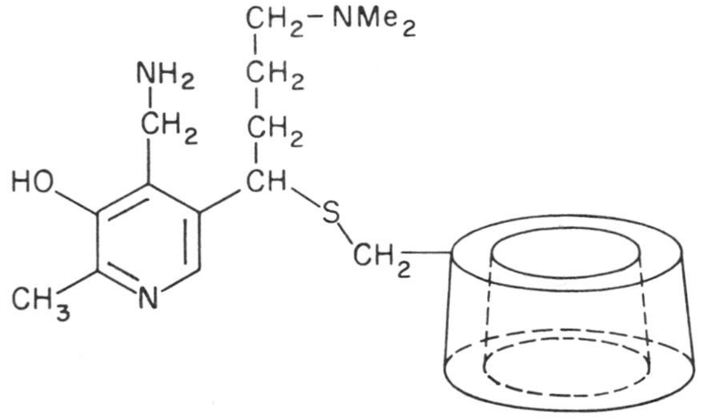

Figure 7. An artificial enzyme combining a coenzyme, binding group, and chirally mounted base catalyst.

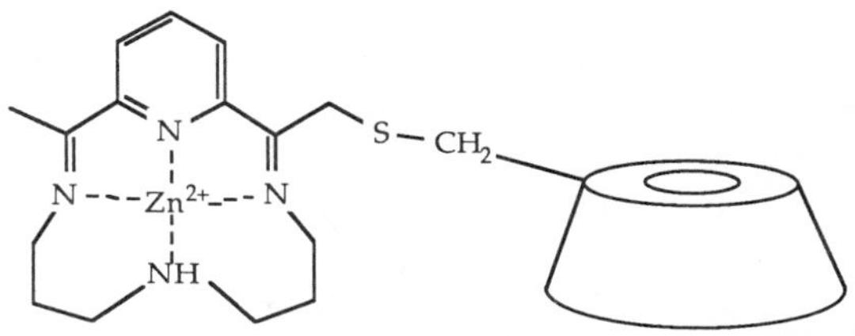

Figure 8. An artificial phosphatase with a binding group and a catalytic zinc complex group.

lyzed reactions on substrates that can be bound into the cyclodextrin or artificial cavity. Furthermore, other coenzyme-like materials, such as nicotinamide rings, have been attached to cyclodextrins, and some selectivities have also been observed. The combination of coenzyme and binding group exemplified by these substrates seems to be an interesting one with considerable scope.

Metal Phosphate Mimics

Many enzymes use metals to catalyze reactions. In recognition of this, our earliest artificial enzyme put a metal-binding group onto a cyclodextrin (Breslow and Overman 1970). In many enzymes, the effective metal is zinc. Rather good ligands are needed to hold zinc in solution at neutral or slightly basic pH; the most effective synthetic ligand that has been described so far is a macrocycle with four nitrogen atoms. We have examined the zinc complex of this material and have found (Gellman et al. 1986) that it is quite a good catalyst for phosphate ester hydrolysis. In particular, it hydrolyzes triaryl phosphates even though these are not significantly bound to metals. For this reason, we were able to improve the hydrolysis of these substrates by attaching the zinc macrocycle to a cyclodextrin ring (S. Singh et al., unpubl.). As expected, this compound (Fig. 8) is an even better catalyst for phosphate ester cleavage because it binds the substrate next to the catalytic metal. Very recently, we have found that compounds in this series are catalysts for the hydrolysis of compounds related to RNA. In these cases, phosphate diesters are involved, and the phosphate anion groups do coordinate with the metals. An active program is under way in our laboratory to develop such zinc catalysts into really effective artificial enzymes for the cleavage of RNA.

ACKNOWLEDGMENTS

I thank my co-workers for their contributions and the National Institutes of Health and Office of Naval Research for support of this work.

REFERENCES

Bender, M.L. and M. Komiyama. 1977. *Cyclodextrin chemistry.* Springer-Verlag, New York.
Breslow, R. 1972. Biomimetic chemistry. *Chem. Soc. Rev.* **1**: 553.

———. 1986. Artificial enzymes and enzyme models. *Adv. Enzymol. Relat. Areas Mol. Biol.* **58**: 1.

Breslow, R. and P. Campbell. 1969. Selective aromatic substitution within a cyclodextrin mixed complex. *J. Am. Chem. Soc.* **91**: 3085.

———. 1971. Selective aromatic substitution by hydrophobic binding of a substrate to a simple cyclodextrin catalyst. *Bioorg. Chem.* **1**: 140.

Breslow, R. and D. Chipman. 1965. Mixed metal complexes as enzyme models. I. Intracomplex nucleophilic catalysis by an oxime anion. *J. Am. Chem. Soc.* **87**: 4195.

Breslow, R. and A.W. Czarnik. 1983. Transaminations by pyridoxamine selectively attached at C-3 in beta-cyclodextrin. *J. Am. Chem. Soc.* **105**: 1390.

Breslow, R. and M. Labelle. 1986. Sequential general base-acid catalysis in the hydrolysis of RNA by imidazole. *J. Am. Chem. Soc.* **108**: 2655.

Breslow, R. and U. Maitra. 1984. On the origin of product selectivity in aqueous Diels-Alder reactions. *Tetrahedron Lett.* **25**: 1239.

Breslow, R. and L.E. Overman. 1970. An "artificial enzyme" combining a metal catalytic group and a hyrophobic binding cavity. *J. Am. Chem. Soc.* **92**: 1075.

Breslow, R. and A. Schepartz. 1987. On the mechanism of peptide cleavage by carboxypeptidase A and related enzymes. *Chem. Lett.* **1**: 1.

Breslow, R. and D. Wernick. 1976. On the mechanism of catalysis by carboxypeptidase A. *J. Am. Chem. Soc.* **98**: 259.

———. 1977. Unified picture of mechanisms of catalysis by carboxypeptidase A. *Proc. Natl. Acad. Sci.* **74**: 1303.

Breslow, R., P. Bovy, and C. Lipsey Hersh. 1980a. Reversing the selectivity of cyclodextrin bisimidazole ribonuclease mimics by changing the catalyst geometry. *J. Am. Chem. Soc.* **102**: 2115.

Breslow, R., M. Hammond, and M. Lauer. 1980b. Selective transamination and optical induction by a beta-cyclodextrin-pyridoxamine artificial enzyme. *J. Am. Chem. Soc.* **102**: 421.

Breslow, R., H. Kohn, and B. Siegel. 1976. Methylated cyclodextrin and a cyclodextrin polymer as catalysts in selective anisole chlorination. *Tetrahedron Lett.* 1645.

Breslow, R., U. Maitra, and D. Rideout. 1983a. Selective Diels-Alder reactions in aqueous solutions and suspensions. *Tetrahedron Lett.* **24**: 1901.

Breslow, R., G. Trainor, and A. Ueno. 1983b. Optimization of metallocene substrates for β-cyclodextrin reactions. *J. Am. Chem. Soc.* **105**: 2739.

Breslow, R., J. Chin, D. Hilvert, and G. Trainor. 1983c. Evidence for the general base mechanism in carboxypeptidase A-catalyzed reactions. Partitioning studies on nucleophiles and H₂0-18 kinetic isotope effects. *Proc. Natl. Acad. Sci.* **80**: 4585.

Breslow, R., J. Doherty, G. Guillot, and C. Lipsey. 1978. Beta-cyclodextrinyl-bisimidazole. A model for rinonuclease. *J. Am. Chem. Soc.* **100**: 3227.

Breslow, R., A.W. Czarnik, M. Lauer, R. Leppkes, J. Winkler, and S. Zimmerman. 1986. Mimics of transaminase enzymes. *J. Am. Chem. Soc.* **108**: 1969.

Brown, F.S. and L.P. Hager. 1967. Chloroperoxidase. IV. Evidence for an ionic electrophilic substitution mechanism. *J. Am. Chem. Soc.* **89**: 719.

Corcoran, R., M. Labelle, A.W. Czarnik, and R. Breslow. 1985. An assay to determine the kinetics of RNA cleavage. *Anal. Biochem.* **144**: 563.

Gellman, S., R. Petter, and R. Breslow. 1986. Catalytic hydrolysis of a phosphate triester by tetracoordinated zinc complexes. *J. Am. Chem. Soc.* **108**: 2388.

Heinrich, N. and F. Cramer. 1965. Inclusion compounds. XVIII. The catalysis of the fission of pyrophosphates by cyclodextrin. A model reaction for the mechanism of enzymes. *J. Am. Chem. Soc.* **87**: 1121.

Hilvert, D. and R. Breslow. 1984. Functionalized cyclodextrins as holoenzyme mimics of thiamine-dependent enzymes. *Bioorg. Chem.* **12**: 206.

Le Noble, W.J., S. Srivastava, R. Breslow, and G. Trainor. 1983. Effect of pressure on two cyclodextrin-promoted ester hydrolyses. *J. Am. Chem. Soc.* **105**: 2745.

Lipsey, C. 1980. "Imidazole cyclodextrins: Models for ribonuclease." Ph.D. thesis, Columbia University, New York.

Lutter, H.-D. and F. Diederich. 1986. Synthesis of a macrobicyclic thiazolium-host and supramolecular catalysis of the benzoin condensation. *Angew. Chem.* **25**: 1125.

O'Krongly, D., S.R. Denmeade, M.Y. Chiang, and R. Breslow. 1985. Efficient triple coupling reaction to produce a self-adjusting molecular cage. *J. Am. Chem. Soc.* **107**: 5544.

Rideout, D. and R. Breslow. 1980. Hydrophobic acceleration of Diels-Alder reactions. *J. Am. Chem. Soc.* **102**: 7816.

Schepartz, A. and R. Breslow. 1987. Hydrolysis of an amide in a carboxypeptidase model using Co(III) and bifunctional catalysts. *J. Am. Chem. Soc.* **109**: 1814.

Tabushi, I. 1982. Cyclodextrin catalysts as a model for enzyme action. *Accts. Chem. Res.* **15**: 66.

Tabushi, I., Y. Kuroda, M. Yamada, H. Higashimura, and R. Breslow. 1985. A-modified B-6-B[omega-amino-ethylamino]-beta-cyclodextrin as an artificial B-6 enzyme for chiral aminotransfer reaction. *J. Am. Chem. Soc.* **107**: 5545.

Trainor, G. and R. Breslow. 1981. High acylation rates and enantioselectivity with cyclodextrin complexes of rigid substrates. *J. Am. Chem. Soc.* **103**: 154.

von Hippel, P.H. and T. Schleich. 1969. Ion effects on the solution structure of biological macromolecules. *Accts. Chem. Res.* **2**: 257.

Weiner, W., J. Winkler, S.C. Zimmerman, A.W. Czarnik, and R. Breslow. 1985. Mimics of tryptophan synthetase and of biochemical dehydroalanine formation. *J. Am. Chem. Soc.* **107**: 4093.

Winkler, J., E. Coutouli-Argyropoulou, R. Leppkes, and R. Breslow. 1983. Artificial transaminase carrying a synthetic macrocyclic binding group. *J. Am. Chem. Soc.* **105**: 7198.

Zimmerman, S.C. and R. Breslow. 1984. Asymmetric synthesis of amino acids by pyridoxamine enzyme analogous utilizing general base-acid catalysis. *J. Am. Chem. Soc.* **106**: 1490.

Zimmerman, S.C., A.W. Czarnik, and R. Breslow. 1983. Intramolecular general base-acid catalysis in transaminations catalyzed by pyridoxamine enzyme analogues. *J. Am. Chem. Soc.* **105**: 1694.

Phosphorus-containing Peptide Analogs as Peptidase Inhibitors

P.A. Bartlett, C.K. Marlowe, P.P. Giannousis, and J.E. Hanson
Department of Chemistry, University of California, Berkeley, California 94720

Peptidases play a variety of roles in living organisms, from the routine work of digestion to highly specific hormonal regulation. They are involved in such diverse processes as the blood-clotting and complement cascades, blood pressure regulation, egg fertilization, posttranslational processing in protein synthesis, tumor invasion, and degenerative diseases such as emphysema and arthritis. Synthetic and naturally occurring peptidase inhibitors have been useful for studying the function of these enzymes and as medicinal agents. Indeed, a successful treatment for hypertension involves the use of an inhibitor of the peptidase that produces the octapeptide pressor hormone angiotensin II from its decapeptide precursor.

The task of devising peptidase inhibitors is straightforward, since their mechanisms are relatively well understood. All peptidases whose mechanisms have been elucidated fall into one of four classes: the serine and cysteine peptidases, whose reactions proceed via a covalent acyl enzyme intermediate, and the zinc and aspartic peptidases, which catalyze the direct addition of water to the amide linkage. Moreover, inhibition strategies appear to be general within each class of peptidase. On the other hand, these generalities of mechanism and inhibition strategies make it more of a challenge to devise low-molecular-weight inhibitors of high specificity.

A general and highly effective approach for the design of an enzyme inhibitor is to devise a molecule that resembles the putative transition state or a high-energy intermediate along the reaction pathway (Wolfenden 1976; Stark and Bartlett 1984). Such a strategy is based on the recognition that the lower activation energy of the enzyme-catalyzed transformation reflects a corresponding increase in the binding energy between the enzyme and the substrate as their complex proceeds from the ground state to the transition state conformation. If a "transition state analog" can take advantage of even part of this additional binding energy, it will be a highly effective inhibitor (Frick et al. 1986; Jones and Wolfenden 1986).

The major change in the structures of the ground and transition states for hydrolysis of a peptidase substrate is the progression in geometry of the carbonyl carbon from trigonal to tetrahedral. Incorporation of a functional group that can adopt the tetrahedral geometry has therefore been crucial to the design of transition state analog inhibitors for these enzymes. For the zinc and aspartic peptidases, which do not involve a co-

valently bound intermediate, a particularly attractive design motif is to incorporate a phosphorus atom in place of the carbonyl carbon of the scissile linkage. The high valency of phosphorus allows a number of heteroatom substituents to be incorporated at this position while retaining a stable tetrahedral geometry. Several naturally occurring inhibitors have evolved on the basis of this strategy; a notable example is phosphoramidon, a phosphoryl dipeptide that is a potent inhibitor of the zinc endopeptidase thermolysin (Komiyama et al. 1975). In early work in this area, a number of simple *N*-phosphoryl amino acids and dipeptides were shown to be effective inhibitors of thermolysin (Kam et al. 1979; Nishino and Powers 1979) and the mechanistically related enzyme carboxypeptidase A (Holmquist 1977; Hofmann and Rottenberg 1980). More recently, in addition to our work reviewed below, phosphonic and phosphinic amino acid analogs have been incorporated into substrate sequences appropriate for a number of other zinc peptidases and have been shown to give rise to potent inhibitors (Galardy 1982; Thorsett et al. 1982; Galardy and Grobelny 1983; Galardy et al. 1983; Petrillo et al. 1983).

Phosphoramidon

PHOSPHORUS-CONTAINING INHIBITORS OF ZINC PEPTIDASES

Carboxypeptidase A

With the recognition that peptidyl phosphoramidates are effective inhibitors of thermolysin and carboxypeptidase A, a logical extension of the concept was the literal extension of the inhibitors in the direction of the P_1 and P_2 sites, i.e., with the incorporation of the tetrahedral phorphorus as an amino acid analog, rather than a phosphoric acid derivative. We therefore synthesized Cbz-Gly^P-Phe (Gly^P represents the phosphonic acid analog of glycine) and evaluated it as an inhibitor of carboxypeptidase A (see Jacobsen and Bartlett 1981a). This compound proved to be a good inhibitor of the peptidase, with a $K_i = 9 \times 10^{-8}$ M. A number of analogs and congeners were compared with this compound, as indicated in Table 1. It is clear that the

Table 1. Inhibition of Carboxypeptidase A

Inhibitor		K_i (nM)[a]	Reference
$\underset{\underset{O^-}{\overset{\overset{S}{\|}}{\text{CH}_3-\text{P}-\text{Phe}}}}{}$	(R_p isomer) (S_p isomer)	8500 5300	Jacobsen and Bartlett (1981b) Jacobsen and Bartlett (1981b)
$\underset{\underset{O^-}{\overset{\overset{O}{\|}}{^-O-\text{P}-\text{Phe}}}}{}$		5000	Kam et al. (1979)
$\underset{\underset{O^-}{\overset{\overset{O}{\|}}{\text{CH}_3-\text{P}-\text{Phe}}}}{}$		1200	Jacobsen and Bartlett (1981b)
$\underset{\underset{O^-}{\overset{\overset{O}{\|}}{\text{Cbz}-\text{NHCH}_2-\text{P}-\text{Phe}}}}{}$ (Cbz-Gly^P-Phe)		90	Jacobsen and Bartlett (1981a)
$\underset{\underset{O^-}{\overset{\overset{O}{\|}}{\text{Cbz}-\text{NHCH}_2-\text{P}-\text{O}-\text{Phe}}}}{}$ (Cbz-Gly^P-(O)-Phe)		60	Jacobsen and Bartlett (1981b)
L-α-Benzylsuccinate		450	Byers and Wolfenden (1973)
3-Benzyl-2-mercaptopropanoate		11	Ondetti et al. (1979)

[a]pH 7.5, 25°C.

presence of the Cbz-amino-methyl moiety is a significant factor in the binding interaction. Other comparisons in Table 1 indicate that there is no significant difference in binding between the phosphonamidate derivative and the phosphonate ester, nor is any advantage to be gained by the incorporation of a sulfur ligand in the form of a thiophosphonamidate, regardless of the configuration at the phosphorus center (see Jacobsen and Bartlett 1981b).

Thermolysin

Phosphonamidate inhibitors. What is not revealed by the results of Table 1 is whether it is the tetrahedral nature of the phosphorus derivatives that accounts for their binding affinity or merely the anionic nature of the phosphonate moiety. To examine this broader question, we turned to thermolysin, a bacterial endopeptidase that is evolutionarily different from, but mechanistically analogous to, carboxypeptidase A. Although it is difficult to predict quantitatively what the binding affinity should be for a given transition state analog, theoretical considerations suggest that for a series of inhibitors and related substrates, there should be a proportionality between the inhibitor K_i and substrate K_m/k_{cat} values (Eq. 1) *if* the inhibitors take advantage of the binding interactions available in the transition state conformation (Westerik and Wolfenden 1972; Bartlett and Marlowe 1983; Thompson 1973).

$$K_i \propto K_m/k_{cat} \quad \text{(Assumptions: } K_S = K_m\text{, rate of} \atop \text{nonenzymatic reaction constant} \atop \text{over substrate series)} \quad (1)$$

To explore the validity of this prediction and of the transition state analog appellation for the phosphonamidate derivatives, we synthesized a series of tripeptide inhibitors of thermolysin of the form Cbz-Gly^P-Leu-(amino acid) (Table 2) (Bartlett and Marlowe 1983). Within the corresponding series of substrates, there is relatively little variation in K_m values; however, there is a span in K_m/k_{cat} values of almost three orders of magnitude (Table 2, columns 3 and 4) (Morihara and Tsuzuki 1970). A clear distinction could therefore be made between correlation of inhibitor K_i with K_m/k_{cat} and K_m alone (Table 2, column 1; Fig. 1, open squares), indicating that these inhibitors are transition state analogs.

Phosphonate ester inhibitors. In addition to the phosphonamidates ($Y = \text{NH}$), we prepared the corresponding phosphonate esters ($Y = \text{O}$), primarily because they are more stable toward hydrolysis and because in our earlier work, we did not find a significant difference in the affinity of carboxypeptidase A for Cbz-Gly^P-Phe and Cbz-Gly^P-(O)-Phe (Table 1). Thermolysin, in contrast, discriminates against the phosphonate esters by a factor of 840, on average, reflecting a loss of 4.0 kcal/mole of binding energy as compared with the phosphonamidates (Bartlett and Marlowe

Table 2. Inhibition of Thermolysin by Cbz-Gly^P-Leu-X

Inhibitor	K_i (nM)[a] $(Y = NH)$	K_i (μM)[b] $(Y = O)$	K_m (mM)[c]	K_m/k_{cat} (μM sec)[c]
Cbz-Gly^P-(Y)-Leu-D-Ala[d]	>1700	—	16.6	3200
Cbz-Gly^P-(Y)-Leu-NH$_2$	760	660	20.6	196
Cbz-Gly^P-(Y)-Leu-Gly	270	230	10.8	165
Cbz-Gly^P-(Y)-Leu-Phe	78	53	2.4	20
Cbz-Gly^P-(Y)-Leu-Ala	16.5	13.0	10.6	13.6
Cbz-Gly^P-(Y)-Leu-Leu	9.1	9.0	2.6	7.0

pH 7.0, 25°C.
[a]Data from Bartlett and Marlowe (1983).
[b]Data from Bartlett and Marlowe (1987a).
[c]For corresponding substrate, see Morihara and Tsuzuki (1970).
[d]Contaminated with about 0.9% of L-Ala isomer.

1987a). The near constancy of this incremental binding loss across the series suggested to us that the inhibitors are all bound in a similar manner and that there is a specific binding interaction available to the amidates that is not available to the esters, most likely a hydrogen bond. Both of these inferences were substantiated by X-ray crystallographic investigations of the complexes of thermolysin with Cbz-Gly^P-Leu-Leu and Cbz-Gly^P-(O)-Leu-Leu (Tronrud et al. 1987). Between the two complexes, both the protein and inhibitor structures are virtually superimposable (largest difference < 0.2 Å), demonstrating that the difference in binding affinity does not result from a different orientation of

the inhibitors in the active site or a change in remote interactions. Moreover, the existence of a hydrogen bond between the phosphonamidate NH and the carbonyl oxygen of Ala-113 was supported by the observation of a 3-Å separation between the two heteroatoms. This hydrogen bond involves two formally uncharged groups, which is expected to result in a modest (0.5-1.0 kcal/mole) contribution to the binding energy (Fersht et al. 1985). That this hydrogen bond contributes 4.0 kcal/mole may reflect the fact that it is highly favored entropically, i.e., the interacting groups are positioned similarly whether or not the hydrogen bond is present.

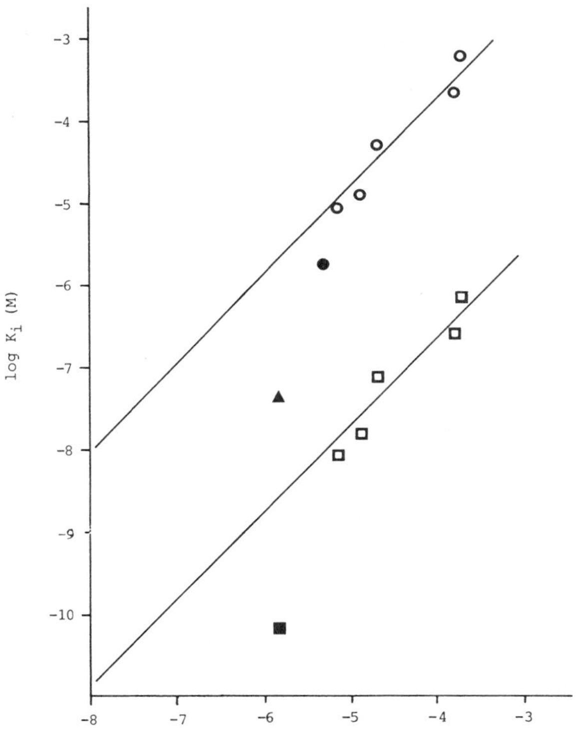

Slow-binding inhibitors. Equation 1 implies that to design a more potent inhibitor of thermolysin (lower K_i), one should look for a better substrate (higher k_{cat}/K_m = lower K_m/k_{cat}) and make the corresponding phosphonamidate or phosphonate analog. With this intention, we synthesized a number of phosphorus-containing tripeptides in which a phosphonic acid analog of a substituted amino acid is incorporated at the P$_1$ position (Table 3; Fig. 1, solid points) (Bartlett and Marlowe 1987b). The behavior of these inhibitors was striking in two respects. First, those inhibitors for which a comparison can be made (Cbz-Phe^P-Leu-Ala, Cbz-Ala^P-(O)-Leu-Ala, and Cbz-Phe^P-(O)-Leu-Ala) are seen to bind *more* tightly to thermolysin than the transition state correlation would predict. Second, *all* of the P$_1$-substituted inhibitors are slow binding.

The tighter than predicted binding of the P$_1$-substituted inhibitors reveals the importance of the assumptions made in deriving Equation 1 (Bartlett and Marlowe 1983), namely, that within the series (1) the substrates must be expected to have the same rate constants for the noncatalyzed transformation and (2) the same step must be rate-limiting for the enzymatic transformations. Neither of these may be true for the P$_1$-substituted inhibitors: The noncatalyzed rate constant for addition of water to the carbonyl group of a substituted amino acid is likely to be lower than that for addition of water to glycine. Moreover, an extrapolation of Figure 1 (solid square and triangle) reveals that thermolysin would have to turn over Cbz-Phe-Leu-Ala at a rate exceeding 10^7 M^{-1}s^{-1} to match the correlation with the inhibitor K_i values. Since the on rate for

Figure 1. Comparison of peptide substrate K_m/k_{cat} values with the K_i values for Cbz-Gly^P-Leu-X ($\square$), Cbz-Gly^P-(O)-Leu-X ($\bigcirc$), and Cbz-X^P-(Y)-Leu-Ala (solid points). Point for Cbz-Gly^P-Leu-D-Ala is not depicted.

Table 3. Inhibition of Thermolysin by Cbz-X^P-(Y)-Leu-Ala

	Phosphonamidates (Y = NH)		Phosphonates (Y = O)	
Inhibitor	K_i (nM)[a]	k_{on} (M^{-1} s^{-1})	K_i (nM)[a]	k_{on} (M^{-1} s^{-1})
Cbz-Ala^P-(Y)-Leu-Ala	—		1800	1250
Cbz-Leu^P-(Y)-Leu-Ala	—		680	480
Cbz-Phe^P-(Y)-Leu-Ala	0.068[b]	1000	45	470
Cbz-D-Ala^P-(Y)-Leu-Ala	—		24,000	2.1
Cbz-D-Leu^P-(Y)-Leu-Ala	—		42,000	2.8
Cbz-D-Phe^P-(Y)-Leu-Ala	480	1300	30,000	400

[a]Data from Bartlett and Marlowe (1987b). Determined at pH 7.0, 25°C by steady-state kinetics, unless otherwise indicated; dash indicates compound not prepared.
[b]Calculated from $K_i = k_{off}/k_{on}$.

the related mansyl substrate is only 3×10^6 M^{-1}s^{-1} (Morgan and Fruton 1978), it is possible that turnover of this substrate is limited by substrate association, not chemical catalysis.

A greater puzzle is the origin of the slow-binding behavior observed for all of the tripeptide analogs depicted in Table 3. Whereas Cbz-Gly^P-Leu-Leu binds normally, with an on rate $\geq 10^5$ M^{-1}s^{-1}, the on rates for those with a substituent α to phosphorus are at least three orders of magnitude below that expected for a diffusion-limited process (Morgan and Fruton 1978; Brouwer and Kirsch 1982). This slow-binding behavior appears to be unrelated to the size of this substituent, its configuration, whether the inhibitor is a phosphonamidate or phosphonate ester, or whether it is a potent or weak inhibitor. Although slow binding is often associated with a two-step binding process and attributed to a protein conformational change required for attainment of the final, "tight" complex (Morrison and Walsh 1987), neither Cbz-Phe^P-Leu-Ala nor Cbz-Phe^P-(O)-Leu-Ala shows evidence for a "loose" intermediate complex with a K_D below 4 mM.

Determination of the structure of the complex of thermolysin with Cbz-Phe^P-Leu-Ala reveals that the protein has not undergone any significant conformational change in comparison with the native enzyme or the complex with the fast-binding inhibitor Cbz-Gly^P-Leu-Leu (Holden et al. 1987). We are therefore inclined to rule out a mechanism for slow binding in which such a conformational change is responsible. On the other hand, the P_1-substituted inhibitor occupies the S_1 and S_2 subsites in a different manner than the Gly^P derivatives do, with rotation around the C_α-N bond of the phosphorus amino acid residue placing the carbamate moiety deeper into the active-site cleft. Nevertheless, this inhibitor conformation is attained by a single bond rotation, and it does not represent an unfavorable conformation. It is therefore difficult to attribute the slow-binding phenomenon to this conformational feature. Binding of the inhibitor in this conformation does, however, require expulsion of an additional water molecule, in comparison to the fast-binding inhibitors. We have therefore explored the possibility that the slow-binding behavior of the P_1-substituted inhibitors may simply reflect a difficult exchange between bound water and bound inhibitor.

A binding sequence in which a specific water molecule must dissociate before the inhibitor can associate with the protein could lead to slow binding even if all of the individual steps are fast, simply because it is a rare form of the enzyme that the inhibitor must encounter. The results of a preliminary investigation of the effect of viscosity on the binding of Cbz-Phe^P-(O)-Leu-Ala are consistent with this interpretation: The rate of association of this inhibitor is almost completely diffusion-limited, despite the fact that $k_{on} = 470$ M^{-1}s^{-1}. Further studies of this effect may provide more understanding of the dynamic and static aspects of protein-ligand association processes.

Carboxypeptidase A Revisited

As indicated above, our work on zinc peptidase inhibitors began with the phosphonic acid analogs of Cbz-Gly^P-Phe, which showed inhibition constants toward carboxypeptidase A on the order of 60–90 nM (Table 1) (Jacobsen and Bartlett 1981a,b). Although these inhibitors are potent, they do not constitute the most tightly bound synthetic inhibitors reported for this enzyme (Ondetti et al. 1979). Tripeptides such as Cbz-Ala-Ala-Phe are more rapidly hydrolyzed by carboxypeptidase A than Cbz-Gly-Phe; therefore, a longer phosphonic acid peptide analog was an attractive target for an improved inhibitor. Since carboxypeptidase A does not appear to discriminate against phosphonate esters (in comparison to the phosphonamidates) the way thermolysin does, we prepared the more stable Cbz-Ala-Ala^P-(O)-Phe.

Cbz-Ala-Ala^P-(O)-Phe

Although this material is not particularly slow binding, compared with some of our thermolysin inhibitors, it is sufficiently tightly bound that its inhibition constant cannot be measured under steady-state conditions (Morrison and Walsh 1987). We were therefore required to determine separately the rates for association and dissociation of the inhibitor from the enzyme. Since the dissociation rate proved to be very slow, it was necessary to find conditions under which the enzyme is stable for extended periods of time. Figure 2 depicts the results from two experiments, in which the equilibrium between enzymes and inhibitor was established in two directions, enabling us to determine the on and off rates and to verify the equilibrium constant. These incubations were carried out in the absence of substrate; the concentration of free enzyme was monitored by removing aliquots and measuring the residual (for k_{on}) or recovering activity (for k_{off}). That the K_i value for Cbz-Ala-Ala^P-(O)-Phe is indeed only 3 pM is underscored by the correspondence between the observed equilibrium constant and the value calculated from the on and off rates. This compound is, by several orders of magnitude, the most potent small-molecule inhibitor reported for carboxypeptidase A. As was the case for the P_1-substituted inhibitors of thermolysin, Cbz-Ala-Ala^P-(O)-Phe is more potent than expected based on extrapolation from Cbz-Gly^P-(O)-Phe, according to the K_i versus K_m/k_{cat} correlation of Equation 1. Again, however, this comparison involves substrates that differ substantially in structure.

Collagenase

Although collagenases as a group are poorly understood from the point of view of substrate specificity and mechanism, they belong to the zinc peptidases and appear to be inhibited by strategies that are effective against the other members of this class (Galardy and Grobelny 1983; Vencill et al. 1985). On the basis of emerging information on the substrate specificity of human neutrophil collagenase (Mookhtiar et al. 1986), the phosphonate-containing peptides listed in Table 4 were designed and synthesized; as indicated, they proved to be good inhibitors of the enzyme (Mookhtiar et al. 1987).

Table 4. Inhibition of Human Neutrophil Collagenase

Inhibitor	K_i (mM)
Cbz-Gly^P-Leu	2.1
Cbz-Gly^P-Leu-NH$_2$	1.3
Cbz-Gly^P-Leu-Ala	0.078
Cbz-Gly^P-Leu-D-Ala	2.6
Cbz-Gly^P-Leu-Gly	6.8
Cbz-Gly^P-Leu-Phe	0.98
Cbz-Gly^P-(O)-Leu-Ala	2.5
Cbz-Pro-Ala-Gly^P-Leu-NH$_2$	0.15
Cbz-Phe-Gly^P-Leu-Ala	0.071
Cbz-Gly^P-Leu-Ala-Gly	0.014

pH 7.5, 30°C. Data from Mookhtiar et al. (1987).

Leucine Aminopeptidase

In contrast to collagenase, the substrate specificity of leucine aminopeptidase is well understood, but the mechanistic details are not (Delange and Smith 1971). It is considered a member of the zinc peptidase class in view of its requirement for this metal and its inhibition by chelating agents and hydroxamic acid amino acid analogs. However, no structural comparison with thermolysin or carboxypeptidase A is available, nor is there a similar correspondence in effective inhibition strategies. The most potent inhibitors reported for leucine aminopeptidase are the naturally occurring dipeptide analog bestatin (Wilkes and Prescott 1985) and the aldehyde (Andersson et al. 1985) and boronic acid (Shenvi 1986) analogs of leucine. In view of the success of phosphonic acid peptide analogs as inhibitors of the more well-defined members of the zinc peptidase class, we synthesized and evaluated an analogous series of derivatives for leucine aminopeptidase (see Table 5) (Giannousis and Bartlett 1987).

Leu^P-(O)-Leu and Phe^P-(O)-Leu were patterned after the corresponding dipeptide substrates, which are hydrolyzed very effectively by the enzyme; the phos-

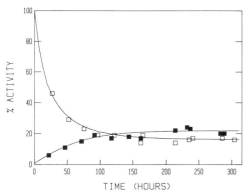

Figure 2. Establishment of equilibrium between Cbz-Ala-Ala^P-(O)-Phe (I) and carboxypeptidase A (E). Conditions: pH 7.5, 25°C, 50 mM Tris-HCl, 0.5 M NaCl, 0.1 mg/ml BSA, 1 μM ZnCl$_2$. Association reaction: 45 pM E + 50 pM I. Dissociation reaction: 45 pM EI complex. Theoretical curves represent $k_{on} = 2.5 \times 10^5$ M^{-1}s^{-1} and $k_{off} = 7.5 \times 10^{-7}$ s^{-1}.

Table 5. Inhibition of Leucine Aminopeptidase

Inhibitor	K_i (μM)
Leu^P-(O)-Leu	58[a]
Phe^P-(O)-Leu	340[a]
Leu^P-(CONH)-Leu, $X = O^-$	56[a]
Leu^P-(CONH)-Leu, $X = NH_2$	40[b]
L-Leu^P	0.23
D-Leu^P	220
L-Phe^P	0.42
D-Phe^P	15.4
Leu^P-H	87
Phe^P-H	59
Bestatin	0.0006[c]
Leu-H	0.06[d]
Leu^B	0.13[e]

pH 8.6, 25°C. Data from Giannousis and Bartlett (1987), unless otherwise indicated.
[a]Mixture of two diastereomers.
[b]Mixture of four diastereomers.
[c]Wilkes and Prescott (1985).
[d]Andersson et al. (1985).
[e]Shenvi (1986).

phonate esters were prepared instead of the phosphonamidates in view of the lability of the latter in the presence of a free α-amino group. In place of the secondary alcohol of bestatin, which may mimic the tetrahedral carbon of the transition state, the carbamoylphosphinates incorporate a tetrahedral phosphorus, as the phosphinate anion as well as neutral amide.

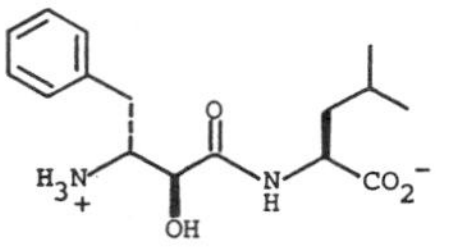

Bestatin 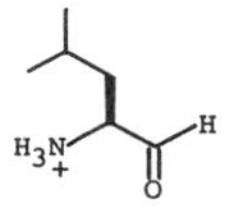   Leu-H 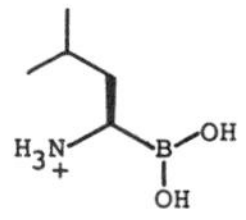   Leu^B

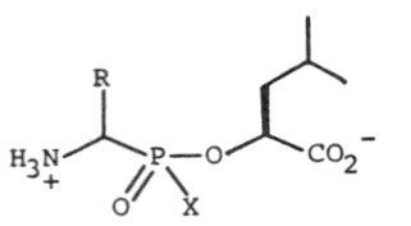

R = iBu: Leu^P-(O)-Leu
R = Bn: Phe^P-(O)-Leu

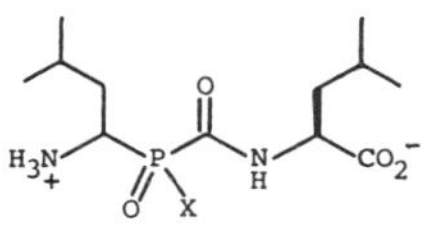

Leu^P-(CONH)-Leu
(X = NH$_2$, O$^-$)

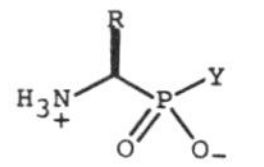

R = iBu, Y = O$^-$: L-Leu^P
R = Bn, Y = O$^-$: L-Phe^P
R = iBu, Y = H: Leu^P-H
R = Bn, Y = H: Phe^P-H

Neither the phosphonate dipeptide analogs nor the phosphorus derivatives similar to bestatin are particularly potent inhibitors of leucine aminopeptidase. In contrast, the simple phosphonic acid analogs of leucine and phenylalanine are good inhibitors of the enzyme ($K_i < 1$ μM). The affinity is strongest for the L-enantiomers, and they proved to be slow binding ($k_{on} \leqslant 500$ M^{-1}s^{-1}). The disparity between the potent inhibition by phosphonates of the classic zinc peptidases and the modest inhibition revealed in Table 5, coupled with the efficacy of leucinal and boroleucine against the serine peptidases, as well as leucine aminopeptidase, suggests that the mechanism of the latter may involve an enzyme-bound nucleophile, rather than direct addition of water to the scissile carbonyl group.

PHOSPHORUS-CONTAINING INHIBITORS OF ASPARTIC PROTEASES

The mechanism of the aspartic proteases, like that of the zinc peptidases addressed above, involves direct addition of water to the scissile carbonyl group. For these enzymes as well, evolutionary or intentional incorporation of a tetrahedral species into an oligopeptide, as a mimic either of the transition state or of the two substrates (peptide plus water), has led to effective inhibitors. Indeed, the most potent inhibitors for the aspartic peptidases have been analogs of the naturally occurring pepsin inhibitor, pepstatin, in which the unusual amino acid statine occupies the P$_1$ and P$_1'$ po-

sitions and presents a secondary hydroxyl group to the catalytic residues in the enzyme active site (Rich 1985). In view of the intermediacy of a tetrahedral adduct in the mechanisms of both the zinc and aspartic peptidases, it appeared likely that tetrahedral phosphorus amino acid analogs should be effective as inhibitors of the latter class as well.

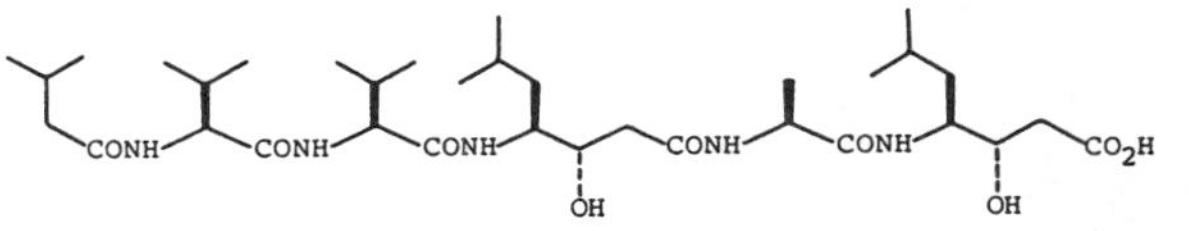

Iva-Val-Val-L-Sta-Ala-L-Sta (Pepstatin)

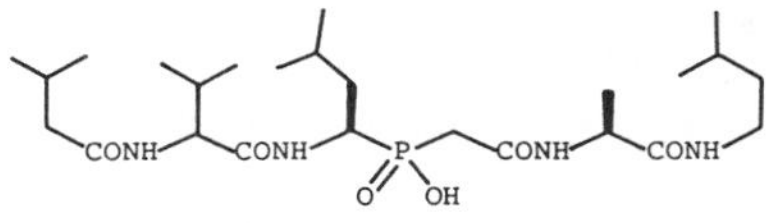

Iva-Val-L-Sta^P-Ala-Iaa

Pepsin

A series of analogs of pepstatin have been investigated by Rich et al. (1985) in order to define the requirements for tight-binding and slow-binding inhibition of pepsin. As indicated in Table 6, the truncated derivative Iva-Val-L-Sta-Ala-Iaa, although not showing the absolute affinity for the enzyme that pepstatin does, nevertheless shows the high affinity and two-step binding mechanism characteristic of the naturally occurring inhibitor.

The "phosphastatine" derivatives listed in Table 6 were synthesized and evaluated as pepsin inhibitors (Bartlett and Kezer 1984). As indicated, the L-derivative of Iva-Val-Sta^P-Ala-Iaa shows not only high affinity, but also unusual kinetic behavior. An initial, reversible complex is formed with a K_D of 7 nM. With time, this complex is converted to a more tightly bound form, whose affinity we have not yet determined accurately ($K_i < 0.07$ nM). Whether this represents a very tight but noncovalent complex or a covalent one has also not been determined, although the fact that the half-life for isomerization of the "loose" to the "tight" complex is on the order of 2 hours makes the former possibility seem remote.

Table 6. Inhibition of Pepsin

Inhibitor	K_D (nM)[a]	K_i (nM)
Iva-D-Sta^P-Ala-Iaa	—	25,000
Iva-L-Sta^P-Ala-Iaa	—	900
Iva-L-Sta-Ala-Iaa	—	350[b]
Iva-Val-D-Sta^P-Ala-Iaa	—	200
Iva-Val-L-Sta^P-Ala-Iaa	7	<0.07
Iva-Val-L-Sta-Ala-Iaa	60	3[b]
Iva-Val-Val-L-Sta-Ala-Sta	13	0.056[b]

pH 3.5, 37°C. Data from Bartlett and Kezer (1984), unless otherwise indicated.
[a]Dash indicates two-step binding not observed.
[b]Rich and Sun (1980); Rich (1985).

Table 7. Inhibition of Penicillopepsin

Inhibitor	K_i (nM)
Iva-Val-Val-Sta-OEt	47[a]
Iva-Val-Val-Sta^P-OEt (pH 4.5)	111[b]
Iva-Val-Val-Sta^P-OEt (pH 3.5)	24[b]
Iva-Val-Val-Sta-Ala-Sta	0.15[a]

[a] Data from Rich (1985).
[b] Data from J.E. Hanson and P.A. Bartlett (unpubl.).

Penicillopepsin

The bacterially derived but mechanistically and structurally related penicillopepsin shows a similar affinity for statine-containing oligopeptides; Iva-Val-Val-Sta-OEt, for example, inhibits this enzyme with a K_i of 47 nM (Rich 1985). Incorporation of phosphastatine into this sequence produces an effective inhibitor; however, the relative effect is considerably less than in the case of pepsin (Table 7). The reduced affinity of penicillopepsin for the phosphastatin derivative can be traced in part to the higher pH at which this enzyme is active in comparison to pepsin. The pK$_a$ of the phosphinic acid is <3; hence, under the conditions of the assay, it is appreciably ionized. In contrast, the actual tetrahedral intermediate resulting from water addition to the enzyme-bound substrate is formally neutral. The fact that the K_i decreases with pH suggests that the enzyme binds only the neutral form of the inhibitor. In contrast to the behavior of the phosphastatine pepsin inhibitor, Iva-Val-Val-Sta^P-OEt shows no unusual binding behavior. Of significant encouragement are the preliminary results of a crystallographic analysis of the complex between the phosphinic acid analog Iva-Val-Val-Sta^P-OEt and penicillopepsin (James et al. 1982; M.N.G. James and A. Sielecki, unpubl.). This investigation has shown that the tetrahedral phosphorus is bound in the active site, as would be expected for a mimic of the tetrahedral intermediate, with the two active-site aspartic acid residues hydrogen-bonded (separately) to the two oxygens of the phosphinic acid moiety. As such, this complex provides a model for the actual transition state or reactive intermediate and support for the indicated mechanism.

CONCLUSIONS

The study of phosphorus-containing peptide analogs has led both to potent inhibitors for a variety of zinc and aspartic peptidases and to insight into some of the details of the enzymatic transformations and of the interactions between these proteins and their ligands. It is also our hope that they will provide an opportunity to elucidate some of the dynamic aspects of ligand-protein association as well, in particular the nature of slow-binding inhibition.

ACKNOWLEDGMENTS

This work was supported by a grant from the National Institutes of Health (CA-22747). We express our appreciation to Professor Brian Matthews and his colleagues for fruitful discussions and their crystallographic studies of the thermolysin inhibitors. We also thank Professor Michael James and his colleagues for their crystallographic studies of our penicillopepsin inhibitor.

REFERENCES

Andersson, L., J. MacNeela, and R. Wolfenden. 1985. Use of secondary isotope effects and varying pH to investigate the mode of binding of inhibitory amino aldehydes by leucine aminopeptidase. *Biochemistry* **24:** 330.

Bartlett, P.A. and W.B. Kezer. 1984. Phosphinic acid dipeptide analogues: Potent, slow-binding inhibitors of aspartic peptidases. *J. Am. Chem. Soc.* **106:** 4282-3.

Bartlett, P.A. and C.K. Marlowe. 1983. Phosphonamidates as transition state analog inhibitors of thermolysin. *Biochemistry* **22:** 4618.

———. 1987a. Evaluation of intrinsic binding energy from a hydrogen bonding group in an enzyme inhibitor. *Science* **235:** 569.

———. 1987b. A possible role for water dissociation in the slow-binding of phosphorus-containing transition state analog inhibitors of thermolysin. *Biochemistry* (in press).

Brouwer, A.C. And J.F. Kirsch. 1982. Investigation of diffusion-limited rates of chymotrypsin reactions by viscosity variation. *Biochemistry* **21:** 1302.

Byers, L.D. and R. Wolfenden. 1973. Binding of the by-product analog benzylsuccinic acid by carboxypeptidase A. *Biochemistry* **12:** 2070.

Delange, R.J. and E.L. Smith. 1971. Leucine aminopeptidase and other N-terminal exopeptidases. In *The enzymes*, 3rd edition (ed. P.D. Boyer), vol. 3, p. 81. Academic Press, New York.

Fersht, A.R., J.-P. Shi, J. Knill-Jones, D.M. Lowe, A.J. Wilkinson, D.M. Blow, P. Brick, P. Carter, M.M.Y. Waye, and G. Winter. 1985. Hydrogen bonding and biological specificity analysed by protein engineering. *Nature* **314:** 235.

Frick, L., R. Wolfenden, E. Smal, and D.C. Baker. 1986. Transition-state stabilization by adenosine deaminase: Structural studies of its inhibitory complex with deoxycoformycin. *Biochemistry* **25:** 1616.

Galardy, R.E. 1982. Inhibition of angiotensin converting enzyme by phosphoramidates and polyphosphates. *Biochemistry* **21:** 5777.

Galardy, R.E. and D. Grobelny. 1983. Inhibition of collagenase from *Clostridium histolyticum* by phosphoric and phosphonic acid amides. *Biochemistry* **22:** 4556.

Galardy, R.E., V. Kontoyiannidou-Ostrem, and Z.P. Kortylewicz. 1983. Inhibition of angiotensin converting enzyme by phosphonic amides and phosphonic acids. *Biochemistry* **22:** 1990.

Giannousis, P.P. and P.A. Bartlett. 1987. Phosphorus amino acid analogs as inhibitors of leucine aminopeptidase. *J. Med. Chem.* (in press).

Hofmann, W. and M. Rottenberg. 1980. A transition state analogous organophosphate inhibitor of carboxypeptidase A. In *Enzyme inhibitors* (ed. U. Brodbeck), p. 19. Verlag Chemie, Basel.

Holden, H.M., D.E. Tronrud, A.F. Monzingo, L.H. Weaver, and B.W. Matthews. 1987. Slow and fast-binding inhibitors of thermolysin display different modes of binding: A crystallographic analysis of extended phosphonamidate transition-state analogs. *Biochemistry* (in press).

Holmquist, B. 1977. Characterization of the "microprotease" from *Bacillus cereus*. A zinc neutral endoprotease. *Biochemistry* **16:** 4591.

Jacobsen, N.E. and P.A. Bartlett. 1981a. A phosphorus-containing dipeptide analog as an inhibitor of carboxypeptidase A. *J. Am. Chem. Soc.* **103:** 654.

———. 1981b. Phosphonate inhibitors of carboxypeptidase A. *ACS Symp. Ser.* **171:** 221.

James, M.N.G., A. Sielecki, F. Salituro, D.H. Rich, and T. Hofmann. 1982. Conformational flexibility in the active sites of aspartyl proteinases revealed by a pepstatin fragment binding to penicillopepsin. *Proc. Natl. Acad. Sci.* **79:** 6137.

Jones, W. and R. Wolfenden. 1986. How rare are the covalent hydrates of purine ribonucleoside and nicotinamide? A method for estimating positions of highly unfavorable equilibria. *J. Am. Chem. Soc.* **108:** 7444.

Kam, C.-M., N. Nishino, and J.C. Powers. 1979. Inhibition of thermolysin and carboxypeptidase A by phosphoramidates. *Biochemistry* **18:** 3032.

Komiyama, T., H. Suda, T. Aoyagi, T. Takeuchi, H. Umezawa, K. Fujimoto, and S. Umezawa. 1975. Inhibitory effect of phosphoramidon and its analogs on thermolysin. *Arch. Biochem. Biophys.* **171:** 727.

Mookhtiar, K.A., F. Wang, and H.E. Van Wart. 1986. Functional constituents of the active site of human neutrophil collagenase. *Arch. Biochem. Biophys.* **246:** 645.

Mookhtiar, K.A., C.K. Marlowe, P.A. Bartlett, and H.E. Van Wart. 1987. Phosphonamidate inhibitors of human neutrophil collagenase. *Biochemistry* **26:** 1962.

Morgan, G. and J.S. Fruton. 1978. Kinetics of the action of thermolysin on peptide substrates. *Biochemistry* **17:** 3562.

Morihara, K. and H. Tsuzuki. 1970. Thermolysin: Kinetic study with oligopeptides. *Eur. J. Biochem.* **15:** 374.

Morrison, J.F. and C.T. Walsh. 1987. The behavior and significance of slow-binding enzyme inhibitors. *Adv. Enzymol. Relat. Areas Mol. Biol.* (in press).

Nishino, N. and J.C. Powers. 1979. Design of potent reversible inhibitors for thermolysin. Peptides containing zinc coordinating ligands and their use in affinity chromatography. *Biochemistry* **18:** 4340.

Ondetti, M.A., M.E. Condon, J. Ried, E.F. Sabo, H.S. Cheung, and D.W. Cushman. 1979. Design of potent and specific inhibitors of carboxypeptidases A and B. *Biochemistry* **18:** 1427.

Petrillo, E.W., Jr., D.W. Cushman, M.E. Duggan, J.E. Heikes, D.S. Karanewsky, M.A. Ondetti, J.E. O'Reilly, G.C. Rovnyak, J. Schwartz, E.R. Spitzmuller, and N.-Y. Wang. 1983. Angiotensin-converting enzyme inhibitors: phosphinic acid analogs of acyl-tripeptides: In *Proceedings of the 8th American Peptide Symposium* (ed. V.J. Hruby and D.H. Rich), p. 541. Pierce Chemical Company, Rockford, Illinois.

Rich, D.H. 1985. Pepstatin-derived inhibitors of aspartic proteinases. A close look at an apparent transition-state analogue inhibitor. *J. Med. Chem.* **28:** 263.

Rich, D.H and E.T.O. Sun. 1980. Mechanism of inhibition of pepsin by pepstatin. Effect of inhibitor structure on dissociation constant and time-dependent inhibition. *Biochem. Pharmacol.* **29:** 2205.

Shenvi, A.B. 1986. α-Aminoboronic acid derivatives: Effective inhibitors of aminopeptidases. *Biochemistry* **25:** 1286.

Stark, G.R. and P.A. Bartlett. 1984. Design and use of potent, specific enzyme inhibitors. *Pharmacol. Therap.* **23:** 45.

Thompson, R.C. 1973. Use of peptide aldehydes to generate transition-state analogs of elastase. *Biochemistry* **12:** 47.

Thorsett, E.D., E.E. Harris, E.E. Peterson, W.J. Greenlee, A.A. Patchett, E.H. Ulm, and T.C. Wassil. 1982. Phosphorus containing inhibitors of angiotensin converting enzyme. *Proc. Natl. Acad. Sci.* **79:** 2176.

Tronrud, D.E., H.M. Holden, and B.W. Matthews. 1987. Structures of two thermolysin inhibitor complexes that differ by a single hydrogen bond. *Science* **235:** 571.

Vencill, C.F., D. Rasnick, K.V. Crumley, N. Nishino, and J.C. Powers. 1985. *Clostridium histrolyticum* collagenase: Development of new thio ester, fluorogenic, and depsipeptide substrates and new inhibitors. *Biochemistry* **24:** 3149.

Westerik, J.O. and R. Wolfenden. 1972. Aldehydes as inhibitors of papain. *J. Biol. Chem.* **247:** 8195.

Wilkes, S.H. and J.M. Prescott. 1985. The slow, tight binding of bestatin and amastatin to aminopeptidases. *J. Biol. Chem.* **260:** 13154.

Wolfenden, R. 1976. Transition state analog inhibitors and enzyme catalysis. *Annu. Rev. Biophys. Bioeng.* **5:** 271.

Catalytic Antibodies

A. TRAMONTANO,* K. JANDA,* A.D. NAPPER,[†] S.J. BENKOVIC,[†] AND R.A. LERNER*
*Department of Molecular Biology, Research Institute of Scripps Clinic, La Jolla, California 92037;
[†]Department of Chemistry, Pennsylvania State University, University Park, Pennsylvania 16802

Immunology is a science of binding. Historically, researchers were interested in the antigenicity of organic compounds as a means of understanding the specificity of immunological reactions (Lerner 1984). More recently, attention has turned to the molecular and genetic mechanisms by which the vast number of different binding specificities is achieved. There are about 10^8 primary binding specificities in the immunological repertoire, and each can generate, by a process of somatic mutation, at least 10^4 different antibodies during maturation of an immune response. During the induction of a response, the concentration of antigen decreases while the concentration of antibody increases. Insofar as the system is selective and antigen-driven, the decreasing concentration of antigen causes the system to drive toward higher binding energy, and during a response, the equilibrium constants for a given antigen can span ten orders of magnitude ($K_{eq} = 10^4$–10^{14}).

This system, with its diversity of binding specificities and affinities, has the potential to be harnessed for applications beyond the simple binding that has been understood as its essence for over 100 years. Essentially, one would like to use the binding energy of an antibody as an enzyme would—to induce chemical transformations. During the last several years, we have been interested in the problem of developing catalytic antibodies (Lerner 1984; Tramontano et al. 1986a,b). This research has as its guidelines the principles by which natural enzymes are thought to increase the rate of chemical transformations. The underlying idea is to design antigens that are expressive of chemical mechanisms so that the induced antibodies perform the reaction implicit in the antigen design.

Ester Hydrolysis

Consider the mechanism of ester hydrolysis reactions. Like any chemical transformation, these proceed along a reaction coordinate with the most unstable species, the transition state at the peak of the energy profile (Fig. 1). According to the Pauling principle of catalysis, one way in which enzymes increase the rate of chemical reactions is by using their binding energy to stabilize selectively reactants at their transition state and thereby allowing a transformation to proceed via a low-energy pathway. By this logic, an antibody that might act as an enzyme should have its maximum binding energy directed toward the transition state. But the immunological partner for the antibody is its antigen. How then should the antigen be designed to elicit a recognition for the transition state of ester hydrolysis? Ester hydrolysis is an example of an acyl transfer reaction (in this case to water) and proceeds from a planar SP^2-hybridized carbon in the ground state through a tetrahedral SP^3-hybridization in the transition state. Along with this change in geometry, there is a developing electrostatic polarization around the acyl group. The transition state is a fleeting intermediate with a lifetime of about 10^{-13} seconds and therefore does not exist on an immunogenic time scale. However, the features of the transition state can be mimicked by a

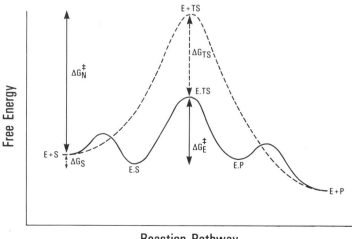

Figure 1. Reaction coordinate for a hypothetical uncatalyzed and catalyzed reaction. The catalyst allows the reaction to proceed by a lower-energy pathway.

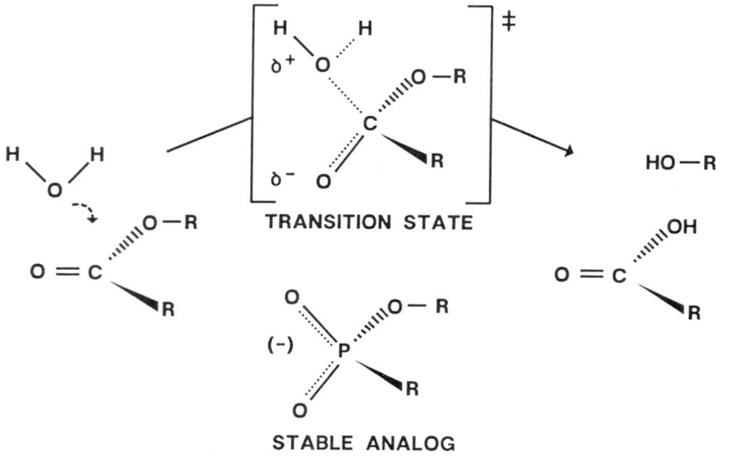

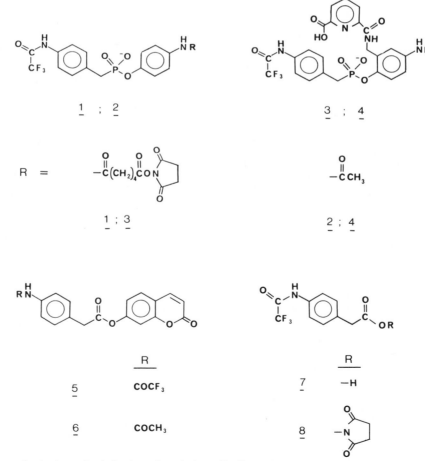

Figure 2. A phosphonate ester is an analog having the developing charge and tetrahedral geometry of the transition state (‡) for hydrolysis of an ester.

stable analog. One possibility for this is an organophosphonate structure (Fig. 2).

A corollary to the Pauling principle catalysis predicts that such a transition state mimic should be a good inhibitor for the enzyme that catalyzes the implicit reaction (Pauling 1948). In fact, phosphonates and phosphonamidates have been shown to be potent inhibitors of some esterases and amidases (Wolfenden 1972, 1978; Lienhard 1973). Our initial studies used aryl phosphonates as antigenic mimics for the transition state of ester hydrolysis (Tramontano et al. 1986a,b). We chose aryl phosphonates in order to direct binding interactions toward the phenolic and benzylic rings in the stereochemical orientation defined by the phosphonyl group. The particular antigen used is shown in Figure 3.

Figure 3. Antigens for induction of catalytic antibodies and substrate for assay of their activity.

The pyridine dicarboxylic acid appendage was included in the initial construct to provide a site for coordination of a metal in later experiments. To detect esterase activity, we designed a substrate (Fig. 3) that allowed a spectrophotometric assay. The acyl portion of the substrate is homologous to a portion of the antigen, and the phenolic coumarin is fluorescent when the ester bond is cleaved. A number of the monoclonal antibodies obtained against the antigen shown in Figure 3 reacted with the coumarin ester, but the reaction was stoichiometric. A probable mechanism of this reaction was proposed in which an imidazole side chain of histidine acts as a nucleophile in an acyl transfer reaction (Tramontano et al. 1986a,b). The main problem with this reaction is that the mechanistic implication of the phosphonate antigen is for water or hydroxide anion as the nucleophile, and replacement by imidazole violates this design principle. This led us to suggest that perhaps the labile coumarin ester is not the appropriate substrate, and once a better substrate is found, this same antibody would be truly hydrolytic. Assuming that there is an imidazole in the binding pocket of the antibody, what is the basis for its participation as a nucleophilic group in this reaction? Classic studies on the mechanism of imidazole catalysis of ester hydrolysis reveal a change in mechanism with changing ester structure. Esters with good leaving groups are hydrolyzed with nucleophilic catalysis by imidazole, whereas

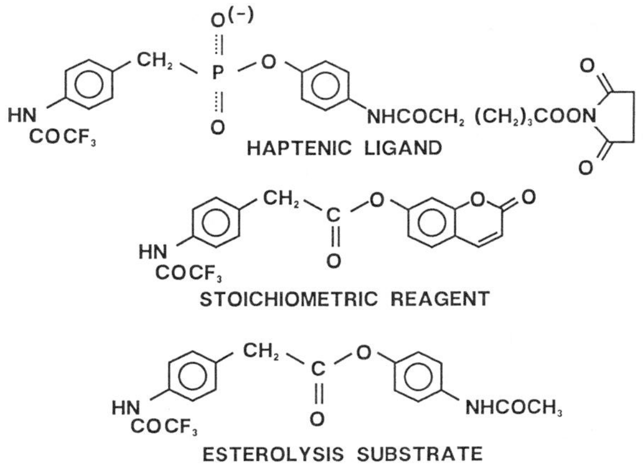

Figure 4. Structural relationships between the immunizing phosphonate antigen, the stoichiometric reagent with the coumarin leaving group, and the catalytic substrate with the acetaminophen leaving group.

those with poor leaving groups proceed by a general base mechanism of catalysis. Thus, as the pK_a of the leaving group increases, the activation energy for collapse of the tetrahedral intermediate into products increases until the expulsion of imidazole to return to ester is much more favorable. Ester hydrolysis may still be catalyzed, but the role of imidazole changes from a nucleophilic to a general base catalyst. Thus, it seemed

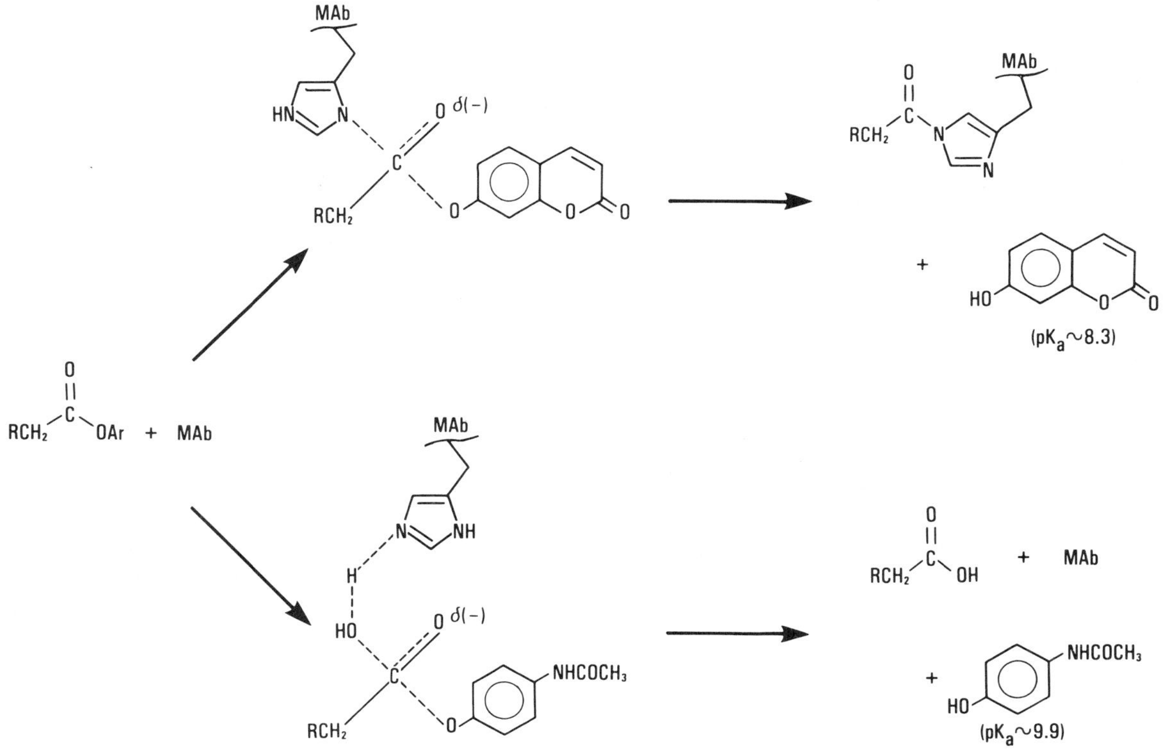

Figure 5. A proposed scheme to account for the divergent chemistry observed in the reaction of an anti-4 monoclonal antibody (MAb) with carboxylic esters 5 and 7. A histidine residue in the combining site is presumed to act as a nucleophilic (upper pathway) or general base (lower pathway) catalyst during the formation and breakdown of a tetrahedral intermediate. The ester with a good leaving group reacts by the upper pathway, since the rate-limiting step, formation of the intermediate, is facile. This pathway cannot be used by the ester with a poor leaving group, since the rate-limiting step, breakdown of the intermediate, is not catalyzed relative to the analogous step in the lower pathway, which may be general-based-catalyzed.

that for the antibody to affect a noncovalent mechanism of catalysis, the leaving group should have a higher pK_a. This would mean that the ester bond is more stable to cleavage. To best exploit the binding interaction with the antibody, the substrate should also be more congruent with the transition state analog. An acetamidophenyl ester, whose relationship to the coumarin ester and the antigen are given in Figure 4, seemed appropriate (Tramontano et al. 1986b). Although these substrates are equivalent in their acyl portion, they differ in the leaving group structure. The

coumarin ester has the phenolic character of the antigen, but the lactone ring system of coumarin shows poor homology with the disubstituted phenol of the hapten. However, the acetamidophenyl ester has homology in both the benzylic and phenolic portions of the antigen. This ester proved to be a good substrate for the antibody, and true catalytic hydrolysis resulted (Fig. 5). As with the coumarin ester, the reaction was competitively inhibited by the antigens or transition state analog. The kinetic parameters of the reaction are shown in Table 1.

Table 1. Kinetic Parameters for Hydrolysis of Carboxylic Esters by Monoclonal Antibody and by Hog Liver Esterase

Substrate	Antibody (6D4) ($t_{1/2}$ min)	Esterase ($t_{1/2}$ min)	K_{uncat}[a] (10^5 sec^{-1})
7	16 ± 3	4 ± 1	2.8
8	55 ± 5	52 ± 5	3.8
9	*	4 ± 1	0.25
10	*	<2[b]	1.63
11	*	5 ± 1	6.10

Hydrolysis of carboxylic esters by monoclonal antibody (from hybridoma 6D4) and by hog liver esterase (Sigma, E.C.3.1.1.1) determined by HPLC on an analytical RP-C18 column (Vy-dac 218TP54) with isocratic elution (65:35 water:acetonitrile; 0.1% trifluoroacetic acid) at a flow rate of 1.0 ml/min and detector set to 245 nm. The initial substrate concentration was 5 μM and that of internal standard (acetophenone) was set at 10 μM in 50 mM phosphate buffer at pH 8.0. Retention times (minutes): acetophenone, 5.0; 7, 8.3; 8, 6.7; 9, 4.1; 10, 11.1 (40% acetonitrile elution); 11, 8.2. The antibody concentration was 15 μg/ml (0.1 μM) and that of esterase was 5.5 μg/ml. The reaction mixtures were kept at 23°C, and aliquots were analyzed at intervals of 2–20 min. Three or more determinations were used to plot a curve from which the half-life of the reaction was estimated. Asterisks indicate that the ester was not consumed faster than the background rate of hydrolysis.
[a]Rate constants were determined spectrophotometrically (at 245 nm) by measuring initial rates at five concentrations of ester.
[b]Reaction rate was too rapid to be measured accurately by HPLC.

Haptens and substrates used in the production and assay of monoclonal antibodies with esterolytic properties. The identity of substituents R and R' are as follows: (1, 3, and 7) R = NHCOCF$_3$, R' = NHCOCH$_3$; (2 and 4) R = NHCOCF$_3$, R' = NHCO(CH$_2$)$_4$COON(COCH$_2$)$_2$; (8) R = NHCOCF$_3$, R' = NHCO(CH$_2$)$_2$COOH; (9) R, R' = NHCOCH$_3$; (10) R = NHCOCF$_3$, R' = H; (11) R = NHCOCH$_3$, R' = NHCOCF$_3$.

Although the rates are slower than those of some natural enzymes, they are still substantial, and one cannot be certain that these are the best substrates. Just as there is diversity in antibodies, the mechanisms by which antibodies catalyze a particular chemical reaction may differ. In addition, one can expect that as the diversity of the mechanism begins to match the diversity of binding, large variations in the rates of reaction will be observed.

Specificity of Catalytic Antibodies

The hallmark of the immune system is its exquisite binding specificity. One would therefore expect that this specificity would be reflected in substrate selectivity for catalytic antibodies. This is indeed the case for the catalytic antibodies studied to date (Table 2).

Catalysis of "Stereospecific Reactions" by Antibodies

As in other proteins, the binding pockets of antibodies are asymmetric. The system we selected offered another test of the enzyme-like qualities of antibodies, namely, a choice between two reaction pathways that in the absence of a chiral reagent would be equal in free energy (enantiomeric) but in the presence of the antibody should be unequal in free energy (diastereomeric) and lead to a stereospecific cyclization. We constructed an antigen for the induction of antibodies capable of a cyclization by ester exchange (Napper et al. 1987). An amide derivative of the phosphonic ester 2-phenoxy-2-oxo-6-(aminomethyl)-1,2-oxaphosphorinane resembles a product-like intermediate along the route of cyclization of the corresponding ester substrate (Fig. 6). The chirality at the carbinol atom introduces a stereochemical choice for the antibody that catalyzes this reaction.

Several monoclonal antibodies were obtained to the diastereomeric transition state analog, and 24 of these were characterized for binding and catalysis. One antibody, selected as a potential catalyst, was studied in more detail. The rates of phenol release from its ester substrate in the presence of antibody (24B11) were determined spectrophotometrically. The initial rates as a function of substrate concentration obeyed Michaelis-Menten kinetics. The kinetic parameters for this reac-

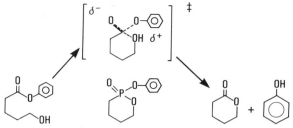

Figure 6. Conversion of a hydroxy ester to a δ-lactone proceeds through a cyclic, product-like, transition state. A cyclic phosphonate ester is a stable representation for this.

tion, indicated a rate acceleration of approximately 167-fold. This degree of rate acceleration is consistent with the reduction of rotational entropy by antibody binding. A striking characteristic of this reaction is its cessation at approximately 50% completion (Fig. 7).

To rule out the possibility of a coincidental product inhibition, a second aliquot of substrate was added to the completed reaction solution, resulting in a second depletion of approximately 50% of the freshly added substrate. It seemed that the antibody catalyzed cyclization of one enantiomer, resulting in a kinetic resolution. To confirm this, the lactone produced by the antibody was isolated and its nuclear magnetic resonance (NMR) spectrum was measured in the presence of chiral lanthanide shift reagent. Clear separation of each of the three single pNMRs for the protons of the CH_3CONH substituent and side chain CH_2 of the lactone (Fig. 8) into two proton signals was achieved for both the antibody-generated and chemically synthesized samples of 5. A portion of the spectrum is shown in Figure 8. The equivalence of peak areas for the synthetic sample, as expected for a racemate, validates the analytical method and indicates that the observed enantiomeric excess (% major peak − % minor peak) generated by the antibody-catalyzed cyclization is 66 ± 4%. Correcting for spontaneous cyclization of the substrate under these conditions, the antibody-catalyzed cyclization of 1 gives one enantiomer in 94 ± 8% excess, given the limits of our present determinations. Experiments with the separate enantiomers should permit a more precise measure of this enantiomeric differentiation which probably is close to absolute.

Table 2. Kinetic Parameters for Hydrolysis of Esters by Monoclonal Antibody

Substrate	K_m $(10^6 M)$	K_i $(10^7 M)$	V_{max} $(10^9 M sec^{-1})$	K_{cat} $(10^2 sec^{-1})$	k_{cat}/k_{uncat}
7	1.90 ± 0.20	1.60 ± 0.40	2.2 ± 0.2	2.7 ± 0.2	960
8	0.62 ± 0.05	0.65 ± 0.25	1.0 ± 0.1	0.8 ± 0.1	210

A Perkin-Elmer λ 4B spectrophotometer, equipped with thermostatted cell holder, was used to measure absorption changes at 245 nm. Cells containing the substrate at concentrations of 0.5–50 μM in phosphate buffer (50 mM, pH 8.0) were preequilibrated at 25°C. The concentration of active immunoglobulin G in a stock solution was found by reacting with coumarin ester 5 and measuring the yield of hydroxycoumarin by fluorescence (Tramontano et al. 1986b). The kinetic run was initiated by addition of an aliquot of the antibody stock solution (in 50 mM phosphate buffer, pH 8.0) calculated to give 100 mM immunoglobulin G. The mixture was allowed to equilibrate for 2–3 min, and the rate was then measured during the subsequent 10 min. The absorption change for complete hydrolysis (Δε 4500) was determined by treatment with esterase. Kinetic parameters were obtained from Lineweaver-Burk plots. Inhibition constants were determined from a plot of the slopes with at least four concentrations of 3. The data were analyzed by linear regression.

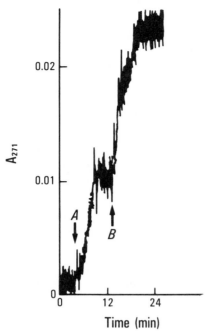

Figure 7. Cyclization of *1* by monoclonal antibody, 24B11. The reaction was followed by monitoring the absorbance at 271 nm due to release of phenol. Antibody (20 μM in 25 mM phosphate buffer, pH 7.0) was preincubated at 25°C. An aliquot of *1* (3.34 mM in phosphate buffer, pH 7.0), calculated to give a 40 μM solution of *1*, was added at points *A* and *B*. The average observed absorbance increase was shown to correspond to consumption of 49 ± 13% of *1* present relative to a phenol standard.

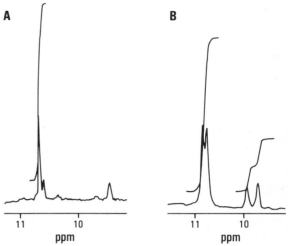

Figure 8. Part of the H NMR (360 MHz, CDC1$_3$) spectrum for the two enantiomers of *5* in the presence of ~1 equivalent of tris[heptafluoropropylhydroxymethylene-*d*-camphorato] europium (III). Chemical shifts are shown in ppm downfield from TMS. Peak assignments and the chemical shift differences between enantiomers ($\Delta\Delta\delta$) are as follows: (*A*) δ 9.45, 9.68 (one of C*H*$_2$NHAc, $\Delta\Delta\delta$ = 0.23), 10.60, and 10.67 (NHCOC*H*$_3$, $\Delta\Delta\delta$ = 0.07); (*B*) δ 9.71, 9.94 (one of C*H*$_2$NHAc, $\Delta\Delta\delta$ = 0.023), 10.74, and 10.82 (NHCOC*H*$_3$, $\Delta\Delta\delta$ = 0.08). The lactone *5* was obtained by cyclization of ester *1* for 55 min at 25°C in 25 mM phosphate buffer, pH 7, in the presence of antibody 24B11 (spectrum A) or in the absence of antibody (spectrum B). Antibody was removed by Centricon filtration, and *5* was isolated from the filtrate by CH$_2$Cl$_2$ extraction, followed by column chromatography on silica. The initial ratio of *1* to 24B11 was 9.2 mM:115 μM.

This work provides an example of an antibody-catalyzed cyclization reaction, but more significantly, a demonstration that the stereochemical control of a reaction course so typical of enzymes extends to these catalysts as well. These experiments further the vision that general catalysts from immunological sources can be tailor-made for reactions that require chemical stereospecificity.

CONCLUDING COMMENTS

This work demonstrates that the binding energy of antibodies can be harnessed for chemical synthesis. We foresee that other chemical reactions will be addressed and that catalytic antibodies should apply to any chemical reaction for which a credible mechanism can be visualized and an appropriate transition state analog synthesized. The real question is how best to proceed at this incipient stage of the research given the vast possibilities. Our approach is to address some important chemical and biochemical problems using catalytic antibodies. Thus, we are currently turning our attention to antibodies capable of hydrolyzing amide bonds as well as those that should catalyze important synthetic reactions. A complementary part of current experiments is to learn how to control the kinds of amino acid side chains that an antibody will employ in response to a certain antigenic challenge. For example, an antibody

may stabilize point charges on an antigen by using side chains in the binding pocket of opposite charge. One can thus think about designing antigens with geometrically spaced point charges so that a geometry of opposite charges is reflected in the antibody-binding pocket. Such a constellation of negative charges might be expected to be able to coordinate an oxidized metal ion which would be important for various catalytic applications.

REFERENCES

Lerner, R.A. 1984. Antibodies of predetermined specificity in biology and medicine. *Adv. Immunol.* **36:** 1.

Lienhard, G.E. 1973. Enzymatic catalysis and transition-state theory. *Science* **180:** 149.

Napper, A.D., S.J. Benkovic, A. Tramontano, and R.A. Lerner. 1987. A stereospecific cyclization catalyzed by an antibody. *Science* **237:** 1041.

Pauling, L. 1948. Chemical achievement and hope for the future. *Am. Sci.* **36:** 51.

Tramontano, A., K.D. Janda, and R.A. Lerner. 1986a. Catalytic antibodies. *Science* **234:** 1566.

———. 1986b. Chemical reactivity at an antibody-binding site elicited by mechanistic design of a synthetic antigen. *Proc. Natl. Acad. Sci.* **83:** 6736.

Wolfenden, R. 1972. Analog approaches to structure of transition-state in enzyme reactions. *Accts. Chem. Res.* **5:** 10.

———. 1978. In *Transition states in biochemical processes* (ed. R.D. Gandour and R.L. Schowen), part IV. Plenum Press, New York.

Antibody Catalysis by Transition State Stabilization

S.J. POLLACK AND P.G. SCHULTZ

Department of Chemistry, University of California, Berkeley, California 94720

A key element in the evolution of enzymatic catalysts is the development of selective ligand-binding sites. The immune system is capable of producing antibodies, which, like enzymes, bind both macromolecules and small synthetic molecules with high specificities and high affinities (Landsteiner 1944; Pressman and Grossberg 1968; Nisonoff et al. 1975). Immunoglobulin combining sites, although lacking the ability to catalyze selective chemical transformations can, unlike enzymes, be rapidly and selectively generated against virtually any molecule of interest (Goding 1986). Consequently, the development of strategies for introducing catalytic activity into the combining sites of antibodies may enable us to generate rationally enzyme-like catalysts with tailored specificities and catalytic properties. We are currently exploring three such strategies: (1) generation of antibodies that selectively stabilize the rate-limiting transition state on a reaction pathway, (2) generation of antibodies that bind and orient substrates in a reactive conformation for intra- or intermolecular reactions, and (3) selective chemical modification of antibody combining sites with synthetic catalytic groups.

Recently, we reported that antibodies elicited to an aryl phosphonate transition state analog selectively catalyze the hydrolysis of the corresponding aryl carbonate (Jacobs et al. 1987). The antibody-catalyzed reaction is characterized by high selectivity, a rate acceleration of 1.7×10^4 above the uncatalyzed reaction, and is first order in hydroxide ion. Moreover, chemical and spectroscopic probes suggest the presence of lysine and tyrosine residues in the antibody combining sites that might act to stabilize the transition state arising via attack of a combining-site-accessible hydroxide ion. These results, although consistent with the notion that antibody combining sites that selectively stabilize the transition state configuration may act as catalysts, do not rule out other mechanisms of catalysis. To define more precisely the nature of antibody-catalyzed reactions, both as a test of Pauling's notion of enzymatic catalysis (Pauling 1948) and as a guide to the design of other catalytic antibodies, we have explored the chemistry of the structurally and genetically well-characterized phosphorylcholine (PC)-binding antibodies (Pollack et al. 1986).

Importantly, this class of antibodies, specific for PC monoesters and diesters, has been characterized with regard to biomolecular structure (Segal et al. 1974; Padlan 1977; Satow et al. 1986), ligand-binding specificity and kinetics (Leon and Young 1971; Pollet et al. 1974; Goetze and Richards 1977, 1978; Bennett and

Glaudemans 1979), and the genetics of antibody expression (Crews et al. 1981; Perlmutter et al. 1984). Inspection of the heavy-chain variable sequences of over 25 PC-binding antibodies reveals a high degree of sequence homology (Gearhart et al. 1981). Moreover, the X-ray crystal structure of a representative PC-binding antibody, the Fab fragment of McPC 603 complexed to PC, has been solved to 2.7-Å resolution (Segal et al. 1974; Satow et al. 1986). In a previous report, we demonstrated that the PC-specific antibody MOPC 167, which binds the transition state analog 4-nitrophenylphosphorylcholine, selectively catalyzes the hydrolysis of the corresponding choline carbonate (Pollack et al. 1986). We report here the properties of a second PC-specific antibody and discuss these properties in relation to the mechanism of the antibody-catalyzed reaction.

MATERIALS AND METHODS

Antibody purification. MOPC 167, T15, and McPC 603 IgA antibodies were purified from ascites fluid by reduction with 5 mM dithiothreitol (DTT), followed by alkylation with iodoacetamide and affinity chromatography on glycyltyrosine-(4-azo-phenylphosphorylcholine)-derivatized Sepharose CL-4B (Chesebro and Metzger 1972). Affinity-purified antibody was then dialyzed exhaustively against assay buffer and judged to be homogeneous by SDS-PAGE (Laemmli 1970). Fab fragments of MOPC 167 and T15 were prepared from the antibodies by treating with papain (Anglister et al. 1984) in the presence of 1 mM DTT. The Fab fragments were purified by affinity chromatography as described above and were judged to be homogeneous by SDS-PAGE.

Substrate synthesis. 4-Nitrophenylphosphorylcholine (2) was purchased from Sigma. 4-Nitrophenyl N-trimethylammonioethyl carbonate chloride (1) was prepared by treating 4-nitrophenylchloroformate with choline chloride (one equivalent) and pyridine (one equivalent) in dry acetonitrile. After 12 hours, the precipitated product was filtered off and washed with acetonitrile. Recrystallization from acetonitrile afforded 1 as a white solid: mp 165–166°C; IR (KBr pellet) 3005, 1755, 1620, 1592, 1518, 1490, 1350, 1310, 1255, 1210 cm^{-1}; ^{1}H NMR (250 MHz, D$_2$O) δ 3.07 (s, 9H and t, 2H, J = 1.9 Hz), 3.67 (t, 2H, J = 2.2 Hz), 7.34 (d, 2H, J = 7.0 Hz), 8.20 (d, 2H, J = 7.0 Hz), ^{13}C NMR (D$_2$O) δ 56.2, 65.0, 66.6, 124.5, 128.0, 148.0, 154.8, 157.3; analysis calculated for C$_{12}$H$_{17}$ClN$_2$O$_5$: C 47.28,

H 5.58, Cl 11.69, N 9.19; found: C 47.41, H 5.63, Cl 11.64, N 9.08.

2-Nitrophenyl *N*-trimethylammonioethyl carbonate chloride (*5*) was prepared from 2-nitrophenylchloroformate and choline chloride in an analogous fashion to the above preparation of *1*. 4-Nitrophenyl *N*-trimethylammonio (1-methyl)-ethyl carbonate iodide (*3*) was prepared by treating *N*-trimethyl-2-ammonio-1-propanol iodide with 4-nitrophenylchloroformate as described above for *1*. The reaction mixture was concentrated to an orange solid. The crude product was triturated with ethanol to give pure *3* as an off-white solid: mp 166–167°C; analysis calculated for $C_{13}H_{19}IN_2O_5$: C 38.05, H 4.63, N 6.83; found: C 37.84, H 4.65, N 6.65.

Ethyl 4-nitrophenyl carbonate (*4*) was prepared by heating 4-nitrophenylchloroformate in ethanol at reflux in the presence of pyridine (one equivalent). The volatiles were removed in vacuo, and the residue was purified by silica gel flash chromatography eluting with methylene chloride to give *4*: mp 54–55°C; analysis calculated for $C_9H_9NO_5$: C 51.18, H 4.27, N 6.64; found: C 51.05, H 4.25, N 6.63.

Assay conditions. The rates of hydrolysis of carbonate substrates in the presence (k_{obs}) and absence (k_{un}) of 2–13 μM antibody were determined by monitoring the increase in absorbance at 400 nm due to 4-nitrophenolate ion release (412 nm for 2-nitrophenolate). Measurements were made in 25 mM NaCl, 25 mM Tris-HCl buffer (pH 7.0) at 30°C. Protein molarity was determined by absorbance at 280 nm with the extinction coefficient ($E_{0.1\%}$) = 1.37 and a molecular weight of 150,000 for IgA. Reactions were initiated by addition of 10 μl of a substrate solution (in CH_3CN, diluted from a 50 mM stock solution in CH_3CN with 1% H_2O, prepared fresh weekly) to 0.5 ml equilibrated reaction medium. Kinetic constants were determined according to the method of initial rates. Hydroxide ion dependence was determined at 30°C in 50 mM Tris-HCl by dialyzing the antibody against buffer of the appropriate pH prior to the assays. K_i values were determined for 4-nitrophenylphosphorylcholine *2* by Dixon plots (Dixon 1953) at 100 μM carbonate *1* for MOPC 167 and 500 μM *1* for T15. Stopped-flow spectrophotometry was carried out in 25 mM NaCl, 25 mM Tris-HCl buffer at 17°C, using a model RA401 Union Giken spectrophotometer linked to On Line Instrument Systems software. The dead time of the instrument was 1 msec.

Chemical modification. Protein modification reactions were carried out with 5–10 μM antibody in the presence or absence of 50 mM 4-nitrophenylphosphorylcholine *2*. Arginine modification was carried out with 500 equivalents of 1,2-cyclohexanedione (Patthy and Smithl 1975); lysine modification, with 3000 equivalents of succinic anhydride (Freedman et al. 1968); tyrosine modification, with 500 equivalents of tetranitromethane (Sokolovsky et al. 1966); and histidine modification, with 700 equivalents of diethyl-

pyrocarbonate (Holbrook and Ingram 1973). Affinity labeling with 4-diazonium phenylphosphorylcholine (3 equivalents) was carried out as described by Chesebro and Metzger (1972). After each modfication reaction, the antibody samples were dialyzed exhaustively against assay buffer, except in the case of the 1,2-cyclohexanedione reaction, which was dialyzed against borate buffer to stabilize the arginine adduct (Patthy and Smithl 1975).

RESULTS

Immunoglobulins T15 and MOPC 167 Catalyze the Hydrolysis of Carbonate *1*

The PC-binding immunoglobulins MOPC 167 and T15 were purified from ascites fluid, after mild reduction, by affinity chromatography on glycyl tyrosine-(4-azophenylphosphorylcholine)-derivatized Sepharose CL-4B (Chesebro and Metzger 1972). Antibody was judged to be homogeneous by SDS-PAGE.

The rates of hydrolysis of carbonate *1* in the presence (k_{obs}) and absence (k_{un}) of MOPC 167 and T15 were determined as a function of substrate concentration (Fig. 1). Carbonate hydrolysis was monitored spectrophotometrically in 25 mM NaCl, 25 mM Tris-HCl buffer (pH 7.0) at 30°C by following the increase in absorbance at 400 nm due to nitrophenolate ion release. Both immunoglobulins were found to catalyze the hydrolysis of carbonate *1* with kinetics consistent with the scheme:

$$[\text{Ig}] + [1] \rightleftharpoons [\text{Ig} \cdot 1] \xrightarrow{k_{cat}} [\text{Ig}] + \text{products}$$

The value of the catalytic constant (k_{cat}) and the Michaelis constant (K_m) were found to be 0.40 min^{-1} and 208 μM for MOPC 167 and 0.32 min^{-1} and 708 μM, respectively, for T15. Preliminary results suggest that the antibody McPC 603 is also catalytic. Stopped-flow experiments were carried out in the presence of 5.3 μM MOPC 167 and 2.5 mM *p*-nitrophenyl *N*-trimethylammonioethyl carbonate *1* in 25 mM NaCl, 25 mM Tris-HCl buffer (pH 7.0) at 17°C. No burst of nitrophenolate anion was observed under these conditions where the instrument dead time is 1 msec. These results are consistent with direct hydrolysis of antibody-complexed carbonate by hydroxide ion or water (Fig. 2).

Catalysis Is Associated with the Immunoglobulin Combining Site

A series of control experiments were carried out. The catalytic activity associated wth T15 and MOPC 167 was destroyed by thermal denaturation of the antibody at 95°C for 10 minutes, followed by rapid cooling to 0°C. MOPC 167 and T15 were also cleaved with papain, and the resulting Fab fragments were isolated by affinity chromatography as described above (Pollet et al. 1974). The Fab fragment, which contains the antibody combining site, accelerated the rate of hy-

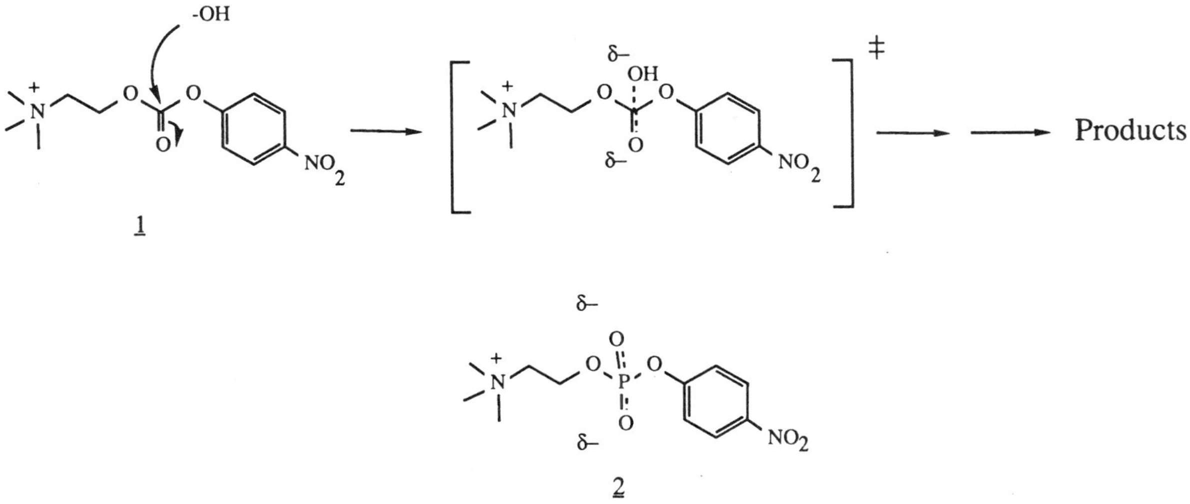

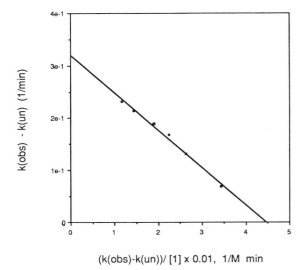

Figure 1. Hydrolysis reaction and transition state analog.

drolysis of carbonate *1* to the same degree as native immunoglobulin. Antibody to staphylococcal enterotoxin B, which has no appreciable binding affinity for nitrophenylphosphorylcholine, did not accelerate the rate of hydrolysis of carbonate *1* above the background rate. MOPC 167 and T15 were also treated with the irreversible affinity label, 4-diazonium phenylphosphorylcholine (Chesebro and Metzger 1972), in the absence and presence of 4-nitrophenylphosphorylcholine. Reaction of each antibody with three equivalents of 4-diazonium phenylphosphorylcholine followed by extensive dialysis resulted in nearly complete loss of catalytic activity (see Table 1). The above results are consistent with catalysis occurring in the immunoglobulin combining site. Chemical modification experiments of the catalytic antibodies have been carried out with maleic anhydride, diethylpyrocarbonate, 1,2-

cyclohexanedione, and tetranitromethane, both in the presence and in the absence of bound inhibitors (Table 1). These experiments point to the presence of a positively charged arginine and a tyrosine residue in the antibody combining site, which may function to stabilize the negatively charged tetrahedral transition state geometry generated by attack of a binding-site-accessible water molecule on the carbonate moiety. No inactivation occurs with lysine- or histidine-specific reagents. These results are consistent with the three-dimensional structure of McPC 603, in which the conserved arginine and tyrosine residues are thought to stabilize the anionic phosphate moiety of PC by hydrogen bonding and electrostatic interactions.

If catalytic activity is associated with the antibody combining site, then the antibody-catalyzed reaction should be competitively inhibited by the addition of the negatively charged tetrahedral transition state analog, 4-nitrophenylphosphorylcholine *2*. The inhibition constant K_i for the formation of the T15 antibody–4-nitrophenylphosphorylcholine *2* complex was determined to be 5.5×10^{-5} M at 30°C in 25 mM NaCl, 25 mM Tris-HCl buffer (pH 7.0). The K_i for the MOPC 167–*2* complex (under the same conditions) was previously reported to be 5.0×10^{-6} M (Fig. 3) (Pollack et al. 1986). These values agree with those reported in the literature (Leon and Young 1971; Kluskens et al. 1975; Goetze and Richards 1978) which demonstrate that 4-nitrophenylphosphorylcholine is bound more tightly by T15 and MOPC 167 than is acetylcholine. If we assume that the K_m for carbonate *1* approximates K_d (*1*), which seems reasonable in light of the relatively low turnover numbers of MOPC 167 and T15, then the differential binding affinity of the antibody to the transition state analog and substrate is consistent with lowering of the free energy of activation for reaction (Wolfenden 1976). However, there is not a clear correlation of K_i, K_m and the rate acceleration of the antibody-catalyzed reaction, implying other factors play a role in catalysis.

Figure 2. Eadie plot of $(k_{obs}-k_{un})$ versus $(k_{obs}-k_{un})/[1]$ for hydrolysis of carbonate *1* by T15.

Table 1. Chemical Modification of MOPC 167 and T15

		% Activity remaining			
		MOPC 167		T15	
Residue	Reagent	(+)NPPC	(−)NPPC	(+)NPPC	(−)NPPC
(Affinity labeling)	diazonium phenyl-phosphorylcholine	83	12	90	14
Lysine	maleic anhydride	85	85	86	88
Arginine	cyclohexane-1,2-dione	100	45	96	40
Tyrosine	tetranitromethane	100	18	100	22
Histidine	diethylpyrocarbonate	100	88	98	94

Hydroxide Ion Dependence of Antibody-catalyzed Hydrolysis

Both the T15 and the MOPC 167 antibody-catalyzed hydrolyses of carbonate *1* are first order in hydroxide ion. The V_{max} of the T15-catalyzed hydrolysis of carbonate *1* exhibited a first-order dependence on hydroxide ion concentration between pH 6.0 and pH 8.0 in 50 mM Tris-HCl at 30°C, whereas the K_m for the antibody-catalyzed reaction remained relatively unaffected. Similar results were reported earlier for the MOPC-167-catalyzed reaction, and both sets of experiments are consistent with the results of Goetze and Richards (1978), which demonstrated little variance in K_a for 4-nitrophenylphosphorylcholine in this pH range (Fig. 4).

The rate of the antibody-catalyzed reaction can be directly compared with the rate of the uncatalyzed reaction, since it has been demonstrated that the V_{max} of both antibody-catalyzed reactions is first order in hydroxide ion concentration, whereas K_m is relatively unaffected. Since the substrate can also be cleaved in the absence of immunoglobulin by direct nucleophilic attack of hydroxide ion, we can compare this rate $v_{uncatalyzed} = k_{uncat} [1] [OH^-]$ with the rate of hydrolysis in the antibody-substrate complex, $v_{complex} = k_{complex}$ [complex] [OH⁻]. Note that we are directly comparing the rate of the antibody-catalyzed reaction with an uncatalyzed reaction which follows the same rate law. This comparison should provide us with an accurate estimation of the degree of transition state stabilization afforded by the antibody combining site relative to the uncatalyzed reaction. The background hydroxide-ion-catalyzed rate can be determined by extrapolating the rate of the uncatalyzed reaction to zero buffer concentration. The ratio of $k_{complex}/k_{uncat}$ is 770 for MOPC 167 and 620 for antibody T15. However, as pointed out earlier, this ratio is probably 15-fold higher, i.e., 11,500 for MOPC 167 and 9200 for T15, since the background rate of hydrolysis of choline carbonate *1* free in solution is 15-fold higher than that of ethyl nitrophenyl carbonate, due to intramolecular assistance of the tetra-alkylammonium ion (Bruice and Benkovic 1966; Pollack et al. 1986). On the basis of the known crystal structure of the highly homologous antibody McPC 603 (Segal et al. 1974), this assistance is probably not occurring in the antibody combining site, where choline is bound in a more extended conformation and the tetra-alkylammonium ion is stabilized by interactions with Glu-35H and Asp-97L.

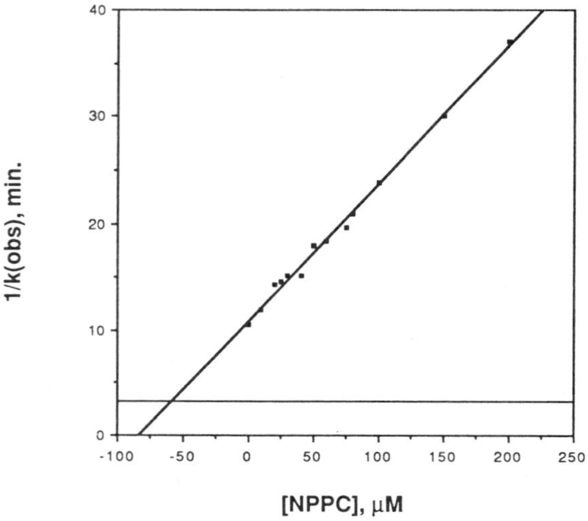

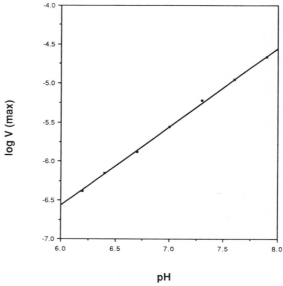

Figure 3. Dixon plot of inhibition of the T15-catalyzed hydrolysis of carbonate *1* by 4-nitrophenylphosphorylcholine.

Figure 4. Plot of V_{max} as a function of pH for the T15-catalyzed hydrolysis of carbonate *1*.

Specificity of Antibody-catalyzed Reaction

Both MOPC 167 and T15 show relatively high substrate specificity. The introduction of a methyl group into the alkyl side chain of 4-nitrophenyl choline carbonate affords a K_m of 2 mM and a k_{cat} of 0.2 min^{-1} for the MOPC-167-catalyzed hydrolysis of 3 (racemate) and a K_m of 1.5 mM and k_{cat} of 0.09 min^{-1} for the T15-catalyzed hydrolysis of 3 (Fig. 5). There is no measurable difference in the k_{cat} and K_m values of MOPC-167-catalyzed hydrolysis of the two enantiomers of carbonate 3 when assayed in separate experiments. Neither T15 nor MOPC 167 catalyzed the hydrolysis of ethyl-4-nitrophenylcarbonate 4. These results are consistent with those in the literature, which suggest that the combining sites of PC-specific antibodies are highly complementary to the choline moiety (Fig. 7).

The antibody MOPC 167 catalyzes the hydrolysis of choline-4-nitrophenyl carbonate 1 and choline-2-nitrophenyl carbonate 5 with a k_{cat} of 0.4 and 0.3 min^{-1}, respectively, suggesting that the aryl ring of 1 does not lie in a well-defined site in MOPC 167. No appreciable rate acceleration in hydrolysis of choline-4-nitrophenyl carbamate or of the phosphodiester bond of 4-nitrophenylphosphorylcholine was observed.

DISCUSSION

Two catalytic antibodies, MOPC 167 and T15, have been characterized from a group of mouse myeloma immunoglobulins that specifically bind PC. In this group, the primary structures of the heavy-chain variable regions of over 28 PC-specific antibodies (Gearhart et al. 1981) have been determined. In addition, the association constants of many of these antibodies to choline and PC monoesters and diesters have been determined, and the immunoglobulin combining sites have been probed by NMR, rotary dispersion, and affinity labeling (Leon and Young 1971; Pollet et al. 1974; Goetze and Richards 1977; Bennett and Glaudemans 1979). Importantly, a three-dimensional structure of a representative PC-binding antibody, McPC 603 Fab and its complex with PC, has allowed direct identification of the combining site residues critical in determining antibody specificity (Segal et al. 1974; Satow et al. 1986). Correlation of the structural information with the protein sequence data suggests that the binding site is highly conserved in immunoglobulins with PC specificity (Padlan 1977). For example, the T15 heavy-chain hypervariable sequence differs from the McPC 603 sequence in only two amino acids in the third hypervariable region (HV3). The

MOPC 167 sequence differs from the McPC 603 structure substantially in the HV3 region, but no differences are found in HV2 or HV1 (Gearhart et al. 1981). Another relevant point is that the genes encoding the light- and heavy-chain sequences of T15 have been cloned, sequenced, and expressed on overproducing vectors, allowing the possibility of site-directed mutagenesis studies (Table 2) (P. Tucker, pers. comm.). The detailed information available on the molecular interactions of PC-specific immunoglobulins and the accessibility of the T15 genes make this an ideal system for studying the molecular basis of antibody catalysis.

Both PC-specific immunoglobulins T15 and MOPC 167 show catalytic activity with a k_{cat} of 0.32 min^{-1} and 0.40 min^{-1}, respectively. These values, although substantially below those of typical enzyme-catalyzed reactions, correspond to rate accelerations above the hydroxide-catalyzed reactions of 9200 and 11,500, respectively. These values are based on a direct comparison of the hydroxide ion hydrolysis of carbonate 1 with the antibody-catalyzed reaction, which is also first order in [OH$^-$]. Antibody-catalyzed rate accelerations of 10^3 to 10^4 (Pollack et al. 1986; Tramontano et al. 1986) are in the same range as those attributable both experimentally and theoretically to transition state stabilization in hydrolytic enzymes (Serpersu et al. 1987; S. Rao, in prep.). Note that it is unlikely that the turnover number of T15 or MOPC 167 is limited by hapten-antibody dissociation since the measured rate for dissociation of PC from McPC 603 is 10 s^{-1} (Goetze and Richards 1977); moreover, PC is bound three orders of magnitude more tightly than choline (Leon and Young 1971). The K_m values of T15 and MOPC 167 for carbonate 1 are 2.1×10^{-4} M and 7.1×10^{-4} M, respectively. Thus, although the PC-specific antibodies preferentially bind phosphate 2, they do have appreciable binding affinity toward the choline moiety of the substrate.

A series of experiments demonstrate that catalysis is associated with the immunoglobulin combining site. The kinetics of the antibody-catalyzed reactions are consistent with the formation of a Michaelis complex, presumably involving the antibody PC combining site. The Fab fragment retains catalytic activity, again suggesting that activity is associated with the variable region. The antibody-catalyzed hydrolysis of carbonate 1 is competitively inhibited by 4-nitrophenylphosphorylcholine, the transition state analog for the hydrolysis of 1. Treatment of MOPC 167 and T15 with the affinity label 4-diazonium phenylphosphorylcholine, which has been demonstrated to label the combining site of immunoglobulin T15 (Chesebro and Metzger 1972), de-

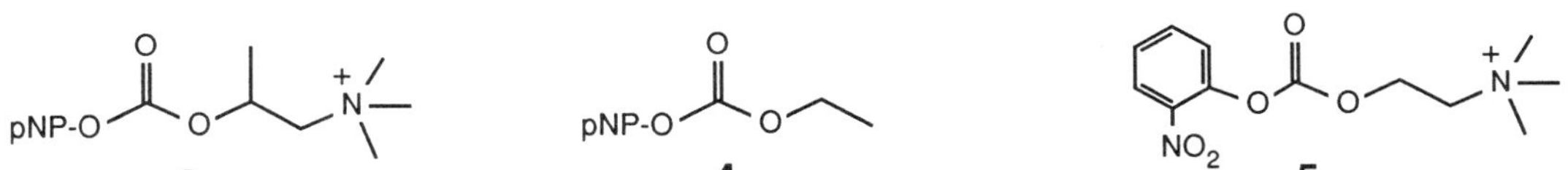

Figure 5. Altered substrates.

Table 2. Protein Sequences of V_H Regions of PC-specific Immunoglobulins

Ig	HV1 31 — — 35	HV2 50 — — — — — — — — 60 — — — — — 67 .	HV3 101 — — — — — — — — — — — — —
McPC 603	D F Y M E	A S R N K G N K Y T T E Y S A S V K	N Y Y G S T W Y F D V
T15	- - - - -	- - - - - A - D - - - - - - - - -	D - - - - S Y - - - - -
HOPC8	- - - - -	- - - - - A - D - - - - - - - - -	D - - - - N Y - - - - -
S107	- - - - -	- - - - - A - D - - - - - - - - -	D - - - - S Y - - - - -
MOPC 167	- - - - -	- - - S - A H D - R - - - - - - -	D A D - - D S Y F G - - B -
C57BL23169	- - - - -	- - - - - A - D - - - - - - - - -	- - - - - S Y - - - - -

Data from Perlmutter et al. (1984). Numbering of residues is sequential from the amino terminus relative to the longest sequence, MOPC 167.

stroys all catalytic activity. Chemical modification experiments demonstrate that arginine and tyrosine residues play a key role in substrate binding and/or catalysis. Structural data in the literature strongly suggest that Arg-52H and Tyr-33H, which are invariant in the PC-binding antibodies, are essential for binding of the anionic phosphate moiety. No evidence for essential lysine or histidine residues in the catalytic site is provided by chemical modification experiments, consistent with the crystallographic data.

Importantly, the T15- and MOPC-167-catalyzed hydrolysis of carbonate *1* shows high selectivity, as do the other catalytic antibodies reported in the literature (Tramontano et al. 1986; Jacobs et al. 1987). Consequently, although the turnover numbers of catalytic antibodies are low, they offer the possibility of developing catalysts with binding sites tailored to the substrate of interest.

The first-order dependence of the antibody-catalyzed reaction on hydroxide ion concentration is consistent with three possible catalytic mechanisms. The antibody combining site may be acting to polarize the bound carbonate functionality toward the transition state geometry via specific binding interactions. The nucleophilic species, a combining-site-accessible hydroxide ion, then hydrolyzes the polarized carbonate in the rate-determining step. In mechanism 2 (Fig. 6), a fortuitously placed combining-site residue may be acting as a general base to activate H_2O for attack on the antibody-complexed substrate. A third possibility involves the initial attack of a nucleophilic combining-site residue, such as invariant Tyr-33H, on the bound carbonate to generate a covalent choline carboalkoxy-antibody intermediate. This intermediate is then hydrolyzed in the subsequent rate-determining step by attack of a combining-site-accessible hydroxide ion. The third mechanism suggests that an initial rapid rate of nitrophenolate ion release should be observable,

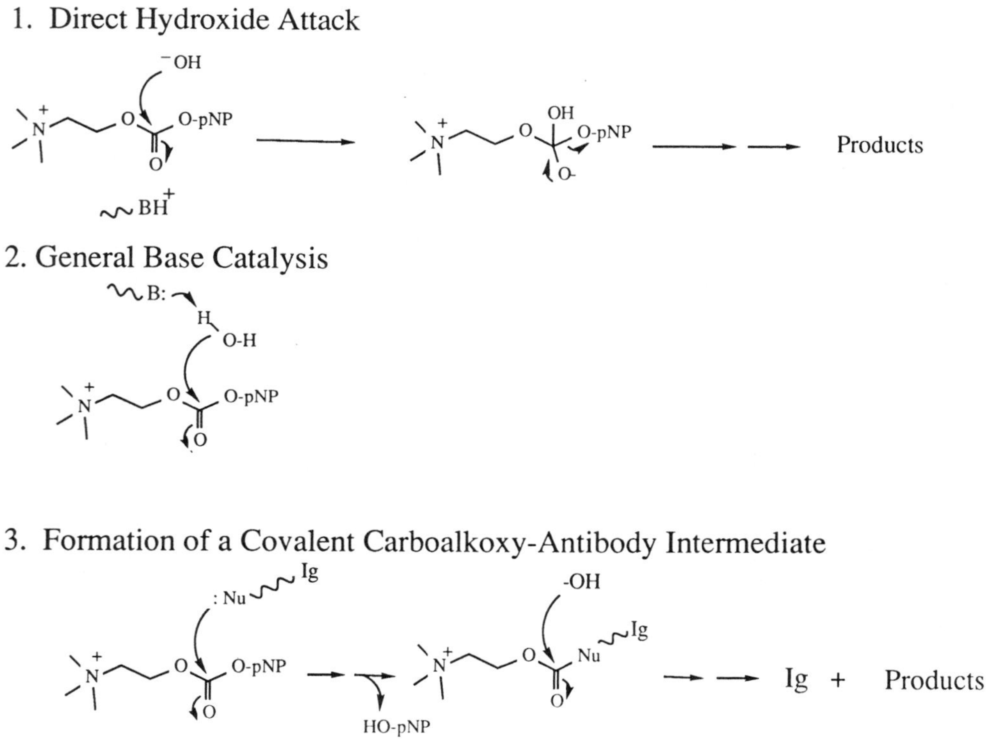

1. Direct Hydroxide Attack

2. General Base Catalysis

3. Formation of a Covalent Carboalkoxy-Antibody Intermediate

Figure 6. Possible mechanisms for antibody-catalyzed carbonate hydrolysis. (*1*) Transition state stabilization with attack by combining-site-accessible hydroxide ion; (*2*) general base catalysis; (*3*) formation of a carboalkoxy-antibody intermediate.

followed by slower breakdown of the carboalkoxy-antibody adduct. Stopped-flow experiments provide no evidence for a sudden burst of nitrophenolate anion release. It is therefore likely that the antibody-catalyzed reaction is proceeding through transition state stabilization and/or general base catalysis. Examination of the three-dimensional structure of the PC-specific immunoglobulin McPC 603 may allow us to distinguish these two mechanistic alternatives. Note that both the McPC 603 and MOPC 167 V_H genes that encode most of the residues that interact with the hapten are derived from the germ-line T15 V_H gene segment and are highly homologous (Gearhart et al. 1981).

Crystallographic studies of McPC 603 reveal a high degree of complementarity between the antibody combining site and PC (Segal et al. 1974; Satow et al. 1986). The hapten is bound in the cavity of McPC 603 with the choline group deep in the interior and the phosphate toward the exterior, in contact with solvent molecules (Fig. 7). The heavy-chain residues Tyr-33H and Arg-52H, which are invariant in all of the PC-binding immunoglobulins sequenced to date, bind the phosphate via hydrogen bonding and electrostatic interactions with the phosphoryl oxygen atoms. The positive charge of the choline moiety is partially neutralized by the light-chain residue Asp-97L and the invariant Glu-35H, which are buried deep in the hapten-binding cavity. In addition, there are van der Waals contacts between the hapten and residues Tyr-33H and Trp-107aH. Charges on the heavy-chain residues Glu-61, Lys-54, and Lys-57 may align the hapten via dipolar interactions as it binds to the cavity. Notable differences among McPC 603, T15, and MOPC 167 (Table 2) include (1) the presence of Asn-101H in McPC 603, which is replaced by Asp-101H in T15 and MOPC 167, and (2) the presence of Asp-106H in MOPC 167, which is lacking in both McPC 603 and T15 and thought to interact to some degree with both the tetraalkylammonium and phosphate moieties of the hapten.

The crystal structure of McPC 603 clearly shows that antibody-complexed PC is accessible to a solvent water molecule or hyroxide ion, the nucleophilic species in both mechanisms 1 and 2. Note that generation of an antibody against a transition state analog does not ensure that nucleophilic amino acid residues will be incorporated into the antibody combining site. The hapten must be appropriately designed to enable the complexed substrate to be accessible to solvent (Jacobs et al. 1987). The combining site of McPC 603 is both sterically and electronically complementary to the tetrahedral negatively charged phosphate moiety of PC. Since this tetrahedral phosphate mimics the transition state for hydroxide-ion-catalyzed hydrolysis of *1* (Bruice and Benkovic 1966; Weaver et al. 1977; Bartlett and Marlowe 1983), the PC antibodies should be capable of stabilizing the transition state configuration for carbonate hydrolysis. Because the ground state structure of *1* differs substantially from the transition state configuration, the differential binding affinity of the immunoglobulin to these two species should be reflected in a lowered free energy of activation for reaction (Pauling 1948; Wolfenden 1976). In fact, the transition state analog 4-nitrophenylphosphorylcholine is bound more tightly than the corresponding substrate by both MOPC 167 and T15. However, the differential binding of T15 and MOPC 167 to carbonate *1* and the transition state analog *2* does not fully account for the magnitude of the rate accelerations. In addition, the ratio of $K_i(2)/K_m(1)$ for T15 is four times that of $K_i(2)/K_m(1)$ for MOPC 167, even though the rate accelerations above the $[OH^-]$ hydrolysis are similar. Therefore, although the crystallographic and binding data strongly suggest that T15 and MOPC 167 selectively stabilize the transition state configuration and thereby reduce the barrier for reaction, other factors are contributing to the rate acceleration.

The conformation of bound substrate or solvent accessibility may influence reaction rate, although the crystallographic data suggest that PC binds in a relatively open cavity. Asp-106H of MOPC 167 was postulated earlier (Schultz and Jacobs 1987) to act as a general base, but since T15 and MOPC 167 have similar turnover numbers, this residue cannot be essential for catalysis. Both Arg-52H and Tyr-33H are located so as to act as a general base, although NMR experiments (Goetze and Richards 1978) indicate that both residues are protonated in the PC antibody complex at pH 7.0. Crystallographic and chemical modification data rule out participation of histidine in catalysis. We have begun to carry out a series of mutagenesis studies on the combining-site residues of the immunoglobulin T15 both to define more precisely the roles these residues play in catalysis and to introduce selectively histidine and cysteine residues to act as general bases and nucleophilic groups. In addition, antibodies are being elicited to uncharged α-difluoroketone and hydroxymethylene transition state analogs to determine the role that electronic and geometric complementarity play in antibody catalysis.

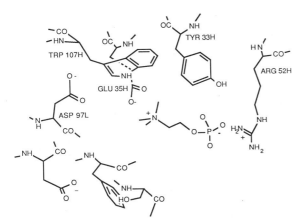

Figure 7. Combining site of the antibody McPC 603. PC is surrounded by the conserved heavy-chain residues Tyr-33, Glu-35, Arg-52, and Glu-61 (numbered).

In summary, the PC-binding antibodies MOPC 167 and T15 bind and catalyze the hydrolysis of carbonate *1*. The combining-site residues of T15 and MOPC 167 are located so as to provide additional binding interactions to the tetrahedral negatively charged transition state configuration relative to the neutral substrate. This study strongly supports the notion that immunoglobulins elicited against transition state analogs can act to stabilize preferentially the transition state configuration (Jacobs et al. 1987). However, it is clear that this is not the only factor contributing to catalysis, and much work remains to be done to define guidelines and strategies for generating catalytic antibodies for reactions of general interest.

ACKNOWLEDGMENT

This work was supported in part by a Presidential Young Investigator Award to P.G.S. from the National Science Foundation (CHE85-43106).

REFERENCES

Anglister, S., T. Frey, and H.M. McConnell. 1984. Magnetic resonance studies of a monoclonal anti-spin-label antibody. *Biochemistry* 23: 1138.

Bartlett, P.A. and C. Marlowe. 1983. Phosphonamidates as transition-state analogue inhibitors of thermolysin. *Biochemistry* 22: 4618.

Bennett, L.G. and C.P. Glaudemans. 1979. Contributions by ionic and steric features of ligands to their binding with phosphorylcholine-specific immunoglobulin IgA H-8 as determined by fluorescence spectroscopy. *Biochemistry* 18: 3337.

Bruice, T. and S. Benkovic. 1966. Acyl transfer reactions involving carboxylic acid esters and amides. In *Bioorganic mechanisms* (ed. R. Breslow and M. Karplus), p. 134. Benjamin Press, New York.

Chesebro, B. and H. Metzger. 1972. Affinity labeling of a phosphorylcholine binding mouse myeloma protein. *Biochemistry* 11: 766.

Crews, S., J. Griffin, H. Huang, K. Calame, and L. Hood. 1981. A single V_H gene segment encodes the immune response to phosphorylcholine: Somatic mutation is correlated with the class of the antibody. *Cell* 25: 59.

Dixon, G. 1953. The determination of enzyme inhibitor constants. *Biochem. J.* 55: 170.

Freedman, M.H., A.L. Grossber, and D. Pressman. 1968. The effects of complete modification of amino groups on the antibody activity of antihapten antibodies. Reversible modification with maleic anhydride. *Biochemistry* 7: 1941.

Gearhart, P.J., N.D. Johnson, R. Douglas, and L. Hood. 1981. IgG antibodies to phosphorylcholine exhibit more diversity than their IgM counterparts. *Nature* 291: 29.

Goding, J.W. 1986. *Monoclonal antibodies: Principles and practice.* Academic Press, New York.

Goetze, A.M. and J.H. Richards. 1977. Magnetic resonance studies of the binding site interactions between phosphorylcholine and specific mouse myeloma immunoglobulin. *Biochemistry* 16: 228.

———. 1978. Molecular studies of subspecificity differences among phosphorylcholine-binding mouse myeloma anti-

bodies using ^{31}P nuclear magnetic resonance. *Biochemistry* 17: 1733.

Holbrook, J.J. and V.A. Ingram. 1973. Ionic properties of an essential histidine residue in pig heart lactate dehydrogenase. *Biochem. J.* 131: 729.

Jacobs, J., P.G. Schultz, R. Sugasawara, and M. Powell. 1987. Catalytic antibodies. *J. Am. Chem Soc.* 109: 2174.

Kluskens, L., W. Lee, and H. Kohler. 1975. Immune response to phosphorylcholine. *Eur. J. Immunol.* 5: 489.

Laemmli, U.K. 1970. Cleavage of structural proteins during assembly of the head bacteriophage T4. *Nature* 227: 680.

Landsteiner, K. 1944. *The specificity of serological reactions.* Harvard University Press, Cambridge, Massachusetts.

Leon, M.A. and N.M. Young. 1971. Specificity for phosphorylcholine of six murine myeloma proteins reactive with *pneumococcus c polysaccharide* and β-lipoprotein. *Biochemistry* 10: 1424.

Nisonoff, A., J. Hopper, and S. Spring. 1975. *The antibody molecule.* Academic Press, New York.

Padlan, E.A. 1977. Structural basis for the specificity of antibody antigen reactions and stuctural mechanisms for the diversification of antigen-binding specificities. *Q. Rev. Biophys.* 10: 35.

Patthy, L. and E.L. Smithl. 1975. Identification of functional arginine residues in ribonuclease A and lysozyme. *J. Biol. Chem.* 250: 565.

Pauling, L. 1948. Chemical achievement and hope for the future. *Am. Sci.* 36: 51.

Perlmutter, R., S Crews, R. Douglas, G. Sorensen, N. Johnson, N. Nivera, P. Gearhart, and L. Hood. 1984. Diversity in phosphorylcholine-binding antibodies. *Adv. Immunol.* 35: 1.

Pollack, S.J., J.W. Jacobs, and P.G. Schultz. 1986. Selective chemical catalysis by an antibody. *Science* 234: 1570.

Pollet, R., H. Edelhoch, S. Rudikoff, and M. Potter. 1974. Changes in optical parameters of myeloma proteins with phosphorylcholine binding. *J. Biol. Chem.* 249: 5188.

Pressman, D. and A. Grossberg. 1968. *The structural basis of antibody specificity.* Benjamin Press, New York.

Satow, Y., G.H. Cohen, E.A. Padlan, and D.R. Davies. 1986. Phosphocholine binding immunoglobulin Fab McPC603, an X-ray diffraction study at 2.7 Å. *J. Mol. Biol.* 190: 593.

Schultz, P.G. and J. Jacobs. 1987. Catalytic antibodies: Generation and characterization. In *Molecular structure and energetics* (ed. J.F. Liebman and A. Greenberg). VCH, Deerfield Beach, Florida. (In press.)

Segal, D.M., E.A. Padlan, G.H. Cohen, S. Rudikoff, M. Potter, and D.R. Davies. 1974. The three-dimensional structure of a phosphorylcholine-binding mouse immunoglobulin Fab and the nature of the antigen binding site. *Proc. Natl. Acad. Sci.* 71: 4298.

Serpersu, E., D. Shortle, and A. Mildvan. 1987. Kinetic and magnetic resonance studies of active site mutants of staphylococcal nuclease: Factors contributing to catalysis. *Biochemistry* 26: 1289.

Sokolovsky, M., J.F. Riordan, and B.L. Vallee. 1966. Tetranitromethane. A reagent for the nitration of tyrosyl residues in proteins. *Biochemistry* 5: 3582.

Tramontano, A., K. Janda, and R. Lerner. 1986. Catalytic antibodies. *Science* 234: 1566.

Weaver, L.H., W.R. Kester, and B.W. Matthews. 1977. A crystallographic study of the complex of phosphoramidon with thermolysin. A model for the presumed catalytic transition state and for the binding of the extended substrate. *J. Mol. Biol.* 114: 119.

Wolfenden, R. 1976. Transition state analogues. *Annu. Rev. Biophys. Bioeng.* 5: 271.

Engineering of Antibodies with a Known Three-dimensional Structure

A. Plückthun, R. Glockshuber, I. Pfitzinger, A. Skerra, and J. Stadlmüller
Genzentrum der Universität München, c/o Max-Planck-Institut für Biochemie, D-8033 Martinsried, West Germany

There are several approaches to the study of catalysis. Most paradigms of enzymology are the fruit of the first approach, the continuous search for new enzymes and their judicious study. This "discovery" approach has led not only to the characterization of enzymes catalyzing new reaction types, but also to the meticulous dissection of the simplest elementary catalytic steps. A second approach, the modification of *one* enzyme by chemical or, nowadays, mainly genetic means (i.e., the perturbation of the catalytic machinery), has recently also begun to provide further insight into the mechanisms of catalysis (for review, see Leatherbarrow and Fersht 1986; Wetzel 1986; Knowles 1987). Most enzymes have probably evolved to a rather high efficiency. The consequence is that modification will, most probably, only reduce their activity or leave it unaffected when they are tested for the reaction and conditions for which they were intended by nature (Albery and Knowles 1977).

The third approach to the study of catalysis involves the "design" of suitable (probably at first rather modest) catalytic entities. The presumption here is that this may provide a very sensitive test of the requirements for efficient catalytic rate enhancements. Moreover, one may hope for the clearer delineation of such rules by a critical comparison of "professional" versus "home-built" catalytic entities. The success of all approaches depends on treating each new or mutant protein as a *new* enzyme to be thoroughly studied.

The principle of this design approach is, of course, by no means new. A multitude of model reactions have been devised for many classes of enzymatic reactions to probe the chemical feasibility of alternative pathways. Many detailed studies that included the binding aspect of catalysis were carried out on cyclodextrins, crown ether derivatives, and similar compounds (see, e.g., Cramer and Mackensen 1966; Bender and Komiyama 1978; Breslow et al. 1978; Tabushi et al. 1980; Breslow and Czarnik 1983; Hilvert and Breslow 1984; Cram and Trueblood 1985; Kellogg 1985; Breslow 1986; Lehn 1986; D'Souza and Bender 1987). The disadvantage of these otherwise elegant model systems is that they do not involve proteins as catalysts. The extrapolation to natural enzymes becomes therefore somewhat longer. In addition, the synthetic effort to produce them is not much diminished after a number of models have been successfully made. It was therefore thought advantageous to carry out investigations directly with a protein. That enzymes do not possess a *vis vitalis* is illustrated by

occasional discoveries of serendipitous catalytic activities in proteins not destined to work as enzymes. Bovine serum albumin, for example, decomposes Meisenheimer complexes, whereas nitrophenyl-binding antibodies and even human serum albumin do not (Taylor and Vatz 1973). In addition, hemoglobin can act as a monooxygenase in a variety of reactions (Ferraiolo et al. 1984; Starke et al. 1984).

In search of a suitable protein with which to carry out such investigations on the engineering of active sites, we decided on antibodies. Antibodies comprise a family of rather stable and similar structures that are able to bind to a very large number of antigens. The essence of antibody structure has been well reviewed (Kabat 1978; Amzel and Poljak 1979; Davies and Metzger 1983). The antibody domains consist of a highly conserved framework of β sheets. The antigen-binding region is made up of six hypervariable loops (three derived from each chain) connecting the β strands within each subunit, and almost all binding interactions are contributed by residues from these loops.

Indeed, fortuitous catalytic (precisely: hydrolytic) activities have been discovered in antibodies as well. Slobin (1966) described the catalysis of the hydrolysis of nitrophenyl acetate, catalyzed in a bimolecular reaction by a base on the protein, but not related to the nitrophenyl-binding properties of the antibodies. Rather, he showed that in these antibodies, binding protected the substrate from hydrolysis. In later studies, specific yet serendipitous reactions were found. Some antibodies reacted only stoichiometrically (Kohen et al. 1980b) and others showed a sluggish turnover (Kohen et al. 1979, 1980a). These experiments demonstrated again that there is at least nothing in the antibody molecule that *prevents* a reaction from turning over in such a hypothetical active site.

One of the most essential features of enzyme catalysis is selective binding. Enzymes must distinguish their substrates from others, and they gain catalytic efficiency by differentiating substrate and product with respect to binding energies (Albery and Knowles 1977). Possibly the most effective contribution of binding to catalysis is, however, the further discrimination of the transition state as the structure to be bound most tightly (for review, see Albery and Knowles 1977; but see also Jencks 1975). This idea of transition state complementarity was already considered by Haldane (1930). Pauling (1946) expressed this concept succinctly and proposed the synthesis of transition state analogs (for review, see Wolfenden 1976) as inhibitors. He had also recognized the fundamental similarity between enzymes and antibodies in binding specific molecules (Pauling 1948). The idea of actually using transition state analogs as haptens for immunization was probably first explicitly stated by Jencks (1969) and has been tested experimentally several times since then with varying degrees of success (Raso and Stollar 1975a,b; Tramontano et al. 1986a,b; Jacobs et al. 1987). We do not know whether it is possible, even in principle, to design transition state analogs that elicit optimal catalytic groups for many reactions in the antihapten antibody as opposed to eliciting just some way of holding on to the hapten.

As a starting point for investigations on binding and catalysis, we decided to use an antibody with a known three-dimensional structure that may be reasonably close to a transition-state-binding protein. Such a system is the phosphorylcholine-binding mouse immunoglobulin A McPC 603 (for reviews, see Potter 1977; Perlmutter et al. 1984). The structure (Segal et al. 1974) and sequence (Rudikoff and Potter 1974; Rudikoff et al. 1981) of this and many analogous proteins (Potter 1977; Kabat et al. 1983; Perlmutter et al. 1984) have been determined. In analyzing binding and catalysis by a macromolecule, we believe it is essential to have complete structural information available. Even though modeling of variants is necessary in this case as well, it remains on firmer ground. The availability of high-quality crystals for X-ray diffraction studies is still a major uncertainty for every new protein, and we therefore decided to choose a protein for which this hurdle has already been passed.

McPC 603 binds phosphorylcholine. Phosphorus compounds, such as phosphonates, phosphonamides, but also phosphate esters, have been recognized as good inhibitors of the enzymatic hydrolysis of suitable carboxyl esters and amides, and they conform to the criteria of transition state analogs (Weaver et al. 1977; Kam et al. 1979; Hofmann and Rottenberg 1980; Jacobsen and Bartlett 1981; Thorsett et al. 1982; Bartlett and Marlowe 1983, 1987; Galardy et al. 1983; Tronrud et al. 1986, 1987). The phosphorus provides all the ligands of the tetrahedral intermediate itself (which is thought to be structurally and energetically similar to the transition states leading to and away from it, by Hammond's principle). It does not require complexation with an enzyme nucleophile to yield the actual analog (as boronates or activated carbonyl compounds would to mimic the tetrahedral intermediate). It should therefore be effective in systems where the attacking nucleophile is not enzyme bound and can be displaced (i.e., where it is water). Indeed, all of the literature examples above concern the inhibition of Zn proteases. Since the antibody makes no specific contact to the bridging oxygen of phosphorylcholine, the choice of atoms around the carbonyl group in a substrate undergoing hydrolysis should be somewhat permissive.

While this work was in progress, Pollack et al. (1986) reported that a related antibody, MOPC 167, already had the spontaneous capability to accelerate the hydrolysis of a suitable carbonate ester. This observation underlined once again the validity of Pauling's concept formulated 40 years ago, and, in addition, demonstrated that the antibody chosen by us with a known three-dimensional structure may indeed provide a promising experimental model for the systematic study of binding and rate acceleration.

We therefore decided to work out an experimental system in which such an antibody may be altered by design and in which active fragments of the antibody and its mutants can be obtained in large amounts for experimental investigations. We describe here the gene synthesis and bacterial expression of the F_V and F_{ab} fragments of the antibody protein. The genes corresponding to the variable domains V_H and V_L were obtained synthetically using the known protein sequence (Rudikoff and Potter 1974; Rudikoff et al. 1981). The gene for the light-chain constant domain C_L was derived from a genomic clone (Altenberger et al. 1981), whereas the gene for the first constant domain of the heavy-chain C_{H1} was obtained from a cDNA clone of a mouse IgA1 (Auffray et al. 1981).

EXPERIMENTAL PROCEDURES

General methods. Bacterial growth was carried out according to the methods described by Miller (1972), and DNA manipulations were based on the procedures described by Maniatis et al. (1982). Plasmid isolation (Birnboim and Doly 1979; Holmes and Quigley 1981; Ish-Horowicz and Burke 1981), transformation of *Escherichia coli* (Dagert and Ehrlich 1979; Hanahan 1983), DNA sequencing (a variation of the method of Chen and Seeburg 1985), polyacrylamide gel electrophoresis of proteins (Laemmli 1970; Fling and Gregerson 1986), and Western blots (Blake et al. 1984) were carried out essentially as described previously.

DNA synthesis. The oligonucleotides were synthesized with an Applied Biosystems Model 380A synthesizer using the phosphoramidite method (Sinha et al. 1984). They were then purified by polyacrylamide gel electrophoresis, phosphorylated with polynucleotide kinase, hybridized, and ligated with T4 ligase using methodology similar to that described elsewhere (Dörper and Winnacker 1983; Rommens et al. 1983).

Affinity chromatography. A phosphorylcholine affinity ligand was synthesized, coupled to a column resin, and used as described elsewhere (Chesebro and Metzger 1972). The myeloma protein McPC 603 was a gift from M. Potter and was purified from ascites. IgG affinity chromatography of protein A fusion proteins was carried out as described elsewhere (Moks et al. 1987).

Protein purification. The purification of the insoluble LacZ fusion proteins was carried out in analogy to the procedure described by Nagai et al. (1985). The fusion protein was recovered from the insoluble part of

French press lysates, solubilized with 8 M urea, and separated from insoluble material by centrifugation. The fusion proteins become highly enriched by this procedure. The urea was removed by dialysis, and the material was subsequently cleaved with the blood-clotting protease factor Xa. The factor X was purified (Fujikawa et al. 1972a) from bovine blood and activated with Russell's viper venom protease to factor Xa as described elsewhere (Fujikawa et al. 1972b).

Cell fractionation. Cell-fractionation experiments were carried out essentially as described previously (Plückthun and Knowles 1987); the protein was not radioactively labeled but was instead detected by Western blotting (Blake et al. 1984).

RESULTS AND DISCUSSION

We chose to investigate the expression of the antibody genes in a bacterial host system because of the ease of genetic manipulations and the feasibility of rather rapid inexpensive fermentations. The present paper describes the expression of the F_V and F_{ab} fragments of the antibody McPC 603 in *E. coli*. Numerous studies on a whole range of antibodies have shown that only the F_{ab} portion is required for binding, and often even the F_V portion suffices (Hochman et al. 1976).

Four genes therefore had to be obtained: one for each of the variable domains (V_L and V_H) to express the F_V fragment alone and one each comprising $V_L C_L$ and $V_H C_H$, respectively, thus making up the exact F_{ab} fragment that had been crystallized (Segal et al. 1974).

The genes for the F_V fragment were obtained synthetically. The design of the sequences according to the known protein sequences (Rudikoff and Potter 1974; Rudikoff et al. 1981) took the following points into consideration: (1) The number of unique restriction sites with sticky ends was maximized. (2) The RNA secondary structure was minimized iteratively, especially in the amino-terminal region. (3) Codons very rare in *E. coli* (Grosjean and Fiers 1982) were avoided. Otherwise, codon usage was not further restricted. The V_H gene was assembled from three subclones (*Eco*RI-*Xma*I, *Xma*I-*Pst*I, and *Pst*I-*Hin*dIII [at position 381]), each ligated from six oligonucleotides around 40–50 bases in length (Fig. 1A). The V_L gene was assembled from two subclones (*Eco*RI-*Sal*I and *Sal*I-*Hin*dIII [at position 360]), each ligated from eight oligonucleotides (Fig. 1B). The various subclones were tested and confirmed by DNA sequencing. Correct gene fragments were ligated, and the DNA sequences of the whole genes were again verified.

The genes for the F_{ab} fragment were obtained by fusing the synthetic genes to cloned genes coding for the constant domains. The $V_H C_H$ gene (Fig. 1A) was obtained by linking a fragment from the cDNA clone of a mouse IgA with an identical C_{H1} sequence as in McPC 603 (Auffray et al. 1981), via synthetic oligonucleotides to the gene for the V_H domain. The corresponding construction of $V_L C_L$ made use of a genomic κ light-chain C_L clone (Altenburger et al. 1981) that was linked to the synthetic gene for the V_L domain via synthetic oligonucleotides (Fig. 1B). Additionally, the carboxy-terminal ends of both genes had to be fitted with a *Hin*dIII site, and in the case of the heavy chain, a stop codon had to be introduced. This was achieved with oligonucleotide fragments and/or appropriate subcloning. The correctness of the DNA constructions was verified by DNA sequencing of both complete F_{ab} genes, i.e., $V_H C_H$ and $V_L C_L$ (Fig. 1). In addition, all four genes were brought under the control of bacterial promoters (e.g., *tac*), and in an in vitro translation experiment, it was demonstrated that the four proteins were of the expected sizes (V_L 115 amino acids; V_H 122 amino acids; $V_L C_L$ 220 amino acids; $V_H C_H$ 222 amino acids).

To aid in the detection of the proteins expressed in vivo, the genuine myeloma protein McPC 603 was purified from ascites by phosphorylcholine affinity chromatography, and antibodies against it were raised in a rabbit. Western blot experiments showed that these antibodies recognized the four recombinant proteins (V_L, V_H, $V_L C_L$, and $V_H C_H$) and that all four proteins could be expressed in vivo, albeit in moderate amounts (Fig. 2).

The expression of antibody genes in bacteria was reported previously (see, e.g., Boss et al. 1984; Cabilly et al. 1984; see also Boss and Wood 1985). In these and other experiments, cytoplasmic expression was intended and rather variable yields were reported. Refolding experiments led only to relatively low yields of recovered activity (Boss and Wood 1985). It must also be noted that the resulting proteins, when highly expressed in the cytoplasm, are likely to carry an uncleaved amino-terminal methionine or even a formylmethionine residue (Sherman et al. 1985). At present, it is not clear if and by how much this may affect the binding properties of an antibody. Preliminary evidence suggests that the variable domains of an immunoglobulin may be rather unstable in *E. coli*, and direct expression may be limited to larger fragments. Expression for preparative purposes was therefore investigated by three different methods: (1) expression of a highly expressed cytoplasmic hybrid protein with a protease-sensitive site, (2) expression as a potentially exportable hybrid protein with a protease-sensitive site, and (3) expression as a fusion with a signal sequence with ensuing transport to the periplasm.

In the first approach, fusions were constructed between a truncated β-galactosidase and the variable domains, linked by a recognition sequence for the blood-clotting protease factor Xa. These hybrid proteins were synthesized in high amounts and were found as inclusion bodies. They could therefore be highly enriched already by centrifugation of the cell lysate and urea extraction of the pellet (Fig. 3A). After solubilization, the hybrid protein was then cleaved with factor Xa, a protease of narrow specificity (Lottenberg et al. 1981). The cleavage mixture was fractionated by ion-exchange chromatography in the presence of a denaturant (8 M urea). By using this procedure, V_L could be obtained in pure form (Fig. 3B), whereas V_H could be obtained

A

B

Figure 1. (See facing page for legend.)

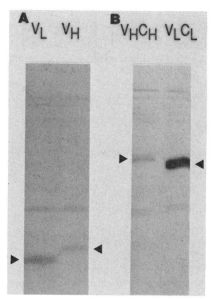

Figure 2. Expression of the proteins V_L, V_H, V_HC_H, and V_LC_L in *E. coli*. (*A*) Western blot of V_L and V_H expressed under the *trp* promoter in *E. coli* B. (*B*) Western blot of V_HC_H and V_LC_L under the control of the *tac* promoter in *E. coli* B.

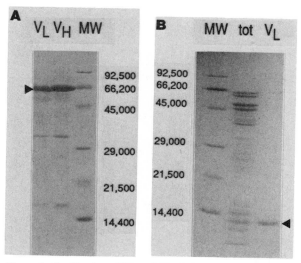

Figure 3. Purification of V_L and V_H. (*A*) Total insoluble protein from *E. coli* harboring *lacZ*-V domain fusions. V_L denotes the fusion of *lacZ* to V_L and V_H denotes the fusion of *lacZ* to V_H. (*B*) Purification of V_L from factor-Xa-cleaved fusion protein. *tot* denotes reaction mixture after partial factor Xa cleavage of fusion protein, and V_L denotes purified V_L protein. Polyacrylamide gels were stained with Coomassie blue.

highly enriched. It is now clear that the specificity of the blood-clotting factor Xa is somewhat more relaxed than originally thought (Nagai and Thogersen 1984) and it cuts within the truncated β-galactosidase as well as (very slowly) within V_H. The resulting variable-domain proteins were renatured by dilution from urea or guanidinium-HCl in the presence of reduced and oxidized glutathione, either each chain separately or both chains in a 1:1 mixture. Amino acid analyses for disulfide formation after iodoacetate derivatization of cysteines (Gurd 1967) suggested that the reoxidation and refolding yields found here have probably not surpassed reported values for antibodies.

In the second approach, fusions were constructed with domains of the *Staphylococcus aureus* protein A (Abrahmsen et al. 1985, 1986). This protein has been shown to be partially secreted to the culture medium of *E. coli* and to be able to direct the transport of a small peptide fused to the carboxyl terminus of protein A out to the culture medium. Protein A consists of one polypeptide chain with five homologous domains. We constructed a vector containing the first domain (called domain E) of protein A in tandem, fused to the variable domains V_H or V_L via a factor Xa recognition sequence. The cells expressed both hybrid proteins, and the V_L-containing fusion was found enriched in the growth medium. In fusions with the heavy chain, however, *E. coli* showed a severe growth defect and partial

cell lysis; the plasmid is unstable. Therefore, further hybrid proteins were constructed, bringing the hybrid proteins under the control of the inducible *tac* promoter. These hybrid proteins contain only one domain E fused to either V_L, V_H, V_LC_L, or V_HC_H via a factor-Xa-sensitive site. These plasmids now remain stable when not induced. The fusions with V_H and V_L were further investigated, and it was shown that the hybrid proteins were partially transported to the medium with expression-dependent (i.e., inducible) partial cell lysis (Fig. 4). Only the mature form of the V_L fusion and small amounts of mostly the precursor form of the V_H fusion were found in the medium. The analysis of cytoplasmic, membrane, and periplasmic fractions (Plückthun and Knowles 1987) suggested that both the mature and precursor form are, to a large extent, found in the insoluble membrane fraction. That the mature size protein is indeed derived from transport through the membrane and subsequent signal peptidase cleavage is suggested by the inhibition of cleavage by the uncoupler carbonyl cyanide *m*-chlorophenyl-hydrazone (CCCP) (Fig. 4) (Enequist et al. 1981). The CCCP sensitivity of maturation makes degradation by cytoplasmic proteases very unlikely. The precise understanding of the appearance of a band of mature size in the cytoplasmic and membrane fractions for both V_H and V_L fusions must await protease accessibility experiments (Minsky et al. 1986), which are in progress.

Figure 1. Nucleotide sequences of the V_LC_L gene (*A*) and of the V_HC_H gene (*B*). Many singular restriction sites are marked. The coding region of the V_L gene ends in alanine at position 355, followed by the sequence TGATAAGCTT, which codes for two stop codons and ends in a *Hind*III site. The coding region of the V_H gene ends in serine at position 376, followed by the same sequence TGATAAGCTT, which codes for two stop codons and ends in a *Hind*III site. Double underlines indicate the hypervariable loops (complementarity determining regions, CDR) according to the definition by Kabat et al. (1983).

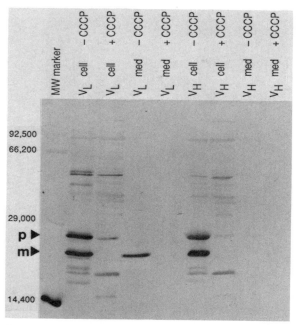

Figure 4. Sensitivity of the processing of protein A–variable domain fusions to the effect of the uncoupler carbonyl cyanide *m*-chlorophenyl hydrazone (CCCP). A Western blot of cellular and growth medium fractions of *E. coli* B is shown. + denotes samples treated with 0.1 mM CCCP as described in Results and Discussion and − denotes untreated. The precursor (p) and mature (m) forms of the hybrid proteins are indicated by arrowheads.

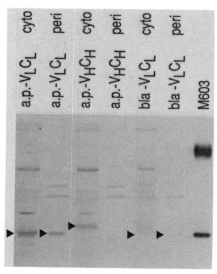

Figure 5. Cell fractionation of *E. coli* expressing V_LC_L or V_HC_H fused precisely to bacterial signal sequences. Western blot of periplasmic (peri) and cytoplasmic (cyto) fractions of fusions to alkaline phosphatase (a.p.) or β-lactamase (bla). M603 denotes the myeloma protein from ascites.

In the third approach, precise fusions were constructed between several signal sequences and V_L, V_H, V_LC_L, and V_HC_H. The transport to the bacterial periplasm is thought to result often in correct folding and in formation of correct disulfide bonds (for a recent review, see Briggs and Gierasch 1986). The antibody molecules are designed for export in eukaryotes via the endoplasmic reticulum. When V_LC_L and V_HC_H were fused precisely to the signal sequences of either alkaline phosphatase or β-lactamase, correct transport and cleavage were seen for the light chain. The heavy-chain fusion was cleaved, yet remained associated with the spheroblast fraction, i.e., was probably either membrane-associated or was released but remained insoluble (Fig. 5). We are now conducting experiments to elucidate the reason for this apparent difference in transport behavior between the two chains. It is conceivable that particular interactions between the light and heavy chain help the transport of the latter in the plasma cell endoplasmic reticulum or that the bacterial transport differs from the eukaryotic enough that the heterologous secretion and release are only possible for the light chain in bacteria, at least under the conditions tested. To eliminate the possibility that a particular interaction between the natural signal sequence and the protein may be critical, we also fused the natural eukaryotic signal sequence to the heavy chain. In this case, however, a very severe growth defect resulted that complicates the analysis of the fate of the protein.

The further optimization of these expression systems to very large scale preparations of protein remains an ongoing quest, since the full characterization of mutations will have to include structure determinations by X-rays of the mutant proteins. Such mutant antibody structures should aid substantially in the further improvement of methods for analyzing and predicting loop conformations.

The antibody domains have proved themselves throughout evolution as stable and suitable in numerous structures designed for particular versatility in recognition problems (realized, for example, in antibodies, MHC complexes, the T-cell receptor, as well as enzymes such as superoxide dismutase). They therefore provide very promising model systems with which to investigate the efficiency of binding ground states and transition states by an "engineering" approach.

ACKNOWLEDGMENTS

We express our gratitude to Dr. R. Mertz (Martinsried) for the synthesis of the oligonucleotides, to Dr. H. Zachau (Munich) for the clone of the mouse κ constant region, to Dr. F. Rougeon (Paris) for the clone of the IgA constant region, and to Dr. M. Potter (Bethesda) for mouse ascites.

REFERENCES

Abrahmsen, L., T. Moks, B. Nilsson, and M. Uhlen. 1986. Secretion of heterologous gene products to the culture medium of *Escherichia coli*. *Nucleic Acids Res.* **14:** 7487.

Abrahmsen, L., T. Moks, B. Nilsson, U. Hellman, and M. Uhlen. 1985. Analysis of signals for secretion in the staphylococcal protein A gene. *EMBO J.* **4:** 3901.

Albery, W.J. and J.R. Knowles. 1977. Efficiency and evolution of enzyme catalysis. *Angew. Chem. Int. Ed. Engl.* **16:** 285.

Altenburger, W., P.S. Neumaier, M. Steinmetz, and H.G. Zachau. 1981. DNA sequence of the constant gene region of the mouse immunoglobulin kappa chain. *Nucleic Acids Res.* **9:** 971.

Amzel, L.M. and R.J. Poljak. 1979. Three-dimensonal structure of immunoglobulins. *Annu. Rev. Biochem.* **48:** 961.

Auffray, C., R. Nageotte, J.L. Sikorav, O. Heidmann, and F. Rougeon. 1981. Mouse immunoglobulin A: Nucleotide sequence of the structural gene for the α-heavy chain derived from cloned cDNAs. *Gene* **13:** 365.

Bartlett, P.A. and C.K. Marlowe. 1983. Phosphonamidates as transition state analogue inhibitors of thermolysin. *Biochemistry* **22:** 4618.

———. 1987. Evaluation of intrinsic binding energy from a hydrogen bonding group in an enzyme inhibitor. *Science* **235:** 569.

Bender, M.C. and M. Komiyama. 1978. *Cyclodextrin chemistry.* Springer-Verlag, Berlin.

Birnboim, H.C. and J. Doly. 1979. A rapid alkaline extraction procedure for screening recombinant plasmid DNA. *Nucleic Acids Res.* **7:** 1513.

Blake, M.S., K.H. Johnston, G.J. Russel-Jones, and E.C. Gotschlich. 1984. A rapid, sensitive method for detection of alkaline phosphatase-conjugated anti-antibody on Western blots. *Anal. Biochem.* **136:** 175.

Boss, M.A. and C.R. Wood. 1985. Genetically engineered antibodies. *Immunol. Today* **6:** 12.

Boss, M.A., J.H. Kenten, C.R. Wood, and J.S. Emtage. 1984. Assembly of functional antibodies from immunoglobulin heavy and light chains synthesized in *E. coli. Nucleic Acids Res.* **12:** 3791.

Breslow, R. 1986. Approaches to artificial enzymes. *Ann. N.Y. Acad. Sci.* **471:** 60.

Breslow, R. and A.W. Czarnik. 1983. Transaminations by pyridoxamine selectively attached at C-3 in β-cyclodextrin. *J. Am. Chem. Soc.* **105:** 1390.

Breslow, R., J.B. Doherty, G. Guillot, and C. Lipsey. 1978. β-Cyclodextrinbisimidazole, a model for ribonuclease. *J. Am. Chem. Soc.* **100:** 3227.

Briggs, M.S. and L.M. Gierasch. 1986. Molecular mechanisms of protein secretion: The role of the signal sequence. *Adv. Protein Chem.* **38:** 109.

Cabilly, S., A.D. Riggs, H. Pande, J.E. Shively, W.E. Holmes, M. Rey, L.J. Perry, R. Wetzel, and H.L. Heyneker. 1984. Generation of antibody activity from immunoglobulin polypeptide chains produced in *Escherchia coli. Proc. Natl. Acad. Sci.* **81:** 3273.

Chen, E.Y. and P.H. Seeburg. 1985. Supercoil sequencing: A fast and simple method for sequencing plasmid DNA. *DNA* **4:** 165.

Chesebro, B. and H. Metzger. 1972. Affinity labeling of a phosphorylcholine binding mouse myeloma protein. *Biochemistry* **11:** 766.

Cram, D.J. and K.N. Trueblood. 1985. Concept, structure and binding in complexation. In *Host guest complex chemistry: Macrocycles* (ed. F. Vögtle and E. Weber), p. 125. Springer-Verlag, Berlin.

Cramer, F. and G. Mackensen. 1966. A model for the action of chymotrypsin. *Angew. Chem. Int. Ed. Engl.* **5:** 601.

Dagert, M. and S.D. Ehrlich. 1979. Prolonged incubation in calcium chloride improves the competence of *Escherichia coli. Gene* **6:** 23.

Davies, D.R. and H. Metzger. 1983. Structural basis of antibody function. *Annu. Rev. Immunol.* **1:** 87.

Dörper, T. and E.L. Winnacker. 1983. Improvements in the phosphoramidite procedure for the synthesis of oligodeoxyribonucleotides. *Nucleic Acids Res.* **11:** 2575.

D'Souza, V.T. and M.L. Bender. 1987. Miniature organic models of enzymes. *Accts. Chem. Res.* **20:** 146.

Enequist, H.G., T.R. Hirst, S. Harayama, S.J.S. Hardy, and L.L. Randall. 1981. Energy is required for maturation of exported proteins in *Escherichia coli. Eur. J. Biochem.* **116:** 227.

Ferraiolo, B.L., G. Onady, and J.J. Mieyal. 1984. Monooxygenase activity of human hemoglobin: Role of quaternary structure in the preponderant activity of the β-subunits within the tetramer. *Biochemistry* **23:** 5528.

Fling, S.P. and D.S. Gregerson. 1986. Peptide and protein molecular weight determination by electrophoresis using a high-molarity Tris-buffer system without urea. *Anal. Biochem.* **155:** 83.

Fujikawa, K., M.E. Legaz, and E.W. Davie. 1972a. Bovine factors X_1 and X_2 (Stuart factor). Isolation and characterization. *Biochemistry* **11:** 4882.

———. 1972b. Bovine factor X_1 (Stuart factor). Mechanism of activation by a protein from Russell's viper venom. *Biochemistry* **11:** 4892.

Galardy, R.E., V. Kontoyiannidou-Ostrem, and Z.P. Kortylewicz. 1983. Inhibition of angiotensin converting enzyme by phosphonic amides and phosphonic acids. *Biochemistry* **22:** 1990.

Grosjean, H. and W. Fiers. 1982. Preferential codon usage in prokaryotic genes: The optimal codon-anticodon interaction energy and the selective codon usage in efficiently expressed genes. *Gene* **18:** 199.

Gurd, F.R.N. 1967. Carboxymethylation. *Methods Enzymol.* **11:** 532.

Haldane, J.B.S. 1930. *Enzymes.* Longmans, Green and Co., London (1965, MIT Press, Cambridge, Massachusetts).

Hanahan, D. 1983. Studies on transformation of *Escherichia coli* with plasmids. *J. Mol. Biol.* **166:** 557.

Hilvert, D. and R. Breslow. 1984. Functionalized cyclodextrins as holoenzyme mimics of thiamine-dependent enzymes. *Bioorg. Chem.* **12:** 206.

Hochman, J., M. Gavish, D. Inbar, and D. Givol. 1976. Folding and interaction of subunits at the antibody combining site. *Biochemistry* **15:** 2706.

Hofmann, W. and M. Rottenberg. 1980. A transition state analogous organophosphate inhibitor of carboxypeptidase A. In *Enzyme inhibitors* (ed. U. Brodbeck), p. 19. Verlag Chemie, Weinheim.

Holmes, D.S. and M. Quigley. 1981. A rapid boiling method for the preparation of bacterial plasmids. *Anal. Biochem.* **114:** 193.

Ish-Horowicz, D. and J.F. Burke. 1981. Rapid and efficient cosmid cloning. *Nucleic Acids Res.* **9:** 2989.

Jacobs, J., P.G. Schultz, R. Sugasawara, and M. Powell. 1987. Catalytic antibodies. *J. Am. Chem. Soc.* **109:** 2174.

Jencks, W.P. 1969. Strain, distortion and conformation change. *Catalysis in chemistry and enzymology,* p. 282. McGraw-Hill, New York.

———. 1975. Binding energy, specificity and enzymic catalysis: The Circe effect. *Adv. Enzymol.* **43:** 219.

Jacobsen, N.E. and P.A. Bartlett. 1981. A phosphonamidate dipeptide analogue as an inhibitor of carboxypeptidase A. *J. Am. Chem. Soc.* **103:** 654.

Kabat, E.A. 1978. The structural basis of antibody complementarity. *Adv. Protein Chem.* **32:** 1.

Kabat, E.A., T.T. Wu, H. Bilofsky, M. Reid-Miller, and H. Perry. 1983. *Sequences of proteins of immunological interest.* U.S. Department of Health and Human Services, Public Health Service, National Institutes of Health, Bethesda, Maryland.

Kam, C.M., N. Nishino, and J.C. Powers. 1979. Inhibition of thermolysin and carboxypeptidase A by phosphoramidates. *Biochemistry* **18:** 3032.

Kellogg, R.M. 1985. Bioorganic modelling—Stereoselective reactions with chiral neutral ligand complexes as model systems for enzyme catalysis. In *Host guest complex chemistry: Macrocycles* (ed. F. Vögtle and E. Weber), p. 283. Springer-Verlag, Berlin.

Kohen, F., Z. Hollander, J.F. Burd, and R.C. Boguslaski. 1979. A steroid immunoassay based on antibody-enhanced hydrolysis of a steroid-umbelliferone conjugate. *FEBS Lett.* **100:** 137.

Kohen, F., J.B. Kim, G. Barnard, and H.R. Lindner. 1980a. Antibody-enhanced hydrolysis of steroid esters. *Biochim. Biophys. Acta* **629:** 328.

Kohen, F., J.B. Kim, H.R. Lindner, Z. Eshhar, and B. Green. 1980b. Monoclonal immunoglobulin G augments hydrolysis of an ester of the homologous hapten. *FEBS Lett.* **111:** 427.

Knowles, J.R. 1987. Tinkering with enzymes: What are we learning? *Science* **236:** 1252.

Laemmli, U.K. 1970. Cleavage of structural proteins during the assembly of the head of bacteriophage T4. *Nature* **227:** 680.

Leatherbarrow, R.J. and A.R. Fersht. 1986. Protein engineering. *Protein Eng.* **1:** 7.

Lehn, J.M. 1986. Recent studies of supramolecular catalysis and transport processes. *Ann. N.Y. Acad. Sci.* **471:** 41.

Lottenberg, R., V. Christensen, C.M. Jackson, and P.L. Coleman. 1981. Assay of coagulation proteases using peptide chromogenic and fluorogenic substrates. *Methods Enzymol.* **80:** 341.

Maniatis, T., E.F. Fritsch, and J. Sambrook. 1982. Molecular cloning: A laboratory manual. Cold Spring Harbor Laboratory. Cold Spring Harbor, New York.

Miller, J.H. 1972. *Experiments in molecular genetics.* Cold Spring Harbor Laboratory. Cold Spring Harbor, New York.

Minsky, A., R. Summers, and J.R. Knowles. 1986. Secretion of β-lactamase into the periplasm of *Escherichia coli*: Evidence for a distinct release step associated with a conformational change. *Proc. Natl. Acad. Sci.* **83:** 4180.

Moks, T., L. Abrahmsen, B. Österlöf, S. Josephson, M. Östling, S.O. Enfors, I. Persson, B, Nilsson, and M. Uhlen. 1987. Large scale affinity purification of human insulin-like growth factor I from culture medium of *Escherichia coli. Biotechnology* **5:** 379.

Nagai, K. and H.C. Thogersen. 1984. Generation of β-globin by sequence-specific proteolysis of a hybrid protein produced in *E. coli. Nature* **309:** 810.

Nagai, K., M.F. Perutz, and C. Poyart. 1985. Oxygen binding properties of human mutant hemoglobins synthesized in *Escherichia coli. Proc. Natl. Acad. Sci.* **82:** 7253.

Pauling, L. 1946. Molecular architecture and biological reactions. *Chem. Eng. News.* **24:** 1375.

———. 1948. Antibodies and specific biological forces. *Endeavour* **7:** 43.

Perlmutter, R.M., S.T. Crews, R. Douglas, G. Sorensen, N. Johnson, N. Nivera, P. Gearhart, and L. Hood. 1984. The generation of diversity in phosphorylcholine-binding antibodies. *Adv. Immunol.* **35:** 1.

Plückthun, A. and J.R. Knowles. 1987. Consequences of stepwise deletions from the signal processing site in β-lactamase. *J. Biol. Chem.* **262:** 3951.

Pollack, S.J., J.W. Jacobs, and P.G. Schultz. 1986. Selective chemical catalysis by an antibody. *Science* **234:** 1570.

Potter, M. 1977. Antigen binding myeloma proteins of mice. *Adv. Immunol.* **25:** 141.

Raso, V. and B.D. Stollar. 1975a. The antibody-enzyme analogy. Characterization of antibodies to phosphopyridoxyl tyrosine derivatives. *Biochemistry* **14:** 584.

———. 1975b. The antibody-enzyme analogy. Comparison of enzymes and antibodies specific for phosphopyridoxyl tyrosine. *Biochemistry* **14:** 591.

Rommens, J., D. MacKnight, L. Pomeroy-Cloney, and E. Jay. 1983. Gene expression: Chemical synthesis and molecular cloning of a bacteriophage T5 (T5P25) early promoter. *Nucleic Acids Res.* **11:** 5921.

Rudikoff, S. and M. Potter. 1974. Variable region sequence of the heavy chain from a phosphorylcholine binding myeloma protein. *Biochemistry* **13:** 4033.

Rudikoff, S., Y. Satow, E. Padlan, D. Davies, and M. Potter. 1981. Kappa chain structure from a crystallized murine F_{ab}: Role of joining segment in hapten binding. *Mol. Immunol.* **18:** 705.

Segal, D.M., E.A. Padlan, G.H. Cohen, S. Rudikoff, M. Potter, and D.R. Davies. 1974. The three-dimensional structure of a phosphorylcholine-binding mouse immunoglobulin F_{ab} and the nature of the antigen binding site. *Proc. Natl. Acad. Sci.* **71:** 4298.

Sherman, F., J.W. Stewart, and S. Tsunasawa. 1985. Methionine or not methionine at the beginning of a protein. *Bioessays* **3:** 27.

Sinha, N.D., J. Biernat, J. McManus, and H. Köster. 1984. Polymer support oligonucleotide synthesis. XVIII: Use of β-cyanoethyl-N,N-dialkylamino-/N-morpholino phosphoamidite of deoxynucleosides for the synthesis of DNA fragments simplifying deprotection and isolation of the final product. *Nucleic Acids Res.* **12:** 4539.

Slobin, L.I. 1966. Preparation and some properties of antibodies with specificity toward p-nitrophenyl esters. *Biochemistry* **5:** 2836.

Starke, D.W., K.S. Blisard, and J.J. Mieyal. 1984. Substrate specificity of the monooxygenase activity of hemoglobin. *Mol. Pharmacol.* **25:** 467.

Tabushi, I., Y. Kuroda, and A. Mochizuki. 1980. The first successful carbonic anhydrase model prepared through a new route to regiospecifically bifunctionalized cyclodextrin. *J. Am. Chem. Soc.* **102:** 1152.

Taylor, R.P. and J.B. Vatz. 1973. Bovine serum albumin as catalyst. Accelerated decomposition of a Meisenheimer complex. *J. Am. Chem. Soc.* **95:** 5819.

Thorsett, E.D., E.E. Harris, E.R. Peterson, W.J. Greenlee, A.A. Patchett, E.H. Ulm, and T.C. Vassil. 1982. Phosphorus-containing inhibitors of angiotensin-converting enzyme. *Proc. Natl. Acad. Sci.* **79:** 2176.

Tramontano, A., K.D. Janda, and R.A. Lerner. 1986a. Chemical reactivity at an antibody binding site elicited by mechanistic design of a synthetic antigen. *Proc. Natl. Acad. Sci.* **83:** 6736.

———. 1986b. Catalytic antibodies. *Science* **234:** 1566.

Tronrud, D.E., H.M. Holden, and B.W. Matthews. 1987. Structures of two thermolysin-inhibitor complexes that differ by a single hydrogen bond. *Science* **235:** 571.

Tronrud, D.E., A.F. Monzingo, and B.W. Matthews. 1986. Crystallographic structural analysis of phosphoramidates as inhibitors and transition-state analogs of thermolysin. *Eur. J. Biochem.* **157:** 261.

Weaver, L.H., W.R. Kester, and B.W. Matthews. 1977. A crystallographic study of the complex of phosphoramidon with thermolysin. A model for the presumed catalytic transition state and for the binding of extended substrates. *J. Mol. Biol.* **114:** 119.

Wetzel, R. 1986. What is protein engineering? *Protein Eng.* **1:** 3.

Wolfenden, R. 1976. Transition state analog inhibitors and enzyme catalysis. *Annu. Rev. Biophys. Bioeng.* **5:** 271.

Conformational Changes and Dynamics of tRNAs: Evidence from Hydrolysis Patterns

A.C. DOCK-BREGEON AND D. MORAS

Laboratoire de Cristallographie Biologique, Institut de Biologie Moléculaire et Cellulaire, 67084 Strasbourg Cedex, France

Splitting of the ribose-phosphate chain of RNA has been reported in different works dealing with mRNA (see, e.g., Berger and Birkenmeier 1979), rRNA (see, e.g., Carbon et al. 1978; Garrett and Olesen 1982), and tRNA (Vlassov et al. 1981; Garret et al. 1984; Romby et al. 1985b). In some of these reports, ribonuclease contamination has been implicated (Berger and Birkenmeier 1979); in others, different experimental conditions have allowed the search for other causes of the degradations observed. This parasite phenomenon is of small amplitude (only a small percentage of the molecules are involved) but occurs even under the mild conditions generally used in biochemical work.

Crystals provide a homogeneous sample of molecules, free from ribonucleases and under controlled conditions of ionic strength, pH, and temperature. Observation of the cleavage of the backbone of crystallized tRNAs has already been reported: Brown et al. (1983) and Rubin and Sundaralingam (1983) have described lead-induced cleavage in tRNA^{Phe}. Degradation patterns in tRNA^{Asp} crystals were shown to be dependent on the conformation of the molecule (Moras et al. 1986).

Analysis of cleavage sites in crystals of tRNAs of known three-dimensional structure may provide some interesting insights into the cleavage mechanism or at least some information about the structural constraints of the reaction. Moreover, since the discovery of self-splicing, a new concept of catalysis where RNA acts as substrate and catalyst is emerging (for review, see Cech and Bass 1986). Since crystal packing could generate a matrix for the hydrolysis reaction in a way that could be related to the splicing process, it was also tempting to analyze this aspect of the hydrolysis data in light of the available information provided by tRNA crystals concerning conformations as well as interactions of these molecules.

EXPERIMENTAL RESULTS

Comparison between Yeast tRNA^{Asp} and tRNA^{Phe}

Two crystal forms for each tRNA have been refined to high resolution (Hingerty et al. 1978; Sussman et al. 1978; Westhof et al. 1985), and some of their solvent molecules have also been located. A comparative analysis of the two tRNA molecules leads to two main

conclusions: First, there is overall structural homology with conservation of all basic interactions, except for an interesting deviation for the Watson-Crick base pair G19-C56. Relevant examples of these structural similarities are shown in Figure 1, where the canonical TψC and anticodon loops are superposed. Despite the sometimes important flexibility of these loops, suggested by the high values of their temperature factors, their conformation is quite conserved.

Second, there are significant differences in the distances between the anticodon and the CCA end. The change is most apparent when the anticodon loops are superposed as shown in Figure 1. In this case, the distance difference between the two CCA ends of the two superposed molecules is larger than 10 Å. The variation results from the successive addition of small local changes located essentially in the stem regions and not from a rotation around the hinge region in the center of the molecule, as a superficial inspection could suggest. These conformational changes occur essentially in tRNA^{Asp} crystals, where molecules form dimers through anticodons' interactions. The correlation between dimerization and conformational changes was demonstrated by chemical labeling of C56 in solution (Moras et al. 1985).

Hydrolysis of tRNAs

Two different basic mechanisms that can explain the hydrolytic reaction lead to two different types of products bearing either a 3'-phosphate end group or a 5'-phosphate end group. It is generally acknowledged that cleavage occurs by an S_N2 attack by a nucleophile, in line with the P–O bond to be broken, and that a trigonal bipyramide configuration is produced for the phosphate in the transition state (Witzel 1963; Brown 1974; Dugas and Penney 1981).

Cleavage at P–O3' or P–O5' results from the opportunity to find a good nucleophile and its proximity in the initial state of the reaction. The greater susceptibility of RNA versus DNA to hydrolysis is related to the presence of the 2'-OH group on the ribose. Oxygen at position 2' may act like a nucleophile, leading to the cleavage of the P–O5' bond through a 2',3'-cyclic phosphate intermediate, if its naturally weak nucleophilicity can be increased.

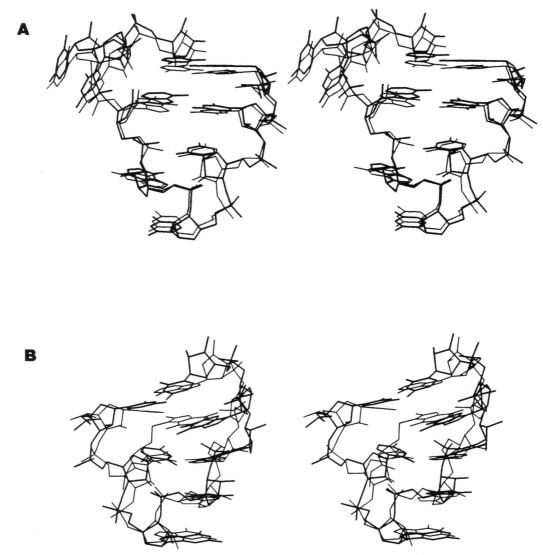

Figure 1. Superposition of loops of tRNA^Phe (light lines) on tRNA^Asp (heavy lines). (*A*) TψC loops; (*B*) anticodon loops. The superposition was obtained by least-squares fitting of backbone coordinates.

Cleavage Sites of tRNAs in Solution

Data concerning the cleavage sites of tRNAs in solution can be found in Vlassov et al. (1981), Riehl et al. (1983), Garret et al. (1984), and Romby et al. (1985b) and more completely in Romby (1986). Figure 2 (from Romby 1986) shows a compilation of the cleavage sites in eight tRNAs. These cuts have been observed in different biochemical experiments (usually chemical or enzymatic structure-probing experiments) in the control lanes of the gel electrophoresis analysis. They appear during incubation of the labeled tRNA, without addition of the chemical probe or the enzyme, in a solution (pH 7.5) containing 10 mM magnesium. The temperature varies from 20°C to 37°C.

Sequence dependence: Cuts appear mostly in YpA sequences. A strong sequence dependence can be observed: Most of the cuts appear in pyrimidine-adenosine sequences. Among 49 cuts observed in Figure 2, 41 precede an adenosine and 37 of them follow a pyrimidine (Fig. 2). YpA sequence preference was reported previously by Witzel (1963) on the basis of experiments with dinucleotides.

Since the cleavage leads to a 3'-phosphate end group, the attacking nucleophile could be the 2'-OH of the ribose on the pyrimidine side, provided that the proton of this 2'-OH group has been removed. An explanation of the sequence specificity could then be found in the involvement of this proton in a hydrogen bond specific to this sequence. Witzel postulated a direct hydrogen bond between 2'-OH and the adjacent N3 (if a purine) or O2 (if a pyrimidine); the latter bond would be stronger, according to the closest distance O2'-O2 inferred from model building. Such a direct hydrogen bonding between O2' and the adjacent base has never been found in tRNA structures. However, the study of

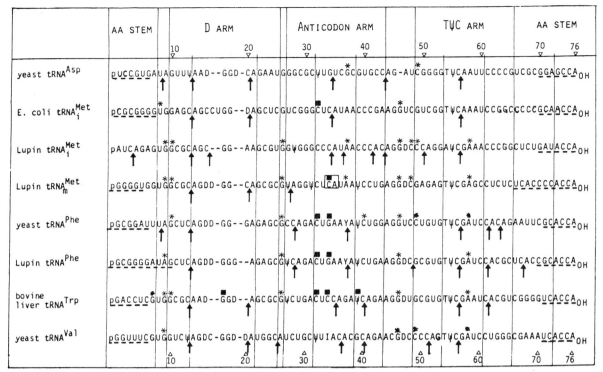

Figure 2. Localization of major spontaneous cuts in several tRNAs. These cuts are observed in control lanes of the sequencing gels used in structure-mapping experiments. End-labeled tRNA was incubated at 20°C or 37°C in buffer containing 10 mm MgCl₂ at pH 7.5. More precise experimental details are described in Romby et al. (1985b). (■) Methylated ribose; (*) modified base; (→) spontaneous cut; (----) region not tested. (Reprinted, with permission, from Romby 1986.)

hydration of tRNA^Phe in monoclinic and orthorhombic forms and of tRNA^Asp in both A and B forms (E. Westhof et al., in prep.) shows that suitable water bridges can be found between 2′-OH of a ribose and O2 of a pyrimidine or N3 of a purine bound to this same ribose, thus opening the possibility for the proton to be captured. There is as yet no visible preference for bridging O2, rather than N3, to O2′.

Location of the cuts in the molecular structure. The YpA cuts occur predominantly in loops, and all YpA sequences in loop regions exhibit cuts. However, stem regions are not insensitive (see e.g., C51-A52 in yeast tRNA^Val and C61-A62 or C28-A29 in yeast tRNA^Phe). Two interesting locations of YpA cuts can be noted with respect to important features of tRNA function. These sites occur just before the conserved residue A14 at the junction of the D loop and D stem and just after C56 in the T loop. In the latter case, position 57 is always a purine, but the cleavage seems to occur whether it is an adenine or a guanine.

The P13-A14 site in yeast tRNA^Asp and the C13-A14 site in yeast tRNA^Phe are shown in Figure 3. A water molecule bridges O4 from U8 to the anionic oxygen of phosphate 14. This water position seems to be constant and related to the stabilization of the reverse-Hoogsteen U8-A14 base pair, and it is suitably placed to play a role in the cleavage reaction. Figure 4 shows the T loop site of cleavage in the two known structures. Here,

a general hydration scheme can also be drawn: Conserved water molecules lie between pseudouridine 55 and thymine 54; others surround the methyl group of thymine 54. These water positions are susceptible to evolve according to the dynamics of the molecule, and slight variations in the surrounding medium can make use of these water molecules to induce cleavage.

Another important site of cleavage is the anticodon loop. Here again, the cleavage affects a fundamental function in the tRNA structure. Methylation on the 2′ position of ribose prevents the cleavage, as verified in lupin tRNA_m^Met at Cm34-A35. Methylation occurs very often in the anticodon loop and can be a general way to protect against hydrolysis. An interesting case is yeast tRNA^Asp, which is cleaved between G34 and U35. This cleavage site is discussed below.

A need for flexibility. The stereochemical condition of the generally acknowledged S_N2 mechanism raises a problem. The attacking O2′ should be in line with the P–O5′ bond to be broken. In the loop regions, this condition can be filled through local flexibility. However, when the cuts are found in the helical parts of the structure, it is necessary to invoke a "breathing" of the tRNA. Figure 5 shows the results of an experiment where 3′-end-labeled tRNA^Asp has been incubated with magnesium or the chelating agent ethylenediaminetetraacetate and then analyzed on a denaturing gel. Two types of cleavage sites are observed: YpA cuts (after

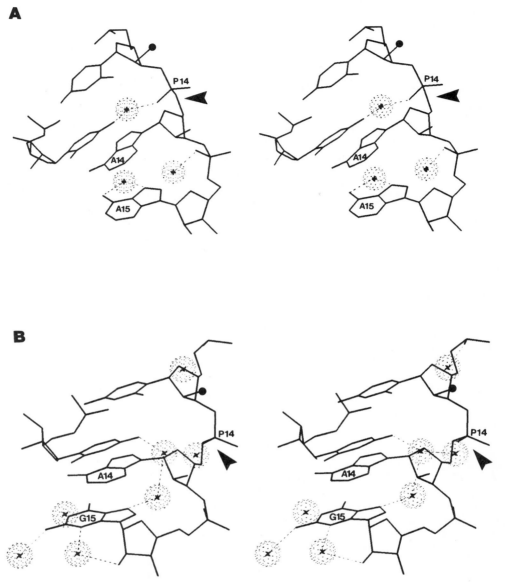

Figure 3. Stereoviews of the site of preferential cleavage between residues 13 and A14. (*A*) tRNA^Asp B form; (*B*) tRNA^Phe monoclinic form. Arrows show which bond is cleaved. Spheres represent water molecules. The coordinates for tRNA^Asp were from Dumas et al. (1985) and those for the monoclinic form of tRNA^Phe were from Westhof and Sundaralingam (1986).

C43 and C56) and anticodon cuts (the principal one after U35). They seem to appear at all pH values from 6.0 to 8.0, but a decrease in intensity is observed at a more acidic pH value of 4.5. When magnesium is present (Fig. 5, lanes 2, 5, 8, and 11), the strongest cuts are found in the anticodon loop, supporting the idea that the cleavage at U35 is catalyzed by a magnesium ion bound in the neighborhood. Indeed, a magnesium ion has been found in the anticodon loop of tRNA^Phe for the orthorhombic crystal form. In tRNA^Asp form A, there is also a possible binding site in this region (P. Dumas et al., in prep.). When magnesium is absent and EDTA present in the incubation medium, YpA cuts after C43 and C56 are enhanced (Fig. 5, lanes 1, 4, 7, and 10). Since the absence of magnesium weakens the

three-dimensional structure of the tRNA, denaturation can occur, the secondary structure can open, especially at the extremities of stems as at position C43, and the flexibility attained allows cleavage to occur.

Cleavage Sites Observed in the Crystals

Degradation patterns observed in the crystals are shown in Figure 6. Crystals were washed several times in a saturated mother liquor to avoid contamination by noncrystallized molecules and then dissolved in the labeling buffer. The labeling reaction was quick enough to minimize new degradations that could appear. These results verify that degradations do occur in the crystals, without ribonuclease or heavy metal ion contamina-

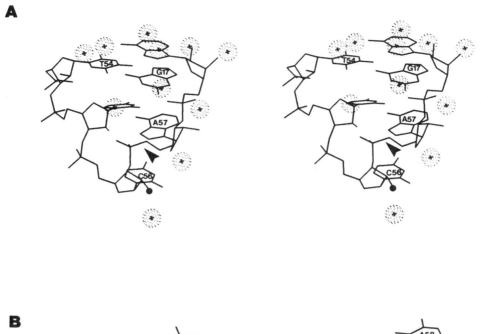

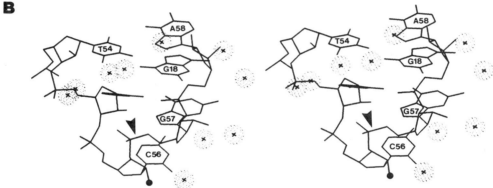

Figure 4. Stereoviews of the site of preferential cleavage between C56 and purine 57 in tRNA^{Asp} B form and tRNA^{Phe} orthorhombic form. Coordinates for tRNA^{Phe} were obtained from Sussman et al. (1978) and Westhof et al. (1987).

tion. We did not find any correlation between the occurrence of cleavage and the intermolecular contacts provided by crystal packing. An interesting point is that no YpA cuts appeared in the crystals. As tRNA unfolding is strictly restricted by crystal packing, this observation supports our hypothesis that the occurrence of YpA cuts is bound to tRNA breathing.

Degradation patterns of tRNA^{Phe} and tRNA^{Met} crystals. Orthorhombic crystals of tRNA^{Phe} (Kim et al. 1973) have been tested for degradations after a stay of several months in their mother liquor (Fig. 6a). The degradation pattern obtained exhibits two major sites of cleavage. The cleavage site after A38 is probably related to the presence of the magnesium site in the anticodon loop and to the particular hydration of pseudouridine P39. It is interesting to note that the CCA end of a symmetrically related molecule comes near the anticodon loop. The cleavage site after U47 is shown in Figure 7. The base U47 makes a bulge out of the core of tRNA^{Phe} and is particularly agitated. A

water molecule bridges the 2'-OH group of residue U47 to the phosphate oxygen of U50, and it may attract the proton of 2'-OH, thus allowing O2' to attack.

Crystallized yeast tRNA^{Met} (Schevitz et al. 1979) shows an important cleavage site in the anticodon loop (Fig. 6b). The packing of these crystals leaves the anticodon loop quite free, and this part of the molecule much agitated. Here again, the local flexibility of the loop can explain the cleavage.

Degradation patterns in tRNA^{Asp} crystals. Lane e in Figure 6 is particularly interesting since it was obtained in a different manner. In this case, tRNA^{Asp} was labeled before crystallization and repurified by electrophoresis in a polyacrylamide-urea denaturing gel, ensuring that there were no degradations previous to crystallization. The cleavage occurs in the anticodon loop after G34 and C36 and leaves 3'-phosphate end groups, like T$_1$ products, as can be seen by comparison with the T$_1$ digest (Fig. 6f). This cleavage site is very close to the magnesium-induced cleavage site described

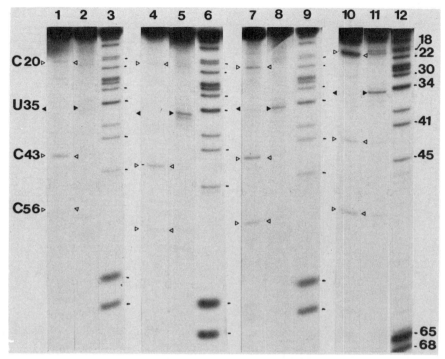

Figure 5. Autoradiograms of degradation patterns of end-labeled yeast tRNA^{Asp} in solution. The tRNA was incubated at 50°C for 30 min either with 1 mM EDTA (lanes *1,4,7,10*) or with 10 mM MgCl$_2$ (lanes *2,5,8,11*) in 50 mM cacodylate buffer at pH 4.5 (lanes *1,2*), pH 6.0 (lanes *4,5*), pH 7.0 (lanes *7,8*), or pH 8.0 (lanes *10,11*). Lanes *3, 6, 9*, and *12* show partial ribonuclease T1 digests to localize the degradation sites.

for tRNA^{Asp} in solution, where we observed a principal hit after U35, and most likely has the same origin. The degradation can propagate along the loop as can be seen (Fig. 6d), when a different crystal form, obtained at lower ionic strength, is tested.

Figure 6c shows the degradation pattern of C222$_1$ crystals of tRNA^{Asp} of known structure, obtained in ammonium sulfate at neutral pH (Giegé et al. 1977). The cleavage in the anticodon loop still occurs, but new, strong cleavage sites appear in the D loop. We already showed that the D-loop cuts are associated with the increased flexibility of the D loop, resulting from the particular conformation of tRNA^{Asp} in the C222$_1$ crystals (Moras et al. 1986). This conformation of the tRNA is due to the existence of an interaction between anticodons of two symmetrically related molecules. The degradations in the D loop do not appear in lane e and are strongly reduced in lane d, indicating less flexibility in the D loop. Indeed, it has been shown (Romby et al. 1985a) that tRNA^{Asp} dimerization through anticodon-anticodon interaction cannot occur in the acidic range of pH, where the crystals used for lane e were grown, and is not favored at low ionic strength, the growth condition of crystals used in experiment d.

The permanent observation of the cleavage in the anticodon loop is apparently inconsistent with the existence of the anticodon-anticodon interaction. However, two remarks can be made. The U-U base pair accommodates some flexibility, as shown by the diffu-

sion of a mercury atom between the two base pairs (Westhof et al. 1985). Second, although the CCA end is disordered, model building and packing considerations lead to a positioning of the terminal adenine close to the groove of the anticodon loop. This situation resembles that observed in tRNA^{Phe} and also suggests again an involvement of the adenine base in the cleavage.

DISCUSSION

A Need for Catalysis

In neutral solution, a polyribonucleotide should be stable, and catalysis is necessary to induce the reaction either by increasing the electrophilicity at the phosphorus atom or by increasing the nucleophilicity of the 2'-OH group of the ribose.

Acid and base catalysis proceeds through addition of H$^+$ or OH$^-$ ions: Either H$^+$ protonates the P–O$^-$ group, leading to the polarization of this bond, an increased electrophilicity at the phosphorus atom, and the possibility for the weak nucleophile 2'-OH to attack, or OH$^-$ removes the proton of the 2'-OH group, thus giving a strongly nucleophilic alcoholate anion. This last chemical path, base catalyzed, is well known as alkaline hydrolysis of RNA. This path is also followed by different ribonucleases, in particular by RNase A, whose mechanisms have been thoroughly studied in light of its available high-resolution X-ray

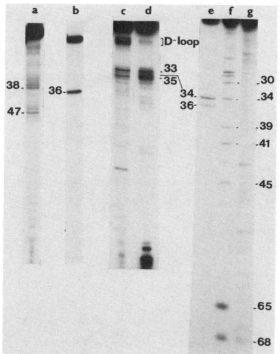

Figure 6. Degradation patterns of crystallized tRNAs. Crystals were dissolved, and tRNA was labeled as described by Moras et al. (1986). (*a*) Yeast tRNA^{Phe} in orthorhombic form; (*b*) yeast tRNA^{fMet}; (*c*) classic tRNA^{Asp} C222$_1$ crystal form obtained in ammonium sulfate; (*d*) yeast tRNA^{Asp} crystallized with polyethylene glycol as precipitating agent (Dock et al. 1984); (*e*) tRNA^{Asp} labeled before crystallization and repurified on a polyacrylamide-urea denaturing gel to eliminate degradated molecules. It was then mixed with cold tRNA, buffer, and ammonium sulfate as in an ordinary setup, except that the pH was between 5.0 and 6.0. This solution was seeded with fragments of a C222$_1$ crystal, and the microcrystals that formed were simply dissolved in water for analysis on gel. T1 ribonuclease digest (*f*) and alkaline hydrolysis (*g*) were carried out to allow localization of the degradations.

structure (Richards and Wyckoff 1971; Brooks et al. 1986).

Other possible catalysts, which can act at about neutral pH, are metal ions. These ions can perturb their surrounding water molecules, which are then potential nucleophiles or potential attracting groups, for the proton at 2′-OH. Metal ions can also act by direct coordination on the phosphate group, thus increasing the electrophilicity of the phosphorus atom (Cooperman 1976; Marzilli et al. 1980). Experiments concerning tRNA cleavage induced by different metal ions have been reported previously, e.g., zinc (Butzow and Eichhorn 1971), europium (Rordorf and Kearns 1976), lead (Werner et al. 1976), and magnesium (Wintermeyer and Zachau 1973). Europium, zinc, and particularly lead are much more effective than magnesium. Lead-induced cleavage of tRNA^{Phe} in both crystal forms has been reported (Brown et al. 1983; Rubin and Sundaralingam 1983), providing some indication of the mechanism involved. Cleavage involves two different parts of the tRNA chain: residues 59 and 60 in the T loop as the lead-binding site and residues D17 and G18 in the D loop as the cleavage site. It is noteworthy that in all of the experiments involving metal-ion-induced cleavage in tRNA^{Phe} reported thus far, the cleavage sites have been located on the D loop and the metal ion has always been supposed to occupy a precise binding site on the tRNA. Why not then consider the catalyst as the metal-ion–tRNA-chain complex? This idea has recently been proved (O. Uhlenbeck, pers. comm.) and is related to the ribosome concept, emerging from the discoveries of self-splicing in *Tetrahymena thermophila* pre-rRNA (Zaug et al. 1983) and maturation of pre-tRNAs by the RNA subunit of ribonuclease P from *Escherichia coli* or *Bacillus subtilis* (Guerrier-Takada et al. 1983, 1986; Gardiner et al. 1985). RNA catalysis can also account for the splicing of mRNA precursors (Sharp 1987).

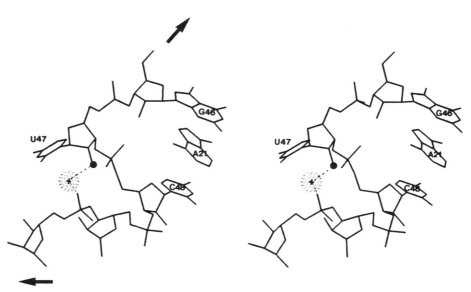

Figure 7. Stereoview of the cleavage site in the orthorhombic crystals of tRNA^{Phe} between U47 and C48. A water molecule is bridging 2′-OH of U47 to a phosphate oxygen of P50.

Additional evidence of magnesium-induced cleavage of tRNA was reported by Wintermeyer and Zachau (1973), who showed that fragments of tRNA[Phe] could be produced after several hours of incubation at pH 9.5 in the presence of magnesium. Our results emphasize the fact that this phenomenon already appears at neutral pH, although notably reduced in intensity. Interestingly, for tRNA[Asp], the principal cleavage site depends on the conformational state of the molecule.

In the vicinity of the cleavage sites, the only evidence suggesting the presence of free bases of proximal molecules, which could act as catalysts in a manner suggested by the ribozyme concept, is the terminal adenines in the anticodon loops. In the case of tRNA[Asp], the quality of the map at the CCA end does not allow us to prove a direct implication of the free purine in the cleavage mechanism.

Based on observations involving tRNA in solution as well as in the crystalline state, our analysis strongly suggests the need for local flexibility in order to adapt the conformation to the correct transition state. Ions and water molecules suitably located can act as catalysts by deprotonating the appropriate hydroxyl group. It is interesting that, when free tRNA molecules exhibit strong dependence on the YpA sequence in their cleavage patterns, only the more flexible loops are cleaved in the crystallized tRNA molecules without obvious sequence correlations. This latter observation applies to all tRNAs analyzed, quite different in both their crystalline and ionic environments. Crystallographic temperature factor distribution correlates with the degradation patterns and supports the explanation through flexibility. Thus, analysis of tRNA hydrolysis brings additional evidence of the intrinsic flexibility of tRNA molecules. This flexibility enables local adaptation as well as more important conformational changes through correlated variations.

ACKNOWLEDGMENTS

This paper is the result of many experiments of the biochemistry and crystallography groups at I.B.M.C. We express our gratitude to R. Giegé, C. Florentz, P. Romby, and E. Westhof for many fruitful discussions. We are especially indebted to P. Romby for Fig. 2.

REFERENCES

Berger, S.L. and C.S. Birkenmeier. 1979. Inhibition of intractable nucleases with ribonucleoside-vanadyl complexes: Isolation of messenger ribonucleic acids from resting lymphocytes. *Biochemistry* 18: 5143.
Brooks, C., A. Brunger, M. Francl, K. Haydock, L.C. Allen, and M, Karplus. 1986. Role of active site residues and solvation in RNase A. *Ann. N.Y. Acad. Sci.* 471: 295.
Brown, D.M. 1974. Chemical reactions of polynucleotides and nucleic acids. In *Basic principles in nucleic acid chemistry*, (ed. P.O.P. Ts'O) vol. 2, p.1. Academic Press, New York.
Brown, R.S., B.E. Hingerty, J.C. Dewan, and A. Klug. 1983. Pb(II)-catalysed cleavage of the sugar-phosphate backbone of yeast tRNA[Phe]. Implications for lead toxicity and self-splicing RNA. *Nature* 303: 543.
Butzow, J.J. and G.L. Eichhorn. 1971. Interaction of metal ions with nucleic acids and related compounds. XVII. On the mechanism of degradation of polyribonucleotides and oligoribonucleotides by Zinc(II) ions. *Biochemistry* 10: 2019.
Carbon, P., C. Ehresmann, B. Ehresmann, and J.P. Ebel. 1978. The sequence of *Escherichia coli* ribosomal 16S RNA determined by new rapid gel methods. *FEBS Lett.* 94: 152.
Cech, T.R. and B.L. Bass. 1986. Biological catalysis by RNA. *Annu. Rev. Biochem.* 55: 599.
Cooperman, B.S. 1976. The role of divalent metal ions in phosphoryl and nucleotidyl transfer. In *Metal ions in biological systems* (ed. H. Sigel), vol. 5, p. 79. Marcel Dekker, New York.
Dock, A.C., B. Lorber, D. Moras, G. Pixa, J.C. Thierry, and R. Giegé. 1984. Crystallization of transfer ribonucleic acids. *Biochimie* 66: 179.
Dugas, H. and C. Penney. 1981. Bioorganic chemistry of the phosphates. In *Bioorganic chemistry* (ed. C. Cantor), p. 108. Springer Verlag, New York.
Dumas, P., J.P. Ebel, R. Giegé, D. Moras, J.C. Thierry and E. Westhof. 1985. Crystal structure of yeast tRNA[Asp]: Atomic coordinates. *Biochimie* 67: 597.
Gardiner, K., T. Marsh, and N. Pace. 1985. Ion dependence of the *Bacillus subtilis* RNase P reaction. *J. Biol. Chem.* 260: 5415.
Garret, M., B. Labouesse, S. Litvak, P. Romby, J.P. Ebel, and R. Giegé. 1984. Tertiary structure of animal tRNA[Trp] in solution and interaction of tRNA[Trp] with tryptophanyl-tRNA synthetase. *Eur. J. Biochem.* 138: 67.
Garrett, R.A. and S.O. Olesen. 1982. Structure of eukaryotic 5S ribonucleic acid: A study of *Saccharomyces cerevisiae* 5S ribonucleic acid with ribonucleases. *Biochemistry* 21: 4823.
Giegé, R., D. Moras, and J.C. Thierry. 1977. Yeast transfer RNA[Asp]: A new high resolution X-ray diffracting crystal form of a transfer RNA. *J. Mol. Biol.* 115: 91.
Guerrier-Takada, C., K. Haydock, L. Allen, and S. Altman. 1986. Metal ions requirements and other aspects of the reaction catalyzed by M1 RNA, the RNA subunit of ribonuclease P from *Escherichia coli*. *Biochemistry* 25: 1509.
Guerrier-Takada, C., K. Gardiner, T. Marsh, N. Pace, and S. Altman. 1983. The RNA moiety of ribonuclease P is the catalytic subunit of the enzyme. *Cell* 35: 849.
Hingerty, B., R.S. Brown, and A. Jack. 1978. Further refinement of the structure of yeast tRNA[Phe]. *J. Mol. Biol.* 124: 523.
Kim, S.H., G. Quigley, F.L. Suddath, A. McPherson, D. Sneden, J.J. Kim, J. Weinzierl, and A. Rich. 1973. X-ray crystallographic studies of polymorphic forms of yeast phenylalanine transfer RNA. *J. Mol. Biol.* 75: 421.
Marzilli, L.G., T.H. Kirstenmacher, and G.L. Eichhorn. 1980. Structural principles of metal ion-nucleotide and metal ion-nucleic acid interactions. In *Nucleic acid-metal ion interaction* (ed. T.G. Spiro), p. 180. Wiley, New York.
Moras, D., A.C. Dock, P. Dumas, E. Westhof, P. Romby, J.P. Ebel, and R. Giegé. 1985. The structure of yeast tRNA[Asp]. A model for tRNA interacting with messenger RNA. *J. Biomol. Struct. Dyn.* 3: 479.
———. 1986. Anticodon-anticodon interaction induces conformational changes in tRNA: Yeast tRNA[Asp], a model for tRNA-mRNA recognition. *Proc. Natl. Acad. Sci.* 83: 932.
Richards, F.M. and H.W. Wyckoff. 1971. Bovine pancreatic ribonuclease. In *The enzymes*, 3rd edition (ed. P.D. Boyer), vol. 4, p. 647. Academic Press, New York.
Riehl, N., R. Giegé, J.P. Ebel, and B. Ehresmann. 1983. Effect of elongation factor Tu on the conformation of phenylalanine-tRNA[Phe]. *FEBS Lett.* 154: 42.
Romby, P. 1986. Instabilité structurale des tRNA. "Contribution à l'étude structurale et fonctionelle de l'acide ribonucléique de transfert," p. 66. Thèse de doctorat ès Sciences, Université Louis Pasteur de Strasbourg.

Romby, P., R. Giegé, C. Houssier, and H. Grosjean. 1985a. Anticodon-anticodon interactions in solution. Studies of the self-association of yeast or *Escherichia coli* tRNA^Asp and of their interactions with *Escherichia coli* tRNA^Val. *J. Mol. Biol.* **184:** 107.

Romby, P., D. Moras, M. Bergdoll, P. Dumas, V.V. Vlassov, E. Westhof, J.P. Ebel, and R. Giegé. 1985b. Yeast tRNA^Asp tertiary structure in solution and areas of interaction of the tRNA with aspartyl-tRNA synthetase. *J. Mol. Biol.* **184:** 455.

Rordorf, B.F. and D.R. Kearns. 1976. Effect of Europium(III) on the thermal denaturation and cleavage of transfer ribonucleic acids. *Biopolymers* **15:** 1491.

Rubin, J.R. and M. Sundaralingam. 1983. Lead ion binding and RNA chain hydrolysis in phenylalanine tRNA. *J. Biomol. Struct. Dyn.* **1:** 639.

Schevitz, R.W., A.D. Podjarny, N. Krishnamachari, J.J. Hughes, P.D. Sigler, and J.L. Sussman. 1979. Crystal structure of an eukaryotic initiator tRNA. *Nature* **278:** 188.

Sharp, P. 1987. Splicing of messenger RNA precursors. *Science* **235:** 766.

Sussman, J.L., S.R. Holbrook, R.W. Warrant, G.M. Church, and S.H. Kim. 1978. Crystal structure of yeast phenylalanine transfer RNA. I. Crystallographic refinement. J. Mol. Biol. **123:** 607.

Vlassov, V.V., R. Giegé, and J.P. Ebel. 1981. Tertiary structure of tRNAs in solution monitored by phosphodiester modification with ethylnitrosourea. *Eur. J. Biochem.* **119:** 51.

Werner, C., B. Krebs, G. Keith, and G. Dirheimer. 1976. Specific cleavages of pure tRNAs by plumbous ions. *Biochim. Biophys. Acta* **432:** 161.

Westhof, E. and M. Sundaralingam. 1986. Restrained refinement of the monoclinic form of yeast phenylalanine transfer RNA. Temperature factors and dynamics, coordinated waters and base-pair propeller twist angles. *Biochemistry* **25:** 4868.

Westhof, E., P. Dumas, and D. Moras. 1985. Crystallographic refinement of yeast aspartic acid transfer RNA. *J. Mol. Biol.* **184:** 119.

———. 1987. Restrained refinement of two crystalline forms of yeast aspartic acid and phenylalanine transfer RNA crystals. *Acta Crystallogr. A* **43:** (in press).

Wintermeyer, W. and H.G. Zachau. 1973. Mg^{2+}-katalisierte, spezifische spaltung von tRNA. *Biochim. Biophys. Acta* **299:** 82.

Witzel, H. 1963. The function of the pyrimidine base in the ribonuclease reaction. *Prog. Nucleic Acid Res.* **2:** 221.

Zaug, A.J., P.J. Grabowski, and T.R. Cech. 1983. Autocatalytic cyclization of an excised intervening sequence RNA is a cleavage-ligation reaction. *Nature* **301:** 578.

Improved Parameters for Prediction of RNA Structure

D.H. Turner,* N. Sugimoto,* J.A. Jaeger,* C.E. Longfellow,* S.M. Freier,[†] and R. Kierzek[‡]

*Department of Chemistry, University of Rochester, Rochester, New York 14627; [†]Molecular Biosystems Inc., San Diego, California 92121; [‡]Institute of Bioorganic Chemistry, Polish Academy of Sciences, 60-704 Poznan, Noskowskiego 12/14, Poland

Complete understanding of the molecular basis of catalysis by an enzyme requires knowledge of the three-dimensional structure of the enzyme. Determining sequences of enzymes is much easier than determining structures. Thus, structure determination is a limiting step in understanding structure-function relationships. This limitation is particularly severe in the case of RNA enzymes because it is extremely difficult to crystallize large RNA molecules. In principle, one way to accelerate our understanding of RNA enzymes is to develop methods for reliably predicting structure from sequence. It should be easier to develop such methods for RNA than for proteins because the local interactions determining RNA structures tend to be stronger than those determining protein structure. For example, short, isolated RNA helixes are more stable than their protein counterparts (Freier et al. 1986b; Shoemaker et al. 1987).

Prediction of secondary structure is one step toward prediction of three-dimensional structure. Tinoco et al. (1971) developed a method for predicting the secondary structure of RNA that is based on minimizing the free-energy change associated with nearest-neighbor interactions. Applications of this method, however, have been hindered by lack of experimental data providing parameters for the nearest-neighbor interactions. Recent improvements in methods for synthesizing oligoribonucleotides (Neilson et al. 1980; Beckett and Uhlenbeck 1984; Markiewicz et al. 1984; Kierzek et al. 1986) make it possible to greatly expand the database for providing nearest-neighbor interactions. We report improved parameters derived from thermodynamic studies of the stability of short RNA duplexes. The results also provide insight into the strengths of fundamental interactions such as stacking and hydrogen bonding. Comparisons with the three-dimensional structure of yeast phenylalanine tRNA suggest that these insights may also be useful for predicting the three-dimensional structure of RNA.

METHODS

Oligoribonucleotide synthesis. Oligoribonucleotides were synthesized on solid support using phosphoramidite procedures (Kierzek et al. 1986) and purified by high-performance liquid chromatography (HPLC) on a Hamilton PRP-1 column (Ikuta et al. 1984). Purities after final deblocking were confirmed by HPLC on a C-8 column.

Thermodynamic parameters. Absorbance versus temperature melting curves were measured in 1 M NaCl, 0.01 M Na cacodylate, and 0.5 mM EDTA (disodium salt) at pH 7, as described by Kierzek et al. (1986). Concentrations were determined from the high-temperature absorbance using extinction coefficients calculated as described by Freier et al. (1983).

Computer predictions of structure. The program of Zuker and Stiegler (1981; Jacobson et al. 1984) was used to predict secondary structures. The program was modified by M. Zuker (pers. comm.) to accept the sequence dependence of GU base pairs (Sugimoto et al. 1986) and was further modified to accept penalties for asymmetric loops, as suggested by Papanicolaou et al. (1984).

RESULTS AND DISCUSSION

Parameters for Base Pairs

The most common motif found in the secondary structures of RNA molecules is the double helix. Thus, accurate predictions for the stabilities of double helixes will be important for predicting the secondary structures of RNA. The nearest-neighbor model approximates the stability of an RNA duplex by the sum of the free-energy increments for all nearest neighbors in the duplex (Tinoco et al. 1971; Borer et al. 1974). For a set of 19 oligomers, the measured free-energy changes, $\Delta G°$, for duplex formation by pairs of oligomers with identical nearest neighbors, but different sequences, differ on the average by 6% (Kierzek et al. 1986). For example, the $\Delta G°$s of duplex formation at 37°C for GUCGAC and GACGUC are −7.1 and −7.4 kcal/mole, respectively. Thus, the nearest-neighbor model should be sufficient to predict to within about 10% the free-energy change of duplex formation for any oligoribonucleotide containing only Watson-Crick base pairs.

Free-energy parameters at 37°C for all ten nearest-neighbor combinations containing only Watson-Crick base pairs have been provided by thermodynamic measurements of duplex formation by 45 oligoribonucleotides (see Table 1) (Freier et al. 1986b). For the 45 oligomers used to derive these parameters, the $\Delta G°$ of duplex formation is predicted to within 4% on average (Freier et al. 1986b). Table 2 lists some additional tests of these and other nearest-neighbor parameters. For example, for duplex formation by the non-self-

Table 1. Free-energy Parameters for RNA Helix Initiation and Propagation

(a) *Free-energy Increments for Base Pairs (kcal/mole)*

3' Base pair	5' Base pair				
	GU	AU	UA	CG	GC
GU	-0.5	-0.5	-0.7	-1.5	-1.3
AU	-0.5	-0.9	-1.1	-1.8	-2.3
UA	-0.7	-0.9	-0.9	-1.7	-2.1
CG	-1.9	-2.1	-2.3	-2.9	-3.4
GC	-1.5	-1.7	-1.8	-2.0	-2.9

(b) *Free-energy Increments for Loops (kcal/mole)*

Type of loop	Size of loop																
	1	2	3	4	5	6	7	8	9	10	12	14	16	18	20	25	30
bulge	3.3	5.2	6.0	6.7	7.4	8.2	9.1	10.0	10.5	11.0	11.8	12.5	13.0	13.6	14.0	15.0	15.8
hairpin	—	—	7.4	5.9	4.4	4.3	4.1	4.1	4.2	4.3	4.9	5.6	6.1	6.7	7.1	8.1	8.9
internal	—	0.8	1.3	1.7	2.1	2.5	2.6	2.8	3.1	3.6	4.4	5.1	5.6	6.2	6.6	7.6	8.4

Free-energy parameters were measured in 1 M NaCl at 37°C (Freier et al. 1986b).

Part a: Free-energy increments for stacking of GC, AU (Freier et al. 1986b), and internal GU pairs (Sugimoto et al. 1986) are given. The first base in the top row corresponds to the 5' nucleotide in a stack. The first base in the left-hand column corresponds to the 3' nucleotide in a stack. For example, ΔG°_{37} for $\overrightarrow{CA}$ / $\overleftarrow{GU}$ is -1.8 kcal/mole. For a bimolecular association of strands, an initiation free-energy change of +3.4 kcal/mole is added. If the two strands in a bimolecular association are self-complementary, an additional symmetry correction of +0.4 kcal/mole is added.

Part b: Most of these parameters are based on untested assumptions and are particularly unreliable. An indication of the sensitivity of structure prediction to these parameters is given in Tables 3 and 4. In Tables 3 and 4, parameter set c corresponds to the above parameters. Parameter set d corresponds to the above parameters with the addition of penalties for certain types of internal loops. As suggested by Papanicolaou et al. (1984), if an internal loop has branches of unequal lengths, $N1$ and $N2$, then an additional free-energy increment was added. This increment is the minimum of 6.0 or $N \times f(M)$ kcal/mole, where $N = N1 - N2$; $M = $ minimum of 5, $N1$, or $N2$; and $f(1) = 0.7$, $f(2) = 0.6$, $f(3) = 0.4$, $f(4) = 0.2$, $f(5) = 0.1$. As suggested by Gralla and Crothers (1973), internal loops closed by two AU pairs are penalized by adding an additional 1.8 kcal/mole relative to parameters in the above Table. As suggested by Pipas and McMahon (1975), internal loops closed by one AU and one GC pair are penalized by adding an additional 0.8 kcal/mole relative to parameters in the above Table. The penalties associated with loop closure by one or two AU pairs compared to closure by two GC pairs are the same as those adopted by Salser (1978). GU pairs closing internal loops are considered equivalent to AU pairs.

Table 2. Predicted and Measured Stabilities of Short RNA Helixes

	Reference	Measured $\Delta G°_{37}$ (kcal/mole)	Predicted $\Delta G°_{37}$ (kcal/mole)
Helixes without loops			
5′ GCGGCG 3′ CGCCGC	a	−10.3	−10.3
5′ GCGGCGA 3′ ACGCCGC	a	−14.5	−13.1
5′ GCAACGA 3′ UCGUUGC	a	−9.2	−9.1
5′ GCGGUCA 3′ ACGCCAG	a	−11.7	−12.7
Helixes with bulge loops			
5′ GCG^{U}GCG 3′ CGC−CGC	a	−6.7	−7.0
5′ GCG−GCG 3′ CGC$_A$CGC	a	−7.0	−7.0
5′ GCA−ACGA 3′ UCGU$_A$UGC	a	−4.9	−5.8
5′ GCG^{AA}GCGA 3′ ACGC—CGC	a	−6.7	−7.9
5′ GCG^{AA}GUCA 3′ ACGC—CAG	a	−6.5	−7.5
5′ GCG—GCG 3′ CGC$_{AAA}$CGC	a	−6.8	−4.3
Helixes with hairpin loops			
5′ CA—GA^{C}m^{UG}m 3′ GUm^{5}Cψ_{AYAA}	b	−1.9[b]	−1.7
5′ AUCCUA 3′ UAGGAU^{T4}	c	−3.7[c]	−3.0
5′ AAAAAA 3′ UUUUUU^{C6}	d	+0.7	−0.2

[a] C.E. Longfellow et al. (unpubl.). Measurements were made in 1 M NaCl.
[b] Clore et al. (1984). Measurements were made in 0.5 M KCl.
[c] $\Delta G°_{37}$ was derived from data in Hilbers et al. (1985). Measurements were made in 0.2 M Na$^+$.
[d] Uhlenbeck et al. (1973). Measurements were made in 1 M NaCl.

complementary oligomers GCGGCG and CGCCGC, the free energy change is predicted by:

$$\Delta G°_{37}(\text{predicted}) = \Delta G°_{37}(\text{initiation}) + \Delta G°(\text{symmetry})$$
$$+ 2\Delta G°_{37}(\text{GC}) + 2\Delta G°_{37}(\text{CG})$$
$$+ \Delta G°_{37}(\text{GG})$$
$$= 3.4 + 0 + 2(-3.4) + 2(-2.0) + (-2.9)$$
$$= -10.3 \text{ kcal/mole}$$

The results in Table 2 indicate that the measured $\Delta G°_{37}$ is −10.3 kcal/mole, in agreement with the prediction. This demonstrates the power of the method since this duplex was not included in the data set used to derive the parameters in Table 1. From the results shown in Table 2, for oligomers having only Watson-Crick base pairs and unpaired terminal nucleotides (dangling ends), the predicted and measured $\Delta G°$s agree to within 10%. Thus, the nearest-neighbor model appears to be a good approximation for RNA duplexes with only Watson-Crick base pairs and unpaired terminal nucleotides.

Parameters for Helixes with Loops

In addition to double helixes, typical RNA secondary structures contain many helixes with loops such as bulges, internal loops, and hairpins. Much less experimental data are available on the stabilities of these motifs. In fact, most parameters currently used are derived from theory, rather than from experiment (Jacobson and Stockmayer 1950; DeLisi and Crothers 1971; Gralla and Crothers 1973; Tinoco et al. 1973). Nevertheless, Table 1 contains tabulations of available parameters in order to permit predictions of RNA secondary structure. One test of these parameters is to predict stabilities of short segments of RNA containing helixes with loops. For example, the anticodon hairpin (loop and stem) from yeast phenylalanine tRNA has the sequence, C-A-G-A-C$_m$-U-G$_m$-A-A-Y-A-ψ-m^{5}C-U-G. For hairpin formation at 1 M NaCl, if ψ is considered equivalent to U,

$$\Delta G°_{37}(\text{predicted}) = \Delta G°_{37}(\text{loop of 7}) + \Delta G°_{37}(\text{CA})$$
$$+ \Delta G°_{37}(\text{AG}) + \Delta G°_{37}(\text{GA})$$
$$= 4.1 + (-1.8) + (-1.7) + (-2.3)$$
$$= -1.7 \text{ kcal/mole}$$

In 0.5 M KCl, the measured $\Delta G°_{37}$ is −1.9 kcal/mole (Clore et al. 1984). Additional comparisons are contained in Table 2. The results suggest that further experimental results are required to provide reliable predictions of stabilities for helixes with loops.

Predictions of Structure from Sequence

Another test of the nearest-neighbor model and of the available parameters is the ability to predict secondary structures of natural RNA sequences (Ninio 1979). The secondary structure of tRNA was deduced from its sequence (Holley et al. 1965) and has been established by X-ray diffraction (Kim et al. 1974; Robertus et al. 1974). Secondary structures for several other RNAs have been deduced from phylogenetic and/or chemical modification data. These include 5S RNA (Erdmann et al. 1985), 16S RNA (Noller 1984; Brimacombe and Stiege 1985; Moazed et al. 1986), and the self-splicing intervening sequence from the rRNA precursor in *Tetrahymena thermophila* (Cech et al. 1983; Michel and Dujon 1983; Waring et al. 1983; Waring and Davies 1984). Secondary structure can be predicted from the sequence by using a computer algorithm to minimize the free-energy change associated with forming the secondary structure (Pipas and McMahon 1975; Ninio 1979; Zuker and Stiegler 1981; Nussinov et al. 1982). Tables 3 and 4 contain comparisons between structures predicted with the program of Zuker and Stiegler (1981; see also Jacobson et al. 1984), and structures deduced from phylogenetic data. Results using parameters collected by Salser (1978) and in Table 1 are reported. In almost all cases, the parameters in Table 1 predict a structure closer to the phylogenetically deduced structure. Evidently, improved parameters lead to improved predictions. The predicted structures, however, often contain roughly only half of the expected helixes. This suggests additional improved parameters will be required to provide reliable predictions of secondary structure.

Ninio (1979) has suggested that comparisons of pre-dicted and known secondary structures can be used to deduce improved parameters. Comparisons of structures used to generate Tables 3 and 4 indicate that deviations between predicted and known structures are often associated with internal loops. The sensitivity of predicted structures to internal loop parameters was therefore tested. Tables 3 and 4 contain the results obtained by adding nine additional parameters for internal loops, and Figures 1 and 2 illustrate two particular comparisons of structure. As suggested by Papanicolaou et al. (1984), seven parameters were added to penalize internal loops that do not have an equal number of unpaired bases on both sides of the loop (see footnotes to Tables 1, 3, and 4). As originally suggested by Gralla and Crothers (1973) and adopted by Pipas and McMahon (1975) and Salser (1978), two more parameters were added to discriminate between internal loops closed by two GC base pairs, two AU base pairs, or one AU base pair and one GC base pair. The results in Tables 3 and 4 show a considerable improvement in the reliability of the predicted structure. This suggests that further experimental results on internal loops may be important for improving predictions of structure.

Unpaired Terminal Nucleotides

In the predictions described above, favorable free-energy increments are only provided by Watson-Crick base pairs and GU mismatches. Studies of oligoribonucleotides, however, indicate that unpaired terminal nucleotides (dangling ends) and mismatches can also contribute to helix stability (Martin et al. 1971; Romaniuk et al. 1978; Alkema et al. 1981; Petersheim and Turner

Table 3. Comparison of Structures Deduced from Computer Prediction and Phylogenetic Data for tRNA and 5S RNA

RNA	Parameter set	phylogenetic helixes predicted[a]	predictions with n helixes[a]	predictions with $(n-1)$ or n helixes[a]
tRNA	b	69	35	58
	c	80	50	75
	d	92	82	90
5S RNA	b	45	21	31
	c	48	16	41
	d	67	40	57

[a]Secondary structure was predicted with the program of Zuker and Stiegler (1981). For tRNA, structure predictions were made on 141 randomly chosen sequences. Modified nucleotides that are unable to base pair were not allowed to base pair. The cloverleaf model with $n = 4$ helixes was taken as the structure deduced from phylogenetic data. For 5S RNA, structure predictions were made on 67 randomly chosen sequences. The structure described by Erdmann et al. (1985) with $n = 5$ helixes was taken as the structure deduced from phylogenetic data. A helix was correct if it did not lack more than two base pairs deduced phylogenetically.

[b]Salser (1978).

[c]Freier et al. (1986b).

[d]Freier et al. (1986b), with asymmetric loops penalized as described by Papanicolaou et al. (1984), internal loops closed by two AU pairs penalized by 1.8 kcal/mole (Gralla and Crothers 1973), loops closed by one AU and one GC pair penalized by 0.8 kcal/mole (Pipas and McMahon 1975) relative to internal loops closed by two GC pairs. See Table 1 for further description.

Table 4. Comparison of Structures Deduced from Computer Prediction and Phylogenetic Data for *T. thermophila* Self-splicing RNA and for *E. coli* 16S rRNA Domains

RNA	Nucleotides	No. of Helixes	Parameter set	Percentage of phylogenetic helixes predicted[a]
IVS	−12 to −1, 2 to 424	14[e]	b	50
			c	57
			d	79
16S Domain 1	27–576	24	b	8
			c	42
			d	46
16S Domain 2	576–912	15	b	53
			c	93
			d	60
16S Domain 3	923–1393	22	b	14
			c	41
			d	55
16S Domain 4	1394–1542	4	b	0
			c	25
			d	75
16S Summary	—	65	b	20
			c	52
			d	54

[a]Secondary structure was predicted with the program of Zuker and Stiegler (1981). For the self-splicing intervening sequence (IVS) from the rRNA precursor of *T. thermophila*, the structure reported by Waring et al. (1986) was taken as the structure deduced from phylogenetic data. The helix denoted P7 in Waring et al. (1986) was disregarded because it represents tertiary pairing. Secondary structure was predicted for the region inclusive of −12 to 424 omitting the G at +1 (Cech et al. 1983). For 16S rRNA, the "naked" structure reported by Moazed et al. (1986) was taken as the structure deduced from phylogenetic data. Secondary structure was predicted separately for each of the domains inclusive of the indicated nucleotides. A helix was defined as a region containing three or more base pairs with no bulge or interior loops containing three or more nucleotides. A helix was correct if it did not lack more than two base pairs deduced phylogenetically.
[b]Salser (1978).
[c]Freier et al. (1986b).
[d]Freier et al. (1986b), with asymmetric loops penalized as described by Papanicolaou et al. (1984), internal loops closed by two AU pairs penalized by 1.8 kcal/mole (Gralla and Crothers 1973), loops closed by one AU and one GC pair penalized by 0.8 kcal/mole (Pipas and McMahon 1975) relative to internal loops closed by two GC pairs. See Table 1 for further description.
[e]Although a total of 16 helixes are present, 2 sets are mutually exclusive as secondary structure pairings (see Fig. 1).

1983a,b; Freier et al. 1983, 1985a,c; Sugimoto et al. 1987a,b). For example, at 10^{-4} M, the melting temperature of the self-complementary duplex formed by GGCCAp is 24°C higher than that formed by GGCCp, and the free-energy changes for duplex formation at 37°C are −9.0 and −5.2 kcal/mole, respectively (Freier et al. 1983). Presumably, this is due to additional stacking interactions at the ends of the helix. Table 5 lists free-energy increments at 37°C for sequences providing the largest and smallest free-energy increments for unpaired terminal nucleotides. These are termed strong and weak stacking sequences, respectively. These increments range from 0 to −1.7 kcal/mole. This is almost as wide a range as the −0.9 to −3.4 kcal/mole for free-energy increments of base pairs (see Table 1). Additional studies of oligoribonucleotides containing terminal mismatches indicate that the free-energy increments for non-GU mismatches are roughly equal to the sum of the constituent dangling ends (Hickey and Turner 1985; Freier et al. 1986a; Sugimoto et al.

1987b). Thus, unpaired terminal nucleotides and mismatches should be important for determining the stabilities of helixes and therefore the structures of large RNA molecules.

An important question is whether the stability increments measured for unpaired terminal nucleotides on oligoribonucleotides are also relevant for the ends of helixes in large RNA molecules. The nearest-neighbor model suggests that they are, since these increments simply provide measures of nearest-neighbor stacking interactions. Further support for this is provided by the crystal structure of yeast phenylalanine tRNA (Kim et al. 1974; Robertus et al. 1974). Figures 3 and 4 show the secondary and three-dimensional structures of this tRNA. In Figure 3, nucleotides corresponding to the strong and weak stacking nucleotides listed in Table 5 are circled and boxed, respectively, in the secondary structure. In Figure 4 (top), the strong stacking bases and adjacent base pairs are shaded in the three-dimensional structure. In each case, the unpaired base is

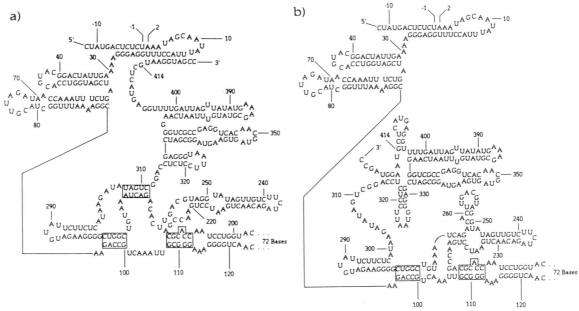

Figure 1. Structure of the self-splicing intervening sequence with short sections of exons from *T. thermophila* as deduced from phylogenetic data (*a*) (Waring et al. 1986) and computer prediction (*b*) of structure from the sequence, with parameters from Freier et al. (1986b) modified to include penalties for asymmetric loops (Papanicolaou et al. 1984) and for internal loops closed by one or two AU pairs (Gralla and Crothers 1973). This prediction was scored as 79% correct.

stacked directly on top of the adjacent base pair and extends the helix. This suggests that strong stacking sequences are helix-extending sequences. In Figure 4 (bottom), the weak stacking bases and adjacent base pairs are shaded. In each case, the unpaired base does not stack on the adjacent base pair. In four out of five cases, the backbone turns sharply at these sequences, suggesting that weak stacking sequences are turn-permitting sequences. The correlation between the thermodynamic parameters for these unpaired nucleotides and the three-dimensional structure of tRNA suggests that these parameters should be included in

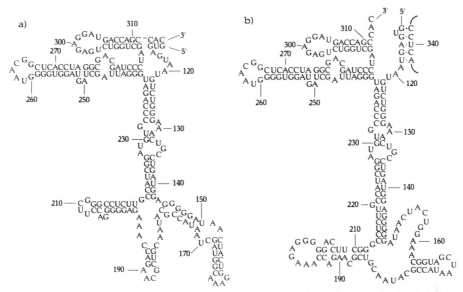

Figure 2. Structure of 16S rRNA between nucleotides 113 and 314 as deduced from phylogenetic data (*a*) (Moazed et al. 1986) and computer prediction (*b*) of the structure from the sequence, with parameters from Freier et al. (1986b) modified to include penalties for asymmetric loops (Papanicolaou et al. 1984) and for internal loops closed by one or two AU pairs (Gralla and Crothers 1973). This section of the computer prediction was scored as 50% correct. The computer-predicted helix between residues 143–148 and 214–219 is not consistent with the structure of Moazed et al. (1986), but it is consistent with the structure of Brimacombe and Stiege (1985).

Table 5. Free-energy Increments for Some Unpaired Terminal Nucleotides

Strong stacking (helix-extending) sequences		Weak stacking (turn-permitting) sequences			
sequence	ΔG°_{37} (kcal/mole)	sequence	ΔG°_{37} (kcal/mole)	sequence	ΔG°_{37} (kcal/mole)
$\overrightarrow{CA}$ / G	−1.7	$\overrightarrow{UC}$ / A	−0.1	$\overrightarrow{AG}$ / C	−0.2
$\overrightarrow{CG}$ / G	−1.7	$\overrightarrow{UU}$ / A	−0.1	$\overrightarrow{GG}$ / C	0.0
$\overrightarrow{CU}$ / G	−1.2	$\overrightarrow{UA}$ / U	−0.2	$\overrightarrow{UG}$ / C	0.0
$\overrightarrow{GA}$ / C	−1.1	$\overrightarrow{CC}$ / G	(−0.2)[a]	$\overrightarrow{CU}$ / A	(−0.2)[a]
$\overrightarrow{CG}$ / C	−1.3	$\overrightarrow{GC}$ / G	−0.2	$\overrightarrow{UU}$ / A	(−0.2)[a]
		$\overrightarrow{UC}$ / G	−0.1		

[a]Values in parentheses have not been measured directly, but are approximated from known parameters.

predictions of secondary structure and may also help predict three-dimensional structure (Sugimoto et al. 1987a).

The lack of crystal structures for RNAs other than tRNAs makes it difficult to obtain further direct evidence for or against helix-extending and turn-permitting sequences. The parameters in Table 5, however, suggest that site-directed mutagenesis experiments could be used to test this concept. In particular, the turn-permitting sequences $\overrightarrow{UU}$ and $\overrightarrow{UC}$ can be mutated to the helix-extending sequence $\overrightarrow{CU}$. If the concept is general, then such a mutation could have a large effect on the stability of the three-dimensional structure of the RNA. Figure 5 shows three examples where this type of mutation might have a large effect.

Hydrogen Bonding in RNA

Another interaction that may be important for determining the structures of RNAs is hydrogen bonding. Recent results on oligoribonucleotides provide insights into the free-energy increments associated with hydrogen bonds in RNA (Freier et al. 1985, 1986c; Sugimoto et al. 1987a; Turner et al. 1987). Comparisons of free-energy increments for unpaired and paired terminal nucleotides on short duplexes indicate that complementary pairing can substantially increase the stability of the duplex. For example, comparisons of duplex stabilities at 37°C for the self-complementary oligomers CCGG and CCGGC indicate that each 3' dangling C adds a free-energy increment of −0.4 kcal/mole to duplex stability. A similar comparison with GCCGG indicates that each 5' dangling G adds −0.2 kcal/mole (see Table 5). In the fully paired duplex, GCCGGC, however, each terminal base pair adds −3.4 kcal/mole to duplex stability. Thus, the pairing interaction of G with C results in a large favorable free-energy change relative to that observed for the individual stacking interactions of the nucleotides as dangling ends. Presumably, this pairing interaction is primarily due to hydrogen bonds. Similar comparisons indicate that the contributions of pairing are quite sequence-dependent (Freier et al. 1985, 1986c; Sugimoto et al. 1987a).

An independent measure of the strength of a hydrogen bond has been obtained by comparing duplex stabilities for oligoribonucleotides containing terminal GC and IC base pairs (Turner et al. 1987). The stacking properties of inosine and guanine as dangling ends

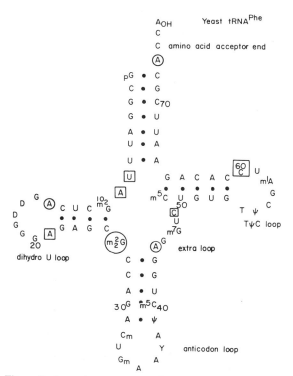

Figure 3. Secondary structure of yeast phenylalanine tRNA with strong stacking nucleotides circled and weak stacking nucleotides boxed.

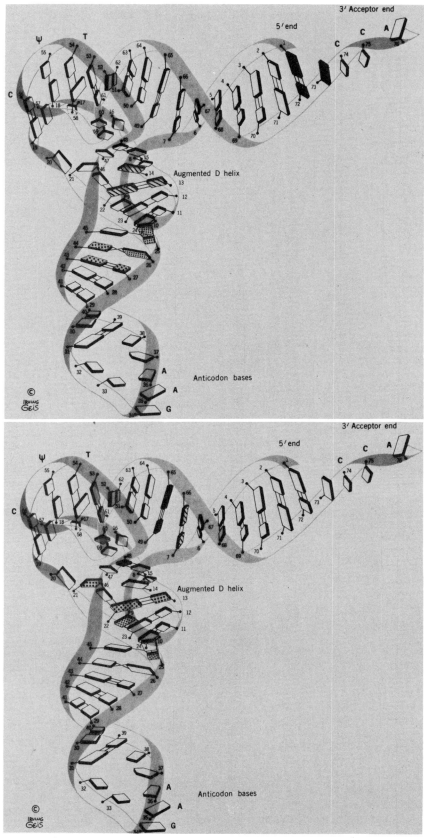

Figure 4. Three-dimensional structure of yeast phenylalanine tRNA. (*Top*) Strong stacking (helix-extending) sequences are shaded. The stacked unpaired terminal nucleotides are A14, m²₂G26, A44, and A73. (*Bottom*) Weak stacking (turn-permitting) sequences are shaded. The unpaired terminal nucleotides not stacked on their adjacent base pairs are U8, A9, A21, C48, and C60. (Adapted, with permission, from Cantor and Schimmel 1980 [illustration copyright by Irving Geis].)

130

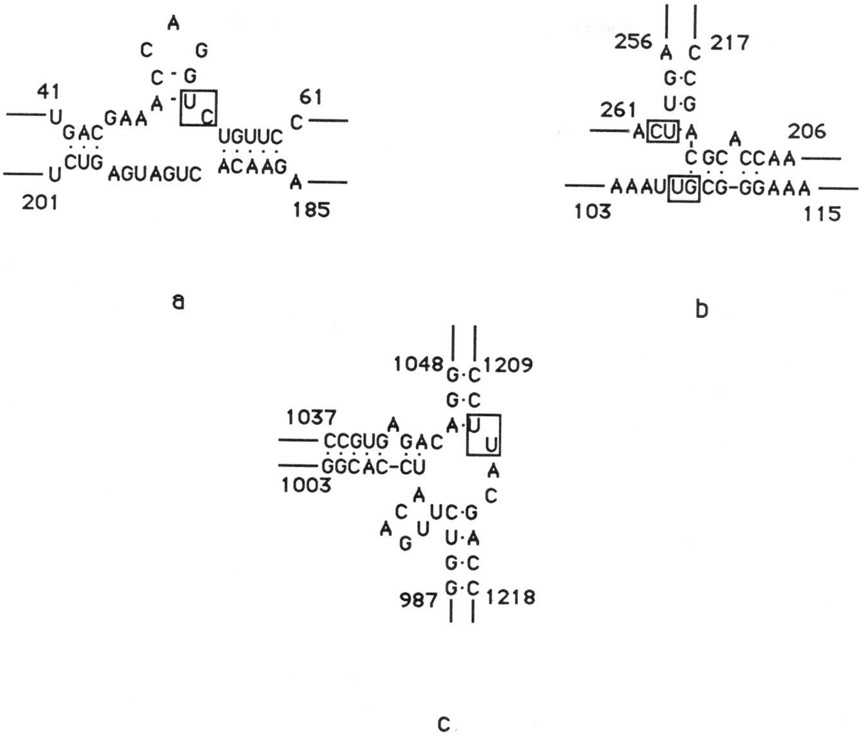

Figure 5. Examples of weak stacking (turn-permitting) sequences in avocado sunblotch viroid (Hutchins et al. 1986) (*a*), self-splicing intervening sequence from *Tetrahymena thermophila* (*b*) (Waring et al. 1986), and 16S ribosomal RNA (*c*) (Moazed et al. 1986).

are similar. Inosine, however, lacks the 2-amino group of guanine and can therefore form only two hydrogen bonds with cytosine. Thus, the difference in stability increments for terminal GC and IC pairs reflects the contribution of a hydrogen bond between amino and carbonyl groups. Comparisons of duplex stabilities for GCCGGC vs. ICCGGC and CGGCCG vs. CGGCCI give free-energy increments of -1.6 and -0.7 kcal/mole, respectively, for this hydrogen bond. Combined with the results described above, this indicates that the free-energy change for a hydrogen bond ranges from roughly -0.5 to -2 kcal/mole in a sequence-dependent manner (Turner et al. 1987). Strong stacking sequences are associated with weak hydrogen bonds and weak stacking sequences are associated with strong hydrogen bonds. The results indicate that a single hydrogen bond can potentially stabilize a structure as much as adding a weak base pair or a stacking interaction.

SUMMARY

Thermodynamic studies of oligoribonucleotides are providing parameters and insights for the fundamental interactions that determine RNA structure. These results can be used to predict the secondary structure of RNA from its sequence. Comparisons of predicted structures with those deduced from phylogenetic data indicate a modest success rate that is improving as more parameters are determined experimentally.

Two major fundamental interactions in RNA are stacking and hydrogen bonding. Both contribute similar increments to free-energy changes for associations of oligoribonucleotides. Thus, parameters for stacking and hydrogen bonding will likely be important for predicting the three-dimensional structures of RNAs and for interpreting RNA-RNA associations. Both applications should be important for providing a full understanding of catalysis by RNA.

ACKNOWLEDGMENTS

We thank Michael Zuker for revising his structure-prediction program to accept the sequence dependence of GU pairs, for help with using his program, and for many stimulating discussions. This work was supported by National Institutes of Health grant GM-22939.

REFERENCES

Alkema, D., R.A. Bell, P.A. Hader, and T. Neilson. 1981. Triplet GpCpA forms a stable RNA duplex. *J. Am. Chem. Soc.* **103:** 2866.

Beckett, D. and O.C. Uhlenbeck. 1984. Enzymatic synthesis of oligoribonucleotides. In *Oligonucleotide synthesis: A practical approach* (ed. M.J. Gait), p. 185. IRL Press, Oxford, England.

Borer, P.N., B. Dengler, I. Tinoco, Jr., and O.C. Uhlenbeck. 1974. Stability of ribonucleic acid double-stranded helices. *J. Mol. Biol.* **86:** 843.

Brimacombe, R. and W. Stiege. 1985. Structure and function of ribosomal RNA. *Biochem. J.* **229:** 1.

Cantor, C.R. and P.R. Schimmel. 1980. *Biophysical chemistry*, part I: *The conformation of biological macromolecules*. W.H. Freeman, New York.

Cech, T.R., N.K. Tanner, I. Tinoco, Jr., B.R. Weir, M. Zuker, and P.S. Perlman. 1983. Secondary structure of the *Tetrahymena* ribosomal RNA intervening sequence: Structural homology with fungal mitochondrial intervening sequences. *Proc. Natl. Acad. Sci.* **80:** 3903.

Clore, G.M., A.M. Gronenborn, E.A. Piper, L.W. McLaughlin, E. Graeser, and J.H. Van Boom. 1984. The solution structure of a RNA pentadecamer comprising the anticodon loop and stem of yeast tRNA^{Phe}. *Biochem. J.* **221:** 737.

DeLisi, C. and D.M. Crothers. 1971. Prediction of RNA secondary structure. *Proc. Natl. Acad. Sci.* **68:** 2682.

Erdmann, V.A., J. Wolters, E. Huysmans, and R. DeWachter. 1985. Collection of published 5 S, 5.8 S and 4.5 S ribosomal RNA sequences. *Nucleic Acids Res.* **13:** r105.

Freier, S.M., D. Alkema, A. Sinclair, T. Neilson, and D.H. Turner. 1985. Contributions of dangling end stacking and terminal base-pair formation to the stabilities of XGGCCp, XCCGGp, XGGCCYp and XCCGGYp helixes. *Biochemistry* **24:** 4533.

Freier, S.M., B.J. Burger, D. Alkema, T. Neilson, and D.H. Turner. 1983. Effects of 3′ dangling end stacking on the stability of GGCC and CCGG double helices. *Biochemistry* **22:** 6198.

Freier, S.M., R. Kierzek, M.H. Caruthers, T. Neilson, and D.H. Turner. 1986a. Free energy contributions of GU and other terminal mismatches to helix stability. *Biochemistry* **25:** 3209.

Freier, S.M., R. Kierzek, J.A. Jaeger, N. Sugimoto, M.H. Caruthers, T. Neilson, and D.H. Turner. 1986b. Improved free-energy parameters for predictions of RNA duplex stability. *Proc. Natl. Acad. Sci.* **83:** 9373.

Freier, S.M., N. Sugimoto, A. Sinclair, D. Alkema, T. Neilson, R. Kierzek, M.H. Caruthers, and D.H. Turner. 1986c. Stability of XGCGCp, GCGCYp, and XGCGCYp helixes: An empirical estimate of the energetics of hydrogen bonds in nucleic acids. *Biochemistry* **25:** 3214.

Gralla, J. and D.M. Crothers. 1973. Free energy of imperfect nucleic acid helices. *J. Mol. Biol.* **78:** 301.

Hickey, D.R. and D.H. Turner. 1985. Effects of terminal mismatches on RNA stability: Thermodynamics of duplex formation for ACCGGGp, ACCGGAp and ACCGGCp. *Biochemistry* **24:** 3987.

Hilbers, C.W., C.A.G. Haasnoot, S.H. de Bruin, J.J.M. Joordens, G.A. Van Der Marel, and J.H. Van Boom. 1985. Hairpin formation in synthetic oligonucleotides. *Biochemie* **67:** 685.

Holley, R.W., J. Apgar, G.A. Everett, J.T. Madison, M. Marquisee, S.H. Merrill, J.R. Penswick, and A. Zamir. 1965. Structure of a ribonucleic acid. *Science* **147:** 1462.

Hutchins, C.J., P.D. Rathjen, A.C. Forster, and R.H. Symons. 1986. Self-cleavage of plus and minus RNA transcripts of avocado sunblotch viroid. *Nucleic Acids Res.* **14:** 3627.

Ikuta, S., R. Chattopadhyaya, and R.E. Dickerson. 1984. Reverse-phase polystyrene column for purification and analysis of DNA oligomers. *Anal. Chem.* **56:** 2253.

Jacobson, A.B., L. Good, M. Simonetti, and M. Zuker. 1984. Some simple computational methods to improve the folding of large RNAs. *Nucleic Acids Res.* **12:** 46.

Jacobson, H. and W.H. Stockmayer. 1950. Intramolecular reaction in polycondensations. I. The theory of linear systems. *J. Chem. Phys.* **18:** 1600.

Kierzek, R., M.H. Caruthers, C.E. Longfellow, D. Swinton, D.H. Turner, and S.M. Freier. 1986. Polymer-supported RNA synthesis and its application to test the nearest-neighbor model for duplex stability. *Biochemistry* **25:** 7840.

Kim, S.H., F.L. Suddath, G.J. Quigley, A. McPherson,

J.L. Sussman, A.H.J. Wang, N.C. Seeman, and A. Rich. 1974. Three-dimensional tertiary structure of yeast phenylalanine transfer RNA. *Science* **185:** 435.

Markiewicz, W.T., E. Biala, and R. Kierzek. 1984. Applications of the tetraisopropyldisiloxane-1,3-diyl group in the chemical synthesis of oligoribonucleotides. *Bull. Pol. Acad. Sci. Chem.* **32:** 433.

Martin, F.H., O.C. Uhlenbeck, and P. Doty. 1971. Self-complementary oligoribonucleotides: Adenylic acid–uridylic acid block copolymers. *J. Mol. Biol.* **57:** 201.

Michel, F. and B. Dujon. 1983. Conservation of RNA secondary structures in two intron families including mitochondrial-, chloroplast- and nuclear-encoded members. *EMBO J.* **2:** 33.

Moazed, D., S. Stern, and H.F. Noller. 1986. Rapid chemical probing of conformation in 16 S ribosomal RNA and 30 S ribosomal subunits using primer extension. *J. Mol. Biol.* **187:** 399.

Neilson, T., P.J. Romaniuk, D. Alkema, D.W. Hughes, J.R. Everett, and R.A. Bell. 1980. The effects of base sequence and dangling bases on the stability of short ribonucleic acid duplexes. *Nucleic Acids Symp. Ser.* **7:** 293.

Ninio, J. 1979. Prediction of pairing schemes in RNA molecules-loop contributions and energy of wobble and non-wobble pairs. *Biochimie* **61:** 1133.

Noller, H.F. 1984. Structure of ribosomal RNA. *Annu. Rev. Biochem.* **47:** 119.

Nussinov, R., I. Tinoco, Jr., and A.B. Jacobson. 1982. Small changes in free energy assignments for unpaired bases do not affect predicted secondary structures in single stranded RNA. *Nucleic Acids Res.* **10:** 341.

Papanicolaou, C., M. Gouy, and J. Ninio. 1984. An energy model that predicts the correct folding of both the tRNA and the 5 S RNA molecules. *Nucleic Acids Res.* **12:** 31.

Petersheim, M. and D.H. Turner. 1983a. Base-stacking and base-pairing contributions to helix stability: Thermodynamics of double-helix formation with CCGG, CCGGp, CCGGAp, ACCGGp, CCGGUp and ACCGGUp. *Biochemistry* **22:** 256.

———.1983b. Proton magnetic resonance melting studies of CCGGp, CCGGAp, ACCGGp, CCGGUp and ACCGGUp. *Biochemistry* **22:** 269.

Pipas, J.M. and J.E. McMahon. 1975. Method for predicting RNA secondary structure. *Proc. Natl. Acad. Sci.* **72:** 2017.

Robertus, J.D., J.E. Ladner, J.T. Finch, D. Rhodes, R.S. Brown, B.F.C. Clark, and A. Klug. 1974. Structure of yeast phenylalanine tRNA at 3 Å resolution. *Nature* **250:** 546.

Romaniuk, P.J., D.W. Hughes, R.J. Gregoire, T. Neilson, and R.A. Bell. 1978. Stabilizing effect of dangling bases on a short RNA double helix as determined by proton nuclear magnetic resonance spectroscopy. *J. Am. Chem. Soc.* **100:** 3971.

Salser, W. 1978. Globin mRNA sequences: Analysis of base pairing and evolutionary implications. *Cold Spring Harbor Symp. Quant. Biol.* **42:** 985.

Shoemaker, K.R., P.S. Kim, E.J. York, J.M. Stewart, and R.L. Baldwin. 1987. Tests of the helix dipole model for stabilization of α-helices. *Nature* **326:** 563.

Sugimoto, N., R. Kierzek, and D.H. Turner. 1987a. Sequence dependence for the energetics of dangling ends and terminal base pairs in ribonucleic acid. *Biochemistry* **26:** 4554.

———. 1987b. Sequence dependence for the energetics of terminal mismatches in ribooligonucleotides. *Biochemistry* **26:** 4559.

Sugimoto, N., R. Kierzek, S.M. Freier, and D.H. Turner. 1986. Energetics of internal GU mismatches in ribooligonucleotide helixes. *Biochemistry* **25:** 5755.

Tinoco, I., Jr., O.C. Uhlenbeck, and M.D. Levine. 1971. Estimation of secondary structure in ribonucleic acids. *Nature* **230:** 363.

Tinoco, I., Jr., P.N. Borer, B. Dengler, M.D. Levine, O.C. Uhlenbeck, D.M. Crothers, and J. Gralla. 1973. Improved estimation of secondary structure in ribonucleic acids. *Nat. New Biol.* **246:** 40.

Turner, D.H., N. Sugimoto, R. Kierzek, and S.D. Dreiker. 1987. Free energy increments for hydrogen bonds in nucleic acid base pairs. *J. Am. Chem. Soc.* **109:** 3783.

Uhlenbeck, O.C., P.N. Borer, B. Dengler, and I. Tinoco, Jr. 1973. Stability of RNA hairpin loops: A_6-C_m-U_6. *J. Mol. Biol.* **73:** 483.

Waring, R.B. and R.W. Davies. 1984. Assessment of a model for intron RNA secondary structure relevant to RNA self-splicing—A review. *Gene* **28:** 277.

Waring, R.B., C. Scazzocchio, T.A. Brown, and R.W. Davies. 1983. Close relationship between certain nuclear and mitochondrial introns. *J. Mol. Biol.* **167:** 595.

Waring, R.B., P. Towner, S.J. Minter, and R.W. Davies. 1986. Splice-site selection by a self-splicing RNA of *Tetrahymena*. *Nature* **321:** 133.

Zuker, M. and P. Stiegler. 1981. Optimal computer folding of large RNA sequences using thermodynamics and auxiliary information. *Nucleic Acids Res.* **9:** 133.

RNA Structure from A to Z

I. Tinoco, Jr., P.W. Davis, C.C. Hardin, J.D. Puglisi, G.T. Walker, and J. Wyatt
Department of Chemistry and Laboratory of Chemical Biodynamics, University of California, Berkeley, California 94720

RNA performs a wide variety of known functions in biological systems, and it probably is involved in an even greater variety of as yet unknown functions. It is the genome in RNA viruses, virusoids, and viroids; in viroids, it sometimes catalyzes its own specific cleavage (Hutchins et al. 1986; Prody et al. 1986). The design and construction of proteins are controlled by messenger RNAs, ribosomal RNAs, and transfer RNAs. These RNAs are formed from their primary transcripts by a processing that can involve RNA enzymes (Cech and Bass 1986) and small nuclear RNAs (Black et al. 1985). Catalytic RNAs (ribozymes) have been shown to operate on polynucleotides (Zaug and Cech 1986) and polysaccharides (Shvedova et al. 1987). Intrinsic RNA components are involved in the signal-recognition particle, which mediates the extrusion of proteins through cell membranes (Zweib and Ullu 1986). RNA also plays important roles in control of replication (Dooley et al. 1985), transcription, and translation (Landick et al. 1985). All of these different RNA functions require different RNA structures. Here, we discuss a variety of structural elements that contribute to the secondary and tertiary structures of RNA.

SECONDARY STRUCTURE

Single Strands

Single-strand regions exist in most RNAs, and therefore their conformations are of interest. Bases in single-strand regions will stack in a right-handed helix, with the order of stacking being $G > A > C > U$. This difference in stacking propensity is such that when two purines are separated by U, they will stack on each other and bulge the U out of the stack (Lee and Tinoco 1980; Altona 1982). The ribose conformations depend on stacking. In mononucleotides, proton nuclear magnetic resonance (NMR) shows that the ribose ring is in fast exchange (shorter than milliseconds) among different conformations. The scalar coupling constants for 1'-2', 2'-3', and 3'-4' protons indicate a strong preference for a 2'-*endo* conformation. However, as base stacking occurs in oligonucleotides, the conformation changes to nearly 100% 3'-*endo*. In monodeoxyribonucleotides, the deoxyribose also prefers a 2'-*endo* conformation, but tends toward 100% 2'-*endo* when the bases are stacked in oligodeoxyribonucleotides (Altona 1982). These differences in sugar conformations are mirrored in the RNA and DNA conformations usually found in solution. In tRNA crystals, the ribose con-

formations are 3'-*endo*, except for nucleotides involved in special tertiary interactions, such as hydrogen-bonded base triples, intercalated bases, and parallel double strands, where 2'-*endo* can be found (Saenger 1984). We use 2'-*endo* to include other conformations on the south side of the pseudorotation circle and 3'-*endo* to include other conformations on the north side (Altona 1982).

Double-stranded A-Form RNA

When an RNA folds to a double-stranded A form, the conformations of the nucleotides do not change much. The ribose conformations remain 3'-*endo*, the glycosidic bonds joining the bases to the riboses have an anticonformation, and the strands wrap around each other in a right-handed double helix. Of course, the hydrogen bonding that determines the base pairs changes the intrastrand base stacking. In fibers of synthetic ribo-polynucleotides (Arnott et al. 1973), the number of base pairs per turn is 11 (A form) or 12 (A' form); similar values are found in tRNA crystals (Saenger 1984). However, there have been no reports on the number of base pairs per turn for RNA in solution, as determined for DNA (Peck and Wang 1981; Rhodes and Klug 1981). NMR can give definite answers about sugar conformations in solution from scalar coupling constants of sugar protons, but sensitive methods for determining the details of base stacking are not yet available. Accurate methods for determining nucleic acid geometry in solution based on NMR, circular dichroism (CD), Raman scattering, or other methods are obviously needed.

Double-stranded helical geometry can be characterized in terms of base pairs per turn, axial rise per base pair, propeller twist of the bases in each pair, base-pair tilt and roll, and displacement, D, of each base pair from the helix axis (Saenger 1984). The tilt and roll axes and the definition of D are illustrated in Figure 1. The values of the parameters are correlated so that if, for example, D is fixed, the range of other variables is limited (Zhurkin et al. 1978). It must also be noted that the structures are dynamic; there may be fluctuations of propeller twist or roll of 5–10°. For duplex RNA, one expects an axial rise per base pair of 2.8–3.0 Å, a tilt angle of 10–15°, and a displacement from the helix axis, D, of 4.4 Å (Saenger 1984). In many ways, the value of D is most important for characterizing the duplex structure. In B-DNA, D is zero; the base pairs are stacked on the helix axis. The

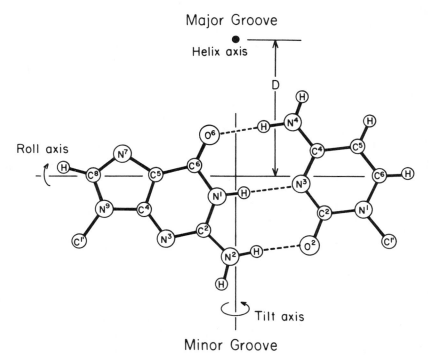

Figure 1. Definition of the displacement, D, one of the most characteristic features that distinguishes A-family duplexes from B-family duplexes. D measures the distance of each base pair from the helix axis. A forms have D near $+4$ Å; this produces a very deep major groove and a shallow minor groove. B forms have D near 0, or less than -1 Å; thus, major and minor grooves have equal depths. Although A forms usually have 3'-*endo* sugars and B forms usually have 2'-*endo* sugars, each sugar conformation allows a wide range of D values.

change to A-RNA (or A-DNA) moves the base pairs more than 4 Å away from the major groove. This produces a deep and narrow major groove and a shallow minor groove, in contrast to B-DNA, which has a wide major groove, with major and minor grooves of similar depth.

When thinking about A-form RNA duplexes (which are most often expected in natural RNAs), we are not limited to Watson-Crick base pairs. A G · U base pair occurs in the amino acceptor stem and a tertiary A · G pair occurs in tRNA^Phe (Saenger 1984); there is also evidence for other non-Watson-Crick base pairs in other tRNAs and in 5S RNAs (Papanicolaou et al. 1984). By analogy with DNA duplexes, these and other base-base oppositions need not distort the helix excessively (Patel et al. 1982b, 1984; Hunter et al. 1986; Arnold et al. 1987).

Double-stranded B-Form RNA

Definitive evidence for a B conformation in a polynucleotide containing only ribonucleotides is lacking; however, B-form structures are known for hybrid polynucleotides. X-ray diffraction of poly(rA) · poly(dT) fibers gives a B-form pattern at high humidity; at lower humidity, an A′ structure is obtained (Zimmerman and Pheiffer 1981). CD spectra of poly(rA) · poly(dT) and poly(rA) · poly(dU) are consistent with heteronomous structures with A-like ribo strands and B-like deoxyribo strands (Steely et al. 1986). Comparison of NMR

and CD spectra of the hybrid oligonucleotide [d(T-C-A-C-A-T) · r(A-U-G-U-G-A)] with its DNA analog suggests that it has a B conformation (Reid et al. 1983). Jayasena and Behe (1987) showed that the CD spectrum of poly(rG-dC) in tetrabutyl ammonium chloride solutions at concentrations above 100 mM is very similar to that of B-form poly[d(G-C)]. In solutions containing less than 10 mM tetrabutyl ammonium chloride, poly(rG-dC) has the CD spectrum of A-form poly-[r(G-C)]. In tetramethyl, ethyl, or propyl ammonium chloride, the conformation of poly(rG-dC) is either A or Z, depending on salt concentration, but it only becomes B form in tetrabutyl ammonium chloride. We have found that in 1 mM tetrabutyl ammonium sulfate, poly[r(A-C) · r(G-U)] has a CD spectrum very similar to that of B-form poly[d(A-C) · d(G-T)]. Further tests are needed to prove that the poly[r(A-C) · r(G-U)] is indeed B form.

Molecular mechanics calculations have been used to obtain energy-minimized duplex structures for the self-complementary hexanucleotide r(CGCGCG) in A, B, and Z forms (Rao and Kollman 1986). The calculations were done with and without counterions, but without solvent. Without counterions, the B form is calculated to have an energy intermediate to that of the A and Z forms. With counterions, the Z form is calculated to be most stable and the B form least stable. More accurate calculations based on free energies and including solvent need to be done, but the results show that a B-form RNA can exist with a reasonable geometry and energy. The calculated B-RNA structure (with 2'-endo riboses) has guanosine 2'-OHs similar to those in A-RNA, but cytidine 2'-OHs are hydrogen-bonded to the N7s of the guanines on the 3' side. The C3'-O3' and phosphodiester conformations vary over a larger range than B-DNA; but these conformations do occur in some tertiary interactions of tRNA.

B-form RNA should not be rejected out of hand. At the very least, it is important to realize that A and B are just designations for families of structures. A double helix may have B-form (2'-endo) sugars but A-form base-pair stacking (D >2 Å). Calculations for DNA show that 2'-endo sugars can form duplexes, with D ranging from about −2 Å to +2 Å for 8–11 bp per turn. DNA with 3'-endo sugars are calculated to allow a range of D from +2 Å to +5 Å for 9–12 bp per turn (Zhurkin et al. 1978). Also, sugar puckers are not rigid. For example, it is well established that nanosecond time scale motions occur in nucleic acids due to pseudorotation of the ribose ring (Levy et al. 1983; Kearns 1984). The stability of possible double helix structures depends on sequence and solvent. For example, dA·dT pairs favor the B family (Alexeev et al. 1987), whereas dG·dC pairs favor the A family (Nishimura et al. 1985a; Sarma et al. 1986). High water activity favors the B family (for various explanations, see Drew and Dickerson 1981; Saenger et al. 1986). Furthermore, even within one family, the conformation of each base pair is different depending on the sequence (Calladine 1982). As more RNA sequences are studied in solution and in crystals, we will eventually learn the rules for how RNA duplex geometry depends on sequence and solvent.

Double-stranded Z-Form RNA

Left-handed Z-RNA is the most recently discovered double-stranded RNA conformation, and the evidence for it is reviewed in some detail. After poly[d(C-G)] was found to undergo a B → Z transition in high salt (Pohl and Jovin 1972), it was obvious to look for a similar transition in poly[r(C-G)]. However, the salt concentrations that caused the transition in DNA did not work for RNA. There was a change in CD at very high salt and ethanol concentrations, but the CD spectrum did not look like that of Z-DNA. The Z-RNA structure for poly[r(C-G)] in 6 M NaClO$_4$ was first established by NMR (Hall et al. 1984). From crystal structure data (Saenger 1984), the following are the main characteristics of the Z form. (1) Guanosines are in syn conformations with 3'-endo riboses, whereas cytidines are anti with 2'-endo riboses. (2) CpG phosphodiesters have very different conformations from GpC phosphodiesters. (3) The duplex is left-handed. A crystal structure containing alternating rC-rG has not been solved, but a crystal of the tetranucleotide duplex r(C-br^{8}G-C-br^{8}G) has a structure similar to that of Z-DNA (Nakamura et al. 1985).

The syn or anti orientation of the bases and the sugar puckers can be determined accurately by proton NMR.

Figure 2 shows the interproton distances expected for Z forms; these distances can be established by nuclear Overhauser effect (NOE) measurements. The NOE depends on magnetic dipole-dipole coupling between nuclei; the magnitude depends on the inverse sixth power of the distance between nuclei. For distances greater than about 5 Å, the effect is too small to detect at present. Figure 2 shows that there is an excellent internal distance standard in the polynucleotide provided by the cytosine H6-H5 distance (2.4 Å), which is independent of conformation. The NOEs can be measured in a two-dimensional NMR experiment, called a NOESY, in which cross-peak volumes are proportional to NOEs between two protons. A small section of a NOESY contour spectrum is given in Figure 3; the cross-peak labeled C6-C5 is our standard of 2.4 Å. Note that the cross-peak for the proton at the 8-position of guanine and its ribose H1' (peak G1'-G8) are of similar size. The cytosine H6 is close to both its own ribose H2' (C2'-C6) and the neighboring guanosine ribose H2' (G2'-C6); the cytosine H5 is also close to the guanosine ribose H2' (G2'-C5). These large NOE peaks are only consistent with a Z geometry. When the guanosines are anti as in A form, the G1'-G8 peak is much smaller. Only the alternating 2'-endo–3'-endo sugar puckers with anti cytidine will allow cytosine H6 to be close both to its own H2' and to a neighboring

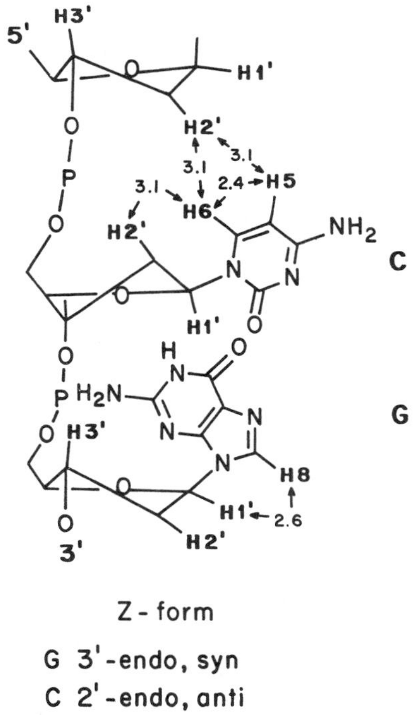

Z - form

G 3'-endo, syn

C 2'-endo, anti

Figure 2. Inter-proton distances that can be used to distinguish Z conformations from right-handed A or B conformations. Note the close distance between the guanine H8 and its H1' ribose proton, which defines a syn conformation. The short cytosine H6 distances to both its own ribose H2' and to the neighboring ribose H2' is only consistent with cytidine anti and 2'-endo and guanosine 3'-endo. The cytosine H5-H6 distance is a constant independent of conformation.

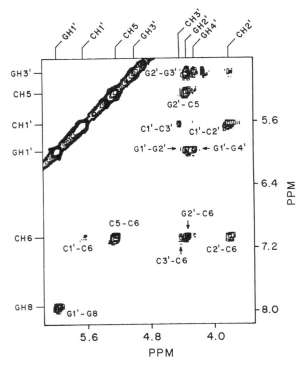

Poly r(G–C), Z-form, 5.7 M NaBr

Figure 3. A portion of a two-dimensional proton NMR spectrum (NOESY contour plot) for Z-form poly[r(C-G)] in 5.7 M NaBr (pH 7) at 25°C. The volumes of the cross-peaks are proportional to the inverse sixth power of the inter-proton distances. The H5-H6 distance (2.4 Å) in cytosine is independent of conformation and serves as a calibration for the peak labeled C5-C6.

H2′. More quantitative measures of r^{-6} averages of interproton distances can be obtained by measuring NOESY peak intensities as a function of mixing times, but this is not necessary for our purposes here.

Further evidence for the sugar puckers comes from H1′-H2′ scalar coupling constants, J. The polynucleotide proton NMR peaks are too broad to measure the splittings, but the Z-form hexanucleotide duplex r(CpGpCpGpCpG) gives $J_{1'-2'}$ of approximately 8 Hz (2′-*endo*) for the cytidines and $J_{1'-2'}$ of less than 1 Hz (3′-*endo*) for the internal guanosines (the terminal G has $J_{1'-2'}$ of ~4 Hz). This is consistent with the Z-form sugar puckers.

Phosphorus NMR gives a clear indication of the zigzag phosphodiester backbone conformation. In A-form poly[r(C-G)], the CpG and GpC ^{31}P chemical shifts differ by only 0.4 ppm; in Z form, they differ by 1.3 ppm, similar to those in Z DNA (Hall et al. 1984). Analogous changes occur in the spectra of the oligonucleotides r(CpGpCpG) and r(CpGpCpGpCpG), but here the number of peaks that shift provide the assignments directly. In the tetranucleotide, one peak shifts downfield when the Z form is induced; therefore, this must be the single GpC phosphorus (Davis et al. 1986). In the hexanucleotide, two peaks shift and three do not, as expected.

Evidence for right- or left-handed double helices comes from CD measurements below 200 nm (Riazance et al. 1985). All right-handed forms of poly(C-G), whether A- or B-form poly[d(C-G)] or A-form poly[r(C-G)], have an intense positive peak near 185 nm and a positive CD between 180 and 200 nm. The left-handed Z forms of poly[r(C-G)] and poly[d(C-G)] both show intense negative CD between 185 and 200 nm, with a negative peak near 190 nm. Theoretical calculations (Williams et al. 1986) for all alternating purine-pyrimidine sequences indicate that the CD in this region should be able to distinguish the left-handed Z form from the right-handed polynucleotides. This is not true for the CD from 220 to 300 nm, which is the region usually studied. In this region, the CD values of poly[r(C-G)] and poly[d(C-G)] are very different and are solvent-dependent; below 200 nm, they are much more similar.

The Raman spectrum shows characteristic changes for an A→Z transition in RNA (Nishimura et al. 1985b; Tinoco et al. 1986; Trulson et al. 1987); the changes are similar to those seen in the B→Z transition in DNA (Benevides and Thomas 1983). The phosphodiester antisymmetric stretch at 813 cm^{-1} in the A-RNA spectrum essentially disappears in the Z-RNA spectrum. The guanine ring breathing mode at 671 cm^{-1} in the A-RNA spectrum shifts to 642 cm^{-1} in the Z-RNA spectrum; the corresponding shift is from 682 cm^{-1} in B-DNA to 625 cm^{-1} in Z-DNA.

We now have a wide variety of spectroscopic methods to monitor the A→Z transition in RNA: proton NMR, phosphorus NMR, CD, and Raman scattering. Each method has advantages and disadvantages. CD requires the least sample and is the easiest to use, and NMR can provide the most information, but requires the most sample and time.

Z-RNA Habitats

The Z form of poly[r(C-G)] is favored by high salt, high temperature, and low water activity. Above 5.5 M NaClO$_4$ or 6 M NaBr, the Z form exists at 25°C; at lower salt concentrations, the solution must be heated to induce the Z conformation. Adding ethanol to the solutions favors the Z form. Salt, ethanol, and increasing temperature are additive; they can all compensate for each other. Divalent cations induce Z at lower concentrations than univalent cations. At room temperature, 3 M Mg(ClO$_4$)$_2$ or 4 M MgCl$_2$ induces the Z form. These Mg^{++} solutions produce a Z-form RNA that has a CD spectrum above 220 nm, very similar to that of Z-form poly[d(C-G)], and thus different from poly[r(C-G)] in Na$^+$ solutions (Cruz et al. 1986). Either the Z-RNA conformations are different in these different solvents or specific ion binding may change the CD spectrum. Many other salts have been tried without success to induce Z-RNA; these include NaCl, LiClO$_4$, LiCl, CsCl, CsF, NH$_4$Br, NiCl$_2$, MnCl$_2$, Co(NH$_3$)$_6$Cl$_3$, urea, and guanidinium chloride. Clearly, it is much harder to induce Z-RNA than to induce

Z-DNA. In studying the A→Z transitions in polynucleotides, it is necessary to realize that the transition can be very slow; sometimes hours are needed to reach apparent equilibrium.

For poly[r(C-G)] in any solvent, the phase changes are always A→Z→single strands with increasing temperature, but the melting of the Z form is too high to observe. However, with oligonucleotides, the duplex to single strands transition can occur near room temperature, and the A→Z transition should occur at even lower temperature. We found that for r(C-G-C-G)$_2$ in 6 M NaClO$_4$, there is an equilibrium between the Z form and single strands at 0°C; at −15°C, a new species appears that is probably the A form (Davis et al. 1986). In r(C-G-C-G-C-G)$_2$ in 4.5 M NaBr, a broad transition occurs between the A and Z forms from 5°C to 25°C; in higher salt concentrations, the Z form is the main duplex structure at room temperature and below. Decreasing the length of the polynucleotide thus lowers the melting temperature of the duplex and allows the Z form to occur at lower temperatures.

Oligonucleotides also allow the study of the kinetics of the transition. NMR shows that the A duplex to single strands equilibrium is fast on an NMR time scale of 1–10 ms.; only one peak is seen for each proton in the two species at equilibrium. The single strands to Z transition and the A→Z transition are much slower on this same time scale; individual peaks are seen for the species at equilibrium. More quantitative data can be obtained from temperature-jump kinetics. At 37°C in 0.1 M NaClO$_4$, the association rate constant for r(C-G-C-G-C-G) single strands to A-form duplex is about 2×10^6 s^{-1} M^{-1}; at the same temperature in 6 M NaClO$_4$, the association rate constant to the Z form is about 0.07×10^6 s^{-1} M^{-1}. The activation energies for association are on the order of 10 kcal/mole for both A and Z forms. Clearly, at 37°C, it is much easier to nucleate an A-form helix from single strands than it is to nucleate a Z-form helix; the rate is 30 times faster. Possibly, the need to rotate the G from *anti* to *syn* is the main contributor to the difference in association rates. In contrast, the dissociation rates of the duplex to single strands is very similar for the A and Z forms.

A modification of poly[r(C-G)] that strongly favors the Z form is bromination; this is also seen for poly[d(C-G)]. Presumably, an 8-bromoguanine (br^{8}G) destabilizes the *anti* guanosine of the A form and favors the *syn* guanosine of the Z form. The brominated polynucleotide (which contains br^{8}G and br^{5}C) is partly Z at 37°C in 0.15 M salt (Hardin et al. 1987). The CD of the brominated polynucleotide changes from that of the unbrominated Z-RNA in Na$^+$ ion solutions (Z$_R$-like spectra) to that of unbrominated Z-RNA in Mg^{++} ion solutions (Z$_D$-like), depending on the extent of bromination and the salt concentration. Low bromination (< 1/3 of the bases modified) and high salt favors Z$_R$ spectra. Proton NMR NOE measurements for guanosine H8-H1′ reveal that unbrominated guanine residues are in the *syn* conformation as required for Z-RNA. Proton and phosphorus NMR,

Raman, and CD measurements all show that both brominated and unbrominated bases undergo a transition to the Z form near physiological conditions. Methylation of the 8-position of guanine also favors the Z form (Uesugi et al. 1984), as expected. It is surprising, however, that unlike Z-DNA, bromination or methylation at the 5-position of cytosine inhibits the A→Z transition (T. Jovin, pers. comm.).

Biological Occurrence of Z-RNA

The ability to form Z-RNA (and Z-DNA) under physiological salt and temperature conditions means that antibodies against the Z conformation can be prepared. The anti-Z antibodies can be used to search for Z-RNA in naturally occurring RNA molecules and in biological samples. Although long sequences of alternating C-G sequences have not been found in natural RNAs, sequences of four to six alternating pyrimidine-purines are common (Woese et al. 1983; Noller 1984). The fact that r(C-G-C-G)$_2$ and r(C-G-C-G-C-G)$_2$ can be in a Z conformation below room temperature (in very high salt) is somewhat encouraging.

Anti-Z-RNA antibodies were induced in rabbits by injection with brominated poly[r(C-G)] (C.C. Hardin et al., in prep.). Rabbits A and B received polynucleotide with 32% br^{8}G and 26% br^{5}C; rabbits C and D received polynucleotide with 49% br^{8}G and 43% br^{5}C. Sera were obtained prior to booster injections at 1-month intervals for a period of 1 year. IgG fractions were prepared by standard methods using a protein A–Sepharose column as the final purification step. The polyclonal anti-Z-RNA antibodies were tested in a filter-binding assay for reactivity with Z-RNA (brominated poly[r(C-G)]) and for cross-reactivity with Z-DNA in the form of poly[d(br^{5}C-G)], poly[d(m^{5}C-G)], and poly[d(C-G)]. Figure 4 shows that at 37°C in a pH 7.5 buffer in 220 mM NaCl, antibodies B6 and C6 bind strongly to Z-RNA; however, their cross-reactivities are very different. Antibody B6 (elicited with the less brominated antigen) recognizes Z-DNA, but antibody C6 does not. The cross-reactivities of anti-Z-RNA antibodies were also tested with Z-DNA in negatively supercoiled M13 DNA by electrophoretic mobility retardation analysis (Zarling et al. 1987), and similar results were obtained. Neither of the anti-Z-RNA antibodies reacts with A-RNA or B-DNA (poly[r(C-G)], poly[r(C-I)], poly[d(C-G)], and poly[d(A)·d(T)]). Clearly, C6 can be used to detect specifically Z-RNA in biological samples.

The cross-reactivity between anti-Z-DNA antibodies and Z-RNA is also of interest (Hardin et al. 1987). Filter-binding assays were done at 37°C with brominated poly[r(C-G)] and a rabbit polyclonal anti-Z-DNA IgG called T4 (Zarling et al. 1984). At 220 mM NaCl (pH 7.5), the anti-Z-DNA antibody recognizes Z-RNA, but with a lower affinity than it has for Z-DNA in the form of poly[d(br^{5}C-G)] at 220 mM NaCl, of poly[d(m^{5}C-G)] at 1.5 M NaCl, or of poly[d(C-G)] at 3 M NaCl. To prove that the same antibody molecules

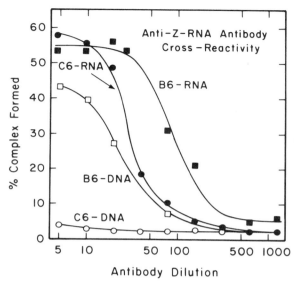

Figure 4. Filter-binding assays for the reactivity and cross-reactivity of two anti-Z-RNA polyclonal antibodies for Z-RNA (brominated poly[r(C-G)]) and Z-DNA (poly[d(br^{5}C-G)]). Antibody B6 was elicited with brominated poly[r(C-G)] containing 32% br^{8}G and 26% br^{5}C; the antigen used to elicit antibody C6 contained 49% br^{8}G and 43% br^{5}C. Reactions were done at 37°C in a 40 mM Tris buffer at pH 7.5 (4 mM EDTA, 220 mM NaCl).

in the polyclonal mixtures were binding to Z-RNA and Z-DNA, competition experiments were done. At 220 mM NaCl, Z-DNA (poly[d(br^{5}C-G)]) successfully competed for antibody with Z-RNA (brominated poly[r(C-G)]). Analogous results were obtained with poly[d(C-G)] in 4 M NaCl, demonstrating that the antibodies specifically recognize the Z conformation and not only modified nucleotides. A-RNA (poly[r(C-G)]) and B-DNA (poly[d(C-G)]) had no effect.

The antibody experiments provide some hints about similarities and differences between Z-RNA and Z-DNA. The cross-reactivity of T4 anti-Z-DNA antibody with Z-RNA and of B6 anti-Z-RNA antibody with Z-DNA indicates that similar conformations exist between Z-RNA and Z-DNA; they have some common epitopes. Also, specific phosphate inhibition of the reactions suggests the recognition of similar phosphodiester backbone determinants in Z-RNA and Z-DNA. However, the lack of recognition of Z-DNA by C6-anti-Z-RNA antibody indicates either that the C6 binding site involves the 2'-OH or that the conformations of Z-RNA and Z-DNA are significantly different. Raman spectra and the different CD spectra above 220 nm for Z-DNA and Z-RNA may also indicate different conformations.

Zarling et al. (1987) have found that anti-Z-RNA antibodies bind specifically in the cytoplasm of fixed protozoan cells. *Crithidia luciliae, Crithidia fasciculata, Trypanosoma bruceii bruceii, Paramecium multimicronucleatum,* and *Tetrahymena thermophila* cells were fixed in ethanol and acetone and then resuspended in buffer containing 150 mM salt. Purified anti-Z-RNA

rabbit polyclonal IgG antibodies were added, and the anti-Z-RNA antibodies were detected by immunofluorescence using fluorescently labeled goat anti-rabbit antibody. Appropriate controls with nonimmune IgGs and with anti-Z-DNA antibodies (which bound in the nucleus) were carried out. All of the cells bound anti-Z-RNA antibody and essentially all of the binding occurred in the cytoplasm. Pretreatment of the cells with ribonuclease A or T$_1$ eliminated the binding. Adriamycin and ethidium prevented binding, but actinomycin D, which binds only to DNA, did not. It is known that ethidium binding by Z-RNA induces a transition to a right-handed conformation (C.C. Hardin et al., in prep.). Z-RNA, but not A-RNA or B-DNA, successfully competed for the anti-Z-RNA antibody binding to the cytoplasm. The evidence is thus very strong that some RNA molecules in the cytoplasm of fixed cells have a left-handed Z-RNA conformation.

The identification of these molecules remains to be done. We have looked for binding between anti-Z-RNA antibody and *E. coli* rRNAs and ribosomes, and no response was observed. The anti-Z-RNA antibody did not interfere with the self-splicing reaction of *Tetrahymena* rRNA in vitro or with M1 RNA-catalyzed maturation of tRNA primary transcripts in vitro. Of course, a cell is a very complex entity and the target RNA may be part of a large protein-RNA particle, or be otherwise sequestered.

Hairpin Loops, Internal Loops, and Bulges

Hairpin loops. There is very little structural information on hairpin loops, internal loops, or bulges in RNA. The crystal structure of tRNA reveals that in the anticodon hairpin loop of seven nucleotides, five nucleotides continue stacking on the 5' end of the double helix, and then two nucleotides make the abrupt turn to link to the 3' end of the helix (Saenger 1984). Proton NOE measurements have confirmed that the detailed conformational features of the anticodon hairpin loop are retained in solution in the absence of the rest of the tRNA molecule (Clore et al. 1984).

Calculations of the distances between phosphates on different strands of an A-form double helix show that the shortest distances (10 Å) occur between phosphates separated by six or seven nucleotides; a separation of five or eight nucleotides leads to a distance of about 13 Å (Haasnoot et al. 1986). These distances can be linked by two nucleotides spanning the major groove of the helix. This is consistent with the tRNA result, in which the 5' end of the stem is extended by stacking of the bases in the anticodon loop. If five nucleotides on the 3' end were stacked on the stem, the distance to be spanned across the minor groove by the remaining two nucleotides would be over 25 Å—an impossible feat. Thus, if stacking is an important contribution to the free energy of hairpin loop stability (relative to the single strand), we expect that RNA loops will have stacked bases on the 5' end of the stem. In B-DNA, the same argument leads to stacked bases on the 3' end of the stem and the linking nucleotides crossing the minor groove. One should keep in mind that nucleotides in loops have a great deal of motional freedom. ^{19}F NMR studies of 5-fluorouracil-substituted tRNA[Val] show that a vector (the F5-H6 vector) in a base within a loop has an average amplitude of motion over a cone of half-angle equal to 45–60°; this is in contrast with values of 30–35° for bases in helical or tertiary structural domains (Hardin and Horowitz 1987). All of the motions are on nanosecond time scales.

A-RNA or B-DNA hairpin loop crystal structures have not yet been solved, and the D and T loops of tRNA are too involved in tertiary structure to be good models, so we must await further X-ray or NMR data to test the stacking hypothesis in loops. We should also remember that bases in loops can base pair with other bases in the loop or form hydrogen-bonded triples with pairs in the stem. Loops with many different sizes and sequences will need to be studied before generalizations can be made.

Bulges. Bulges are unpaired nucleotides that occur on only one strand of a double-stranded helix; the other strand has a continuous sequence of paired bases. The most common size bulge proposed for natural RNA is one or two nucleotides. Model building for a one-base bulge indicates that the base pairs on either side of the bulge can stack and that the unbonded nucleotide can swing out of the helix. Another possible model is for the unbonded base to intercalate between the neighboring base pairs. There are no data for RNA, but in DNA, NMR studies (Patel et al. 1982a; Morden et al. 1983) have shown that both cases occur depending on sequence.

Interior loops. Essentially no data are available on interior loops. Formally, an interior loop contains two or more unbonded bases with at least one unbonded base on each strand. Thus, a base-base mismatch can be considered an interior loop of two. As discussed earlier, some mismatches will perturb the duplex very little, whereas others may have a large effect. It will be necessary to study, either experimentally or theoretically, a wide range of examples to learn the rules of secondary structure.

TERTIARY STRUCTURE

The distinction between which structural elements constitute secondary structure and which constitute tertiary structure is arbitrary. We chose single strands, double-stranded duplexes, hairpin loops, internal loops, and bulges as secondary structural elements. Any additional interactions among these structural elements constitutes tertiary structure. This means, for example, that base pairings between two loops or between a loop and a single-strand region are tertiary interactions. All base triples are tertiary structures. These definitions are consistent with computer algorithms currently in use to calculate secondary RNA folding (Zuker and Steigler 1981; Williams and Tinoco

1986). The algorithms make an exhaustive search of all possible Watson-Crick base-paired structures that involve secondary structures as defined above and calculate the lowest free energies. The methods depend on the additivity of the free energies for the secondary structural elements; this simple additivity would be lost with a wider definition of secondary structure. A complete search among all possible secondary structures would no longer be possible.

Most of the evidence for tertiary interactions comes from tRNA; its three-dimensional structure reveals many tertiary structural elements, including pairing between loops, base triples, and intercalation of a base from one secondary structural element between two neighboring bases in another. An additional type of tertiary structure, the pseudoknot, has been found at the end of various RNAs (Pleij et al. 1985; van Belkum et al. 1987).

Base Triples

A base triple is an approximately planar group of three bases involving at least one hydrogen bond joining each pair. There are 20 combinations of four bases taken three at a time; they include the four combinations of identical bases, the 12 cases with two identical bases, and the four cases with all three bases different. Of course, each combination can have different orientations of the three bonded bases. In yeast tRNA[Phe], there are three triples: two involve a G bonding to the G of a Watson-Crick G:C, and the other is an A bonding to the A of a Watson-Crick A:U (Saenger 1984). Other triples are inferred from sequences of naturally occurring tRNAs (Kim 1978) or from mutants of tRNA[Phe] (J. Sampson and O. Uhlenbeck, pers. comm.). The list of known or inferred base triples in tRNAs are (AA:U and GA:U), (AG:C, GG:C, UG:C, GG:U and UG:U), and (AC:G and GC:G). In each case, the Watson-Crick base pair (or wobble) is designated with a colon; the last two triples in the list are the least certain. Poly(A) · poly(U)$_2$ triple helices occur with one of the U strands forming Watson-Crick base pairs and the other involved in Hoogsteen pairing (UA:U). Extrapolation from these structures suggests that any base can be added to either side of a Watson-Crick or wobble base pair to provide further stabilization.

Pseudoknots

Pseudoknots were defined in the folding of RNA by Studnicka et al. (1978), as illustrated in Figure 5 (top). A knot requires that a hairpin loop with at least one turn in the stem have one of the ends pass completely through the loop; pulling on both ends will leave a knotted strand. Knots are probably rare in RNA structure. A pseudoknot in a folded RNA has a hairpin loop plus a single strand folded back to form base pairs with the bases in the loop; it is topologically the same as a single strand, because a complete turn is not formed either in the stem or in the loop. On the basis of

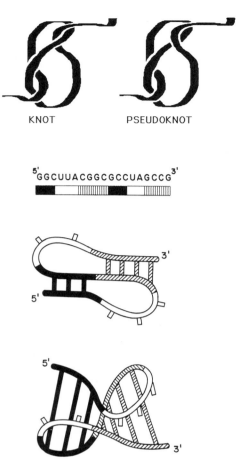

Figure 5. (*Top*) A sketch of the difference between a knot and a pseudoknot. Pulling on the ends of a knot produces a knotted strand; pulling on the ends of a pseudoknot leaves a single strand. (*Bottom*) A 19-mer oligonucleotide folded to form a pseudoknot. The two stems can stack coaxially to form a duplex of 7 bp.

chemical reactivity, enzymatic structure mapping, and sequence comparisons, a Dutch group (Rietveld et al. 1982; Pleij et al. 1985, 1986; van Belkum et al. 1987) has proposed that a pseudoknot occurs at the 3' ends of some plant viral RNAs. Their pseudoknots have the base-paired bases in the loop stacked on the hairpin stem; thus, all of the base pairs are stacked to form a continuous helix. The pseudoknot thus consists of two stems and two loops, with the stems stacked coaxially on each other. The unbonded bases of one loop cross the major groove, whereas those of the other loop cross the minor groove. Possible roles for pseudoknots have been proposed in ribosome function and in RNA self-splicing (Goringer and Wagner 1986; Pleij et al. 1986).

We have synthesized an oligonucleotide that is capable of forming a pseudoknot in the hope of being able to use NMR to study its structure in detail. A 19-mer was synthesized with T7 RNA polymerase using the method developed by Uhlenbeck's group (Lowary et al. 1986; J.F. Milligan et al., in prep.). The reaction was primed with pG to avoid having a triphosphate on

the 5' end. The sequence is 5'-r(GGC)UUA[CGGC] (GCC)UA[GCCG]-3'; two types of parentheses are used to show which sequences can pair (see Fig. 5, bottom). A three-dimensional representation of the pseudoknot is shown in Figure 6.

Evidence for a pseudoknotted conformation of the 19-mer is based on absorbance melting curves and on susceptibility to enzymatic hydrolysis. The enzyme reactions were done under conditions where less than 10% of the oligonucleotide molecules were cut. At 22°C or 37°C (0.50 mM $MgCl_2$, 10 mM NaCl in a 5 mM [pH 7] Tris buffer), snake venom V1 nuclease, which is specific for double strands, cuts at 15 of the 18 phosphodiester bonds (see Fig. 7). The only ones not cut are the two end nucleotides and the A_{15}-G_{16} link in a loop. These cuts require that most of the molecule be in a conformation that is similar to a double strand. As a control to test the ability of the enzyme to cut in loop regions, a hairpin with 7 bp in the stem and a loop of 4 bases was tried under identical conditions. The stem was cut, and there were only weak cuts in the loop region. Single-stranded A_6C was not cut at all by nuclease V1. Furthermore, a mutant 19-mer whose 5' end starts with GAG and thus cannot form a pseudoknot is no longer cut at links 2, 3, and 4; however, cuts at the 3' stem still occur. This is consistent with the single hairpin expected for the 3' end of the molecule. In contrast, under these same conditions, S1 nuclease, which is specific for single strands, only makes seven cuts, a strong cut at the 5' nucleotide and weak cuts in the loops (see Fig. 7). The S1 nuclease completely hydrolyzes a test oligonucleotide, A_6C, and cuts all four bases in the loop of our test hairpin under these same conditions. Thus, the results from both enzymes are consistent with a pseudoknot at 22°C and 37°C.

The enzymatic reactions all contained 5'-labeled oligonucleotide at a strand concentration of 1.5 μM or less. At higher concentrations, dimerization of the 19-mer occurred. This was clearly evident on a (BioRad TSK 125) sieving column that separates molecules by size. Increasing the salt concentration (e.g., to 50 mM NaCl) causes significant dimerization as seen on the sieving column. Only conditions of salt and oligonucleotide concentrations that gave less than 1% dimer were used in our experiments.

Absorbance melting curves were not very accurate because of the small concentrations needed to prevent dimerization of the oligonucleotide. However, a melting curve with a T_m between 70°C and 75°C, with about a 10% hyperchromicity, was obtained. Enzymatic data at 37°C and 22°C give very similar results; the 19-mer is a pseudoknot at both temperatures. Better melting curves and more enzymatic data are required to determine whether the pseudoknot melts in an all-or-none manner; the nature of the melting may well depend critically on the Mg^{++} and Na^+ concentrations.

NMR experiments are needed on this and other oligonucleotides to establish their folded structures; however, the use of oligonucleotides to determine the details of pseudoknot structure is very promising.

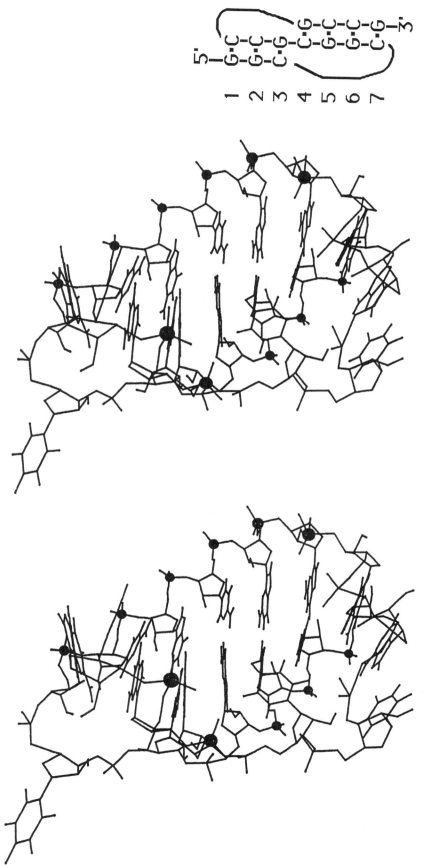

Figure 6. A computer graphics stereo pair of a three-dimentional structure of the pseudoknotted 19-mer shown in Fig. 5. The model was made on an Evans and Sutherland molecular graphics system starting with an A-RNA duplex of 7 bp. The two loops were added, and the resulting structure was adjusted to avoid close contacts; only small changes in the A-RNA duplex were required. A diagram of the 19-mer is also shown to illustrate the numbering system.

ENZYMATIC DIGESTION
37°C, pH 7, 0.50 mM Mg⁺⁺

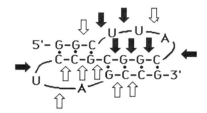

V1 CUTS
Double strand specific

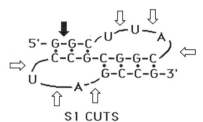

S1 CUTS
Single strand specific

Figure 7. Locations of enzymatic cuts in the 19-mer at 37°C in a pH 7 buffer (5 mM Tris, 10 mM NaCl, 0.50 mM MgCl$_2$). The oligonucleotide concentration was 1.5 μM or less; these are conditions where dimerization of the oligonucleotide does not occur. Double-strand-specific (V1) and single-strand-specific (S1) enzymes were used to produce less than one cut per oligonucleotide. Reactions of the 5'-labeled oligonucleotides were analyzed on a denaturing polyacrylamide gel and detected by autoradiography. Closed arrows indicate the major cuts for the digestion. Both V1 and S1 nuclease patterns are consistent with a pseudoknot structure; a single strand and a hairpin were used as controls.

CONCLUSIONS

Conformational details of secondary and tertiary structures in RNA are just beginning to be established. The structure of phenylalanine tRNA was our main text in this subject for many years; now other structures such as Z-RNA and pseudoknots have been found. The great improvements in organic and enzymatic synthesis methods for RNA will encourage further rapid progress in structure determination. For each new structure, there may be a new biological function.

ACKNOWLEDGMENTS

We thank all the people of the Uhlenbeck laboratory, in particular D. Groebe, J. Milligan, J. Sampson, and O. Uhlenbeck, for helpful instruction, advice, and encouragement. Mr. Wilson Ross was very helpful with the computer graphics. Drs. M. Behe, T. Jovin, and D. Zarling kindly made their results available prior to publication. Dr. W. Studier kindly provided a plasmid containing the T7 RNA polymerase gene, and Dr. R. Adamiak kindly provided the r(CGCGCG). This work was supported in part by National Institutes of Health grant GM-10840 and by the U.S. Department of Energy, OHER grant DE-FG03-82ER60406. C.C.H. was supported by a National Institutes of Health fellowship (GM-11638).

REFERENCES

Altona, C. 1982. Conformational analysis of nucleic acids. Determination of backbone geometry of single-helical RNA and DNA in aqueous solution. *Recl. Trav. Chim. Pays-Bas. Belg.* **101:** 413.

Alexeev, D.G., A.A. Lipanov, and I.Y. Skuratovskii. 1987. Poly(dA)·poly(dT) is a double helix with a distinctly narrow minor groove. *Nature* **325:** 821.

Arnold, F.H., S. Wolk, P. Cruz, and I. Tinoco, Jr. 1987. Structure, dynamics, and thermodynamics of mismatched DNA oligonucleotide duplexes d(CCCAGGG)$_2$ and d(CCCTGGG)$_2$. *Biochemistry* **26:** 4068.

Arnott, S., D.W.L. Hukins, S.D. Dover, W. Fuller, and A.R. Hodgson. 1973. Structures of synthetic polynucleotides in the A-RNA and A'-RNA conformations of polyadenylic·polyuridylic acid and polyinosinic acid·polycytidylic acid. *J. Mol. Biol.* **81:** 107.

Benevides, J.M. and G.J. Thomas, Jr. 1983. Characterization of DNA structures by Raman spectroscopy: High-salt and low-salt forms of double helical poly(dG-dC) in H$_2$O and D$_2$O solutions and applications to B, Z and A-DNA. *Nucleic Acids Res.* **11:** 5747.

Black, D.L., B. Chabot, and J.A. Steitz. 1985. U2 as well as U1 small nuclear ribonucleoproteins are involved in pre-messenger RNA splicing. *Cell* **42:** 737.

Calladine, C.R. 1982. Mechanics of sequence-dependent stacking in B-DNA. *J. Mol. Biol.* **161:** 343.

Cech, T.R. and B. Bass. 1986. Biological catalysis by RNA. *Annu. Rev. Biochem.* **55:** 599.

Clore, G.M., A.M. Gronenborn, E.A. Piper, L.W. McLaughlin, E. Graeser, and J.H. van Boom. 1984. The solution structure of a RNA pentadecamer comprising the anticodon loop and stem of yeast tRNA^{Phe}. *Biochem. J.* **221:** 737.

Cruz, P., K. Hall, J. Puglisi, P. Davis, C.C. Hardin, M.O. Trulson, R.A. Mathies, I. Tinoco, Jr., W.C. Johnson, Jr., and T. Neilson. 1986. The left-handed Z-form of double-stranded RNA. In *Biomolecular stereodynamics* (ed. R.H. Sarma and M.H. Sarma), vol. 4, p. 179. Adenine Press, Albany, New York.

Davis, P.W., K. Hall, P. Cruz, I. Tinoco, Jr., and T. Neilson. 1986. The tetranucleotide rCpGpCpG forms a left-handed Z-RNA double-helix. *Nucleic Acids Res.* **14:** 1279.

Dooley, T.P., J. Tamm, and B. Polisky. 1985. Isolation and characterization of mutants affecting functional domains of Col E1 RNA1. *J. Mol. Biol.* **186:** 87.

Drew, H.R. and R.E. Dickerson. 1981. Structure of a B-DNA dodecamer. III. Geometry of hydration. *J. Mol. Biol.* **151:** 535.

Goringer, H.U. and R. Wagner. 1985. Does 5S RNA from *E. coli* have a pseudoknotted structure? *Nucleic Acids Res.* **14:** 7473.

Haasnoot, C.A.G., C.W. Hilbers, G.A. van der Marel, J.H. van Boom, U.C. Singh, N. Pattabiraman, and P.A. Kollman. 1986. On loopfolding in nucleic acid hairpin-type structures. *J. Biomol. Struct. Dyn.* **3:** 843.

Hall, K., P. Cruz, I. Tinoco, Jr., T.M. Jovin, and J.H. van de Sande. 1984. "Z-RNA"—A left-handed RNA double helix. *Nature* **311:** 584.

Hardin, C.C. and J. Horowitz. 1987. Mobility of individual 5-fluorouridine residues in 5-fluorouracil-substituted *Escherichia coli* valine transfer RNA: A ^{19}F NMR relaxation study. *J. Mol. Biol.* (in press).

Hardin, C.C., D.A. Zarling, J.D. Puglisi, M.O. Trulson, P.W. Davis, and I. Tinoco, Jr. 1987. Stabilization of Z-RNA by chemical bromination and its recognition by anti-Z-DNA antibodies. *Biochemistry* **26:** 5191.

Hunter, W.N., T. Brown, N.N. Anand, and O. Kennard. 1986. Structure of an adenine·cytosine base pair in DNA and its implications for mismatch repair. *Nature* **320:** 552.

Hutchins, C.J., P.D. Rathjen, A.C. Forster, and R.H. Symons. 1986. Self-cleavage of plus and minus RNA transcripts of avocado sunblotch viroid. *Nucleic Acids Res.* **14:** 3627.

Jayasena, S.D. and M.J. Behe. 1987. Influence of tetraalkyl ammonium ions on the structure of poly(rG-dC)·poly(rG-dC): Unexpected transitions among the Z, A, and B conformations. *Nucleic Acid Res.* **15:** 3907.

Kearns, D. 1984. NMR studies of conformational states and dynamics of DNA. *Crit. Rev. Biochem.* **15:** 287.

Kim, S.-H. 1978. Crystal structure of yeast tRNA^{Phe} and general structural features of other tRNAs. In *Transfer RNA: Structure, properties and recognition* (ed. P.R. Schimmel et al.), p. 83. Cold Spring Harbor Laboratory, Cold Spring Harbor, New York.

Landick, R., J. Carey, and C. Yanofsky. 1985. Translation activates the paused transcription complex and restores transcription of the *trp* operon leader region. *Proc. Natl. Acad. Sci.* **82:** 4663.

Lee, C.-H. and I. Tinoco, Jr. 1980. Conformation studies of 13 trinucleoside diphosphates by 360 MHz NMR spectroscopy. A bulged base conformation. I. Base protons and H1′ protons. *Biophys. Chem.* **11:** 283.

Levy, G.C., D.J. Kraik, A. Kumar, and R.E. London. 1983. A critical evaluation of models for complex molecular dynamics: Applications to NMR studies of double-stranded and single-stranded DNA. *Biopolymers* **22:** 2703.

Lowary, P., J. Sampson, J. Milligan, D. Groebe, and O. Uhlenbeck. 1986. A better way to make RNA for physical studies. In *Structure and dynamics of RNA* (ed. P.H. van Knippenberg and C.W. Hilbers), p. 69. Plenum Press, New York.

Morden, K.M., Y.G. Chu, F.H. Martin, and I. Tinoco, Jr. 1983. The unpaired cytosine in the deoxyoligonucleotide duplex dCA$_3$CA$_3$G·dCT$_6$G is outside of the helix. *Biochemistry* **22:** 5557.

Nakamura, Y., S. Fujii, H. Urata, S. Uesugi, M. Ikehara, and K. Tomita. 1985. Crystal structure of a left-handed RNA tetramer, r(C-br^{8}G)$_2$. *Nucleic Acids Symp. Ser.* **16:** 29.

Nishimura, Y., C. Torigoe, and M. Tsuboi. 1985a. An A-form poly(dG)·poly(dC) in H$_2$O solution. *Biopolymers* **24:** 1841.

Nishimura, Y., M. Tsuboi, S. Uesugi, M. Ohkubo, and M. Ikehara. 1985b. Salt induced conformational transition between A and Z forms of r(CGCGCG) as revealed by a Raman spectroscopic study. *Nucleic Acids Symp. Ser.* **16:** 25.

Noller, H.F. 1984. Structure of ribosomal RNA. *Annu. Rev. Biochem.* **53:** 119.

Papanicolaou, C., M. Gouy, and J. Ninio. 1984. An energy model that predicts the correct folding of both the tRNA and the 5S RNA molecules. *Nucleic Acids Res.* **12:** 31.

Patel, D.J., S.A. Kozlowski, S. Ikuta, and K. Itakura. 1984. Deoxyguanosine-deoxyadenosine pairing in the d(C-G-A-G-A-A-T-T-C-G-C-G) duplex. Conformation and dynamics at and adjacent to the dG·dA mismatch site. *Biochemistry* **23:** 3207.

Patel, D.J., S.A. Kozlowski, L.A. Marky, J.A. Rice, C. Broka, K. Itakura, and K.J. Breslauer. 1982a. Extra adenosine stacks into the self-complementary d(CGCAGAATTCGCG) in solution. *Biochemistry* **21:** 445.

Patel, D.J., S.A. Kozlowski, L.A. Marky, J.A. Rice, C. Broka, J. Dallas, K. Itakura, and K.J. Breslauer. 1982b. Structure, dynamics, and energetics of deoxyguanosine thymidine wobble base pair formation in the self-

complementary d(CGTGAATTCGCG) duplex in solution. *Biochemistry* **21:** 437.

Peck, L.J. and J.C. Wang. 1981. Sequence dependence of the helical repeat of DNA in solution. *Nature* **292:** 375.

Pleij, C.W.A., K. Rietveld, and L. Bosch. 1985. A new principle of RNA folding based on pseudoknotting. *Nucleic Acids Res.* **13:** 1717.

Pleij, C.W.A., A. van Belkum, K. Rietveld, and L. Bosch. 1986. Pseudoknots in RNA: A novel folding principle. In *Structure and dynamics of RNA* (ed. P.H. van Knippenberg and C.W. Hilbers), p. 87. Plenum Press, New York.

Pohl, F.M. and T.M. Jovin. 1972. Salt-induced co-operative conformational change of a synthetic DNA: Equilibrium and kinetic studies with poly-(dG-dC). *J. Mol. Biol.* **67:** 375.

Prody, G.A., J.T. Bakos, J.M. Buzayan, I.R. Schneider, and G. Bruening. 1986. Autolytic processing of dimeric plant virus satellite RNA. *Science* **231:** 1577.

Rao, S.N. and P.A. Kollman. 1986. Conformations of the 8-methylated and unmethylated ribohexamer r(CGCG-CG)$_2$. *J. Am. Chem. Soc.* **108:** 3048.

Reid, D.G., S.A. Salisbury, T. Brown, D.H. Williams, J.-J. Vasseur, B. Rayner, and J.-L. Imbach. 1983. Use of interproton nuclear Overhauser effects to assign the nuclear magnetic resonance spectra of oligodeoxynucleotides and hybrid duplexes in aqueous solution. *Eur. J. Biochem.* **135:** 307.

Rhodes, D. and A. Klug. 1981. Sequence-dependent helical periodicity of DNA. *Nature* **292:** 378.

Riazance, J.H., W.A. Baase, W.C. Johnson, Jr., K. Hall, P. Cruz, and I. Tinoco, Jr. 1985. Evidence for Z-form RNA by vacuum UV circular dichroism. *Nucleic Acids Res.* **13:** 4983.

Rietveld, K., R. van Poelgeest, C.W.A. Pleij, J.H. van Boom, and L. Bosch. 1982. The tRNA-like structure at the 3′ terminus of turnip yellow mosaic virus RNA. Differences and similarities with canonical tRNA. *Nucleic Acids Res.* **10:** 1929.

Sarma, M.H., G. Gupta, and R.H. Sarma. 1986. 500-MHz ^{1}H NMR study of poly(dG)·poly(dC) in solution using one-dimensional nuclear Overhauser effect. *Biochemistry* **25:** 3659.

Saenger, W. 1984. *Principles of nucleic acid structure.* pp. 228–336. Springer-Verlag, New York.

Saenger, W., W.N. Hunter, and O. Kennard. 1986. DNA conformation is determined by economics in the hydration of phosphate groups. *Nature* **324:** 385.

Shvedova, T.A., G.A. Korneeva, and T.V. Venkstern. 1987. Catalytic activity of the nucleic acid component of the 1,4-α-glucan branching enzyme from rabbit muscles. *Nucleic Acids Res.* **15:** 1745.

Steely, Jr., H.T., D.M. Gray, and R.L. Ratliff. 1986. CD of homopolymer DNA·RNA hybrid duplexes and triplexes containing A·T or A·U base pairs. *Nucleic Acids Res.* **14:** 10071.

Studnicka, G.M., G.M. Rahn, I.W. Cummings, and W.A. Salzer. 1978. Computer method for predicting the secondary structure of single-stranded RNA. *Nucleic Acids Res.* **5:** 3365.

Tinoco, I., Jr., P. Cruz, P. Davis, K. Hall, C.C. Hardin, R.A. Mathies, J.D. Puglisi, M.O. Trulson, W.C. Johnson, Jr., and T. Neilson. 1986. Z-RNA: A left-handed double helix. In *Structure and dynamics of RNA* (ed. P.H. van Knippenberg and C.W Hilbers), p. 56. Plenum Press, New York.

Trulson, M.O., J.D. Puglisi, P. Cruz, I. Tinoco, Jr., and R.A. Mathies. 1987. Raman spectroscopic studies of left-handed forms of RNA. *Biochemistry* (in press).

Uesugi, S., M. Ohkubo, H. Urata, M. Ikehara, Y. Kobayashi, and Y. Kyogoku. 1984. Riboligonucleotides, r(C-G-C-G) analogues containing 8-substituted guanosine residues, form left-handed duplexes with Z-form-like structure. *J. Am. Chem. Soc.* **106:** 3675.

van Belkum, A., J. Bingkun, K. Rietveld, C.W.A. Pleij, and

L. Bosch. 1987. Structural similarities among valine accepting tRNA-like structures in tymoviral RNAs and elongator tRNAs. *Biochemistry* **26:** 1144.

Williams, Jr., A.L. and I. Tinoco, Jr. 1986. A dynamic programming algorithm for finding alternative RNA secondary structures. *Nucleic Acids Res.* **14:** 299.

Williams, Jr., A.L., C. Cheong, I. Tinoco, Jr., and L.B. Clark. 1986. Vacuum ultraviolet circular dichroism as an indicator of helical handedness in nucleic acids. *Nucleic Acids Res.* **14:** 6649.

Woese, C.R., R.R. Guttell, R. Gupta, and H.F. Noller. 1983. Detailed analysis of the higher-order structure of 16S-like ribosomal ribonucleic acids. *Microbiol. Rev.* **47:** 621.

Zarling, D.A., C.J. Calhoun, C.C. Hardin, and A.H. Zarling. 1987. Cytoplasmic Z-RNA. *Proc. Natl. Acad. Sci.* **84:** 6117.

Zarling, D.A., D.J. Arndt-Jovin, M. Robert-Nicoud, L.P. McIntosh, R. Thomae, and T.M. Jovin. 1984. Immuno-globulin recognition of synthetic and natural left-handed Z DNA conformations and sequences. *J. Mol. Biol.* **176:** 369.

Zaug, A. and T.R. Cech. 1986. The intervening sequence RNA of *Tetrahymena* is an enzyme. *Science* **231:** 470.

Zhurkin, V.B., Y.P. Lysov, and V.I. Ivanov. 1978. Different families of double-stranded conformations of DNA as revealed by computer calculations. *Biopolymers* **17:** 377.

Zimmerman, S.B. and B.H. Pheiffer. 1981. A RNA·DNA hybrid that can adopt two conformations: An X-ray diffraction study of poly(rA)·poly(dT) in concentrated solution or in fibers. *Proc. Natl. Acad. Sci.* **78:** 78.

Zuker, M. and P. Steigler. 1981. Optimal computer folding of large RNA sequences using thermodynamics and auxiliary information. *Nucleic Acids Res.* **9:** 133.

Zweib, C. and E. Ullu. 1986. Identification of dynamic sequences in the central domain of 7SL RNA. *Nucleic Acids Res.* **14:** 4639.

Structures Involved in *Tetrahymena* rRNA Self-splicing and RNA Enzyme Activity

M.D. Been,*[†] E.T. Barfod,* J.M. Burke,[‡] J.V. Price,*[§] N.K. Tanner,*[††]
A.J. Zaug,* and T.R. Cech*

*Department of Chemistry and Biochemistry, University of Colorado, Boulder, Colorado 80309;
[†]Department of Chemistry, Williams College, Williamstown, Massachusetts 01267

In eukaryotic genes, coding sequences in the DNA are often interrupted by stretches of noncoding DNA. These intervening sequences (IVSs), or introns, are transcribed along with the flanking coding sequences (exons) to give a large precursor RNA. RNA splicing is the process by which the IVSs are removed from the precursor and the exons are ligated.

Three major classes of RNA splicing can be delineated on the basis of splicing mechanism. Nuclear tRNA precursors undergo splicing by separable cleavage and rejoining reactions, which are catalyzed by traditional enzymes, including endonucleases and ligases (Filipowicz and Shatkin 1983; Greer et al. 1983). Group I RNA precursors include examples from fungal mitochondrial pre-mRNAs and pre-rRNAs, the nuclear pre-rRNA of *Tetrahymena* and *Physarum*, and several bacteriophage pre-mRNAs (Michel and Dujon 1983; Waring et al. 1983; Chu et al. 1986). They undergo splicing by a two-step transesterification mechanism (Fig. 1) and exemplify intramolecular catalysis; i.e., splicing is accomplished by the folded structure of the IVS RNA (Cech et al. 1981; Kruger et al. 1982; Cech and Bass 1986). In some cases, RNA catalysis is only partial, such that splicing requires proteins in addition to the folded structure of the RNA (Lazowska et al. 1980; Garriga and Lambowitz 1986). The final class of RNA-splicing reactions encompasses the bulk of nuclear mRNAs and the mitochondrial and chloroplast group II mRNAs. In these cases, splicing occurs by formation of a branched RNA known as the lariat (Padgett et al. 1984; Ruskin et al. 1984). Nuclear mRNA splicing occurs in a large complex of proteins and small nuclear RNAs, and evaluation of the relative contribution of the protein and RNA components to catalysis has just begun (Padgett et al. 1986; Maniatis and Reed 1987). Group II mRNA IVSs have a conserved structure (Michel and Dujon 1983) that mediates lariat formation in a self-splicing reaction (Peebles et al. 1986; van der Veen et al. 1986).

Following the discovery of self-splicing group I RNAs, we have been working to establish structure-function relationships for this class of RNA-splicing reactions. The immediate goal has been to understand the biochemical mechanism of an important step in gene expression. The long-term goal is to understand mechanisms of RNA catalysis: Does RNA catalysis simply recapitulate catalytic strategies already understood for protein enzymes, or will novel mechanisms of catalysis be uncovered?

The chemistry of self-splicing RNA and RNA en-

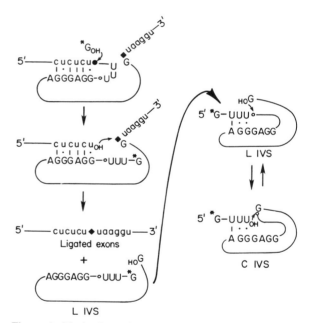

Figure 1. Mechanism of self-splicing and auto-cyclization. The 3′ end of the 5′ exon (cucucu) binds to a 5′-exon-binding site within the IVS (GGAGGG), which positions the 5′ splice site (●) for nucleophilic attack by the 3′-OH of GTP (*G) or guanosine. The GTP becomes covalently attached to the 5′ end of the IVS. The 5′ exon, still bound to the binding site, now has a free 3′-OH and undergoes nucleophilic attack at the 3′ splice site (◆). The 5′ exon becomes covalently attached to the 3′ exon, and the ligated exons are released. After its excision, the IVS RNA refolds and $U^{13}U^{14}U^{15}$ pairs with a purine sequence adjacent to the 5′-exon-binding site (see text; Fig. 3); pairing to $G^{26}G^{27}A^{28}$ is illustrated. The cyclization site (○) is thus positioned for nucleophilic attack by the 3′-OH of the 3′-terminal guanosine of the IVS (G^{414}). Circular IVS (C IVS) is formed, and a free 15-mer is released from the 5′ end. In the reverse reaction, the 3′-OH of U^{15} acts as the nucleophile and attacks at the phosphate following G^{414}. Lowercase letters indicate exon sequences, and uppercase letters indicate intervening sequence.

Present addresses: [†]Department of Biochemistry, Duke University Medical Center, Durham, North Carolina 27710; [§]Biology Department, Princeton University, Princeton, New Jersey 08544; [††]Division of Biology, Caltech, Pasadena, California 91125.

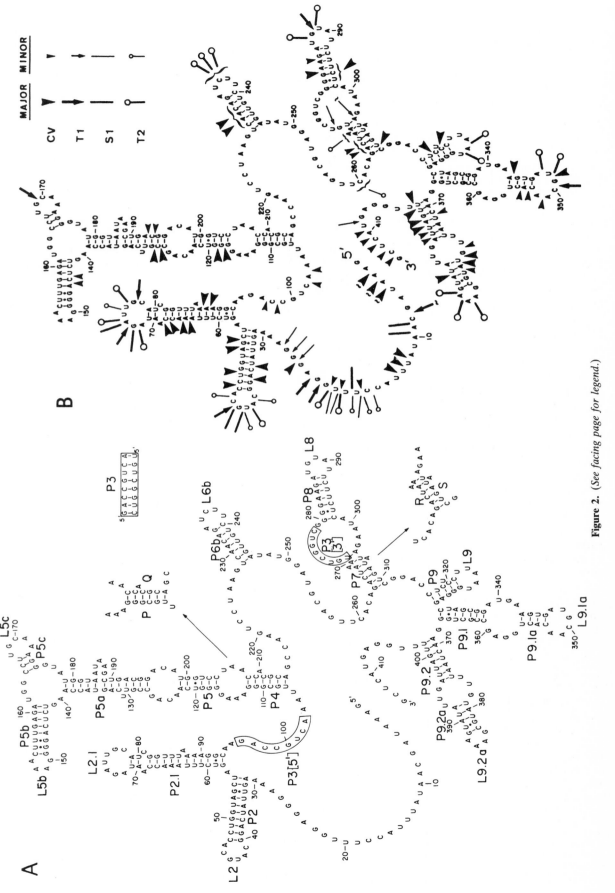

Figure 2. (*See facing page for legend.*)

zymes has been reviewed recently (Cech 1987). In this paper, we review our current understanding of the RNA structures that are responsible for self-splicing of the *Tetrahymena* IVS RNA and ideas about how these structures contribute to catalysis.

IVS Secondary Structure

The secondary-structure model of the IVS RNA is shown in Figure 2A. It was derived from computer-modeling studies and represents the most stable folding consistent with a limited amount of data on nuclease accessibility of the intact IVS RNA (Cech et al. 1983). Phylogenetic comparisons of the rRNA IVSs of different species of *Tetrahymena* have been made, and the results are consistent with this model (Wild and Sommer 1980; Nielsen and Engberg 1985). The model includes base-paired elements P2, P4, P5, P7, P8, and P9, which characterize group I IVSs (Davies et al. 1982; Michel et al. 1982). P1 involves 5′ exon sequences and therefore is not present in the excised IVS RNA. P3 is not part of the secondary structure model but is a possible tertiary structure interaction (upper right corner of Fig. 2A).

Secondary structure models for the *Tetrahymena* rRNA IVS and adjacent exons have been proposed by Michel and Dujon (1983) and by Waring et al. (1983). Their models, which are based on computer modeling and homology with fungal mitochondrial IVSs, are very similar to our model and, in addition, include conserved base-paired element P6 (nucleotides [nt] 215–216 paired with 257–258) not predicted in our model.

We have collected additional data on nuclease cleavage of the IVS RNA under a variety of conditions. IVS RNA was labeled at its 5′ end with ^{32}P or at its 3′ end with [^{32}P]pCp. The RNA was probed with double-strand-specific cobra venom nuclease (Vasilenko et al. 1983) and with single-strand-specific RNase T1, RNase T2, and nuclease S1 (Wurst et al. 1978) under nondenaturing conditions (5 mM $MgCl_2$, 200 mM NaCl, 10 mM Tris, pH 7.5). Under these conditions, most of the IVS (>80%) was capable of cyclizing. The RNA was digested at temperatures from 0°C (where no cyclization occurs) to 42°C (cyclization temperature). Because the first 15 nucleotides of the IVS are released during the cyclization reaction at 42°C, IVS RNA that was ^{32}P-labeled at the 5′ end was generally blocked at the 3′ end with unlabeled pCp and T4 RNA ligase. No difference in the cleavage pattern was noticed between 3′ blocked and unblocked RNAs.

The cumulative nuclease cleavage data are shown in Figure 2B. On the basis of the pattern of nuclease cleavage, the structure is largely invariant from 0°C to 42°C. The nuclease cleavage data reveal the average structure of what could be a dynamic molecule. This may be the reason why nucleotides within the region C^{17}-A^{28} and within A^{347}-A^{352} are cut by both single-strand-specific and double-strand-specific nucleases. The C^{17}-A^{28} region would be expected to be dynamic because it is part of the internal guide sequence (IGS) (Davies et al. 1982; Waring and Davies 1984); in the excised IVS, alternative portions of the IGS may interact with sequences at the cyclization sites (see below). We do not know why nucleotides within A^{347}-A^{352} are cut by both types of enzymes; however, it is noted that U^{340}-A^{352} could form a 12-bp stem, with U^{75}-A^{87} containing a single-base-pair mismatch. The secondary structure determined from the circular form of the IVS, based on the susceptibility of the RNA to chemical modification and nuclease digestion, is consistent with the proposed structure shown in Figure 2 (Inoue and Cech 1985). Cleavage of the IVS RNA by methidium-propyl-EDTA · Fe(II), a double-strand-specific reagent, also supports the model shown (Tanner and Cech 1985).

Although the 3′-terminal G_{OH} is not shown locked in an interaction, the experimental evidence indicates that it is base-paired, at least part of the time. Nucleotides U^{409}-G^{414} are lightly digested by cobra venom nuclease. This region is also the site of a psoralen monoadduct (N.K. Tanner, unpubl.). There is no obvious continuous sequence within the IVS that can form Watson-Crick base pairs with this region. Non-Watson-Crick base-pair interactions are certainly possible but are difficult to identify. Thus, we do not yet know how the 3′ end of the IVS is held in position to react with the cyclization site following U^{15} (Zaug et al. 1983; Tanner and Cech 1987).

Deletion Analysis of the IVS

Group I IVSs vary in size from 258 to 2641 nucleotides (Michel and Cummings 1985; Trinkl and Wolf 1986). Comparison of the available secondary structures reveals an identical core arrangement, dictated by the conserved pairings that define group I IVSs (Michel and Dujon 1983; Waring et al. 1983). The differences in size between the different IVSs are found in additional helices or variations in the length of conserved helices. In some cases, the extra sequences contain open reading frames not found in the *Tetrahymena* IVS.

Helices that are common to all of the self-splicing

Figure 2. Secondary structure of the *Tetrahymena* IVS. (*A*) The RNA secondary-structure model is shown as published by Cech et al. (1983), except that paired regions not consistent with the results of Inoue and Cech (1985) are shown single-stranded. Base-paired regions (Ps) and hairpin loops (Ls) are labeled according to Burke et al. (1987), which is similar to the nomenclature of Waring and Davies (1984). Conserved sequence elements P, Q, R, and S and the tertiary interaction P3 are drawn displaced from the main figure. (*B*) Cumulative nuclease cleavage data for 5′- and 3′-end-labeled IVS. Sites of cleavage of the RNA under nondenaturing conditions by double-strand-specific cobra venom nuclease (CV) and by the single-strand-specific nucleases T1, S1, and T2 are indicated. 3′-end-labeled IVS was not tested with nuclease S1. Brackets indicate regions where the exact site of cleavage was not determined. ∼ indicates cleavages seen only at higher levels of digestion; we do not know if these cleavages are occurring on intact molecules.

IVSs may be those that are required for activity. Removal of the nonconserved helices would yield a minimal IVS of about 100 nucleotides. For the *Tetrahymena* rRNA IVS (Fig. 2A), this would mean that it may be possible to remove helices P2, P2.1, P5a, P5b, P5c, P6b, P9.1, P9.1a, P9.2, and P9.2a and retain splicing activity.

Convenient restriction enzyme sites allowed nucleotides 332–409 to be deleted to form a 335-nucleotide IVS (Δ332–409) in which the two 3'-terminal stems composed of P9.1, P9.1a, P9.2, and P9.2a were removed (E. Barfod and T. Cech, unpubl.). RNA transcribed from Δ332–409 self-splices and cyclizes under normal conditions. A deletion of one more nucleotide (Δ331–409) results in decreased splicing activity. However, under conditions of higher temperature and MgCl$_2$ concentrations, there is accumulation of the IVS-3' exon, the splicing intermediate (Fig. 1).

Nuclease BAL-31 has been used to make a library of deletions centered at position 236. An IVS with a deletion of P6b (Δ224–252) retains self-splicing activity (Price et al. 1985; Price and Cech 1985; Waring et al. 1985). However, deletions that extend farther from position 236, and remove nucleotides 218–223 in the 5' direction or nucleotides 253–258 in the 3' direction, disrupt self-splicing. Michel and Dujon (1983) and Waring et al. (1985) have proposed that these nucleotides are involved in elements P6 and P6a, the former of which is universal among group I IVSs; perhaps this proposed structural element is necessary for self-splicing, and thus its disruption eliminates self-splicing activity.

A library of nuclease BAL-31 deletions centered at position 42 addresses the requirement for L2 and P2 (Price et al. 1985; Price and Cech 1985). Deletions removing L2 and part of P2 do not prevent self-splicing. RNA containing a larger deletion (Δ28–58) that removes all of P2 is unable to self-splice. However, this deletion also eliminates a few nucleotides beyond the base of the helix and therefore does not directly indicate a requirement for the presence of P2 for self-splicing activity.

The minimum requirements for a self-splicing group I IVS are yet to be defined. Clearly, an IVS in the 100–150-nucleotide size range, which retained high splicing activity, would be useful in many physical and biochemical studies. The deletion approach is one of several that will provide information to allow the design of a smaller self-splicing group I IVS.

Core Structure Sequences and Their Interactions

Conserved internal sequence elements P, Q, R, and S are found within group I IVSs at locations remote from the splice sites in the primary structure (Waring and Davies 1984). Base pairing between portions of P and Q to form paired region P4, and between portions of R and S to form P7, is thought to be common to all group I IVS secondary structures (Fig. 2A). Other elements of the group I core structure, such as P3, are conserved in their location relative to P4 and P7 but are not highly conserved in nucleotide sequence. Using oligonucleotide-directed mutagenesis, in vitro transcription, and splicing, experiments have been conducted to examine the role of several parts of the core structure in self-splicing of the *Tetrahymena* IVS (Burke et al. 1986; Williamson et al. 1987). The structure and properties of each mutant are summarized in Table 1.

In the IVS secondary structure model (Fig. 2A), the P3 pairing is proposed to consist of 7 bp (nt 96–103 pairing with 271–278). Among group I IVSs, only two residues are conserved in sequence, a G at the 5' end of P3[3'] (G^{272} in the *Tetrahymena* IVS) and a C at the 3' end of P3[5'] (C^{102}). The existence of P3 has been tested (Williamson et al. 1987). Two-base mutations were constructed in P3[3'] (G272A:C274G) and P3[5'] (G100C:C102U) designed to destabilize the putative P3 pairing. In addition, the compensatory P3 mutant (G100C:C102U:G272A:C274G) was constructed. In this mutant, the ability to form 7 bp is restored, although the nucleotide sequence varies from wild type at four positions.

Results of splicing experiments demonstrate that P3 exists and is essential for self-splicing activity. Under self-splicing conditions (200 μM GTP, 2 mM MgCl$_2$, 30 mM Tris-HCl [pH 7.5], 100 mM [NH$_4$]$_2$SO$_4$, 30°C or 42°C), the P3[5'] and P3[3'] mutations each result in a

Table 1. Mutants in P3 and Sequence Elements R and S

Sequence element	Base changes	Splicing	Hydrolysis	Comments
P3[3']	G272A:C274G	−	−	disrupts P3
P3[5']	G100C:C102U	−	−	disrupts P3
P3	G100C:C102U:G272A:C274G	+	+	restores P3
R	C266G:A268C	−	−	disrupts P7
S	U307G:G309C	−	−	disrupts P7
P7	C266G:A268C:U307G:G309C	+	+	restores P7
R	C266G:A268U	+	+	disrupts P7
S	U307A:G309C	−	−	disrupts P7
P7	C266G:A268U:U307A:G309C	+	+	restores P7
R (J6/7)	U259A:A261C	+	+	increases K_M for GTP
S (J8/7)	A301C:A302G:G303C	−	+	loss of transesterification

Notation for nucleotide sequence changes is as follows: A301C indicates that the A residue at IVS position 301 was changed to C. Hydrolysis indicates site-specific hydrolysis at 3' splice site. J6/7 and J8/7 are joining segments as defined by Burke et al. (1987).

loss of self-splicing activity. Activity is restored in the compensatory P3 mutant. Kinetic analysis showed that the activity of the compensatory P3 mutant (k_{cat}/K_M) was nearly identical to that of wild type (93% of wild type at 30°C and 110% of wild type at 42°C). The P3[5′] and P3[3′] mutations greatly reduce activity in GTP addition at the 5′ splice site, exon ligation (measured by *trans*-splicing with CpU; Inoue et al. 1985), and 3′-splice-site hydrolysis (Inoue et al. 1986). All of these activities are restored in the compensatory P3 mutant. We conclude that the P3 pairing is essential for all IVS self-catalyzed reactions. On the basis of this single group of mutants, it appears that although the RNA secondary structure involving these mutants is critical for self-splicing, the precise nucleotide sequence may be of lesser importance. These results extend an earlier genetic analysis of a yeast mitochondrial group I IVS by Weiss-Brummer et al. (1983).

A similar series of experiments was carried out to examine the contributions of elements R (nt 259–270) and S (nt 301–312) to IVS structure and function. The highly conserved GACUA (nt 264–268) near the 3′ end of R is proposed to form 5 bp with the highly conserved UAGUC (nt 307–311) near the 3′ end of S. In contrast, structure-mapping data and IVS structural models suggest that the highly conserved nucleotides at the 5′ ends of elements R (J6/7, nt 259–261) and S (J8/7, nt 301–306) are largely single-strand regions of the IVS.

Several pre-rRNA variants containing mutations in P7 were constructed and characterized. Two-base mutations in elements R (C266G:A268C) and S (U307G:G309C) are each predicted to disrupt 2 of the 5 bp in P7. A compensatory P7 4-base mutant (C266G:A268C:U307G:G309C) is predicted to restore pairing. Splicing results confirm that P7 exists and is essential for IVS activity. The R (C266G:A268C) and S (U307G:G309C) mutations each result in the loss of all self-catalyzed processing activity, whereas the compensatory P7 (C266G:A268C:U307G:G309C) mutations restore self-splicing. Unlike the P3 compensatory mutant, the activity of the P7 compensatory mutant differs from wild type in two important respects. First, the splicing activity of the P7 compensatory mutant (k_{cat}/K_M) is only 6% of that of wild type at 42°C. Second, splicing of the P7 compensatory mutant requires a higher temperature than wild type, suggesting that the compensatory mutations cause an increase in splicing activation energy. A second series of related mutations at the same sites were constructed (Table 1). Results for element S (U307A:G309C) and compensatory P7 (C266G:A268U:U307A:G309C) mutants were similar to those for their counterparts above. Unexpectedly, the element R (C266G:A268U) mutant showed increased activity relative to wild type (k_{cat}/K_M = 260% of wild type at 30°C, 350% at 42°C). Point mutations in this region will be constructed and characterized.

A two-base mutation (U259A:A261C) was constructed in J6/7, the nonpairing segment of sequence element R. Somewhat surprisingly, this mutation of two highly conserved bases does not drastically affect splicing. However, significant kinetic effects are observed. The J6/7 mutation results in an increase in K_M for the GTP substrate, from 29 μM (wild type) to 120 μM (U259A:A261C mutant); however, k_{cat} is unchanged. Therefore, the primary effect of the U259A:A261C mutation is to decrease GTP binding. The calculated difference in binding free energy, 0.9 kcal/mole, is on the order of that expected from the loss of a single hydrogen bond or base-stacking interaction. Reductions of GTP-binding affinity by the mutation might reflect direct interactions between U^{259} or A^{261} and GTP. Alternatively, structural changes induced by these substitutions could indirectly alter the IVS structure such that a nearby binding site is distorted.

Mutations were constructed to address the function of J8/7, the highly conserved nonpairing segment of sequence element S, in self-splicing. Simultaneous substitutions at three sites (A301C:A302C:G303C mutant) eliminates self-splicing; however, hydrolysis at the 3′ site proceeds normally, yielding 5′ exon-IVS and free 3′ exon. The mutations block three distinct transesterification reactions—GTP addition at the 5′ splice site, CpU addition at the 3′ splice site, and cyclization of the 5′ exon-IVS. Unlike mutations in P7 and P3, activity is not restored by increased Mg^{++} concentrations. These results suggest that J8/7 may participate in the catalysis of transesterification.

Specification of the 5′ Splice Site

The 5′ splice-site duplex. The IGS is located between the 5′ splice site and P2. It has the potential to base pair with sequences near the 5′ splice site and often with the exon sequence near the 3′ splice site to give paired regions P1 and P10, respectively. These interactions were proposed to be involved in the process of splice-site selection and alignment (Davies et al. 1982; Waring and Davies 1984). There is supporting evidence from genetics (Perea and Jacq 1985) and in vitro splicing studies (Inoue et al. 1985; Been and Cech 1986; Waring et al. 1986) for the structure involving pairing with the 5′ splice site. Evidence for base pairing with the 3′ splice site is less conclusive; for the *Tetrahymena* IVS, deleting the portion of the IGS that can pair with the 3′ splice site does not eliminate in vitro splicing activity, although activity is decreased (Been and Cech 1985).

Specific base substitutions were introduced into the sequences that are proposed to base pair (Fig. 3). Substitutions at positions −2, −3, and −4 in the exon (c-2g, u-3g, c-4g, c-4u; see genotype designation, Table 2) all reduce splicing activity. Substitutions in the IVS at positions 23, 24, and 25 (G23C, G23U, G23A, A24C, G25C, G25U, and G25A) also reduce activity and appear to do so to a greater extent than the exon mutations. Substitutions at positions 26 and 27 (G26C and G27C) reduce activity to a lesser degree, and a substitution at position 28 (A28C) appears to have no effect on splicing activity.

Four double substitutions were generated as a test for a base-pairing requirement in this structure. Pre-

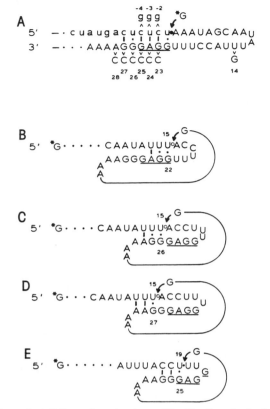

Figure 3. (*A*) Secondary structure of the 5'-splice-site duplex. The 5' exon sequence is indicated in lowercase letters and is numbered in reverse from the 5' splice site; the IVS (uppercase) is numbered according to the convention used for the excised IVS, which contains a 5' noncoded G, and thus the sequence encoded in the DNA begins with number 2. The positions of bases that were changed are indicated. We consider the underlined 5'-GGAG-3' sequence to be the most critical for reaction at the 5' splice site. (*B*) Secondary structure for the cyclization site duplex if it used the 5'-exon-binding site (see text). (*C,D,E*) Three potential secondary structures that could be involved in cyclization site selection.

cursor c-2g:G23C RNA splices marginally faster than wild type, whereas u-3g:A24C, c-4g:G25C, and c-4u:G25A RNAs have more activity than those with single substitutions, but are slower than wild type. The ability to suppress the effects of individual base substitutions in combinations that restore complementarity supports the hypothesis that the duplex is required for accurate splicing activity. A similar conclusion was reached independently by Waring et al. (1986).

Deletion of 5' exon sequences. The requirement for exon sequences has also been studied by replacing exon sequences with plasmid sequences (Price et al. 1987). Precursor RNA, with 9 nucleotides of the natural *Tetrahymena* 5' exon and 26 nucleotides of the natural 3' exon, is able to self-splice accurately and efficiently. When the natural 5' exon is shortened to 4 nucleotides, splicing remains accurate but occurs with reduced efficiency. When only 2 nucleotides of the 5' exon remain, splicing is no longer observed. This is what might

be expected according to the proposed role for the IGS (Waring et al. 1983), wherein the 6 nucleotides preceding the 5' splice site (CUCUCU) are able to bind to the 5' exon binding site (GGAGGG). Not predicted were aberrant splicing products that occurred in increasing amounts as the size of the natural 5' exon sequence was reduced.

Some of the aberrant products were found to be the result of GTP addition to novel sites in the exon sequences. One of the sites of GTP addition was similar to the 5' splice site in that it was preceded by the sequence CUCU, but it occurred 52 nucleotides downstream from the 3' splice site in plasmid sequences following the 3' exon. This observation led to a model whereby the GTP-addition site served as a cryptic 5' splice site (Fig. 4). The model predicted that the sequence CUCU would be transferred to the 3' splice site in a reaction analogous to exon ligation, producing a small circular fragment of the 3' exon. A small circular RNA was identified and characterized and found to support the model (Price et al. 1987). Thus, the selection of the 5' splice site is somewhat independent of its location in the RNA and depends more heavily on the sequence and the accessibility of the candidate site.

U · G interaction at the 5' splice site. It has been proposed that in group I IVSs, the conserved U preceding the 5' splice site is paired to a conserved G within the IVS and is part of the 5'-splice-site duplex (P1) described above (Davies et al. 1982; Michel and Dujon 1983; Inoue et al. 1986). This proposal was tested by making substitutions of the 5'-splice-site U (u^{-1}) and the putative base-pairing G (G^{22}) by site-directed mutagenesis (E. Barfod and T. Cech, unpubl.). The U at position −1 has been changed to C, G, and A. The G at position 22 has been changed to A and U. For all of the mutants, splicing is less efficient than for wild type, and the reactions require elevated concentrations of GTP. The u-1c mutant has the most normal phenotype, since it splices to some extent under standard reaction conditions and yields only accurately ligated exons.

Mutants u-1a and u-1g have more complex phenotypes. They do not splice appreciably under standard conditions, but they produce some ligated exons at 42°C in the presence of higher concentrations of Mg^{++} and GTP. With both mutants, GTP attack occurs at two sites: at the normal splice site following the mutated base and after the U at position −3 in the 5' exon. Ligated exons resulting from attack at the normal position contain the mutated nucleotide accurately joined to the 3' exon. This indicates that both steps in splicing (Fig. 1) can proceed with nucleotides other than U at position −1. Ligated exons resulting from attack 3' to u^{-3} contain the truncated 5' exon joined to the normal 3' exon. For the u-1g mutant, 70–80% of the product is initiated by attack following u^{-3}. For u-1a, the proportion of products is evenly distributed between the two sites of attack. Alternative duplex alignments that could yield these products are shown in Figure 5.

Mutation of the conserved G^{22} shows a similar pat-

Table 2. Summary of Splicing and Circularization Reactions for Various Mutants

	Genotype[a]	Splicing	Circularization	
			position 15	position 19
1.	Wild type	+++	+++	+++
2.	c-2g	−[b]	n.d.[c]	n.d.
3.	u-3g	+/−	n.d.[c]	n.d.
4.	c-4g	+/−	n.d.[c]	n.d.
5.	c-4u	+	n.d.[c]	n.d.
6.	G23C	+/−	n.d.[c]	n.d.
7.	G23A	+/−	n.d.[c]	n.d.
8.	G23U	+/−	n.d.[c]	n.d.
9.	A24C	−	n.d.[c]	n.d.
10.	G25C	−	n.d.	n.d.
11.	G25A	+/−	n.d.	n.d.
12.	G25U	+/−	n.d.	n.d.
13.	c-2g:G23C	++++	++++	+++
14.	u-3g:A24C	++	++	++
15.	c-4g:G25C	++	+/−	−
16.	c-4u:G25A	++	n.d.	n.d.
17.	G26C	++	+/−	−
18.	G27C	++	+/−	−
19.	G28C	+++	+/−	++++
20.	U14G	+++	−	++++
21.	U14G:G27C	++	++++	−
22.	U14G:A28C	+++	++++	+
23.	C18G:G26C	++	+	++

Activity for wild type is assigned three pluses. For the mutants: no activity, minus; barely detectable activity, plus/minus; intermediate activity, one or two pluses; and activity greater than wild type, four pluses. n.d. indicates not determined. Splicing conditions: 0.2 mM GTP, 100 mM $(NH_4)_2SO_4$, 5 mM $MgCl_2$, 40 mM HEPES (pH 7.5), 30°C. Cyclization conditions: 100 mM $(NH_4)_2SO_4$, 10 mM $MgCl_2$, 40 mM HEPES (pH 7.5), 42°C.

[a]Genotype notation: c-2g indicates a c to g substitution in the 5′ exon at position −2. Likewise, G23C indicates a G to C substitution in the IVS at position 23.

[b]Ligated exons produced are due largely to splicing to a secondary splice site between positions −2 and −3 in the 5′ exon.

[c]A product comigrating with the position of circle in polyacrylamide gels is produced with these mutations. It is assumed, but not proven, to be due to hydrolysis at the 3′ splice site followed by circle formation either to the 5′ splice site or to one of the circularization sites (Inoue et al. 1986).

tern. Both G22U and G22A mutants yield ligated exons resulting from attack at the normal splice site. These results can be explained by rearrangements of the reaction duplex to maintain a U · G base pair (Fig. 5). Alternatively, it is possible for G22A that splicing occurs next to a U · A base pair and for G22U that splicing occurs next to an unpaired base. The results from mutagenesis at positions −1 and 22 are consistent with the u^{-1}/G^{22} interaction being the preferred structure in the splicing reaction.

Specification of the Cyclization Sites

Cyclization of the excised L IVS is in many respects similar to the first step in splicing (Zaug et al. 1983; Been and Cech 1985; Sullivan and Cech 1985; Inoue et al. 1986; Tanner and Cech 1987). Those similarities suggest a common mechanism and perhaps a common binding site for the 5′ splice site and the cyclization sites (Fig. 3A,B). We tested the common-binding-site model by examining the effect of substitutions in the 5′-exon-binding site on the cyclization reaction. The results (Table 2) suggest that splicing and cyclization involve different binding sites. Substitutions at position

23 or 24 (c-2g:G23C and u-3g:A24C) do not prevent cyclization following the U at position 15 or 19 in the IVS, even though a second base substitution in the exon is required to suppress the effect on splicing. On the other hand, the identity of bases at positions 25–28 appears to be important in the cyclization reaction. Base substitutions at position 25, 26, or 27 (G25C, G26C, and G27C) reduce cyclization to the position following U^{15} and appear to eliminate activity following U^{19}. The substitution at position 28 (A28C) changes the preferred cyclization site from a position following U^{15} to one following U^{19} (Been and Cech 1987).

Three double substitutions were generated in an attempt to define potential duplex structures involved in cyclization. A substitution at position 14 (U14G) prevents cyclization to the position after U^{15} but is suppressed when a C is substituted for the purine at position 27 or 28 (U14G:G27C and U14G:A28C). Likewise, C18G:G26C cyclizes to the position after U^{19} but G26C does not. The results from experiments with the double substitutions do not define a unique binding site for the cyclization reaction; instead, it appears that multiple alignments involving largely Watson-Crick base pairing can function to direct the cyclization reac-

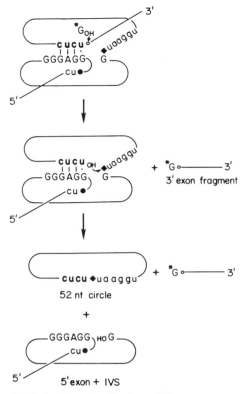

Figure 4. Mechanism of cyclization of 3' exon sequences. In plasmids pJE443 and pJE441 (Price et al. 1987), portions of the normal exon preceding the 5' splice site have been deleted. Because the remaining 5' exon sequences are so short (4 nt and 2 nt, respectively), they no longer bind efficiently to the 5'-exon-binding site. Instead, an alternative site (cucu, bold-face letters) at positions 49–52 of the 3' exon can bind competitively and function as a cryptic 5' splice site. First, the phosphate bond (○) to the right of the cryptic site (analogous to the phosphate bond at the 5' splice site) is transferred to GTP (*G). The released RNA, containing the distal part of the 3' exon covalently attached to the GTP, is observed when [^{32}P]GTP is used as the substrate for guanosine addition to ^{3}H-labeled RNA. The cucu (in the proximal part of the 3' exon) remains bound to the 5'-exon-binding site, and its free 3'-OH can now attack the phosphate at the normal 3' splice site (♦), becoming covalently attached to position 1 of the 3' exon. Since the cryptic 5' splice site was itself located in the 3' exon, the product is a 52-nt circle. A third product of this reaction is the 5' exon-IVS, which remains after release of the 52-nt circle. Lowercase letters indicate exon sequences; uppercase letters indicate IVS.

tion (Fig. 3C–E). Alternative structures suggest that the IGS is not fixed in position but may be able to shift or slide in some manner. We hypothesize that this "sliding guide" sequence can function much as a template strand, in that it can move relative to the active site of the ribozyme (Been and Cech 1987).

Specification of the 3' Splice Site

Very little is known about the mechanism of 3'-splice-site recognition. As mentioned above, Waring et al. (1983) have proposed that the IGS within the IVS aligns the splice sites. According to this model, nucleotides 2–8 of the 3' exon are paired to nucleotides 14–20 in the IGS. However, deleting nucleotides 14–21 of the IGS does not prevent self-splicing activity in vitro (Been and Cech 1985). Thus, it seems that although the IGS plays an essential role in the recognition and positioning of the 5' splice site, some other mechanism is employed for recognition of the 3' splice site. One possibility could be that the 3' splice site is held in the vicinity of the active site by being tethered to some internal structure by a specific number of nucleotides. However, correct choice of the 3' splice site is seen with pre-rRNA that contains insertions of 8 or 40 nucleotides at position 409 (5 nt upstream of the 3' splice site) (Price et al. 1985) and with a deletion of 78 of the 83 nucleotides preceding the 3' splice site (Δ332–409, see above).

Another possibility is that the last few nucleotides at the 3' end of the IVS, including the terminal guanosine (G^{414}), define the 3' splice site. This could account for the specificity seen in site selection for two mechanistically similar reactions, reverse cyclization (Sullivan and Cech 1985) and intermolecular exon ligation (Inoue et al. 1985), both of which involve nucleophilic attack after G^{414} by short pyrimidine oligonucleotides. As mentioned above, there is evidence that the 3' end of the IVS is base-paired. Recently, a binding site that recognizes the sequences at the 3' end of the IVS and positions the 3'-terminal G$_{OH}$ for the cyclization reaction has been demonstrated (Tanner and Cech 1987). Most of the productive binding interactions can be obtained from the last two nucleotides (CG). The same process could be used to recognize and position the 3' splice site.

Enzymatic Activities of the IVS RNA

After its excision from the *Tetrahymena* pre-rRNA, the linear IVS RNA undergoes a cascade of cyclization and self-cleavage reactions (Zaug et al. 1984). The final product, the L − 19 IVS RNA, is missing the first 19 nucleotides of the IVS that contain the major and minor sites of cyclization. Therefore, it cannot undergo any further intramolecular reactions. The L − 19 IVS RNA still retains activity, however, and can catalyze cleavage-ligation reactions on exogenous RNA substrates (Zaug and Cech 1986a). The L − 19 IVS RNA is regenerated in each reaction cycle, so that it works with multiple turnover. It acts as an enzyme.

One of the enzymatic activities of the L − 19 IVS RNA resembles that of RNA polymerase (Fig. 6A). Early in the reaction with C$_5$ as a substrate, the L − 19 IVS RNA catalyzes the reaction 2 C$_5$ → C$_4$ + C$_6$. One C$_5$ is used as a "monomer" unit to donate a pC moiety, and the other C$_5$ acts as a primer to be extended. The C$_4$ is analogous to the pyrophosphate produced during the normal RNA polymerase reaction. As C$_6$ accumulates, it begins to be used as a substrate, resulting in

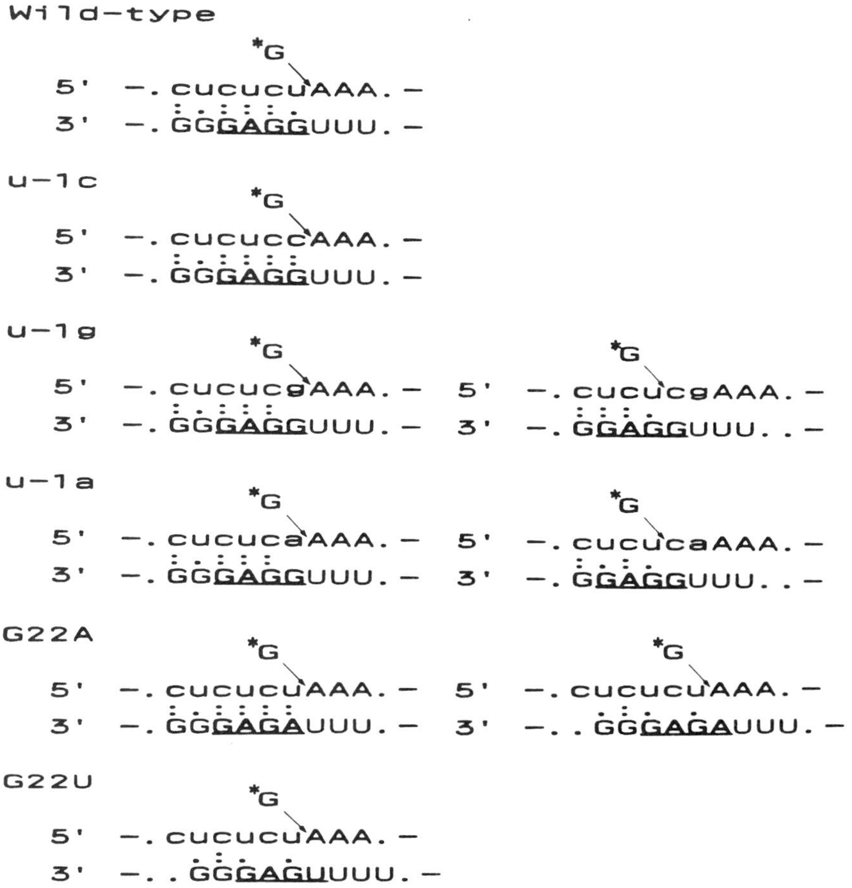

Wild-type
*G
5' —. CUCUCUAAA. —
3' —. GGGAGGUUU. —
u-1c
*G
5' —. CUCUCCAAA. —
3' —. GGGAGGUUU. —
u-1g
*G
5' —. CUCUCgAAA. —
3' —. GGGAGGUUU. —
*G
5' —. CUCUCgAAA. —
3' —. GGAGGUUU. . —
u-1a
*G
5' —. CUCUCaAAA. —
3' —. GGGAGGUUU. —
*G
5' —. CUCUCaAAA. —
3' —. GGAGGUUU. . —
G22A
*G
5' —. CUCUCUAAA. —
3' —. GGGAGAUUU. —
*G
5' —. CUCUCUAAA. —
3' —. . GGGAGAUUU. —
G22U
*G
5' —. CUCUCUAAA. —
3' —. . GGGAGUUUU. —

Figure 5. Some potential alternative secondary structures at the 5′ splice site for mutants with substitutions at either position −1 or 22.

A
(I)
GOH
GGGAGG 5'
C5
(II)
CCCCpC
GGGAGG 5'
C4
(III)
GpC
GGGAGG 5'
C5
(IV)
GpC
CCCCC OH
GGGAGG 5'
C6
B
5'——CUCUCUA——3'
+ *GOH
L - 19
IVSβ RNA
3'
5'
GGGAGG
*GOH
5'——CUCUCUA——3'
GGGAGG
5'——CUCUCUOH
+ *GA——3'

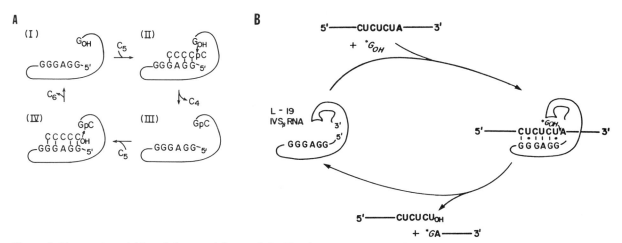

Figure 6. Enzymatic activities of shortened forms of the *Tetrahymena* IVS RNA. (*A*) Poly(C) polymerase activity (Zaug and Cech 1986a). The L − 19 IVS RNA enzyme (I) is shown with the oligopyrimidine-binding site (GGAGGG) near its 5′ end and G^{414} with a free 3′-OH group at its 3′ end. The complex folded core structure of the molecule is simply represented by a curved line. The enzyme binds its substrate (C_5) by Watson-Crick base pairing to form the noncovalent enzyme-substrate complex (II). Nucleophilic attack by G^{414} leads to formation of the covalent intermediate (III). If C_5 binds to the intermediate (III) in the manner shown in IV, transesterification can occur to give the new product C_6 and regenerate the enzyme (I). (Reprinted, with permission, from Been and Cech 1986.) (*B*) Sequence-specific endoribonuclease activity (Zaug et al. 1986). The L − 19 IVS RNA is subjected to periodate oxidation and β-elimination to remove its 3′-terminal guanosine residue. The resulting RNA enzyme (L − 19 IVSβ RNA) binds an RNA substrate (boldface letters and thick lines) and a free guanosine nucleoside or nucleotide (*G) and catalyzes the cleavage of the RNA substrate by transesterification. (Reprinted, with permission, from Cech et al. 1987.)

production of C_7. Continuation of this cycle gives products as large as C_{30} after 1 hour. Thus, the L − 19 IVS RNA can act as a poly(C) polymerase. The K_M for C_5 is 42 μM, and the turnover number is ~100/hr (Zaug and Cech 1986a). The reaction mechanism (Fig. 6A) involves steps that are intermolecular versions of pre-rRNA self-splicing and other self-processing reactions. More specifically, formation of the covalent intermediate (II → III) is analogous to IVS RNA cyclization, and resolution of the intermediate (IV → I) is analogous to exon ligation or the reversal of cyclization.

The substrate specificity of this RNA enzyme can be altered by site-specific mutagenesis of the sequence GGAGGG in the active site. Changing the guanosine-rich active site to an adenosine-rich sequence (GAAAAG) changes the substrate from oligo(C) to oligo(U) (Been and Cech 1986). Thus, the RNA enzyme is not restricted to being a poly(C) polymerase. Yet, the RNA enzyme differs from natural RNA polymerases in that it uses an internal template to direct the polymerization reaction, whereas natural RNA polymerases are dependent on an external template. It might be possible to detach the template of the RNA enzyme from its catalytic domain and get it to function with an external template. If so, the ribozyme could conceivably act as a primitive RNA replicase (Cech 1986; Szostak 1986; Zaug and Cech 1986a).

The L − 19 IVS RNA also uses phosphate monoesters as substrates. The RNA enzyme dephosphorylates C_5p by transferring the 3′-phosphate to the 3′-terminal guanosine of the enzyme. Phosphorylation of the enzyme is reversible by C_5-OH and other oligo(pyrimidines); thus, the RNA enzyme acts as a phosphotransferase. At pH 4–5, the phosphoenzyme undergoes slow hydrolysis to yield inorganic phosphate; thus, the RNA is also an acid phosphatase (Zaug and Cech 1986b).

Finally, the L − 19 IVS RNA can act as a sequence-specific endoribonuclease (Fig. 6B) by a guanylyl transfer mechanism analogous to the first step of self-splicing (Fig. 1). Because it uses a free guanosine nucleotide, the endoribonuclease activity does not require the 3′-terminal guanosine of the IVS RNA enzyme; in this respect, it differs from the poly(C) polymerase activity of the same enzyme. The wild-type L − 19 IVS RNA cleaves other RNA molecules after sequences that resemble CUCU, the sequence that precedes the 5′ splice site of the Tetrahymena pre-rRNA. Site-specific mutations in the active site of the L − 19 IVS RNA alter the sequence specificity in a predictable manner. Ribozymes that cleave after the sequences CUGU, CGCU, and GUCU have been synthesized and tested. Thus, a large set of ribozymes that act like RNA restriction endonucleases can be synthesized (Zaug et al. 1986).

ACKNOWLEDGMENTS

We thank Alice Sirimarco for preparing the manuscript. This work was supported by grants to T.R.C. from the American Cancer Society (NP-374) and the National Institutes of Health (GM-28039) and to J.M.B. from the National Institutes of Health (GM-36981) and the National Science Foundation (DMB-8502691).

REFERENCES

Been, M.D. and T.R. Cech. 1985. Sites of circularization of the Tetrahymena rRNA IVS are determined by sequence and influenced by position and secondary structure. Nucleic Acids Res. 13: 3389.
———. 1986. One binding site determines sequence specificity of Tetrahymena pre-rRNA self-splicing, trans splicing, and RNA enzyme activity. Cell 47: 207.
———. 1987. Selection of circularization sites in a group I IVS RNA requires multiple alignments of an internal template-like sequence. Cell 50: 951.
Burke, J.M., M. Belfort, T. Cech, R.W. Davies, R. Schweyen, D. Shub, J. Szostak, and H. Tabak. 1987. Structural conventions for group I introns. Nucleic Acids Res. (in press).
Burke, J.M., K.D. Irvine, K.J. Kaneko, B. Kerker, A.B. Oettgen, W. Tierney, C. Williamson, A.J. Zaug, and T.R. Cech. 1986. Role of conserved sequence elements 9L and 2 in self-splicing of the Tetrahymena ribosomal RNA precursor. Cell 45: 167.
Cech, T.R. 1986. A model for the RNA-catalyzed replication of RNA. Proc. Natl. Acad. Sci. 83: 4360.
———. 1987. The chemistry of self-splicing RNA and RNA enzymes. Science 236: 1532.
Cech, T.R. and B.L. Bass. 1986. Biological catalysis by RNA. Annu. Rev. Biochem. 55: 599.
Cech, T.R., A.J. Zaug, and M.D. Been. 1987. Multiple enzymatic activities of an intervening sequence RNA from Tetrahymena. In Molecular biology of RNA: New perspectives (ed. M. Inouye), p. 37. Academic Press, New York.
Cech, T.R., A.J. Zaug, and P.J. Grabowski. 1981. In vitro splicing of the ribosomal RNA precursor of Tetrahymena: Involvement of a guanosine nucleotide in the excision of the intervening sequence. Cell 27: 487.
Cech, T.R., N.K. Tanner, I. Tinoco, Jr., B.R. Weir, M. Zuker, and P.S. Perlman. 1983. Secondary structure of the Tetrahymena ribosomal RNA intervening sequence: Structural homology with fungal mitochondrial intervening sequences. Proc. Natl. Acad. Sci. 80: 3903.
Chu, F.K., G.F. Maley, D.K. West, M. Belfort, and F. Maley. 1986. Characterization of the intron in the phage T4 thymidylate synthase gene and evidence for its self-excision from the primary transcript. Cell 45: 157.
Davies, R.W., R.B. Waring, J.A. Ray, T.A. Brown, and C. Scazzocchio. 1982. Making ends meet: A model for RNA splicing in fungal mitochondria. Nature 300: 719.
Filipowicz, W. and A.J. Shatkin. 1983. Origin of the splice junction phosphate in tRNAs processed by HeLa cell extract. Cell 32: 547.
Garriga, G. and A.M. Lambowitz. 1986. Protein dependent splicing of a group I intron in ribonucleoprotein particles and soluble fractions. Cell 46: 669.
Greer, C.L., C.L. Peebles, P. Gegenheimer, and J. Abelson. 1983. Mechanism of action of a yeast RNA ligase in tRNA splicing. Cell 32: 537.
Inoue, T. and T.R. Cech. 1985. Secondary structure of the circular form of the Tetrahymena rRNA intervening sequence: A technique for RNA structure analysis using chemical probes and reverse transcriptase. Proc. Natl. Acad. Sci. 82: 648.
Inoue, T., F.X. Sullivan, and T.R. Cech. 1985. Intermolecular exon ligation of the rRNA precursor of Tetrahymena: Oligonucleotides can function as 5′ exons. Cell 43: 431.
———. 1986. New reactions of the ribosomal RNA precursor of Tetrahymena and the mechanism of self-splicing. J. Mol. Biol. 189: 143.

Kruger, K., P.J. Grabowski, A.J. Zaug, J. Sands, D.E. Gottschling, and T.R. Cech. 1982. Self-splicing RNA: Autoexcision and autocyclization of the ribosomal RNA intervening sequence of *Tetrahymena*. *Cell* **31**: 147.

Lazowska, J., C. Jacq, and P.P. Slonimski. 1980. Sequence of introns and flanking exons in wild type and box3 mutants of cytochrome *b* reveals an interlaced splicing protein coded by an intron. *Cell* **22**: 333.

Maniatis, T. and R. Reed. 1987. The role of small nuclear ribonucleoprotein particles in pre-mRNA splicing. *Nature* **325**: 673.

Michel, F. and D.J. Cummings. 1985. Analysis of class I introns in a mitochondrial plasmid associated with senescence of *Podospora anserina* reveals extraordinary resemblance to the *Tetrahymena* ribosomal intron. *Curr. Genet.* **10**: 69.

Michel, F. and B. Dujon. 1983. Conservation of RNA secondary structures in two intron families including mitochondrial-, chloroplast-, and nuclear-encoded members. *EMBO J.* **2**: 33.

Michel, F., A. Jacquier, and B. Dujon. 1982. Comparison of fungal mitochondrial introns reveals extensive homologies in RNA secondary structure. *Biochemie* **64**: 867.

Nielsen, H. and J. Engberg. 1985. Sequence comparisons of the rDNA introns of six different species of *Tetrahymena*. *Nucleic Acids Res.* **13**: 7445.

Padgett, R.A., P.J. Grabowski, M.M. Konarska, S. Seiler, and P.A. Sharp. 1986. Splicing of messenger RNA precursors. *Annu. Rev. Biochem.* **55**: 1119.

Padgett, R.A., M.M. Konarska, P.J. Grabowski, S.F. Hardy, and P.A. Sharp. 1984. Lariat RNAs as intermediates and products in the splicing of messenger RNA precursors. *Science* **225**: 898.

Peebles, C.L., P.S. Perlman, K.L. Mecklenberg, M.L. Petrillo, J.H. Tabor, K.A. Jarrell, and H.-L. Cheng. 1986. A self-splicing RNA excises an intron lariat. *Cell* **44**: 213.

Perea, J. and C. Jacq. 1985. Role of the 5′ hairpin structure in the splicing accuracy of the fourth intron of the yeast cob-box gene. *EMBO J.* **4**: 3281.

Price, J.V. and T.R. Cech. 1985. Coupling of *Tetrahymena* ribosomal RNA splicing to β-galactosidase expression in *Escherichia coli*. *Science* **228**: 719.

Price, J.V., J. Engberg, and T.R. Cech. 1987. 5′ Exon requirement for self-splicing of the *Tetrahymena thermophila* pre-ribosomal RNA and identification of a cryptic 5′ splice site in the 3′ exon. *J. Mol. Biol.* **196**: 49.

Price, J.V., G.L. Kieft, J.R. Kent, E.L. Sievers, and T.R. Cech. 1985. Sequence requirements for self-splicing of the *Tetrahymena thermophila* pre-ribosomal RNA. *Nucleic Acids Res.* **13**: 1871.

Ruskin, B., A.R. Krainer, T. Maniatis, and M.R. Green. 1984. Excision of an intact intron as a novel lariat structure during pre-mRNA splicing *in vitro*. *Cell* **38**: 317.

Sullivan, F.X. and T.R. Cech. 1985. Reversibility of cyclization of the *Tetrahymena* rRNA intervening sequence: Implication for the mechanism of splice-site choice. *Cell* **42**: 639.

Szostak, J.W. 1986. Enzymatic activity of the conserved core of a group I self-splicing intron. *Nature* **322**: 83.

Tanner, N.K. and T.R. Cech. 1985. Self-catalyzed cyclization of the intervening sequence RNA of *Tetrahymena*: Inhibition by methidium propyl · EDTA and localization of the major dye binding sites. *Nucleic Acids Res.* **13**: 7759.

———. 1987. Guanosine binding required for cyclization of the self-splicing intervening sequence ribonucleic acid from *Tetrahymena thermophila*. *Biochemistry* **26**: 3330.

Trinkl, H and K. Wolf. 1986. The mosaic cox1 gene in the mitochondrial genome of *Schizosaccharomyces pombe*: Minimal structural requirements and evolution of group I introns. *Gene* **45**: 289.

van der Veen, R., A.C. Arnberg, G. van der Horst, L. Bonen, H.F. Tabak, and L.A. Grivell. 1986. Excised group II introns in yeast mitochondria are lariats and can be formed by self-splicing *in vitro*. *Cell* **44**: 225.

Vasilenko, S.K., A.S. Butorin, S.P. Maev, F.I. Vityugov, L.G. Boldyreva, and V.K. Rait. 1983. Specificity of nuclease from Oxus Cobra (*Najanaja oxiana*) venom for polyribonucleotide macro-structure. *Mol. Biol.* **17**: 818.

Waring, R.B. and R.W. Davies. 1984. Assessment of a model for intron RNA secondary structure relevant to RNA self-splicing—A review. *Gene* **28**: 277.

Waring, R.B., C. Scazzocchio, T.A. Brown, and R.W. Davies. 1983. Close relationship between certain nuclear and mitochondrial introns. *J. Mol. Biol.* **167**: 595.

Waring, R.B., P. Towner, S.J. Minter, and R.W. Davies. 1986. Splice-site selection by a self-splicing RNA of *Tetrahymena*. *Nature* **321**: 133.

Waring, R.B., J.A. Ray, S.W. Edwards, C. Scazzocchio, and R.W. Davies. 1985. The *Tetrahymena* rRNA intron self-splices in *E. coli*: *In vivo* evidence for the importance of key base-paired regions of RNA for RNA enzyme function. *Cell* **40**: 371.

Weiss-Brummer, B., J. Holl, R.J. Schweyen, G. Rodel, and F. Kaudewitz. 1983. Processing of yeast mitochondrial RNA: Involvement of intramolecular hybrids in splicing of cob intron 4 RNA by mutation and reversion. *Cell* **33**: 195.

Wild, M.A. and R. Sommer. 1980. Sequence of a ribosomal RNA gene intron from *Tetrahymena*. *Nature* **283**: 693.

Williamson, C.L., W.M. Tierney, B.J. Kerker, and J.M. Burke. 1987. Site-directed mutagenesis of core sequence elements 9R′, 9L, 9R, and 2 in self-splicing RNA. *J. Biol. Chem.* (in press).

Wurst, R.M., J.N. Vournakis, and A.M. Maxam. 1978. Structure mapping of 5′-^{32}P labeled RNA with S1 nuclease. *Biochemistry* **17**: 4493.

Zaug, A.J. and T.R. Cech. 1986a. The intervening sequence RNA of *Tetrahymena* is an enzyme. *Science* **231**: 470.

———. 1986b. The *Tetrahymena* intervening sequence RNA enzyme is a phosphotransferase and an acid phosphatase. *Biochemistry* **25**: 4478.

Zaug, A.J., M.D. Been, and T.R. Cech. 1986. The *Tetrahymena* ribozyme acts like an RNA restriction endonuclease. *Nature* **324**: 429.

Zaug, A.J., P.J. Grabowski, and T.R. Cech. 1983. Autocatalytic cyclization of an excised intervening sequence RNA is a cleavage-ligation reaction. *Nature* **301**: 578.

Zaug, A.J., J.R. Kent, and T.R. Cech. 1984. A labile phosphodiester bond at the ligation junction in a circular intervening sequence RNA. *Science* **224**: 574.

Implications of Intermolecularly Catalyzed Reactions by the *Tetrahymena* Ribozyme

P.S. KAY AND T. INOUE

The Salk Institute for Biological Studies, San Diego, California 92138

One class of intervening sequences (IVSs), group I introns, are known to reside in the precursors of nuclear RNA, mitochondrial rRNA, and mRNA, and some chloroplast tRNA molecules. They are defined by a set of conserved structural elements (Davies et al. 1982; Michel et al. 1982; Michel and Dujon 1983; Waring et al. 1983). For several group I IVS precursors, splicing occurs in vitro in the absence of any proteins and is mediated by the IVS itself (Kruger et al. 1982; Garriga and Lambowitz 1984; Van der Horst and Tabak 1985; Chu et al. 1986; Gott et al. 1986; Tabak et al. 1987). In this class of IVSs, splicing initiates with guanosine addition to the 5′ end of the IVS, releasing the 5′ exon. The 5′ exon then joins to the 3′ exon, releasing the IVS as a linear molecule. Since the IVS RNA catalyzes its own excision from the precursor, the reaction is termed self-splicing.

The precursor rRNA of *Tetrahymena* contains a group I intron of 413 nucleotides. This RNA can be spliced accurately and efficiently in vitro in the presence of a divalent cation (Mg^{++} or Mn^{++}) and a monomeric guanosine derivative (Kruger et al. 1982). In the first step of self-splicing, the reaction scheme can be presented as

$$\cdots UCUpA \cdots + G_{OH} \xrightarrow{IVS} \cdots UCU_{OH} + GpA \cdots$$
5′ splice site   5′ exon

and the second step as

$$\cdots UCU_{OH} + \quad GpU \cdots \xrightarrow{IVS} \cdots UCUpU \cdots + G_{OH}$$
5′ exon   3′ splice site   ligated exons

The IVS RNA thus appears to perform a set of transformations by repetition of a single transesterification reaction. In fact, nearly all of the reported reactions catalyzed by the *Tetrahymena* IVS can be viewed as an analog of a single transesterification reaction or the combination of three classes of reactions (Inoue et al. 1986; Kay and Inoue 1987a):

$$\cdots YYUpN \cdots + G_{OH} \rightleftharpoons \cdots YYU_{OH} + GpN \cdots$$
$$\downarrow IVS$$
$$G_{OH} + pN \cdots$$

where Y is a pyrimidine and N is any nucleoside. These three classes involve either transesterification by guanosine, transesterification by oligopyrimidine, or "specific hydrolysis," which produces a 3′-OH group

and a 5′ phosphate at the newly created termini. We have tested this hypothesis and discovered that a newly prepared large fragment of the IVS RNA of *Tetrahymena*, termed L − 21 *Sca*I IVS, can mediate a simple transesterification reaction between the substrate GpN (N = A, C, G, or U) and the nucleophile CpU. The reaction is reversible and can be written as

$$YUpN + G_{OH} \overset{IVS}{\rightleftharpoons} YU_{OH} + GpN$$

where Y is a pyrimidine and N is any nucleoside. Thus, nearly all transesterification reactions mediated by the *Tetrahymena* IVS can be described as the forward or reverse of this single reaction. For example, the forward reaction represents the first step of self-splicing and the reverse reaction represents the second step (Kay and Inoue 1987a).

This newly prepared IVS was also found to be capable of catalyzing a specific hydrolysis reaction. When the substrate GpN (N = A, C, G, or U) was incubated under mildly alkaline conditions in the presence of Mg^{++}, the phosphodiester bond was hydrolyzed in a unique manner to produce G_{OH} and pN. The 3′ splice site of the precursor rRNA is preceded by a guanosine and is known to be hydrolyzable in an analogous manner (Inoue et al. 1986). These results confirm that the phosphodiester bond of GpN is chemically equivalent to the 3′ splice site when reacted with the IVS RNA. In all cases, group I self-splicing requires initiation by nucleophilic attack of a guanosine molecule. Although the U preceding the 5′ splice site is universal, the nucleotide preceding the U need not be a pyrimidine. The G residue preceding the 3′ splice site is universal. Thus, the transesterification scheme can be generalized for all group I self-splicing IVSs as

$$XUpN + G_{OH} \rightleftharpoons XU_{OH} + GpN$$

where X can represent any of the four nucleotides, and each IVS has a binding site for its own particular XU sequence (Kay and Inoue 1987a).

In this paper, we further discuss the nature of L − 21 *Sca*I IVS RNA, which possesses the fundamental transesterification activities and specific hydrolysis activity of the *Tetrahymena* IVS. L − 19 IVS RNA, lacking 19 nucleotides from the excised full-length linear IVS RNA of *Tetrahymena* pre-rRNA, acts as an RNA catalyst and has been shown to behave as a nucleotidyl transferase, a phosphodiesterase, a phosphotransferase, and an acid phosphatase (Zaug and Cech 1986a,b). Thus, a comparison of the activity of L − 21 ScaI IVS RNA to that of L − 19 IVS RNA was performed under a variety of conditions.

EXPERIMENTAL PROCEDURES

Materials. T4 polynucleotide kinase (3′ phosphatase-free) and calf intestinal phosphatase were purchased from Boehringer-Mannheim; restriction enzymes, from New England Bio-Labs; T4 polynucleotide kinase, from U.S. Biochemical Corp.; and RNase T1, from Pharmacia. Unlabeled dinucleotides and nucleoside triphosphates, sodium periodate, aniline, and RNase P1 were purchased from Sigma, and labeled nucleoside triphosphates were purchased from ICN Radiochemicals. T7 RNA polymerase was prepared as described previously (Davanloo et al. 1984) and purified according to a procedure originally developed for SP6 RNA polymerase (Butler and Chamberlin 1982).

Preparation of L − 19 IVS RNA. pT7-TT1A3 DNA was cut with EcoRI endonuclease and transcribed in a 5-ml reaction volume containing 125 μg of DNA, 1 mM each of the four NTPs (including 200 μCi of [^{3}H]UTP), 15 mM MgCl$_2$, 10 mM dithiothreitol, 2 mM spermidine, 40 mM Tris (pH 7.5), and 12,500 units of T7 polymerase. The transcription mix was incubated at 37°C for 2 hours, and NaCl was then added to a final concentration of 240 mM. The reaction mix was incubated for an additional 30 minutes to promote excision and cyclization of the IVS RNA (Zaug and Cech 1986a). The reaction was stopped upon addition of Na$_2$EDTA (to a final concentration of 20 mM), and T7 polymerase was extracted with phenol. The transcription products were ethanol-precipitated, redissolved in a 500-μl reaction volume containing 20 mM MgCl$_2$ and 50 mM CHES (2-[cyclohexylamino]ethansulfonic acid) and incubated at 42°C for 1 hour to promote site-specific hydrolysis of the circular IVS RNA (Zaug and Cech 1986a). The resultant major product, L − 19 IVS RNA, was ethanol-precipitated, separated by electrophoresis in a 5% polyacrylamide–8 M urea gel, cut and eluted from the gel, and purified by ethanol precipitation and chromatography on Sephadex G-10-120.

Preparation of L − 21 ScaI IVS RNA. pT7-TT1A3 DNA was cut with ScaI endonuclease and transcribed in a 5-ml reaction volume as described above. The transcription mix was incubated at 37°C for 2 hours. The reaction was stopped upon addition of Na$_2$EDTA (to a final concentration of 20 mM), and T7 polymerase was extracted with phenol. The transcription products were ethanol-precipitated, redissolved in a 500-μl reaction volume containing 50 mM MgCl$_2$, 50 mM HEPPS (pH 7.5), 5 mM GTP, and 5 mM CpU and incubated at 42°C for 2 hours. The resultant major product, L − 21 ScaI IVS RNA, was ethanol-precipitated, separated by electrophoresis in a 5% polyacrylamide–8 M urea gel, cut and eluted from the gel, and purified by ethanol

precipitation and chromatography on Sephadex G-10-120.

β-Eliminated forms of the IVS RNA. Either L − 19 IVS RNA or L − 21 ScaI IVS RNA (100–200 pmoles) was incubated in a 50-μl reaction volume with 0.5 mg of NaIO$_4$ at 25°C for 2 hours in the dark. To stop the reaction, 20 μl of 10% ethylene glycol was added, and the mixture was diluted tenfold with water. The resultant oxidized product was ethanol-precipitated and redissolved in a 200-μl aniline solution (PhNH$_2$:H$_2$O, 1:33; pH adjusted to 5.2 with HCl) and incubated at 45°C for 30 minutes. The resultant β-eliminated product was purified by ethanol precipitation and chromatography on Sephadex G-10-120 (Kay and Inoue 1987b).

RESULTS

Time Course of the Transesterification Reactions

Under our standard conditions, 5′-end-labeled [^{32}P]pCpUpA or [^{32}P]pGpA (unless otherwise stated, the 5′ phosphate of oligonucleotides is labeled) was allowed to react with nonlabeled pG or nonlabeled CpU, respectively, in the presence of L − 21 ScaI IVS RNA (Kay and Inoue 1987a). The reactions represent the forward (equivalent to the first step of splicing) or the reverse (equivalent to the second step of splicing) direction of the transesterification reactions catalyzed by the IVS. Both reactions were conducted by incubating different concentrations of the nucleophile with 5 μM of the electrophile and 2.0 μM of L − 21 ScaI IVS. The time courses of the reactions are given in Figure 1. For both reactions, the yields increased linearly relative to the reaction time. The rate of the transesterification between CpU and [^{32}P]pGpA is much faster than that between pG and [^{32}P]pCpUpA. With 1 mM of pG as a nucleophile, the reaction rate of the cleavage of [^{32}P]pCpUpA approaches the V_{max}, whereas with 1 mM of CpU, the rate of the cleavage of [^{32}P]pGpA has not yet attained V_{max}.

Magnesium Dependence

To investigate the magnesium dependence of the transesterification reactions, [^{32}P]pGpA or [^{32}P]-pCpUpA was allowed to react with nonlabeled CpU or nonlabeled pG, respectively, in the presence of L − 21 ScaI IVS RNA. The results are shown in Figure 2a. In the range of 0 to 50 mM of MgCl$_2$ concentrations, the yields of both reactions increase relative to the increase of concentration of MgCl$_2$. No reactions were detected in the absence of MgCl$_2$. For the reaction between [^{32}P]pGpA and CpU, the effect of higher MgCl$_2$ concentrations was further investigated and is depicted in Figure 2b. In the 0 to ~100 mM range, the yield increased relative to the increase of MgCl$_2$. At ~100 mM or higher, however, no increase in the yield was observed. A similar result was observed for the specific hydrolysis of [^{32}P]pGpA with varying concentrations of MgCl$_2$ (Fig. 2c).

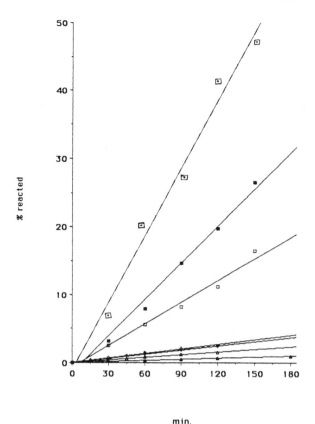

Figure 1. Time course of the pG/CpUpA and CpU/GpA reactions. L − 21 *Sca*I IVS RNA (2.0 μM) was incubated with either [^{32}P]pCpUpA (5.0 μM) and pG or [^{32}P]pGpA (5.0 μM) and CpU. The reaction was carried out in 50 mM MgCl$_2$, 50 mM HEPPS (pH 7.5) at 42°C. (▫) [CpU] 5 mM; (■) 1 mM; (□) 0.1 mM; (◇) [pG] 5 mM; (◆) 1 mM; (△) 0.5 mM; (▲) 0.05 mM.

Comparison of the Reactivities of L − 19 IVS RNA and L − 21 *Sca*I IVS RNA

The reactions catalyzed by L − 19 IVS are initiated by the nucleophilic attack of the guanosine (G^{414}) located at its 3′ end (Cech 1987). L − 21 *Sca*I IVS, which we utilize as a catalyst, does not have a guanosine at its 3′ end. However, both IVSs are terminated with *cis* 2′,3′-hydroxy groups that are known to be good nucleophiles and can attack a phosphodiester bond (Kay and Inoue 1987b). To compare the activities of the IVSs under the same conditions, the reactivities of L − 19 IVS and L − 21 *Sca*I IVS and the corresponding β-eliminated form of the IVSs were tested in the reaction of [^{32}P]pGpA with CpU. When the β-eliminated form of L − 19 IVS (L − 19 IVS$_\beta$) was used as a catalyst instead of L − 19 IVS, the yield of pG was found to be markedly increased. However, when the β-eliminated form of L − 21 *Sca*I IVS was employed instead of L − 21 *Sca*I IVS, no difference was observed for the activity of the catalyst (Fig. 3a). The activity of L − 19 IVS$_\beta$ was determined (by scintillation counting) to be comparable to those of both forms of L − 21 *Sca*I IVSs.

When provided with an oligocytidylate as a sub-

strate, L − 19 IVS acts as a nucleotidyltransferase and a phosphodiesterase (Zaug and Cech 1986a). The reaction proceeds by the initial nucleophilic attack of G^{414} at a phosphodiester bond of an oligocytidylate, followed by the transesterification by another oligocytidylate molecule at the newly created phosphodiester bond preceded by the 3′ end of the IVS. To examine the 3′-end nucleophilicities of the four IVSs, [^{32}P]pC$_{7OH}$ was incubated with L − 19 IVS, L − 19 IVS$_\beta$, L − 21 *Sca*I IVS, or L − 21 *Sca*I IVS$_\beta$, all under the same conditions (Fig. 3b). L − 19 IVS demonstrated the dismutation reaction with high efficiency. The rest of the IVS RNAs lacking G^{414} also showed minor dismutation activity. Although these data suggest that the reaction for the IVS RNAs lacking G^{414} is not due to the nucleophilic activity of the 3′ end of the IVSs, it is still possible that a small amount of some contaminant IVS RNA possessing 3′-end nucleophilicity is present.

To investigate further the activity of L − 21 *Sca*I IVS$_\beta$, a 3′-end phosphorylated oligocytidylate, pC$_5$p (lacking the nucleophilic *cis* diol at its 3′ terminus), was prepared and employed as a substrate. [^{32}P]pC$_5$p was incubated in the presence and absence of an externally added nucleophile, C$_5$OH, with L − 21 *Sca*I IVS$_\beta$. Thus, if L − 21 *Sca*I IVS$_\beta$ or some RNA copurified with it possessed 3′-end nucleophilicity, the cleavage of a phosphodiester bond of [^{32}P]pC$_5$p should be observed even in the absence of [^{32}P]C$_5$OH. As judged from the band corresponding to [^{32}P]pC$_3$OH in Figure 4a, the cleavage of pC$_5$p was observed only in the presence of C$_5$OH. This result suggests that the reaction proceeds via the direct attack of C$_5$OH at a phosphodiester bond of pC$_5$p. However, another interpretation is possible: C$_5$OH first reacts with L − 21 *Sca*I IVS$_\beta$ to create a new 3′-end terminus, which then serves as a nucleophile to cleave pC$_5$p. To test this hypothesis, L − 21 *Sca*I IVS$_\beta$ was first preincubated with C$_5$OH and then allowed to react with pC$_5$p. The results (Fig. 4a) show that reactivity of L − 21 *Sca*I IVS$_\beta$ was enhanced when preincubated by itself. However, its preincubation with C$_5$OH did not obviously enhance the activity of L − 21 *Sca*I IVS$_\beta$. When this preincubation technique was applied in the reaction of [^{32}P]pGpA with C$_5$OH, again a minor enhancement of the activity of the L − 21 *Sca*I IVS$_\beta$ was detected in the reaction without C$_5$OH, but no significant difference was observed in the transesterification with C$_5$OH (Fig. 4b).

DISCUSSION

The transesterification reaction between GpA and CpU and its reverse reaction can be interpreted as representing the self-splicing of *Tetrahymena* pre-rRNA (Kay and Inoue 1987a). In fact, the reactions are analogous to the self-splicing reaction and are not kinetically limited (as demonstrated in time-course experiments). The reactions proceed with nucleophiles in the micromolar range, and the yields of both reactions increase linearly relative to the reaction time. However, the velocities of the two reactions are very differ-

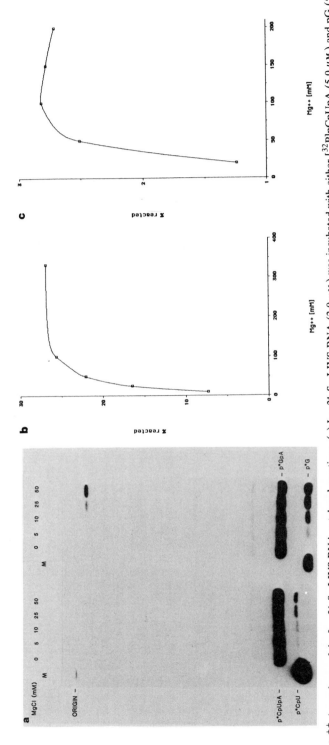

Figure 2. Mg^{++} dependence of the L − 21 *Sca*I IVS RNA-catalyzed reactions. (*a*) L − 21 *Sca*I IVS RNA (2.0 μM) was incubated with either [^{32}P]pCpUpA (5.0 μM) and pG (5.0 mM) or [^{32}P]pGpA (5.0 μM) and CpU (5.0 mM). The reaction was carried out in varying MgCl$_2$ concentrations and 50 mM HEPPS (pH 7.5) at 42°C for 2 hr. M denotes authentic markers; asterisks indicate the labeled phosphates. (*b*) L − 21 *Sca*I IVS RNA (2.0 μM) was incubated with [^{32}P]pGpA (2.5 μM) and CpU (5.0 mM). The reaction was carried out in varying MgCl$_2$ concentrations and 50 mM HEPPS (pH 7.5) at 42°C for 1 hr. (*c*) L − 21 *Sca*I IVS RNA (2.0 μM) was incubated with [^{32}P]pGpA (2.5 μM). The reaction was carried out in varying MgCl$_2$ concentrations and 50 mM EPPS (pH 8.5) at 42°C for 30 min. For *b* and *c*, the products of the reactions were separated on 20% polyacrylamide/8 M urea gels and visualized by autoradiography. The fraction reacted was determined for each reaction by liquid scintillation counting the corresponding gel slices.

162

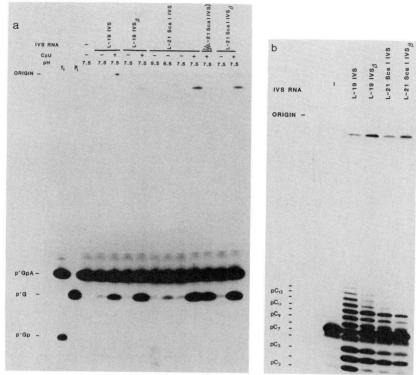

Figure 3. Reactions of L − 19 and L − 21 *Sca*I IVS RNAs. (*a*) [^{32}P]pGpA (5 μM) was incubated with an IVS RNA (0.6 μM) in the presence of CpU (5 mM) or no cofactor. 1/2(L − 21 *Sca*I IVS) denotes incubation with 0.3 μM IVS RNA. The reaction was carried out in 50 mM MgCl$_2$ and 50 mM HEPPS (pH 7.5), HEPPS (pH 8.5), or CHES (pH 9.5) at 42°C for 2 hr. T1 denotes treatment of [^{32}P]pGpA with RNase T1; P1 denotes treatment of [^{32}P]pGpA with RNase P1. Note that the reaction of [^{32}P]pGpA with L − 21 *Sca*I IVS RNA at pH 9.5 resulted in the degradation of the starting material. (*b*) [^{32}P]pC$_7$ (10 μM) was incubated either alone as a control or with an IVS RNA (1.6 μM) in 20 mM MgCl$_2$ and 50 mM Tris (pH 7.5) at 42°C for 1 hr. The band near the origin represents addition of labeled [^{32}P]pC$_n$ at or near the 5′ end of the IVS RNA.

ent under the same conditions. This might indicate that the binding of GpA to the IVS is better than that of CpUpA. At present, it is too premature to interpret these data for their relevance to the self-splicing reaction.

The reactions can proceed under physiological MgCl$_2$ concentrations. For both reactions, the formation of the products was detected in the presence of 10 mM MgCl$_2$ or less. These MgCl$_2$ concentrations conform to the standard conditions employed in the self-splicing of *Tetrahymena* pre-rRNA (Bass and Cech 1984). However, in the reaction between CpU and pGpA, the production of pG is relative to the increase in the concentration of MgCl$_2$. The yield reaches its maximum at ~ 100 mM and then remains constant up to 700 mM. This can be interpreted to mean that the IVS requires relatively high concentrations of MgCl$_2$ to bind the oligonucleotides in order to perform the reaction. Since the short oligonucleotides are provided intermolecularly as either the nucleophile or electrophile in this reaction, it is plausible that the stability of the interaction of these externally added nucleotides to the IVS can determine the reaction rate.

The activities of L − 19 IVS RNA and L − 21 *Sca*I IVS RNA as well as their β-eliminated forms were compared in the reaction between CpU and pGpA. As anticipated, it was found that no covalent intermediate

was formed during the course of the reaction. Furthermore, it was found that the reaction was inhibited in the presence of L − 19 IVS RNA. Because L − 19 IVS RNA possesses a 3′-end guanosine (G^{414}) (which is known to act as the nucleophile in the transesterification reactions mediated by this IVS), the result could be attributed to the competition between G^{414} and pGpA for a guanosine-binding site in the IVS. The activities of the four IVS RNAs were compared in the dismutation reaction of pC$_7$. L − 19 IVS RNA was found to be the most active among the four IVSs. Although the three other IVSs showed minor activity in this reaction, it was not clear whether the reactions observed were catalyzed by themselves or by some IVS RNA copurified with them. If the reactions were not due to the 3′-end nucleophilicity of the IVSs, this would indicate that the reactions proceed between pC$_7$ via direct transesterification and that such a "pyrimidine exchange" reaction could exist.

Most of the transesterification reactions catalyzed by the IVS follow a rule that guanosine as a nucleophile cleaves a phosphodiester bond preceded by a pyrimidine, and pyrimidine as a nucleophile cleaves a phosphodiester bond preceded by a guanosine (Inoue et al. 1986). As far as we know, this is the first example indicating that a pyrimidine can attack a phosphodiester bond preceded by a pyrimidine. Recently, we

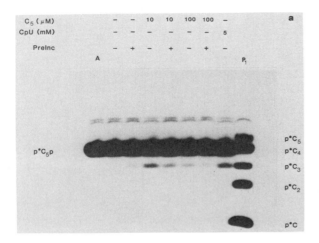

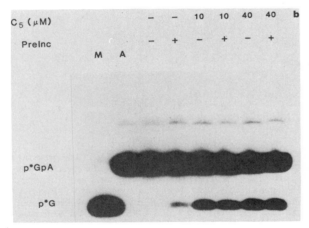

Figure 4. Reactions of L − 21 *Sca*I IVS$_\beta$ RNA. (*a*) L − 21 *Sca*I IVS$_\beta$ RNA (0.6 μM) was incubated with [^{32}P]pC$_5$p in the presence of C$_5$, CpU, or no cofactor. The reaction was carried out in 50 mM MgCl$_2$ and 50 mM HEPPS (pH 7.5) at 42°C for 1 hr. (PreInc) Preincubation of the IVS RNA with or without C$_5$ at 42°C for 2 hr; (A) incubation of [^{32}P]pC$_5$p with RNase P1. (*b*) L − 21 *Sca*I IVS$_\beta$ RNA (1.6 μM) was incubated with [^{32}P]pGpA in the presence of C$_5$ or no cofactor. The reaction was carried out in 50 mM MgCl$_2$ and 50 mM HEPPS (pH 7.5) at 42°C for 1 hr. (PreInc) Preincubation of the IVS RNA with or without C$_5$ at 42°C for 2 hr; (M) authentic marker; (A) incubation of [^{32}P]pGpA without L − 21 *Sca*I IVS$_\beta$ RNA.

discovered that L − 21 *Sca*I IVS can catalyze the transesterification reaction between a monomeric guanosine derivative and GpN (P.S. Kay and T. Inoue, in prep.). Although further investigation is needed, the implication of these findings to the mechanism of the *Tetrahymena* IVS RNA catalysis can be summarized as follows: The core of the IVS RNA catalyst might be designed essentially to mediate transesterification between a *cis*-diol and a phosphodiester bond, whereas the specific binding of guanosine and an oligopyrimidine assists to promote these reactions efficiently. Thus, this would indicate that the recognition of the bases at the reaction sites is not the minimum requirement for the transesterification reactions of self-splicing group I IVSs.

ACKNOWLEDGMENTS

This work was supported by grants from the National Institutes of Health and the Alfred Krupp von Bohlen und Halbach-Stiftung. We thank Sylvia Bailey for manuscript preparation.

REFERENCES

Bass, B.L. and T.R. Cech. 1984. Specific interaction between the self-splicing RNA of *Tetrahymena* and its guanosine substrate: Implications for biological catalysis by RNA. *Nature* **308:** 820.

Butler, E.T. and M.J. Chamberlin. 1982. Bacteriophage SP6-specific RNA polymerase: Isolation and characterization of the enzyme. *J. Biol. Chem.* **257:** 5772.

Cech, T.R. 1987. The chemistry of self-splicing RNA and RNA enzymes. *Science* **236:** 1532.

Chu, F.K., G.F. Maley, D.K. West, M. Belfort, and F. Maley. 1986. Characterization of the intron in the phage T4 thymidylate synthase gene and evidence for its self-excision from the primary transcript. *Cell* **45:** 157.

Davanloo, P., A.H. Rosenberg, J.J. Dunn, and F.W. Studier. 1984. Cloning and expression of the gene for bacteriophage T7 RNA polymerase. *Proc. Natl. Acad. Sci.* **81:** 2035.

Davies, R.W., R.B. Waring, J.A. Ray, T.A. Brown, and C. Scazzocchio. 1982. Making ends meet: A model for RNA splicing in fungal mitochondria. *Nature* **300:** 719.

Garriga, G. and A.M. Lambowitz. 1984. RNA splicing in *Neurospora* mitochondria: Self-splicing of a mitochondrial intron *in vitro*. *Cell* **38:** 631.

Gott, J.M., D.A. Shub, and M. Belfort. 1986. Multiple self-splicing introns in bacteriophage t4: Evidence from autocatalytic GTP labeling of RNA *in vitro*. *Cell* **47:** 81.

Inoue, T., F.X. Sullivan, and T.R. Cech. 1986. New reactions of the ribosomal RNA precursor of *Tetrahymena* and the mechanism of self-splicing. *J. Mol. Biol.* **189:** 143.

Kay, P.S. and T. Inoue. 1987a. Catalysis of splicing-related reactions between dinucleotides by a ribozyme. *Nature* **327:** 343.

———. 1987b. Reactivity of modified ribose moieties of guanosine: New cleavage reactions mediated by the IVS of *Tetrahymena* precursor rRNA. *Nucleic Acids Res.* **15:** 1559.

Kruger, K., P.J. Grabowski, A.J. Zaug, J. Sands, D.E. Gottschling, and T.R. Cech. 1982. Self-splicing RNA: Autoexcision and autocyclization of the ribosomal RNA intervening sequence of *Tetrahymena*. *Cell* **31:** 147.

Michel, F. and B. Dujon. 1983. Conservation of RNA secondary structure in two intron families including mitochondrial-, chloroplast- and nuclear-encoded members. *EMBO J.* **2:** 33.

Michel, F., A. Jacquier, and B. Dujon. 1982. Comparison of fungal mitochondrial introns reveals extensive homologies in RNA secondary structure. *Biochemie* **64:** 867.

Tabak, H.F., G. Van der Horst, A.M.J.E. Kamps, and A.C. Arnberg. 1987. Interlocked RNA circle formation by a self-splicing yeast mitochondrial Group I intron. *Cell* **48:** 101.

Van der Horst, G. and H.F. Tabak. 1985. Self-splicing of yeast mitochondrial precursor RNA. *Cell* **40:** 759.

Waring, R.B., C. Scazzocchio, T.A. Brown, and R.W. Davies. 1983. Close relationship between certain nuclear and mitochondrial introns. *J. Mol. Biol.* **167:** 595.

Zaug, A.J. and T.R. Cech. 1986a. The intervening sequence RNA of *Tetrahymena* is an enzyme. *Science* **231:** 470.

———. 1986b. The *Tetrahymena* sequence ribonucleic acid enzyme is a phosphotransferase and an acid phosphatase. *Biochemistry* **25:** 4478.

Internal Guide Sequence and Reaction Specificity of Group I Self-splicing Introns

R.W. Davies,[*][†] R.B. Waring,[*][‡] and P. Towner[*]

*Department of Biochemistry and Applied Molecular Biology, UMIST, Manchester M60 IOD, United Kingdom;
†Allelix Inc., Mississauga, Ontario L4V 1P1, Canada

The existence of RNA catalysis in present day biochemistry was demonstrated first and incontrovertibly by the discovery that accurate splicing of the large rRNA precursor of *Tetrahymena thermophila* occurred in the absence of protein (Cech et al. 1981; Kruger et al. 1982). The intron excised during this self-splicing reaction is a member of a widespread class of introns known as group I introns. This class of introns is common in mitochondrial genomes of fungi, being transcribed into both rRNA and mRNA precursors, and is also found in nuclear genomes of protozoa, in chloroplast genomes of plants, and in bacteriophage. All group I introns are RNA catalysts in various stages of dependence on nuclear or organellar ("maturases") proteins. The *Tetrahymena* pre-rRNA (*Tet*) intron remains the best-studied RNA catalyst, and group I introns may prove to have been the prototypes of all other classes of introns (except those near tRNA anticodons). Their retention of catalytic capacity after excision has led to the fascinating possibility that similar molecules may have given rise to the first replication and protein synthesis systems (Cech 1986; Been et al.; Weiner and Maizels; both this volume).

The sequence of RNA-catalyzed reactions in which the *Tet* intron is involved is (1) RNA self-splicing (Fig. 2), resulting in intron excision and ligation of the 5' and 3' exons and consisting of two subreactions, and (2) a series of two cyclization and specific hydrolysis reactions yielding finally the "L − 19" form of linear intron, which still retains catalytic activity if presented with the right substrate such as oligocytidylate (Zaug and Cech 1986).

All of these reactions are transesterification reactions in which one phosphodiester bond is broken for each one formed. As shown in Figure 1, the RNA self-splicing reaction is actually two separate transesterification reactions. The first is "5' cutting," in which a nucleophilic attack via the 3'-OH of a specifically bound guanosine cofactor on the phosphodiester bond at the 5' splice junction generates a cut 5' exon, the guanosine cofactor being added to the 5' end of the intron-3' exon molecule. In the second subreaction, the phosphodiester bond at the 3' splice junction is broken, and a new phosphodiester bond is formed as the exons are ligated together. In the subsequent cyclization reac-

tion, the free 3' G_{OH} at the end of the linear free intron attacks a site 15 bases from the 5' end, yielding an L − 15 circle and a 15-base fragment. Specific hydrolysis can occur at the cyclization site, followed by a

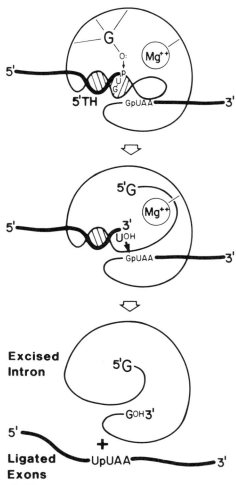

Figure 1. Diagrammatic representation of the two separate transesterification (cleavage/ligation) reactions that constitute RNA self-splicing. 5'TH (5' target helix; Waring et al. 1986) is a functional designation for the P1 pairing region; here, IGS bases are paired with 5' exon bases and bases at the 5' end of the intron. Part of this base-paired region is retained after the 5' cleavage, holding the free 3'-OH of the 5' exon in place to attack the 3' splice junction in the 3' cleavage/ligation reaction that completes RNA splicing. Also shown are Mg^{++} ions, necessary for both subreactions, and the guanosine cofactor that is needed only for 5' cleavage/ligation.

‡Present address: Department of Pharmacology, UMDNJ, Piscataway, N.J. 08854.

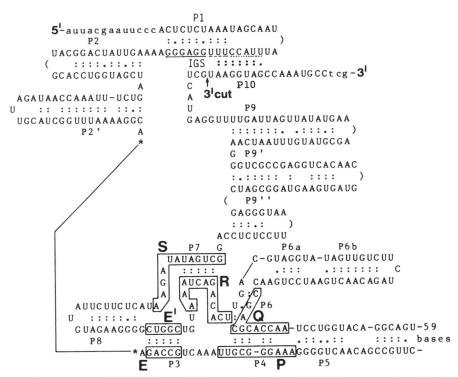

Figure 2. RNA secondary structure of the *Tet* intron. All base-paired regions (P1–P10) shown are found in all or most group I introns, with the exceptions of the stems P2′, P9′, and P9″. The primary sequences of group I introns are characterized by four conserved RNA sequences called P, Q, R, and S, which are always in the same order. Parts of P and Q are involved in conserved base pairing with one another, as are parts of R with parts of S. The only other conserved features of the primary sequence are the conservation of a G at position 22 and a G at position 414, which is the 3′ end of the excised intron. However, large sections of the intron are conserved with regard to secondary structure, in the sense that certain stem-loop structures always occur at certain positions relative to the P-Q and R-S pairings, even though they may vary in size and complexity. Also, one particular long-range base pairing (called E-E′) is always found between sequences in well-defined positions relative to P, Q, R, and S. Typically, ten conserved regions of base pairing can be identified, P1 to P10. For a detailed consideration of the structure, see Waring and Davies (1984).

second cyclization reaction to give an L − 19 circle, which again can hydrolyze, producing the final L − 19 molecule (Zaug et al. 1985; Zaug and Cech 1986). The only two requirements for most of these RNA-catalyzed reactions to occur are (1) a particular RNA structure and (2) Mg++ ions. In addition, the very first reaction, 5′ cleavage/ligation, requires the presence of a guanosine derivative.

There are two central questions to be asked about self-splicing RNAs: What is the mechanism of catalysis? How is the reaction kept so specific for particular phosphodiester bonds? The range of reactions that can be catalyzed has been demonstrated by Cech and co-workers (Cech 1986; Been et al., this volume), and a plausible mechanism of catalysis has been proposed (Zaug et al. 1985). It seems likely that significant advances in understanding catalysis depend strongly on the determination of a three-dimensional structure of the RNA catalyst. On the other hand, a partial definition of the basis of splice-junction specificity is possible by genetic and biochemical experiments, working from secondary structure predictions. The work described here addresses primarily this question, using the *Tet* intron as a convenient experimental system.

In studying how the intron selects its substrates, the

splice junctions, we have of necessity provided evidence for interactions between particular base sequences and defined some components of the active site. If, as seems likely, it is difficult to make hydrophobic pockets with RNA, then RNA-structure-dependent positioning of metal ions and attacking hydroxy groups and possible structure-dependent stress on particular phosphodiester bonds are all that remains as a basis for catalysis; thus, by identifying the key elements of sequence and their interactions as determinants of specificity, we also begin to learn about catalysis.

The RNA structure of group I introns is the key to their function as catalysts and to the specificity of the reactions catalyzed. All the evidence available support quite exactly our proposed model (Davies et al. 1982), the *Tet* intron version of which is shown in Figure 2. The RNA structure can be divided into two sections: a "core" region, including P-Q, R-S, and E-E′, that has been shown experimentally (Szostak 1986) to contain all of the structures necessary for catalysis, and two base-paired regions in which contiguous sequences of the intron pairs with exon sequences, proposed (Davies et al. 1982) to be important for "alignment" of the 5′ and 3′ splice junctions.

The intron sequence that pairs sequentially with 5′

and 3' exon sequences is known as the internal guide sequence (IGS). This sequence is always similarly placed relative to the P2 base-paired region, always occurs before P, Q, R, and S, and contains the conserved G^{22}. In addition, it plays a crucial role in many of the RNA-catalyzed reactions that the *Tet* intron undergoes. We discuss here recent experimental evidence from our laboratory that sheds light on the role of the IGS in 5' cleavage/ligation, 3' cleavage/ligation, and cyclization.

METHODS

The procedures described fully by Waring et al. (1985, 1986) were used throughout. All mutations discussed here (except $C^{-4}U$) were made by oligodeoxyribonucleotide-directed in vitro mutagenesis as described by Zoller and Smith (1984). The system used to detect mutations affecting splicing (Waring et al. 1985) was plaque color of M83.TET.14, a derivative of phage M13mp8.3, with the *Tet* intron (with 7 and 17 bases of flanking 5' and 3' exons, respectively) inserted so that the synthesis of the β-galactosidase α-fragment is prevented unless the intron excises itself in vivo in *Escherichia coli*. For in vitro splicing reactions, the insert in M83.TET.14 was shuttled into pSP65, and templates were cut with various restriction enzymes to yield the 3' end of the message (usually *Pvu*II) transcribed with SP6 polymerase. The *Pvu*II precursor RNA starts 24 bases before the first base of the intron and ends 214 bases after the last base of the intron (plus one or two randomly added bases; Waring et al. 1986).

RESULTS AND DISCUSSION

The strong conservation of potential base pairing between the IGS and 5' exon and 3' exon sequences close to the splice junctions (Fig. 2) is most easily explained if these base pairings are important, directly or indirectly, in ensuring the specificity of the reaction. Moreover, by providing the substrates of the 5' and 3' cleavage/ligation reactions in the correct three-dimensional position, and possibly in some special state, these pairings would contribute directly to catalysis. We have investigated the roles of P1 (IGS-5' exon) and P10 (IGS-3' exon) base-paired regions by making mutations in each partner strand that would seriously weaken these pairings, observing the in vivo and in vitro splicing phenotypes, and then combining mutations to reconstruct base pairings as strong as the originals but with altered base sequences. If the splicing phenotype of the RNA molecules containing the repaired base-paired region is significantly closer to wild type than the single mutations (second-site suppression), we can conclude that the base-paired region occurs and make conclusions about its function from the biochemical effects of the mutations. We have been able to show that the IGS plays a central role in 5' cleavage/ligation and cyclization and an important role in 3' cleavage/ligation. A detailed presentation of some of this work has been or will be made elsewhere (Waring et al. 1986; R.B. Waring and R.W. Davies, in prep.).

5' Cleavage/Ligation

The P1 pairing is conserved throughout group I introns, and within it, the conserved G^{22} in the IGS always pairs with the last base of the 5' exon (U in all but one case). Therefore, the P1 pairing *contains* the 5' splice junction; it was renamed the 5' target helix (5'TH) by Waring et al. (1986) in light of their results, which are summarized here.

Mutations in the 5' exon partner strand (5THex; Fig. 3A) or the IGS partner strand (5THint; Fig. 3A) that weaken base pairing without directly affecting the splice junction have strong defects in 5' cleavage/ligation, the strength of the defect being proportional to the loss of base-pairing potential. The phenotypes of mutations in either strand are very similar (Fig. 4), as would be expected if the disruption of the pairing was the source of the phenotypic change (rather than interference with RNA folding via the formation of alternative base pairings, or direct interference with catalysis); both the double mutants 5THint and 5THex are almost completely defective in 5' cleavage/ligation. As shown in Figure 3A, 5THint and 5THex were designed to be complementary when both are present at once and to restore the original number of hydrogen bonds. When 5THint and 5THex are present in the same RNA molecule (5THsup), a significant level of intron excision and exon ligation is reached (Fig. 4). Therefore, second-site suppression of the mutant phenotypes occurs, proving that the P1 (5'TH) pairing plays a crucial function in 5' cleavage/ligation. However, suppression is not complete. Although the steady-state level of the intervening sequence (IVS) and ligated exon production approaches wild type, the rate of RNA splicing in vitro is 50–100-fold slower. The number of hydrogen

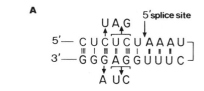

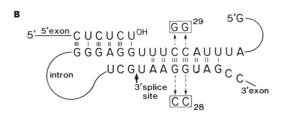

Figure 3. Mutations in the P1 (5'TH) and P10 base-paired regions. (*A*) P1 mutations: The $U^{-3}C^{-2}$ to $A^{-3}G^{-2}$ mutant is called 5THex, and $A^{24}G^{23}$ to $U^{24}C^{23}$ is called 5THint, according to Waring et al. (1986). (*B*) P10 mutations: Mutant 29 is $C^{17}C^{18}$ to $G^{17}G^{18}$, and in mutant 28, the 3' exon bases $G^{+4}G^{+5}$ are changed to $C^{+4}C^{+5}$. Bases are numbered from 5' to 3' as they occur in the linear excised intron, i.e., with the G cofactor added to the 5' end as base 1; 5' exon bases are numbered from −1 and 3' exon bases are numbered from +1, starting at the respective splice junction.

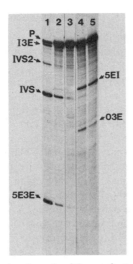

Figure 4. Gel electrophoresis of the products of in vitro RNA-splicing reactions. Reaction conditions and pSP65 precursor transcripts were described by Waring et al. (1986). (*1*) Wild-type +GTP; (*2*) mutant 29 +GTP; (*3*) wild-type −GTP; (*4*) mutant 29 −GTP + 4 mM spermidine; (*5*) 5THex −GTP + 4 mM spermidine. (P) Precursor; (I3E) intron joined to 3′ exon; (IVS2) linear excised intron with aberrant 3′ end; (IVS) excised linear intron; (5EI) 5′ exon fused to the intron; (03E) circular 3′ exon; (5E3E) ligated 5′ and 3′ exons.

bonds is the same, and thus the sequence alteration in the 5′TH (P1) must cause this. This indicates that the tertiary interactions between bases in 5′TH and other parts of the molecules are important for correct positioning of the phosphodiester bond at the 5′ splice junction. These tertiary interactions must underlie the ability of the core RNA enzyme to bind and cleave its 5′ substrate when this is provided on a separate molecule (Szostak 1986). Another interesting, and nonexclusive, possibility is that the UpA bond at the 5′ splice junction is in a special state and that altering the stacking interactions nearby alters this state.

The importance of the IGS in 5′ cleavage/ligation is clear. Further support was brought by Been and Cech (1986). The experiments of Waring et al. (1986) also showed that the part of the IGS that pairs with 5′ exon bases also plays a crucial part in the 3′ cleavage/ligation reaction (Davies et al. 1982). A GTP-independent (3′ cleavage-like) side reaction occurs with some mutations in this part of the IGS, since the sequence alteration can provide an improved base-pairing partner for the 3′ end of the mRNA. The 3′-OH at the end of the mRNA is then used by the RNA catalyst as if it were the end of the cut 5′ exon; i.e., it is ligated to the 5′ end of the 3′ exon. The occurrence of the products of the 3′-end-invasion side reaction (5EI, intron with the 5′ exon still attached; 03E, circular 3′ exon) is diagnostic of any condition under which P1 is weakened or faced with competition. Thus, the 5′-exon-pairing IGS region not only is involved in forming the target of 5′ cleavage/ligation, but also holds the cut 5′ exon correctly for its 3′-OH to attack the phosphodiester bond at the 3′ splice junction in the 3′ cleavage/ligation reaction.

These results are also interesting because they identify the IGS, or at least that part of it that pairs with the cut 5′ exon, as the receptor or binding site for externally supplied oligonucleotides of reasonable complementarity. Inoue et al. (1985) showed that oligonucleotides such as CpU (which pairs with IGS bases $G^{22}G^{23}$) could replace the 5′ exon and become ligated to the 3′ exon. Thus, the *Tet* intron with a weakened P1, or in the absence of the 5′ exon, becomes a *trans*-acting catalyst, with its specificity determined by the IGS.

3′ Cleavage/Ligation

The spatial relationship of the attacking and target groups in 3′ cleavage/ligation (5′ exon $3'_{OH}$; 3′ splice junction GpU) must be very similar to that between the attacking and target groups of 5′ cleavage/ligation (cofactor G_{OH}, 5′ splice junction UpA). Thus, the 3′ splice junction *must* be very close to the 3′ end of the 5′ exon within the active site for the 3′ cleavage/ligation reaction to occur. Three mechanisms, which are in no way mutually exclusive, could account for this: (1) The last G^{414} of the intron could become bound in the G cofactor-binding site (Kay and Inoue 1987a,b). (2) G^{414} and/or bases close to it could be involved in non-Watson-Crick hydrogen bonding with noncontiguous bases in the active site. (3) The P10 pairing might bring the G^{414} pU into the correct position.

The P10 pairing is found in most, but not all, group I introns (Waring and Davies 1984) and is a reasonably strong base-paired region of the *Tet* intron. Thus, despite early indications from our own work and that of Been and Cech (1985) that exon bases involved in P10 could be altered or deleted without drastically affecting self-splicing, we have investigated whether second-site suppression could be used to support the formation of the P10 pairing and have studied the phenotypes of some mutations in P10 in detail. The data will be presented in full in a forthcoming publication (R.B. Waring and R.W. Davies, in prep.).

Mutation 29 (Fig. 3B) alters bases C^{17} C^{18} to G^{17} G^{18}, C^{17} and C^{18} being in the portion of the IGS (Davies et al. 1982) that should be involved in P10. Similarly, 3′ exon bases G^{+4} G^{+5} that should be involved in P10 were changed to $C^{+4}C^{+5}$ (mutant 28). Both mutants 28 and 29 have *E. coli* in vivo phenotypes recognizably different from wild type, whereas the combination 28 + 29 is more like wild type. The in vitro phenotype of mutant 28 is very similar to wild type, except for the rate of use of secondary splice sites. Mutant 29 has a very distinctive in vitro phenotype, as shown in Figure 4. The production of 5E1 and 03E molecules in a GTP-independent reaction was described for the 5THint mutation above and is due to enhanced mRNA 3′-end pairing with IGS bases because P1 is destabilized. 5THex, which has a wild-type IGS but a weakened P1, can be made to produce 5EI and 03E in the presence of spermidine (Fig. 4), whereas wild type cannot. This is precisely what happens with mutant 29. Therefore, mutant 29 must directly or indirectly interfere with the formation or stability of the P1 base pairing. However mutant 29 exerts its effect, combining 29 with 28 in one RNA molecule suppresses the mutant 29 effect (R.B. Waring and R.W. Davies in prep.), showing that these bases really do pair.

P10 is thus a real base-paired region, but it plays a housekeeping role in the RNA structure, preventing the formation of incorrect structures at either the 5' end or the 3' end, rather than a direct role in the active site. Nevertheless, P10 does make a significant contribution to ensuring that G^{414}pU is chosen as the phosphodiester bond at the 3' splice junction.

Cyclization

In the first cyclization reaction, the free 3' G_{OH} of the excised intron attacks a phosphodiester bond near the 5' end of the molecule in an RNA-catalyzed reaction, producing a circular intron and a 15-base fragment. Cech and co-workers have studied this reaction in some detail (Inoue et al. 1986), have shown that cyclization always occurs on the 3' side of a tripyrimidine stretch, and have suggested that this tripyrimidine stretch pairs transiently with bases (initially, A^{24} G^{23} G^{22} was proposed; Inoue et al. 1985; Sullivan and Cech 1985) in the IGS before cleavage. The mutants 5THint (C^{23} U^{24}), 5THex (A^{-3} G^{-2}), and 29 (G^{17} G^{18}) clearly occur in regions intimately involved in this process according to this model, and as Figure 5 shows, the spectrum of cyclization products made by these mutants does shed some light on the specificity requirements of this reaction.

Cyclization of the excised intron occurs normally during a splicing reaction involving the wild-type precursor (Fig. 5, track WTa). This track is overexposed in order to visualize the cyclization products of rarer RNA species used as precursors in the other tracks; but as

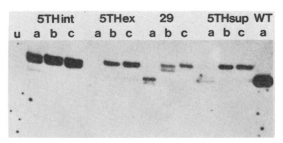

Figure 5. Circular products of RNA-splicing reactions. The top section of a 7 M urea–6% polyacrylamide gel is shown, since the circles run well above the precursor band and all splicing products. All circles were produced under the standard splicing conditions (at 37°C) as described by Waring et al. (1986) and not under conditions designed to particularly favor cyclization. All tracks labeled *a* are incubations of the precursor pSP65 transcript; all *b* and *c* tracks are incubations of gel-purified 5EI molecules produced by the various mutants; track *u* is the unincubated 5THint precursor. The band in the 29 *a* track and the faint bottom band in the 5THint *a* track are the normal L − 15 circle.

extensively documented by Cech and co-workers (Zaug et al. 1985), the wild-type band is actually a doublet consisting of the L − 15 and L − 19 circles. The exact position of the L − 15 band can be seen in track 5THsup a (cyclization of 5THsup is like wild type, but slow because excision is slow). The mutant 29 precursor yields L − 15 circles, but no L − 19 circles, these being replaced by a circular species that migrates slightly faster, and is therefore smaller (Fig. 5, track 29a). The loss of the L − 19 circle is to be expected if tripyrimidine stretches pair with the IGS, since mutant 29 changes the relevant tripyrimidine stretch C^{17} C^{18} U^{19} to GGU, and the L − 15 tripyrimidine stretch is unaffected. The only tripyrimidine stretch available to account for the slightly smaller circle made by mutant 29 is U^{19} U^{20} U^{21}, which would yield an L − 21 molecule. The importance of this is that (as well as supporting the general model of Cech and co-workers) the occurrence of L − 21 is incompatible with the tripyrimidine pairing with A^{24} G^{23} G^{22}, since the minimum number of bases needed to make a turn in RNA is three, and U^{21} is immediately adjacent to G^{22}.

In Figure 5 (tracks b and c), cyclization of purified 5EI (3'-cleaved intron with the 5' exon still attached) molecules from the various mutants is demonstrated. 5THint 5EI gives rise to two major cyclization species. Note that these two bands predominate in 5THint precursor cyclization, although here (track 5THint, a), a small amount of the L − 15 circle is seen; this reflects the relative amounts of 5EI and IVS generated. The two larger circles decay by hydrolysis (data not shown) to linear RNA species, one exactly the length of linear excised intron and the other 7 ± 2 bases longer. The cyclization of a 5EI molecule differs from cyclization of the IVS because the 5' exon is present, allowing the formation of P1 and other alternative 5'-end-pairings and providing new tripyrimidine stretches. It is clear that the formation of P1 or P1-like base-paired regions suppresses the use of the normal L − 15 cyclization site after U^{15}. The most likely cyclization site for the L + 7 molecule is immediately 3' to the (non-*Tetrahymena*) C^{-10} C^{-9} C^{-8} sequence in the hybrid pSP65 5' exon. Since the smaller hydrolysis product is the same size as linear IVS, the new cyclization site for this molecule must be the 5' splice junction, i.e., 3' to the tripyrimidine U^{-3} C^{-2} U^{-1}. That this is the case is shown in Figure 5 by 5THex tracks b and c, where the L − 0 circle is not produced, clearly because 5THex changes U^{-3} C^{-2} to A^{-3} G^{-2} U^{-1}, destroying the tripyrimidine. What does this tripyrimidine pair with? The U^{-3} C^{-2} U^{-1} tripyrimidine is intact in 5THint, but the bases with which it pairs in the P1 (5'TH) base pairing are changed from A^{24} G^{23} G^{22} to U^{24} C^{23} G^{22}. Therefore, although the capacity for base pairing in the P1 region suppresses L − 15 cyclization, P1 is not the structure used as a target for alternative cyclization; instead, the U^{-3} C^{-2} U^{-1} tripyrimidine can only pair with the IGS bases G^{27} G^{26} G^{25} or the A run immediately 3' to this. The probable use of C^{-10} C^{-9} C^{-8} as the tripyrimidine to generate the L + 7 circle indicates the use of G^{27} G^{26}

G^{25} rather than any As. Presumably, the three AU base pairs in the intron-intron part of P1 ($A^1 A^2 A^3/U^{21} U^{20} U^{19}$) remain in place, whereas the exon pyrimidine tract pairs in various ways with the IGS. Why particular tripyrimidines are preferred is not obvious; close inspection does reveal faint bands that probably correspond to use of alternative tripyrimidines in the 5′-exon pyrimidine stretch, but $U^{-3} C^{-2} U^{-1}$ predominates. The 5THsup 5EI behaves like 5THex 5EI, because the 5′ exon strand of 5THsup is like that of 5THex, disrupting the $U^{-3} C^{-2} U^{-1}$ tripyrimidine. Note that, although the 5THsup intron strand contains the 5THint mutant sequence, the 5THsup precursor produces the L − 15 circle perfectly well, showing again that the $A^{24} G^{23} G^{22}$ sequence is not the cyclization binding site within the IGS. Thus, in accord with more recent suggestions of Cech and co-workers (Been and Cech 1986), the segment of the IGS that acts as the tripyrimidine-binding site in cyclization is $G^{27} G^{26} G^{25}$.

The circular products of an RNA-splicing reaction involving mutant 29 5EI are different in the presence and absence of GTP. Without GTP, only L + 7 is produced, whereas in the presence of GTP, L + 7 and L − 0 circles are found. No L − 15 or L − 19 circles are produced; the L − 19 tripyrimidine is destroyed by mutant 29, and as described above, P1 and possibly other 5′-end structures are epistatic to the pairing needed for L − 15 cyclization. Why cyclization should occur at the 5′ splice junction in the presence of GTP, but not without it, is a very interesting question. We suggest (R.B. Waring and R.W. Davies, in prep.) that the phenotype of 29 may be due to the formation of a alternative 5′-end base-paired structure that is competitive with P1. This alternative structure would prevent access to the tripyrimidine involved in L − 0 cycli-

zation, but allow access to the L + 7 tripyrimidine (Fig. 6A). Thus, predominance of the alternative structure leads to only L + 7 circles being produced, as is seen in the absence of GTP. The P1 pairing of mutant 29 is wild type and, dependent on the preferred modes of local denaturation and renaturation, could favor the presentation of any of the local tripyrimidine stretches to the $G^{27} G^{26} G^{25}$ site. As with 5THint, the preferred tripyrimidine is that adjacent to the 5′ splice junction, so that L − 0 circles are generated; however, this is GTP-dependent. An explanation for this would be provided if the binding of the guanosine cofactor directly (via hydrogen bonding between P1 bases and cofactor) or indirectly (via conformational adjustments, allowing hydrogen bonds between P1 bases and others) favored the formation of P1. Since it seems likely from the experiments of Inoue and co-workers (Kay and Inoue 1987 a,b and this volume) that the G cofactor and the intron 3′-end G^{414} occupy similar sites for the two subreactions, it makes functional sense if a "5′TH (P1) helix-bound G cofactor" state were favored until the 5′TH splice junction is cleaved, whereupon the disruption of the 5′TH would directly or indirectly weaken the G cofactor binding, allowing the 3′ end of the intron to enter the vacated site. We may have found the first evidence for part of the mechanism of the RNA-splicing reaction which has been little studied.

Internal Guide Sequence

The IGS is the determinant of specificity for the *Tet* and all other group I introns. Figure 7 shows the sequence of the IGS of the *Tet* intron, and indicates regions of known function. The IGS has been already shown to be important in (1) the formation of 5′TH

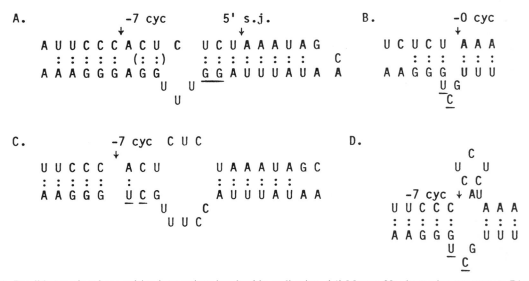

Figure 6. Possible transient base-pairing interactions involved in cyclization. (*A*) Mutant 29; alternative structure to P1 at the 5′ intron-exon junction (R.B. Waring and R.W. Davies, in prep.), with the $C^{-10} C^{-9} C^{-8}$ tripyrimidine paired ready for cyclization. (*B*) Mutant 5THint; possible transient structure for cyclization at the L − 0 site (5′ splice junction). (*C,D*) Mutant 5THint; possible transient structures for cyclization at the L − 7 site.

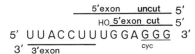

Figure 7. Functional regions of the IGS of the intron in the large rRNA precursor of *T. thermophila*. (cyc) Putative site of binding of tripyrimidine tracts for cyclization.

(P1) and thus the selection of the 5' splice junction (Waring et al. 1986); (2) the presentation of the cut 3'-OH end of the 5' exon in the 3' cleavage/ligation reaction (Waring et al. 1986); (3) enhancing the probability of correct 3' splice junction choice by forming the P10 pairing (R.B. Waring and R.W. Davies, in prep.); (4) forming the cyclization target pairing with a tripyrimidine stretch; (5) forming the binding site for oligonucleotides to act as *trans*-supplied 5' exon (Inoue et al. 1985; Garriga et al. 1986); (6) forming the binding site for cyclization reversal by oligonucleotides (Sullivan and Cech 1985); and (7) forming the binding site for oligocytidylate in the RNA-catalyzed polymerization reaction (Zaug and Cech 1986).

As well as playing a crucial role in the RNA-splicing reaction, the IGS thus acts as the key specificity determinant in the variety of enzymatic reactions catalyzed by this RNA enzyme, and as such may have played a central role in the history of all organisms.

ACKNOWLEDGMENTS

We thank Allelix Inc. for generous support to R.W.D. and P.T. during the latter part of this work, UMIST for hospitality in its laboratories, and the Medical Research Council for the initial funding of this work through a grant to R.W.D. and Dr. C. Scazzocchio.

REFERENCES

Been, M.D. and T.R. Cech. 1985. Sites of circularization of the *Tetrahymena* rRNA IVS are determined by sequence and influenced by position and secondary structure. *Nucleic Acids Res.* **13**: 8389.
———. 1986. One binding site determines sequence specificity of *Tetrahymena* pre-rRNA self-splicing, *trans*-splicing, and RNA enzyme activity. *Cell* **47**: 207.

Cech, T.R. 1986. A model for the RNA catalysed replication of RNA. *Proc. Natl. Acad. Sci.* **83**: 4360.
Cech, T.R., A.J. Zaug, and P.J. Grabowski. 1981. *In vitro* splicing of the ribosomal RNA precursor of *Tetrahymena*: Involvement of a guanosine nucleotide in the excision of the intervening sequence. *Cell* **27**: 487.
Davies, R.W., R.B. Waring, J.A. Ray, T.A. Brown, and C. Scazzocchio. 1982. Making ends meet: A model for RNA splicing in fungal mitochondria. *Nature* **300**: 719.
Garriga, G., A.M. Lambowitz, T. Inoue, and T.R. Cech. 1986. Mechanism of recognition of the 5' splice-site in self-splicing group I introns. *Nature* **322**: 86.
Inoue, T., F.X. Sullivan, and T.R. Cech. 1985. Intermolecular exon ligation of the rRNA precursor of *Tetrahymena*: Oligonucleotides can function as 5' exons. *Cell* **43**: 431.
———. 1986. New reactions of the ribosomal RNA precursor of *Tetrahymena* and the mechanism of self-splicing. *J. Mol. Biol.* **189**: 142.
Kay, P.S. and T. Inoue. 1987a. Reactivity of modified ribose moieties of guanosine: New cleavage reactions mediated by the IVS of *Tetrahymena* precursor RNA. *Nucleic Acids Res.* **15**: 1559.
———. 1987b. Catalysis of splicing-related reactions between dinucleotides by a ribozyme. *Nature* **327**: 343.
Kruger, K., P.J. Grabowski, A.J. Zaug, J. Sands, D.E. Gottschling, and T.R. Cech. 1982. Self-splicing RNA: Autoexcision and autocyclisation of the ribosomal RNA intervening sequence of *Tetrahymena*. *Cell* **31**: 147.
Sullivan, F.X. and T.R. Cech. 1985. Reversibility of cyclisation of the *Tetrahymena* rRNA intervening sequence: Implication for the mechanism of splice site choice. *Cell* **42**: 639.
Szostak, J.W. 1986. Enzymatic activity of the conserved core of a group I self-splicing intron. *Nature* **322**: 83.
Waring, R.B. and R.W. Davies. 1984. Assessment of a model for intron RNA secondary structure relevant to RNA self-splicing — A review. *Gene* **28**: 277.
Waring, R.B., P. Towner, S.J. Minter, and R.W. Davies. 1986. Splice-site selection by a self-splicing RNA of *Tetrahymena*. *Nature* **321**: 133.
Waring, R.B., J.A. Ray, S.W. Edwards, C. Scazzocchio, and R.W. Davies. 1985. The *Tetrahymena* rRNA self-splices in *E. coli*: *In vivo* evidence for the importance of key base-paired regions of RNA for RNA enzyme function. *Cell* **40**: 371.
Zaug, A.J. and T.R. Cech. 1986. The intervening sequence RNA of *Tetrahymena* is an enzyme. *Science* **231**: 470.
Zaug, A.J., J.R. Kent, and T.R. Cech. 1985. Reactions of the intervening sequence of the *Tetrahymena* rRNA precursor; pH dependence of cyclization and site-specific hydrolysis. *Biochemistry* **24**: 6211.
Zoller, M.J. and M. Smith. 1984. Oligonucleotide-directed mutagenesis: A simple method using two oligonucleotide primers and a single-stranded DNA template. *DNA* **3**: 479.

Genetic Dissection of an RNA Enzyme

J.A. Doudna, A.S. Gerber, J.M. Cherry, and J.W. Szostak

Department of Molecular Biology, Massachusetts General Hospital, Boston, Massachusetts 02114

The Group I Introns

The group I introns are characterized by short conserved sequences and a highly conserved secondary structure. Several members of this class of introns have been shown to be capable of self-splicing in vitro, without the participation of any proteins. The best-characterized example of a self-splicing group I intron is the intron from the nuclear rRNA genes of *Tetrahymena thermophila*, originally shown to be self-splicing by Cech and his colleagues (Kruger et al. 1982; Zaug et al. 1983).

The group I introns show a remarkably wide phylogenetic distribution. They are found in fungal mitochondria, chloroplasts, nuclear genes of ciliates, and T-even bacteriophages. The ability to compare widely differing sequences has been a great help in studies of the secondary structure of these introns. Similar models of the secondary structure of the group I introns were proposed by three groups on the basis of limited phylogenetic comparison data (Davies et al. 1982; Cech et al. 1983; Michel and Dujon 1983). Figure 1 shows the conserved core of the *Tetrahymena* enzyme, drawn according to Waring and co-workers (1983). Many group I introns have subsequently been examined, and all are consistent with this core secondary structure. Some details of this structure are completely invariant; e.g., there are always four bases between P3 and P4 and between P6 and P7. P4 and P7 are always 5 bp long. In contrast, the loops are highly variable. In some cases, long open reading frames are located in the loops (L3, L4, and L5).

The Splicing Reactions

Splicing as it occurs in the intact intron is a cascade of three transesterification reactions (Zaug et al. 1983). First, the 3'-OH of a free guanosine attacks the phosphate between the 5' exon and the intron. The guanosine displaces the 5' exon, becoming linked by a 5'-3' phosphodiester bond to the first nucleotide of the intron, and leaving the 5' exon terminated in a 3'-OH. It is this 3'-OH which, in the second step of the reaction, attacks the phosphate of the intron–3' exon junction. This time, the intron is displaced and the 5' exon becomes linked to the 3' exon. In the final step, the 3'-OH of the free linear intron attacks an internal site in the intron, generating a circular RNA molecule and a short linear fragment from the 5' end of the intron. Zaug et al. (1983) have shown that this circular form of the intron retains many of the catalytic activities of the intact intron.

All three of these reactions may occur within a very similar sequence and secondary structure context. In the first reaction, the sequence flanking the exon-intron junction is paired with a sequence just inside the intron called the internal guide sequence (IGS), forming a short stem-loop. This pairing interaction has been shown to be essential by genetic studies, in which mutations that disrupt the pairing decrease activity, and second site mutations that restore pairing also restore activity (Waring et al. 1986). Thus, in this reaction, the guanosine is attacking a region of double-stranded RNA. In the second reaction, both exons may be aligned by pairing with the IGS. A potential pairing of

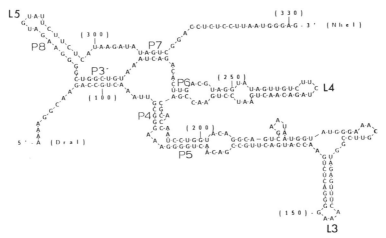

Figure 1. Secondary structure of the conserved core of the *Tetrahymena* intron.

the 3' exon and the IGS is found in the majority of group I introns, but many introns do not show this pairing, and a direct genetic test of its role in splicing has not yet been reported. In this reaction, the last nucleotide of the intron is a guanosine, which is thus in the analogous position to the attacking free guanosine in the first reaction. Reaction II may be simply the reverse of reaction I (Zaug et al. 1983). The circularization reaction may also occur in a similar context, supporting the idea that all three reactions involve essentially the same substrate, and may be catalyzed by the same enzyme.

Catalytic and Substrate Domains

Kruger et al. (1982) originally showed that the *Tetrahymena* intron was capable of self-splicing by transcribing the cloned intron in vitro with *Escherichia coli* RNA polymerase. The RNA transcript these authors generated was capable of self-splicing without any protein component, requiring only mono- and divalent cations and guanosine as a cosubstrate.

Since the middle half of the intron contains all of the conserved sequences and secondary structures, that region of the RNA seemed most likely to constitute the catalytic domain of the intron. The exon-intron junctions, in this view, are substrates that the catalytic domain (the "core enzyme") recognizes while carrying out the cascade of phosphoester transfer reactions that result in removal of the intron and formation of the mature transcript. To begin to test this idea, we carried out a deletion analysis of the intron, using the T7 RNA polymerase system to generate RNA in vitro. We began with a plasmid containing the entire intron and some flanking exon sequences cloned downstream from a T7 promoter. As expected, full-length transcripts from this plasmid were capable of self-splicing. The role of the sequences 3' to the conserved core of the intron was easily tested by making runoff transcripts on templates that had been truncated at various sites within the intron by restriction enzyme cleavage. Cleavage at sites further than 20 nucleotides downstream from the core retained self-splicing activity, but cleavage at a site within the core led to the generation of an inactive transcript. These experiments showed that approximately 80 nucleotides at the 3' end of the 413-nucleotide intron are not required for catalytic activity (Szostak 1986).

We then wanted to know if any sequences 5' to the conserved core could be deleted. We made a series of deletions that removed the exon-intron junction and extended for various distances into the intron. Since these deletions removed the natural substrate for the RNA enzyme, we added to the reactions a second RNA molecule, which was a 119-nucleotide transcript covering the exon-intron junction and extending 62 nucleotides into the intron. We assayed the site-specific cleavage of this second RNA in the presence of the catalytic domain RNA. Again, we found that deletions extending quite close to the conserved core of the

intron retained splicing activity, supporting the idea that the conserved core of the intron contains the catalytic domain.

The two-component reaction described above has many advantages for the study of the catalytic mechanisms. The substrate and enzyme RNAs may be altered independently and enzyme-substrate interactions can be studied more readily. The substrate in particular is small enough to be made by the direct transcription of synthetic oligonucleotides (see below). The catalytic domain is inactive by itself and remains unaltered during the in vitro transcription process. In addition, the reaction is considerably simplified, since only the first step of the splicing process is occurring. Reaction kinetics are thus easier to interpret. We generally follow the reaction by observing the incorporation of labeled GTP into RNA fragments of the correct size, as determined by mobility on denaturing polyacrylamide gels.

In this paper, we describe deletions and substitution mutations in the catalytic and substrate domains of the self-splicing intron. These mutations further define the essential regions of the enzyme and its substrate.

MATERIALS AND METHODS

Oligonucleotides were synthesized on a Biosearch Model 8750 DNA synthesizer and purified by polyacrylamide gel electrophoresis. Enzyme RNA was synthesized by runoff transcription of plasmid templates digested with a restriction enzyme. Substrate RNA was synthesized by runoff transcription of oligonucleotide templates containing the 23-base T7 RNA polymerase promoter sequence at the 3' end. An 18-base region of the promoter was made double-stranded by annealing the complementary 18-mer to the template strand. Transcription reactions were carried out using 200–600 nM concentrations of template. RNA was purified by polyacrylamide gel electrophoresis. *Trans*-splicing assays were performed using 0.2 μM enzyme, 2 μM substrate, 2 μM [α-^{32}P]GTP, and 20 mM MgCl$_2$. The enzyme used to test substrate mutants was the transcript of *Nhe*I-cut pAG100 (see Results). After incubation at 58°C for 15 minutes, products were analyzed by polyacrylamide gel electrophoresis and autoradiography.

RESULTS

Modifications of the Core Enzyme

We have previously described the construction of a plasmid containing the middle portion of the *Tetrahymena* rRNA intron inserted downstream from a promoter for T7 RNA polymerase (Szostak 1986). This plasmid, pSZ243, can be used to generate a fragment of RNA that will catalyze the site-specific attack of a guanosine on a separate small RNA fragment containing the exon-intron junction. When pSZ243 is cleaved with the restriction enzyme *Nhe*I, and transcribed with T7 RNA polymerase, a 275-nucleotide long transcript is generated, consisting of 28 nucleotides at the 5' end derived from the transcribed portion of the T7 promoter and polylinker sequences, and 247 nucleotides derived from the intron (from the DraI site to the NheI site). To facilitate the mutational analysis of the core enzyme, we have made several modifications of plasmid pSZ243. These changes include the deletion of nonessential sequences at the 5' and 3' ends of the transcript and the introduction of restriction site sequences in places where the intron sequence is not conserved. These changes allow the rapid generation of mutants at specific sites and, more critically, facilitate construction of double and triple mutants to test specific tertiary interactions.

As shown in Figure 1, the core enzyme secondary structure consists of a number of base-paired regions alternating with non-base-paired connecting segments and loops. The three loops, L3, L4, and L5, do not show any sequence conservation, when a variety of group I introns are compared. In addition, some deletions of sequences in L3 and L4 retain self-splicing activity (Price et al. 1985). It therefore seemed likely that these sequences could be altered to encode restriction enzyme sites, without affecting the catalytic activity of the core enzyme. This would divide the transcript into four segments: 5' to L3, L3 to L4, L4 to L5, and L5 to the 3' end. These segments would be small enough to synthesize chemically. Mutant enzymes could then be made by replacement of these short restriction fragments with chemically synthesized fragments of altered sequence.

In the first step in this series of modifications, we changed the sequence of three nucleotides in L3 to generate a SalI restriction site and deleted ten nucleotides of extraneous vector sequences from the 5' end of the transcribed region. This was done by purifying the large EcoRI-BglII fragment of pSZ243 and replacing the missing segment (corresponding to the 5' end to L4) with synthetic DNA. This region was synthesized as two segments. The first, from the EcoRI site at the 5' end to the new SalI site in L3, consisted of two complementary 68-mers, and the second, from the new SalI site to the BglII site in L4, consisted of two complementary 84-mers. The synthetic oligomers were annealed and mixed with the vector fragment of pSZ243 in the presence of kinase and ligase. Plasmids were recovered in E. coli, and isolates with the correct restriction map were sequenced. One plasmid with the correct sequence, pSZ250, was used for further experiments. DNA from this plasmid was digested with NheI, and T7 transcripts were made and purified; this RNA was catalytically active.

In the second step, L5 was modified and extraneous restriction sites distal to the intron sequence were removed. This was accomplished by purifying the large BglII-HindIII fragment of pSZ243 and replacing the missing information with synthetic oligonucleotides as above. In this case, we changed one nucleotide of L5 to generate an NsiI site (this change was not incorporated into our final version of the enzyme). The synthetic DNA again consisted of two pairs of annealed oligonu-

cleotides. The fragment from the BglII site to the new NsiI site was made from a 57-mer annealed with a 49-mer; the fragment from the new NsiI site to the HindIII site was made from a 52-mer annealed with a 60-mer. This latter fragment consisted of the intron sequence up to the NheI site, followed by a BamHI site, which, in turn, was followed by the 5' overhanging end of the HindIII site. However, the HindIII site was not regenerated, and a SalI site present in the original plasmid was deleted. One plasmid with the correct restriction map and DNA sequence, pSZ248, was tested for the catalytic activity of the T7 transcript. The transcript was catalytically active.

In the third step, the modifications present in the vector sequence in pSZ248 and in the core enzyme sequence in pSZ250 were combined. The large EcoRI-NheI fragment of pSZ248 and the small EcoRI-NheI fragment of pSZ250 were purified and ligated together to generate the plasmid pSZ253. This plasmid contains a SalI site in L3, with no other SalI sites present on the plasmid. Since the entire EcoRI-NheI fragment derives from pSZ250, the RNA transcript is unchanged.

In the fourth and final step, the sequences of both L4 and L5 were modified to introduce HindIII and BglII sites at these locations. For this construction, the SalI-NheI fragment of pSZ253 was purified and ligated with two annealed pairs of synthetic oligonucleotides. The oligonucleotides were designed to change the BglII site present in L4 to a HindIII site and to change the L5 sequence to introduce a BglII site at that position. The first pair of annealed oligonucleotides consisted of two 84-mers extending from the SalI site to the new HindIII site. The second set was composed of two 80-mers, extending from the HindIII site through L5 to the NheI site at the 3' end of the core enzyme sequence. The sequence of these oligonucleotides changes the L5 sequence to a BglII site. In addition, 18 nucleotides are deleted from the 3' end of the enzyme, immediately preceding the NheI site. A plasmid with the correct restriction map and DNA sequence was named pAG100 and has been used for all subsequent experiments. The sequence changes are summarized in Figure 2.

We have compared the activity of pAG100 transcripts to that of the earlier derivatives pSZ241-NheI (the unmodified intron truncated at the NheI site) and pSZ243-NheI (the unmodified conserved core of the intron). In this experiment (Fig. 3), we used the 91.1 transcript, described below, as a substrate. Although the pAG100 transcripts showed approximately the same level of activity as the pSZ241 transcript, the pSZ243 RNA showed much more activity than either. This was surprising, because in an earlier study using a different and larger substrate RNA, enzyme RNAs made from pSZ241 and pSZ243 showed approximately the same level of activity (Szostak 1986). Another surprising result was the apparent increase in specificity of the pAG100 enzyme relative to the other versions of the enzyme. The pAG100-BamI transcript, which is six nucleotides longer than the pAG100-NheI transcript,

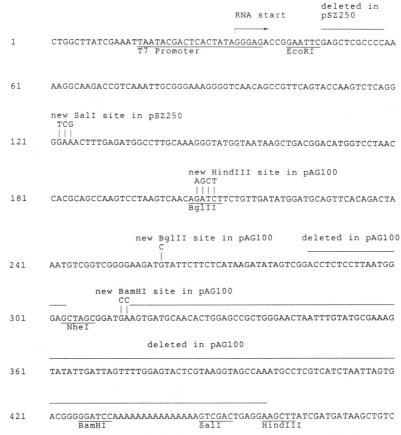

```
                                    RNA start              deleted in
                                                           pSZ250
  1    CTGGCTTATCGAAATTAATACGACTCACTATAGGGAGACCGGAATTCGAGCTCGCCCCAA
                           T7 Promoter              EcoRI


 61    AAGGCAAGACCGTCAAATTGCGGGAAAGGGGTCAACAGCCGTTCAGTACCAAGTCTCAGG


       new SalI site in pSZ250
       TCG
       |||
121    GGAAACTTTGAGATGGCCTTGCAAAGGGTATGGTAATAAGCTGACGGACATGGTCCTAAC


                               new HindIII site in pAG100
                               AGCT
                               ||||
181    CACGCAGCCAAGTCCTAAGTCAACAGATCTTCTGTTGATATGGATGCAGTTCACAGACTA
                               BglII


                 new BglII site in pAG100          deleted in pAG100
                 C
                 |
241    AATGTCGGTCGGGGAAGATGTATTCTTCTCATAAGATATAGTCGGACCTCTCCTTAATGG


              new BamHI site in pAG100
              CC
              ||
301    GAGCTAGCGGATGAAGTGATGCAACACTGGAGCCGCTGGGAACTAATTTGTATGCGAAAG
         NheI


                        deleted in pAG100

361    TATATTGATTAGTTTTGGAGTACTCGTAAGGTAGCCAAATGCCTCGTCATCTAATTAGTG


421    ACGGGGGATCCAAAAAAAAAAAAAAAAGTCGACTGAGGAAGCTTATCGATGATAAGCTGTC
              BamHI                       SalI        HindIII
```

Figure 2. Alterations in the pSZ243 sequence to generate pAG100.

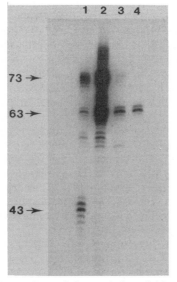

Figure 3. Comparison of the catalytic activities of four versions of the core enzyme. Each reaction contained 0.4 μM enzyme RNA, 2 μM substrate RNA, and 2 μM [α-^{32}P]GTP. The substrate RNA used in each case was the 91.1 transcript (a 73-mer RNA). (Lane *1*) pSZ241-*Nhe*I transcript; (lane *2*) pSZ243-*Nhe*I transcript; (lane *3*) pAG100-*Nhe*I transcript; (lane *4*) pAG100-*Bam*HI transcript.

shows much less processing of the substrate at incorrect sites than any of the other RNAs. We are currently determining which of the alterations in pAG100 are responsible for its decreased activity and increased specificity relative to pSZ243.

Mutational Analysis of the RNA Substrate

Our original substrate RNA was synthesized as a runoff transcript from pSZ241 cleaved with the restriction enzyme *Dra*I. This yields a 119-nucleotide RNA species consisting of 25 nucleotides of vector sequences at the 5′ end, followed by 32 nucleotides of the 5′ exon and the first 62 nucleotides of the intron. This RNA species contains the 5′ exon-intron junction, and upon incubation with [α-^{32}P]GTP in the presence of the RNA enzyme, it yields a 63-nucleotide labeled product, corresponding to cleavage at the junction and addition of guanosine at the 5′ end of the intron.

To remove extraneous 5′ sequences from this substrate, a DNA template oligonucleotide was synthesized that encoded an 82-nucleotide RNA substrate. This species lacks 12 nonconserved nucleotides from the exon, in addition to the 25-nucleotide vector sequence. Figure 4 shows the secondary structure of the

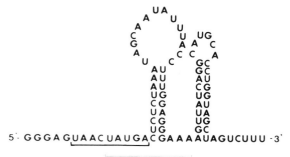

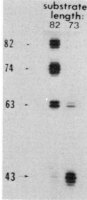

Figure 4. Secondary structures of modified substrates and products of RNA-catalyzed transesterification of these substrates. (*Top*) 82-mer substrate secondary structure. The first five nucleotides are derived from the transcribed portion of the T7 RNA polymerase promoter, followed by 15 nucleotides of exon sequence and 62 nucleotides of the intron. The UG base pair at the exon-intron junction is the site of RNA-enzyme-catalyzed guanosine attack. The bracket indicates the nine nucleotides deleted to make the 73-mer substrate. (*Bottom*) Products of RNA-enzyme-catalyzed transesterification of the 82-mer and the 73-mer.

transcripts of this template and the products observed after incubation with enzyme and $[\alpha\text{-}^{32}\text{P}]$GTP. The band at 63 corresponds to the cleavage at the expected site. The band at 82 corresponds to apparent end-labeling of the substrate, perhaps by guanosine exchange. The bands at 74 and 43 probably result from cleavage/guanosine addition at alternate sites in the substrate. This substrate was used as the parent for further deletions. The removal of nine nucleotides from the 5' single-strand region yielded a 73-nucleotide substrate spliced preferentially at an alternate site, such that the bands at 41–45 are the primary products of the splicing reaction (Fig. 4). Deletion of eight nucleotides from the A loop of this 73-mer yielded a 65-mer substrate, with a cleavage pattern identical to that of the 73-mer, except that all bands were eight nucleotides shorter. Specificity of splicing at the correct site was restored in a 73-mer in which the 3 bp at the bottom of the P1 stem were simply reversed (Fig. 5). This transcript has been named 91.1 after the number of the oligonucleotide from which it was synthesized.

Several mutants with deleted or altered P2 stems have been synthesized and tested. Deletion of the entire P2 stem and loop from the 73-mer yielded a 49-mer that showed barely detectable splicing by the enzyme. Substrates identical to the 49-mer but with one, two, or three additional A residues in the 3' tail region were synthesized and tested. We wanted to correct for the difference in length of the 3' tail caused by deletion of the P2 stem. However, these substrates were also inert.

Two mutants with small deletions in the P2 stem were synthesized and tested. One contained a deletion of the AU base pair at the bottom of the stem and the other contained a deletion of the two GC base pairs at the top of the stem. Both of these substrates showed no detectable splicing by the enzyme.

Mutants in which the spacing of the stems is altered are spliced much less efficiently than wild type. A mutant with an additional A residue in the 3' tail and a mutant with an A residue deleted between the stems both had low levels of spliced products after incubation with $[\alpha\text{-}^{32}\text{P}]$GTP in the presence of enzyme.

Modeling the Attack of Guanosine on the Substrate RNA

We have used computational chemistry methods in conjunction with computer graphics to model the attack of the guanosine on the double-stranded RNA substrate. We assumed that the reaction proceeds via an in-line nucleophilic substitution (S_N2) mechanism. Although there is no direct evidence for this mechanism in the case of the group I introns, all known enzyme-catalyzed phosphoester transfer reactions use this mechanism. We wanted to see if this mechanism imposed significant constraints on the location of the guanine base of the attacking guanosine, as part of our efforts to understand the nature of the guanosine-binding site.

The modeling was done by building the substrate double-stranded RNA and then docking the guanosine cosubstrate into a position consistent with an S_N2 reaction. We placed the O3' of the ribose moiety of the guanosine opposite and in line with the P-O3' bond of the 5' exon (the leaving group), oriented so that the angle between the attacking C3'-O3' and the attacked P is within the normal limits for a C–O–P bond angle.

The RNA A-form double-helical atomic coordinates were generated with the program CHARMm (Polygen, Inc.) using bond and torsion angle parameters extracted from one strand of a large helical region (residues 63–73) within the crystal structure of yeast phenylalanine tRNA refined by Jack et al. (1976) (Brookhaven database code name 4TNA). These A-form RNA helical parameters were averaged before inclusion in the CHARMm parameters file. The guanosine atomic coordinates are also from an averaged guanosine in the *anti* conformation with the ribose C-3' end from A-form RNA helix.

The two components of the reaction model were visualized on an Evans and Sutherland PS340 graphics computer, with the graphics program HYDRA (R. Hubbard, York University, England). Figure 6 is a stereo pair of the result of docking the guanosine

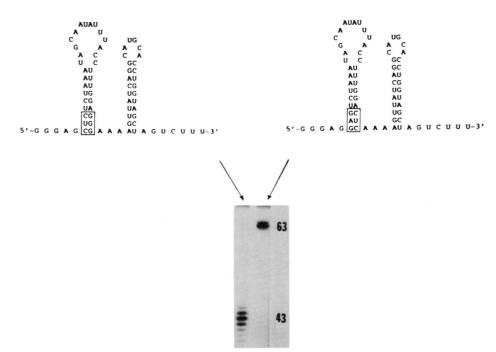

Figure 5. Altered specificity of splicing of two 73-mers. The wild-type sequence is shown at the left; this substrate is spliced preferentially at an alternate site by the enzyme to give the indicated products. Specificity of splicing was restored to the expected site when the 3 bp at the base of the first stem were reversed, as shown.

monophosphate at the site of attack on the substrate RNA helix. Although only one position is shown here, the guanosine could, of course, be in any position defined by rotation about the incipient P-O 3′ bond. It is clear from a study of these possible guanosine positions that the guanine base cannot interact with the bases of the RNA substrate. Interactions of the ribose and/or the guanine with the sugar-phosphate backbone of the RNA substrate cannot be excluded. Nevertheless, it is clear that most, if not all, of the guanosine-binding site must lie within the catalytic domain of the RNA enzyme.

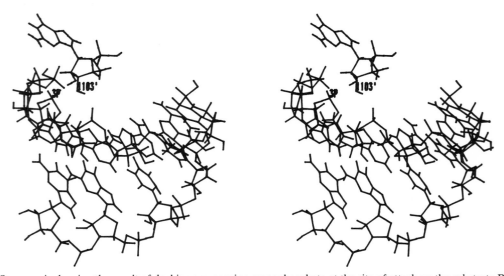

Figure 6. Stereo pair showing the result of docking a guanosine monophosphate at the site of attack on the substrate RNA helix. The guanosine is oriented so that the O3′ (labeled 1103′) is 2.5 Å from the attacked phosphorus (labeled 3P). The angle formed between 11C3′ and 1103′-3P is 110°. This orientation is just one possible arrangement of the guanosine cosubstrate relative to the substrate helix that is consistent with an S_N2 reaction mechanism. The helix shown is just 5 bp of the substrate "A" stem (5′-CUAAA-3′, 5′-UUUGG-3′).

DISCUSSION

Construction of a Modified Core Enzyme

Although they show wide phylogenetic distribution, the group I self-splicing introns have a high degree of sequence and structural homology. This has allowed us to identify invariant, conserved, and nonconserved nucleotides and structural elements in this class of introns. We have applied this analysis to our study of the group I rRNA intron from *T. thermophila*.

We showed previously that the core intron can function in *trans* to catalyze the attack of a free guanosine residue at a specific site in an exogenous substrate containing the 5′ exon-intron junction (Szostak 1986). This reaction is equivalent to reaction I of the three-step self-splicing mechanism. The separation of substrate and enzyme has simplified synthesis and mutational analysis of both species.

We set out to modify the intron sequence to remove nonessential 5′ and 3′ regions and to introduce restriction sites at convenient locations. This has been achieved in several steps (see Results). The intron with these sequence modifications is encoded on the plasmid pAG100. Runoff transcripts from pAG100 cut with the restriction enzymes *Nhe*I or *Bam*HI retain catalytic activity. Comparison of the activity of the different mutant introns with that of the wild type reveals that both specificity and level of activity vary. The nature of these variations is currently under investigation.

Analysis of Altered RNA Substrates

We previously described a 119-nucleotide RNA substrate synthesized by runoff transcription of *Dra*I-cut pSZ241. We wanted to eliminate extraneous 5′ sequences from the substrate to shorten it so that it could be synthesized by transcription of a synthetic oligonucleotide. This was achieved by deleting the first 37 nucleotides at the 5′ end of the original substrate. An oligonucleotide template encoding this species was transcribed to yield an 82-mer that was efficiently

spliced by the core enzyme. Products corresponding to splicing at alternate sites are also apparent.

The effects of deletion and substitution mutations in this substrate species suggest functional roles for various regions in the substrate. Removal of nine nucleotides from the 5′ single-strand region of the 82-mer generates a 73-mer that is preferentially spliced at an alternate site, such that the primary product of the splicing reaction is a 43-mer, rather than the expected 63-mer. Specificity was almost completely restored to the correct site when 3 bp at the base of the P1 stem were simply reversed. This suggests that substrates can have alternate forms of pairing that are recognized by the enzyme. Substrates altered such that alternate pairing is destabilized would restore specificity of splicing to the expected site.

The size of the P1 loop is apparently unimportant for substrate recognition by the enzyme, since eight nucleotides can be deleted with no detectable effect on splicing. However, the spacing between the two stems and the length of the 3′ single-strand region are quite important, since small changes have drastic effects on splicing. In addition, the B stem appears to have an important role in substrate recognition by the enzyme. Complete removal of the stem, as well as small deletions within it, lead to virtually inert substrates. The role of the P2 stem and loop is the subject of current investigation.

Early Evolution of RNA Replicases and Group I Introns

Sharp (1985) proposed that a simple RNA replicase could act by splicing short oligonucleotides together on an RNA template. This is essentially the same as reaction II carried out by the self-splicing *Tetrahymena* intron, in which the two exons are aligned by pairing with the IGS (the "template" strand) and spliced together. This is a transesterification reaction and is the same reaction that is carried out by present-day RNA polymerases. As shown in Figure 7, it is easy to imagine

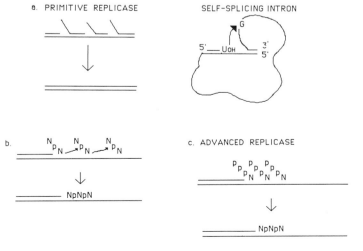

Figure 7. Model for evolution of a template-directed ribozyme RNA polymerase from a primitive ribozyme. (*a*) The primitive ribozyme might have catalyzed ligation of oligonucleotides partially annealed to a template (Sharp 1985), analogous to reaction II catalyzed by the *Tetrahymena* intron. (*b,c*) Gradual transition to a more sophisticated replicase that uses single nucleotides as substrates.

a series of intermediate versions of these reactions illustrating a gradual transition from a primitive replicase, using short random oligonucleotides as substrates, to a more sophisticated polymerase that uses activated nucleosides as substrates. The primitive replicase would presumably not show any sequence specificity toward its template or primer. Highly specific RNA processing enzymes, and ultimately the present-day group I introns, could have evolved by the addition of substrate specificity to the primitive replicase. Almost all group I introns have a U:G base pair formed between the last base of the 5' exon and the IGS, and the last base of the intron is a G. Presumably these almost invariant features are recognized by the enzyme and account, at least in part, for the specificity of the splicing process.

REFERENCES

Cech, T.R., N.K. Tanner, I. Tinoco, Jr., B.R. Weir, M. Zuker, and P.S. Perlman. 1983. Secondary structure of the *Tetrahymena* ribosomal RNA intervening sequences: Structural homology with fungal mitochondrial intervening sequences. *Proc. Natl. Acad. Sci.* **80:** 3903.

Davies, R.W., R.B. Waring, J.A. Ray, T.A. Brown, and C. Scazzocchio. 1982. Making ends meet: A model for RNA splicing in fungal mitochondria. *Nature* **300:** 719.

Jack, A., J.E. Ladner, and A. Klug. 1976. Crystallographic refinement of yeast phenylalanine transfer RNA at 2.5 angstroms resolution. *J. Mol. Biol.* **108:** 619.

Kruger, K., P.J. Grabowski, A.J. Zaug, J. Sands, D.E. Gottschling, and T.R. Cech. 1982. Self-splicing RNA: Autoexcision and autocyclization of the ribosomal RNA intervening sequence of *Tetrahymena*. *Cell* **31:** 147.

Michel, R. and B. Dujon. 1983. Conservation of RNA secondary structures in two intron families including mitochondrial-, chloroplast-, and nuclear-encoded members. *EMBO J.* **2:** 33.

Price, J.V., G.L. Kieft, J.R. Kent, E.L. Sievers, and T.R. Cech. 1985. Sequence requirements for self-splicing of the *Tetrahymena thermophila* pre-ribosomal RNA. *Nucleic Acids Res.* **13:** 1871.

Sharp, P.A. 1985. On the origin of RNA splicing and introns. *Cell* **42:** 397.

Szostak, J.W. 1986. Enzymatic activity of the conserved core of a group I self-splicing intron. *Nature* **322:** 83.

Waring, R.B., C. Scazzocchio, T.A. Brown, and R.W. Davies. 1983. Close relationship between certain nuclear and mitochondrial introns: Implications for the mechanism of RNA splicing. *J. Mol. Biol.* **167:** 595.

Waring, R.B., P. Towner, S.J. Minter, and R.W. Davies. 1986. Splice-site selection by a self-splicing RNA of *Tetrahymena*. *Nature* **321:** 133.

Zaug, A.J., P.J. Grabowski, and T.R. Cech. 1983. Autocatalytic cyclization of an excised intervening sequence RNA is a cleavage-ligation reaction. *Nature* **301:** 578.

Genetic Delineation of Functional Components of the Group I Intron in the Phage T4 *td* Gene

M. BELFORT,[*][†] P.S. CHANDRY,[*][‡] AND J. PEDERSEN-LANE[*]

[*]*Wadsworth Center for Laboratories and Research, New York State Department of Health, Albany, New York 12201;*
[†]*School of Public Health Sciences of the State University of New York, New York State Department of Health, Albany, New York 12201;* [‡]*Department of Microbiology and Immunology, Albany Medical College, Albany, New York 12208*

Group I introns are extremely widespread, occurring in nuclear or organellar genes of a variety of plants, slime molds, protists, and fungi as well as in bacteriophage genomes (for review, see Cech 1986). The classification of these evolutionarily diverse introns into a single group was based on their ability to adopt a similar core secondary structure (Davies et al. 1982; Michel et al. 1982; Michel and Dujon 1983). It is believed that this distinctive RNA structure imparts the catalytic character to these molecules (Cech et al. 1983; Michel and Dujon 1983; Waring and Davies 1984), which play an instrumental role in their own splicing reactions. Regardless of whether these reactions proceed spontaneously or require accessory factors, group I splicing occurs by a common mechanism (Cech 1986; Garriga and Lambowitz 1986). The distinguishing feature of the splicing pathway, which proceeds by a series of transesterification reactions, occurs at its first step. The reaction is initiated at the 5′ splice site via nucleophilic attack by the 3′-OH of a guanosine nucleotide that becomes covalently joined to the 5′ end of the intron (Cech et al. 1981).

Genetic studies on group I intervening sequences developed concurrently with the notion that these elements were catalytic entities. Thus, *cis*-dominant mutations that prevent intron excision were identified in several *Saccharomyces cerevisiae* mitochondrial introns (Anziano et al. 1982; De La Salle et al. 1982; Weiss-Brummer et al. 1982). Since then, fungal and phage genetics, on the one hand, and site-directed mutagenesis targeted to the *Tetrahymena* rRNA gene, on the other, have implicated several pairings to be of major functional importance in the group I splicing reaction. These are the P1[1] helix (Been and Cech 1986; Waring et al. 1986; Hall et al. 1987), the P3 (Weiss-Brummer et al. 1983) and P4 pairings (Waring et al. 1985; Williamson et al. 1987), the P7 interaction (Hensgens et al. 1983; Holl et al. 1985; Burke et al. 1986), and the P9 helix (Hall et al. 1987). The P1 element is formed by the base pairing of an exon 1 sequence with a guide sequence in the intron, whereas the P3, P4, and P7 pairings are formed by the interactions within the intron. P4 and P7 are paired elements formed by association of the conserved P/Q and R/S sequences,

respectively. The functional roles of other phylogenetically conserved elements of the core structure remain to be established in terms of RNA catalysis.

The existence of a group I intron in the *td* gene of T4 (Chu et al. 1984) facilitates the use of prokaryotic genetics to study group I splicing in the natural cellular context. Fortunately, the *td* gene is endowed with an extraordinary wealth of phenotypes. First, a T4*td*[+] phage, with a functional *td* gene that encodes thymidylate synthase (TS), can be readily distinguished from a T4*td*[−] phage (TS-defective) by characteristic plaque morphologies (Simon and Tessman 1963). These properties have been exploited to implicate the intron extremities as the two domains that are functional in splicing (Hall et al. 1987). Thus, fewer than 220 nucleotides at each end, flanking the central open reading frame (ORF) of the 1016-bp[2] intron, constitute the catalytic core of the molecule. Second, the cloned *td* gene complements TS-defective *thyA*[−] *Escherichia coli*, imparting on such a host the ability to grow in the absence of thymine (Mileham et al. 1980; Belfort et al. 1983b; Chu et al. 1984) and providing a selection for a functional *td* gene. Third, *low* TS levels confer a selective advantage on cells when grown in the presence of folate analogs, such as trimethoprim, and thymine (Okada et al. 1961). We therefore reasoned that these latter growth conditions would provide a positive selection for *td* mutations, including those that cause defects in splicing.

A genetic study to dissect the catalytic components of *td* pre-mRNA has been initiated, taking advantage of those phenotypes that reflect *td* function as well as *td* dysfunction. First, linker insertion and deletion mutants were generated to probe the role of the central intron elements in splicing and to provide a splicing-proficient deletion construct for subsequent point mutagenesis studies. Second, 13 nondirected splicing-defective mutants were isolated and characterized. These random chemically induced mutations, which were isolated strictly on the basis of phenotype, are scattered throughout the two functional domains of the intron. Although some mutations are in phylogenetically conserved elements previously shown to be of

---

[1]The nomenclature recommended by Burke et al. (1987) has been adopted. For a diagram of the *td* core structure, see Fig. 7B.

[2]The intron length was previously considered to be 1017. Resequencing has, however, revealed a single T at residue 93 of the intron rather than a doublet.

functional importance in fungal mitochondrial and *Tetrahymena* precursors (P1, P4, and P7), others are in elements to which no role in splicing has previously been ascribed (P5, P6, P7.2, P8, and P9.2). Relating these structural changes to aberrations in catalytic performance will provide a useful adjunct to functional studies of an RNA enzyme.

MATERIALS AND METHODS

Media. TBYET is tryptone broth (1.0% Bacto-tryptone and 0.5% NaCl) supplemented with 0.5% yeast extract and 50 μg/ml of thymine. The composition of the minimal medium, which was supplemented with 0.1% Norit-A-treated casamino acids and 0.2% glucose, has been described previously (Belfort et al. 1983b). Solid medium was prepared by adding 1.5% Bacto-agar. Ampicillin was added at 100 μg/ml. TTM medium used for selection of TS-defective clones is minimal medium supplemented with thymine (50 μg/ ml) and trimethoprim (20 μg/ml).

Bacterial and bacteriophage strains. *E. coli* strain Rue 10 is a *thyA* derivative (Rubin et al. 1980) of HB101 (Bolivar and Backman 1979). D1210*thyA*, JM103*thyA*, and JM83*thyA* are *thyA* derivatives isolated in this laboratory from D1210 (HB101 *lacI^q*) (Brosius and Holy 1984), JM103 (Δ*lac-pro*, *supE*, *thi*, *endA*, *strA*, *sbc*B15, *hsd*R4, F′*tra*D36, *proAB$^+$*, *lacI^q*ZΔM15), and JM83 (Δ*lac-pro*, *ara*, *strA*, *thi*, φ80 *lacI^q*ZΔM15) (Vieira and Messing 1982), respectively. M13-Td derivatives are described in Figure 6.

Plasmids. pUC-Td has a 2.85-kb *Eco*RI fragment containing the entire *td* gene in the *Eco*RI site of pUC9 (Fig. 1) (Chu et al. 1984). pUC-TdX1 and pUC-TdX3 were generated after partial digestion of pUC-Td with *Aha*III, isolation of unit-length linear fragments, and recircularization via *Xba*I linkers (5′-CTCTAGAG-3′). *Aha*III was chosen because it is a blunt-end cutter and has no sites within the exons, and several sites within the intron, near the ends of the intron ORF. *Xba*I was used to screen for plasmids that had acquired *Xba*I sites and to map the site of insertion. The large *Xba*I-*Bam*HI fragment of pUC-TdX1 and the small *Xba*I-*Bam*HI fragment of pUC-TdX3 (double-headed dashed arrows in Fig. 1) were ligated to form pUC-TdΔ1-3. Sequencing across the deletion joint confirmed the presence of an 8-bp *Xba*I linker at the site of the 631-bp deletion, between residues 934 and 1566 within the intron (for residue numbers, see Fig. 2).

A 2-kb *Eco*RI-*Hpa*I *td* fragment, containing intact exons, was transferred from pUC-TdΔ1-3 into the *Eco*RI-*Sma*I interval of vector pKK223-3 (Brosius and Holy 1984) to generate pKK-TdΔ1-3. This construct has the modified *td* gene under the control of the p*tac* promoter, with the *rrnB* T$_1$T$_2$ transcriptional terminators of the vector at the 3′ end of the *td* fragment. This 2-kb fragment and the 2.85-kb *Eco*RI fragment from pUC-Td were cloned into transcription vector pBSM13 (Stratagene, Inc.) under the control of the

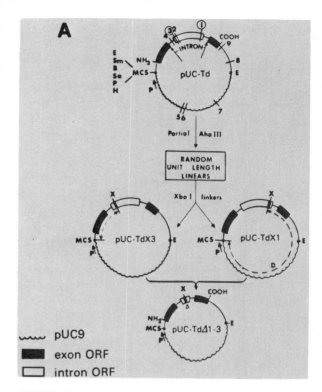

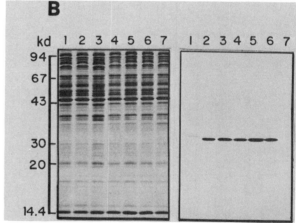

Figure 1. Expression of the modified *td* gene. (*A*) Intron insertion and deletion constructs. Cloning of *Xba*I (X) linkers into the *Aha*III sites (labeled *1–9*) of pUC-Td is described in Methods. Linker insertions occur at sites 1 and 3 (circled) in the intron in constructs pUC-TdX1 and pUC-TdX3, respectively. These two latter plasmids were used to generate the intron deletion construct pUC-TdΔ1-3. (MCS) Multiple cloning site; (E) *Eco*RI; (Sm) *Sma*I; (B) *Bam*HI; (Sa) *Sal*I; (P) *Pst*I; (H) *Hin*dIII. p*lac* (p) drives transcription of the *td* insert in the direction of the short arrow. (*B*) TS expression by the modified *td* gene. TS was monitored in crude extracts of stationary-phase plasmid-containing JM83*thyA* by ternary complex formation with [³H]FdUMP and 5,10-CH₂-H₄Pte-Glu. Proteins were separated on 12.5% SDS-polyacrylamide gel and visualized by Coomassie staining (*left* panel). A molecular-weight calibration is shown at the far left. The TS/5-10-CH₂-H₄PteGlu/[³H]FdUMP ternary complexes are evident in the fluorogram of the gel (*right* panel). Extracts were prepared from cells containing the following plasmids: pUC-thyA (lane *1*), pUC-Td (lanes *2* and *6*), pUC-TdX1 (lane *3*), pUC-TdX3 (lane *4*), pUC-TdΔ1-3 (lane *5*), and pUC9 (lane *7*). Note that *E. coli* TS (faint band in lane *1*) migrates more slowly than T4 TS (lanes *2–6*).

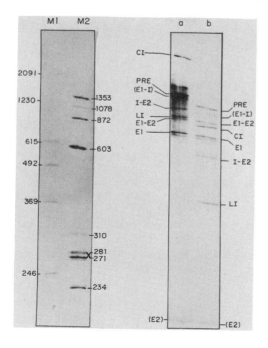

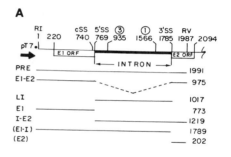

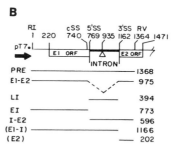

Figure 2. In vitro reaction products of pBS-Td and pBS-TdΔ1-3. The products of an in vitro transcription reaction with pBS-Td (lane *a*) and pBS-TdΔ1-3 (lane *b*) were separated on a 5% acrylamide gel alongside denatured, labeled DNA size markers (lanes M1 and M2). The labeled RNA bands correspond to the transcripts diagramed at the right for pBS-Td (*A*) and pBS-TdΔ1-3 (*B*). (PRE) Runoff precursor transcript; (E1-E2) ligated exons; (LI) linear intron; (CI) circular intron; (E1) exon I intermediate; (I-E2) intron-exon II intermediate; (E1-I) exon I-intron; (E2) exon II. The latter two, shown in parentheses, are presumptive hydrolysis products (Inoue et al. 1986). The theoretical number of residues comprising each transcript is indicated at the right of *A* and *B*. These calculations were based on transcription starting at −5 (dot at top left of maps). Residue numbers are indicated above each map. Intron lengths in pBS-Td and pBS-TdΔ1-3 are 1016 bp and 393 bp, respectively, with the linear intron being extended by 1 residue with the added G in each case. (RI) *Eco*RI; (cSS) cryptic 5′ splice site; (5′SS) 5′ splice site; (3) start point of Δ1-3 deletion; (1) end point of Δ1-3 deletion; (Δ) site of deletion in *B*; (3′SS) 3′ splice site; (RV) *Eco*RV, the site of plasmid linearization. Bands (no labels) below E1 in *a* and *b* result from cleavage at the cryptic 5′ splice site (corresponding bands above LI and I-E2 are apparent on darker exposures; Chandry and Belfort 1987). The identity of the RNA species was corroborated by mobilization of appropriate bands, following directed RNase H cleavage targeted with intron, exon I, and exon II oligonucleotides (data not shown).

phage T7 promoter to form pBS-TdΔ1-3 and pBS-Td, respectively. The *E. coli rrnB* T$_1$ transcriptional terminator was cloned from pKK232-8 (Brosius 1984) on a 170-bp *Eco*RI fragment via *Xba*I linkers into the *Xba*I site at the deletion joint in the intron of pUC-TdΔ1-3. pUC-TdΔ1-3-T$^+$ and pUC-TdΔ1-3-T$^-$ contain the terminator in transcriptional and reverse orientation, respectively. pUC-*thyA* contains the 1.2-kb *thyA* fragment with *Hin*dIII linkers (Belfort et al. 1983a) in the *Hin*dIII site of pUC9.

TS assays. Ternary complex formation between TS, [6-^{3}H]fluorodeoxyuridylate ([^{3}H]FdUMP) and 5,10-methylenetetrahydrofolate (5,10-CH$_2$H$_4$PteGlu) and subsequent separation and fluorography were carried out as described previously (Belfort et al. 1983b). For each sample, 10 μg of protein was treated for ternary complex formation and subsequently applied to the gel. Enzyme activity in these samples was approximately 1 mU as determined by the tritium release assay described by Roberts (1966) with [5-^{3}H]dUMP as substrate. One unit of activity is defined as the amount of enzyme required to convert 1 μmole of dUMP to dTMP per minute at 30°C.

In Vitro transcription. Linearized templates were treated with proteinase K, extracted with phenol-chloroform, and precipitated with ethanol. DNA (1 μg) was incubated at 37°C for 30 minutes with 10 units of T7 polymerase and 10 nmoles of ATP, GTP, and UTP, and 1 nmole of [^{32}P]CTP (5 μCi/nmole). The reaction was performed in 50 mM Tris-HCl (pH 8), 8 mM MgCl$_2$, 2 mM spermidine, 50 mM NaCl, and 30 mM dithiothreitol, in a total volume of 25 μl. One unit of RNase-free DNase I was added, and the incubation was continued for 15 minutes. After heat denaturation in formamide, the samples, each containing 5 × 10^4 acid-insoluble cpm, were loaded on a 5% acrylamide gel.

Mutagenesis and trimethoprim selection. CsCl gradient-purified pKK-TdΔ1-3 was mutagenized with hydroxylamine. Mutagenesis and subsequent dialysis were carried out as described previously (Belfort and Pedersen-Lane 1984). D1210*thyA* was then transformed with mutagenized plasmid and plated onto TTM media supplemented with ampicillin (TTM + Amp). Plates were incubated overnight at 37°C. Thy$^-$ transformants were purified by two passages on TTM + Amp plates at 37°C.

NH₂TS assay. Transformants were grown at 37°C until mid-log phase in TBYET supplemented with ampicillin. Isopropylthio-β-galactoside (IPTG) was then added to a concentration of 2 mM. Cultures were induced for the indicated times, and the cells were pelleted and then washed with TM (10 mM Tris-HCl [pH 7.4], 10 mM MgCl₂). Washed pellets were lysed in stop-load buffer and separated on a 10% bis-acrylamide gel (Laemmli 1970), which was stained with Coomassie blue.

Dot-blot assay. Transcription was induced in transformants with IPTG as detailed above. Total cellular RNA was extracted as described previously (Belfort et al. 1985), and 800 ng of RNA was spotted onto Hybond-N filters (Amersham Corp.). The filters were UV-irradiated for 5 minutes to fix the RNA. Hybridization with 5′ ³²P-end-labeled oligonucleotides was carried out according to the method of Hall et al. (1987). Filters were washed three times for 30 minutes each in 6× SSC (1× SSC is 0.15 M NaCl, 0.015 M Na citrate) at 23°C before autoradiography.

Genetic mapping. Cells containing *td* mutant plasmids were grown overnight at 37°C in TBYET plus ampicillin. The cells were then diluted 1:100 in the same media and grown to early log phase at 37°C. Recombinant M13 phage (see Fig. 6) were added to cells at a multiplicity of infection of about one, and the mixture was shaken for 3 hours at 37°C. Infected cells were dripped across selective minimal media plates containing ampicillin but lacking thymine and incubated at 43–44°C overnight. Positive marker rescue was indicated by the growth of Thy⁺ recombinant colonies.

Double-stranded dideoxy sequencing. Supercoiled plasmid DNA was isolated from cells by a twofold scale-up of the alkaline lysis procedure described by Maniatis et al. (1982). After RNase treatment, the plasmid preparation was reextracted with phenol-chloroform and precipitated with 0.5 volumes of 7.5 M NH₄OAc and 2 volumes of 100% ethanol. After a 70% ethanol rinse and drying, the pellet was resuspended in 15 μl of TE. The double-stranded supercoiled DNA was then sequenced according to the procedure of Bartlett et al. (1986), using *td*-specific oligonucleotides as sequencing primers.

RESULTS

Expression of the *td* Gene Containing Intron Modifications

To initiate the intron mutagenesis study, we created linker insertions within the intron. This was achieved as described in Figure 1A by placing synthetic octometric *Xba*I sites at strategic positions near the ends of the intron ORF, thereby disrupting the reading frame. The two constructs pUC-TdX1 and pUC-TdX3, with inserts at opposite ends of the ORF, were both able to complement *thyA E. coli* for growth on minimal medium lacking thymine (not shown). Furthermore, they produced

wild-type levels of TS of apparently normal size (32 kD) by the FdUMP-binding assay (Fig. 1B). These results not only indicate the suitability of these insertion plasmids as intermediates for constructing an intron deletion, but also demonstrate the nonessential nature of the intron ORF for *td* gene expression (i.e., for splicing) in vivo.

TS⁻ cells transformed with plasmid pUC-TdΔ1-3, constructed by deleting 631 intron residues between the *Xba*I linker insertions of pUC-TdX1 and pUC-TdX3, are also phenotypically Thy⁺ (see below). This deletion construct actually produces higher TS levels than the parental *td* clone both in vivo and in vitro (Fig. 1B; West et al. 1986). The ability of pUC-TdΔ1-3 to support TS production is in agreement with genetic experiments with T4 *td* mutants (Hall et al. 1987), which indicated the dispensability of the central portion of the intron to *td* gene expression.

Splicing Proficiency of the *td*Δ1-3 Construct

Since it was our intention to generate splicing-defective point mutations in the *td*Δ1-3 construct, whose intron is only 393 bp long (385 *td* residues plus 8 linker nucleotides), it was of importance to examine the RNA products of the modified gene. The in vitro transcription analysis shown in Figure 2 indicates that *td*Δ1-3 pre-mRNA splices normally, with an efficiency similar to that of wild type. In addition to ligated exons of similar size to wild type, both linear and circular intron species appropriately reduced in size were detected. For both wild-type and *td*Δ1-3 RNAs, exon I and intron-exon II splicing intermediates were also apparent, as were exon I-intron and free exon II, the presumptive products of the splicing-independent hydrolysis reaction at the 3′ splice site (Inoue et al. 1986). Additionally, cleavage products that result from activation of a cryptic 5′ splice site in exon I (29 residues from the authentic 5′ splice site) are evident from both the parental and modified templates (Chandry and Belfort 1987). In all cases, the precursors, cleavage, and splice products were present in similar relative amounts for the two templates, indicating that the efficiency of the processing reactions is similar.

The accuracy of the splicing reaction for *td*Δ1-3 RNA was verified by the following criteria: (1) Intron RNA that had been labeled with [³²P]GTP in a self-splicing reaction (Ehrenman et al. 1986) was sequenced with base-specific ribonucleases and shown to have an authentic 5′ end. (2) The splice junction of the exon ligation product was confirmed by primer-extension analysis with an exon II primer (sequence as for wild type; Belfort et al. 1985). (3) The cyclization junction of the intron was verified with a 5′ intron primer by primer-extension analysis (sequence as for wild type; Ehrenman et al. 1986). (4) Finally, the production of active TS both in vivo (Fig. 1B) and in vitro from *td*Δ1-3 (West et al. 1986) confirms the fidelity of the RNA-processing reactions with the intron deletion construct.

Phenotypes of *td*[+] and *td*[−] Transformants

Although phenotypes based on TS function have been useful in mutagenesis studies of the *E. coli thyA* gene (Belfort and Pedersen-Lane 1984), we needed to test growth phenotypes based on *td* expression. Whereas *E. coli thyA* TS-defective mutants are not able to grow in the absence of thymine (Fig. 3A, track 1), a *thyA* host transformed with a *td*Δ1-3 construct grows well on similar media (Fig. 3A, track 2). On the other hand, abolishing *td* expression, in this particular case by inserting the *rrnB* T₁ transcriptional terminator in functional orientation into the intron in *td*Δ1-3, again resulted in a Thy⁻ phenotype (Fig. 3A, track 3). Partial activity of the *rrnB* T₁ terminator in reverse orientation results in incomplete restoration of phenotype, as evidenced by weaker growth on −THY media (Fig. 3A, track 4). These growth phenotypes correlate with *td*-encoded TS production by these clones. TS activity in

mU/mg protein was < 0.1, 4.3, 0.1, and 2.4 for IPTG-induced clones shown in tracks 1, 2, 3, and 4, respectively. The correlation of plating phenotype with enzymatic activity for *td* transformants is similar to those observed with the cloned *thyA* gene (Belfort and Pedersen-Lane 1984). These results provided assurance that the folate selection with trimethoprim would prove useful in a saturation mutagenesis study of the *td* gene.

Selection of *td* Mutants

Mutations were created by nondirected in vitro hydroxylamine mutagenesis of pKK-TdΔ1-3. D1210*thyA* transformants harboring mutated plasmids were selected by their ability to grow on media containing trimethoprim, thymine, and ampicillin (TTM) at 37°C. On the basis of this positive selection for *td* dysfunction, 100 TS⁻ mutants were isolated (42 of these are shown in Fig. 3B). It should be noted that the Thy⁻ control, lacking the *td* gene, grew on trimethoprim-containing TTM media at both 37°C and 42°C, in contrast to the Thy⁺ control containing the unmutagenized parental *td*⁺ plasmid that was selected against on TTM. On the other hand, the Thy⁺ (but not the Thy⁻) control grew on media lacking thymine (−THY). A range of phenotypes was found among the TTM-selected mutants. Many mutants were unable to grow in the absence of thymine at 37°C and fewer yet survived 42°C on −THY plates. Mutants that grew on both TTM and −THY media at both temperatures are leaky Thy⁻ mutants, producing enough TS to grow in the absence of exogenous thymine, but too little to become sensitive to trimethoprim (Belfort and Pedersen-Lane 1984). Many of the splicing-defective mutants belong to this latter class (see Fig. 3C and below), producing active TS, albeit at very low levels.

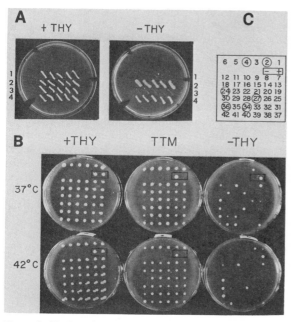

Figure 3. Plating phenotypes of wild-type and mutant clones. (*A*) Correlation of *td* expression with the ability of clones to grow in the absence of thymine. Transformants were patched onto minimal media in the presence (+THY) or absence (−THY) of thymine and incubated at 37°C for 16 hr (*left*) or 26 hr (*right*). Rue10 host cells were transformed with pUC9 (*1*), pUC9-TdΔ1-3 (*2*), pUC9-TdΔ1-3-T⁺ (*3*), and pUC9-TdΔ1-3-T⁻ (*4*). (*B,C*) Growth phenotype of *td* mutants. The mutant clones are D1210*thyA* cells transformed with the mutagenized pKK-TdΔ1-3 plasmid. Cells were grown in microtiter dishes as 0.2-ml cultures in TBYET supplemented with ampicillin. A 48-pin inoculator was used to print the array onto minimal media–ampicillin plates in the absence (−THY) or presence (+THY) of thymine or onto TS⁻-selective TTM media. Plates were incubated overnight at the indicated temperatures. Numbering of the array, representing the mutants SC1-SC42, is shown in *C*, with the splicing-defective mutants circled. Boxed areas indicate the controls. The Thy⁻ control (−) is D1210 *thyA* transformed with pKK223-3 vector, and the Thy⁺ control (+) contains the unmutagenized pKK-TdΔ1-3 plasmid.

Screening Assays for Splicing-defective *td* Mutants

Two assays were used to screen this heterogeneous mutant collection for those mutants with defects in splicing. First, we developed an assay that takes advantage of the fact that *td* RNA encodes two translation products, representing the stages before and after splicing (Fig. 4A,B) (Belfort et al. 1986). Exon I of the unspliced pre-mRNA is translated into NH₂TS, whereas mature, spliced mRNA encodes the full-length protein, TS. The distinguishing characteristics of a splicing-defective mutant would therefore be the accumulation of NH₂TS and very low TS levels. The protein profiles of the 100 *td* mutants were examined (Fig. 4A). Mutants with a variety of different ratios of TS to NH₂TS were found as well as mutants with translation products of altered molecular weight. Thirteen mutants with appropriately high NH₂TS/TS ratios were selected for further study.

A splicing-defective mutation is not the only possible explanation for cells producing NH₂TS alone. A nonsense codon in the mRNA might, for example, yield a protein of approximately the same molecular weight as

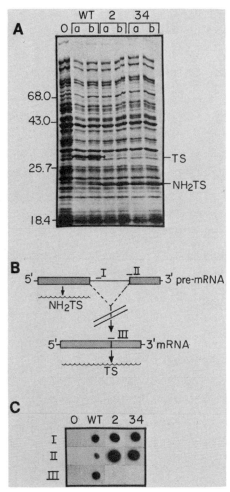

Figure 4. Screening assays. (*A*) NH₂TS assay. D1210*thyA* transformed with pKK223-3 vector (0), pKK-TdΔ1-3 (WT), or splicing-deficient derivatives of pKK-TdΔ1-3, SC2 (2) and SC34 (34) were treated with 2 mM IPTG for 1 (*a*) or 2 (*b*) hr. The 0 control was treated for 2 hr. Coomassie staining demonstrated the presence of two induced protein bands: TS encoded by the mRNA and NH₂TS encoded by exon I of the pre-mRNA. Molecular-weight standards are given in kilodaltons. (*B*) Products of the *td* gene. Stippled boxes represent exon sequences, which are separated by the intron. Products that accumulate when splicing is defective are indicated above the diagonal lines (pre-mRNA and NH₂TS), whereas mature gene products (mRNA and TS) appear below the diagonal lines. The numbered bars represent the three oligonucleotides that were used as probes in *C*. Probe I is a 22-mer complementary to the 5' intron, 49 residues from the 5' splice site; probe II is a 25-mer complementary to the intron/exon II junction of the pre-mRNA; and probe III is a 24-mer complementary to the splice junction in the mRNA. (*C*) Oligonucleotide hybridization assay. RNA was isolated after 1 hr of induction with 2 mM IPTG from D1210*thyA* transformed with pKK223-3 (0), pKK-TdΔ1-3 (WT), and pKK-TdΔ1-3 mutants SC2 (2) and SC34 (34). RNA was immobilized and probed with ³²P-labeled oligonucleotides shown in *B*.

that of NH₂TS, and no TS. The RNA phenotype of the selected mutants was therefore examined to confirm their splicing defects. Total RNA was spotted onto

filters and probed with ³²P-labeled oligonucleotides (Fig. 4B,C). An oligonucleotide specific for the intron/exon II junction of pre-mRNA (II) and for the splice junction of mRNA (III) demonstrated a large buildup of pre-mRNA and only trace amounts of mRNA in mutants, as compared with that in wild type. Such RNA assays confirmed the splicing-defective nature of all 13 of the mutants identified by the NH₂TS assay. Furthermore, they suggested an accumulation of precursors that resists cleavage at the 3' splice site for all 13 mutants.

Primer-extension Analysis at the 5' Splice Site

To examine the first step of splicing, RNA extracted from cells transformed with *td* mutant plasmids was used as a template for cDNA synthesis, with a primer that anneals to the intron 49 nucleotides from the 5' splice site. For wild type, cDNAs correspond to the linear intron, with stops in all lanes at its 5' end, and the circular intron, where the cDNA continues into the 3' end of the intervening sequence (Fig. 5A). In contrast, for the mutants, exemplified in Figure 5A by SC79, the sequence reads from the 5' end of the intron into exon I of the pre-mRNA, indicating that cleavage is impaired at the 5' splice site. This is the case for all 13 mutants, as shown in Figure 5B, where reduced cleavage at the 5' splice site is apparent from the diminished intensity of the cDNA banding in this region. Furthermore, the banding pattern for all mutants except SC99, which is a missplicing mutant (Chandry and Belfort 1987), is similar to that for SC79. These data were corroborated by generating dideoxynucleotide sequence ladders as for SC79 (data not shown). Additionally, when RNAs were labeled with [³²P]GTP under self-splicing conditions, the radioactive 394-nucleotide linear intron band was reduced in intensity relative to wild type for each of the mutants (data not shown). These results are therefore in agreement that each of the 13 mutants is defective in the first step of the group I splicing pathway.

Genetic Mapping and Sequence Determination

One of the advantages of working in a prokaryotic system lies in the ease of genetic mapping through marker rescue. JM103*thyA* (Rec⁺ and F⁺) containing a mutant *td* plasmid was infected with one of a set of M13 clones containing portions of the gene (Fig. 6A). The mapping of SC34 demonstrated the appearance of Thy⁺ recombinants in infections with M13 clones that allow rescue of wild-type sequences (Fig. 6B). To reduce background, it was important to select for Thy⁺ recombinants at 43–44°C, temperatures at which most of the splicing-defective mutants are Thy⁻. Utilizing this system, the mutants were mapped to within 1 of 7 deletion intervals (Fig. 6A), eliminating the need to sequence the entire intron and the surrounding exon regions for each mutant.

Mutations were sequenced directly from the double-

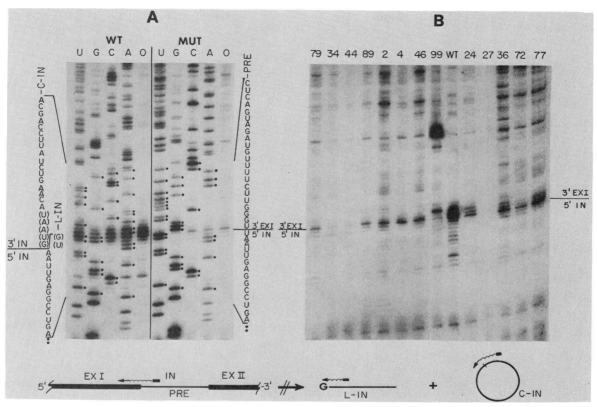

Figure 5. Primer-extension analysis at the 5' splice site. (*A*) Dideoxy sequence analysis of the exon I/intron junction region of *td*. Total RNA from D1210*thyA* transformed with pKK-TdΔ1-3 (WT) or with splicing-defective mutant SC79 (MUT) was isolated 1 hr after induction with 2 mm IPTG. Primer-extension sequencing reactions were performed in the absence (0) or presence of the four ddNTPs (A, C, G, and U represent the complementary nucleotides) with an intron primer that anneals 49 nucleotides from the 5' splice site. Reading upward, the sequences diverge at the 5' end of the intron. Sequences correspond to linear (L-IN) or circular (C-IN) intron for WT and to pre-mRNA (PRE) for the mutant (diagramed below, with primer represented by a solid box, and the extension products by a wavy arrow). Nucleotides that are obscured on the gel are bracketed. (*B*) Primer-extension screening of mutant RNAs. RNA was prepared as described above from splicing-defective mutants SC79, SC34, SC44, SC89, SC2, SC4, SC46, SC99, SC24, SC27, SC36, SC72, and SC77 as well as from pKK-TdΔ1-3 (WT). cDNA synthesis in the absence of ddNTPs was primed with the same primer as in *A*. The primer extension of SC27 was repeated (data not shown) and was shown to have the same banding pattern as the other mutants that appear similar to SC79. SC99 was the only mutant that exhibited atypical bands.

stranded plasmid template. Once the deletion interval was determined for a mutation, an oligonucleotide with specificity for a downstream sequence was used as the primer for dideoxynucleotide sequencing. Table 1 lists the deletion intervals and nucleotide change(s) for each mutant, and Figure 7A shows the linear distribution of the mutations.

Although all 13 mutants are defective at the 5' splice site, only 4 mutations are in the 5' domain. Of these, SC99 is in the upstream exon, and SC77, SC46, and SC89 are in the intron. The nine 3' mutations SC36, SC34, SC27, SC72, SC2, SC44, SC79, SC24, and SC4 span the region from the end of the intron ORF to within 10 nucleotides of the 3' splice site. Of these, SC2 and SC44 are identical, despite their independent origin, and SC4 harbors 2 mutations, 11 residues apart. The wide distribution of mutations indicates that there are multiple elements involved in targeting the 5' splice site and/or effecting cleavage at this site.

DISCUSSION

The discovery of a group I intron in the *td* gene of phage T4 (Chu et al. 1984, 1986, 1987; Ehrenman et al. 1986) has underscored the phylogenetic diversity of these genetic elements. Although the existence of introns in prokaryotes is consistent with RNA as the primordial nucleic acid, the evolutionary origin of bacteriophage introns remains unclear. In particular, the variable occurrence of group I intervening sequences in the closely related T-even phages (Pedersen-Lane and Belfort 1987), and the striking similarities between the prokaryotic and eukaryotic group I introns, raises the possibility of horizontal transfer of these elements (Michel and Dujon 1986; Shub et al. 1987). Regardless of their evolutionary origins, the existence of bacteriophage introns makes available the tools of prokaryotic genetics for the study of self-splicing RNAs.

As the first step in the functional analysis of the *td*

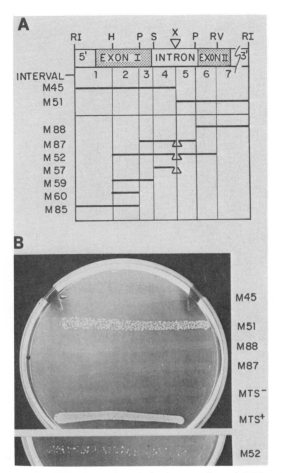

Figure 6. Deletion mapping of *td* point mutations. (*A*) Map of deletion constructs in phage M13. The map depicts the *td*Δ1-3 construct (*top*) with the 631-nucleotide intron deletion represented by an inverted triangle (for coordinates, see Fig. 2B). The M13-Td derivatives were made using the indicated restriction sites: *Eco*RI (RI), *Hin*dIII (H), *Pvu*II (P), *Stu*I (S), *Xba*I (X), and *Eco*RV (RV). The M13 deletion constructs were made using fragments with the full-length intron, except for constructs M45 and M51, which are *td*Δ1-3 derivatives. The indentation in the line represents the sequences in M52, M57, and M87 that are not present in the *td*Δ1-3. M13mp10 was used as vector, except that M87 and M88 used M13mp8 and M85 used M13mp9. (*1–7*) Seven intervals to which a mutation can be mapped by marker rescue with the listed constructs. (*B*) Marker-rescue mapping of SC34. The mutation was mapped to interval 5 utilizing TS⁻ host JM103*thyA* transformed with SC34 and infected with the indicated M13-Td derivatives. TS⁺ recombinant colonies were selected on minimal media at 43°C. Controls for the marker-rescue mapping are M13 containing a wild-type TS insert (MTS⁺) and M13 containing no insert (MTS⁻).

intron, a series of linker insertion mutations was generated within the intron ORF. These insertions disrupted the ORF without measurably affecting *td* function, suggesting that expression of the ORF is not essential for splicing in vivo. Furthermore, the linker mutants were instrumental in constructing the deletion *td*Δ1-3, which is missing 631 central residues of the 1016-nucleotide intron, including most of the intron

ORF (Fig. 1). In agreement with genetic studies that suggested the nonessential nature of these 631 intron residues in *td* expression (Hall et al. 1987), *td*Δ1-3 is fully splicing-proficient. This was reflected in the efficiency and accuracy of RNA processing and in the level of active TS production (Figs. 1 and 2) (Ehrenman et al. 1986; West et al. 1986; J. Galloway Salvo et al., unpubl.).

The positive and negative genetic selections associated with TS uniquely lend the *td* gene to saturation mutagenesis of a group I intron (Fig. 3). Thus, nondirected point mutations were isolated in a *td*Δ1-3 construct to define residues and secondary structures that are functionally important in splicing. To facilitate this approach, screening methods were devised to permit the splicing-defective mutants to be distinguished from other variants resulting from nondirected mutagenesis. A functional assay based on the overproduction of NH₂TS, the translation product of pre-mRNA, provided a rapid and simple screen for splicing-defective mutants (Fig. 4A). The RNA phenotype of 13 of the 100 hydroxylamine-generated *td* mutants selected on the basis of the NH₂TS assay was verified to be splicing-defective, utilizing an RNA-deoxyoligonucleotide hybridization assay (Fig. 4B) previously described by Hall et al. (1987). The buildup of pre-mRNA in the mutants was indicated with an intron-exon II probe, suggesting impaired cleavage for all the mutants at the 3′ splice site.

Surprisingly, primer-extension analysis demonstrated that each of the 13 mutants is also defective in cleavage at the authentic 5′ splice site. Since the mutants are blocked at the first step in the RNA processing pathway, they all accumulate intact pre-mRNA. Of the 13 mutants, SC99, harboring an exon I mutation, is the most unusual. Although it accumulates less pre-mRNA than the other mutants, atypical cleavage and splice products are formed in this mutant through use of a cryptic splice site in the upstream exon (Chandry and Belfort 1987).

Interestingly, the mutations affecting 5′ cleavage are spread throughout four deletion intervals (Figs. 6 and 7). Thus, mutations scattered throughout both the 3′ and 5′ domains of the intron can have a profound effect on recognition and/or cleavage at the 5′ splice site. The absence from our collection of mutations affecting only later steps of the splicing pathway may well be related to mechanistic features of the reactions and/or to the nature of the phenotypic selections. From a mechanistic standpoint, if most of the elements required for cleavage at the 3′ splice site and exon ligation are also essential for the first step of splicing, a population of random mutants would be highly enriched for those impaired at the 5′ splice site. One also needs to consider that mutational events that reduce activity at the 5′ splice site might have the strongest phenotypes, since subsequent steps in the concerted group I pathway would also be expected to be impaired. Since splicing-defective mutants have leaky plating phenotypes, because of a low level of active TS production (Fig. 3),

Table 1. Map Positions and Sequence Changes of Mutations Causing Splicing Defects

Mutant	Deletion interval	Nucleotide[a]	Intron residue[b]	Change
SC99[c]	3	766	−3	G to A
SC77	4	819	51	G to A
SC46	4	835	67	G to A
SC89	4	847	79	C to T
SC36	5	1634	866	C to T
SC34	5	1641	873	C to T
SC27	5	1659	891	G to A
SC72	5	1666	898	G to A
SC2[d]	5	1700	932	G to A
SC44[d]	5	1700	932	G to A
SC79	5	1736	968	G to A
SC4[e]	6	1765	997	G to A
		1775	1007	G to A
SC24	6	1768	1000	C to T

[a]Nucleotide numbers are based on the undeleted wild-type *td* gene. Intron coordinates are as follows: 769 is the first coded nucleotide of the intron; residues 934 and 1566 form the deletion joint of *td*Δ1-3.

[b]Residue numbering begins at the first coded nucleotide of the intron (769).

[c]SC99 is an exon I mutant, 3 nucleotides upstream of the 5′ splice site.

[d]SC2 and SC44 are independent isolates that have the same base change.

[e]SC4 contains two base changes.

those mutants with the most dramatic splicing impediments would be the most likely to pass the trimethoprim selection. It will be of interest to isolate mutations in a single-copy gene (as opposed to the multicopy plasmid used in this study) to provide mutants with more subtle and varied phenotypes.

The data from these as well as other studies suggest that substantially more of the central region of the intron than that deleted in *td*Δ1-3 is dispensable to splicing. First, the linear distribution of mutations shown in Figure 7A reveals that although mutations cluster in the first 80 residues and the last 150 residues of the intron, none occur within the central 150 residues of *td*Δ1-3. Second, the distribution of an independent collection of *td* mutations, generated in T4 with an intact *td* intron, is similar. Thus, the 17 splicing-defective mutations that have been sequenced in the T4 collection lie scattered throughout the 5′ and 3′ intron domains, with none more centrally located than SC89 and SC36, on the 5′ and 3′ sides, respectively (Hall et al. 1987; K. Ehrenman et al., in prep.). Third, a secondary structure model independently generated by F. Michel (Shub et al. 1987) defines the core *td* group I structure on the basis of the first 93 residues and the last 167 residues of the intron. This structure, which is based on conserved sequence and structural elements, suggests that the functional core of the *td* intron is confined to about 260 nucleotides. This is within the size range estimated from the mutational studies and also corresponds to the smallest naturally occurring group I intron found to date (258 bp) in the *cox*1 gene of *Schizosaccharomyces pombe* (Trinkl and Wolf 1986).

The mutations are shown in the context of the Michel secondary structure model in Figure 7B. Ten of the mutations disrupt pairings predicted by the model. These occur in the P1, P4, P5, P6, P7, P7.2, P8, P9, and P9.2 elements. Although a combination of genetic approaches has implicated a role for the P1, P3, P4, P7, and P9 pairings in group I splicing (see introduction to this paper), this work provides the first evidence for the functional involvement of P5, P6, P7.2, P8, and P9.2 in the process. These results are particularly noteworthy given that the P7.1 and P7.2 elements and multiple P9 pairings are not typical features of the core structure of group I introns (Michel et al. 1982; Waring and Davies 1984). Interestingly, both P7.1 and P7.2 elements as well as all three P9 elements are also found to occur in the two other T4 introns, in the *nrd*B and *sun*Y genes (Gott et al. 1986; Shub et al. 1987). Mutations in these elements clearly establish their critical role in splicing. Whereas second-site revertants will be required to confirm the proposed structures, primary mutations in these elements will be instrumental in establishing their functional role in this special subclass of group I introns.

Mutant SC4 harbors two base changes (Table 1; Fig. 7). Although the phenotypes of the individual mutations have not yet been established, it should be noted that neither mutation is in a predicted helical region. The other two mutations that are in apparently unpaired regions are SC72 and SC36. SC72 is in the loop of the P7.2 element, whereas SC36 lies in the last codon of the intron ORF, in the critical region between the P6 stem and the residues of the R element that pair with S (P7). SC36 therefore provides evidence that the 3′ end of the ORF forms part of the active splicing structure as suggested by the model. This has interesting implications for the mutual exclusivity of translation and splicing, where ribosomes are thought to prevent formation of the RNA conformation required for splicing (Shub et al. 1987).

One role for unpaired residues may be to interact directly with extrinsic components of the reaction (e.g., the guanosine nucleotide or Mg^{++}). Indeed, unpaired bases immediately upstream of the P7 pairing residues of the R element have been implicated in substrate binding (Williamson et al. 1987). Alternatively, critical

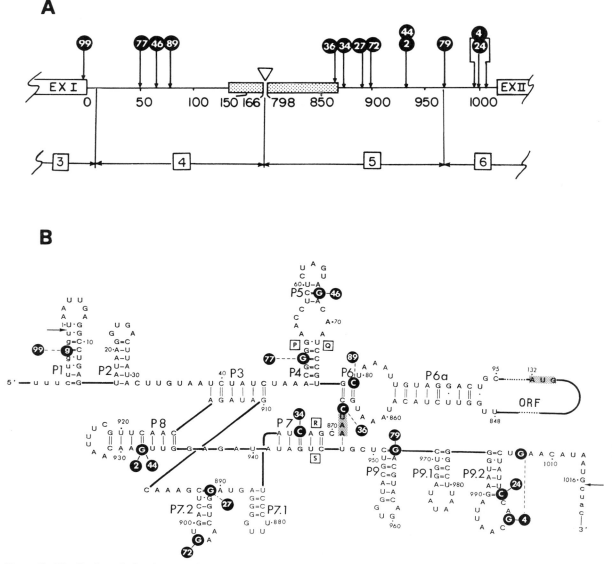

Figure 7. Distribution of *td* point mutations on linear and secondary structure maps. (*A*) Linear map of the intron of *td*Δ1-3. Open boxes represent the exons. Numbering commences at the first coded intron residue and is based on the undeleted wild-type *td* gene. The inverted triangle depicts the location of the 631-nucleotide deletion within the intron ORF (stippled boxes). Intron residue number and type of nucleotide change for each of the 13 mutations (closed circles) are shown in Table 1. Four of the seven deletion intervals (Fig. 6) are demarcated below the map (numbered 3–6 in boxes). (*B*) Secondary structure model of the *td* intron. The proposed secondary structure generated by F. Michel (Shub et al. 1987) is numbered as in the linear map. The display of the intron and numbering of conserved structural elements conform to recently revised conventions (Burke et al. 1987). Arrows represent 5′ and 3′ splice sites. The intron sequence appears in uppercase letters, whereas exon residues are represented by lowercase letters. The discontinuous open loop from residue 95 includes the ORF with start codon (shaded) at intron residue number 132. The end of the ORF extends into the structure, with its UAA stop codon (shaded) 3′ to the P6 stem. Mutation numbers are represented in closed circles, whereas conserved pairings within group I introns have been given P numbers according to the nomenclature of Waring and Davies (1984). The P7.1 and P7.2 helices, characteristic of subclass IA of the group I introns, correspond to the δ elements of Michel et al. (1982). Conserved complementary sequences P/Q and R/S, which make up the P4 and P7 pairings, respectively, are boxed.

residues that are not in double-stranded regions of the secondary structure may be involved in tertiary structure foldings. The *td* system is uniquely suited to the isolation of spontaneous intragenic suppressors. Such compensatory pseudorevertants hold the key to verifying the secondary structure model and to entering the unexplored terrain of tertiary interactions.

ACKNOWLEDGMENTS

We are deeply thankful to Francois Michel for providing us with the secondary structure model of the *td* intron. We thank James Reston for assistance with the genetic mapping and Dwight Hall for his comments on the manuscript. This work was supported by grants from the National Institutes of Health (GM-33314) and the National Science Foundation (DM-B8502961 and DM-B8505527).

REFERENCES

Anziano, P.Q., D.K. Hanson, H.R. Mahler, and P.S. Perlman. 1982. Functional domains in introns: Trans-acting and *cis*-acting regions of intron 4 of the *cob* gene. *Cell* **30:** 925.

Bartlett, J.A., R.K. Gaillard, Jr., and W.K. Joklik. 1986. Sequencing of supercoiled plasmid DNA. *Biotechniques* **4:** 308.

Been, M.D. and T.R. Cech. 1986. One binding site determines sequence specificity of *Tetrahymena* self-splicing, *trans*-splicing and RNA enzyme activity. *Cell* **47:** 207.

Belfort, M. and J. Pedersen-Lane. 1984. Genetic system for analyzing *Escherichia coli* thymidylate synthase. *J. Bacteriol.* **140:** 371.

Belfort, M., G. Maley, J. Pedersen-Lane, and F. Maley. 1983a. Primary structure of the *Escherichia coli thy*A gene and its thymidylate synthase product. *Proc. Natl. Acad. Sci.* **80:** 4914.

Belfort, M., A. Moelleken, G.F. Maley, and F. Maley. 1983b. Purification and properties of T4 phage thymidylate synthase produced by the cloned gene in an amplification vector. *J. Biol. Chem.* **258:** 2045.

Belfort, M., J. Pedersen-Lane, D. West, K. Ehrenman, G. Maley, F. Chu, and F. Maley. 1985. Processing of the intron-containing thymidylate synthase (*td*) gene of phage T4 is at the RNA level. *Cell* **41:** 375.

Belfort, M., J. Pedersen-Lane, K. Ehrenman, F.K. Chu, G.F. Maley, F. Maley, D.S. McPheeters, and L. Gold. 1986. RNA splicing and *in vivo* expression of the intron-containing *td* gene of bacteriophage T4. *Gene* **41:** 93.

Bolivar, F. and K. Backman. 1979. Plasmids of *Escherichia coli* as cloning vectors. *Methods Enzymol.* **68:** 245.

Brosius, J. 1984. Plasmid vectors for the selection of promoters. *Gene* **27:** 151.

Brosius, J. and A. Holy. 1984. Regulation of ribosomal RNA promoters with a synthetic lac operator. *Proc. Natl. Acad. Sci.* **81:** 6929.

Burke, J.M., M. Belfort, T.R. Cech, R.W. Davies, R.J. Schweyen, D.A. Shub, J.W. Szostak, and H.F. Tabak. 1987. Structural conventions for group I introns. *Nucleic Acids Res.* **15:** 7217.

Burke, J.M., K.D. Irvine, K.J. Kaneko, B.J. Kerber, A.B. Oettgen, W.M. Tierny, C.L. Williamson, A.J. Zaug, and T.R. Cech. 1986. Role of conserved sequence elements 9L and 2 in self-splicing of the *Tetrahymena* ribosomal RNA precursor. *Cell* **45:** 167.

Cech, T.R. 1986. The generality of self-splicing RNA: Relationship to nuclear mRNA splicing. *Cell* **44:** 207.

Cech, T.R., A.J. Zaug, and P.J. Grabowski. 1981. *In vitro* splicing of the ribosomal RNA precursor of *Tetrahymena*: Involvement of a guanosine nucleotide in the excision of the intervening sequence. *Cell* **27:** 487.

Cech, T.R., N.K. Tanner, I. Tinoco, Jr., B.R. Weir, M. Zuker, and P.S. Perlman. 1983. Secondary structure of the *Tetrahymena* ribosomal RNA intervening sequence: Structural homology wth fungal mitochondrial intervening sequences. *Proc. Natl. Acad. Sci.* **80:** 3903.

Chandry, P.S. and M. Belfort. 1987. Activation of a cryptic 5′ splice site in the upstream exon of the phage T4 *td* transcript: Exon context, missplicing and mRNA deletion in a fidelity mutant. *Genes Dev.* (in press).

Chu, F.K., G.F. Maley, and F. Maley. 1987. Mechanism and requirements of in vitro RNA splicing of the primary transcript from the T4 bacteriophage thymidylate synthase gene. *Biochemistry* **26:** 3050.

Chu, F.K., G.F. Maley, F. Maley, and M. Belfort. 1984. An

intervening sequence in the thymidylate synthase gene of bacteriophage T4. *Proc. Natl. Acad. Sci.* **81:** 3049.

Chu, F.K., G.F. Maley, D.K. West, M. Belfort, and F. Maley. 1986. Characterization of the intron in the phage T4 thymidylate synthase gene and evidence for its self-excision from the primary transcript. *Cell* **45:** 157.

Davies, R.W., R.B. Waring, J.A. Ray, T.A. Brown, and C. Scazzocchio. 1982. Making ends meet: A model for RNA splicing in fungal mitochondria. *Nature* **300:** 719.

De La Salle, H., C. Jacq, and P.P. Slonimski. 1982. Critical sequences within mitochondrial introns: Pleiotropic mRNA maturase and cis-dominant signals of the *box* intron controlling reductase and oxidase. *Cell* **28:** 721.

Ehrenman, K., J. Pedersen-Lane, D. West, R. Herman, F. Maley, and M. Belfort. 1986. Processing of phage T4 *td*-encoded RNA is analogous to the eukaryotic group I splicing pathway. *Proc. Natl. Acad. Sci.* **82:** 5875.

Garriga, G. and A.M. Lambowitz. 1986. Protein-dependent splicing of a group I intron in ribonucleoprotein and soluble fractions. *Cell* **46:** 669.

Gott, J.M., D.A. Shub, and M. Belfort. 1986. Multiple self-splicing introns in bacteriophage T4: Evidence from autocatalytic GTP labeling of RNA *in vitro*. *Cell* **10:** 81.

Hall, D.H., C.M. Povinelli, K. Ehrenman, J. Pedersen-Lane, F. Chu, and M. Belfort. 1987. Two domains for splicing in the intron of the phage T4 thymidylate synthase (*td*) gene established by non-directed mutagenesis. *Cell* **48:** 63.

Hensgens, L.A.M., L. Bonen, M. De Haan, G. Van der Horst, and L.A. Grivell. 1983. Two intron sequences in yeast mitochondrial *COXI* gene: Homology among URF-containing introns and strain-dependent variation in flanking exons. *Cell* **32:** 379.

Holl, J., G. Rödel, and R.J. Schweyen. 1985. Suppressor mutations identify *box9* as a central nucleotide sequence in the highly ordered structure of intron RNA in yeast mitochondria. *EMBO J.* **4:** 2081.

Inoue, T., F.X. Sullivan, and T. Cech. 1986. New reactions of the ribosomal RNA precursor of *Tetrahymena* and the mechanism of self-splicing. *J. Mol. Biol.* **189:** 143.

Laemmli, U.K. 1970. Cleavage of structural proteins during assembly of the head of bacteriophage T4. *Nature* **227:** 680.

Maniatis, T., E.F. Fritsch, and J. Sambrook. 1982. *Molecular cloning: A laboratory manual*, p. 368. Cold Spring Harbor Laboratory, Cold Spring Harbor, New York.

Michel, F. and B. Dujon. 1983. Conservation of RNA secondary structures in two intron families including mitochondrial-, chloroplast-, and nuclear-encoded members. *EMBO J.* **2:** 33.

———. 1986. Genetic exchanges between bacteriophage T4 and filamentous fungi. *Cell* **46:** 323.

Michel, F., A. Jacquier, and B. Dujon. 1982. Comparison of fungal mitochondrial introns reveals extensive homologies in RNA secondary structure. *Biochimie* **64:** 867.

Mileham, A.J., H.R. Revel, and N.E. Murray. 1980. Molecular cloning of the T4 genome; organization and expression of the *frd*-DNA ligase region. *Mol. Gen. Genet.* **179:** 227.

Okada, T., K. Yanagisawa, and F.J. Ryan. 1961. A method for securing thymineless mutants from strains of *E. coli*. *Z. Vererbungsl.* **92:** 403.

Pedersen-Lane, J. and M. Belfort. 1987. Variable occurrence of the *nrd*B intron in the T-even phages suggests intron mobility. *Science* **237:** 182.

Roberts, D. 1966. An isotopic assay for thymidylate synthetase. *Biochemistry* **5:** 3546.

Rubin, E.M., G.A. Wilson, and F.E. Young. 1980. Expression of thymidylate synthetase activity in *Bacillus subtilis* upon integration of a cloned gene from *Escherichia coli*. *Gene* **10:** 227.

Shub, D.A., J.M. Gott, M.-Q. Xu, B.F. Lang, F. Michel, J. Tomaschewski, J. Pedersen-Lane, and M. Belfort. 1987. Structural conservation between three homologous introns of phage T4 and the group I introns of eukaryotes. *Proc. Natl. Acad. Sci.* (in press).

Simon, E.H., and I. Tessman. 1963. Thymidine-requiring mutants of phage T4. *Proc. Natl. Acad. Sci.* **50:** 526.

Trinkl, H. and K. Wolf. 1986. The mosaic *cox*I gene in the mitochondrial genome of *Schizosaccharomyces pombe*: Minimal structural requirements and evolution of group I introns. *Gene* **45:** 289.

Vieira, J. and J. Messing. 1982. The pUC plasmids, an M13mp7-derived system for insertion mutagenesis and sequencing with synthetic universal primers. *Gene* **19:** 259.

Waring, R.B. and R.W. Davies. 1984. Assessment of a model for intron RNA secondary structure relevant to RNA self-splicing — A review. *Gene* **28:** 277.

Waring, R.B., P. Towner, S.J. Minter, and R.W. Davies. 1986. Splice-site selection by a self-splicing RNA of *Tetrahymena*. *Nature* **321:** 133.

Waring, R.B., J.A. Ray, S.W. Edwards, C. Scazzocchio, and R.W. Davies. 1985. The *Tetrahymena* rRNA intron self-splices in *E. coli*: *In vivo* evidence for the importance of key base-paired regions of RNA for RNA enzyme function. *Cell* **40:** 371.

Weiss-Brummer, B., G. Rödel, R.J. Schweyen, and F. Kaudewitz. 1982. Expression of the split gene *cob* in yeast: Evidence for a precursor of a "maturase" protein translated from intron 4 and preceding exons. *Cell* **29:** 527.

Weiss-Brummer, B., J. Holl, R.J. Schweyen, G. Rödel, and F. Kaudewitz. 1983. Processing of yeast mitochondrial RNA: Involvement of intramolecular hybrids in splicing of *cob* intron 4 RNA by mutation and reversion. *Cell* **33:** 195.

West, D.K., M. Belfort, G.F. Maley, and F. Maley. 1986. Cloning and expression of an intron-deleted phage T4 *td* gene. *J. Biol. Chem.* **261:** 13446.

Williamson, C.L., W.M. Tierny, B.J. Kerker, and J.M. Burke. 1987. Site-directed mutagenesis of core sequence elements 9R', 9L, 9R and 2 in self-splicing *Tetrahymena* pre-rRNA. *J. Biol. Chem.* (in press).

A Family of Autocatalytic Group I Introns in Bacteriophage T4

D.A. SHUB, M.-Q. XU, J.M. GOTT, A. ZEEH, AND L.D. WILSON
Department of Biological Sciences, State University of New York, Albany, New York 12222

The first intron to be discovered in a prokaryotic mRNA was found in the *td* gene of bacteriophage T4 (see Belfort et al., this volume). The presence of an intron in this gene, which encodes thymidylate synthase, was detected by sequence comparisons at the DNA and protein levels. Thus, a stop codon was encountered in the DNA sequence before the end of the protein-coding sequence (Chu et al. 1984). Subsequent experimentation revealed that the intron in the *td* gene was excised autocatalytically from precursor RNA (Belfort et al. 1985). The splicing mechanism resembled that used by group I introns of eukaryotes: a series of transesterification reactions triggered by nucleophilic attack by guanosine (or GTP) at the 5′ splice site (Ehrenman et al. 1986; Chu et al. 1987). The primary intron excision product was linear, containing a non-coded G at the 5′ end (Ehrenman et al. 1986).

Although the discovery of an intron in phage T4 was entirely unexpected, it encouraged us (in collaboration with M. Belfort, Wadsworth Center for Laboratories and Research, N.Y. State Department of Health) to look for additional group I introns in the T4 genome. Further examples would permit sequence and structural comparisons that might lend insight into their evolutionary origin. Additionally, we hoped that their locations within the T4 genome would infer a possible regulatory function in prokaryotic gene expression. We took advantage of the fact that, since G is added to the 5′ end of the intron, autocatalytic group I introns could be specifically labeled in vitro for use as probes for DNA blotting experiments (Garriga and Lambowitz 1984). If group I introns were in more than just the *td* gene, multiple RNA species should be labeled when total RNA is extracted from T4-infected cells and incubated with $[\alpha\text{-}^{32}P]$GTP in vitro. When used as a probe for a Southern blot of T4 DNA, this RNA should hybridize to several DNA bands.

RESULTS

When T4 RNA was end-labeled with $[\alpha\text{-}^{32}P]$GTP under self-splicing conditions and used as a probe for Southern blots of T4 DNA, three bands hybridized (Gott et al. 1986). One band could be assigned to the *td* gene and another band was mapped to *nrdB*, the gene for the small subunit of ribonucleoside diphosphate reductase (Gott et al. 1986). In vitro transcription of the *nrdB* region revealed an intron (Gott et al. 1986), which we subsequently determined to be 598 nu-

cleotides (Shub et al. 1987). Sjöberg et al. (1986) independently showed that the T4 coding region homologous to the *Escherichia coli nrdB* gene was interrupted by about 600 bp of nonhomologous DNA.

The third putative intron mapped to a region of the T4 genome that is relatively silent genetically. A brief description of how we determined the identity of the third split gene follows.

The *sunY* Intron

The third restriction fragment that hybridized to the GTP end-labeled T4 RNA probe was usually barely detectable on the autoradiogram (Gott et al. 1986). However, this weak band could be mapped in each case to the same region of the T4 genome (Fig. 1), between the *Xba*I restriction sites at 44.2 and 49.1 kb. This *Xba*I fragment was isolated from an agarose gel and various portions were cloned into pBSM13 + . Figure 2 presents a summary of the results when DNA from each of the clones was subjected to dot-blot analysis with the same GTP end-labeled probe. The 2.1-kb *Xba*I-*Pst*I clone (pMPX401) hybridized to the autocatalytically labeled RNA, whereas the *Kpn*I-*Xba*I fragment did not; we did not succeed in cloning the central *Kpn*I-*Pst*I fragment. Additional hybridization experiments with subclones from the *Pst*I-*Xba*I region showed that the 5′ end of the intron falls within a small *Hin*dIII restriction fragment located at about 45 kb (Fig. 2b). The DNA sequence of this region (Tomaschewski and Rüger 1987) shows that there are a total of 13 unassigned open reading frames (ORFs) between genes *49* and *55*, three of which are in the vicinity of this putative intron (Fig. 3). In vitro transcription (from the T3 promoter) of pMPX401, or a derivative containing a 1.3-kb *Acc*I-*Xba*I insert (pMAX1), gave typical group I splicing products (data not shown) when the plasmid was linearized at the *Rsa*I site or beyond (Fig. 3). Each reaction contained a species approximately 1.0 kb smaller than the runoff transcript, as well as a species expected for ligated exons. In addition, a slowly migrating species was present, characteristic of circular RNA. However, when the plasmid was cut with *Ssp*I, the two major products were the runoff transcript and a species that was smaller by the size of exon I. It is known that group I introns can undergo excision at the 5′ splice site even when they lack sequences at the 3′ end (Szostak 1986; Doudna et al., this volume).

Sequencing of RNAs made in vivo and in vitro al-

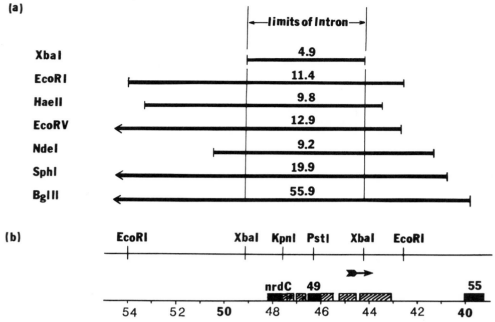

Figure 1. Localization of the *sunY* intron. (*a*) Restriction fragments in the 40–54-kb region showing hybridization to total T4 RNA, end-labeled with [α-³²P]GTP in vitro. The region of overlap of all of the fragments is denoted as the limits of the intron. Numbers indicate sizes of the restriction fragments in kilobases. Those fragments shown only partially are represented by arrows. (*b*) Schematic representation showing correlation between the restriction map and the T4 genetic map. Closed boxes represent known genes in the region of 40–54 kb. Hatched boxes represent unassigned open reading frames. The arrow indicates direction of transcription in this region.

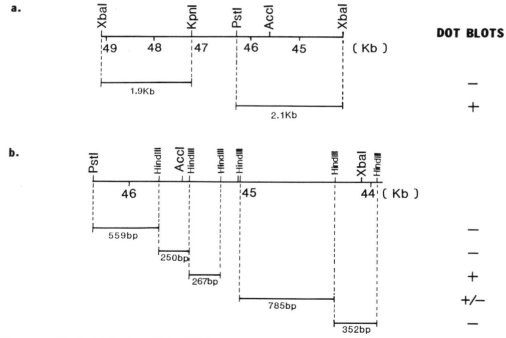

Figure 2. Summary of dot hybridization with [α-³²P]GTP end-labeled T4 RNA probe. Restriction fragments from the 44–49-kb region, cloned into pBSM13 (Stratagene Cloning Systems), were tested for hybridization to RNA extracted from T4-infected cells at 7 min and end-labeled in vitro with [α-³²P]GTP. Cloned fragments are indicated by bars under the restriction map. Their extent of hybridization to the RNA probe is indicated on the left by strong (+), weak (+/−), or no (−) hybridization compared with control plasmids lacking a T4 DNA insert.

194

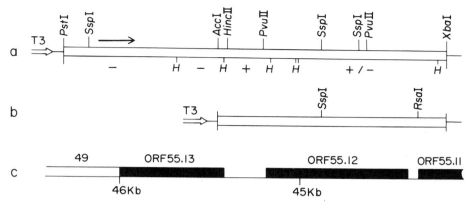

Figure 3. Plasmids used for in vitro transcription of the *sunY* region. (*a*) pMPX401: The 2.1-kb *Pst*I-*Xba*I fragment from the 4.9-kb *Xba*I fragment (Fig. 1a) was inserted into the multiple cloning site of pBSM13 + . Relevant restriction sites are shown (H indicates *Hin*dIII), with the extent of dot hybridization to end-labeled T4 RNA indicated as in Fig. 1b. Arrow indicates the direction of transcription from the phage T3 promoter. (*b*) pMAX1: The insert in pMPX401 was reduced to 1.3 kb by deleting the DNA between the unique *Pst*I and *Acc*I restriction sites. Arrow indicates the direction of transcription from the phage T3 promoter. (*c*) Positions of unassigned ORFs in the vicinity of the *sunY* intron are indicated by closed rectangles, and the position of gene *49* is shown by an open rectangle.

lowed us to determine the precise boundaries of the intron (Shub et al. 1987). It comprises 1033 nucleotides and connects ORFs 55.13 and 55.11 with ORF 55.12 contained within the intron. Since it is our intention to understand the role that introns play in T4 reproduction, we have given the gene that contains this intron the provisional name *sunY* (*s*plit gene, *un*known function, *why*).

Structures of the T4 Introns

Since their splicing mechanism resembled that of the group I introns, we attempted to fit the sequences of the T4 introns to the secondary structure pattern typical of group I intron RNAs (Michel et al. 1982; Cech et al. 1983; Waring and Davies 1984). Figure 4 shows that the T4 introns fit the group I model in every detail (Shub et al. 1987). They belong to the group IA subclass (Michel et al. 1982), which is characterized by the insertion of additional nucleotides between P7 and P3 and by systematic variations in the phylogenetically conserved sequences (P, Q, R, S) (Waring and Davies 1984; Michel and Cummings 1985). Interestingly, the T4 introns closely resemble an intron within the large rRNA of *Chlamydomonas* chloroplasts (Rochaix et al. 1985). Although this rRNA intron shares little sequence homology with the T4 introns, the degree of structural homology is striking. In each, the extra sequence between P7 and P3 can be represented as two stem loops (the group IA introns of fungal mitochondria generally have one such helix [Michel et al. 1982; Waring and Davies 1984]), and each of these introns has an ORF entirely bounded by intron sequences. Furthermore, the ORFs of the *Chlamydomonas*, *nrdB*, and *td* introns reside in the P6 loop (an unusual position for intron ORFs of mitochondrial fungi). The *sunY* intron ORF occurs in another uncommon location, a loop near the 3′ end of the intron (Fig. 4). In all cases, however, the

ORF extends beyond the loop and terminates within the core structure of the intron. The regulatory implications of this gene arrangement are discussed below.

DISCUSSION

It has been suggested that the absence of introns from eubacteria is the result of selection for minimum genome size in rapidly proliferating microorganisms (Darnell and Doolittle 1986). Certainly, bacteria have efficient mechanisms to eliminate DNA that does not confer a selective advantage. Therefore, the observation of introns in bacteriophage T4 strongly suggests that there is a selective advantage for their maintenance. The pressure for efficient genome design is even greater for viruses than for their bacterial hosts: Since the amount of DNA in a viral genome is fixed by the internal volume of the capsid, any DNA sequence takes the place (literally) of potential alternative sequences. Alternative splicing could make the genome more efficient by allowing the same DNA sequences to code for several different peptides. Likewise, regulation of splicing could be used to regulate gene expression, which would also favor the retention of introns. We suggest that regulation of a biochemical pathway induced during T4 infection is accomplished by the regulation of splicing.

Although one of the introns described in phage T4 is in a gene of unknown function (*sunY*), the other two (*nrdB* and *td*) are in genes specifying components of the same biochemical pathway: synthesis of deoxyribonucleotide precursors for DNA synthesis. Furthermore, the enzymes encoded by these split genes are both coupled to consumption of reducing equivalents (NADPH). Although these functional similarities in the products of the split genes may be fortuitous, we regard them as suggestive of a role for splicing in regulation of the pathway. This pathway is not abso-

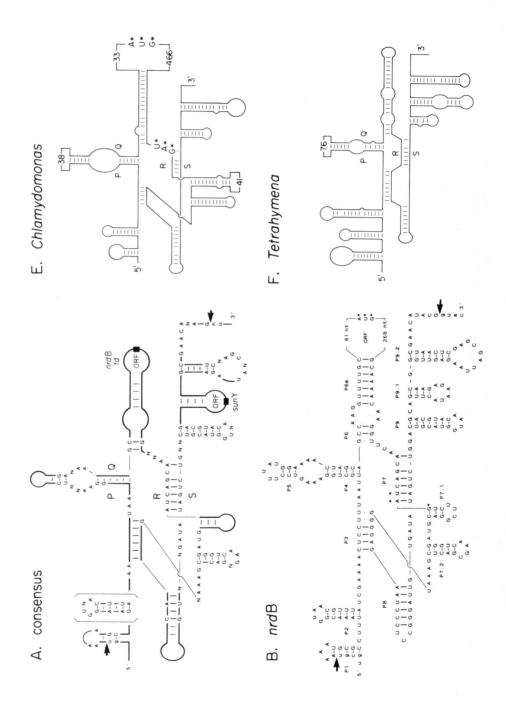

A. consensus

B. *nrdB*

E. *Chlamydomonas*

F. *Tetrahymena*

196

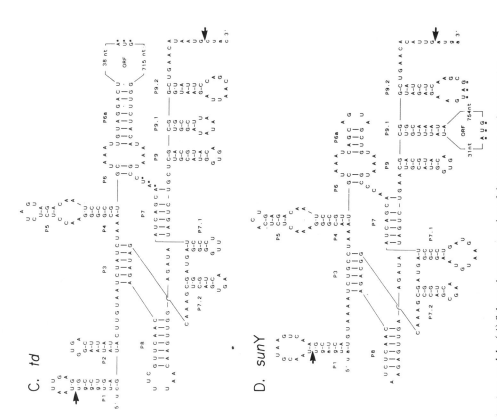

Figure 4. Secondary structure models. (*A*) Schematic representation of the sequence and structural elements conserved among the T4 introns. Nucleotides common to RNAs from each of the three intron-containing T4 genes are shown, with conserved spacings between them indicated by Ns and conserved base pairings indicated by lines between the phosphodiester backbone. Thin lines represent connections between adjacent nucleotides, and thick lines indicate varying lengths of nonconserved nucleotides. P, Q, R, and S refer to sequences that are highly conserved among group I introns (Michel et al. 1982; Waring and Davies 1984). Splice sites are indicated by arrows between the exon sequences (lowercase) and intron nucleotides (uppercase). Closed rectangles represent the intron ORFs, which extend from stems that are conserved in structure, but not in sequence. Although well conserved between the *td* and *nrdB* genes, the P2 stem is absent from the *sunY* gene and is therefore shown in brackets. (*B–D*) Predicted secondary structures for intron sequences from the *nrdB*, *sunY*, and *td* genes, respectively. The pairings P1 through P9.2 refer to structural elements characteristic of group I introns (Michel et al. 1982; Waring and Davies 1984). The nomenclature and intron displays are according to recent revised conventions (Burke et al. 1987). The initiator AUG and stop codons of each intron ORF are indicated by asterisks (*). Numbers indicate the number of nucleotides between given structural elements. (*E–F*) Schematic illustrations of the phosphodiester backbone and base pairings predicted for the rRNA introns from *C. reinhardii* (Rochaix et al. 1985) and *Tetrahymena thermophila* (Cech et al. 1983). Conserved sequences P, Q, R, and S and the position of the *C. reinhardii* intron ORF are shown.

197

lutely required for phage replication, since in its absence, a burst of about 20 phages can be obtained by the recycling of nucleotides derived from the degradation of the host chromosome. However, when the pathway is intact, the rate of phage DNA synthesis and the burst size are increased severalfold. Thus, the ability to convert excess ribonucleotides (rRNA synthesis is repressed after infection) to deoxyribonucleotides is advantageous for T4 when it infects a host cell that is growing under optimal conditions; i.e., when the growth rate is sufficient to support the synthesis of more than 20 phage equivalents of capsid and assembly proteins. However, when the host is growing poorly, induction of the pathway may deplete the cell of badly needed GTP, ATP, and reducing equivalents, thus reducing the overall phage yield.

T4 did not evolve in a host growing exponentially in the stable environment of the broth in a laboratory shaker flask. Rather, the bacterial cells must deal with the rapidly changing environment of their animal host. Cellular metabolism takes violent swings from nutritional feast to famine (depending on the time since the previous meal) and from anaerobic to aerobic growth (as the bacteria are eliminated in the feces). We would be surprised if T4 fails to optimize the expression of its genes in accord with the metabolic state of the cells it infects. We propose that the existence of autocatalytically spliced group I introns in genes of related function provides two potential mechanisms for metabolic regulation. Moreover, since mitochondria and chloroplasts are derived from bacterial ancestors, we hope that insight into intron function derived from T4 will be directly applicable to the role of introns in these organelles.

Feedback Inhibition

The group I intron of the *Tetrahymena* large rRNA gene has all the characteristics of a true enzyme (for reviews, see Cech 1987; Been et al., this volume). In particular, this ribozyme has an active site for guanosine (or its 5' phosphates), which can be competitively inhibited by guanosine analogs (Bass and Cech 1986). The autocatalytic T4 introns use the same mechanism, with total dependence on GTP for in vitro splicing of the *td* intron (Chu et al. 1987) as well as the *nrdB* and *sunY* introns (D.A. Shub et al., unpubl.). Bacteria have an elaborate system, whereby imbalances in metabolism are signaled via the accumulation of high concentrations of small molecules that are altered forms of normal metabolites. These *alarmones* (Stephens et al. 1975) are typically nucleotides, and several are guanosine derivatives, e.g., guanosine tetraphosphate, which is involved in general growth rate regulation and starvation for amino acids (for review, see Cashel and Rudd 1987), and ZTP, which accumulates during folate limitation (Bochner and Ames 1982). Clearly, there are other alarmones yet to be discovered, and it would not surprise us if some of them are competitive (or even allosteric) inhibitors of the T4 intron ribozymes.

Splice Attenuation

The placement of ORFs within the T4 introns suggests a regulatory coupling of splicing and translation analogous to the attenuation of transcriptional termination in bacteria. In that well-documented scheme (Landick and Yanofsky 1987), an ORF overlaps a series of secondary structure elements that are required for transcriptional termination. Depending on the relative rates of movement of the RNA polymerase on DNA and the ribosome on the nascent mRNA, alternative mutually exclusive secondary structures in the RNA determine whether termination occurs. The ORFs within the self-splicing T4 introns could be performing an analogous role. If the ORFs can be tranlated, ribosomes will travel into, and terminate within, important regions of the intron core structure. For *nrdB* and *td*, the ORFs terminate within the highly conserved R sequence (disrupting P7), whereas for *sunY*, the ORF terminates within P9.2, a highly conserved element at the 3' ends of the T4 introns (Fig. 4). Since mutations in both P7 and P9.2 block splicing of the *td* gene (Belfort et al., this volume), we would expect translation of the ORFs to delay splicing, at least until the ribosomes clear the pre-mRNA. In analogy with the attenuation model, it is possible to draw competing secondary structures in some cases, which might prevent formation of the correct pairings even after departure of the ribosome. Unstructured bacterial mRNA is highly unstable, especially in the absence of translation. One could imagine that if a significant amount of exon 2 sequences were made before splicing occurred, the untranslated portion would be especially vulnerable to degradation. Thus, the rate of translation of the intron ORFs could be a sensitive regulator of expression of the products of the split genes.

For splice attenuation to function as a regulatory mechanism, translation of the intron ORFs must be sensitive to the metabolic state of the cell. We do not know the mechanism for this, but the answer may lie in the structure of the translational initiation regions of the ORFs. Figure 5 shows the sequences preceding the initiator AUG of the T4 intron ORFs. The initiation regions of the *td* (Chu et al. 1986) and *sunY* ORFs are sequestered in a rather stable secondary structure. The first AUG of the *nrdB* ORF is only three residues from the Shine-Dalgarno sequence, which suggests that it is not an efficient initiation site (Stormo et al. 1982). Interestingly, a structure reminiscent of the other ORFs exists just upstream of this region, where a sequestered Shine-Dalgarno sequence is suitably spaced with respect to a potential initiator UUG. If this is a functional translation initiation site, a frameshift (Craigen and Caskey 1987; Weiss et al., this volume) would be required to translate the complete intron ORF.

Several other T4 genes are transcribed in early polycistronic mRNAs, where upstream sequences sequester their initiation sites (Macdonald et al. 1984; McPheeters et al. 1986). At late times, these genes are transcribed into monocistronic mRNAs, free of inhibitory

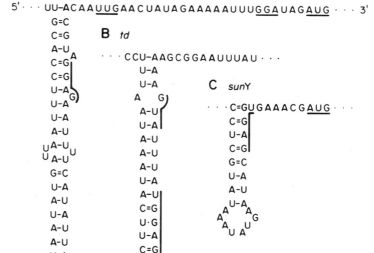

Figure 5. Secondary structures preceding the T4 intron ORFs. Possible stable secondary structures preceding the *nrdB* (*A*), *td* (*B*), and *sunY* (*C*) intron ORFs are shown. Potential initiator codons and Shine-Dalgarno sequences are indicated by solid lines.

secondary structure. McPheeters et al. (1986) proposed that this arrangement exists to allow the early expression of these late genes, under conditions of cellular stress. We have been led to exactly the same hypothesis for the expression of the intron ORFs. According to this scheme, the ORFs contained within the introns cannot be translated under normal conditions, allowing splicing to occur. However, if under poor physiological conditions, translation of the ORFs is stimulated, splicing would be blocked.

Whether or not these models are correct in detail, we would be surprised if evolution has not taken advantage of what (to us) seems like such a logical opportunity. Thus, primitive introns could provide a mechanism for the metabolic regulation of gene activity in either the RNA (Gilbert 1986) or RNP worlds (Maizels and Weiner, this volume).

ACKNOWLEDGMENTS

We thank Marlene Belfort and members of her research group for advice and encouragement throughout the course of this work, B. Franz Lang and Francois Michel for help with intron secondary structure models, and Jörg Tomaschewski and Wolfgang Rüger for the sequence of the *sunY* region prior to publication. This work was supported by grants from the National Science Foundation (DMB-8609066) and the National Institutes of Health (GM-3774601).

REFERENCES

Bass, B.L. and T.R. Cech. 1986. Ribozyme inhibitors: Deoxyguanosine and dideoxyguanosine are competitive inhibitors of self splicing of the *Tetrahymena* ribosomal ribonucleic acid precursor. *Biochemistry* **25:** 4473.

Belfort, M., J. Pedersen-Lane, D. West, K. Ehrenman, G. Maley, F. Chu, and F. Maley. 1985. Processing of the intron-containing thymidylate synthase (*td*) gene of phage T4 is at the RNA level. *Cell* **41:** 375.

Bochner, B. and B. Ames. 1982. ZTP (5-amino 4-imidazole carboxamide riboside 5'-triphosphate): A proposed alarmone for 10-formyl-tetrahydrofolate deficiency. *Cell* **29:** 929.

Burke, J.M., M. Belfort, T.R. Cech, R.W. Davies, R.J. Schweyen, D.A. Shub, J.W. Szostak, and H.F. Tabak. 1987. Structural conventions for group I introns. *Nucleic Acids Res.* **15:** 7217.

Cashel, M. and K.E. Rudd. 1987. The stringent response. In *Escherichia coli and Salmonella typhimurium: Cellular and molecular biology* (ed. F.C. Neidhardt), p. 1410. American Society for Microbiology, Washington, D.C.

Cech, T.R. 1987. The chemistry of self-splicing RNA and RNA enzymes. *Science* **236:** 1532.

Cech, T.R., N.K. Tanner, I. Tinoco, Jr., B.R. Weir, M. Zucker, and P. Perlman. 1983. Secondary structure of the *Tetrahymena* ribosomal RNA intervening sequence: Structural homology with fungal mitochondrial intervening sequences. *Proc. Natl. Acad. Sci.* **80:** 3903.

Chu, F.K., G.F. Maley, and F. Maley. 1987. Mechanism and requirements of in vitro RNA splicing of the primary transcript from the T4 bacteriophage thymidylate synthase gene. *Biochemistry* **26:** 3050.

Chu, F.K., G.F. Maley, F. Maley, and M. Belfort. 1984. An intervening sequence in the thymidylate synthase gene of bacteriophage T4. *Proc. Natl. Acad. Sci.* **81:** 3149.

Chu, F.K., G.F. Maley, D.K. West, M. Belfort, and F. Maley. 1986. Characterization of the intron in the phage T4 thymidylate synthase gene and evidence for its self-excision from the primary transcript. *Cell* **45:** 157.

Craigen, W.J. and C.T. Caskey. 1987. Translational frameshifting: Where will it stop? *Cell* **50:** 1.

Darnell, J.E. and W.F. Doolittle. 1986. Speculations on the early course of evolution. *Proc. Natl. Acad. Sci.* **83:** 1271.

Ehrenman, K., J. Pedersen-Lane, D. West, R. Herman, F. Maley, and M. Belfort. 1986. Processing of phage *td* encoded RNA is analogous to the eukaryotic group I splicing pathway. *Proc. Natl. Acad. Sci.* **83:** 5875.

Garriga, G. and A.M. Lambowitz. 1984. RNA splicing in *Neurospora* mitochondria: Self-splicing of a mitochondrial intron in vitro. *Cell* **39:** 631.

Gilbert, W. 1986. The RNA world. *Nature* **319:** 618.

Gott, J.M., D.A. Shub, and M. Belfort. 1986. Multiple self-splicing introns in bacteriophage T4: Evidence from autocatalytic GTP labeling of RNA in vitro. *Cell* **47:** 81.

Landick, R. and C. Yanofsky. 1987. Transcriptional attenuation. In Escherichia coli *and* Salmonella typhimurium: *Cellular and molecular biology* (ed. F.C. Neidhardt), p. 1276. American Society for Microbiology, Washington, D.C.

Macdonald, P.M., E. Kutter, and G. Mosig. 1984. Regulation of a bacteriophage T4 late gene, *soc*, which maps in the early region. *Genetics* **106:** 17.

McPheeters, D.S., A. Christensen, E.T. Young, G. Stormo, and L. Gold. 1986. Translational regulation of expression of the bacteriophage T4 lysozyme gene. *Nucleic Acids Res.* **14:** 5813.

Michel, F. and D.J. Cummings. 1985. Analysis of class I introns in a mitochondrial plasmid associated with senescence of *Podospora anserina* reveals extraordinary resemblance to the *Tetrahymena* ribosomal intron. *Curr. Genet.* **10:** 69.

Michel, F., A. Jacquier, and B. Dujon. 1982. Comparison of fungal mitochondrial introns reveals extensive homologies in RNA secondary structure. *Biochimie* **64:** 867.

Rochaix, J.D., M. Rahire, and F. Michel. 1985. The chloroplast ribosomal intron of *Chlamydomonas reinhardii* codes for a polypeptide related to mitochondrial maturases. *Nucleic Acids Res.* **13:** 975.

Shub, D.A., J.M. Gott, M.-Q. Xu, B.F. Lang, F. Michel, J. Tomaschewski, J. Pedersen-Lane, and M. Belfort. 1987. Structural conservation between three homologous introns of phage T4 and the group I introns of eukaryotes. *Proc. Natl. Acad. Sci.* **84:** (in press).

Sjöberg, B.-M., S. Hahne, C.Z. Mathews, C.K. Mathews, K.N. Rand, and M.J. Gait. 1986. The bacteriophage T4 gene for the small subunit of ribonucleotide reductase contains an intron. *EMBO J.* **5:** 2031.

Stephens, J.C., S.W. Artz, and B.N. Ames. 1975. Guanosine 5'-diphosphate 3'-diphosphate (ppGpp): Positive effector for histidine operon transcription and general signal for amino-acid deficiency. *Proc. Natl. Acad. Sci.* **72:** 4389.

Stormo, G.D., T.D. Schneider, and L.M. Gold. 1982. Characterization of translational initiation sites in *E. coli*. *Nucleic Acids Res.* **10:** 1971.

Szostak, J.W. 1986. Enzymatic activity of the conserved core of a group I self-splicing intron. *Nature* **322:** 83.

Tomaschewski, J. and W. Rüger. 1987. Nucleotide sequence and primary structures of gene products coded for by the T4 genome between map positions 48.266 kb and 39.166 kb. *Nucleic Acids Res.* **15:** 3632.

Waring, R.B. and R.W. Davies. 1984. Assessment of a model for intron RNA secondary structure relevant to RNA self-splicing—A review. *Gene* **28:** 277.

Long-range Intron-Exon and Intron-Intron Pairings Involved in Self-splicing of Class II Catalytic Introns

F. MICHEL AND A. JACQUIER

Centre de Génétique Moléculaire du CNRS, Laboratoire Associé à l'Université
Pierre et Marie Curie, 91190 Gif-sur-Yvette, France

Secondary structure models for the two unrelated families of organelle introns were proposed in 1982 (Michel et al. 1982; for class I, see Davies et al. 1982). Shortly afterward, the *Tetrahymena* self-splicing intervening sequence was recognized as a typical member of class I (Burke and RajBhandary 1982; Cech et al. 1983; Michel and Dujon 1983; Waring et al. 1983), and speculation on the possible catalytic properties of its organelle counterparts began.

The 1982 models were based on a small number of sequences, and the model for class II was regarded as merely tentative, having been deduced from the comparison of only two sequences. Nevertheless, both the class I and class II original models have successfully withstood the test of time, for all subsequently determined sequences readily lent themselves to secondary structure modeling when the set of "rules" proposed in the 1982 papers was followed (for review of the evidence for class I, see Waring and Davies 1984; for class II, see Michel and Dujon 1983; Schmelzer et al. 1983; Osiewacz and Esser 1984; Lang et al. 1985; Matsuura et al. 1986; Jacquier and Michel 1987).

The original class I secondary structure models of Michel et al. (1982) and Davies et al. (1982) incorporated some of the neighboring exon sequences. In all members of class I, there exists a short sequence stretch, usually (but not always) located not far downstream from the intron 5' end, that can pair with the last nucleotides of the 5' exon. Furthermore, as first noted by Davies et al. (1982), in many, although not all, class I sequences, pairing can be extended on the distal side by incorporating the first few nucleotides of the 3' exon. The intronic component of that structure would thus constitute a "guide" sequence, whose function would be to ensure that the two exons are properly aligned for the ligation step. Proof that the last nucleotides of the exon 5' to class I introns actually pair with complementary intron nucleotides was provided first by genetic means (Perea and Jacq 1985) and then by site-directed mutagenesis and analysis of its consequences on the ability to self-splice in vitro (Been and Cech 1986; Garriga et al. 1986; Waring et al. 1986). In contrast, exon sequences were excluded from the 1982 and subsequent class II models. No short-range pairing could be identified that would involve both exon and intron sequences and be conserved by evolution. In addition, and contrary again to the situation for class I, class II intron-exon junctions seemed to be readily

defined by primary sequence alone: Most class II introns begin with GUGYG and end in AY.

Only recently has it become necessary to reconsider the possibility of interactions between class II introns and their exons. Organelle class II introns appear to share the same splicing pathway and intermediates as their counterparts (and possible relatives) in nuclear pre-mRNAs (Peebles et al. 1986; van der Veen et al. 1986). As is true for the nuclear introns, some type of interaction should therefore be postulated between the two proposed splicing intermediates, the 5' exon and an intron lariat with the 3' exon still attached, which otherwise would diffuse away from each other between the two steps of the splicing reaction. The problem is that, at least for those members of class II that self-splice in vitro (i.e., in the absence of any other macromolecule), the interaction between the 5' exon and the intron must be direct. Direct proof that class II introns recognize their 5' exons was provided by the "*trans*-splicing" experiments of Jacquier and Rosbash (1986), in which coincubation of the 5' exon and intron-3' exon transcripts resulted in the efficient production of spliced exons and free, linear introns.

Prompted by these results, we have addressed the question of how mutual recognition of class II introns and their 5' exons is ensured. We now show that (1) it relies on multiple pairings between the introns and their 5' exons and (2) in a fraction of class II members, one of the intron-exon pairings could be extended by incorporating the first nucleotide or first few nucleotides of the 3' exon, just like in class I. In addition, we report that, on the intron side of the 3' exon-intron junction, the last intron nucleotide is involved in a solitary base pair, together with a nucleotide that is part of the intron's core, several hundred residues further upstream. Some aspects of this work were dealt with previously (Jacquier and Michel 1987) but will be discussed again in a functional prespective.

MATERIALS AND METHODS

Sources of intron sequence. The class II introns whose sequences were used in this work are listed in Figure 1 in abbreviated form. Mitochondrial introns are *Zma*I (intron in the cytochrome oxidase subunit I gene of *Zea mays*; Fox and Leaver 1981); *Sca*1, *Sca*2, and *Sca*5 (first, second, and fifth introns in the cytochrome oxidase subunit I gene of *Saccharomyces cerevisiae*;

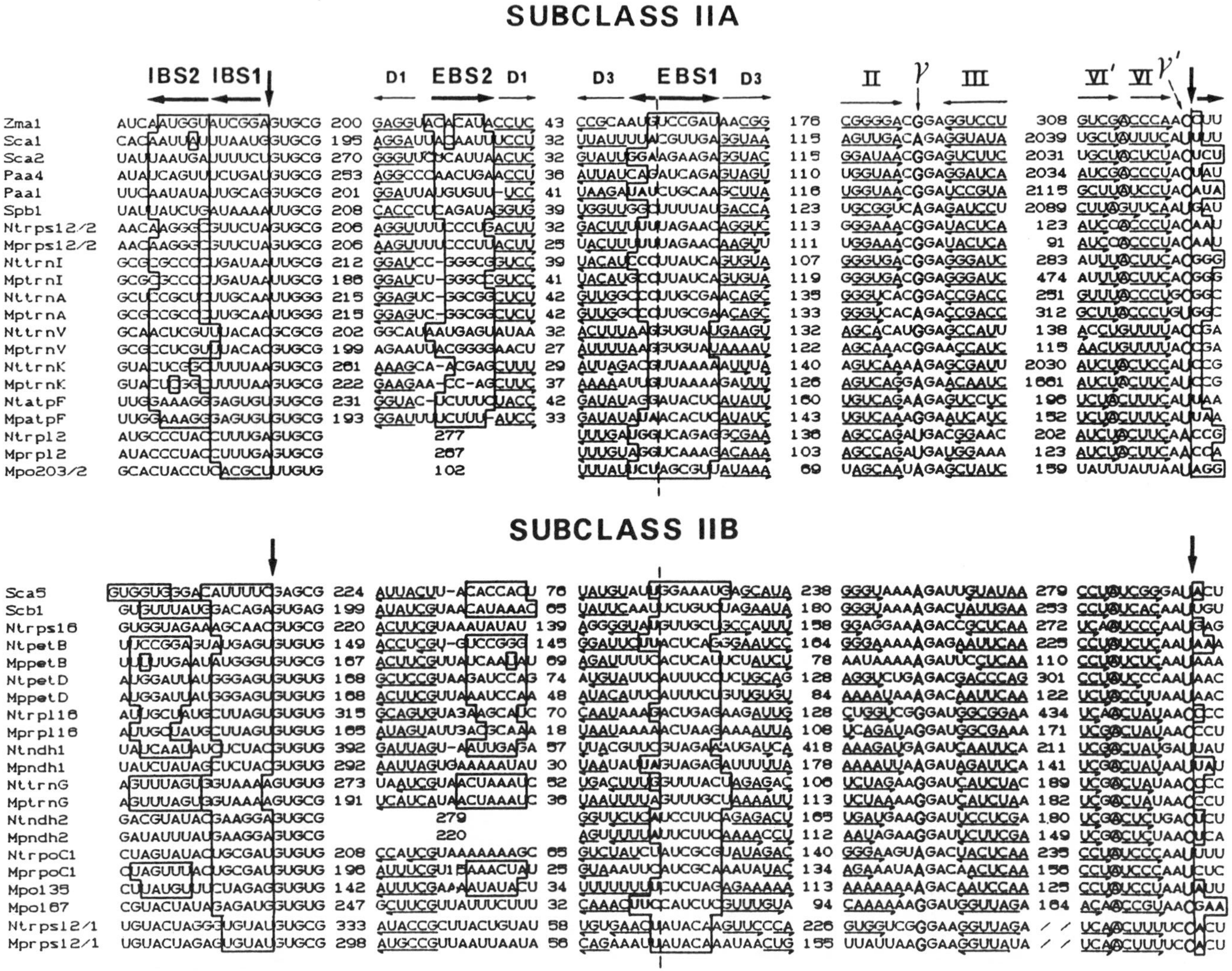

SUBCLASS IIA

	IBS2 IBS1		D1 EBS2 D1		D3 EBS1 D3		II γ III		VI' VI' γ'

Row labels (top to bottom): Zma1, Sca1, Sca2, Paa4, Paa1, Spb1, Ntrps12/2, Mprps12/2, NttrnI, MptrnI, NttrnA, MptrnA, NttrnV, MptrnV, NttrnK, MptrnK, NtatpF, MpatpF, Ntrpl2, Mprpl2, Mpo203/2

SUBCLASS IIB

Row labels (top to bottom): Sca5, Scb1, Ntrps16, NtpetB, MppetB, NtpetD, MppetD, Ntrpl16, Mprpl16, Ntndh1, Mpndh1, NttrnG, MptrnG, Ntndh2, Mpndh2, Ntrpoc1, Mprpoc1, Mpo135, Mpo187, Ntrps12/1, Mprps12/1

Figure 1. Long-range base pairings involving the splice junctions of organelle class II introns. For intron sources and abbreviations, see Materials and Methods. Vertical arrows represent intron-exon junctions. The IBS and EBS sequence elements are boxed. The right part of the EBS1 sequence (to the right of the vertical dashed line) is complementary to the IBS1 sequence, its leftmost part is complementary to the first or first few nucleotides of the 3' exon. D1, D3, II, III, and VI refer to components of the secondary structure of class II introns (see Fig. 2; a leftward arrow indicates a 5' helix branch and a rightward arrow indicates a 3' helix branch). The circled, bulging A on the 3' side of stem VI is the proposed site of lariat formation, by analogy to the situation in *S. cerevisiae* introns a5 and b1 (Schmelzer and Schweyen 1986; van der Veen et al. 1986; Jacquier and Michel 1987). Numbers of nucleotides separating blocks of sequences are indicated. Note that the 5' and 3' sections of the rps12/1 intron are encoded on separate transcription units (Ohyama et al. 1986; Shinozaki et al. 1986).

Bonitz et al. 1980); *Paa*1 and *Paa*4 (first and fourth introns in the corresponding gene of *Podospora anserina*; Osiewacz and Esser 1984); *Scb*1 (first intron in the cytochrome *b* gene of *S. cerevisiae*; Schmelzer et al. 1983); and *Spb*1 (intron in the corresponding gene of *Schizosaccharomyces pombe*; Lang et al. 1985). Chloroplast introns: Mp*xxx* represents introns in the chloroplast genome of *Marchantia polymorpha* (Ohyama et al. 1986); and Nt*xxx* represents the corresponding introns in the chloroplast genome of *Nicotiana tabacum* (Shinozaki et al. 1986).

Construction of plasmids and site-directed mutageneses. Our "wild-type" reference was plasmid Δ52 (Jacquier and Michel 1987), which carries the last 52 nucleotides of the exon 5′ to *S. cerevisiae* intron a5, the entire intron, and 189 nucleotides of its 3′ exon inserted downstream from the SP6 promoter of plasmid pSP64. Isolation of Δ52 plasmids carrying point mutations −5AA and −12AC (5′ exon), 238GT and 241GT (intron), and +1C (3′ exon), as well as 5′ exon deletion mutants Δ13 and 24, was described recently (Jacquier and Michel 1987). Point mutations 587G and 887C were obtained directly in a Δ52 plasmid context by using the mutagenesis technique of Inouye and Inouye (1986). They were then transferred in a Δ24 context by triple ligation, taking advantage of the unique *Hin*dIII and *Eco*RI sites of the pSP64 plasmid and its derivatives and the *Sau*3A site at position 190 of intron a5. We proceeded in the same way to combine mutants 238GT and 241GT with the Δ13 deletion. The 3′ exon mutant E3-1 was obtained by transferring the *Hin*dIII-*Bam*HI fragment of plasmid +1C into plasmid pSP64. The 3′ exon mutant E3-2 resulted from substitution of the *Bam*HI-*Eco*RI fragment of plasmid +1C by the *Bgl*II(1837)-*Eco*RI(1890) fragment of *S. pombe* intron b1 (Lang et al. 1985).

RNA synthesis and analysis. Procedures for in vitro RNA transcription and *trans*- and *cis*-splicing experiments were described elsewhere (Jacquier and Michel 1987).

RESULTS

Long-range Base Pairings Involving the Splice Junctions of Class II Introns as Revealed by Comparative Sequence Analysis

When we started this project, secondary structure models based on comparative sequence analysis had been proposed for parts at least of ten class II introns (Michel et al. 1982; Michel and Dujon 1983; Schmelzer et al. 1983; Osiewacz and Esser 1984; Lang et al. 1985; Matsuura et al. 1986), and many more were available in preliminary form (Fig. 2; F. Michel, in prep.). Using these models as a starting point, we carried out a systematic search for conserved base pairings that would involve, on the one hand, some of the sequence stretches surrounding the intron splice junctions and, on the other hand, single-strand terminal or internal

loops in the secondary structure models of these introns. The outcome of that search is summarized in Figure 1. The four potential pairings identified are described below.

First, the last six (sometimes five or seven) nucleotides of the 5′ exon (IBS1, intron-binding site 1) are always complementary to a stretch of six nucleotides (EBS1, exon-binding site 1) that constitute part of the single-strand terminal loop of a base-paired stem located at the periphery of domain ID (see Fig. 2 for our labeling of domains and individual helices in class II models).

Second, in most class II introns, a second potential pairing can be identified between another section of domain ID (EBS2) and a short stretch (five to six nucleotides) of the 5′ exon (IBS2), located from zero to three nucleotides upstream of IBS1. Concerning the precise location of the EBS2 sequence, two subclasses of introns must be distinguished; definition of these subclasses actually rests on a much wider array of rather subtle, but constant, differences in local secondary structure and sequence (F. Michel, in prep.; see also Fig. 1 and compare the secondary structure models of *S. cerevisiae* introns a5 and b1 [subclass IIB] in Fig. 2 with those of introns a1 and a2 [subclass IIA] in Michel et al. 1982. In subclass IIA introns, the EBS2 site coincides with the single-strand terminal loop of helix D1, which arises from the same internal loop as helix D3. In subclass IIB introns, all that is left of helix D1 is precisely that loop, which lies immediately distal to a helix with a rather well-conserved primary sequence (Fig. 1 and 2).

Third, in subclass IIA introns, the nucleotide immediately 5′ to the EBS1 sequence can always pair with the first nucleotide of the 3′ exon (Fig. 1): The 30 subclass IIA sequences available at present (not all shown in Fig. 1) yield 11 G-C pairs, 7 C-G pairs, 5 A-U pairs, 5 U-A pairs, and 2 G-U pairs for these two sites. In 17 of these sequences, complementarity (excluding G-U pairs) extends to the next site, or even next two sites, upstream of EBS1 and downstream from the 3′ intron-exon junction, respectively. In subclass IIA introns, the D3 single-strand loop could therefore be used to align precisely the 5′ and 3′ exons for the ligation step, exactly as was proposed for the "RNA guide" identified by Davies et al. (1982) in class I introns. In contrast, we have little evidence in favor of the EBS1 sequence element serving such a function in subclass IIB introns: In only about half of them (14 out of 25) can the EBS1-IBS1 pairing be extended to include at least the first nucleotide of the 3′ exon (Fig. 1). This might relate to the fact that the section of EBS1 that pairs with the 5′ exon is located more dissymmetrically within the D3 terminal loop in subclass IIA than in subclass IIB, thus facilitating access to the rest of that loop.

Finally, almost all class II introns have a pyrimidine as their last residue, C and U being nearly as frequent. We noticed that there is one site (γ in Fig. 1) within the short single-strand stretch that joins domains II and III,

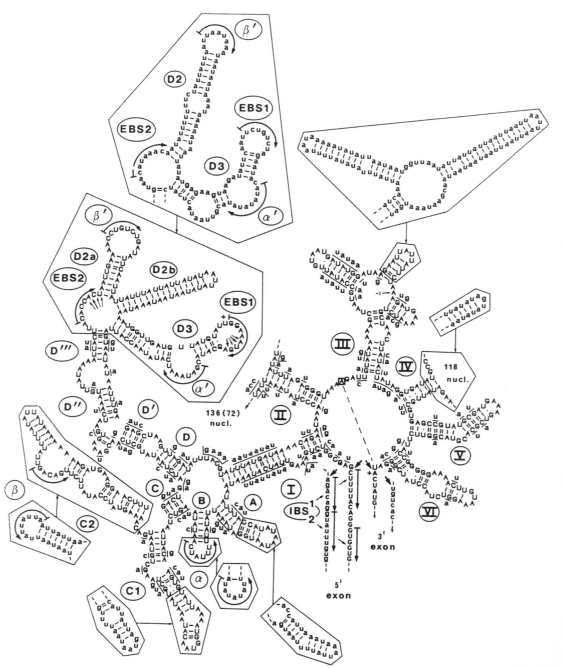

Figure 2. Secondary structure models of introns a5 and b1. The sequence of intron a5 (uppercase letters) is from Bonitz et al. (1980) and the sequence of intron b1 (lowercase letters; only those nucleotides that differ from their counterparts in intron a5 are shown) is from Schmelzer et al. (1983), except at position 175 (a G, as in Lazowska et al. 1983). Short, straight arrows point to 5′ and 3′ intron-exon junctions. Long curved arrows indicate proven or putative long-distance pairings, whether between intron and exon (EBS and IBS sites) or within the intron (the latter are designated by Greek letters; the α-α′ pairing is very well supported by comparative evidence [see Fig. 8 in Jacquier and Michel 1987], whereas the β-β′ pairing involves two highly variable sections and is merely tentative). The γ-γ′ tertiary base pair, which joins the last nucleotide of the intron to the squared A in the segment connecting domains II and III, is indicated by a dashed line. A possible extension of the IBS1-EBS1 pairing that would involve the first nucleotide of the a5 3′ exon (see Fig. 1 and text) is suggested by + signs.

where G and A alternate with about equal frequencies. Remarkably, in all introns whose last nucleotide is a C, the γ site is filled by a G, whereas all introns in which that G is replaced by an A happen to have a U as their last nucleotide. Even more striking, in the only class II intron to end with an A (the one in the gene for ribosomal protein L2 of the chloroplasts of higher plants), the γ site happens to be filled with a U (Fig. 1).

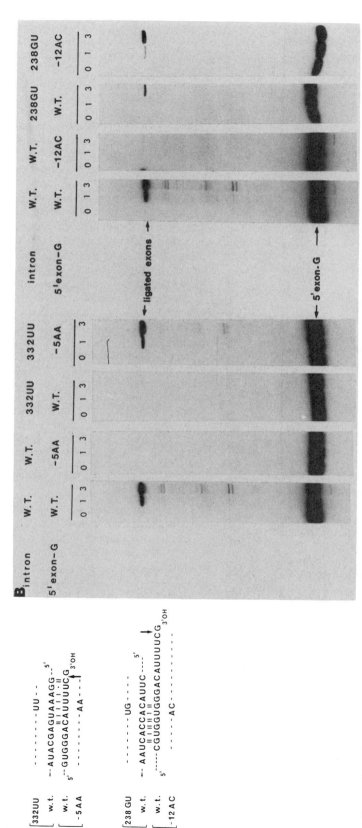

A

EBS1 $\begin{bmatrix} 332UU \\ w.t. \end{bmatrix}$ `- - - - - - UU - -`

IBS1 $\begin{bmatrix} w.t. \\ -5AA \end{bmatrix}$

```
           - -AUACGAGUAAAGG- - - 5'
             | | || | | |  ||   ||
        5' - -GUGGGACAUUUUC G
           - - - - - - -AA - - -↑ 3'OH
```

EBS2 $\begin{bmatrix} 238GU \\ w.t. \end{bmatrix}$ `- - - - - - UG - - - -`

IBS2 $\begin{bmatrix} w.t. \\ -12 AC \end{bmatrix}$

```
        - -AAUCACCACAUUC- - - - 5'
          || ||| || || |        ↓
    5' - - - - -CGUGGUGGGACAUUUUUC G 3'OH
        - - - - - - -AC - - - - - -
```

Figure 3. *Trans*-splicing with mutants in the IBS and EBS sequences. (*A*) IBS1-EBS1 and IBS2-EBS2 pairings and the mutations introduced in each of these four elements. The arrow points to the 5′ splice site. The exonic sequence shown is that of a 5′ exon-G transcript. (*B*) Time course of *trans*-splicing reactions between either wild-type or mutant 5′ exon-G molecules and either wild-type or mutant intron-3′ exon transcripts (see Materials and Methods). Aliquots (1 μl of each reaction) were taken at 0, 1, and 3 hr and loaded on a 6% acrylamide–urea gel (Jacquier and Michel 1987).

205

Mutations at Either the IBS1 (and EBS1) or IBS2 (and EBS2) Sites Affect the Ability to Perform *Trans*-splicing

As shown in Figure 3A, we have introduced mutations within each of the four sequence elements predicted to be involved in the mutual recognition of *S. cerevisiae* intron a5 and its 5' exon. This intron was the first member of class II for which the ability to perform self-splicing in vitro was demonstrated (Peebles et al. 1986; van der Veen et al. 1986), and it was also used by Jacquier and Rosbash (1986) in their *trans*-splicing experiments. To ensure that we would severely disrupt the EBS1-IBS1 and EBS2-IBS2 pairings, each of our four mutations affected two neighboring sites. Moreover, the −5AA (IBS1) and 322UU (EBS1) mutants were chosen so that combining them would restore the EBS1-IBS1 pairing, although with a different sequence, and the same strategy was adopted for mutants −12AC (IBS2) and 238GU (EBS2). (Since both the IBS2 and EBS2 sequences are repetitive, they could be paired in several different ways, but the one shown in Fig. 3 is the most stable.)

A 5' exon transcript carrying mutation −5AA is completely unable to participate in the *trans*-splicing reaction of Jacquier and Rosbash (1986) when incubated with a wild-type transcript of intron a5 and its 3' exon (Fig. 3B). An intron-3' exon transcript carrying mutation 322UU is hardly more efficient when confronted with a wild-type exon. Its residual activity might be ascribed to the fact that a double UU mismatch should be less damaging than a double AA mismatch (generated by the −5AA mutation). However, the point here is that coincubating a −5AA exon with a 322UU intron results in fully normal levels of *trans*-splicing (Fig. 3B), and this proves not only that EBS1-IBS1 pairing actually occurs, but that it is required in *trans*-splicing.

The same type of analysis was done in Figure 3C for the EBS2-IBS2 pairing. Although *trans*-splicing is completely inhibited by mutation −12AC, the 238GU mutation results only in partial impairment of the reaction. But the important point again is that by combining it with 12AC, the mutated exon's ability to participate in the reaction is fully restored, which proves that EBS2-IBS2 pairing actually occurs.

Cis-splicing of Mutants with Altered EBS2-IBS2 Pairings

We have already shown that mutation −5AA in the IBS1 sequence completely blocks the normal, *cis*-splicing reaction, although this reaction can be restored to its wild-type level by combining the −5AA mutant with the 332UU mutant (Jacquier and Michel 1987). However, in contrast to its effects on *trans*-splicing, −12AC in the IBS2 element does not markedly affect the ability of intron a5 to perform *cis*-splicing, and this is true for all EBS2 and IBS2 mutants we have investigated (Fig. 7B in Jacquier and Michel 1987). Only by combining

them with deletion mutants of the 5' exon can effects be observed. These consist primarily of enhanced production of a new splicing product, which we showed was the predicted, but until then elusive, intermediate of the splicing reaction, i.e., an intron lariat with the 3' exon still attached. Our interpretation was that accumulation of that intermediate results from its decreased affinity for the 5' exon when the EBS2-IBS2 pairing is destabilized due to mutations in either the EBS2 or the IBS2 sequences.

One would predict then that partial deletion of the IBS2 site will result in the same phenotype, i.e., accumulation of large amounts of the intron-3' exon lariat. This is shown to be the case in Figure 4B. Incubation under self-splicing conditions of Δ13 transcripts (in which the EBS2-IBS2 pairing should be reduced to only 3 bp due to extensive deletion of the a5 5' exon; see Fig. 4A) yields almost as much intron-3' exon lariat as intron lariat. Conversely, the ratio of inron-3' exon lariat to intron lariat can be considerably decreased by combining the Δ13 mutant with intron mutant 241GU in the EBS2 sequence (lanes 3 and 4), which restores two out of the three missing base pairs, even though their constituent nucleotides differ from the wild-type nucleotides (Fig. 4A). More of a surprise is the fact that combining the Δ13 exon with intron mutant 238GU results in much the same phenotype as that of Δ13 alone, even though nothing should now be left of the IBS2-EBS2 pairing (Fig. 4A). One possible interpretation is that, because they are repetitive, the modified EBS2 and IBS2 sequences can still pair, although in an altered and less efficient way when compared to the wild type (Fig. 4A). Such a possibility would also account for the different phenotypes of our Δ13 mutant and the +11 (= Δ11) mutant of van der Veen et al. (1987), in which nearly all of the IBS2 element was deleted and which shows no splicing activity at all (see also discussion in Jacquier and Michel 1987).

Does the a5 3' Exon Contain Any Information Essential to Splicing?

Contrary to its *S. cerevisiae* b1 sibling, intron a5 is one of the subclass IIB introns in which the first nucleotide of the 3' exon (here an A) could pair with that immediately upstream of the EBS1 sequence (here a U). In an attempt to determine whether this pairing plays some part in the splicing process, we mutated the first residue of the a5 3' exon to C (Fig. 5A). As shown in Figure 5B, this results in no detectable phenotype. In addition (data not shown), combining this +1C mutant with EBS1 mutant 332UU results in no distinct phenotype compared with that of 332UU alone, even though the two mutations should alter the same structure according to the RNA guide hypothesis.

The +1C mutation happens to create a GGATCC (*Bam*HI) site at the 3' intron-exon junction. Cleavage by *Bam*HI followed by in vitro transcription and incubation under splicing conditions leads to a very efficient

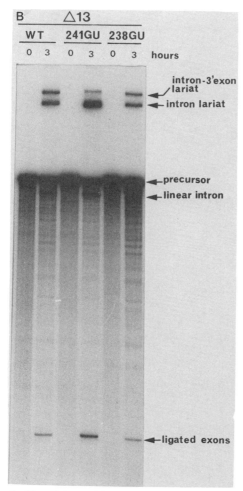

A
Δ52 exon   5' gaaua/45n/ACGUGGUGGGACAUUUUC 3'
                         ‖ ‖ ‖‖‖ ‖‖
wild-type intron   3' AAUCACCACAUUC 5'

Δ13 5' exon   5' gaauacaagcuugcGUGGGACAUUUUC 3'
                              ‖ ‖ ‖‖
wild-type intron   3' AAUCACCACAUUC 5'

Δ13 5' exon   5' gaauacaagcuugcGUGGGACAUUUUC 3'
                              ‖ ‖ ‖‖
241GU intron   3' AAUCUGCACAUUC 5'

Δ13 5' exon   5' uugcGUGGGACA 3'   5' uugcGUGGGACA 3'
                        ‖‖   ‖‖‖‖‖
238GU intron   3' CACCUGAUUC 5'   or   5' AAUCACCUGAUUC 3'

B   **△13**

WT   241GU   238GU

0   3   0   3   0   3   hours

intron-3'exon
/lariat
← intron lariat

← precursor
← linear intron

← ligated exons

Figure 4. *Cis*-splicing activity of a partial deletion of the IBS2 sequence combined with either wild-type or mutant versions of the EBS2 sequence. (*A*) Possible pairings between a Δ13 5' exon (Jacquier and Michel 1987) and either wild-type or mutant versions of the EBS2 sequence. *S. cerevisiae*-derived segments are in uppercase letters and those derived from pSP64 are in lowercase letters. (*B*) RNAs were synthesized by SP6 transcription, in the presence of [α-³²P]UTP, of *Eco*RI digests of the original Δ13 plasmid (lane W.T.), or Δ13 plasmids carrying mutations 241GU and 238GU, respectively. An aliquot of each transcript was incubated for 0, 1, or 3 hr at 45°C in standard splicing buffer and analyzed on a 4% acrylamide gel. For the identification and designation of the various products of the reaction, see Jacquier and Michel (1987).

production of intron lariats (Fig. 5B, lanes 7–9). The 3' exon sequences therefore play no part in the first step of the reaction, consisting of cleavage at the 5' intron-

exon junction and simultaneous formation of the 2',5'-phosphodiester bond between the first intron nucleotide and the bulging A, eight nucleotides upstream of the 3' intron-exon junction (Peebles et al. 1986; Schmelzer and Schweyen 1986; van der Veen et al. 1986; Jacquier and Michel 1987).

We also took advantage of the *Bam*HI site to substitute the 3' exon of intron a5 with different sequences by in vitro recombination. The effects of two such substitutions are shown in Figure 5B. Mutation E3-1 (see Materials and Methods) has clear-cut effects, yielding about equal amounts of two products, whose mobilities are compatible with those of the intron lariat and a lariat intermediate with a 195-nucleotide-long 3' exon, respectively. Such an outcome is expected if mutation E3-1 severely decreases the rate of the second step of the splicing reaction (consisting of cleavage at the 3' intron-exon junction and simultaneous ligation of the exons). This should result in a corresponding increase in the lifetime of the intermediate splicing complex and, consequently, in the concentration of intron-3' exon lariat; the underlying assumption is that cleavage at the 3' intron-exon junction is not the limiting step in the in vitro splicing process. Close examination of the sequence of the E3-1 mutant provides a ready interpretation for its inability to perform efficient cleavage at the 3' intron-exon junction. Because the substituted 3' exon of the E3-1 mutant happens to be complementary to the 3' branch of helix VI, substituting it for the wild-type one could lead to formation of the alternative structure shown in Figure 5A, which is very unlikely to allow cleavage at the 3' intron extremity; note, however, that this competitor structure is such a good mimic of the real one that it might support formation of the lariat bond at its normal site on the bulging A nucleotide of helix VI.

In contrast to the exon of mutant E3-1, the E3-2 3' exon was designed to interfere as little as possible with the predicted structures at the 3' end of intron a5. As shown in Figure 5B, lanes 10–12, E3-2 transcripts are nearly as efficient as wild-type transcripts in catalyzing the splicing of their exons. However, the reaction also yields detectable amounts of a product with the mobility expected for the E3-2 lariat intermediate (the E3-2 exon is 54 nucleotides long; see Fig. 5), which we interpret again as reflecting a somewhat decreased ability for cleaving the 3' intron-exon junction. We are currently testing the behavior of a number of other 3' exon substitutes with the aim of determining whether the wild-type a5 3' exon is optimal, and if so, why.

The Rate of Cleavage at the 3' Intron-Exon Junction Depends on the Last Intron Nucleotide Being Able to Pair with the One at the γ Site

To investigate the role of the γ-γ' pairing in the splicing process, we introduced mutations at both of the sites involved, i.e., positions 587 (γ) and 887 (last nucleotide of intron a5). But neither mutation 587G, which replaces the wild-type A-U pair by a G-U pair,

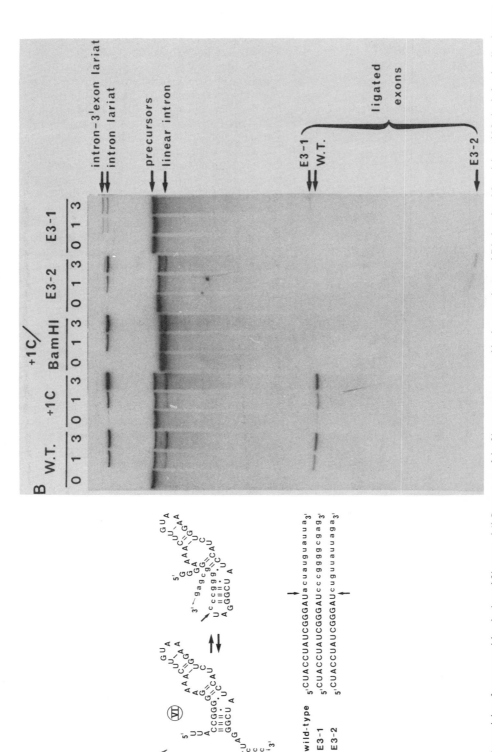

Figure 5. Splicing activity of mutants with substituted 3′ exons. (*A*) Sequences of the 3′ exons. (*A*) Sequences of the 3′ exon mutants used in the experiment of *B* below (see Materials and Methods for details of construction), together with two possible competing structures for helix VI in mutant E3-1. Arrows point to the 3′ intron-exon junction. (*B*) RNAs were synthesized by SP6 transcription, in the presence of [α-³²P]UTP, of the following DNAs: (lanes W.T. and +1C) Plasmids Δ52 and +1C digested by *Eco*RI; (lanes +1C/*Bam*HI) plasmid +1C digested by *Bam*HI; (lane E3-1) plasmid E3-1 digested by *Pvu*II; (lane E3-2) plasmid E3-2 digested by *Eco*RI. An aliquot of each transcript was incubated for 0, 1, and 3 hr at 45°C in standard splicing buffer and analyzed on a 4% acrylamide gel.

nor mutation 887C, which results in an A-C mismatch (assuming the γ-γ' pair to be a classic one), had any detectable effect on splicing in vitro. One possible explanation was that destruction of the γ-γ' pairing has only moderate effects on the rate of cleavage at the 3' junction cleavage, and these could not be detected, because cleavage at the 5' intron-exon junction was the limiting step in the splicing process. We therefore transferred our mutations in a Δ24 context, our reasoning being that the phenotype of mutants with an unstable intermediate splicing complex should be sensitive even to rather subtle variations in the rate of the second step of the splicing reaction. This is indeed the case, as shown in Figure 6. Introduction of mutation 887C in Δ24 transcripts leads to a fourfold increase in the ratio of intron-3' exon lariat over intron lariat, which we interpret as reflecting a corresponding decrease in the rate of cleavage at the 3' intron-exon junction. (Since Δ24 5' exon transcripts cannot participate in *trans*-splicing [Jacquier and Michel 1987], dissociation of the intermediate complex is therefore irreversible, and the ratio of intron to intron-3' exon lariats should be determined solely by the relative rates of the reactions that liberate these products, i.e., cleavage at the 3' junction and dissociation of the complex between intron-3' exon and 5' exon, respectively.) But once again, the main point is that mutation 587G compensates

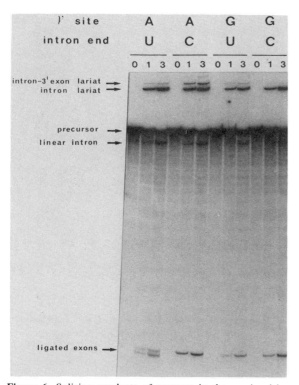

Figure 6. Splicing products of mutants in the γ-γ' pairing. RNAs were synthesized by SP6 transcription, in the presence of [α-³²P]UTP, of *Eco*RI-digested plasmids carrying the mutations indicated at the top of the figure. An aliquot of each transcript was incubated for 0, 1, and 3 hr at 45°C in standard splicing buffer and analyzed on a 4% acrylamide gel.

mutation 887C, and doubly mutated transcripts yield even lower amounts of intron-3' exon lariat than wild-type transcripts, i.e., replacing the γ-γ' (A-U) pair of intron a5 by a G-C pair *increases* the rate of cleavage at the 3' intron-exon junction (~2.5-fold).

DISCUSSION

Figure 7 summarizes the state of our knowledge concerning structural elements involved in specific steps of the splicing pathway of class II introns, on the basis of the data presented here and elsewhere (Jacquier and Michel 1987). The available evidence is critically reviewed below.

Stability of the Intermediate Splicing Complex Is Ensured by Multiple Intron-Exon Interactions

Recognition and binding of their 5' exons by class II introns are necessary to prevent the two molecules from diffusing away from each other after cleavage at the 5' intron-exon junction. It was only reasonable to assume that the EBS1-IBS1 and EBS2-IBS2 intron-exon pairings, which are universal or nearly so in class II members (Fig. 1), would play a major part at that particular stage of the splicing reaction. That this inference was correct was checked by (at least partially) disrupting the EBS-IBS helices in *S cerevisiae* intron a5 EBS1 mutation 332UU (Jacquier and Michel 1987), and, when placed in specific 5' exon contexts, the various mutations we introduced in the EBS2 and IBS2 sequence elements (see, e.g., Fig. 4) all resulted in a partially aborted splicing reaction, through accumulation of a new splicing product. We also showed that this product is the expected reaction intermediate, i.e., a lariat with the 3' exon still attached. Two distinct interpretations might yet have been contemplated: Accumulation of the intron-3' exon and 5' exon splicing intermediates could be due either to weakened intermolecular bonds, leading to premature dissociation of the complex, or to a delay in the second step of the splicing process, i.e., cleavage at the 3' intron-exon junction. That the former explanation is the most likely to be correct is shown by the fact that the same mutations that result in production of the intron-3' exon lariat also prevent *trans*-splicing between 5' exon and intron-3' exon transcripts (Fig. 3).

The presence of the IBS1 and IBS2 elements, i.e., of the last 16 nucleotides of the upstream exon, is nevertheless not sufficient to ensure full recognition by the a5 intron of its 5' exon. Only exons with more than 35 nucleotides will engage in *trans*-splicing (Jacquier and Michel 1987). In addition, *cis*-splicing with mutants retaining 24 or even 35 nucleotides of the a5 5' exon still yields detectable amounts of the intron-3' exon lariat. Mutations in the EBS2 and IBS2 sequences do not manifest themselves in *cis* unless partially truncated 5' exons are used. All this points to some sort of information being used in intron-exon recognition that lies somewhere between positions −35 and −52. Either

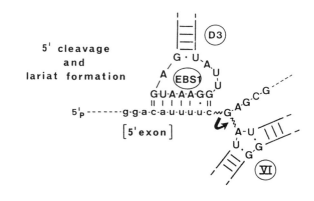

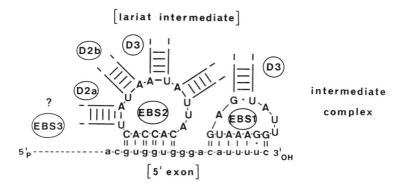

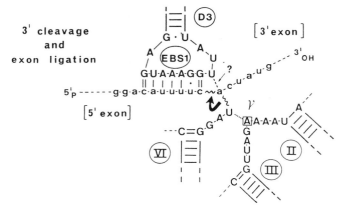

Figure 7. Structural elements involved at specific stages of the class II self-splicing process. Nucleotides that are part of *S. cerevisiae* intron a5 are in uppercase letters and exonic sequences are in lowercase letters.

there is some sequence element that acts indirectly by facilitating access to the IBS sites or the a5 5′ exon includes a third intron-binding site, whose intron counterpart was missed by our comparative sequence analyses because the interaction was specific to intron a5. Whatever the final answer, it is worth noting that covalent attachment of the a5 intron to its 5′ exon drives the latter into a more accessible conformation, since both point mutations and exon truncations have much more severe effects in *trans* than in *cis*.

Cleavage at the 5′ and 3′ Intron-Exon Junctions Involves Long-distance Base Pairings

It was already known from *trans*-splicing experiments (Jacquier and Rosbash 1986) that cleavage at the a5 5′ intron-exon junction necessitates neither a covalent link between the 5′ exon and sequences beyond the first intron nucleotide (a G) nor even formation of the lariat bond between that G and the bulging A of helix VI (even though the two reactions are normally coupled). The inescapable conclusion was that the intron-exon junction was made labile primarily by an interaction between the 5' exon and some unknown, presumably remote element of intron a5. We have now identified that interaction: Contrary to the other mutations we introduced in intron a5 and its exons, mutations 332UU in EBS1 and −5AA in IBS1 have marked effects on the rate of the first step of the splicing process, estimated from the rate of production of intron and intron-3' exon lariats in *cis* (Jacquier and Michel 1987). Cleavage at the 5' intron extremity appears therefore to rest on formation of the EBS1-IBS1 helix, which always extends down to the intron-exon boundary (except perhaps in the chloroplast tRNA glycine introns, where a terminal G-A pair would have to be invoked; see Fig. 1). The questions now, which can be answered only by additional mutageneses, are (1) Is there a strict requirement in vitro for the last nucleotide of the 5' exon taking part in the EBS1-IBS1 pairing or are some mismatches tolerated at that site? (2) Would *trans*-splicing work with 5' exon-*N* transcripts, where *N* would be just any nucleotide?

Cleavage at the 3' intron-exon junction also depends in part on one of the nucleotides next to the intron-exon boundary becoming involved in a long-distance base pairing, but the base pair (γ-γ') appears to be a solitary one and the nucleotide involved is on the intron (not exon) side of the junction. Moreover, the γ-γ' pairing is not strictly necessary for the second step of the reaction to occur: Substitution of the normal A-U pair by an A-C pair is clearly detrimental but does not prevent production of spliced exons (Fig. 6). Also, at least one of the nucleotides at the γ and γ' sites must be subject to some other constraint than merely base pairing with its partner, since only rarely do class II introns end with a nucleotide other than C or U. One may wonder, for example, whether it will suffice to put a C at the γ site and G at the γ' site to obtain a viable version of intron a5 that would end in AG, like its counterparts in nucleus-encoded pre-mRNAs.

Specificity of Exon Recognition by Class II Introns: An Evolutionary Perspective

Even though some class II introns encode proteins related to the reverse transcriptases of retroviruses (Michel and Lang 1985), whether they are bona fide transposable elements remains highly debatable (for discussion, see Flavell 1985). Nevertheless, the facts are that present-day members of class II occupy a wide variety of exonic environments, as is evident from Figure 1. If we are to reach any deep understanding of the duplication/diversification process experienced by their ancestors, the extent of interdependence of class II introns and their exons must be correctly assessed.

Although it is obvious by now that recognition by class II introns of their 5' exons is highly specific, much less information is available concerning possible interactions with 3' exons. In subclass IIA, the nucleotide immediately upstream of EBS1 is clearly constrained to

remain complementary to the first nucleotide of the downstream exon (Fig. 1), which is readily accounted for by the "guide hypothesis" of Davies et al. (1982), originally proposed for class I introns. Whether some subclass IIB members make use of such a device is doubtful, given the lack of good statistical evidence, on the one hand, and our failure to affect splicing by changing from A to C the nucleotide immediately downstream from the 3' intron-exon junction of intron a5 (Fig. 5). Clearly, the a5 3' exon cannot be replaced by just any sequence, as shown by the effects of the E3-1 or even E3-2 substitutions (Fig. 5). At present, this cannot be interpreted as evidence of interactions between intron a5 and its downstream exon, a possibility also unsupported so far by comparative sequence analyses. What might be envisioned, on the other hand, is base pairing between the 5' and 3' exons of class II introns, which, by competing with the EBS1-IBS1 and EBS2-IBS2 pairings, would help drive the reaction forward, ensuring that the ligated exons become liberated as soon as splicing is completed. Partial complementarity of the upstream and downstream exons is clearly a fact for those class II introns that inserted themselves into the anticodon loop of a number of chloroplast tRNA genes. The 5' and 3' exons of intron a5 could pair in a number of different ways, and we are presently attempting to determine whether any of these potential pairings plays some part in the splicing process.

Coevolution of class II introns and their exonic environment may be governed by chance events alone, or alternatively, it might turn out to be the outcome of organized transposition processes. Whatever the final answer, a critical piece of information lies in the exact number of mutations needed to adapt a class II intron to new surroundings. Inspection of Figure 1 suggests that there are very few constraints on the sequence of the EBS1 and IBS1 elements, except for the need to pair with each other. All that may be worth noting is that in subclass IIA, the first nucleotide of the downstream exon is not normally a G, except in those introns (the chloroplast tRNA IIe and tRNA Ala introns and *S. pombe* intron b1) that start with a U (Fig. 1). This may be easily rationalized by invoking the need for that nucleotide to pair with the one immediately upstream of EBS1, and the possible necessity to avoid filling the latter site with a C (except in introns that do not start with a G), failing which the EBS1-IBS1 pairing would extend beyond the 5' intron-exon junction; note, however, that no such restrictions appear to hold in subclass IIB.

The possibility nevertheless remains that some sites of the EBS1 and IBS1 sequences, especially those closest to the intron-exon junction, must be filled by particular nucleotides in a given class II intron. Whether that is the case can be ascertained only by additional mutageneses, but it seems unlikely at present that some of the highly conserved core elements of class II introns will turn out to interact directly with the EBS1 or EBS2 elements. Rather, the type of organization shown by class II introns, with the elements responsible for exon specificity being relegated at the far end of a large structural domain, would seem to be destined to favor coevolution of intron and "substrate" by minimizing contact with the invariant core elements.

ACKNOWLEDGMENTS

We thank our colleagues L. Colleaux, A. Perrin, and C. Monteilhet for pleasant discussions. We are especially grateful to B. Dujon for his comments and criticisms. This work was supported by grant 861007 from INSERM.

REFERENCES

Been, M.D. and T.R. Cech. 1986. One binding site determines sequence specificity of *Tetrahymena* pre-rRNA self-splicing, *trans*-splicing, and RNA enzyme activity. *Cell* **47:** 207.

Bonitz, S.G., G. Coruzzi, B.E. Thanlenfeld, A. Tzagoloff, and G. Macino. 1980. Assembly of the mitochondrial membrane system: Structure and nucleotide sequence of the gene coding for subunit 1 of yeast cytochrome oxidase. *J. Biol. Chem.* **255:** 11927.

Burke, J.M. and U.L. RajBhandary. 1982. Intron within the large rRNA gene of *N. crassa* mitochondria: A long open reading frame and a consensus sequence possibly important in splicing. *Cell* **31:** 509.

Cech, T.R., N.K. Tanner, I. Tinoco, Jr., B.R. Weir, M. Zuker, and P.S. Perlman. 1983. Secondary structure of the *Tetrahymena* ribosomal RNA intervening sequence: Structural homology with fungal mitochondrial intervening sequences. *Proc. Natl. Acad. Sci.* **80:** 3903.

Davies, R.W., R.B. Waring, J.A. Ray, T.A. Brown, and C. Scazzocchio. 1982. Making ends meet: A model for RNA splicing in fungal mitochondria. *Nature* **300:** 719.

Flavell, A. 1985. Introns continue to amaze. *Nature* **316:** 574.

Fox, T.D. and C.J. Leaver. 1981. The *Zea mays* mitochondrial gene coding cytochrome oxidase subunit II has an intervening sequence and does not contain TGA codons. *Cell* **26:** 315.

Garriga, G., A.M. Lambowitz, T. Inoue, and T.R. Cech. 1986. Mechanism of recognition of the 5' splice site in self-splicing group I introns. *Nature* **322:** 86.

Jacquier, A. and F. Michel. 1987. Multiple exon-binding sites in class II self-splicing introns. *Cell* **50:** 17.

Jacquier, A. and M. Rosbash. 1986. Efficient *trans*-splicing of a yeast mitochondrial RNA group II intron implicates a strong 5' exon-intron interaction. *Science* **234:** 1099.

Inouye, S. and M. Inouye. 1986. Oligonucleotide-directed mutagenesis using double-stranded plasmid DNA. In *DNA and RNA synthesis* (ed. S. Narang). Academic Press, New York.

Lang, B.F., F. Ahne, and L. Bonen. 1985. The mitochondrial genome of the fission yeast *Schizosaccharomyces pombe*: The cytochrome b gene has an intron closely related to the first two introns in the *Saccharomyces cerevisiae* cox1 gene. *J. Mol. Biol.* **184:** 353.

Lazowska, J., A. Gargouri, and P.P. Slonimski. 1983. The corrected sequence of the first intron of the *cob-box* gene in the yeast strain 777-3A. In *Mitochondria 1983* (ed. R.J. Schweyen et al.), p. 405. Walter de Gruyter, Berlin.

Matsuura, E.T., J.M. Domenico, and D.J. Cummings. 1986. An additional class II intron with homology to reverse transcriptase in rapidly senescing *Podospora anserina*. *Curr. Genet.* **10:** 915.

Michel, F. and B. Dujon. 1983. Conservation of RNA secondary structures in two intron families including mitochondrial-, chloroplast-, and nuclear-encoded members. *EMBO J.* **2:** 33.

Michel, F. and B.F. Lang. 1985. Mitochondrial class II introns encode proteins related to the reverse transcriptases of retroviruses. *Nature* **316:** 641.

Michel, F., A. Jacquier, and B. Dujon. 1982. Comparison of fungal mitochondrial introns reveals extensive homologies in RNA secondary structure. *Biochimie* **64:** 867.

Ohyama, K., H. Fukuzawa, T. Kohchi, H. Shirai, T. Sano, S. Sano, K. Umesono, Y. Shiki, M. Takeuchi, Z. Chang, S. Aota, H. Inokuchi, and H. Ozeki. 1986. Chloroplast gene organization deduced from complete sequence of liverwort *Marchantia polymorpha* chloroplast DNA. *Nature* **332:** 572.

Osiewacz, H.D. and K. Esser. 1984. The mitochondrial plasmid of *Podospora anserina*: A mobile intron of a mitochondrial gene. *Curr. Genet.* **8:** 299.

Peebles, C.L., P.S. Perlman, K.L. Mecklenburg, M.L. Petrillo, J.H. Tabor, K.A. Jarrell, and H.-L. Cheng. 1986. A self-splicing RNA excises an intron lariat. *Cell* **44:** 213.

Perea, J. and C. Jacq. 1985. Role of the 5' hairpin structure in the splicing accuracy of the fourth intron of the yeast *cob-box* gene. *EMBO J.* **4:** 3281.

Schmelzer, C. and R.J. Schweyen. 1986. Self-splicing of group II introns in vitro: Mapping of the branch point and mutational inhibition of lariat formation. *Cell* **46:** 557.

Schmelzer, C., C. Schmidt, K. May, and R.J. Schweyen. 1983. Determination of functional domains in intron bI1 of yeast mitochondrial RNA by studies of mitochondrial mutations and a nuclear suppressor. *EMBO J.* **2:** 2047.

Shinozaki, K., M. Ohme, M. Tanaka, T. Wakasugi, N. Hayashida, T. Matsubayashi, N. Zaita, J. Chunwongse, K. Obokata, K. Yamaguchi-Shinozaki, C. Ohto, K. Torozawa, B.Y. Meng, M. Sugita, H. Deno, T. Kamogashira, K. Yamada, J. Kusuda, F. Takaiwa, A. Kato, N. Tohdoh, H. Shmida, and M. Sugiura. 1986. The complete nucleotide sequence of tobacco chloroplast genome: Its gene organization and expression. *EMBO J.* **5:** 2043.

van der Veen, R., A.C. Arnberg, and L.A. Grivell. 1987. Self-splicing of a group II intron in yeast mitochondria: dependence on 5'-exon sequences. *EMBO J.* **6:** 1079.

van der Veen, R., A.C. Arnberg, G. van der Horst, L. Bonen, H.F. Tabak, and L.A. Grivell. 1986. Excised group II introns in yeast mitochondria are lariats and can be formed by self-splicing in vitro. *Cell* **44:** 225.

Waring, R.B. and R.W. Davies. 1984. Assessment of a model for intron RNA secondary structure relevant to RNA self-splicing — A review. *Gene* **28:** 277.

Waring, R.B., C. Scazzocchio, T.A. Brown, and R.W. Davies. 1983. Close relationship between certain nuclear and mitochondrial introns. *J. Mol. Biol.* **167:** 595.

Waring, R.B., P. Towner, S.J. Minter, and R.W. Davies. 1986. Splice-site selection by a self-splicing RNA of *Tetrahymena*. *Nature* **321:** 133.

Reactions Mediated by Yeast Mitochondrial Group I and II Introns

H.F. Tabak, G. Van der Horst, A.J. Winter, J. Smit, R. Van der Veen,
J.H.J.M. Kwakman, L.A. Grivell, and A.C. Arnberg*

*Section for Molecular Biology, Laboratory of Biochemistry, University of Amsterdam, Kruislaan 318, 1098 SM
Amsterdam, The Netherlands; *Laboratory of Biochemistry, University of Groningen,
Nijenborgh 16, 9747 AG Groningen, The Netherlands*

Mitochondria of *Saccharomyces cerevisae* contain a circular genome of about 80 kbp that encodes rRNAs, tRNAs, an RNA involved in tRNA processing, and proteins that function in the respiratory chain complexes or in RNA splicing. Three genes, coding for large rRNA, apocytochrome *b*, and subunit I of cytochrome oxidase, are interrupted by intervening sequences, whose properties have been revealed by DNA sequence analysis and genetic studies. Most contain long open reading frames, often in-phase with the preceding exon, together with short sequences that are well conserved among several introns. Genetic and Northern blot analyses showed that splicing of the fourth cytochrome *b* intron was blocked in a mutant with a disturbed intronic reading frame. Splicing could be restored, however, by providing a wild-type allele in *trans*, suggesting that the intron internal reading frame is translated into a diffusable (protein) product ("maturase"), involved in excision of the intron by which it is coded (for review, see Dujon 1981; Tabak and Grivell 1986). Direct proof for this proposal was reported by Banroques et al. (1986), who adapted the reading frame of the fourth intron of the apocytochrome *b* gene to the "cytoplasmic" genetic code and supplied the modified gene with a mitochondrial import signal. A yeast strain with a mutation in the reading frame of this fourth intron was indeed restored to respiratory competence after the introduction of the DNA construct into the cell, indicating that correct splicing had taken place.

Mutations in the short conserved sequences also block intron splicing, but they are *cis*-dominant in a complementation test, indicating the importance of intron RNA sequences per se in splicing. From analysis of second-site suppressor mutants, it became clear that some of these sequences interact with each other via base pairing, suggesting a contribution in the formation of intron secondary structure (Holl et al. 1985). On the basis of these results and a comparison of intron RNA sequences, secondary structure models were proposed and a distinction was made between two families of introns, group I and group II (Michel and Dujon 1983). A particularly interesting feature of the group I RNA structure is the possible base pairing of the exon borders with a complementary intron sequence, the so-called internal guide sequence (IGS) (Davies et al. 1982).

Insight into the role of the folding of group I introns came from an independent line of research on an intron present in the nuclear genome of *Tetrahymena thermophila*. This intron mediates its own excision from ribosomal precursor RNA (self-splicing) and behaves in many ways like an enzyme (Cech et al. 1981). Sequence comparison showed that the *Tetrahymena* intron is a member of the group I family (Cech et al. 1983), and it was subsequently shown that some of the fungal mitochondrial introns (including group II introns) also display self-splicing in vitro (Garriga and Lambowitz 1984; Van der Horst and Tabak 1985; Peebles et al. 1986; Van der Veen et al. 1986).

The mechanisms of the group I and II self-splicing reactions are compared in Figure 1. All of the yeast mitochondrial group I introns obey the rules established for the self-splicing *Tetrahymena* intron (Cech 1986): The 3'-OH of a guanosine nucleotide attacks the 5' splice site and adds to the 5' end of the intron RNA. The 5' exon–3'-OH subsequently opens the 3' splice site and adds to the 3' exon. The 3'-terminal G of the excised intron attacks an internucleotide bond at the

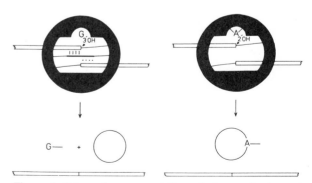

Figure 1. Schematic representation of the mechanism of group I and group II self-splicing reactions. Black spheres symbolize the RNA tertiary structure with the reaction center, in which the splice sites are supposed to take position in the middle. The 5'-exon border is shown base-paired with the internal splice guide (thick bar), and the guanosine nucleotide is shown hydrogen-bonded in the reactive center of the group I intron RNA (*left*). The major part of the intron RNA accumulates in circular form. In the group II reaction (*right*), the attacking nucleotide (*A*), represented in the reactive center, is part of the intron RNA itself. Excised intron RNA accumulates as a lariat.

beginning of the intron, which circularizes itself while a short 5′ segment is eliminated. For every bond broken, a new one is made (transesterification), and no external source of energy is required. Self-splicing of group II introns occurs independently of a guanosine nucleotide (Peebles et al. 1986; Van der Veen et al. 1986). In this case, the 2′-OH of an intron-internal adenine ribonucleotide presumably serves as the attacking group to open the 5′ splice site. The 5′ exon–3′-OH attacks the 3′ splice site in a manner analogous to the group I reaction. The fate of the excised intron RNA, however, is different. It accumulates in the form of a lariat with the 5′-intron terminal nucleotide linked via a 2′-5′ phosphodiester bond to the intron-internal A. The branch point is located close to the 3′ splice site, resulting in a short tail. Excised group II introns purified from mitochondrial RNA preparations appear in the electron microscope as circular molecules (Arnberg et al. 1980). Primer extension with reverse transcriptase on such seemingly circular molecules leads to a strong stop at the position of the branch point, indicating that the circles are actually lariats. Lariats therefore also exist in vivo and are bona fide products of mitochondrial group II splicing (Grivell et al. 1983).

The simple techniques to synthesize experimental precursor RNAs with group I or group II introns in vitro allow one to investigate the reactions in detail and to study the effects of deletions, insertions, and nucleotide substitutions on self-splicing. Here, we describe our results on three group I introns and one group II intron derived from yeast mitochondrial DNA.

METHODS

The construction of recombinant DNA clones with yeast mitochondrial inserts behind the SP6 promoter has been described previously (Van der Horst and Tabak 1985; Van der Veen et al. 1986). In some cases, the mitochondrial DNA inserts were recloned behind the T7 promoter. Deletions and point mutations were introduced by standard techniques (Maniatis et al. 1982), and procedures for analysis of RNA-splicing products have been described previously (Van der Horst and Tabak 1985; Arnberg et al. 1986; Tabak et al. 1987). A more detailed account of the clones shown in Figure 2 will be presented elsewhere.

Two-dimensional polyacrylamide gel electrophoresis was carried out as follows: A 4% slab gel was electrophoresed in the first dimension. After completion, one glass plate was removed, and the strip containing the lane with separated RNA products was cut free and transferred to a second glass plate precooled at −70°C, changing its orientation by 90°. This plate was mounted with gel spacers and a second glass plate. An 8% gel was poured on top of the gel strip and electrophoresis was resumed. Self-splicing conditions for group II precursor RNA were 100 mM Tris-HCl (pH 7.5), 70 mM MgCl₂, and 200 mM (NH₄)₂ SO₄ at 45°C.

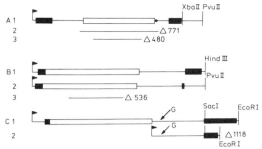

Figure 2. Schematic representation of the recombinant DNA clones used for in vitro synthesis of group-I-intron-containing precursor RNAs. (■) Exons; (□) intron internal reading frames. The closed circle following the reading frame in the rRNA intron (A1) indicates the dodecamer sequence motif. Lines underneath show the introduced deletions and their length in base pairs. Lines extending from exons to the right and left are vector sequences. Bars with closed triangles show the position of the promoter (T7 or SP6). (*A*) Clones containing the complete intron of the large rRNA gene behind the SP6 promoter (pSP65-C21) or the T7 promoter (pT7-C21) and derivatives with deletions of 771 (pT7-C21Δ771) or 480 bp (pT7-C21Δ480). (*B*) Clones containing the intron aI5α of the cytochrome oxidase subunit I gene with a large part of the 3′ exon (pT7-aI5α/1), a shorter part of the 3′ exon (pSP-aI5α/2), and a derivative with a deletion of 536 bp (pSP-aI5αΔ536). (*C*) Clones containing the intron aI3 of the cytochrome oxidase subunit I gene (pT7-aI3) and its truncated version (pT7-aI3Δ1118).

RESULTS

The rI Intron Present in the Large rRNA Gene

The gene coding for large rRNA is split by an intron of 1143 nucleotides (Fig. 2A). It contains a free-standing reading frame that codes for a DNA endonuclease implicated in intron dispersal during mating between intron-containing and intronless strains (Jacquier and Dujon 1985; Macready et al. 1985; Colleaux et al. 1986). The end of this reading frame is marked by a dodecamer sequence also found elsewhere in the mitochondrial genome at positions of transcription termination or RNA processing (see Osinga et al. 1984). Among the intron-containing RNA products present in isolated mitochondria, one finds both linear and circular forms with features that support the existence of a mitochondrial splicing pathway similar to that established for the large rRNA intron of *Tetrahymena*. Moreover, some RNA molecules end at the dodecamer sequence, suggesting a complex transcription and/or processing pathway operative in the coordinate expression of the two interlaced genes located in this genomic region (Tabak et al. 1984).

Experimental precursor RNA containing the large rRNA group I intron shows self-splicing in vitro (Van der Horst and Tabak 1985). Apart from the RNA products predicted on the basis of the group I self-splicing mechanism, a number of unexpected products were found, including (1) a 3′ exon with an extra G covalently attached to its 5′ end, resulting from attack at the 3′ splice site; (2) a complete precursor RNA in which the 5'-terminal G has been replaced by a guanosine nucleotide from the reaction mixture; and (3) lariats. The precursor end labeling is only manifested by RNA synthesized from a DNA insert cloned behind the SP6 promoter. A similar runoff precursor RNA transcribed from the T7 promoter is not end-labeled by incubation with $[\alpha\text{-}^{32}\text{P}]\text{GTP}$, suggesting the importance of the RNA sequence at the 5' end. The G exchange reaction also occurs at the 5' end of excised linear intron RNA. SP6-promoter-derived precursor RNA and intron RNA both possess the sequence 5'-GAA-3' at their 5' ends; this sequence also occurs at the 3' splice site (intron G/AA exon). Since this 5'-GAA-3' sequence can base pair with the IGS, it is possible to explain the reactions that give rise to products 1 and 2 (see above) as variations on the basic group I self-splicing reaction (Van der Horst and Tabak 1987). The lariats formed during the self-splicing reaction have been studied by electron microscopy and have been shown to consist of various subpopulations (Arnberg et al. 1986). This has precluded a biochemical characterization and identification of the branch points in the lariats thus far. Contour length measurements suggest that an appreciable number of lariats correspond in length to complete precursor RNA. We therefore wondered whether the 5'-terminal exchange reaction and lariat formation were based on the same

molecular mechanism. This is unlikely, however, since precursor RNA synthesized from the T7 promoter, of which the 5'-terminal nucleotide cannot be exchanged, does give rise to lariats upon self-splicing (see below; Fig. 4A).

We have constructed large deletions spanning the region of the intron containing the open reading frame (see Fig. 2A) to test the prediction (Michel and Dujon 1983) that this RNA region does not contribute to the self-splicing reaction and to investigate whether a simpler collection of lariats would result if part of the intron is deleted. Both types of RNA precursors are still active in self-splicing, as is evident from analysis by two-dimensional polyacrylamide gel electrophoresis. The simplest pattern of RNA products arises from self-splicing of the precursor RNA with the shortest deletion (Δ480; Fig. 3A). At least four RNAs show abnormal migration and remain in the second dimension above the diagonal formed by the linear RNAs. Some of these may consist of the circular and lariat forms we observed in the electron microscope (see below). Surprisingly, a more complicated picture emerges from self-splicing of the precursor RNA with the largest deletion (Δ771; Fig. 3B). Linear RNA products, such as the excised linear intron RNA, ligated exons, and the precursor RNA itself, migrate in the second dimension according to their length along the

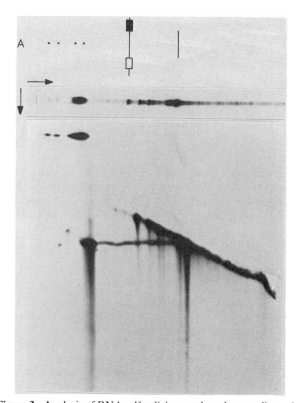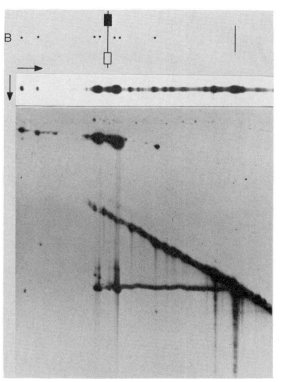

Figure 3. Analysis of RNA self-splicing products by two-dimensional polyacrylamide gel electrophoresis obtained from ribosomal precursor RNAs containing large intron-internal deletions. Sketches next to the RNA products separated in the first dimension indicate the position of splicing products. (□) 5' exon; (■) 3' exon. Line between boxes indicates the intron. Asterisks symbolize RNA products with topological constraint. (*A*) pT7-C21Δ480; (*B*) pT7-C21Δ771. For experimental details, see Methods.

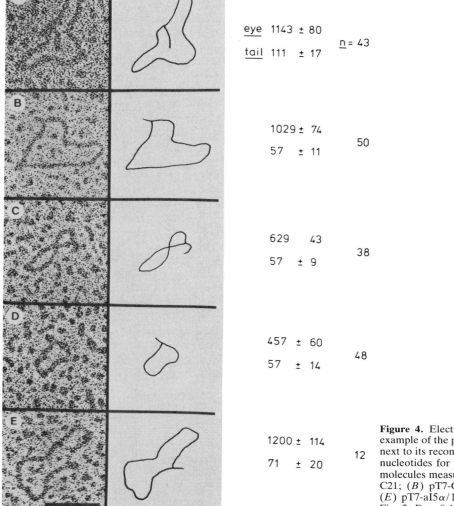

eye 1143 ± 80
                        n = 43
tail 111 ± 17

1029 ± 74
                        50
  57 ± 11

629   43
                        38
 57 ± 9

457 ± 60
                        48
 57 ± 14

1200 ± 114
                        12
  71 ± 20

Figure 4. Electron micrographs of lariats. An example of the predominant lariat class is shown next to its reconstruction. The average length in nucleotides for eye and tail and the number of molecules measured (*n*) are indicated. (*A*) pT7-C21; (*B*) pT7-C21Δ480; (*C,D*) pT7-C21Δ771; (*E*) pT7-aI5α/1. For details about clones, see Fig. 2. Bar, 0.1 μm.

diagonal. Quite a number of RNA products with topological constraint hardly move at all in the second dimension. Some of these have the same electrophoretic mobility as linear intron RNA when released from their topological constraints. Part of the circular or lariat intron RNA molecules (Fig. 3A,B) linearize during electrophoresis in the first dimension and during the preparation to start the second dimension, giving rise to spots and a horizontal streak underneath the diagonal and pointing toward the position of the linear intron RNA. We ascribe this to site-specific cleavage during electrophoresis and handling of the RNA preparation, rather than to random degradation. In an electron microscopy survey of the RNA-splicing products, lariats and circles were again observed, confirming the results obtained by two-dimensional gel analysis. Examples of the major lariat class are shown for each deletion mutant with their respective length measurements (Fig. 4B–D). The results show that both shortened precursor RNAs are still fully active in self-

splicing and unexpectedly give rise to various RNA molecules with topological constraint. We hope that their shorter length and separation in two-dimensional gel electrophoresis will make them more amenable to biochemical analysis.

The Cytochrome Oxidase Subunit I Gene Intron aI5α

The gene coding for subunit I of cytochrome oxidase is interrupted by both group I and group II introns, varying in number from strain to strain. Group I intron aI5α of strain KL14-4A was cloned behind the T7 promoter for synthesis of intron-containing precursor RNA (see Fig. 2B). Upon incubation under standard self-splicing conditions, a number of products arise, demonstrating the capacity to self-splice (Fig. 5a,b). In a provisional analysis including sequence determination by primer extension with reverse transcriptase (not shown), we found the expected products: a circularized

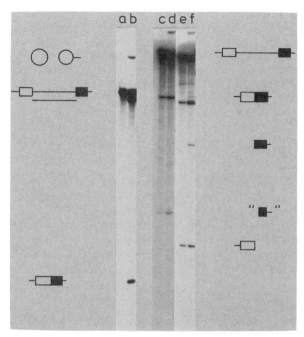

Figure 5. Self-splicing RNA products obtained from aI5α group-I-intron-containing precursor RNA. Sketches represent the position of RNA products. (□) 5' exon; (■) 3' exons. Hyphenated black box indicates the 3' exon opened at the cryptic splice site. (*a, b*) Input and self-splicing products of a 15-min reaction of pT7-aI5α/1 separated on a 3.3% polyacrylamide gel; (*c, d*) input and self-splicing products of a 30-min reaction of pT7-aI5α/1 separated on a 5% polyacrylamide gel; (*e, f*) input and splicing products of pSP-aIαΔ536 under conditions similar to those in *d*.

intron RNA and ligated exons. Again, aberrant products were also observed. Inspection under the electron microscope of RNA species migrating more slowly than precursor RNA showed not only circular RNA molecules, but also lariats (Fig. 4E). Furthermore, no product was found with the size of the 3' exon. Instead, an RNA species appeared that migrated consistently slightly faster than predicted for its length (Fig. 5, lane d vs. f). Primer extension with reverse transcriptase using this RNA as a template identified it as a truncated form of the 3' exon lacking nucleotides at its 5' end. The same molecule can be labeled with $[\alpha\text{-}^{32}P]GTP$ when unlabeled precursor RNA is allowed to splice in the presence of $[\alpha\text{-}^{32}P]GTP$. Partial T1 nuclease digestion on the end-labeled RNA product (not shown) indicates that the G attack is directed at a 3'-exon internal position and takes place within a sequence identical to that found at the 5' splice site. Precursor RNA transcribed from a clone in which this sequence is deleted (see Fig. 2, B2) undergoes G-mediated opening at the authentic 3' splice site, giving rise to a normal 3' exon (Fig. 5f). We therefore propose that a cryptic 5' splice site is efficiently recognized under the in vitro conditions of self-splicing.

Intron aI5α is a typical group I mitochondrial intron, with a large reading frame in-phase with the preceding exon. All of the group I sequence elements are located

in the 3' part of the intron, except for the postulated IGS, which is found close to the 5' splice site. We therefore investigated whether it is possible to delete a large part of the intron-internal reading frame, leaving the IGS intact, without affecting the self-splicing reaction. We show in Figure 5 (lanes e and f) that this is indeed the case: Upon incubation of precursor RNA, shortened by 536 nucleotides (Fig. 2, B3), all of the expected RNA products arise, some only smaller, corresponding to the size of the deletion. The small difference in length between the ligated exon products (Fig. 5, lane d vs. f) is due to the fact that the precursor RNAs were transcribed from different promoters (see Fig. 2B).

The Cytochrome Oxidase Subunit I Gene Intron aI3

We have recently demonstrated that group I intron aI3 containing precursor RNA follows a very intricate pathway of self-splicing under in vitro conditions (Tabak et al. 1987). Precursor and intron RNAs can be opened by G attack at an intron-internal position (see Fig. 2C), and apart from the fully excised intron RNA, two subintronic segments can be formed, accumulating in part as interlocked circles of 1083 and 431 nucleotides. All the group-I-specific sequence elements are located in the distal 431-nucleotide section, suggesting that it contains the functional part of the intron. A recombinant DNA clone containing only this region (Fig. 2, C2) was derived from the original full-length intron clone (Fig. 2, C1) to test this prediction. The unidentified reading frame (URF) containing part of the intron and 5' exon was removed, and the remaining fragment was inserted behind the T7 promoter. In the 3' exon (at positions 2 and 5), two nucleotides were altered by site-directed mutagenesis to create a *Sac*I cleavage site. The coding DNA strand of *Sac*I cut DNA ends with a 5' C that codes for the last guanosine nucleotide of the intron RNA. The 3'-protruding end of the DNA was removed by treatment with DNA polymerase I (Klenow fragment) to prevent abortive transcription continuing on the opposite DNA strand. Transcription leads to a runoff RNA terminating with the 3'-intron guanosine nucleotide. Upon incubation, this RNA gives rise to products (Fig. 6 a,b) identical in size and electrophoretic behavior to that of the linear and circular 431-nucleotide RNAs produced from the original full-length intron clone (Fig. 6c). RNA structures of unidentified nature migrating more slowly than circular 431-nucleotide RNA and precursor RNA are also formed. Together, these reactions indeed attest to the reactivity of this 3' segment of the aI3 intron RNA. Mutations in the 3' exon to create the *Sac*I site, at least one of which being expected to interfere with the postulated interaction of the 3' exon with the IGS, do not effect the self-splicing of full-length precursor RNA (Fig. 6c). This is in line with similar observations made with *Tetrahymena* precursor RNA (Been and Cech 1986).

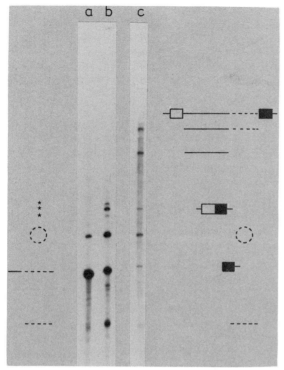

Figure 6. Self-splicing products obtained from precursor RNA transcribed from a truncated group aI3 intron. (a, b) Input and RNA-splicing products of a 30-min reaction of T7-aI3Δ1118 precursor RNA (see Fig. 2, C2); (c) splicing products of full-length pT7-aI3 as a control (see Fig. 2, C1). Sketches indicate positions of RNA products. The 5′ part of the intron is indicated by a continuous line, and the 3′ part is indicated by a dashed line. For further information, see Fig. 5.

The Cytochrome Oxidase Subunit I Gene Intron aI5γ

Intron aI5γ of the cytochrome oxidase subunit I gene is an example of the group II introns. These introns lack the short sequence elements characteristic of group I, and the predicted secondary structure is quite different (Michel and Dujon 1983). The accuracy of these predictions, however, still must be verified by direct biochemical tests. An interesting feature of group II introns is a hairpin located close to the 3′ splice site, which contains the adenine nucleotide to which the 2′-5′ bond of the lariat is made (Van der Veen et al. 1986). This hairpin with the unpaired adenine nucleotide in a bulge is strongly conserved. Nucleotide alterations in and around the hairpin present in the group II intron of the apocytochrome b gene lead to a deficiency in splicing (Schmelzer and Schweyen 1986). To identify sequences involved in catalysis, we have constructed mutant forms of the aI5γ intron. One mutant has a particularly interesting phenotype. It contains an extra uridine nucleotide inserted 25 nucleotides upstream of branch-point A, so that this nucleotide, which normally bulges out, is brought into a base pair. The mutant precursor RNA tested in vitro for self-splicing activity under standard conditions displayed no

activity. However, after increasing the concentration of Mg^{++} and NH_4^+ ions, products of self-splicing activity appear (Fig. 7). They consist predominantly of the ligated exons and the linear form of the intron. Only after prolonged exposure of the autoradiogram could trace amounts of the lariat form of the excised intron be observed. Work is in progress to establish whether the RNA present in the linear intron band is indeed linear. We interpret these results as evidence of a reaction in which splicing occurs in the absence of lariat formation. The alternative—that lariats are formed, but rapidly degraded—cannot be formally excluded, but we consider it unlikely, since time course experiments give no indication for short-lived intermediates (not shown). The conditional nature of this mutant and the deviation from the normal course of the group II self-splicing reaction are remarkable considering the fact that the nucleotide alteration was introduced in a highly conserved region of the intron.

DISCUSSION

Yeast mitochondrial group I introns are rather large, since they often contain reading frames specifying proteins, in addition to the conserved sequence elements implicated in the process of RNA self-splicing. In the case of the intron present in the gene coding for the large rRNA, expression of the intronic reading frame is not essential for maturation of rRNA. In a petite mu-

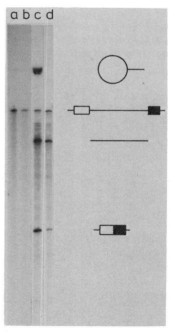

Figure 7. Self-splicing products obtained from a mutant precursor form containing the aI5γ group II intron. (a, c) Input and RNA-splicing products of a 60-min reaction of wild-type precursor RNA (pSP64/6); (b, d) input and splicing products of mutant precursor RNA (pSP-aI5γ + T856). For symbols, see Fig. 5. Products were separated on a 4% polacrylamide gel.

tant, which lacks mitochondrial protein synthesis, large rRNA is normally produced (Tabak et al. 1981). The demonstration that this gene codes for a DNA endonuclease confirms and clarifies this conclusion (Colleaux et al. 1986). In most of the other cases, however, genetic experiments have indicated that the intronic reading frames, often occurring in-phase with the preceding exon, do have a function in intron excision. Biochemical evidence supports this in a more direct way. Splicing of the *Neurospora crassa* group I intron of the large rRNA is dependent in vitro on the addition of a mitochondrial protein extract, and the protein(s) responsible could be partially purified on the basis of the protein-supported splicing reaction (Garriga and Lambowitz 1986). In the case of the *S. cerevisiae* group I introns, we encounter a rather puzzling situation. We have shown that most group I introns show self-splicing under the conditions chosen for the in vitro experiments, indicating that the RNA alone is self-sufficient for splicing. Yet, in a petite mutant, the introns aI3 and aI5α are not spliced out from precursor RNA, presumably because the intronic reading frames cannot be expressed (the continued splicing of large ribosomal precursor RNA in a petite mutant could be supported by import into the organelle of proteins encoded by the nuclear genome). Two possible functions for such proteins can be considered: (1) Conditions in mitochondria deviate from those employed in the in vitro experiments, and the group I introns may not self-splice in vivo. The protein then supplements the RNA catalytic properties of the intron. (2) The in vitro self-splicing process is far from reliable, and we have described the formation of various aberrant RNA products. Their formation is schematically summarized in Figure 8. In mitochondria, such aberrant splicing reactions could be

suppressed by association of protein(s) with the intron RNA core structure. The fact that aberrant splicing is not observed in petite mutants may indicate that both mitochondrion-encoded and nucleus-encoded protein(s) assist in intron excision and that lack of one protein does not result in the formation of abnormal products.

The observation that the proteins specified by the group I introns are not necessary for self-splicing in vitro suggests that we can also dispense with the RNA section corresponding to these reading frames. Indeed, as we have shown here, deleting large parts of these reading frames from precursor RNA does not detract from the "catalytic" properties of the introns.

Interesting RNA products of aberrant group I self-splicing are lariats (Arnberg et al. 1986). Not only do they arise during splicing of large ribosomal precursor RNA, but they have also been observed in the electron microscope among the self-splicing products of aI3- and aI5α-containing precursor RNAs (experiment not shown). The formulation of a mechanism whereby lariats can arise requires a more detailed biochemical characterization of the branch point with respect to both the nature of the chemical bond involved and its position in the precursor RNA sequence. The observation that lariats are still present after splicing of large ribosomal precursor RNA containing partial intron deletions will be of great help for such an investigation. The fact that group I introns can produce lariats that are normal products of group II splicing suggests that despite principal differences between the two mechanisms of self-splicing, some relationships exist as well. This is strengthened by our observation that introduction of a single point mutation in a group II intron results in a self-splicing reaction in which linear intron RNA molecules accumulate instead of lariats. Although proof that self-splicing in this mutant proceeds via a linear intermediate is incomplete, we consider this very likely, however, when we compare our results with those obtained by Jacquier and Rosbash (1986) on *trans*-splicing reactions with the same group II intron. Using two precursor half-molecules inactive by themselves, these authors were able to dissect the group II self-splicing process into partial splicing reactions, and they showed that the formation of the lariat was not an essential prerequisite for either of these. Taken together, these results suggest that group II self-splicing can proceed via linear RNA intermediates in the test tube. Why a reaction proceeding via a lariat structure is preferred in mitochondria cannot yet be answered due to our limited insight in the reaction mechanism.

It is interesting that, from a more detailed study of the various aberrant and partial reactions, a picture emerges in which group I and group II self-splicing mechanisms are less different than initially thought. Moreover, it is also remarkable that the processing of nuclear precursor RNAs synthesized by RNA polymerase II proceeds via a splicing pathway, which is identical in terms of RNA intermediates (lariats) to that followed by group-II-intron-containing precursor RNA.

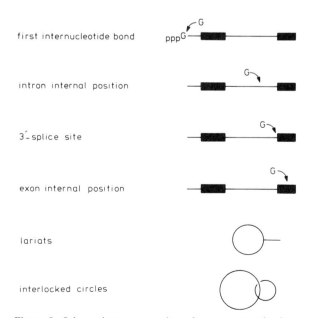

Figure 8. Schematic representation of some yeast mitochondrial group I aberrant splicing reactions and products.

The only difference is that group II intron excision is mediated by *cis*-acting RNA sequence elements within the intron itself, whereas nuclear introns are removed by *trans*-splicing factors. One may therefore wonder whether splicing of group I, group II, and nuclear intron RNA has descended from a common ancestral pathway in which introns were exclusively removed in an RNA-mediated process. It is possible to envisage that only at a later stage proteins were recruited to assist in RNA splicing. The *Tetrahymena* group I intron still strongly resembles this hypothetical progenitor RNA. No protein factor has been found (thus far) that is required for its excision in vivo. Other group I and group II introns, present, for example, in fungal mitochondrial genomes, became dependent on *trans*-acting factors (proteins) for their excision, in addition to the contribution of the intron RNA itself. Nuclear introns may represent the end of the line in this development. They have lost these *cis*-acting RNA sequences involved in self-splicing completely to become entirely dependent on a splicing machinery acting in *trans*. Some of these *trans*-acting factors, however, consist of ribonucleoprotein particles (snRNPs), the RNA components of which can in some cases base pair with the 5' splice site or lariat branch site, respectively (Zhuang and Weiner 1986; Parker et al. 1987). We therefore consider it possible that the snRNAs may have evolved from the *cis*-acting RNA elements originally present in a hypothetical self-splicing progenitor RNA (Arnberg et al. 1986).

ACKNOWLEDGMENTS

We are grateful to Professor P. Borst and Drs. R. Benne and P. Sloof for stimulating discussions. We thank Ms. Y. Mul for her contribution in the two-dimensional gel analysis of RNA products, Dr. R. Benne for his thoughtful comments on the manuscript, and Ms. G.J.M. Schlots for typing the manuscript. This work was supported in part by grants from the Netherlands Foundation for Chemical Research (SON) with financial aid from the Netherlands Organization for the Advancement of Pure Research (ZWO).

REFERENCES

Arnberg, A.C., G. Van der Horst, and H.F. Tabak. 1986. Formation of lariats and circles in self-splicing of the precursor to the large ribosomal RNA of yeast mitochondria. *Cell* 44: 235.

Arnberg, A.C., G.J.B. Van Ommen, L.A. Grivell, E.F.J. Van Bruggen, and P. Borst. 1980. Some yeast mitochondrial RNAs are circular. *Cell* 19: 313.

Banroques, J., A. Delahodde, and C. Jacq. 1986. A mitochondrial RNA maturase gene transferred to the yeast nucleus can control mitochondrial mRNA splicing. *Cell* 46: 837.

Been, M.D. and T.R. Cech. 1986. One binding site determines sequence specificity of *Tetrahymena* pre-rRNA self-splicing, trans-splicing, and RNA enzyme activity. *Cell* 47: 207.

Cech, T.R. 1986. RNA as an enzyme. *Sci. Am.* 254: 64.

Cech, T.R., A.J. Zaug, and P.J. Grabowski. 1981. In vitro splicing of the ribosomal RNA precursor of *Tetrahymena*: Involvement of a guanosine nucleotide in the excision of the intervening sequence. *Cell* 27: 487.

Cech, T.R., N.K. Tanner, I. Tinoco, B.R. Weir, M. Zuker, and P.S. Perlman. 1983. Secondary structure of the *Tetrahymena* rRNA IVS: Structural homology with fungal mitochondrial intervening sequence. *Proc. Natl. Acad. Sci.* 80: 3903.

Colleaux, L., L. d'Auriol., M. Betermier, G. Cottarel, A. Jacquier, F. Galibert, and B. Dujon. 1986. Universal code equivalent of a yeast mitochondrial intron reading frame is expressed into *E. coli* as a specific double strand endonuclease. *Cell* 44: 521.

Davies, R.W., R.B. Waring, J.A. Ray, T.A. Brown, and C. Scazzocchio. 1982. Making ends meet: A model for RNA splicing in fungal mitochondria. *Nature* 300: 719.

Dujon, B. 1981. Mitochondrial genetics and functions. In *Molecular biology of the yeast,* Saccharomyces: *Life cycle and inheritance* (ed. J.H. Strathern et al.), p. 505. Cold Spring Harbor Laboratory, Cold Spring Harbor, New York.

Garriga, G. and A.M. Lambowitz. 1984. RNA splicing in *Neurospora* mitochondria: Self-splicing of a mitochondrial intron in vitro. *Cell* 38: 631.

———. 1986. Protein-dependent splicing of a group I intron in ribonucleoprotein particles and soluble fractions. *Cell* 46: 669.

Grivell, L.A., L. Bonen, and P. Borst. 1983. Mosaic genes and RNA processing in mitochondria: In *Genes: Structure and expression* (ed. A.M. Kroon), p. 279. Wiley, Chichester.

Holl, J., G. Rödel, and R.J. Schweyen. 1985. Suppressor mutations identify box 9 as a central nucleotide sequence in a highly ordered structure of intron RNA in yeast mitochondria. *EMBO J.* 4: 2081.

Jacquier, A. and B. Dujon. 1985. An intron encoded protein active in a gene conversion process that spreads an intron into a mitochondrial gene. *Cell* 41: 383.

Jacquier, A. and M. Rosbash. 1986. Efficient trans-splicing of a yeast mitochondrial RNA group II intron implicates a strong 5'-exon-intron interaction. *Science* 234: 1099.

Macready, I.G., R.M. Scott, A.R. Zinn, and R.A. Butow. 1985. Transposition of an intron in yeast mitochondria requires a protein encoded by that intron. *Cell* 41: 395.

Maniatis, T., E.F. Fritsch, and J. Sambrook. 1982. *Molecular cloning: A laboratory manual.* Cold Spring Harbor Laboratory, Cold Spring Harbor, New York.

Michel, F. and B. Dujon. 1983. Conservation of RNA secondary structure in two intron families including mitochondrial-, chloroplast- and nuclear encoded members. *EMBO J.* 2: 33.

Osinga, K.A., E. De Vries, G. Van der Horst, and H.F. Tabak. 1984. Processing of yeast mitochondrial messenger RNAs at a conserved dodecamer sequence. *EMBO J.* 3: 829.

Parker, R., P.G. Siliciano, and C. Guthrie. 1987. Recognition of the TACTAAC box during mRNA splicing in yeast involves basepairing to the U_2-like snRNA. *Cell* 49: 229.

Peebles, C.L., P.S. Perlman, K.L. Meeklenburg, M.L. Petrillo, J.H. Tabor, K.A. Jarrell, and H.L. Cheng. 1986. A self-splicing RNA excises an intron lariat. *Cell* 44: 213.

Schmelzer, C. and R.J. Schweyen. 1986. Self-splicing of group II introns in vitro: Mapping of the branch point and mutational inhibition of lariat formation. *Cell* 46: 537.

Tabak, H.F. and L.A. Grivell. 1986. RNA catalysis in the excision of yeast mitochondrial introns. *Trends Genet.* 2: 51.

Tabak, H.F., G. Van der Horst, A.M.J.E. Kamps, and A.C. Arnberg. 1987. Interlocked RNA circle formation by a self-splicing yeast mitochondrial group I intron. *Cell* 48: 101.

Tabak, H.F., G. Van der Horst, K.A. Osinga, and A.C. Arnberg. 1984. Splicing of large ribosomal precursor RNA and processing of intron RNA in yeast mitochondria. *Cell* **39:** 623.

Tabak, H.F., J. Van der Laan, K.A. Osinga, J.P. Schouten, J.H. Van Boom, and G.H. Veeneman. 1981. Use of a synthetic DNA oligonucleotide to probe the precision of RNA splicing in a yeast mitochondrial petite mutant. *Nucleic Acids Res.* **9:** 4475.

Van der Horst, G. and H.F. Tabak. 1985. Self-splicing of yeast mitochondrial, ribosomal and messenger RNA precursors. *Cell* **40:** 759.

————. 1987. New RNA mediated reactions by yeast mitochondrial group I introns. *EMBO J.* **6:** 2139.

Van der Veen, R., A.C. Arnberg, G. Van der Horst, L. Bonen, H.F. Tabak, and L.A. Grivell. 1986. Excised group II introns in yeast mitochondria are lariats and can be formed by self-splicing in vitro. *Cell* **44:** 225.

Zhuang, Y. and A.M. Weiner. 1986. A compensatory base change in the U_1 snRNA suppresses a 5'-splice site mutation. *Cell* **46:** 827.

Group II Intron Self-splicing: Development of Alternative Reaction Conditions and Identification of a Predicted Intermediate

C.L. Peebles,* E.J. Benatan,* K.A. Jarrell[†] and P.S. Perlman[†]

*Department of Biological Sciences, University of Pittsburgh, Pittsburgh, Pennsylvania 15260;
[†]Department of Molecular Genetics, Ohio State University, Columbus, Ohio 43210

Many introns found in fungal mitochondria, plant mitochondria, and chloroplasts have been classified as either group I or group II on the basis of sequence homologies and proposed secondary structures (Michel and Dujon 1983). Members of each group undergo self-splicing in vitro (Kruger et al. 1982; Garriga and Lambowitz 1984; Van der Horst and Tabak 1985; Peebles et al. 1986; Schmelzer and Schweyen 1986; Van der Veen et al. 1986). The boundary sequences of group II introns resemble those of nuclear introns, and it has been suggested that the latter two types follow essentially the same pathway of splicing (Cech 1986; Padgett et al. 1986; Peebles et al. 1986; Van der Veen et al. 1986). For example, self-splicing of the group II intron *oxi3* intron-5-γ (I5γ) from yeast mitochondria proceeds readily in vitro to yield spliced exons (E5-E3) and excised intron (intervening sequence) lariat (IVS-Lar) products (Peebles et al. 1986; Van der Veen et al. 1986). These two products correspond to the final products of in vitro splicing of nuclear pre-mRNA introns (Grabowski et al. 1984: Padgett et al. 1984; Ruskin et al. 1984). If the reaction pathway of group II self-splicing is indeed similar to that proposed for nuclear introns, there are at least two distinct stages. Stage 1 is cleavage of the 5′ splice junction and lariat formation, and stage 2 is cleavage at the 3′ splice junction and exon joining. The intermediate contains both the free 5′ exon and a large lariat composed of the intron and 3′ exon. Such RNAs are prominent among the products of in vitro splicing of nuclear introns (Grabowski et al. 1984; Padgett et al. 1984; Ruskin et al. 1984). The key prediction of this pathway as applied to group II self-splicing is that there is a similar two-part intermediate (Cech 1986). Neither a free 5′ exon (E5) nor a large lariat with the intron and 3′ exon (IVS-E3-Lar) was characterized in the initial reports of group II self-splicing (Peebles et al. 1986; Schmelzer and Schweyen 1986; Van der Veen et al. 1986).

Recently, we have undertaken an analysis of modified reaction conditions with the intent of identifying intermediates or by-products of self-splicing reactions. Several alternative buffer formulations have been developed that enhance the overall reaction rate, and some of these also dramatically alter the pattern of products (K.A. Jarrell et al., in prep.). Part of that study focused on characterizing several products of the reaction as it occurs under the new conditions. These products included IVS-Lar, broken lariat (IVS-BL), and true linear intron (IVS-Lin). The latter two forms comigrate on polyacrylamide gels, so gel mobility alone is not sufficient to distinguish which form is the product of a particular reaction (Peebles et al. 1986). Additional products included a separate 5′ exon (E5), 3′ exon (E3), a shortened form of E5 (E5s), and spliced exons (E5-E3). Finally, a linear intermediate of splicing was analyzed and found to contain intron and 3′ exon sequences (IVS-E3-Lin). In a reaction requiring E5, IVS-E3-Lin undergoes splicing efficiently (K.A. Jarrell et al., in prep.). (This reaction is similar to the "*trans*-splicing" system described previously [Jacquier and Rosbash 1986].) If E5 is absent, IVS-E3-Lin cleaves itself to yield a fragment of E3 termed E3-291. That cleavage event occurs at a sequence similar to the 5′ splice junction (K.A. Jarrell et al., in prep.).

The alternative reaction conditions have also revealed several reactions that do not occur readily in low salt. These include partial reactions clearly related to splicing, such as cleavage at the 5′ splice junction of transcripts lacking part of the intron. We have also identified a series of secondary reactions, such as spliced exon reopening. That reaction is catalyzed by the intron product and accounts for the appearance of the separate E5 and E3. Thus, the alternative reaction conditions have proved useful for separating the steps of the splicing reaction and for analyzing the reactivity of partial transcripts (K.A. Jarrell et al., in prep.).

In this paper, we describe additional experiments crucial to our development of these alternative conditions. Further characterization of some of the products formed under these conditions is also presented. In addition, we present evidence for IVS-E3-Lar, one predicted component of the intermediate for group II splicing. Since the other, E5, has recently been identified as a product that may be formed either by exon reopening or by hydrolysis—either under high-salt conditions as an intermediate of a *trans*-splicing reaction (Jacquier and Rosbash 1986; K.A. Jarrell et al., in prep.)—only IVS-E3-Lar represents distinctive evidence for the intermediate. Here, we provide three lines of evidence for the IVS-E3-Lar. The putative large lariat contains a nuclease-resistant trinucleotide and a 2′-5′ bond that is sensitive to debranching treatment. Its gel mobility and debranching products indicate that it contains the intron and 3' exon of the transcript from which it is derived.

EXPERIMENTAL PROCEDURES

Preparation of transcripts and splicing products. Plasmid DNAs were prepared and digested with restriction endonucleases before use as transcription templates, as described previously (Peebles et al. 1986; K.A. Jarrell et al., in prep.). In this study, plasmids pKM2 and pJD1 were used. RNA was purified by electrophoresis through 4% polyacrylamide gels containing 8 M urea, 90 mM Tris, 50 mM boric acid, 2.5 mm Na_2EDTA, and 0.1% SDS. Excised gel slices were soaked in buffer overnight to elute RNA which was then precipitated with ethanol. Agarose gels (1.5%) contained the same buffer with no urea. Radioactivity was determined by counting gel slices without scintillation fluid.

Splicing reactions. Transcripts were incubated at 45°C for various times in reaction mixtures modified from the standard conditions (Peebles et al. 1986) as indicated in the figure legends.

Filter hybridizaton. The procedure and oligonucleotides used were described previously (Peebles et al. 1986).

Nuclease P1 digestion and thin-layer chromatography. These procedures were done according to Konarska et al. (1985).

RNase T1 digestion and oligonucleotide analysis. RNA fractions containing 5–10 μg of tRNA carrier were treated with RNase T1 and analyzed on a 20% polyacrylamide gel as described previously (Perlman et al. 1987).

Debranching treatments. HeLa cell S-100 extract was obtained from M. Green or M. Edmonds, and debranching was performed according to the protocol of Ruskin and Green (1986).

RESULTS

Development of New Reaction Conditions for Group II Self-splicing

Our original investigation of self-splicing by the group II intron, *oxi3* I5γ, showed that this reaction occurs in a simple salt solution containing Mg^{++} ions, spermidine, a buffer near neutral pH, and an incubation temperature of 45°C (Peebles et al. 1986). Several products appeared after 1 hour, including E5-E3, IVS-Lar, and some IVS-BL. Notably absent were RNAs with the properties of the predicted bipartite intermediate 5' exon plus a large lariat containing the intron and the 3' exon. In an effort to either accelerate or perturb the reaction, modified reaction conditions were developed. First, the concentration of Mg^{++} was varied over a broad range, 0.01–0.5 M (Fig. 1A). It can be seen that the self-splicing reaction displays an optimum for this cofactor of about 0.10 M. At the lowest concentration, 0.01 M Mg^{++}, the addition of spermidine is required to allow efficient splicing. However, some splicing is detectable even at the extremes of Mg^{++} concentration. Although the rate varies significantly, the pattern of products formed is little affected by these changes in conditions. Finally, it should be noted that spermidine has no effect on the rate or products observed at the higher concentrations of Mg^{++}. The titration experiment shown here was carried out with no added spermidine (Fig. 1A). The anion provided by the Mg^{++} salt has little effect on these results; essentially the same response was obtained with sulfate, chloride, and acetate salts.

The ability of splicing to proceed in high ionic strength, such as 0.25 M $MgCl_2$, was surprising to us, since we had found that addition of as little as 0.1 M potassium acetate completely inhibited the reaction under the original conditions of 0.01 M Mg^{++} and 2 mM spermidine. We next investigated the response to monovalent cation salts under the condition of 0.10 M Mg^{++}. The splicing reaction proceeded readily over a broad range of NaCl concentrations; unexpectedly, there was a dramatic shift in the pattern of products (Fig. 1B). The reaction was evident throughout the range of 0–2.0 M added salt. The yields of IVS-Lar and E5-E3 increased as the concentration of added salt approached 1.0 M; additional products are also evident and these predominate at 2.0 M. The most abundant novel products have been characterized elsewhere and include the separate E3, E5, and IVS-Lin (K.A. Jarrell et al., in prep.). There is also an effect on the overall reactivity of the RNA as the concentration of NaCl is increased, as judged either from the rate of disappearance of the intact transcript or from the accumulation of products. Several other salts have been tested, and most promote the same change in the pattern seen here with NaCl. The most potent salt we have found for activation of the new pattern of products is KCl. A few salts, such as LiCl and Na_2SO_4, hardly affect either the pattern or the rate of splicing in 0.1 M $MgCl_2$ (S.L. Romiti and C.L. Peebles, unpubl.). In contrast, $(NH_4)_2SO_4$ stimulates the rate of splicing relative to the low-salt reaction condition, but hardly affects the pattern of products, except at the higher concentrations (Fig. 1C). Time course experiments indicate that 0.5 M $(NH_4)_2SO_4$ enhances the rate significantly; half of the RNA reacts by 8 minutes, compared to 2 hours under the original low-salt conditions (C.L. Peebles, unpubl.).

Earlier investigations of group II self-splicing have not explicitly addressed the effect of pH on either the rate or the product distribution. For the case of a group I intron, splice-site hydrolysis and intron circle reopening reactions have been found that are highly sensitive to the pH of the reaction—both are greatly accelerated by somewhat alkaline conditions (Zaug et al. 1984, 1985; Inoue et al. 1986). Since we are attempting to expand the known repertoire of group II reactions,

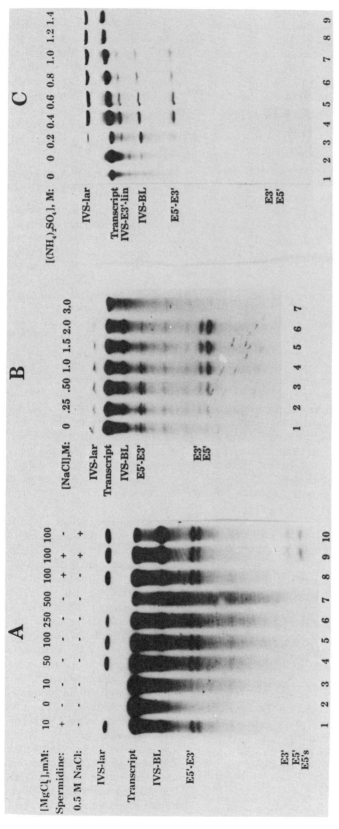

Figure 1. Development of modified self-splicing reaction conditions. Transcripts were prepared in vitro from linearized plasmid DNA templates, either pKM2 (*A,B*) or pJD1 (*C*) as described previously (Peebles et al. 1986). (*A*) Purified transcripts were incubated for 60 min at 45°C in reaction buffers with various additions to the standard mixture as indicated. (*B*) Reaction mixtures with the indicated additions of NaCl were incubated for 30 min at 45°C. (*C*) Reaction mixtures with the indicated concentrations of $(NH_4)_2SO_4$ were incubated for 10 min at 45°C.

225

experiments were conducted at a series of pH values in either $(NH_4)_2SO_4$ or KCl reaction buffers. The rate of splicing in $(NH_4)_2SO_4$ was estimated by determining the radioactivity in the IVS-Lar product after incubation (Fig. 2). There is a clear increase in the rate of the reaction with an increase in the pH. This effect is only about twofold per unit change in pH. The rate of the reaction in KCl varies with changes of pH similarly (C. Harris-Kerr and C.L. Peebles, unpubl.). However, little significant change in the pattern of products could be discerned as the pH was varied, except that above pH 9, the RNA was substantially hydrolyzed. These results indicate that there is a pH-sensitive component of the reaction center for self-splicing but that hydroxide ion may not participate directly in the reaction pathway, since the change in reaction rate is much less than tenfold per unit change in pH. As no evidence was found for rapid splice junction hydrolysis with higher pH, the mechanism by which group II introns activate the splice junctions for attack is apparently different from that used by group I introns.

Several other variables were also examined in these studies of group II splicing, including variations in temperature, additions of organic solvents, and changes in the identity of the buffering species. Under either $(NH_4)_2SO_4$- or KCl-containing reactions, the optimum temperature remained near 45°C; however, the profile of the temperature response became broader in high salt than it is in low salt. For example, at 40°C or 50°C in $(NH_4)_2SO_4$, self-splicing retains at least 50% of the maximum rate (C. Harris-Kerr and C.L. Peebles, unpubl.). In contrast, splicing in low salt is reduced to less than 10% of the maximum at those temperatures (Peebles et al. 1986). Addition of organic solvents inhibited splicing as the concentration approached 20%; among those tested were ethanol, dimethylsulfoxide, for-

mamide, and acetonitrile. In none of these experiments were novel products observed. Several different buffering species were also examined near pH 7.5; splicing proceeded at reasonable rates in Tris-HCl, HEPES, MES, and PIPES. The rate in Tris-HCl was slightly greater, so that buffer has been used for most experiments. We find that the ionic detergent SDS is tolerated up to at least 1.0% under these high-salt reaction conditions, and its addition protects the RNA from the action of traces of contaminating RNases (S.L. Romiti and C.L. Peebles, unpubl.).

New Products Appear Under Alternative Reaction Conditions

After exploration of several parameters, we have chosen two reaction conditions for most of our subsequent experiments. These represent the extremes with respect to the yield of spliced exons (Fig. 3A). In 0.5 M $(NH_4)_2SO_4$, more than 80% of the reacted transcript can be accounted for as IVS-Lar plus E5-E3. As detailed below, smaller amounts of IVS-Lin or IVS-BL in addition to separate E5 and E3 are present. A novel RNA, IVS-E3-Lin, can be seen migrating between the transcript and IVS-Lin; filter hybridization analysis shows that it contains sequences from the IVS and E3 (Fig. 4). More detailed analysis has established that it is a linear RNA extending from the first nucleotide of the intron through the 3′ end of the transcript (K.A. Jarrell et al., in prep.). In 0.5 M KCl, the main products are separate E3 and E5 and true linear IVS. Significant amounts of IVS-Lar and IVS-E3-Lin are also obtained, whereas there is virtually no E5-E3. An additional product related to the 5′ exon, E5s, is also seen. The structures and reactivities of these products will be described in detail (K.A. Jarrell et al., in prep.). In brief, IVS-Lar and E5-E3 are identical to the products formed in the low-salt reaction. The separate exon products were initially identified by a filter hybridization experiment (Fig. 4). Further analyses showed that they contain precisely the 5′-exon and 3′-exon sequences with 3′-OH and 5′-PO_4 termini, respectively (K.A. Jarrell et al., in prep.). A second, shorter form of the 5′ exon (E5s) is about 25 nucleotides smaller than E5 but still binds to the oligonucleotide complementary to the 19 nucleotides adjacent to the splice junction (Fig. 4). We have also shown that the E5 and E5s molecules share a common 3′ end by S1-nuclease protection experiments (K.A. Jarrell et al., in prep.).

Finally, we have demonstrated that E5s can replace E5 for reconstitution of a splicing intermediate with IVS-E3-Lin and yields a spliced exon product shorter than that with E5 (S.L. Romiti and C.L. Peebles, unpubl.). This indicates that the 3′ end of E5s is intact and functionally identical to that of E5; some material has been removed from the 5′ end of E5 to account for the reduced size of E5s. This novel 5′ end is formed during the splicing reaction and does not exist in the input transcripts. We suspect that the transcript or the E5 product is cleaved at a specific site during incubation

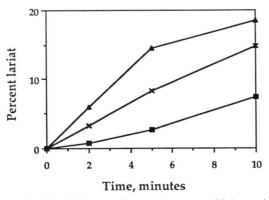

Figure 2. Self-splicing reaction rate increases with increasing pH. Transcripts were incubated in reaction mixtures containing 0.1 M $MgCl_2$, 0.5 M $(NH_4)_2SO_4$, and either 40 mM PIPES (pH 6.4), 40 mM Tris-HCl (pH 7.5), or Tris-HCl (pH 8.3). Samples were incubated for various intervals at 45°C and analyzed on a 4% polyacrylamide gel. Slices containing products were excised, and radioactivity was determined. Net production of IVS-Lar is shown. (■) pH 6.4; (×) pH 7.5; (▲) pH 8.3.

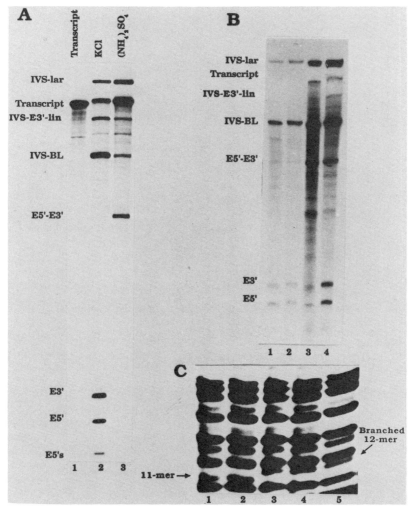

Figure 3. Alternative reaction conditions yield distinctive product distributions. (*A*) Transcript RNA (unincubated, lane *1*) was mixed with reaction buffer and incubated for 10 min at 45°C in 0.1 M MgCl$_2$, 0.1% SDS, and 40 mM Tris-HCl (pH 7.5) plus either 0.5 M KCl (lane *2*) or 0.5 M (NH$_4$)$_2$SO$_4$ (lane *3*). Products were displayed on a 4% polyacrylamide gel. (*B*) Products from either KCl- or (NH$_4$)$_2$SO$_4$-containing reactions were freed of salts by gel filtration and ethanol precipitation. Samples were either analyzed directly (lanes *1* and *3*) or incubated a second time in the other reaction buffer (lanes *2* and *4*) before analysis. (*C*) Isolated IVS-Lin (lanes *1* and *2*) and IVS-Lar (lanes *3–5*) were digested with RNase T1, and the pattern of oligonucleotides was displayed on a 20% polyacrylamide gel. Prior to digestion, samples were incubated in either 0.5 M KCl (lanes *1* and *3*) or 0.5 M NH$_4$Cl (lane *4*) containing reaction buffer for 2 hr at 45°C. The migration position of the branched 12-mer unique to IVS-Lar is indicated at the right, and the 11-mer unique to IVS-Lin is indicated at the left.

by the action of the intron ribozyme (K.A. Jarrell et al., in prep.).

How do the separate exon products arise? One possibility is that they result from site-specific hydrolysis by the intron acting on E5-E3. An alternative possibility is that they are not really end products but are in equilibrium with the E5-E3 material. The yield of separate exons under different salt conditions would then be a reflection of the position of that equilibrium at the moment that the reaction is stopped. In this case, products formed in KCl (or [NH$_4$]$_2$SO$_4$) would undergo a shift in their pattern if they received a second incubation in (NH$_4$)$_2$SO$_4$ (or KCl) (see Fig. 3B). The products formed in KCl are stable when incubated in (NH$_4$)$_2$SO$_4$, whereas E5-E3 from (NH$_4$)$_2$SO$_4$ under-

goes some exon reopening in KCl. The amounts of the other products remain unchanged, showing that these are indeed stable final products of the reaction. We conclude that E5 and E3 are formed by hydrolysis and cannot be ligated by the action of the intron. There is also no sign that the IVS-Lar is unstable in KCl, arguing against the idea that it can carry out its own "debranching" to account for the accumulation of IVS-Lin. This idea has been tested more directly in the experiment shown in Figure 3C.

The possibility exists that IVS-Lin is derived from IVS-Lar by specific hydrolysis at the branchpoint and that reaction might occur most readily under KCl incubation conditions. In this model, the IVS-E3-Lin would likewise be derived from a lariat form. Preparations of

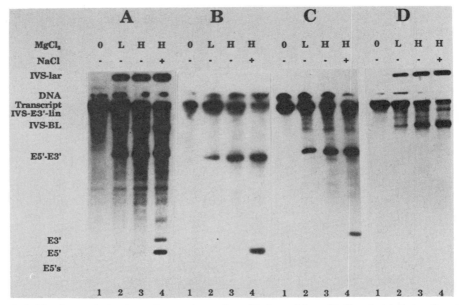

Figure 4. Filter hybridization analysis of reaction products of modified conditions. Uniformly labeled radioactive or unlabeled RNA was incubated for 1 hr in either 10 mM Tris-HCl (pH 7.5), 1 mM Na₃EDTA (lane *1*); 40 mM Tris-HCl (pH 7.5), 2 mM spermidine, 10 mM MgCl₂ (lane *2*); the same as *2* except 0.1 M MgCl₂ (lane *3*); or the same with 0.1 M MgCl₂ plus 0.5 M NaCl (lane *4*). Samples were analyzed on a 4% polyacrylamide gel, transferred to a filter, and hybridized with oligonucleotides complementary to the transcript. The four lanes of *A* contained radioactive RNA and were not hybridized; the four lanes of *B* were hybridized with an oligonucleotide complementary to 19 nucleotides in the 5′ exon adjacent to the splice junction; the four lanes of *C* were hybridized with an oligonucleotide complementary to positions 55–73 from the 3′ splice junction; and the four lanes of *C* were hybridized with an oligonucleotide complementary to positions 172–190 of the IVS (Peebles et al. 1986).

IVS-Lar contain some IVS-BL, and more IVS-BL accumulates upon extensive incubation of the IVS-Lar. IVS-Lin and IVS-BL comigrate, so it is possible that some of that material is really IVS-Lin. Branched and unbranched forms of the IVS can be sensitively distinguished by RNase T1 analysis; a characteristic branched 12-mer replaces a unique 11-mer in the oligonucleotide pattern (Perlman et al. 1987; K.A. Jarrell et al., in prep.). Both IVS-Lar and IVS-Lin were incubated in reaction buffer containing KCl and cut with RNase T1. The 11-mer is present, and no 12-mer appears after incubation and digestion of the IVS-Lin samples. The oligonucleotide pattern for IVS-Lar contains the branched 12-mer and no 11-mer either before or after incubation (Fig. 3C). This shows that there is no "self-debranching" of the lariat in either KCl or NH₄Cl.

We also examined the excised intron products formed under both alternative conditions for branchpoint trinucleotide after nuclease P1 digestion and thin-layer chromatography (Fig. 5). We expect the IVS-Lar product to be all branched molecules, since its characteristic mobility is determined by its partially circular structure. Indeed, both alternative conditions yield lariat with similar high mole fractions of resistant trinucleotide (0.87, [NH₄]₂SO₄; 0.82 KCl). The content of branchpoint trinucleotide in the IVS-Lin/BL fractions gives a measure of how much broken lariat is present in a particular preparation. These contain much lower mole fractions of trinucleotide (0.54, [NH₄]₂SO₄; 0.24,

KCl). This shows that a substantial majority of the excised intron is IVS-Lin after the KCl reaction, although as much as one fifth of the total may be

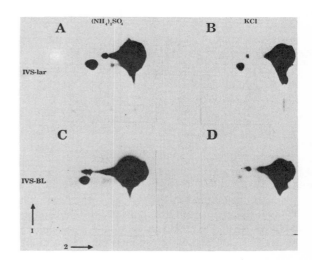

Figure 5. Branchpoint trinucleotide content of excised intron products from the alternative reaction conditions. Radioactive transcripts were prepared using 5′ [α-³²P]UTP and incubated in either 0.5 M KCl or 0.5 M (NH₄)₂SO₄ for 30 min at 45°C. Excised intron products (IVS-Lar and IVS-Lin/BL) were isolated and digested with nuclease P1 before two-dimensional thin-layer chromatography (Konarska et al. 1985). Branchpoint and 5′UMP products were excised, and radioactivity was determined. Product positions are illustrated in the diagram in Fig. 7C.

branched. In $(NH_4)_2SO_4$-containing reactions, virtually all of the IVS product is branched; no more than 5% appears to be IVS-Lin.

Identification of a Novel, Larger Lariat RNA

These alternative reaction conditions for group II self-splicing have enabled us to separate several of the steps in the reaction (K.A. Jarrell et al., in prep.). Stage 1 is release of E5, normally coupled with lariat formation. Stage 2 is attack of the 3' end of E5 on the phosphodiester at the 3' splice junction. E5 may be released without branch formation; this is relatively rare in $(NH_4)_2SO_4$ but is preferred in KCl. The linear intermediate, IVS-E3-Lin, can participate in stage 2, as shown by reconstitution with E5 to yield E5-E3. The IVS-Lin product results from this pathway. IVS-Lar results from the pathway proceeding through a large lariat intermediate containing IVS and E3 sequences. Such an RNA had not been previously identified biochemically for this system, although some structures have been found in electron micrographs that are candidates for IVS-E3-Lar molecules (Van der Veen et al. 1986). If substantial amounts of IVS-E3-Lar were present, it should appear as a species migrating more slowly than IVS-Lar. Filter hybridization analyses using oligonucleotides complementary to either E3 or IVS failed to detect material migrating in that part of the gel (Fig. 4). Since identification of that intermediate is a prerequisite for further studies of its properties, we undertook a series of experiments to detect the large lariat even though we expected that the upper limit on its abundance was about 0.2% of the total RNA in splicing reactions.

Our strategy was based on the fact that nonlinear RNAs display lower mobility on denaturing polyacrylamide gels than do linear RNAs with the same number of nucleotides (Padgett et al. 1984; Ruskin et al. 1984). For example, we originally identified the IVS-Lar as a slow-moving product of self-splicing (Peebles et al. 1986). Both IVS-Lar and the predicted IVS-E3-Lar have circular parts of 880 nucleotides. IVS-E3-Lar would have a linear portion of about 300 nucleotides (or longer, depending on the length of the 3' exon) and would be expected to migrate more slowly than IVS-Lar, which has a linear tail of only seven nucleotides. Repeated experiments failed, however, to identify IVS-E3-Lar directly as a radioactive species. We reasoned that IVS-E3-Lar might be very rare and could be masked by other material. We next separated reaction products by electrophoresis through two different types of gels: denaturing polyacrylamide and nondenaturing agarose. In the latter system, the mobility of both linear and nonlinear molecules is a function of their number of nucleotides. For example, IVS-Lar comigrates with both IVS-Lin and IVS-BL (Fig. 6, lanes 4 and 7). The large lariat would be expected to migrate with IVS-E3-Lin. Most of the slowly migrating RNA consists of large

heterogeneous transcripts, since it still migrates slowly when analyzed on the agarose gel (Fig. 6, lanes 1–3). Only one fraction contains a discrete species that migrates with the appropriate marker, IVS-E3-Lin (Fig. 6, lanes 2 and 6). The novel nonlinear species is apparently IVS-E3-Lar. Repetition of this two-dimensional gel analysis using a transcript with a longer E3 reveals a larger IVS-E3-Lar with a mobility on agarose matching that of the longer IVS-E3-Lin (E.J. Benatan and C.L. Peebles, unpubl.). Both IVS-Lar and IVS-E3-Lar have anomalous mobilities on denaturing acrylamide, indicating their partially circular structure. Since IVS-E3-Lar migrates more slowly on agarose than IVS-Lar and decreases mobility with increases in E3 length, IVS-E3-Lar and IVS-Lar are distinct nonlinear RNAs.

Branched RNAs such as IVS-Lar and nuclear intron lariats contain a nuclease-resistant structure due to the presence of the 2'-5' linkage that closes the circular part (Wallace and Edmonds 1983; Konarska et al. 1985; Peebles et al. 1986; Van der Veen et al. 1986). The IVS-E3-Lar contains such a P1-nuclease-resistant product that is not found in the IVS-E3-Lin (Fig. 7A,B). The identification of the nuclease-resistant product as a trinucleotide was confirmed by electrophoresis through a 25% polyacrylamide gel, where it comigrates with the linear trinucleotide pGAC and with the branchpoint trinucleotide pA(2'G,3'C) derived from IVS-lariat (Fig. 7D). The presence of this branchpoint-derived

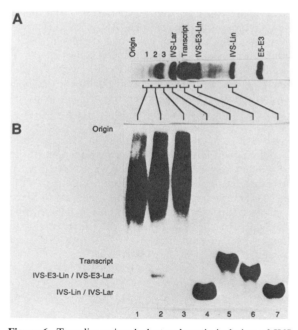

Figure 6. Two-dimensional electrophoretic isolation of IVS-E3-Lar. Radioactive transcripts were prepared and splicing was carried out in 0.5 M $(NH_4)_2SO_4$ at 45°C for 20 min. (*A*) RNA was separated by electrophoresis through a 4% polyacrylamide gel. Several fractions were excised as indicated on the autoradiogram. (*B*) Eluted RNA was applied on a 1.5% agarose gel and dried, and the autoradiogram is displayed.

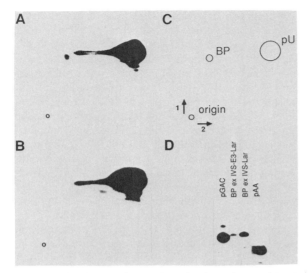

Figure 7. Nuclease-resistant branchpoint trinucleotide is found in IVS-E3-Lar. IVS-E3-Lar (*A*) and IVS-E3-Lin (*B*) were isolated and digested with nuclease P1. The products were analyzed by two-dimensional thin-layer chromatography. (*C*) Positions of the origin of chromatography (origin), 5'UMP (pU), and the trinucleotide branchpoint (BP). The trinucleotide products were eluted and subjected to analysis (*D*) on a 25% polyacrylamide gel in parallel with linear oligonucleotide markers, [^{32}P]pGAC and [^{32}P]pAA.

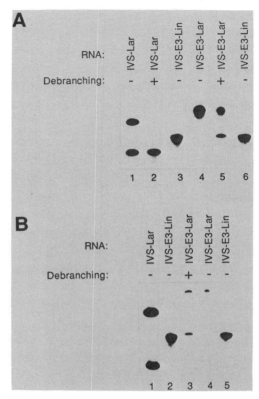

Figure 8. Debranching analysis of IVS-E3-Lar. Transcripts were prepared using as templates linear plasmid DNAs digested with either *Hin*dIII (*A*) or *Pvu*II (*B*) to yield RNAs with E3 of 294 or 386 nucleotides, respectively. IVS-Lar, IVS-E3-Lin, and IVS-E3-Lar were eluted and subjected to treatment with a HeLa cell S-100 fraction (Debranching) before analysis on 4% polyacrylamide gels. Addition (+) or omission (−) of extract (Debranching) is indicated.

trinucleotide shows that the putative large lariat is a branched molecule.

Extracts of mammalian cells contain a debranching activity that hydrolyzes the 2'-5' linkage of lariat RNAs under conditions that leave linear RNAs intact (Ruskin and Green 1986). IVS-Lar is sensitive to this treatment and yields a linear intron product (Peebles et al. 1986). Treatment of an IVS-E3-Lar fraction with the debranching extract converts about half of the radioactivity to a faster-migrating form; the resistant material is probably a mixture of transcripts (Fig. 8). The product released by debranching IVS-E3-Lar comigrated with IVS-E3-Lin on polyacrylamide gels. The length of the debranched large lariat matched the length of the IVS-E3-Lin derived from the same transcript (Fig. 8). This pattern of debranching products confirms that the large lariat contains the intron and the 3' exon. Since there is a single new product after the debranching treatment, the 2'-5' bond presumably closes a circular structure, rather than attaching one leg of a Y-shaped molecule.

DISCUSSION

Role of the Large Lariat RNA

A summary of the evidence supports our identification of the IVS-E3-Lar. The large lariat migrates more slowly on denaturing polyacrylamide gels than IVS-Lar and migrates through agarose gels with IVS-E3-Lin. The large lariat contains a branched circular

structure as shown both by the appearance of a P1-nuclease-resistant trinucleotide and by its sensitivity to debranching. The size of the debranching product is consistent with an RNA containing the intron and 3' exon. Our interpretation of these data is that the large lariat represents the predicted self-splicing intermediate. Only a small quantity of IVS-E3-Lar is available; in these experiments, it represents no more than 0.05% of the input RNA. A detailed structural analysis and a demonstration that it can react further in vitro have become practical with the discovery of a way to prepare IVS-E3-Lar in larger amounts (Jacquier and Michel 1987). These investigators constructed a derivative with a shortened E5; this transcript reacts and accumulates the large lariat. They have shown that this RNA readily reacts further in the presence of full-length E5 to yield E5-E3 and IVS-Lar.

The existence of the IVS-E3-Lar provides important support for the two-stage reaction scheme mentioned above. Since E5 can be formed by a specific hydrolysis reaction, the intermediate cannot be identified by its appearance. In contrast, the IVS-E3-Lar is characteristic of that intermediate, since it is not known to form in any other reaction. Whether splicing occurs via a linear intermediate or a lariat intermediate, E5 is thought to remain bound to IVS-E3 until splicing occurs. Since very little IVS-E3-Lar is found at any given time, it seems likely that stage 2 is fast relative to stage 1. IVS-E3-Lin is also a functional splicing intermediate (Jacquier and Rosbash 1986; K.A. Jarrell et al., in prep.). Since IVS-E3-Lin is much more abundant in vitro than IVS-E3-Lar, stage 2 may be quite slow relative to stage 1 when the linear form is involved. In that case, one advantage of forming a lariat intermediate may be to position the 3' end of E5 close to the 3' splice junction.

Modified Conditions Accelerate Splicing and Promote Alternative Reactions

Several reaction pathways are available to group II introns in vitro. Our model is designed to account for the final products obtained under different conditions utilized in this study. The standard splicing pathway predominates in low salt or in the presence of $(NH_4)_2SO_4$ and is thought to proceed through two transesterification steps: (1) attack of the 2'-OH from the branch site on the phosphodiester at the 5' splice junction and (2) attack of the 3'-OH of the 5' exon on the phosphodiester at the 3' splice junction. This pathway is strictly analogous to that proposed for nuclear pre-mRNA splicing. There is also a clear parallel with the pathway for group I introns; the main difference is that the 3'-OH of the guanosine cofactor attacks the 5' junction in that case. Step 1 of the group II pathway yields an intermediate composed of E5 and IVS-E3-Lar. The existence of this intermediate had been inferred from the production of IVS-Lar. We have detected this large lariat as a rare product of splicing the full-length transcript. We argue that E5 remains bound to the lariat form of IVS-E3 throughout the reaction by specific contacts between IVS and E5. Such an interaction has been defined for group I introns and involves base pairing between the 5' junction and a site within the intron termed the internal guide sequence (IGS). For group II introns, a similar interaction has been demonstrated and probably serves to position the 3'-OH of E5 for attack at the 3' junction to yield the final products, IVS-Lar and E5-E3, in step 2 (Jacquier and Michel 1987; Van der Veen et al. 1987). In low salt, this is the only detectable pathway. In the presence of high concentrations of $(NH_4)_2SO_4$, this pathway still predominates and proceeds more rapidly.

An alternative pathway is evident when high concentrations of various other salts are present in the reaction. Step 1 is attack (perhaps by water) at the 5' junction to release E5 and IVS-E3-Lin. Since about half of the excised IVS is linear and the rest is lariat (in NaCl), this pathway accounts for about half of the products. The rate of the reaction is not strongly pH-dependent; a twofold increase per unit increase in pH is observed (Fig. 2). This reaction, probably hydrolysis,

competes with branch formation. As before, E5 remains bound to IVS and attacks the phosphodiester of the 3' junction to yield IVS-Lin and E5-E3. The total rate of utilization of the transcript remains nearly unchanged, comparing $(NH_4)_2SO_4$ and NaCl conditions; instead, the relative rates of hydrolysis and branch formation vary. In NaCl, these are roughly equal; but in $(NH_4)_2SO_4$, branch formation occurs much more frequently than hydrolysis. The important outcome of step 1 is the formation of E5 for step 2; splicing can occur whether or not a branch has been formed in step 1. These observations are consistent with the idea that the slow step in this self-splicing reaction is E5 release; step 2 is then relatively rapid. The fact that the 5' junction can be attacked either by the 2'-OH of the branch site or by water indicates that part of the mechanism for directing the 5' junction to react involves some form of site-specific activation of that phosphodiester bond. This is in contrast to the situation in group I splicing, where the 5' junction is not particularly susceptible to hydrolysis.

The kinetics of accumulation of IVS-E3-Lin in KCl suggest that this intermediate may be longer lived than IVS-E3-Lar. Since about half of IVS is found as lariat and the rest as linear when the reaction nears completion, it appears that the rates of step 1 hydrolysis and branch formation are similar. In this case, the relative amounts of the intermediate forms would be determined primarily by their relative rates of consumption by step 2. The IVS-E3-Lar is rare (0.05% of the RNA), whereas IVS-E3-Lin represents as much as 5% of the RNA. Our interpretation is that lariat formation plays a significant kinetic role in step 2 of the reaction, perhaps by constraining the 5' end of the intron with the bound E5 to remain close to the 3' end of the IVS and thereby facilitating step 2.

This reaction scheme depends on secondary reactions—exon reopening and site-specific hydrolysis—to explain the final products observed. We propose that the extent of exon reopening is determined by its rate relative to the rate of dissociation of E5-E3 from IVS. In $(NH_4)_2SO_4$, little of either separate exon product can be detected, so reopening must be slow relative to dissociation. In KCl, separate exons are prominent, so it seems that the rate of reopening is large relative to that of dissociation. If E5-E3 were released and rebound, dilution of the reaction or addition of nonradioactive E5-E3 should have resulted in the accumulation of radioactive E5-E3. In these experiments, there was essentially no change in the pattern of products over a 500-fold range of RNA concentration (K.A. Jarrell and P.S. Perlman, unpubl.). As there is no evidence for (and ample evidence against) site-specific hydrolysis at the 3' junction, the simple interpretation is that E5-E3 is formed and remains bound until reopening occurs. Formation of the other products, such as E5s, can best be explained by proposing that the intron can recognize sequences and activate them for attack by water. Further analysis of these reactions are required to substantiate this idea.

IVS-E3-Lin Is a True Splicing Intermediate

When splicing initiates by hydrolysis instead of branch formation, IVS-E3-Lin results. We have determined its structure and examined its reaction products (K.A. Jarrell et al., in prep.). The results of our analysis indicate that it is a true intermediate. It appears early during the time course of the reaction and declines later as the transcript is consumed. A significant fraction of the excised IVS accumulates as true linear; this could happen only if a similar amount of linear intermediate were to complete step 2, since we have shown that IVS-Lar cannot debranch itself (Fig. 3). The best evidence that IVS-E3-Lin is an intermediate is that isolated IVS-E3-Lin can associate with E5 productively to yield E5-E3. In KCl, E3 release is seen, and we interpret this as an indication that splicing had occurred and was followed by reopening. This argument depends on the observed reaction products of IVS-E3-Lin alone: E3-291 and an IVS-E3 fragment. Significantly, no E3 was produced, implying that hydrolysis cannot occur on the intact 3′ junction. Since no E3-291 is seen among the products of reactions initiated with full-length transcript, all of the IVS-E3-Lin must be consumed by splicing, which is followed by reopening. We conclude that the 3′ junction must be attacked exclusively by the 3′-OH of E5 under the influence of IVS if it is to react at all. The conclusion that IVS-E3-Lin is a true intermediate also establishes that branched intron or branch formation per se is not essential for exon joining at step 2 as shown earlier by Jacquier and Rosbash (1986).

The value of developing the alternative reaction conditions has been to accelerate the splicing reaction and to reveal a number of additional capacities of the intron for rearranging the structure of RNA. We have used these conditions to prepare a variety of novel reaction products that we have characterized (this paper and K.A. Jarrell et al., in prep.). These conditions have also proved most useful for the analysis of mutant forms of the intron that retain the ability to catalyze either partial or secondary reactions. Finally, these conditions have enabled us to prepare and study both the separate exons and the IVS-E3 intermediates to establish that group II self-splicing really does proceed through a two-stage reaction.

ACKNOWLEDGMENTS

We thank the members of our laboratory and our collaborators in the laboratory of Dr. Philip S. Perlman at Ohio State University for continued support and critical discussions of these experiments. Many of these experiments were conducted with the excellent technical assistance of Mr. Steven L. Romiti. We thank Drs. B. Ruskin and M.R. Green (Harvard University) for supplying us with debranching procedures and extracts. We also thank Dr. Mary Edmonds of this department and Dr. John Woolford of Carnegie-Mellon University for criticism of portions of this manuscript. This work was supported by grants from the National Institutes of Health to C.L.P. (GM-37166) and P.S.P. (GM-31480).

REFERENCES

Cech, T.R. 1986. The generality of self-splicing RNA: Relationship to nuclear mRNA splicing. *Cell* **44:** 207.

Garriga, G. and A.M. Lambowitz. 1984. RNA splicing in *Neurospora* mitochondria: Self-splicing of a mitochondrial intron in vitro. *Cell* **39:** 631.

Grabowski, P.J., R.A. Padgett, and P.A. Sharp. 1984. Messenger RNA splicing in vitro: An excised intervening sequence and a potential intermediate. *Cell* **37:** 415.

Inoue, T., F.X. Sullivan, and T.R. Cech. 1986. New reactions of the ribosomal RNA precursor of *Tetrahymena* and the mechanism of self-splicing. *J. Mol. Biol.* **189:** 143.

Jacquier, A. and F. Michel. 1987. Multiple exon-binding sites in class II self-splicing introns. *Cell* **50:** 17.

Jacquier, A. and M. Rosbash. 1986. Efficient *trans*-splicing of a yeast mitochondrial RNA group II intron implicates a strong 5′ exon-intron interaction. *Science* **234:** 1099.

Konarska, M.M., P.J. Grabowski, R.A. Padgett, and P.A. Sharp. 1985. Characterization of the branch site in lariat RNAs produced by splicing of mRNA precursors. *Nature* **313:** 552.

Kruger, K., P.J. Grabowski, A.J. Zaug, J. Sands, D.E. Gottschling, and T.R. Cech. 1982. Self-splicing RNA: Autoexcision and autocyclization of the ribosomal RNA intervening sequence of *Tetrahymena*. *Cell* **31:** 147.

Michel F. and B. Dujon. 1983. Conservation of RNA secondary structures in two intron families including mitochondrial-, chloroplast-, and nuclear-encoded members. *EMBO J.* **2:** 33.

Padgett, R.A., P.J. Grabowski, M.M. Konarska, S. Seiler, and P.A. Sharp. 1986. Splicing of messenger RNA precursors. *Annu. Rev. Biochem.* **55:** 1119.

Padgett, R.A., M.M. Konarska, P.J. Grabowski, S.F. Hardy, and P.A. Sharp. 1984. Lariat RNAs as intermediates and products in the splicing of messenger RNA precursors. *Science* **225:** 898.

Peebles, C.L., P.S. Perlman, K.L. Mecklenberg, M.L. Petrillo, J.H. Tabor, K.A. Jarrell, and H.-L. Cheng. 1986. A self-splicing RNA excises an intron lariat. *Cell* **44:** 213.

Perlman, P.S., K.A. Jarrell, R.C. Dietrich, C.L. Peebles, S.L. Romiti, and E.J. Benatan. 1987. Mitochondrial gene expression in yeast: Further studies of a self-splicing group II intron. In *Extrachromosomal elements in lower eukaryotes* (ed. R.B. Wickner et al.), p. 39. Plenum Press, New York.

Ruskin, B. and M.R. Green 1986. An RNA processing activity that debranches RNA lariats. *Science* **229:** 135.

Ruskin, B., A.R. Krainer, T. Maniatis, and M.R. Green. 1984. Excision of an intact intron as a novel lariat structure during pre-mRNA splicing in vitro. *Cell* **38:** 317.

Schmelzer, C. and R.J. Schweyen. 1986. Self-splicing of group II introns in vitro: Mapping of the branchpoint and mutational inhibition of lariat formation. *Cell* **46:** 557.

Van der Horst, G. and H.F. Tabak. 1985. Self-splicing of yeast mitochondrial ribosomal and messenger RNA precursors. *Cell* **40:** 759.

Van der Veen, R., A.C. Arnberg, and L.A. Grivell. 1987. Self-splicing of a group II intron in yeast mitochondria: Dependence on 5′ exon sequences. *EMBO J.* **6:** 1079.

Van der Veen, R., A.C. Arnberg, G. Van der Horst, L. Bonen, H.F. Tabak, and L.A. Grivell. 1986. Excised group II introns in yeast mitochondria are lariats and can be formed by self-splicing in vitro. *Cell* **44:** 225.

Wallace, J.C. and M. Edmonds. 1983. Polyadenylated nuclear RNA contains branches. *Proc. Natl. Acad. Sci.* **80:** 950.

Zaug, A.J., J.R. Kent, and T.R. Cech. 1984. A labile phosphodiester bond at the ligation junction in a circular intervening sequence RNA. *Science* **224:** 574.

———. 1985. Reactions of the intervening sequence of the *Tetrahymena* rRNA precursor: pH dependence of cyclization and site-specific hydrolysis. *Biochemistry* **24:** 6211.

Characteristics of Ribonuclease P from Various Organisms

N. Lawrence, D. Wesolowski, H. Gold, M. Bartkiewicz,* C. Guerrier-Takada,
W.H. McClain,[†] and S. Altman
*Department of Biology, Yale University, New Haven, Connecticut 06520; [†]Department of Bacteriology,
University of Wisconsin, Madison, Wisconsin 53706*

Ribonuclease P (RNase P) is an endoribonuclease required for the maturation of the 5' termini of tRNAs from their precursors (for review, see Altman et al. 1986). This enzyme, which engages in a single cleavage event to generate a 5' phosphate in its tRNA products in vivo and in vitro, has been best characterized in extracts of *Escherichia coli*. It has a catalytic RNA subunit (M1 RNA) and a protein subunit (C5 protein; Guerrier-Takada et al. 1983). Under certain conditions in vitro, the RNA subunit alone can carry out the cleavage of tRNA precursors. This reaction, catalyzed by M1 RNA, has all the features of a true enzymatic reaction, and its mechanism differs from those of the reactions governed by other RNA enzymes (Table 1). Although RNase P generates the same end groups in its products as do group I self-splicing introns during the cleavage step performed by these introns, the RNase P reaction is not a transesterification (for review, see Cech and Bass 1986; Been et al.; Forster et al.; Epstein and Gall; all this volume), nor has a covalent linkage been detected, transient or otherwise, between the enzyme and substrate. The RNase P reaction is also clearly different from the autocleavage reactions performed by virusoid RNA or transcripts of newt satellite DNA. In these latter cases, the end groups in the cleavage products are 5'-OH and 3'-P. If we assume that these catalytic RNAs were present in primitive biochemical systems, then several different catalytic mechanisms governed by RNAs participated in the earliest stages of evolution.

*Permanent address: Institute of Biochemistry and Biophysics, Polish Academy of Sciences, Warsaw, Poland.

MATERIALS AND METHODS

Culture conditions. *Halobacterium volcanii* strain DS2 (ATCC 29605) was grown in medium containing 125 g NaCl, 45 g $MgCl_2 \cdot 6H_2O$, 10 g $MgSO_4 \cdot 7H_2O$, 10 g KCl, 1.34 g $CaCl_2 \cdot 2H_2O$, 3 g yeast extract, and 5 g Bactotryptone (per liter) (Daniels et al. 1985). Cells were grown at 30°C with vigorous shaking to a reading of 530 (2.7×10^8 cells/ml) on a Klett-Summerson photoelectric colorimeter. The cells were harvested by centrifugation and then frozen and stored at −70°C.

Preparation of RNase P. Crude extracts (S30) were prepared by grinding frozen cells, harvested from 2 liters of culture medium, with alumina according to the conditions described by Robertson et al. (1972). The S30 extract was diluted 1:4 with Buffer A (50 mM Tris-HCl [pH 7.5], 60 mM NH_4Cl, 10 mM Mg[OAc]$_2$, 6 mM 2-mercaptoethanol) and loaded onto a DEAE-Sephadex A50 column (bed vol. 100 ml) equilibrated with Buffer A (Stark et al. 1978). The column was washed with 250 ml of Buffer A containing 0.3 M NH_4Cl. A 600-ml continuous gradient of Buffer A containing NH_4Cl concentrations ranging from 0.3 to 0.7 M was passed through the column and collected in 20-ml fractions. The fractions were then assayed for RNase P activity as described below. The active fractions were pooled and precipitated by the addition of 0.55 g $(NH_4)_2SO_4$ per milliliter of eluate. The resulting precipitate was resuspended and dialyzed against Buffer A.

Assay of RNase P activity. Radioactive substrate (pTyr) for RNase P was prepared by transcription in vitro according to the procedures of Melton et al.

Table 1. Some Properties of Catalytic RNAs

RNA	End groups[a]	Cofactor[b]	Mechanism
Group I introns	5'-P, 3'-OH	yes	transesterification
M1 RNA	5'-P, 3'-OH	no	?
Viroid/virusoid	5'-OH, 3'-P	no	?

For further information, see Been et al., Forster et al., Sampson et al., and Epstein and Gall (all this volume) as well as McCorkle and Altman (1987).

[a]The end groups are those produced during the cleavage step of self-splicing reactions or the usual cleavage reaction of other RNA species.

[b]All agents listed require metal ions. This column refers to the use of a nucleotide cofactor.

(1984), using plasmid DNA (pGem1/HB-3) harboring a gene for *E. coli* tRNA[Tyr] as a template (C. Guerrier-Takada et al., in prep.). RNase P activity was assayed according to the procedures of Guerrier-Takada et al. (1986), except that the standard assay buffer was replaced with Buffer B (50 mM Tris-HCl [pH 7.5], 55 mM MgCl$_2$).

Cesium sulfate density gradient centrifugation. The buoyant densities of *H. volcanii* RNase P and *E. coli* RNase P were determined from Cs$_2$SO$_4$ step gradients according to the procedures of Akaboshi et al. (1980) with the following variations. The step gradients were prepared by layering 1.6 ml each of 45% (w/w), 37%, and 31% Cs$_2$SO$_4$ solutions made in Buffer C (50 mM Tris-HCl [pH 7.5], 10 mM MgCl$_2$, 100 mM NH$_4$Cl). RNase P purified through a DEAE-Sephadex column (0.4 ml) was then layered on the gradient and centrifuged at 58,000 rpm in a Beckman SW65 rotor for 20 hours at 4°C. Fractions of five drops each were collected by puncturing the bottom of the tubes with an 18-gauge hypodermic needle. Aliquots of each fraction were then assayed for RNase P activity according to the methods described above.

Inactivation of RNase P by micrococcal nuclease. RNase P (5.0 µl) purified through the DEAE-Sephadex column was mixed with 2.0 µl of 100 mM Tris-HCl (pH 8.0), 2.0 µl of 10 mM CaCl$_2$, and 1.0 µl of micrococcal nuclease (MN; 12 units/µl). The mixture was incubated at 37°C for 30 minutes; 2.0 µl of 40 mM EGTA (ethyleneglycol-bis[β-aminoethyl ether] N, N'-tetraacetic acid) was added to inactivate the MN, and 5.0 µl of the mix was then assayed for RNase P activity as described above.

Heterologous reconstitution of RNase P from subunits from H. volcanii and E. coli. The RNAs present in *H. volcanii* RNase P purified through a DEAE-Sephadex column were removed with LiCl/EDTA according to the methods of Vioque and Altman (1986). The supernatant-containing protein was then used for reconstitution with M1 RNA from *E. coli* made in vivo (Reed et al. 1982); 12.5 µl of *H. volcanii* protein (2.6 µg/µl)

was mixed with 2.5 µl M1 RNA (33.6 ng/µl), 5.0 µl of 10 M urea, and 30 µl H$_2$O. The mixture was dialyzed against 1.0 liter of Buffer C for 3 hours with one change, and 20 µl of the mix was then assayed for RNase P activity.

RESULTS

Sources and Substrates

RNase P-like activities and substrates for the reaction have been identified in extracts of several organisms (for summaries, see Krupp et al. 1986; Altman et al. 1987); i.e., various tRNA precursors, when used as substrates, were cleaved by these extracts to generate products that contain the tRNA sequences and the appropriate 5′ termini of the mature tRNA. We have shown, for example, that substrates from *E. coli*, yeast mitochondria, and HeLa cell nuclei are all cleaved by activities from *E. coli* and HeLa cell nuclei, although these cleavages occur at different rates (Gold and Altman 1986). Some common feature in all of the substrates is recognized by the RNase P activities from these and other organisms. Earlier work with mutants in which the secondary and/or tertiary structures of the tRNA moiety of tRNA precursors were disrupted led to the conclusion that the structure in solution of the various substates was the critical feature recognized by RNase P (for review, see Altman 1975). We have recently extended our characterization of RNase P-like activities from different organisms to include the archaebacteria by characterizing an activity found in extracts of *H. volcanii*.

We used the precursor to tRNA[Tyr] from *E. coli* as a test substrate and found that *H. volcanii* contained an activity that produced the same cleavage products in this substrate, with the same end groups (data not shown), as does authentic RNase P from *E. coli*. This newly characterized RNase P activity has some of the important features that have been exhibited by RNase P activities from other sources. It can be inactivated by pretreatment with micrococcal nuclease (Fig. 1) as can, for example, activities from *E. coli* (Stark et al. 1978),

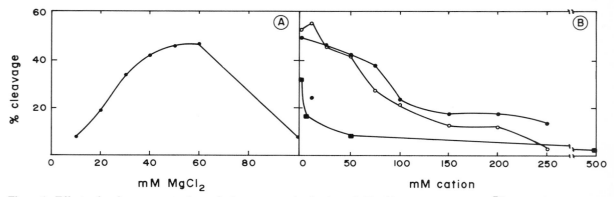

Figure 1. Effects of various concentrations of salts on processing in vitro of pTyr (the precursor to tRNA[Tyr]) by RNase P from *H. volcanii*. (*A*) Effect of MgCl$_2$ at various concentrations on the extent of cleavage of pTyr by RNase P from *H. volcanii*. (*B*) Effect of KCl (○), NaCl (■), and NH$_4$Cl (●) at various concentrations on the extent of cleavage of pTyr by RNase P from *H. volcanii*.

Bacillus subtilis (Gardiner and Pace 1980), *Schizosaccharomyces pombe* (Krupp et al. 1986), *Xenopus laevis* (Gold 1988), HeLa cell nuclei (Koski 1978; Gold 1988), and HeLa cell mitochondria (Doersen et al. 1985). This sensitivity to micrococcal nuclease is a strong indication that each RNase P-like enzymatic activity has an essential RNA component. The buoyant density of the activity from *H. volcanii* is compatible with that of an RNA-protein complex (Table 2). In contrast to the bacterial enzymes, the mammalian activities have a much lower ratio of RNA to protein. We have also found discrete RNA species that copurify with the enzymatic activity from *H. volcanii* (data not shown). The hydrodynamic properties of the activity from *H. volcanii* suggest that the RNase P from this source is somewhat larger than that from *E. coli* or from HeLa cells (Table 2). The activity from *H. volcanii* is inhibited by monovalent cations (Fig. 2), and the optimal concentration of Mg^{++} is 55 mM. In both these respects, properties of the RNase P activity from *H. volcanii* differ from the properties of RNase P from *E. coli* (Fig. 2) (Guerrier-Takada et al. 1986). It is noteworthy that monovalent cations inhibit *H. volcanii* RNase P, since this organism requires 2 M NaCl in its culture medium for growth.

Hybrid Enzymes and Gene Sequences

Another indication of the conserved functional features of RNase P activities from various sources is their ability to form hybrid enzymes in reconstitution experiments in vitro with subunits from other organisms. Separated protein and RNA components from RNase P from one organism can be mixed in vitro under conditions where neither subunit shows any activity with the RNA or protein component from RNase P from another organism, and the enzymatic activity can be recovered. In some cases, these hybrids have been reconstituted with partially purified preparations only. We have now succeeded in making such hybrids with the protein component of RNase P from *H. volcanii* and M1 RNA from *E. coli* (Fig. 3), although the reciprocal experiment has not yet yielded positive results. Nevertheless, the range of organisms that yield active hybrid enzymes by the addition of the protein component from their analog of RNase P to M1 RNA from *E. coli* now includes *H. volcanii* (Fig. 3, lane 2; M1 RNA alone has no activity in vitro under these conditions), *B. subtilis* (Guerrier-Takada et al. 1983), *E. coli* (Kole et al. 1980), of course, and HeLa cells (Gold and Alt-

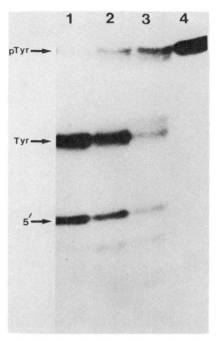

Figure 2. Inactivation of RNase P from *H. volcanii* by pretreatment with micrococcal nuclease (MN). (*1*) Control pretreatment, $CaCl_2$ present but MN absent; (*2*) control pretreatment, MN present but $CaCl_2$ absent; (*3*) pretreatment with MN in the presence of $CaCl_2$; (*4*) substrate, precursor tRNA alone. Positions of the substrate (pTyr) and the cleavage fragments that contain the mature tRNA sequence (Tyr) and the extra 5'-proximal fragment are indicated.

man 1986). These results illustrate the ability of the subunits to interact across widely separated species lines. However, the nucleotide sequences of the genes for the RNA and protein subunits of the various RNase P activities are not highly conserved.

No positive signal in Southern hybridization experiments is observed when the genes from *E. coli* for M1 RNA or for C5 protein are used as probes for genomes outside the gram-negative group (Reed 1984; Gold and Altman 1986). Within the gram-negative group, we have isolated several genes analogous to the gene for M1 RNA from *E. coli* by complementation of a temperature-sensitive mutant in *E. coli* (Lawrence et al. 1987). Comparison of the analogous sequences has facilitated construction of a possible secondary structure for M1 RNA, but many more sequences will have to be determined from a wide range of organisms before those features of the structure of M1 RNA that account for its highly conserved function are identified.

Table 2. Physical Properties of RNase P Activities from Different Sources

Property	*E. coli*	HeLa nuclei[a]	*H. volcanii*[a]	Veal heart
$\rho(g/ml)$[b]	1.55[c]	1.28	1.61	1.33[c]
$s_{20,w}$	12[d]	15	18	—

[a]Data reported in this paper.
[b]Measured in cesium sulfate density gradients. The density of protein is 1.24 g/ml and that of single-stranded RNA is greater than 1.66 g/ml in these gradients.
[c]Data from Akaboshi et al. (1980).
[d]Data from Robertson et al. (1972).

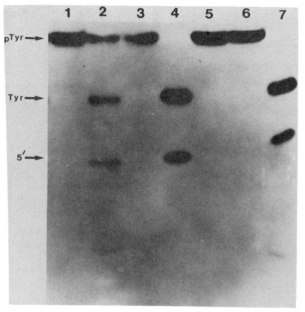

Figure 3. Heterologous reconstitution of RNase P activity with the protein subunit of RNase P from *H. volcanii* and M1 RNA from *E. coli*. Subunits were reconstituted by mixing in 1.0 M urea, dialyzing against Buffer C (10 mM MgCl$_2$), and then assayed in the same buffer. (*1*) *H. volcanii* protein alone; (*2*) *H. volcanii* protein and M1 RNA from *E. coli*; (*3*) M1 RNA from *E. coli* alone (M1 RNA has no activity in vitro under these conditions); (*4*) M1 RNA from *E. coli* assayed in the presence of 100 mM MgCl$_2$; (*5*) *H. volcanii* protein alone (pretreated by boiling for 5 min and then chilling on ice); (*6*) *H. volcanii* protein (pretreated as in lane 5) and M1 RNA from *E. coli*; (*7*) *H. volcanii* RNase P. The positions of the substrate (pTyr) and the cleavage fragments that contain the mature tRNA sequence (Tyr) and the extra 5′-proximal fragment are indicated.

A Small Substrate for RNase P

Some progress has been made in determining what aspects of the substrates for RNase P are essential for

cleavage by the enzyme. These results come from studies of a "minimal" tRNA precursor substrate.

We have known for some time that at least one substrate for RNase P in vivo is not a standard tRNA precursor molecule. This substrate, the precursor to 4.5S RNA from *E. coli* (Bothwell et al. 1976; Bourgaize and Fournier 1987), consists of a long stem-and-loop structure, with an "extra" 5′ sequence that is released upon cleavage by RNase P (Fig. 4). We have recently synthesized a truncated tRNA precursor molecule (Fig. 4) that contains only the aminoacyl and T stems of the tRNA moiety and the T loop, with the 5′ extra sequence covalently linked to nucleotide 1 of the usual mature tRNA sequence (W.H. McClain et al., in prep.). This molecule, which has a hairpin structure resembling the precursor to 4.5S RNA, is cleaved by M1 RNA at a rate comparable to that of the standard tRNA precursor substrate. This novel substrate is also cleaved by the RNase P holoenzyme from *E. coli* and by the partially purified RNase P from *H. volcanii*, to yield the appropriate 5′ terminus of the usual mature tRNA sequence. Further work is required to investigate systematically what aspects of this structure are preserved in other tRNA precursors and are essential for recognition and cleavage by RNase P. Nevertheless, the minimal hairpin substrate may represent a recognition element sought by all RNase P activities, and its existence could account, in part, for the ability ot this enzyme to cross species lines to cleave other substrates.

Antibodies to RNase P Activity

Another indication of the conserved nature of the characteristics of RNase P is provided by experiments with polyclonal antibodies from human sera. We tested the ability of the RNase P from HeLa cells, a small nuclear RNP (snRNP), to cross-react with antibodies against the abundant Sm-snRNPs that contain U1 and U2 snRNAs (Lerner and Steitz 1979). Anti-Sm anti-

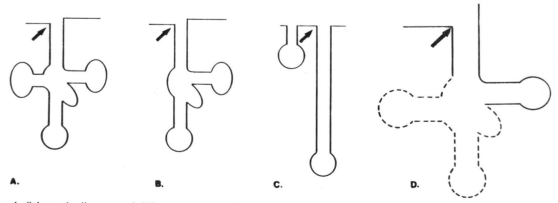

Figure 4. Schematic diagrams of different substrates for RNase P from *E. coli*. In each case, the solid outline indicates the phosphodiester backbone. Arrows point to the site of RNase P or M1 RNA cleavage. Regions indicated by parallel lines are hydrogen-bonded. (*A*) Precursor to *E. coli* tRNA[Phe] (Normanly et al. 1985); (*B*) derivative of the molecule shown in *A* with the D loop and stem truncated to create a tRNA moiety resembling a mitochondrial tRNA (W.H. McClain et al., in prep.); (*C*) precursor to *E. coli* 4.5S RNA (Bothwell et al. 1976); (*D*) derivative of the molecule shown in *A* in which both the D loop and the stem and the anticodon loop and stem are missing (dashed lines), and the 5′ side of the aminoacyl stem is covalently joined to the 5′ side of the T stem (W.H. McClain et al., in prep.).

bodies do not precipitate (or inactivate) RNase P activity. Indeed, RNase P is found in the flowthrough of anti-Sm affinity columns, and discrete RNA species copurify with that activity (Gold and Altman 1986). This observation demonstrates that RNase P does not share antigenic determinants with the Sm-snRNPs. A more extensive screening of sera from patients with systemic lupus erythematosus (SLE) has identified certain sera with the ability to inactivate and precipitate the RNase P activity from HeLa cells (H.A. Gold et al., in prep.). The anti-RNase P antibodies also cross-react with preparations of RNase P from sources other than HeLa cells. For example, both the purified holoenzyme from *E. coli* and the partially purified RNase P from *H. volcanii* can be inactivated by anti-RNase P antibodies (H.A. Gold et al., in prep.). Presumably, some feature of the protein subunit of the RNase P activities supplies the antigenic determinant. We do know, from examination of the sequences that encode them, that the protein subunits of the enzyme from *E. coli* and *B. subtilis* (Ogasawara et al. 1985) have an identical region of amino acids, but whether or not this region is the one recognized by the antibodies is not known.

The Protein Subunit

The protein subunit of RNase P from *E. coli* can be dispensed with in vitro; however, it is essential for the viability of *E. coli* in vivo. Furthermore, addition of the protein to a reaction mixture in vitro can increase enormously the rate at which M1 RNA can cleave certain substrates. This increase is especially conspicuous in the case of those substrates that lack the 3′-terminal CCA sequence or of a "nonstandard" substrate, such as the precursor to 4.5S RNA from *E. coli*. Addition of the protein subunit enhances the rate of cleavage about 100-fold for the precursor to tRNA^{fMet} from HeLa cells, a substrate that lacks the 3′-terminal CCA sequence (Guerrier-Takada et al. 1984). Observations of this kind have led us to suggest that the protein subunit of *E. coli* plays an important role in regulating the activity of RNase P in vivo.

CONCLUSION

Several lines of evidence indicate that RNase P (and/or the RNA subunit thereof) represents an ancient solution to the problem of processing gene transcripts, in particular tRNA gene transcripts, in vivo. The functional features of this enzyme and its substrates are represented in all cell types examined thus far and have been preserved in the solution conformation of both enzyme and substrate. Although some model substrates have been constructed that indicate what the features of the "minimal" substrate must be, the features that determine recognition of its substrates by RNase P, and the mechanism of the reaction are still not understood in any detail.

ACKNOWLEDGMENTS

M.B. was supported in part by the Rudolph Anderson Fund of the Yale University Graduate School, W.H.M. is supported by National Institutes of Health grant AI-10257, and S.A. is supported by National Institutes of Health grant GM-19422 and National Science Foundation grant DMB-8418931.

REFERENCES

Akaboshi, E., C. Guerrier-Takada, and S. Altman. 1980. Veal heart ribonuclease P. has an essential RNA component. *Biochem. Biophys. Res. Commun.* **96:** 831.

Altman, S. 1975. Biosynthesis of transfer RNA in *Escherichia coli. Cell* **4:** 21.

Altman, S., H.A. Gold, and M. Bartkiewicz. 1987. Ribonuclease P. as a snRNP. In *Small nuclear ribonucleoproteins* (ed. M.L. Bernstiel). Springer-Verlag, Berlin. (In press.)

Altman, S., M. Baer, C. Guerrier-Takada, and A. Vioque. 1986. Enzymatic cleavage of RNA by RNA. *Trends Biochem. Sci.* **11:** 515.

Bothwell, A.L.M., R.L. Garber, and S. Altman. 1976. Nucleotide sequence and *in vitro* processing of a precursor molecule to *Escherichia coli* 4.5S RNA. *J. Biol. Chem.* **251:** 7709.

Bourgaize, D.B. and M.J. Fournier. 1987. Initiation of translation is impaired in *E. coli* cells deficient in 4.5S RNA. *Nature* **325:** 281.

Cech, T.R. and B.L. Bass. 1986. Biological catalysis by RNA. *Annu. Rev. Biochem.* **55:** 599.

Daniels, C.J., J.D. Hofman, J.G. MacWilliam, W.F. Doolittle, C.R. Woese, K.R. Luehrsen, and G.E. Fox. 1985. Sequence of 5S ribosomal RNA gene regions and their products in the archaebacterium *Halobacterium volcanii. Mol. Gen. Genet.* **198:** 243.

Doersen, C.J., C. Guerrier-Takada, S. Altman, and G. Attardi. 1985. Characterization of an RNase P activity from HeLa cell mitochondria. *J. Biol. Chem.* **260:** 5942.

Gardiner, K. and N. Pace. 1980. RNase P of *Bacillus subtilis* has an essential RNA component. *J. Biol. Chem.* **255:** 7507.

Gold, H.A. 1988. "Studies of HeLa cell ribonuclease P." Ph.D. thesis, Yale University, New Haven, Connecticut.

Gold, H.A. and S. Altman. 1986. Reconstitution of RNase P activity using inactive subunits from *E. coli* and HeLa cells. *Cell* **44:** 243.

Guerrier-Takada, C., W.H. McClain, and S. Altman. 1984. Cleavage of tRNA precursors by the RNA subunit of *E. coli* ribonuclease P (M1 RNA) is influenced by 3′-proximal CCA in the substrates. *Cell* **38:** 219.

Guerrier-Takada, C., K. Haydock, L. Allen, and S. Altman. 1986. Metal ion requirements and other aspects of the reaction catalyzed by M1 RNA, the RNA subunit of ribonuclease P from *Escherichia coli. Biochemistry* **25:** 1509.

Guerrier-Takada, C., K. Gardiner, T. Marsh, N. Pace, and S. Altman. 1983. The RNA moiety of ribonuclease P is the catalytic subunit of the enzyme. *Cell* **35:** 849.

Kole, R., M.F. Baer, B.C. Stark, and S. Altman. 1980. *E. coli* RNase P has a required RNA component in vivo. *Cell* **79:** 881.

Koski, R. 1978. "Characterization of human KB cell ribonuclease P · Hsa and ribonuclease NU." Ph.D thesis, Yale University, New Haven, Connecticut.

Krupp, G., B. Cherayil, D. Frendeway, S. Nishikawa, and D. Soll. 1986. Two RNA species copurify with RNase P from the fission yeast *Schizosaccharomyces pombe. EMBO J.* **5:** 1697.

Lawrence, N.P., A. Richman, R. Amini, and S. Altman. 1987. Heterologous enzyme function in *E. coli* and the selection of genes for the catalytic RNA subunit of RNase P. *Proc. Natl. Acad. Sci.* **84:** (in press).

Lerner, M.R. and J.A. Steitz. 1979. Antibodies to small nuclear RNAs complexed with protein are produced by patients with systemic lupus erythematosus. *Proc. Natl. Acad. Sci.* **76:** 5495.

McCorkle, G.M. and S. Altman. 1987. RNA's as catalysts. *J. Chem. Educ.* **64:** 221.

Melton, D.A., P.A. Krieg, M.R. Rebagliati, T. Maniatis, K. Zinn, and M.R. Green. 1984. Efficient in vitro synthesis of biologically active RNA and RNA hybridization probes from plasmids containing a bacteriophage SP6 promoter. *Nucleic Acids Res.* **12:** 7035.

Normanly, J., J.-M. Masson, L.G. Kleina, J. Abelson, and J.H. Miller. 1986. Construction of two *Escherichia coli* amber suppressor genes: tRNA $_{CUA}^{Phe}$ and tRNA $_{CUA}^{Cys}$. *Proc. Natl. Acad. Sci.* **83:** 6548.

Ogasawara, N., S. Moriya, K. von Meyenburg, F.G. Hansen, and H. Yoshikawa. 1985. Conservation of genes and their organization in the chromosomal replication origin region of *Bacillus subtilis* and *Escherichia coli*. *EMBO J.* **4:** 3345.

Reed, R.E. 1984. "A study of the RNA component of *E. coli* RNase P." Ph.D. thesis, Yale University, New Haven, Connecticut.

Reed, R.E., M.F. Baer, C. Guerrier-Takada, H. Donis-Keller, and S. Altman. 1982. Nucleotide sequence of the gene encoding the RNA subunit (M1 RNA) of ribonuclease P from *Escherichia coli*. *Cell* **30:** 627.

Robertson, H.D., S. Altman, and J.D. Smith. 1972. Purification and properties of a specific *Escherichia coli* ribonuclease which cleaves a tyrosine transfer ribonucleic acid precursor. *J. Biol. Chem.* **247:** 5243.

Stark, B.C., R. Kole, E. Bowman, and S. Altman. 1978. Ribonuclease P: An enzyme with an essential RNA component. *Proc. Natl. Acad. Sci.* **75:** 3717.

Vioque, A. and S. Altman. 1986. Affinity chromatography with an immobilized RNA enzyme. *Proc. Natl. Acad. Sci.* **83:** 5904.

Structure and Catalytic Function in Ribonuclease P

N.R. Pace, C. Reich, B.D. James, G.J. Olsen, B. Pace, and D.S. Waugh
Department of Biology and Institute for Molecular and Cellular Biology,
Indiana University, Bloomington, Indiana 47405

Ribonuclease P (RNase P) is the enzyme responsible for removing the 5′ precursor segments from tRNA during its maturation. RNase P is particularly interesting because its catalytic element is an RNA, not a protein (Guerrier-Takada et al. 1983; Gardiner et al. 1985). Although the recognition of RNase P as a catalytic RNA was preceded by the discovery of a self-splicing intron in some *Tetrahymena* 26S rRNA precursors (Kruger et al. 1982), the RNase P RNA differs in an important way: It engages in *inter*molecular reactions. In contrast, the self-splicing intron activity in vivo is a series of *intra*molecular rearrangements that collectively result in the excision of the intron and the ligation of the flanking exons (for review, see Cech 1985). RNase P therefore offers not only a model for RNA catalytic mechanisms, but also a system for exploring the nature of specific RNA-RNA recognition that almost certainly goes beyond the familiar Watson-Crick base-pairing interactions.

The RNase P of *Escherichia coli* was one of the first RNA-processing enzymes to be analyzed in vitro (Altman and Smith 1971). It was shown subsequently by Altman and his colleagues to consist of two components, an RNA (M1 RNA) and a protein (C5 protein) (Stark et al. 1978). The ribonucleoprotein nature of RNase P has proved to have a wide phylogenetic distribution. *Bacillus subtilis*, a eubacterium distantly related to *E. coli*, also possesses an RNase P with protein and RNA elements (Gardiner and Pace 1980). RNA subunits have been implicated in RNase P activities from other organisms, e.g., *Schizosaccharomyces pombe* (Kline et al. 1981) and both the nuclei and mitochondria of human cells (Doersen et al. 1985; Gold and Altman 1986). It is not completely clear whether RNase P is always associated with an RNA element; the corresponding activity from *Xenopus* oocytes seems to lack RNA (Castano et al. 1986). Further characterizations of RNase P from diverse organisms will be important for establishing functional commonalities that may underlie variability in the structure of the enzyme. Thus far, however, only the eubacterial enzymes have been inspected in much detail.

The RNase P RNA Is the Enzyme

The RNase P holoenzymes of *B. subtilis* and *E. coli* are similar in their general properties. The proteins have a molecular weight of 15,000–17,000, and the RNAs are about 400 nucleotides in chain length. The RNase P proteins from each of these organisms will complement the RNA from the other, so they clearly have some homologous functions (Guerrier-Takada et al. 1983).

Although RNase P undoubtedly functions in vivo as a ribonucleoprotein particle, the catalytic element is the RNA moiety. This was discovered during tests of the optimum ionic environment for the enzyme reaction in vitro (Guerrier-Takada et al. 1983). High cation concentrations could supplant a requirement for the protein in the intrinsically RNA-catalyzed reaction. The salt concentration required to activate the RNase P is high, optimally about 800 mM NH_4Cl and 100 mM $MgCl_2$ for the *B. subtilis* RNA (C. Reich et al., in prep.). The optimum salt concentration varies to some extent depending on the enzyme RNA and on the character of the pre-tRNA substrate (C. Reich, unpubl.). Proof that the RNase P is indeed the catalytic element in this reaction is rigorous: In vitro transcripts from the cloned *E. coli* (Guerrier-Takada and Altman 1984) and *B. subtilis* (Reich et al. 1986) RNase P RNA genes are catalytically active under high-salt protein-independent conditions.

The most straightforward explanation for the requirement for high salt concentrations in the RNase P RNA ("RNA alone") reaction is that the cations decrease the electrostatic repulsion between the enzyme and substrate RNAs, each of which carries one negative charge per nucleotide phosphate. Without this counterion effect, the charge repulsion between enzyme and substrate would prevent the intimate contact required for binding and catalysis. Thus, part of the role of the RNase P protein presumably is to provide charge titration. The protein is quite small relative to the RNase P RNA, so its effect is likely to be localized, perhaps just to the tRNA binding region.

Although ionic screening is one interpretation of the ability of high salt concentrations to alleviate the requirement for the protein in the RNase P reaction, not all the data are straightforwardly explained by this notion. For example, if the salt effects were simply a matter of ionic screening, it would be anticipated that alkali metal cations with small radii would be more effective at low concentrations than would larger cations. The reason is that the ions with smaller radii bind to nucleic acid phosphates more tightly than the larger ones, in the order $Li^+ > Na^+ > K^+ > Rb^+ > Cs^+$ (Ross and Scruggs 1964). However, the observed order of effectiveness of the ions in promoting the RNase P reaction is clearly different: $Rb^+, Cs^+, K^+, NH_4^+ > Li^+, Na^+$ (Gardiner et al. 1985). It may be that only the larger cations can achieve a packing geometry with the RNA surfaces that results in activity. It is also conceivable that electrostatic shielding of phosphate residues is not the only role of monovalent cations in the RNA-alone activity.

Some experimental results have been interpreted to indicate that conformational transitions in substrate or enzyme RNAs may be involved in the RNase P RNA reaction (Gardiner et al. 1985; Altman and Guerrier-Takada 1986), but the findings are equally interpretable in electrostatic terms. For instance, mildly denaturing solvents (ethanol, dimethyl sulfoxide, and ethylene glycol) potentiate the reaction at lower salt concentrations than required in fully aqueous media (Gardiner et al. 1985). This might suggest that polynucleotide structural fluidity is important in the reaction, perhaps permitting the enzyme RNA to conform to the various pre-tRNAs and other low-molecular-weight RNA substrates. Alternatively, this effect can be explained from the electrostatic viewpoint, since the solvents reduce the dielectric constant of the reaction medium. This would, by Coulomb's law, enhance the electrostatic interaction potential. Therefore, the screening cations would bind more tightly to the polynucleotides and thereby exert their influence at lower concentrations in the presence of solvents.

Role of Ionic Strength and Protein in the RNase P Reaction

The ability of high ionic strength to substitute for the RNase P protein might be exerted in the substrate-binding process, the catalytic mechanism, or both. This has been evaluated by inspection of the dependence of the kinetic parameters, K_m and k_{cat}, on the ionic strength or on the presence of the protein in the reaction medium (Reich et al. 1987). Figure 1 shows an autoradiogram of a typical kinetic assay for RNase P and describes the nature of the enzyme and that of the substrate RNAs, produced by in vitro transcription from genes cloned adjacent to phage T7 promoters. The dependence of the RNA-alone reaction on ionic strength, at various substrate concentrations, is summarized in Figure 2A. It is evident that changes in monovalent and divalent salt concentrations seem to influence the binding step (K_m); the catalytic rate (V_{max}) is essentially unchanged over the salt range tested.

These data are consistent with the notion that elevated salt concentrations counteract repulsion between the enzyme and substrate; binding is more facile at high ionic strength. However, the turnover number (k_{cat}) of the RNA-alone reaction is remarkably low, only about 1 mole of substrate per minute per mole of enzyme RNA.

Figure 2B compares the kinetic parameters of the RNA-alone reaction with those of the holoenzyme under their respective optimal ionic conditions. It is clear that the RNase P RNA and holoenzyme bind the substrate equally well; the K_m values are the same. This

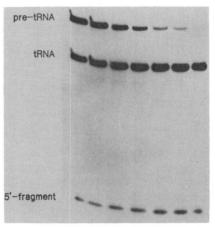

Figure 1. An example of an RNase P activity assay. In general, RNase P activity was assayed at 37°C by incubating uniformly ^{32}P-labeled precursor tRNA^{Asp} with RNase P RNA, either alone (as shown) or in the presence of saturating amounts of purified RNase P protein ("holoenzyme"). The autoradiograph shows the time course for the cleavage of pre-tRNA^{Asp}, by *B. subtilis* RNase P RNA. Sampling times are, from left to right, 1, 3, 5, 10, 15, 20, and 30 min. The results of this assay are plotted as E + S in Fig. 4A. Both substrate and enzyme RNAs were produced by in vitro transcription of the corresponding genes cloned adjacent to T7 promoters (Reich et al. 1986). RNA-alone reactions were carried out at high salt concentrations (typically 50 mM Tris-HCl [pH 8.0], 800 mM NH$_4$Cl, 100 mM MgCl$_2$); holoenzyme reactions were carried out in 50 mM Tris-HCl (pH 8.0), 100 mM NH$_4$Cl, and 15 mM MgCl$_2$. Following ethanol precipitation, reaction products were resolved on 8% polyacrylamide gels containing 8 M urea. After fixing and drying the gels, product bands were located by autoradiography, excised, and counted. Reaction rates were expressed as moles of substrate cleaved per mole of enzyme per minute.

is consistent with the notion that high ionic strength and the RNase P protein play the same role in the reaction: titrating anionic repulsion between the substrate and enzyme RNAs. However, in addition, the V_{max} of the reaction in the presence of the protein, at low ionic strength, is approximately 20-fold greater than in its absence in the RNA-alone reaction at high ionic strength.

The RNase P protein could enhance the overall catalytic rate of the processing reaction in several ways. For example, it could increase the number of enzymatically active RNase P RNA molecules, it could increase the rate of pre-tRNA binding or cleavage, or it might promote more rapid dissociation of the enzyme-product complex following cleavage.

The holoenzyme and RNA-alone reactions in the experiments shown in Figure 2 were carried out at the same nominal concentrations of RNase P RNA. However, it was conceivable that oligomerization of the RNA was required to form an active enzyme in the absence of the protein. Thus, equimolar concentrations of RNase P RNA would not correspond to equal concentrations of active enzyme in the two types of reactions. Indeed, it has been reported that dimerization of the *E. coli* RNase P RNA is required for activity in the

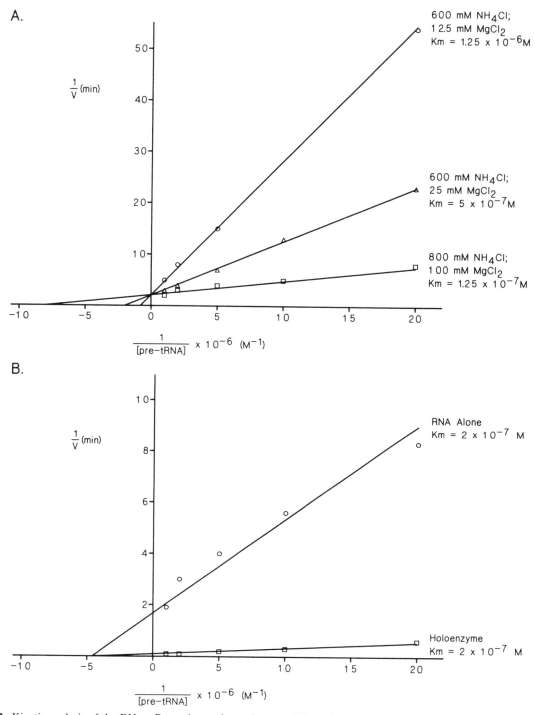

Figure 2. Kinetic analysis of the RNase P reaction under various conditions. (*A*) Double reciprocal (Lineweaver-Burk) plot of RNase P RNA activity shown as a function of substrate concentration, under the specified ionic conditions. Reactions were carried out in 50 mM Tris-HCl (pH 8.0) for 15 min and analyzed as described in Fig. 1. (*B*) Double reciprocal plot of RNase P RNA and holoenzyme activities shown as a function of substrate concentration. Ionic conditions were optimal for both reactions, namely, 800 mM NH_4Cl and 100 mM $MgCl_2$ for RNA alone, and 100 mM NH_4Cl and 15 mM $MgCl_2$ for holoenzyme.

absence of the protein (Guerrier-Takada et al. 1986). This conclusion was based on the observation that the activity of the RNA alone seemed to have a second-order dependence on the concentration of the catalytic RNA. We have not been able to confirm this result. As shown in Figure 3 for the RNase P RNAs of both *E. coli* and *B. subtilis*, the enzymatic activity is directly proportional to the amount of RNA added to the reac-

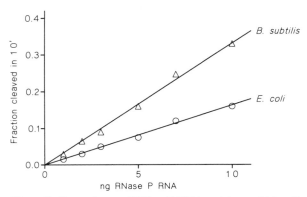

Figure 3. Dependence of RNase P RNA activity on RNase P RNA concentration, for the *B. subtilis* and *E. coli* RNAs. Pre-tRNA^{Asp} (36 ng, ~1 pmole) was incubated at 37°C with different amounts of RNase P RNA, varying from 1 to 10 ng (~0.0075–0.075 pmole). The extent of the reactions are reported as the fraction of substrate cleaved in 10 min.

tions. Thus, we see no reason to invoke the formation of dimer or higher-order RNase P RNA oligomers in the RNA-alone reaction. It remains possible that the protein activates RNase P RNA molecules that are

inactive under the high-salt conditions, but the following results make this unlikely.

To explore the steps in the overall RNase P reaction that are accelerated by the protein, we inspected the early courses of reactions containing a substrate:enzyme ratio of only 2:1 (Reich et al. 1987). Thus, it was possible to compare the first round of cleavage of the substrate by the holoenzyme and the RNA alone. The influence of the protein on the release of the cleaved product was tested by saturating the enzyme with mature tRNA prior to the addition of the pre-tRNA substrate. A lengthy residence time for the product would be seen as a reduction in the rate of the first round of cleavage, beyond that caused by addition of mature tRNA and substrate simultaneously. The results of such experiments with the *B. subtilis* RNase P RNA and holoenzyme are shown in Figure 4. It is evident that the first round of cleavage by the RNA is rapid in the absence of competing tRNA; it is even more rapid than observed in the holoenzyme reaction. Clearly, the stimulation of the overall reaction velocity (k_{cat}) by the protein is not at the steps of binding or cleaving the substrate. After the initial burst of processing, the rates of both the holoenzyme and RNA-alone reac-

A. RNA alone

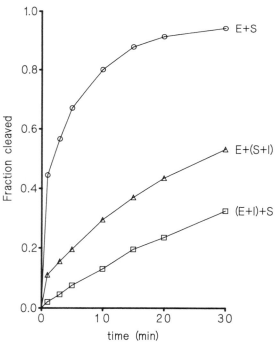

B. Holoenzyme

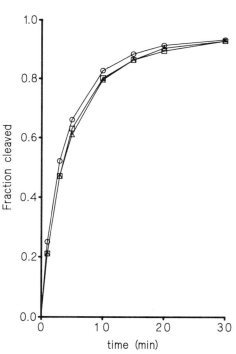

Figure 4. Early course of the RNase P reaction in the presence or absence of mature tRNA competitor. Precursor tRNA^{Asp} (S), inhibitor bulk tRNA (I), and either RNase P RNA or holoenzyme (E) were preincubated for 15 min at 37°C, either alone or in the combinations shown in parentheses. At zero time, reactions were started by combining either enzyme and substrate (○), or enzyme and substrate + tRNA (△), or enzyme + tRNA and substrate (□). RNA-alone reactions were carried out in 50 mM Tris-HCl (pH 8.0), 2 M NH$_4$Cl, and 100 mM MgCl$_2$. For holoenzyme, conditions were 50 mM Tris-HCl (pH 8.0), 100 mM NH$_4$Cl, and 15 mM MgCl$_2$. Concentrations of reactants were [S] = 3×10^{-8} M, [E] = 1.5×10^{-8} M, and [I] = 10^{-7} M. At the indicated times, aliquots were removed and precipitated with ethanol. The extent of the reaction was determined as described in Fig. 1 and is reported as the fraction of substrate cleaved. (*A*) RNA-alone reactions; (*B*) holoenzyme reactions.

tions are reduced; however, the extents of reduction are complicated by product inhibition, and thus are not interpretable in a straightforward way. The fact that the first round of cleavage is more rapid in the RNA-alone reaction is not consistent with the possibility that there are fewer active enzymes at high salt concentrations (see above).

In the presence of mature tRNA competitor, the RNA-alone and holoenzyme reactions behave differently. The course of the RNA-alone reaction is exactly as expected if the product did not dissociate readily from the enzyme following cleavage: Presaturation of the enzyme with mature tRNA abolishes the initial burst of cleavage. The residual reaction is slow, limited by tRNA (product) dissociation. In contrast, the holoenzyme reaction is hardly influenced by the mature tRNA at the concentrations tested, even if added prior to the substrate. The rate at which the product dissociates from the holoenzyme must be rapid, compared to that occurring in the RNA-alone reaction.

In light of the kinetic data available, the role of the RNase P protein in the reaction and the ability of high salt concentrations to substitute for the protein seem qualitatively understood. A model explaining the data is diagrammed in Figure 5. As discussed above, counter-ion screening of anionic repulsion between the substrate and enzyme RNAs is necessary for contact to occur. In the case of the RNA-alone reaction, this is reflected in the progressive decrease in K_m values (increase in binding efficiency), with an increase in mono- and divalent cation concentrations. The RNase P protein, which is strongly basic, also would serve as a cation screen. It seems likely that the protein does not establish specific contacts with the substrate, contributing binding energy, since the K_m values of the RNase P

RNA and holoenzyme are the same at their respective ionic optima.

The higher V_{max} value of the holoenzyme reaction apparently is due to a more rapid dissociation of the enzyme-product complex than occurs during the RNA-alone reaction. This is evident from the finding that preloading the RNase P RNA, but not the holoenzyme, with mature tRNA abolishes the rapid first round of binding and cleavage of the substrate. The difference in the dissociation rates can be interpreted in ionic terms. Because the RNase P protein is small in comparison to the catalytic RNA, it could provide only a localized titration of the repulsion between the enzyme and product RNA phosphates. Consequently, at the relatively low ionic strength that is optimal for the holoenzyme, some of the repulsion between the RNAs would remain, driving product dissociation. In contrast, at the high cation concentrations required for the RNA-alone activity, the general charge neutralization also would quench those repulsive elements. The product would therefore be more tightly locked onto the RNA than onto the holoenzyme.

In summary, the data indicate that the RNase P protein is the cellular solution to the delivery of a high concentration of cations to a specific region of the RNase P RNA, presumably where it contacts the pre-tRNA substrate. It is also possible that the protein counters repulsion between domains of the RNase P RNA, stabilizing the active conformation. We believe that electrostatic insulation will prove to be a common theme for the function of proteins in ribonucleoprotein complexes. For instance, in the ribosome or in small nuclear RNPs (snRNPs), many of the proteins may constitute local pools of counterions, lowering the intrinsic repulsion between polynucleotide chains.

On the Mechanism of RNase P Action

RNase P generates 5'-P and 3'-OH termini, as do most specific processing nucleases composed of protein. Our knowledge of RNA-catalyzed reaction mechanisms is rudimentary; however, it is clear that catalysis by RNase P differs from that carried out by the self-splicing of introns so far characterized.

The excision of both group I and group II self-splicing introns occurs through a series of transesterifications (for review, see Cech and Bass 1986). The reactions of group I introns are initiated by the 3'-OH of guanosine, or a guanosine-containing nucleotide. RNase P does not use this mode of action. It has no requirement for a cosubstrate, and periodate oxidation of the 3' ends of both RNase P and substrate RNAs, which destroys their 2'-OH and 3'-OH groups, does not inactivate the reaction (Marsh and Pace 1985). The initial cleavage of group II introns occurs through an attack of the intron-exon boundary by a 2'-OH group in the intron, producing a covalent conjugate between the interior of the intron and its 5' end, a "lariat" (Padgett et al. 1986). Thus far, searches for a covalent association between RNase P RNA and its substrate, employ-

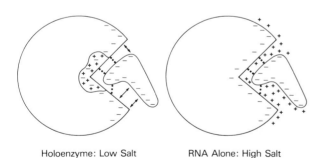

Holoenzyme: Low Salt
[E·tRNA] ⇌ E+tRNA

RNA Alone: High Salt
[E·tRNA] ⇌ E+tRNA

Figure 5. Schematic summary of salt and RNase P protein influence in the RNA-catalyzed reaction. As discussed in the text, we suggest that the RNase P protein titrates local anionic repulsion in the RNA enzyme so that the pre-tRNA may bind. The effect of the protein might be on the RNase P RNA, allowing it to adopt an active conformation, or it might directly counter repulsion between enzyme and substrate RNAs. In the case of the holoenzyme, because the charge titration by the protein is local, intrinsic repulsion between the RNAs remains, driving dissociation following cleavage of the substrate. In the RNA-alone reaction, high ionic strength screens the anionic repulsion in a general, rather than a local, manner, so that product dissociation is slowed. (Adapted from Reich et al. 1987.)

ing the *B. subtilis* (T.L. Marsh and D.S. Waugh, unpubl.) or *E. coli* (Guerrier-Takada et al. 1986) systems, have been unsuccessful. These results, albeit negative, make it likely that water, rather than a 2′-OH group, effects strand scission in the tRNA precursor.

The reactions carried out by hydrolases composed of protein are well studied and are commonly catalyzed by amino acid functional groups that donate or capture protons, as needed to drive catalysis. An analogous proton-exchange scheme is shown for the RNase P reaction in Figure 6. It is likely that the enzyme RNA activates a water molecule to participate in the reaction, rather than utilizing a free hydroxyl ion. This is suggested by the fact that the RNase P reaction rate is not directly proportional to hydroxide ion concentration over the active pH range (Marsh and Pace 1985). Nucleic acid groups are assumed to serve as proton sinks in the reaction shown. The role could be played by either nucleic acid bases or phosphodiester chain elements, both of which can serve in proton transfer and catalyze general acid/general base reactions (Pace and Marsh 1985).

Structure of RNase P RNA

Understanding the mechanism of the RNase P RNA will require knowledge of its secondary and tertiary structures. Such information is crucial to the interpretation of experiments that perturb the RNA structure. Fairly detailed secondary structure models for the RNase P RNAs of *B. subtilis* and *E. coli* have been derived using a phylogenetic comparative approach to identify base-paired sequences (James et al. 1987).

Evaluating higher-order RNA structure is a process of progressive refinement. The first step attempts to predict secondary structure from nucleotide sequence, using thermodynamic estimates for helix stabilities to define possible complementary pairings. However, computational approaches to predicting helical structure from nucleotide sequences are not well developed (Papanicolaou et al. 1984). There are several reasons

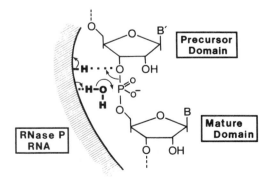

Figure 6. Hypothetical mechanism for the hydrolysis of tRNA precursors by RNase P. The hatched boundary indicates the RNase P surface. B and B′ are bases. The phosphodiester bond connecting the precursor and mature domains of the pre-tRNA is depicted. (Adapted from Marsh and Pace 1985.)

for the inability to predict secondary structure reliably. One reason is that the available estimates of free-energy values for base pairings are inexact; they are based on data from limited collections of oligonucleotides and apply to specific in vitro conditions. Moreover, there are no reliable estimates for the stabilities of noncanonical base pairs (A-G, A-C, etc.) or for the effects of local sequence context. Helix discontinuities, such as unpaired bases, are other common elements in natural RNAs that cannot yet be treated thermodynamically with good credibility. Finally, the existing computational methods for evaluating secondary structure from nucleotide sequence cannot account for helix stabilizing or destabilizing constraints imposed by tertiary structure.

Although thermodynamic predictions of sequence pairing are inexact, they provide models for experimental evaluation. There are two broad approaches toward testing RNA-folding models. One approach uses structure-specific enzymes and chemicals to identify duplex and single-strand segments in the RNA under native conditions (Vournakis et al. 1981). However, interpreting the results of such experiments requires a reliable structure model, and, in any case, the results do not identify the pairing partners of duplex segments. At this time, the best a priori method for evaluating the secondary structures of large RNAs is the phylogenetic comparative approach (Fox and Woese 1975; Noller and Woese 1981). Possible helices in an RNA, as indicated by the occurrence of complementary sequences, are tested by seeking the equivalent pairing possibilities in the homologous RNA from another organism in which the sequence varies. Helical regions are indicated by covariance of complementary bases in compared sequences; nucleotide substitutions compensate one another to maintain complementarity.

The sequences of the *E. coli* (Reed et al. 1982; Sakamoto et al. 1983) and *B. subtilis* (Reich et al. 1986) RNase P RNAs were the first available for structural comparisons. We were surprised when they proved to be so dissimilar that homologous sequences could not be identified over most of the lengths of the molecules: The sequences could not be aligned (Reich et al. 1986). In contrast, the 16S rRNAs from these organisms display substantial sequence similarity (Reich et al. 1986). It is evident that the primary structure of RNase P RNA evolves very rapidly in comparison to that of 16S rRNA. The inability to align homologous nucleotides in the two RNase P RNA sequences unambiguously meant, however, that comparison of these sequences could not be used for an initial determination of helical pairings. The identification of compensatory changes that indicate structures demands that only homologous nucleotides be considered. Hence, it was necessary to inspect the RNase P RNA sequences of organisms more closely related to either *B. subtilis* or *E. coli*, seeking less profound differences than occur between the RNAs of those organisms.

The choice of appropriate organisms for phylogenetic comparative analysis of the RNase P RNA structure requires a quantitative view of evolutionary relatedness, now available from comparative studies of rRNA sequences (for review, see Pace et al. 1986). From this perspective, *B. subtilis* and *E. coli* are fairly distant from one another. They are members of different eubacterial "phyla": *B. subtilis* is a member of the "gram-positive and relatives" group, and *E. coli* is one of the "purple bacteria and relatives" group. For analysis of the gram-positive and purple bacterial RNase P RNA structures, we sequenced the corresponding genes from organisms within those phyla and having 5S rRNA sequence similarities of 75–80% with *B. subtilis* or *E. coli*. These included the gram-positive bacteria *Bacillus megaterium*, *Bacillus brevis*, and *Bacillus stearothermophilus*, and the purple bacterium relative *Pseudomonas fluorescens*.

As detailed elsewhere (James et al. 1987), the intraphylum comparisons provided evidence for a number of helices. Some sequences were invariant within the two phyla. These more conserved sequences were valuable landmarks in establishing the interphylum sequence alignment. There emerged a core of primary and secondary structures that are common to the two phyla. Additionally, the RNase P RNAs of each of the phyla contain structural elements not present in the other. The proposed foldings of the *B. subtilis* and *E.*

coli RNase P RNAs are shown in Figure 7. These models are minimally structured; some of the sequences shown as unpaired are complementary. However, we cannot be certain that they pair in vivo because the sequences are constant among all the organisms considered; there is no sequence covariation to support the helices. Information on the structures of these highly conserved sequence elements will require the inspection of additional, diverse RNase P RNAs.

In view of the overall low sequence similarity, the commonality of the core features of the RNase P RNAs of the two phyla encourages confidence that the structures are correct. The structures provide a framework for the further analysis of the catalytic RNA. Moreover, the sequence and secondary structural elements that are common to the RNase P RNAs from the two phyla must contain the important elements involved in precursor tRNA binding and cleavage and in the interaction with the RNase P protein.

Coaxial stacking of helical elements is a common structural theme in the rRNAs and tRNAs; it orders helical units, providing superstructure in large molecules. The relative positions of the evolutionarily conserved helices in the RNase P RNA structure suggest that they form two coaxial stacks. One would consist of the helices that, in *B. subtilis*, are formed by nu-

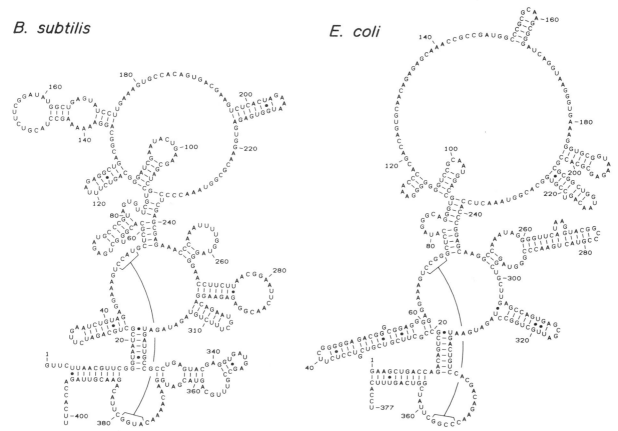

Figure 7. Secondary structure models for the *B. subtilis* and *E. coli* RNase P RNAs based on phylogenetic comparisons (see text). (Adapted from James et al. 1987.)

cleotides 5-13/386-394, 15-22/321-328, and 23-40/36-43. The second coaxial stack would be formed by the *B. subtilis* nucleotide pairings 52-55/376-379, 57-61/240-244, and 86-90/235-239, and perhaps capped by the helix composed of residues 91-96/107-112 (or 132-133/233-234). The sequences and structures within and adjacent to these two coaxial stacks are the most evolutionarily conservative in the molecule, so they likely contain the enzymatically active elements.

In addition to their common features, the RNase P RNAs contain structural elements that seem to be unique to one or the other of the phyla. Even within a phylum, some features are highly variable in structure, e.g., in hairpin length (James et al. 1987). Because they are so evolutionarily volatile, it seems unlikely that these variable structures have a direct role in the RNase P reaction. The variable elements might relate to additional, group-specific functions of the RNase P RNAs. It is noteworthy that the length variations in the molecules tend to be localized in hairpins and sequences that are peripheral in the foldings. The internal loops or long-range pairs constituting the structure that is common to the phyla inspected tend to be constant in length, with substantial sequence conservation.

Some Mutational Analyses of RNase P RNA

We anticipate that the RNase P RNA structural elements that are conserved between the phyla will prove to be the seat of the enzymatic activity. Mutational analyses carried out so far are generally consistent with this notion (D.S. Waugh, unpubl.). Moreover, at least one important site of interaction between the RNase P RNA and the protein is located in the conserved portion of the RNAs. During the course of site-directed modifications of the *B. subtilis* RNase P RNA gene (cloned adjacent to a phage T7 promoter to provide an in vitro expression system), the nucleotide sequence corresponding to residues 236–239 in the RNA (UCGA, see Fig. 7) was tandemly duplicated (D.S. Waugh, unpubl.). This duplication would be expected to disrupt the coaxial stacking of helix 86-90/235-239 with helix 91-96/107-112 and alter the positioning of the adjacent conserved sequence (*B. subtilis* nucleotides ~223–234). As shown in Figure 8, the transcript of this modified gene is as active as the native RNase P RNA in the RNA-alone reaction at high ionic strength. However, its activity is not appreciably stimulated by the RNase P protein under the holoenzyme reaction conditions. The most straightforward interpretation of this result is that the disrupted sequence is an important contact for the protein; however, there are other possibilities. For instance, the insertion might perturb the local conformation in a manner that affects the interaction with the protein but not catalysis.

In a second type of mutational analysis, important catalytic elements were sought by constructing RNase P RNAs from which sequences of varying lengths were omitted (D.S. Waugh, unpubl.). Some of the constructs were completely inactive. However, considering the

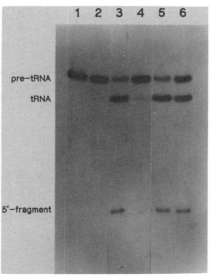

Figure 8. Site-directed mutation of an RNase P RNA site that influences RNase P protein interaction. A small sequence (5'-TCGA-3') was duplicated within the *Xho*I site of the *B. subtilis* RNase P RNA gene (nucleotides 236 through 239) by cleavage with the restriction enzyme, filling the single-strand termini using the Klenow fragment of DNA polymerase, and ligating the blunt ends. T7 RNA polymerase runoff transcripts (Reich et al. 1986) of both mutant and wild-type RNase P RNAs were assayed for enzymatic activity in the absence (odd-numbered lanes) or in the presence (even-numbered lanes) of partially purified *B. subtilis* RNase P protein as described in Fig. 1. (*1,2*) No RNase P RNA; (*3,4*) RNase P RNA containing the tetranucleotide duplication; (*5,6*) wild-type RNase P RNA.

collection of deleted RNA constructs that are at least partially active, it was possible to remove every residue in the *B. subtilis* RNase P RNA without completely abolishing the activity. The reaction rates of some of the active constructs were reduced many orders of magnitude below that of the wild-type RNA; nevertheless, they catalyzed the correct cleavage of the pre-tRNA. This result indicates that the catalytic mechanism of RNase P does not depend absolutely on a single nucleotide or local sequence. Rather, the structure required for activity likely consists of mulitiple elements, arranged by the folding of the RNA. This view of the RNase P RNA catalytic center is analogous to that commonly seen in protein enzymes: Active sites result from the tertiary structural positioning of amino acids that may be distributed widely in the sequence (Creighton 1983).

Why is RNase P Made of RNA?

The question of course arises: Why is the catalytic element of RNase P an RNA molecule? We know that proteins can specifically recognize RNAs and that cells generally use proteins as catalysts. Indeed, the other known specific processing nucleases that act intermolecularly, e.g., those involved in rRNA maturation, are proteins. One often-proposed explanation for the

RNA nature of RNase P is that it may be a historical accident, a remnant of early life forms, from the time before the protein-synthesizing machinery was fully established. This view suggests that the early commitment of RNA to an essential function precluded the subsequent assumption of the role by a protein. This explanation for the RNA composition of RNase P as a historical accident seems unlikely, however, since the RNase P structure is so highly variable (see above). An evolutionarily constrained remnant of the earliest life on earth might be expected to be much more conservative in its architecture, at least as conservative as the rRNAs or tRNAs.

An alternative, to us more likely, explanation is that RNase P remains an RNA because it plays some role that proteins cannot so readily perform. One possibility is that the RNase P RNA provides structure to, and coordinates, several elements in a multienzyme, tRNA-processing complex analogous to the ribosome, and it happens to be a nuclease, as well, in the interests of cellular economy. All tRNA precursors must undergo multiple processing steps, such as terminal cleavages and methylations. It is attractive to consider that this would occur in a multienzyme complex. Another possibility derives from the fact that RNase P has a nearly unique role among enzymes—it must handle many different, yet specific, substrates: the 50 or so distinct tRNAs produced by cells. All the tRNAs have the same general form, the L-shaped tertiary structure, but they differ in minor details, a consequence of different sequences, loop sizes, precursor-specific sequences, etc. RNase P must accommodate all of these, perhaps by molding, "induced fit," to the substrates. Proteins, too, are capable of interacting with all tRNAs. For instance, elongation factor Tu binds selectively to all aminoacylated tRNAs; nucleotidyl transferase catalyzes the addition of the 3'-terminal CCA sequence to all tRNAs. On the other hand, RNase P must accommodate variable precursor-specific sequences and any resulting variability in higher-order structure in the vicinity of the substrate bonds. Perhaps RNase P activity is therefore embodied in RNA because of a requirement for structural fluidity in the active site. Proteins offer a greater wealth of chemically functional groups than do polynucleotides, but RNA structure may be intrinsically more mobile than that of proteins.

ACKNOWLEDGMENTS

This work was supported by National Institutes of Health grant GM-34527 to N.R.P. We thank Ms. Anna Wyatt for assistance in preparing the manuscript.

REFERENCES

Altman, S. and C. Guerrier-Takada. 1986. M₁ RNA, the RNA subunit of *Escherichia coli* ribonuclease P, can undergo a pH-sensitive conformational change. *Biochemistry* **25:** 1205.

Altman, S. and J.D. Smith. 1971. Tyrosine tRNA precursor molecule polynucleotide sequences. *Nat. New Biol.* **233:** 35.

Castano, J.G., R. Ornberg, J.G. Koster, J.A. Tobian, and M. Zasloff. 1986. Eukaryotic pre-tRNA 5' processing nuclease: Copurification with a complex cylindrical particle. *Cell* **46:** 377.

Cech, T.R. 1985. Self-splicing RNA: Implications for evolution. *Int. Rev. Cytol.* **93:** 3.

Cech, T.R. and B.L. Bass. 1986. Biological catalysis by RNA. *Annu. Rev. Biochem.* **55:** 599.

Creighton, T.E. 1983. *Proteins.* W.H. Freeman, New York.

Doersen, C., C. Guerrier-Takada, S. Altman, and G. Attardi. 1985. Characterization of an RNase P activity from HeLa cell mitochondria: Comparison with the cytosol RNase P activity. *J. Biol. Chem.* **260:** 5942.

Fox, G. and C. Woese. 1975. 5S RNA secondary structure. *Nature* **256:** 505.

Gardiner, K. and N.R. Pace. 1980. RNase P from *Bacillus subtilis* has a RNA component. *J. Biol. Chem.* **255:** 7507.

Gardiner, K.J., T.L. Marsh, and N.R. Pace. 1985. Ion dependence of the *Bacillus subtilis* RNase P reaction. *J. Biol. Chem.* **260:** 5415.

Gold, H.A. and S. Altman. 1986. Reconstitution of RNase P activity using inactive subunits from *E. coli* and HeLa cells. *Cell* **44:** 243.

Guerrier-Takada, C. and S. Altman. 1984. Catalytic activity of an RNA molecule prepared by transcription in vitro. *Science* **223:** 285.

Guerrier-Takada, C., K. Haydock, L. Allen, and S. Altman. 1986. Metal ion requirements and other aspects of the reaction catalyzed by M₁ RNA, the RNA subunit of ribonuclease P from *Escherichia coli*. *Biochemistry* **25:** 1509.

Guerrier-Takada, C., K. Gardiner, T. Marsh, N. Pace, and S. Altman. 1983. The RNA moiety of ribonuclease P is the catalytic subunit of the enzyme. *Cell* **35:** 849.

James, B.D., G.J. Olsen, J. Liu, and N.R. Pace. 1987. The secondary structure of ribonuclease P RNA, the catalytic element of a ribonucleoprotein enzyme. *Cell* (in press).

Kline, L., S. Nishikawa, and D. Söll. 1981. Partial purification of RNase P from *Schizosaccharomyces pombe*. *J. Biol. Chem.* **256:** 5058.

Kruger, K., P. Grabowski, A. Zaug, J. Sands, D. Gottschling, and T.R. Cech. 1982. Self-splicing RNA: Autoexcision and autocyclization of the ribosomal RNA intervening sequence of *Tetrahymena*. *Cell* **31:** 147.

Marsh, T.L. and N.R. Pace. 1985. Ribonuclease P catalysis differs from ribosomal RNA self-splicing. *Science* **229:** 79.

Noller, H.F. and C.R. Woese. 1981. Secondary structure of 16S ribosomal RNA. *Science* **212:** 403.

Pace, N.R. and T.L. Marsh. 1985. RNA catalysis and the origin of life. *Origins Life* **16:** 97.

Pace, N.R., G.J. Olsen, and C.R. Woese. 1986. Ribosomal RNA phylogeny and the primary lines of evolutionary descent. *Cell* **45:** 325.

Padgett, R.A., P.J. Gradowski, M.M. Konarska, S. Seiler, and P.A. Sharp. 1986. Splicing of messenger RNA precursors. *Annu. Rev. Biochem.* **55:** 1119.

Papanicolaou, C., M. Gouy, and J. Ninio. 1984. An energy model that predicts the correct folding of both the tRNA and the 5S RNA molecules. *Nucleic Acids Res.* **12:** 31.

Reed, R.E., M. Baer, C. Guerrier-Takada, H. Donis-Keller, and S. Altman. 1982. Nucleotide sequence of the gene encoding the RNA subunit (M₁ RNA) of ribonuclease P from *Escherichia coli*. *Cell* **30:** 627.

Reich, C., G.J. Olsen, B. Pace, and N.R. Pace. 1987. The role of the protein moiety of ribonuclease P, a ribonucleoprotein enzyme. *Science* (in press).

Reich, C., K.J. Gardiner, G.J. Olsen, B. Pace, T.L. Marsh, and N.R. Pace. 1986. The RNA component of the *Bacillus subtilis* RNase P: Sequence, activity, and partial secondary structure. *J. Biol. Chem.* **261:** 7888.

Ross, P.D. and R.L. Scruggs. 1964. Electrophoresis of DNA. III. The effect of several univalent electrolytes on the mobility of DNA. *Biopolymers* **2:** 231.

Sakamoto, H., N. Kimuro, F. Nagawa, and Y. Shimura. 1983. Nucleotide sequence and stability of the RNA component of RNase P from a temperature-sensitive mutant of *E. coli*. *Nucleic Acids Res.* **11:** 8237.

Stark, B.C., R. Kole, E.J. Bowman, and S. Altman. 1978. Ribonuclease P: An enzyme with an essential RNA component. *Proc. Natl. Acad. Sci.* **75:** 3717.

Vournakis, J.N., J. Celantano, M. Finn, R.E. Lockard, T. Mitra, G. Pavlakis, A. Troutt, M. Vandenberg, and R.M. Wurst. 1981. Sequence and structure analysis of end-labeled RNA with nucleases. In *Gene amplification and analysis: Structural analysis of nucleic acids* (ed. J.G. Chirikjian and T.S. Papas), vol. 2, p. 268. Elsevier/North-Holland, New York.

Structural and Ionic Requirements for Self-cleavage of Virusoid RNAs and *trans* Self-cleavage of Viroid RNA

A.C. FORSTER, A.C. JEFFRIES, C.C. SHELDON, AND R.H. SYMONS
Department of Biochemistry, University of Adelaide, Adelaide, S.A. 5000, Australia

Certain circular and low-molecular-weight, single-stranded plant pathogenic RNAs can self-cleave at specific sites in vitro in the presence of Mg^{++} (Buzayan et al. 1986a; Hutchins et al. 1986; Prody et al. 1986; Forster and Symons 1987a). This property is considered to be important in their replication in vivo by a rolling-circle mechanism. All of these self-cleavage reactions generate 5'-OH and 2',3'-cyclic phosphodiester termini in what is essentially a transphosphorylation reaction involving attack by the free 2'-OH group on the 3',5'-phosphodiester linkage (Fig. 1A). These self-cleavage reactions are clearly different from the self-splicing reactions involved in the removal of introns from rRNA and mRNA precursors that produce excised fragments with 5'-phosphate and 3'-OH termini (Cech and Bass 1986; Sharp 1987).

Self-cleavage occurs in the plus and minus RNAs derived from the 247-nucleotide avocado sunblotch viroid (ASBV) (Hutchins et al. 1986), the 359-nucleotide linear satellite RNA of tobacco ringspot virus (sTRSV) (Buzayan et al. 1986a; Prody et al. 1986), and the 324-nucleotide virusoid (circular satellite RNA) of lucerne transient streak virus (vLTSV) (Forster and Symons 1987a). Similar hammerhead-shaped secondary structures were proposed for the self-cleavage site of plus and minus ASBV RNAs (Fig. 1B), plus and minus vLTSV RNAs (Fig. 1C), and plus sTRSV (Hutchins et al. 1986; Forster and Symons 1987a). Although the minus sequence of sTRSV self-cleaves (Buzayan et al. 1986a), a hammerhead structure cannot be formed at its active site (Forster and Symons 1987a).

In the case of plus vLTSV, 5'- and 3'-deletion analyses of in-vitro-synthesized RNA transcripts indicated that only 51 nucleotides within the hammerhead structure (Fig. 1D) are necessary for rapid and complete self-cleavage to occur upon addition of Mg^{++} (Forster and Symons 1987b). For longer plus and minus vLTSV RNAs, heating and snap cooling were essential prior to the addition of Mg^{++} for self-cleavage to occur. The data indicated that these longer RNAs were in inactive configurations and that the heating–snap-cooling step was required to convert some of the inactive configurations to active ones (Forster and Symons 1987a,b). This situation contrasts with that for plus and minus RNA transcripts of ASBV and sTRSV, where self-cleavage occurs without prior heating and snap cooling (Buzayan et al. 1986a; Hutchins et al. 1986; Prody et al. 1986).

In this paper, we report further characterization of the self-cleavage reactions of plus and minus RNA transcripts of vLTSV and show that 61 nucleotides of minus sequence are sufficient for self-cleavage. In addition, we provide data on the self-cleavage of minus RNA transcripts of ASBV by showing that two separate RNA fragments can act in *trans* to give specific self-cleavage.

MATERIALS AND METHODS

Reagents. SP6 RNA polymerase, T4 polynucleotide kinase, $[\alpha\text{-}^{32}P]UTP$, and $[\gamma\text{-}^{32}P]ATP$ were obtained from BRESA, Adelaide, and T7 RNA polymerase was obtained from Promega Biotec. T4 RNA ligase was obtained from Pharmacia; restriction enzymes, from New England Bio-Labs and Toyobo; RNase T1, from Sigma; and RNase U2, from Calbiochem. RNase PhyM from *Physarum polycephalum* was purified as described by Donis-Keller (1980). Synthetic oligodeoxynucleotides were prepared on an Applied Biosystems Model 380B DNA synthesizer by S. Rogers and D. Skingle.

Plasmid constructions. Two plasmids containing partial-length (273 nucleotides) plus and minus sequences of vLTSV-A in the plasmid pSP64 were prepared by P. Keese as described by Forster and Symons (1987a). These plasmids contained the sequence corresponding to nucleotides 55–3 of vLTSV-A (Australian isolate). In addition, a synthetic double-stranded DNA fragment, with *Hin*dIII and *Bam*HI sticky ends, containing 56 nucleotides of vLTSV-A sequence (nucleotides 163–218), was prepared by annealing two 61-mer oligodeoxynucleotides. The sequence of the 61-mer containing the plus vLSTV sequence (italicized) is 5'-AGCT*TACGTC....ACGTAC*G-3'. The double-strand fragment was cloned by J. Cassady into the pSP64 plasmid vector restricted with *Hin*dIII and *Bam*HI. The orientation of the insert produced plus vLTSV RNA sequences on transcription.

In vitro synthesis of plus and minus vLTSV-A RNAs on plasmid templates. Nonradioactive transcription reactions containing 0.1 $\mu g/\mu l$ template DNA, 0.5 unit/μl SP6 RNA polymerase, 40 mM Tris-HCl (pH 7.5), 6 mM $MgCl_2$, 0.1 $\mu g/\mu l$ bovine serum albumin (BSA), 10 mM dithiothreitol (DTT), and 0.5 mM of each of the four NTPs were incubated at 40°C for 1–2 hours. Radioactive transcription mixtures contained 0.025 mM UTP and up to 5 $\mu Ci/\mu l$ of $[\alpha\text{-}^{32}P]UTP$. Reaction mixtures were fractionated as described below.

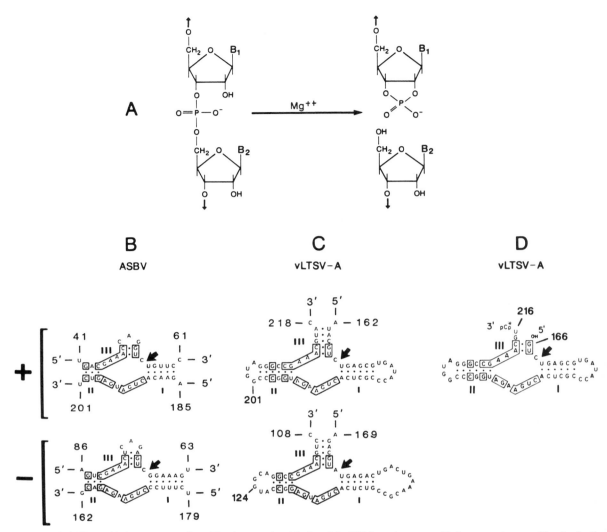

Figure 1. (*A*) The self-cleavage reaction. The internucleotide bond in RNA undergoes self-cleavage at a specific site in the presence of Mg⁺⁺ or some other polyvalent cations to give 2′,3′-cyclic phosphate and 5′-OH termini. The reaction is not reversible in vLTSV (Forster and Symons 1987a) and also probably not in ASBV. (*B,C*) Secondary structural models for the active sites for plus and minus ASBV (Hutchins et al. 1986) and vLTSV RNAs (Forster and Symons 1987a). Arrows indicate self-cleavage sites, and boxed areas indicate nucleotides strictly conserved between the proposed hammerhead structures (Forster and Symons 1987a). Recent data suggest that the depicted base pairs involving the conserved GAAAC may not be present in the active structures (Forster and Symons 1987b). (*D*) Structural model for the 51-nucleotide fragment of plus vLTSV-A (residues 166–216) that cleaves rapidly and completely in the presence of Mg⁺⁺ (Forster and Symons 1987b). The 3′-terminal pCp is the radioactive label added to the unlabeled fragment with T4 RNA ligase; asterisk indicates labeled phosphate.

In vitro synthesis of RNA from a synthetic DNA template. The procedure follows that of Lowary et al. (1986) and Zaug et al. (1986). A 16-mer oligodeoxynucleotide was annealed to the 3′ end of an 81-mer oligodeoxynucleotide to provide a double-stranded DNA T7 RNA polymerase promoter and a single-stranded DNA template. A solution containing equimolar concentrations (500 nM) of each oligonucleotide was heated to 75°C in 10 mM Tris-HCl (pH 8.0) and then cooled gradually to 30°C over about 1 hour. Transcription reactions containing 50 nM template DNA, 1.5 units/μl T7 RNA polymerase, 40 mM Tris-HCl (pH 7.5), 6 mM MgCl₂, 0.1 μg/μl BSA, 10 mM DTT, 0.5 mM of each of the four NTPs, and about 1 μCi/μl of [α-³²P]UTP were incubated at 40°C for 1 hour and then analyzed by gel electrophoresis (see below).

Gel electrophoresis and purification of RNAs. Transcription mixtures or self-cleavage reactions were added to an equal volume of loading solution (95% formamide, 10 mM sodium-EDTA, 0.02% xylene cyanol FF, 0.02% bromophenol blue), heated at 80°C for 30 seconds, and snap-cooled on ice before loading on 35 × 20 × 0.05-cm, 7 M urea–polyacrylamide gels that were run in 90 mM Tris-borate (pH 8.3) and 2 mM EDTA. Autoradiography was carried out at −70°C with an intensifying screen for the detection of labeled

RNAs. Nonradioactive products were detected by staining with 0.05% toluidine blue and brief destaining in water. When required, RNAs were eluted from gel slices in 0.1% SDS, 1 mM EDTA, and 10 mM Tris-HCl (pH 7.5) for several hours at 37°C, precipitated by the addition of 3 M sodium acetate (pH 5) to 0.3 M and 2.5 volumes of cold ethanol, stored at 0°C or −20°C, and later centrifuged.

RESULTS

Further Characterization of the Self-cleavage Reactions of Plus and Minus vLTSV RNAs

To account for the self-cleavage data obtained with 336-nucleotide long plus and minus RNA transcripts containing 84% of the LTSV virusoid sequence, we propose that the reaction pathway in Figure 2 summarizes the sequence of events for self-cleavage (Forster and Symons 1987a). Full-length transcripts purified by gel electrophoresis, elution, and ethanol precipitation are in an inactive configuration, C_I, which does not self-cleave upon addition of Mg^{++}. Heating and snap cooling these transcripts in 1 mM EDTA converts them to a mixture of structures: those with an inactive conformation and those with an active conformation, C_A, which self-cleaves to completion upon addition of Mg^{++}. The self-cleavage reaction is not reversible (Forster and Symons 1987a).

Evidence that different conformational forms of the 336-nucleotide plus and minus RNA transcripts exist was shown by gel electrophoresis at 4°C under nondenaturing conditions (for a similar analysis of different conformations of the potato spindle tuber viroid, see Riesner et al. 1979). The patterns observed for the inactive, untreated, purified transcripts (Fig. 3, lanes 1 and 4) resembled the inactive, heated, and slowly cooled RNAs (Fig. 3, lanes 3 and 6) (Forster and Symons 1987a), but differed significantly from the partially active, heated, and snap-cooled RNAs (Fig. 3, lanes 2 and 5). The heated and slowly cooled RNAs are expected to be in their most thermodynamically stable conformations. The patterns in Figure 3 indicate the complexity of the conformational forms of the plus and minus RNAs after these three different treatments.

To define the temperature requirements for self-cleavage of plus and minus RNAs, the RNAs were heated to temperatures below the standard 80°C for 1 minute in 1 mM EDTA before snap cooling on ice and incubation at 25°C for 10 minutes in 5 mM $MgCl_2$, 0.5 mM EDTA, and 50 mM Tris-HCl (pH 7.5). Results showed that the 336-nucleotide RNAs preheated at

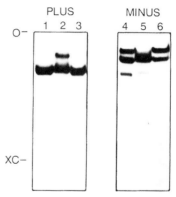

Figure 3. Evidence for different conformational forms of the 336-nucleotide plus and minus RNA transcripts of vLTSV DNA clones. ^{32}P-labeled transcripts were prepared from partial-length DNA clones of vLTSV as described previously (Forster and Symons 1987a). These transcripts contained 273 nucleotides of vLTSV (residues 55–3), with 3′- and 5′-terminal vector sequences totaling 63 nucleotides. (1,4) Purified RNA transcripts with no further treatment; (2,5) RNAs in 1 mM EDTA heated at 80°C for 1 min and then placed on ice for 5 min; (3,6) RNAs in 1 mM EDTA heated to 80°C and allowed to cool gradually to room temperature over 4 hr and then placed on ice. For analysis, 5-μl samples were mixed with 5 μl of ice-cold 20% glycerol, 10 mM EDTA, 0.04% xylene cyanol FF, and 0.04% bromophenol blue, and loaded on a single 10% polyacrylamide gel (90 mM Tris-borate, 2 mM EDTA, pH 8.3) at 4°C. Electrophoresis was carried out at 20 mA (900–1400 V) for 2 hr at 4°C.

65°C or 50°C self-cleaved as efficiently as when heated at 80°C, but no self-cleavage occurred after preheating at 37°C (data not shown). Although the active structures of the heated and snap-cooled RNAs were stable on ice for at least 10 minutes, the active structures of the minus RNAs, but not the plus RNAs, were unstable at 25°C (5 min). The self-cleavage reactions occurred to the same extent whether or not the incubations with Mg^{++} were carried out at the standard 25°C or at 4°C for 10 minutes.

Further data characterizing the self-cleavage reaction are given in Figure 4. The effect of the presence of various concentrations of NaCl during the preheating step on subsequent self-cleavage after snap cooling and the addition of Mg^{++} is shown in Figure 4A. The extent of self-cleavage was determined by separation of the self-cleavage products by gel electrophoresis (Forster and Symons 1987a) and scintillation counting. Self-cleavage of the plus transcript decreased with increasing concentrations of NaCl and was eliminated at 200 mM NaCl. The effect was more pronounced with the minus RNA transcript, and self-cleavage was eliminated at 50 mM NaCl. Similarly, the presence of 5 mM $MgCl_2$ and 50 mM Tris-HCl (pH 7.5) during the preheating and snap-cooling steps almost abolished self-cleavage. These effects were not due to inhibition of self-cleavage during the 25°C incubation because neither NaCl nor $MgCl_2$/Tris-HCl inhibited self-cleavage of RNAs heated and snap-cooled in 1 mM EDTA. Hence, the data indicate that increasing concentrations of salt

$$C_I \xrightleftharpoons{\triangle} C_A \xrightarrow{Mg^{++}} 5'F + 3'F$$

Inactive	Active	Self-cleavage
Conformation	Conformation	Fragments

Figure 2. Reaction pathway for the self-cleavage of plus and minus RNAs of vLTSV.

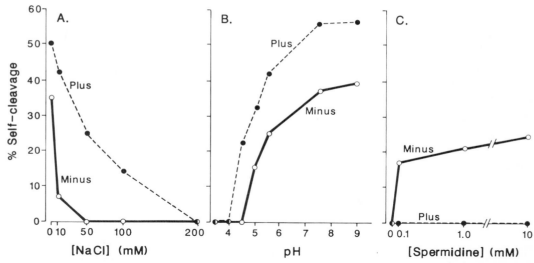

Figure 4. Effect of conditions during the preheating and snap-cooling step and the subsequent self-cleavage incubation on the ability of plus and minus vLTSV RNA transcripts to self-cleave. ^{32}P-labeled RNA transcripts were prepared from partial-length DNA clones of vLTSV as described in Fig. 3. Standard conditions to test for self-cleavage were to heat the purified RNA in 1 mM EDTA (pH ~ 6) at 80°C for 1 min, snap-cool on ice for 5 min, adjust the solution to 5 mM $MgCl_2$, 50 mM Tris-HCl (pH 7.5) at 0°C with an equal volume, and then incubate at 25°C for 10 min. The extent of self-cleavage was then determined by gel electrophoresis (Forster and Symons 1987a). (*A*) RNAs preheated and snap-cooled in the presence of various concentrations of NaCl. (*B*) Effect of pH during the 25°C incubation. Sodium acetate/acetic acid buffers (50 mM) were used at pH values from 3.5 to 5.5, and Tris-HCl buffers were used at pH values of 7.5 and 9.0. (*C*) Effect of various concentrations of spermidine trihydrochloride as a replacement for $MgCl_2$ in the 25°C incubation.

interfere with the conversion of inactive conformations to active ones by preventing the melting out of secondary structures during the heating step and/or the formation of active conformations during the snap cooling.

Self-cleavage reactions of heated and snap-cooled RNAs were usually carried out at pH 7.5. Self-cleavage showed little variation between pH 7.5 and pH 9.0 but decreased as the pH in reaction mixtures was lowered (Fig. 4B). It was eliminated in minus RNA at pH 4.5 and in plus RNA at pH 4.0. The inhibitory effect at low pH is probably due to destruction of the active structures by protonation and/or a direct role of OH⁻ in the self-cleavage reaction.

It was previously shown that Na⁺ could not substitute for Mg⁺⁺ in the self-cleavage reactions (Forster and Symons 1987a). In this study, a range of divalent cations were investigated as alternatives to Mg⁺⁺. At a concentration of 1 mM, Ca⁺⁺ and Mn⁺⁺ gave efficient self-cleavage of both plus and minus RNAs, whereas Ba⁺⁺ was only effective with minus RNA. Co⁺⁺, Ni⁺⁺, and Zn⁺⁺ did not cause self-cleavage. At a concentration of 5 mM, Ca⁺⁺ gave lower self-cleavage than at 1 mM and this decreased further at higher concentrations. This is in contrast to Mg⁺⁺, where the extent of self-cleavage was independent of concentration between 1 mM and 100 mM.

Spermine tetrahydrochloride at concentrations from 0.1 mM to 10 mM did not cause self-cleavage of either plus or minus RNAs. An experimental difficulty was the partial precipitation of RNA by spermine tetrahydrochloride at concentrations of 1 mM and higher. In

contrast, spermidine trihydrochloride concentrations from 0.1 mM to 10 mM gave significant self-cleavage of minus RNA but were completely ineffective with plus RNA (Fig. 4C). These data show that no specific cation is necessary for self-cleavage, but there is an absolute requirement for a polyvalent cation. Such ions are presumably essential for stabilization of the active structures.

Additional Support for the Hammerhead Model and the Minimal Sequences Necessary for Self-cleavage in Plus vLTSV

Deletion analysis from both the 5′ and the 3′ termini of the 336-nucleotide plus vLTSV transcript showed that the sequences in the hammerhead model (Fig. 1C) were sufficient for self-cleavage (Forster and Symons 1987b). The 52-nucleotide fragment (residues 166–216), isolated from a polyacrylamide gel containing a ladder of fragments produced by the chemical degradation of a 3′ terminally labeled truncated plus transcript, cleaved rapidly to completion at the self-cleavage site upon addition of Mg⁺⁺. In contrast, the 51- and 50-nucleotide fragments were completely inactive (Forster and Symons 1987b). The proposed structure of this 52-nucleotide fragment is shown in Figure 1D.

It was possible, albeit unlikely, that the cleavage of the 52-nucleotide fragment was catalyzed by unlabeled fragments of the same size produced during the chemical degradation of the 3′ terminally labeled transcript. To provide further evidence that this was not the case, a synthetic DNA template for T7 RNA polymerase was prepared (Lowary et al. 1986; Zaug et al. 1986) to provide a 58-nucleotide full-length transcript consisting of 53 nucleotides of plus vLTSV (residues 164–216; Fig. 1C) and 5 nucleotides from the promoter region. This transcript contained 51 of the 52 nucleotides in the 52-nucleotide RNA that is capable of cleavage. On transcription of this synthetic DNA template, the two predicted self-cleavage products were present (in equimolar amounts), with only trace amounts of the full-length transcript. Hence, self-cleavage had gone almost to completion in the transcription reaction mixture in the absence of extraneous RNA fragments (Forster and Symons 1987b). Furthermore, when the residual full-length transcript was purified, it gave the two predicted self-cleavage products under self-cleavage conditions (results not shown).

As an extension of this work, a synthetic, double-stranded 61-mer was cloned into the HindIII and BamHI sites of the pSP64 plasmid vector (Fig. 5A). The cloned insert contained 56 vLTSV nucleotides (residues 163–218; Fig. 1C). Transcription with SP6 RNA polymerase of the intact plasmid and of the plasmid cut with EcoRI, RsaI, and HpaII gave the plus RNA transcription products shown in Figure 5B. As expected, the uncut plasmid gave long products plus the 17-mer produced by self-cleavage at the 5′ end of the transcript (see Fig. 5A). The first 11 nucleotides of this 17-mer are derived from transcription of vector sequences plus four nucleotides of the cloned insert and are unrelated to vLTSV sequences. The next six nucleotides correspond to residues 163–168 of vLTSV. Transcripts derived from the plasmid cut with EcoRI and RsaI produced no full-length transcript but only the expected two self-cleavage products. In contrast, the HpaII-cut plasmid only provided a single full-length transcript of 50 nucleotides, with no self-cleavage products.

These results provide even further confirmation that only those nucleotides in the proposed plus hammerhead structure are necessary for self-cleavage. For the RsaI transcript, only 54 vLTSV nucleotides were present. The lack of self-cleavage activity of the HpaII transcript is consistent with previous data (Forster and Symons 1987b). This RNA terminates at residue 201 in the hairpin loop of stem II (Fig. 1C).

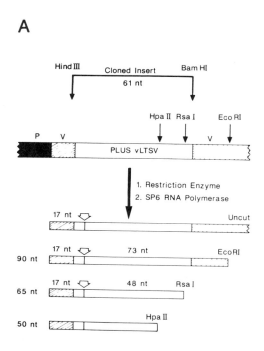
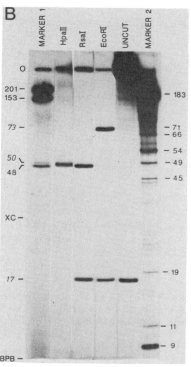

Figure 5. Self-cleavage of plus RNA transcripts of a cloned, synthetic 56-nucleotide sequence of vLTSV. The cloned 61-mer insert in the pSP64 plasmid vector contained 56 vLTSV nucleotides (residues 163–218) plus extra nucleotides to provide the HindIII and BamHI sites for cloning. (A) Diagram of the DNA template and of the SP6 RNA polymerase products generated by transcription of the template either uncut or linearized with EcoRI, RsaI, or HpaII. (P) Promoter; (V) vector sequences. Open arrow indicates site of self-cleavage to give a 5′-terminal 17-nucleotide fragment. Length of each RNA transcript is given at left-hand end; lengths of self-cleavage fragments are given above RNAs. (B) Analysis of RNA transcription reactions by electrophoresis on a 20% polyacrylamide–7 M urea gel in 90 mM Tris-borate and 2 mM EDTA (pH 8.3), and autoradiography. The 3′ self-cleavage fragment from the RsaI template is expected to be identical to the 48-nucleotide RNA in the Marker 1 track. (Marker 1) Plus RNA transcripts prepared from a partial-length vLTSV DNA clone in pSP64 linearized with RsaI (see Forster and Symons 1987b). (Marker 2) RNA fragments prepared by the partial digestion with RNase U2 of the 5′ ³²P-labeled 3′ self-cleavage fragment of the 336-nucleotide plus RNA (Forster and Symons 1987a,b).

It should be noted that the 5' ^{32}P-labeled 61-nucleotide synthetic DNA containing the sequence of the plus hammerhead structure (see Materials and Methods) does not self-cleave under conditions that self-cleave vLTSV (results not shown).

Minimal Sequences Necessary for the Self-cleavage of Minus vLTSV

The approach taken here was similar to that used for the plus sequences of vLTSV (for details, see Forster and Symons 1987b). The chemical deletion method for 3' terminally labeled transcripts proved to be very useful for scanning a large fragment to determine the minimum number of nucleotides required for self cleavage (Forster and Symons 1987b). The principle of the method (Fig. 6A) was to (1) 3'-end-label a purified nonradioactive transcript capable of self-cleavage to give a fixed reference point at its 3' end, (2) randomly cleave the transcript in the absence of Mg^{++} to generate a series of radiolabeled fragments with 5'-terminal deletions, (3) subject the fragments to self-cleavage

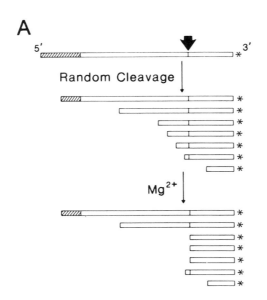

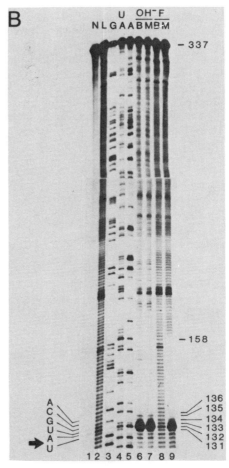

Figure 6. Self-cleavage analysis of 5' terminally deleted fragments of a 3'-end-labeled 336-nucleotide minus vLTSV RNA transcript. The nonradioactive full-length 336-nucleotide RNA transcript was prepared from a partial-length DNA clone of vLTSV in the pSP64 plasmid vector and 3'-end-labeled with 5' [^{32}P]pCp using T4 RNA ligase as described previously (Forster and Symons 1987a). (A) General method used for 5'-deletion analyses (from Forster and Symons 1987b). 3'-end-labeled RNA was randomly cleaved in the absence of Mg^{++} to generate a series of 5' terminally deleted radiolabeled fragments, which were then subjected to self-cleavage conditions in the presence of Mg^{++}. Heavy arrow indicates the self-cleavage site. (B) Analysis by gel electrophoresis of 5'-deletion and self-cleavage reaction mixtures. (Lanes 6,7) Purified end-labeled RNA transcript was heated at 100°C for 3 min in 50 mM NaHCO$_3$/Na$_2$CO$_3$ (pH 9) and 1 mM EDTA, and the resulting RNA fragments were ethanol-precipitated and redissolved in 1 mM EDTA. One aliquot was incubated in 5 mM MgCl$_2$, 0.5 mM EDTA, and 50 mM Tris-HCl (pH 7.5) for 1 min at 25°C (lane 7, labeled M), and another aliquot was incubated under the same conditions in the absence of MgCl$_2$ (lane 6, labeled B). (Lanes 8,9) End-labeled RNA transcript was dissolved in deionized formamide containing 1 mM MgCl$_2$ and heated at 80°C for 5 min. Excess EDTA was added, the solution was diluted, and the fragments were precipitated with ethanol. Fragments were then treated with pH 7.5 buffer (lane 8) or with buffer containing 5 mM MgCl$_2$ (lane 9) as in lanes 6 and 7, except that the incubation time was 10 min. (Lane 1) No treatment of 3'-end-labeled RNA transcript. (Lanes 2-5) Markers produced by enzymatic sequencing of the end-labeled RNA (see Fig. 3 in Forster and Symons 1987a). (Lane 2) Ladder produced by heating in formamide and 1 mM MgCl$_2$. (Lane 3) RNA treated with RNase T1 and labeled G; (lane 4) RNA treated with *P. polycephalum* RNase and labeled U/A; (lane 5) RNA treated with RNase U2 and labeled A. Reactions were terminated with gel-loading solution containing EDTA and formamide, electrophoresed on an 80-cm 6% polyacrylamide–7 M urea–30% formamide gel, and then autoradiographed. The top portion of the gel did not contain any bands and has been omitted.

conditions, and (4) analyze the products by denaturing gel electrophoresis.

For this work, a full-length 336-nucleotide minus RNA transcript was prepared from a pSP64 DNA clone containing 273 vLTSV nucleotides by transcription with SP6 RNA polymerase and purified from the self-cleavage products by gel electrophoresis (for full details of the clone and transcription, see Forster and Symons 1987a). The purified, nonradioactive transcript was 3′-end-labeled with 5′ [³²P]pCp using T4 RNA ligase. No self-cleavage occurred during the labeling reaction, presumably because the RNA was in its inactive conformation. The labeled RNA was then heated at 100°C (pH 9) in the absence of Mg⁺⁺ or at 80°C in formamide containing Mg⁺⁺ to generate a series of 5′-deleted fragments, which were then subjected to self-cleavage conditions in the presence of Mg⁺⁺. Reaction mixtures were fractionated on a denaturing polyacrylamide gel together with enzymatic RNA sequencing reaction mixtures as markers (Fig. 6B). Lane 8 (RNA heated in formamide) contained the 5′ terminally deleted labeled fragments in roughly equimolar proportions to provide a ladder. In lane 9 (same fragments treated with Mg⁺⁺), the intensity of the large and small fragments was the same as that in lane 8, but fragments between 135 and 158 nucleotides long were absent. The presence of this "window" in the ladder, and a major band at the position expected for the 3′-self-cleavage fragment of 132 nucleotides, was indicative of self-cleavage. In contrast to these results, deletion fragments produced by heating at 100°C in aqueous pH 9 buffer gave almost the same window as in lane 9 whether or not these fragments were incubated with Mg⁺⁺ (lanes 6 and 7). These results were reproducible with different preparations of RNA and were independent of the ethanol precipitation and incubation steps. Hence, self-cleavage of minus RNA fragments appeared to be occurring during the pH 9 ladder treatment (in the absence of Mg⁺⁺) under conditions in which the plus RNA fragments were inert (Forster and Symons 1987b). Increasing the concentration of EDTA in the sodium carbonate/bicarbonate pH 9 buffer from 1 to 25 mM did not significantly alter the pattern (results not shown). This suggests that a polyvalent cation is not necessary for self-cleavage of the minus fragments, but we cannot rule out the possibility that there were trace amounts of contaminating polyvalent cations that were released from chelation by the 100°C heating step.

The minus fragments that cleaved efficiently were between 135 and 158 nucleotides long (Fig. 6B). Thus, minus fragments containing from 3 to 26 nucleotides on the 5′ side of the self-cleavage site cleaved efficiently, whereas larger fragments cleaved poorly or not at all under the conditions used. As with the plus RNA, it appears that the minus RNA requires only the lower 2 bp of stem III of the hammerhead structure for efficient self-cleavage (Fig. 1C). The efficient cleavage of certain 5′ deletion fragments of the plus RNA after the addition of Mg⁺⁺ and without prior heating and snap cooling was also observed (Forster and Symons 1987b), although the reaction was slower with minus RNA than

with plus RNA. Hence, these window fragments are all in active conformations (Fig. 2). Fragments longer than about 158 nucleotides do not form active conformations under the same conditions, presumably because the extra sequences favor alternative, inactive conformations. The data support the proposal that structural switching of the minus RNA mirrors that of the plus RNA (Forster and Symons 1987a).

The study of the effect of 3′ deletions on self-cleavage was limited by the lack of suitable restriction enzyme sites in the cloned minus vLTSV sequence. The NcoI site was the only one suitable, and the pSP64 clone cleaved with this enzyme provided an RNA transcript that terminated at nucleotide 124 (Fig. 1C) in the hairpin loop of stem II. This RNA, as expected, did not self-cleave during in vitro synthesis or during incubation with Mg⁺⁺ after heating and snap cooling (data not given). Hence, to obtain self-cleaving minus transcripts of minimal length, we turned to T7 RNA polymerase transcription of synthetic DNA, which had already been used successfully for the preparation of a plus transcript that self-cleaved (Forster and Symons 1987b).

Self-cleavage of a 64-nucleotide Minus vLTSV RNA in Transcription Reactions Using a Synthetic DNA Template

A synthetic DNA template for T7 RNA polymerase was constructed (Fig. 7A) according to the method of Lowary et al. (1986; see also Zaug et al. 1986). This template was designed to direct the synthesis of a 64-nucleotide full-length RNA transcript containing, after three 5′-terminal G residues required for the promoter sequence, 61 nucleotides of the minus vLTSV sequence from residues 169 to 107 (Fig. 7A,B). Hence, the RNA transcript contained all of the nucleotides of the proposed hammerhead structure and was expected to self-cleave to give a 5′-terminal 10-nucleotide fragment and a 3′-terminal 54-nucleotide fragment.

Transcription of the synthetic DNA template with T7 RNA polymerase in the presence of [α-³²P]UTP gave two major products with mobilities that corresponded to the predicted self-cleavage fragments (Fig. 7C, lane 2). The 64-nucleotide full-length RNA transcript, which showed anomalous migration relative to the markers, self-cleaved to the two predicted products after purification (results not shown). The two products (Fig. 7C, lane 2) were in approximately equimolar proportions as determined by liquid scintillation counting. Transcription of both of the synthetic DNA templates in Figure 7C in the presence of a lower concentration of UTP (0.025 mM instead of 0.5 mM) resulted in the same products as in Figure 7C, lanes 1 and 2, plus a product in both transcriptions that had the same intensity as the large (3′-terminal) product and that migrated about one nucleotide faster (results not shown). This indicates that termination of transcription at the 5′ ends of the synthetic DNA templates is dependent on UTP concentration.

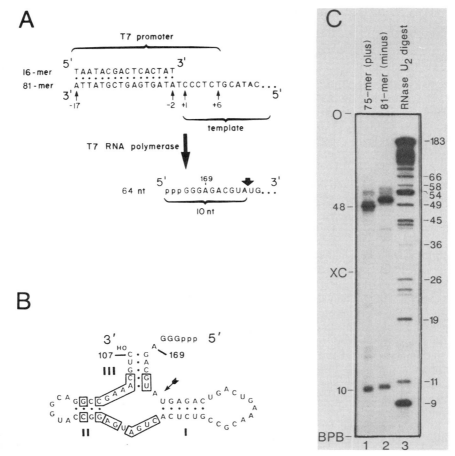

Figure 7. Synthesis of a self-cleaving, minus vLTSV RNA transcribed from a synthetic DNA template. (*A*) Diagram of the DNA template and of the full-length product generated by transcription of the template with T7 RNA polymerase. The 23-nucleotide conserved sequence of the class III promoter for T7 RNA polymerase is located at the 3' end of the 81-mer. The site of initiation of transcription is labeled +1. The first minus vLTSV residue in the 64-nucleotide RNA transcript is an A, labeled residue 169 (see also Fig. 1C). The site of self-cleavage is indicated by a short, thick arrow. (*B*) Primary and proposed secondary structure for the complete RNA transcript produced from the template in *A*. Nucleotide numbers refer to those in the full-length minus vLTSV molecule (Keese et al. 1983). The self-cleavage site is indicated by the arrow and stems are numbered. (*C*) Analysis of transcription reaction by electrophoresis on a 20% polyacrylamide–7 M urea gel and autoradiography. (Lane 2) Minus vLTSV RNA transcripts of the template in *A*. (Lane 1) RNA markers produced by transcription of a synthetic 75-mer DNA template containing the plus vLTSV hammerhead sequence (Forster and Symons 1987b). The 10-nucleotide RNA has the same 5' and 3' termini and number of nucleotides as the expected 5'-terminal self-cleavage fragment in lane 2 and only differs in containing a 3'-terminal C instead of an A. (Lane 3) Marker RNase U2 digest; same as Marker 2 in Fig. 5B. Presumably, the discrepancy in mobilities of the predicted 54-nucleotide self-cleavage fragment and the 54-nucleotide marker fragment is due to differences in sequence.

Trans Self-cleavage of Minus ASBV

The plus and minus hammerhead structures proposed for the active sites in vLTSV are formed from a short continuous sequence at one end of the rod-like molecule (Fig. 1C; Forster and Symons 1987a). In contrast, the plus and minus hammerhead structures for ASBV each consist of two short sequences from opposite sides of the central region in the circular rod-shaped molecule (Fig. 1B; Hutchins et al. 1986). These two short sequences are separated by about 80 nucleotides of continuous sequence on one side of the hammerhead structures and about 130 nucleotides on the other side. Since only the sequences that make up the plus and minus hammerhead structures in vLTSV

are required for self-cleavage activity, it seemed likely that a short sequence of ASBV could act in *trans* to cause self-cleavage of another short sequence.

We report here a preliminary investigation into self-cleavage activity in *trans* using long sections of the minus ASBV molecule. A diagram of the proposed structure of the two long fragments that showed significant self-cleavage activity in the presence of Mg++ is given in Figure 8A. One fragment (T in Fig. 8A) was the 3'-terminal fragment obtained from a self-cleavage reaction of an in-vitro-synthesized RNA transcript prepared on a dimeric minus cDNA clone of ASBV in the pSP65 plasmid vector (Hutchins et al. 1986). This fragment was 183 nucleotides long and contained 20 nucleotides of vector sequence at its 3' terminus; it is the

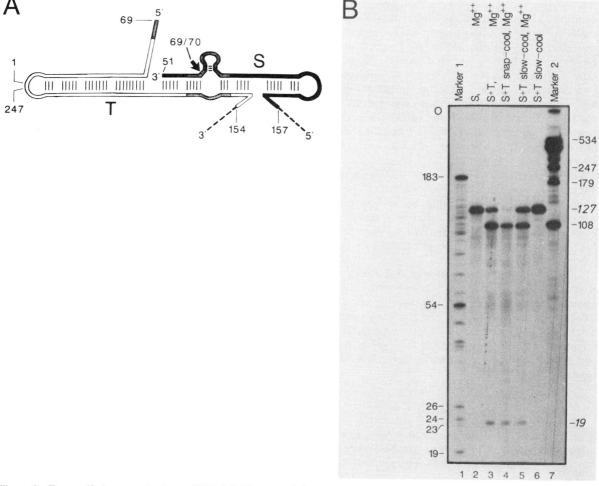

Figure 8. *Trans* self-cleavage of minus ASBV. (*A*) Diagram of the two minus ASBV fragments and the proposed self-cleavage structure. Nonradioactive *trans*-acting fragment T and radiolabeled substrate fragment S were prepared as described in the text. Residue numbers for this minus sequence are the same as those of the plus sequence (Symons 1981). Fragment T was 183 nucleotides long and contained 20 nucleotides of vector sequence at its 3' terminus. Fragment S was 127 nucleotides long, with 20 nucleotides of vector sequence at its 5' terminus. Gray areas represent the nucleotides in the minus hammerhead structure in Fig. 1B. Arrow indicates the self-cleavage site between residues 69 and 70. Black and white areas, respectively, indicate other ASBV sequences in fragments S and T. Vector sequences are dashed. The overall rod-shaped structure is considered to be similar to that of circular ASBV (Symons 1981). (*B*) Analysis of *trans* self-cleavage reactions by gel electrophoresis. Nonradioactive fragment T (*A*) (labeled 3'E in Fig. 1b of Hutchins et al. 1986) was isolated from a transcription of a *Hin*dIII-linearized dimeric minus ASBV DNA clone in the pSP65 plasmid vector (Hutchins et al. 1986). ³²P-labeled fragment S (*A*) was prepared from the same dimeric DNA clone as described above, linearized with *Bst*NI. Fragment S was added to an excess of fragment T in 50 mM Tris-HCl (pH 8.5) and then either left at room temperature for 1 hr (lane *3*) or heated to 80°C for 1 min and then snap-cooled on ice (lane *4*) or heated to 75°C and then cooled gradually to 30°C over 1 hr (lanes *5* and *6*). Lane *2* contained only fragment S. All RNAs except those in lane *6* were then incubated at 40°C for 2 hr in 50 mM MgCl₂ and 40 mM Tris-HCl (pH 8.5). Reactions were terminated with gel-loading solution containing EDTA and formamide, electrophoresed on a 35-cm 10% polyacrylamide–7 M urea gel, and then autoradiographed. (Marker 1) Same as Marker 2 in Fig. 5B. Presumably, the discrepancy in mobilities of the predicted 19-nucleotide self-cleavage fragment and the 19-nucleotide marker fragment is due to differences in sequence. (Marker 2) RNA transcripts prepared from a dimeric minus ASBV DNA clone in pSP65, linearized with *Hin*dIII as described by Hutchins et al. (1986). The 108-nucleotide RNA is identical to the predicted 5' self-cleavage fragment of fragment S (lanes *3–5*).

fragment labeled 3'E in Figure 1b in Hutchins et al. (1986) and contained residues 69–154 of minus ASBV. The second fragment (Fig. 8A, S) was obtained by transcription of the same dimeric minus cDNA clone of ASBV in pSP65 after linearization with *Bst*NI; it spanned residues 157–51 of minus ASBV and contained 20 residues of vector sequence at its 5' terminus to give a total of 127 nucleotides. Together, these two

fragments contained the entire 247 nucleotides of minus ASBV, plus an additional 23 nucleotides of repeated ASBV sequence.

In the experiment of Figure 8B, fragment T was not labeled; fragment S was labeled with ³²P. As expected, fragment S on its own was incapable of self-cleavage (Fig. 8, lane 2). The fragments were annealed under different conditions and incubated at 40°C for 2 hours, and the reaction mixtures were then analyzed by denaturing polyacrylamide gel electrophoresis. In the presence of Mg^{++}, almost complete self-cleavage occurred after prior heating at 80°C for 1 minute and snap cooling (Fig. 8B, lane 4), whereas prior heating and slow cooling gave about 50% self-cleavage (lane 5). However, prior mixing of the two fragments at room temperature was efficient to give extensive self-cleavage (lane 3), indicating that the sequences in the two fragments that make up the active hammerhead structure (Fig. 1B) were accessible and not locked in stable, alternative conformations.

The expected sizes of the two self-cleavage products, 108 and 19 nucleotides, are consistent with those of the marker RNAs in lanes 1 and 7. No self-cleavage occurred in the absence of Mg^{++} after the fragments were heated and slowly cooled (lane 6) or in the presence of Mg^{++} when fragment T was replaced by *Escherichia coli* tRNA (not shown).

These initial experiments showed that a *trans*-acting RNA fragment could cause efficient self-cleavage of another fragment, and they provide the basis for a more comprehensive analysis of this type of reaction. It would be of considerable interest to define the minimum sequences required for this type of reaction and to determine if the *trans*-acting RNA can act catalytically.

DISCUSSION

Sequences in the Hammerhead Structures of Plus and Minus vLTSV RNAs Are Necessary and Sufficient for Self-cleavage

The data presented on the self-cleavage of both plus and minus vLTSV RNAs extend those presented previously (Forster and Symons 1987a,b) and provide conclusive evidence that only those sequences in the hammerhead structures of Figure 1C are required for self-cleavage. In the case of plus vLTSV, only the lower 2 bp of stem III of the hammerhead structure (Fig. 1C,D) are required, and 51 nucleotides of vLTSV sequence are all that are necessary for rapid and complete self-cleavage in the presence of Mg^{++} (Forster and Symons 1987b). For minus vLTSV, the 5'-deletion analyses of Figure 6, the 3'-deletion analysis described in Results, and the in vitro transcription studies of Figure 7 also indicate that only the lower 2 bp of stem III (Fig. 1C), and most of the 60 nucleotides in the hammerhead structure, are necessary and sufficient for self-cleavage. These data confirm the proposal (Forster and Symons 1987a) that about one third of the vLTSV-A sequence is required for self-cleavage.

The complete self-cleavage of short plus and minus vLTSV RNA fragments without heating and snap cooling contrasts with partial or no self-cleavage of larger fragments without heating and snap cooling (Fig. 6) (Forster and Symons 1987a,b). However, heating and snap cooling these larger fragments at low salt concentration can convert up to one half of the RNA to

active conformations. We believe that these active forms self-cleave rapidly and completely on the addition of Mg^{++}, whereas other data indicate that there is no equilibrium between the active and inactive conformations during incubation with Mg^{++} (Forster and Symons 1987a).

In the case of purified plus and minus RNA transcripts of DNA clones of ASBV, self-cleavage occurred upon addition of Mg^{++} without the necessity for prior heating and snap cooling (Hutchins et al. 1986). In addition, the extent of self-cleavage increased with the time of incubation in the presence of Mg^{++} (P. Rathjen et al., unpubl.). Hence, with long ASBV transcripts, there is probably an equilibrium between inactive and active conformations, even in the presence of Mg^{++}, that would be expected to stabilize secondary and tertiary interactions.

How Can the Mechanism of Self-cleavage be Determined?

Given that the active sites of plus and minus vLTSV RNAs are hammerhead structures (Fig. 1C), they provide an attractive system for mechanistic analyses because of their small size and the simplicity of their reactions. Normal Watson-Crick base pairing, as well as other secondary and tertiary interactions, will need to be defined to explain the lowering of the activation energy at a specific internucleotide bond to allow nonhydrolytic cleavage that results in 5'-OH and 2',3'-cyclic phosphate termini.

Important basic information on the sequence requirements for self-cleavage can be obtained by in vitro mutagenesis. The effect on self-cleavage of base changes, insertions, and deletions can be rapidly assessed by the production of RNA transcripts from synthetic DNA templates.

The probable mechanism of a nonbiological RNA-mediated reaction, the Pb^{++}-catalyzed cleavage of tRNA^{Phe}, has been determined by X-ray crystallography (Brown et al. 1985). Structural studies by this approach and by nuclear magnetic resonance require milligrams of RNA (Wemmer and Reid 1985). Techniques for the chemical synthesis of long RNA chains are not yet available, and thus production of sequences of vLTSV need to be done by large-scale enzymatic synthesis. A major problem that would have to be circumvented is the rapid self-cleavage of RNA in the transcription reactions.

What Is the Role of the Self-cleavage Reaction In Vivo?

On the basis of the presence of various oligomeric plus and minus forms of viroids, virusoids, and sTRSV in vivo, a rolling-circle mechanism for their replication is considered likely (Branch and Robertson 1984; Hutchins et al. 1985, 1986; Buzayan et al. 1986b; Forster and Symons 1987a). An essential feature of such a mechanism is the specific cleavage of RNA transcripts produced by an unidentified RNA polymerase on the circular RNA template to give linear monomeric molecules that can then be circularized. It is likely that this cleavage occurs by a nonenzymatic self-cleavage reaction as characterized in vitro for plus and minus ASBV, vLTSV, and sTRSV RNAs.

One approach to investigate this possibility is to look at the effect of site-directed mutagenesis on the infectivity of DNA clones and/or their RNA transcripts. Infectious DNA clones and RNA transcripts have been prepared for sTRSV (Gerlach et al. 1986) and vLTSV (E.C. Dunlop et al., unpubl.). A correlation between the ability of RNA transcripts to self-cleave in vitro and infectivity would provide strong circumstantial support for self-cleavage in vivo, although self-cleavage of virusoid minus RNA may not be essential for replication (Forster and Symons 1987a).

Self-cleavage in *trans* and RNA Restriction Enzyme Activity

The demonstration that two fragments of minus ASBV can act in *trans* to enable specific self-cleavage (Fig. 8) suggests that short sequences of the hammerhead structures of ASBV, vLTSV, and sTRSV may be able to act like stringent, specific restriction enzymes. For example, the lower sequence of the plus or minus ASBV hammerhead structure (Fig. 1B) by itself, or linked to a larger molecule, could bind to the upper sequence in another molecule to enable catalytic self-cleavage. Such an RNA restriction endonuclease would differ from the *Tetrahymena* RNA restriction endonuclease, which requires the addition of a G residue as an essential part of its cleavage mechanism (Zaug et al. 1986).

The presumptive ability of small RNA fragments to act in *trans* provides a simple system for detailed characterization of the reaction. It would be interesting to determine whether a DNA fragment can replace a *trans*-acting RNA to form a DNA enzyme. It should be possible to prepare model RNA enzymes and substrates by incorporation of the appropriate sequences into larger molecules. However, the ability of long RNAs to form more than one conformation (as demonstrated here and in Forster and Symons 1987a,b) would require careful design of both RNA enzyme and substrate to allow formation of the active self-cleavage structure. Such data would contribute to our understanding of the possible roles for RNA catalysts in evolution (Cech 1985).

ACKNOWLEDGMENTS

We thank Jennifer Cassady for her experimental contribution and Tamara Edmonds for assistance. This work was supported by the Australian Research Grants Scheme and the Commonwealth Special Research Centre for Gene Technology.

REFERENCES

Branch, A.D. and H.D. Robertson. 1984. A replication cycle for viroids and other small infectious RNAs. *Science* **223:** 450.

Brown, R.S., J.C. Dewan, and A. Klug. 1985. Crystallographic and biochemical investigation of the lead (II)-catalysed hydrolysis of yeast phenylalanine tRNA. *Biochemistry* **24:** 4785.

Buzayan, J.M., W.L. Gerlach, and G. Bruening. 1986a. Nonenzymatic cleavage and ligation of RNAs complementary to a plant virus satellite RNA. *Nature* **323:** 349.

Buzayan, J.M., W.L. Gerlach, G. Bruening, P. Keese, and A.R. Gould. 1986b. Nucleotide sequence of satellite tobacco ringspot virus RNA and its relationship to multimeric forms. *Virology* **151:** 186.

Cech, T.R. 1985. Self-splicing RNA: Implications for evolution. *Int. Rev. Cytol.* **93:** 3.

Cech, T.R. and B.L. Bass. 1986. Biological catalysis by RNA. *Annu. Rev. Biochem.* **55:** 599.

Donis-Keller, H. 1980. Phy M: An RNase activity specific for U and A residues useful in RNA sequence analysis. *Nucleic Acids Res.* **8:** 3133.

Forster, A.C. and R.H. Symons. 1987a. Self-cleavage of plus and minus RNAs of a virusoid and a structural model for the active sites. *Cell* **49:** 211.

———. 1987b. Self cleavage of virusoid RNA is performed by the proposed 55-nucleotide active site. *Cell* **50:** 9.

Gerlach, W.L., J.M. Buzayan, I.R. Schneider, and G. Bruening. 1986. Satellite tobacco ringspot RNA: Biological activity of DNA clones and their *in vitro* transcripts. *Virology* **151:** 172.

Hutchins, C.J., P.D. Rathjen, A.C. Forster, and R.H. Symons. 1986. Self-cleavage of plus and minus RNA transcripts of avocado sunblotch viroid. *Nucleic Acids Res.* **14:** 3627.

Hutchins, C.J., P. Keese, J.E. Visvader, P.D. Rathjen, J.L. McInnes, and R.H. Symons. 1985. Comparison of multimeric plus and minus forms of viroids and virusoids. *Plant Mol. Biol.* **4:** 293.

Keese, P., G. Bruening, and R.H. Symons. 1983. Comparative sequence and structure of circular RNAs from two isolates of lucerne transient streak virus. *FEBS Lett.* **159:** 185.

Lowary, P., J. Sampson, J. Milligan, D. Groebe, and O.C. Uhlenbeck. 1986. A better way to make RNA for physical studies. In *Structure and dynamics of RNA* (ed. P.H. van Knipperberg and C.N. Hilbers), p. 69. Plenum Press, New York.

Prody, G.A., J.T. Bakos, J.M. Buzayan, I.R. Schneider, and G. Bruening. 1986. Autolytic processing of dimeric plant virus satellite RNA. *Science* **231:** 1577.

Riesner, D., K. Henco, U. Rokohl, G. Klotz, A.K. Kleinschmidt, H. Domdey, P. Jank, H.J. Gross, and H.L. Sanger. 1979. Structure and structure formation of viroids. *J. Mol. Biol.* **133:** 85.

Sharp, P.A. 1987. Splicing of messenger RNA precursors. *Science* **235:** 766.

Symons, R.H. 1981. Avocado sunblotch viroid: Primary sequence and proposed secondary structure. *Nucleic Acids Res.* **9:** 6527.

Wemmer, D.E. and B.R. Reid. 1985. High resolution NMR studies of nucleic acids and proteins. *Annu. Rev. Phys. Chem.* **36** 105.

Zaug, A.J., M.D. Been, and T.R. Cech. 1986. The *Tetrahymena* ribozyme acts like an RNA restriction endonuclease. *Nature* **324:** 429.

Transcripts of Newt Satellite DNA Self-cleave In Vitro

L.M. EPSTEIN* AND J.G. GALL[†]

*Department of Biological Science, Florida State University, Tallahassee, Florida 32306;
[†]Carnegie Institution of Washington, Department of Embryology, Baltimore, Maryland 21210

The eastern newt, *Notophthalmus viridescens*, has an abundant supply of material for studying the evolution and function of repetitive DNA. The haploid genome of this organism contains 45 pg of DNA, approximately 15 times the amount in the human genome. Much of the newt genome consists of repetitive sequences, some of which exist as tandemly repeated "satellite" DNA. Two satellite sequences from the newt have been studied in detail; these have been named satellite 1 and satellite 2.

The organization and transcription of satellite 1 have been described previously (Diaz et al. 1981; Gall et al. 1983). Tandem repeats of this 220-bp sequence are localized mainly to pericentric heterochromatin on each of the 11 newt chromosomes. This sequence is transcribed on lampbrush chromosomes during oogenesis, probably as a result of "readthrough" from nearby histone gene clusters. However, this transcription does not result in the accumulation of discrete satellite-1 transcripts (K. Mahon, unpubl.).

The properties of satellite 1 contrast with the remarkable features of satellite 2, the subject of this paper. This 330-bp sequence is not localized to discrete, heterochromatic chromosomal regions. Rather, tandem repeats of satellite 2 are dispersed uniformly throughout the genome (Epstein et al. 1986). In addition, transcripts homologous to satellite 2 are found in the nuclei and cytoplasm of a variety of tissues. These transcripts correspond in size to the entire satellite-2 repeat unit or to whole multiples of the repeat.

Although we realized it would be difficult to investigate their function, we felt encouraged to study the formation of these unusual transcripts. One model that accounts for transcripts with the size of a tandemly repeated DNA sequence is that large multimeric transcripts are cleaved to produce monomers. We present evidence for this model by demonstrating that satellite-2 transcripts undergo self-catalyzed cleavage in vitro at a specific phosphodiester bond located once within each satellite-2 repeat. This reaction is especially intriguing because it has many similarities to the self-cleavage of a number of infectious RNAs found in plants.

Although satellite-2 transcripts are able to self-cleave in vitro, it has not been demonstrated that this mechanism is used in vivo. If cleavage is involved in the production of cellular satellite-2 transcripts, the reaction is modified so as to occur at a site 46 or 47 nucleotides away from the in vitro cleavage site. We speculate that the ancestor of satellite-2 sequences was

an infectious RNA that had the ability to self-cleave in a manner analogous to that of the plant RNAs and that the newt has evolved cellular factors to modify that reaction for its own purposes.

RESULTS AND DISCUSSION

In Vivo Satellite-2 Transcripts

The diversity of transcripts homologous to satellite 2 can be seen in the Northern analysis shown in Figure 1. The probes for this analysis were specific for one or the other strand of satellite 2 and were derived from genomic satellite-2 clones in the single-stranded phage vector M13. Each probe hybridized to a 330-bp ladder in *Bgl*II-digested DNA (lanes 1 and 5). This pattern results from the occurrence of a single *Bgl*II recognition site in some, but not all, of the tandem satellite-2 repeats. The various steps in the ladder represent monomeric, dimeric, and larger multimeric satellite-2

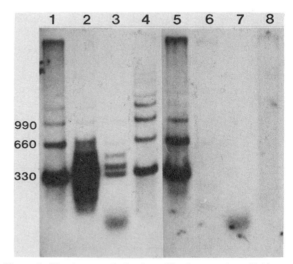

Figure 1. Northern analysis of satellite-2 transcripts. Gel lanes contain 0.3 µg of *Bgl*II-digested *Notophthalmus* DNA (lanes *1* and *5*), 15 µg of total ovary RNA (lanes *2* and *6*), 55 ng of germinal vesicle RNA (lanes *3* and *7*), and 15 µg of total liver RNA (lanes *4* and *8*). Lanes *1–4* were probed with the A strand of a cloned satellite-2 repeat; lanes *5–8* were probed with the B strand. The apparent hybridization to a low-molecular-weight RNA in lanes *3* and *7* is due to nonspecific binding of both probes to an excess of yeast tRNA used as a carrier in the isolation of germinal vesicle RNA. Sizes in bases.

fragments and served as size markers for the transcripts that hybridized to the satellite-2 probes.

One of the satellite-2 strands (arbitrarily designated the A strand) hybridized to discrete transcripts in each of the tissue RNA preparations. The majority of these transcripts correspond in size precisely to monomeric or multimeric DNA repeat units. Monomer transcripts were predominant in the ovary (lane 2), whereas the transcripts in somatic tissues, such as the liver (lane 4), were mostly dimers and larger multimers. Some transcripts that do not correspond to perfect repeat unit lengths were also seen. They were especially prominent in germinal vesicle RNA (lane 3).

The abundant, monomer-sized transcripts in total ovary RNA were sequenced by primer-extension reactions in the presence of dideoxynucleotide chain terminators (Epstein et al. 1986). The primers used in this analysis were complementary to four different regions in the consensus sequence of eight independent satellite-2 genomic clones. Most of the lengths of the ovary transcripts were sequenced, and the almost complete lack of ambiguities in the sequencing gels indicated that the transcripts were homogeneous. In contrast, the eight cloned genomic repeats were characterized by numerous single nucleotide substitutions, insertions, and deletions relative to their consensus sequence. We concluded that the transcripts were derived from a homogeneous subset of genomic satellite-2 repeats.

Of the 282 nucleotides that were sequenced in the transcripts, there were only seven differences from the DNA consensus sequence. We postulate that at some time in the past, functional satellite-2 DNA gave rise to many copies that were dispersed throughout the newt genome and became nonfunctional by the gradual accumulation of mutations. If the mutations were more or less random, the consensus sequence of the diverged copies would closely approximate the conserved functional sequence and the RNA it encodes.

The functional satellite-2 copies were apparently present early in the evolution of newts. Unlike other simple-sequence, tandemly repeated DNAs (for re-

view, see Brutlag 1980), satellite 2 is highly conserved between distantly related species. DNA homologous to satellite 2 is present in the genomes of all salamandrid species examined to date (K. Mahon; Z. Wu; H.C. Macgregor; G. Barsacchi-Pilone; all unpubl.), and the sequence of a cloned repetitive DNA from the European newt, *Triturus cristatus carnifex*, is 75% homologous to the *Notophthalmus* consensus sequence (Epstein et al. 1986). Satellite 2 is also transcribed in a number of different species. The transcripts from two species of *Triturus* (*T. c. carnifex* and *T. vulgaris meridionalis*) have been examined and were found to have the same size and 5′ ends as the *Notophthalmus* transcripts (G. Barsacchi-Pilone, unpubl.). As might be expected, preliminary data indicate that the *Triturus* and the *Notophthalmus* transcripts have similar sequences.

In Vitro Cleavage of Satellite-2 Transcripts

We reasoned that if monomeric transcripts were produced by site-specific cleavage, then multimeric transcripts synthesized in vitro should be cleaved after injection into newt oocytes. To examine this possibility, transcripts were synthesized using the plasmid pSP6-D6 as a template for SP6 polymerase. pSP6-D6 consists of a dimer-size satellite-2 DNA fragment inserted next to the SP6 RNA polymerase promoter (Fig. 2). When this plasmid was digested with *Hin*dIII, SP6 polymerase promoted the synthesis of a 723-nucleotide transcript (Fig. 3, lane 5), corresponding to a 660-nucleotide satellite-2 dimer plus adjacent vector sequences. We noticed that smaller fragments were also produced during, or immediately following, the transcription reaction. One of these fragments was the size of a monomer, and the sum of the lengths of this fragment and two of the other fragments equaled the full-length transcript. These are the characteristics we expected for site-specific cleavage products of injected transcripts, and we were encouraged to investigate the possibility

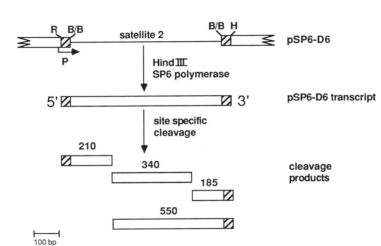

Figure 2. Diagram of pSP6-D6, its SP6 transcript, and the products of self-cleavage of the transcript. The 723-bp insert consists of two tandem repeats of satellite 2 (thin line) flanked by 50 bp of M13 polylinker (hatched boxes). Numbers above cleavage products represent sizes in nucleotides. (P) SP6 RNA polymerase promoter; (R) *Eco*RI; (H) *Hin*dIII; (B/B) sites generated when *Bgl*II-digested newt DNA was inserted into the *Bam*HI site of M13mp10 prior to subcloning into pSP6-5. For details of the construction of pSP6-D6, see Epstein and Gall (1987).

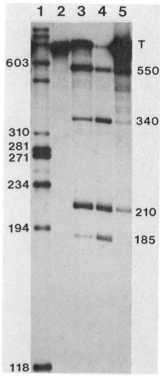

Figure 3. Self-cleavage of pSP6-D6 transcripts. The products of the SP6 RNA polymerase transcription of pSP6-D6 were electrophoresed on a 6% acrylamide–8 M urea gel (lane 5). The full-length transcript was gel-purified (lane 2) and incubated at 34°C for 18 hr in either *Tetrahymena* rRNA self-splicing buffer (lane 3) or a modified SP6 RNA polymerase buffer (lane 4). For the components of these buffers, see Epstein and Gall (1987). Lane 1 is *Hae*III-digested φX DNA (sizes in bases).

that the synthetic transcripts are self-cleaving in the absence of any cellular factors.

Gel-purified full-length transcripts were incubated either in SP6 RNA polymerase buffer or in the buffer used by Cech (1985) for the *Tetrahymena* rRNA self-splicing reaction. In both buffers, most of the transcripts were cleaved into fragments 550, 340, 210, and 185 nucleotides long (Fig. 3, lanes 3 and 4). From a detailed primer-extension analysis of these fragments (Epstein and Gall 1987), we concluded that the fragments were formed by self-cleavage at the two sites in the pSP6-D6 transcript as illustrated in Figure 2. The 550-nucleotide fragment was formed by cleavage at only one of these sites.

The only component of these buffers absolutely required for cleavage was Mg^{++}. In our hands, optimal cleavage occurred in 133 mM 4-morpholine ethane sulfonic acid (MES) (pH 6.9), 30 mM $MgCl_2$, and 10 mM NaCl. By determining the activity of the cleavage products as substrates for T4 RNA ligase and T4 kinase, we determined that cleavage results in fragments with 5′-OH groups and 3′-phosphate groups. In collaboration with H. Robertson and A. Branch (Rockefeller University), we found that at least some of the 3′-phos-

phate groups have 2′,3′-cyclic phosphate linkages. This was deduced when monomer-sized cleavage fragments were efficiently circularized by wheat-germ RNA ligase. This enzyme is specific for RNA substrates with 2′,3′-cyclic phosphates (Konarska et al. 1982).

Relationship to Other Catalytic RNAs

The self-catalyzed cleavage of satellite-2 transcripts differs from the reactions of the self-splicing group I introns found in nuclear rRNA (Zaug et al. 1983; Cech 1985) and mitochondrial mRNA and rRNA (Garriga and Lambowitz 1984; Van der Horst and Tabak 1985). These reactions require a guanosine nucleotide cofactor, which is added to the 5′ end of the intron during splicing, and result in excised introns with 5′-phosphate and 3′-OH groups. Group II introns of yeast are also able to undergo self-splicing (Peebles et al. 1986; Schmelzer and Schweyen 1986; Van der Veen et al. 1986). Although this reaction does not require a guanosine cofactor, it is nevertheless more similar to the group I splicing reaction than to the satellite-2 self-cleavage reaction. In the group II reaction, a nucleotide within the intron attacks the 5′ splice site to initiate splicing. The resulting excised intron has a lariat structure with a free 3′-OH group. This structure is also found in the products of nuclear mRNA processing, a reaction that is not self-catalytic but requires the interaction of several small nuclear ribonucleoprotein particles (for review, see Sharp 1987). These various observations led to the proposal that all classes of introns are spliced by an evolutionarily related mechanism (Cech 1986). Satellite-2 transcripts do not appear to utilize this same mechanism.

The satellite-2 self-cleavage reaction is similar to the self-catalyzed cleavage of a number of infectious RNAs found in plants, including the avocado sunblotch viroid (Hutchins et al. 1986), the satellite of the tobacco ringspot virus (Prody et al. 1986), and the virusoid from lucerne transient streak virus (Forster and Symons 1987). Multimeric forms of these 247–359-nucleotide RNAs cleave in vitro in the presence of a divalent cation to produce monomers with 5′-OH and 2′,3′-cyclic phosphate groups. Cleavage is believed to be an important step during the cellular replication of these RNAs (Branch and Robertson 1984), although cleavage in vivo has not been demonstrated.

Hutchins et al. (1986) proposed a novel structure for the self-cleavage sites of the infectious plant RNAs (Fig. 4A). The boxed nucleotides are invariant in each of these RNAs and in a number of other virusoids that are believed to be cleaved during in vivo replication. The lateral stem structures are also conserved in these RNAs, but the nucleotide composition of the stems varies. It has recently been demonstrated that small, synthetic RNA molecules consisting solely of this proposed cleavage site are self-cleaving (Sampson et al., this volume).

Satellite-2 transcripts can be folded into an identical structure (Fig. 4B), and in vitro cleavage occurs at a

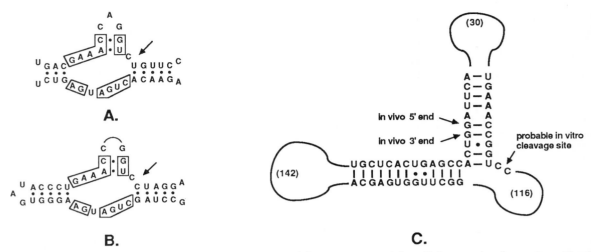

Figure 4. Proposed secondary structures of self-cleaving RNAs. (*A*) Structure around the self-cleavage site of avocado sunblotch viroid as suggested by Hutchins et al. (1986). Arrow denotes self-cleavage site. (*B*) Satellite-2 transcript folded into same structure as in model of Hutchins et al. (1986). (*C*) Another possible secondary structure for satellite-2 RNA, drawn as a closed circle. Where it is known, the sequence is that of the ovary transcript; elsewhere the consensus genomic sequence is shown. Numbers in parentheses indicate number of nucleotides omitted. (Reprinted, with permission, from Epstein and Gall 1987.)

site within this proposed structure. Therefore, in addition to having similar reaction requirements and resulting in products with similar end groups, self-cleavage in all these cases may depend on similar sequence and structure motifs.

Comparison of In Vivo Transcripts and In Vitro Cleavage Products

Despite the efficiency of in vitro self-cleavage of satellite-2 transcripts at a site conserved between distantly related organisms, cleavage does not occur at this site in vivo. The 5′ end of the in vitro cleavage product is 46 or 47 bases downstream from the 5′ end of the ovary transcript. This relationship is shown in Figure 4C, where an alternative structure is diagrammed for the satellite-2 monomer. This structure is interesting because it reduces the distance between the ends of the in vivo and in vitro transcripts to less than one-half turn of the double helix in a moderately stable hairpin loop. If this were the favored structure of satellite-2 transcripts, one can imagine that cellular factors could modify the reaction so that cleavage occurs at the in vivo site. It is also possible that cleavage of satellite-2 transcripts is regulated by conformational switches between the two structures shown in Figure 4, B and C. A conformational switch between the self-cleavage structure and a more stable rod-like structure may be involved in regulating cleavage of the virusoid from lucerne transient streak virus in vivo (Forster and Symons 1987). Although it has not been demonstrated that cellular factors influence the conformation of satellite-2 transcripts, it is clear that the environment within the ovary is somehow preventing cleavage of these transcripts at a site that is cleavable in vitro.

Origin of Satellite-2 DNA

The similarities between satellite-2 transcripts and the infectious plant RNAs led to the interesting speculation that satellite-2 DNA might have arisen from an infectious agent. The infecting RNA could have been incorporated into the genome by way of a cDNA intermediate. Such reverse flow of genetic information, termed retroposition, is probably responsible for many pseudogenes and repetitive elements in the eukaryotic genome (Rogers 1985; Weiner et al. 1986). Further retroposition events involving transcripts from the integrated copies would explain the genomic distribution of satellite-2 repeats.

Whatever the mechanism for dispersal of satellite-2 repeats, some of these copies have diverged in sequence, and transcripts from many of the repeats have lost the ability to undergo efficient self-cleavage. In addition to pSP6-D6, three other clones have been constructed containing dimer-sized genomic satellite-2 fragments. Transcripts from these clones have reduced ability to cleave at one or both of their cleavage sites (Fig. 5). If it is assumed that cleavage is required to help stabilize satellite-2 transcripts, the homogeneity of the ovarian transcripts can be explained. Only those DNA repeats that have maintained the sequence or overall structure conducive to cleavage will contribute to the stable RNA population.

If satellite-2 sequences did evolve from an ancestral RNA infection, the modification to cleavage that occurs in vivo represents an adaptation that the newt has evolved to utilize the RNA for its own purposes. Whatever this purpose is, it may have developmental importance, since there is a difference in the size of the transcripts generated in ovarian and nonovarian tissues (Fig. 1). Alternatively, the newt may have modified the

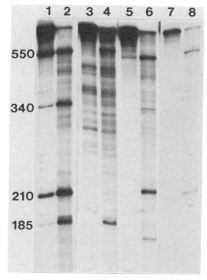

Figure 5. Self-cleavage of transcripts from four different satellite-2 clones. SP6 RNA polymerase transcripts from four independent satellite-2 dimer clones were allowed to self-cleave at 40°C for 4 hr (lanes *1,3,5,7*) or for 18 hr (lanes *2,4,6,8*). (*1,2*) pSP6-D6; (*3,4*) pSP6-D4; (*5,6*) pSP6-D5; (*7,8*) pSP6-D7. Sizes of the pSP6-D6 cleavage products are indicated in nucleotides. Due to a slightly different cloning history, pSP6-D5 has different M13 polylinker sequences from the other three clones, and, thus, its cleavage fragments differ in size.

cleavage reaction as a protective measure. By altering the reaction so as to generate permuted monomers, the activity of the RNA molecules may have been diminished. Further studies concentrating on the factors involved in the generation of the in vivo transcripts should help resolve these questions.

ACKNOWLEDGMENTS

We are indebted to Andrea Branch and Hugh Robertson, who carried out the wheat-germ ligase experiments. We are especially grateful to Guiseppina Barsacchi-Pilone, Herbert Macgregor, Kathleen Mahon, Jennifer Varley, and Zhengan Wu for sharing their original, unpublished observations. Finally, we thank Tom Cech and Olke Uhlenbeck for invaluable discussions. This work was supported by National Institutes of Health research grant GM-33397. J.G.G. is an American Cancer Society Professor of Developmental Genetics.

REFERENCES

Branch, A.D. and H.D. Robertson. 1984. A replication cycle for viroids and other small infectious RNAs. *Science* **223:** 450.

Brutlag, D.L. 1980. Molecular arrangement and evolution of heterochromatic DNA. *Annu. Rev. Genet.* **14:** 121.

Cech, T.R. 1985. Self-splicing RNA: Implications for evolution. *Int. Rev. Cytol.* **93:** 3.

———. 1986. The generality of self-splicing RNA: Relationship to nuclear mRNA splicing. *Cell* **44:** 207.

Diaz, M.O., G. Barsacchi-Pilone, K.A. Mahon, and J.G. Gall. 1981. Transcripts from both strands of a satellite DNA occur on lampbrush chromosome loops of the newt *Notophthalmus*. *Cell* **24:** 649.

Epstein, L.M. and J.G. Gall. 1987. Self-cleaving transcripts of satellite DNA from the newt. *Cell* **48:** 535.

Epstein, L.M., K.A. Mahon, and J.G. Gall. 1986. Transcription of a satellite DNA in the newt. *J. Cell Biol.* **103:** 1137.

Forster, A.C. and R.H. Symons. 1987. Self-cleavage of plus and minus RNAs of a virusoid and a structural model for the active sites. *Cell* **49:** 211.

Gall, J.G., M.O. Diaz, E.C. Stephenson, and K.A. Mahon. 1983. The transcription unit of lampbrush chromosomes. In *Gene structure and regulation in development* (ed. S. Subtelny and F.C. Kafatos), p. 137. A.R. Liss, New York.

Garriga, G. and A.M. Lambowitz. 1984. RNA splicing in *Neurospora* mitochondria: Self-splicing of a mitochondrial intron in vitro. *Cell* **39:** 631.

Hutchins, C.J., P.D. Rathjen, A.C. Forster, and R.H. Symons. 1986. Self-cleavage of plus and minus RNA transcripts of avocado sunblotch viroid. *Nucleic Acids Res.* **14:** 3627.

Konarska, M., W. Filipowicz, and H.J. Gross. 1982. RNA ligation via 2'-phosphomonoester, 3',5'-phosphodiester linkage: Requirement of 2',3'-cyclic phosphate termini and involvement of a 5'-hydroxyl polynucleotide kinase. *Proc. Natl. Acad. Sci.* **79:** 1474.

Peebles, C.L., P.S. Perlman, K.L. Mecklenburg, M.L. Petrillo, J.H. Tabor, K.A. Jarrell, and H.-L. Cheng. 1986. A self-splicing RNA excises an intron lariat. *Cell* **44:** 213.

Prody, G.A., J.T. Bakos, J.M. Buzayan, I.R. Schneider, and G. Breuning. 1986. Autolytic processing of dimeric plant virus satellite RNA. *Science* **231:** 1577.

Rogers, J.H. 1985. The origin and evolution of retroposons. *Int. Rev. Cytol.* **93:** 187.

Schmelzer, C. and R.J. Schweyen. 1986. Self-splicing of group II introns in vitro: Mapping of the branch point and mutational inhibition of lariat formation. *Cell* **46:** 557.

Sharp, P.A. 1987. Splicing of messenger RNA precursors. *Science* **235:** 766.

Van der Horst, G. and H.F. Tabak. 1985. Self-splicing of yeast mitochondrial ribosomal and messenger RNA precursors. *Cell* **40:** 759.

Van der Veen, R., A.C. Arnberg, G. Van der Horst, L. Bonen, H.F. Tabak, and L.A. Grivell. 1986. Excised group II introns in yeast mitochondria are lariats and can be formed by self-splicing in vitro. *Cell* **44:** 225.

Weiner, A.M., P.L. Deininger, and A. Efstratiadis. 1986. Nonviral retroposons: Genes, pseudogenes, and transposable elements generated by the reverse flow of genetic information. *Annu. Rev. Biochem.* **55:** 631.

Zaug, A.J., P.J. Grabowski, and T.R. Cech. 1983. Autocatalytic cyclization of an excised intervening sequence RNA is a cleavage-ligation reaction. *Nature* **301:** 578.

Characterization of Two RNA-catalyzed RNA Cleavage Reactions

J.R. SAMPSON, F.X. SULLIVAN, L.S. BEHLEN, A.B. DIRENZO, AND O.C. UHLENBECK
Department of Chemistry and Biochemistry, University of Colorado, Boulder, Colorado 80309

The discovery that RNA molecules can have enzymatic activities has led to the speculation that the first self-replicating systems developed with RNA molecules alone (Darnell and Doolittle 1986; Gilbert 1986). This paper presents experiments on two very different modern examples of specific RNA self-cleavage reactions that provide insight into the possible mechanism of primitive ribonucleases. The first example is the self-cleavage reaction that occurs in the hammerhead domain (Hutchins et al. 1986) involved in processing the RNA genomes of certain plant viroids and satellite viruses. The second example is the Pb^{++}-dependent cleavage within the D loop of yeast tRNA^{Phe} (Dirheimer et al. 1972). In both cases, cleavage of the phosphodiester bond is the result of a transesterification reaction, where the 2'-OH attacks the internucleotide linkage to form termini with a 2',3'-cyclic phosphate and a 5'-OH. We show that in both cases, the large rate enhancement is a consequence of the RNA chain folding into a domain that promotes the reactions. We also find that it is possible to assemble active self-cleaving domains by combining two separate RNA fragments that are joined together by short RNA helices. Specific cleavage is only observed when both fragments are present in the reaction mixture. Under conditions where strand exchange between the fragments is rapid, many rounds of cleavage occur when an excess of the cleaved strand is present. Thus, the uncleaved strand acts as a catalyst in the specific cleavage of the other strand. The fact that certain short RNA fragments can act as specific ribonucleases would aid in the generation of unique RNA molecules in the prebiotic world.

EXPERIMENTAL PROCEDURES

RNA for self-cleavage reactions was prepared by in vitro runoff transcription of plasmid or synthetic DNA templates by T7 RNA polymerase. The advantages of this system for preparing RNA for physical or biochemical studies are discussed by Lowary et al. (1986). Oligoribonucleotides of less than 30 residues were prepared using synthetic DNA templates of the type shown in Figure 1A. Since only the promoter portion of the template need be double-stranded, only one DNA fragment has to be synthesized for each RNA desired. Under optimal reaction conditions, several hundred moles of RNA can be made per mole of template (Milligan et al. 1987).

To prepare transcripts that contain the sequence of yeast tRNA^{Phe}, six synthetic DNA fragments were cloned into a high-copy-number plasmid to give p67YFO (Fig. 1B) (Sampson and Uhlenbeck 1987). The yeast tRNA^{Phe} gene is flanked by the T7 promoter and a *Bst*NI restriction site such that in vitro transcription of *Bst*NI-digested p67YFO results in a 76-nucleotide RNA fragment having the exact sequence of yeast tRNA^{Phe} but without any modified nucleotides. A number of different mutations in the tRNA^{Phe} gene have been prepared in a similar way using other DNA fragments. In vitro transcription of *Mnl*I-digested p67YFO gave an unmodified RNA having the sequence of the 5' half of tRNA^{Phe} (residues 1–35). The 3' half

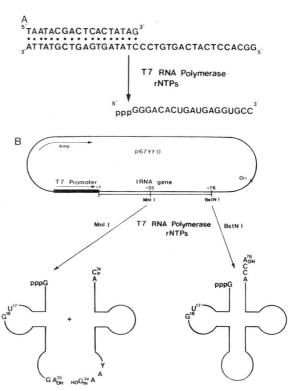

Figure 1. Synthesis of self-cleaving RNAs. (*A*) Synthesis of X1 by transcription of a synthetic DNA template using T7 RNA polymerase (Milligan et al. 1987). (*B*) Preparations of the full-length unmodified tRNA^{Phe} and the 5' half molecule were prepared by runoff transcription of linearized plasmid DNA using T7 RNA polymerase (Sampson and Uhlenbeck 1987). The 3' half molecule was isolated from native tRNA^{Phe}.

molecule of tRNA[Phe] (residues 34–74) was prepared by RNase A digestion of native yeast tRNA[Phe] as described by Wittenberg and Uhlenbeck (1985).

tRNA transcripts and hammerhead oligomers stored in neutral H_2O were heated to 90°C for 1 minute before use to avoid aggregation. tRNA half molecules were annealed by heating to 90°C and slow-cooled to 25°C in 10 mM Tris-HCl. Hammerhead self-cleavage reactions were initiated by the addition of the lower strand, and tRNA cleavage reactions were initiated by the addition of Pb^{++}. Reactions were terminated by the addition of an equal volume of 8 M urea–EDTA dye mix. Reaction products were separated by electrophoresis on 20% polyacrylamide–7 M urea gels and located by autoradiography. The bands were excised from the gel and counted. The extent of reaction was determined from the percentage of starting material converted to specific cleavage products. For the multiple turnover reaction with the tRNA half molecules, the radioactivity corresponding to the nonspecific cleavage products in the absence of the 3' half molecule were subtracted.

RESULTS

The Hammerhead Domain

As part of their rolling-circle replication mechanism, a specific site of RNA cleavage occurs in the single-stranded RNA genomes of certain plant viroids, virusoids, and satellite viruses (Branch et al. 1981). Bruening and co-workers have shown that the mature termini of the 359-nucleotide satellite tobacco ringspot virus (sTRSV) are generated autocatalytically by incubating either naturally derived genome dimers or transcripts of cDNA clones in neutral buffers at physiological temperatures (Prody et al. 1986). This autocatalytic cleavage reaction was shown to be reversible and only require about 100 nucleotides of the sTRSV genome (Buzayan et al. 1986). Symons and co-workers discovered four additional examples of the self-cleavage reaction in both the plus and minus strands of the avocado sunblotch viroid (ASBV) (Hutchins et al. 1986) and the lucerne transient streak virusoid (Forster and Symons 1987). A consensus hammerhead structure was found to be present in all five self-cleaving RNAs. As shown in Figure 2A, this proposed self-cleaving domain consists of 13 conserved nucleotides and 3 RNA double helices that can be formed from nucleotides contiguous on the RNA sequence or from two distant parts of the RNA chain. The cleavage site indicated by the arrow occurs between two nonconserved nucleotides but is at a constant position with respect to the rest of the structure. This consensus structure derived from the plant pathogen sequences was successful in accurately predicting the site of self-cleavage of a newt satellite DNA (Epstein and Gall 1987).

The cleavage properties of a pair of oligoribonucleotides (Fig. 2B, 01 and 02) designed to combine and form the self-cleaving domain have recently been

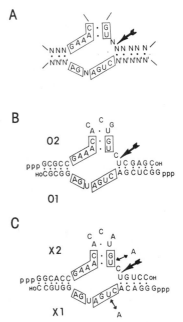

Figure 2. Secondary structure of the hammerhead domain. (*A*) Consensus hammerhead structure modified to include an additional self-cleaving sequence. (*B*) T7 transcripts 01 and 02 base paired to form a secondary structure consistent with the consensus structure. (*C*) T7 transcripts X1 and X2 base paired that also conform with the consensus secondary structure. X1* and X2* are identical to X1 and X2, respectively, except for the U to A substitutions at the positions indicated. Boxed nucleotides are conserved in all self-cleaving domains of this type.

characterized in considerable detail (Uhlenbeck 1987). Cleavage only occurs when both oligomers are incubated together, confirming that the hammerhead domain is both necessary and sufficient for cleavage. The reaction occurs rapidly ($t_{1/2} = 5$ min) and to a great extent ($>90\%$ cleavage) under physiological conditions (50 mM Tris-HCl [pH 7.5], 10 mM $MgCl_2$). Identification of the reaction products confirmed that cleavage occurs at the expected site, giving 2',3'-cyclic phosphate and 5'-OH termini. The reaction showed only a very modest increase in the rate of cleavage with pH unlike the base-catalyzed hydrolysis of RNA. It appears that divalent ion (Mg^{++}, Mn^{++}, or Ca^{++}) is needed for the reaction, and optimal rates require above 10 mM. Unlike the self-cleaving reactions of sTRSV and ASBV, spermidine or high salt cannot substitute for the divalent ion (Prody et al. 1986; Forster and Symons 1987). The reaction rate increases with temperature until 50°C and then rapidly decreases, presumably as a result of denaturation of the structure of the domain.

Figure 2C presents a second pair of oligoribonucleotides (X1 and X2) that were also designed to fit the consensus self-cleaving domain. Like the 01-02 pair, the central portion of the X1-X2 pair closely resembles the minus strand of ASBV, but the right and left helices differ from 01-02 and from any natural self-cleaving

RNA. As shown in Figure 3 for both pairs of oligomers, cleavage only occurs when both strands are present. Judging from the lengths of the X1 and X2 reaction products, cleavage occurs at the expected site for this pair. When the noncomplementary pairs are mixed (X2 with 01 or 02 with X1), no cleavage occurs. These experiments provide additional evidence for the hammerhead secondary structure and show that it is essential for cleavage. The right and left helices must form in order for cleavage to occur, but more than one sequence can be accommodated as the consensus structure predicts.

Since DNA-RNA helices have a structure very similar to that of RNA helices, it is conceivable that the two lower strands (01 and X1) would be active as DNA oligomers. As shown in Figure 3, no cleavage occurs when deoxy-01 was incubated with 02. This was also true for the deoxy X1-X2 pair. Presumably, the nonhelical portion of the domain requires the presence of one or more riboses for activity.

It is likely that the hammerhead domain folds into a precise three-dimensional structure involving tertiary interactions. Tertiary interactions in tRNA usually involve nucleotides considered to be single-stranded in the secondary structure that interact either with one

another to form non-Watson-Crick pairing interactions or with base pairs to form triple-strand interactions. Due to the structural constraints in the folding of the tRNA chain, nucleotides involved in tertiary interactions are usually conserved or semiconserved. This suggests that many of the conserved nucleotides in the self-cleaving domain may be also involved in tertiary interactions and thus be essential for reaction. This possibility was tested by preparing variants of X1 and of X2, where one of the conserved nucleotides is changed (Fig. 2C). Figure 3 shows that neither of these variants was active in the self-cleaving reaction when combined with the active cofragment. Although this result is consistent with the idea that the altered nucleotides are involved in tertiary interactions, it is also possible they are important for other aspects of the self-cleavage reaction.

Lead-induced Cleavage of Yeast tRNA[Phe]

Incubation of low (0.3 mM) concentrations of Pb^{++} with yeast tRNA[Phe] at pH 7.4 and 37°C results in rapid ($t_{1/2} > 5$ min) cleavage between D_{17} and G_{18} to give 2',3'-cyclic phosphate and 5'-OH termini (Werner et al. 1976). Longer incubation results in additional slower, nonspecific cleavages in the tRNA chain, reflecting the known ability of Pb^{++} to cleave RNA (Farkas 1968). Although this cleavage reaction does not have any known physiological relevance and is less specific than the reaction involving the hammerhead domain, it is an interesting topic of study due to the availability of the tRNA[Phe] crystal structure and the precise localization of the Pb^{++} ion-binding sites.

Klug and co-workers have studied the Pb^{++} cleavage reaction using X-ray crystallography (Brown et al. 1983, 1985). By soaking Pb^{++} into tRNA[Phe] crystals at pH 5 and at pH 7.4, these authors were able to obtain a difference map between the cleaved and uncleaved forms. The only structural difference between the molecules was that the phosphate at the cleavage site was delocalized in the cleaved tRNA. In addition, the diffraction data clearly implicated one of the tightly bound Pb^{++} atoms in the cleavage reaction. This lead atom, Pb(1), lies about 6 Å from the cleavage site and is less than 3 Å from (and presumably directly coordinated with) the 04 of U_{59} and the N3 of C_{60}. Pb(1) is also about 3.5 Å (and presumably coordinated through water) from the N3 of U_{59}, the N4 and 02 of C_{60}, and the OR of P_{19}. In binding to tRNA[Phe], Pb(1) displaces one tightly bound Mg^{++} located a few angstroms away. On the basis of the position of Pb(1) with respect to the cleavage site, Brown et al. (1985) proposed that the most likely mechanism for cleavage involves $(PbOH)^+$ ion abstracting the hydrogen from the 2'-OH of ribose-17, thereby facilitating nucleophilic attack on phosphorous-18. Since less rearrangement of the backbone would be required for an equitorial attack on the phosphate followed by a pseudo-rotation, Brown et al.

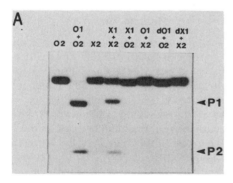

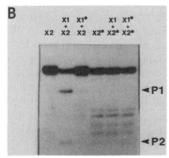

Figure 3. Structural requirements in the hammerhead domain necessary for self-cleavage. (*A*) 15 nM ^{32}P-labeled oligonucleotides 02 or X2 was incubated in the presence or absence of 100 nM unlabeled oligonucleotides 01, X1, deoxy-01 (d01), or deoxy-X1 (dX1) in 50 mM HEPES (pH 7.5), 10 mM MgCl$_2$, 0.1 mM EDTA at 50°C for 4 hr. P1 and P2 correspond to the 5' and 3' cleavage products, respectively. (*B*) ^{32}P-labeled oligonucleotides X2 or X2* were incubated in the presence or absence of unlabeled X1 or X1* as described in *A*. The sequence of each oligomer is given in Fig. 2.

(1985) favored this mechanism over the more conventional in-line attack.

Our laboratory has been studying the physical and biochemical properties of a totally unmodified tRNA^{Phe} obtained by in vitro transcription (Sampson and Uhlenbeck 1987). We have found that in many respects, this tRNA is very similar to the fully modified counterpart. Above 10 mM MgCl$_2$, the transcribed tRNA^{Phe} and the naturally occurring yeast tRNA^{Phe} aminoacylate by yeast phenylalanine synthetase with virtually the same kinetics. Analysis of the nuclear magnetic resonance (NMR) spectrum of the transcript in H$_2$O indicated that most of the tertiary interactions were present (K. Hall, unpubl.). Thus, it is not surprising that incubation of the transcript with Pb^{++} results in cleavage at the same site found for tRNA^{Phe}. Since we have been preparing a number of variant transcripts containing specific nucleotide substitutions for structure-function studies, it was of interest to assay these variants for their ability to cleave with Pb^{++}.

As would be expected from the precise coordination of the Pb^{++} ion in the crystal structure, cleavage is highly sensitive to the RNA structure in the neighborhood of the cleavage site. Figure 4 shows the cleavage properties of a number of tRNA^{Phe} variants. Although we do not know the structure of these variant tRNAs, their cleavage properties can often be explained in terms of local changes in the structure.

Two variants that change single-stranded nucleotides in the neighborhood of the cleavage site are G$_{20}$→U and U$_{16}$U$_{17}$→C$_{16}$C$_{17}$. Both of these variants cleave normally. This can be explained by the fact that these three nucleotides are not involved in any tertiary interactions and are not directly coordinated to Pb^{++}. Thus, it is likely that these variants have a structure identical to that of the wild-type transcript and therefore bind Pb^{++} and cleave normally. It is interesting to note that tRNA resembles the hammerhead domain in the sense that the nucleotide 5' to the cleavage site can be substituted without affecting cleavage.

The situation is more complex for variants of the tertiary Watson-Crick base pair between G$_{19}$ and C$_{56}$ that is located about 6 Å from the Pb(1) site. This base pair is conserved in all nonmitochondrial tRNAs. Both the G$_{19}$→C and C$_{56}$→G single-base variants cleave very poorly after U$_{17}$ and show enhanced cleavage at another site. Presumably, the absence of a normal tertiary interaction either destabilizes the tRNA or alters the folding in such a way that normal cleavage does not occur. Since the OR of phosphate-19 is coordinated to Pb(1), it is possible that the loss of structure prevents proper orientation of the (PbOH)$^+$ necessary for cleavage. As would be expected, the C$_{19}$G$_{56}$ double mutant that restores the base pair cleaves normally. These experiments agree well with the ability of these tRNAs to interact with yeast phenylalanine synthetase. The two single mutants show slower rates of aminoacylation, whereas the double mutant aminoacylates at the same rate as the wild type (Uhlenbeck et al. 1987).

A second tertiary interaction we studied was the

trans G$_{15}$C$_{48}$ pair that also lies about 6 Å from Pb(1) and is present in 70% of all tRNAs. Since a trans A U pair is virtually isomorphic and is found in the corresponding positions in the remaining 30% of tRNAs, it is not surprising that the A$_{15}$U$_{48}$ double mutant cleaves normally. However, the mismatched data are less easily explained, since A$_{15}$C$_{48}$ cleaves at U$_{17}$, whereas G$_{15}$U$_{48}$ does not. Since both of these single mutants can be folded into possible trans purine-pyrimidine base pairs, and lie well away from Pb(1), the structural basis for these data is unclear. These results emphasize the need for structural data on variant tRNAs before interpretation is complete.

To extend the analogy between the tRNA and hammerhead cleavage reactions, the Pb^{++} cleavage reaction was studied in an intermolecular configuration by preparing a transcript that terminated in the anticodon loop and studying its cleavage in the presence of the 3' half molecule of yeast tRNA^{Phe} (residues 34–74). As shown in Figure 5, specific cleavage only occurs when both half molecules are present and the rate of cleavage of the annealed halves is about half of that for the intact transcript. This relatively small difference may simply be the result of incomplete annealing of the tRNA half molecules. We conclude that the folding of tRNA^{Phe} near the Pb(1) site is not substantially altered by breaking the tRNA chain in the anticodon loop.

Multiple Turnovers

Although it has not been studied in detail, the rate of strand exchange in short RNA helices would be expected to be quite rapid near the melting temperature. Since the bimolecular self-cleaving domains studied here are partially held together by helices, it seems likely that conditions could be found where they change pairing partners in the same time scale as the cleavage rate. If an excess of the cleaved strand is present under these conditions, the uncleaved strand should be able to combine with it and induce cleavage many times. An example of multiple turnovers in the 01 + 02 hammerhead system is shown in Figure 6. When 832 pmoles of 02 are combined with 11 pmoles of 01, cleavage occurs at a constant rate until more than 40% of the 02 is cleaved. This means that each 01 molecule has participated in an average of 25 cleavage events. This multiple turnover reaction has been extensively characterized (Uhlenbeck 1987). At a constant, low 01 concentration, the initial rate of 02 cleavage saturates at high 02 concentrations. The data were found to fit well to Michaelis-Menton kinetics, giving a $K_m = 0.5$ μM and a $k_{cat} = 0.5$/min. This k_{cat} is similar to what has been reported for the Tetrahymena intron splicing reaction ($k_{cat} = 2$/min) and for Escherichia coli M1 RNA ($k_{cat} = 1$/min) (Guerrier-Takada et al. 1983; Zaug and Cech 1986). In addition, at saturating 02 concentration, the initial rate of cleavage is directly proportional to 01 concentration. Thus, 01 behaves as an enzyme capable of specifically cleaving 02. When present in small amounts, 01 greatly enhances the reaction rate without

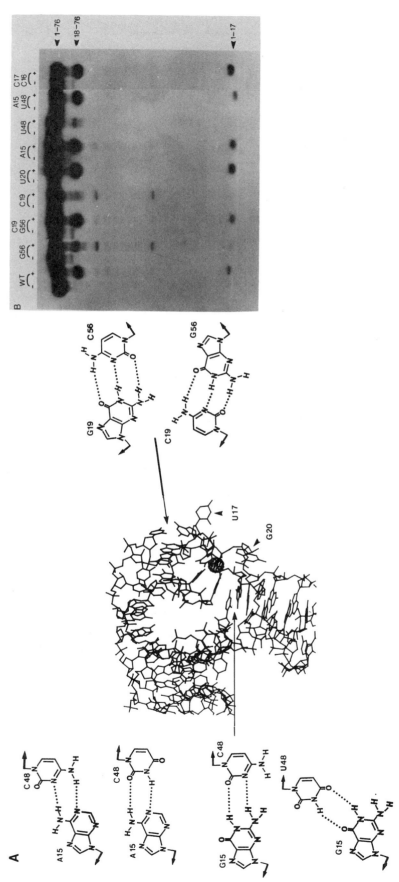

Figure 4. Pb^{++}-dependent cleavage of various tRNA^{Phe} mutants. (*A*) Tertiary structure of yeast tRNA^{Phe} in the neighborhood of the Pb^{++}-cleavage site. Pb(1) is indicated by the sphere. Nucleotides that have been changed are indicated and possible base-pairing arrangements for several variants are given. (*B*) 2.0 μM ^{32}P-labeled tRNA transcripts was incubated in 15 mM Tris-HCl, 15 mM MgCl$_2$ with (+) or without (−) 0.4 mM PbOAc for 1 min at 42°C to produce cleavage products. WT is the wild-type transcript; nucleotides that have been changed in each mutant transcript are indicated.

271

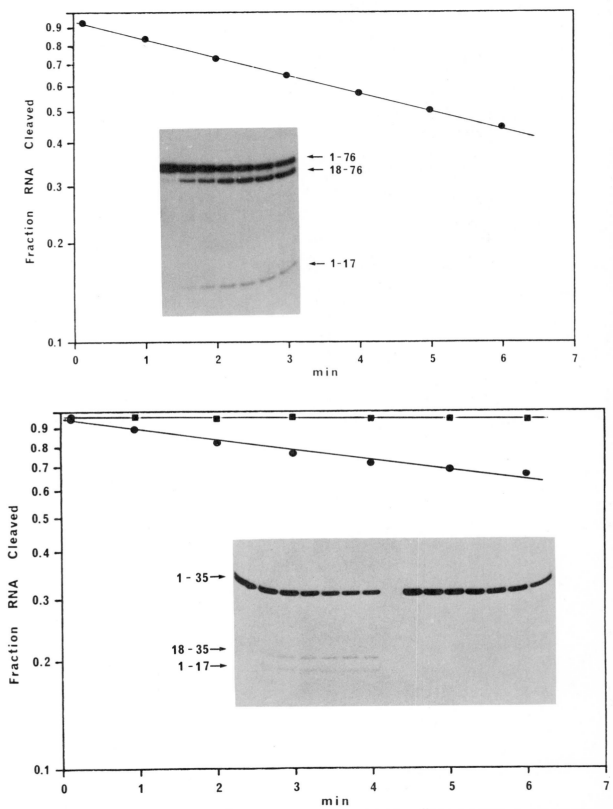

Figure 5. Pb^{++}-dependent cleavage of $tRNA^{Phe}$ and the 5' half molecule. (*A*) 1.0 μM ^{32}P-labeled tRNA transcript (1-76) was incubated in 10 mM Tris-Cl (pH 7.4), 10 mM $MgCl_2$, 0.2 mM PbOAC at 37°C for the indicated times to produce the cleavage products 1-17 and 18-76. (*B*) 1.0 μM ^{32}P-labeled 5' half transcript (1-35) was incubated in the presence (●) or absence (■) of 1.0 μM unlabeled native 3' half molecule under the same conditions as *A* to produce the cleavage products 1-17 and 18-35.

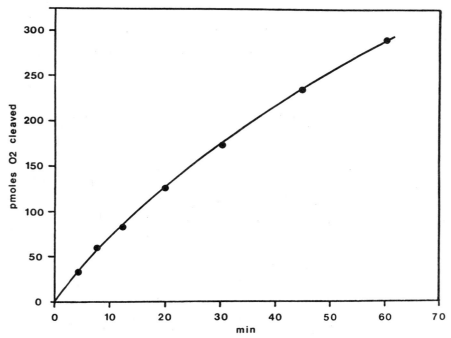

Figure 6. Enzymatic cleavage of 02 by 01. ^{32}P-labeled 02 (832 pmoles) was incubated with 11 pmoles of unlabeled 01 in 40 μl of 50 mM Tris-Cl (pH 7.5) and 10 mM MgCl$_2$ at 55°C for the indicated times.

being consumed. At 19 nucleotides, 01 is the smallest RNA enzyme found to date.

The first demonstration of multiple turnovers in the tRNA half molecule system is shown in Figure 7. To allow rapid strand exchange while maintaining the tRNA structure, the Mg^{++} ion concentration and temperature were adjusted from the conditions given in Figure 5. In addition, the Pb^{++} concentration was lowered in order to suppress secondary Pb^{++} cleavage sites in the isolated 5' half molecule. When 400 pmoles of

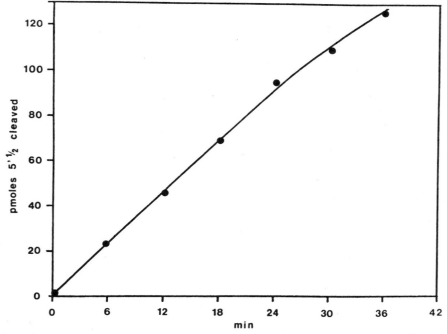

Figure 7. Pb^{++}-dependent enzymatic cleavage of the tRNA 5' half molecules by the 3' half molecule. ^{32}P-labeled 5' half tRNA transcript (400 pmoles) was incubated in the presence or absence of 40 pmoles of unlabeled native tRNA 3' half molecule in 40 μl of 10 mM Tris-Cl (pH 7.4), 4 mM MgCl$_2$, 50 μM PbOAC at 60°C for the indicated times.

the transcribed 5' half molecule was incubated with 40 pmoles of the tRNA^{Phe} 3' half molecule, cleavage occurred at a constant rate for 36 minutes, by which time 120 pmoles of specific cleavage products appeared. Thus, each 3' half molecule participated in an average of three cleavage events. The rate of this reaction corresponds to 0.1 pmole 5' half cleaved/min/3' half or about 20% of the k_{cat} for the hammerhead domain. Although this reaction needs further characterization, it is clear that the 3' half of the tRNA^{Phe} shows enzyme-like properties by promoting the specific cleavage of the 5' half molecule in the presence of Pb^{++}.

DISCUSSION

Of the two types of self-cleaving RNAs we have described, it is clear that the hammerhead domain is the more sophisticated. It is characterized by very precise and extraordinarily rapid cleavage. Although it is difficult to obtain a reliable rate of nonspecific cleavage of RNA under the same reaction conditions, it has been estimated that the rate of cleavage of the hammerhead is at least four orders of magnitude greater (Uhlenbeck 1987). Due to the efficiency of the reaction, it is not surprising that several modern examples of the hammerhead domain are used for RNA processing steps in the replication of simple RNA genomes. It is likely that this type of reaction is less common than Pb^{++} cleavage. Only two examples of nonhammerhead self-cleaving reactions have been found thus far and both serve as natural RNA processing sites (Watson et al. 1984; Buzayan et al. 1986).

The Pb^{++}-assisted cleavage reaction of tRNA^{Phe} appears to be a more primitive example of a self-cleaving RNA and therefore is potentially a better example of a prebiotic reaction. The reaction is much less specific. Conditions at which the rate of tRNA cleavage was comparable to that of the hammerhead cleavage resulted in cleavage at other sites in the tRNA. We estimate that nonspecific cleavage of RNA is only 10–100-fold slower than that found for the specific site in tRNA^{Phe}. Pb^{++}-promoted cleavage of RNA is quite common, since the mechanism simply involves the specific binding of the reactive Pb^{++} ion such that it is oriented properly with respect to the polynucleotide chain. Due to a pK$_a$ of about 7 for the (PbOH)$^+$ ion, Pb^{++} is the most effective cation for promoting such a reaction. However, similar specific cleavage of tRNA^{Phe} by Zn^{++} and even Mg^{++} at high pH and temperature has been reported (Wintermeyer and Zachau 1973). Interestingly, Mg^{++} cleaves tRNA^{Phe} at a different site, between D$_{16}$ and D$_{17}$. Presumably, other ions capable of cleaving RNA, such as lanthanum (Eichhorn and Butzow 1965), also can promote specific RNA cleavage. In addition, other tRNA sequences incubated with Pb^{++} do not cleave in the D loop but show preferential cleavage sites elsewhere in the molecule, presumably as a result of altered Pb^{++} binding (Werner et al. 1976). In light of this large number of possible cleavage sites and lower specificity of cleavage, it is not surprising that

there are no known examples where this type of reaction is used in a modern RNA processing reaction.

Although it is tempting to speculate that the hammerhead domain is a highly evolved form of a divalent ion cleavage domain, there is little evidence to support this. Although the 01-02 cleavage reaction appears to have a divalent ion requirement, the hammerhead cleavage domains in sTRSV and ASBV do not. In addition, the two reactions show a very different pH dependence of cleavage, suggesting that a substantially different mechanism is involved. It seems more likely that the hammerhead cleavage domain evolved independently. The fact that it appears in both plants and animals suggests a comparatively early origin.

A clear conclusion from our experiments is that the ability of RNA to promote self-cleavage is a consequence of the folding of the polyribonucleotide chain. Point mutations in both self-cleaving domains resulted in loss of activity even when the mutation was far away from the cleavage site. In the case of the tRNA cleavage reaction, it is clear that the proper folding of the RNA, rather than the nucleotide sequence, is crucial for the specific cleavage activity, since several structurally isomorphic substitutions cleaved normally. It is interesting that the sizes of both self-cleaving domains are relatively small. The minimal size for an active hammerhead domain has been estimated to be about 30 nucleotides (Uhlenbeck 1987). Since it is likely that the tRNA cleavage reaction could occur without at least part of the anticodon and acceptor stems, a cleavage domain of fewer than 50 nucleotides is possible. Considering the fact that a hairpin loop of 10–15 nucleotides is the minimal size for an RNA molecule with nonrandom structure, these self-cleaving domains are not very large. This emphasizes the ease with which RNA chains can achieve structural complexity with relatively few nucleotides.

Although both self-cleaving reactions studied here were originally reported to be intramolecular reactions, we were able to convert them to intermolecular reactions quite easily. In both cases, the strategy involved breaking the chain at a site that did not disturb the structure of the self-cleaving domain. An active self-cleavage structure could then form by recombining the two half molecules into a complex stabilized by two RNA helices. In the case of the hammerhead system, these helices were essential for cleavage, since no cleavage occurred with the 01-X2 and X1-02 pairs. A very similar strategy was used to convert the intramolecular transesterification reactions of the *Tetrahymena* intron (Szostak 1986; Zaug and Cech 1986) and the type II self-splicing intron (Jaquier and Rosbach 1986) into the corresponding intermolecular reactions. This general capacity to convert RNA intramolecular reactions to intermolecular reactions reflects the propensity of RNA to maintain its overall structure even when the polynucleotide chain is broken at one or more sites. Thus, no mechanistic difference exists between the intra- and intermolecular reactions.

Our demonstration of turnover in each type of

bimolecular cleavage reaction domain suggests that a similar reaction may have been operative in prebiotic catalytic RNA processing reactions. The mechanism would involve the joining of two RNA fragments to form a self-cleaving domain through the annealing of short RNA helices. Subsequent cleavage would be followed by the displacement of the cleaved products by a fresh substrate strand through a strand-exchange mechanism. If the substrate part of the self-cleaving domain were embedded within a longer RNA, the enzyme part could define the terminus of a prebiotic RNA molecule in a true RNA processing reaction. Since the enzyme portion could turn over many times, a low concentration of one sequence could generate identical termini on a large variety of different RNA molecules. The definition of unique termini on RNA molecules is an important preliminary step to developing defined genomes with precise replication pathways. In addition, unique termini would permit the development of specific chemistry using the ends of RNA.

It is interesting that the formation and dissociation of short intramolecular RNA helices appear to be an essential component of the mechanism of these primitive ribozymes. It is likely that the efficiency of the cleavage reaction will depend on the stability of the helices and thus their degree of complementarity. The formation and dissociation of short, often imprecise intramolecular RNA helices is also a characteristic of several modern RNA processing reactions. The internal guide sequence in the *Tetrahymena* self-splicing reaction base pairs with the intron-exon boundary, and at least two of the small nuclear RNAs pair with pre-mRNA during the nuclear mRNA splicing mechanism (Zhuang and Weiner 1986; Parker et al. 1987). We note that the formation and dissociation of small RNA helices are also an essential component of the translation mechanism, emphasizing the importance of this type of interaction.

ACKNOWLEDGMENT

This work was supported by grants from the National Institutes of Health (GM-36944 and GM-37552).

REFERENCES

Branch, A.D., H.D. Robertson, and E. Dickson. 1981. Longer-than-unit-length viroid minus strands are present in RNA from infected plants. *Proc. Natl. Acad. Sci.* **78:** 6381.

Brown, R.S., J.C. Dewan, and A. Klug. 1985. Crystallographic and biochemical investigation of the lead (II)-catalyzed hydrolysis of yeast phenylalanine tRNA. *Biochemistry* **24:** 4785.

Brown, R.S., B.E. Hingerty, J.C. Dewan, and A. Klug. 1983. Pb(II)-catalyzed cleavage of the sugar-phosphate backbone of yeast tRNA^{Phe}—Implications for lead toxicity and self-splicing RNA. *Nature* **303:** 543.

Buzayan, J.M., W.L. Gerlach, and G. Bruening. 1986. Nonenzymatic cleavage and ligation of RNAs complementary to a plant virus satellite RNA. *Nature* **323:** 349.

Darnell, J.E. and W.F. Doolittle. 1986. Speculations on the early course of evolution. *Proc. Natl. Acad. Sci.* **83:** 1271.

Dirheimer, G., J.P. Ebel, J. Bonnet, J. Gangloff, G. Keith, B. Krebs, B. Kuntzel, A. Roy, J. Weissenbach, and C. Werner. 1972. Structure primaire des tRNA. *Biochimie* **54:** 127.

Eichhorn, G.L. and J.J. Butzow. 1965. Interactions of metal ions with polynucleotides and related compounds. *Biopolymers* **3:** 79.

Epstein, L.M. and J.G. Gall. 1987. Self-cleaving transcripts of satellite DNA from the newt. *Cell* **48:** 535.

Farkas, W.R. 1968. Depolymerization of ribonucleic acid plumbous ion. *Biochim. Biophys. Acta* **155:** 401.

Forster, A.C. and R.H. Symons. 1987. Self-cleavage of plus and minus RNAs of a virusoid and a structural model for the active sites. *Cell* **49:** 211.

Gilbert, W. 1986. The RNA world. *Nature* **391:** 618.

Guerrier-Takeda, C., K. Gardiner, T. Marsh, N. Pace, and S. Altman. 1983. The RNA moiety of ribonuclease P is the catalytic subunit of the enzyme. *Cell* **35:** 849.

Hutchins, C.J., P.D. Rathjen, A.C. Forster, and R.H. Symons. 1986. Self-cleavage of plus and minus RNA transcripts of avocado sunblotch viroid. *Nucleic Acids Res.* **14:** 3627.

Jacquier, A. and M. Rosbash. 1986. Efficient trans-splicing of a yeast mitochondrial RNA group II intron implicates a strong 5' exon-intron interaction. *Science* **234:** 1099.

Lowary, P., J.R. Sampson, J. Milligan, D. Groebe, and O.C. Uhlenbeck. 1986. A better way to make RNA for physical studies. In *Structure and dynamics of RNA* (ed. P.H. van Knipperberg and C.N. Hilbers), p. 69. Plenum Press, New York.

Milligan, J.F., D.R. Groebe, G.W. Witherall, and O..C Uhlenbeck. 1987. Oligoribonucleotide synthesis by transcription of synthetic DNA. *Nucleic Acids Res.* (in press).

Parker, R., P.G. Siliciano, and C. Guthrie. 1987. Recognition of the TACTAAC box during mRNA splicing in yeast involves base pairing to the U2-like snRNA. *Cell* **49:** 229.

Prody, G.A., J.T. Bakos, J.M. Buzayan, I.R. Schneider, and G. Bruening. 1986. Autolytic processing of dimeric plant satellite RNA. *Science* **231:** 1577.

Sampson, J.R. and O.C. Uhlenbeck. 1987. Biochemical and physical characterization of an unmodified yeast tRNA^{Phe} transcribed *in vitro*. *Proc. Natl. Acad. Sci.* (in press).

Szostak, J.W. 1986. Enzymatic activity of conserved core of a group I self-splicing intron. *Nature* **322:** 83.

Uhlenbeck, O.C. 1987. A small catalytic oligoribonucleotide. *Nature* **328:** 596.

Uhlenbeck, O.C., H. Wu, and J.R. Sampson. 1987. Recognition of RNA by proteins. In *New perspectives on the molecular biology of RNA* (ed. M. Inouye). Academic Press, New York. (In press.)

Watson, N., M. Gurevitz, J. Ford, and D. Apirion. 1984. Self-cleavage of a precursor RNA from bacteriophage T4. *J. Mol. Biol.* **172:** 301.

Werner, C., B. Krebs, G. Keith, and G. Dirheimer. 1976. Specific cleavages of pure tRNAs by plumbous ions. *Biochim. Biophys. Acta* **432:** 161.

Wintermeyer, W. and H.G. Zachau. 1973. Mg^{2+} katalysierte spezifische spaltung von tRNA. *Biochim. Biophys. Acta* **299:** 82.

Wittenberg, W.L. and O.C. Uhlenbeck. 1985. Specific replacement of functional groups of uridine-33 in yeast phenylalanine transfer ribonucleic acid. *Biochemistry* **24:** 2705.

Zaug, A.J. and T.R. Cech. 1986. The intervening sequence of *Tetrahymena* is an enzyme. *Science* **231:** 470.

Zhuang, Y. and A.M. Weiner. 1986. A compensatory base change in U1 snRNA suppresses a 5' splice site mutation. *Cell* **46:** 827.

Splicing of Messenger RNA Precursors

P.A. Sharp, M.M. Konarksa, P.J. Grabowski, A.I. Lamond, R. Marciniak, and S.R. Seiler

*Center for Cancer Research, and Department of Biology, Massachusetts Institute of Technology,
Cambridge, Massachusetts 02139*

A decade has passed since the first description of RNA splicing and introns. In the interim, introns have been characterized in all lineages of eukaryotic organisms. The macromolecular structures of small nuclear ribonucleoprotein particles (snRNPs) and self-splicing RNAs have been discovered. The biochemical mechanisms responsible for splicing of tRNAs, nuclear mRNA precursors, and self-splicing RNAs have been partially analyzed. These results have focused renewed attention on the role of RNA in biological systems and the evolutionary origin of genes.

Intron Sequences

Introns within nuclear genes encoding polypeptides have consensus sequences at their 5' and 3' splice sites (sequences shown in Fig. 1, where *n* ranges from 10 to 20). The GU and AG dinucleotide sequences immediately adjacent to the splice sites are almost invariant among different introns. Mutations altering these highly conserved bases inactivate processing of the intron (for review, see Padgett et al. 1986). The same type of consensus sequence is observed in introns of vertebrates, plants, and single-cell eukaryotes such as yeast. The most pronounced variation in these sequences between different types of organisms is that the polypyrimidine tract is not as extensive in yeast as in vertebrate organisms. The introns of yeast are typically small ($\sim$ 50–150 N), and sequences bracketing the branch site are much more highly conserved in yeast than in vertebrates. Thus, sequences at the branch site might constitute the major determinant in specifying the 3' splice site in yeast.

The consensus sequence containing the branch site in yeast is UACUAACA, where the italicized A residue

is the site of branch formation (Langford and Gallwitz 1983; Pikielny et al. 1983). Mutations that change any base in these sequences either reduce the efficiency or totally block the splicing reaction (Langford et al. 1984; Newman et al. 1985). The branch site sequences in vertebrate introns are not as highly conserved, forming a consensus of $^{U}_{C}N^{U}_{C}UGA^{A}_{C}$ (see Fig. 1). This site is typically located between 20 and 50 nucleotides upstream of the 3' splice site. Deletion of the natural branch site from a vertebrate intron normally results in a three- to fivefold decrease in the rate of splicing, with the utilization of another adenosine moiety for branch formation (Rautmann and Breathnach 1985; Ruskin et al. 1985; Aebi et al. 1986). In some cases, the sequences surrounding the cryptic branch site fit poorly to the consensus sequences (Padgett et al. 1985). Thus, comparing the situation in yeast and vertebrates, recognition of the 3' splice site in yeast is probably primarily specified by the branch site sequences, whereas in introns of vertebrates, the equivalent specificity is probably located in sequences at the 3' splice site.

Introns in vertebrate genes can be 100,000 nucleotides in length. The limited tract of consensus sequences at the two splice sites is unlikely to contain sufficient information to specify uniquely a site of cleavage and ligation over this length of RNA. Thus, for long introns, additional information must be present either in flanking exons or within the introns. The nature of this additional information is not known. For example, it is possible that binding sites for additional factors could be present within sequences of long introns. A few introns are processed in a cell-type-specific fashion; i.e., a particular intron might be excised when the RNA is expressed in one cell type but not processed in a second cell type (Breitbart et al. 1987). Thus,

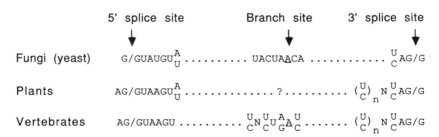

Figure 1. Consensus sequences for the 5' and 3' splice sites of vertebrates (Padgett et al. 1986), plants (Brown 1986), and yeast (Teem et al. 1984) are from tabulations of sequences aligned by positioning GU and AG at the two boundaries. The data for fungi are primarily sequences from genes of *S. cerevisiae*. The branch-site consensus sequence for vertebrates is from Reed and Maniatis (1985). N represents any nucleotide.

SHARP ET AL.

trans-acting factors involved in splicing must vary between cell types.

Mechanism of Splicing of Precursors to mRNAs

At the moment, it is thought that all introns within nuclear precursors to mRNAs, regardless of length or of species origin, are excised by the mechanism outlined in Figure 2. There are two interesting aspects of this mechanism. First, lariat RNAs are generated that have a branch site (Grabowski et al. 1984; Padgett et al. 1984; Ruskin et al. 1984). The excised intron is released as a lariat RNA and is rapidly degraded in vivo. The half-life of excised introns is on the order of a few seconds. Sequences within the vast majority of introns appear to serve no other function within cells than to link two exons that will ultimately be joined by splicing. This lack of physiological function for introns is supported by the rapid evolution of internal intron sequences, which occurs at a rate comparable to that

observed for silent nucleotide positions within codons (Perler et al. 1980). The second interesting aspect of the splicing mechanism is the generation of an intermediate. The intermediate is produced by cleavage at the 5′ splice site with concomitant formation of the branch. The 5′ exon (E1) is subsequently joined to the 3′ exon (E2) by reaction at the 3′ splice site.

The actual chemistry of the cleavage and ligation reactions at either the 5′ or 3′ splice site has not been established. However, it has been shown that the phosphate moieties at both sites are conserved during the reactions (Konarska et al. 1985). Thus, the data are consistent with both of these reactions being transesterifications. For example, reaction at the 5′ splice site could occur by the mechanism of conversion of the 2′-OH group at the branch site to a nucleophile (RO^-), which could then attack the phosphate group. The phosphodiester bond to the 5′ exon would be displaced, producing the intermediate RNAs. A similar transesterification mechanism could be responsible for the reaction at the 3′ splice site.

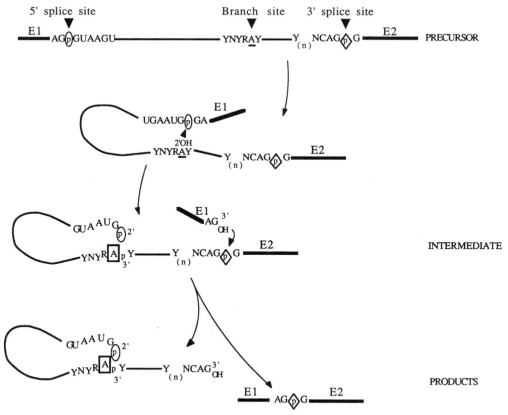

Figure 2. Splicing mechanism of the mRNA precursor. A prototype precursor RNA is drawn with the intervening sequences or intron sequences spanning from the indicated 5′ and 3′ splice sites. The intervening sequences are flanked by the 5′ exon (E1) and 3′ exon (E2). Consensus sequences are indicated at the splice sites and branch site (Y, pyrimidine; R, purine; and N, any base). The fate of the phosphate moieties at the 5′ and 3′ splice sites during the reaction can be deduced from following the circled p and the p surrounded by a diamond, respectively. The two RNAs of the intermediate are diagramed on the third line. At the bottom of the figure, the two products of the reaction, the lariat form of the excised intervening sequences and the spliced exons, are shown.

Potential Relationship of Splicing of mRNA Precursors to Self-splicing RNAs

Several features of the mechanism for splicing of nuclear precursors to mRNAs suggest that this process is related to that of self-splicing RNAs (Fig. 3) (Cech 1985a,b; Sharp 1985). Self-splicing RNAs can be assigned to two groups on the basis of conserved sequences within the intron (Cech and Bass 1986). Group I RNAs bind a guanosine cofactor for reaction at the 5′ splice site (Cech et al. 1981), whereas group II RNAs utilize a 2′-OH group within the intron for reaction at this site (Peebles et al. 1986; Van der Veen et al. 1986). Due to the nature of the reactants and the absence of high-energy cofactors, all reactions by self-splicing introns must occur by a transesterification process. As discussed above, the two steps of the nuclear splicing process could also involve transesterification reactions. All three splicing processes involve two steps, an initial reaction at the 5′ splice site, with generation of a noncovalently bound 5′ exon, and then a subsequent reaction at the 3′ splice site. Finally, the nuclear splicing process and the group II self-splicing process share the obvious similarity of branch formation. In view of these similarities, it is reasonable to hypothesize that the nuclear splicing process is evolutionarily related to that of the self-splicing RNAs. In fact, the nuclear splicing process might also be RNA catalyzed. If this is the case, the catalytic RNA cannot be formed exclusively from intron sequences, since these can be deleted or substituted without loss of activity (Wieringa et al. 1984). The catalytic RNA structure would probably be formed instead by snRNAs, which are now known to be components of the spliceosome.

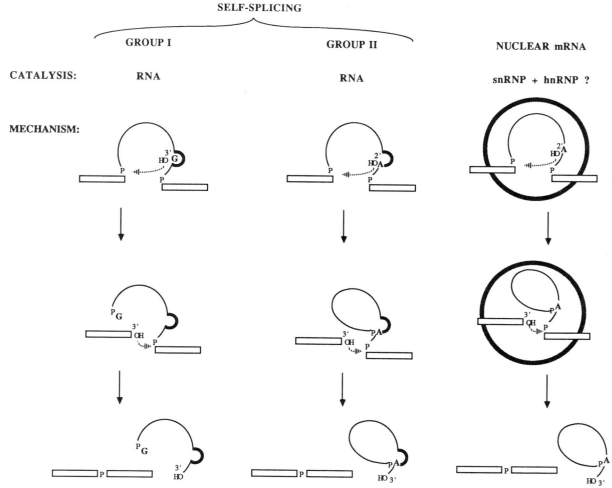

Figure 3. Comparison of self-splicing and nuclear mRNA splicing mechanisms. The first column outlines the splicing mechanism of self-splicing introns of the group I type. This process is catalyzed by RNA structures within the intron (dark semicircle) utilizing a guanosine (G) cofactor. The second column outlines the splicing mechanism of self-splicing introns of the group II type. This process is also catalyzed by RNA structures within the intron (dark semicircle) but utilizing instead of a cofactor an adenosine residue (A) within the intron to form a lariat RNA. The third column outlines the mRNA precursor splicing mechanism diagramed in Fig. 1. The large heavy circle represents a multicomponent complex, the spliceosome, which promotes the splicing reaction. The fate of the phosphates at the 5′ and 3′ splice sites is indicated.

Spliceosome

The concept that a common multicomponent complex might be responsible for the cleavage and ligation steps in the splicing of all nuclear introns is embodied in the term spliceosome or splicing body. The first indication that a complex was involved in splicing was the structure of the intermediate. It seemed logical that the two RNAs of this intermediate, the 5' exon and lariat intervening sequence (IVS) 3' exon, would remain bound together in a single entity. When examined, using reactions containing extracts of either mammalian or yeast cells, these two RNAs cosedimented in velocity gradients as complexes at 60S (Grabowski et al. 1985) and 40S (Brody and Abelson 1985), respectively. This suggested that the spliceosome was a relatively large complex.

Dating from the recognition of complementarity between RNA sequences at the 5' end of the most abundant metazoon snRNA, U1 snRNA, and the consensus sequences at the 5' splice site, it was anticipated that one or more snRNPs would be components in the spliceosome (Lerner et al. 1980; Rogers and Wall 1980). snRNP particles contain, in addition to a set of five to eight polypeptides, a highly modified short RNA (snRNA), which has a trimethyl cap. All snRNPs share a common set of five polypeptides, whereas the more abundant particles, U1 and U2 snRNPs, also possess unique polypeptides. Affinity chromatography has been used to purify the spliceosome and define its snRNA components (Grabowski and Sharp 1986). When purified from a glycerol gradient fraction, the mammalian spliceosome contains the snRNAs U2, U4, U5, and U6. An additional small RNA (called X) was also purified by affinity chromatography with the spliceosome complex formed on adenovirus substrate (Grabowksi and Sharp 1986). The nature of this RNA has not yet been determined; however, it is interesting that purification of the equivalent type of spliceosome formed on a substrate RNA containing sequences from the second intron of rabbit β-globin did not enrich for an X-type RNA (A.I. Lamond and P.J. Grabowski, unpubl.). Therefore, spliceosomes may consist of a common core of snRNPs, with possibly additional components that are substrate-specific.

Spliceosome-type complexes can also be resolved by electrophoresis in native polyacrylamide gels (Konarska and Sharp 1986, 1987; Pikielny and Rosbash 1986). The higher resolution of this methodology permits the detection of a number of different splicing-related complexes. The snRNA composition of these complexes has been analyzed either by transfer of RNA from the native gel to a membrane and hybridization with probes specific for each snRNA or by elution of RNA from a particular band, labeling with radioactivity, and electrophoresis in 8 M urea–polyacrylamide gels. Each complex resolved by gel electrophoresis can then be characterized by (1) its mobility during electrophoresis, (2) its kinetics of synthesis and turnover, (3) its snRNA composition, (4) the structure of the substrate RNA it contains (precursor RNA, intermediate RNAs, spliced exons, and excised lariat RNAs), and (5) the effect of alterations in the sequence of the substrate RNA on its synthesis or turnover. A tentative pathway of sequential assembly of different complexes can be constructed from these data; however, it is important to note that the experimental results do not establish a firm precursor-product relationship between the various complexes. The validity of the pathway will emerge as more biochemical and genetic experiments are completed.

A schematic of the pathway of assembly of complexes involved in splicing is shown in Figure 4. The most rapidly formed complex, when substrate RNA is added to a reaction, contains no snRNPs, but is rather composed of an assortment of proteins bound to the RNA in a relatively sequence-independent fashion. Some of these proteins are components of the classic 30S heterogeneous nuclear RNP (hnRNP) particles (Konarska and Sharp 1987). It is not clear whether specific proteins in these complexes play a critical role in splicing, although we have shown that antibodies to the hnRNP C protein will inhibit splicing in vitro (Choi et al. 1986). Since the rapidly forming complexes are heterogeneous and form on any RNA added to the reaction in an ATP-independent fashion, it is difficult to investigate their role in splicing. The second most rapidly forming complex that can be resolved by gel electrophoresis has U2 snRNP bound to sequences upstream of the 3' splice site (Black et al. 1985; Konarska and Sharp 1986). This complex does not contain U1 snRNA or other snRNAs, but its formation is probably promoted by U1 snRNP recognition of sequences at the 5' splice site (Lamond et al. 1987). Kinetically, the next complex to form contains substrate RNA and the set of U2, U4, U5, and U6 snRNPs. This complex corresponds to the spliceosome as isolated by affinity chromatography. Again, U1 snRNP is not stably bound to this complex. U4 snRNP is probably subsequently released from this complex either before or around the time of cleavage at the 5' splice site. Substrate RNA with mutations at the 5' splice site, either GU → AU or GU → GA, proceeds through cleavage at the 5' splice site and lariat formation, but it stops at this stage (Newman et al. 1985; Reed and Maniatis 1985; Aebi et al. 1986). A complex accumulates in reactions with those mutant substrate RNAs that contains the intermediate RNAs and U2, U5, and U6 snRNPs (A.I. Lamond and M.M. Konarksa, unpubl.). Thus, it is likely that U4 snRNP is released before cleavage at the 3' splice site. The products of the splicing reaction are generated as two distinct types of complexes. The excised intervening sequences are released complexed to U2, U5, and U6 snRNPs (Konarska and Sharp 1987). In vivo, this complex probably rapidly dissociates, and the intron sequences are degraded. The spliced exons are released not bound to snRNP but probably complexed to hnRNP proteins. In vivo, the spliced exons are subsequently transported through a nuclear pore to the cytoplasm.

Through the work of a number of laboratories, and

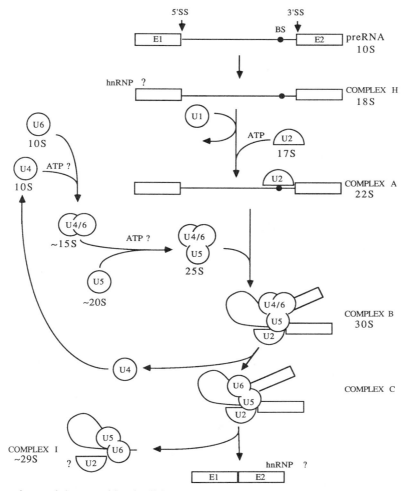

Figure 4. Schematic pathway of the assembly of splicing complexes. Top line shows a structure of a pre-RNA substrate that contains two exons (E1 and E2) separated by an IVS. 5'SS, 3'SS, and BS indicate 5' and 3' splice sites and branch site, respectively. Complex H represents a potential hnRNP-type of complex assembled on pre-RNA. Complex A is formed by binding of U2 snRNP to sequences upstream of the 3' splice site of pre-RNA. Complex B represents a probable structure of the spliceosome. Complex C is generated from complex B by release of U4 snSRNP and primarily contains the intermediate RNAs. Splicing products—the excised lariat IVS associated with snRNPs (complex I) and the spliced exons E1-E2, probably released in an hnRNP complex—are shown on the bottom line. The relative positions of snRNPs with respect to themselves and to pre-RNA sequences in complexes U4/5/6, B, C, and I are arbitrary. (Modified from Konarska and Sharp 1987; A.I. Lamond et al., unpubl.)

particularly that of C. Guthrie, the number and structure of snRNAs in the yeast *Saccharomyces cerevisiae* have been defined (see Fig. 5). Both affinity chromatography and gel electrophoresis assays have been used to analyze the snRNP composition of spliceosomes in yeast (Pikielny and Rosbash 1986; Pikielny et al. 1986; Cheng and Abelson 1987). The results of these experiments are strikingly consistent with the scheme shown in Figure 4 for the mammalian spliceosome. In particular, the snRNP composition of various splicing complexes is similar if not identical. The yeast analog of U1 snRNP (snR19) is not as stably bound to the spliceosome as the other snRNPs. A pre-spliceosome complex contains the yeast equivalent of U2 snRNP (snR20) and a spliceosome complex contains the yeast equivalent of U2, U4, U5, and U6 snRNPs (snR20, snR14, snR7, and snR6). Finally,

snR14 is released from the spliceosome complex that contains the intermediate RNAs in a fashion similar to that of U4 snRNP. Thus, both the constituents of the spliceosome and its pathway of formation are apparently conserved from fungi to vertebrates. A corollary of this conservation is that probably all nuclear introns within mRNA precursors are processed by formation of a spliceosome containing this core set of snRNPs.

An important aspect of the scheme outlined in Figure 4 is the release of U4 snRNP. The U4 particle shares common features with U1, U2, and U5 snRNPs in that it contains a set of core proteins (possessing the Sm antigenic determinant) and an RNA with a trimethyl cap. Unlike the other particles, the snRNP containing U4 also contains U6 snRNA (Bringmann et al. 1984; Hashimoto and Steitz 1984). The latter snRNA is different in that it is transcribed by RNA polymerase III

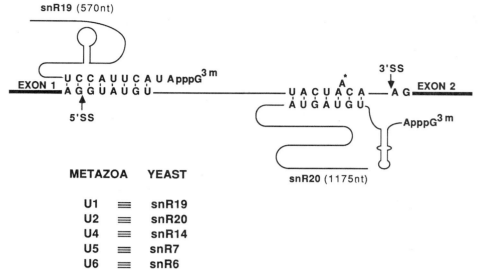

Figure 5. snRNAs of *S. cerevisiae* have been analyzed for trimethyl cap content and binding to the Sm antigen after injection into *Xenopus* oocytes (Riedel et al. 1987). The suggested equivalence between individual metazoa and yeast snRNAs is based on sequence and functional homology: U1 = snR19 (Kretzner et al. 1987; Siliciano et al. 1987a), U2 = snR20 (Ares 1986), U4 = snR14 (Siliciano et al. 1987b), U5 = snR7 (Patterson and Guthrie 1987), and U6 = snR6 (Siliciano et al. 1987b). Shown at the top of the figure is the complementarity between snR19 and 5′ splice site sequences (Kretzner et al. 1987; Siliciano et al. 1987a) and snR20 and the conserved sequences at the branch site (Parker et al. 1987).

(not polymerase II) and does not possess a trimethyl cap (Kunkel et al. 1986; Reddy et al. 1987). A tract of sequences in U6 snRNA is complementary to U4 snRNA (Rinke et al. 1985). The unique character of U6 snRNA is also conserved in yeast (Siliciano et al. 1987b). The fact that U4 snRNP is released from the spliceosome while U6 snRNA remains associated suggests that the interaction of these two snRNAs is dynamic (Konarska and Sharp 1987). The splicing of every intron probably involves the assembly of the snRNPs in the spliceosome from fully dissociated particles. The pathway of assembly of snRNPs into the spliceosome shown in Figure 4 was deduced from the analysis of snRNP-snRNP complexes resolved by gel electrophoresis from splicing reactions. The formation of some of these multi-snRNP complexes is apparently effected by incubation with ATP. Thus, the assembly and dissociation of these snRNP-snRNP complexes may be dependent on hydrolysis of a high-energy cofactor.

CONCLUSIONS

The similarities between the RNA self-splicing reactions and the nuclear splicing reaction suggest that the latter process might be RNA-catalyzed. The catalytic RNA for this reaction would have to be formed from the conserved set of snRNAs assembled in the spliceosome (Sharp 1985; Arnberg et al. 1986). It is likely that only U2, U5, and U6 snRNAs are present in the spliceosome when reactions at the 5′ and 3′ splice sites occur. The total lengths of these three RNAs sums to over 400 N and this is more than sufficient complexity for formation of a catalytic RNA. The common feature

of branch formation by group II self-splicing introns and nuclear splicing suggests that the catalytic process in these two pathways might be similar. This implies that some of the conserved sequence structures of group II introns might be present in the combination of sequences of the snRNAs in the spliceosome. However, to date, these hypothetical common sequences or structures have not been identified.

The hypothesis that the nuclear splicing process is evolutionarily related to self-splicing introns suggests an interesting scheme for the origin of introns (Sharp 1985). The attraction of this scheme is that it provides for coevolution of introns and the splicing process. It seems improbable that splicing arose as a process in anticipation of the insertion of introns. Similarly, introns within coding sequences would obviously be lethal in the absence of a splicing process for their removal. A second attractive feature of this scheme is the bridge it provides between the evolution of genes in an RNA world before the appearance of DNA and the current gene structure in eukaryotes.

In brief, the scheme proposes that short protein-encoding exons evolved as sequences within RNAs bracketed by self-splicing introns (Fig. 6). These exons could be joined by intramolecular splicing to form mRNAs for larger proteins. Alternatively, inter-molecular or *trans*-splicing of the exon-containing RNAs could occur to generate novel combinations of exons. *Trans*-splicing of two group-II-type introns has been suggested as an essential step in the synthesis of the mRNA for a ribosomal protein of a chloroplast (Fukuzawa et al. 1986; Koller et al. 1987). This process probably occurs by the association of complementary sequences within the two introns, since tracts of con-

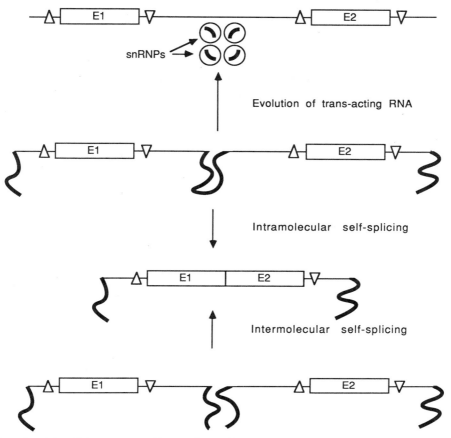

Figure 6. Evolution of nuclear splicing process and introns from self-splicing introns. Heavy curved lines represent RNA structure and complementarity within the intron responsible for self-splicing. At the bottom of the figure, two RNAs are bound through this complementarity to form a catalytic structure that will *trans*-splice the flanking exons. ($\triangle$,∇) Sequences originally recognized in the self-splicing reaction at the boundary of the exons that are hypothetically conserved in the consensus sequences at the 5' and 3' splice sites. The circles containing heavy curved lines represent snRNPs that are shown as being formed from fragments of the self-splicing intron.

served complementary sequences are common to all self-splicing introns and, indeed, essential for formation of the catalytic structure. Thus, the joining of exons by *trans*-splicing might have been a common event in an RNA world with a high abundance of self-splicing introns. Exons that encode either functional domains of polypeptides or correctly folding domains, which could be readily combined into many larger proteins in a functional fashion, would obviously have been selected in such an RNA world (Gilbert 1978, 1986).

As the ability to synthesize deoxynucleotides and to replicate DNA evolved, it was probably selectively advantageous to evolve a splicing process, where a common set of *trans*-acting factors could splice all the introns within an organism. A limited set of genes encoding these *trans*-acting factors could then be transmitted to each generation, freeing the major fraction of the sequences within an intron from the constraint of specifying a self-splicing RNA. It seems probable that the *trans*-acting splicing factors arose by fragmentation of the self-splicing intron and distribution of segments of the catalytic RNA to the snRNPs found within

spliceosomes (see also Tabak et al., this volume). Some sequences of the original self-splicing introns were probably retained by introns, e.g., those at the boundaries of the intron and flanking the branch site. These would correspond to the conserved consensus sequences at the 5' and 3' splice sites and the branch site of contemporary genes. In fact, the sequences at the 5' and 3' splice sites of group II self-splicing introns GU and AU, respectively, are related to those of introns within nuclear genes encoding mRNAs, GU and AG, respectively (Cech 1985b). In this view, the nuclear splicing process is RNA-catalyzed by the snRNAs within the spliceosome, and these snRNAs are evolutionarily derived from fragmented self-splicing introns. It is of course possible that the nuclear splicing process originally evolved from self-splicing introns, but in the interim, catalytic proteins have taken over the role of catalytic RNAs. Only further analysis of the nuclear splicing reaction will determine which of these alternatives is the best description.

An interesting suggestion of the scheme outlined in Figure 6 is that intron structure was a fundamental feature of the original gene structure. This is consistent with the hypothesis of Gilbert (1986) that exons found in genes of contemporary vertebrates and plants encode functional or structural domains and that this structure reflects the evolution of the gene. A major obstacle to accepting the view that genes originally evolved with intron structure is that the genes of contemporary prokaryotic organisms do not contain introns that are processed by the nuclear mechanism, and prokaryotic-type organisms are thought to be the progenitors of eukaryotic organisms. Thus, how could the hypothetical primitive intron structure of genes have been transmitted through prokaryotic organisms?

ACKNOWLEDGMENTS

The authors gratefully acknowledge Dr. Konarksa, our co-author, for drawing all the figures. This work was supported by grants from the National Institutes of Health (GM-34277), from the National Cancer Institute (PO1-CA-42063), and partially from the NCI Cancer Center support (core) (P30-CA-14051), and from the National Science Foundation (DCB-8502718).

REFERENCES

Aebi, M., H. Horing, R.A. Padgett, J. Reiser, and C. Weissmann. 1986. Sequence requirements for splicing of higher eukaryotic nuclear pre-mRNA. *Cell* **47:** 555.

Ares, M., Jr. 1986. U2 RNA from yeast is unexpectedly large and contains homology to vertebrate U4, U5 and U6 small nuclear RNAs. *Cell* **47:** 49.

Arnberg, A.C., G. Van der Horst, and H.F. Tabak. 1986. Formation of lariats and circles in self-splicing of the precursor to the large ribosomal RNA of yeast mitochondria. *Cell* **44:** 235.

Black, D.L., B. Chabot, and J.A. Steitz. 1985. U2 as well as U1 small nuclear ribonucleoproteins are involved in premessenger RNA splicing. *Cell* **42:** 737.

Breitbart, R.E., A. Andreadis, and B. Nadal-Ginard. 1987. Alternative splicing: A ubiquitous mechanism for the generation of multiple protein isoforms from single genes. *Annu. Rev. Biochem.* **56:** 467.

Bringmann, P., B. Appel, J. Rinke, R. Reuter, H. Theissen, and R. Lührmann. 1984. Evidence for the existence of snRNAs U4 and U6 in a single ribonucleoprotein complex and for their association by intermolecular base pairing. *EMBO J.* **3:** 1357.

Brody, E. and J. Abelson. 1985. The "spliceosome": Yeast premessenger RNA associates with a 40S complex in a splicing-dependent reaction. *Science* **228:** 963.

Brown, J.W.S. 1986. A catalogue of splice junction and putative branch point from plant introns. *Nucleic Acids Res.* **14:** 9549.

Cech, T.R. 1985a. Self-splicing RNA: Implications for evolution. *Int. Rev. Cytol.* **93:** 3.

———. 1985b. RNA splicing: Three themes with variations. *Cell* **34:** 713.

Cech, T.R. and B.L. Bass. 1986. Biological catalysis by RNA. *Annu. Rev. Biochem.* **55:** 599.

Cech, T.R., A.J. Zaug, and P.J. Grabowski. 1981. In vitro splicing of the ribosomal RNA precursor of *Tetrahymena*: Involvement of a guanosine nucleotide in the excision of the intervening sequence. *Cell* **27:** 487.

Cheng, S.-C. and J. Abelson. 1987. Spliceosome assembly in yeast. *Genes Dev.* (in press).

Choi, Y.D., P.J. Grabowski, P.A. Sharp, and G. Dreyfuss. 1986. Heterogeneous nuclear ribonucleoproteins: Role in RNA splicing. *Science* **231:** 1534.

Fukuzawa, H., T. Kohchi, H. Shinai, K. Ohyama, K. Unesono, H. Inokuchi, and H. Ozeki. 1986. Coding sequences for chloroplast ribosomal protein S12 from the liverwort *Marchantia polymorpha* are separated far apart on the different DNA strands. *FEBS Lett.* **198:** 11.

Gilbert, W. 1978. Why genes in pieces? *Nature* **271:** 501.

———. 1986. The RNA world. *Nature* **319:** 618.

Grabowski, P.J. and P.A. Sharp. 1986. Affinity chromatography of splicing complexes: U2, U5, and U4 + U6 small nuclear ribonucleoprotein particles in the spliceosome. *Science* **233:** 1294.

Grabowski, P.J., R.A. Padgett, and P.A. Sharp. 1984. Messenger RNA splicing *in vitro*: An excised intervening sequence and a potential intermediate. *Cell* **37:** 415.

Grabowski, P.J., S.R. Seiler, and P.A. Sharp. 1985. A multicomponent complex is involved in the splicing of messenger RNA precursors. *Cell* **42:** 345.

Hashimoto, C. and J.A. Steitz. 1984. U4 and U6 RNAs coexist in a single small nuclear ribonucleoprotein particle. *Nucleic Acids Res.* **12:** 3283.

Koller, B., H. Fromm, E. Galun, and E. Edelman. 1987. Evidence for *in vivo* trans-splicing of pre-mRNAs in tobacco chloroplasts. *Cell* **48:** 111.

Konarska, M.M. and P.A. Sharp. 1986. Electrophoretic separation of complexes involved in the splicing of precursors to mRNAs. *Cell* **46:** 845.

———. 1987. Interactions between small nuclear ribonucleoprotein particles in formation of spliceosomes. *Cell* **49:** 763.

Konarska, M.M., P.J. Grabowski, R.A. Padgett, and P.A. Sharp. 1985. Characterization of the branch site in lariat RNAs produced by splicing of mRNA precursors. *Nature* **313:** 552.

Kretzner, L., B.C. Rymond, and M. Rosbash. 1987. *Saccharomyces cerevisiae* U1 RNA is large and has limited primary sequence homology to metazoon U1 snRNA. *Cell* **50:** 593.

Kunkel, G.R., R.L. Maser, J.P. Calvet, and T. Pederson. 1986. U6 small nuclear RNA is transcribed by RNA polymerase III. *Proc. Natl. Acad. Sci.* **83:** 8575.

Lamond, A.I., M.M. Konarksa, and P.A. Sharp. 1987. A mutational analysis of spliceosome assembly: Evidence for splice site collaboration during spliceosome formation. *Genes Dev.* **1:** 532.

Langford, C.J. and D. Gallwitz. 1983. Evidence for an intron-contained sequence required for the splicing of yeast RNA polymerase II transcripts. *Cell* **33:** 519.

Langford, C.J., F.-J. Klinz, C. Donath, and D. Gallwitz. 1984. Point mutations identify the conserved, intron-contained TACTAAC box as an essential splicing signal sequence in yeast. *Cell* **36:** 645.

Lerner, M.R., J.A. Boyle, S.M. Mount, S.L. Wolin, and J.A. Steitz. 1980. Are snRNPs involved in splicing? *Nature* **283:** 220.

Newman, A.J., R.-J. Lin, S.C. Cheng, and J. Abelson. 1985. Molecular consequences of specific intron mutations on yeast mRNA splicing in vivo and in vitro. *Cell* **42:** 335.

Padgett, R.A., P.J. Grabowski, M.M. Konarska, S. Seiler, and P.A. Sharp. 1986. Splicing of messenger RNA precursors. *Annu. Rev. Biochem.* **55:** 1119.

Padgett, R.A., M.M. Konarksa, P.J. Grabowski, S.F. Hardy, and P.A. Sharp. 1984. Lariat RNAs as intermediates and products in the splicing of mRNA precursors. *Science* **225:** 898.

Padgett, R.A., M.M. Konarksa, M. Aebi, H. Hornig, C. Weissmann, and P.A. Sharp. 1985. Nonconsensus branch-site sequences in the in vitro splicing of transcripts of mutant rabbit β-globin genes. *Proc. Natl. Acad. Sci.* **82:** 8349.

Parker, R., P.G. Siliciano, and C. Guthrie. 1987. Recognition of the TACTAAC box during mRNA splicing in yeast involves base pairing to the U2-like snRNA. *Cell* **49:** 229.

Patterson, B. and C. Guthrie. 1987. An essential yeast snRNA with a U5-like domain is required for splicing in vivo. *Cell* **49:** 613.

Peebles, C.L., P.S. Perlman, K.L. Mecklenburg, M.L. Petrillo, J.H. Tabor, K.A. Jarrell, and H.-L. Cheng. 1986. A self-splicing RNA excises an intron lariat. *Cell* **44:** 213.

Perler, F., A. Efstratiadis, P. Lomedico, W. Gilbert, R. Kolodner, and J. Dodgson. 1980. The evolution of genes: The chicken preproinsulin gene. *Cell* **20:** 555.

Pikielny, C.W. and M. Rosbash. 1986. Specific small nuclear RNAs are associated with yeast spliceosomes. *Cell* **45:** 869.

Pikielny, C.W., B.C. Rymond, and M. Rosbash. 1986. Electrophoresis of ribonucleoproteins reveals an ordered assembly pathway of yeast splicing complexes. *Nature* **324:** 341.

Pikielny, C.W., J.L. Teem, and M. Rosbash. 1983. Evidence for the biochemical role of an internal sequence in yeast nuclear mRNA introns: Implications for U1 RNA and metazoon mRNA splicing. *Cell* **34:** 395.

Rautmann, G. and R. Breathnach. 1985. A role for branch points in splicing in vivo. *Nature* **315:** 430.

Reddy, R., D. Henning, G. Das, M. Harless, and D. Wright. 1987. The capped U6 small nuclear RNA is transcribed by RNA polymerase III. *J. Biol. Chem.* **262:** 75.

Reed, R. and T. Maniatis. 1985. Intron sequences involved in lariat formation during pre-mRNA splicing. *Cell* **41:** 95.

Riedel, N., S. Wolin, and C. Guthrie. 1987. A subset of yeast snRNAs contains functional binding sites for the highly conserved Sm antigen. *Science* **235:** 328.

Rinke, J., B. Appel, M. Digweed, and R. Lührmann. 1985. Localization of a base-paired interaction between small

nuclear RNAs U4 and U6 in intact U4/U6 ribonucleoprotein particles by psoraden crosslinking. *J. Mol. Biol.* **185:** 721.

Rogers, J. and R. Wall. 1980. A mechanism for RNA splicing. *Proc. Natl. Acad. Sci.* **77:** 1877.

Ruskin, B., J.M. Greene, and M.R. Green. 1985. Cryptic branch point activation allows accurate *in vitro* splicing of human β-globin intron mutants. *Cell* **41:** 833.

Ruskin, B., A.R. Krainer, T. Maniatis, and M.R. Green. 1984. Excision of an intact intron as a novel lariat structure during pre-mRNA splicing *in vitro*. *Cell* **38:** 317.

Sharp, P.A. 1985. On the origin of RNA splicing and introns. *Cell* **42:** 397.

Siliciano, P.G., M.H. Jones, and C. Guthrie. 1987a. *S. cerevisiae* has a U1-like snRNA with unexpected properties. *Science* (in press).

Siliciano, P.G., D.A. Brow, H. Roiha, and C. Guthrie. 1987b. An essential snRNA from *S. cerevisiae* has properties predicted for a U6-like snRNA. *Cell* **50:** 585.

Teem, J.L., N. Abovich, N.F. Kaufer, W.F. Schwindinger, J.R. Warner, A. Levy, J. Woolford, R.J. Leer, M.M.C. van Raamsdonk-Duin, W.H. Mager, R.J. Planta, L. Schultz, J.D. Friesen, H. Fried, and M. Rosbash. 1984. A comparison of yeast ribosomal protein gene DNA sequences. *Nucleic Acids Res.* **12**(22): 8295.

Van der Veen, R., A.C. Arnberg, G. Van der Horst, L. Bonen, H.F. Tabak, and L.A. Grivell. 1986. Excised group II introns in yeast mitochondria are lariats and can be formed by self-splicing in vitro. *Cell* **44:** 225.

Wieringa, B., E. Hofer, and C. Weissmann. 1984. A minimal intron length but no specific internal sequence is required for splicing the large rabbit β-globin intron. *Cell* **37:** 915.

Different Small Nuclear Ribonucleoprotein Particles Are Involved in Different Steps of Splicing Complex Formation

D. Frendewey,* A. Krämer,† and W. Keller†
Division of Molecular Biology, Institute of Cell and Tumor Biology,
German Cancer Research Center, D-6900 Heidelberg, Federal Republic of Germany

Splicing of the introns in messenger RNA precursors (pre-mRNA) is an important part of the chain of post-transcriptional processing reactions that these primary transcripts have to undergo in the nuclei of eukaryotic cells (for reviews, see Padgett et al. 1986; Green 1986). Conceptually, all known types of RNA splicing can be subdivided into several distinct steps: Specific internal sequences must be recognized and the molecules must be folded such that distant splice sites are brought into proximity and become precisely aligned. This is a prerequisite for the ensuing catalysis of the two-step cleavage-ligation reactions that give rise to spliced RNA. In the case of self-splicing RNAs (for reviews, see Cech 1986, 1987; Cech and Bass 1986; Been et al., this volume), recognition-alignment, as well as the provision of an RNA catalyst, is accomplished by the folding of the molecules via *intra*molecular base pairing into specific structures.

The distinguishing feature that sets nuclear pre-mRNA splicing apart, in particular from the closely related lariat-forming group II mechanism (Jacquier and Michel 1987; Michel and Jacquier; Peebles et al.; Tabak et al.; all this volume), is the participation of small nuclear ribonucleoprotein particles (snRNPs) as *trans*-acting specificity determinants (for reviews on snRNPs, see Reddy and Busch 1983; Steitz et al. 1983; Brunel et al. 1985; Birnstiel 1987).

Studies with in vitro splicing systems prepared from yeast (*Saccharomyces cerevisiae*) or human (HeLa) cells have shown that the splicing reaction is preceded by the formation of large, multicomponent complexes, termed spliceosomes (Brody and Abelson 1985; Frendewey and Keller 1985; Grabowski et al. 1985). These and subsequent reports have indicated that the key events in spliceosome assembly involve the ordered interaction of snRNPs with the pre-mRNA substrate (for review, see Maniatis and Reed 1987; Sharp 1987; Sharp et al., this volume). Although the precise details of the assembly pathway are not yet known, there is general agreement that the formation of spliceosomes occurs in several discrete steps, requires auxiliary protein factors (which are not further considered here),

and involves the participation of all the major nucleoplasmic U-type snRNPs present in HeLa cell extracts, U1, U2, U4, U5, and U6 (Bindereif and Green 1986, 1987; Grabowski and Sharp 1986; Konarska and Sharp 1986, 1987) or their yeast counterparts snR19, snR20, snR14, snR7, and snR6, respectively (Ares 1986; Pikielny and Rosbash 1986; Pikielny et al. 1986; Cheng and Abelson 1987; Kretzner et al. 1987; Parker et al. 1987; Patterson and Guthrie 1987; Rymond et al. 1987; Siliciano et al. 1987a,b).

The sites of interaction of different snRNPs with model pre-mRNAs under the conditions of splicing have been mapped by immunoprecipitation/nuclease-protection analyses with snRNP-specific antibodies (Chabot et al. 1985). It was shown that U1 snRNP binds to the 5' splice site, U2 snRNP binds to the branch-point sequence (Black et al. 1985), and another snRNP, most likely U5, binds to the 3' splice site region (Chabot et al. 1985). These findings were later extended by applying the same methods to splicing complexes after their isolation by velocity sedimentation (Chabot and Steitz 1987a,b). In contrast, no unique pre-mRNA binding site could be detected for the U4 and the U6 particles, even though these snRNPs are involved in splicing complex formation (see below) and in the splicing reaction (Berget and Robberson 1986; Black and Steitz 1986).

Genetic complementation experiments (Zhuang and Weiner 1986; Zhuang et al. 1987) have provided compelling evidence that the recognition of 5' splice sites by U1 snRNP is governed by the formation of intermolecular base pairs with short, complementary sequences at the 5' end of U1 RNA, as had been postulated (Lerner et al. 1980; Rogers and Wall 1980). Similarly, Parker et al. (1987) have shown by genetic suppression studies that the yeast U2 RNA analog snR20 (or LSR 1; Ares 1986) interacts with the site of subsequent branch formation in pre-mRNAs by forming intermolecular base pairs. As discussed below, this base pairing may not be required for the initial binding of U2 snRNP to the intron, but it may serve to select a suitable nucleotide for branch formation at a later step. In any event, as in self-splicing RNAs, the generation of short, complementary RNA:RNA helices appears to be a general principle in the assembly of a splicing-competent structure. However, RNA:RNA base pairing is certainly not the only mode of intron recognition

---

Present address: *Cold Spring Harbor Laboratory, Cold Spring Harbor, New York 11724; † Biocenter of the University of Basel, CH-4056 Basel, Switzerland.

in nuclear pre-mRNA splicing. For example, the selection of the 3' splice site, probably one of the earliest events in splicing complex formation, is mediated by the binding of a specific protein that may be a component of the U5 snRNP (Gerke and Steitz 1986; Tazi et al. 1986).

To obtain further insights on the pathway of splicing complex assembly, we have attempted to study this process by applying the method of selective inactivation of snRNPs in splicing extracts by site-directed cleavage of their RNA moieties with RNase H and complementary oligonucleotides. This technique has been used previously to demonstrate the participation of the U1, U2, U4, and U6 snRNPs in splicing (Krämer et al. 1984; Black et al. 1985; Krainer and Maniatis 1985; Berget and Robberson 1986; Black and Steitz 1986). The results indicate that inactivation of these snRNPs interferes with splicing complex formation; it also inhibits their binding to the pre-mRNA substrate. The results also show that two different domains of the U2 RNA are required at different levels of spliceosome formation, implying that U2 snRNP has a dual function in this process.

METHODS

Preparation of pre-mRNA substrates. The construction of plasmids containing the promoter for SP6 RNA polymerase (Melton et al. 1984) and various portions of sequences derived from the major late transcription unit of adenovirus 2 has been described elsewhere (Frendewey and Keller 1985; Krämer 1987). In vitro transcription of linearized templates to generate capped ^{32}P-labeled RNAs and their purification is detailed elsewhere (Frendewey and Keller 1985). Three different types of pre-mRNA substrates were used; these are designated RNA 1, RNA 10, and RNA 12. RNA 1 and RNA 10 correspond to the same species described in Frendewey and Keller (1985). RNA 12 is described in Krämer (1987). A schematic representation of their composition is given in Figure 5 (top).

Incubation conditions for splicing and formation of splicing complexes. HeLa cell nuclear extracts were prepared according to Dignam et al. (1983) as modified by Heintz and Roeder (1984). As noted (Black and Steitz 1986), such extracts are less prone to lose splicing activity upon the preincubation period required to carry out site-directed RNase H cleavages of U-snRNAs (see below). The preincubation mixtures contained 15 μl of nuclear extract, 2.5 μl of Buffer D (Dignam et al. 1983), 1.5 μl of 50 mM MgCl$_2$, 1 μl of 10 mM MgATP, and 5 μl of 0.1 M creatine phosphate. Incubation in the presence or absence of oligodeoxynucleotides was carried out for 60 minutes at 30°C. The splicing reaction was initiated by the addition of 25 μl of a mixture containing substrate RNA (~6–60 fmoles; 10,000–100,000 Cerenkov cpm), 7.5 μg of tRNA (*Escherichia coli*), 7.5 μl of Buffer D, and 1 μl of 10 mM MgATP. Reaction mixtures were incubated at

30°C for the times indicated in the figures and stopped by quick freezing. For direct analysis of reaction products, 10-μl portions were removed, treated with proteinase K, extracted with phenol/chloroform, and electrophoresed in 12% acrylamide–8 M urea gels followed by autoradiography (Frendewey and Keller 1985).

Oligodeoxynucleotide-directed RNase H cleavage. Synthetic oligonucleotides used for site-directed cleavage of snRNAs, given with their target sequences, were U1, 5'-TTCAGGTAAGTACTCA-3', nucleotides 2–11 of U1 RNA; U2a, 5'-AGGCCGAGAAGC-GAT-3', nucleotides 1–15 of U2 RNA; U2b, 5'-CAG-ATACTACACTTG-3', nucleotides 28–42 of U2 RNA; U4, 5'-GGGTATTGGGAAAAGTTTTC-3', nucleotides 64–83 of U4 RNA. Oligonucleotides U1, U2a, and U2b have been described by Black et al. (1985). The control oligonucleotide is complementary to a region in a putative U7 RNA from HeLa cells and has the sequence 5'-UCUGAAAAA-3'. Nuclear extract was treated with oligonucleotides during the preincubation period (see above). U2a, U2b, U4, and the control oligonucleotide were used at a final concentration of 10 mM and U1 was used at 40 mM. Incubation was carried out for 45 minutes at 30°C, followed by the addition of 4 μl (80 μg) of RNase-free DNase I and further incubation for 15 minutes. Splicing reactions were initiated by addition of 21 μl of a mixture containing RNA substrate, tRNA, MgATP, and Buffer D (see above).

Gel electrophoresis of splicing complexes. One-dimensional electrophoresis of splicing complexes was carried out in 4% polyacrylamide gels (acrylamide:bisacrylamide 80:1; Konarska and Sharp 1986) in 25 mM Tris-OH, 25 mM boric acid, and 1 mM EDTA (pH 8). Gel dimensions were 15 × 15 cm × 1.5 mm. Before loading, gels were pre-run for 45–60 minutes at 150–200 V at room temperature. Samples (5 μl) of reaction mixtures were mixed with 1 μl of heparin (sodium salt, 1 mg/ml) and left at room temperature for 10 minutes. Before loading, a trace of bromophenol blue and xylene cyanol was added. Electrophoresis was carried out for 2 hours at 200 V until the xylene cyanol marker reached the bottom. Radioactivity was visualized by autoradiography on Kodak XAR-5 film at −70°C with intensifying screens. In some cases, the electrophoresis conditions were varied, as indicated (Fig. 5).

Two-dimensional electrophoresis was performed as follows: Samples were treated with heparin as described above and run first in a nondenaturing composite gel (Goodwin and Dahlberg 1982) of 4% polyacrylamide (acrylamide:bisacrylamide 250:1) and 0.5% agarose. Electrophoresis was carried out as described above. After brief autoradiography, single-lane gel strips were cut out and soaked in 5 ml of a solution of 0.5 mg/ml proteinase K and 0.1% SDS in Tris-borate-EDTA buffer (TBE; Maniatis et al. 1982) for 15 minutes at 37°C. Second-dimension denaturing gels were 12% polyacrylamide (acrylamide:bisacrylamide, 19:1)–8.3 M urea in TBE. The gels were pre-run at 30 mA for

1 hour with a solution of 8.3 M urea in the wells. Electrophoresis was at 800 V and was followed by autoradiography.

RNase A protection assay. The procedures for the detection of RNA-binding components by RNase A protection mapping in splicing extracts after oligonucleotide-directed RNase H cleavage of snRNAs have been described previously (Krämer 1987). Specific conditions are given in Figure 6.

RESULTS

Electrophoretic Properties of Splicing Complexes

Spliceosomes were discovered by investigating the sedimentation behavior of radiolabeled pre-mRNA upon prior incubation with nuclear extracts under splicing conditions (Brody and Abelson 1985; Frendewey and Keller 1985; Grabowski et al. 1985). Since then, gel electrophoresis under nondenaturing conditions has proved to be superior in resolution and convenience for the analysis of spliceosomes and splicing-related complexes (Konarska and Sharp 1986, 1987; Pikielny and Rosbash 1986; Pikielny et al. 1986; Cheng and Abelson 1987; Lamond et al. 1987). We have adapted this method to characterize the complexes formed with the pre-mRNA substrates routinely used in our laboratory.

Figure 1 shows an example of the complexes formed with RNA 1, an SP6-generated pre-mRNA derived from the major late transcription unit of adenovirus 2 (Frendewey and Keller 1985). Without incubation in the splicing extract, the pre-mRNA migrates to the bottom of the gel. Upon mixing with nuclear extract, the pre-mRNA instantaneously forms a complex (termed H) that migrates as a diffuse and heterogeneous zone with a mobility slower than that of naked RNA. By 5 minutes of incubation, a new band appears that is larger than H, and at 10 minutes, an even larger complex is formed. The two retarded bands are called complex A and complex B to comply with the terminology of Konarska and Sharp (1986, 1987). With time, the intensity of H diminishes and that of band B increases; complex A appears to plateau at around 20 minutes of incubation.

It should be noted that the samples were treated with heparin (~0.2 mg/ml) prior to electrophoresis to prevent the retention of material in the sample slots (Konarska and Sharp 1986). In the absence of heparin, the relative separation of the three bands is the same, but their electrophoretic mobility is slightly slower than that observed with prior heparin treatment (results not shown). This would be expected if proteins that are associated with complex H, A, and B, but are not necessary for their structural integrity, were removed by the polyanion. In our experience, the addition of heparin at concentrations above 1 mg/ml leads to disruption of the A and B complexes.

Figure 2 shows a two-dimensional analysis of the radioactive RNAs present in complexes H, A, and B. A 60-minute splicing reaction was fractionated in a 4%

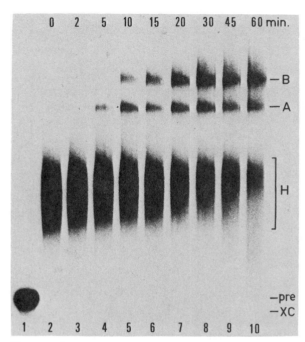

Figure 1. Separation of splicing complexes by nondenaturing gel electrophoresis. [^{32}P]RNA 1 was incubated under splicing conditions as described in Methods. At the indicated times, the reactions were stopped by freezing. Aliquots of 5 μl were mixed with 1 μl (1 μg) of heparin, incubated at room temperature for 10 min, and electrophoresed on a 4% polyacrylamide gel. (*1*) Control incubation at 30°C for 60 min without nuclear extract; (*2*) reaction stopped immediately after the addition of pre-mRNA; (*3–10*) reactions incubated at 30°C for the times indicated at top. Positions of the A, B, and H complexes are indicated at right. (pre) Position of free pre-mRNA; (XC) position of the xylene cyanol dye.

polyacrylamide–0.5% agarose composite gel. After disrupting the complexes in the gel strip by treatment with proteinase K and SDS (see Methods), the RNAs were separated in a second dimension on a denaturing 8 M urea–polyacrylamide gel. Inspection of the second-dimension gel pattern shows that pre-mRNA is present in all three complexes. In addition to precursor, the B complex contains the products of the first cleavage-ligation reaction, exon 1 and the intron-exon 2 lariat RNAs. Thus, the appearance of the B complex correlates with the formation of an active splicing complex. The final products of the splicing reaction appear to have been released from the B complex. The intron lariat is found in a large structure that migrates between complexes A and B (Fig. 2, closed arrow). Some intron lariat is also associated with a complex that runs faster than H but slower than free RNA (Fig. 2, open arrow). Spliced exon 1–exon 2 RNA (indicated by a square bracket) migrates in a similar position near the bottom of the first-dimension gel. The diffuse appearance of the signal coming from this RNA suggests that the spliced RNA may exist in the form of a ribonucleoprotein containing variable amounts of protein. The partitioning of the intron lariat between two structures is interesting. The larger and more abundant form most

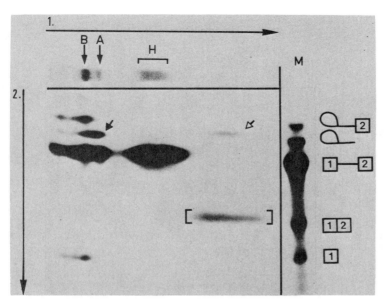

Figure 2. Two-dimensional gel electrophoretic analysis of splicing complexes. (*1*) A 60-min splicing reaction with [^{32}P]RNA 1 was electrophoresed in the first dimension on a 4% polyacrylamide–0.5% agarose gel to separate the splicing complexes. This separation is shown at the top. The positions of the A, B, and H complexes are indicated. (*2*) After treatment to disrupt the complexes (see Methods), the first-dimension gel strip was layered on top of a 12% polyacrylamide–8 M urea gel and electrophoresed in the second dimension. Extracted RNA from a splicing reaction was also applied to the second-dimension gel as reference (lane M on the right). Identification of RNAs is given schematically at the right of the autoradiogram. See text for further details.

likely corresponds to complex I (Konarska and Sharp 1987), a postsplicing complex that still has snRNPs bound to it; the smaller, less abundant form is probably an RNP, which contains no snRNPs.

The results shown in Figures 1 and 2 can be correlated with our previous sedimentation analysis of splicing complexes (Frendewey and Keller 1985). The H complex represents the 22S structure that forms immediately upon the addition of pre-mRNA to nuclear extract. Any RNA substrate that we have tested will form an H complex regardless of its ability to be spliced or not (see below). Complex A corresponds to the 35S complex observed in sucrose gradients. It appears early during a splicing reaction and requires the presence of a 3′ splice site sequence in the RNA substrate as well as low concentrations (10–50 μM) of ATP (G. Lahr and D. Frendewey, unpubl.). Complex B corresponds to the species sedimenting at 50S in sucrose gradients and represents the structure in which the splicing reaction takes place; it is the active spliceosome. Kinetic experiments carried out in the presence of different concentrations of ATP (G. Lahr and D. Frendewey, unpubl.) have suggested that complex B is formed by the conversion of complex A. This requires a splicing-competent pre-mRNA substrate and higher concentrations of ATP (100–400 μM).

Inhibition of Splicing by snRNP Inactivation

To test the function of the U1, U2, and U4/U6 snRNPs in spliceosome assembly, we specifically inactivated these particles by oligonucleotide-directed cleavage with RNase H. U5 snRNP is not amenable for this type of analysis because its RNA is not accessible to oligonucleotide-directed RNase H cleavage (Chabot et al. 1985). Figure 3 shows the sequence and proposed secondary structures of the five U-snRNAs that participate in pre-mRNA splicing. Black lines indicate the

regions targeted for RNase H cleavage by complementary deoxyoligonucleotides. The results of a splicing assay with nuclear extracts after RNase H cleavage are shown in Figure 4a. As can be seen, treatment of nuclear extract with oligonucleotides U1, U2a, U2b, and U4 caused severe inhibition of in vitro splicing. This is in agreement with results obtained previously by other investigators with similar or identical oligonucleotides (Black et al. 1985; Krainer and Maniatis 1985; Berget and Robberson 1986; Black and Steitz 1986). The U1 oligonucleotide at a concentration of 40 mM caused a greater than 95% inhibition of splicing (Fig. 4a, lane 3), and the inhibition with the U2a, U2b, and U4 oligonucleotides was essentially complete at 10 mM (lanes 4–6). The control oligonucleotide also led to a considerable inhibition of splicing (~30%, as compared to a reaction without oligonucleotide; Fig. 4, lanes 2 and 7). However, in all experiments, the inhibition observed with the specific oligonucleotides was always much higher than that of the controls.

Visualization of the snRNAs in the oligonucleotide-treated reactions (Fig. 4b) shows that the cleavage was snRNA-specific and at the expected sites. In addition, all digestions resulted in the essentially complete loss (>95%) of the targeted RNA, as judged from ethidium bromide staining. Analysis on sucrose gradients of oligonucleotide/RNase-H-treated nuclear extracts has shown that the snRNPs cleaved with the U1, U2a, and U2b oligonucleotides still sedimented at 10S–12S, indicating that the removal of parts of their RNA components did not cause complete disruption of the particles (results not shown). We do not know whether the 5′ region (nucleotides 1–27) of U2 RNA remains associated with U2 snRNP after cleavage with the U2b oligonucleotide. Treatment with the U4 oligonucleotide caused the dissociation of the U4-U6 double particle (Hashimoto and Steitz 1984; Rinke et al. 1985) into separately sedimenting U4 and U6 snRNPs (results not shown).

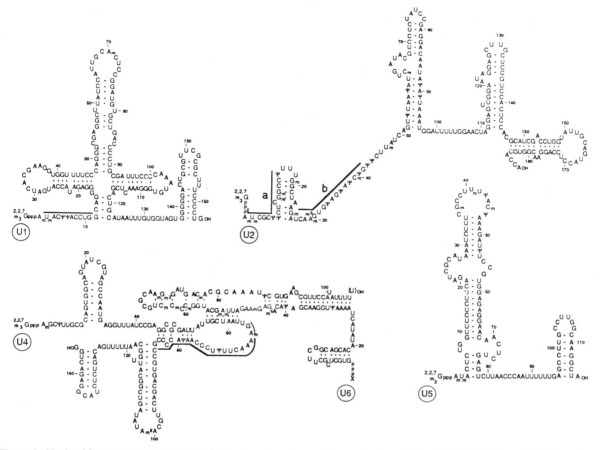

Figure 3. Nucleotide sequences and proposed secondary structures of the nucleoplasmic U-snRNAs. Solid lines indicate regions that were cleaved by complementary deoxyoligonucleotides and RNase H. The U1, U4, and U5 sequences are human, and the U2 and U6 sequences are from the rat (Reddy 1986). The U1 structure was adapted from Mount and Steitz (1981); U2, from Keller and Noon (1985); U4/U6, from Rinke et al. (1985); and U5, from Branlant et al. (1983). This figure was kindly provided by D. Black and J.A. Steitz (Yale University).

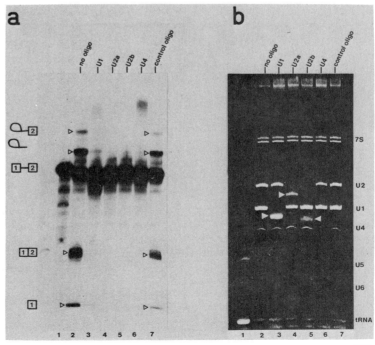

Figure 4. Effect of oligonucleotide-directed RNase H cleavage of U1, U2, and U4 snRNAs on pre-mRNA splicing. (*a*) [^{32}P]RNA 1 was incubated for 90 min under splicing conditions in nuclear extracts that had been pretreated with the indicated oligonucleotides. RNA was prepared and separated by electrophoresis on a 12% polyacrylamide–8 M urea gel. Radioactive RNAs were visualized by autoradiography and are identified schematically at the left. (*1*) Control reaction in the absence of nuclear extract; (*2*) control reaction in which the nuclear extract had been preincubated in the absence of oligonucleotide; (*3–7*) reactions with nuclear extract pretreated with oligonucleotides as indicated on top. (*b*) The same gel shown in panel *a* was stained with ethidium bromide and photographed under UV light. Small RNA species are indicated at the right; arrowheads indicate the cleavage products.

Selective snRNP Inactivation Affects Distinct Steps in Spliceosome Assembly

The fact that site-specific snRNA cleavage causes the inhibition of both steps of the in vitro splicing reaction suggests that the snRNPs must be intact for the correct assembly of active spliceosomes that occurs before the onset of the reaction. This was tested by native gel electrophoresis. Targeted cleavage of the snRNPs in splicing extracts was carried out as described above; radiolabeled substrate RNA was added, and the reaction mixtures were incubated under splicing conditions

for 45 minutes. Complexes were subsequently separated by electrophoresis. Because we knew that different types of complexes were formed with a complete pre-mRNA, compared with RNAs that are lacking either the 5′ or the 3′ splice site (Frendewey and Keller 1985), we tested the effects of site-specific snRNP inactivation with three different RNA substrates, the composition of which is shown schematically in Figure 5 (top).

RNA 1 is a complete, splicing-competent pre-mRNA that consists of two exons separated by a short intron. It is the same RNA that was used for the experiments

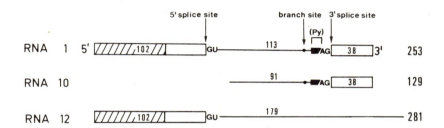

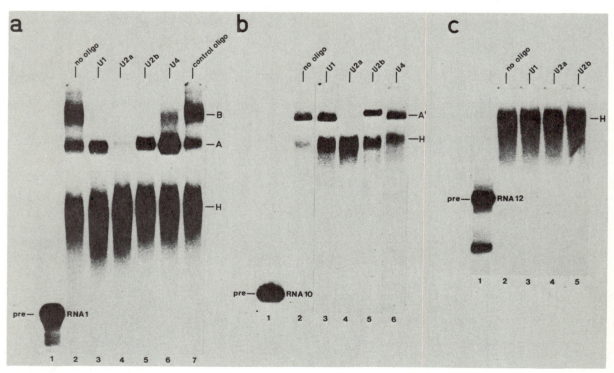

Figure 5. Effect of oligonucleotide-directed RNase H cleavage of U1, U2, and U4 snRNAs on splicing complex formation. A schematic representation of pre-mRNAs is shown at the top. Exons are indicated by open boxes, intron sequences by a solid line. Shaded areas within the chimeric first exons show SP6 vector sequences. In the intron, the dot represents the adenosine residue at the branch site, and the closed box indicates the polypyrimidine tract. Numbers within the exons and above the introns show the lengths, in nucleotides, of these sequences within the respective pre-mRNAs; numbers at the right refer to the total lengths of the transcripts. For further details, see Frendewey and Keller (1985) and Krämer (1987). (a) RNA 1 as substrate. Aliquots from the splicing reaction described in Fig. 4 were removed after 45 min and frozen; 5 μl of each was treated with heparin and fractionated on a 4% gel as described in Fig. 1. Complexes were visualized by autoradiography. Lanes 1–7 are the same as those in Fig. 4. (b) RNA 10 as substrate; 45-min splicing reactions were performed with RNA 10. Each reaction (5 μl) was fractionated without heparin treatment on a 3% acrylamide–0.5% agarose gel. Lanes 1–6 are the same as those in Fig. 4, except that [³²P]RNA 10 is the substrate. Complexes A and H are identified at the right. (c) RNA 12 as substrate. Reactions and gel analysis are the same as in b. Lanes 1–5 are the same as those in Fig. 4, except that RNA 12 is the substrate. RNA 12 forms a slow-migrating complex that behaves like an H complex and is labeled as such at the right.

presented in Figures 1 through 4 above. Upon incubation in splicing extract, which was mock-incubated or treated with the control oligonucleotide, RNA 1 associates with components to form complexes H, A, and B, as expected (Fig. 5a, lanes 2 and 7). In contrast, site-specific inactivation of the U1, U2, or U4 snRNPs results in a nearly complete inhibition of spliceosome (complex B) formation (lanes 3–6). Thus, the inhibition of splicing caused by the cleavage of the U1, U2, and U4 RNAs (Fig. 4) is due to a block of spliceosome assembly.

Examination of the results in more detail indicates that particular regions or domains of the snRNAs are involved in distinct steps of the assembly pathway. Removal of approximately ten nucleotides from the 5′ end of U1 RNA prevents the conversion of complex A to complex B (Fig. 5a, lane 3); this shows that the 5′-proximal region of U1 RNA is absolutely necessary for spliceosome formation, but that it is not required to generate a presplicing complex A. In contrast to this, the 5′-terminal part of U2 RNA is required at an earlier stage. Removal of the 5′-terminal 15 nucleotides causes a complete abolition of complex B as well as a nearly total loss of the A complex (Fig. 5a, lane 4). Thus, the 5′ end of U2 snRNA is needed to assemble the presplicing complex or, more specifically, to convert complex H into complex A.

A different effect was observed when oligonucleotide U2b was used to direct the cleavage of an internal segment of the U2 RNA (nucleotides 28–42). Under these conditions, the formation of the presplicing complex A was not affected, whereas spliceosome formation (complex B) was blocked (Fig. 5, lane 5). The differential effect of the two U2 RNA oligonucleotides suggests a dual function of the U2 snRNP in spliceosome assembly. The 5′-terminal portion of its RNA is necessary for the U2 snRNP to participate in the early events that convert the H complex to a presplicing complex A, and internal sequences between nucleotides 28 and 42 are needed for U2 snRNP function in the conversion of complex A into complex B, the active spliceosome.

Disruption of the U4 RNA results in a block of spliceosome formation (complex B) but has no effect on the generation of the presplicing complex A (Fig. 5a, lane 6). (The diffuse zone of material migrating slightly faster than complex B in this lane appears to be a gel artifact; it was not observed in other experiments.)

In summarizing the results, it appears that the snRNA domains complementary to oligonucleotides U1, U2b, and U4 (Fig. 3) are all involved in the same step of spliceosome assembly, namely, the conversion of complex A to complex B. In contrast, the U2 sequence at the 5′ end (complementary to oligonucleotide U2a) is needed to generate the presplicing complex A.

This conclusion is corroborated by an experiment in which RNA 10 was employed as substrate for complex formation. RNA 10 has an intact 3′ splice site, including the wild-type branch point and polypyrimidine tract

and a downstream exon, but it is lacking exon 1 and a 5′ splice site (Fig. 5, top). Upon incubation under splicing conditions, RNA 10 makes a 35S complex (Frendewey and Keller 1985). When analyzed by electrophoresis on nondenaturing gels, RNA 10 only shows two retarded bands, as compared to the three complexes seen with RNA 1. This is shown in Figure 5b (note that the electrophoretic mobility of complexes in Fig. 5 cannot be directly compared between panels a, b, and c, because different electrophoresis conditions were used in each case). The band with the faster electrophoretic mobility (Fig. 5b, lanes 2–6) corresponds to the H complex observed with RNA 1 (Fig. 5a) because it forms instantaneously upon incubation with nuclear extract and does not require splicing-specific conditions (results not shown). The slower migrating band (A′) represents an A-type complex; it forms within 5 minutes of incubation, requires low levels (10–50 μM) of ATP, and is absent upon incubation in snRNP-depleted nuclear extract (results not shown). Oligonucleotide-directed snRNP cleavage with U1, U2b, and U4 does not affect the formation of complex A′ with RNA 10 (Fig. 5b, lanes 2, 5, and 6). In contrast, prior treatment of the extract with oligonucleotide U2a results in a complete inhibition of the assembly of complex A′ (Fig. 5b, lane 4). The results with RNA 10 complement those obtained with RNA 1 and indicate that the U2a domain is essential for the formation of a presplicing-type complex.

The third RNA substrate we have analyzed is RNA 12. As illustrated (Fig. 5, top), this RNA has a normal upstream exon and 5′ splice site but lacks a 3′ splice site region and the downstream exon. Upon incubation with control and oligonucleotide-treated extracts, RNA 12 does not form any of the splicing-related complexes (Fig. 5c). The retarded band in lanes 2–5 corresponds to an unspecific complex H. This complex forms immediately upon incubation and does not require splicing-specific conditions (results not shown).

Taken together, the experiments shown in Figure 5 illustrate that formation of a presplicing complex (A) requires the presence of a 3′ splice site region and a downstream exon on the RNA substrate; in addition, domain U2a of the U2 snRNP must be intact. To generate a splicing complex (B), a splicing-competent pre-mRNA is needed that contains all the sequence elements known to be essential for splicing and the snRNPs U1, U2, and U4/6 have to be intact. In the absence of a 3′ splice site region on the pre-mRNA, no specific complex can be observed under the conditions of native gel electrophoresis.

RNase A Protection Mapping

We have employed an RNA "footprinting" assay for locating the sites of interaction of components in the splicing extract with adenovirus-derived pre-mRNAs by mapping the fragments of RNA remaining after digestion with RNase A to the known sequence of the RNA substrates. This method has previously proved useful in studying stable RNA contacts with factors during the in vitro splicing of globin pre-mRNA (Ruskin and Green 1985). The results of this investigation have been reported in detail elsewhere (Krämer 1987). Under the conditions of in vitro splicing, two regions of the pre-mRNA become resistant to RNase A degradation. As shown in Figure 6, the protected fragments encompass the 5' splice site (fragments A and B) and a region upstream of the 3' splice site in the vicinity of the branch point (fragments C–I). In a time course experiment, the interaction near the branch point precedes that at the 5' splice site. The protection in the branch-point region is independent of the presence of a 5' splice site sequence in the pre-mRNA. In contrast, RNase protection of the 5' splice site strictly depends on the presence of an intact branch point/polypyrimidine tract/3' splice site. These results parallel those obtained by gel electrophoresis and are consistent with the idea that protection from RNase A arises primarily as a consequence of snRNP binding to the pre-mRNA during splicing complex assembly.

Figure 6 also shows the pattern of RNase-protected fragments obtained after incubation of RNA 1 with nuclear extracts in which snRNPs had been cleaved by specific oligonucleotides and RNase H. When the 5' end of U2 RNA is removed, no RNase-A-resistant fragments mapping at the 5' splice site are detected, and fragments derived from the branch-point region are highly reduced in abundance (lane 3) when compared to the control reaction (lane 7). In contrast, after degradation of an internal region (nucleotides 28–42) of U2 or U4 (nucleotides 64–83), or after removal of the 5' end of U1 RNA, protection of the branch-point region is not affected (lanes 4–6). However, the protection of the 5' splice site is lost in all of these reactions. These results demonstrate that the 5' end of U2 RNA must be intact for protection of the branch-point region. Likewise, an intact 5' end of U1 RNA is essential for protection at the 5' splice site. Interestingly, when the internal region of U2 RNA is removed, the particle retains its ability to interact with the branch-point region. However, the removal of the internal U2 RNA segment interferes with a stable interaction of components at the 5' splice site. The finding that degradation of U4 RNA does not prevent an association in the branch-point region implies that the U4 snRNP is required for a step that occurs after the binding of U2 snRNP near the branch site. Since the 5' splice site is not protected after the inactivation of the U4 snRNP, it appears that this particle participates in a process that leads to a stable interaction with the 5' splice site.

DISCUSSION

We have investigated the role of different snRNPs and snRNP domains in splicing complex formation after targeted degradation of snRNA sequences with complementary oligonucleotides and RNase H. The association of labeled pre-mRNAs with components in splicing extracts was analyzed by electrophoresis in nondenaturing gels and by mapping the sites of interac-

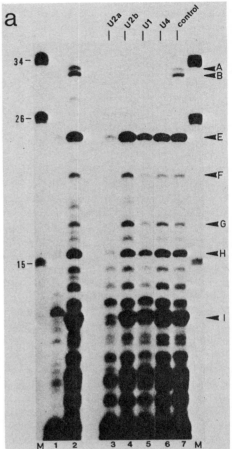

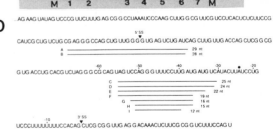

Figure 6. Protection of RNA 1 from RNase A digestion in nuclear extracts after site-specific hydrolysis of U1, U2, and U4 RNAs. (*a*) Splicing reactions were performed in nuclear extracts for 30 min after hydrolysis of U1, U2, and U4 RNA sequences with specific oligonucleotides. RNA was then digested with 5 μg of RNase A per milliliter for 15 min at 30°C. The resulting RNA fragments were size-fractionated on a 20% denaturing polyacrylamide gel (Krämer 1987). The oligonucleotides used are indicated at the top of lanes *3–7*. Lanes *1* and *2* show standard protection reactions without addition of an oligonucleotide in the absence or presence of nuclear extract, respectively. Fragments specifically protected from RNase A digestion are indicated at the right. (M) DNA size markers generated by *Hpa*II digestion of pBR322. (*b*) Location of the protected fragments within the sequence of RNA 1. The sequence of the first 15 nucleotides of RNA 1 is unknown. The nucleotide sequence is arranged according to fragments generated by RNase T1 digestion. The dot above the adenosine 24 nucleotides upstream of the 3' splice site denotes the branch point. Numbers above the intron sequence refer to the distance from the 3' splice site. The lengths of the protected fragments (lines below the RNA sequence) are indicated. (Protected fragments C and D are only protected at lower RNase A concentrations [Krämer 1987].)

tion on the pre-mRNA with an RNase-A-protection assay. In accordance with previous reports (Konarska and Sharp 1986, 1987; Christofori et al. 1987), we find that a pre-mRNA derived from the adenovirus-2 major late transcription unit gives rise to two specifically retarded bands (A and B) upon gel electrophoresis. Band A and band B correspond to two previously observed forms of complexes that sediment in sucrose gradients at 35S and at 50S, respectively (Frendewey and Keller 1985). The kinetics of their appearance and the requirement of distinct sequences in the pre-mRNA for their formation, combined with the results of RNase-protection mapping (Krämer 1987) indicate that the complexes result from the assembly of spliceosomes in two major steps. The "subspliceosomal" complex A precedes the appearance of the active spliceosome (complex B) by a few minutes. The generation of complex A requires the presence of a functional 3' splice site region on the RNA substrate, whereas a 5' splice site is dispensable. Concomitant with A complex formation, a region in the intron near the point of subsequent branch formation becomes resistant to digestion with RNase A.

Complex B can only be made with pre-mRNA substrates that contain a functional 5' splice site and a 3' splice site. In addition to the region protected from RNase A digestion near the branch point characteristic of complex A, an additional region of protection spanning the 5' splice site is found in complex B. Two-dimensional electrophoresis of splicing complexes has demonstrated that the products of the first step of the pre-mRNA splicing reaction, exon 1 and the intron-exon 2 lariat, are exclusively associated with complex B, thus identifying complex B as the structure in which the splicing reaction takes place. In contrast, the final products of the splicing reaction, exon 1–exon 2 RNA and most of the intron lariat, are released from the splicing complex, as becomes evident after denaturing gel electrophoresis of the reaction products present in the splicing complexes.

The analysis of splicing complexes by native gel electrophoresis after selective inactivation of snRNPs in the splicing extract showed that the removal of the 5' terminus of U1 RNA, or of an internal region of U2 RNA, or of an internal region of U4 RNA (which causes the disruption of the U4/U6 particle) resulted in an apparent block in the conversion of the presplicing complex to the active spliceosome. This conclusion is supported by the results obtained by RNase-A-protection mapping that showed that an interaction of components with the 5' splice site region is precluded in all of these cases. Thus, the inhibition of splicing observed upon snRNA digestion can be correlated with an arrest in splicing complex assembly.

A Dual Function for U2 snRNP?

Site-directed cleavage of two different RNA domains of U2 RNA in splicing extracts has unveiled an interesting differential effect on splicing complex formation.

Degradation of an internal segment (targeted by oligonucleotide U2b [Fig. 3]) had no effect on the formation of the presplicing complex but prevented its conversion to the spliceosome (see above). In marked contrast, removal of the 5' portion of U2 RNA (targeted by oligonucleotide U2a) led to an almost complete abolition of the formation of presplicing complexes. In agreement with this, the appearance of protected pre-mRNA fragments in the branch-point region by RNase A mapping was also drastically reduced. These results could be explained by assuming that the 5' region of U2 RNA (the "U2a domain") is required for the initial binding of U2 snRNP to its cognate site in the 3' splice site region. The internal region of U2 RNA (the "U2b domain"), however, is dispensable for this primary interaction but must be intact to allow the further assembly of an active spliceosome.

At first sight, our results appear to be at odds with the recent report of Parker et al. (1987), who have demonstrated that a region within the U2b domain of the yeast U2 RNA analog (nucleotides 33–39 in snR20) interacts with the branch site of pre-mRNAs by forming complementary base pairs. (This region is absolutely conserved in sequence between human and yeast U2 RNAs [Ares 1986].) Parker et al. have also put forward strong arguments in favor of base pairing between mammalian U2 RNA (nucleotides 33–38 within domain U2b) and branch sites. When written with a mammalian branch-point consensus sequence (Green 1986), the base pairing proposed is

Position		-5	-4	-3	-2	-1	0	$+1$
Mammalian consensus	$5'-$	Py	N	C	U	Pu	$\underline{A}$	$C-3'$
U2 snRNA sequence	$3'-$	A	$\cdot$ U	$\cdot$ G	$\cdot$ A	$\cdot$ U		$\cdot$ G $-5'$

This scheme is particularly attractive because it proposes a bulged branch-point A residue (underlined), a feature also present in proposed secondary structures for self-splicing group II introns (Michel and Dujon 1983; Peebles et al. 1986; Schmelzer and Schweyen 1986; Van der Veen et al. 1986). By comparing branch sites of yeast pre-mRNAs, it was noted (Guthrie et al. 1986; Parker et al. 1987) that base pairing with snR20 can often be extended to three positions beyond the bulged A residue. Comparison of this model with 25 known metazoan branch sites shows that if the two nucleotides at positions $+2$ and $+3$ beyond the bulged nucleotide are included, it is always possible to form five or more base pairs with U2 RNA (D. Frendewey et al., unpubl.).

To explain our finding that the U2b domain is not needed for the initial interaction of U2 snRNP with the pre-mRNA, we propose that this snRNP may have two different binding modes. Its initial binding may be dictated by an interaction with the 3'-splice-site-binding component (Gerke and Steitz 1986; Tazi et al. 1986), in agreement with the observations (Black et al. 1985;

Reed and Maniatis 1985; Ruskin and Green 1985; Ruskin et al. 1985; Krämer 1987) that a certain distance between the intron-exon border and the branch point is a prerequisite for splicing to occur and that binding of U2 snRNP depends on the presence of a polypyrimidine tract/3' splice site signal. The proposed base pairing between sequences in the U2b domain and a suitable branch-point sequence could then be a secondary event and may be triggered by conformational changes imposed upon the splicing complex during the conversion from complex A to complex B.

We do not know why the 5' region of U2 RNA (domain U2a) is needed for the initial binding of the snRNP to pre-mRNA. There are no obvious sequence complementarities discernible between this region of U2 RNA and conserved sequence elements in mammalian introns. Therefore, the binding may be governed by some other type of interaction (e.g., protein-RNA, or protein-protein to an adjacent intron-binding component). There is, however, a conspicuous sequence complementarity to U1 RNA. As noted by Black et al. (1985), of the nucleotides between positions 5 and 14 of U2 RNA, nine are complementary to nucleotides 11–20 of U1 RNA (this includes six G:C pairs, one A:U pair, and two G-U pairs; see Fig. 3 for sequences). Thus, it is conceivable that this or other sequence complementarities between U1 and U2 RNA (for further discussion, see Black et al. 1985; Kretzner et al. 1987) could play a role in transient base-pairing interactions between these particles in the course of spliceosome assembly. The existence of U1:U2 snRNP interactions is supported by several lines of evidence. For example, in vitro studies have shown that RNA fragments containing both 5' and 3' splice site sequences of globin pre-mRNA can be precipitated by antibodies directed against either U1 or U2 snRNP (Black et al. 1985; Bindereif and Green 1987; Chabot and Steitz 1987a,b). Note that unlike native gel electrophoresis or RNase-A-protection mapping used here, immunoprecipitation combined with RNase T1 digestion can detect relatively "weak" interactions, such as U1 snRNP binding at a 5' splice site or the binding of the 3'-splice-site-recognition factor at early times of an in vitro splicing reaction. Also, a certain amount of U1 and U2 snRNPs are coprecipitated from *Xenopus* oocytes with antibodies specific for the individual snRNPs (Mattaj et al. 1986). In addition, in a fraction of total isolated snRNPs, part of the U1 and U2 RNAs can be cross-linked to each other by psoralen (R. Lührmann, pers. comm.). It has also recently been reported that U1 snRNP is required at an early step of splicing complex formation (Zillmann et al. 1987). U1:U2 interaction could provide a mechanism for bringing a 5' splice site into proximity with its cognate 3' splice region complex. Joining of the remaining snRNPs and structural rearrangements would then result in the generation of an active spliceosome. The question of how individual snRNPs communicate with each other and with their respective pre-mRNA binding sites in the intricate choreography involved in

spliceosome assembly and disassembly will certainly receive much attention in the near future.

In summary, there is no doubt that snRNPs are key elements for building the complicated structure of spliceosomes. It has been widely discussed that snRNPs may have originated from ancestral self-splicing introns and that the catalytic activity for the cleavage-ligation reactions in nuclear pre-mRNA splicing may reside in snRNA (Cech 1985, 1986; Been et al.; Sharp et al.; both this volume; Maniatis and Reed 1987; Sharp 1985, 1987). The discovery of catalytic RNA and, in particular, the recent demonstration that very short RNA helices can be endowed with enzymatic activity (Forster and Symons 1987; Uhlenbeck 1987; Forster et al.; Sampson et al.; both this volume) make this a real possibility. In this scheme, the protein constituents of snRNPs would be relegated to ancillary functions. The answers to these and many other remaining questions must come from future experiments.

ACKNOWLEDGMENTS

We are indebted to Albert E. Dahlberg (Brown University, Providence, R.I.) for his guidance and many helpful suggestions on gel electrophoresis procedures. We thank Silke Bienroth for helping with the analysis of splicing complexes and Marion Frick for providing HeLa cell extracts and for skillful technical assistance. W.K. would like to thank Alan Weiner for discussions and help during the Symposium. We thank Iain Mattaj for critically reading the manuscript, Signe Mähler for preparing the illustrations, and Ursula Joa for typing. This work was supported by grants from the Deutsche Forschungsgemeinschaft and the Fonds der Chemischen Industrie.

REFERENCES

Ares, M. 1986. U2 RNA from yeast is unexpectedly large and contains homology to vertebrate U4, U5, and U6 small nuclear RNAs. *Cell* **47:** 49.

Berget, S.M. and B.L. Robberson. 1986. U1, U2, and U4/U6 small nuclear ribonucleoproteins are required for in vitro splicing but not polyadenylation. *Cell* **46:** 691.

Bindereif, A. and M.R. Green. 1986. Ribonucleoprotein complex formation during pre-mRNA splicing in vitro. *Mol. Cell. Biol.* **6:** 2582.

———. 1987. An ordered pathway of snRNP binding during mammalian pre-mRNA splicing complex assembly. *EMBO J.* **6:** 2415.

Birnstiel, M.L., ed. 1987. *Structure and function of major and minor small nuclear ribonucleoprotein particles.* Springer-Verlag, Berlin.

Black, D.L. and J.A. Steitz. 1986. Pre-mRNA splicing in vitro requires intact U4/U6 small nuclear ribonucleoprotein. *Cell* **46:** 697.

Black, D.L., B. Chabot, and J.A. Steitz. 1985. U2 as well as U1 small nuclear ribonucleoproteins are involved in pre-messenger RNA splicing. *Cell* **42:** 737.

Branlant, C., A. Krol, E. Lazar, B. Haendler, M. Jacob, L. Galego-Dias, and C. Pousada. 1983. High evolutionary conservation of the secondary structure and of certain nucleotide sequences of U5 RNA. *Nucleic Acids Res.* **11:** 8359.

Brody, E. and J. Abelson. 1985. The "spliceosome": Yeast pre-messenger RNA associates with a 40S complex in a splicing-dependent reaction. *Science* **228**: 963.

Brunel, C., J. Sri-Widada, and P. Jeanteur. 1985. snRNPs and scRNPs in eukaryotic cells. *Prog. Mol. Subcell. Biol.* **9**: 1.

Cech, T.R. 1985. Self-splicing RNA: Implications for evolution. *Int. Rev. Cytol.* **93**: 3.

———. 1986. The generality of self-splicing RNA: Relationship to nuclear mRNA splicing. *Cell* **44**: 207.

———. 1987. The chemistry of self-splicing RNA and RNA enzymes. *Science* **236**: 1532.

Cech, T.R. and B.L. Bass. 1986. Biological catalysis by RNA. *Annu. Rev. Biochem.* **55**: 599.

Chabot, B. and J.A. Steitz. 1987a. Multiple interactions between the splicing substrate and small nuclear ribonucleoproteins in spliceosomes. *Mol. Cell. Biol.* **7**: 281. ———. 1987b. Recognition of mutant and cryptic 5′ splice sites by the U1 small nuclear ribonucleoprotein in vitro. *Mol. Cell. Biol.* **8**: 698.

Chabot B., D.L. Black, D.M. LeMaster, and J.A. Steitz. 1985. The 3′ splice site of pre-messenger RNA is recognized by a small nuclear ribonucleoprotein. *Science* **230**:1344.

Cheng, S.-C. and J. Abelson. 1987. Yeast spliceosome assembly in yeast. *Genes Dev.* **1**: 1014.

Christofori, G., D. Frendewey, and W. Keller. 1987. Two spliceosomes can form simultaneously and independently on synthetic double-intron messenger RNA precursors. *EMBO J.* **6**: 1747.

Dignam, J.D., R.M. Lebovitz, and R.G. Roeder. 1983. Accurate transcription initiation by RNA polymerase II in a soluble extract from isolated mammalian nuclei. *Nucleic Acids Res.* **11**: 1475.

Forster, A.C. and R.H. Symons. 1987. Self-cleavage of virusoid RNA is performed by the proposed 55-nucleotide active site. *Cell* **50**: 9.

Frendewey, D. and W. Keller. 1985. Stepwise assembly of a pre-mRNA splicing complex requires U-snRNPs and specific intron sequences. *Cell* **42**: 355.

Gerke, V. and J.A. Steitz. 1986. A protein associated with small nuclear ribonucleoprotein particles recognizes the 3′ splice site of premessenger RNA. *Cell* **47**: 973.

Goodwin, G.H. and A.E. Dahlberg. 1982. Electrophoresis of nucleoproteins. In *Gel electrophoresis of nucleic acids: A practical approach* (ed. D. Rickwood and B.D. Hames), p. 213. IRL Press, Oxford, England.

Grabowski, P.J. and P.A. Sharp. 1986. Affinity chromatography of splicing complexes: U2, U5, and U4/U6 small nuclear ribonucleoprotein particles in the spliceosome. *Science* **233**: 1294.

Grabowski, P.J., S.R. Seiler, and P.A. Sharp. 1985. A multicomponent complex is involved in the splicing of messenger RNA precursors. *Cell* **42**: 345.

Green, M.R. 1986. Pre-mRNA splicing. *Annu. Rev. Genet.* **20**: 671.

Guthrie, C., N. Riedel, R. Parker, H. Swerdlow, and B. Patterson. 1986. Genetic analysis of snRNAs and RNA processing in yeast. *UCLA Symp. Mol. Cell. Biol. New Ser.* **33**: 301.

Hashimoto, C. and J.A. Steitz. 1984. U4 and U6 RNAs coexist in a single small nuclear ribonucleoprotein particle. *Nucleic Acids Res.* **12**: 3283.

Heintz, N. and R.G. Roeder. 1984. Transcription of human histone genes in extracts from synchronized HeLa cells. *Proc. Natl. Acad. Sci.* **81**: 2713.

Jacquier, A. and F. Michel. 1987. Multiple exon-binding sites in class II self-splicing introns. *Cell* **50**: 17.

Keller, E.B. and W.A. Noon. 1985. Intron splicing: A conserved internal signal in introns of *Drosophila* pre-mRNAs. *Nucleic Acids Res.* **13**: 4971.

Konarska, M.M. and P.A. Sharp. 1986. Electrophoretic separation of complexes involved in the splicing of precursors to mRNAs. *Cell* **46**: 845.

———. 1987. Interactions between small nuclear ribonucleoprotein particles in formation of spliceosomes. *Cell* **49**: 763.

Krainer, A.R. and T. Maniatis. 1985. Multiple factors including the small nuclear ribonucleoproteins U1 and U2 are necessary for pre-mRNA splicing in vitro. *Cell* **42**: 725.

Krämer, A. 1987. Analysis of RNase A resistant regions of adenovirus 2 major late precursor-mRNA in splicing extracts reveals an ordered interaction of nuclear components with the substrate RNA. *J. Mol. Biol.* **196**: 559.

Krämer, A., W. Keller, B. Appel, and R. Lührmann. 1984. The 5′ terminus of the RNA moiety of U1 small nuclear ribonucleoprotein particles is required for the splicing of messenger RNA precursors. *Cell* **38**: 299.

Kretzner, L., B.C. Rymond, and M. Robash. 1987. *Saccharomyces cerevisiae* U1 RNA is large and has limited primary sequence homology of metazoan U1 snRNA. *Cell* **50**: 593.

Lamond, A.I., M.M. Konarska, and P.A. Sharp. 1987. A mutational analysis of spliceosome assembly: Evidence for splice site collaboation during spliceosome formation. *Genes Dev.* **1**: 532.

Lerner, M.R., J.A. Boyle, S.M. Mount, S.L. Wolin, and J.A. Steitz. 1980. Are snRNPs involved in splicing? *Nature* **283**: 220.

Maniatis, T. and R. Reed. 1987. The role of small nuclear ribonucleoprotein particles in pre-mRNA splicing. *Nature* **325**: 673.

Maniatis, T., E.F. Fritsch, and J. Sambrook. 1982. *Molecular cloning: A laboratory manual.* Cold Spring Harbor Laboratory, Cold Spring Harbor, New York.

Mattaj, I.W., W.J. Habets, and W.J. van Venrooij. 1986. Monospecific antibodies reveal details of U2 snRNP structure and interaction between U1 and U2 snRNPs. *EMBO J.* **5**: 997.

Melton, D.A., P.A. Krieg, M.R. Rebagliatti, T. Maniatis, K. Zinn, and M.R. Green. 1984. Efficient in vitro synthesis of biologically active RNA and RNA hybridization probes from plasmids containing a bacteriophage SP6 promoter. *Nucleic Acids Res.* **12**: 7035.

Michel, F. and B. Dujon. 1983. Conservation of RNA secondary structure in two intron families including mitochondrial-, chloroplast-, and nuclear-encoded members. *EMBO J.* **2**: 33.

Mount, S.M. and J.A. Steitz. 1981. Sequence of U1 RNA from *Drosophila melanogaster*: Implications for U1 secondary structure and possible involvement in splicing. *Nucleic Acids Res.* **9**: 6351.

Padgett, R.A., P.J. Grabowski, M.M. Konarska, S.R. Seiler, and P.A. Sharp. 1986. Splicing of messenger RNA precursors. *Annu. Rev. Biochem.* **55**: 119.

Parker, R., P.G. Siliciano, and C. Guthrie. 1987. Recognition of the TACTAAC box during mRNA splicing in yeast involves base-pairing to the U2-like snRNA. *Cell* **49**: 229.

Patterson, B. and C. Guthrie. 1987. An essential yeast snRNA with a U5-like domain is required for splicing in vivo. *Cell* **49**: 613.

Peebles, C.L., P.S. Perlman, K.L. Mecklenburg, M.L. Petrillo, J.H. Tabor, K.A. Jarell, and H.-L. Cheng. 1986. A self-splicing RNA excises an intron lariat. *Cell* **44**: 213.

Pikielny, C.W. and M. Rosbash. 1986. Specific small nuclear RNAs are associated with yeast spliceosomes. *Cell* **45**: 869.

Pikielny, C.W., B.C. Rymond, and M. Rosbash. 1986. Electrophoresis of ribonucleoproteins reveals an ordered assembly pathway of yeast splicing complexes. *Nature* **324**: 341.

Reddy, R. 1986. Compilation of small RNA sequences. *Nucleic Acids Res.* (suppl.) **14**: r61.

Reddy, R. and H. Busch. 1983. Small nuclear RNAs and RNA processing. *Prog. Nucleic Acid Res. Mol. Biol.* **30**: 127.

Reed, R. and T. Maniatis. 1985. Intron sequences involved in lariat formation during pre-mRNA splicing. *Cell* **42**: 95.

Rinke, J., B. Appel, M. Digweed, and R. Lührmann. 1985. Localization of a base-paired interaction between small nuclear RNAs U4 and U6 in intact U4/U6 ribonucleoprotein particles by psoralen crosslinking. *J. Mol. Biol.* **185:** 721.

Rogers, J. and R. Wall. 1980. A mechanism for RNA splicing. *Proc. Natl. Acad. Sci.* **77:** 1877.

Ruskin, B. and M.R. Green. 1985. Specific and stable intron-factor interactions are established early during in vitro pre-mRNA splicing. *Cell* **43:** 131.

Ruskin, B., J.M. Greene, and M.R. Green. 1985. Cryptic branchpoint activation allows accurate in vitro splicing of human beta-globin intron mutants. *Cell* **41:** 833.

Rymond, B.C., D.D. Torrey, and M. Rosbash. 1987. A novel role for the 3' region of introns in pre-mRNA splicing of *Saccharomyces cerevisiae. Genes Dev.* **1:** 238.

Schmelzer, C. and R.J. Schweyen. 1986. Self-splicing of group II introns *in vitro*: Mapping of the branch point and mutational inhibition of lariat formation. *Cell* **46:** 557.

Sharp, P.A. 1985. On the origin of RNA splicing and introns. *Cell* **42:** 397.

———. 1987. Splicing of messenger RNA precursors. *Science* **235:** 766.

Siliciano, P.G., M.H. Jones, and C. Guthrie. 1987a. *S. cerevisiae* has a U1-like snRNA with unexpected properties. *Science* **237:** 1484.

Siliciano, P.G., D.A. Brow, H. Roiha, and C. Guthrie. 1987b. An essential snRNA from *Saccharomyces cerevisiae* has

properties predicted for U4, including interaction with the U6-like snRNA. *Cell* **50:** 585.

Steitz, J.A., S.L. Wolin, J. Rinke, I. Pettersson, S.M. Mount, E.A. Lerner, M. Hinterberger, and E. Gottlieb. 1983. Small ribonucleoproteins from eukaryotes: Structures and roles in RNA biogenesis. *Cold Spring Harbor Symp. Quant. Biol.* **47:** 893.

Tazi, J., C. Alibert, J. Témsamani, I. Reveillaud, G. Cathala, C. Brunel, and P. Jeanteur. 1986. A protein that specifically recognizes the 3' splice site of mammalian pre-mRNA introns is associated with a small nuclear ribonucleoprotein. *Cell* **47:** 755.

Uhlenbeck, O.E. 1987. A small catalytic oligoribonucleotide. *Nature* **328:** 596.

Van der Veen, R., A.C. Arnberg, G. van der Horst, L. Bonen, H.F. Tabak, and L.A. Grivell. 1986. Excised group II introns in yeast mitochondria are lariats and can be formed by self-splicing in vitro. *Cell* **44:** 225.

Zhuang, Y. and A.M. Weiner. 1986. A compensatory base change in U1 snRNA suppresses a 5' splice site mutation. *Cell* **46:** 827.

Zhuang, Y., H. Leung, and A.M. Weiner. 1987. The natural 5' splice site of simian virus 40 large T antigen can be improved by increasing the base complementarity to U1 RNA. *Mol. Cell. Biol.* **7:** 3018.

Zillmann, M., S.D. Rose, and S.M. Berget. 1987. U1 small nuclear ribonucleoproteins are required early during spliceosome assembly. *Mol. Cell. Biol.* **7:** 2877.

Replication and Evolution of Short-chained RNA Species Replicated by Qβ Replicase

C.K. Biebricher

Max-Plank-Institut für Biophysikalische Chemie, D-3400 Göttingen, Federal Republic of Germany

RNA genomes are quite common for viruses, but extremely rare in cellular organisms—RNA plasmids (Wickner 1986) may be regarded as inherited relics of viral infections—and thus RNA replication does not occur in the normal processing of cellular genetic information. The best-understood copying mechanism of viral RNA is the RNA-dependent RNA replication system of RNA coliphages (lentiviridae). It utilizes a single enzyme, called a replicase, and differs fundamentally in several respects from DNA replication:

1. The template and the products of RNA replication are single-stranded RNA; double-stranded RNA has no template activity, although it can bind to replicase (Weissmann 1974; Biebricher et al. 1982).
2. The replicase is highly specific in its choice of template; in vivo it replicates plus and minus strands of the viral RNA while ignoring the vast excess of cellular RNA (Haruna and Spiegelman 1965). The specificity makes use of the tertiary structure of the RNA, since a different folding of the same RNA sequence may destroy its activity as template (Biebricher et al. 1982). Therefore, the RNA template cannot be regarded as a mere substrate; it shares the catalytic role with the replicase by complementing it structurally to form an active site for several crucial steps in the replication cycle (Biebricher et al. 1983).
3. Autocatalytic amplification requires template activity of both plus and minus strands. Replication thus involves two cross-catalytic cycles; each reproducing species consists of two different RNA types with complementary sequences.

RNA that is accepted by the replicase can be readily replicated in vitro; Qβ replicase is a rather stable enzyme and can be purified to homogeneity. Spiegelman and co-workers (Mills et al. 1967; Levisohn and Spiegelman 1969) showed that RNA replicated in vitro by extraneously added replicase undergoes an evolution process that can only be interpreted as mutation and selection. Since gene expression, packaging, and other processes required in the in vivo infection cycle are neither possible nor necessary, RNA molecules are selected under these conditions only for their ability to be replicated as efficiently as possible by Qβ replicase, i.e., to catalyze together with the replicase their own replication. Because there is no need for translation, all of the extrinsic genomic information (Dickerson et al. 1986) of the virus is dispensable.

"Template-free" synthesis with Qβ replicase produces self-replicating RNA species with nucleotide chain lengths from 70 to 250. These RNA species prove to be particularly suitable for the study of in vitro evolution processes.

METHODS

Crucial for the experimental procedure is careful purification of the Qβ replicase to complete removal of RNA templates (Sumper and Luce 1975; Biebricher et al. 1986). Two preparations of Qβ replicase can be obtained from infected bacteria, a core enzyme containing the viral subunit complexed to the elongation factors of protein biosynthesis, (EF)Tu · Ts (Blumenthal et al. 1972), and a holoenzyme that has an additional host subunit, the ribosomal protein S1 (Wahba et al. 1974). Both preparations yield effective catalysts; some differences in kinetic behavior are found between the two preparations.

Particular care has been taken to produce RNA preparations that are really pure at the molecular level; one strand of an advantageous RNA present as an impurity will grow out after a few generations. Physical separation steps must thus always be followed by re-cloning of the RNA. Most of the techniques have been described in detail previously (Biebricher et al. 1981a,b, 1982, 1984, 1985, 1986); procedures used for cloning of RNA into DNA and details of the analysis of the quasi-species distribution will be published later.

RESULTS

Kinetics of RNA Replication

Comparison of the nucleotide sequences of several self-replicating RNA species (Mills et al. 1973; Mills et al. 1975; Schaffner et al. 1977; Mekler 1981) does not reveal common features except for a C cluster at the 3' ends and a corresponding G cluster at the 5' ends (Kamen 1969; Rensing and August 1969). The high template selectivity of Qβ replicase shows that this feature alone could not be sufficient for recognition. Also common to all self-replicating RNA is an unusually strong secondary structure (Mills et al. 1977) evidenced by high melting points (Biebricher et al. 1982). Clearly, recognition of a template by replicase is not dependent on an isolated recognition box; instead, it has to be controlled kinetically by the lifetimes of the initiation complexes. As a first step, the RNA template must undergo complex formation with replicase. Any RNA binds to some degree to replicase; however, effective templates bind practically irreversibly to replicase, whereas other RNA-replicase complexes rapidly redissociate. Strong binding alone, however, is not sufficient for initiation: The 3' end must also form a pocket with the two nucleoside-triphosphate-binding sites of the replicase in order to allow geminal association of the initiating GTP molecules. A new replica chain is then started by the initial "priming" phosphodiester formation. Chain elongation then proceeds by successive association of triphosphate, followed by phosphodiester formation. It is very likely that there is a transient stretch of double strands between replica and template at the replication fork, because selection of substrates observes Watson-Crick base pairing (Weissmann 1974). As chain elongation proceeds, replica and template are released in their single-stranded forms; the mechanism of strand separation is not understood. The completed replica chain is terminated by uninstructed adenylation at the 3' end (Weber and Weissmann 1970) and then released (Dobkin et al. 1979). The remaining inactive template-enzyme complex cannot return to the priming configuration; instead, it is reactivated only after first dissociating into RNA and free enzyme, a step that is rate-limiting for most experimental conditions (Biebricher et al. 1981b, 1983).

Incorporation profiles (Fig. 1) of replication show two main growth phases: (1) an *exponential growth* phase, where replicase is in excess and both replica and, after dissociation of the replication complex, template strands are able to start further replication rounds, and (2) a *linear growth* phage, where enzyme is saturated with template. Further growth in the linear phase depends on (the rate-determining step of) recycling the enzyme by releasing both template and replica. In the late linear growth phase, the incorporation levels off due to product inhibition and substrate exhaustion.

The replication rate in the linear growth phase ρ is defined as $d[I_o]/[E_c]dt$, where $[I_o]$ is the total concentration of free and enzyme-bound template RNA and $[E_c]$ is the concentration of enzyme bound to RNA. Since the enzyme is saturated with template in the linear phase, $[E_c] \approx [E_o]$, i.e., the template-bound enzyme concentration is almost the total enzyme concentration. The value of ρ can be determined easily from the slope of the incorporation profiles. In the exponential growth phase, the overall replication rate κ is defined as $d[I_o]/[I_o]dt$. It may be determined from the slope of a semilogarithmic plot of the incorporation profile. However, it can be measured with higher accuracy and greater convenience from the time lag increase in the profiles at different dilutions of the template (Fig. 1).

Replication seems to proceed about threefold more rapidly in the exponential growth phase than in the linear growth phase. This cannot be attributed to multiple replication forks present on one template strand of such short chain length. Instead, the linear growth rate is determined by the rate of enzyme reactivation, whereas under conditions of enzyme excess, the released replica can start a new replication round immediately (Biebricher et al. 1981b, 1983).

A simplified three-step replication mechanism consisting of two cross-catalytic cycles (Fig. 2) has been found that describes the essential features of the replication process quite well (for discussion of a more detailed mechanism, see Biebricher et al. 1983). Most

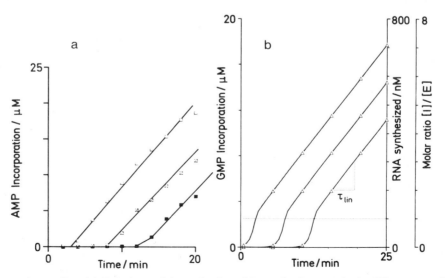

Figure 1. Incorporation profiles. (*a*) Experimental determination of the replication rates in the different growth phases; 10^{10}, 10^7, and 10^4 strands, respectively, of the MNV-11 template were added to incubation mixtures containing 150 nM Qβ holoenzyme. The overall rate in the linear phase ρ was determined by calculating the rate of RNA synthesis per mole of enzyme. The overall rate in the exponential phage κ was calculated from the shift of the profile by the time required for a 1000-fold greater exponential amplification of template. (*b*) Computer-simulated profiles. The predicted transition from exponential growth to linear growth is also found experimentally (Biebricher et al. 1981b).

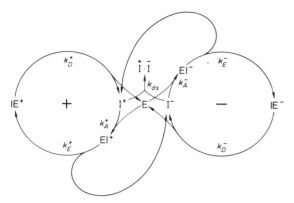

Figure 2. Simplified three-step replication mechanism. Reverse reactions are neglected. (k_A) Rate of template binding of enzyme; (k_E) rate of producing and releasing a replica strand; (k_D) rate of reactivation by dissociation of the inactive enzyme-template complex; (k_{ds}) rate of double-strand formation from free complementary strands.

relevant rate-constant values can be determined from experiments; for others, plausible values can be found. Computer simulations by numerical integration of the pertinent differential equations yield incorporation profiles in excellent agreement with those determined experimentally (Fig. 1). Under conditions of coherent exponential growth and of steady-state concentrations of replication intermediates, compact equations can be found that describe the replication process adequately and show the relevant functional dependences.

Complementary single strands of a sequence complexity (in this case, equal to sequence length) as small as 100–200 can be expected to combine to double strands at quite high rates. In the exponential phase, complexing of the RNA to enzyme apparently protects the strands from immediate double-strand formation, but in the linear phase, irreversible double-strand formation of the accumulating free RNA strands takes place, annihilating the template activity of both strands (Biebricher et al. 1984). In the late linear phase, synthesis of new template strands is balanced by loss of template by double-strand formation; the concentrations of free single strands reach steady-state concentrations, and only the concentration of double strands increases. In the exponential growth phase, incorporation ends up predominantly in enzyme-bound RNA ($\mathrm{d}[pp]/\{(n-1)dt\} \approx \mathrm{d}[E_c]/dt$), in the early linear phase in free strands ($\mathrm{d}[pp]/\{(n-1)dt\} \approx \mathrm{d}[I]/dt$), and in the late linear phase exclusively in double-stranded RNA ($\mathrm{d}[pp]/\{(n-1)dt\} \approx 2 \times \mathrm{d}[II]/dt$) (Fig. 3), where $\mathrm{d}[pp]/dt$ is the pyrophosphate production, n is the chain length of the RNA, $[I]$ is the concentration of the free single-stranded RNA, and $[II]$ is the concentration of double-stranded RNA.

Double-strand formation also causes equal incorporation into plus and minus strands even though the intrinsic replication rates may differ in the plus and minus cycles; a lower replication rate for one strand is balanced by a higher share of enzyme bound to it (Biebricher et al. 1984).

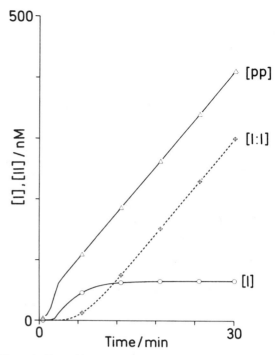

Figure 3. Fate of incorporated nucleotides. In the exponential phase, incorporation ends up predominantly in enzyme-bound RNA (E_c), in the early linear phase in single-stranded RNA (I), and in the late linear phase in double-stranded RNA (II). The computer simulations shown are confirmed by experimental evidence. (Modified from Biebricher 1986.)

Competition among Different Species

Different species replicating in the same sample need not interfere directly with each other's growth. However, they do share the same environment, including replicase, substrate, inhibitors, and other factors affecting growth. As in other cases of vegetative growth (Moser 1957), the relative population change of species i, $(\mathrm{d}[^iI]/(^iI]dt)$, was found to be a suitable criterion for its success in selection; species with the highest so-defined selection value become enriched in a replicating population.

Selection pressure is fundamentally different in different growth phases. In the exponential phase, where enzyme and substrate are in large excess and loss terms can be neglected, RNA species grow just as they would in different compartments, and their selection values are equal to the overall replication rates in the exponential phase. The fastest-growing species outraces the others; when the system is kept in the exponential growth phase indefinitely by serial dilution of aliquots into fresh solution containing substrate and replicase, the slower species are eventually diluted out, as in any typical example of evolution success by higher fecundity. In the linear growth phase, however, the resource of free enzyme becomes growth-limiting, and the selection success of an RNA species depends on its competition for free enzyme. Selection value and replication rate of a species are not correlated; in fact, often the more slowly growing species wins the competition. In-

302 BIEBRICHER

stead, the rate of binding free enzyme is critical for selection success; additionally, the competition is also strongly affected by the rate of template loss by double-strand formation. Despite this complicated behavior, it is possible to calculate the selection behavior quantitatively (Fig. 4). There are several rather surprising features of selection in the linear growth phase: (1) In the steady state of one species, another one present only as a few copies grows up exponentially; the concentration ratios of the species then change rapidly. (2) Negative selection values of one species may temporarily appear, when the decreasing amounts of template searching for a replicase molecule no longer compensate loss by double-strand formation. (3) Eventually, a stable coexistence of unrelated RNA species may be reached, where the species reach steady-state concentrations dependent only on their rates of enzyme binding and double-strand formation (Biebricher et al. 1985; Biebricher 1986).

Generally, selection in the exponential phase favors species with shorter chain lengths, since reactivation

proceeds more rapidly at lower chain length, whereas in the linear phase, species with longer chains are selected due to their lower rates of double-strand formation; longer chains also usually have higher enzyme-binding rates as well. Calculation of the selection values is complicated by the presence of plus and minus strands of each species, which also compete with each other; however, as described above, competition between complementary strands is restricted by the feedback of cross-catalysis. Further complications arise when the sequences of two species are related to such an extent that the rate of forming hybrid double strands becomes important. This is, of course, always the case when the competing RNA species are members of a mutant distribution.

Sequence Heterogeneity

In the competition experiments described above, mutational processes were disregarded. From the average misincorporation rate for Qβ replicase (3×10^{-4};

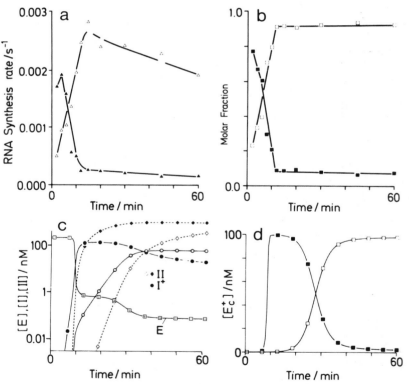

Figure 4. Growth of MDV-1 in the steady state of MNV-11. (*a,b*) Experimental determination. MNV-11 was grown until the double-strand steady state was obtained. MDV-1 was added at concentration of 1/1000 of the enzyme concentration. Synthesis of MNV-11 (open symbols) and MDV-1 (closed symbols) was measured by pulse-labeling experiments and electrophoretic separation of the products. (*a*) Rates of production (d[I_o]/dt) of the RNA species; (*b*) mole fraction of MNV-11 and MDV-1 produced. Note that the more slowly replicating MDV-1 grows out very rapidly by displacing MNV-11 from the enzyme. In the exponential phase (not shown), MNV-11 is selected. (*c,d*) Computer simulation of the competition between a species with a fourfold standard rate of reactivation (closed symbols) and another one with a fourfold standard rate of template binding. At time 0, the concentrations of both species are equal. In the exponential phase, the white species wins due to its lower overall rate of replication; it saturates the enzyme and enters the steady state of double-strand formation. The black species continues to grow exponentially at a lower rate and competes successfully for the enzyme. Finally, a stable coexistence is reached. When competion of double strands for free enzyme is also taken into account, the characteristic product inhibition effect seen in the experimental determination also appears at long times. (Modified from Biebricher et al. 1985.)

Batschelet et al. 1976; Domingo et al. 1978) and the chain lengths of the self-replicating RNA species, one might expect high replication fidelity. Experimentally, however, self-replicating RNA species are found to contain extremely high sequence heterogeneities, so that direct sequencing of the RNA with read-off methods becomes virtually impossible with some RNA species. There is no reason to assume a particularly high misincorporation rate of Qβ replicase in vitro or with certain self-replicating RNA species.

Mutant frequencies, i.e., the relative population numbers of mutants, however, are not determined by mutation rates alone. Selection forces play a dominant role in a replication system with inherent error propagation. Selection among mutants and species differs in two important respects: (1) Experimentally, mutants are very difficult to distinguish from one another, whereas separation of species is easy, and (2) the sequences of mutants are very similar and thus formation of double strands proceeds with little or no discrimination against heterologous strands.

In the exponential growth phase, double-strand formation of any kind can be neglected. The differential equations can be written (Eigen 1971 and this volume)

$$\mathrm{d}x_i/dt = (W_{ii} - \bar{E}[t])x_i(t) + \sum_{k \neq i} W_{ik}x_k(t)$$

where x_i is the relative population of mutant i, W_{ki} is the rate of obtaining replica k from replicating template i, and $\bar{E}$ is the average productivity. Evaluation of the different terms is relatively straightforward in the RNA replication system. The propagation rate for sequence i, W_{ii}, is equal to the overall replication rate $^i\kappa$ corrected for the production of incorrect copies, i.e.,

$$W_{ii} = {}^i\kappa - \sum_{i \neq k} W_{ki} \approx {}^i\kappa \bar{q}^n$$

where n is the chain length and $\bar{q}$ is the average incorporation fidelity per nucleotide. Decomposition of RNA in the exponential growth phase is negligible; thus, the RNA concentration would rapidly increase and saturate the enzyme unless loss terms by serial dilution or flux in a flow reactor balance the growth. The rates of producing incorrect copies W_{ki} are also dependent on the replication rate $^i\kappa$ multiplied by a mutation probability. The limited data available so far indicate that mutation rates depend mainly on the type of mutation, e.g., base transitions have values of 10^{-3}, whereas base transversions occur much less frequently. Modulation of the mutation rates by the sequence context, e.g., nearest-neighbor effects, appears to be limited; multiple error copies often can be considered to have arisen by independent mutation events (Eigen and Biebricher 1987). It can be readily seen from the equation above that so-called "hot-spot" mutations, i.e., mutant frequencies x_i that are particularly high, are mainly caused by $^i\kappa$ values exceeding or at least approaching the average production $\bar{E}$. The first (prop-

agation) term becomes small compared to the second (mutation) term (1) shortly after cloning, when the mutant populations x_i are still small, and (2) with mutants containing lethal or crippling mutations; in both cases, small x_i values result. The equation above assumes deterministic behavior, whereas stochastic behavior may seem more appropriate, since mutation events are rather rare. In principle, steady-state population numbers, i.e., a stable mutant distribution called a quasi-species, are only reached after an infinite number of replication rounds and with infinite population sizes. However, in the RNA replication system, we are dealing with (large populations $\approx 10^{11}/\mu$l, rapid replication with duplication times less than 1 minute, and low chain length limiting the combination possibilities; e.g., there are only 7310 possible mutants of MNV-11 containing two base transitions), an at least temporary steady state is reached, where all mutants with low Hamming distance from the master sequence are represented deterministically.

The mutant production equation is also valid in the linear growth phase. However, whereas in the exponential growth phase all W values are constants, this is not true in the linear growth phase. The probability of mutation events during a replication round is not affected, but for the evaluation of the W values, the κ values have to be replaced by the selection values mentioned above (for a detailed discussion, see Biebricher et al. 1985). In the linear growth phase, the selection values are dependent on the different mutant concentrations and are thus variables instead of constants. The selection pressure is different in the growth phases, and the quasi species formed in the two phases are probably quite different. The set of nonlinear differential equations cannot be solved analytically, but computer simulation by numerical integration remains possible. In the linear growth phase, competition between mutants is substantially different from competition between species, since loss terms by formation of heterologous double strands become crucial: No peaceful coexistence between closely related mutants is possible (Biebricher et al. 1985). On the other hand, alterations of sequence parts involved in the nucleation process of double-strand formation or alterations favoring different conformations of plus and minus strands provide protection from heterologous double-strand formation and thus selection advantages.

Experimental determination of quasi-species distributions is still in its beginnings. Fingerprinting investigations of different species have revealed an unusually high number of minor spots due to sequence heterogeneity. Schaffner et al. (1977), while sequencing one RNA species, also took all sequence alterations represented to more than 5% into account. The quasi-species distribution (which could not be determined in detail) was found to be centered around three related master sequences differing by four and seven base exchanges, where the structural effects are apparently cancelled. The "missing links" containing single mutation events, however, could not be detected (x_i values were too low), since the structure is disrupted in at least one of the complementary strands, thus abolishing template activity. Deletion of a five-nucleotide stretch was also observed.

We have found base insertions and deletions to be frequent errors during replication of MNV-11, particularly at the ends of the sequence. Presumably, the short stretch of base pairing at the replication fork allows slippage at certain sequences. A size distribution of single strands was found (Biebricher 1987); read-off sequencing methods consequently gave unsatisfactory results due to sequence superpositioning. Careful sizing of the strands before sequencing improved the results only partially, since deletions and insertions can compensate each other. Treatment of double-stranded MNV-11 with ribonuclease A introduced nicks into the double strand that yielded after melting an array of RNA fragments. The sequences of these RNA pieces were homogeneous, indicating that nicking occurred at mismatches.

Both fingerprinting and mismatching analyses give only information about error frequencies at different positions of the sequences, and no information at all of what the actual mutant populations look like. To determine a quasi-species distribution directly, we cloned an RNA quasi-species into DNA and sampled the sequences of a large number of clones. Figure 5 shows the MNV-11 sequence and indicates the positions where errors have been detected. Since DNA replication is much more accurate and lacks the bias of $Q\beta$ replicase, we anticipate eventually compiling a complete picture of the MNV-11 quasi-species population. Transcription of the DNA back into RNA should furthermore allow preparation of (at least initially) homogeneous mutant RNA, which will allow a determination of the effects of individual mutations on replication efficiency and selection values.

RNA Synthesis without Template Instruction

When serially diluted RNA template is added to incorporation mixtures, the lag times required for am-

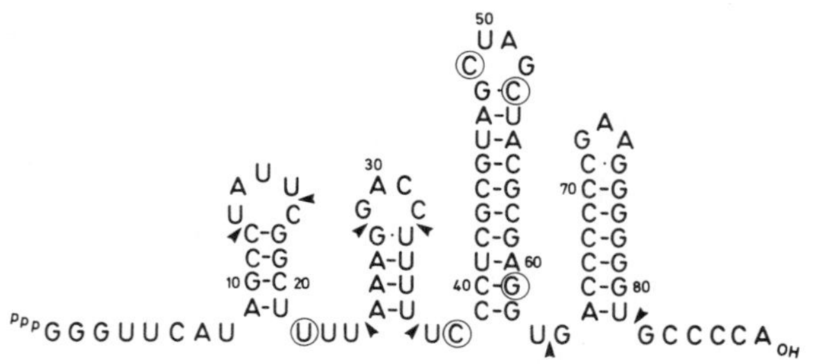

Figure 5. Nucleotide sequence of MNV-11 plus strand, determined by the chain-termination method (Sanger et al. 1977) from DNA clones obtained by retrotranscription of MNV-11 (Maniatis et al. 1982). RNA sequencing by the nuclease method (Donis-Keller et al. 1977) shows nucleotide ambiguity by mutation at the circled positions. Arrows indicate the positions where double-stranded MNV-11 is nicked by RNase treatment. The structure shown is confirmed by the nuclease data except for the stem at positions 25–36, which is unstable.

plification to macroscopic appearance are initially increased by constant time periods, showing that the overall replication rates in the exponential growth phase are independent of template concentration. As shown above, incorporation profiles are reproducible and the products are—disregarding mutation—copies of the template used. When the dilution reaches a certain threshold, corresponding to complete removal of template, the profiles change radically: The lag times become very extended and scatter, the profiles are irreproducible, and the products do not resemble the input template (Fig. 6). In addition, the products cannot be copies of self-replicating RNA present as impurity in the enzyme preparation (Biebricher et al. 1981b, 1986). The material must therefore have been produced de novo (Sumper and Luce 1975). (Participation of oligonucleotides present in the incorporation mixture cannot be ruled out.) At low enzyme or substrate concentrations or at elevated ionic strength, no de novo synthesis takes place; RNA molecules can be readily cloned under these conditions.

Other DNA and RNA polymerases are also capable of de novo synthesis (Kornberg et al. 1964; Krakow and Karstadt 1967). Even though the products of the different polymerases are different, the mechanism is probably similar for all polymerases. In a first step, nucleoside triphosphates are condensed to oligonucleotides more or less randomly. Once a self-replicating RNA, however poorly it may replicate, is formed, it is amplified rapidly in the usual template-instructed mechanism. Incorporation profiles show kinks, and new electrophoresis bands appear and replace others. Apparently, an evolutionary optimization process takes place, since the fingerprints of the new bands are closely related, whereas de novo products of different incorporation samples are completely different (Biebricher et al. 1981a). The phase of condensing nucleoside triphosphates could be observed directly with $Q\beta$ replicase when one (pyrimidine) nucleoside triphosphate was left out of the mixture, thus preventing amplification: Nucleoside triphosphates were then condensed, at a rate five orders of magnitude slower than template-instructed nucleotide incorporation, to generate a mixture of oligonucleotides of the composition $pppGpR(pN)_n$ peaking at chain lengths of 5–20, with a tail of longer material (Biebricher et al. 1986).

The process of optimization of early de novo products is also irreproducible; different but sequentially related optimization products were observed in different ("geographically isolated") test tubes, indicating that rare events are involved (Biebricher 1983). The mechanism of optimization is not clear. Probably insertions are involved, because nucleotides were found to be added slowly and nonrandomly to the 3' end of templates if initiation of new chains was suppressed by replacing GTP with ITP.

The biological significance of these noninstructed processes is not yet understood. Because they were found to proceed about five orders of magnitude more slowly even under conditions of high substrate and

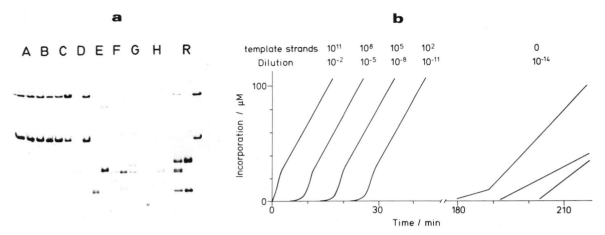

Figure 6. Template-instructed and template-free incorporation profiles. Serial dilutions of MDV-1 ($\sim 10^{12}$ strands/μl) were added to incubation mixtures. (*a*) Electropherogram of products after incubation overnight. Each dilution of MDV-1 was incubated in duplicate. Dilutions: (*A*) 10^{-8}; (*B*) 10^{-9}; (*C*) 10^{-10}; (*D*) 10^{-11}; (*E*) 10^{-12}; (*F*) 10^{-13}; (*G*) 10^{-14}; (*H*) without template addition; (*R*) MNV-11, SV-11, and MDV-1 as references. Note the stochastic behavior at *D*, where only a few strands are present per sample. (*b*) Kinetic profiles at serial dilutions of template. Conditions are similar to those of the experiments shown in Fig. 1.

enzyme concentrations, at less optimal conditions, these side reactions, including de novo synthesis, must be so slow that they could not be detected. I would thus argue that these processes are rare side reactions such as occur in any enzymatic reaction. Autocatalytic amplification of rare advantageous products can make those reactions detectable. Noninstructed RNA synthesis by Qβ replicase might also occur in vivo: the heterogeneous "6S" RNA found in infected cells (Banerjee et al. 1969) might be produced by a de novo process; there is no evidence that this RNA is derived from viral or bacterial genetic material.

DISCUSSION

The minimal requirements for efficient replication by Qβ replicase are not known. Necessary conditions are (1) a C cluster at the 3' end and a corresponding G cluster at the 5' end; (2) a stable secondary structure to lower the rate of double-strand formation after replication; and (3) possibly stable stems near the ends to prevent reformation of double strands between the single-stranded ends of replica and template during the replication process itself (Mills et al. 1987).

The requirements for tertiary structure, possibly the most important structural feature for competitive success, are unknown. Electrooptic measurements of several RNA species (Biebricher et al. 1982) have revealed similarities that might be interpreted as rigid "flower structures," which would also be compatible with electron microscopy observations. The resolution of structure by these experimental methods is too weak and can at best provide hints about the real structure.

Characterization of self-replicating RNA species has been so far restricted to the optimized species that can be readily prepared in large amounts. De novo experi-

ments provide an ample source of nonoptimized RNA templates, but the inherent irreproducibility of the de novo process itself and the difficulty of faithful amplification of poor templates have so far not allowed the preparation of sufficient quantities of such RNA species. The technology is now on hand: After cloning into DNA and amplification of the DNA, sufficient amounts of the RNA can be prepared by transcription. The optimization during amplification of de novo products leads to species with relatively well-defined sequences, which indicates that nearly every position of the chain has sufficient influence on the selection value to avoid sequence degeneracy. We also have no idea about the probability of finding—no matter how poorly—a self-replicating sequence. Experiments with cellular RNA have indicated that some RNAs, e.g., tRNA, are weakly bound by replicase and therefore ignored. Other RNAs, e.g., rRNA, are bound rather strongly, and we found evidence that Qβ replicase is working on it by condensing nucleotides to the 3' end, but it is unable to convert any resulting sequence to a self-replicating RNA species.

The catalytic activity of the RNA is apparently restricted to its role of complementing the replicase to form an active enzyme. Of the RNA species we investigated, none showed detectable self-splicing or other nucleotidyl transferase activities (Cech and Bass 1986; Been et al., this volume) in the absence of replicase under any of the conditions tested.

ACKNOWLEDGMENTS

The excellent assistance of Mr. R. Luce and Ms. M. Druminski is gratefully acknowledged. I am indebted to Drs. M. Eigen and W.C. Gardiner for stimulating discussions and many suggestions.

REFERENCES

Banerjee, A.K., U. Rensing, and J.T. August. 1969. Replication of RNA viruses. Replication of a natural 6 S RNA by the Qβ RNA polymerase. *J. Mol. Biol.* **45**: 181.

Batschelet, E., E. Domingo, and C. Weissmann. 1976. The proportion of revertant and mutant phage in a growing population, as a function of mutation and growth rate. *Gene* **1**: 27.

Biebricher, C.K. 1983. Darwinian selection of RNA molecules *in vitro*. *Evol. Biol.* **16**: 1.

———. 1986. Darwinian evolution of self-replicating RNA. *Chem. Scr.* **26B**: 51.

———. 1987. Replication and selection kinetics of short-chained RNA species. *UCLA Symp. Mol. Cell. Biol.* **54**: 9.

Biebricher, C.K., S. Diekmann, and R. Luce. 1982. Structural analysis of self-replicating RNA synthesized by Qβ replicase. *J. Mol. Biol.* **154**: 629.

Biebricher, C.K., M. Eigen, and W.C. Gardiner. 1983. Kinetics of RNA replication. *Biochemistry* **22**: 2544.

———. 1984. Kinetics of RNA replication: Plus-minus asymmetry and double-strand formation. *Biochemistry* **23**: 3186.

———. 1985. Kinetics of RNA replication: Competition and selection among self-replicating RNA species. *Biochemistry* **24**: 6550.

Biebricher, C.K., M. Eigen, and R. Luce. 1981a. Product analysis of RNA generated *de novo* by Qβ replicase. *J. Mol. Biol.* **148**: 369.

———. 1981b. Kinetic analysis of template-instructed and *de novo* RNA synthesis by Qβ replicase. *J. Mol. Biol.* **148**: 391.

———. 1986. Template-free RNA synthesis by Qβ replicase. *Nature* **321**: 89.

Blumenthal, T., T.A. Landers, and K. Weber. 1972. Bacteriophage Qβ replicase contains the protein biosynthesis elongation factors EF Tu and EF Ts. *Proc. Natl. Acad. Sci.* **69**: 1313.

Cech, T.R. and B.L. Bass. 1986. Biological catalysis by RNA. *Annu. Rev. Biochem.* **55**: 599.

Dickerson, R.E., M.L. Kopka, and P. Pjura. 1986. Pathways of information readout in DNA. *Chem. Scr.* **26B**: 139.

Dobkin, C., D.R. Mills, F.R. Kramer, and S. Spiegelman. 1979. RNA replication: Required intermediates and the dissociation of template, product, and Qβ replicase. *Biochemistry* **18**: 2038.

Domingo, E., D. Sabo, T. Taniguchi, and C. Weissmann. 1978. Nucleotide sequence heterogeneity of an RNA phage population. *Cell* **13**: 735.

Donis-Keller, H., A.M. Maxam, and W. Gilbert. 1977. Mapping adenines, guanines, and pyrimidines in RNA. *Nucleic Acids Res.* **4**: 2527.

Eigen, M. 1971. Selforganization of matter and the evolution of biological macromolecules. *Naturwissenschaften* **58**: 465.

Eigen, M. and C.K. Biebricher. 1987. Sequence space and quasispecies distribution. In *RNA genetics* (ed. E. Domingo et al.), vol. 3. CRC Press, Boca Raton, Florida. (In press.)

Haruna, I. and S. Spiegelman. 1965. Recognition of size and sequence by an RNA replicase. *Proc. Natl. Acad. Sci.* **54**: 1189.

Kamen, R. 1969. Infectivity of bacteriophage R17 RNA after sequential removal of 3′ terminal nucleotides. *Nature* **221**: 321.

Kornberg, A., L.L. Bertsch, J.F. Jackson, and H.G. Khorana. 1964. Enzymatic synthesis of DNA. XVI. Oligonucleotides as templates and the mechanism of their replication. *Proc. Natl. Acad. Sci.* **51**: 315.

Krakow, J.S. and M. Karstadt. 1967. *Azotobacter vinelandii* RNA polymerase. Unprimed synthesis of rIC copolymer. *Proc. Natl. Acad. Sci.* **58**: 2094.

Levisohn, R. and S. Spiegelman. 1969. Further extracellular Darwinian experiments with replicating RNA molecules: Diverse variants isolated under different selective condicions. *Proc. Natl. Acad. Sci.* **63**: 807.

Maniatis, T., E.F. Fritsch, and J. Sambrook. 1982. *Molecular cloning: A laboratory manual.* Cold Spring Harbor Laboratory, Cold Spring Harbor, New York.

Mekler, P. 1981. "Determination of nucleotide sequences of the bacteriophage Qβ genome: Organization and evolution of an RNA virus." Ph.D. thesis, University of Zurich, Switzerland.

Mills, D.R., F.R. Kramer, and S. Spiegelman. 1973. Complete nucleotide sequence of a replicating RNA molecule. *Science* **180**: 916.

Mills, D.R., R.L. Peterson, and S. Spiegelman. 1967. An extracellular Darwinian experiment with a self-duplicating nucleic acid molecule. *Proc. Natl. Acad. Sci.* **58**: 217.

Mills, D.R., C. Priano, and F.R. Kramer. 1987. Requirement for secondary structure formation during coliphage RNA replication. *UCLA Symp. Mol. Cell. Biol.* **54**: 35.

Mills, D.R., F.R. Kramer, C. Dobkin, T. Nishihara, and S. Spiegelman. 1975. Nucleotide sequence of microvariant RNA: Another small replicating molecule. *Proc. Natl. Acad. Sci.* **72**: 4252.

Mills, D.R., T. Nishihara, C. Dobkin, F.R. Kramer, P.E. Cole, and S. Spiegelman. 1977. The role of template structure in the recognition mechanism of Qβ replicase. In *Nucleic acid–protein recognition* (ed. H.J. Vogel), p. 533. Springer-Verlag, New York.

Moser, H. 1958. Structure and dynamics of bacterial populations maintained in the chemostat. *Cold Spring Harbor Symp. Quant. Biol.* **22**: 121.

Rensing, U. and J.T. August. 1969. The 3′-terminus and the replication of phage RNA. *Nature* **224**: 853.

Sanger, F., S. Nicklen, and A.R. Coulson. 1977. DNA sequencing with chain-terminating inhibitors. *Proc. Natl. Acad. Sci.* **74**: 5463.

Schaffner, W., K.J. Rüegg, and C. Weissmann. 1977. Nanovariant RNAs: Nucleotide sequence and interaction with bacteriophage Qβ replicase. *J. Mol. Biol.* **117**: 877.

Sumper, M. and R. Luce. 1975. Evidence for *de novo* production of self-replicating and environmentally adapted RNA structures by bacteriophage Qβ replicase. *Proc. Natl. Acad. Sci.* **72**: 162.

Wahba, A.J., M.J. Miller, A. Niveleau, T.A. Landers, G.G. Carmichael, K. Weber, D.A. Hawley, and L.I. Slobin. 1974. Subunit I of Qβ replicase and 30 S ribosomal protein S1 of *Escherichia coli*. Evidence for the identity of the two proteins. *J. Biol. Chem.* **249**: 3314.

Weber, H. and C. Weissmann. 1970. The 3′-termini of bacteriophage Qβ plus and minus strands. *J. Mol. Biol.* **51**: 215.

Weissmann, C. 1974. The making of a phage. *FEBS Lett. (suppl.)* **40**: S10.

Wickner, R.B. 1986. Double-stranded RNA replication in yeast: The killer system. *Annu. Rev. Biochem.* **55**: 373.

New Concepts for Dealing with the Evolution of Nucleic Acids

M. EIGEN

Max-Planck-Institut für Biophysikalische Chemie, Goettingen, West Germany

If we are asked where the transition from nonlife to life occurred, we must first refer to the conceptual level of DNA, of RNA, or of any of their self-replicating precursors. If we take any class of chemical compounds that are composed of a finite number of monomeric types, which we may call symbols, and if these symbols are lined up in linear sequences, thereby representing messages that can be "read" through specific interactions (i.e., complementary base pairing), then our class of compounds embodies a new property that goes beyond chemistry: This property is *information*. Such a quality can no longer be called typical for chemistry; it is characteristic of biology.

The property of self-reproduction—unique to DNA, to RNA, or to any analogous precursor polymer—has two consequences. (1) The information stored in the sequence of symbols is conserved in replication; this provides a genetic memory that resists the destruction to which all chemical compounds are subject. (2) The inherently autocatalytic nature of replication is the basis of selective evaluation and hence the basis of evolutionary optimization.

The first consequence of self-reproduction (i.e, replication, providing conservation of genetic information despite a steady chemical destruction) is obvious, whereas the second consequence is not as clear and therefore deserves some explanation. If we denote by c_i the concentration of template i and by k_i its growth constant, the rate of self-reproduction can be expressed by $dc_i(t)/dt = k_i c_i(t)$, which in the absence of growth limitation means:

$$c_i(t) = c_i(t = 0) \exp(k_i t) \qquad (1)$$

Now consider competition among many templates l present in the system. We are interested in relative, rather than absolute, population numbers or concentrations, i.e., $x_i = c_i/\Sigma_l c_l$. If we write the above differential equation in terms of relative concentrations x_i, we obtain the nonlinear differential equation:

$$dx_i(t)/dt = \{k_i - \bar{k}(t)\} x_i(t) \qquad (2)$$

where $\bar{k}(t) = \Sigma_l k_l x_l(t)$ is a function of time representing the average growth constant. Equation 2 tells us that it is replication that causes natural selection, because for any $k_i < \bar{k}(t)$, the rate dx_i/dt will be negative and hence x_i will decay, whereas for any $k_j > \bar{k}(t)$, the rate of dx_j/dt will be positive and x_j will increase. In this way, the average $\bar{k}(t)$ will increase steadily until $\bar{k}(t)$ reaches

k_m, where the index m refers to the type exhibiting maximum growth rate. Once this state is reached, all x_k values except x_m will have decayed to zero, and hence the compound m ($x_m = 1$) is the only survivor (regardless of whether the system as a whole grows or whether it reaches a steady state). Note that the extremum principle $\bar{k}(t) \rightarrow k_m$ describes a new category of chemical behavior (we may call it selection) entirely different from the category of material behavior called equilibration. Equilibration will always yield finite concentration ratios:

$$x_i/x_m = \exp - (\Delta G_{im}/RT) \qquad (3)$$

where ΔG_{im} is the free enthalpy difference between states i and m.

Since the extremum principle behind equilibration is of a more general nature than that for natural selection—it holds for any type of reaction (near equilibrium)—we require for selection that the replicating system stay sufficiently far from equilibrium. In fact, all nucleic acids in natural, i.e., in aqueous, environments are synthesized from energy-rich monomers and decay into energy-deficient products and hence represent metastable intermediates that are far from chemical equilibrium. Since all living beings come about by reproduction, which is eventually related to replication of their genomic DNA, they are subject to natural selection, although the processes involved are generally of much more subtle nature than expressed by the simple equations given above.

Even for simple RNA replicator systems, Equation 2 can only show that natural selection is a consequence of replication. For any realistic description, one would at least have to include mutation terms. In classic population genetics of vegetatively reproducing organisms such as prokaryotes (or viruses), mutation is generally introduced as a small perturbation, superimposed upon reproduction. As a result, the following five statements have become popular in evolutionary biology:

1. The target of selection is the wild type, which is the best-adapted type under given natural conditions. Hence, fitness is a property of single types.
2. Selectively neutral mutants grow up independently of population size. Hence, there is a steady random drift of sequence composition in the population.
3. Unique sequences signalize homogeneous wild-type populations. Nonhomogeneous populations are the result of hot spots of mutation.

4. Mutants appear randomly. There is no special bias that induces the preferred appearance of mutants that are better adapted.

5. Evolutionary optimization is due to random search for the best-adapted type.

This interpretation of Darwinian behavior, if correct, would be very difficult to represent quantitatively. The enormously large number of possible mutants of even relatively short sequences is prohibitive for any random search algorithm. A sequence of length 300 (encoding a protein of only 100 amino acid residues) possesses no less than about 10^{23} possible ten-error mutants. If any such mutant were required in the optimization procedure, its probability of occurrence by chance would be hopelessly small. Hence, evolution according to a random mutation algorithm would have to be based on small error mutations and thereby would soon get stuck on minor local fitness peaks, unless fitness were, in general, to increase monotonically with decreasing distance to the target sequence of optimal fitness.

In this paper, it is shown that taking correct account of mutations leads to results that modify the above statements considerably. In particular, it is shown that for molecular (including viral) populations of sufficiently large size (typical for laboratory experiments), the following statements are more appropriate:

1. The target of selection is not the single wild type, but rather the total mutant distribution, called quasi species.

2. Neutral mutants modify the quasi-species distribution to a considerable extent but, in sufficiently large populations, generally do not lead to random drift.

3. Despite the appearance of a unique sequence, the underlying wild type is usually present only in relatively small numbers. The sequence in the population appears to be uniform, since it is a defined consensus sequence. So-called "hot spots" in sequences are more likely to be due to the presence of nearly neutral mutants than to greatly increased mutation rates.

4. Nearly neutral mutants not only are present, but also form more frequently than deleterious ones, because fitness is clustered in connected mutant domains.

5. Evolutionary optimization is biased by the mutant population and proceeds along continuous routes of increasing fitness through intermediates that are nearly neutral.

New concepts favoring this modified interpretation of Darwinian behavior are described below.

NEW CONCEPTS THAT APPLY TO NUCLEIC ACID SEQUENCES

Sequence Space

DNA and RNA sequences are an invaluable source of evolutionary information and, given the wealth of data already available, comparative sequence analysis has become the most powerful tool of evolutionary research. To organize the data and to characterize possible kinships, it is important to have an appropriate space of representation. Phylogenetic analysis usually starts from the assumption of consecutive divergence and therefore tries to organize the data so as to make them fit an optimal tree-like topology. Inherent in such a procedure is the supposition of a metric space of distances. The distance is the number of positions that, in any pair of partially homologous (aligned) sequences, are differently occupied. Partial homology of sequences may be the result either of common ancestry or of convergent adaptation. Distances depend not only on mutation rates, but also on the probability of acceptance or fixation after mutation has occurred. Mutation rates often differ for transitions and transversions, and, most certainly, fixation rates depend on the functional relevance of the particular position that has mutated. We therefore cannot expect that a distance metric will generally be uniform.

In a bundle-like divergence, one may easily test the uniformity of distance metric by vertical analysis of a set of aligned sequences. For every position in the alignment, one can determine a consensus occupation, i.e., the symbol (A, U, G, or C) that appears most frequently. We then record how many sequences at a particular position deviate from the consensus sequence. In the histogram in Figure 1, the abscissa shows how many sequences deviate from the consensus at a given position and the ordinate indicates for how many positions this is the case. An abscissa value of zero thus means that all sequences are identically occupied at some positions, and the ordinate value shows for how many positions this is true. An ordinate value corresponding to about three quarters of the aligned sequences indicates complete randomization, i.e., accidental agreements with any of the four nucleotides. The histogram in Figure 1 refers to three families of tRNA sequences (Eigen and Winkler-Oswatitsch 1981a,b) and shows that a large number of positions are entirely invariant, probably owing to the presence of some bias, whereas the other positions show all degrees of variance up to complete randomization. In contrast, a computer simulation with a uniform probability of substitution at each position gives a Gaussian distribution with well-defined mean and variance.

We therefore prefer to use a space of representation for which the distance metric is left open. Such a space has been introduced in "informatics" (Hamming 1980) and was proposed for the representation of nucleic acids (Rechenberg 1973). The following requirements for such a space should be met (Eigen 1985, 1986; Schuster 1986; Schuster and Swetina 1987).

1. Each sequence should be represented by a discrete position in this space. Since there are 4^ν possible sequences of length ν, the capacity must be adequately high. (To give an example: our universe, or better, a sphere with a radius of 10^{10} light years comprises about 10^{108} cubes of 1-Å edge lengths. A nucleic acid molecule of only 180 nucleotides has equally many possible different sequences, i.e., $4^{180} \approx 10^{108}$.)

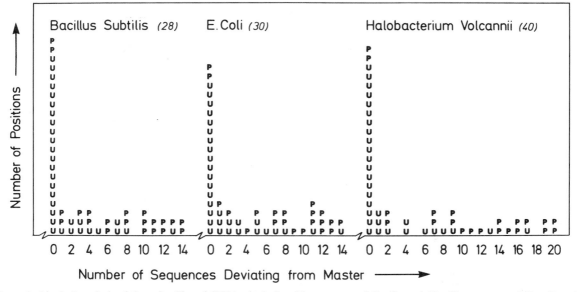

Figure 1. Vertical analysis of three families of tRNAs, including 28 sequences of *Bacillus subtilis*, 30 sequences of *E. coli*, and 40 sequences of *Halobacterium volcanii*. U refers to unpaired positions, and P refers to base-paired positions that were counted as one position. The sequences were given in binary, i.e., *R-Y* notation. Note (1) the disproportionately large number of constant positions (zero deviation from master) and (2) the nonhomologous variability of the rest of the positions, ranging from zero deviation to complete randomization (M. Eigen et al., in prep.).

2. The space must correctly reflect kinships among *all* sequences. Hence, sequences that differ at only one position must be arranged such that they are nearest neighbors. It is easily seen that such a space requires many dimensions, depending on the sequence length ν.

The space is otherwise not constrained to a particular metric. Distances, for instance, are counted like street-block distances, without defining their length. Figure 2 shows with an example of binary sequences how such a space may be built up in an iterative way by doubling each former arrangement. For binary sequences, the dimension of the sequence space then equals the sequence length ν, comprising 2^ν possible alternatives. It is easily seen that for quarternary sequences such as nucleic acids, the dimension is 2ν, allowing for a mapping of 4^ν different sequences. One possible way to represent a quarternary sequence space is to start with the hypercube in Figure 2, in which each point specifies only a sequence given in R,Y notation (R is purine and Y is pyrimidine) and then to attach to each of the points another ν-dimensional binary space, where each point specifies for the particular R,Y sequence which of the two bases represent $R(G,A)$ or $Y(C,U)$. An alternative means of representation might consist of an interlocked set of self-similar tetrahedra. The four equivalent corners of each tetrahedron are attached to the four bases A,U,G,C.

Figure 2 gives us some idea of the features of multidimensional hypercubes that are important for our purposes.

1. The capacity of representation is adequate. Remember that a dimension of 360 is sufficient to map the 10^{108} cubes of 1-Å edge lengths that would fill a three-dimensional sphere having a radius of 10^{10} light years.

2. Despite the large capacity of representation, detour-free distances always remain smaller than the dimension (detour-free means the most direct and loop-free connection between two points). Again, the above example may help us to imagine this: In the 360-dimensional hypercube mapping the universe, the largest distance is equivalent to 360 Å, rather than to 10^{10} light years as in three-dimensional representation.

3. The connectivity in multidimensional spaces is enormous, especially if jumps are allowed. If k-fold jumps (k-error mutants) are allowed, one may reach from any point of the hypercube a total of $\binom{\nu}{k}$ different neighboring states; in the above example, with $k = 10$, this is about 10^{19} states.

Fitness Topography

The peculiar properties of multidimensional hypercubes, such as large capacity, short distances, and high connectivity, would be of only little importance if the evolutionary process (which may be described now as a search process in sequence space) were entirely random in nature. In such a case, a major part of all alternatives would have to be checked before the target—an optimal sequence—could be reached. We must therefore look for properties that might provide guidance in such a search process. Short distances will then prove to be of great advantage, whereby the high connectivity may provide an escape from possible traps.

In the simple Darwinian picture, survival would mean that a given population occupies a local fitness peak in sequence space. Mutation may make such a

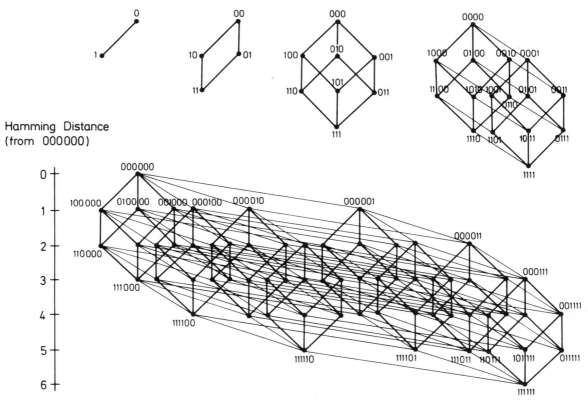

Figure 2. Recursive representation of sequence space. In each successive step, the former diagram is doubled, and positions corresponding to each other in the doubled diagram are connected. The lines in this representation connect only nearest neighbors (disregarding multiple mutations) (M. Eigen et al., in prep.).

distribution somewhat diffuse, but selection means that it is definitely localized in a certain region of sequence space.

To calculate the population structure, we have to know the fitness landscape. Fitness, of course, depends on the evolutionary target and on the environmental conditions under which evolutionary adaptation occurs. Hence, it may change with time; but, at any instant, a certain topography of fitness values for all points on the hypercube will exist.

How must we imagine such a topography? It certainly will not be random (Eigen 1986). Altitudes on earth are not randomly distributed either. As Mandelbrot (1983) has shown, even in the absence of any long-range order, height distributions on earth are of a fractal nature. Altitudes do not usually change abruptly; a peak is not a singularity in altitude, but rather a more or less smooth distribution with continuous variation. High peaks are separated further than are the lower peaks situated between them. There are large planes with no peaks at all, and mountain regions with many peaks of various sizes in a self-similar distribution. A fitness landscape should also have the same nature because there is a similarity relationship: Similar primary sequences will cause similar spatial structures, which in turn may produce similar functional qualities. Experiments utilizing site-directed mutagenesis have shown that this is generally true. Minor changes in gene sequences cause, in most cases, only minor changes in

functional (e.g., enzymatic) properties. There are, of course, critical positions whose correct occupation is absolutely obligatory. Likewise, in mountain landscapes, we may also find abrupt changes in altitude.

The connective nature of fitness landscapes provides gradients for evolutionary optimization. The usual strategy in mountain climbing is to start from a pass and then to follow a ridge up to the peak. The same may be true for evolutionary optimization, but the major difference is that the fitness landscape refers to a multidimensional space. Mandelbrot (1983) has shown that in a mountainous landscape of sufficiently high dimension, a raindrop falling at any site will always eventually reach the ocean. The high connectivity in the hypercube, especially if mutational jumps are allowed, has been shown to increase greatly the number of routes that lead to the highest peaks. Here, the enormous connectivity of points that may be reached by way of mutational jumps prevents the process from getting stuck on any minor fitness peak.

The Concept of Quasi Species

Little is known about the detailed shapes of fitness landscapes, required in order to calculate a population structure and its distribution in sequence space. The examples given below refer to some simple types of fitness structures.

How does fitness or value topography map into

population topography? To calculate relative population numbers x_i (cf. above), we must start from the kinetic equations dx_i/dt for each of the sequence states and take into account all possible mutation terms. The equations (Eigen 1971; Eigen and Schuster 1979; Schuster and Sigmund 1985; Eigen and Biebricher 1987) are of the form:

$$dx_i/dt = \{W_{ii} - \bar{E}(t)\}x_i + \sum_{1 \neq i} W_{il}x_1 \qquad (4)$$

which can be transformed to

$$dy_i/dt = \{\lambda_i - \bar{\lambda}(t)\}y_i \qquad (5)$$

(Thompson and McBride 1974; Jones et al. 1976), which is formally identical to Equation 1. $\bar{\lambda}(t) \equiv \bar{E}(t)$ is the average of all eigenvalues and represents the average excess production of the total system (similar to $\bar{k}(t)$ in Eq. 1). Equation 3 again describes selection as a consequence of self-reproduction, but unlike Equation 1, it no longer refers to single types as characterized by the individual relative population variables x_i. The population variable y_i refers rather to what we call a quasi species, i.e., a mutant "clan" that is ordered around one or a degenerate set of selected master sequences, containing weighted contributions from all mutants present in the distribution. Selection again means that only one such mutant distribution survives, namely, the one associated with a maximum eigenvalue λ_m:

$$\bar{\lambda}(t) \rightarrow \lambda_m \qquad (6)$$

This distribution, and not a single type, is the target of selection. To know the population structure, one has to solve explicitly the system of kinetic equations (Eq. 4) (Rumschitzki 1987). The rate coefficients W_{ii} reflect in their absolute values the detailed structure of the fitness landscape. The matrix of rate coefficients is related to the error or mutation matrix, with the diagonal terms referring to zero error, i.e., to exact self-reproduction. For uniform error models, this matrix can be built up iteratively in the same way that was shown for the binary sequence space model in Figure 2.

Let us consider some concrete systems that have been simulated on the computer. They show, more than abstract mathematical considerations can, the physical nature of selection. The essential quantities that determine the population structure of a selected quasi-species distribution are the following. The sequence length ν, which has been (but need not be) assumed to be uniform, is, so to speak, a measure of the amount of information contained in the sequence. This information must not get lost in successive replications. Hence, there must be an average fidelity $\bar{q}$ for reproducing a single nucleotide ($0 < \bar{q} < 1$) that is the geometric mean of the probabilities of correct reproduction taken over all positions in the sequence. The average error rate per position then is $(1 - \bar{q})$, referring to misincorporation of any of the three alternative (noncomplementary) nucleotides. For the total se-

quence, the expectation value of errors is $\nu(1 - \bar{q})$ and the quality of reproduction, i.e., the probability of error-free reproduction Q_{ii}, is given by $\bar{q}^\nu$. For stable selection, there must be an error threshold that depends on the fitness of the master sequence relative to its mutant competitors and that can be expressed by a superiority coefficient $\sigma > 1$. The error threshold relationship then is approximately (Eigen 1971; McCaskill 1984)

$$\nu(1 - \bar{q}) < \ln \sigma \qquad (7)$$

This threshold relationship indicates that selection may be regarded as a kind of phase transition in sequence space. Violation of Equation 7 means the accumulation of errors in successive replications and thereby the "melting" of information. Indeed, it has been shown that $\ln \{\bar{q}/(1 - \bar{q})\}$ may be treated as the analog of an inverse temperature. Equation 7 then shows that there is a critical temperature (similar to the Curie temperature in ferromagnetism) where the phase transition occurs (Leuthäusser 1986).

The phase-transition-like behavior is clearly demonstrated by the computer simulations illustrated in Figure 3 (Swetina and Schuster 1982). The diagrams show relative population numbers x_i as functions of error rate $(1 - \bar{q})$. The example in Figure 3 refers to binary sequences of length $\nu = 50$. The master sequence (index 0) has a (diagonal) replication rate coefficient $W_o = 10$, whereas for all its mutant competitors (indices 1, 2, etc. refer to error classes, i.e., numbers of errors in sequence) $W_i = 1$ (all mutants being degenerate). Only at error rate $(1 - \bar{q}) = 0$ is the result a clear "survival of the fittest" ($x_o = 1$; $x_{i \neq o} = 0$). With increasing error rate, the relative population number of the master sequence decreases sharply, although the quasi species remains stable. Near the threshold at $(1 - \bar{q}) = (\ln 10)/50 = 0.046$, the master sequence drops to very low population numbers (cf. semilogarithmic plot in Fig. 3); however, sequence analysis would still clearly reveal the same uniform sequence as the consensus sequence of the symmetrically distributed quasi species. Only by crossing the threshold would the sequence sharply randomize and thereby disappear, and only then is its information irretrievably lost. Crossing the threshold means that all $2^{50} \approx 10^{15}$ sequences, including the former master sequence, drop to the same low relative expectance value of about 10^{-15} and hence, for a finite population size, appear only sporadically.

The above example illustrates well the physical nature of selection, which may be understood as a condensation of a sequence distribution in a particular, although extended, region of sequence (or information) space. However, it is otherwise quite unrealistic, in particular with respect to the assumed symmetrical value landscape. In real systems, there will not be just one clearly defined master sequence, nor will the mutants be degenerate or symmetric with respect to their individual fitness values. Let us therefore briefly consider another, still oversimplified, simulation experi-

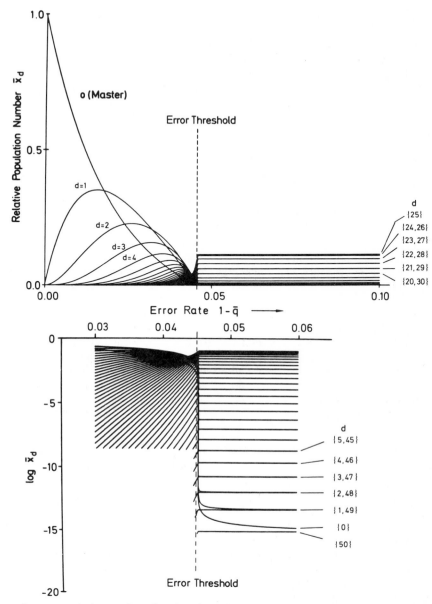

Figure 3. Relative stationary population numbers $\bar{x}_d$ as functions of mean error rate $(1 - \bar{q})$. The index d refers to the mutation or Hamming distance d (see text). The top diagram records population numbers and the bottom diagram records their logarithms. The population numbers of mutants with Hamming distance $d > 0$ refer to the whole mutant class, i.e., to the sum of all mutants in class d. Note the clearly defined error threshold, which characterizes selection as a kind of phase transition in sequence space (Swetina and Schuster 1982).

ment (Swetina and Schuster 1982) which shows more clearly it is the whole mutant distribution, and not just the master sequence, that is evaluated by natural selection.

Again, all sequences have a length of $\nu = 50$ and, for simplicity, are assumed to be binary. This time, we have two sequences at the extreme mutation distance (Hamming distance) $d = 50$ that are nearly equally fit, W_o being 10 and W_{50} being 9. If all mutants were degenerate, we would clearly obtain (below error threshold) a sharp selection of the sequence with index 0, and this would still be true if the difference between

W_o and W_{50} were much smaller. However, the 50 one-error mutants of the sequence with index 50 (we may give them the index 49 because they are 49-error mutants of sequence 0) are assumed to be better adapted than the rest of mutants, i.e., $W_{49} = 5$, while $W_i (i \neq 0,$ 49, 50) = 1. In other words, the best-adapted sequence $(W_o = 10)$ is surrounded by 50 one-error mutants $(W_o = 1)$ that are not as well adapted as the 50 one-error mutants $(W_{49} = 5)$ of a far distant $(d = 50)$ and slightly inferior sequence $(W_{50} = 9)$. The result of the competition is that at zero error rate, sequence 0 clearly wins and remains dominant with increasing error rate until its error threshold is reached. So far, the result is quite analogous to the one shown in Figure 3. However, at the error threshold of sequence 0, a new quasi species builds up around sequence 50, which, under these conditions, is still stable until, with increasing error rate, it reaches a second threshold, at which the whole distribution finally becomes random.

This experiment shows clearly that the target of selection is not necessarily the fittest single type, but rather the fittest quasi species, in which the master sequence and all mutant sequences are rated with respect to their fitness. It now becomes obvious that we must redefine the term "wild type." The result also raises the question of how to define "neutral" types. So far, one has regarded two types as being neutral if their relative fitnesses differ by less than $1/N$, N being the effective population size (Kimura and Ohta 1971; Kimura 1983). Our theory does not have to define neutrals in this way, since every mutant is rated according to its true relative fitness. As the above example shows, a relative fitness difference of 0.1 at large population sizes (which for molecular distributions usually are of

the order of magnitude of 10^{10}) may be sufficient to cause neutrality or even an entire change of fitness, depending on error rate. Indeed, we must ask, Does neutrality exist at all at population sizes typical for molecular, viral, or microorganismic distributions? It would require not only (nearly) identical types, but also practically identical fitness landscapes around the identical types. In our experiments, transitions are always extremely sharp, such that at typical molecular population sizes, coexistence of two distant neutral types was never found. Neutral drift should thus be limited to relatively small populations and large genome sizes, i.e., to higher organisms. Only then is mutation a truly stochastic and irreproducible event. On the other hand, the importance of nearly neutral types for evolution is stressed in our model even more than in neutral theory.

The third example, in particular, will confirm the above statement. In Figure 4, two nonoverlapping regions of sequence space are depicted. We consider a sequence of about 300 positions, i.e., of the size of a small gene. If each digit accounts for two positions in the sequence, the states of each region will refer to all

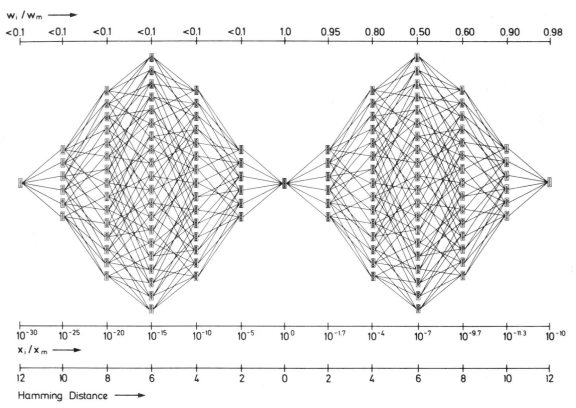

Figure 4. Two regions of 12-error mutants and their precursors in sequence space are represented. Each symbol refers to two positions; hence, the six symbols quoted cover a range up to $d = 12$. In the left-hand region, the selection value drops sharply to less than 10% of the master value and remains at a low level (plane region in value landscape). The right-hand region represents a typical mountain landscape. The selection value drops from the master value to some valley position (half of the master value) at $d = 6$ and increases again to a second peak at $d = 12$. The top row of numbers records the relative selection values, and the bottom row records the corresponding relative population numbers (with respect to master). Note that the relative population numbers in the left-hand half drop quickly to unrealizable values, whereas in the right-hand half, they remain realizable. A 12-error mutant in the right-hand diagram is bound to appear deterministically, whereas in the left-hand diagram, it will never show up. (Note the many orders of magnitude.)

precursors of a particular 12-error mutant (cf. the bottom line, which records the Hamming distance). (We chose this representation with six digits because the detailed network with 12 digits would be too difficult to survey.) A binary sequence of 300 digits has $\binom{300}{12} \sim 10^{21}$ such 12-error regions, of which only 25 regions are nonoverlapping. Hence, what is shown in Figure 4 is only a small section of the total 12-error neighborhood of the master sequence. The two regions now differ in that the left region has a fitness landscape for which all $W_i < 0.1\ W_o$, whereas the right region shows a typical "mountain region" value profile (the fitness values are given in the line above the diagram). The numbers on the line below the diagram then give the relative population numbers of the various sequence states. In the left-hand region, which represents a fitness plane, the population number decreases for every two mutation steps by about a factor 10^5 (for each mutation: 300), whereas in the right-hand region, the mountain site, and thus the relatively high fitness of the mutants, modifies the population numbers considerably. A 12-error mutant in the left-hand region has an expectation value, relative to the master sequence, of 10^{-30}, whereas the expectation value of the 12-error mutant in the right-hand region lies only 10 to 11 orders of magnitude below that of the master sequence. If selective advantage were to require a mutation at 12 positions, the particular mutant in a plane region, given a typical laboratory sample of, for example, 10^{12} sequences, would practically never appear, whereas in the mountain region it would occur with almost deterministic predictability. An advantageous 12-error mutant would certainly not be situated in the midst of a planar fitness landscape. Rather, it would be expected in the mountain region and, as is seen, there is systematic guidance through the population of intermediates that increases the likelihood of appearance of an advantageous mutant over a disadvantageous mutant by many orders of magnitude. The truly surprising fact is how large the effect turns out to be. One may also say that evolution will, almost deterministically, proceed only in connected mountain ridges in the fitness landscape. Note that this important guidance only becomes effective in the multidimensional landscape of sequence space. It requires a sufficiently large population in which the relevant mutant states are populated. A few out of a total of 10^{12} sequences are sufficient to effect this guidance. To find such relatively rare mutants, one would have to carry out systematic cloning experiments and try to establish a topographic map of the value landscape.

Statistical Geometry

The concept of sequence space may also be applied to comparative sequence analysis. It was shown that cumulative distances among any pair of sequences may be misleading if the distance metric is not uniform for all positions. Yet most methods of comparative sequence analysis in use are based on distances. One

possible way out of these difficulties would be to identify positions that show uniform divergences and to modify the distance analysis correspondingly. One step in this direction was taken by Kimura (1980), who devised a formula for evolutionary distance that takes into consideration possible differences in transition and transversion rates. Another straightforward approach for determining correct topologies of divergence is a method that we have called statistical geometry (M. Eigen et al.; A.M. Dress et al.; both in prep.).

Statistical geometry tries to combine horizontal and vertical (i.e., position-specific) analyses of a set of aligned sequences. It starts from subsets of, for example, four sequences that are projected into sequence space. It is "geometry," since the four-sequence correlations can be represented by geometric figures, the various connecting lines of which refer to positionally different classes of distances representing differing degrees of divergence. It is "statistical," since it considers all possible quartets of sequences and thereby determines average geometries. Note that a set of 40 sequences involves $\binom{40}{4} \approx 10^5$ different quartets. The method is outlined for the lucid example of quartets of binary (R,Y) sequences in Figure 5. Eight individual distances, or three classes of distances, are distinguished by this analysis. The optimal topology is obtained as a result subject to mathematical criteria. (Note that tree analysis usually starts from the assumption of a tree topology, the most parsimonious den-

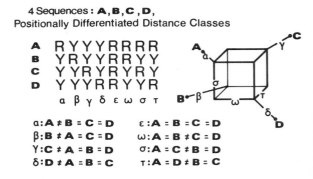

4 Sequences : **A , B , C , D ,**
Positionally Differentiated Distance Classes

A	R Y Y Y R R R R	
B	Y R Y Y R R Y Y	
C	Y Y R Y R Y R Y	
D	Y Y Y R R R Y Y R	
	α β γ δ ε ω σ τ	

α : **A ≠ B = C = D**   ε : **A = B = C = D**
β : **B ≠ A = C = D**   ω : **A = B ≠ C = D**
γ : **C ≠ A = B = D**   σ : **A = C ≠ B = D**
δ : **D ≠ A = B = C**   τ : **A = D ≠ B = C**

Distance Classes ⟨averages⟩

Mean Branch Length : · · · · · · · · · 1/4(α + β + γ + δ)
Deviations from   ⎧ l = Max (ω, σ, τ)
Tree- and Bundlelikeness · · · · · · · ⎨ m = Inf (ω, σ, τ)
Tree : l + S > 2m , Bundle : l + S ≈ 2m , ⎩ S = Min (ω, σ, τ)
Number of Homologies : · · · · · · · · · ε

Figure 5. The method of statistical geometry is illustrated with an example of four binary (R,Y) sequences. Eight distance classes (α, β, γ, δ, ω, σ, and τ) can be put into three categories: (1) All sequences agree (ϵ); (2) all but one sequence agree (α, β, γ, and δ); and (3) there is a mutually exclusive, pairwise agreement of two sequences (ω, σ, and τ). The situation can be represented geometrically as a projection into a subspace of sequence space (cf. Fig. 2). The topology then results from the relative magnitudes of the class distances as specified above. Such an analysis is to be carried out for all $\binom{n}{4}$ sequence combinations that are possible in a set of n sequences, yielding reliable figures for the average class distances.

drogram of which is then searched for by suitable optimization algorithms.) Referring to Figure 5, we may distinguish three obvious cases of statistical results:

1. If the averages of all three box dimensions (ω, σ, τ) remain small with respect to the averages of the protrusions (α, β, γ, δ), then the divergence is bundle-like, with a small degree of randomization. For an ideal bundle, $\omega = \sigma = \tau = 0$; otherwise, $\omega > \sigma > \tau > 0$.

2. If one box parameter is essentially larger than the two others, in particular, if the sum of the largest and smallest box dimensions is considerably larger than twice the medium box dimensions (i.e., $\omega + \tau - 2\sigma \gg 0$), then we are dealing with a tree-like (i.e., consecutive) divergence, again with small randomization if $\sigma, \tau \ll \alpha, \beta, \gamma, \delta$, whereas an ideal tree requires σ and τ to be zero.

3. Finally, if the box dimensions are comparable to, or even larger than, the protrusions and if, in particular, $\omega + \tau - 2\sigma \approx 0$, then the distribution is randomized. The precursor may have been either a bundle, a tree, or a quasi-species-like network.

Figure 6 shows an example of four ribosomal 5S RNA sequences that diverged quite early in evolution. The dendrogram based on distances (Fig. 6, top) suggests an ideal tree-like divergence with a relatively small nodal distance. However, the sequence-space analysis (Fig. 6, bottom) reveals that the ideal distance dendrogram results from some error compensation. The true randomization may be taken from the box dimensions, which reveal themselves as more bundle-like than tree-like, suggesting a nodal distance that is so small compared with the branches of independent divergence that it falls within the limits of randomization. Any point within the box, most probably a fairly central position, could be the earliest common node (Eigen et al. 1985).

An even more detailed specification of positionally differentiable distance classes is obtained for quartets of quarternary (A,U,G,C) sequences. The geometric figures obtained are then of a more sophisticated structure, but they are still well defined, so that statistical averages of all edge-classes can be obtained. These refer to the five poker combinations, i.e., for sequences A, B, C, and D, four of a kind: A = B = C = D; three of a kind: A = B = C $\neq$ D; one pair: A = B $\neq$ C $\neq$ D; two pairs: A = B $\neq$ C = D; and no pair A $\neq$ B $\neq$ C $\neq$ D.

Statistical geometry is an obvious application of the concept of sequence space to comparative sequence analysis, and it may be extended to higher correlations. In an age of sequence libraries, this method may prove to have many important applications (cf. the example below).

APPLICATIONS

This paper was intended mainly to review some new concepts that deal with the evolution of nucleic acids. Such a review would be incomplete without reference

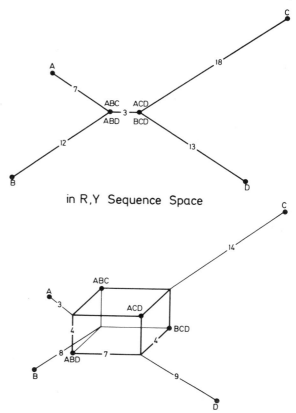

Figure 6. Four 5S rRNA sequences are compared in the upper half by plain RY-distance space analysis and in the lower half by RY sequence space analysis. The four sequences (two archaebacterial, one eubacterial, and one from a blue-green alga) have diverged during a quite early phase of evolution, and hence there is much noise superimposed on their early divergence. The distance analysis does not reflect this situation correctly, whereas the sequence space analysis shows that any early internodal distance is entirely obliterated by noise. The true nodes may be at any position within the box (Eigen et al. 1985). (*A*) *Bacillus pasteurii*; (*B*) *Halobacterium salinarium*; (*C*) *Anacystis nidulans*; (*D*) *Methanococcus vannielli*.

to experimental work that has been undertaken in order to test the new ideas. For a review of experimental approaches to artificial and natural RNA quasi species, see Biebricher (this volume). A brief survey of three types of applications is presented below. These applications refer to past, present, and future.

Reconstructing the Evolutionary Past

Nearly a thousand sequences of tRNA are known today (Sprinzl et al. 1987). They may be grouped into two categories: (1) about 15 families of tRNAs belonging to given species, such as *Escherichia coli, Bacillus subtilis, Halobacterium volcanii,* chloroplasts, mitochondria, yeast, *Drosophila,* and mammals, each family comprising between 20 and 45 individual tRNAs; and (2) about 24 individual tRNAs (defined by their anticodon) for which phylogenies can be reconstructed that include more than 15 (up to 40) species.

Obviously, divergence of tRNA within families should be largely bundle-like. It started in the time during which the genetic code was established and only the initial period could possibly reflect some tree-like divergence—if the genetic code originated in a successive fashion. The major time span, including about 3×10^9 years of phylogenetic divergence, must have produced a simultaneous and independent accumulation of mutations that proved to be acceptable. Phylogeny of a given tRNA, on the other hand, should be tree-like, offering the possibility of determining some early reference sequence. With 24 early reference sequences, we have another family (which existed about 3×10^9 years ago). It could now be compared with present families. Hence, a dating of the origin of the genetic code relative to the origin of early and present cells should be possible.

The data shown in Figure 1 suggested that the distance metric of tRNA sequences is highly nonuniform. We therefore used statistical geometry to produce kinship topologies (Eigen and Winkler-Oswatitsch 1981a,b). The results turned out to be quite self-consistent. Three categories of the 73 (i.e., 76 minus the anticodon) homologous positions of tRNAs could be established (referring to R, Y sequence notation): There are 25 invariant positions that agree in nearly all sequences studied and that refer to a possibly convergent evolution, biased by functional requirements. The rest of the 48 positions fall into two categories: 29 moderately variable positions and 19 highly variable positions. Owing to base-pairing requirements, they reduce to 20 moderately and 10 highly variable independent positions. The 20 moderately variable positions can be entirely reconstructed and, in terms of relative distances, dated. The 10 highly variable positions turn out to be completely randomized, not only in all present families, but also, to the same extent, in the precursor family of the 24 sequences mentioned. They probably refer to the initial divergence of a quasi-species distribution that was used for assignment of different amino acids to different adaptors. Remarkably, they contain a well-measurable residual tree-likeness that refers to a successive establishment of the genetic code. The relative divergences of the moderately variable positions suggest that the distance between origin of the code and divergence of first cells is only about one third to one fourth of the total distance of divergence of present families. Since error rate must have been higher in the early phases of evolution than in the later phases (where error-correcting mechanisms had been optimized and adapted to the large size of genomes), the time of origin of the genetic code dates back no more (and probably considerably less) than 4×10^9 years (supposing the first phylogenetic divergences appeared about 3×10^9 years ago). This may not surprise the biologists, but for the first time, it is a result that is based on experimental facts.

Quasi-species Distributions in the Present-day Natural Environment

Viruses seem to be the best candidates for a study of quasi species in a natural environment. Experimental evidence has been reviewed recently (Biebricher and Eigen 1987; Eigen and Biebricher 1987). By cloning single particles of the bacteriophage Qβ in *E. coli* cultures, Weissmann and co-workers demonstrated that in the amplified clones, sequences were uniform but slightly different from the wild type (Domingo et al. 1978). Weissmann concluded from his data that the extent of the presence of wild-type individuals is less than 5%. By serial dilution, one usually singles out those particles present in largest abundance. They will most probably be one- or two-error mutants that happen to be nearly neutral, since otherwise they would have had no chance to form a uniform distribution centered around the cloned mutant.

The formation of revertants makes it generally difficult to analyze cloned mutants. To obtain sufficient material for fingerprint or sequence analysis, the clones must be amplified through many generations. During this process, a mutant quasi species builds up that soon contains revertants that may outgrow the cloned mutant. This method will therefore only generate relatively well-adapted mutants. Sequence analysis requires approximately 10^9 particles, which is equivalent to 30 generations of clone amplification, or several hours to days. A mutant with only 10% reduced replication rate after 30 generations lags behind by about one order of magnitude in population number.

It is important to distinguish between mutant frequency [as expressed by relative population variables x_i] and mutation frequency or mutation rate [as expressed by $(1 - \bar{q})$]. The reason for a frequent appearance of particular mutants may be a high mutation rate at certain positions (hot spots); however, it may just as well mean that the particular mutants are nearly neutral and therefore are coselected. As the examples described above (see The Concept of Quasi Species) have shown, the latter effect may account for many orders of magnitude in population numbers of certain mutants. All data available for mutation rates of single-stranded RNA viruses indicate that the average error rate $(1 - \bar{q})$ is close to its threshold value, which through Equation 7 is related to the number of nucleotides (ν) in the viral genome. For phage Qβ, the sequence length ν is 4200 and $(1 - \bar{q})$ has been found to be 3×10^{-4} (Batschelet et al. 1976; Domingo et al. 1976). Similar results were reported for foot-and-mouth disease virus (Domingo et al. 1980) and vesicular stomatitis virus (Holland et al. 1982; Spindler et al. 1982; O'Hara et al. 1984; Schubert et al. 1984). For influenza virus with a total genome size (8 RNA units) of $\nu \approx 14,000$, an error rate $(1 - \bar{q})$ of 7×10^{-5} has been found (Parvin et al. 1986). Here, the method could only detect mutants that were nearly neutral, which may mean either that a large number of the mutants of this virus (at least at the site of the genome that has been analyzed) are indeed neutral or that the σ-value (cf. Eq. 7) is relatively large. Differences in σ (the parameter that expresses the superiority of the wild type over its mutants) have to be taken into account. The error threshold is not simply given by the reciprocal genome length, although $(1 - \bar{q})$ is often close to $1/\nu$. If σ is only slightly larger than 1, $(1 - \bar{q})_{max}$ may be appreciably smaller than $1/\nu$, and if σ is much larger than 1, $(1 - \bar{q})_{max}$ may be larger than $1/\nu$. The presence of nearly neutral mutants may strongly influence σ. Such effects may account for the differences in the mutation rates found for influenza and poliovirus (although their genome sizes are similar).

The recent findings of relatively large mutation rates in viruses (Schubert et al. 1984; Buonagurio et al. 1986) at first caused some surprise. However, it turns out that these rates are quite in agreement with the predictions of the quasi-species model. In other words, these high mutation rates, which cause so much trouble when humans try to develop an efficient immune protection toward virus diseases, are quite "natural."

The Future: Evolution of Genes in the Laboratory

S. Spiegelman was the first to carry out evolution experiments using RNA templates. He incubated in the test tube a cell-free mixture containing the four nucleoside triphosphates and the enzyme Qβ replicase, isolated from infected *E. coli* cells, along with suitable RNA templates that could be recognized specifically by the enzyme (Mills et al. 1967; Spiegelman 1970). In particular, he tried to adapt templates to the presence of ethidium bromide, a drug that interferes with the incorporation of nucleotides in replication (Kramer et al. 1974). Although he was able to increase the specific replication rates of Qβ RNA variants to values considerably exceeding those found under natural conditions, which already must have been subject to optimization, the results of drug adaptation, as Figure 7 (left) shows, were quite poor. In successive steps of three one-error mutations, he finally obtained a mutant that under the conditions of his experiments turned out to be just a factor 2 more efficient than the wild-type sequence. As extrapolation to zero concentration of ethidium bromide shows, this mutant under natural conditions is not much less efficient than the wild type and hence must be present in any sufficiently large wild-type population. Sumper and Luce (1975) and Biebricher et al. (1981a,b) found that Qβ replicase under special conditions is able to synthesize RNA de novo (Biebricher et al. 1986). If incubated in the presence of ethidium bromide, de novo products appear that are much more efficient than wild type under those conditions. Some of them are even drug-addicted, as Figure 7 (right) shows.

Of course, when Spiegelman carried out his experiments, the theory of replication and the quasi-species model were not yet in existence; otherwise, it would have been apparent that the experiments were not carried out under optimal conditions. The midi-variant that was used in Spiegelman's experiments comprises 220 nucleotides (Mills et al. 1973), whereas the error rate of Qβ replicase is only 3×10^{-4} (Batschelet et al. 1976). Hence, the error rates were far below threshold. Only 3% of the replication rounds resulted in mutants, and 97% of the replicas obtained were error-free.

It is obvious that the best conditions for progressive

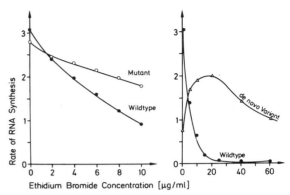

Figure 7. Evolutionary experiments in the test tube. The left-hand diagram illustrates an experiment carried out by S. Spiegelman and co-workers (Kramer et al. 1974). Midi-variant of Qβ RNA was adapted to the presence of ethidium bromide, which interferes with replication. In three successive one-error mutation steps, a three-error mutant was obtained that shows the performance depicted above. It appears to be almost neutral vis-a-vis the wild type in the absence of ethidium bromide, and it is only moderately superior to the wild type at higher ethidium bromide concentrations. The right-hand diagram depicts the behavior of a variant that was obtained by synthesis de novo (using Qβ replicase) in the presence of ethidium bromide. This variant is not only highly superior to the wild type, it is even drug-addicted and works best at a finite concentration of ethidium bromide (Sumper et al. 1975).

evolution are obtained near the error threshold. As shown in Figure 3, the error threshold is like a melting point, a point where information melts away. One may work out programs that control the error rate and allow something like annealing or zone melting. The error threshold is thereby surpassed in a controlled way, such that the system is not destabilized, but such that a maximum number of mutants is produced. Mutation rates can be controlled through variation of the ratios of nucleoside triphosphate concentrations. The dilution rate then must be adapted to these variations. The whole procedure requires automation, since generation times are in the range of 1 minute. Incubation can be triggered by temperature jumps from 0°C to 37°C that can be brought about within 1 second. Figures 8 and 9 show that such a machine has now become a reality. It works in the following way. A low-temperature store contains a large number (10^2 to 10^3) of sample plates providing sample volumes of 1–10 μl. The sample holes are filled with incubation mixtures containing enzyme (e.g., Qβ replicase) and substrates (nucleoside triphosphates at various concentrations) that have been precalculated to allow for an optimal annealing program. The plates are moved by step-motor-driven carriers (1) to a position at which dilution and addition of templates (carried out by a micropipette) occurs (0°C); (2) to the incubation position (37°C), where the reaction is monitored by a y-shaped light guide, connected with a laser fluorimeter; and (3) upon a signal triggered by the fluorescence measurement, back to the 0°C position for serial transfer of sample to the next plate, and finally to low-temperature storage. This procedure is

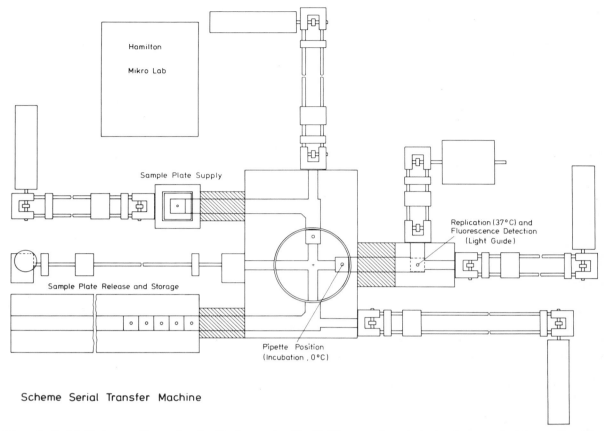

Scheme Serial Transfer Machine

Figure 8. Serial dilution machine as described in the text (see Fig. 9). The central part is the "active center" of the machine. The pipette position (where serial dilution takes place) is at 0°C, and the fluorescence detection position (where growth and competition takes place) is at 37°C. The sample jumps back and forth between both temperatures, with relaxation times of about 1 sec. Not shown is the laser fluorimeter and the device for providing a water-saturated atmosphere at 0°C and 37°C (Otten 1987).

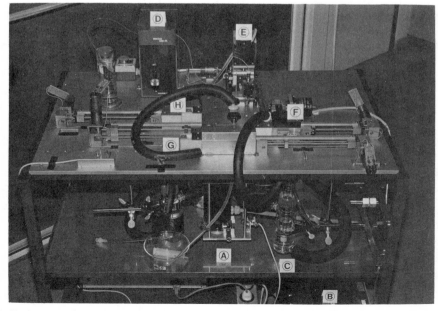

Figure 9. Serial dilution machine described in Fig. 8 (Otten 1987). (A,B) Step motor and controller; (C) humidity for water-saturated atmosphere (0°C, 37°C); (D) Hamilton Micro Lab; (E) pipette; (F) measuring position; (G) sample plate release; (H) sample plate inlet.

iterated, allowing evolutionary adaptation over a large number of generations.

The next step toward an evolutionary biotechnology is to clone large numbers of single mutants that, by controlled mutation rate, are hierarchically ordered with respect to their mutation distances. The cloning plates (e.g., with 10^3 sample holes) are then monitored by a multichannel glass fiber fluorimeter, and the procedure is iterated in a manner similar to that carried out in the serial dilution machine. However, selection is now done at will, guided by the comparative results. Thus, the fitness landscape is checked, and the process may be guided to fitness values optimized with respect to any desired function, without the requirement for natural selection, i.e., coupling the functional advantage to replication.

In recent years, it has proved possible to solve many of the technical problems associated with this type of evolutionary technology. Otten (1987) constructed the prototype of an evolution machine and deserves special mention. The Qβ experiments are now being carried out by G. Bauer, B. Lindemann, and A. Schwienhorst, after many of the prerequisites had been worked out in test-tube experiments by C. Biebricher and R. Luce (Biebricher 1983, 1987; Biebricher et al. 1985).

ACKNOWLEDGMENTS

I thank Ruthild Winkler-Oswatitsch for the design of the drawings and for valuable suggestions and Paul Woolley for revising the English manuscript.

REFERENCES

Batschelet, E., E. Domingo, and C. Weissmann. 1976. The proportion of revertant and mutant phage in a growing population as a function of mutation and growth rate. *Gene* **1**: 27.

Biebricher, C.K. 1983. Darwinian selection of RNA molecules in vitro. *Evol. Biol.* **16**: 1.

———. 1987. Replication and selection kinetics of short-chained self-replicating RNA molecules. *UCLA Symp. Mol. Cell. Biol.* **54**: 9.

Biebricher, C.K. and M. Eigen. 1987. Kinetics of RNA replication by Qβ replicase. In *RNA genetics* (ed. E. Domingo et al.), vol. 1. CRC Press, Boca Raton, Florida. (In press.)

Biebricher, C.K., M. Eigen, and W.C. Gardiner. 1985. Kinetics of RNA replication: Competition and selection among self-replicating RNA species. *Biochemistry* **24**: 6550.

Biebricher, C.K., M. Eigen, and R. Luce. 1981a. Product analysis of RNA generated de novo by Qβ replicase. *J. Mol. Biol.* **148**: 369.

———. 1981b. Kinetic analysis of template-instructed and de novo RNA synthesis by Qβ replicase. *J. Mol. Biol.* **148**: 391.

———. 1986. Template-free RNA synthesis of Qβ replicase. *Nature* **321** No 6065: 89.

Buonagurio, D.A., S. Nakada, J.D. Parvin, M. Krystal, P. Palese, and W.M. Fitch. 1986. Evolution of human influenza A viruses over 50 years: Rapid, uniform rate of change in NS gene. *Science* **232**: 980.

Domingo, E., M. Dávila, and J. Ortín. 1980. Nucleotide sequence heterogeneity of the RNA from a natural population of foot-and-mouth disease virus. *Gene* **11**: 333.

Domingo, E., A. Flavell, and C. Weissmann. 1976. In vitro site-directed mutagenesis: Generations and properties of an infectious extra-cistronic mutant of bacteriophage Qβ. *Gene* **1**: 3.

Domingo, E., D. Sabo, T. Taniguchi, and C. Weissmann. 1978. Nucleotide sequence heterogeneity of an RNA phage population. *Cell* **13**: 735.

Eigen, M. 1971. Self-organisation of matter and the evolution of biological macromolecules. *Naturwissenschaften* **58**: 465.

———. 1985. Macromolecular evolution: Dynamical ordering in sequence space. *Ber. Bunsen-Ges. Phys. Chem.* **89**: 658.

———. 1986. The physics of molecular evolution. *Chem. Scr.* **26B**: 13.

Eigen, M. and C.K. Biebricher. 1987. Sequence space and quasi-species distribution. In *RNA genetics* (ed. E. Domingo et al.), vol. 3. CRC Press, Boca Raton, Florida. (In press.)

Eigen, M. and P. Schuster. 1979. *The hypercycle—A principle of natural self-organisation.* Springer-Verlag, Heidelberg.

Eigen, M. and R. Winkler-Oswatitsch. 1981a. Transfer RNA: The early adaptor. *Naturwissenschaften* **68**: 217.

———. 1981b. Transfer RNA; an early gene? *Naturwissenschaften* **68**: 282.

Eigen, M., B. Lindemann, R. Winkler-Oswatitsch, and C.H. Clarke. 1985. Pattern analysis of 5S rRNA. *Proc. Natl. Acad. Sci.* **82**: 2437.

Hamming, R.W. 1980. *Coding and information theory.* Prentice Hall, Englewood Cliffs, New Jersey.

Holland, J., K. Spindler, F. Horodyski, E. Grabau, S. Nichol, and S. Van de Pol. 1982. Rapid evolution of RNA genomes. *Science* **215**: 1577.

Jones, B.L., R.H. Enns, and S.S. Rangnekar. 1976. On the theory of selection of coupled macromolecular systems. *Bull. Math. Biol.* **38**: 15.

Kimura, M. 1980. A simple method for estimating evolutionary rates of base substitutions through comparative studies of nucleotide sequence. *J. Mol. Evol.* **16**: 111.

———. 1983. *The neutral theory of molecular evolution.* Cambridge University Press, Cambridge, England.

Kimura, M. and T. Ohta. 1971. *Theoretical aspects of population genetics.* Princeton University Press, Princeton, New Jersey.

Kramer, F.R., D.R. Mills, P.E. Cole, T. Nishihara, and S. Spiegelman. 1974. Evolution in vitro: Sequences and phenotype of a mutant RNA resistant to ethidium bromide. *J. Mol. Biol.* **89**: 719.

Leuthäusser, I. 1986. An exact correspondence between Eigen's evolution model and a two-dimensional Ising system. *J. Chem. Phys.* **84**: 1884.

Mandelbrot, B.B. 1983. *The fractal geometry of nature.* W.H. Freeman, New York.

McCaskill, J.S. 1984. A localisation threshold for macromolecular quasi-species from continuously distributed replication rates. *J. Chem. Phys.* **80(10)**: 5194.

Mills, D.R., F.R. Kramer, and S. Spiegelman. 1973. Complete nucleotide sequence of a replicating RNA molecule. *Science* **180**: 916.

Mills, D.R., R.L. Peterson, and S. Spiegelman. 1967. An extra-cellular Darwinian experiment with a self-duplicating nucleic acid molecule. *Proc. Natl. Acad. Sci.* **58**: 217.

O'Hara, P.J., F.M. Horodyski, S.T. Nichol, and J.J. Holland. 1984. Vesicular stomatitis virus mutants resistant to defective-interfering particles accumulate stable 5′-terminal and fewer 3′-terminal mutations in a stepwise manner. *J. Virol.* **49**: 793.

Otten, H. 1987. "Ein Beitrag zur Durchführung von kontrollierten Evolutionsexperimenten mit biologischen Makromolekülen." Ph.D. thesis, Braunschweig-Göttingen.

Parvin, J.D., A. Moscona, W.T. Pan, J. Lieder, and P. Palese. 1986. Measurement of the mutation rates of animal viruses: Influenza A virus and polio virus type I. *J. Virol.* **59**: 377.

Rechenberg, I. 1973. Evolutionsstrategie. *Problemata* From-mann-Holzboog, Stuttgart-Bad Canstatt.

Rumschitzki, D. 1987. Spectral properties of Eigen's evolution matrices. *J. Math. Biol.* **24:** 667.

Schubert, M., G.G. Harmison, and E. Meier. 1984. Primary structure of the vesicular stomatitis virus polymerase (L) gene: Evidence for a high frequency of mutations. *J. Virol.* **51:** 505.

Schuster, P. 1986. The physical basis of molecular evolution. *Chem. Scr.* **26B:** 27.

Schuster, P. and K. Sigmund. 1985. Dynamics of evolutionary optimization. *Ber. Bunsen-Ges. Phys. Chem.* **89:** 668.

Spiegelman, S. 1970. The development and use of an extracellular RNA replicating system. *Harvey Lect.* **64:**1.

Spindler, K.R., F.M. Horodyski, and J.J. Holland. 1982. High multiplicities of infection favor rapid and random evolution of vesicular stomatitis virus. *Virology* **119:** 96.

Sprinzl, M., T. Hartmann, F. Meissner, J. Moll, and T. Vorderwuelbecke. 1987. Compilation of tRNA sequences and sequences of tRNA genes. *Nucleic Acids Res.* **15:** r53.

Sumper, M. and R. Luce. 1975. Evidence for de novo production of self-replicating and environmentally adapted RNA structures by bacteriophage Qβ replicase. *Proc. Natl. Acad. Sci.* **72:** 162.

Swetina, J. and P. Schuster. 1982. Self-replication with error—A model for polynucleotide replication. *Biophys. Chem.* **16:** 329.

Thompson, C.L. and J.L. McBride. 1974. On Eigen's theory of the selforganisation of matter and the evolution of biological macromolecules. *Math. Biosci.* **21:** 127.

Evolution of the RNA Coliphages: The Role of Secondary Structures during RNA Replication

C. PRIANO,* F.R. KRAMER,[†] AND D.R. MILLS*

*Institute of Cancer Research and Department of Genetics and Development, College of
Physicians & Surgeons, Columbia University, New York, New York 10032; [†]Department of
Molecular Genetics, Public Health Research Institute, New York, New York 10016

The process of RNA-directed RNA synthesis is central to the survival of the RNA bacteriophages (Loeb and Zinder 1961). Despite their apparent simplicity, these infectious agents have evolved a highly sophisticated mechanism of propagation that obviates the need for a DNA intermediate (Cooper and Zinder 1962; Doi and Spiegelman 1962; Haywood and Sinsheimer 1963). The phage RNA provides a dual function during lytic infection. Upon entering a host, it serves as a polycistronic messenger RNA (Ohtaka and Spiegelman 1963), directing translation of phage-specific proteins. Later, the same RNA serves as a template for its own replication by a phage-induced RNA-directed RNA replicase (Haruna and Spiegelman 1965a). Using the single-stranded viral RNA as template, the RNA replicase synthesizes a single-stranded, antiparallel complement (Spiegelman et al. 1969; Weissmann et al. 1969). This complementary RNA, in turn, serves as a template for the production of new single-stranded phage RNA molecules (Feix et al. 1968). The mechanism by which the phage RNA chromosome functions as a template for RNA-directed RNA synthesis during reproduction of bacteriophage Qβ has been the subject of extensive investigation.

The genome of the bacteriophage Qβ is a single-stranded linear RNA that contains 4220 nucleotides (Mekler 1981). Approximately 75% of the viral RNA is involved in specific secondary structure. The phage genes are encoded in three cistrons that are translated in the same reading frame. From the 5' end of the RNA, these cistrons encode the maturation protein, the coat protein, and one of the four subunits that comprise mature Qβ replicase (Blumenthal and Carmichael 1979).

Qβ replicase is highly selective for its own RNA templates. It promotes the autocatalytic synthesis of Qβ RNA (Haruna and Spiegelman 1965a), the genomic RNA of the closely related group III RNA bacteriophages (Miyake et al. 1971), and several smaller, naturally occurring "variant RNAs" (Banerjee et al. 1967; Kacian et al. 1972; Mills et al. 1975; Schaffner et al. 1977; C. Priano et al., in prep.). It does not replicate other viral RNAs, nor any known *Escherichia coli* RNA or DNA (Haruna and Spiegelman 1965b). The specific template requirements of Qβ RNA replication have been studied extensively in in vitro systems using a number of the variant RNAs as model templates for Qβ replicase.

Three variant templates for Qβ replicase, midivariant type 1 (MDV-1) RNA (Kacian et al. 1972; microvariant RNA (Mills et al. 1975), and cordycepin tolerant (CT) RNA (C. Priano et al., in prep.), have been isolated from Qβ replicase reactions that were incubated in the absence of exogenous template, and their nucleotide sequences have been completely determined (Mills et al. 1973, 1975; Kramer and Mills 1978; C. Priano et al., in prep.). The mechanism of their replication has been studied in detail (Kacian et al. 1972; Mills et al. 1978, 1980, 1987; Dobkin et al. 1979; Kramer and Mills 1981; Bausch et al. 1983; Nishihara et al. 1983; C. Priano et al., in prep.) and has been shown to be fundamentally similar to that of the replication of Qβ RNA. The mechanism of RNA synthesis is illustrated in Figure 1. The replicase first binds to a highly structured internal region of the template RNA (Nishihara et al. 1983). The synthesis of the product strand is then initiated at the 3' end of the template, and the product strand is polymerized in the 5' to 3' direction. Although the replicase relies on base pairing for the synthesis of the product strand, the mechanism of replication is such that, in general, both the product and the template are single-stranded. After completion

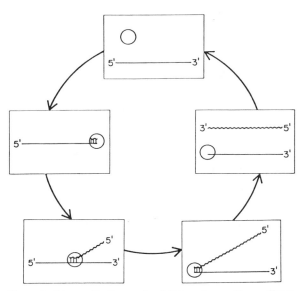

Figure 1. The replication cycle of Qβ replicase. The replicase (circle) synthesizes a single-strand product from a single-strand template.

of product-strand elongation, both the product strand and the template strand are released from the replication complex as single-stranded RNAs (Dobkin et al. 1979). The replicase is then free to bind to any RNA for use as a template in the next cycle of replication.

In this paper, we compare the synthesis of MDV-1 RNA, microvariant RNA, and CT RNA. We studied the secondary structures that they can form, the kinetics of their synthesis, the variability in their rates of chain elongation, and the propensity of their complementary strands to reassociate, both in solution and while involved in replication complexes during RNA synthesis. The results suggest that the formation of secondary structures during chain elongation of bacteriophage RNA is required for efficient autocatalytic replication.

METHODS

General procedures. Qβ replicase was isolated from bacteriophage Qβ-infected *E. coli* Q13 according to the method of Eoyang and August (1971), with the hydroxyapatite step omitted. Melting of RNA was carried out by heating to 100°C for 3 minutes in a specified solution and then chilling rapidly to 0°C by swirling in an ice bath. Phenol extraction was carried out by mixing equal volumes of an aqueous solution with phenol (saturated with 0.1% 8-hydroxyquinoline [Mallinckrodt] and 50 mM Tris-HCl at pH 7.8) and then separating phases by centrifugation.

Precipitation of RNA from solutions containing either 400 mM NaCl or 2 M ammonium acetate was carried out by adding 2.5 volumes of absolute ethanol, chilling the solution for either 60 minutes at −16°C (if NaCl was present) or 15 minutes at 0°C (if ammonium acetate was present), and then concentrating the RNA by centrifugation. RNA pellets were washed with 70% ethanol and dried in a vacuum.

Polyacrylamide gel electrophoresis. Denaturing gel electrophoresis was carried out on 10% polyacrylamide gels containing 7 M urea that were cast and run in 50 mM Tris-borate (pH 8.3) and 2 mM EDTA. Nondenaturing gel electrophoresis was carried out on 8% polyacrylamide gels that were cast and run in 50 mM Tris-borate (pH 8.3) and 1 mM MgCl₂. All gels were pre-run at 500 V for 2 hours. ³²P-labeled RNA was located by autoradiography. RNA was eluted from gel slices by shaking for 16 hours at 4°C in 20 mM Tris-HCl (pH 7.5), 3 mM EDTA, and 400 mM NaCl (GE buffer).

Standard RNA synthesis. RNA was synthesized at 37°C in reactions containing 84 mM Tris-HCl (pH 7.5), 12 mM MgCl₂, 0.4 mM of each ribonucleoside triphosphate (P-L Biochemicals), one of which was radioactively labeled with ³²P (Amersham), 40 μg/ml Qβ replicase, and 50 ng/ml of single-stranded template RNA. Reactions were terminated by adding one volume of GE buffer. The terminated reaction was extracted with phenol, and RNA was purified by chromatography through a Sephadex G-50 (Pharmacia) column

that was equilibrated and run in GE buffer plus 1 mg/ml SDS. The RNA in the excluded fraction was precipitated with ethanol. RNA was further purified by denaturing gel electrophoresis, and complementary plus and minus strands were then separated by nondenaturing gel electrophoresis. Prior to each electrophoresis, RNA was dissolved in 50 mM Tris-borate (pH 8.3), 2 mM EDTA, 7 M urea, 1 mg/ml xylene cyanol, and 1 mg/ml bromophenol blue (melting buffer) to a final concentration of less than 20 μg/ml (for CT RNA and microvariant RNA) or less than 200 μg/ml (for MDV-1 RNA). RNA was melted in this solution prior to applying it to the gel. RNA was eluted from the gel and precipitated with ethanol.

Kinetics of RNA synthesis. Reactions contained 40 μl of 84 mM Tris-HCl (pH 7.5), 12 mM MgCl₂, 0.1 mM of each ribonucleoside triphosphate, 250 pmoles of [α-³²P]GTP (400 Ci/mmole; Amersham), and 56 μg/ml of Qβ replicase. For exponential RNA synthesis, the molar amount of initiating template was lower than that of the replicase. For linear RNA synthesis, the molar amount of initiating template was higher than that of the replicase. Reactions were incubated at 37°C. At fixed intervals, 3-μl aliquots were removed and absorbed onto Whatman 3MM filters. Each filter was submerged into 500 ml of 3% (v/v) phosphoric acid, 20 mM sodium pyrophosphate, and 3 mM EDTA at 0°C to precipitate the RNA on the filter. Filters were rinsed in the same solution to remove unincorporated radioactivity, then rinsed with 95% ethanol, and air dried.

Analysis of RNA elongation intermediates. Elongation intermediates of each RNA were synthesized in two-step reactions. In the first step, product-strand elongation was allowed to proceed only 9–13 nucleotides by omitting one nucleoside triphosphate from an RNA synthesis reaction. Each reaction contained 40 μl of 84 mM Tris-HCl (pH 7.5), 12 mM MgCl₂, 0.1 mM ATP, 2.4 μM [α-³²P]GTP (400 Ci/mmole; Amersham), either 25 μM UTP (CT RNA or microvariant RNA synthesis) or 25 μM CTP (MDV-1 RNA synthesis), 500 nM Qβ replicase, and 500 nM template RNA. Each reaction was incubated at 37°C for 5 minutes. In the second reaction step, chain elongation was allowed to continue at 0°C. After the initial reaction was completed, its contents were mixed with an equal volume of a solution containing 84 mM Tris-HCl (pH 7.5), 12 mM MgCl₂, 0.1 mM ATP and GTP, and 0.2 mM UTP and CTP. Chase reactions were also performed in which the temperature of the elongation reaction was raised to 37°C, and incubation was continued for 5 minutes.

At various times during chain elongation, aliquots were removed, and the reaction in each was terminated by adding 100 μl of 50 mM Tris-borate (pH 8.3), 34 mM EDTA, and 12.5 g/liter SDS. Each aliquot was deproteinized by extraction with phenol; 50 μl of 6 M ammonium acetate (pH 6.5) and 20 μg of unlabeled yeast RNA were added, and the RNA was precipitated with ethanol. The RNAs were dissolved in 10 μl of melting buffer. The RNA was melted and then analyzed by denaturing gel electrophoresis.

Isolation of RNA duplexes during RNA synthesis.
RNA synthesis reactions (40 µl) were initiated under
exponential growth conditions (see above), and the
kinetics of RNA synthesis were measured as described.
For electrophoretic analysis, 2-µl aliquots were removed at various times and diluted into 50 µl of
50 mM Tris-borate (pH 8.3), 20 mM EDTA, 80% formamide, 5 g/liter of SDS, 1 mg/ml of xylene cyanol, and
50 µg/ml of unlabeled yeast RNA, at 0°C; 25 µl was
applied directly onto an 8% nondenaturing polyacrylamide gel, without melting the RNA. The RNA in
the remaining 25 µl was melted and then applied to the
gel. Electrophoresis was conducted at 30 mA. Portions
of the gel containing RNA were excised, and the
amount of Cerenkov radiation in each was determined.

Determination of reassociation rate constants. Each
RNA was radioactively labeled in standard RNA synthesis reactions (see above), and the complementary
plus and minus strands were separated by nondenaturing gel electrophoresis. Separated plus and minus
strands were incubated together, and the extent of
hybridization that occurred was measured at various
times during incubation. The hybridization buffer contained 84 mM Tris-HCl (pH 7.5), 1 mM MgCl$_2$, 0.1 mM
of each ribonucleoside triphosphate, 2.5 mM ammonium sulfate, 25 mM EDTA, 125 µM β-mercaptoethanol, and 1% glycerol. Either 0.8, 8, or 80 pmoles
of plus-strand RNA were dissolved in 64 µl of a 1.25-
fold concentration of the hybridization buffer. An equivalent amount of the complementary minus strand was
dissolved in 16 µl of distilled water. Both solutions
were prewarmed by incubation at 37°C for 1 minute.
The plus-strand solution was then divided into four
16-µl portions, and 4 µl of the minus-strand solution
was added. Incubation was continued at 37°C in closed
0.5-ml polypropylene tubes to minimize evaporation.
Following incubation, each reaction was added to 5 µl
of 250 mM Tris-borate (pH 8.3), 5 mM MgCl$_2$, 125
mg/ml ficoll, 5 mg/ml xylene cyanol, and 1 mg/ml
unlabeled yeast RNA at 37°C. The entire volume was
loaded immediately onto an 8% nondenaturing polyacrylamide gel containing 1 mM MgCl$_2$. Electrophoresis was carried out at 30 mA. Portions of the gel
containing RNA were excised, and the amount of
Cerenkov radiation in each was determined.

RESULTS

RNA Templates

The nucleotide sequences of MDV-1 RNA (221 nucleotides), microvariant RNA (115 nucleotides), and
CT RNA (77 nucleotides) possess many self-complementary regions that are capable of forming hairpin
structures. Figure 2 shows the structure of each RNA
predicted by computer analysis to be the most stable
(Zuker and Stiegler 1981). These structures have been
confirmed experimentally by several means: They have
been directly visualized (Klotz et al. 1980), utilizing
hollow-cone, dark-field electron microscopy; chemical
agents that modify nucleotides in single-strand regions

have been used to identify specific structures (Mills et
al. 1980); band compression in RNA sequencing gels
(Kramer and Mills 1978) has been used to identify
regions that form secondary structures (Mills and
Kramer 1979; C. Priano et al., in prep.); and the tertiary structure of each RNA was probed by subjecting it
to mild cleavage with ribonuclease T1 (F.R. Kramer et
al.; C. Priano et al; both in prep.).

Description of RNA Replication Kinetics

RNA replication by Qβ replicase occurs in two
phases. Under conditions of replicase excess, when
both the template and the product strands can serve as
template for each round of replication, RNA synthesis
proceeds at an exponential rate (Haruna and Spiegelman 1965c). When the number of active template molecules exceeds the number of active replicase molecules,
synthesis proceeds at a linear rate. The kinetics of RNA
synthesis were compared for MDV-1 RNA, microvariant RNA, and CT RNA under the two different
sets of conditions.

Kinetics during Linear RNA Synthesis

Figure 3 shows the kinetics of linear RNA synthesis
for all three templates under competitive and noncompetitive conditions. The rates of RNA synthesis that
were determined for RNAs within a given reaction are
summarized in Table 1. The data show that (1) the
linear rate of MDV-1 RNA synthesis was unaffected by
the presence of other replicating RNAs, (2) the linear
rate of microvariant RNA synthesis was reduced when
MDV-1 RNA was present but was unaffected by the
presence of CT RNA, and (3) the synthesis of CT RNA
was completely inhibited in the presence of either microvariant RNA or MDV-1 RNA. In general, these
results indicate that under conditions of linear RNA
synthesis, Qβ replicase preferentially associates with
replicating MDV-1 RNA molecules. Since RNA templates compete for available Qβ replicase molecules
during linear RNA synthesis, binding affinities were
examined directly by analyzing how Qβ replicase molecules were distributed among different combinations of
templates (data not shown). The results of these binding experiments indicated that binding of CT RNA was
indeed inhibited by the presence of a second template,
thereby explaining the reduced rate of linear synthesis
under competitive reaction conditions. However, microvariant RNA and MDV-1 RNA were shown to have
equal binding affinities. This result was inconsistent
with the kinetic data. Even though the intrinsic binding
affinities of microvariant RNA and MDV-1 RNA were
the same, the MDV-1 RNA population was preferentially replicated during competitive linear synthesis.

Kinetics of Exponential RNA Synthesis

An examination of the kinetics of exponential synthesis for the three RNA templates presented an additional paradox. Since RNAs do not compete for repli-

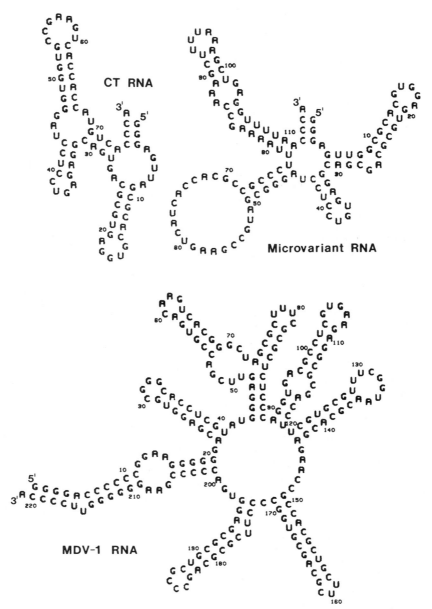

Figure 2. Comparison of the nucleotide sequences and secondary structures of the plus strands of CT RNA, microvariant RNA, and MDV-1 RNA.

case molecules during exponential replication, each RNA was synthesized under noncompetitive conditions (Fig. 4). The results of these analyses are summarized in Table 2. Two significant observations were made: First, it took less time for the MDV-1 RNA population to double in number than it did for the microvariant RNA and the CT RNA populations. This result was surprising because smaller molecules should take less time to replicate than larger RNAs. This observation might be explained if the intrinsic rate of product chain elongation is sufficiently lower for CT RNA and for microvariant RNA than it is for MDV-1 RNA, thereby causing a drastic reduction in the overall rate of population doubling for the smaller molecules. The second

observation was that more moles of RNA were present at the time of enzyme saturation during synthesis of CT RNA and microvariant RNA than during synthesis of MDV-1 RNA. This result was also unexpected since enzyme saturation should occur at equivalent molar concentrations of template for all replicating RNAs. These data suggest that inactive CT RNA and microvariant RNA molecules were accumulating during the exponential phase of synthesis.

Analysis of RNA Chain Elongation

We began investigating the reasons for the contradictory kinetic results by examining the intrinsic rates of

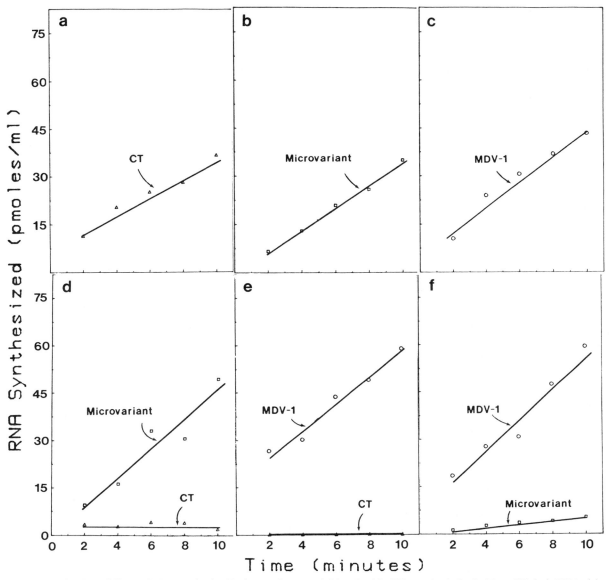

Figure 3. Kinetics of linear RNA synthesis. Each reaction was initiated with 500 pmoles/ml of either CT (+) RNA (*a*), microvariant (+) RNA (*b*), MDV-1 (−) RNA (*c*), equimolar amounts of CT (+) RNA and microvariant (+) RNA (*d*), equimolar amounts of CT (+) RNA and MDV-1 (−) RNA (*e*), or equimolar amounts of microvariant (+) RNA and MDV-1 (−) RNA (*f*).

product-strand elongation for each of the three RNA templates. Qβ replicase synthesizes RNA at a variable rate (Mills et al. 1978). During elongation, the progress of the replicase is temporarily interrupted at a small

Table 1. Kinetic Analysis of Linear RNA Synthesis

RNA	Rate of RNA synthesis ([pmole/ml]/min)					
	a	b	c	d	e	f
CT	3.0	—	—	0	0	—
Microvariant	—	3.4	—	4.8	—	0.7
MDV-1	—	—	3.9	—	4.2	4.6

The rate of RNA synthesis for each RNA in reactions a through f (Fig. 3). A dash indicates that an RNA was not present as template in a reaction.

number of specific sites and then resumes spontaneously with a finite probability (Mills et al. 1978). Since the time spent between these pause sites is negligible compared with the time spent at pause sites, the mean time of chain elongation is well approximated by the sum of the mean times spent at each pause site. Nucleotide sequence analysis indicates that pauses occur just after the synthesis of sequences that form hairpin structures in the partial product (Mills et al. 1978). Thus, the effect of replicase pausing on the RNA chain elongation rate is expected to be different for various RNA templates.

The chain elongation of CT RNA, microvariant RNA, and MDV-1 RNA was observed by analyzing the electrophoretic distribution of partially synthesized

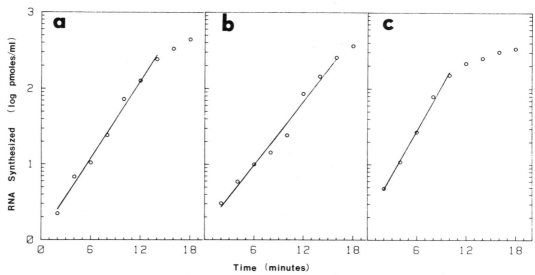

Figure 4. Kinetics of exponential RNA synthesis. Each reaction was initiated with 20 pmoles/ml of either CT (+) RNA (*a*), microvariant (+) RNA (*b*), or MDV-1 (−) RNA (*c*). The slope of the straight line on the semilogarithmic plot is inversely proportional to the population doubling time.

product strands during one single round of RNA synthesis. Each RNA was synthesized in similar reactions containing an equivalent amount of Qβ replicase and saturating amounts of template RNA. Each reaction was carried out in two stages (Mills et al. 1978). In the first stage, replication was permitted to proceed until the first pyrimidine triphosphate was required. In the second stage, the missing pyrimidine triphosphate was added to the reactions, and samples were removed at various times. Figure 5 shows the electrophoretic analysis of the partially synthesized RNAs. Numerals indicate prominant elongation intermediates for each RNA. Whereas several pauses occurred during elongation of MDV-1 (−) RNA (Mills et al. 1978), only one major pause occurred during elongation of CT (+) RNA and microvariant (+) RNA. Furthermore, it took less time for completed CT RNA and microvariant RNA molecules to be produced than it did for completed MDV-1 RNA molecules. Whereas most of the CT RNA and microvariant RNA products were completed between 2 and 5 minutes, less than half of the MDV-1 RNA products reached full size by 10 minutes. These data intensified the dilemma that was presented by the kinetic analyses; i.e., MDV-1 RNA should exhibit a lower exponential growth rate not only because of its larger size, but also because of its lower rate of chain elongation.

Table 2. Kinetic Analysis of Exponential RNA Synthesis

RNA	T_d (sec)	T_s (min)	C_s (pmole/ml)
CT	105	14	240
Microvariant	129	16	254
MDV-1	94	10	150

T_d is the doubling time, T_s is the time of enzyme saturation, and C_s is the RNA concentration at saturation.

Reassociation of Complementary RNA Strands

We investigated the possibility that inactive duplex RNAs are created in replication complexes during RNA synthesis, thereby accounting for the unexpected kinetic data. We first examined the relative rates of reassociation between the complementary strands of each RNA. Double-stranded CT RNA, microvariant RNA, and MDV-1 RNA were prepared, melted apart, and then incubated together under conditions similar to those that occur during RNA synthesis. At various times during the incubation, the proportion of complementary strands that reassociated was analyzed by polyacrylamide gel electrophoresis. Figure 6 shows the resulting reassociation curves ($C_o t$) that were obtained. The reassociation constants determined for each RNA (Table 3) indicate that the complementary strands of MDV-1 RNA are about 50 times less likely to hybridize than those of microvariant RNA, and 330 times less likely to hybridize than those of CT RNA. These results imply that as the RNA concentration increases during replication, the complementary strands of CT RNA and of microvariant RNA are much more likely to form duplexes than are the complementary strands of MDV-1 RNA. This occurrence would explain the competition that was observed during the linear replication of microvariant RNA and MDV-1 RNA (Fig. 3). Since RNA duplexes are inactive as templates for Qβ replicase (Nishihara et al. 1983), the more prevalent formation of microvariant RNA duplexes would cause the relative proportion of single-stranded MDV-1 RNA template molecules to increase continually compared with that of microvariant RNA.

In addition to the probability of RNA double strands forming in solution, the results of the reassociation experiments further suggest that complementary strand hybridization occurs in the replication complex at different rates for different RNAs. Since the localized

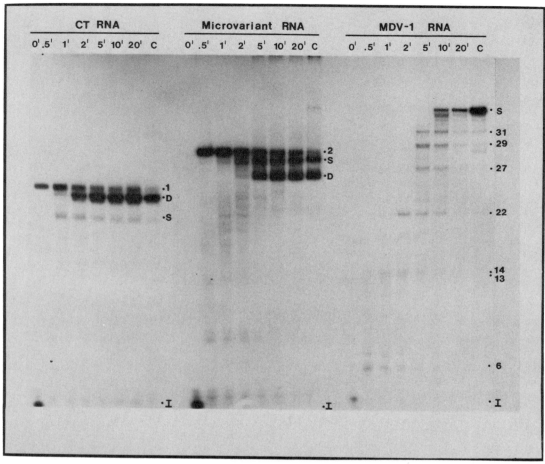

Figure 5. Analysis of chain elongation. (I) Initiation complex formed in the first reaction stage; (S) full-size single-stranded RNA; (D) full-size double-stranded RNA. Numerals identify prominent elongation intermediates. Lane C shows the full-size RNA products of 37°C chase reactions.

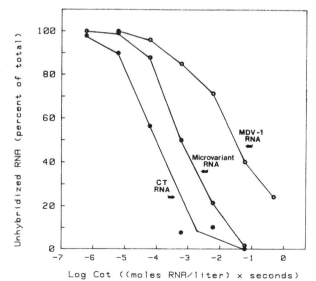

Figure 6. Kinetics of complementary strand reassociation. For CT RNA (closed circles), microvariant RNA (half-open circles), and MDV-1 RNA (open circles), the average fraction of RNA that reassociated was plotted as a function of the logarithm of C_0t.

concentration of a template and a product RNA involved in a replication complex is very high, the conditions mimic those that occur when there is a high concentration of RNA in solution. Thus, there would be a greater probability that, compared with MDV-1 RNA, the complementary strands of CT RNA and of microvariant RNA will hybridize to each other while associated with the replicase in the replication complex.

Duplex Formation in Replication Complexes

To determine whether RNA duplexes were actually forming in replication complexes, we directly examined the occurrence of double-stranded RNAs during the

Table 3. Reassociation Rate Constants

RNA	$C_0t_{1/2}$	k
CT	9.0×10^{-5}	11,000
Microvariant	6.0×10^{-4}	1,700
MDV-1	3.0×10^{-2}	33

$C_0t_{1/2}$ is the value of C_0t, in (moles of RNA/liter) × seconds, at which 50% of the reassociation occurred. k is the association rate constant ($\text{M}^{-1} \text{sec}^{-1}$).

exponential phase of synthesis for each of the RNA templates. RNA synthesis reactions were initiated under conditions for exponential growth. At various times, samples were removed, and the proportion of duplex RNA isolated, compared with the total amount of RNA present, was analyzed by polyacrylamide gel electrophoresis (Fig. 7). The relative proportion of double strands that occurred was consistently higher for CT RNA, lower for microvariant RNA, and lowest for MDV-1 RNA. Control experiments were performed to ensure that these RNA duplexes were not artificially created on the gel. When the RNA in a sample was first melted, the complementary strands remained separated during electrophoresis (data not shown). Furthermore, RNA duplex formation was not a result of the deproteinization of replication complexes (Feix et al. 1968). If this were the case, the proportion of duplex RNA that occurred would have decreased during linear RNA synthesis, in parallel with a decreased proportion of total RNA involved in replication complexes.

The results shown in Figure 7 therefore indicate that RNA duplexes resulted either from the hybridization of free complementary strands in solution or from the hybridization of complementary strands in replication complexes. If the RNA in duplex form resulted from RNAs in replication complexes, then the proportion of double-stranded RNA would remain constant with time. This was the case with MDV-1 RNA (Fig. 7). If the RNA in duplex form resulted from the collision of free complementary strands in solution, then the proportion of double-stranded RNA would increase with time, as the total RNA concentration increased. This was observed with CT RNA and microvariant RNA, although the increase occurred above a base level of about 30% for microvariant RNA and about 50% for CT RNA. These data suggest that both types of duplex formation were occurring simultaneously.

Using the reassociation constants determined for each RNA (Table 3), we were further able to calculate the proportion of duplex RNA that would be expected to occur as a result of solution hybridization during the exponential synthesis of each of the RNA templates. We then compared these values with the actual proportion of duplex RNA isolated from the reactions described in Figure 7 (Table 4). The difference between the actual (A) and the expected (E) fractions of duplex RNA represents the fraction of total RNA that was formed into duplexes while in replication complexes. These data show that for each RNA, this rate of duplex formation was virtually constant over time, indicating that a fixed proportion of RNA was converted to duplex form in replication complexes in each cycle of replication. These proportions were estimated to be 32% for CT RNA, 30% for microvariant RNA, and 17% for MDV-1 RNA. Thus, a major cause of duplex formation during the exponential phase of synthesis for each RNA was hybridization while in replication complexes. Since duplex RNAs are inactive as templates for $Q\beta$ replicase (Nishihara et al. 1983), these different hybridization propensities contribute significantly to differences in replication efficiencies such that the replication of MDV-1 RNA results in a relatively higher proportion of active template molecules after each cycle of replication.

DISCUSSION

Effect of Duplex Formation during RNA Replication

There are two ways in which inactive double-stranded RNA molecules are generated during replication. During exponential RNA synthesis, when the RNA concentration is relatively low, the major cause of duplex formation is hybridization in replication complexes, which occurs at a fixed rate that is characteristic of the RNA species. As the RNA concentration increases during linear RNA synthesis, a higher proportion of duplex formation is expected to occur from solution hybridization, according to a fixed rate of reassociation (Biebricher and Eigen 1985). These results are consistent with the observed kinetics of RNA synthesis. Since double-stranded RNAs are not active as templates for $Q\beta$ replicase (Nishihara et al. 1983), the formation of a fixed proportion of duplex RNAs during each cycle of exponential synthesis, in addition to the smaller amounts of duplex RNAs formed by solution hybridi-

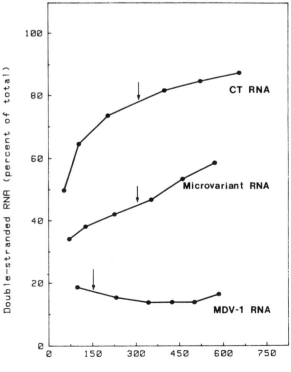

Figure 7. Proportion of total RNA in double-stranded form during RNA synthesis. Arrow indicates the total amount of RNA present at the transition from the exponential phase of synthesis to the linear phase of synthesis.

Table 4. Actual vs. Expected Occurrence of Duplex RNA

t (min)	RNA (pM)	E	A	A–E	RNA (pM)	E	A	A–E	RNA (pM)	E	A	A–E
10	50	0.17	0.50	0.33	71	0.05	0.34	0.29	98	0.00	0.19	0.19
14	104	0.29	0.65	0.36	126	0.08	0.38	0.30	232	0.00	0.15	0.15
18	204	0.45	0.74	0.29	226	0.14	0.42	0.28				

t is time of synthesis; RNA is the RNA concentration at time t; E is the fraction of RNA expected to occur as duplex; and A is the actual fraction of RNA that was isolated as duplex. $E = (1 - [1/1 + kCt_a])$, where t_a is the mean lifetime, in seconds, of the total RNA present, and k is the reassociation rate constant for the template RNA (Table 3). t_a is the population doubling time (247 sec for CT RNA; 287 sec for microvariant RNA; and 158 sec for MDV-1 RNA) times $1/(\ln 2)$ (C. Peskin, Courant Institute of Mathematical Sciences, New York University, pers. comm.).

zation, results in a decreased population doubling rate. Furthermore, the molar amount of RNA present at the time of enzyme saturation would be greater than expected, due to the accumulation of these inactive duplexes. Solution hybridization also contributes to the competition that was observed between MDV-1 RNA and microvariant RNA during the linear phase of synthesis. As the concentration of each RNA increases during the reaction, the relative proportion of single-stranded MDV-1 RNA templates continually increases compared with that of microvariant RNA templates, which reassociate at a higher rate.

The propensity of a replicating RNA population to form inactive duplexes while in replication complexes has a dramatic effect on the efficiency of RNA amplification during exponential synthesis. Exponential amplification is maximal when no double-strand formation occurs. When duplexes form in the replication complex, available template molecules are removed and the rate of exponential increase becomes reduced. If the proportion of double strands that occurs in each replication cycle is as high as 50%, there would be no net increase of available single strands in subsequent rounds of synthesis, so that total RNA synthesis would proceed at a linear rate. Furthermore, if the proportion of duplex formation that occurs in each round of synthesis is greater than 50%, the number of available single strands in subsequent rounds of synthesis would continually decrease and approach zero. Thus, the intrinsic propensity to form double strands while associated with the replicase can have severe effects on the continual propagation of an RNA population.

Role of RNA Secondary Structure in Preventing Duplex Formation

It is probable that the formation of secondary structures during RNA chain elongation is central to the generation of active single-strand templates for Qβ replicase. The lack of replicase pausing that occurred during the synthesis of CT RNA and microvariant RNA suggests that the formation of strong secondary structures was minimal. It was these RNAs that exhibited a higher rate of duplex formation in replication complexes compared with that of MDV-1 RNA. It is likely that the more stable structures that form in MDV-1 RNA result in a greater prevention of hybridization between the complementary strands in repli-

cation complexes by reducing the probability of an interstrand nucleation event occurring.

Evolution of RNA Secondary Structure

The results of several mutational analyses of CT RNA, microvariant RNA, and MDV-1 RNA indicate that there is a prevailing drive toward the preservation of hairpin structures to ensure maximal template efficiency (Kramer et al. 1974 and in prep.; C. Priano et al., in prep.). Most nucleotide substitutions that are evolutionarily selected occur in single-strand regions of these molecules. The few that have been seen in double-strand regions occurred as base-pair substitutions, thereby preserving the integrity of their hairpin stem. This persistent selection toward strong secondary structure is by no means trivial, since the formation of secondary structures during RNA replication dramatically slows down the rate of chain elongation by causing the replicase to pause (Mills et al. 1978). Because of the severe impeding effect of pausing on the overall rate of RNA synthesis, few structures would be expected to form in a growing RNA unless their presence confers an overriding selective advantage. The maintenance of the single-strand state in replication complexes, made possible by the formation of strong secondary structures, provides this advantage by preventing the formation of inactive double strands.

Evolution of the RNA Phage Genome

The RNA coliphages have evolved small, highly structured, single-strand genomes (Min Jou et al. 1972; Fiers et al. 1975, 1976). The secondary structures that are present in these genomes are apparently functional in protein recognition and binding (Blumenthal and Carmichael 1979) and in the control of protein synthesis (Lodish and Robertson 1969; Robertson and Lodish 1970). In addition, these stable intrastrand duplexes may serve to protect the viral RNAs from degradation. The results of our experiments suggest that the extensive RNA structures present in these replicating RNAs have evolved not only as a means of providing functional surfaces and stability, but also as a means of maintaining single-strandedness during replication. Since the production of duplex RNAs during infection is detrimental to the survival of these organisms, it is probable that the biological necessity to generate single-strand progeny provided the primary drive toward the evolution of structures in these genomes. Hence, despite the high cost of a reduced replication rate, only those viral RNAs that retain their structures through evolution are able to give rise to viable progeny.

ACKNOWLEDGMENTS

This work was supported by National Science Foundation grant PCM-82-15902, American Cancer Society grant MV-191B, and National Institutes of Health grants GM-32044, GM-33345, and CA-23767.

REFERENCES

Banerjee, A.K., L. Eoyang, K. Hori, and J.T. August. 1967. Replication of RNA viruses. IV. Initiation of RNA synthesis by the Qβ RNA polymerase. *Proc. Natl. Acad. Sci.* **57:** 986.

Bausch, J.N., F.R. Kramer, E.A. Miele, C. Dobkin, and D.R. Mills. 1983. Terminal adenylation in the synthesis of RNA by Qβ replicase. *J. Biol. Chem.* **258:** 1978.

Biebricher, C.K. and M. Eigen. 1985. Kinetics of RNA replication: Competition and selection among self-replicating RNA species. *Biochemistry* **24:** 6550.

Blumenthal, T. and G.G. Carmichael. 1979. RNA replication: Function and structure of Qβ-replicase. *Annu. Rev. Biochem.* **48:** 525.

Cooper, S. and N.D. Zinder. 1962. The growth of an RNA bacteriophage: The role of DNA synthesis. *Virology* **18:** 405.

Dobkin, C., D.R. Mills, F.R. Kramer, and S. Spiegelman. 1979. RNA replication: Required intermediates and the dissociation of template, product and Qβ replicase. *Biochemistry* **10:** 2038.

Doi, R.H. and S. Spiegelman. 1962. Homology test between the nucleic acid of an RNA virus and the DNA in a host cell. *Science* **138:** 1270.

Eoyang, L. and J.T. August. 1971. Qβ RNA polymerase from phage Qβ-infected *E. coli*. In *Procedures in nucleic acid research* (ed. G.L. Cantoni and D.R. Davies), vol. 2, p. 829. Harper and Row, New York.

Feix, G., R. Pollet, and C. Weissmann. 1968. Replication of viral RNA. XVI. Enzymatic synthesis of infectious viral RNA with noninfectious Qβ minus strands as template. *Proc. Natl. Acad. Sci.* **59:** 145.

Fiers, W., R. Contreras, F. Duerinck, G. Haegeman, D. Iserentant, J. Merregaert, W. Min Jou, F. Molemans, A. Raeymaekers, A. Van den Berghe, G. Volckaert, and M. Ysebaert. 1976. Complete nucleotide sequence of bacteriophage MS2 RNA: Primary and secondary structure of the replicase gene. *Nature* **260:** 500.

Fiers, W., R. Contreras, F. Duerinck, G. Haegeman, J. Merregaert, W. Min Jou, A. Raeymaekers, G. Volckaert, M. Ysebaert, J. Van de Kerckhove, F. Nolf, and M. Van Montagu. 1975. A-protein gene of bacteriophage MS2. *Nature* **256:** 273.

Haruna, I. and S. Spiegelman. 1965a. Recognition of size and sequence by an RNA replicase. *Proc. Natl. Acad. Sci.* **54:** 1189.

———. 1965b. Specific template requirements of RNA replicases. *Proc. Natl. Acad. Sci.* **54:** 579.

———. 1965c. Autocatalytic synthesis of a viral RNA *in vitro*. *Science* **150:** 884.

Haywood, A.M. and R.L. Sinsheimer. 1963. Inhibition of protein synthesis in *E. coli* protoplasts by actinomycin D. *J. Mol. Biol.* **6:** 247.

Kacian, D.L., D.R. Mills, F.R. Kramer, and S. Spiegelman. 1972. A replicating RNA molecule suitable for a detailed analysis of extracellular evolution and replication. *Proc. Natl. Acad. Sci.* **69:** 3038.

Klotz, G., F.R. Kramer, and A.K. Kleinschmidt. 1980. Conformational details of partially base-paired small RNAs in the nanometer range. *Electron Microsc.* **2:** 530.

Kramer, F.R. and D.R. Mills. 1978. RNA sequencing with radioactive chain-terminating ribonucleotides. *Proc. Natl. Acad. Sci.* **75:** 5334.

———. 1981. Secondary structure formation during RNA synthesis. *Nucleic Acid Res.* **9:** 5109.

Kramer, F.R., D.R. Mills, P.E. Cole, T. Nishihara, and S. Spiegelman. 1974. Evolution *in vitro*: Sequence and phenotype of a mutant RNA resistant to ethidium bromide. *J. Mol. Biol.* **89:** 719.

Lodish, H.F. and H.D. Robertson. 1969. Cell-free synthesis of bacteriophage f2 maturation protein. *J. Mol. Biol.* **45:** 9.

Loeb, T. and N.D. Zinder. 1961. A bacteriophage containing RNA. *Proc. Natl. Acad. Sci.* **47:** 282.

Mekler, P. 1981. Ph.D. thesis, University of Zurich, Switzerland.

Mills, D.R. and F.R. Kramer. 1979. Structure-independent nucleotide sequence analysis. *Proc. Natl. Acad. Sci.* **76:** 2232.

Mills, D.R., C. Dobkin, and F.R. Kramer. 1978. Template-determined, variable rate of RNA chain elongation. *Cell* **15:** 541.

Mills, D.R., F.R. Kramer, and S. Spiegelman. 1973. Complete nucleotide sequence of a replicating RNA molecule. *Science* **180:** 916.

Mills, D.R., C. Priano, and F.R. Kramer. 1987. Requirement for secondary structure formation during coliphage RNA replication. *UCLA Symp. Mol. Cell. Biol.* **54:** 35.

Mills, D.R., F.R. Kramer, C. Dobkin, T. Nishihara, and P. Cole. 1980. Modification of cytidines in a Qβ replicase template: Analysis of conformation and localization of lethal nucleotide substitutions. *Biochemistry* **19:** 228.

Mills, D.R., F.R. Kramer, C. Dobkin, T. Nishihara, and S. Spiegelman. 1975. Nucleotide sequence of microvariant RNA: Another small replicating molecule. *Proc. Natl. Acad. Sci.* **72:** 4252.

Min Jou, W., G. Haegeman, M. Ysebaert, and W. Fiers. 1972. Nucleotide sequence of the gene coding for the bacteriophage MS2 coat protein. *Nature* **237:** 82.

Miyake, T., I. Haruna, T. Shiba, Y.H. Itoh, K. Yamane, and I. Watanabe. 1971. Grouping of RNA phages based on the template specificity of their RNA replicases. *Proc. Natl. Acad. Sci.* **68:** 2022.

Nishihara, T., D.R. Mills, and F.R. Kramer. 1983. Localization of the Qβ replicase recognition site in MDV-1 RNA. *J. Biochem.* **93:** 669.

Ohtaka, Y. and S. Spiegelman. 1963. Translational control of protein synthesis in a cell-free system directed by a polycistronic viral RNA. *Science* **142:** 493.

Robertson, H.D. and H.F. Lodish. 1970. Messenger characteristics of nascent bacteriophage RNA. *Proc. Natl. Acad. Sci.* **67:** 710.

Schaffner, W., K.J. Rüegg, and C. Weissmann. 1977. Nanovariant RNAs: Nucleotide sequence and interaction with bacteriophage Qβ replicase. *J. Mol. Biol.* **117:** 877.

Spiegelman, S., N.R. Pace, D.R. Mills, R. Levisohn, T.S. Eikhom, M.M. Taylor, R.L. Peterson, and D.H.L. Bishop. 1969. The mechanism of RNA replication. *Cold Spring Harbor Symp. Quant. Biol.* **33:** 101.

Weissmann, C., G. Feix, and H. Slor. 1969. *In vitro* synthesis of phage RNA: The nature of the intermediates. *Cold Spring Harbor Symp. Quant. Biol.* **33:** 83.

Zuker, M. and P. Stiegler. 1981. Optimal computer folding of large RNA sequences using thermodynamics and auxiliary information. *Nucleic Acids Res.* **9:** 133.

Evidence Implicating a tRNA Heritage for the Promoters of Positive-strand RNA Synthesis in Brome Mosaic and Related Viruses

L.E. MARSH AND T.C. HALL
Department of Biology, Texas A&M University, College Station, Texas 77843-3258

Many animal viruses, and the majority of plant viruses, have an RNA-based genome. Far less is known about molecular mechanisms of replication for these viruses than is the case for viruses having a DNA genome, one reason being that RNA-based genomes have been inherently less amenable to experimental manipulation. Recently, however, considerable strides have been made in understanding this process at the molecular level for brome mosaic virus (BMV), which infects cereal grasses (Bujarski et al. 1986; Bujarski and Kaesberg 1986; French et al. 1986; Miller et al. 1986; Dreher and Hall 1987; French and Ahlquist 1987; Marsh et al. 1987).

BMV is a tripartite positive-strand RNA virus (Fig. 1), the genomic RNAs also functioning as mRNAs. It has only four known cistrons, one each on genomic RNAs 1 and 2 and two on genomic RNA 3. Only the 5′ cistron of dicistronic RNA 3 is translated; the 3′ cistron encodes the viral coat protein being translated from RNA 4, which is expressed as a subgenomic component. RNAs 3 and 4 are encapsidated within a single virion (an icosahedron containing 186 copies of the coat protein molecule), whereas RNAs 1 and 2 are encapsidated separately (Lane and Kaesberg 1971). All four RNAs have a common 3′ sequence that is aminoacylatable with tyrosine both in vitro and in vivo (Hall et al. 1972; Hall 1979; Loesch-Fries and Hall 1982), for which a tRNA-like structure has been proposed (Rietveld et al. 1983; Pleij et al. 1985).

Three technical advances have contributed to rapid progress with the BMV system: (1) the development of a template-dependent and template-specific in vitro replicase system (Hardy et al. 1979; Bujarski et al. 1982; Miller and Hall 1983), (2) the ability to transcribe cDNA clones in vitro (Ahlquist and Janda 1984; Dreher et al. 1984), and (3) the availability of full-length cDNAs capable of yielding infectious transcripts (Ahlquist et al. 1984c). Using the in vitro replicase system in a novel hybrid-arrested replication reaction, Ahlquist et al. (1984b) showed that the promoter for synthesis of negative-strand RNAs was located within the 3′ tRNA-like structure. The replicase system has also allowed deletion mutation analysis of this promoter (Bujarski et al. 1985). To our knowledge, this was the first analysis at the molecular level of a promoter on an RNA virus that infects eukaryotic cells. RNAs bearing deletions and point mutations have also been assayed for aminoacylation and nucleotidyl transferase activities in vitro to determine those regions that are discrete from, and those that overlap with, negative-strand promoter functions (Dreher et al. 1984; Bujarski et al. 1985; Miller et al. 1986; Dreher and Hall 1987).

The replicase also proved to be competent in the synthesis of positive-strand subgenomic RNA 4 in vitro (Miller et al. 1985). This characteristic of the replicase has permitted a functional analysis of deletion and point mutations of the internal subgenomic promoter (Marsh et al. 1987 and in prep.), providing the first definitive characterization of a subgenomic promoter.

The ability to transcribe infectious viral RNA from cDNA has allowed some of the deletion and point mutations in the tRNA-like structure to be tested in vivo, from which correlations with the results obtained in vitro can be drawn (Bujarski et al. 1986; T.W.

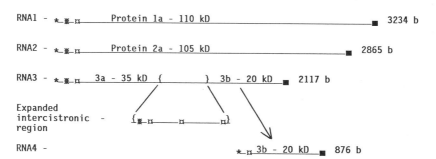

Figure 1. Linear representation of the BMV genome. Genomic positive-sense RNAs 1, 2, and 3 and subgenomic RNA 4 of BMV are shown together with the proteins they encode. Cross-hatched and open box symbols show the approximate positions of the homology with the ICRs 1 and 2 of tRNAs. Asterisk indicates the 5′ m⁷GpppG cap, and the closed box indicates the 3′ tRNA-like structure. The intercistronic region of dicistronic RNA 3 is expanded below RNA 3.

Dreher et al., in prep.). This approach has also shown that replication of BMV is, in part, dependent on sequences in the intercistronic region (French and Ahlquist 1987). It also led to a demonstration of recombination between the genomic RNAs of BMV in the region of the shared tRNA-like structure, probably through a template-switching mechanism (Bujarski and Kaesberg 1986).

Deletion analysis of the subgenomic promoter revealed the presence of a core sequence and three modulating regions: a region determining correct initiation (primarily the bases immediately downstream from the base at which the subgenomic RNA is initiated), a short (A-U) tract upsteam that is required for substantial yield, and a region corresponding to the intercistronic poly(A), which probably serves to facilitate access of the replicase to the promoter core (Marsh et al. 1987 and in prep.).

Comparison of these subgenomic promoter sequences (especially the promoter core sequence) with other regions of the BMV genome, and with the genomes of related viruses, has revealed remarkable homologies with ICRs (internal control regions) 1 and 2 (also known as A and B boxes) known to be involved in the promotion and control of transcription in eukaryotic tRNAs (Sharp et al. 1985). To our knowledge, these homologies have not previously been recognized; they raise exciting concepts for the evolution of this important group of RNA viruses.

MATERIALS AND METHODS

Sequence comparisons were made using the UW-GCG programs produced by the University of Wisconsin Genetics Computer Group running on a DEC MicroVAX II. For consistency, all sequences are given as DNA sequences, even in the case of the viral RNAs which are shown as cDNA sequences.

RESULTS

Homologies between the 5' Termini of BMV Genomic RNAs and ICRs 1 and 2 of tRNAs

A comparison of the 5' sequences for BMV RNAs 1, 2, and 3 with the consensus ICR sequences compiled by Sharp et al. (1985) from 115 tRNA genes reveals a remarkably high degree of homology (Table 1). In the case of ICR 2, homology with the tRNA consensus (GGTTCGANTCC) ranges from 91% (10 of 11 bases for RNA 3) to 82% (9 of 11 bases for RNAs 1 and 2). It is important to note that many instances can be found among tRNA sequences where the variable (N) nucleotide is deleted, as is found in the RNA 1 and RNA 2 sequences. BMV RNAs 1 and 2 differ from RNA 3 and the tRNA consensus in having an A substituted for a G at the sixth position. However, this change is found in about 20% of the tRNA sequences cited by Sharp et al. (1985) and is therefore a somewhat conservative change.

Immediately upstream of the ICR 2 region, a strong sequence resemblance is also found at the 5' ends of the genomic RNAs to the portion (underlined: see Table 1) of the extended ICR 1 consensus sequence GTGGCNNAGT■■GGT■■AGNGC (the closed square indicates an optional position for tRNAs) of Sharp et al. (1985), which contains the more general consensus sequence for polymerase III type-1 genes: TRRYNNARYGG. The consensus sequence for the ICR 1 boxes of BMV RNAs is 1 base shorter than that of the tRNAs, presumably because one of the two variable positions has been deleted. Also, to align the C residue at position 6 of the BMV sequence with the highly conserved C at position 5 in the tRNA consensus sequence, the two sequences must be staggered with respect to each other. The A at position 3 of the BMV consensus sequence is a conservative change, since 36% of the tRNAs possess this alternative, whereas the A at position 4 is less conservative in that this G is almost invariant, only one tRNA in the compiled sequences showing this deviation (Sharp et al. 1985). A C in the variable positions is quite conservative, 36% of the tRNAs having C in the first variable position and 44% in the second. The C prior to the final double GG in the BMV consensus is found at that position in only 14% of the tRNAs.

ICR 2 Homologies Present at the 5' Ends of Other Tripartite Viruses

Rezian et al. (1985) noted that homology exists between the 5' termini of cucumber mosaic virus (CMV) and BMV genomic RNAs. Table 2 reveals that the 5' sequences of the genomic RNAs of both of these viruses, and also of alfalfa mosaic virus (AMV), contain homology with the ICR 2 consensus sequence of tRNAs discussed above. As in the case of the BMV RNAs, homology with ICR 1 is not immediately obvious.

The CMV RNA consensus ICR 2 (see Table 2) GGTTCAACCCC, differs somewhat from that of the tRNAs. An A is substituted for the G at position 6, which is a conservative change similar to that seen in BMV RNAs 1 and 2. A less-conservative change is the presence of a C at the variable position 8; only about 10% of tRNAs have C at this position. The C for T substitution at position 9 is also a conservative change, 28% of the tRNAs sequenced showing this variation. The ICR 2 homology in CMV RNA 3 is found considerably internal to its 5' terminus, apparently as a consequence of its 92-base untranslated leader. This leader contrasts with the extremely short untranslated sequences of the other viral genomic RNAs.

The AMV consensus sequence, AGT − CAA − TCC has weaker homology with the tRNA ICR 2 consensus, GGTTCGANTCC. The AMV RNA sequence has 1 base deleted with respect to the BMV RNA consensus sequence and 2 bases with respect to the tRNA consensus sequence. As in the case of BMV and CMV RNAs, the variable position is deleted; additionally,

Table 1. BMV 5'-terminal Homology with ICRs 1 and 2 (A and B Boxes)

```
                    10              20           30                40               50
RNA1   GTAGA...C.CA.CGGAACGAGGTTCAA.TCCCTTGTTCGACCACGGTTCTGCTACT
       |||||    | | | |||     ||||||||   |||
                                         30                40               50
RNA2   GTAAA...C.CA.CGGAACGAGGTTCAA.TCCCTTGTTCGACCCACGGTTTGCGCAA
       |||||    | | | |||     ||||||||   |||
                                              40              50
RNA3   GTAAAATAC.CAACTAATTCTCGTTCGATTCCGGCGAACATTCTATTTTACC
       |||||     | | ||         || |||

Consensus
BMV    GTAAA...C.CA.CGG          GGTTCAA.TCC
       ||||    | | | ||          |||||| |||
tRNA   GTGG....CNNAGTGG          GGTTCGANTCC
```

ICR 1 consensus for all polymerase III type-1 genes   TRRYNNARYGG
ICR 2 consensus for all polymerase III type-I genes   GtTCRA

The 5' sequences of (cDNAs to) BMV RNAs 1, 2 (Ahlquist et al. 1984a), and 3 (Ahlquist et al. 1981b) shown above are aligned to maximize regions of homology with ICR 1 (single underline) and ICR 2 (double underline). Spaces inserted to maximize alignment (|) to the BMV RNA consensus are denoted by a dot. The derivation of the tRNA consensus sequences is given in the text.

Table 2. ICR 2 Homologies in the 5' Termini of AMV and CMV RNAs

A. CMV (strain Q) ICR 2 homologies

```
        10        20        30        40        50        60
RNA1 GTTTTATTTACAAGAGCGTACGGTTCAACCCCTGCCTCCTCTGTAAAACTACCCCTTTGAA
        10        20        30        40        50        60
RNA2 GTTTTATTCTCAAGAGCGTATGGTTCAACCCCTGCCTCCTCTGTGAAATTACCCTAGTTTT
        90       100       110       120       130
RNA3 --ATTACGAAGGTTATGGCTTTCCAAGGTCCCAGTAGGACGTTAACTCAACAGTCCTCGG
```

B. AMV (S strain) ICR 2 homologies

```
        10        20        30        40        50        60
RNA1 GTTTTTATCTTACACACGCTTGTGCAAGATAGTTAATCCATTTATTTTTTCCTTGTATTT
        10        20        30        40        50        60
RNA2 GTTTTTATCTTTTCGGCGATTCAAAAGATAAGTTTCAGAGTCTAATCTTTTCAATATGTTC
        10        20        30        40        50        60
RNA3 GTTTTCATCTTACACACGCTTGTGCAAGATAGTTAATCATTCCAATTCAACTCAATTAAC
```

C. Summary of ICR 2 homologies

```
CMV:                          AMV:
RNA1 GGT..TCAA.CCCC           RNA1 AGTT.AA.TCC
RNA2 GGT..TCAA.CCCC           RNA2 AGT.CTAATCT
RNA3 GCTTTCCAAGGTCC           RNA3 AAT.CA.TTCC

Consensus:
tRNA  GGTTCGANTCC
BMV   GGTTCAA.TCC
CMV   GGTTCAACCCC
AMV   AGT.CAA.TCC
```

Regions of homology with the ICR 2 sequence (double underline) are shown for the 5' sequences of the genomic RNAs of CMV (A) (Gould and Symons 1982; Rezian et al. 1984, 1985) and AMV (B) (Koper-Zwarthoff et al. 1980; Ravelonandro et al. 1983); a summary of these homologies is shown in C. Sequences corresponding to the conserved AAGA box in the subgenomic promoter of BMV RNA 3 (Marsh et al. 1987) are denoted by a single underline.

the third (or fourth) position is missing from the AMV RNA sequence. The A at position 1 of the AMV RNA consensus sequence is found in 12% of the tRNAs. As is the case for BMV and CMV RNAs, AMV RNAs have an A for G change at position 6. The 5′ terminus of TSV (tobacco streak virus) RNA 3 (Cornelissen et al. 1984) also possesses a sequence that has apparent homology with the tRNA ICR 2 consensus sequence (data not shown).

Homologies between Viral 5′ Sequences, Subgenomic Promoters, and ICRs

Although CMV and AMV RNAs do not have recognizable sequence homology with the ICR 1 sequences of tRNAs, they show a tantalizing resemblance (see Table 3) to sequences that we have demonstrated experimentally to be involved in the subgenomic promoter of BMV RNA 3 responsible for generation of subgenomic RNA 4 (Marsh et al. 1987). Two sequence blocks, AAGA and GTCCTAA, are conserved between the core sequence of the subgenomic promoter of BMV RNA 3 and core sequences that we have postulated for other plant virus subgenomic promoters (Marsh et al. 1987 and in prep.). The sequence order of these blocks is conserved between BMV RNA and the other putative subgenomic promoters. Furthermore, the sequence GTCCTAA is conserved between the subgenomic promoter of BMV RNA 3 and the postulated subgenomic promoters of the alphaviruses (Ou et al. 1982; Marsh et al. 1987), which contain the sequence CGGTCCTAA.

CMV RNAs 1 and 2 possess the sequence block AAGA immediately 5′ of the ICR 2 homology, whereas all of the genomic RNAs of AMV also have this block slightly 5′ of the ICR 2 homology. The consensus ICR 2 homology in BMV and CMV RNAs begins with GGTTCAA. The presence of the AAGA sequences immediately 5′ of the ICR 2 homologous blocks in AMV and CMV RNAs thus gives the 5′ ends of these genomic RNAs homology with the core sequence of the subgenomic promoter of BMV RNA 3 (Table 3). However, these 5′ termini lack sequences strictly homologous to those immediately upstream and downstream from the actual initiation site of subgenomic RNA 4.

Additional ICR Homologies within the BMV RNA 3 Intercistronic Region

Examination of the plus strands of BMV RNAs for further similarities to the ICRs of tRNAs reveals four places within the intercistronic region of dicistronic RNA 3 having homology with the ICR 2 of tRNAs (Fig. 1). One of these, starting at nucleotide 1100, has been recognized as having homology with the 5′ end of BMV and CMV RNAs (Rezian et al. 1985): French and Ahlquist (1987) noted that replication of BMV RNA 3 in vivo was in part dependent on the intercistronic region, and consequently implicated this sequence as being involved in its replication. However, these authors also commented that the only homology found between the 5′ end of the BMV RNAs and the intercistronic region of BMV RNA 3 was that starting at position 1100. In fact, a more extensive homology occurs slightly upstream, starting at nucleotide 1004, where approximately the first 40 bases of the untrans-

Table 3. Comparison of BMV, CMV, and AMV 5′ Sequences to the BMV RNA 3 Subgenomic Promoter Core Sequence

BMV RNAs 1 and 2 ICR 2 homology	A A C G A . . . . G G T T C . A A T C C
	| | | * | | * | | | | * |
BMV subgenomic promoter core	A A . G A T C T A T G T C C T A A T T C
CMV RNA 1 5′ ICR 2 homology	A A G A G C G T A C G G T T C . A A C C C
	| | | | * | | | * | | * | | | * * |
BMV subgenomic promoter core	A A G A T C . T A T . G T C C T A A T T C
CMV RNA 2 5′ ICR 2 homology	A A G A G C G T A T G G T T C . A A C C C
	| | | | * | | | | | | * | | | * * |
BMV subgenomic promoter core	A A G A T C . T A T . G T C C T A A T T C
CMV RNA 3 5′ ICR 2 homology	A A G G T . T A T G G C T T T C C . A A G G T C
	| | | * | | | | | | | | | | | * | |
BMV subgenomic promoter core	A A G A T C T A T G . . . . T C C T A A . T T C
AMV RNA 1 5′ ICR 2 homology	A A G A T . . A . G T T . . A A T C C
	| | | | | | | | * | | | * |
BMV subgenomic promoter core	A A G A T C T A T G T C C T A A T T C
AMV RNA 2 5′ ICR 2 homology	A A G A T A A G T T T C A G A . G T C . T A A . T C
	| | | * | | | * | | | | | | | | |
BMV subgenomic promoter core	A A G A . T C T . A T G T C C T A A T T C
AMV RNA 3 5′ ICR 2 homology	A A G A . . T A . G T . . T A A T . C A
	| | | | | | | | | | | | | |
BMV subgenomic promoter	A A G A T C T A T G T C C T A A T T C A

An asterisk denotes a mismatch.

lated 5′ end of BMV RNA 3 are duplicated. This duplication contains homology with both ICR 1 and ICR 2 (see Table 4). The third and fourth regions of homology are present in the subgenomic promoter region, where two sequence blocks having homology with ICR 2 occur. One region of homology (starting at position 1229) corresponds to the core sequence of the subgenomic promoter (Marsh et al. 1987), upstream of the site at which the subgenomic RNA initiates (see Fig. 1). The homology within this region is actually closer to the ICR 2 region at the 5′ end of the viral RNAs discussed above than it is to the tRNA ICR 2 consensus sequence. Another block homologous to ICR 2 occurs at the 5′ end of the subgenomic transcript in approximately the same relative position as the ICR 2 homology at the 5′ ends of the genomic RNAs. Although there is a general resemblance between the 5′ end of the subgenomic RNA 4 and that of the genomic RNAs, there is no obvious ICR 1 homology at its 5′ end.

DISCUSSION

tRNA-like Features of the BMV Genome

Previous studies from our laboratory have characterized several tRNA-like functions of BMV RNAs. These include the ability to accept tyrosine with an efficiency similar to that of a tRNA (Hall et al. 1972), and to interact with nucleotidyl transferase to repair its $3′\text{-CCA}_{OH}$ terminus (Bujarski et al. 1986). Secondary and tertiary structures have been proposed (Rietveld et al. 1983; Pleij et al. 1985) for the 3′-terminal region of BMV RNA that strongly resemble those generally accepted for tRNAs, except that the 5′ coding region of the virus is a very long extension departing from the "extra arm"; the acceptor stem is formed by a pseudoknot structure (Pleij et al. 1985). Investigations using native and mutant RNA templates obtained by in vitro transcription of cDNAs have identified various regions within the 3′ structure that are responsible for the tRNA-like functions (Dreher and Hall 1987). These templates have also been used to define regions within the 3′ terminus involved in recognition by the viral replicase (Bujarski et al. 1985, 1986; Dreher and Hall 1987) and initiation of replication (Miller et al. 1986). From these studies, it is evident that the tRNA-like region functions as an efficient and specific promoter for negative-strand synthesis of the viral RNAs. We have not yet identified any ICR-like regions within the 3′ end of BMV RNAs; however, if it is accepted that primitive life forms had an RNA genome, then some mechanism for copying tRNAs that involved the formation of complementary strands must have existed. Possibly, the negative-strand promoter reflects such a primitive mechanism that was adapted during the evolution of the self-replicating structure now seen as a viral genomic component.

Our studies with the cell-free replicase have also provided rigorous evidence as to how the subgenomic RNA 4 is generated from a promoter internal to BMV RNA 3 (Miller et al. 1985; Marsh et al. 1987) and have shown that this promoter consists of a core sequence flanked by three modulating sequences (L.E. Marsh et al., in prep.). We have been intrigued by the lack of similarity between the negative-strand promoter and the subgenomic promoter; the finding reported here that the subgenomic promoter contains elements strongly resembling ICR 2 (and, to a degree, ICR 1) is highly suggestive that the viral positive-strand replication system uses such elements. Although homology between the 5′ termini of the genomic RNAs of BMV and CMV was recently identified by Rezian et al. (1985), the homology of these regions with ICRs does not appear to have previously been recognized. From the data presented in Tables 1 and 2, it is clear that canonical regions recognized in polymerase III transcription are present at the 5′ end of the genomic RNAs of BMV and, to a lesser degree, CMV and AMV. With this in mind, careful reevaluation of the role of host polymerase functions in the replication of these viruses may be important. It has long been thought that host components are involved in viral replication (Hall et al. 1987), and the present evidence implicates components of polymerase III as potential candidates. Sequences in the RNA-2-coding regions of BMV, CMV, and AMV have homologies with retroviral and other RNA-dependent polymerases (Kamer and Argos 1984), but whether such homologies can be extended to regions encoding components of the polymerase III system in eukaryotic genomes is not known. No DNA phase for the RNA viruses described here has been identified, but the possibility that RNA-dependent replication occurs within the nucleus (or organelles) of infected cells has not been rigorously excluded. Interestingly, we have failed to copy correctly terminated genomic negative-strand templates with our replicase (T.W. Dreher and T.C. Hall, unpubl.), and it is tempting to think that host nuclear or organelle components may be required. This thought is supported by the fact that all four encapsidated BMV RNAs bear a 5′ m^7GpppG residue that is presumably added by capping enzymes typically present in the nucleus of eukaryotic cells. Certainly, far more copious production of positive-strand molecules from negative-strand molecules occurs in the host than vice versa; results from cell-free experiments are in marked contrast since, to our knowledge, there are no reliable reports of genomic positive strands being produced from template negative strands. It is conceivable, if unlikely, that the mechanism for genomic positive-strand synthesis differs markedly from that for genomic negative-strand synthesis, the ability of our replicase to generate positive-strand subgenomic RNAs representing a cytoplasmic amplification system important in the production of adequate quantities of viral coat protein. Evaluation of the concepts discussed above can be assisted by careful investigation of the subcellular location and quantity of each viral positive- and negative-strand RNA and virally encoded protein during infection.

Table 4. Comparison of BMV RNA 3 5′ and Intercistronic ICR Homologies

BMV intercistronic sequences:

```
          1000                        1040                         1060
TAGAATTAAATAGGTAAATCCGGTCTAACAAGCTCGGTCCATTTCGTAGAGTTAAGCAAGCTGGGGAGAC
                     1080                   1100                  1120
CCCCGACAGCCGTTTGGATCAGCGCTCGGCTCGTTTGGGTTCAATTCCCTTACCTTACAACGGCGTGT
      1140                         1180                        1200
TGAGATAGGTCCTCGGGGGAGGTTATCCATGTTTGTGGATATTCTATGTGTGTCTGAGTTCTATTATTA
                   1220                   1240                1260
AAAAAAAAAAAAAAAAAGATCTATGTCCTAATTCAGCGTATTAATAATGTCGACTTCAGGAACTGG
                                          ↑
```

ICR 1 Comparison

```
RNA 3 5′ end ICR 1:    GTAAAATAC . CAA . CTAA
                       | | | | | |   | | * * | | | |
RNA 3 intercistronic:  GTAA . AT . C . CGGTCTAA
                       | | * *   | * | | * *
tRNA ICR 1:            GTGG . . . . CNNAGT■■GG
```

ICR 2 Comparison

5′-end consensus:	GGTTCAA . TCC
Intercistronic #1:	AGCTCGG . TCC
Intercistronic #2:	GGTTCAATTCC
Intercistronic #3:	GTCCTAA . TTC
Intercistronic #4:	GT . CGACTTC
tRNA consensus:	GGTTCGANTCC

The intercistronic region of BMV RNA 3 (Ahlquist et al. 1981b; Dasgupta and Kaesberg 1982) shown includes the initiation site (↑) for subgenomic RNA 4. Regions of ICR 1 and 2 homology are denoted as in Table 1; Asterisk denotes a mismatch and closed box indicates an optional base in tRNAs.

337

Implications of ICR Sequences in Viral RNA

The evidence presented above argues strongly for conservation within this group of RNA viruses of sequences having remarkable homology with the ICRs 1 and 2 of tRNAs. The degree of homology with ICR 1 is lower than that with ICR 2, and the spacing between these sequences is considerably shorter than is found in tRNAs. The relative order of these sequences is, however, correct. Differences in spacing also occur for ICRs 1 and 3 (A and C boxes) of 5S RNA, which are closer together (Pieler et al. 1987), although not as close as found for the viral sequences. The overall similarity of the ICR-like sequences of BMV, CMV, and AMV RNAs to tRNA ICRs suggests that they and the tRNAs have descended from a common ancestor, BMV having evolved the least and AMV the most in terms of sequence change at the 5′ end of the viral genomic RNAs. The 5′ ends of these viruses seem to have coevolved with the subgenomic promoter of BMV (see Table 4), with the exception that the ICR-2-like sequences lack the downstream initiation site present in the subgenomic promoter region (Marsh et al. 1987). We have found (L.E. Marsh et al., in prep.) that deletions in the subgenomic promoter region downstream from the initiation site extending toward the initiation site enhance end-to-end copying that initiates (about 600 bases upstream of the correct initiation site) at the 5′ end of the supplied RNA template. Thus, the viral subgenomic promoter, like the tRNA promoters, is capable of stimulating initiation upstream of the promoter core sequence. However, in the case of the wild-type subgenomic RNA, modulating sequences direct correct initiation to a position downstream from the promoter core. Thus, by analogy, the ICR-2-like sequences at the 5′ ends of the genomic RNAs correspond to the core sequence of the subgenomic promoter, except that they direct initiation at the 5′ end.

Evidence for an Evolutionary Fusion in RNA 3

Our observation that the 5′ end of BMV RNA 3 is duplicated at the intercistronic region (Table 3), together with the recent observation that BMV is capable of undergoing genetic recombination through a template-switching mechanism (Bujarski and Kaesberg 1986), supports the speculative hypothesis that this dicistronic genomic RNA is evolutionarily descended from a fusion of two monocistronic RNAs. The experimental results referred to above, in which deletions into the region controlling correct initiation resulted in enhanced upstream initiation, imply that a promoter newly internalized within an intercistronic region by a fusion event would still be able to participate in promotion of synthesis of positive genomic RNA even though it was no longer located at the 5′ end. These deletions provide additional supportive evidence in that they cause increased initiation at both upstream and downstream cryptic sites (and decreased initiation at the correct site). Similarly, when truncated templates are used in vitro for generation of subgenomic RNA, de-

creased initiation at the correct site and increased initiation at downstream cryptic sites are observed (L.E. Marsh et al., in prep.). These latter two results imply that an early evolutionary step following internalization of a 5′ genomic promoter would be the conversion, through point mutations, of a downstream cryptic initiation site into an efficient subgenomic initiation site. Through such steps, an internalized genomic promoter could become an effective subgenomic promoter. In BMV, this latter step may have been preceded by a duplication of the internalized promoter, allowing the upstream copy to function still in promoting genomic replication, whereas the more 3′ internalized promoter has been specialized by evolution for subgenomic transcription. This hypothesis is corroborated by the results of French and Ahlquist (1987), showing that the replication of BMV RNA 3 in vivo is at least partially dependent on its intercistronic region. Indeed, the sequence cited by French and Ahlquist (1987) as being involved in genomic replication is among several sequences within this region for which we have shown ICR 2 homology (Table 4). However, attributing such activity to the slightly more 5′ site (which has both ICR 1 and 2 homologies) seems to be at least as likely and is equally consistent with their data. The site of potential ICR 2 homology on the 5′ end of the RNA 4 transcript would not appear to be required for either genomic replication or RNA 4 transcription in that it is centered around a SalI site immediately downstream from the subgenomic initiation site; downstream deletion mutants constructed using this site retained substantial activity (60–70% of wild type) as templates in transcription (Marsh et al. 1987). However, such mutant templates do not retain complete wild-type activity; thus, this latter site of ICR 2 homology may retain a modulating role.

In multipartite viruses, the genomic RNAs are encapsidated separately, and systemic infection requires that a given cell must be infected simultaneously with at least one particle for each genomic RNA. Thus, BMV and other tripartite genome viruses presently require infection simultaneously with three particles. The common ancestral virus of these tripartite genome viruses (bromoviruses, cucumoviruses, ilarviruses, and the alfalfa mosaic virus group) may have had four genomic RNAs, requiring simultaneous infection with four particles. Indeed, successful infection by AMV requires the presence of RNA 4 (or coat protein) in addition to the three genomic RNAs (Bol et al. 1971; Alblas and Bol 1978). Reduction of the number of particles required for infection would appear to enhance greatly the probability of obtaining a successful systemic infection and provide a selective advantage for fusing smaller genomic RNAs. An extension of this argument implies that many other viruses, including animal viruses such as the alphaviruses, are the result of a similar fusion process. Indeed, the larger, polycistronic, positive-strand RNA viruses (e.g., tobacco mosaic virus, tobacco rattle virus, and barley stripe mosaic virus), which have several subgenomic RNAs, may be the result of such multiple fusion events.

Origin of ICR Regions in RNA Viruses

Two divergent theories can be derived for the origin of the ICR homologies found in these tripartite genome viruses. In one, acquisition is of relatively recent evolutionary origin. Such would be in accord with the fascinating phenomena observed in vivo by Monroe and Schlesinger (1983), where two independent isolates of alphavirus defective-interfering (DI) RNAs were observed to have acquired cellular tRNA^{Asp} sequences at their 5' ends. The selective advantage to the DI RNAs may well have been in acquiring the ICRs present in the tRNA sequences. In both isolates, ICR 2 was intact, but in one, ICR 1 lacks 3 bases at its 5' end (Fig. 2) and in the other, a few more bases are absent. By analogy with the recombination events that presumably created these DI RNAs, and in light of the recently demonstrated ability of BMV to undergo recombination (Bujarski and Kaesberg 1986), one can hypothesize that an ancestral viral genomic RNA of a virus with a quadripartite genome acquired such a cellular tRNA and then converted the 5' end of other three genomic RNAs through further recombination. Such a process could also be implicated in the evolution of the lengthy (over 200-nucleotide) region of homology at the 3' end of each of the genomic RNAs of BMV and other tripartite genome viruses (Symons 1979; Gunn and Symons 1980a,b; Ahlquist et al. 1981a).

In considering whether such sequences could actually be involved in the replication and transcription of the RNAs of viruses such as BMV, it must be recognized that BMV, and probably most other positive-strand RNA viruses, has a cistron (that of RNA 2 in BMV) that retains homology with polymerases of other viruses and other RNA-dependent polymerases. Thus, the active polymerase in replication of the viral RNAs was probably not cellular polymerase III, but the viral evolutionary homolog. In light of the number of factors involved in plant cellular polymerase III complexes,

and the small number of viral cistrons (four), cellular factors are probably substantially involved in the actual replication complex. Thus, these sequences may interact with factors other than the replicase alone, i.e., cellular factors that are components of the replicase complex. Furthermore, in light of the sequence homology between the subgenomic promoters of BMV and the alphaviruses (Marsh et al. 1987), these viruses appear to share a common ancestry. Therefore, it is possible that the DI RNAs acquired the tRNA sequences in order to utilize the tRNA transcriptional signals that were compatible with the viral replicative machinery, which already shared commonality with tRNA transcription at the mechanistic level.

An alternative hypothesis for the origin of ICRs in viral genomes is that they reflect an ancient replication strategy. If it is assumed that life was once RNA-based, then early genomes must also have functioned as coding regions. Like tRNAs and other nucleic acid components of the protein-synthesizing system, the genome must have been capable of promoting its own replication from within its sequence. As DNA-based genomes evolved, tRNAs maintained the internal signals promoting positive-strand synthesis, but no longer required internal signals for promoting synthesis of the complementary negative strand. In BMV, CMV, and AMV, the 3' promoter within the tRNA-like structure may resemble that recognized by the primitive polymerase. We have already mentioned that the RNA 2-coding sequence of these viruses exhibits homology with other RNA-dependent polymerases (including those of retroviruses). It is conceivable that polymerase III is descended from a primitive RNA-dependent replicase by adaption for DNA-based transcription of functional RNAs. An evolutionary relatedness of these viral replicases and polymerase III may allow the viral replication system to co-opt host transcriptional functions which recognize ICRs for the active synthesis of viral positive strands.

In summary, BMV RNAs have several features that can be considered primitive: They contain tRNA-like signals at the 5' and 3' ends that control replication without a DNA intermediate; they have multiple tRNA functions including recognition by aminoacyl-tRNA synthetase and nucleotidyl transferase; and they have mRNA functions that encode at least part of the proteins catalyzing their replication. Many of these features parallel those currently conceived as being characteristic of early RNA-based life forms (Pace and Marsh 1985; Cech and Bass 1986).

Why Do These Viruses Retain an RNA Genome?

If nucleic-acid-based life originated through RNA-based reaction, it is not unrealistic to believe that successful aspects of this process may have survived to the present day. DNA-based heredity appears to have proven superior primarily because of its relative stability and consequent suitability for higher levels of complexity, RNA genomes persisting and evolving princi-

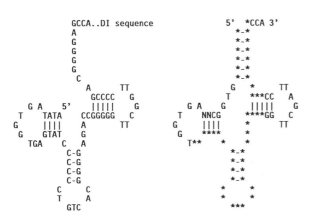

Figure 2. Comparison of 5' region of Sindbis DI RNA and canonical tRNA. (*Left*) The structure corresponds to the tRNA^{Asp} 5' end of a Sindbis DI RNA (Monroe and Schlesinger 1983). (*Right*) The structure corresponds to a canonical tRNA in which bases corresponding to ICR sequences are denoted by uppercase letters and other bases by asterisks.

pally as parasitic systems. In the plant viruses discussed here, this may relate to the constant need for the viruses to adapt to changes or differences in the host. For example, BMV is clearly dependent on several host functions, including the probable involvement of host factors in replication. In nature, the hosts will contain an isozymic spectrum of such enzymes: The lack of a proofreading mechanism, coupled with a relatively high error rate, may allow for rapid adaption of the viral genome as the infection process proceeds within a given host. As a result, two apparently opposing events occur: Regions of genomes of RNA viruses are rigidly conserved (by functional selection) and the overall genome is subject to rapid drift (beneficial mutations being positively selected). Superimposed on this drift is the ability of these RNAs to recombine (Bujarski and Kaesberg 1986). This latter process probably serves to both conserve the more fundamental functions and allow the coupling of separate beneficial mutations.

Molecular studies are revealing the basic processes involved in positive-strand RNA viral infections. The homologies recognized here provide new insight into replication strategies of these viruses and suggest alternative directions for virus research, particularly to investigating subcellular locations of the various replication and protein synthetic functions. They also stimulate conjecture as to whether the replication strategies of these viruses represent new adaptations of previously used catalytic functions or whether they represent ancient processes frozen in time.

ACKNOWLEDGMENTS

The authors gratefully acknowledge insight gained from discussions with Theo Dreher and Rick DeRose, and thank Mike Benedik for assistance with computing facilities. This work was supported by National Institutes of Health grant AI-22345.

REFERENCES

Ahlquist, P. and M. Janda. 1984. cDNA cloning and *in vitro* transcription of the complete brome mosaic virus genome. *Mol. Cell. Biol.* **4:** 2876.

Ahlquist, P., R. Dasgupta, and P. Kaesberg. 1981a. Near identity of 3' RNA secondary structure in bromoviruses and cucumber mosaic virus. *Cell* **23:** 183.

———. 1984a. Nucleotide sequence of brome mosaic virus genome and its implications for viral replication. *J. Mol. Biol.* **172:** 369.

Ahlquist, P., V. Luckow, and P. Kaesberg. 1981b. Complete nucleotide sequence of brome mosaic virus RNA3. *J. Mol. Biol.* **153:** 23.

Ahlquist, P., J.J. Bujarski, P. Kaesberg, and T.C. Hall. 1984b. Localization of the replicase recognition site within brome mosaic virus by hybrid-arrested RNA synthesis. *Plant Mol. Biol.* **3:** 37.

Ahlquist, P., R.M. French, M. Janda, and L.S. Loesch-Fries. 1984c. Multicomponent RNA plant virus infection derived from cloned viral cDNA. *Proc. Natl. Acad. Sci.* **81:** 7066.

Alblas, F. and J.F. Bol. 1978. Coat protein is required for infection of cowpea protoplasts with alfalfa mosaic virus. *J. Gen. Virol.* **41:** 653.

Bol, J.F., L. van Vloten-Doting, and E.M.J. Jaspars. 1971. A functional equivalence of top component *a* RNA and coat protein in the initiation of infection by alfalfa mosaic virus. *Virology* **46:** 73.

Bujarski, J.J. and P. Kaesberg. 1986. Genetic recombination between RNA components of a multipartite plant virus. *Nature* **321:** 528.

Bujarski, J.J., T.W. Dreher, and T.C. Hall. 1985. Deletions in the 3'-terminal tRNA like structure of brome mosaic virus RNA differentially affect aminoacylation and replication *in vitro*. *Proc. Natl. Acad. Sci.* **82:** 5636.

Bujarski, J.J., S.F. Hardy, W.A. Miller, and T.C. Hall. 1982. Use of dodecyl-β-D-maltoside in the purification and stabilization of RNA polymerase from brome mosaic virus infected barley. *Virology* **119:** 465.

Bujarski, J.J., P. Ahlquist, T.C. Hall, T.W. Dreher, and P. Kaesberg. 1986. Modulation of replication, aminoacylation and adenylation *in vitro* and infectivity *in vivo* of BMV RNAs containing deletions within the multifunctional 3' end. *EMBO J.* **5:** 1769.

Cech, T.R. and B.L. Bass. 1986. Biological catalysis by RNA. *Annu. Rev. Biochem.* **55:** 599.

Cornelissen, B.J.C., H. Janssen, D. Zuidema, and F.J. Bol. 1984. Complete nucleotide sequence of tobacco streak virus RNA 3. *Nucleic Acids Res.* **12:** 2427.

Dasgupta, R. and P. Kaesberg. 1982. Complete nucleotide sequence of the coat protein messenger RNAs of brome mosaic virus and cowpea chlorotic mottle virus. *Nucleic Acids Res.* **10:** 703.

Dreher, T.W. and T.C. Hall. 1987. Mutational analysis of the functions of the tRNA-like region of brome mosaic virus RNA. *UCLA Symp. Mol. Cell. Biol.* **54:** 317.

Dreher, T.W., J.J. Bujarski, and T.C. Hall. 1984. Mutant viral RNAs synthesized *in vitro* show altered aminoacylation and replicase template activities. *Nature* **311:** 171.

French, R. and P. Ahlquist. 1987. Intercistronic as well as terminal sequences are required for efficient amplification of brome mosaic virus RNA3. *J. Virol.* **61:** 1457.

French, R., M. Janda, and P. Ahlquist. 1986. Bacterial gene inserted in an engineered RNA virus: Efficient expression in monocotyledonous plant cells. *Science* **231:** 1294.

Gould, A.R. and R.H. Symons. 1982. Cucumber mosaic virus RNA 3: Determination of the nucleotide sequence provides the amino acid sequences of protein 3A and viral coat protein. *Eur. J. Biochem.* **126:** 217.

Gunn, M.R. and R.H. Symons. 1980a. Sequence homology at the 3'-termini of the four RNAs of alfalfa mosaic virus. *FEBS Lett.* **109:** 145.

———. 1980b. The RNAs of bromoviruses: 3'-terminal sequences of the four brome mosaic virus RNAs and comparison with cowpea chlorotic mottle virus RNA 4. *FEBS Lett.* **115:** 77.

Hall, T.C. 1979. Transfer RNA-like structures in viral genomes. *Int. Rev. Cytol.* **60:** 1.

Hall, T.C., T.W. Dreher, and L.E. Marsh. 1987. Replicase and replication: Strategies for brome mosaic virus. *UCLA Symp. Mol. Cell. Biol.* **48:** 295.

Hall, T.C., D.S. Shih, and P. Kaesberg. 1972. Enzyme-mediated binding of tyrosine to brome mosaic virus ribonucleic acid. *Biochem. J.* **129:** 969.

Hardy, S.F., T.L. German, L.S. Loesch-Fries, and T.C. Hall. 1979. Highly active template-specific RNA-dependent RNA polymerase from barley leaves infected with brome mosaic virus. *Proc. Natl. Acad. Sci.* **76:** 4956.

Koper-Zwarthoff, E.C., F.T. Brederode, G. Veeneman, J.H. van Boom, and J.F. Bol. 1980. Nucleotide sequences at the 5'-termini of the alfalfa mosaic virus RNAs and the intercistronic junction in RNA 3. *Nucleic Acids Res.* **8:** 5635.

Kamer, G. and P. Argos. 1984. Primary structural comparison of RNA dependent polymerases from plant, animal, and bacterial viruses. *Nucleic Acids Res.* **12:** 7269.

Lane, L.C. and P. Kaesberg. 1971. Multiple genetic components in bromegrass mosaic virus. *Nat. New Biol.* **232:** 40.

Loesch-Fries, L.S. and T.C. Hall. 1982. *In vivo* aminoacylation of brome mosaic and barley stripe mosaic virus RNAs. *Nature* **298:** 771.

Marsh, L.E., T.W. Dreher, and T.C. Hall. 1987. Mutational analysis of the internal promoter for transcription of subgenomic RNA4 of BMV. *UCLA Symp. Mol. Cell. Biol.* **54:** 327.

Miller, W.A. and T.C. Hall. 1983. Use of micrococcal nuclease in the purification of highly template dependent RNA-dependent RNA polymerase from brome mosaic virus-infected barley. *Virology* **125:** 236.

Miller, W.A., T.W. Dreher, and T.C. Hall. 1985. Synthesis of brome mosaic virus subgenomic RNA *in vitro* by internal initiation on (−) sense genomic RNA. *Nature* **313:** 68.

Miller, W.A., J.J. Bujarski, T.W. Dreher, and T.C. Hall. 1986. Minus-strand initiation by brome mosaic virus replicase within the 3′ tRNA-like structure of native and modified RNA templates. *J. Mol. Biol.* **187:** 537.

Monroe, S.S. and S. Schlesinger. 1983. RNAs from two independently isolated defective-interfering particles of Sindbis virus contain a cellular tRNA at their 5′ ends. *Proc. Natl. Acad. Sci.* **80:** 3279.

Ou, J.H., C.M. Rice, L. Dalgarno, E.G. Strauss, and J.H. Strauss. 1982. Sequence studies of several alphavirus genomic RNAs in the region of the start of the subgenomic RNA. *Proc. Natl. Acad. Sci.* **79:** 5235.

Pace, N.R. and T.L. Marsh. 1985. RNA catalysis and the origin of life. *Origins Life* **16:** 97.

Pieler, T., J. Hamm, and R.G. Roeder. 1987. The 5S gene internal control region is of three distinct sequence elements, organized as two functional domains with variable spacing. *Cell* **48:** 91.

Pleij, C.W.A., K. Rietveld, and L. Bosch. 1985. A new principle of RNA folding based on psuedoknotting. *Nucleic Acids Res.* **13:** 1717.

Ravelonandro, M., T. Godfrey-Colburn, and L. Pinck. 1983. Structure of the 5′-terminal untranslated region of the genomic RNAs from two strains of alfalfa mosaic virus. *Nucleic Acids Res.* **11:** 2815.

Rezian, M.A., R.H.V. Williams, and R.H. Symons. 1985. Nucleotide sequence of cucumber mosaic virus RNA1: Presence of a sequence complementary to part of the viral satellite RNA and homology with other viral RNAs. *Eur. J. Biochem.* **150:** 331.

Rezian, M.A., R.H.V. Williams, K.H.J. Gordon, A.R. Gould, and R.H. Symons. 1984. Nucleotide sequence of cucumber mosaic RNA 2 reveals a translation product significantly homologous to corresponding proteins of other viruses. *Eur. J. Biochem.* **143:** 277.

Rietveld, K., C.W.A. Pleij, and L. Bosch. 1983. Three-dimensional models of the tRNA-like 3′ termini of some plant viral RNAs. *EMBO J.* **2:** 1079.

Sharp, S.J., J. Shaack, L. Cooley, D.J. Burke, and D. Söll. 1985. Structure and transcription of eucaryotic tRNA genes. *CRC Crit. Rev. Biochem.* **19:** 107.

Symons, R.H. 1979. Homology at the 3′-terminus of the four RNAs of cucumber mosaic virus. *Nucleic Acids Res.* **7:** 825.

Molecular Events Leading to Poliovirus Genome Replication

A.V. PAUL, C.-F. YANG, S.-K. JANG, R.J. KUHN,* H. TADA, M. NICKLIN,
H.-G. KRÄUSSLICH, C.-K. LEE, AND E. WIMMER
Department of Microbiology, School of Medicine, State University of New York, Stony Brook, New York 11794

There are more than 500 human viruses, and most of them contain RNA genomes. In fact, RNA viruses outnumber DNA viruses in all those eukaryotic systems that are plagued by these etiological agents. The reason for this preponderance of RNA viruses is not known. In contrast to DNA viruses, however, the RNA viruses have for the most part evolved to replicate outside the nucleus of the host cells, and they are thus independent of cellular replication functions such as DNA polymerases, RNA transcriptases, and processing enzymes. Free of such links, the replicative machineries of RNA viruses were allowed to adapt to parasitic life in every aspect imaginable. As a consequence of this, a multitude of replicative strategies exist, and we know of plus-stranded, minus-stranded, ambisense, mono-partite and multipartite, naked and enveloped, spherical, and elongated RNA viruses.

Much is written in this volume about the constraints with which an RNA genome of a self-replicating entity is burdened: the chemical instability of the ribonucleotide linkage, the multitude of RNA processing (or degrading) enzymes that an RNA molecule is likely to encounter in the host cell, and, most severely, the lack of proofreading, editing, and repair mechanisms in RNA synthesis. These constraints are thought to be the reason that genomes of RNA viruses are much smaller than those of DNA viruses. The limitation in size dictated that genetic information be condensed and, as a consequence, that regulatory sequences be reduced or eliminated (Reanney, this volume). Poliovirus is a case of a mammalian RNA virus whose genetic content has been reduced to a minimum. In the simplest term, the genome of this virus can be viewed as mRNA encoding a single polypeptide (a "polyprotein"). This mRNA acquired additional skills as, for example, the ability to replicate and subsequently to encoat itself with a protecting shell of proteins.

Poliovirus, a small, naked particle with a diameter of only 28 nm, consists of 60 copies each of four capsid proteins (VP1, VP2, VP3, and VP4) enclosing a single-stranded RNA genome of plus-strand polarity (Rueckert 1985). The 5′ end, interestingly, has its 5′-terminal phosphate residue esterified to the O^4-hydroxyl group of a tyrosine residue, the latter being an amino acid of a small protein called VPg (Fig. 1). The 3′ terminus, on the other end, is polyadenylylated (Kuhn and Wimmer 1987; Semler et al. 1987 and references therein).

Poliovirus belongs to one of the largest families of human pathogens, the Picornaviridae. These viruses cause a bewildering array of disease syndromes ranging from fatal paralysis, encephalitis, meningitis, conjunc-

---

*Present address: Division of Biology 156-29, California Institute of Technology, Pasadena, California 91125.

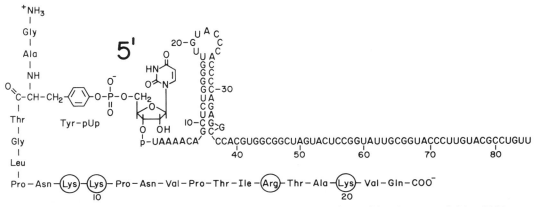

Figure 1. Structure of the 5′ terminus of poliovirus RNA. The oligonucleotide ($n = 85$) is a fragment of virion RNA generated by RNase III of *Escherichia coli* (Larsen et al. 1981). VPg is linked to the RNA via an energy-rich phosphodiester between the O^4-hydroxyl group of tyrosine and a uridylate residue. The position of tyrosine relative to the amino terminus appears to be essential, as determined by site-directed mutagenesis in this region (R.J. Kuhn et al., in prep.). VPg is a cleavage product of the poliovirus polyprotein (see Fig. 2). Basic amino acids have been circled. (Reprinted, with permission, from Kitamura et al. 1981.)

tivitis, hepatitis, myocarditis, and pancreatitis to the common cold. The incidence of human infections with picornaviruses is high, and serious long-term effects have been noticed. Even poliomyelitis remains a serious health problem in many parts of the world, although two excellent poliovirus vaccines have been developed (Horstmann et al. 1984).

mRNA Function of the Poliovirus Genome

The genome of poliovirus is a heteropolymer of 7441 nucleotides plus a poly(A) tail ($n = 60 \pm 30$). Nucleotides (6627) of the heteropolymeric RNA form an open reading frame of 2209 codons specifying the "polyprotein" (see Fig. 2). The events of adsorption, penetration, and uncoating of the virus in the initial stages of infection are poorly understood. However, once the viral RNA has entered the cytoplasm of the host cell, it associates with ribosomes and allows translation to commence 743 nucleotides downstream from the 5' end.

In view of the arguments presented above, it is surprising that an RNA virus would retain such a long sequence of a 5' noncoding region (5'NCR). It contains eight seemingly unused initiation codons before translation begins at the ninth AUG triplet. Several studies have already indicated that the sequence and secondary structures of the 5'NCR might play an important role in viral replication (Harris 1979; Larsen et al. 1981; Varta-

petian et al. 1983; Evans et al. 1985; Racaniello and Meriam 1986; Semler et al. 1986; Nomoto et al. 1987; Kuge and Nomoto 1987 and references therein). Inversions, deletions, and point mutations have been found to have a deleterious effect on viral replication without apparent reason. Clearly, the 5'NCR could harbor signals for genome replication, encapsidation, or scanning-independent initiation of translation. Only the hairpin near the 5' end (Fig. 1) has been proved to exist in solution (Larsen et al. 1981); other higher-order structures have yet to be identified. Computer-aided modeling, based on structures seen in the electron microscope, has been carried out for parts of the viral genome (Currey et al. 1986), but a thorough and exhaustive structural analysis of the 5'NCR remains to be done to accommodate the phenotypic changes seen so far. The function of the hairpin structure seen in Figure 1 is unknown, but a point mutation in its stem has rendered the mutant virus temperature-sensitive (Racaniello and Meriam 1986).

A peculiar observation was made several years ago that remains unexplained: The 5'-terminal VPg is absent from viral RNA serving as mRNA, although mRNA and virion RNA have identical sequences (Pettersson et al. 1977; Nomoto et al. 1977b). Indeed, viral RNA from which VPg has been removed by proteolytic degradation, or synthetic viral RNA transcribed from plasmids with phage T7 RNA polymerase, is infectious (Nomoto et al. 1977a; van der Werf et al. 1986). Thus,

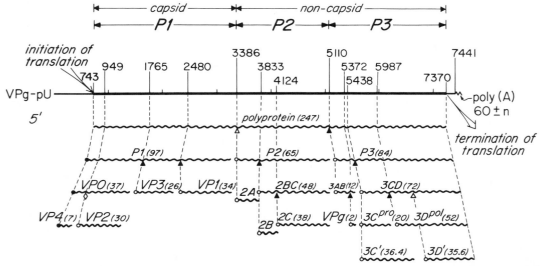

Figure 2. Gene organization and polypeptide processing of poliovirus. Virion RNA, terminated at the 5' end with the genome-linked protein VPg and at the 3' end with poly(A), is shown as a solid line, the translated region being more pronounced than the noncoding regions. Arrows indicate the sites at which initiation (743) and termination (7370) of translation occur. The numbers above the virion RNA line refer to the first nucleotide of the codon specifying the amino-terminal amino acid of each virus-specific protein. The coding region has been divided into three regions (P1, P2, and P3), corresponding to major cleavage products of the polyprotein. The newly adapted nomenclature of picornavirus proteins is presented according to Rueckert and Wimmer (1984). Polypeptides are presented as wavy lines. Numbers in parentheses are molecular weights calculated from the amino acid sequences. Carboxy-terminal "trimming" does not occur. (○) Glycine in all cases except for VP2, where it is serine. The carboxy-terminal amino acid of 3CD is phenylalanine. (●) Amino terminus is known to be blocked (Dorner et al. 1982) with myristic acid (Chow et al. 1987; Paul et al. 1987). (▲) Gln-Gly; (△) Tyr-Gly; (◇) Asn-Ser cleavage sites. Polypeptides 3C' and 3D' are products of an alternative cleavage mode of 3CD, the biological significance of which is unknown. (Modified from Kitamura et al. 1981.)

VPg is not necessary for the function of viral RNA during the initial stages of infection, although all viral RNA formed during replication is VPg-linked (see Fig. 3). Ambros and Baltimore (1980) have described a cellular activity thought to be responsible for the "unlinking" of VPg from viral RNA, but the enzyme has not yet been further characterized. Once removed, the small protein VPg appears to be rapidly degraded in the cytoplasm (Dorner et al. 1981 and references therein).

Protein Synthesis: Proteolytic Processing of the Polyprotein

Proteolytic processing of the polyprotein of picornaviruses is one of the most fascinating aspects of this family of viruses (for reviews, see Nicklin et al. 1986; Toyoda et al. 1986a; Wimmer et al. 1987). Most eukaryotic plus-strand RNA viruses synthesize and process polyproteins, but in comparison to picornaviruses, other systems are less well understood. It should be pointed out that all viral polyproteins known are initially processed by virus-encoded proteinases that are elements of the polyproteins themselves. In contrast, cellular polyproteins, e.g., the precursors to neuropeptides, are cleaved by cellular proteinases that are encoded by separate cellular genetic elements (see Marx 1987).

Poliovirus polyprotein processing occurs in three stages. The primary cleavage takes place during polyprotein synthesis. It is carried out by proteinase 2A and leads to the rapid separation of the capsid precursor P1 from nonstructural proteins (P2 and P3; see Fig. 1). The secondary cleavages are catalyzed by proteinase 3C that, after intramolecular liberation, acts in *trans* to cut at Q-G pairs. The tertiary cleavage occurs during morphogenesis of the virion (cleavage of VP0 to VP4 and VP2 at an N-S pair; See Fig. 1). As an exciting possibility, this cleavage may be an intramolecular event that involves elements of the viral RNA (Arnold et al. 1987). As first suggested by Rossmann et al. (1985), the Ser-10 in VP2 may be the amino acid that, after activation by a proton-abstractor (a base of the nucleic acid), may catalyze cleavage between the as-

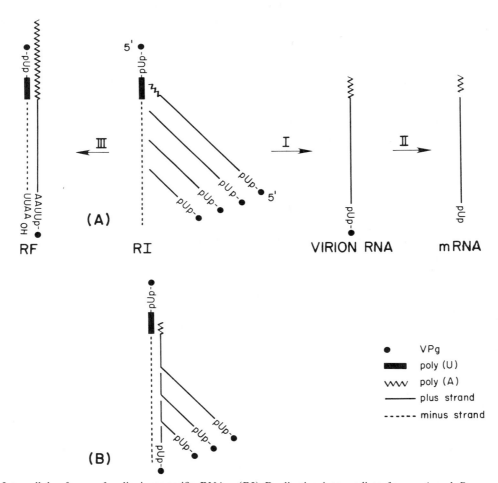

Figure 3. Intracellular forms of poliovirus-specific RNAs. (RI) Replicative intermediate forms, *A* and *B* representing two possible structures of this polynucleotide; (RF) replicative form, the terminal structures of which have been described by Larsen et al. (1980). (Redrawn from Kitamura et al. 1980.)

paragine and serine, the latter being the amino-terminal amino acid of VP2 (Larsen et al. 1982). Other specific considerations regarding the processing events are described below.

1. 2A and 3C can act in *cis* as well as in *trans* (Kräusslich et al. 1987; Nicklin et al. 1987; Ypma-Wong and Semler 1987). The nature of the active site has been predicted by comparison of amino acid sequences of several picornaviruses (Argos et al. 1984) and contains Cys-147 and His-161. This prediction received support by site-directed mutagenesis experiments (Ivanoff et al. 1986). Studies with inhibitors support the notion that 3C of encephalomyocarditis virus (EMCV) and of poliovirus is a sulfhydryl proteinase (Pelham 1978; Palmenberg and Rueckert 1982; Gorbalenya and Svitkin 1983; M.J.H. Nicklin and E. Wimmer, unpubl.). Extensive enzymology with 3C, however, has not been performed due to a lack of purified enzyme and substrate. From comparisons of amino acid sequences of picornavirus polypeptides, we suggest that 2A is also a sulfhydryl protease (Toyoda et al. 1986b), but experiments to support this claim have not been carried out.

2. All picornaviruses studied produce 3C, but an active 2A appears to be a product of the polyprotein of enteroviruses and rhinoviruses only.

3. The proteinases cleave with high specificity: Poliovirus 3C proteinase does not cleave precursor proteins of EMCV and vice versa (M.J.H. Nicklin and A.C. Palmenberg, unpubl.). This specificity of $3C^{pro}$ is remarkable in view of the fact that the cleavage signal recognized by $3C^{pro}$ of both poliovirus and EMCV is mainly Q-G. $3C^{pro}$ of poliovirus does not even cleave all 13 Q-G sites present in its own polyprotein. Instead, it recognizes only 8–9 Q-G sites; but, surprisingly, those Q-G pairs that are cleaved have surrounding amino acid sequences that differ from each other. We have speculated, however, that an additional determinant of recognition may be the amino acid at position −4 relative to the Q-G cleavage site; in poliovirus, this amino acid is most often an alanine residue (Nicklin et al. 1986; Toyoda et al. 1986a). It is unlikely that the selection of the proper Q-G sites is based solely on accessibility. $3C^{pro}$ may require Q-G pairs in structurally flexible contexts surrounding the active Q-G sites, as has been proposed recently by Arnold et al. (1987). The high specificity of $3C^{pro}$ may be an explanation for the observation that no cellular proteins have yet been identified that are cleaved by $3C^{pro}$; the same may be true for $2A^{pro}$ (Korant et al. 1980; Lee et al. 1985; Lloyd et al. 1985, 1986).

4. Synthetic peptides corresponding to poliovirus sequences (with Y-G or Q-G pairs in the center) that are cleaved specifically by the 2A or 3C proteinases have not been found.

5. Poliovirus is the only virus whose $3C^{pro}$ cleavage sites are exclusively Q-G pairs. In other picornaviruses, the $3C^{pro}$ cleavage sites can vary considerably but are generally Glx-Gly, where the glycine can be replaced by S, T, A, V or M residues (Q-G, Q-S, Q-T, Q-A, Q-V, Q-M; and E-G, E-S) (Nicklin et al. 1986; Palmenberg 1987). Site-directed mutagenesis of individual amino acids and the use of mutagenesis cartridges (R.J. Kuhn et al., in prep.) will allow us to assess what sequences can function as cleavage signals for 3C.

6. Poliovirus rapidly and effectively turns off host-cell protein synthesis (Ehrenfeld 1982), and this event is accompanied by the cleavage of a large polypeptide (termed p220, corresponding to its relative molecular weight of 220×10^3) from the cell's cap-binding complex. Neither $2A^{pro}$ nor $3C^{pro}$ cleaves p220 directly; however, on the basis of genetic and biochemical experiments, polypeptide 2A appears to "activate" the degradation of p220 (Bernstein et al. 1985; Kräusslich et al. 1987). In agreement with this finding, infection with EMCV (a virus whose 2A is not homologous in function to the 2A of poliovirus) does not induce the cleavage of this p220 cellular polypeptide (Mosenkis et al. 1985).

7. The Y-G-specific cleavage in polypeptide 3CD that yields 3C' and 3D' (Fig. 1) may be fortuituous and of no biological significance other than lowering the yield of $3C^{pro}$ and $3D^{pol}$ (3D polymerase). Site-directed mutation of the tyrosine residue of this Y-G site in 3CD to a phenylalanine residue (F-G) did not abolish the infectivitiy of the altered genome. Surprisingly, 3C' and 3D' were still produced from this altered cleavage site (C.-K. Lee and E. Wimmer, in prep.). On the other hand, alteration of the cleavage site from TY-G to AY-G completely abolished the production of 3C' and 3D' without detectable effects on virus growth (C.-K. Lee and E. Wimmer, in prep.).

8. Polypeptide 3AB, a membrane-associated protein (Semler et al. 1982; Takegami et al. 1983a), is relatively stable in pulse-chase experiments of infected cells, although it contains an "active" Q-G site. It has been speculated that 3AB is processed to 3A and VPg only after a tyrosine residue in the 3B portion of 3AB has been uridylylated (Takegami et al. 1983b; Takeda et al. 1986: Kuhn and Wimmer 1987).

9. Substrates for 2A and 3C have been synthesized in rabbit reticulocyte lysates (RRLs) and have been used to define some aspects of the cleavage activity and to develop assays for 2A and 3C (Kräusslich et al. 1987; Nicklin et al. 1987; Ypma-Wong and Semler 1987). It has become apparent that the relationship between substrate and proteinase is complex in that some truncated, virus-specific polypeptides, although containing bona fide cleavage sites, are no longer processed by the enzyme.

10. The polyprotein of poliovirus contains only one

VPg segment, whereas that of foot-and-mouth disease virus (FMDV) contains three VPg segments that are tandemly arranged (Forss and Schaller 1982). The three VPg segments in the FMDV polyprotein differ considerably in their amino acid sequences. The reason for the tandem repeat of VPgs (all of which are used in genome synthesis) is unknown.

Viral RNA as Template in Genome Replication

There is no doubt that poliovirus RNA replication follows the general pathway of all lytic RNA viruses: Genomic RNA is transcribed into complementary RNA that, in turn, serves as a template for virion RNA synthesis. Since poliovirion RNA is of plus-strand polarity (the same polarity as mRNA), the flow of information proceeds from plus strands to minus strands to plus strands. In this, it resembles the replication of phage Qβ genomic RNA (see other papers in this volume). In contrast to earlier expectations, however, there may be *no* additional similarities between Qβ and poliovirus genome replication. Apart from fundamental differences in genome structures, these agents have evolved to encode very different RNA polymerases: The polymerase of Qβ can initiate RNA synthesis de novo, whereas that of poliovirus is a strictly primer-dependent enzyme (for recent reviews, see Kuhn and

Wimmer 1987; Semler et al. 1987; Wimmer et al. 1987).

Mere inspection of the poliovirus genome (Figs. 1 and 2) leaves us with the following unsolved puzzle: The termini of the RNA are so different that it is difficult to imagine how a single enzyme can recognize them and start replication. It is possible and even likely that there are "internal" recognition signals for the "replicase." Even after recognition has occurred, the poliovirus RNA polymerase might need a primer that has to function at template structures that are chemically very different. Moreover, the termini of the template RNAs must be restored during replication. We now know that poly(A) of poliovirus RNA is genetically coded (Dorsch-Hasler et al. 1975); i.e., polyadenylylation occurs simply by transcription of the 5′-terminal poly(U) of minus strands. The mechanism of attachment of VPg, on the other hand, is obscure (see below).

Viral RNA structures found in the infected cells are shown in Figure 3, and the pathways by which these structures are thought to arise are shown in Figure 4 (Kuhn and Wimmer 1987; Semler et al. 1987 and references therein). The replicative intermediate (RI), long known to be the structure involved in single-stranded RNA synthesis, may exist in the cell in one of two possible forms: predominantly single-stranded (Fig. 3A) or predominantly double-stranded (Fig. 3B). Evidence has been presented supporting either structure

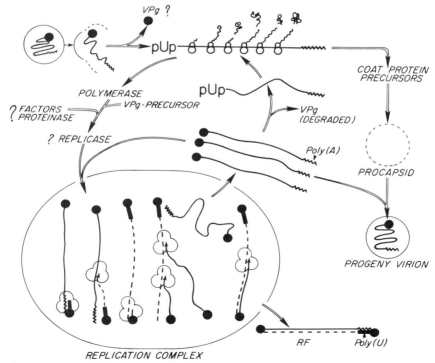

Figure 4. Schematic representation of the growth cycle of poliovirus with emphasis on RNA replication. The replication complex is membrane-bound. (RI) Replicative intermediate forms; (RF) replicative form (see Fig. 3). (Redrawn from Kitamura et al. 1980.)

(Nilsen et al. 1981; Richards et al. 1984 and discussion and references therein). Structure B requires that long stretches of double-stranded RNA be unwound during strand elongation, a process requiring much energy and possibly the help of an RNA helicase, a function not yet discovered for any RNA replicating systems. Structure A, on the other hand, requires functions keeping the complementary strands apart. In Qβ RNA replication, this is achieved by stable secondary structures within the nascent strands that are formed immediately after their formation. Formation of similar secondary structures, however, seems to play less of a role in eukaryotic viral RNA replication. For example, brome mosaic virus or sindbis virus contain plus-stranded RNA genomes in which segments have been replaced by foreign genes (e.g., *cat* gene) without loss of the ability of the RNA to replicate in vivo (French et al. 1986; Levis et al. 1987).

Another virus-specific RNA structure found in infected cells is double-stranded RNA, also called replicative form (RF; Fig. 3). Poliovirus RF is *not* generated during isolation of viral RNA from infected cells but is a by-product of viral replication (Larsen et al. 1980). RF may even be an intermediate in minus-strand synthesis (for discussion, see Takeda et al. 1986), although evidence supporting this view is lacking. Poliovirus RF is infectious. Transfection does not lead to progeny virus in enucleated cells, an observation suggesting the need for nuclear function(s). In contrast, transfections with single-stranded RNA do not require that the host cell contains a nucleus (see Detjen et al. 1978).

Other virus-specific RNA molecules found in the infected cell are virion RNA and mRNA (Figs. 3 and 4), two identical polynucleotides that differ in their 5' ends (see above). Why VPg is removed from viral mRNA is not clear. One hypothesis states that VPg would interfere with the attachment of the 40S ribosomal subunit, and thus inhibit the process of "scanning" (Kozak 1983). Since poliovirus mRNA is not capped, we cannot rule out the possibility that the attachment of functional ribosomal subunits occurs at a specific nucleotide sequence *within* the 5'NCR, a process that would defy Kozak's scanning mechanism. Indeed, in an in vitro system using multicistronic synthetic RNAs, we have obtained compelling evidence supporting "internal" attachment of ribosomal subunits (S.-K. Jang et al., unpubl.).

Flanegan and his colleagues have reported that an additional species of RF molecules can be found in poliovirus-infected HeLa cells. These are thought to be covalently linked at one end of the RNA, and it has been implied that they are intermediates in the hairpin replication of viral RNA (Young et al. 1985; see below). Virus-specific, double-stranded RNA molecules of unusual structure have been found before in picornavirus-infected cells (Romanova and Agol 1979; Senkevich et al. 1980 and references therein), but the significance of these structures has never been established (see discussion in Takeda et al. 1986).

Mechanism of RNA Replication

A genetic analysis of picornavirus RNA replication has not been possible because picornavirus mutants, for unknown reasons, do not form complementation groups (Cooper 1977).

In the absence of genetic information, numerous biochemical studies have been performed whose objective was to separate and purify components of the infected cell that are involved in viral RNA synthesis. The ultimate goal of all these experiments is to reconstitute in vitro a replication complex. We define replication of RNA in vitro as the synthesis of progeny RNA that has the same polarity as the input template RNA. Starting with virion RNA, this implies the pathway: plus strands → minus strands → plus strands. The synthesis of complementary RNA is, of course, not replication, although in many publications this distinction has not been made.

Despite numerous efforts during the last 25 years, no replication system of picornavirus RNA has been developed in vitro. It should be noted that most investigators concerned with the replication of any RNA viral genome have tried to reproduce the classic experiments of S. Spiegelman and his collaborators: the incubation of a "purified viral protein" with genomic RNA (bacteriophage Qβ RNA) and nucleotide precursors that yielded authentic phage RNA synthesized de novo (Spiegelman and Hayashi 1964). However, the purified viral protein used in the replication reaction turned out to be a subtle complex of the phage-encoded RNA polymerase with three bacterial proteins, the latter normally being involved in the translation of cellular mRNA. This important discovery by Kamen, Weissmann, and Weber and their colleagues that cellular proteins unrelated to nucleic acid metabolism are recruited by a viral RNA-synthesizing machinery has enormously influenced all subsequent research on RNA viral replication (for review, see Kamen 1975). It suddenly appeared possible that any cytoplasmic polypeptide of the host cell has the potential to be involved in picornavirus RNA replication, either in a complex with the virus-encoded RNA polymerase or as a separate entity. This kind of reasoning, in fact, has led investigators to search for host-cell components that might be involved in poliovirus replication. No convincing evidence has been presented so far that such host factors play a role in poliovirus RNA synthesis in vivo.

Poliovirus-specific RNA synthesis is catalyzed by a virus-encoded, RNA template-dependent RNA polymerase, $3D^{pol}$ (Flanegan and Baltimore 1977; Flanegan and van Dyke 1979 and references therein). This enzyme maps at the carboxyl terminus of the polyprotein (Fig. 2). Whereas the role of $3D^{pol}$ in RNA chain elongation has been firmly established, the following properties of the enzyme have posed as yet unsolved problems: (1) $3D^{pol}$ is primer-dependent, a feature that is unusual for virus-encoded RNA polymerases (but similar to the RNA polymerase of influenza virus). The mechanism of initiation of RNA synthesis is still obscure. (2) Purified $3D^{pol}$, when used in conjunction with an oligonucleotide primer (or host factor), shows little, if any, specificity for poliovirus RNA (for review, see Kuhn and Wimmer 1987; Semler et al. 1987). Yet RNA replication in infected cells must be discriminatory and indeed is confined to viral RNA strands. Signal recognition and/or sequestering of viral RNA, possibly in membranous complexes, may facilitate specificity. (3) Purified $3D^{pol}$, even when supplemented with a synthetic primer oligonucleotide, does not replicate RNA but merely synthesizes complementary RNA. Moreover, the enzyme does not link VPg onto the RNA products (for discussion, see Wimmer et al. 1987).

Two different strategies have been followed to study the mechanism of RNA replication in vitro. The first involved the purification of polypeptide(s) from infected (or uninfected) host cells. The various fractions were analyzed separately or in combinations, and the ability of such reconstituted mixtures was analyzed to synthesize bona fide viral RNA. The second strategy is a study of a membranous replication complex isolated from infected cells (see Fig. 4) that is capable of synthesizing authentic virion RNA. This subject has been extensively reviewed recently (Kuhn and Wimmer 1987; Semler et al. 1987) and will only be summarized here.

The first model involves soluble systems of RNA synthesis. The isolation of $3D^{pol}$ from infected HeLa cells and its characterization were facilitated by a simple assay: chain elongation of oligo(U) bound to poly(A), the latter serving as template for poly(U) synthesis (Flanegan and Baltimore 1977). The poly(A) template could be replaced by any polyadenylylated RNA (e.g., poliovirus RNA), but RNA transcription was always strictly dependent on the presence of an oligo(U) primer. A host factor (HF) was subsequently isolated (identified to be a protein kinase; Dasgupta et al. 1980; Morrow et al. 1985) that could replace oligo(U) and induce $3D^{pol}$ to transcribe poliovirus RNA without added primer. The mechanism by which HF functions in the priming of RNA synthesis in vitro is currently being disputed (Lubinski et al. 1986; Hey et al. 1987). Andrews and Baltimore (1986a,b), on the other hand, have recently proposed that the active ingredient of HF is a terminal uridylylate transferase (TUT) that adds uridylate residues to the template RNA, thereby promoting snapback structures that allow intramolecular priming of $3D^{pol}$. This mechanism of initiation of RNA synthesis had been suggested earlier by Young et al. (1985) (see Fig. 5), who found double-stranded RNA molecules covalently linked (at one of their termini) among the in vitro polymerization products. Flanegan's model of initiation is shown in Figure 5 and predicts that VPg (or a precursor thereof) cleaves the hairpin, thereby linking itself to the viral RNA (Flanegan et al. 1987; for discussions, see Kuhn and Wimmer 1987; Semler et al. 1987; Wimmer et al. 1987).

The second model of initiation suggests that uridylylated VPg (or its precursor) serves as a primer for the

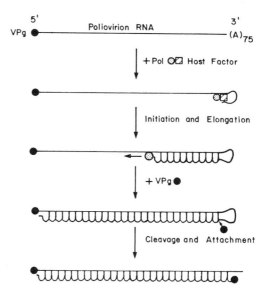

Figure 5. Self-priming by template RNA. A host factor (either a protein kinase or a terminal uridylate transferase) produces a hairpin at the 3' end of the template RNA that serves as a primer for $3D^{pol}$. After some elongation has taken place, VPg (or its precursor) will cleave the hairpin, thereby attaching itself to the 5' end of the nascent RNA strand. If nicking does not occur, an end-linked RF molecule is formed; as shown here, the homopolymeric segments of the RF would be covalently bound. We have named those structures homo-linked RF (Takeda et al. 1986; Kuhn and Wimmer 1987). Hairpin-mediated initiation and complete transcription of minus-strand template would yield hetero-linked RF molecules. (Drawing kindly provided by J.B. Flanegan, University of Florida, Gainesville.)

RNA polymerase $3D^{pol}$ (Nomoto et al. 1977b; Wimmer 1982), a mechanism resembling priming of adenovirus DNA synthesis by the deoxycytidylylated terminal protein (Stillman 1983 and references therein). The VPg-pU priming model is shown in Figure 6 (Takegami et al. 1983a).

A major consideration for any model of poliovirus genome replication is the fact that all virus-specific RNA synthesis occurs on membranes. A membranous replication complex can be isolated (called crude replication complex, CRC) from infected HeLa cells that is capable of synthesizing in vitro virion RNA, i.e., VPg-linked and polyadenylylated (Takegami et al. 1983b; Takeda et al. 1986, 1987; Toyoda et al. 1987). Moreover, CRC, when incubated only with $[\alpha^{-32}P]$UTP, synthesizes VPg-pU that can be chased into VPg-pUpU and, to some extent, into viral RNA (Takegami et al. 1983a; Takeda et al. 1986, 1987; Toyoda et al. 1987). Synthesis of uridylylated VPg or of single-stranded RNA in CRC is inhibited by nonionic detergent (0.5% NP-40), whereas chain elongation by $3D^{pol}$ is not. This observation suggests that membranes may be necessary for proper initiation of RNA synthesis to occur.

The activity catalyzing uridylylation of VPg, if it occurs at all, is obscure. In vitro genetic data implicated $3D^{pol}$ to be involved in this process (Toyoda et al. 1987), but there are other candidates as well, most

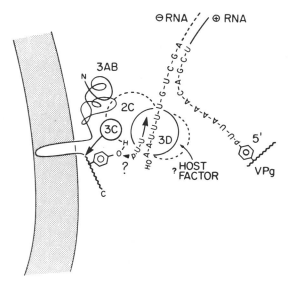

Figure 6. Model of VPg-pUpU-primed initiation of RNA synthesis. 3AB is the membrane-bound poliovirus protein whose carboxyl terminus (wavy line) is VPg, 3C is the virus-encoded proteinase (responsible for the cleavage between 3A and 3B), 3D the primer-dependent RNA polymerase, and 2C an auxiliary viral protein, mutations of which (g^r) lead to an altered phenotype of RNA synthesis in vivo. The shaded area depicts a smooth membrane. The possibility of the involvement of a host factor is indicated, although there is no evidence to support that such a factor is functioning in the membrane-bound replication complex. This model can account for the initiation of both plus- and minus-strand RNAs. (Modified from Takegami et al. 1983a.)

notably 2C. This polypeptide, a nonstructural protein mapping in the P2 region of the viral genome (Fig. 2), is thought to be involved in viral RNA synthesis. This is based on the observation that RNA synthesis of wild-type virus is inhibited by 2 mM guanidine in vivo and that point mutations, leading to guanidine resistance, map to 2C (Pincus and Wimmer 1986 and references therein).

Considering the profound difference of the 3' termini of the template strands where initiation of RNA synthesis occurs—poly(A) on plus strands and heteropolymeric sequence on minus strands—it is conceivable that initiation of plus and minus strands follows two different mechanisms (Takeda et al. 1986). The studies with CRC are confined to initiation of plus strands, since CRC synthesizes mainly RNA of this polarity. Studies with purified proteins, on the other hand, have been concerned only with minus-strand synthesis. It would be surprising, however, if a virus as small as poliovirus would have evolved the extravagance of dual mechanisms for RNA replication.

Why is the poliovirus RNA polymerase primer-dependent when the majority of RNA transcriptases, viral and cellular alike, can initiate RNA synthesis de novo? We have recently speculated that 3D^{pol} of poliovirus mechanistically resembles reverse transcriptase or even DNA polymerases (Wimmer 1982); i.e., poliovirus RNA polymerase may have evolved from a

DNA polymerase having learned to read and synthesize RNA. Alternatively, 3D^{pol} may resemble progenitor catalytic activities to DNA polymerases, a hypothesis that immediately poses the question of whether poliovirus, or any RNA viruses for that matter, preceded DNA replicating systems or evolved from a DNA ancestorial system (Baltimore 1980; Reanney 1984). This question, of course, remains unanswered, although an analysis of the dinucleotide frequencies and codon usage of poliovirus RNA favors the hypothesis of DNA origin (Rothberg and Wimmer 1981).

REFERENCES

Ambros, V. and D. Baltimore. 1980. Purification and properties of a HeLa cell enzyme able to remove the 5'-terminal protein from poliovirus RNA. *J. Biol. Chem.* **255:** 6739.

Andrews, N.C. and D. Baltimore. 1986a. Lack of evidence for VPg priming of poliovirus RNA synthesis in the host factor-dependent *in vitro* replicase reaction. *J. Virol.* **58:** 212.

———. 1986b. Purification of a terminal uridylyl-transferase that acts as host factor in the *in vitro* poliovirus replicase reaction. *Proc. Natl. Acad. Sci.* **83:** 221.

Argos, P., G. Kamer, M.J.H. Nicklin, and E. Wimmer. 1984. Similarity in gene organization and homology between proteins of animal picornaviruses and a plant comovirus suggest common ancestry of these virus families. *Nucleic Acids Res.* **12:** 7251.

Arnold, E., M. Luo, G. Vriend, M.G. Rossman, A.C. Palmenberg, G.D. Parks, M.J.H. Nicklin, and E. Wimmer. 1987. Implication of the picornavirus capsid structure for proteolytic processing. *Proc. Natl. Acad. Sci.* **84:** 21.

Baltimore, D. 1980. Evolution of RNA viruses. *Ann. N.Y. Acad. Sci.* **354:** 492.

Bernstein, H.D., N. Sonenberg, and D. Baltimore. 1985. Poliovirus mutant that does not selectively inhibit host cell protein synthesis. *Mol. Cell. Biol.* **5:** 2913.

Chow, M., J.F.E. Newman, D. Filman, J.M. Hogle, D.J. Rowlands, and F. Brown. 1987. Myristylation of picornavirus capsid protein VP4 and its structural significance. *Nature* **327:** 482.

Cooper, P.D. 1977. Genetics of picornaviruses. In *Comprehensive virology* (ed. M. Fraenkel-Conrat and R. Wagner), vol. 9, p. 133. Plenum Press, New York.

Currey, K.M., B.M. Peterlin, and J.V. Maizel, Jr. 1986. Secondary structure of poliovirus RNA: Correlation of computer-predicted with electron microscopically observed structure. *Virology* **148:** 33.

Dasgupta, A., P. Zabel, and D. Baltimore. 1980. Dependence of the activity of poliovirus replicase on a host cell protein. *Cell* **19:** 423.

Detjen, B.M., J. Lucas, and E. Wimmer. 1978. Poliovirus single-stranded RNA and double-stranded RNA: Differential infectivity in enucleate cells. *J. Virol.* **27:** 582.

Dorner, A.J., P.G. Rothberg, and E. Wimmer. 1981. The fate of VPg during *in vitro* translation of poliovirus RNA. *FEBS. Lett.* **132:** 219.

Dorner, A.J., L.F. Dorner, G.R. Larsen, E. Wimmer, and C.W. Anderson. 1982. Identification of the initiation site of poliovirus polyprotein synthesis. *J. Virol.* **42:** 1017.

Dorsch-Hasler, K., Y. Yogo, and E. Wimmer. 1975. Replication of picornaviruses. I. Evidence from *in vitro* RNA synthesis that poly(A) of the poliovirus genome is genetically coded. *J. Virol.* **16:** 1512.

Ehrenfeld, E. 1982. Poliovirus-induced inhibition of host-cell protein synthesis. *Cell* **28:** 435.

Evans, D.M.A., G. Dunn, P.D. Minor, G.C. Schild, A.J. Cann, G. Stanway, J.W. Almond, K. Currey, and J.V.

Maizel, Jr. 1985. Increased neurovirulence associated with a single nucleotide change in a noncoding region of the Sabin type 3 poliovaccine genome. *Nature* **314:** 548.

Flanegan, J.B. and D. Baltimore. 1977. Poliovirus-specific primer-dependent RNA polymerase able to copy poly(A). *Proc. Natl. Acad. Sci.* **74:** 3677.

Flanegan, J.B. and T.A. Van Dyke. 1979. Isolation of a soluble and template dependent poliovirus RNA polymerase that copies virion RNA *in vitro. J. Virol.* **32:** 155.

Flanegan, J.B., D.C. Young, G.J. Tobin, M.M. Stokes, C.D. Murphy, and S.M. Oberste. 1987. Mechanism of RNA replication by the poliovirus RNA polymerase, HeLa cell host factor, and VPg. *UCLA Symp. Mol. Cell. Biol.* **54:** 273.

Forss, S. and H. Schaller. 1982. A tandem repeat gene in a picornavirus. *Nucleic Acids Res.* **10:** 6441.

French, R., M. Janda, and P. Ahlquist. 1986. Bacterial gene inserted in an engineered RNA virus: Efficient expression in monocotyledonous plant cells. *Science* **231:** 1294.

Gorbalenya, A.E. and Y.V. Svitkin. 1983. Encephalomyocarditis virus protease: Purification and role of the SH groups in processing of the precursor of structural proteins. *Biochemistry* (Engl. Transl. BioKhimiya) **48:** 442.

Harris, T.J.R. 1979. The nucleotide sequence of the 5' end of foot-and-mouth virus RNA. *Nucleic Acids Res.* **7:** 1765.

Hey, T.D., O.C. Richards, and E. Ehrenfeld. 1987. Host factor-induced template modification during synthesis of poliovirus RNA *in vitro. J. Virol.* **61:** 802.

Horstmann, D.M., T.C. Quinn, and F.C. Robbins. 1984. International Symposium of Poliomyelitis Control. *Rev. Infect. Dis.* (suppl. 2) **6.**

Ivanoff, L.A., T. Towatari, J. Ray, B.D. Korant, and S.R. Petteway, Jr. 1986. Expression and site-specific mutagenesis of the poliovirus 3C protease in *Escherichia coli. Proc. Natl. Acad. Sci.* **83:** 5392.

Kamen, R.I. 1975. Structure and function of the QB RNA replicase. In *RNA phages* (ed. N.D. Zinder), p. 203. Cold Spring Harbor Laboratory, Cold Spring Harbor, New York.

Kitamura, N., C.J. Adler, P.G. Rothberg, J. Martinko, S.G. Nathenson, and E. Wimmer. 1980. The genome-linked protein of picornaviruses. VII. Genetic mapping of poliovirus VPg by protein and RNA sequence studies. *Cell* **21:** 295.

Kitamura, N., B.L. Semler, P.G. Rothberg, G.R. Larsen, C.J. Adler, A.J. Dorner, E.A. Emini, R. Hanecak, J.J. Lee, S. Van Der Werf, C.W. Anderson, and E. Wimmer. 1981. Primary structure, gene organization, and polypeptide expression of poliovirus RNA. *Nature* **291:** 547.

Korant, B.D., J. Langner, and J. Powers. 1980. Protein synthesis and cleavage in picornavirus-infected cells. In *Biosynthesis, modification and processing of cellular and viral protein* (ed. G. Koch and D. Richter), p. 257. Academic Press, New York.

Kozak, M. 1983. Comparison of initiation of protein synthesis in procaryotes, eucaryotes, and organelles. *Microbiol. Rev.* **47:** 1.

Kräusslich, H.G., M.J.H. Nicklin, H. Toyoda, D. Etchison, and E. Wimmer. 1987. Poliovirus proteinase 2A induces cleavage of eucaryotic initiation factor 4F polypeptide p220. *J. Virol.* **61:** 2711.

Kuge, S. and A. Nomoto. 1987. Construction of viable deletion and insertion mutants of the Sabin strain of type I poliovirus: Function of the 5' noncoding sequence in viral replication. *J. Virol.* **61:** 1478.

Kuhn, R.J. and E. Wimmer. 1987. The replication of picornaviruses. In *The molecular biology of positive strand RNA viruses* (ed. D.J. Rowlands et al.), p. 17. Academic Press, New York.

Larsen, G.R., B.L. Semler, and E. Wimmer. 1981. Stable hairpin structure within the 5'-terminal 85 nucleotides of poliovirus RNA. *J. Virol.* **37:** 328.

Larsen, G.R., A.J. Dorner, T.J.R. Harris, and E. Wimmer.

1980. The structure of poliovirus replicative form. *Nucleic Acids Res.* **8:** 1217.

Larsen, G.R., C.W. Anderson, A.J. Dorner, B.L. Semler, and E. Wimmer. 1982. Cleavage sites within the poliovirus capsid protein precursors. *J. Virol.* **41:** 340.

Lee, K.A.W., I. Edery, R. Hanecak, E. Wimmer, and N.C. Sonenberg. 1985. Poliovirus protease 3C (P3-7c) does not cleave P220 of the eucaryotic mRNA cap binding protein complex. *J. Virol.* **55:** 489.

Levis, R., H. Huang, and S. Schlesinger. 1987. Engineered defective interfering RNAs of Sindbis virus express bacterial chloramphenicol acetyltransferase in avian cells. *Proc. Natl. Acad. Sci.* **84:** 4811.

Lloyd, R.E., D. Etchison, and E. Ehrenfeld. 1985. Poliovirus protease does not mediate cleavage of the 220,000-Da component of the cap binding protein complex. *Proc. Natl. Acad. Sci.* **82:** 2723.

Lloyd, R.E., H. Toyoda, D. Etchison, E. Wimmer, and E. Ehrenfeld. 1986. Cleavage of the cap binding protein complex polypeptide p220 is not affected by the second poliovirus protease 2A. *Virology* **150:** 299.

Lubinski, J.M., G. Kaplan, V.R. Racaniello, and A. Dasgupta. 1986. Mechanism of *in vitro* synthesis of covalently linked dimeric RNA molecules by the poliovirus replicase. *J. Virol.* **58:** 459.

Marx, J.L. 1987. A new wave of enzymes for cleaving prohormones. *Science* **235:** 285.

Morrow, C.D., G.F. Gibbons, and A. Dasgupta. 1985. The host protein required for *in vitro* replication of poliovirus is a protein kinase that phosphorylates eukaryotic initiation factor 2. *Cell* **40:** 913.

Mosenkis, J., S. Daniels-McQueen, S. Janovec, R. Duncan, J.W.B. Hershey, J.A. Grifo, W.C. Merrick, and R.E. Thach. 1985. Shutoff of host translation by encephalomyocarditis virus infection does not involve cleavage of the eucaryotic initiation factor 4F polypeptide that accompanies poliovirus infection. *J. Virol.* **54:** 643.

Nicklin, M.J.H., H. Toyoda, M.G. Murray, and E. Wimmer. 1986. Proteolytic processing in the replication of polio and related viruses. *Biotechnology* **4:** 33.

Nicklin, M.J.H., H.G. Kräusslich, H. Toyoda, J.J. Dunn, and E. Wimmer. 1987. Poliovius polypeptide precursors: Expression *in vitro* and processing by 3C and 2A proteinases. *Proc. Natl. Acad. Sci.* **84:** 4002.

Nilsen, T.W., D.L. Wood, and C. Baglioni. 1981. Cross-linking of viral RNA by 4'-aminomethyl-4',5',8 trimethylpsoralen in HeLa cells infected with encephalomyocarditis virus and the *ts* G114 mutant of vesicular stomatitis virus. *Virology* **109:** 82.

Nomoto, A., B. Detjen, R. Pozzatti, and E. Wimmer. 1977a. The location of the polio genome protein in viral RNAs and its implication for RNA synthesis. *Nature* **268:** 208.

Nomoto, A., N. Kitamura, F. Golini, and E. Wimmer. 1977b. The 5'-terminal structures of poliovirion RNA and poliovirus mRNA differ only in the genome-linked protein VPg. *Proc. Natl. Acad. Sci.* **74:** 5345.

Nomoto, A., M. Kohara, S. Kuge, N. Kawamura, M. Arita, T. Komatsu, S. Abe, B.L. Semler, E. Wimmer, and H. Itoh. 1987. Study on virulence of poliovirus type 1 using *in vitro* modified viruses. *UCLA Symp. Mol. Cell. Biol.* **54:** 437.

Palmenberg, A.C. 1987. Comparative organization and genome structure in picornaviruses. *UCLA Symp. Mol. Cell. Biol.* **54:** (in press).

Palmenberg, A.C. and R.R. Rueckert. 1982. Evidence for intramolecular self-cleavage of picornaviral replicase precursors. *J. Virol.* **41:** 244.

Paul, A.V., A. Schultz, S.E. Pincus, S. Oroszlan, and E. Wimmer. 1987. Capsid protein VP4 of poliovirus is N-myristoylated. *Proc. Natl. Acad. Sci.* (in press).

Pelham, H.R.B. 1978. Translation of encephalomyocarditis virus RNA *in vitro* yields an active proteolytic processing enzyme. *Eur. J. Biochem.* **85:** 457.

Pettersson, R.F., J.B. Flanegan, J.K. Rose, and D. Baltimore. 1977. 5'-Terminal nucleotide sequence of poliovirus polyribosomal RNA and virion RNA are identical. *Nature* **268**: 270.

Pincus, S.E. and E. Wimmer. 1986. Production of guanidine resistant and dependent poliovirus from cloned cDNA: Demonstration that mutations in polypeptide 2C are directly responsible for altered guanidine sensitivity. *J. Virol.* **60**: 793.

Racaniello, V.R. and C. Meriam. 1986. Poliovirus temperature-sensitive mutant containing a single nucleotide deletion in the 5'-noncoding region of the viral RNA. *Virology* **155**: 498.

Reanney, D. 1984. The molecular evaluation of viruses. In *The microbe* (ed. B.W.J. Mahy and J.R. Pattison), part I, p. 175. Cambridge University Press, Cambridge, England.

Richards O.C., S.C. Martin, H.G. Jense, and E. Ehrenfeld. 1984. Structure of poliovirus replicative intermediate RNA. Electron microscope analysis of RNA cross-linked *in vivo* with psoralen derivative. *J. Mol. Biol.* **173**: 325.

Romanova, L.I. and V.I. Agol. 1979. Interconversion of linear and circular forms of double-stranded RNA of encephalomyocarditis virus. *Virology* **93**: 574.

Rossmann, M.G., E. Arnold J.W. Erickson, E.A. Frankenberger, J.P. Griffith, H.-J. Hecht, J. Johnson, G. Kamer, M. Luo, A.G. Mosser, R.R. Rueckert, B. Sherry, and G. Vriend. 1985. Structure of a human common cold virus and functional relationship to other picornaviruses. *Nature* **317**: 145.

Rothberg, P.G. and E. Wimmer. 1981. Mononucleotide and dinucleotide frequencies, and codon usage in poliovirion RNA. *Nucleic Acids Res.* **9**: 6221.

Rueckert, R.R. 1985. Picornaviruses and their replication. In *Virology* (ed. B.M. Fields et al.), p. 705. Raven Press, New York.

Rueckert, R.R. and E. Wimmer. 1984. Systematic nomenclature of picornavirus proteins. *J. Virol.* **50**: 957.

Semler, B.L., V.H. Johnson, and S. Tracy. 1986. A chimeric plasmid from cDNA clones of poliovirus and coxsackievirus produces a recombinant virus that is temperature sensitive. *Proc. Natl. Acad. Sci.* **83**: 1777.

Semler, B.L., R.J. Kuhn, and E. Wimmer. 1987. Replication of the poliovirus genome. In *RNA genetics* (ed. E. Domingo et al.). CRC Press, Boca Raton, Florida. (In press).

Semler, B.L., C.W. Anderson, R. Hanecak, L.F. Dorner, and E. Wimmer. 1982. A membrane-associated precursor to poliovirus VPg identified by immunoprecipitation with antibodies directed against a synthetic heptapeptide. *Cell* **28**: 405.

Senkevich, T.G., I.M. Cumakov, G.Y. Lipskaya, and V.I. Agol. 1980. Palindrome-like dimers of double-stranded RNA of encephalomyocarditis virus. *Virology* **102**: 339.

Spiegelman, S. and M. Hayashi. 1964. The present status of the transfer of genetic information and its control. *Cold Spring Harbor Symp. Quant. Biol.* **28**: 161.

Stillman, B.W. 1983. The replication of adenovirus DNA with purified proteins. *Cell* **35**: 7.

Takeda, N., C.-F. Yang, R.J. Kuhn, and E. Wimmer. 1987. Uridylylation of the genome-linked protein of poliovirus *in vitro* is dependent upon an endogenous RNA template. *Virus Res.* (in press).

Takeda, N., R.J. Kuhn, C.-F. Yang, T. Takegami, and E. Wimmer. 1986. Initiation of poliovirus plus-strand RNA synthesis in a membrane complex of infected HeLa cells. *J. Virol.* **60**: 43.

Takegami, T., R.J. Kuhn, C.W. Anderson, and E. Wimmer. 1983a. Membrane-dependent uridylylation of the genome-linked protein VPg of poliovirus. *Proc. Natl. Acad. Sci.* **80**: 7447.

Takegami, T., B.L. Semler, C.W. Anderson, and E. Wimmer. 1983b. Membrane fractions active in poliovirus RNA replication contain VPg precursor polypeptides. *Virology* **128**: 33.

Toyoda, H., M.J.H. Nicklin, M.G. Murray, and E. Wimmer. 1986a. Proteolytic processing of the poliovirus polyprotein by two virus encoded proteinases. In *Protein engineering: Application in science, medicine, and industry* (ed. M. Inouye and R. Sarma) p. 319. Academic Press, New York.

Toyoda, H., C.-F. Yang, N. Takeda, A. Nomoto, and E. Wimmer. 1987. Analysis of RNA synthesis of type 1 poliovirus using an *in vitro* molecular genetic approach. *J. Virol.* (in press).

Toyoda, H., M.J.H. Nicklin, M.G. Murray, C.W. Anderson, J.J. Dunn, F.W. Studier, and E. Wimmer. 1986b. A second virus-encoded proteinase involved in proteolytic processing of poliovirus polyprotein. *Cell* **45**: 761.

van der Werf, S., J. Bradley, E. Wimmer, F.W. Studier, and J.J. Dunn. 1986. Synthesis of infectious poliovirus RNA by purified T7 RNA polymerase. *Proc. Natl. Acad. Sci.* **83**: 2330.

Vartapetian, A.B., A.S. Mankin, E.A. Skripkin, K.M. Chumakov, V.D. Smirnov, and A.A. Bogdanov. 1983. The primary and secondary structure of the 5' end region of encephalomyocarditis virus RNA: A novel approach to sequencing long RNA molecules. *Gene* **26**: 189.

Wimmer, E. 1982. Genome-linked proteins of viruses. *Cell* **28**: 199.

Wimmer, E., R.J. Kuhn, S. Pincus, C.-F. Yang, H. Toyoda, M. Nicklin, and N. Takeda. 1987. Molecular events leading to picornavirus genome replication. In *Virus replication and genome interactions: 7th John Innes Symposium* (ed. J.W. Davis et al.), p. 1. John Innes Institute, Norwich, England.

Young, D.C., D.M. Tuschall, and J.B. Flanegan. 1985. Poliovirus RNA-dependent RNA polymerase and host cell protein synthesize product RNA twice the size of poliovirion RNA *in vitro*. *J. Virol.* **54**: 256.

Ypma-Wong, M.F. and B.L. Semler. 1987. *In vitro* molecular genetics as a tool for determining and differential cleavage specificities of the poliovirus 3C proteinase. *Nucleic Acids Res.* **15**: 2069.

Transcription and Replication of Influenza Virion RNA in the Nucleus of Infected Cells

R.M. Krug, C. St. Angelo, B. Broni, and G. Shapiro
Graduate Program of Molecular Biology, Memorial Sloan-Kettering Cancer Center, New York, New York 10021

Influenza virus is a negative-strand RNA virus with a segmented genome. Consequently, the virion contains the enzyme system that transcribes the virion RNA (vRNA) segments into mRNAs. The mRNAs are not full-length copies of the vRNAs (Hay et al. 1977a,b), so that a different type of transcription is needed in the infected cell to generate full-length copies, or template RNAs, for replication. The synthesis of template RNAs and their subsequent copying into vRNAs require the synthesis of one or more virus-specific proteins (Barrett et al. 1979; Hay et al. 1982). All steps of virus-specific RNA synthesis occur in the nucleus of infected cells (Herz et al. 1981; Shapiro et al. 1987). Here, we describe some of our recent results on the mechanism of transcription and replication of influenza vRNAs.

RESULTS AND DISCUSSION

Viral mRNA Synthesis

Influenza virus employs a novel mechanism for the synthesis of its viral mRNAs. Viral mRNA synthesis requires initiation by host-cell primers, specifically capped (m^7GpppNm-containing) RNA fragments derived from host-cell RNA polymerase II transcripts (Bouloy et al. 1978; Plotch et al. 1979, 1981; Krug 1981). Because this occurs in the nucleus of infected cells (Herz et al. 1981), viral mRNA synthesis requires the continuous functioning of the cellular RNA polymerase II and is inhibited by α-amanitin (Mark et al. 1979). The host-cell primers are generated by a viral cap-dependent endonuclease that cleaves the capped cellular RNAs 10–13 nucleotides from their 5' ends preferentially at a purine residue (Plotch et al. 1981). Transcription is initiated by the incorporation of a G residue onto the 3' end of the resulting fragments, directed by the penultimate C residue of the vRNAs. Viral mRNA chains are then elongated until a stretch of 4–7 uridine residues is reached 17–22 nucleotides before the 5' ends of the vRNAs, where transcription terminates and polyadenylate (poly[A]) is added to the mRNAs (Hay et al. 1977a,b; Robertson et al. 1981). Viral mRNA synthesis is catalyzed by viral nucleocapsids (Inglis et al. 1976; Plotch et al. 1981), which consist of the individual vRNAs associated with four viral proteins, the nucleocapsid (NP) protein, and the three P (PB1, PB2, and PA) proteins (Inglis et al. 1976; Ulmanen et al. 1981). The P proteins are re-

sponsible for viral mRNA synthesis, and some of their roles have been determined by analyses of the in vitro reaction catalyzed by virion nucleocapsids. UV-light-induced cross-linking experiments showed that the three P proteins are in the form of a complex that starts at the 3' ends of the vRNA templates and moves down the templates in association with the elongating mRNAs during transcription (Braam et al. 1983). The PB2 protein in this complex recognizes and binds to the cap of the primer RNA (Ulmanen et al. 1981; Braam et al. 1983), as verified by the in vitro behavior of the nucleocapsids from PB2 temperature-sensitive mutants (Ulmanen et al. 1983). The PB1 protein, which is initially found at the first residue (a G residue) added onto the primer, moves as part of the P protein complex to the 3' ends of the growing viral mRNA chains, indicating that it most likely catalyzes each nucleotide addition (Braam et al. 1983). On the basis of the relative positions of PB1 and PB2 on the nascent chains, it was concluded that the P protein complex most likely has the PB1 protein at its leading edge and the PB2 protein at its trailing edge. Figure 1 shows a model of the functions and movements of the P proteins during viral mRNA synthesis.

The analysis of the transcription reaction catalyzed by virion nucleocapsids left unresolved many important questions about the mechanism of viral mRNA synthesis and the role of the P proteins. Thus, it was not determined how the complex of the three P proteins is assembled at the 3' ends of the vRNA templates where transcription initiates. It is also not known which P protein(s) is the endonuclease. Although PA is in the P protein complex, no specific role for PA in viral mRNA synthesis has been found. In fact, PA may not have a role in viral mRNA synthesis, since experiments with temperature-sensitive virus mutants with defects in the PA gene indicate that the principal role of the PA protein in infected cells is most probably in viral RNA replication, rather than in viral mRNA synthesis (Krug et al. 1975; Mahy et al. 1981; Mowshowitz 1981).

To address these questions, it was necessary to establish a better in vitro system, in which the individual P proteins could be added separately and in various combinations to the appropriate templates, i.e., one or more vRNAs associated with NP proteins. Attempts by several laboratories to solubilize active P proteins from virion nucleocapsids have not been successful. Consequently, we employed an expression system to produce large amounts of each of the three P proteins (and

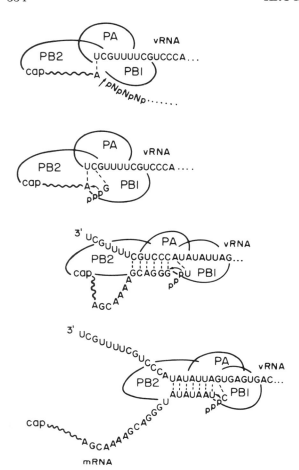

Figure 1. Model of the functions and movements of the three P proteins during capped RNA-primed viral mRNA synthesis. The sequence shown is that of the vRNA and mRNA coding for the NP protein. (Reprinted, with permission, from Braam et al. 1983.)

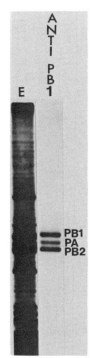

Figure 2. Formation of a complex containing the three P proteins in Spodoptera cells. Cells infected with all three baculovirus P recombinants were labeled with [^{35}S]methionine from 38 to 39 hr postinfection and were fractionated into cytoplasmic and nuclear extracts as described previously (Beaton and Krug 1986). The proteins in the nuclear extract were resolved on a 8% polyacrylamide gel containing 4 M urea (lane E). An equivalent aliquot of the nuclear extract was adjusted to 50 mM Tris-HCl, 5 mM EDTA, 0.5% Triton X-100, and 50 mM NaCl. Immunoprecipitation with an anti-PB1 antiserum was then carried out as described previously (Detjen et al. 1987), except that SDS was omitted from all solutions. The immune complexes were then solubilized by heating at 100°C in gel-loading buffer, and the labeled proteins were resolved on a 8% polyacrylamide gel containing 4 M urea (anti-PB1 lane).

also the NP protein) (St. Angelo et al. 1987). The DNA copies of these influenza virus genes were inserted into baculoviruses under the control of the polyhedrin promoter. Insect cells (Spodoptera cells) that were infected with the baculovirus recombinants containing the P genes synthesized high levels of the P proteins (St. Angelo et al. 1987).

As the first test for function, we determined whether the three expressed P proteins were able to form a complex with one another. As discussed above, the P proteins that are associated with transcribing nucleocapsids are in the form of a complex (Braam et al. 1983). In addition, infected cells contain a large pool of P protein complexes that are not associated with nucleocapsids (Detjen et al. 1987). We infected insect cells simultaneously with all three baculovirus P recombinants. The cells were labeled for 1 hour at 38 hours postinfection, and the proteins in the nuclear extract from these cells were resolved by gel electrophoresis (Fig. 2, lane E). The three P proteins can be discerned against the background. To determine whether these proteins were in the form of a complex, we subjected

the nuclear extract to immunoprecipitation with an antiserum directed against the PB1 protein. If this antiserum precipitated the PB1 protein and one or both of the other P proteins, this would indicate that the immunoprecipitated P proteins were in a complex. Under the conditions of immunoprecipitation employed (0.5% Triton X-100 and no SDS), the anti-PB1 antiserum precipitated not only the PB1 protein, but also the PB2 and PA proteins (Fig. 2). In the absence of the PB1 proteins, neither PB2 or PA was precipitated by the PB1 antiserum (St. Angelo et al. 1987). PB2 antiserum also precipitated all three P proteins (data not shown). These results indicate that the three P proteins expressed in insect cells do form a complex with each other and that the ability to form a complex is an intrinsic property of these three P proteins that does not require the participation of other influenza virus gene products. When immunoprecipitation was carried out under harsher conditions (i.e., in the presence of 0.1% SDS), the PA protein was not found in the complex (St. Angelo et al. 1987), indicating that the PA protein was less stably associated with the other two P proteins. These results, in conjunction with the finding of nonnucleocapsid P protein complexes in infected cells, strongly suggest that it is a complex of the three P proteins, rather than a particular one of the P proteins, that recognizes and binds to the 3' ends of the vRNAs to initiate mRNA synthesis. Experiments are in progress to reconstitute P protein complexes that are active in one or more steps of viral mRNA synthesis.

Template RNA Synthesis

The first step in the replication of influenza vRNA is the switch from viral mRNA synthesis to the synthesis of template RNAs, i.e., full-length copies of vRNA that then serve as templates for vRNA replication. This switch requires (1) a change from the capped RNA-primed initiation of transcription used during mRNA synthesis to unprimed initiation and (2) antitermination at the poly(A) site, 17–22 nucleotides from the 5' ends of vRNAs, that is used during mRNA synthesis (Hay et al. 1977a, 1982). Because the switch from mRNA to template RNA synthesis requires protein synthesis in vivo (Barrett et al. 1979; Hay et al. 1982), it is likely that one or more newly synthesized virus-specific proteins are needed for unprimed synthesis and/or antitermination.

To identify these proteins and to determine their roles, we employed an in vitro system that catalyzes the synthesis of template RNA as well as of viral mRNA (Beaton and Krug 1986). Nuclear extracts prepared from HeLa cells at 4 hours postinfection catalyzed one of the steps involved in the switch from mRNA to template RNA synthesis, the antitermination step. In these experiments, M13 single-stranded DNA specific for transcripts copied off the NS vRNA (the smallest vRNA) was used to measure the NS1 mRNA and NS template RNA synthesized by the nuclear extracts. This assay includes a digestion with RNase T2, which removes the poly(A) and the 5'-capped primer-donated region from the NS1 mRNA. As a result, the NS template RNA is about 20 nucleotides larger than the NS1 mRNA and hence has a slower mobility than the NS1 mRNA during gel electrophoresis. In the absence of an added primer, these extracts synthesized only low levels of NS1 mRNA and NS template RNA (Fig. 3, lane 1). However, addition of a high concentration (0.4 mM) of the dinucleotide ApG, which had been shown to act as a primer for viral mRNA synthesis catalyzed by virion nucleocapsids (McGeoch and Kitron 1975; Plotch and Krug 1977), greatly stimulated the synthesis of both NS1 mRNA and NS template RNA catalyzed by these nuclear extracts (Fig. 3, lane 2) (Beaton and Krug 1986). Consequently, these nuclear extracts contained the factor(s) that causes antitermination at the poly(A) site used during viral mRNA synthesis, but they were deficient in unprimed initiation of template RNA synthesis and in the capped primers needed for viral mRNA synthesis. The addition of ApG circum-

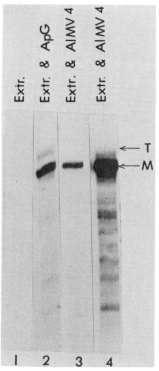

Figure 3. Synthesis of template RNAs by infected cell nuclear extracts. A nuclear extract from infected HeLa cells (4 hr postinfection) was incubated under the conditions described previously (Beaton and Krug 1986) in the absence of a primer (lane *1*), in the presence of 0.4 mM ApG (lane *2*), or in the presence of alfalfa mosaic virus RNA 4 containing a m^{7}GpppGm cap (lane *3*). Lane *4* shows a longer exposure of lane *3*. The RNA products were analyzed for NS1 mRNA (M) and NS template RNA (T) as described previously (Beaton and Krug 1986). (Reprinted, with permission, from Beaton and Krug 1986.)

vented the inefficient unprimed initiation and hence allowed the analysis of the mechanism of antitermination. In contrast to ApG, the addition of a capped RNA primer stimulated the synthesis of only NS1 mRNA; little or no NS template RNA was synthesized (Fig. 3, lane 3). Consequently, viral RNA transcripts that initiated with a capped primer were not antiterminated by the nuclear factor(s) that antiterminated the ApG-initiated viral transcripts.

To determine whether the factor(s) was associated with the viral nucleocapsids, the nuclear extract was separated by ultracentrifugation into a supernatant fraction and a pellet fraction that contained particles larger than 20S, including viral nucleocapsids (Beaton and Krug 1986). The pellet fraction synthesized NS1 viral mRNA but little or no NS template RNA (Fig. 4, lane 1), indicating the virtual absence of the antitermination factor in the pellet. The supernatant fraction by itself had little activity in either viral mRNA or template RNA synthesis (Beaton and Krug 1986) (data not shown). When the supernatant was added to the pellet in the presence of ApG, NS template RNA synthesis was restored (Fig. 4, lane 2), indicating that the super-

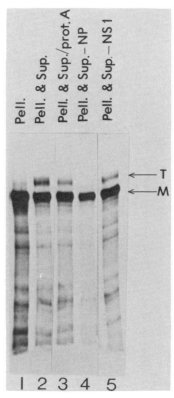

Figure 4. Viral NP molecules not associated with viral nucleocapsids are required for template RNA synthesis. The supernatant fraction from an infected cell nuclear extract was either untreated (lane 2), incubated with protein A–Sepharose alone (lane 3), incubated with protein A–Sepharose containing pooled NP monoclonal antibodies (lane 4), or incubated with protein A–Sepharose containing pooled NS1 monoclonal antibodies (lane 5). Each of these supernatants was incubated with the nuclear pellet in the presence of ApG, and the amount of synthesis of NS1 mRNA (M) and NS template RNA (T) was determined. Lane 1 shows the products made by the nuclear pellet alone in the presence of ApG. (Reprinted, with permission, from Beaton and Krug 1986.)

natant fraction contained the factor(s) required for antitermination at the poly(A) site.

The identity of this factor was determined by depleting the supernatant of individual virus-specific proteins (Beaton and Krug 1986). Depletion was carried out by incubating the supernatant with protein A–Sepharose containing a specific antiserum directed against an individual virus-specific protein. The protein A–Sepharose was then removed by centrifugation, and the resulting supernatant was then added to the pellet fraction in the presence of ApG. After incubation with protein A–Sepharose containing pooled monoclonal antibodies directed against the viral NP protein, the supernatant lost its ability to antiterminate, as NS1 mRNA and not NS template RNA was synthesized (Fig. 4, lane 4). The control experiment indicated that the NP protein had been quantitatively removed from the supernatant (Beaton and Krug 1986). In contrast, antitermination activity was retained in supernatants that had been incubated with protein A–Sepharose

alone (Fig. 4, lane 3) or with protein A–Sepharose containing pooled monoclonal antibodies directed against the NS1 protein (Fig. 4, lane 5), the predominant viral nonstructural protein that accumulates in the nucleus. These results thus indicate that there is a pool of NP protein molecules free of nucleocapsids that is required for antitermination during template RNA synthesis.

The mechanism by which the NP protein causes antitermination has not been determined. The most likely possibility is that NP acts by binding to the viral RNA transcript. It has been shown that template RNAs in infected cells are in the form of nucleocapsids containing NP (Krug 1972; Hay et al. 1977a), so that it can be presumed that the templates synthesized in vitro also become coated with NP to form nucleocapsids. Indeed, with another negative-strand RNA virus, vesicular stomatitis virus (VSV), the NP protein is also required for antitermination in vitro, and the resulting RNAs are in the form of nucleocapsids (Patton et al. 1983, 1984; Peluso and Moyer 1983). In this case, there is only a single vRNA template that has a termination signal near its 3′ end. In the absence of NP protein, RNA synthesis terminates, yielding a small 47-nucleotide-long RNA, and the transcriptase then reinitiates at the cap site of the first downstream mRNA sequence. However, most likely as a consequence of the binding of NP to a sequence in the nascent 47-nucleotide-long RNA, antitermination occurs and a full-length template RNA is made. This binding site is also apparently the site for the initiation of nucleocapsid assembly (Blumberg et al. 1981). With influenza virus, there are eight vRNA templates, all of which have termination signals at their 5′ ends, rather than at their 3′ ends (Hay et al. 1977a, 1982). One possibility is that, as with VSV, the NP protein initially binds to the nascent transcripts at a sequence close to the site of termination, both causing antitermination and initiating nucleocapsid assembly. However, the eight viral RNA transcripts do not have a common sequence in this region. An alternative possibility is that NP binds at, or close to, the common 12-nucleotide-long sequence at the 5′ ends of the nascent transcripts. Subsequent addition of NP molecules to the growing chains would allow readthrough when the termination site is reached. The latter hypothesis would provide an explanation for the observation that influenza virus RNA transcripts initiated with a capped primer were not antiterminated in the presence of the NP molecules that were active in the antitermination of ApG-initiated transcripts (Beaton and Krug 1986). Perhaps the 5′-terminal cap structure and/or the primer-donated sequence preceding the common 5′ sequence of the viral transcripts blocks the binding of the NP protein. An alternative explanation would be that a P-transcription complex that initiates with a capped RNA primer might be different from the complex found after unprimed or ApG-primed initiation and that this different structure might not allow recognition of the antitermination signal.

In any case, it is clear that the type of initiation used by the transcriptase largely determines the choice between mRNA synthesis and the first step of replication, which is not the case for VSV. The termination of all capped RNA-primed transcripts at the poly(A) site likely ensures that these transcripts, which contain host sequences at their 5' ends, are used only as mRNAs and not as templates for vRNA replication. It is conceivable that if these transcripts had copies of the 5' ends and of the 3' ends of the vRNAs, they might inadvertently be recognized as templates by the replicating enzymes. Because the type of initiation is so pivotal, it is essential to establish an in vitro system that catalyzed unprimed initiation as well as antitermination. Recently, using nuclear extracts from HeLa cells at later times of infection, we have achieved some unprimed initiation of template RNA in vitro. These results will be described elsewhere (G. Shapiro and R. Krug, in prep.).

Virion RNA Synthesis

Little is known about the second step in vRNA replication, i.e., the copying of template RNA into vRNA. This synthesis almost certainly occurs without a primer, since the vRNAs contain a triphosphorylated 5' end (Young and Content 1971). It might then be anticipated that the P protein complexes involved in vRNA synthesis would differ from those involved in capped RNA-primed viral mRNA synthesis. The copying of template RNA into vRNA is an important point of regulation during the early phase of viral infection, as the selective copying of certain template RNAs into their vRNAs determines which viral proteins are preferentially synthesized at early times of infection (Hay et al. 1977a; Smith and Hay 1982; Sharpiro et al. 1987). A significant part of this control mechanism is directed at the preferential synthesis of the NP and NS1 proteins early and at delaying the synthesis of the membrane protein, a major structural protein that forms a layer under the lipid envelope of the virus. The NP and NS1 proteins are synthesized early presumably because they are needed for template RNA and/or vRNA synthesis. As noted above, NP molecules not associated with nucleocapsids have been shown to be required for the antitermination step that occurs as part of the switch from viral mRNA to template RNA synthesis (Beaton and Krug 1986), and studies with viral temperature-sensitive mutants in the NP gene indicate that the NP protein is also most likely needed for vRNA synthesis (Krug et al. 1975; Scholtissek 1978; Mahy et al. 1981). However, it has not yet been established that the NS1 protein is involved in template RNA and/or vRNA synthesis. To identify the proteins involved in vRNA synthesis and to determine their roles, it will be necessary to establish an in vitro system that catalyzes the initiation and elongation of vRNA chains. Recently, we have shown that nuclear extracts from HeLa cells at late times of infection synthesize vRNA chains in vitro.

These results will be described elsewhere (G. Shapiro and R. Krug, in prep.).

In summary, the basic mechanism of the unique process of capped RNA-primed viral mRNA synthesis and some of the roles of the viral P proteins in this process are known. Future studies will need to resolve the remaining unanswered questions about the roles of the P proteins in viral mRNA synthesis. With regard to the switch from viral mRNA to template RNA synthesis, it is known that the NP protein is required for antitermination and that this protein can only act on transcripts that are initiated without a capped RNA primer. However, the mechanism by which the NP protein causes antitermination has not been established, nor has it been ruled out that other viral proteins are involved. In addition, the proteins involved in the unprimed initiation of template RNAs have not been identified. Finally, the viral proteins involved in the unprimed initiation and elongation of vRNA chains have not been identified, and the mechanism of the selective initiation of specific vRNAs at early times of infection has not been determined.

ACKNOWLEDGMENTS

We thank Eveyon Maldonado for typing the manuscript. The investigations carried out by the authors were supported by U.S. Public Health Service grants CA-08747 and AI-11772. Monoclonal antibodies to the NP and NS1 proteins were kindly provided as ascites fluids by Robert Webster.

REFERENCES

Barrett, T., A.J. Wolstenholme, and B.W.J. Mahy. 1979. Transcription and replication of influenza virus RNA. *Virology* **98**: 211.

———. 1986. Transcription antitermination during influenza viral template RNA synthesis requires the nucleocapsid protein and the absence of a 5' capped end. *Proc. Natl. Acad. Sci.* **83**: 6282.

Blumberg, B.M., M. Leppert, and D. Kolakofsky. 1981. Interaction of VSV leader RNA and nucleocapsid protein may control VSV genome replication. *Cell* **23**: 837.

Bouloy, M., S.J. Plotch, and R.M. Krug. 1978. Globin mRNAs are primers for the transcription of influenza RNA *in vitro*. *Proc. Natl. Acad. Sci.* **75**: 4886.

Braam, J., I. Ulmanen, and R.M. Krug. 1983. Molecular model of a eucaryotic transcription complex: Functions and movements of influenza P proteins during capped RNA primed transcriptions. *Cell* **34**: 609.

Detjen, B.M., C. St. Angelo, M.G. Katze, and R.M. Krug. 1987. The three influenza virus polymerase (P) proteins not associated with viral nucleocapsids in the infected cell are in the form of a complex. *J. Virol.* **61**: 16.

Hay, A.J., J.J. Skehel, and J. McCauley. 1982. Characterization of influenza virus RNA complete transcripts. *Virology* **116**: 517.

Hay, A.J., B. Lomniczi, A.H. Bellamy, and J.J. Skehel. 1977a. Transcription of the influenza virus genome. *Virology* **83**: 337.

Hay, A.J., G. Abraham, J.J. Skehel, J.C. Smith, and P. Fellner. 1977b. Influenza virus messenger RNAs are incomplete transcripts of the genome RNAs. *Nucleic Acids Res.* **4**: 4197.

Herz, C., E. Stavnezer, R.M. Krug, and T. Gurney, Jr. 1981. Influenza virus, an RNA virus, synthesizes its messenger RNA in the nucleus of infected cells. *Cell* **26**: 391.

Inglis, S.C., A.R. Carroll, R.A. Lamb, and B.W.J. Mahy. 1976. Polypeptides specified by the influenza virus genome. I. Evidence for eight distinct gene products specified by fowl plague virus. *Virology* **74**: 489.

Krug, R.M. 1972. Cytoplasmic and nucleoplasmic viral RNPs in influenza virus-infected MDCK cells. *Virology* **50**: 103.

———. 1981. Priming of influenza viral RNA transcription by capped heterologous RNAs. *Curr. Top. Microbiol. Immunol.* **93**: 125.

Krug, R.M., M. Ueda, and P. Palese. 1975. Temperature-sensitive mutants of influenza WSN virus defective in virus-specific RNA synthesis. *J. Virol.* **16**: 790.

Mahy, B.W.J., T. Barrett, S.T. Nichol, C.R. Penn, and A.J. Wolstenholme. 1981. Analysis of the functions of influenza virus genome RNA segments by use of temperature-sensitive mutants of fowl plague virus. In *The replication of negative strand viruses* (ed. D.H.L. Bishop and R.W. Compans), p. 379. Elsevier, New York.

Mark, G.E., J.M. Taylor, B. Broni, and R.M. Krug. 1979. Nuclear accumulation of influenza viral RNA and the effects of cyclohexamide actinomycin D and alpha amanitin. *J. Virol.* **29**: 744.

McGeoch, D. and N. Kitron. 1975. Influenza virion RNA-dependent RNA polymerase: Stimulation by guanosine and related compounds. *J. Virol.* **15**: 686.

Mowshowitz, S.L. 1981. RNA synthesis of temperature-sensitive mutants of WSN influenza virus. In *The replication of negative strand viruses* (ed. D.H.L. Bishop and R.W. Compans), p. 317. Elsevier, New York.

Patton, J.T., N.L.E. Davis, and G. Wertz. 1983. Cell-free synthesis and assembly of vesicular stomatitis virus nucleocapsids. *J. Virol.* **45**: 155.

———. 1984. N protein alone satisfies the requirement for protein synthesis during RNA replication of vesicular stomatitis virus. *J. Virol.* **49**: 303.

Peluso, R.W. and S.A. Moyer. 1983. Initiation and replication of vesicular stomatitis virus genome RNA in a cell-free system. *Proc. Natl. Acad. Sci.* **80**: 3198.

Plotch, S.J. and R.M. Krug. 1977. Influenza virion transcriptase: Synthesis *in vitro* of large, polyadenylic acid-containing complementary RNA. *J. Virol.* **21**: 24.

Plotch, S., M. Bouloy, and R.M. Krug. 1979. Transfer of 5′ terminal cap of globin mRNA to influenza viral complementary RNA during transcription *in vitro*. *Proc. Natl. Acad. Sci.* **76**: 1618.

Plotch, S.J., M. Bouloy, I. Ulmanen, and R.M. Krug. 1981. A unique cap (mGppXm)-dependent influenza virion endonuclease cleaves capped RNAs to generate the primers that initiate viral RNA transcription. *Cell* **23**: 847.

Robertson, J.S., M. Schubert, and R.A. Lazzarini. 1981. Polyadenylation sites for influenza virus mRNA. *J. Virol.* **38**: 157.

Scholtissek, C. 1978. The genome of the influenza virus. *Curr. Top. Microbiol. Immunol.* **80**: 139.

Shapiro, G.I., T. Gurney, Jr., and R.M. Krug. 1987. Influenza viral gene expression: Control mechanisms at early and late times of infection and nuclear-cytoplasmic transport of virus-specific RNAs. *J. Virol.* **61**: 764.

Smith, G.L. and A.J. Hay. 1982. Replication of the influenza virus genome. *Virology* **118**: 96.

St. Angelo, C., G.E. Smith, M.D. Summers, and R.M. Krug. 1987. Two of the three influenza viral polymerase (P) proteins expressed using baculovirus vectors form a complex in insect cells. *J. Virol.* **61**: 361.

Ulmanen, I., B.A. Broni, and R.M. Krug. 1981. Role of two of the influenza virus core P proteins in recognizing cap 1 structures (m⁷GpppNm) on RNAs and in initiating viral RNA transcription. *Proc. Natl. Acad. Sci.* **78**: 7355.

———. 1983. Influenza virus temperature-sensitive cap (m⁷GpppNm)-dependent endonuclease. *J. Virol.* **45**: 27.

Young, R.J. and J. Content. 1971. 5′-Terminus of influenza virus RNA. *Nature* **230**: 140.

Coronavirus: A Jumping RNA Transcription

M.M.C. Lai, S. Makino, L.H. Soe, C.-K. Shieh, J.G. Keck, and J.O. Fleming
Departments of Microbiology and Neurology, University of Southern California
School of Medicine, Los Angeles, California 90033

DNA- and RNA-dependent RNA polymerases usually recognize specific promoter sequences and initiate RNA transcription at some distances downstream from the promoter. Initiation of transcription requires only complementary nucleoside triphosphates, although oligonucleotides could, under some conditions, act as primers for transcription (Niyogi and Stevens 1965; Minkley and Pribnow 1973). An exception to this general rule is the RNA-dependent RNA polymerase of influenza virus, which utilizes capped mRNAs derived from host cells as a primer for transcription (Plotch et al. 1981). The completed RNA transcripts in mammalian cells are frequently processed by a mechanism of RNA splicing, by which a leader RNA from the 5' end is fused to downstream RNA sequences (Padgett et al. 1986). In this process, segments of intron sequences are removed. This RNA splicing can be mediated either by specific nuclear components (Padgett et al. 1986) or by RNA molecules themselves, such as in the case of *Tetrahymena* pre-rRNA (Cech and Bass 1986). Thus, the catalytic functions of RNA transcription and processing involve either proteins or RNA as an enzyme.

Coronavirus, an RNA-containing virus, utilizes a transcription mechanism that combines RNA priming and processing into a single step. Transcription is mediated by a virus-specified RNA polymerase, which transcribes a specific leader RNA from the viral RNA sequence. The leader RNA is subsequently utilized as a primer for transcription of mRNAs at downstream sites. As a result, mRNAs containing leader RNA derived from a distant site are generated, without utilizing conventional RNA-splicing mechanisms. Thus, free leader RNA is an integral part of coronavirus RNA transcription.

Coronaviruses are enveloped viruses containing a single-stranded RNA genome of 6×10^6 to 8×10^6 daltons (Lomniczi and Kennedy 1977; Lai and Stohlman 1978). Various coronaviruses infect many domestic animals, causing respiratory and gastrointestinal tract illnesses (Wege et al. 1982). The prototype coronavirus is mouse hepatitis virus (MHV), which often latently infects mice. Upon viral infection of a susceptible cell, the viral RNA genome is first translated into an RNA-dependent RNA polymerase (Brayton et al. 1982), which, in turn, transcribes the viral RNA into a full-length negative-strand RNA template (Lai et al. 1982). This latter RNA species is subsequently transcribed into a full-length positive-strand genomic RNA and six subgenomic mRNA species, which have a 3'-coterminal nested-set structure; i.e., the sequence of each mRNA is contained within the next larger RNA (Lai et al. 1981). Each mRNA, except the smallest mRNA, is physically polycistronic, but functionally monocistronic; namely, only the 5'-unique portion of each mRNA, which does not overlap with the next smaller mRNA, is used to synthesize a protein product (Rottier et al. 1981; Leibowitz et al. 1982). The viral genome contains seven genes, encoding three structural proteins (a spike glycoprotein E2, a matrix glycoprotein E1, and a nucleocapsid phosphoprotein N) and possibly four nonstructural proteins. The gene encoding the RNA polymerase is the 5'-most gene that, as revealed by the sequence of another coronavirus, avian infectious bronchitis virus (IBV), encompasses 18 kb, with a coding potential for up to 700 kD of proteins (Boursnell et al. 1987).

Another unusual feature of coronavirus mRNAs is the presence of an identical leader sequence of roughly 70 nucleotides at the 5' end of each mRNA and the genomic RNA (Lai et al. 1983, 1984; Spaan et al. 1983). Two lines of evidence suggest that the leader RNA is not derived by conventional RNA splicing mechanisms: (1) Coronavirus replicates in the cytoplasm (Brayton et al. 1981; Wilhelmsen et al. 1981), whereas conventional RNA splicing takes place in the nucleus, and (2) UV transcriptional mapping studies suggest that subgenomic mRNAs are transcribed independently and are not derived by cleavage of a large RNA precursor (Jacobs et al. 1981). We have previously proposed several models for MHV mRNA transcription: RNA template looping out, leader-primed transcription, and posttranscriptional *trans*-splicing (Baric et al. 1983). Indirect biochemical evidence suggests that the leader-primed transcriptional mechanism is the most likely one utilized by coronavirus (Baric et al. 1983). This model proposes that a leader RNA species is synthesized from the 3' end of the negative-strand RNA template, detaches from the template, and later binds to the same or a different template at the initiation sites of the various subgenomic mRNAs. This leader RNA then serves as the primer for mRNA transcription (Fig. 1).

We have already obtained direct biochemical data in support of this transcription model: (1) Free leader RNA species of 50–90 nucleotides have been detected in the cytoplasm of MHV-infected cells. These RNA species are discrete and reproducible in size. Some of the leader RNAs are dissociated from the RNA template and free in the cytoplasm (Baric et al. 1985). (2)

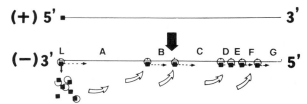

Figure 1. Model of leader-primed transcription of MHV subgenomic mRNAs. (■) Free leader RNAs; (○) RNA polymerase. The seven genes of MHV are represented by letters A through G (Lai et al. 1981). L represents the leader sequence.

A temperature-sensitive mutant has been isolated that synthesizes only the small leader RNAs, and not the mRNAs, at the nonpermissive temperature, suggesting that the transcription of leader RNA and mRNAs are discontinuous and may involve different viral proteins (Baric et al. 1985). The second viral protein required for mRNA transcription may be a modified RNA polymerase or a protein that binds the leader RNA to the template RNA. (3) The leader RNA sequences on the mRNAs can be freely exchanged between two MHVs infecting the same cells. Thus, up to 50% of the mRNAs of each virus could contain the leader sequences derived from the co-infecting virus (Makino et al. 1986a). This result suggests that the leader RNA is a separate transcriptional unit, which dissociates from the RNA template before participating in initiating mRNA transcription. (4) Expression of antisense leader RNA delayed the kinetics of RNA synthesis of a superinfecting MHV (Lai et al. 1987), suggesting that the leader RNA is required for mRNA transcription. (5) Sequence homology of 7–18 nucleotides occurs between the 3' end of the leader RNA and the initiation sites of various mRNAs. Thus, the intergenic regions on the negative-strand RNA template provides a complementary sequence for the leader RNA to bind (Shieh et al. 1987). Sequence analysis further suggested that the leader RNA is cleaved by an endonuclease activity before RNA transcription can proceed on this primer (Shieh et al. 1987). This activity is reminiscent of the influenza virus RNA polymerase (Plotch et al. 1981).

Another unusual feature of coronavirus RNA synthesis is that the virus undergoes RNA recombination at a very high frequency (Makino et al. 1986b; Keck et al. 1987). RNA recombination is very rare among RNA phages or RNA viruses (Horiuchi 1975). The only other viruses that can undergo RNA recombination are picornaviruses (King et al. 1982). The unusually high frequency, approaching 10% under some circumstances (Makino et al. 1986b), of coronavirus RNA recombination suggests that discontinuous RNA transcripts might be generated during coronavirus RNA synthesis. These incomplete RNA intermediates may rejoin the original template or a different RNA template to continue RNA synthesis, resulting in RNA recombination in the latter case. Indeed, such RNA intermediates have been detected in MHV-infected

cells (Baric et al. 1987). This finding suggests that coronavirus RNA synthesis involves an additional form of discontinuous, jumping transcription.

To understand the mechanism of leader-primed transcription and RNA recombination, we have further examined the structure of MHV-specific and -defective mRNA species in MHV-infected cells. We have demonstrated that MHV uses a "jumping" discontinuous transcription for mRNA synthesis. In addition, by analysis of RNA recombinants, we have shown that transcriptional jumping occurs frequently. Thus, RNA polymerase of MHV possesses unique properties of discontinuous and nonprocessive transcription.

MATERIALS AND METHODS

Viruses and cells. A59, JHM, and MHV-2 strains of MHV were used in this study. The viruses were grown in DBT cells, a mouse brain tumor cell line (Hirano et al. 1974). Defective-interfering (DI) particles of JHM at passage 18 were also used (Makino et al. 1985). The conditions of virus growth have been described previously (Lai et al. 1981; Makino et al. 1984a).

Isolation of recombinants. Recombinants were isolated by a modification of published procedures (Makino et al. 1986b; Keck et al. 1987). The use of neutralizing monoclonal antibodies followed the procedures of Fleming et al. (1986). The amount of monoclonal antibodies used was such that the virus titer was reduced by $4 \log_{10}$ units after treatment of viruses with antibodies. A mixture of two monoclonal antibodies, J.2.2 and J.7.2, was used (Fleming et al. 1986). The percentage of surviving viruses in a natural virus stock would thus be 10^{-8}. Therefore, essentially only recombinant viruses were selected under these conditions.

Molecular cloning of DI RNAs. The intracellular RNAs isolated from DI virus-infected cells were separated by agarose gel electrophoresis. The DI-specific RNAs were extracted from the gel and used for cDNA cloning as described previously (Shieh et al. 1987), except that oligo(dT) was used as a primer. The colonies obtained were screened with the cDNA clones representing the 5' end of the wild-type MHV genome (Shieh et al. 1987), since previous studies suggested that the DI-specific RNAs contained intact 5'-end sequences (Makino et al. 1985). The clones containing the intact 5'-end leader sequences were selected with the leader-specific cDNA (Lai et al. 1984). The clones obtained were sequenced by the Maxam-Gilbert method (1980) and Sanger's dideoxy termination sequencing method (Sanger et al. 1977).

Oligonucleotide fingerprinting. ^{32}P-labeled RNAs isolated from purified viruses were digested with RNase T1 and separated by two-dimensional polyacrylamide gel electrophoresis as described previously (Lai et al. 1981).

Primer extension. A 5'-end-labeled synthetic oligonucleotide (18-mer) complementary to nucleotides 123–140 from the 5' end of the JHM genomic RNA was hybridized to JHM intracellular genome-sized RNA in the presence of methylmercury according to the method of Maniatis et al. (1982). The primer-template hybrid was then extended with reverse transcriptase as described previously (Lai et al. 1984). Reaction products were analyzed by electrophoresis on 6% polyacrylamide gels containing 8 M urea.

RESULTS

Analysis of Sequences Involved in Leader RNA Binding

The leader-primed transcription model indicates that the free leader RNA generated from the 5' end of the RNA genome binds to a complementary site on the negative-strand RNA template at the initiation points of various mRNAs. Sequence analysis of the JHM strain of MHV showed the presence of 7–18 homologous nucleotides between the 3' end of the free leader RNA and the intergenic sequences of several mRNAs (Shieh et al. 1987). The consensus recognition sequence among the mRNAs analyzed is UCUAAAC, which is conserved among several coronaviruses of different species, including porcine transmissible gastroenteritis virus (Kapke and Brian 1986), bovine coronavirus (Lapps et al. 1987), and human coronavirus OC43 (T. Kamahora, unpubl.). To determine whether there is heterogeneity of leader RNA sequences at the 5' end of the genome, we performed primer-extension studies using a specific primer that is

complementary to nucleotides 123–140 from the 5' end of the genome, thus representing sequences downstream from the 5' leader RNA. This primer was hybridized to the genomic RNA and extended with reverse transcriptase. A single cDNA product of 140 nucleotides was obtained (Fig. 2, left), indicating the size homogeneity of the 5'-end sequences. The nucleic acid sequence was determined from this cDNA product and was shown to be identical to that obtained previously from cDNA clones (Fig. 2, right) (Shieh et al. 1987). It is notable that three UCUAA repeats are present within the region involved in leader fusion. The number of this repeat varies with different MHV strains (data not shown).

Another interesting feature of the 5'-end sequence is that the consensus sequence UCUAAAC present at position 70–76 from the 5' end of the RNA genome is imperfectly repeated two nucleotides downstream at position 79–85 (UAUAAAC). This structure may have a functional significance in that the downstream repeat sequence could serve as the initiation site for intracellular genome-size mRNA 1, which is indistinguishable in size from the virion genomic RNA. If this is the case, mRNA 1 will be expected to be shorter than the genomic RNA by nine nucleotides. We have attempted but failed to demonstrate the presence of such a nine-nucleotide-shorter "genome-length" RNA in MHV-infected cells. This failure could have been due to the low amount of such an RNA species. This interpretation is consistent with the low amount of the gene product (RNA polymerase) of mRNA 1. We therefore analyzed the 5' ends of other intracellular RNA species derived from MHV-DI-infected cells to search for the utilization of the UAUAAAC as a leader RNA jumping site.

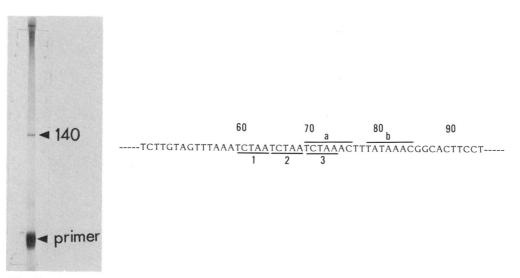

Figure 2. The 5'-end sequence of the intracellular MHV RNA genome as determined by primer-extension studies. (*Left*) A synthetic oligodeoxyribonucleotide (18-mer) complementary to nucleotides 123–140 from the 5' end of the JHM genomic RNA (Shieh et al. 1987) was ^{32}P-labeled at the 5' end, hybridized to the genome-size RNA isolated from JHM-infected cells, and primer-extended with reverse transcriptase. The products were electrophoresed on 6% polyacrylamide gels containing 8 M urea. (*Right*) The DNA sequence of this primer-extended product was determined by the Maxam-Gilbert (1980) method. Only the sequences at the leader junction regions are shown. The repeat sequences are marked.

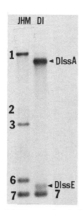

Figure 3. Intracellular RNA species in DI virus-infected cells. ^{32}P-labeled RNA from DI virus (passage 18)-infected cells and wild-type JHM-infected cells were electrophoresed in 1% agarose gel without denaturation.

Structure and 5′-end Sequence of DI RNAs

MHV has been shown to produce DI particles after serial passages in tissue culture at high multiplicities of infection (Makino et al. 1984a). These viruses synthesize novel intracellular RNAs that are distinct from the wild-type mRNA species of MHV (see Makino et al. 1985). Oligonucleotide fingerprinting analysis indicated that these novel DI RNAs contain sequences derived from several discontiguous parts of the genomic RNA, suggesting that they are products of multiple jumping during transcription. To understand the mechanism of RNA transcriptional jumping, we determined the 5′-end sequences of some of these DI RNA species. The RNA species studied are the DIssA and DIssE RNAs generated at passage 18 of DI virus (Fig. 3). For this purpose, we performed cDNA cloning of the DIssA and DIssE RNAs purified by agarose gel electrophoresis. The cDNA clones obtained were then sequenced by both the Maxam-Gilbert method (1980) and Sanger's dideoxy sequencing method (Sanger et al. 1977). Only the sequences at the 3′ end of the leader RNA of these RNA species are shown (Fig. 4). The 3′-end leader sequences of DIssE, DIssA, and wild-type JHM genomic RNAs are heterogeneous at the junctions between the leader sequence and the rest of the genomic sequences. DIssE contains four UCUAA repeats, in contrast to the three repeats in the wild-type JHM genome and DIssA RNA. Furthermore, both

DIssE and DIssA RNAs deleted the nine nucleotides UUUAUAAAC, which contain the second of the two consensus repeats. The sequences were further confirmed by primer-extension studies using DIssA and DIssE RNAs (data not shown). This result is consistent with the interpretation that these repeat consensus sequences are involved in transcriptional jumping. It was probable that during the generation of DI RNA, the leader RNA was synthesized, dissociated from the template, and reassociated with the transcriptional initiation sites for mRNA 1, i.e., the downstream repeat consensus sequence, thus deleting the nine nucleotides. The variation in the number of UCUAA repeats could be another result of imprecise binding of the leader RNA to the template RNA. The finding that precisely these repeat sequences were involved in the deletion or addition of sequences further suggests that transcriptional jumping involves recognition of specific sequences. DIssE has three additional single-base substitutions within the 5′-leader region, probably generated during viral passages (data not shown).

Generation of Multiple RNA Recombinants

It could be argued that generation of DI RNA is a rare event and does not reflect the normal mechanism of transcription. To provide further evidence that MHV transcription is discontinuous, generating incomplete RNA transcripts that could frequently dissociate and reassociate with the RNA template, we examined the outcome of mixed infection with two different strains of MHVs. If RNA transcription does involve frequent interruption and dissociation of RNA transcripts, it is expected that RNA recombinants can be generated as a result of RNA transcripts jumping to a homologous site on the RNA template of the different virus. To select for RNA recombinants, we utilized two selectable markers, the temperature-sensitive mutations and the neutralization or fusion-inducing ability of the virus. The latter property is determined by the gene (gene C) encoding the spike protein (E2) of the virus. Two selection schemes were employed. The first one was the coinfection of the susceptible cells with a temperature-sensitive mutant of A59, which grows and induces cell fusion only at permissive temperature (32°C), and a wild-type MHV-2 strain, which grows at both 32°C and 39°C, but does not cause cell fusion at either temperature. Viruses that cause cell fusion at

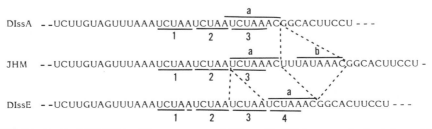

Figure 4. The 5′-end sequences of DI RNAs. The sequences of DI-specific RNAs were obtained from cDNA clones of the purified DIssE and DIssA RNAs. Only the 3′ ends of the leader sequences are shown.

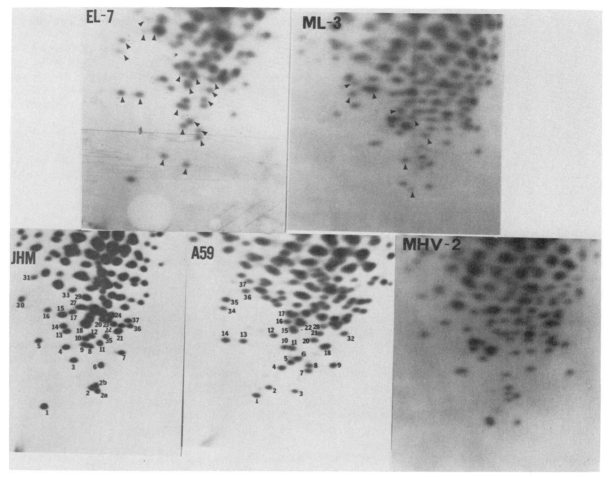

Figure 5. Oligonucleotide fingerprints of the genomic RNA of the recombinant virus EL-7 and its parental viruses A59 and JHM, and also of the recombinant virus ML-3 and its parental viruses A59 and MHV-2. The spots denoted by arrowheads are derived from A59. The rest of the spots are derived from the other parent (JHM or MHV-2).

39°C were selected. The second method was coinfection of the cells with a temperature-sensitive mutant of A59 and wild-type JHM strain. The viruses released at 39°C were treated with neutralizing monoclonal antibodies specific for JHM (Fleming et al. 1986). The surviving viruses thus represent recombinant viruses. From both selection schemes, numerous recombinant viruses have been obtained. Two representative recombinants are presented here. Figure 5 shows the oligonucleotide fingerprint of the RNA genomes of the recombinant EL-7, and its parental viruses A59 and JHM. It is evident that this recombinant contains oligonucleotides derived from both parents. Since the map positions of these oligonucleotides have been determined previously (Lai et al. 1981; Makino et al. 1984b), it was possible to determine the recombination sites of this recombinant from these fingerprints. It is significant that wherever an oligonucleotide derived from one parent is present, the corresponding oligonucleotide in the same position on the genomic map of the other parent is missing. Thus, this recombinant represents a product of homologous recombination. The crossover sites of this recombinant are depicted in Figure 6. It can

be seen that this recombinant contains three crossovers. The crossover within gene *C* was probably the result of the specific selection pressures applied, since the neutralization by monoclonal antibodies was directed specifically toward the gene product, the spike protein, of gene *C*. The other two crossover events had not been selected for. The presence of such unselected crossover events suggests that the recombination frequency is very high. The second recombinant presented is the recombinant, ML-3, between A59 and MHV-2 (Figs. 5 and 6). Similar to the recombinant EL-7, this virus also has multiple crossovers, some of which were

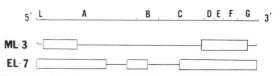

Figure 6. Genetic maps of EL-7 and ML-3. The data were obtained by comparing the oligonucleotide maps of the recombinants and their parental viruses (Fig. 5). The boxed areas represent sequences derived from A59 and the rest of genome derived from either JHM or MHV-2.

unselected for. We have isolated at least five other recombinants with such unselected recombination events. This result further suggests a high frequency of recombination events and is thus consistent with the frequent transcriptional jumping of coronaviruses.

DISCUSSION

The results presented in this paper provide additional evidence that coronavirus RNA transcription is discontinuous, generating incomplete RNA transcripts that can dissociate and reassociate frequently with the RNA template. As a result, RNA transcription involves frequent jumping, which takes place in two forms. The first form is the jumping of the leader RNA from the 5' end of genomic RNA to the initiation sites of subgenomic RNAs. This jumping leads to the leader-RNA-primed transcription of subgenomic mRNAs. It utilizes specific binding sequences, which include two to three UCUAA repeats. These sequences are present near the 3' end of the leader RNA, which is transcribed from the 5' end of the genomic RNA, and also at the initiation points of various mRNA species. The binding is generally precise, but it frequently involves incorrect repeats, resulting in the generation of DI RNAs with different numbers of repeat sequences. The binding of the leader RNA to the incorrect repeat has also been observed frequently in the synthesis of regular subgenomic mRNA species (S. Makino et al., unpubl.). These data further support the notion that the leader RNA jumping is a regular feature of MHV RNA transcription. The result of such a leader RNA jumping is the synthesis of mRNA containing a leader sequence, without using conventional RNA splicing. The second type of transcriptional jumping is suggested by the high frequency of RNA recombination and involves binding of the partially completed RNA transcripts to the original sites or homologous sites on a different viral RNA genome. Biochemical evidence has already been obtained that provides the basis for such a transcriptional jumping model. We have shown that incomplete RNA transcripts of various sizes could be detected in MHV-infected cells (Baric et al. 1987). The sizes of these transcripts correspond to the positions of possible hairpin loops on the RNA template or RNA transcripts. Furthermore, these transcripts are dissociated from the RNA template (Baric et al. 1987). These findings, coupled with the high frequency of RNA recombination, suggest that RNA transcription of MHV proceeds in a discontinuous and nonprocessive manner, being interrupted at the sites of hairpins, and resulting in the release of partial RNA transcripts. These RNA transcripts could rejoin the RNA template to continue transcription or participate in recombination. It should be mentioned that the high frequency of RNA recombination is demonstrated not only by the multiple crossovers in the genome of a recombinant virus, but also by the number of recombinants present in the progeny of a mixed viral infection (Makino et al. 1986b). The biochemical nature of the leader RNA and incomplete RNA transcripts in the infected cells is not yet clear. It is very likely that these RNA species are bound to the RNA polymerase during these transcription processes.

The RNA polymerase of MHV thus exhibits very peculiar properties of frequent jumping during transcription. What is the biochemical nature of MHV RNA polymerase? Although the size of the gene encoding the MHV RNA polymerase has not been reliably determined, the corresponding gene in IBV has been completely sequenced. The gene is 18 kb in size and has a capacity to encode proteins of up to 700 kD (Boursnell et al. 1987). Two slightly overlapping open reading frames were found. The extremely large size of the putative RNA polymerase is consistent with the complex functions required for coronavirus RNA synthesis. So far, no satisfactory in vitro transcription system has been established, and the RNA-polymerase-like proteins have not been identified in coronavirus-infected cells, except that the RNA polymerase activities have been demonstrated (Brayton et al. 1982, 1984). In vitro translation of coronavirus genomic RNA yielded proteins of roughly 200 kD, which are presumably part of the RNA polymerase (Denison and Perlman 1986). An amino-terminal cleavage product, p28, of this protein has been detected in MHV-infected cells (Denison and Perlman 1987). The biochemical nature and functions of these proteins have not been determined. The study of these RNA polymerases should be able to provide additional insights into the mechanism of RNA transcription.

ACKNOWLEDGMENTS

We thank Carol Flores for excellent typing of the manuscript. This work was supported by U.S. Public Health Service grants AI-19244 and NS-18146 from the National Institutes of Health, grant RG-1449 from the National Multiple Sclerosis Society, and grant PCM-4507 from the National Science Foundation. L.H.S. is a postdoctoral fellow of the Bank of America–Giannini Foundation.

REFERENCES

Baric, R.S., S.A. Stohlman, and M.M.C. Lai. 1983. Characterization of replicative intermediate RNA of mouse hepatitis virus: Presence of leader RNA sequence on nascent chains. *J. Virol.* **48:** 633.

Baric, R.S., C.-K. Shieh, S.A. Stohlman, and M.M.C. Lai. 1987. Analysis of intracellular small RNAs of mouse hepatitis virus: Evidence for discontinuous transcription. *Virology* **156:** 342.

Baric, R.S., S.A. Stohlman, M.K. Razavi, and M.M.C. Lai. 1985. Characterization of leader-related small RNAs in coronavirus-infected cells: Further evidence for leader-primed mechanism of transcription. *Virus Res.* **3:** 19.

Boursnell, M.E.G., T.D.K. Brown, I.J. Foulds, P.F. Green, F.M. Tomley, and M.M. Binns. 1987. Completion of the sequence of the genome of the coronavirus avian infectious bronchitis virus. *J. Gen. Virol.* **68:** 55.

Brayton, P.R., R.G. Ganges, and S.A. Stohlman. 1981. Host cell nucleus and murine hepatitis virus replication. *J. Gen. Virol.* **56:** 457.

Brayton, P.R., S.A. Stohlman, and M.M.C. Lai. 1984. Further characterization of mouse hepatitis virus RNA-dependent RNA polymerases. *Virology* **133**: 197.

Brayton, P.R., M.M.C. Lai, C.D. Patton, and S.A. Stohlman. 1982. Characterization of two RNA polymerase activities induced by mouse hepatitis virus. *J. Virol.* **42**: 847.

Cech, T.R. and B.L. Bass. 1986. Biological catalysis by RNA. *Annu. Rev. Biochem.* **55**: 599.

Denison, M.R. and S. Perlman. 1986. Translation and processing of mouse hepatitis virus virion RNA in a cell-free system. *J. Virol.* **60**: 12.

———. 1987. Identification of putative polymerase gene product in cells infected with murine coronavirus A59. *Virology* **157**: 565.

Fleming, J.O., M.D. Trousdale, F.A.K. El-Zaatari, S.A. Stohlman, and L.P. Weiner. 1986. Pathogenicity of antigenic variants of murine coronavirus JHM selected with monoclonal antibodies. *J. Virol.* **58**: 869.

Hirano, N., K. Fujiwara, S. Hino, and M. Matumoto. 1974. Replication and plaque formation of mouse hepatitis virus (MHV-2) in mouse cell line DBT culture. *Arch. Gesamte Virusforsch.* **44**: 298.

Horiuchi, K. 1975. Genetic studies of RNA phages. In *RNA phages* (ed. N. Zinder), p. 29. Cold Spring Harbor Laboratory, Cold Spring Harbor, New York.

Jacobs, L., W.J.M. Spaan, M.C. Horzinek, and B.A.M. van der Zeijst. 1981. The synthesis of the subgenomic mRNAs of mouse hepatitis virus is initiated independently: Evidence from UV transcription mapping. *J. Virol.* **42**: 755.

Kapke, P.A. and D.A. Brian. 1986. Sequence analysis of the porcine transmissible gastroenteritis coronavirus nucleocapsid protein gene. *Virology* **151**: 41.

Keck, J.G., S.A. Stohlman, L.H. Soe, S. Makino, and M.M.C. Lai. 1987. Multiple recombination sites at the 5'-end of murine coronavirus RNA. *Virology* **156**: 331.

King, A.M.Q., D. McCahon, W.R. Slade, and J.W.I. Newman. 1982. Recombination in RNA. *Cell* **29**: 921.

Lai, M.M.C. and S.A. Stohlman. 1978. The RNA of mouse hepatitis virus. *J. Virol.* **26**: 236.

Lai, M.M.C., C.D. Paton, and S.A. Stohlman. 1982. Replications of mouse hepatitis virus: Negative-stranded RNA and replicative form RNA are of genome length. *J. Virol.* **44**: 487.

Lai, M.M.C., R.S. Baric, P.R. Brayton, and S.A. Stohlman. 1984. Characterization of leader RNA sequences on the virion and mRNAs of mouse hepatitis virus, a cytoplasmic virus. *Proc. Natl. Acad. Sci.* **81**: 3626.

Lai, M.M.C., C.D. Patton, R.S. Baric, and S.A. Stohlman. 1983. Presence of leader sequences in the mRNA of mouse hepatitis virus. *J. Virol.* **46**: 1027.

Lai, M.M.C., P.R. Brayton, R.C. Armen, C.D. Patton, C. Pugh, and S.A. Stohlman. 1981. Mouse hepatitis virus A59: Messenger RNA structure and genetic localization of the sequence divergence from the hepatotropic strain MHV-3. *J. Virol.* **39**: 823.

Lai, M.M.C., S. Makino, R.S. Baric, L. Soe, C.-K. Shieh, J.G. Keck, and S.A. Stohlman. 1987. Leader RNA-primed transcription and RNA recombination of murine coronaviruses. 1987. *UCLA Symp. Mol. Cell. Biol.* **54**: 285.

Lapps, W., B.G. Hogue, and D.A. Brian. 1987. Sequence analysis of the bovine coronavirus nucleocapsid and matrix protein genes. *Virology* **157**: 47.

Leibowitz, J.L., S.R. Weiss, E. Paavola, and C.W. Bond.

1982. Cell-free translation of murine coronavirus RNA. *J. Virol.* **43**: 905.

Lomniczi, B. and I. Kennedy. 1977. Genome of infectious bronchitis virus. *J. Virol.* **24**: 99.

Makino, S., N. Fujioka, and K. Fujiwara. 1985. Structure of the intracellular defective viral RNAs of defective interfering particles of mouse hepatitis virus. *J. Virol.* **54**: 329.

Makino, S., S.A. Stohlman, and M.M.C. Lai. 1986a. Leader sequences of murine coronavirus mRNAs can be freely reassorted: Evidence for the role of free leader RNA in transcription. *Proc. Natl. Acad. Sci.* **83**: 4204.

Makino, S., F. Taguchi, and K. Fujiwara. 1984a. Defective interfering particles of mouse hepatitis virus. *Virology* **133**: 9.

Makino, S., J.G. Keck, S.A. Stohlman, and M.M.C. Lai. 1986b. High-frequency RNA recombination of murine coronaviruses. *J. Virol.* **57**: 729.

Makino, S., F. Taguchi, N. Hirano, and K. Fujiwara. 1984b. Analysis of genomic and intracellular viral RNAs of small plaque mutants of mouse hepatitis virus, JHM strain. *Virology* **139**: 138.

Maniatis, T., E.F. Fritsch, and J. Sambrook. 1982. *Molecular cloning: A laboratory manual.* Cold Spring Harbor Laboratory, Cold Spring Harbor, New York.

Maxam, A.M. and W. Gilbert. 1980. Sequencing end-labeled DNA with base-specific chemical cleavages. *Methods Enzymol.* **65**: 499.

Minkley, E.G. and D. Pribnow. 1973. Transcription of the early region of bacteriophage T7: Selective initiation with dinucleotides. *J. Mol. Biol.* **77**: 255.

Niyogi, S.K. and A. Stevens. 1965. Studies of the ribonucleic acid polymerase from *Escherichia coli*. IV. Effect of oligonucleotides on the ribonucleic acid polymerase reaction with synthetic polyribonucleotides as templates. *J. Biol. Chem.* **240**: 2593.

Padgett, R.A., P.J. Grabowski, M.M. Konarska, S. Seiler, and P.A. Sharp. 1986. Splicing of messenger RNA precursors. *Annu. Rev. Biochem.* **55**: 1119.

Plotch, S.J., M. Bouloy, I. Ulmanen, and R.M. Krug. 1981. A unique cap (m⁷GpppXm)-dependent influenza virion endonuclease cleaves capped RNAs to generate primers that initiate viral RNA transcription. *Cell* **23**: 847.

Rottier, P.J.M., W.J.M. Spaan, M.C. Horzinek, and B.A.M. van der Zeijst. 1981. Translation of three mouse hepatitis virus strain A59 subgenomic RNAs in *Xenopus laevis* oocytes. *J. Virol.* **38**: 20.

Shieh, C.-K., L.H. Soe, S. Makino, M.-F. Chang, S.A. Stohlman, and M.M.C. Lai. 1987. The 5'-end sequence of the murine coronavirus genome: Implications for multiple fusion sites in leader-primed transcription. *Virology* **156**: 321.

Sanger, F., S. Nicklen, and A.R. Coulson. 1977. DNA sequencing with chain-terminating inhibitors. *Proc. Natl. Acad. Sci.* **74**: 5463.

Spaan, W., H. Delius, M. Skinner, J. Armstrong, P. Rottier, S. Smeekens, B.A.M. van der Zeijst, and S.G. Siddell. 1983. Coronavirus mRNA synthesis involves fusion of noncontiguous sequences. *EMBO J.* **2**: 1939.

Wege, H., S. Siddell, and V. ter Meulen. 1982. The biology and pathogenesis of coronaviruses. *Curr. Top. Microbiol. Immunol.* **99**: 165.

Wilhelmsen, K.C., J.L. Leibowitz, C.W. Bond, and J.A. Bond. 1981. The replication of murine coronaviruses in enucleated cells. *Virology* **110**: 225.

The Switch from Transcription to Replication of a Negative-strand RNA Virus

G.W. WERTZ,* M.B. HOWARD,* N. DAVIS,[†] AND J. PATTON[‡]

*Department of Microbiology, University of Alabama at Birmingham Medical School, Birmingham, Alabama 35294

Replication of the RNA genomes of the negative-strand Rhabdoviridae requires de novo protein synthesis. However, transcription of these same templates does not. In this paper, we describe experiments that identify the proteins involved in switching the polymerase activity from transcription to replication, and we address their possible functions.

The system we have used to study the proteins involved in viral RNA replication is that of vesicular stomatitis virus (VSV), the prototype of the rhabdovirus group. VSV is one of the simplest of the enveloped, nonsegmented, negative-strand RNA viruses. The genome of VSV codes for five proteins, all of which are structural components of the virion. The RNA genome is always found in the form of a viral nucleocapsid, coated with the major nucleocapsid protein (N) and associated with the phosphoprotein (NS) and the RNA-dependent RNA polymerase (L). The remaining viral proteins are the matrix protein (M), which is located on the inside surface of the viral membrane, and the glycoprotein (G), which is embedded in the membrane. Infection initiates with adsorption of the virus to the cell membrane, followed by uptake into vacuoles and uncoating to release the viral nucleocapsid to the cytoplasm, where the subsequent molecular events of infection take place.

The first event in viral multiplication is transcription of the negative-strand genome by the nucleocapsid-associated RNA-dependent RNA polymerase. The active template for all RNA synthetic events is not the naked RNA; rather, it is the RNA encapsidated with the N protein in a helical nucleocapsid structure containing the NS and L proteins that constitute the RNA polymerase (Emerson and Yu 1975).

In this form, the negative-strand RNA genome of VSV serves as a template for two types of RNA synthetic reactions: (1) transcription, which yields a leader RNA and five polyadenylated mRNAs, and (2) replication, which yields a complete, all-inclusive positive-strand copy of the genome, the template for synthesis of the negative-strand genome. A major distinction between these two RNA synthetic processes is that replication requires continuous viral protein synthesis, whereas transcription does not (Wertz and Levine

1973). Thus, transcription is the first RNA synthetic event, and only after the mRNA products of transcription are translated to yield protein does RNA replication begin. The RNA synthetic events occurring in VSV-infected cells are diagramed in Figure 1.

Transcription initiates at the 3' end of the genome and occurs in an obligatory sequential fashion that reflects the physical arrangement of the five viral genes (Abraham and Banerjee 1976; Ball and White 1976). The products of transcription do not constitute a complete copy of the genome, and the exact mechanism by which the discrete transcripts are produced is unknown (Ball and Wertz 1981). A full-length, positive-strand copy of the genome, whose synthesis is the first step in replication, is synthesized from the infecting nucleocapsid templates only after the onset of protein synthesis. Inhibition of viral protein synthesis at any time results in rapid cessation of replication and a return to the transcriptive pattern of RNA synthesis (Wertz and Levine 1973). Unlike the mRNAs, the full-length positive strand is neither capped nor polyadenylated; furthermore, both the full-length positive-strand and negative-strand products of RNA replication are found only in the form of N-coated nucleocapsid structures, never as naked RNA (Soria et al. 1974).

It has been known for 14 years that protein synthesis is required for VSV RNA replication to occur, but which VSV proteins were required was not known. We asked the question, What proteins need to be synthesized in order to change the RNA synthetic activity of the nucleocapsid templates from transcription of discrete mRNAs to replication of full-length RNA? To answer this question, we developed an in vitro replication system that carries out replication of VSV RNA as a function of ongoing viral protein synthesis programmed in a reticulocyte lysate. This system, consisting of viral nucleocapsids and a micrococcal-nuclease-treated rabbit reticulocyte lysate, replicates VSV RNA when protein synthesis is programmed by the addition of viral mRNA. In the work described in this paper, we used nucleocapsids of a VSV-defective interfering particle (DI-T), which contain only the 5' 20% of the standard genome (Leamnson and Reichmann 1974), as templates in the in vitro system (see Fig. 2). This was done to yield a system in which genome-length RNA replication can be analyzed in the absence of any mRNA synthesis (Wertz 1983). These DI nucleocapsids do not synthesize mRNAs because they lack complete information for any of the structural genes; only a

Present addresses: [†]Department of Microbiology, North Carolina State University, Raleigh, North Carolina 27607; [‡]Department of Biology, University of South Florida, Tampa, Florida 33620.

REPLICATION OF VSV

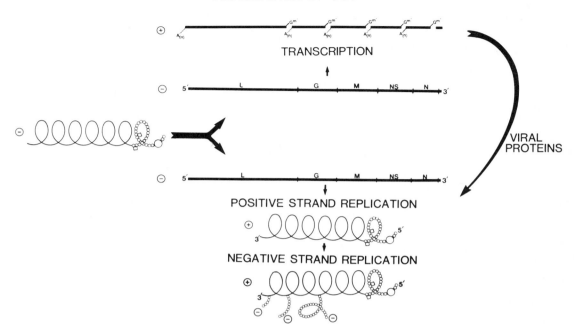

Figure 1. VSV RNA synthetic reactions.

46-nucleotide leader RNA is transcribed in the absence of protein synthesis (Leamnson and Reichmann 1974; Emerson et al. 1977). In the presence of viral protein synthesis, termination does not occur at the end of the leader gene, but the polymerase reads through this junction to replicate a full-length copy of the DI genome (Fig. 3) (Wertz 1983). Since no mRNAs are made by the DI nucleocapsids, protein synthesis and hence RNA replication in this system can be controlled by the addition of exogenous mRNA. Therefore, by adding individual VSV mRNAs to program the expression of individual viral proteins, it has been possible to investigate the requirement for each of the VSV proteins in RNA replication. The results of these experiments are described below.

METHODS

Components of the in vitro replication system. A detailed description of the components constituting the replication system has been reported elsewhere (Davis and Wertz 1982). Reaction mixtures contained micrococcal-nuclease-treated reticulocyte lysate, ribonucleoside triphosphates, creatine kinase, amino acids, salts, dithioerythritol, purified VSV DI nucleocapsids,

1 μCi of [^{3}H]UTP per microliter, and 0.4 μCi of [^{35}S]methionine per microliter in a final volume of 25 μl. Intracellular nucleocapsid templates were prepared from BHK cells coinfected for 13 hours with VSV (multiplicity of infection = 2) and DI particles at a ratio that gave 99% inhibition of standard virus yield (Wertz 1983). Reactions were programmed for protein synthesis by the addition of either polyadenylated RNA isolated from VSV-infected cells or individual hybrid-selected VSV RNAs as indicated. Reactions were typically incubated for 3 hours at 30°C.

RESULTS

N Protein Alone Supports Replication

The protein requirement for replication was analyzed by programming the in vitro system described above with individual VSV mRNAs that had been purified by hybridization selection with cDNA clones to selected

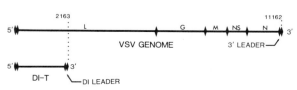

Figure 2. Map of VSV and VSV DI-T RNA.

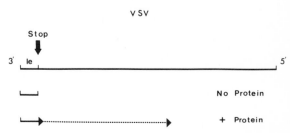

Figure 3. Effect of protein synthesis on RNA products from the DI-T template.

genes. The goal of these experiments was to determine whether addition to the in vitro system of a single species of viral mRNA to program synthesis of the N, NS, or M proteins in the presence of enzymatically competent nucleocapsids (containing the NS and L proteins) would promote the synthesis of genome-length RNA. In these experiments, the syntheses of viral RNA and protein were monitored simultaneously by double-labeling with both [³H]UTP and [³⁵S]methionine. The quantities of RNA and protein synthesized were determined by densitometric scanning of fluorograms of dried gels. The amount of genome-length RNA synthesized in the presence of varying concentrations of individually synthesized proteins was compared with the level of replication in the presence of varying concentrations of all five VSV proteins.

These experiments demonstrated that N mRNA added to the in vitro system to program synthesis of N protein alone was necessary and sufficient for synthesis of genome-length RNA. Neither the NS nor the M protein by itself was able to support the synthesis of genome-length RNA (Patton et al. 1984a).

Quantitation of the levels of genome synthesis and N protein expression for reactions containing either total mRNA or N mRNA alone demonstrated that the amount of genome synthesis was directly proportional to the amount of N protein synthesis in either set of reactions (Fig. 4). These data showed that synthesis of N protein alone was sufficient to fulfill the requirement for protein synthesis in replication.

Newly Synthesized RNA Assembles into Nucleocapsids

In infected cells, newly replicated RNA rapidly assembles with protein to form nucleocapsids. The assembly to form nucleocapsids renders the RNA re-

sistant to degradation by ribonucleases and causes the RNA to band in CsCl at a density of 1.3 g/cm³. We assayed whether or not the newly replicated RNA produced in vitro assembled with newly synthesized N protein to form nucleocapsids by three tests: (1) Did the replication products assemble with newly synthesized N protein as assayed by velocity sedimentation? (2) Were the products RNase-resistant? (3) Would they band in CsCl at the density of authentic nucleocapsids? The products of replication in vitro programmed by synthesis of N protein alone had all three properties (Patton et al. 1984a).

Ability of Pretranslated N Protein to Support Replication

N protein has been reported to exist in a pool in infected cells and to be drawn from that pool to support replication (Hsu et al. 1979). In an effort to mimic conditions in the infected cell, we synthesized N protein in the in vitro system prior to addition of nucleocapsid templates and then added the DI templates to the in vitro reaction that contained a pool of "presynthesized" N protein. The efficiency of replication as a function of concentration of N was measured. Both RNA and protein synthesis were monitored by double labeling as described above. As observed above, a linear relationship between increasing concentration of N protein and increasing amounts of genome RNA product was observed, but only over a low concentration range. However, in contrast to the results in which RNA replication and protein synthesis were concomitant, it was found that when the concentration of presynthesized N increased above a certain range, the efficiency of RNA synthesis per unit of N protein actually declined.

The N protein presynthesized in the in vitro system at high concentrations was analyzed by velocity sedimentation analysis in glycerol gradients. At high concentrations, N protein was shown to sediment to the bottom of the gradients, indicating aggregation. Unaggregated N protein, on the other hand, bands at a characteristic position in the middle of the gradient (data not shown). This aggregation of presynthesized N protein at high concentrations correlated with the inability of the N protein to support replication. These findings were in direct contrast to the results described above in which N protein synthesis and replication occurred simultaneously. Under the conditions of simultaneous synthesis, newly synthesized N protein is immediately used to support replication and formation of progeny nucleocapsids. Thus, under these conditions, free N protein never accumulates to high concentrations in a soluble protein pool and thus does not reach concentrations great enough to aggregate. We conclude that under conditions of low N concentration or simultaneous protein synthesis and RNA replication, N can function alone to support replication. At high concentrations, however, N protein aggregates and in that state is unable to support replication.

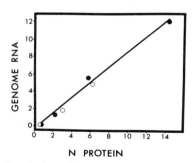

Figure 4. Correlation of genome-length RNA synthesis and N-protein expression. RNA and protein products were analyzed by gel electrophoresis, and fluorograms of the gels were analyzed by densitometry. Exposure times were chosen to give band intensities in the linear range. The relative absorbance units of ³⁵S-labeled N protein for a given reaction are plotted vs. the total amount of genome-length RNA (plus and minus strands) synthesized in that reaction. Results are shown from reactions to which varying amounts of total VSV mRNA (●) or hybrid-selected N mRNA (○) were added. The line has been fitted with a correlation coefficient of 0.995 to the results from reactions containing total VSV mRNA, using a least-squares analysis. (From Patton et al. 1984a.)

Are Proteins Other Than N Required for Optimal Replication?

The experiments described above (first section of Results) showed that N protein synthesis alone was necessary and sufficient to support replication. However, in view of the results showing that high concentrations of N (which was observed in an aggregated state) failed to support replication, we asked whether N protein alone was optimal for replication. Is another protein required to keep N protein available to support replication in the infected cell? A clue to this came from the observation of Bell et al. (1984) and Peluso and Moyer (1984), who observed complexes of N and NS proteins in infected cells. In further experiments (Davis et al. 1986), we demonstrated that in the in vitro system where replication is supported by the synthesis of all five VSV proteins in a manner that is linear with increasing protein concentration, N protein could be found in a complex with the phosphoprotein, NS.

Having observed that N and NS could exist in complexes, we carried out experiments to test directly whether NS protein could function to maintain N protein in a state capable of supporting replication. To do this, the ability of equivalent amounts of N protein to support replication under conditions where replication and N protein synthesis were carried out simultaneously (Fig. 5, N CON) or where N protein was presynthe-

sized (Fig. 5, N PRE) was compared. As shown in Figure 5, the same quantity of presynthesized N protein supported only 37% the level of RNA replication as N protein synthesized concomitantly for the reasons described above. If, however, increasing amounts of NS mRNA were added to N mRNA and the two were presynthesized concurrently, then the presynthesized N protein supported replication with an efficiency equal to or greater than that of N alone when translation and replication were concomitant (Fig. 5).

These data therefore demonstrate that NS protein functions to keep N protein in a state appropriate to support replication. The optimal concentration of N to NS is a molar ratio of approximately 2N:1NS. Furthermore, as shown in the last lane of Fig. 5, when the molar amount of NS exceeds that of N, then the efficiency of replication decreases. Similar results have been obtained under conditions of concurrent synthesis (Patton et al. 1984b). Therefore, these data show that NS functions positively in replication by keeping N in a state suitable to support replication; yet at molar ratios exceeding 1:1, NS inhibits replication.

DISCUSSION

The results described above demonstrate that N protein synthesis alone is sufficient to support the transition from a transcriptive event, the synthesis of only the DI leader RNA, to replication of full-length DI genomic RNA of both positive and negative polarities. However, under conditions where increasing concentrations of N protein are synthesized in the absence of replicating templates, the N protein aggregates and either supports replication inefficiently (Fig. 5) or not at all (data not shown). Presynthesis of the N protein in the presence of the NS protein, on the other hand, maintains the N in a form capable of supporting replication even at high concentrations. In effect, in the presence of NS, the efficiency of RNA replication per unit of N protein is "rescued" and, at a molar ratio of approximately 2N to 1NS, can exceed the level of efficiency for concomitant protein synthesis and RNA synthesis for N alone.

On the basis of these findings, we propose a model whereby NS protein regulates replication by controlling the availability of N protein (see Fig. 6). In this model, N protein alone can support replication if the N protein is at a low concentration. At high concentrations, N protein aggregates and, in the aggregated condition, is no longer able to support replication. NS protein can function to prevent the aggregation of N protein by formation of complexes with N that maintain it in a state usable for replication. The concentration ratio of N to NS is critical to the efficiency of replication, and a molar ratio of 2N:1NS is optimal. However, when the molar amount of NS exceeds that of N, replication is inhibited.

We propose that NS protein may be the factor that controls the balance between VSV RNA replication and transcription and that it does so by controlling the

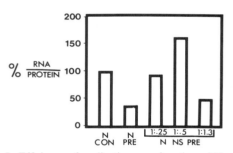

Figure 5. Efficiency of replication as a function of N protein synthesized alone or in the presence of varying concentrations of NS protein. The different conditions used in the in vitro replication reactions and the mRNA species added to the reactions are as indicated. (N CON) Replication reaction containing [^{35}S]UTP, hybrid-selected N mRNA, and DI-T nucleocapsids incubated concomitantly (CON) at 30°C for 2 hr; (N PRE) replication reaction containing [^{35}S]methionine and hybrid-selected N mRNA translated for 60 min (pretranslated) at 30°C prior to the addition of [^{3}H]UTP, anisomycin, and DI-T nucleocapsids, with further incubation for 2 hr; (N, NS, and PRE) replication in which increasing concentrations of hybrid-selected NS mRNA were pretranslated with hybrid-selected N mRNA under the same conditions as indicated for the reaction of N PRE. mRNA concentrations were adjusted so that the proteins were synthesized at a N:NS molar ratio of 1:0.25 (lane N), 1:0.5 (lane NS), and 1:1.3 (lane PRE). Fluorograms of polyacrylamide gels of [^{35}S]methionine-labeled protein and agarose-urea gels of [^{3}H]UTP-labeled RNA were analyzed by densitometry. The percentages of the relative levels of RNA per unit protein are plotted for each reaction. The level of replication in reactions where protein and RNA synthesis were concomitant (CON) was the standard to compare the levels of replication observed in the other four reactions.

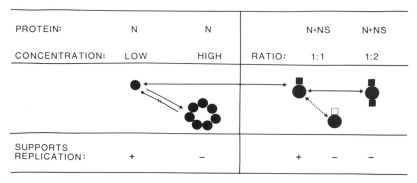

Figure 6. Model for the interactions of the VSV N and NS proteins with respect to RNA replication. N protein monomers can support replication; aggregates formed at high concentrations of N are inactive in replication. Association of N with NS at a ratio of 1:1 or less prevents aggregation and maintains N in a functional state. Complexes of N and NS with increased ratios of NS to N do not support replication. Alternatively, an alteration in the NS protein may render the N:NS complex unable to support replication. (●) N; (■) NS; (□) altered NS.

availability of N protein to support replication. This proposal is consistent with the observation (Hsu et al. 1979) that N and NS exist in infected cells in a soluble pool from which N, but not NS, is drawn to support formation of progeny nucleocapsids.

Finally, NS protein is known to exist in a variety of phosphorylated forms. We are presently investigating the possible role of these various forms in determining whether NS makes N available for replication.

ACKNOWLEDGMENTS

This work was supported by U.S. Public Health Service grant AI-12464 from the National Institute of Allergy and Infectious Diseases.

REFERENCES

Abraham, G. and A.K. Banerjee. 1976. Sequential transcription of the genes of vesicular stomatitis virus. *Proc. Natl. Acad. Sci.* **73:** 1504.

Ball, L.A. and G.W. Wertz. 1981. VSV RNA synthesis; how can you be positive? *Cell* **26:** 143.

Ball, L.A. and C.N. White. 1976. Order of transcription of genes of vesicular stomatitis virus. *Proc. Natl. Acad. Sci.* **73:** 442.

Bell, J.C., E.G. Brown, D. Takayesu, and L. Prevec. 1984. Protein kinase activity associated with immunoprecipitates of the vesicular stomatitis virus phosphoprotein NS. *Virology* **132:** 229.

Davis, N.L. and G.W. Wertz. 1982. Synthesis of vesicular stomatitis virus negative-strand RNA *in vitro*: Dependence on viral protein synthesis. *J. Virol.* **41:** 821.

Davis, N.L., H. Arnheiter, and G.W. Wertz. 1986. Vesicular stomatitis virus N and NS proteins form multiple complexes. *J. Virol.* **59:** 751.

Emerson, S.U. and Y.-H. Yu. 1975. Both NS and L proteins are required for *in vitro* RNA synthesis by vesicular stomatitis virus. *J. Virol.* **15:** 1348.

Emerson, S.U., P.M. Dierks, and J.T. Parsons. 1977. *In vitro* synthesis of a unique RNA species by a T particle of vesicular stomatitis virus. *J. Virol.* **239:** 708.

Hsu, C.H., D. Kingsbury, and K. Murti. 1979. Assembly of vesicular stomatitis virus nucleocapsids *in vivo*: A kinetic analysis. *J. Virol.* **32:** 304.

Leamnson, R. and M.E. Reichmann. 1974. The RNA of defective vesicular stomatitis virus particles in relation to viral cistrons. *J. Mol. Biol.* **85:** 551.

Patton, J.T., N.L. Davis, and G.W. Wertz. 1984a. N protein alone satisfies the requirement for protein synthesis during RNA replication of VSV. *J. Virol.* **49:** 303.

———. 1984b. Role of VSV proteins in RNA replication. In *Nonsegmented negative strand viruses* (ed. D.H.L. Bishop and R.W. Compans), p. 147. Academic Press, New York.

Peluso, R.W. and S.A. Moyer. 1984. Vesicular stomatitis proteins required for the *in vitro* replication of defective interfering particle genome RNA. In *Nonsegmented negative strand viruses* (ed. D.H.L. Bishop and R.W. Compans), p. 153. Academic Press, New York.

Soria, M., S. Little, and A. Huang. 1974. Characterization of vesicular stomatitis virus nucleocapsids. I. Complementary 40S RNA molecules in nucleocapsids. *Virology* **61:** 270.

Wertz, G.W. 1983. Replication of vesicular stomatitis virus defective interfering particle RNA *in vitro*: Transition from synthesis of defective interfering leader RNA to synthesis of full-length defective interfering RNA. *J. Virol.* **46:** 513.

Wertz, G.W. and M. Levine. 1973. RNA synthesis of vesicular stomatitis virus and a small plaque mutant: Effects of cycloheximide. *J. Virol.* **12:** 253.

The Translational Requirement for La Crosse Virus S-mRNA Synthesis

D. Kolakofsky, C. Bellocq, and R. Raju
Department of Microbiology, University of Geneva Medical School, CH-1211 Geneva 4, Switzerland

La Crosse virus (LAC) is a member of the California encephalitis serogroup of the insect-transmitted bunyavirus family. These viruses grow in both insect and animal cells, but the fate of the infection is dramatically different depending on the species. The natural host for LAC is the mosquito *Aedes triseriatus*. In mosquitoes or in mosquito cells in culture, the viral infection is asymptomatic, whereas in mammals or mammalian cells in culture, the viral infection is associated with cytopathic effects. The genome of these viruses consists of three segments of single-stranded RNA of negative polarity, each contained within a separate nucleocapsid (NC), which are labeled small (S), medium (M), and large (L). The viral NCs have helical symmetry and appear in the electron microscope as circular and super-coiled structures (Obijeski et al. 1976).

The mechanism by which bunyaviruses initiate transcription of their mRNAs is remarkably similar to that of influenza viruses (see Krug 1981). Bunyavirus S-mRNAs in vivo contain 5′ nontemplated extensions of about 15 nucleotides in length that are heterogeneous in sequence, presumably the result of a host primer used to initiate transcription (Bishop et al. 1983; Patterson and Kolakofsky 1984). In vitro, purified LAC virions were found to contain a transcriptase that is dependent on natural mRNAs such as alfalfa mosaic virus (AMV) RNA 4, which were shown to act as primers, and a methylated cap-dependent endonuclease that cleaves AMV RNA 4 at the positions expected from the length of the 5′ extensions found on the transcripts made in vitro (Patterson et al. 1984; Bellocq et al. 1987). Bunyaviruses, like influenza viruses, thus snatch capped oligonucleotides from host mRNAs to prime their mRNA synthesis. However, unlike influenza viruses, LAC transcription takes place in the cytoplasm (Rossier et al. 1986), where it uses a stable pool of mRNAs as substrates for primers. The 3′ end of the LAC S-mRNA, which is apparently not polyadenylated, has been mapped to approximately position 886, 100 nucleotides before the end of its genomic template.

Although bunyavirus mRNA synthesis in vivo is independent of host mRNA synthesis, it is unusually sensitive to drugs that disrupt protein synthesis. This finding was first reported by Abraham and Pattnaik (1983) for bunyawera and akabane viruses and has since been confirmed for LAC and Germiston virus (Raju and Kolakofsky 1986; Gerbaud et al. 1987). Since a translational requirement for mRNA synthesis appeared to conflict with the transcriptional activity of purified LAC virions, the nature of the S-genome transcripts generated by purified virions was reexamined. We found that only incomplete transcripts were made under these conditions, the longest having extended 175 nucleotides from the start of the template. However, when this in vitro transcription was coupled to protein synthesis by the addition of rabbit reticulocyte lysate, complete S-mRNA was now the most prominent product made, and the synthesis of the incomplete transcripts was either undetectable or greatly reduced. Drugs that inhibit protein synthesis also inhibited complete mRNA synthesis and, in most cases, led to the reappearance of the incomplete transcripts. The incomplete S transcripts found in vitro could also be detected in virus-infected cells in which protein synthesis had been inhibited by drugs, but not in untreated control cultures (see Bellocq et al. 1987; Raju and Kolakofsky 1987).

In the absence of ongoing protein synthesis, LAC mRNA synthesis therefore initiates normally but terminates prematurely at well-defined sites. These premature termination sites are suppressed in the presence of ongoing protein synthesis, and complete S-mRNA synthesis thus appears to be coupled to translation in some way. The direct coupling of transcription to translation is of course impossible for eukaryotic cell transcription because these events take place on different sides of the nuclear membrane, but no such limitation exists in the special case of a virus that makes its mRNA in the cytoplasm. In addition, direct coupling of transcription to translation is well known in bacteria, where the terms polarity and attenuation are used to describe mechanisms by which the concurrent translation of the nascent mRNA chain is used to modulate termination of RNA polymerase at premature termination sites (Yanofsky 1981; von Hippel et al. 1984; Platt 1986).

Concurrent Translation of the Nascent mRNA Chain Is Required for the Polymerase to Read Past Position 175

The evidence that concurrent translation is required for complete S-mRNA synthesis both in vivo and in vitro is so far based entirely on the use of drugs. We have used several drugs that have different mechanisms of action, such as pactamycin, cycloheximide, and puromycin, and they all inhibit complete mRNA synthesis under conditions where they do not inhibit the initiation of the viral polymerase and the synthesis of the beginning of the mRNA chain.

This situation resembles the polarity effect in bacteria, where ρ-dependent termination sites exist within the coding regions of some mRNAs, but termination does not take place as long as the nascent mRNA chain is being concurrently translated. In polarity, the translational requirement is not for the protein product, but to prevent ρ factor from binding to the nascent mRNA chain, a prerequisite for termination. In the case of LAC mRNA synthesis, there similarly does not appear to be a translational requirement for a particular translation product. For example, there does not appear to be a translational requirement for an unstable or otherwise limiting host factor, since complete S-mRNA synthesis in vitro is unaffected by micrococcal nuclease pretreatment of the reticulocyte lysate, which has effectively eliminated endogenous translation (Bellocq et al. 1987). If there were a translational requirement for a viral protein, which in an extreme case could represent only the amino-terminal fragments of the proteins, then this requirement could only be for a "priming of the pump"-type of mechanism. However, cycloheximide treatment of infected cultures when the viral proteins have accumulated to significant levels still leads to an immediate cessation of new mRNA synthesis (Raju and Kolakofksy 1986). Since there does not appear to be translational requirement for the translation product itself, then it is most likely for the movement of ribosomes along the nascent viral mRNA chain, in analogy to both polarity or attenuation. However, our drug experiments do not rule out the possibility that it could also be for ribosome movement on host mRNAs. For example, it is not impossible that there is a translational requirement for a stable host factor whose availability to the transcription complex is itself controlled by the presence or absence of ongoing protein synthesis. Further interpretations based on drug effects alone are always limited, since these drugs often have multiple effects, some of which are hard to explain.

We therefore sought another way to prevent translation of the nascent mRNA that did not involve inhibitors of protein synthesis. One approach was to saturate the capacity of the lysate for protein synthesis by adding exogenous mRNAs, so that ribosomes would be unavailable to translate the viral transcript. Increasing amounts of AMV RNA 4 were therefore added to a virion polymerase reaction carried out in the presence of a reticulocyte lysate. For some reactions, [^{35}S]-methionine labeling was used to follow AMV coat protein synthesis, whereas for other reactions, the amounts of incomplete and complete S-mRNAs were estimated by Northern blots. As shown in Figure 1, when no exogenous mRNA is added to the lysate, the predominant transcript is complete S-mRNA, whereas the incomplete transcript that terminates at position 175 is made in lesser amounts. When increasing amounts of AMV RNA 4 are included in the reactions, the amount of complete S-mRNA decreases and reaches baseline levels when the capacity of the lysate

to respond to additional AMV RNA 4 has been saturated. The amount of transcripts that terminate at position 175, on the other hand, increases. The presence of saturating amounts of exogenous mRNA thus prevents polymerase molecules from transcribing beyond position 175 even in the presence of active protein synthesis, but on the exogenous mRNA. This would appear to eliminate the possibility that the translational requirement is for a stable host factor whose availability is controlled by active protein synthesis. In addition, premature termination at position 175 can be achieved in a coupled in vitro system without the use of drugs by using sufficient exogenous mRNA to out-compete all other mRNAs for ribosomes. Since translation of the reticulocyte lysate mRNAs is clearly not part of the translational requirement for complete S-mRNA synthesis, it must then be the lack of ribosomes on the nascent mRNA chain that is responsible for premature termination.

Substitution of Inosine for Guanosine Residues in the Nascent mRNA Chain Allows the Polymerase to Read Past Position 175 in the Absence of Translation

The experiment described above suggests that the translational requirement is for ribosomes moving down the mRNA chain in concert with the polymerase, analogous to the coupling of transcription to translation, which characterizes polarity and attenuation. According to these models, active ribosomes and/or their associated factors would be required to prevent interactions of the nascent mRNA from taking place, which, if not prevented, then lead to premature termination. In both polarity and attenuation, termination is thought to be the result, at least in part, of a particular sequence of the nascent chain forming a specific interaction, either with ρ factor (polarity) or with a complementary sequence within the nascent chain for ρ-independent termination (attenuation). Since premature termination of LAC S-mRNA synthesis takes place efficiently when purified virions alone are used, it is unlikely that these interactions involve a host termination factor such as ρ. In this case, RNA:RNA interactions involving the nascent mRNA chain are more likely to be involved.

To examine whether RNA:RNA interactions are involved in premature transcription termination, the effect of substituting inosine for guanosine residues in the mRNA made in vitro was examined. Substitution of inosine for guanosine would be expected to weaken possible RNA:RNA interactions, and this substitution has previously been shown to result in polymerase readthrough of the trp operon attenuator under conditions where the polymerase normally terminates efficiently (Lee and Yanofsky 1977). However, when we completely replaced GTP with ITP in the uncoupled LAC polymerase reaction, we found that very little RNA was made, due to lack of initiation. (GTP, although the penultimate coded nucleotide, is the first nucleotide added to the capped primer during mRNA

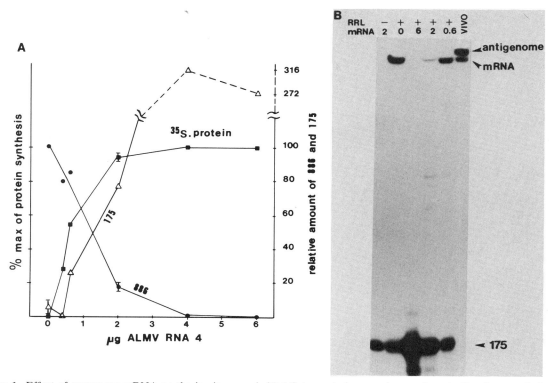

Figure 1. Effect of exogenous mRNA on the in-vitro-coupled LAC transcription reaction products by Northern analysis. LAC transcription reactions were carried out in the presence of a rabbit reticulocyte lysate to which increasing amounts (micrograms) of AMV RNA 4 were added as shown at the top of panel B. The reaction products were pelleted through a CsCl density gradient, separated on a 4% polyacrylamide gel, and electroblotted onto a ζ probe membrane that was annealed with a (−) riboprobe representing nucleotides 1–195. The autoradiograms from two separate experiments were quantitated by densitometry. The autoradiogram from one of these experiments shown in panel B is a longer exposure. The results are plotted in panel A along with the amount of AMV coat protein made in each reaction. The relative amounts of transcripts that terminate at position 175 or 886 are plotted relative to themselves only. The lane marked VIVO in panel B refers to total cytoplasmic RNA from LAC-infected cells used to mark the positions of S-mRNA and S antigenome RNA.

synthesis.) We therefore examined the effect of progressively replacing the GTP with ITP in the uncoupled virion polymerase reaction where the polymerase does not normally read past position 175. Northern blot analysis and a (−) riboprobe representing nucleotides 196–764 were used to examine the results. To monitor the relative incorporation of guanosine and inosine under these conditions, [^{32}P]UTP-labeling was used in parallel reactions, and the nearest-neighbor transfer of the isotope was determined.

As shown in Figure 2, when only GTP was present in the in vitro reaction, riboprobe 196–764 detected no products, as expected. However, when the GTP in the reaction was progressively replaced with ITP, some of the polymerases read past position 175 and terminated heterogeneously, yielding a series of bands approximately 400–900 nucleotides in length. The longest RNA detected comigrates with in vivo S-mRNA, and its amount relative to the total chains initiated clearly increases with the amount of I substituted for G. When only ITP was present, the riboprobe still detected complete S-mRNA, which was now the most prominent product of the reaction; however, the number of chains initiated here was severely reduced.

The level of polymerase readthrough of position 175 was more accurately measured by RNase mapping using a (−) riboprobe containing nucleotides 43–195 (not shown). When the RNA products of a polymerase reaction containing only GTP were used to protect this probe against RNase attack, we found that 95% of the chains terminated at position 175 and 5% extended past position 195. However, when ITP replaced 88% of the GTP in the reaction, then 80% of the RNAs made extended past position 195 by this test.

To examine whether the effect of increasing ratios of ITP/GTP in the reaction on polymerase readthrough was due to the inosine incorporation in the nascent chain as opposed to a nonspecific effect, such as the binding of a modified nucleotide to the polymerase and the subsequent alteration of its termination properties, we tested the effect of the total replacement of the UTP with BrUTP in the reaction. (BrU incorporation would be expected to increase base pairing of the nascent chain.) BrUTP was found to be as efficiently incorporated by the LAC polymerase as UTP, but such product RNA did not extend past position 175 any more frequently than its control. Similar results were obtained with rTTP, which, like BrUTP, is expected to

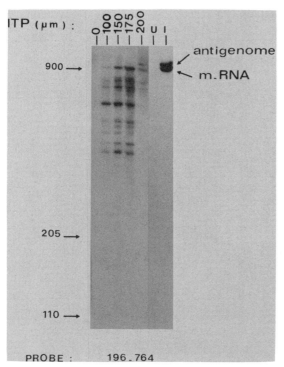

Figure 2. Effect of ITP substitution for GTP in the uncoupled LAC transcription reaction products by Northern analysis. Virion transcription reactions were carried out without reticulocyte lysate using 2 μg of AMV RNA 4, containing various amounts of ITP as indicated. The total amount of both ITP and GTP was always 200 μM. The reaction products were then examined by Northern blotting with a (−) riboprobe representing nucleotides 196–764. The lanes marked U and I refer to 10 μg of total cytoplasmic RNA from uninfected and LAC-infected cells, respectively. Numbers on the left refer to the length in nucleotides of the various RNAs.

strengthen base pairing. Furthermore, total replacement of the UTP with BrUTP when ITP replaced 88% of the GTP in the reaction led to a limited but reproducible decrease (approximately half) in the fraction of the chains that extended past position 175. Since the incorporation of nucleoside analogs that increase base-pairing interactions does not allow increased polymerase readthrough, but rather counteracts the effect induced by inosine incorporation, it seems reasonable that inosine incorporation into the nascent chains acts on polymerase readthrough by weakening RNA:RNA interactions.

The Nascent Chain Is Probably Interacting with Its Template to Cause Premature Termination

The above experiments suggest that RNA:RNA interactions are important in LAC premature termination, and in this respect, the translational requirement more closely resembles attenuation. However, when the first 175 nucleotides of the mRNA sequence are examined for complementarity, this region is predicted to be devoid of strong structure, and in particular, no G-C-rich stem similar to the terminator stem of

the *trp* operon could be formed. Nevertheless, it is not impossible that a weaker or different structure could serve the same purpose. In the case of the *trp* operon, Fisher and Yanofsky (1984) demonstrated that complementary oligonucleotides that specifically prevent formation of the terminator stem could by themselves cause the polymerase to read through the attenuator. We therefore argued that if LAC premature termination involves RNA:RNA interactions within the first 175 nucleotides, these structures should be even more susceptible to interference by complementary oligonucleotides than the *trp* operon leader RNA. To test this possibility, five oligonucleotides complementary to positions 82–179 were added either individually or in various combinations to the uncoupled virion polymerase reaction, and the resulting products were examined by RNase mapping for evidence of increased readthrough of position 175. However, even at concentrations of up to 13 μM, and varying both the temperature and the NTP concentrations to slow the progress of the polymerase, these oligonucleotides did not enhance polymerase readthrough even marginally, although all of the oligonucleotides could be shown to anneal efficiently to the complete S-mRNA chain. These results suggested that if base-pairing interactions of the nascent chain are involved in termination at position 175, these interactions are then more likely to occur with the RNA genome template. In this case, the DNA oligonucleotides would have to compete with perfect RNA matches, which are intramolecular as well, and they would be predicted to be inefficient.

The template for LAC RNA synthesis, i.e., (−) genomic RNA, is found not as free RNA, but only tightly complexed with N protein as nucleocapsids, both intracellularly and in virions (Obijeski et al. 1976). These NCs are remarkably resistant to high salt, since they band in CsCl density gradients without prior fixation, and their buoyant density here (1.31 g/ml), which is very similar to that of other helical NCs (e.g., Sendai virus or tobacco mosaic virus) suggests that the complex is composed of more than 90% N protein by weight. During RNA synthesis, the N protein is assumed to be displaced from the template RNA so that the polymerase can read the bases. Since the completed mRNA is released free of the template, the contacts between the nascent chain and the template that were formed during elongation must be broken as the polymerase moves downstream, and this may result from the N protein resuming its position on the template RNA. The N protein would thus serve the same function here as the noncoding strand of DNA during DNA transcription. Our data suggest that in the absence of concurrent translation, the nascent chain may be base pairing with the template so that the polymerase terminates prematurely at position 175 and that these interactions are prevented or broken by translating ribosomes that follow the polymerase.

We would thus like to examine whether such interactions between the nascent mRNA and its template upstream of the polymerase take place during mRNA synthesis, but it is not clear how this can be approached experimentally. As a first step in this direction, however, we can examine whether sequences upstream of position 175 within genomic NCs are free to anneal to complementary oligonucleotides, under conditions where mRNA synthesis does not take place. To assay for these possible interactions, a source of RNase H was also included so that the formation of RNA:DNA hybrids could be monitored by the specific cleavage of the NC RNA.

Four (+) 20-mers, complementary to positions 105–184, were individually incubated with NP-40-permeabilized virions and wheat-germ extract (the source of RNase H), and the reactions were then examined by Northern blots. Unlike the reticulocyte lysate, the wheat-germ extract by itself does not support LAC transcription, which remains dependent on the addition of mRNA (not shown). As shown in Figure 3, when either no oligonucleotides or a noncomplementary oligonucleotide (PC) was added, no evidence of any degradation of the (−) genomic RNA could be detected. However, when the complementary oligonucleotides were added, specific cleavage of the genomic RNA indicated that at least three of the oligonucleotides could anneal to the template, but to very different extents. When quantitated by densitometry, oligonucleotide 145–164 was found to have annealed the best, 27% of the template being specifically cleaved; oligonucleotides 105–124 and 125–144 induced 13% and 4% cleavage, whereas only oligonucleotide 165–184 showed no evidence of any specific cleavage. To ensure that all of the oligonucleotides were equally competent to anneal to RNase H and cause it to degrade unencapsidated (−) RNA, these

oligonucleotides were tested against a radiolabeled (−) riboprobe representing positions 1–195. As expected, all of the (+) oligonucleotides equally led to the specific cleavage of the (−) riboprobe (not shown). The above experiment demonstrates that some of the sequences within genomic NCs are partially accessible to annealing with complementary oligonucleotides, whereas other sequences are inaccessible. Furthermore, the ability or inability of sequences within NCs to anneal would appear to be a property of the NC structure rather than of the RNA itself, since all the oligonucleotides could be shown to anneal efficiently to unencapsidated RNA.

A Model for the Translational Requirement for Complete S-mRNA Synthesis

The experiments presented here have shown that concurrent translation of the nascent mRNA chain is required to prevent the polymerase from terminating prematurely. In the absence of translation, the replacement of G with I residues in the nascent chain can also suppress premature termination. It is therefore likely that RNA:RNA interactions of the nascent mRNA chain are involved in premature termination and that concurrent translation is then required to prevent these interactions. These interactions could of course occur between the nascent chain and its template or could be intramolecular interactions of the nascent chain alone. Attempts to demonstrate the latter possibility using oligonucleotides complementary to the nascent chain were uniformly negative, whereas we were able to show that some of the sequences within genomic NCs are available for annealing with complementary oligonucleotides and, by implication, that these template sequences are also available for interaction with the nascent mRNA chain.

Although some of the individual experiments are still open to other interpretations, the data as a whole are consistent with the model presented in Figure 4, which is similar in many respects to that of polarity. As in models of prokaryotic DNA transcription, we suspect that the polymerase moves down its template discontinuously, pausing along the way. Pausing is considered essential for termination, as it allows for other events involved in termination to take place before the polymerase can continue downstream. All termination sites are therefore also pause sites, but in bacteria, only a minority of these pause sites are also termination sites (von Hippel et al. 1984). In the case of LAC genome transcription, since the mRNA is initiated on a capped primer, it is immediately ready to load ribosomes. Furthermore, if any pause sites upstream of position 175 are not also termination sites, they would allow the ribosome to catch up to the polymerase, so that the ribosome and the polymerase could then proceed downstream in synchrony. Ribosomes immediately following the polymerase would prevent interactions between the nascent chain and its template, eliminating both pausing and premature termination. In the ab-

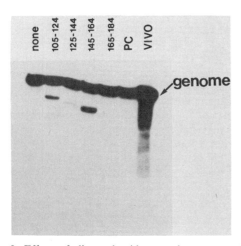

Figure 3. Effects of oligonucleotides complementary to LAC S (−) genomic RNA on the ability of RNase H to cleave NC RNA. Purified virions containing 0.05% NP-40 were incubated with the various oligonucleotides indicated plus wheat-germ extract (the source of RNase H). The RNAs were then isolated and examined on Northern blots with a (+) riboprobe representing nucleotides 196–764. VIVO refers to total cytoplasmic RNA from infected cells used as a marker; PC refers to a Sendai-virus-specific oligonucleotide.

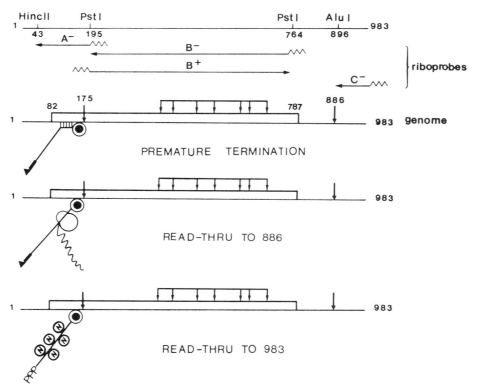

Figure 4. A model for the translational requirement for complete LAC S-mRNA synthesis. At the top is a partial restriction map of the S genome segment and the various riboprobes used. Below this is the (−) genomic template. The boxed area from position 82 to 787 indicates the N-protein-coding region. The arrow at position 175 indicates the premature transcription termination site that can be read through only when the nascent mRNA chain is being concurrently translated; the arrow at 886 shows the termination site for complete S-mRNA. Downstream from position 175, a series of premature termination sites that similarly require concurrent translation for polymerase readthrough also exist, which are only detected when termination at position 175 is incomplete. The viral polymerase is indicated by an open circle with a block dot inside. The nascent mRNA chain is shown attached to the polymerase with a triangle and thick bar at its 5′ end, representing the capped oligonucleotide derived from host-cell mRNA. In the absence of concurrent translation, the nascent mRNA will hybridize to its genomic template at certain sites, causing the polymerase to stall and terminate at position 175. When the nascent mRNA is being concurrently translated, the ribosome's movement behind the polymerase prevents the interaction of the nascent mRNA and its template, the polymerase does not stall and reads through position 175 and all subsequent premature termination sites, and terminates at position 886.

sence of concurrent translation or in situations where the ribosome lags too far behind the polymerase, the nascent chain may interact with its template, causing the polymerase to pause and also terminate if this site is also a termination site. Concurrent translation of the nascent mRNA chain would thus prevent polymerase termination in the coding region of the mRNA chain, but it would be unable to prevent interactions leading to complete S-mRNA termination at position 886.

It is tempting to speculate that these interactions of the nascent mRNA chain with its template are, at least in part, responsible for premature termination, since such a model may also explain some of the other puzzling features of premature termination. For example, although the termination site at position 175 is the first site that the polymerase stops at in the absence of concurrent translation, it is clearly not the only site. When low levels of cycloheximide or puromycin, which only partially inhibit protein synthesis, are used, some of the polymerase molecules read through position 175, but they do not complete the chains because of premature termination at a series of sites after approximately

position 400 (Bellocq et al. 1987). Similarly, when replacement of I for G in vitro is used to cause the polymerase to read through position 175, the polymerase rarely completes the chain, again because of termination at about position 400 and beyond. There thus appears to be one strong site at position 175 and a series of other sites after approximately position 400 that also require concurrent translation for polymerase readthrough, but curiously, the region between positions 175 and approximately 400 does not contain such sites. Similarly, transcription of the first 175 nucleotides of the mRNA chain, is not dependent on concurrent translation, nor can transcription of the last 100 nucleotides be dependent, since translation terminates at position 787. In accordance with this hypothesis, we note that there appear to be no termination sites in the last 100 nucleotides of the mRNA chain, as judged from the absence of bands in this region when readthrough is effected by substitution of I for G (Fig. 2). The multitude of these premature termination sites and their unusual distribution suggest that the determinants for termination are complex. These termination sites would in this model be the result of certain regions of the template RNA interacting with the nascent chain leading to polymerase pausing, and would also depend on whether the site on which the polymerase is stalled is compatible with termination.

These interactions between the nascent chain and the (−) genomic template would presumably also occur during antigenome synthesis, which, unlike the situation for mRNAs, is initiated with ATP and therefore does not contain a cap group for ribosome loading. In this case, it may be the assembly of N protein on the nascent antigenome chain that is responsible for preventing these interactions, since recent evidence indicates that the site for NC assembly is situated at the 5′ end of the genome and antigenome chains. Furthermore, since N protein assembly is independent of the coding and noncoding regions of the chain, it could also prevent the interactions responsible for termination at position 886 during antigenome synthesis.

LAC and Its Natural Host

Since many viruses are classic examples of self-regulatory systems, the question of why productive LAC transcription should be coupled to translation is intriguing. This situation appears to be unique to this group of (−) RNA viruses, and it is perhaps a feature that is unique to these viruses that may provide a clue. The natural host of LAC is the mosquito, and its entire life cycle, including over-wintering by transovarial transmission, can take place in the insect (Thompson 1983; Turell and LeDuc 1983). Although the virus is cytopathic for mammals and occasionally causes encephalitis in humans, in the mosquito, the infection is both persistent and asymptomatic. LAC thus appears to be extremely well adapted to its natural host, and its persistence in the population may require mechanisms which ensure that intracellular replication has a minimum of deleterious effects on the host cell. This may be particularly important during transovarial transmission. According to Tesh (1980), "embryonic development of mosquitoes commences immediately upon oviposition and proceeds without interruption until a fully formed embryo (a pharate larva) is produced. In mosquitoes of the tribe Aedini, the life cycle is normally suspended upon completion of embryonic development. This interruption occurs because hatching of the pharate larva from the egg is not spontaneous: it depends on a variety of environmental factors. The period of larval inactivity (diapause) may last for days, weeks, or months, depending on the environmental conditions. Presumably the virus must also become latent in the insect until hatching occurs." The dependence of LAC transcription on ongoing protein synthesis may be one way of ensuring that viral mRNA levels remain balanced with host mRNA during periods of the developmental cycle when both host transcription and translation are basically shut down. It has previously been noted that bunyaviruses of the California encephalitis serogroup have relatively few adverse effects on larval development as compared to other RNA viruses, such as flaviviruses or sigma virus of *Drosophila*, which are also transmitted transovarially (Tesh 1980).

ACKNOWLEDGMENTS

We thank John Bol (Leiden) for the AMV RNA 4, and David Ward (New Haven) for providing us with several nucleoside triphosphate analogs to test. We also thank Nicholas Acheson and Martinez Hewlett for helpful discussions. This work was supported by a grant from the Swiss National Science Foundation.

REFERENCES

Abraham, G. and A.K. Pattnaik. 1983. Early RNA synthesis in Bunyawera virus-infected cells. *J. Gen. Virol.* **64:** 1277.

Bellocq, C., R. Raju, J. Patterson, and D. Kolakofsky. 1987. Translational requirement of La Crosse virus S-mRNA synthesis: In vitro studies. *J. Virol.* **61:** 87.

Bishop, D.H.L., M.E. Gay, and Y. Matsuoko. 1983. Nonviral heterogeneous sequences are present at the 5′ ends of one species of snowshoe hare bunyavirus S complementary RNA. *Nucleic Acids Res.* **11:** 6409.

Fisher, R. and C. Yanofsky. 1984. Use of complementary DNA oligomers to probe trp leader transcript secondary structures involved in transcription pausing and termination. *Nucleic Acids Res.* **12:** 3295.

Gerbaud, S., N. Pardigon, P. Vialat, and M. Bouloy. 1987. The S segment of Germiston bunyavirus genome: Coding strategy and transcription. In *Biology of negative strand viruses* (ed. D. Kolakofsky and B.W.J. Mahy), p. 191. Elsevier, Amsterdam.

Krug, R.M. 1981. Priming of influenza viral RNA transcription by capped heterologous RNAs. *Curr. Top. Microbiol. Immunol.* **93:** 125.

Lee, F. and C. Yanofsky. 1977. Transcription termination at the trp operon attenuators of *Escherichia coli* and *Salmonella typhimurium*: RNA secondary structure and regulation of termination. *Proc. Natl. Acad. Sci.* **74:** 4365.

Obijeski, J.F., D.H.L. Bishop, E.L. Palmer, and F.A. Murphy. 1976. Segmented genome and nucleocapsid of La Crosse virus. *J. Virol.* **20:** 664.

Patterson, J.L. and D. Kolakofsky. 1984. Characterization of La Crosse virus small-genome transcripts. *J. Virol.* **49:** 680.

Patterson, J.L., B. Holloway, and D. Kolakofsky. 1984. La Crosse virions contain a primer-stimulated RNA polymerase and a methylated cap-dependent endonuclease. *J. Virol.* **52:** 215.

Platt, T. 1986. Transcription termination and the regulation of gene expression. *Annu. Rev. Biochem.* **55:** 339.

Raju, R. and D. Kolakofsky. 1986. Inhibitors of protein synthesis inhibit both La Crosse virus S-mRNA and S genome synthesis in vivo. *Virus Res.* **5:** 1.

———. 1987. Translational requirement of La Crosse virus S-mRNA synthesis: In vivo studies. *J. Virol.* **61:** 96.

Rossier, C., J. Patterson, and D. Kolakofsky. 1986. La Crosse virus small genome mRNA is made in the cytoplasm. *J. Virol.* **58:** 647.

Tesh, R.B. 1980. Experimental studies on the transovarial transmission of Kunjin and San Angelo viruses in mosquitoes. *Am. J. Trop. Med. Hyg.* **29** (4): 657.

Thompson, W.H. 1983. Vector-virus relationships. In *California serogroup viruses*, p.57. A.R. Liss, New York.

Turell, M.J. and J.W. LeDuc. 1983. In *California serogroup viruses*, p.43. A.R. Liss, New York.

von Hippel, P.H., D.G. Bear, W.D. Morgan, and J.A. McSwiggen. 1984. Protein-nucleic acid interactions in transcription: A molecular analysis. *Annu. Rev. Biochem.* **53:** 389.

Yanofsky, C. 1981. Attenuation in the control of expression of bacterial operons. *Nature* **289:** 751.

Molecular Dynamics: Applications to Proteins

M. Karplus, A.T. Brünger,* R. Elber,[†] and J. Kuriyan[‡]

Department of Chemistry, Harvard University, Cambridge, Massachusetts 02138

Molecular dynamics of macromolecules of biological interest began in 1977 with the publication of a paper on the simulation of a small protein, the bovine pancreatic trypsin inhibitor (McCammon et al. 1977). Although the trypsin inhibitor is rather uninteresting from a dynamical viewpoint—its function is to bind to trypsin—experimental and theoretical studies of this model system, the "hydrogen atom" of protein dynamics, served to initiate explorations in this field.

The most important consequence of the first simulations of biomolecules was that they introduced a conceptual change (Karplus and McCammon 1981, 1983). Although to chemists and physicists it is self-evident that polymers like proteins and nucelic acids undergo significant fluctuations at room temperature, the classic view of such molecules in their native state had been static in character. This followed from the dominant role of high-resolution X-ray crystallography in providing structural information for these complex systems. The remarkable detail evident in crystal structures led to an image of biomolecules with every atom fixed in place. D.C. Phillips, who determined the first enzyme crystal structure, wrote, "the period 1965–75 may be described as the decade of the rigid macromolecule. Brass models of DNA and a variety of proteins dominated the scene and much of the thinking" (Phillips 1981). Molecular dynamics simulations have been instrumental in changing the static view of the structure of biomolecules to a dynamic picture. It is now recognized that the atoms of which biopolymers are composed are in constant motion at ordinary temperatures. The X-ray structure of a protein provides approximate average atomic positions, but the atoms exhibit fluid-like motions of sizable amplitudes about these averages. Crystallographers have acceded to this viewpoint and have come so far as to sometimes emphasize the parts of a molecule they do not see in a crystal structure as evidence of motion or disorder (Marquart et al. 1980). Thus, the knowledge of protein dynamics subsumes the static picture, in that use of the average positions still allows discussion of many aspects of biomolecule function in the language of structural chemistry. However, the recognition of the importance of fluctuations opens the way for more sophisticated and accurate interpretations.

Simulation studies on biomolecules have the possibility of providing the ultimate detail concerning motional phenomena (Brooks et al. 1987). The primary limitation of simulation methods is that they are approximate. It is here that experiment plays an essential role in validating the simulations; that is, comparisons with experimental data can serve to test the accuracy of the calculations and to provide criteria for improving the methodology. When experimental comparisons indicate that the simulations are meaningful, their capacity for providing detailed results often makes it possible to examine specific aspects of the atomic motions far more easily than by making measurements.

In what follows, a brief introduction to molecular dynamics will be given, followed by applications that illustrate its utility for increasing our understanding of proteins, including enzymes, and for interpreting experiments in a more effective way.

Methodology

To study theoretically the dynamics of a macromolecular system, it is essential to have a knowledge of the potential energy surface, which gives the energy of the system as a function of the atomic coordinates. The potential energy can be used directly to determine the relative energies of the different possible structures of the system; the relative populations of such structures under conditions of thermal equilibrium are given in terms of the potential energy by the Boltzmann distribution law (McQuarrie 1976). The mechanical forces acting on the atoms of the systems are simply related to the first derivatives of the potential with respect to the atom positions. These forces can be used to calculate dynamical properties of the system, e.g., by solving Newton's equations of motion to determine how the atomic positions change with time (Hansen and McDonald 1976; McQuarrie 1976). From the second derivatives of the potential surface, the force constants for small displacements can be evaluated and used to find the normal modes (Levy and Karplus 1979); this serves as the basis for an alternative approach to the dynamics in the harmonic limit (Levy and Karplus 1979; Brooks and Karplus 1983).

Although quantum mechanical calculations can provide potential surfaces for small molecules, empirical energy functions of the molecular mechanics type are the only possible source of such information for proteins and the surrounding solvent. Since most of the

Present addresses: *Department of Molecular Biophysics and Biochemistry, Yale University, New Haven, Connecticut 06511; [†]Department of Chemistry, University of Illinois at Chicago, Chicago, Illinois 60680; [‡]Laboratory of Biochemistry and Bioorganic Chemistry, Rockefeller University, New York, New York 10021.

motions that occur at ordinary temperatures leave the bond lengths and bond angles of the polypeptide chains near their equilibrium values, which appear not to vary significantly throughout the protein (e.g., the standard dimensions of the peptide group first proposed by Pauling [Pauling et al. 1951]), the energy function representation of the bonding can have an accuracy on the order of that achieved in the vibrational analysis of small molecules. Where globular proteins differ from small molecules is that the contacts among nonbonded atoms play an essential role in the potential energy of the folded or native structure. From the success of the pioneering conformational studies of Ramachandran and co-workers (Ramachandran et al. 1963) that made use of hard-sphere nonbonded radii, it is likely that relatively simple functions (Lennard-Jones nonbonded potentials supplemented by electrostatic interactions) can adequately describe the interactions involved.

The energy functions used for proteins are generally composed of terms representing bonds, bond angles, torsional angles, van der Waals interactions, and electrostatic interactions. The resulting expression has the form (Brooks et al. 1983)

$$E(\bar{R}) = \frac{1}{2} \sum_{\text{bonds}} K_b(b - b_0)^2 + \frac{1}{2} \sum_{\substack{\text{bond} \\ \text{angles}}} K_\theta(\theta - \theta_0)^2$$
$$+ \frac{1}{2} \sum_{\substack{\text{torsional} \\ \text{angles}}} K_\phi[1 + \cos(n\phi - \delta)] \quad (1)$$
$$+ \sum_{\substack{nb \text{ pairs} \\ r<8A}} \left(\frac{A}{r^{12}} - \frac{C}{r^6} + \frac{q_1 q_2}{Dr} \right)$$

The energy is a function of the Cartesian coordinate set, $\bar{R}$, specifying the positions of all the atoms involved, but the calculation is carried out by first evaluating the internal coordinates for bonds (b), bond angles (θ), dihedral angles (ϕ), and interparticle distances (r) for any given geometry, R, and using them to evaluate the contributions to Equation 1, which depend on the bonding energy parameters K_b, K_θ, K_ϕ, Lennard-Jones parameters A and C, atomic charges q_i, dielectric constant D, and geometrical reference values b_0, θ_0, n, and δ. For most simulations use has been made of a representation that replaces aliphatic groups (CH_3, CH_2, CH) by single extended atoms. Although the earliest studies employed the extended atom representation for all hydrogens, present calculations treat hydrogen-bonding hydrogens explicitly. In the most detailed simulations every protein atom (including aliphatic hydrogens) and explicit solvent molecules (e.g., a three-site or five-site model for each water molecule) are included (Brooks et al. 1983).

Given a potential energy function, one may take any of a variety of approaches to study protein dynamics. The most detailed information is provided by molecular dynamics simulations, in which one uses a computer to solve the Newtonian equations of motion for the atoms of the protein and any surrounding solvent (McCam-

mon et al. 1977, 1979; van Gunsteren and Karplus 1982). With currently available computers, it is possible to simulate the dynamics of small proteins for periods of up to a nanosecond. Such periods are long enough to characterize completely the librations of small groups in the protein and to determine the dominant contributions to the atomic fluctuations. To study slower and more complex processes in proteins, it is generally necessary to use other than the straightforward molecular dynamics simulation method. A variety of dynamical approaches, such as stochastic dynamics (Chandrasekhar 1943), harmonic dynamics (Levy and Karplus 1979; Brooks and Karplus 1983), and activated dynamics (Northrup et al. 1982), can be introduced to study particular problems.

Since molecular dynamics simulations have been used most widely for studying protein motions, we briefly describe the methodology. To begin a dynamical simulation, one must have an initial set of atomic coordinates and velocities. These are usually obtained from the X-ray coordinates of the protein by a preliminary calculation that serves to equilibrate the system (Brooks et al. 1983). The X-ray structure is first refined using an energy minimization algorithm to relieve local stresses due to nonbonded atomic overlaps, bond-length distortions, etc. The protein atoms are then assigned velocities at random from a Maxwellian distribution corresponding to a low temperature, and a dynamical simulation is performed for a period of a few psec. The equilibration is continued by alternating new velocity assignments (chosen from Maxwellian distributions corresponding to successively increased temperatures) with intervals of dynamical relaxation. The temperature, T, for this microcanonical ensemble is measured in terms of the mean kinetic energy for the system composed of N atoms as

$$\frac{1}{2} \sum_{i=1}^{N} m_i \langle v_i^2 \rangle = \frac{3}{2} N k_B T$$

where m_i and v_i^2 are the mass and average velocity squared of the ith atom, and k_B is the Boltzmann constant. Any residual overall translational and rotational motion for an isolated protein can be removed to simplify analysis of the subsequent conformational fluctuations; in a solution simulation, the protein can diffuse through the solvent. The equilibration period is considered finished when no systematic changes in the temperature are evident over a time of about 10 psec (slow fluctuations could be confused with continued relaxation over shorter intervals). It is necessary also to check that the atomic momenta obey a Maxwellian distribution and that different regions of the protein have the same average temperature. The actual dynamical simulation, which provides coordinates and velocities for all the atoms as a function of time, is then performed by continuing to integrate the equations of motion for the desired time period. The available simulations for proteins range from 25 psec to 1 nsec. Several different algorithms for integrating the equations of motion in Cartesian coordinates are being used in protein molecular dynamics calculations. Most common are the Gear predictor-corrector algorithm (Verlet 1967), familiar from small molecule trajectory calculations (McCammon et al. 1979), and the Verlet algorithm, widely used in statistical mechanical simulations (van Gunsteren and Berendsen 1977).

Internal Motions and the Underlying Potential Surface

For native proteins with a well-defined average structure, two extreme models for the internal motions have been considered; Figure 1 provides a schematic illustration of these two possibilities. In one, the fluctuations are assumed to occur within a single multidimensional well that is harmonic or quasiharmonic as a limiting case (Karplus and Kushick 1981; Brooks and Karplus 1983; Levitt et al. 1985). The other model assumes that there exist multiple minima or substrates; the internal motions correspond to a superposition of oscillations within the wells and transitions among them (Austin et al. 1975; Frauenfelder et al. 1979; Debrunner and Frauenfelder 1982; Levy et al. 1982; Swaminathan et al. 1982; Brooks and Karplus 1983). Experimental data have been interpreted with both models, but it has proved difficult to distinguish between them (Agmon and Hopfield 1983; Ansari et al. 1985).

To characterize the protein potential surface structurally and energetically, we use a 300 psec molecular dynamics simulation of the protein myoglobin at 300 K; details of the simulation method have been presented (Levy et al. 1985). Myoglobin was chosen for study because it has been examined by a variety of methods and the two motional models have been applied to it (Austin et al. 1975; Frauenfelder et al. 1979; Levy et al. 1982; Agmon and Hopfield 1983; Bialek and Goldstein 1985). It is ideally suited for the present analysis, because its well-defined secondary structure (a series of α helices connected by loops) facilitates a detailed characterization of the dynamics.

The topography of the potential surface underlying the dynamics can be explored by finding the local ener-gy minima associated with coordinate sets sequential in time (Stillinger and Weber 1982, 1984). Thirty-one coordinate sets (one every 10 psec) were selected and their energy was minimized with a modified Newton-Raphson algorithm suitable for large molecules (Brooks et al. 1983). Since the coordinate sets all corresponded to different minima, structures separated by shorter time periods were examined to determine how long the trajectory remains in a given minimum. Seven additional coordinate sets (one every 0.05 psec) were chosen and their behavior on minimization was examined; if two coordinate sets converged, they corresponded to the same minimum; if they diverged, they corresponded to different minima (Fig. 2). The measure for the distance between two structures is their rms coordinate difference after superposition.

Analysis of the short time dynamics (Fig. 3) demonstrates that convergence occurs for intervals up to 0.15 ± 0.05 psec. Thus, the 300 psec simulation samples on the order of 2000 different minima; this is a sizable number, but it may nevertheless be small relative to the total (finite) number of minima available to such a complex system in the neighborhood of the native average structure (i.e. conformations that are nativelike and significantly populated at room temperature). The rms differences among the minimized structures reach a maximum value of approximately 2 Å at about 100 psec. Thus, the difference vector $(\underline{R}_K - \underline{R}_{K'})$, where $\underline{R}_K$ represents the coordinates of all the atoms in a nativelike conformation K, is restricted to a volume bounded by a radius of 2 Å.

Comparison of the energies of the minimized structures shows that the width of the energy distribution is on the order of 20 K (40 cal/mole) per degree of freedom. Since the difference in energy between the "inherent" structures (Stillinger and Weber 1982, 1984) is small, they are significantly populated at room temperature. Furthermore, the large number of such structures sampled by the room-temperature simulation suggests that the effective barriers separating them are low and that the protein is undergoing frequent transitions from one structure to another. The fluctuations within a well can be described by a harmonic

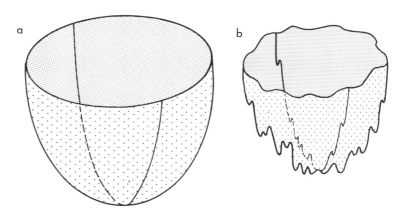

Figure 1. Schematic diagram of two limiting potential surfaces: (*a*) harmonic; (*b*) multiple minima (substates). A two-dimensional projection is used for simplicity.

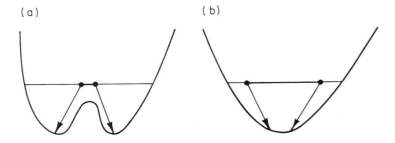

Figure 2. Schematic representation of the rms difference criterion for different minima. (*a*) rms after the minimization is larger than the initial rms, implying that the two conformations correspond to different minima; (*b*) rms after the minimization is smaller than the initial rms, implying that the two conformations correspond to the same minimum.

or quasiharmonic model, whereas the transitions among the wells cannot. Estimates based on the time development of the rms atomic fluctuations for main-chain atoms at room temperature (Swaminathan et al. 1982) indicate that 20–30% of the rms fluctuations are contributed by oscillations within a well and 70–80% arise from transitions among wells; for side chains the contribution from transitions among the multiple wells is expected to be larger. Since energy differences among some of the wells are small, molecules may be trapped in metastable states at low temperatures, in analogy to third law violations in crystals (e.g., crystals of CO) and models for the glassy state (Ziman 1979; Stillinger and Weber 1982, 1984; Toulouse 1984; Ansari et al. 1985; Stein 1985). A number of experiments suggest that the transition temperature for myoglobin is about 200 K (Austin et al. 1975; Debrunner and Frauenfelder 1982; Parak et al. 1982; Ansari et al. 1985). Because large-scale, collective motions that involve the protein surface are important in the fluctuations (Swaminathan et al. 1982), it is possible that the observed transition is due to the freezing of the

solvent matrix (Parak et al. 1982; Swaminathan et al. 1982).

Because the details of the native structure of a protein play an essential role in its function, it is important to determine the structural origins of the multiminimum surface obtained from the dynamics analysis. The general features of the structure (helices and turns) are preserved throughout the simulation, and the differences in position are widely distributed. The motions are associated primarily with loop displacements or relative displacements of helices that individually behave as nearly rigid bodies. Rearrangements within individual loops are the elementary step in the transition from one minimum to another; they are coupled with associated helix displacements. Which loop or turn changes in a given time interval appears to be random. Specific loop motions may be initiated by side-chain transitions in the helix contacts, main-chain dihedral angle transitions of the loops themselves, or a combination of the two. As the time interval between two structures increases, more loop transitions have occurred. At room temperature, the transition probabilities are such that for an interval 100 psec or longer between two structures, some transitions will have taken place in all of the flexible loop regions. However, since the rms differences between structures continue to increase up to 200 psec, the configuration space available to the molecule includes a range of structures for the loop regions that are not completely sampled in 100 psec (Fig. 4).

To characterize the helix motions that are coupled with the loop rearrangements, the internal structural changes of the helices were separated from their relative motions. Individual helices and loops were superimposed and the rms differences for the main chain calculated for the set of structures; the rms difference for the internal structure of the helices is generally less than 1 Å. The corresponding results for the loop regions show that they undergo much larger internal structural changes, on the order of 2.5 Å.

In analyzing the relative motion of the helices, it is of particular interest to examine the behavior of helix pairs that are in van der Waals contact; these are helix pairs A-H, B-E, B-G, F-H, and G-H, for all of which at least three residues from each helix are interacting. Each helix was fitted to a straight line and the fluctuations of the distance between the helix centers of mass and the relative orientations of the lines were

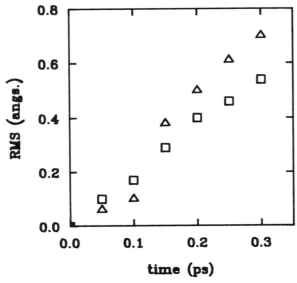

Figure 3. Root-mean-square difference correlation function $\langle rms(0), rms(t)\rangle$ between structures as a function of the time interval between them. Results are for 0.05 psec time interval structures; the squares are from the trajectory and the triangles are the minimized structure results.

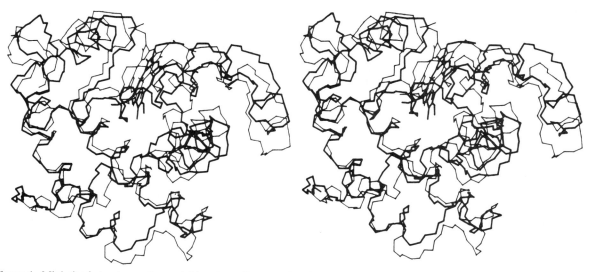

Figure 4. Minimized structures of myoglobin; stereodiagrams showing two superposed structures separated by a time interval of 100 psec along the trajectory.

compared. The relative translations found in this case have rms values of 0.3–0.7 Å and the relative rotations have rms values of 1–14°; the maximum differences are 1.3–2.2 Å and 5–39°, respectively.

The dynamical results for the helix motions can be compared with structural data from two sources; the first is derived from proteins of a given sequence in different environments (e.g., two different crystal forms, deoxy and oxy hemoglobin; Chothia and Lesk 1985) and the second from homologous proteins with different sequences (e.g., the globins; Lesk and Chothia 1980). The maximum dynamical displacements are, in fact, larger than those observed in different X-ray structures of a given protein. The values are of the same order as the differences (2–3 Å, 15–30°; there are some larger changes) found in comparing a series of different globins with known crystal structures and sequence homologies in the range 16–88%. Thus, the range of conformations sampled by a single myoglobin trajectory is similar to that found in the evolutionary variation among crystal structures of the globin series. This suggests a molecular plasticity that is likely to have played an important role in the evolution of protein sequences.

The comparison of the various globin structures (Lesk and Chothia 1980) suggested that the range of helix packings is achieved primarily by changes in side-chain volumes resulting from amino acid substitutions. In the dynamics, it is the correlated motions of side chains that are in contact, plus the rearrangements of loops, that make possible the observed helix fluctuations. Different positions within wells and transitions between wells for side chains (e.g., ±60°, 180° for χ_1) are involved. This is in accord with the results of high-resolution X-ray studies that show significant disorder in side-chain orientations (Smith et al. 1986; Kuriyan et al. 1987). Furthermore, correlated dihedral angle

changes differentiate the various minima. Since more than one set of side-chain orientations is consistent with a given set of helix positions, the known globin crystal structures probably represent only a small subset of the possible local minima.

Myoglobin at normal room temperatures samples a very large number of different minima that arise from the inhomogeneity of the system. This is expected to have important consequences for the interpretation of myoglobin function and, more generally, for the functions of other proteins, including enzymes. There are solidlike microdomains (the helices), whose main-chain structure is relatively rigid, and liquidlike regions (the loops and the side-chain clusters at interhelix contacts) that readjust as the helices move from one minimum to another. Since the minima have similar energies, myoglobin is expected to be glasslike at low temperatures. Freezing in of the liquidlike regions could result in a transition to the glassy state (Stein 1985).

Use of Nuclear Magnetic Resonance Data for Protein Folding

Nuclear magnetic resonance (NMR) is an experimental technique that has played an essential role in the analysis of the internal motions of proteins (Campbell et al. 1978; Gurd and Rothgeb 1979; Karplus and McCammon 1981). Like X-ray diffraction, it can provide information about individual atoms; unlike X-ray diffraction, NMR is sensitive not only to the magnitude but also to the time scales of the motions. Most nuclear relaxation processes are dependent on atomic motions on the nanosecond to picosecond time scale. Although molecular tumbling is generally the dominant relaxation mechanism for proteins in solution, internal motions contribute as well; for solids, the internal motions are of primary importance. In addition, NMR parameters, such as nuclear spin-spin coupling constants and chemical shifts, depend on the protein environment. In many cases, different local conformations exist, but the interconversion is rapid on the NMR time scale, here on the order of milliseconds, so that average values are observed. When the interconversion time is on the order of the NMR time scale or slower, the transition rates can be studied by NMR; an example is provided by the reorientation of aromatic rings (Campbell et al. 1976).

In addition to supplying data on the dynamics of proteins, NMR can also be used to obtain structural information. With recent advances in techniques, it is now possible to obtain a large number of approximate interproton distances for proteins by the use of nuclear Overhauser effect measurements (Noggle and Schirmer 1971). If the protein is relatively small and has a well-resolved spectrum, a large portion of the protons can be assigned and several hundred distances for these protons can be determined by the use of two-dimensional NMR techniques (Wagner and Wüthrich 1982). Clearly, these distances can serve to provide structural information for proteins, analogous to their earlier use for organic molecules (Honig et al. 1971; Noggle and Schirmer 1971). Of great interest is the possibility that enough distance information can be measured to actually determine the high-resolution structure of a protein in solution. This could serve to supplement results from X-ray crystallography, particularly for proteins that are difficult to crystallize.

The nuclear Overhauser effect (NOE) corresponds to the selective enhancement of a given resonance by the irradiation of another resonance in a dipolar coupled spin system. Of particular interest for obtaining motional and distance information are measurements that provide time-dependent NOEs from which the cross-relaxation rates σ_{ij} can be determined directly or indirectly by solving a set of coupled equations. Motions on the picosecond time scale are expected to introduce averaging effects that decrease the cross-relaxation rates by a scale factor relative to the rigid model. A lysozyme molecular dynamics simulation (Ichiye et al. 1986) has been used to calculate dipole vector correlation functions (Olejniczak et al. 1984) for proton pairs whose distance is not fixed by the structure of a residue. The results show that the presence of these motions will cause a general decrease in most NOE effects observed in a protein. However, because the distance depends on the sixth root of the observed NOE, motional errors of a factor of two in the latter lead to only a 12% uncertainty in the distance. Thus, the decrease is usually too small to produce a significant change in the distance estimate from the measured NOE value. This is consistent with the excellent correlation found between experimental NOE values and those calculated using distances from a crystal structure (Poulsen et al. 1980). Specific NOEs can, however, be altered by the internal motions to such a degree that the effective distances obtained are considerably different

from those predicted for a static structure. Such possibilities must, therefore, be considered in any structure determination based on NOE data. This is true particularly for cases involving averaging over large-scale fluctuations.

Because of the inverse sixth power of the NOE distance dependence, experimental data so far are limited to protons that are separated by less than 5 Å. Thus, the information required for a direct protein structure determination is not available. To overcome this limitation, it is possible to introduce additional information provided by empirical energy functions (Brooks et al. 1983). One way of proceeding is to do molecular dynamics simulations with the approximate interproton distances introduced as restraints in the form of skewed biharmonic potentials (Clore et al. 1985; Brünger et al. 1986) with the force constants chosen to correspond to the experimental uncertainty in the distance.

A model study of the small protein crambin, which is composed of 46 residues, was made with realistic NOE restraints (Brünger et al. 1986). Investigators used 240 approximate interproton distances less than 4 Å, including 184 short-range distances (i.e., those connecting protons in two residues that are less than five residues apart in the sequence) and 56 long-range distances. The molecular dynamics simulations converged to the known crambin structure (Hendrickson and Teeter 1981) from different initial extended structures. The average structure obtained from the simulations with a series of different protocols had rms deviations of 1.3 Å for the backbone atoms, and 1.9 Å for the side-chain atoms. Individual converged simulations had rms deviations in the range 1.5–2.1 Å and 2.1–2.8 Å for the backbone and side-chain atoms, respectively. Furthermore, it was shown that a dynamics structure with significantly large deviations (5.7 Å) could be characterized as incorrect, independent of a knowledge of the crystal structure, because of its higher energy and the fact that the NOE restraints were not satisfied within the limits of error. The incorrect structure resulted when all NOE restraints were introduced simultaneously, rather than allowing the dynamics to proceed first in the presence of only the short-range restraints, followed by introduction of the long-range restraints. Also of interest is the fact that, although crambin has three disulfide bridges, it was not necessary to introduce information concerning them to obtain an accurate structure.

The folding process as simulated by the restrained dynamics is very rapid (see Fig. 5). At the end of the first 2 psec, the secondary structure is essentially established while the molecule is still in an extended conformation. Some tertiary folding occurs even in the absence of long-range restraints. When they are introduced, it takes about 5 psec to obtain a tertiary structure that is approximately correct and another 6 psec to introduce the small adjustments required to converge to the final structure.

It is of interest to consider the relation between the results obtained in the restrained dynamics simulation

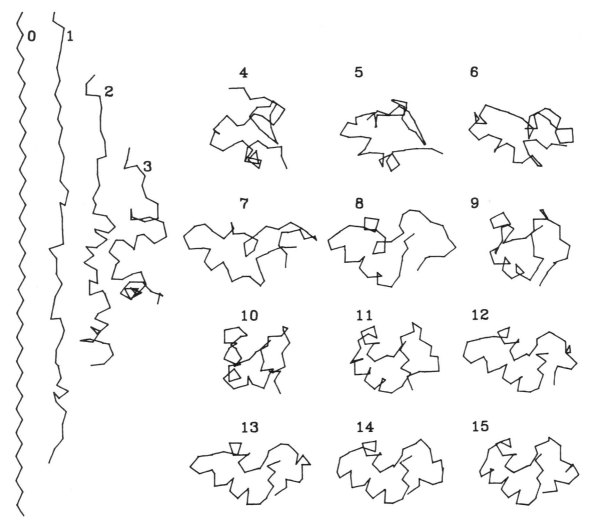

Figure 5. Folding of crambin backbone by restrained molecular dynamics. Starting with the initial structure, snapshots are shown at 1 psec intervals; only the Cα backbone is included in the figure.

and actual protein folding. That correctly folded structures are achieved only when the secondary structural elements are at least partly formed before the tertiary restraints are introduced is suggestive of the diffusion-collision model of protein folding (Bashford et al. 1984). Clearly, the specific pathway has no physical meaning since it is dominated by the NOE restraints. Also, the time scale of the simulated folding process is 12 orders of magnitude faster than experimental estimates. About 6 to 9 orders of magnitude of the rate increase are due to the fact that the secondary structure is stable once it is formed, in contrast to real protein folding where the secondary structural elements spend only a small fraction of time in the native conformation until coalescence has occurred. The remainder of the artificial rate increase presumably arises from the fact that the protein follows a single fairly direct path to the folded state in the presence of the NOE restraints, instead of having to go through a complex search process.

X-ray Refinement by Simulated Annealing

Crystallographic structure determinations by X-ray or neutron diffraction generally proceed in two stages. First, the phases of the measured reflections are estimated and a low- to medium-resolution model of the protein is constructed and second, more precise information about the structure is obtained by refining the parameters of the molecular model against the crystallographic data (Wyckoff et al. 1985). The refinement is performed by minimizing the crystallographic R factor, which is defined as the difference between the observed ($|F_{obs}[h, k, l]|$) and calculated ($|F_{calc}[h, k, l]|$) structure factor amplitudes,

$$R = \sum_{h,k,l} \|F_{obs}(h, k, l)| - |F_{calc}(h, k, l)\| \Big/ \sum_{h,k,l} |F_{obs}(h, k, l)| \quad (2)$$

where h, k, l are the reciprocal lattice points of the crystal.

Conventional refinement involves a series of steps, each consisting of a few cycles of least-squares refinement with stereochemical and internal packing constraints or restraints (Sussman et al. 1977; Jack and Levitt 1978; Konnert and Hendrickson 1980; Moss and Morffew 1982) that are followed by manual rebuilding of the model structure by use of interactive computer graphics. Finally, solvent molecules are included and alternative conformations for some protein atoms may be introduced. The standard refinement procedure is time consuming, because the limited radius of convergence of least-squares algorithms (approximately 1 Å) necessitates the periodic examination of electron density maps computed with various combinations of F_{obs} and F_{calc} as amplitudes, and with phases calculated from the model structure. Also, the least-squares refinement process is easily trapped in a local minimum so that human intervention is necessary.

Simulated annealing (Kirkpatrick et al. 1983), which makes use of Monte Carlo or molecular dynamics (Brünger et al. 1987a) simulations to explore the conformational space of the molecule, can help to overcome the local-minimum problem. This has been demonstrated in the application of molecular dynamics to structure determination with nuclear magnetic resonance (NMR) data (see previous section). In contrast to the NMR application (Brünger et al. 1986), the initial model for crystallographic refinement cannot be arbitrary. It has to be relatively close to the correct geometry to provide an adequate approximation to the phases of the structure factors.

To employ molecular dynamics in crystallographic refinement, an effective potential

$$E_{sf} = S \sum_{h,k,l} (|F_{obs}[h, k, l]| - |F_{calc}[h, k, l]|)^2 \quad (3)$$

was added to the empirical energy potential given in Equation 1. The effective potential E_{sf} describes the differences between the observed structure factor amplitudes and those calculated from the atomic model; it is identical to the function used in standard least-squares refinement methods (Jack and Levitt 1978). The scale factor S was chosen to make the gradient of E_{sf} comparable in magnitude to the gradient of the empirical energy potential of a molecular dynamics simulation with S set to zero.

As in the case of the NMR analysis (see previous section), simulated annealing refinement was also tested on crambin, for which high-resolution X-ray diffraction data and a refined structure, determined by resolved anomalous phasing and conventional least-squares refinement with model building, are available (Hendrickson and Teeter 1981). The initial structure for the molecular dynamics refinement was obtained from the NMR structure determination (see previous section); the orientation and position of the NMR-derived crambin molecule in the unit cell was determined by molecular replacement (Brünger et al.

1987b). The rms differences for residue positions of this initial structure and the final manually refined structure (Hendrickson and Teeter 1981) are as large as 3.5 Å, with particularly large differences for residues 34–40; the R factor of the initial structure was 0.56 at 2 Å resolution. Molecular dynamics refinement at 3000 K starting with 4 Å resolution data for 2.5 psec, extending to 3 Å resolution for 2.5 psec, and finally to 2 Å resolution for 5 psec, followed by several cycles of minimization, reduces the atomic rms deviations to 0.34 and 0.56 Å for the backbone and side-chain atoms, respectively. During the molecular dynamics refinement, some atoms in residues 35–40 moved by more than 3 Å. The essential point is that the refinement of the crambin structure was achieved starting from the initial NMR structure without human intervention. The R factor (0.294) of the molecular dynamics refined structure is somewhat higher than the R factor (0.258) of the manually refined structure without solvent and with constant temperature factors; minor model building would correct this difference. Other annealing protocols using higher temperatures (e.g., 7000 to 9000 K) yield structures that are still closer to the manually refined structure. The refinement required approximately 1 hour of central processing unit time on a CRAY-1; structure factor calculations accounted for about half this time. The latter portion of the calculation has been considerably reduced in time by use of fast Fourier transform methods (A. Brünger, in prep.).

As a control, the initial NMR-derived structure was refined without rebuilding by a restrained least-squares method (Konnert and Hendrickson 1980), starting at 4 Å resolution and then increasing the resolution to 3 Å, and finally to 2 Å. The R factor dropped to 0.381, but the very bad stereochemistry and large deviation from the manually refined structure indicate that this structure has not converged to the correct result; residues 34–40 have not moved and substantial model building would be required to correct the structure. Thus, restrained least-squares refinement in the absence of model building did not produce the large conformational changes that occurred in molecular dynamics refinement by simulated annealing.

CONCLUSION

Molecular dynamics is now playing an important role in the study of the properties of macromolecules of biological interest. It can also be used effectively in the analysis of experimental data and, in particular, has been shown to provide a new approach to structure determination by NMR and X-ray crystallography. Because molecular dynamics simulations are relatively new, they have so far been employed primarily by theoreticians. It is to be hoped that experimentalists, as well, will begin to use molecular dynamics as a research tool for obtaining a deeper understanding of the biomolecules with which they work.

ACKNOWLEDGMENTS

We thank our collaborators who have contributed to the work described here. They include G.M. Clore, C.M. Dobson, A.M. Gronenborn, T. Ichiye, R.M. Levy, E.T. Olejniczak, and G.A. Petsko. The work was supported in part by grants from the National Science Foundation and the National Institutes of Health.

REFERENCES

Agmon, M. and J.J. Hopfield. 1983. CO Binding to heme proteins: A model for barrier height distributions and slow conformational changes. *J. Chem. Phys.* **79:** 2042.

Ansari, A., J. Berendzen, S.F. Bowne, and H. Frauenfelder, I.E.T. Iben, T.B. Sauke, E. Shyamsunder, and R.D. Young. 1985. Protein states and proteinquakes. *Proc. Natl. Acad. Sci.* **82:** 5000.

Austin, R.H., K.W. Beeson, L. Eisenstein, H. Frauenfelder, and I.C. Gunsalus. 1975. Dynamics of ligand binding to myoglobin. *Biochemistry* **14:** 5355.

Bashford, D., D.L. Weaver, and M. Karplus. 1984. Diffusion-collision model for the folding kinetics of the λ-repressor operator-binding domain. *J. Biomol. Struct. Dyn.* **1:** 1243.

Bialek, W. and R.F. Goldstein. 1985. Do vibrational spectroscopies uniquely describe protein dynamics? The case for myoglobin. *Biophys. J.* **48:** 1027.

Brooks, B.R. and M. Karplus. 1983. Harmonic dynamics of proteins: Normal modes and fluctuations in bovine pancreatic trypsin inhibitor. *Proc. Natl. Acad. Sci.* **80:** 6571.

Brooks, B.R., R.E. Bruccoleri, B.D. Olafson, D.J. States, S. Swaminathan, and M. Karplus. 1983. CHARMM: A program for macromolecular energy, minimization, and dynamics calculations. *J. Computational Chem.* **4:** 187.

Brooks, C.B., M. Karplus, and B.M. Pettitt. 1987. Proteins: A theoretical perspective of dynamics structure and thermodynamics. *Adv. Chem. Phys.* (in press).

Brünger, A.T., J. Kuriyan, and M. Karplus. 1987a. Crystallographic R factor refinement by molecular dynamics. *Science* **235:** 458.

Brünger, A.T., G.M. Clore, A.M. Gronenborn, and M. Karplus. 1986. Three-dimensional structure of proteins determined by molecular dynamics with interproton distance restraints: Application to crambin. *Proc. Natl. Acad. Sci.* **83:** 3801.

Brünger, A.T., R.L. Campbell, G.M. Clore, A.M. Gronenborn, M. Karplus, G.A. Petsko, and M.M. Teeter. 1987b. Solution of a protein crystal structure with a model obtained from NMR interproton distance restraints. *Science* **235:** 1049.

Campbell, I.D., C.M. Dobson, and R.J.P. Williams. 1978. Structures and energetics of proteins and their active sites. *Adv. Chem. Phys.* **39:** 55.

Campbell, I.D., C.M. Dobson, G.R. Moore, S.J. Perkins, and R.J.P. Williams. 1976. Temperature dependent molecular motion of a tyrosine residue of ferrocytochrome C. *FEBS Lett.* **70:** 96.

Chandrasekhar, S. 1943. Stochastic problems in physics and astronomy. *Rev. Mod. Phys.* **15:** 1.

Chothia, C. and A.M. Lesk. 1985. Helix movements in proteins. *Trends Biochem. Sci.* **10:** 116.

Clore, G.M., A.M. Gronenborn, A.T. Brünger, and M. Karplus. 1985. Solution conformation of a heptadecapeptide comprising the DNA binding helix F of the cyclic AMP receptor protein of *Escherichia coli*: Combined use of ¹H nuclear magnetic resonance and restrained molecular dynamics. *J. Mol. Biol.* **186:** 435.

Debrunner, P.G. and H. Frauenfelder. 1982. Dynamics of proteins. *Annu. Rev. Phys. Chem.* **33:** 283.

Frauenfelder, H., G.A. Petsko, and D. Tsernoglou. 1979. Temperature-dependent X-ray diffraction as a probe of protein structural dynamics. *Nature* **280:** 558.

Gurd, F.R.N. and J.M. Rothgeb. 1979. Motions in proteins. *Adv. Protein Chem.* **33:** 73.

Hansen, J.P. and I.R. McDonald. 1976. *Theory of simple liquids.* Academic Press, New York.

Hendrickson, W.A. and M.M. Teeter. 1981. Structure of the hydrophobic protein crambin determined directly from the anomalous scattering of sulphur. *Nature* **290:** 107.

Honig, B., B. Hudson, B.D. Sykes, and M. Karplus. 1971. Ring orientation in β-ionone and retinals. *Proc. Natl. Acad. Sci.* **68:** 1289.

Ichiye, T., B.D. Olafson, S. Swaminathan, and M. Karplus. 1986. Structure and internal mobility of proteins: A molecular dynamics study of hen egg white lysozyme. *Biopolymers* **25:** 1909.

Jack, A. and M. Levitt. 1978. Refinement of large structures by simultaneous minimization of energy and R factor. *Acta Crystallogr. Sect. B Struct. Crystallogr. Cryst. Chem.* **A34:** 931.

Karplus, M. and J.N. Kushick. 1981. Method for estimating the configurational entropy of macromolecules. *Macromolecules* **14:** 325.

Karplus, M. and J.A. McCammon. 1981. The internal dynamics of globular proteins. *Crit. Rev. Biochem.* **9:** 293.

———. 1983. Dynamics of proteins: Elements and function. *Annu. Rev. Biochem.* **53:** 263.

Kirkpatrick, S., C.D. Gelatt, Jr., M.P. Vecchi. 1983. Optimization by simulated annealing. *Science* **220:** 671.

Konnert, J.H. and W.A. Hendrickson. 1980. A restrained-parameter thermal-factor refinement procedure. *Acta Crystallogr. Sect. B Struct. Crystallogr. Chem.* **A36:** 344.

Kuriyan, J., M. Karplus, and G.A. Petsko. 1987. Estimation of uncertainties in X-ray refinement results by use of perturbed structures. *Proteins* (in press).

Lesk, A.M. and C. Chothia. 1980. How different amino acid sequences determine similar protein structures: The structure and evolutionary dynamics of the globins. *J. Mol. Biol.* **136:** 225.

Levitt, M., C. Sander, and P.S. Stern. 1985. Protein normal-mode dynamics: Trypsin inhibitor, crambin, ribonuclease and lysozyme. *J. Mol. Biol.* **181:** 423.

Levy, R.M. and M. Karplus. 1979. Vibrational approach to the dynamics of an α-helix. *Biopolymers* **18:** 2465.

Levy, R.M., D. Perahia, and M. Karplus. 1982. Molecular dynamics of an α-helical polypeptide: Temperature dependence and deviation from harmonic behavior. *Proc. Natl. Acad. Sci.* **79:** 1346.

Levy, R.M., R.P. Sheridan, J.W. Keepers, G.S Dubey, S. Swaminathan, and M. Karplus. 1985. Molecular dynamics of myoglobin at 298°K: Results from a 300 ps computer simulation. *Biophys. J.* **48:** 509.

Marquart, M., D. Deisenhofer, R. Huber, and W. Palm. 1980. Crystallographic refinement and atomic models of the intact immunoglobulin molecule kol and its antigen-binding fragment at 3.0 Å and 1.9 Å resolution. *J. Mol. Biol.* **141:** 369.

McCammon, J.A., B.R. Gelin, and M. Karplus. 1977. Dynamics of folded proteins. *Nature* **267:** 585.

McCammon, J.A., P.G. Wolynes, and M. Karplus. 1979. Picosecond dynamics of tyrosine side chains in proteins. *Biochemistry* **18:** 927.

McQuarrie, D.A. 1976. *Statistical mechanics.* Harper and Row, New York.

Moss, D.S. and A.J. Morffew. 1982. Restrain: A restrained least squares refinement program for use in protein crystallography. *Comput. Chem.* **6:** 1.

Noggle, J.H. and R.E. Schirmer. 1971. *The nuclear Overhauser effect.* Academic Press, New York.

Northrup, S.H., M.R. Pear, C.-Y. Lee, J.A. McCammon, and M. Karplus. 1982. Dynamical theory of activated processes in globular proteins. *Proc. Natl. Acad. Sci.* **79:** 4035.

Olejniczak, E.T., C.M. Dobson, R.M. Levy, and M. Karplus. 1984. Motional averaging of proton nuclear Overhauser effects in proteins. Predictions from a molecular dynamics simulation of lysozyme. *J. Am. Chem. Soc.* **106:** 1923.

Parak, F., E.W. Knapp, and D. Kucheida. 1982. Protein dynamics. Mössbauer spectroscopy on deoxymyoglobin crystals. *J. Mol. Biol.* **161:** 177.

Pauling, L., R.B. Corey, and H.R. Branson. 1951. The structure of proteins: Two hydrogen-bonded helical configurations of the polypeptide chain. *Proc. Natl. Acad. Sci.* **37:** 305.

Phillips, D.C. 1981. Closing remarks. In *Biomolecular stereodynamics* (ed. R.H. Sarma), p. 497. Adenine, New York.

Poulsen, F.M., J.C. Hoch, and C.M. Dobson. 1980. A structural study of the hydrophobic box region of lysozyme in solution using nuclear Overhauser effects. *Biochemistry* **19:** 2597.

Ramachadran, G.N., C. Ramakrishnan, and V. Sasisekharan. 1963. Stereochemistry of polypeptide chain configurations. *J. Mol. Biol.* **7:** 95.

Smith, J.L., W.A. Hendrickson, R.B. Honzatko, and S. Sheriff. 1986. Structural heterogeneity in protein crystals. *Biochemistry* **25:** 5018.

Stein, D.L. 1985. A model of protein conformational substrates. *Proc. Natl. Acad. Sci.* **82:** 3670.

Stillinger, F.H. and T.A. Weber. 1982. Hidden structure in liquids. *Physical Rev.* **A25:** 978.

———. 1984. Packing structures and transitions in liquids and solids. *Science* **225:** 983.

Sussman, J.L., S.R. Holbrook, G.M. Church, and S.-H. Kim. 1977. A structure-factor least-squares refinement procedure for macromolecular structures using constrained and restrained parameters. *Acta Crystallogr. Sect. B Struct. Crystallogr. Cryst. Chem.* **A33:** 800.

Swaminathan, S., T. Ichiye, W.F. van Gunsteren, and M. Karplus. 1982. Time dependence of atomic fluctuations in proteins: Analysis of local and collective motions in bovine pancreatic trypsin inhibitor. *Biochemistry* **21:** 5230.

Toulouse, G. 198. Progré récents dans la physique des systémes désordonnés. *Helv. Physiol. Pharmacol. Acta* **57:** 459.

van Gunsteren, W.F. and M.J.C. Berendsen. 1977. Algorithms for macromolecular dynamics and constraint dynamics. *Mol. Physics* **34:** 1311.

van Gunsteren, W.F. and M. Karplus. 1982. Effect of constraints on the dynamics of macromolecules. *Macromolecules* **15:** 1528.

Verlet, L. 1967. Computer "experiments" on classical fluids. I. Thermodynamical properties of Lennard-Jones molecules. *Physical Rev.* **159:** 98.

Wagner, G. and K. Wüthrich. 1982. Amide proton exchange and surface conformation on the basic pancreatic trypsin inhibitor in solution. *J. Mol. Biol.* **160:** 343.

Wyckoff, H.W., C.H.W. Hirs, and S.N. Timasheff. 1985. Diffraction methods for biological macromolecules, part B. *Methods Enzymol.* **115:** 3.

Ziman, J.M. 1979. *Models of disorder.* Cambridge University Press, London.

The C-peptide Helix from Ribonuclease A Considered as an Autonomous Folding Unit

K.R. Shoemaker, R. Fairman, P.S. Kim,* E.J. York,[†] J.M. Stewart,[†] and R.L. Baldwin

Department of Biochemistry, Stanford University School of Medicine, Stanford, California 94305;
[†]Department of Biochemistry, University of Colorado School of Medicine, Denver, Colorado 80262

One of the basic goals of work on the mechanism of protein folding is to define autonomous folding units: those individual segments of a protein which, if excised, contain sufficient structural information to specify their own folding. Surprisingly little is known about this subject. A common opinion is that entire domains are the units of folding. A domain is defined as (1) a continuous segment of polypeptide chain that is folded on itself, as judged by inspection of the protein's X-ray structure, and (2) a folded segment that makes only marginal contacts with neighboring segments. Domains are usually found to contain 100–150 amino acid residues. The nature of protein structure is such that a domain can be divided into two subdomains and each subdomain can be further divided, if the definition of a subdomain is based on part 1 above (Rose 1979), without part 2.

Autonomous folding units might, however, prove to be substantially smaller than entire domains. Gilbert's hypothesis that new proteins can be made by reshuffling exons (Gilbert 1978, 1985) implies that each exon product is an autonomous folding unit (cf. Gō 1981) and the peptide segments encoded by exons are often as small as 30–40 residues. The definition of an autonomous folding unit is tied to the criteria used for stability of the folded structure. Our criteria for an autonomous folding unit are as follows: (1) The structure shown by the excised fragment should be sufficiently stable in aqueous solution to be detected, and should occur by a monomolecular reaction. (2) This structure must closely resemble the structure in the intact protein.

Other types of experiments on autonomous folding units may lead to alternative definitions. It seems likely that peptide reshuffling experiments, based on the methods of genetic engineering, will be used in future work to analyze autonomous folding units. Studies of sequence homology between limited regions of different proteins have been used to suggest folding units and to examine the role of exon boundaries in fixing these folding units (Doolittle 1985). Another approach to the analysis of folding units is to examine the ability of a protein fragment to bind a specific ligand such as heme (Craik et al. 1981), ATP (Knight and McEntee 1986;

Barden and Kemp 1987), α-bungarotoxin (Wilson et al. 1985), or DNA (Bruist et al. 1987).

Autonomous folding units should be larger than pentapeptides, according to the results of Kabsch and Sander (1984), who find that a given pentapeptide sequence can occur as part of an α helix in one protein and part of a β sheet in a different protein. On the other hand, Wright and co-workers have reported formation of a β turn, a four-residue structure, within a nonapeptide fragment of hemagglutinin in aqueous solution (Dyson et al. 1985). Thus, sequences as short as β turns may be autonomous folding units. Only a small fraction of a protein may consist of autonomous folding units. At an early stage in the folding process, only a few segments may be folded and other residues may play a passive role.

Evidence That the C-peptide Helix Is an Autonomous Folding Unit

Residues 3–13 are helical in bovine pancreatic ribonuclease A (RNase A) and only a few of these residues bind the helix to the rest of the protein (Wlodawer and Sjölin 1983). Peptides containing this sequence show partial helix formation in aqueous solution (Brown and Klee 1971; Bierzynski et al. 1982; Kim and Baldwin 1984). The helix has been studied in C-peptide (residues 1–13 of RNase A, terminating in homoserine lactone at residue 13), in S-peptide (residues 1–20 of RNase A), and in chemically synthesized analogs of these peptides.

The following observations suggest that the C-peptide helix is an autonomous folding unit. (1) The C-peptide helix is much more stable than predicted by the Zimm-Bragg equation[1] when host-guest data on synthetic polypeptides (Sueki et al. 1984) are used to provide the Zimm-Bragg parameters. Consequently, the C-peptide helix may be stabilized by specific side-chain interactions and its side-chain structure may be similar to that of the 3–13 helix in RNase A. (2)

---

[1]Shoemaker et al. (1985) give the predicted stability of a 13-residue polyalanine helix and show that the C-peptide helix is about 30 times more stable than expected. They corrected an earlier estimate by Bierzynski et al. (1982), who used an approximate form of the Zimm-Bragg equation. Current studies of alanine peptides that are made water-soluble by inserting a few Lys and Glu residues show that these helices are also more stable than predicted from host-guest data (S. Marquese and R.L. Baldwin, in prep.).

---

*Present address: Whitehead Institute, Nine Cambridge Center, Cambridge, Massachusetts 02142.

Additional evidence that side-chain interactions stabilize the C-peptide helix is given by the strong pH dependence of helicity (Bierzynski et al. 1982). The curve of helicity versus pH, with a maximum at pH 5 and apparent pKs near 3.5 and 6.5, suggests that charged amino acid side chains are critical for helix stability. (3) The helix is localized in S-peptide and does not extend to the carboxy-terminal end, as shown by different types of NMR experiments (Rico et al. 1983; Kim and Baldwin 1984). There is a "helix-stop" signal in S-peptide whose nature remains to be determined. In synthetic polypeptides the average length of a helical sequence at the midpoint of the helix-coil transition is about 100 residues. Thus, localization of the helix in S-peptide gave the first definite indication that it is an autonomous folding unit.

Helix formation by isolated C-peptide occurs monomolecularly, as shown by molecular weight measurements (Brown and Klee 1971), by lack of concentration dependence (Bierzynski et al. 1982), and by gel filtration experiments (Shoemaker et al. 1987). Although the C-peptide helix is only marginally stable, helix formation can be studied readily near 0°C in the absence of organic cosolvents. Moreover, the helicity of C-peptide can be increased by certain amino acid substitutions without increasing the number of residues (Shoemaker et al. 1987).

Invariant Residues and Models for the Determination of the 3–13 Helix

Amino acid sequences for ribonucleases homologous to bovine pancreatic RNase A are known from 38 mammalian species. If we assume that residues 3–13 form the α helix in all 38 ribonucleases, then a study of the invariant residues and their roles in different helix prediction schemes might reveal features of the 3–13 helix involved in its behavior as an autonomous folding unit. The most striking feature of the invariant residues, which are shown in Figure 1, is their large number: in the sequence 1–15, Glu-2, Ala-5, Lys-7, Phe-8, Arg-10, Gln-11, His-12, and Asp-14 all are invariant and some other residues are replaced only by closely related amino acids. Reasons for the invariance of some of these residues have been proposed: His-12 is essential for catalytic activity; Gln-11 aids in substrate binding; Phe-8, His-12, and Asp-14 are needed for tight binding of S-peptide to S-protein (Blackburn and Moore 1982).

The relation between the invariant residues and the helix prediction schemes of Chou and Fasman (1974), Burgess et al. (1974), and Lim (1974) has been discussed by Lenstra et al. (1977). None of these schemes attempts to predict whether the 3–13 helix should be stable in C-peptide, and Lim's method is explicitly based on finding a cluster of side chains, when the peptide is in a helical conformation, that could bind the helix to the protein. Lenstra et al. (1977) suggest that the success of these different predictive schemes is closely correlated with the invariance of the hydrophobic residues. On the other hand, interactions involving ionizing groups contribute to the behavior of the 3–13 helix as an autonomous folding unit (see below). The problem of predicting from sequence which residues can form α helices that are autonomous folding units may be a separate problem from that of predicting α helices in proteins.

Based on studies of the C-peptide helix, we suggest the following model for α helices that are autonomous folding units: they are stabilized by specific intrahelical side-chain interactions which may function also to provide start and stop signals for localizing the helix. Other plausible mechanisms for start and stop signals can be suggested, notably the use of proline residues (Perutz et al. 1965). The concept that α helices might be stabilized by specific side-chain interactions was foreseen by Sela, Katchalski, and co-workers (Ramachandran et al. 1971; Schechter et al. 1971; Goren et al. 1979) who synthesized two types of peptides with simple repeating sequences in order to look for this effect. Maxfield and Scheraga (1975) found statistical evidence in protein α helices for an interaction between Glu and any basic amino acid four residues away (see also Sundaralingam et al. 1985).

Proposed Side-chain Interactions in the C-peptide Helix

In recent work, three types of specific side-chain interactions have been proposed to explain the stability of the C-peptide helix (Fig. 2). (1) Interaction between the α-helix macrodipole and charged groups near the ends of the helix was suggested by Shoemaker et al. (1985) after finding that Glu-2$^-$ and His-12$^+$ are the charged groups responsible for the pH dependence of C-peptide helicity. This interaction is studied in more detail in recent work (Shoemaker et al. 1987). (2) A H-bonded ion pair between Glu-2$^-$ and Arg-10$^+$ is

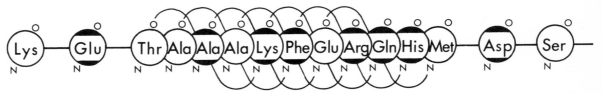

Figure 1. Sequence of the first 15 amino acids in bovine pancreatic RNase A. Darkened residues are invariant in ribonucleases from 38 mammalian species (Blackburn and Moore 1982). In 2 of 38 species, residue 11 is listed as either Gln or Glu with the other 36 as Gln, and also residue 14 is listed as either Asp or Asn in 2 species, with the other 36 as Asp.

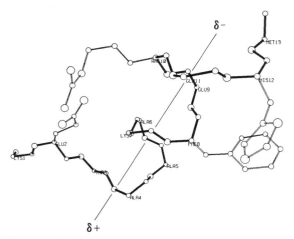

Figure 2. Residues 1–13 of RNase A illustrating the H-bonded ion pair between Glu-2⁻ and Arg-10⁺, a possible aromatic interaction between Phe-8 and His-12, and the α-helix macrodipole. All other side chains have been omitted for simplicity. The coordinates of RNase A are from Wlodawer and Sjölin (1983) and are deposited in the Brookhaven Protein Data Bank.

known to be present in RNase A (Wlodawer and Sjölin 1983), and it has been suggested that it should also be present in C-peptide and S-peptide (Rico et al. 1984, 1986; A. Bierzynski, pers. comm.). (3) Phe-8 and His-12 are positioned in RNase A so that they might make an aromatic interaction of the type discussed by Burley and Petsko (1985) and Blundell et al. (1986) for Tyr, Phe, and Trp. The existence of an aromatic interaction between Phe-8 and His-12 in C-peptide and S-peptide has been proposed (Bermejo et al. 1986; Bierzynski et al. 1986; Rico et al. 1986). It has been suggested further that His-12⁺ interacts more strongly with Phe-8 than does His-12⁰ (A. Bierzynski, pers. comm.), thereby providing a possible explanation for the effect of pH titration of His-12 on the helicity of C-peptide.

Interaction of the Helix Dipole with Charged Groups

The dipoles of the peptide groups add across H bonds so that the α helix has a large dipole moment that is proportional to helix length (3.4 Debye units per residue; Wada 1976). Calculations using point charges indicate that the electrostatic field around an α helix with no formal charges can be represented to a good first approximation by an extended line dipole whose positive and negative poles are near the amino and carboxyl termini, respectively (Hol et al. 1978; Sheridan et al. 1982). A more detailed picture is given by noting that four NH and four CO groups at the amino and carboxyl termini, respectively, of an α helix are not H-bonded and that the partial charges of the helix dipole actually reside on these NH and CO groups. Consequently, a negatively charged group near the amino terminus is helix-stabilizing, but becomes helix-destabilizing if placed near the carboxyl terminus, whereas the opposite is true of a positively charged

group. In X-ray structures of proteins, there are many examples of negatively charged ligands bound close to the amino termini of α helices (Hol 1985). The distribution of charged groups in protein α helices is highly asymmetric, with acidic and basic residues found close to the amino and carboxyl termini, respectively (Chou and Fasman 1974, 1978), and this finding has been explained as reflecting the helix-stabilizing effects of these charged groups (Blagdon and Goodman 1975).

Recent experiments have shown that the charge on the amino-terminal residue of C-peptide affects the stability of the helix according to the qualitative predictions of the helix dipole model (Shoemaker et al. 1987). The naturally occurring residue, Lys-1, which has two positive charges, is helix-destabilizing relative to Ala, whereas succinyl-Ala-1, with one negative charge, is helix-stabilizing. Removing the positive charge on the α-NH₃⁺ group of Ala-1 by pH titration is helix-stabilizing, whereas protonation of succinyl-Ala-1⁻ is helix-destabilizing. Increasing the concentration of NaCl increases helicity for Lys-1⁺⁺ and decreases helicity for succinyl-Ala-1⁻, as expected for screening of charged-group interactions with the helix dipole.

In early work it was found that the α-COOH form of C-peptide shows much lower helicity than the lactone form (Kim et al. 1982; see also Rico et al. 1986). pH titration of the α-COOH group in C-peptide carboxylate affects the chemical shift of the amide proton of His-12, which is too far away to be affected by a through-bond interaction (Bundi and Wüthrich 1979), and the same effect was found in N-acetyl-Gly-His-Gly (Kim et al. 1982). They suggested that an ion pair is formed between the α-COO⁻ group and the protonated side chain of His-12 and that it shifts the helix-coil equilibrium toward the unfolded form. From the work of Shoemaker et al. (1987), it is evident that interaction of the α-COO⁻ group with the helix dipole offers an alternative explanation. To test this point, we synthesized the analog of C-peptide (peptide III[Glu-2→Ala, Arg-10→Ala, α-CONH₂→α-COOH]) whose pH titration of helix content is shown in Figure 3. The peptide lacks Glu-2 so that only the α-COOH group is titrated between pH 2 and pH 5. As Figure 3 shows, protonation of the α-COO⁻ group is helix-stabilizing. Comparison of this peptide to one without a free α-COOH group does not involve comparing the carboxylate form versus the lactone form, so there is no question of whether the lactone stabilizes the helix by some other mechanism.

Next we reinvestigated the NMR evidence for an ion pair interaction between the α-COO⁻ group and the protonated side chain of His-12. Figure 4 shows pH titration of the chemical shifts of some protons in Gly-Gly-Phe-Ala. Titration of the α-COOH group between pH 2 and pH 5 causes substantial changes in the chemical shift of the Gly-2 αCH₂ resonance and of the Phe-3 β,β′CH₂ resonances. These groups are too far from the α-COOH group to experience through-bond effects (Bundi and Wüthrich 1979). Instead, the changes in chemical shifts apparently are caused by a ring current

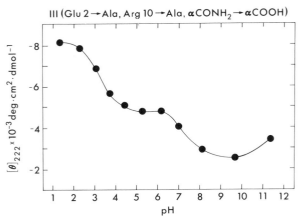

Figure 3. pH titration of helicity for peptide III(Glu-2→ Ala, Arg-10→Ala, α-CONH$_2$→ α-COOH), which has only a free α-COOH group ionizing in the pH range 2–5. (The sequence of reference peptide III is given in Fig. 5 legend.) The figure shows an increase in helicity as the pH is reduced from 5 to 2 and the α-COO$^-$ group is protonated. The effect of titrating His-12 (between pH 9 and pH 6) can also be seen. The mean residue ellipticity at 222 nm was measured at 3°C, 0.1 M NaCl. For experimental methods, see Shoemaker et al. (1985, 1987). The change in $[\theta]_{222}$ for complete helix formation by C-peptide at 3°C is near 30,000 deg cm^2 dmol^{-1}, when the baseline value for 0% helix is estimated as +3,000 deg cm^2 dmol^{-1} (Mitchinson and Baldwin 1986; K.R. Shoemaker et al., in prep.).

effect. The rotamer populations for the Phe-3 αCH— β,β'CH$_2$ bond were calculated from measurements of the coupling constants and equations given by Kopple et al. (1973) and by Pachler (1964) and Feeney (1976), with similar results. The fraction of rotamer III (gauche-gauche) is small and independent of pH between 1 and 4.5 (f[III] = 0.08–0.09 according to Kopple et al. or 0.11–0.12 according to Pachler and Feeney), whereas in this pH range f(II) falls from 0.36 to 0.26 (Kopple et al. 1973) or to 0.27 (Pachler 1964 and Feeney 1976), and f(I) rises accordingly. The α-COOH group is farthest from the aromatic ring of Phe-3 in rotamer I.

For the peptide Gly-Gly-Phe-Ala, there cannot be an ion pair between the α-COO$^-$ group and a neighboring side chain. We conclude that the ion pair explanation is also unlikely for N-acetyl-Gly-His-Gly, for which similar NMR results were obtained (Kim et al. 1982). Therefore, the NMR results for both peptides probably arise from a ring current effect that reflects the rotamer populations of the aromatic side chain (Phe or His). Having thus ruled out the His-12$^+$ $\cdots$ α-COO$^-$ interaction, we conclude that the increase in helicity of peptide III(Glu-2→ Ala, Arg-10→ Ala, α-CONH$_2$→ α-COOH) that occurs as the α-COO$^-$ group is protonated (Fig. 3) can be explained as arising from a charged-group:helix dipole interaction.

The Glu-2$^-$ $\cdots$ Arg-10$^+$ Ion Pair

There is a well-defined H-bonded ion pair between the side chains of Glu-2$^-$ and Arg-10$^+$ in the highly refined structure of RNase A from combined X-ray and

neutron diffraction data (Wlodawer and Sjölin 1983). The interaction has been studied in experiments based on reconstitution of S-peptide and chemically synthesized analogs of S-peptide with S-protein (Hofmann et al. 1970; Marchiori et al. 1972). It is of major interest to determine whether or not the Glu-2$^-$ $\cdots$ Arg-10$^+$ ion pair is present in the C-peptide helix, both because of its unusual nature (formed between residues that are spaced eight residues apart) and because it fixes the amino-terminal boundary of the helix between Glu-2 and Thr-3. It is sterically improbable to make this ion pair if Glu-2 is part of the helix, as can be shown with space-filling models.

One would like to analyze the Glu-2$^-$ $\cdots$ Arg-10$^+$ interaction by the methods that have been used successfully to show that Glu-2$^-$ and His-12$^+$ are responsible for the pH dependence of helicity: chemical modification or deletion of Glu-2 (Rico et al. 1984); replacement of Glu-2 or His-12 by Ala (Shoemaker et al. 1985); and synthesis of C-peptide analogs in which only Glu-2 or His-12 titrates in the pH range of interest (Shoemaker et al. 1987). There are, however, several problems with these approaches. First, Glu-2$^-$ could stabilize the helix by interacting with the helix dipole (Shoemaker et al. 1985, 1987). Therefore, experiments showing that Glu-2$^-$ is a helix-stabilizing residue do not establish that there is a Glu-2$^-$ $\cdots$ Arg-10$^+$ ion pair. Second, the high pK of Arg-10 makes it difficult to employ pH titration.

The strategy used here is to study an analog of C-peptide with the replacement Arg-10→ Ala. If the Glu-2$^-$ $\cdots$ Arg-10$^+$ ion pair exists and stabilizes the C-peptide helix, then the Arg-10→ Ala replacement should have two consequences. (1) The helix content at pH 5 should drop with Arg-10→ Ala. (2) The pH titration of Glu-2 without Arg-10 should no longer affect helicity by this mechanism, although Glu-2$^-$ might instead stabilize the helix by interacting with the helix dipole. For illustration, consider first the effect of the replacement Glu-2→ Ala. Figure 5a shows the pH titration of the reference peptide (III), and Figure 5b shows the titration of III(Glu-2→ Ala). There is a large drop in helicity at pH 5 and the acid limb of the titration curve disappears with Glu-2→ Ala.

The effects of the replacement Arg-10→ Ala are shown in Figure 5c. There is no significant change in helicity at pH 5, but the acid limb of the titration curve again disappears. The latter effect shows that Glu-2$^-$ and Arg-10$^+$ do interact, but does not establish whether the interaction is direct or indirect. The first effect suggests that, if there is a Glu-2$^-$ $\cdots$ Arg-10$^+$ ion pair which contributes to helix stability, then breaking this interaction by Arg-10→ Ala still allows Glu-2$^-$ to stabilize the helix by interacting with the helix dipole. If so, why doesn't pH titration of Glu-2$^-$ to Glu-2^0 cause a drop in helicity (Fig. 5c)? Several explanations are possible, depending on the relative importance of the following effects as Glu-2$^-$ → Glu^0: (1) loss of the helix-stabilizing interaction of Glu-2$^-$ with the helix dipole; (2) intrinsic s value effects (Sueki et al. 1984); (3) a "helix-lengthening" reaction to include

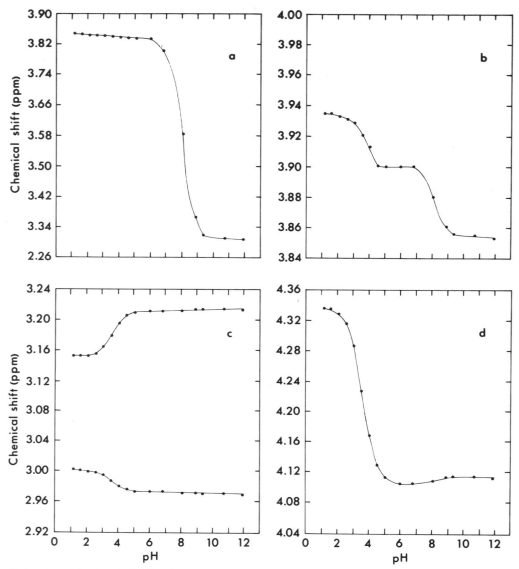

Figure 4. pH titration of the chemical shifts of some protons in the tetrapeptide Gly-Gly-Phe-Ala (0.01 M NaCl, 20°C, D_2O). The figure shows that substantial titration shifts are observed for some resonances (see *b* and *c*) of groups that are too far from the α-COOH group to be influenced by through-bond effects. Chemical shifts are reported relative to the internal standard sodium 3-trimethylsilyl-(2,2,3,3-$^2H_4$)propionate (TSP), and were corrected for the pH dependence of the TSP resonance. Measurements were made on a 500-MHz GE-Nicolet instrument. pH values in D_2O refer to uncorrected meter readings. There are likely to be negligible through-bond effects from the pH titration of the α-COOH group for protons beyond 5 bonds of the α-COOH group (Bundi and Wüthrich 1979). The number of bonds from the α-COO$^-$ group to the αCH$_2$ of Gly-1 (*a*) is 11, to the αCH$_2$ of Gly-2 (*b*) is 8, to the $\beta\beta'$CH$_2$ resonances of Phe-3 (*c*) is 6, and to the αCH of Ala-4 (*d*) is 2. The titration shift for the αCH resonance of Ala-4 is upfield, as expected for a through-bond effect. In contrast, the shift for one of the Phe-8 $\beta\beta'$CH$_2$ resonances is downfield, indicative of a through-space interaction.

acetyl-Ala-1 and Glu-2. Experiments are in progress to address the role of each of these effects.

In summary, our results indicate that the Glu-2$^-$ $\cdots$ Arg-10$^+$ ion pair is present in the C-peptide helix, but that our understanding of this interaction is still obscure, at least by the methods employed so far.

Aromatic Interaction between Phe-8 and His-12

The approach used here is to study peptide III with the replacement Phe-8 → Ala. If an aromatic interac-

tion between Phe-8 and His-12 makes an important contribution to helix stability, then the helicity might drop with Phe-8 → Ala much as it drops with His-12 → Ala (Fig. 6a). Figure 6b shows that there is a moderate drop in helicity with Phe-8 → Ala. Also, NMR data (K.R. Shoemaker et al., in prep.) indicate that a Phe-8 $\cdots$ His-12 interaction can be detected.

If the aromatic interaction exists and is stronger with His-12$^+$ than with His^0 (A. Bierzynski, pers. comm.), then the alkaline limb might disappear with Phe-8 → Ala, as it does with His-12 → Ala (Fig. 6a). There

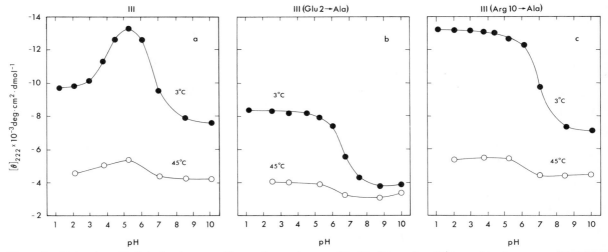

Figure 5. pH titration of helicity for three peptides used to study a possible Glu-2⁻ · · · Arg-10⁺ ion pair: reference peptide III (*a*) (Shoemaker et al. 1987), III(Glu-2→Ala) (*b*), and III(Arg-10→Ala) (*c*). The figure shows the effects on helix content of replacing Glu-2 or Arg-10 by Ala. Conditions: see Fig. 3. The sequence of III is acetyl-A-E-T-A-A-A-K-F-L-R-A-H-A-CONH₂.

are comparable decreases in the magnitudes of both the alkaline and acid limbs of the titration curve (Fig. 6b), showing that the change in the alkaline limb does not necessarily result from loss of a Phe-8 · · · His-12 interaction.

We conclude that a Phe-8 · · · His-12 aromatic interaction makes only a moderate contribution to C-peptide helicity and that it does not completely explain the role of His-12 in determining the pH dependence of C-peptide helix content. As with Glu-2⁻, both helix dipole and intrinsic s value effects also need to be considered.

CONCLUDING REMARKS

A search for specific side-chain interactions that stabilize the C-peptide helix has thus far shown the following. (1) The interaction of charged groups near the ends of the helix with the α-helix macrodipole may either stabilize or destabilize the helix. For example, this interaction explains the destabilizing effects of charged α-NH₃⁺ and α-COO⁻ groups, and explains why Lys-1⁺⁺ destabilizes the helix. (2) Glu-2⁻ may control helicity by forming a Glu-2⁻ · · · Arg-10⁺ ion pair as it does in RNase A. This interaction is especially

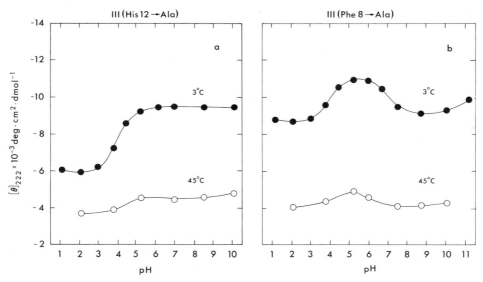

Figure 6. pH titration of helicity for two peptides used to study a possible aromatic interaction between Phe-8 and His-12: III(His-12→Ala) (*a*) and III(Phe-8→Ala) (*b*). See Fig. 5 for III. The figure shows the effects on helix content of replacing Phe-8 or His-12 by Ala. Conditions: see Fig. 3.

important among the specific side-chain interactions because it fixes the amino-terminal boundary of the helix. (3) A helix-stabilizing role for His-12 is served by an aromatic interaction with Phe-8 and/or a helix dipole interaction. (4) It is known that there is also a "helix stop" in the S-peptide sequence that fixes the carboxy-terminal boundary of the helix (Rico et al. 1983; Kim and Baldwin 1984), but the nature of this stop signal remains to be determined. (5) Additional specific side-chain interactions that contribute to C-peptide helix content remain to be identified.

Although the magnitudes of these interactions are not large (each interaction stabilizes the helix only by a factor of 2 or 3), the interactions are important in two respects. First, they help to raise helicity into the range where it is measurable. For example, without the helix-stabilizing effects of Glu-2$^-$ and His-12$^+$, the helicity of C-peptide is so low that the ability of C-peptide to form a helix in aqueous solution would not have been discovered (Fig. 2 of Bierzynski et al. 1982). Reference peptide III does show measurable helicity in the absence of Glu-2 (Fig. 5b) or His-12 (Fig. 6a), but only because III contains other helix-enhancing replacements. Second, although these interactions are small in magnitude, they are important in allowing the C-peptide helix to function as an autonomous folding unit. This effect is particularly striking in the case of the Glu-2$^-\cdots$Arg-10$^+$ ion pair, which sets the amino-terminal boundary of the helix.

Because of competing interactions, determination of specific side-chain interactions in a helix formed by a peptide fragment of a protein is not simple. This point is made clear by the above discussion of the Glu-2$^-\cdots$Arg-10$^+$ ion pair and the Phe-8$\cdots$His-12 interaction. For this reason, it is important that it is possible to analyze Glu$^-\cdots$Lys$^+$ ion pairs in peptides of de novo design. These peptides have simple, repetitive sequences based on an alanine backbone (S. Marqusee and R.L. Baldwin, in prep.). This approach should simplify the problem of analyzing specific side-chain interactions in α helices.

ACKNOWLEDGMENTS

We thank Virginia MacCosham for technical assistance, and Jannette Carey, Homme Hellinga, Fred Hughson, Susan Marqusee, John Osterhout, and David Schultz for helpful discussion. This work was supported by National Institutes of Health grant GM-31475.

REFERENCES

Barden, J.A. and B.E. Kemp. 1987. NMR of a synthetic peptide spanning the triphosphate binding site of adenosine 5′-triphosphate in actin. *Biochemistry* 26: 1471.

Bermejo, F.J., M. Rico, J. Santoro, J. Herranz, E. Gallego, and J.L. Nieto. 1986. Quantum-chemical calculations of a proposed Phe$_n$-His$_{n+4}$ stabilizing interaction in peptide α-helices. *J. Mol. Struct.* 142: 339.

Bierzynski, A., P.S. Kim, and R.L. Baldwin. 1982. A salt bridge stabilizes the helix formed by isolated C-peptide of RNase A. *Proc. Natl. Acad. Sci.* 79: 2470.

Bierzynski, A., M. Dadlez, M. Sobociński, and G. Kupryszewski. 1986. Conformational study of two synthetic peptides with sequence analogies to the N-terminal fragment of RNase A. *Biophys. Chem.* 25: 127.

Blackburn, P. and S. Moore. 1982. Pancreatic ribonuclease. In *The enzymes* (ed. P.D. Boyer), vol. 15, p. 317. Academic Press, New York.

Blagdon, D.E. and M. Goodman. 1975. Mechanisms of protein and polypeptide helix initiation. *Biopolymers* 14: 241.

Blundell, T., J. Singh, J. Thornton, S.K. Burley, and G.A. Petsko. 1986. Aromatic interactions. *Science* 234: 1005.

Brown, J.E. and W.A. Klee. 1971. Helix-coil transition of the isolated amino terminus of ribonuclease. *Biochemistry* 10: 470.

Bruist, M.F., S.J. Horvath, L.E. Hood, T.A. Steitz, and M.I. Simon. 1987. Synthesis of a site-specific DNA-binding peptide. *Science* 235: 777.

Bundi, A. and K. Wüthrich. 1979. Use of amide ^{1}H-NMR titration shifts for studies of polypeptide conformation. *Biopolymers* 18: 299.

Burgess, A.W., P.K. Ponnuswamy, and H.A. Scheraga. 1974. Analysis of conformations of amino acid residues and prediction of backbone topography in proteins. *Isr. J. Chem.* 12: 239.

Burley, S.K. and G.A. Petsko. 1985. Aromatic-aromatic interaction: A mechanism of protein structure stabilization. *Science* 229: 23.

Chou, P.Y. and G.D. Fasman. 1974. Conformational parameters for amino acids in helical, β-sheet, and random coil regions calculated from proteins. *Biochemistry* 13: 211.

———. 1978. Prediction of the secondary structure of proteins from their amino acid sequence. *Adv. Enzymol.* 47: 45.

Craik, C.S., S.R. Buchman, and S. Beychok. 1981. O$_2$ binding properties of the product of the central exon of β-globin gene. *Nature* 291: 87.

Doolittle, R.F. 1985. The genealogy of some recently evolved vertebrate proteins. *Trends Biochem. Sci.* 10: 233.

Dyson, H.J., K.J. Cross, R.A. Houghten, I.A. Wilson, P.E. Wright, and R.A. Lerner. 1985. The immunodominant site of a synthetic immunogen has a conformational preference in water for a type-II reverse turn. *Nature* 318: 480.

Feeney, J. 1976. Improved component vicinal coupling constants for calculating side-chain conformations in amino acids. *J. Magnet. Res.* 21: 473.

Gilbert, W. 1978. Why genes in pieces? *Nature* 271: 501.

———. 1985. Genes-in-pieces revisited. *Science* 228: 823.

Gō, M. 1981. Correlation of DNA exonic regions with protein structural units in haemoglobin. *Nature* 291: 90.

Goren, H.J., M. Fridkin, E. Katchalski-Katzir, and N. Lotan. 1979. Conformational changes of poly(L-histidyl-L-alanyl-α-L-glutamic acid) in solution. Transition pathways and conformational intermediates. *Biopolymers* 18: 981.

Hofmann, K., J.P. Visser, and F.M. Finn. 1970. Studies on polypeptides. XLIV. Potent synthetic S-peptide antagonists. *J. Am. Chem. Soc.* 92: 2900.

Hol, W.G.J. 1985. The role of the α-helix dipole in protein function and structure. *Prog. Biophys. Mol. Biol.* 45: 149.

Hol, W.G.J., P.T. van Duijnen, and H.J.C. Berendsen. 1978. The α-helix dipole and the properties of proteins. *Nature* 273: 443.

Kabsch, W. and C. Sander. 1984. On the use of sequence homologies to predict protein structure: Identical pentapeptides can have completely different conformations. *Proc. Natl. Acad. Sci.* 81: 1075.

Kim, P.S. and R.L. Baldwin. 1984. A helix stop signal in the isolated S-peptide of ribonuclease A. *Nature* 307: 329.

Kim, P.S., A. Bierzynski, and R.L. Baldwin. 1982. A competing salt bridge suppresses helix formation by the isolated C-peptide carboxylate of ribonuclease A. *J. Mol. Biol.* 162: 187.

Knight, K.L. and K. McEntee. 1986. Nucleotide binding by a 24-residue peptide from the RecA protein of *Escherichia coli. Proc. Natl. Acad. Sci.* 83: 9289.

Kopple, K.D., G.R. Wiley, and R. Tauke. 1973. A dihedral angle-vicinal proton coupling constant correlation for the α-β bond of amino acid residues. *Biopolymers* **12**: 627.

Lenstra, J.A., J. Hofsteenge, and J.J. Beintema. 1977. Invariant features of the structure of pancreatic ribonuclease. A test of different predictive models. *J. Mol. Biol.* **109**: 185.

Lim, V.I. 1974. Algorithms for prediction of α-helical and β-structural regions in globular proteins. *J. Mol. Biol.* **88**: 873.

Marchiori, F., G. Borin, L. Moroder, R. Rocchi, and E. Scoffone. 1972. Relation between structure and function in some partially synthetic ribonucleases S'. I. Kinetic determinations. *Biochim. Biophys. Acta* **257**: 210.

Maxfield, F.R. and H.A. Scheraga. 1975. The effect of neighboring charges on the helix forming ability of charged amino acids in proteins. *Macromolecules* **8**: 491.

Mitchinson, C. and R.L. Baldwin. 1986. The design and production of semisynthetic ribonucleases with increased thermostability by incorporation of S-peptide analogues with enhanced helical stability. *Proteins: Struct. Funct. Genet.* **1**: 23.

Pachler, K.G.R. 1964. Nuclear magnetic resonance study of some α-amino acids. II. Rotational isomerism. *Spectrochim. Acta* **20**: 581.

Perutz, M.F., J.C. Kendrew, and H.C. Watson. 1965. Structure and function of haemoglobin. II. Some relations between polypeptide chain configuration and amino acid sequence. *J. Mol. Biol.* **13**: 669.

Ramachandran, J., A. Berger, and E. Katchalski. 1971. Synthesis and physicochemical properties in aqueous solution of the sequential polypeptide poly(tyr-ala-glu). *Biopolymers* **10**: 1829.

Rico, M., E. Gallego, J. Santoro, F.J. Bermejo, J.L. Nieto, and J. Herranz. 1984. On the fundamental role of the Glu-2$^-$ ··· Arg-10$^+$ salt bridge in the folding of isolated ribonuclease A S-peptide. *Biochem. Biophys. Res. Commun.* **123**: 757.

Rico, M., J.L. Nieto, J. Santoro, F.J. Bermejo, J. Herranz, and E. Gallego. 1983. Low-temperature ^{1}H-NMR evidence of the folding of isolated ribonuclease S-peptide. *FEBS Lett.* **162**: 314.

Rico, M., J. Santoro, F.J. Bermejo, J. Herranz, J.L. Nieto, E. Gallego, and M.A. Jiménez. 1986. Thermodynamic parameters for the helix-coil thermal transition of ribonuclease S-peptide and derivatives from ^{1}H-NMR data. *Biopolymers* **25**: 1031.

Rose, G.D. 1979. Hierarchic organization of domains in globular proteins. *J. Mol. Biol.* **134**: 447.

Schechter, B., I. Schechter, J. Ramachandran, A. Conway-Jacobs, and M. Sela. 1971. The synthesis and circular dichroism of a series of peptides possessing the structure (L-tyrosyl-L-alanyl-L-glutamyl)$_n$. *Eur. J. Biochem.* **20**: 301.

Sheridan, R.P., R.M. Levy, and F.R. Salemme. 1982. α-helix dipole model and electrostatic stabilization of 4-α-helical proteins. *Proc. Natl. Acad. Sci.* **79**: 4545.

Shoemaker, K.R., P.S. Kim, E.J. York, J.M. Stewart, and R.L. Baldwin. 1987. Tests of the helix dipole model for stabilization of α-helices. *Nature* **326**: 563.

Shoemaker, K.R., P.S. Kim, D.N. Brems, S. Marqusee, E.J. York, I.M. Chaiken, J.M. Stewart, and R.L. Baldwin. 1985. Nature of the charged-group effect on the stability of the C-peptide helix. *Proc. Natl. Acad. Sci.* **82**: 2349.

Sueki, M., S. Lee, S.P. Powers, J.B. Denton, Y. Konishi, and H.A. Scheraga. 1984. Helix-coil stability constants for the naturally occurring amino acids in water. 22. Histidine parameters from random poly[(hydroxybutyl)glutamine-co-L-histidine]. *Macromolecules* **17**: 148.

Sundaralingam, M., W. Drendel, and M. Greaser. 1985. Stabilization of the long central helix of troponin C by intrahelical salt bridges between charged amino acid sidechains. *Proc. Natl. Acad. Sci.* **82**: 7944.

Wada, A. 1976. The α-helix as an electric macrodipole. *Adv. Biophys.* **9**: 1.

Wilson, P.T., T.L. Lentz, and E. Hawrot. 1985. Determination of the primary amino acid sequence specifying the α-bungarotoxin binding site on the α subunit of the acetylcholine receptor from *Torpedo californica*. *Proc. Natl. Acad. Sci.* **82**: 8790.

Wlodawer, A. and L. Sjölin. 1983. Structure of ribonuclease A: Results of joint neutron and X-ray refinement at 2.0-Å resolution. *Biochemistry* **22**: 2720.

The Evolution of Protein Structures

C. Chothia[*][†] and A.M. Lesk[*][‡]

*MRC Laboratory of Molecular Biology, Cambridge CB2 2QH, England; †Christopher Ingold Laboratory, University College London, London WC1H OAJ, England; ‡Biocomputing Programme, European Molecular Biology Laboratory, Heidelberg, Federal Republic of Germany

As proteins evolve, their amino acid sequences change. These changes can be large—so large that members of the same protein family may have less than one-fifth of the residues at homologous sites are identical. In most instances, the large sequence changes result in no more than a modification of functional properties. How do very different sequences give proteins with similar structures and functions? To answer this question we analyzed in detail the atomic structure of homologous proteins. We determined the effects of the sequence differences on the structures of these proteins. The analyses showed that sequence changes are accommodated by changes in structure.

In this paper, we describe in outline the structural changes that occur during evolution and discuss how their nature and extent are determined by the intrinsic properties of proteins. We also show how, in distantly related proteins, where the structural differences are large, their basic functional properties are maintained by the changes in different parts of the protein being coupled so as to conserve the geometry of the active site.

DIVERGENCES IN AMINO ACID SEQUENCES PRODUCE DIVERGENCES IN STRUCTURE

The comparison of related proteins, especially those with residue identities less than 30%, shows that although some regions have the same fold, other regions have quite different folds. The regions that retain the same fold include major elements of secondary structure and peptides that form the active site. The regions with quite different folds can include peripheral elements of secondary structure and peptides that link major elements. The differences in fold are often the result of insertions or deletions of amino acids in these regions. The exact extent of the regions with the same fold in homologous proteins—which we call the common core—can be found by superposing their atomic coordinates, region by region, and determining which residues occupy the same position in three dimensions.

We determined the size of the common core in 32 pairs of homologous structures: representatives of eight different protein families (Chothia and Lesk 1986). The results of these calculations are shown in Figure 1A. They show that as protein sequences diverge, the structures tend to have increasingly large regions with quite different folds. For proteins whose residue identity is 20%, the common core usually comprises only about half of each molecule.

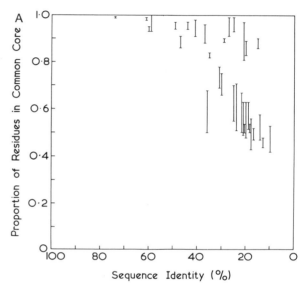

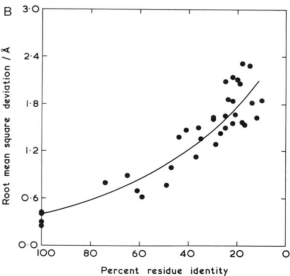

Figure 1. (A) The proportion of residues in the common core of homologous proteins (the regions with the same fold) plotted against the sequence identities of the residues in the common core. If two homologous proteins with n_1 and n_2 residues have c with the same fold, the proportions of each sequence in the common core are c/n_1 and c/n_2. For 32 pairs of homologous proteins from 8 protein families we plot the values of c/n_1 and c/n_2 linked by a bar. (B). The rms deviation in the position of the main-chain atoms of residues in the common cores of homologous pairs of proteins is plotted against their residue identities. (Reprinted, with permission, from Chothia and Lesk 1986.)

Although the common cores of homologous proteins have the same fold, the differences in their amino acid sequences produce some differences in structure. The overall extent of the differences can be measured by optimally superposing the common cores and calculating the root mean square (rms) difference in the position of their main-chain atoms, Δ. The common cores of the 32 pairs of homologous proteins have rms differences of 0.6–2.3 Å.

There will be a contribution to Δ from experimental error and from the effects of different molecular environments. These contributions can be estimated and distinguished by determining the rms difference in the coordinates of proteins for which structures have been determined in different crystal forms, or which have more than one molecule in the asymmetric unit of the crystal. The rms differences in coordinates of such proteins are 0.25–0.40 Å. These differences are about one-half to one-seventh of the differences between homologous structures.

The sizes of the differences in the structures of the common cores, Δ, are approximately related to the proportion of nonidentical residues, H, by the equation $\Delta = 0.40e^{1.87H}$ (Fig. 1B). This is a general relationship holding for all the protein families studied. Note, however, that the percentage of residues in the core varies with sequence homology and with protein family (Chothia and Lesk 1986). The exponential form of the relationship arises because closely related proteins differ primarily in surface residues, whereas distantly related proteins differ in both surface and buried residues. The mutation of buried residues usually produces larger structural changes than the mutation of surface residues.

EVOLUTIONARY CHANGE AND THE STRUCTURAL PROPERTIES OF PROTEINS

Conservation of Hydrophobicity and Hydrophilicity of Mutated Residues and of Protein Surfaces

A major contribution to the stability of proteins is the burial of hydrophobic side chains in protein interiors (Kauzmann 1959; Baldwin 1986). The comparison of the first protein structures, horse hemoglobin and sperm whale myoglobin, showed that during evolution the hydrophobic character of buried side chains was conserved. Perutz et al. (1965) identified some 33 sites that are buried in the two structures and that were occupied only by hydrophobic residues in the globin sequences then known. Later work, both on a much larger number of globin structures and sequences and on other protein families, confirmed their conclusions.

The sites in the globins at which the hydrophobicity of residues is conserved includes all those that on average have less than 10 Å^2 of accessible surface area, and certain of those with between 10 and 20 Å^2 (Lesk and Chothia 1980; Bashford et al. 1987). In a protein of N residues, where N is between 50 and 320, a good approximation of the number of such buried sites, N_b, is

given by the equation $N_b^{1/3} = N^{1/3} - 2.0$ (Janin 1979). This implies that the proportion of sites that are internal and that conserve their hydrophobicity is 20% for proteins of 100 residues and 33% for proteins of 300 residues. For those distantly related proteins in which large regions have quite different folds, certain of the residues that are buried in one structure will be on the surface in others. This means that the proportions of sites at which hydrophobicity is conserved will be lower.

The analysis of a large number of the globin sequence now known (226) shows that there are also constraints on the residue at some 32 surface sites (Bashford et al. 1987). At these sites there are charged, polar, Gly or Ala residues, but no medium or large hydrophobic residues, in 96–100% of the known sequences. These sites have high accessible surface areas in the known globin structures, mostly in excess of 50 Å^2. The conservation maintains protein solubility, prevents aggregation, and may facilitate the folding process.

The contribution to stability of protein structures made by hydrophobicity will be proportional to the surface area that becomes buried on folding. The surface area of an unfolded protein and the fractions of the surface that are buried and that remain accessible on folding are a function of molecular weight (M) (Chothia 1975; Janin 1976; Teller 1976). A recent survey of the accurately determined structures of monomeric proteins showed that the equation $A_s = 6.3M^{0.73}$ gives accessible surface area (A_s) within a few percent of those observed (Miller et al. 1987).

We have seen above how, as protein sequences diverge to low homologies, a substantial fraction of the polypeptide chain may take up a different fold (Fig. 1A). In most cases these regions differ not only in conformation, but in size; they are the regions where large insertions or deletions may occur. These structural changes take place within the restraint of maintaining the relationship between molecular weight and the proportions of the surface that become buried and that remain accessible.

For example, in Figure 2 we plot observed accessible surface area against molecular weight for four sets of homologous proteins. The four sets are T4, goose and hen egg lysozyme; tuna cytochrome c and bacterial cytochrome c; *Streptomyces griseus* protease B and bovine chymotrypsinogen; and plant plastocyanin and bacterial azurin. In these homologous proteins the common core forms approximately half of each structure (Chothia and Lesk 1986). Although these proteins differ in both conformation and size, the refolding of the various regions has occurred in a manner that maintains the relationship between accessible surface area and molecular weight (Fig. 2).

Allowed Conformations and Conformational Change

The extent to which the main-chain regions of helices and β sheets can respond to mutations by local con-

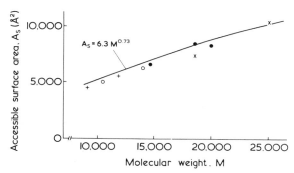

Figure 2. The conservation of the relation between accessible surface area and molecular weight during evolution. We plot here the accessible surface areas of two cytochromes (+), plastocyanin/azurin (○), three lysozymes (●), and two serine proteases (×). These homologous proteins are distantly related. They differ in size, have only about half of their structures in the same fold and have residue identities of 25% or less. For monomeric proteins the equations $A_s = 6.3 M^{0.73}$ gives A_s values to within a few percent of those observed (Miller et al. 1987).

formational change is governed by their intrinsic flexibility. Protein structures, refined at very high resolution, have given accurate descriptions of their conformations. Recently, two surveys have been made of the main-chain and side-chain torsion angles observed in these structures (Moult and James 1986; Ponder and Richards 1987). They confirm the dominating influence on conformation of the polypeptide chain of steric hindrance (Ramachandran and Sasisekharan 1968; Janin et al. 1978).

In α helices the observed ϕ, ψ values tightly cluster about $-65°$, $-41°$ with standard deviations of $\sim 6°$. In β sheets the observed ϕ, ψ values are not so localized and spread over the whole of the region normally allowed for extended polypeptide chains. This difference in conformational properties underlies their response to mutation.

The main-chain regions of helices change little in response to the changes in environment produced by mutations. If homologous helices in distantly related proteins are optimally superposed, the rms differences in position of main-chain atoms are usually 0.25–0.45 Å. Larger differences commonly occur only in residues at the ends of helices or in the few cases where helices are kinked by different amounts.

β sheets, on the other hand, can use their greater conformational flexibility to make local accommodation of mutations (Lesk and Chothia 1982). The local differences in the conformation of β sheets in distantly related proteins are shown by the high rms difference in the coordinates of their main-chain atoms: 1.5 Å (Lesk and Chothia 1986). Strands on the edge of β sheets also have the flexibility to accommodate insertions by the formation of β bulges (Richardson 1981).

Side chains, except for those that are long, usually have one of a small number of distinct conformations (Janin et al. 1978). Deviations from the mean torsion angles of these conformations are small: the standard

deviations of χ_1 are in most cases close to 10°, and that of χ_2 is commonly close to 15° (Moult and James 1986; Ponder and Richards 1987).

The comparison of side chains in homologous proteins shows that conserved residues have very similar conformations: 85% of the χ_1 and χ_2 values differ by less than 30°. The conservation of conformation by mutated residues is less common: only 60% have χ_1 values that differ by less than 30° (Table 1; Lesk and Chothia 1986). These results can be explained by the following argument. Most side chains in a protein make multiple interactions with the rest of the protein: each occupies a cage defined by its contacts with the main chain and the side chains of its nearest neighbors. Conserved residues, in general, have only part of their environment changed by a mutation and will only modify their conformations slightly in response to it. A mutated side chain, however, may not fit in the cage in the conformation of the old residue and so may switch to a different, more appropriate conformation.

Close Packing and the Relative Movement of Secondary Structures

Protein interiors are close packed: the mean volume occupied by a residue in the interior of proteins is the same as the volume of the residue in crystals of its amino acid. Cavities the size of water molecules or greater are rare and form no more than 1–2% of a protein's total volume (Klapper 1971; Richards 1974; Chothia 1975; Rashin et al. 1986).

Most of the residues buried within proteins occur at the interfaces between secondary structures. Close packing of the interiors means that mutations that alter the size of buried residues will perturb the packing of secondary structures: either their local conformation or their relative orientation or both will change in response. In this section, we discuss changes in packing geometry due to mutation. (Changes in local conformation were discussed in the previous section.)

The analysis of the three-dimensional structures of homologous proteins has provided detailed descrip-

Table 1. Differences in the χ Values of Homologous Residues

Range of torsion angle differences (degrees)	Proportion of residues in each range		
	conserved residues		mutated residues
	χ_1	χ_2	χ_1
0–20	0.82	0.73	0.52
20–40	0.05	0.14	0.07
40–60			0.04
60–80	0.05	0.08	0.04
80–100			0.05
100–120			0.11
120–140	0.09	0.05	0.10
140–160			0.04
160–180			0.02

Data taken from Lesk and Chothia (1986).

tions of the differences in the relative orientation of packed secondary structures. These differences arise from mutations at the interfaces between the secondary structures. Data on helix-helix packings have been obtained from the globins (Lesk and Chothia 1980) and cytochromes c (Chothia and Lesk 1985); data on helix-sheet packings from flavodoxins (Smith et al. 1983), and data on sheet-sheet packings from immunoglobin domains (Lesk and Chothia 1982) and azurin/plastocyanin (Chothia and Lesk 1982).

The differences in packing geometry can be defined by the following procedure. First, if A and B are two secondary structures that pack together in one protein and A′ and B′ are the homologous pair in a related protein, A′ is superposed on A. Any difference in packing geometry is then given by the additional shift and rotation required to superpose B′ onto B (Fig. 3).

In globins of low homology, differences in the geometry of packed helices of up to 7Å and 30° are observed, and differences of 3–5 Å are common (Fig. 3). For sheet-sheet packings, differences of 3.5–4.5 Å

are observed in plastocyanin/azurin and the virus coat proteins. In the two flavodoxins the helices that pack on the central β sheet differ by 2–3 Å (Smith et al. 1983).

The general nature of the larger of these structural differences can be rationalized in terms of the differences in the sizes of the residues that form the interface between secondary structures (Lesk and Chothia 1980).

Although in proteins of low homology the geometry of secondary structure packings can differ by several angstroms, the general pattern of residue-residue contacts is conserved. Homologous residues make homologous contacts (Fig. 3). This is because the free energies of native proteins are small; usually only 8–15 kcal per mole lower than those of the unfolded state (Privalov 1979). This means that the individual mutations, which cumulatively have created the large geometrical differences, can only involve energies of a few kilocalories. The small energies available for the accommodation of a mutation make most unlikely any alteration of the pattern of residue contacts and the consequent rearrangement of secondary structures.

The maintenance of the pattern of residue contacts limits the differences that can occur in the packing geometries. For example, in helix-helix packings the intercalation of side chains and the separation of residues on the face of a helix (Fig. 4) limit differences to shifts of 6–8 Å (Lesk and Chothia 1980).

The Refolding of the Regions between the Major Secondary Structures

Short and medium-sized turns have a restricted number of low-energy conformations because of the steric

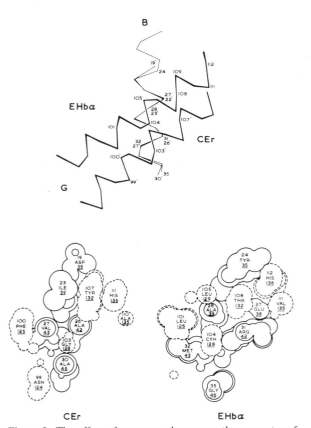

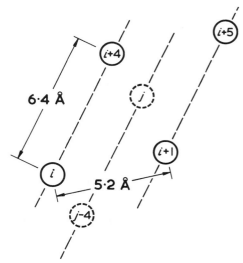

Figure 3. The effect of sequence changes on the geometry of close packed α helices. (*Top*) Cα atoms in B and G helices of the α subunit of horse hemoglobin and of an insect globin. The B helices are superposed. The G helices in the two proteins differ in their position relative to B. The differences in position arise from differences in the residues that form the helix-helix interface. (*Bottom*) Sections cut through space-filling models of the helix interfaces. Homologous residues have the same underlined numbers. (Reprinted, with permission, from Lesk and Chothia 1980.)

Figure 4. The packing of residues at part of a helix-helix interface. The circles labeled i, i + 1, i + 4, and i + 5 represent the position of four Cβ atoms on one helix; j and j + 4 represent the Cβ atoms on a second helix. The exact position of j will depend on the size and shape of the side chains of j and the four i residues. If mutations produce very large changes in these residues, j could move 6–8 Å without significantly changing the pattern of residue contacts.

limits on main-chain torsion angles. In certain cases, the length of the turn and the particular position of Gly, Pro, Asn, or Asp residues determine the conformation of the turn (Venkatachalam 1968; Lewis et al. 1973; Sibanda and Thornton 1985; Efimov 1986a,b). Mutation, insertion, or deletion in such turns will usually switch the conformations from one of these standard types to another.

Large turns in distantly related proteins can have very different conformations. Jones and Thirup (1986), however, found that such regions can be constructed from large substructures taken from quite unrelated proteins. This suggests that the number of conformations commonly available to large turns is also restricted. The nature of the restrictions and the number of allowed conformations remain to be determined.

Turn regions can play a role in the evolutionary changes in the major secondary structures. This is found in proteins formed by packed β sheets. In certain of these structures, such as the immunoglobins and serine proteases, the lateral insertion between the β sheets of a side chain from an external loop can compensate for reduction in the volume within the β sheets (Lesk and Chothia 1982; and unpubl. work).

CONSERVATION OF THE GEOMETRY OF ACTIVE SITES DURING EVOLUTION

The preceding sections have described how protein structures accommodate the sequence changes that have occurred during evolution. Changes in sequence produce changes in structure whose nature depends on the intrinsic properties of proteins. However, sequence changes that are readily accommodated by the protein might well produce changes in structure deleterious to function. Function will select from among the structurally possible changes only those whose effects are neutral or advantageous. The manner in which functional selection operates on structural changes can be found from the analysis of the active sites in distantly related proteins.

During the evolution of the globins, the divergences in their sequences have produced changes in the relative disposition of the helices. The geometries of the packed helices in distantly related globins differ by up to 7 Å and 30° and shifts of 3–6 Å are common (see above). But the residues that form the heme pocket in distantly related globins differ by much less (1–2 Å). The geometry of the heme pocket is conserved by the changes in helix packing having been coupled (Fig. 5). Thus, the sequence changes that have occurred during evolution and the consequent large structural changes have had only small effects on geometry of the residues that form the heme pocket (Lesk and Chothia 1980); small effects that may, of course, produce significant changes in functional properties.

A more complex form of coupled helix movements is found in the cytochrome c family (Chothia and Lesk 1985).

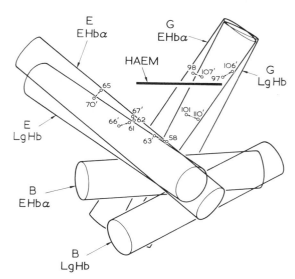

Figure 5. The arrangement of the helices and contact residues that form part of the heme pocket in the α subunit of horse hemoglobin (EHbα) and in lupin leghemoglobin (LgHb). The hemes in the two proteins are superposed. The positions of the B, G, and E helices are shown by cylinders. The positions of homologous pairs of residues that are in contact with the heme are indicated by open circles joined by arrows. The coupling of the shifts at the E-B and B-G helix interfaces keeps the residues that form the heme pocket in the same relative positions. (Reprinted, with permission, from Lesk and Chothia 1980.)

The bacterial and mammalian serine proteases are distantly related structures: only about half of their polypeptide chains have the same fold, and the residue identities in this half are 20–25%. These proteins, however, conserve the geometry of their catalytic residues and of those that form the primary substrate-binding sites. In a bacterial and a mammalian protease, 62 atoms, spread over a region some 15 × 20 Å, have an rms difference in position of 0.39 Å (Sielecki et al. 1979; Read et al. 1983).

The electron transport proteins, plastocyanin and azurin, have Cu-binding sites. Two of four residues that form the ligands of the Cu atom, a cysteine and a methionine, are in adjacent strands of a β sheet. A third ligand, histidine, is in the loop that links strands. Azurin has, relative to plastocyanin, two insertions before the histidine and one deletion after it:

Plastocyanin: C S P   H Q G A G M
Azurin: C T F P G H   S A   L M

The coupling of these insertions and deletions with changes in the conformation of the loop conserves the position of the histidine ligand (Fig. 6; Chothia and Lesk 1982).

In these proteins the necessity to maintain function makes evolutionary changes in protein structure interdependent: possible changes are restricted by their cumulative effect on the geometry of the active sites.

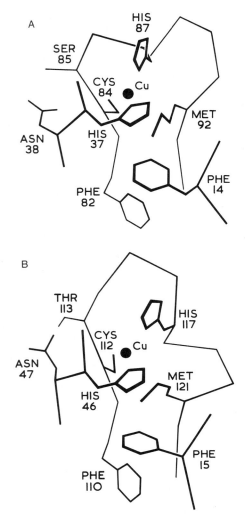

Figure 6. The Cu-binding site in the distantly related proteins plastocyanin (*A*) and azurin (*B*). The Cu ligands His-87 in plastocyanin and His-117 in azurin are in surface loops. These loops differ in size in the two proteins (see text). The differences in size are coupled with differences in conformation, so that in the two proteins the four atoms that bind the copper have the same geometry: the rms difference in their position in the two structures is 0.19 Å. (Reprinted, with permission, from Chothia and Lesk 1982.)

ACKNOWLEDGMENTS

We thank John Cresswell for the figure drawings, and The Royal Society, National Science Foundation, and the National Institute of General Medical Science for support.

REFERENCES

Baldwin, R.L. 1986. Temperature dependence of the hydrophobic interaction in protein folding. *Proc. Natl. Acad. Sci.* **83:** 8069.

Bashford, D., C. Chothia, and A.M. Lesk. 1987. Determinants of a protein fold: Unique features of the globin amino acid sequences. *J. Mol. Biol.* **196:** 199.

Chothia, C. 1975. Structural invariants in protein folding. *Nature* **254:** 304.

Chothia, C. and A.M. Lesk. 1982. Evolution of proteins formed by β-sheets. I. Plastocyanin and azurin. *J. Mol. Biol.* **160:** 309.

———. 1985. Helix movements and the reconstruction of the haem pocket during the evolution of the cytochrome *c* family. *J. Mol. Biol.* **182:** 151.

———. 1986. The relation between the divergence of sequence and structure in proteins. *EMBO J.* **5:** 823.

Efimov, A.V. 1986a. Standard conformations of polypeptide chains in the irregular regions of proteins. *Mol. Biol. (Mosc.)* **20:** 250.

———. 1986b. Standard structures in protein molecules. *Mol. Biol. (Mosc).* **20:** 329.

Janin, J. 1976. Surface area of globular proteins. *J. Mol. Biol.* **105:** 13.

———. 1979. Surface and inside volumes in globular proteins. *Nature* **277:** 491.

Janin, J., S. Wodak, M. Levitt, and B. Maigret. 1978. Conformation of amino acid side-chains in proteins. *J. Mol. Biol.* **125:** 357.

Jones, T.A. and S. Thirup. 1986. Using known substructures in protein model building and crystallography. *EMBO J.* **5:** 819.

Kauzmann, W. 1959. Some factors in the interpretation of protein denaturation. *Adv. Protein Chem.* **14:** 1.

Klapper, M.H. 1971. On the nature of the protein interior. *Biochim. Biophys. Acta* **229:** 557.

Lesk, A.M. and C. Chothia. 1980. How different amino acid sequences determine similar protein structures: The structure and evolutionary dynamics of the globins. *J. Mol. Biol.* **136:** 225.

———. 1982. Evolution of proteins formed by β-sheets. II. The core of the immunoglobulin domains. *J. Mol. Biol.* **160:** 325.

———. 1986. The response of protein structures to amino-acid sequence changes. *Philos. Trans. R. Soc. Lond. A Math. Phys. Sci.* **A317:** 345.

Lewis, P.N., F.A. Momany, and H.A. Scheraga. 1973. Chain reversals in proteins. *Biochim. Biophys. Acta* **303:** 211.

Miller, S., J. Janin, A.M. Lesk, and C. Chothia. 1987. Interior and surface of monomeric proteins. *J. Mol. Biol.* **196:** 641.

Moult, J. and M.N.G. James. 1986. An algorithm for determining the conformation of polypeptide segments in proteins by systematic search. *Proteins-Struct. Funct. Genet.* **1:** 146.

Perutz, M.F., J.C. Kendrew, and H.C. Watson. 1965. Structure and function of haemoglobin II. Some relations between polypeptide chain configuration and amino acid sequence. *J. Mol. Biol.* **13:** 669.

Ponder, J.W. and F.M. Richards. 1987. Tertiary templates for proteins: Use of packing criteria in the enumeration of allowed sequences for different structural classes. *J. Mol. Biol.* **193:** 775.

Privalov, P.L. 1979. Stability of proteins: Small globular proteins. *Adv. Protein Chem.* **33:** 167.

Ramachandran, G.N. and V. Sasisekharan. 1968. Conformation of polypeptides and proteins. *Adv. Protein Chem.* **23:** 284.

Rashin, A.A., M. Iofin, and B. Honig. 1986. Internal cavities and buried waters in globular proteins. *Biochemistry* **25:** 3619.

Read, R.J., M. Fujinaga, A.R. Sielecki, and M.N.G. James. 1983. Structure of the complex of *Streptomyces griseus* protease B and the third domain of the turkey ovomucoid inhibitor at 1.8-Å resolution. *Biochemistry* **22:** 4420.

Richards, F.M. 1974. The interpretation of protein structures: Total volume, group volume distribution and packing density. *J. Mol. Biol.* **82:** 1.

Richardson, J.S. 1981. The anatomy and taxonomy of protein structure. *Adv. Protein Chem.* **34:** 167.

Sibanda, B.L. and J.M. Thornton. 1985. β-Hairpin families in globular proteins. *Nature* **316:** 170.

Sielecki, A.R., W.A. Hendrickson, C.G. Broughton, L.T.J. Delbaere, G.D. Brayer, and M.N.G. James. 1979. Protein structure refinement: *Streptomyces griseus* serine protease A at 1.8 Å resolution. *J. Mol. Biol.* **134:** 781.

Smith, W.W., K.A. Pattridge, M.L. Ludwig, G.A. Petsko, D. Tsernoglou, M. Tanaka, and K.T. Yasunobu. 1983. Structure of oxidized flavodoxin from *Anacystis nidulans*. *J. Mol. Biol.* **165:** 737.

Teller, D.C. 1976. Accessible area, packing volumes and interaction surfaces of globular proteins. *Nature* **260:** 729.

Venkatachalam, C.M. 1968. Stereochemical criteria for polypeptides and proteins. V. Conformation of a system of three linked peptide units. *Biopolymers* **6:** 1425.

β Turns in Early Evolution: Chirality, Genetic Code, and Biosynthetic Pathways

J. Jurka and T.F. Smith

Dana Farber Cancer Institute and Department of Biostatistics,
Harvard School of Public Health, Boston, Massachusetts 02115

β Turns are defined as secondary structures in which four consecutive amino acid residues fold the polypeptide chain back upon itself by nearly 180° (Lewis et al. 1971, 1973). Turns are stabilized by energetically favorable interactions not present to the same degree in non-turns. In this sense, they should be considered to be distinguishable structures analogous to the α helix and β sheet.

More than a decade ago, Orgel (1977) discussed plausible presence of β turns in the early protein structures stabilized by the antiparallel β-pleated sheet. Recently, β turns have been proposed as a dominant element in the early evolution of life (Jurka and Smith 1987) that influenced formation of the genetic code and biosynthetic pathways of amino acids. In this hypothesis, β turns have been considered as autonomous elements somewhat independent of the context of any other protein structure. The following key assumptions underlie the idea: (1) The β turns studied currently are indistinguishable in terms of physicochemical properties from those synthesized billions of years ago; (2) the genetic code co-evolved with biosynthetic pathways of amino acids (Wong 1975); (3) in the evolving biosynthetic pathways, synthesis of precursors was likely to precede synthesis of products. This assumption is used to elucidate ancestor-descendant relations from the precursor-product relations between amino acids.

DATA AND ANALYSIS

Physicochemical Properties of β Turns

β Turns are intrinsically polar structures, and they appear to be stable in a variety of environments, including strong solvents (Rose et al. 1985). Several types of β turns have been distinguished (Venkatachalam 1968; Lewis et al. 1973). Two types of β turns (type I and type II) and their mirror images (type I' and II') predominate both in short peptides and proteins. Based on amino acid conformation at positions 2 and 3, Venkatachalam (1968) made an important distinction between homochiral and heterochiral sequences. Homochiral sequences were predicted to favor I(LL) and I'(DD) and heterochiral sequences were predicted to favor II(LD) and II'(DL) types of β turns. Glycine, having no side chain, was predicted to fit either the L or the D position. Heterochiral forms of turns have been found more often than the homochiral forms, in both synthetic and natural peptides (Toniolo 1980; Rose et

al. 1985). In globular proteins, type I of β turns predominates and is followed by types II, II', and I' (Milner-White and Poet 1987). It is not clear why in proteins type II turns are more than twice as common as the equivalent type II' (see Table 11 in Smith and Pease 1980). An interesting possibility is that type II turns are more compatible with L residues than type II'. If true, this could promote optical enrichment of type II β turns with L-amino acids and type II' with D-amino acids during early evolution.

As expected, glycine predominantly occupies "D" positions in both type II and II' β turns in globular proteins, and this is reflected in the amino acid composition at positions 2 and 3 of these turns. At these positions, glycine is four times as common as either of the next two most common amino acids, alanine and serine (Table 1a). The abundance of glycine is thus explained by the inherent sterical constraints in β turns. It can also be assumed that preferences for amino acids other than glycine are determined by the physicochemical properties of β turns, in particular by their intrinsic polarity. As can be seen from Table 1b, the first five amino acids listed account for almost 50% of the total number of amino acids in the β turns of 29 proteins. The amino acids most common in the contemporary β turns were likely to be most preferred by the earliest β turns.

Evolutionary Relationships

The amino acid composition of β turns shows some correlations to structure of the genetic code. In the genetic code arginine, aspartic acid, asparagine, glutamic acid, glycine, lysine, and serine are coded for by the RRN type of codon (R being either purine nucleotide and N representing any nucleotide). Serine and arginine are also assigned to four non-RRN codons (Table 1b). With the exception of glutamic acid and arginine, these amino acids are among the most common in β turns (Table 1). Among non-RRN amino acids, most abundant are alanine, proline, and threonine. Note that none of the RRN amino acids are β-sheet formers (Chou and Fasman 1978), but rather are either indifferent or β-sheet breakers. Histidine and proline are the only β-sheet breakers outside the RRN group. Given that early β turns had amino acid preferences similar to the contemporary ones, it can be concluded that the assignment of amino acids to the

Table 1. Frequencies of Amino Acids in β Turns and their Codon Types

| Position 2 and 3 of type II(II′)[a] | | Overall[b] | | |
amino acid	number of	amino acid	number of	codon type
Gly	40	Gly	194	GGN
Ala	10	Ser	155	AGY, UCN
Ser	10	Asp	118	GAY
Asn	9	Asn	106	AAY
Asp	8	Lys	103	AAR
Lys	5	Ala	85	GCN
Pro	5	Pro	79	CCN
Arg	4	Thr	79	ACN
Met	3	Leu	62	CUN, UUR
Phe	3	Tyr	62	UAY
Thr	3	Val	53	GUN
Cys	2	Glu	51	GAR
Val	2	Gln	46	CAR
Gln	1	Arg	40	AGR, CGN
Glu	1	His	36	CAY
His	1	Cys	33	UGY
Tyr	1	Ile	32	AUY, AUA
Ile	0	Phe	30	UUY
Leu	0	Trp	22	UGG
Trp	0	Met	13	AUG

Modified from Jurka and Smith (1987). R – purine, Y – pyrimidine, N – any base.

[a] Frequencies of amino acids at positions 2 and 3 of type II(II′) β turns from globular proteins (after Smith and Pease 1980).

[b] The overall amino acid frequencies at all four positions of β turns for 29 proteins as compiled by Chou and Fasman (1978).

RRN type of codon was affected by selection for the β turns.

The amino acid composition of β turns is also correlated with the precursor-product relationships in the biosynthetic pathways of amino acids. Two groups of amino acids can be distinguished with regard to their position in biosynthetic pathways (Wong 1975). The first group, hereafter referred to as a core group, includes alanine, aspartic acid, glutamic acid, glycine, and serine. These amino acids are mutually interconvertible with each other via metabolic cycles, as indicated by double-headed arrows in Figure 1. Single-headed arrows indicate unidirectional precursor-product relationships. As precursors to other amino acids, the core amino acids were likely to exist earlier in the evolution of biosynthetic pathways than their products. The core amino acids, with the exception of alanine, are assigned to the RRN codons. Therefore, selection for the RRN-encoding and β-turn-preferred amino acids may have been linked early in the history of life before final fixation of the genetic code.

There are two important amino acids outside the RRN code that require separate consideration: (1) alanine, placed at the very beginning of the biosynthetic pathways, and present in large amounts in the simulated prebiotic syntheses; and (2) proline, which is fundamental for the formation of many modern β turns. In terms of their abundance in β turns, alanine and proline immediately follow the RRN amino acids (Table 1b); however, biosynthesis of proline seems to be implemented later than biosynthesis of its precursor glutamic acid, which is assigned to the GAR codons.

Alanine and proline can be included in the above proposal if one assumes that they were used for synthesis of β-turn-forming peptides before the evolution of

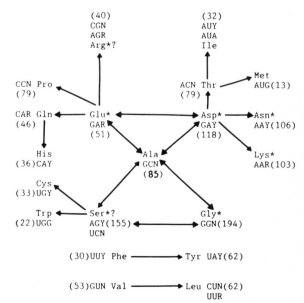

Figure 1. Evolutionary map of the genetic code (Wong 1975) with the amino acid composition of β turns (Chou and Fasman 1978) in parentheses. Biosynthetic interconversions and precursor-product relations are indicated by double-headed and single-headed arrows, respectively. Amino acids assigned to codons with purines in the first two positions are indicated by asterisks, followed by question marks if more than one type of codon is present. (R) Purine; (Y) pyrimidine; (N) any base.

the majority of the precursor-product relations in biosynthetic pathways of amino acids. This requires considering the family of codons coding for these amino acids as members of the code that has originated even earlier than the RRN code. The family includes: GCN(Ala), GGN(Gly), (CCN)Pro, and CGN(Arg). The amino acids coded for by the first two codons are readily available under simulated prebiotic conditions. Proline has been found in concentrations ranging from 0.3% of the glycine content in an electric discharge synthesis to 22% in the Murchison meteorite synthesis (Weber and Miller 1981). There is no established prebiotic synthesis of arginine; however, it has been suggested that arginine replaced ornithine in the genetic code at an advanced stage of evolution (Jukes 1973). Trace amounts of ornithine have been found in electric discharge experiments. Early expansion of biosynthetic pathways coincided with the addition of adenine to the G and/or C code, which gave rise to the RRN code. At a certain time, catabolism of proline became included in biosynthetic pathways without affecting its original assignment to CCN codons. The introduction of arginine could be more dramatic if it indeed replaced its hypothetical predecessor encoded by the CGN codons. Following this logic, the "youngest" amino acids are those included after the appendage of uracil to the genetic code. These "young" amino acids are mostly nonpolar and crucial for the formation of tertiary structures of globular proteins. Possible mechanisms for the early evolution of globular proteins have been outlined elsewhere (Jurka 1977; Jurka et al. 1982).

DISCUSSION

Beginning with the early work by Woese et al. (1966), it was observed that polar and nonpolar amino acids are clearly separated within the genetic code. After Sonneborn (1965), it has repeatedly been suggested that this separation reflects evolutionary adaptation to minimize damaging effects of mutations on protein structures (Epstein 1966; Goldberg and Wittes 1966; Volkenstein 1966; Wolfenden et al. 1979). The above hypothesis opens a way for an alternative explanation. The separation between amino acids with different polarities can be considered as a historical record of evolution leading from the inherently polar β turns to globular protein structures with a polar surface and a nonpolar interior. It was only after the evolution of the globular protein structure that this historically established structural dichotomy of the genetic code began playing a conservative role.

The biological role of β turns in early evolution remains to be established. Possibilities range from their role in specific binding of substrates diluted in the environment to catalysis of the intracellular metabolism. One of the prospective areas for experimental exploration may be interactions of β turns with metals. Extensive research on metal ion complexes with dipeptides (Siegel and Martin 1982) has established solid foundations for similar studies on longer, β-turn-form-

ing peptides. Possible involvement of β turns in contemporary biological function is increasingly well studied. So far, few definite examples of the functional role of β turns exist. However, based on indirect evidence, their participation in biological processes seems to be extensive (for a review, see Smith and Pease 1980).

In summary, the amino acids that are most abundant in β turns are found to be assigned to a well-defined part of the genetic code. This group of amino acids contains key biosynthetic precursors to other amino acids. Evolution of the early genetic code and biosynthetic pathways of amino acids was likely to be driven by selection for β turns. Globular proteins appear to prefer type II β turns over type II′ β turns. The testable prediction is that it reflects different compatibility of these turns with the L residues.

ACKNOWLEDGMENT

We acknowledge Ms. Karen Gruskin for critically reading the manuscript.

REFERENCES

Chou, P.Y. and G.D. Fasman. 1978. Prediction of the secondary structure of proteins from their amino acid sequence. *Adv. Enzymol.* **47**: 45.

Epstein, C.J. 1966. Role of the amino acid "code" and of selection for conformation in the evolution of proteins. *Nature* **210**: 25.

Goldberg, A.L. and R.E. Wittes. 1966. Genetic code: Aspects of organization. *Science* **153**: 420.

Jukes, T.H. 1973. Arginine as an evolutionary intruder into protein synthesis. *Biochem. Biophys. Res. Commun.* **53**: 709.

Jurka, J.W. 1977. On replication of nucleic acids in relation to the evolution of the genetic code and of proteins. *J. Theor. Biol.* **68**: 515.

Jurka, J. and T.F. Smith. 1987. β-Turn-driven early evolution: The genetic code and biosynthetic pathways. *J. Mol. Evol.* **25**: 15.

Jurka, J., Z. Kolosza, and I. Roterman. 1982. Globular proteins, GU wobbling, and the evolution of the genetic code. *J. Mol. Evol.* **19**: 20.

Lewis, P.N., F.A. Momany, and H.A. Scheraga. 1971. Folding of polypeptide chains in proteins: A proposed mechanism of folding. *Proc. Natl. Acad. Sci.* **68**: 2293.

———. 1973. Folding of polypeptide chains in proteins. *Biochim. Biophys. Acta* **303**: 211.

Milner-White, E.J. and R. Poet. 1987. Loops, bulges, turns and hairpins in proteins. *Trends Biochem. Sci.* **12**: 189.

Orgel, L.E. 1977. β-Turns and the evolution of protein synthesis. In *The organization and expression of the eukaryotic genome. Proceedings of the International Symposium,* May 1976, Teheran (ed. E.M. Bradbury and K. Javaherian), p. 499. Academic Press, London.

Rose, G.D., L.M. Gierasch, and J.A. Smith. 1985. Turns in peptides and proteins. *Adv. Protein Chem.* **37**: 100.

Siegel, H. and B.R. Martin. 1982. Coordinating properties of the amide bond. Stability and structure of metal ion complexes of peptides and related ligands. *Chem. Rev.* **82**: 385.

Smith, J.A. and L.G. Pease. 1980. Reverse turns in proteins. *Crit. Rev. Biochem.* **8**: 315.

Sonneborn, R.M. 1965. Degeneracy of the genetic code: Extent, nature, and genetic implications. In *Evolving genes and proteins* (ed. V. Bryson and H.J. Vogel), p. 377. Academic Press, New York.

Toniolo, C. 1980. Intramolecularly hydrogen-bonded peptide conformations. *Crit. Rev. Biochem.* **9:** 1.

Venkatachalam, C.M. 1968. Stereochemical criteria for polypeptides and proteins. V. Conformation of a system of three linked peptide units. *Biopolymers* **6:** 1425.

Volkenstein, M.V. 1966. The genetic coding of protein structure. *Biochim. Biophys. Acta* **110:** 421.

Weber, A.L. and S.L. Miller. 1981. Reason for the occurrence of the twenty coded protein amino acids. *J. Mol. Evol.* **17:** 273.

Woese, C.R., D.H. Dugre, W.C. Saxinger, and S.A. Dugre. 1966. The molecular basis for the genetic code. *Proc. Natl. Acad. Sci.* **55:** 966.

Wolfenden, R.V., P.M. Cullis, and C.C.F. Southgate. 1979. Water, protein folding, and the genetic code. *Science* **206:** 575.

Wong, T.F. 1975. A co-evolution theory of the genetic code. *Proc. Natl. Acad. Sci.* **72:** 1909.

Gene Duplication and the Origin of Repetitive Protein Structures

A.D. McLachlan

MRC Laboratory of Molecular Biology, Cambridge, England CB2 2QH

EVOLUTION TRACED THROUGH CHANGING STRUCTURES

Sequence and Structure

Molecular evolution is a tantalizing science because we have to rely on the proteins still extant in organisms that are alive today to deduce the development of life from simpler beginnings. There are many missing links in this history, and we often cannot be sure what really happened in the past. One way to piece together the history of proteins is from their amino acid sequences, gene sequences, and intron-exon junctions. But these sequences can evolve fast and then they soon diverge beyond recognition. They cannot always take us back very far. X-ray analysis of proteins gives us structural clues that reach back into the even more distant past. This is for the simple reason that the three-dimensional folding pattern of the protein backbone evolves extremely slowly and an ancestral pattern can still be picked out long after the amino acid sequence has thrown off all trace of its origin. X-ray structures give a gallery of historical snapshots from which we can see how some of the most efficient types of enzyme action developed.

The design of a typical successful enzyme involves at least four elements: a stable structural core or framework to separate the reactants from their watery surroundings, a binding site that recognizes the substrate and holds it in place, a set of properly positioned reactive groups, and last, the possibility of allosteric control mechanisms. The solved crystal structures suggest that the two most difficult stages in the evolution of enzymes were the early ones: to learn to fold into a framework and then to make a binding pocket. Once these problems were solved for a particular enzyme type, such as the primitive serine protease, the organic chemistry of the active sites and their control mechanisms could develop in several different ways to produce a whole gene family of related proteins.

Thus, the earliest steps of enzyme evolution, when the framework was first laid down, were probably the same as in nonenzymes. We can therefore learn about this stage of evolution by studying the architecture of all kinds of protein molecules.

Architectural Motifs

Natural selection has preserved those forms of protein architecture that make the best use of stable structural elements, based on the α-helix and β-sheet hydrogen bonding patterns and the exclusion of water from a hydrophobic core. The optimal packing together of these elements builds up typical geometrical motifs that generate a few major classes of protein domain (Levitt and Chothia 1976): all-helix, all-sheet, and helices that alternate with parallel strands of sheet (parallel α/β). Some of the simpler combinations of secondary structure arose quite independently in many different molecules: four-helix bundles, twisted β-hairpins, Greek keys, and the like. But these small motifs are often too unstable by themselves to form a good framework for an enzyme. The next key step in enzyme evolution was to put together the smaller motifs into large stable domains that could resist proteolysis and denaturation and could form binding sites for large substrates. Parallel α/β domains tended to grow by addition of new α/β units at the edges, but all-β domains often achieved a closed structure by fusing together several interlocked subdomains.

The compact structural domains that exist today are the few survivors out of many earlier attempts, and they have been selected not only through their functional efficiency, but also for historical reasons. Out of all the potentially foldable geometric forms, the successful proteins have been those that went forward fastest in the race to improve. They are therefore well represented by the products of those special evolutionary processes that are the most rapid and effective creators of new and improved domain structures.

Repetitive Elements

The ancestral relationships between protein domains are often hard to trace because of "missing links." But there is one particular mode of evolution that can be followed more easily. This is tandem gene duplication, which produces two or more copies of the same protein fold within a single polypeptide chain. Tandem duplication often produces pseudosymmetric structures with internal symmetry axes, and these structures themselves have special functional advantages. They combine the stability of a single chain with some of the structural flexibility of a multiple-subunit enzyme made of nearly identical units.

Proteins with repetitive structures have many different uses: cooperative ligand binding, substrate clefts that open and close, domains built of subdomains, linear assemblies with large-scale molecular spacings, and multiheaded active sites. We shall look at some examples later in this paper.

THE DEVELOPMENT OF COMPLEX STRUCTURES

Short-term Evolution by Piecemeal Growth

In the early days of protein structure analysis, about 1970, most of the known enzyme structures could be described in rather simple terms. They had a nearly rigid structural core of helix and β sheet held together by a network of hydrogen bonds and tightly packed with internal hydrophobic residues. The outside surface of the molecule was covered with polar and charged groups. The active site consisted of a hollowed-out binding region surrounded by reactive groups attached to the core. The evolution within a closely related protein family, such as chymotrypsin, elastase, and trypsin, seemed to follow a pattern of piecemeal growth, in which small surface loops might be added or removed from time to time, but the core remained invariable. The chain might grow at the amino or carboxyl ends, and the active site residues might change to allow an adaptation of the catalytic function, but the overall architecture remained fixed. A typical enzyme would evolve from the interior outward, always retaining a biological function, which changed as a result of small structural steps (McLachlan 1972).

This view of protein evolution now looks much too conservative and short term. It does nothing to account for the complexity and variety of many molecular structures. As we move up the evolutionary scale from primitive organisms to higher organisms, we find many examples of a trend toward greater complexity in protein molecules. Individual molecules become bigger and more complicated in structure: enzymes like alcohol dehydrogenase, virus proteins like influenza hemagglutinin, and fibrous proteins like collagen and keratin. Single proteins also give rise to families where a great variety of molecules have descended by gene duplication from a common ancestor. Other proteins have clearly been constructed by joining several gene products in series. Evolution by point mutations and deletions alone is much too restricted and too slow to have produced the proteins that we observe today.

Major Genetic Events

The origin of new proteins depends on major genetic events that can combine or rearrange preexisting fragments and develop more elaborate functions from them. The genetic mechanisms by which changes take place in proteins can be divided into two main classes.

(1) Minor steps. These are single point mutations, as allowed by the genetic code, or small deletions and insertions of just a few amino acids at loops in the structure. Although even such small steps may lead to great changes in the activity of an enzyme by allowing new ligands to bind or subunits to aggregate, the overall domain structure is left almost unaltered and is still recognizable after many such steps have occurred. For example, in the evolution of the hemoglobins, the arrangement of the α helices has remained almost un-changed, despite considerable adjustments to the positions of helix-helix contacts and to the angles between the helices.

(2) Major steps. Radical reorganization of the genetic material takes place, leading to a new or modified protein of very different character. Massive deletions, insertions of whole new domains, new splicing and chain initiation sites in the introns or exons, tandem duplication, and even cyclic permutations may take place. The major steps are evolutionary discontinuities that provide the opportunity for structural rearrangements on a larger scale. They realize new possibilities that were latent in the original component structural elements. Without major steps, many proteins would reach an evolutionary stagnation point in which every point mutation was slightly harmful.

The results of X-ray crystallography show that many protein families are closely related to one another. Even though there must be many as yet unknown structural motifs and families still to be discovered, it is already clear that the most successful motifs are used over and over again with many variations and combinations. What is it that distinguishes these motifs from others?

The process of evolution depends on the interplay between two factors. The first is the *opportunity* provided by random genetic events. The second is the *improvement in fitness* as tested out by natural selection, where the protein is assessed in its natural environment in the organism. In the evolution of proteins, we find that certain pathways of change are rather common, so that there are preferred routes of evolution that seem to produce distinct advantages.

EVOLUTIONARY EXPERIENCE ACCUMULATES STEP BY STEP

Every organism carries in its genes a great deal of precise genetic information that is coded in its nucleic acids. As pure information, the content is neutral, in the sense that the statistical entropy or binary information content is the same for a highly developed protein as it is for a random coil polypeptide of the same length. The distinctive feature of the genetic information in a viable organism is that it is expressed in terms of the structures of protein molecules, which must operate in their natural environments. Every protein has gradually become adapted by the step-by-step improvement and refinement of its function over millions of years, so that its DNA carries the memory of the organism's evolutionary experience throughout the past. The adaptation has been acquired in the operating environment of the protein, and is only effective within this customary context. Therefore, the genetic information only has its full value within the whole organism and its world. Because adaptation takes so long, the acquired experience is an extremely valuable quantity. Any evolutionary mechanism that produces a new protein function must also preserve those functions that exist already. For this reason, it is unlikely that viable new proteins evolve ready-made from random DNA or from pseudogenes. Instead, they develop by accretion, adding new functions on top of old ones, and new structural features that lean on an old, established framework. Hence, we find that the most common trick of evolution is to use an old protein structure or a piece of structure in some new and unexpected way, but without destroying the existing useful properties of the molecule. Thus, evolution is extremely conservative in its structural aspects. The most successful pathways of change are those in which new functions can be acquired most rapidly and reliably. In structural terms this often means evolution by putting existing parts together in new ways.

New functions are learned by trial and error, through a sequence of increasingly developed ancestors. For example, an enzyme must learn first how to fold itself into a stable domain, then how to bind a substrate, how to place catalytic groups correctly on its surface, how to aggregate several subunits together, and then how to regulate itself by means of effector molecules that bind between the subunits and control the quaternary structure. The evolutionary pathway will be a series of unpredictable jumps, but it is a branching process in which there are only a limited number of possible options at each stage. In general, the most successful evolutionary pathway is likely to be one in which the functions that were learned most recently do not upset those that are already established. Those protein molecules that successfully fix their simpler functions before going on to more elaborate adaptation will tend to evolve more consistently than those that try to achieve a giant leap forward.

SYMMETRY AND THE DEVELOPMENT OF COOPERATIVE OXYGEN BINDING IN HEMOGLOBIN

The hemoglobin molecule illustrates the stepwise evolution of oxygen binding and the relationship between cooperative oxygen binding and a symmetrical structure.

The respiratory proteins that use heme to carry oxygen are a very ancient family, whose lineage can be traced back from man and the mammals to insects, the leghemoglobin of plants, and even to bacteria (*Vitreoscilla*). X-ray analysis shows that all these molecules are built up from the same basic arrangement of α helices grouped around a heme pocket, but their functions have developed from very simple beginnings in the primitive species to a subtle and elaborate regulatory mechanism in human hemoglobin (Perutz 1970; Fermi et al. 1984; Shaanan 1983). We can trace part of the evolution of this mechanism and see how it has built up step-by-step as a result of successive small improvements.

The early globins are single-chain proteins that simply carry a heme group buried in a pocket of hydrophobic amino acids. The pocket protects it from oxidation and allows reversible binding of oxygen. Sperm whale myoglobin is typical of this stage. Fishes have adapted to a wide range of conditions by making several single-chain variants with different oxygen affinities. Later hemoglobins have acquired the power to bind four oxygen molecules cooperatively, to respond to the acidity and carbon dioxide content of the red cell (through the Bohr effect), and to regulate their oxygen affinity by means of the level of organic phosphate in the blood.

(1) The first step toward cooperative behavior is seen in lamprey hemoglobin, where the chains associate and dissociate according to the oxygen pressure. The dissociation is brought about through conformational changes transmitted to the protein surface by movements of the iron atom in the heme. This developed into a dimer-tetramer equilibrium system with four identical chains in a symmetrical structure.

(2) Gene duplication gave rise to two kinds of subunit α and β that acquired the power to aggregate in two different ways in the oxy and deoxy states (Monod's relaxed and tense forms).

(3) An elaborate system of salt bridges formed between the ends of the chains, allowing the molecules to respond to CO_2 and hydrogen ions.

(4) Some mammals acquired the power to bind 2,3-diphosphoglycerate as a regulator in a cavity between the two β chains. Several species then developed special fetal hemoglobins that were modified so as not to bind diphosphoglycerate, and hence had a higher oxygen affinity.

The development followed a number of well-marked stages. Each of them could only usefully begin after the previous step was concluded. For example, although many primitive hemoglobins show a response to pH, the very efficient mechanism for doing this in human hemoglobin today could not develop in its present form before the separation of the α and β chains.

Subunit Association and Cooperative Effects

Monod et al. (1965) proposed that ligands generally produce cooperative effects in proteins indirectly, by altering the mutual interactions between subunits. In hemoglobin, the high-affinity oxy quaternary structure corresponds to their "relaxed" (R) state, since the four chains are weakly linked and dissociate easily. The low-affinity deoxy form is their strongly associated and "tense" (T) state and is constrained by the salt bridges and subunit contacts. The difference in oxygen affinity between the forms is produced by lowering the affinity of the deoxy structure. In fact, the oxy tetramer, the free chains, and the monomeric hemoglobins all have high affinity, and it is the deoxy form in the T state that is unique, having unusually low affinity. Diphosphoglycerate binds only to the T form and stabilizes the low-affinity state. It delays the R → T transition till late in the oxygen-binding sequence.

A tetramer of four identical protein subunits will normally have 222 symmetry, and there will be three kinds of contact regions, across the three two-fold axes.

Why is this tetrahedral arrangement so common, and what advantages does it offer? Monod distinguishes two types of pairing between subunits, isologous and heterologous. Isologous pairing gives contacts in complementary pairs across a two-fold symmetry axis. It is the mode most likely to evolve, as one mutation can lead to two contact regions in a single step. Many proteins form dimers, perhaps for this reason.

The path of evolution to a tetramer could then be as follows: First the dimer forms, giving one bonding region and one two-fold axis. Later on, pairs of dimers couple, initially giving a 222 tetramer with two strong and two weak bonding regions. At this point the evolution of hemoglobin took a new path toward a structure with lower symmetry. Two steps were necessary. One was to differentiate two kinds of subunit, α and β. There was then only one exact symmetry axis, and two approximate ones. The new bonding regions were of four types: $\alpha1-\beta1=\alpha2-\beta2$, $\alpha1-\beta2=\alpha2-\beta1$, $\alpha1-\alpha2$, and $\beta1-\beta2$. The second step was to form an asymmetrical quaternary structure from these four nearly identical subunits. This can be done in a tetramer by sliding two adjacent subunits in opposite directions parallel to a two-fold symmetry axis.

In a tetramer of precisely identical subunits, the direction of sliding would be indeterminate, but in hemoglobin the differences between the α and β chains produce the required sense of direction. The oxy form is close to 222 symmetry, but deoxy is asymmetric. The advantage of an asymmetric tetramer is seen if we consider that the subunits in a protein behave in a first approximation like rigid bodies. In a proper 222 tetramer, any rearrangement that conserves the full symmetry requires four symmetry-related motions, and, in general, all three types of bonds rearrange simultaneously. It is difficult to evolve such a concerted motion, but easy to develop a symmetry-breaking rearrangement that does not disturb the strong contacts ($\alpha1-\beta1$ or $\alpha2-\beta2$ in hemoglobin). The molecule needed only to adapt itself to allow alternative modes of packing at one pair of interfaces ($\alpha1-\beta2$ or $\alpha2-\beta1$). The loss of 222 symmetry allows large relative movements of the chains and alters the interactions between the salt bridges at their ends. The reshaping of the tetramer also allows the formation of a central binding site for a single molecule of 2,3-diphosphoglycerate in a crevice between the β chains.

THE EVOLUTIONARY ADVANTAGES OF TANDEM DUPLICATION

Tandem duplication has occurred in so many proteins that the process clearly has considerable advantages. There are at least three ways in which duplication can be useful. (Here we also include triplication, quadruplication, and other more complicated events.) (1) The repeated units effectively form a locked-together dimeric structure with properties like those of a multi-subunit enzyme: increased stability, new cooperative functions, and formation of binding

sites in a cleft. (2) Growth of long repetitive structures, such as the fibrous proteins, where a series of slightly different variations on a basic motif can be used to build up precisely determined large aggregates by a vernier method. Examples are tropomyosin, myosin, and paramyosin. (3) Production of multiple binding sites in series, which produce either more efficient or more specific binding effects. Examples are the multiple binding sites in serum albumin and the specific DNA-binding "fingers" of the TFIIIA transcription factor. We shall now describe some of these proteins in more detail.

REPEATED STRUCTURES THAT HAVE EVOLVED FROM DIMERS

The Doubled Iron-sulfur Cluster of Ferredoxin

The idea has been put forward (Jukes 1966) that in the earliest stages of evolution the primitive proteins began with the production of repeating amino acid sequences composed of a large number of similar segments. Thus, a large protein could be built up by repeating a small number of basic motifs, which might form structural building blocks for the whole large structure. It was assumed that the repeating amino acid sequence is coded for by a repeating DNA sequence, which is itself formed by duplicating again and again short pieces from the original sequence. Bacterial proteins might then be expected to be more primitive and repetitive than those from mammals.

Actually, the observations up till now show the opposite: the most striking repetitive and complicated protein structures are found in the products of recent evolution, such as the plasma proteins, rather than in the ancient primitive molecules. However, the possibility remains that the primitive proteins did indeed evolve by repetition, but that later structural changes have covered up most traces of these early and simple structural forms. (The four-helix bundle protein hemerythrin, the iron-carrier rubredoxin, and the NAD-binding domain of lactate dehydrogenase may be examples of such a history.)

The bacterial ferredoxins have been cited as evidence for this theory, since the second half of the amino acid sequence is an almost exact duplicate of the first, and each half has a regular periodic arrangement of cysteines. Ferredoxin of *Peptococcus aerogenes* contains two identical clusters of iron and sulfur buried within a small protein. The amino acid sequence consists of two repeating pieces of 27 amino acids each, and was recognized as an example of tandem duplication long before the crystal structure was solved. A surprising fact about the structure (Adman et al. 1973) is that the two halves of the chain do not form separate globular iron-sulfur clusters, as might have been expected. Instead, each cluster uses both sequence halves in a cooperative way and the repeated chain fold has two-fold symmetry, like that of a dimer. If we assume that the ancestral half-sequence could form a single globular cluster by itself, then the present-day structure could only have evolved by undergoing a radical rearrangement. It is more natural to assume that the two halves of today's chain were originally two parts of a molecular dimer in solution, and that these halves adapted themselves to fit together long before the chain length doubled (Weeds and McLachlan 1974). The sequence of evolutionary steps was probably: (1) single cluster, (2) dimer cluster, (3) double-chain pair. The gene duplication event that led to the double-chain pair was therefore taking advantage of a structural adaptation that had already taken place—the ability to fold cooperatively about a local dyad axis.

The small double-headed protease inhibitor, Bowman-Birk inhibitor of the peanut, reflects almost the same evolutionary history (Suzuki et al. 1987). Here the sequence repeat builds two reactive sites at opposite ends of the molecule, which act completely independently. The backbone is made of two β hairpins placed back-to-back around a dyad axis and crosslinked by disulfide bridges.

This pattern of dimerization followed by duplication seems to be a common strategy of evolution (McLachlan and Walker 1977) and has been proposed independently by Tang et al. (1978) to account for the spectacular double-lobed structure of penicillopepsin. Much larger proteins that show a two-lobed structure are the calcium-binding protein parvalbumin from muscle (Kretsinger and Nockolds 1973) and the carrier protein rhodanese (Bergsma et al. 1975).

Paired Calcium Sites in Parvalbumin

In 1972, Kretsinger crystallized and solved the structure of a small calcium-binding protein from fish muscle, called parvalbumin (Kretsinger and Nockolds 1973). The results were interesting, because this protein was the first crystal structure from the important calmodulin family of calcium-regulated proteins, and the molecule had a simple and rather symmetrical structure. The two calcium sites, which are close together at one end of the molecule, have very similar amino acid sequences and are formed from two similar structural motifs of the type (helix A:site S:helix B), where a pair of α helices fold back on one another and form a cage of negatively charged oxygens at the turn. The protein shows unmistakable signs of tandem duplication, as the pair of calcium sites are arranged around a local two-fold symmetry axis and have almost the same conformation. A significant feature of the parvalbumin structure is that the paired sites are coupled together by a short strand of antiparallel β sheet with two buried Ile residues in contact across the two-fold axis. This feature shows that the folding of the two sites is interdependent: neither can fold properly unless its two-fold partner is also folded. Two other helices in the molecule do not form a third site, but their arrangement suggested that they were remnants of an ancient one. Later Collins found a still more interesting sequence in troponin C, which showed that gene quadru-

plication has taken place in this family, and there are two pairs of calcium sites in many of the calmodulins. Thus the calcium-controlling system of calmodulin must have developed by stages. A primordial calcium-binding unit (helix A:site S:helix B) developed the power to form a dimer, then doubled its length to a two-site protein. After some modifications, it duplicated again to give the prototype of calmodulin, with four sites and the characteristic dumb-bell construction of two lobes joined by a long helix (Babu et al. 1985). This long helix is made by placing the last B helix of lobe I end-to-end with the first A helix of lobe II.

Similar Lobes but No Sequence Homology in Rhodanese

The thiosulfate-ion binding protein rhodanese (Bergsma et al. 1975) has two almost identical lobes within one protein chain, paired around a two-fold axis. The X-ray structure suggests that the molecule evolved by gene duplication, but there is no readily detectable similarity between the amino acid sequences of the two halves. This example shows that there is no "stereochemical code" for protein folding; the same structural pattern can be produced by sequences which are, to all appearances, totally different. However, since the path of the polypeptide chain alters much more slowly during evolution than the amino acid sequence, we are able to detect the traces of an ancient gene duplication in the folding pattern, even when the amino acid sequences have diverged too far for any relationship to be recognized.

A general problem in tracing such ancient events is that we do not know how easy it is for the same small structural motif to evolve from different beginnings. Thus the pseudosymmetric four-helix bundle proteins are a numerous class, and it is highly probable that they have evolved from more than one ancestor; this structural pattern is favored by the geometric rules of helix packing. A similar problem occurs in the alternating helix/parallel sheet class of proteins, where there are certain well-known regularities in the molecular architecture, such as the right-handed rule for chain connections between parallel β strands. Here the structural motifs found in many of the dehydrogenases and protein kinases are rather similar; not so similar that a common ancestor is demanded, nor so different that one is excluded. In these families we may need to discover further missing links before any definite path of structural evolution becomes clearly established.

One interesting special example is the NAD-binding protein domain in lactate dehydrogenase (Rossmann and Argos 1977), which has a dyad-like topology, being built out of two similar helix-sheet units, each made of two α helices pressed against three β-sheet strands.

A Symmetrical Ligand-binding Pocket

If the first requirement in evolving an enzyme is to produce a good binding site for the substrate, then the molecules which succeed in evolving a site most rapidly are the most likely to survive and become the well-developed enzymes in the cell. One of the best ways to produce a cleft is to use the gap between two globular subunits that associate about a dyad axis. If these units are held together in a single chain, as a result of tandem duplication, the binding site is likely to be even more stable. The L-arabinose-binding protein (Gilliland and Quiocho 1981) illustrates this mode of evolution. There are two lobes (the P and Q domains) with very similar β-α-β architectures. The arabinose-binding site lies between the two halves. One interesting feature of the interface between the lobes is that it is made by the crossing-over arms of two dyad-related α helices, arranged so that the last helix of the P domain rests against the β-sheet strands of the Q domain, and vice versa. This cross-over suggests how clefts could evolve that easily open and close by rocking on a small contact region.

The Pseudosymmetrical Active Center Pocket in Hexokinase

Hexokinase is a two-lobed structure that has a deep cleft between the lobes, on the edge of which lies the sugar-binding site, where ATP reacts with the sugar (Anderson et al. 1978). Although hexokinase has a very complicated fold, Rossmann and Argos (1977) noticed a repeated structural motif in the alternating helix-sheet region of the molecular core. Later analysis (McLachlan 1979b) showed that a substantial core, consisting of five β strands (a–e) and three α helices (X,Y,Z) formed a dyad-related region centered about the cleft. It seems very probable that this enzyme evolved from a dimer by gene duplication. An interesting feature of the architecture, again, is that the Z helices cross over like two linking arms from the face of one β sheet to the other. Helix Z1 rests against the face of lobe II and helix Z2 against the face of lobe I. The crossed helices help to form part of a flexible pivot that allows the cleft to open and close when sugar is bound. If hexokinase originally evolved by tandem duplication, much has happened since then, as a large assembly of six more helices has been inserted into one lobe between the three β strands (abc) and the helical section (XdYe).

DUPLICATED SUBDOMAINS WITHIN β-SHEET DOMAINS

The "domain" is generally considered to be the fundamental unit of protein assembly and folding. Although there is no generally agreed-upon formal definition of domains, they can easily be recognized in practice as closed globular structures, well supported by a closed system of hydrogen bonds, and built around a well-packed interior of hydrophobic groups. Many domains appear to be independent self-sufficient structures that can fold autonomously without the support of the rest of the protein. Often it is clear that multidomain proteins have evolved by fusing together a num-

ber of totally distinct gene products (for example, the blood-clotting protein thrombin contains a vitamin-K-binding domain, several "kringle" domains, and a complete serine protease). The existence of large domains raises the question of how they evolved, since they must originally have been formed from simpler structures. Some β-sheet protein structures suggest that the evolutionary unit in the early development of their domains was a dimer or trimer of clustered subdomains (McLachlan 1980a).

Chymotrypsin Domains and Subdomains

The original X-ray analysis of chymotrypsin (Birktoft and Blow 1972) showed that the backbone of the protein consists largely of two hydrophobic cores of antiparallel β sheet. The cores are twisted cylinders or hydrogen-bonded barrels and have rather similar hydrogen-bonding patterns, as if they had been formed by gene duplication from one ancestral domain, even though there is now no sequence homology between them.

When these domain backbones are compared quantitatively by superposing their α-carbon atoms, it is found that they match rather well, with 46 carbons fitting within a root-mean-square distance of 2.4 Å. This gives some support to the notion of gene duplication. More interestingly, the analysis shows that each domain is itself a pseudosymmetric structure (McLachlan 1979a), made up of two interlocked twisted fragments of β sheet, which come together across local two-fold axes, one through each domain. Thus, it looks as though an ancestral domain originally began as a dimer of two smaller "subdomains" that evolved a good set of isologous contacts between one another. Later, a tandem duplication converted the dimer into a single domain. Several of the exon boundaries lie between the subdomains (Craik et al. 1982).

If we ask why the domain has evolved in such a complicated way, the answer may be that it takes much less time to adapt the mutual folding of two three-stranded partners of 23 amino acids within a dimer than it does to build up a six-stranded barrel of 46 amino acids by small accretions.

Each of the subdomains in the chymotrypsin barrel is a three-stranded β-sheet fragment that twists in such a way as partially to bury the interior residues inside the corner. The two subdomains come together in an interlocking way so that the hydrogen-bonding core is completed and all the interior groups are buried. The final domain is very resistant to unfolding.

The relationship of the chymotrypsin domains to the evolution of enzyme activity is less straightforward. The domains are not related by a dyad, but by a screw dyad, and so the functional groups of the active site do not come from the corresponding parts of the two barrels. We can guess that perhaps the enzyme originated when the two domains came together and formed a surface groove suitable for binding a polypeptide chain.

The Symmetrical Active Center of Pepsin

The pepsin family of proteases have a highly symmetrical architecture of two large β-sheet domains, held together by strands of antiparallel β sheet that connect them across the middle of the molecule. Below this connecting sheet lies the active site cleft in which two symmetrically related aspartate residues, one from each domain, form the reactive center. The domains have homologous sequences around the active site portion and have clearly evolved by gene duplication (Tang et al. 1978). Later it was noticed by Andreeva and Gustchina, and by Blundell et al. (1979) that each domain possesses a local pseudosymmetry. The domain is a compact globule of tightly interwoven twisted β sheets that forms a bilayer of two topologically equivalent subdomains. The upper layer is made of two central opposed hairpins, a common type of motif; but the lower layer has an unusual interlinked, almost knotted, nucleus of four strands. The pepsin family has probably evolved by two stages of duplication; first to form this unusual domain, then to make the complete enzyme of two domains.

Another completely different β-sheet protein that seems to have evolved by precisely the same route is the eye-lens protein γ-crystallin (Blundell et al. 1981), which contains two symmetrically related domains, each built up of paired "Greek key" subdomains.

The Antibody Combining Site and Subdomains in the Antibody V Domain

The proteins of the immunoglobulin and HLA antigen families are built up from a series of linked compact variable (V) and constant (C) domains, which clearly evolved from a common ancestral domain with a two-layered β-sheet structure. The V domain has eight main strands linked by a short connecting strand, whereas the C domain has a smaller seven-stranded sheet (Poljak et al. 1976).

The V domain has a pseudosymmetrical topology, in which the first four β strands (two from each layer of the sandwich) form one subdomain, and the last four strands form the second. The two half-domains interlock to complete the whole domain, and they are related by a good two-fold axis, but there is no sequence homology between them. The antibody combining site itself is a hollowed-out molecular surface formed by putting together the concave sheet surfaces of a pair of V domains, one from a heavy chain and one from a light chain. These two coupled V domains are again related to one another by an approximate two-fold axis.

These observations suggest a possible pathway for the early evolution of the immunoglobulin family by tandem gene duplication (McLachlan 1980b). An ancestral precursor subdomain P of four β-sheet strands first formed a dimer (the V-domain precursor) that paired with another dimer to form a tetrameric precursor of the combining site, with 222 symmetry. Later steps were: the conversion of this dimer to a single chain to make the V domain proper, the loss of a β-sheet strand to make the C domain, which pairs with another C domain on a different outer surface, and the separation into light and heavy chains. This scheme postulates that a good V-domain combining site evolved at an early stage before the other functions of the C domains developed.

GENE TRIPLICATION SOMETIMES PRODUCES THREE-FOLD SYMMETRY

Monod et al. (1965) suggested that identical subunits would most often associate to form a dimer, but there are a few examples of proteins where gene triplication has produced a three-fold pseudosymmetry.

The soybean trypsin inhibitor (Kunitz) is built from a six-stranded barrel of antiparallel twisted β sheet arranged in a "trefoil" pattern that has a repetitive hydrogen-bonding pattern (McLachlan 1979c). Here the reactive site that binds to trypsin is not related to the symmetry axis.

The B chain of ricin (Rutenber et al. 1987) is even more striking. Here there are two duplicated lobes, as in pepsin, but the design of each lobe is based on a three-fold arrangement of small twisted β-sheet subdomains. The subdomains form a closed domain, and there are significant amino acid sequence repeats centered on invariant tryptophan residues.

A remarkable example of six-fold symmetry appears in the β-sheet barrel of influenza virus neuraminidase (Varghese et al. 1983), which is made of six similar interlocking four-stranded sheet motifs. The active center is placed off-center on one of these fragments.

All these structures suggest to us that complex β-sheet structures can be formed by putting together a number of smaller units that have the power to fold collaboratively. In many cases this "partial folding unit" appears to be a twisted ribbon of three or four β-sheet strands. Ptitsyn (Ptitsyn and Finkelstein 1980) has proposed that the fundamental units of β-sheet folding are the β hairpin and the four-stranded "Greek key" motif.

REPEATED MOTIFS IN α-HELIX BUNDLES

Several small proteins are built from a motif of four closely packed α helices (A,B,C,D) that run alternately up and down and lie almost parallel. Among them, hemerythrin and myohemerythrin have a pseudodyad axis, which rotates A,B into C,D and relates all four of the histidines that bind to two iron atoms at the oxygen combining site (Stenkamp et al. 1978). There is a weak sequence repeat that matches the structural pattern. The progesterone-binding protein uteroglobin (Morize et al. 1987) also has an internal dyad.

A more elaborate helix bundle is the tobacco mosaic virus coat protein. Here the four helices are tied together on the outer ring of the virus rod by a symmetrical box of antiparallel β-sheet strands, and the nucleic acid binds to an interior flexible loop that connects helix C with D. The salt bridges that hold the coat units together in the virus disk have a rather symmetrical arrangement (McLachlan et al. 1980), which suggests that the protein may have evolved by tandem duplication from a dimer of two-helix hairpin precursors. The precursor might originally have bound to RNA in the origin of replication of the virus. This origin RNA may also have coded for its own protein-binding loop.

REGULAR CHARGE PATTERNS AND THE ASSEMBLY OF MYOSIN

When muscles contract, the tension is generated by myosin cross-bridges on the thick filaments, which pull against the actin subunits of the opposed thin-filament lattice. The myosin molecule consists of two parts: the two active heads that contain the enzyme activity, and a long rod of paired α helices, which serves both to transmit the tension and to build up the assembly of regularly spaced rods that constitute the thick filament itself.

The filaments are bipolar, with the rods arranged in two parallel arrays that diverge both ways from the central bare zone. The heads project from the surface with an axial stagger of 143 Å. This stagger can be understood in terms of a series of repeated patterns that run along the length of the coiled coil amino acid sequence (McLachlan and Karn 1982).

The helix has an underlying and typical short-range period of 7 residues, based on the motif (a,b,c,d,e,f,g), in which residues at positions a and d are usually hydrophobic, and those at other positions are polar. As envisaged by Crick, the hydrophobic groups interlock when the two helices come together in a twisted coiled coil. Superposed on the hydrophobic period of 7 is a longer 28-residue gene duplication near-repeat that is characteristic of the myosin family. It has been found in both smooth and striated muscle, in mammals, worms, and even in the primitive *Dictyostelium* and *Acanthamoeba*. The whole nematode myosin rod is built from 40 28-residue zones, which produce a distinctive pattern of surface charges along the 1600-Å length of the helix. A typical zone contains alternating bands of positive and negative charge, three of each kind, each with a period of 28/3 residues. These bands have developed so that strong electrostatic attractions occur when two zones are staggered along the axis by a distance of 14 residues or 21 Å. Thus, on sliding two parallel coiled coils past one another, we find the best interactions at staggers of 14,42,70,98,... residues.

Superposed on the 28-residue repeat is a longer period of 197 residues, produced by modulating the pattern over seven consecutive zones and introducing extra "skip residues" in the sequence at special positions (McLachlan 1983). The result of this modulation is to produce favorable electrostatic linkages between 196-residue units which are half-staggered by 98 residues or 143 Å.

In vertebrate muscles, the thick filament contains a long helical repeat distance of 429 Å that corresponds to a stagger of $3/2 \times 197$ residues. Paramyosin, a closely related protein, also contains 28-residue zones of the same character, and is actually homologous to the LMM portion of the myosin rod. Paramyosin assembles into fibers with the remarkable Bear-Selby net pattern, which has characteristic spacings of 3/2 and $5/2 \times 197$ residues.

The myosin family illustrates how several cycles of gene duplication and sequence modulation can generate stable long-range patterns of structural assembly in a simple way.

MULTISITE PROTEINS

A rather simpler type of repeated protein is one where the structural units have no cooperative connection, but are simply strung together in line to give a large number of similar functional sites. A typical example is the ovomucoid protease inhibitor of Japanese quail (Laskowski and Kato 1980), which contains six slightly different copies of a simple reactive center (Papamokos et al. 1982). These have different specificities against serine proteases, but act independently. Wheat germ agglutinin is a lectin made up of four linearly arranged similar domains grouped around a local dyad (Wright 1987). A larger type of structure is the human apolipoprotein-A-I (Boguski et al. 1986), which is made of a large number of α-helical rods. Each rod is 11 or 22 residues long and has an amphipathic surface, hydrophobic on one side, which enables it to bind to lipid micelles.

Serum Albumin Sites Produced by Gene Triplication

Serum albumin has a remarkable power to bind a huge variety of drugs and other molecules, especially bilirubin, aspirin, fatty acids, and hormones. The protein has many binding sites or pockets, which have been produced by tandem duplications of a largely α-helical motif.

The amino acid sequence has striking regularities. Brown and Meloun found that it consists of a series of 18 disulfide-bridged loops. These are grouped into 9 double loops of the type

–Cys . . . . . . –Cys–Cys– . . . –Cys–

in which the first section is long and the second is short. The sequence is repetitive and consists of three homologous domains, each of about 195 amino acids. Each individual domain itself shows a strong internal repeat in its own three double loops. Here the first and third double loops are very similar, but the middle one has been truncated by deleting approximately 30 of the 44 amino acids in the long section. Here the three-dimensional structure is not yet known, but it is clear that a successful binding pocket has been multiplied and elaborated into a highly effective system of flexible binding sites (McLachlan and Walker 1977).

DNA-BINDING "FINGERS"

The transcription factor protein, TFIIIA, from frog oocytes, illustrates how tandem gene duplication can produce a long beadlike repeated structure that has the capacity to recognize and bind to a specific long segment of genetic DNA.

TFIIIA is required to initiate the transcription of the 5S RNA gene in immature oocytes. It binds specifically to a "control region" about 50 bp long in the coding sequence of the 5S gene, and also binds to the 5S RNA itself. This bound form is stored in the oocyte as a large 7S particle.

The amino acid sequence of the protein deduced from a cDNA clone (Ginsberg et al. 1984) shows that the part of the molecule that binds to 5S RNA contains a repeated sequence of nine units each approximately 30 amino acids long. The repeated region contains an unusual motif of the type

$$\ldots \text{Cys}----\text{Cys}\ldots \text{His}----\text{His}\ldots$$

which binds a zinc ion. The zinc is essential for the structural stability and transcription activity of the protein, and it is believed that the 30-residue unit contains a tightly folded tetrahedral zinc-binding site formed by the Cys and His side chains, with a small elongated "finger" of protein between, about 12 residues long (Miller et al. 1985). Each finger is of a suitable size to bind into the major groove of half a turn of DNA (5.25 bp). Thus the nine fingers are just sufficient to take hold of the 50-bp control region. The DNA sequence of the control region has a periodic pattern of G bases that may match the binding to TFIIIA.

The role of the fingers as structural units is supported by the arrangement of exons in the TFIIIA messenger. These divide off the sequence between the linkers that join one finger to the next (Tso et al. 1986). The same type of finger motif is found in many other control proteins, such as the Kruppel and Serendipity genes of Drosophila.

The binding of TFIIIA to the 5S RNA control region has been mapped out by "footprinting" methods that measure the protection of the bases from chemical attack. These include digestion by micrococcal nuclease and methylation of the guanine N-7 positions by dimethyl sulfoxide. It is found that the protected bases come in groups at intervals of approximately 5 bp, which suggests that the fingers do indeed bind to DNA in half-turns (Fairall et al. 1986).

Given that TFIIIA contains nine similar protein units in series, one may ask how these units are related in space when they are attached to DNA. The simplest and most symmetrical mode of binding would be one in which the nine protein units followed the twist of the major groove (as the minor groove is too narrow to accommodate protein) and each unit made an equivalent type of contact with the edges of the stacked bases. The other possibility is an "alternating" model, where the transcription factor lies all on one side of the DNA double helix and the connection between one finger and the next has to jump across the phosphate backbone at intervals. In an alternating model, the protein enters the major groove alternately from the front or the back side. The methylation protection experiments strongly favor the alternating model, because the sites of strongest protection occur at intervals of 10 or 11 bases. Thus, we have the unexpected possibility that a succession of very similar protein units has "broken symmetry" in its binding to DNA and adopts an alternating quaternary structure.

REFERENCES

Adman, E.T., L.C. Sieker, and L.H. Jensen. 1973. The structure of a bacterial ferredoxin. J. Biol. Chem. 248: 3987.

Anderson, C.M., R.E. Stenkamp, R.C. McDonald, and T.A. Steitz. 1978. A refined model of the sugar binding site of yeast hexokinase B. J. Mol. Biol. 123: 207.

Babu, Y.S., J.S. Sack, T.J. Greenhough, C.E. Bugg, A.R. Means, and W.J. Cook. 1985. Three-dimensional structure of calmodulin. Nature 315: 37.

Bergsma, J., W.G.J. Hol, J.N. Jansonius, K.H. Kalk, J.H. Ploegman, and J.D. Smit. 1975. The double domain structure of rhodanese. J. Mol. Biol. 98: 637.

Birktoft, J.J. and D.M. Blow. 1972. Structure of crystalline α-chymotrypsin. V. The atomic structure of tosyl-α-chymotrypsin at 2 Å resolution. J. Mol. Biol. 68: 187.

Blundell, T.L., B.T. Sewell, and A.D. McLachlan. 1979. Four-fold structural repeat in the acid proteases. Biochim. Biophys. Acta 580: 24.

Blundell, T., P. Lindley, L. Miller, D. Moss, C. Slingsby, I. Tickle, W. Turnell, and G. Wiston. 1981. The molecular structure and stability of the eye lens: X-ray analysis of γ-crystallin II. Nature 289: 771.

Boguski, M.S., M. Freeman, N.A. Elshourbagy, J.M. Taylor, and J.I. Gordon. 1986. On computer-assisted analysis of biological sequences: Proline punctuation, consensus sequences, and apolipoprotein repeats. J. Lipid Res. 27: 1011.

Craik, C.S., O. Laub, G.I. Bell, S. Sprang, R. Fletterick, and W.J. Rutter. 1982. The relationship of gene structure to protein structure. UCLA Symp. Mol. Cell Biol. 26: 35.

Fairall, L., D. Rhodes, and A. Klug. 1986. Mapping of the sites of protection on a 5S RNA gene by the Xenopus transcription factor IIIA. A model for the interaction. J. Mol. Biol. 192: 577.

Fermi, G., M.F. Perutz, B. Shaanan, and R. Fourme. 1984. The crystal structure of human deoxyhaemoglobin at 1.74 Å resolution. J. Mol. Biol. 175: 159.

Gilliland, G.L. and F.A. Quiocho. 1981. Structure of the L-arabinose binding protein from Escherichia coli at 2.4 Å resolution. J. Mol. Biol. 146: 341.

Ginsberg, A.M., B.O. King, and R.G. Roeder. 1984. Xenopus 5S gene transcription factor, TFIIIA: Characterization of a cDNA clone and measurement of RNA levels throughout development. Cell 39: 479.

Jukes, T.H. 1966. Molecules and evolution. Columbia University Press, New York.

Kretsinger, R.H. and C.E. Nockolds. 1973. Carp muscle calcium-binding protein. II. Structure determination and general description. J. Biol. Chem. 248: 3313.

Laskowski, M. Jr., and I. Kato. 1980. Protein inhibitors of proteinases. Annu. Rev. Biochem. 49: 593.

Levitt, M. and C. Chothia. 1976. Structural patterns in globular proteins. Nature 262: 552.

McLachlan, A.D. 1972. Repeating sequences and gene duplication in proteins. J. Mol. Biol. 64: 417.

———. 1979a. Gene duplications in the structural evolution of chymotrypsin. J. Mol. Biol. 128: 49.

———. 1979b. Gene duplication in the evolution of the yeast hexokinase active site. *Eur. J. Biochem.* **100:** 181.

———. 1979c. Three-fold structural pattern in the soybean trypsin inhibitor (Kunitz). *J. Mol. Biol.* **133:** 557.

———. 1980a. Pseudo-symmetric structural elements and the folding of domains. In *Protein folding* (ed. R. Jaenicke), p. 79. Elsevier/North Holland, Amsterdam.

———. 1980b. Early evolution of the antibody domain. In *Protides of biological fluids, 28* (ed. H. Peeters), p. 29. Pergamon Press, New York.

———. 1983. Analysis of gene duplication repeats in the myosin rod. *J. Mol. Biol.* **169:** 15.

McLachlan, A.D. and J. Karn. 1982. Periodic charge distributions in the myosin rod amino-acid sequence match crossbridge spacings in muscle. *Nature* **299:** 226.

McLachlan, A.D. and J.E. Walker. 1977. Evolution of serum albumin. *J. Mol. Biol.* **112:** 543.

McLachlan, A.D., A.C. Bloomer, and P.J.G. Butler. 1980. Structural repeats and evolution of tobacco mosaic virus coat protein and RNA. *J. Mol. Biol.* **136:** 203.

Miller, J., A.D. McLachlan, and A. Klug. 1985. Repetitive zinc-binding domains in the protein transcription factor IIIA from *Xenopus* oocytes. *EMBO J.* **4:** 1609.

Monod, J., J. Wyman, and J.P. Changeux. 1965. On the nature of allosteric transitions: A plausible model. *J. Mol. Biol.* **12:** 88.

Morize, I., E. Surcouf, M.C. Vaney, Y. Epelboin, M. Buehner, F. Fridlansky, E. Milgrom, and J.P. Mornon. 1987. Refinement of the C222₁ crystal form of oxidised uteroglobin at 1.34 Å resolution. *J. Mol. Biol.* **194:** 725.

Papamakos, E., E. Weber, W. Bode, and R. Huber. 1982. Crystallographic refinement of Japanese quail ovomucoid, a Kazal-type inhibitor, and model-building studies of complexes with serine proteases. *J. Mol. Biol.* **158:** 515.

Perutz, M.F. 1970. Stereochemistry of cooperative effects in haemoglobin. *Nature* **228:** 726.

Poljak, R.J., L.M. Amzel, and R.P. Phizackerley. 1976. Studies on the three-dimensional structure of immunoglobulins. *Prog. Biophys. Mol. Biol.* **31:** 67.

Ptitsyn, O.B. and A.V. Finkelstein. 1980. Self-organisation of proteins and the problem of their three-dimensional structure prediction. In *Protein folding* (ed. R. Jaenicke), p. 101. Elsevier/North-Holland, Amsterdam.

Rossmann, M.G. and P. Argos. 1977. The taxonomy of protein structure. *J. Mol. Biol.* **109:** 99.

Rutenber, E., M. Ready, and J.D. Robertus. 1987. Structure and evolution of ricin B chain. *Nature* **326:** 624.

Shaanan, B. 1983. Structure of human oxyhaemoglobin at 2.1 Å resolution. *J. Mol. Biol.* **171:** 31.

Stenkamp, R.E., L.C. Sieker, L.H. Jensen, and J.E. McQueen. 1978. Structure of methemerythrin at 2.8 Å resolution: Computer graphics fit of an averaged electron density map. *Biochemistry* **17:** 2499.

Suzuki, A., Y. Tsunogae, I. Tanaka, T. Yamane, T. Ashida, S. Norioka, S. Hara, and T. Ikenaka. 1987. The structure of Bowman-Birk type protease inhibitor A-II from peanut at 3.3 Å resolution. *J. Biochem.* **101:** 267.

Tang, J., M.N.G. James, I.N. Hsu, J.A. Jenkins, and T.L. Blundell. 1978. Structural evidence for gene duplication in the evolution of the acid proteases. *Nature* **271:** 618.

Tso, J.Y., D.J. Van Den Berg, and L.J. Korn. 1986. Structure of the gene from *Xenopus* transcription factor TFIIIA. *Nucleic Acids Res.* **14:** 2187.

Varghese, J.N., W.G. Laver, and P.M. Colman. 1983. Structure of the influenza virus glycoprotein antigen neuraminidase at 2.9 Å resolution. *Nature* **303:** 35.

Weeds, A.G. and A.D. McLachlan. 1974. Structural homology of myosin alkali light chains, troponin C and carp calcium binding protein. *Nature* **252:** 646.

Wright, C.S. 1987. Refinement of the crystal structure of wheat germ agglutinin isolectin 2 at 1.8 Å resolution. *J. Mol. Biol.* **194:** 501.

Internal Packing and Protein Structural Classes

J.W. PONDER AND F.M. RICHARDS

Department of Molecular Biophysics and Biochemistry, Yale University, New Haven, Connecticut 06511

Protein folding is one of the most important and intriguing of the unsolved problems at the interface between chemistry and biology. The ability of polypeptide chains to fold into unique compact conformations with a vast array of biological functions is rare, if not unique, among high polymers. At this time there is no reason to believe that the chemical interactions currently recognized in small molecules are not directly applicable to proteins, and that the types of these interactions represent the full range that needs to be considered. Of course, the large size of macromolecules and the covalent connectivity will change the relative importance of the various interactions. Some effects barely detectable in small molecules may become dominant in large ones. Of particular interest in the protein folding problem is the observation that similar chain conformations may be seen for a whole series of amino acid sequences that may show little or no sequence homology. The central issue is: "What is the three-dimensional code?"

Drexler (1981) has suggested that it may be useful to express the folding problem in inverted form. Rather than ask the usual question, "What is the tertiary structure of a polypeptide chain of specified sequence?", ask the reverse, "What is the full list of sequences compatible with a given structure?" Pabo (1983) has pointed out that the elaboration of this suggestion may be useful for experiments in protein design as well as providing an approach to the folding problem. Although an answer to Drexler's second question would not remove the need for an answer to the first, it might provide some useful insights.

We are attempting to develop an algorithm that will provide a list of sequences that are compatible with a given structure. The list is called a tertiary template for the target structure. This phrase was introduced by Blundell and Sternberg (1985), and our use is a generalization of their definition. Our focus in the development of the algorithm has been a long-standing interest in intramolecular packing as a characteristic of proteins. Although this parameter can be evaluated in known structures (Richards 1974), its predictive use in the folding problem has remained elusive, even though it should play a major role. The use of packing considerations in the development of the templates is described below.

Background, Assumptions, and Structural Constraints

(1) The tertiary structures of known proteins appear to fall into general classes, as described by Levitt and Chothia (1976), Schulz and Schirmer (1979), and Richardson (1981). Although new classes will certainly be added to those presently known, we assume that the total number is finite and not very large. In recent years, the number of new classes has been rising much less rapidly than the number of new structures.

(2) We assume that the residues of any protein can be divided into two groups; those that are internal, i.e., only in contact with other protein atoms, and those that are external, i.e., partly or wholly in contact with solvent. We further assume that, for the purposes described below, precise division is not important. In general, there will be no simple relations between the sequence positions of either set of residues.

(3) We assume that the internal residues are responsible for the fold of the peptide chain and thus the protein class that it represents. Given an appropriate set of internal residues, the external residues affect the structure only permissively through the global free energy. The electrostatic or other properties of the external residues may affect the stability of the folded structure, but the geometry of the fold will be controlled entirely by the internal residues.

(4) Insertions and deletions in the peptide chains of different members of the class will be restricted to regions of the external set. The immediate expression of biological function will take place most obviously through the external residues that come into direct contact with the ligands. However, to the extent that global aspects of the structure, such as its dynamic behavior, are important, the internal residues will also be involved in function.

(5) Examination of known protein structures by many workers over a period of years has established the broad validity of the following general statements.

(a) The covalent geometry found in relevant small molecules may be used for proteins without significant change.

(b) As with all matter, atomic overlaps are prohibited. The best-known biochemical example is adherence of the actual structures to the Ramachandran map, which defines the allowed conformations of the peptide chain (Ramachandran and Sasisekharan 1968).

(c) Close packing results in small cavity volumes (Richards 1977).

(d) Buried hydrogen-bonding groups normally

---

[a]This paper is a modified version of Ponder and Richards (1987) with a few additional comments at the end.

occur as donor-acceptor pairs (Chothia 1976; Baker and Hubbard 1984).

(e) Groups with formal charges are located predominantly on the surface in contact with solvent (Janin 1979; Rashin and Honig 1984).

These appear to be strong statements that should severely restrict possible structures. However, it has been very difficult so far to apply these rules in a more than qualitative fashion.

The Procedure

The details of the algorithm in its current state of development are given by Ponder and Richards (1987). Only a brief outline is provided here.

(a) The *main chain* is considered to consist of the N, CA, C, O, and CB atoms. These are kept fixed in positions defined by the reference X-ray structure. The CB is removed only when it is in an interior position and is being tested as a possible Gly location.

(b) *Hydrogen atoms* are explicitly included on all carbon and nitrogen atoms in order to maximize the usefulness of the van der Waals overlap constraint in defining the packing. This has been commonly found necessary in other molecular packing studies.

(c) Ideally, the van der Waals contact and packing density portions of the algorithm would operate on all interior residues at once. This poses much too large a computational task. In practice, small interior volumes containing 5–8 residues are used in a single calculation and are referred to as *packing units*. The members of a unit are selected by visual inspection of the protein backbone structure on an interactive graphics terminal and are chosen in such a way that the side chains will point approximately toward the common centroid. Only then will the packing constraints described below operate efficiently. Sequence enumeration is performed for each of these packing units separately. This restriction is not as severe as it may first appear, since an overlapping group of such units may be processed and the results combined into one master template.

(d) The major computational difficulty of a packing study appears to be the conformational flexibility of the side chains. The number of angles involved is shown schematically in Figure 1. To address this problem we have reinvestigated the distribution of side-chain χ angles described some time ago by Janin et al. (1978). Using the 1985 version of the Protein Data Bank and selecting the most carefully refined high-resolution structures, we have found that the rotamer approximation for the angle distributions is much better now than in 1978 (see Fig. 2). The mean positions are very similar, but in all cases the standard deviations are markedly smaller. If we exclude for the moment Met, Lys, and Arg, all of the other 17 amino acids are adequately represented by fewer than 70 rotamers. These angles, and those represented by one standard deviation on either side, provide the *rotamer library*, and are used to represent the allowed conformations of the side chains.

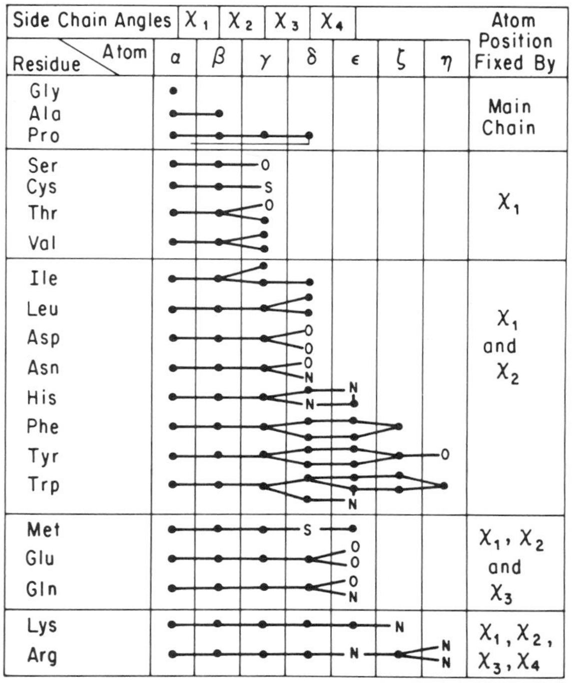

Figure 1. Flexibility of amino acid side chains. The figure shows the χ angle values required to fix the positions of side-chain atoms in each residue type. (Reprinted, with permission, from Ponder and Richards 1987.)

(e) The *van der Waals parameters* used are listed and discussed by Ponder and Richards (1987). Potential hydrogen-bonding groups were identified and treated separately.

(f) The high mean *packing density* found in all globular proteins is a strong structural constraint. The mean residue volumes found in a group of proteins have been calculated by Chothia (1975). Assigning these mean volumes to each residue, the total volume of the packing unit is taken as the sum of the individual residue volumes. We require that any proposed sequence fill the packing unit volume nearly as well as the native sequence. An input parameter allows adjustment of the precise percentage of native volume that will be considered acceptable.

(g) With the structure consisting solely of main-chain atoms (see a), the program goes sequentially through all the residues of the packing unit under study, the *main-chain/side-chain check*. At each position the full rotamer library is substituted one at a time and checked for steric overlap with other parts of the main chain. The restricted rotamer list for each position is filed for later use. Positions that must be occupied by Gly and those that must be Gly if another specified site is non-Gly are recorded. Potential hydrogen bonds to the main chain are also stored. Although there is wide variability in the number of rotamers permitted in the various positions, overall the restrictions introduced by the main chain reduce the number of candidate rotamer

VALINE ROTAMER DISTRIBUTION

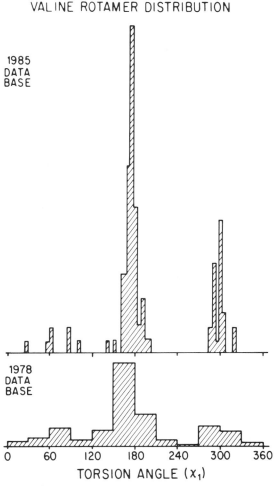

Figure 2. Comparison of 1985 and 1978 valine rotamer distributions. The upper section shows χ_1 values for the 151 Val residues in the 19-protein data base used in the current work. The lower section is a similar presentation for the 238 Val residues in the sample used by Janin et al. (1978). Sample sizes have been normalized so the total areas enclosed under each curve are equal. Similar narrowing of the 1985 distributions relative to 1978 values is observed for other amino acids. (Reprinted, with permission, from Ponder and Richards 1987.)

(i) The *combinatorial enumeration of allowed rotamer sequences* can now proceed. A proposed sequence is checked for steric overlap by table lookup. The packing density constraint is then introduced. A combinatorial tree search is applied in the generation of all nonredundant sequences. Both the allowed rotamer sequences and the corresponding decoded amino acid sequences are stored on disk files.

(j) For most proteins, a set of packing units will be required to cover all of the internal residues. If the units are picked to have overlapping residues, a mutually acceptable list of sequences can be selected from the lists for each unit computed separately. This final list is the *tertiary template*.

(k) Partial information from the full template can be presented in two-dimensional form, a *compositional template*, see Figure 3. The amino acid types are listed on the ordinate and the residue positions in the sequence on the abscissa. For a given sequence position,

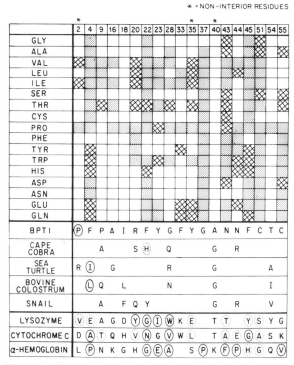

Figure 3. Compositional tertiary template for bovine pancreatic trypsin inhibitor (BPTI). The upper section shows permitted residue position/amino acid type combinations. Dotted combinations are forbidden in both the main-chain plus CB and the full-chain templates. Cross-hatched areas are allowed only in the main-chain plus CB template. Open areas indicate combinations allowed in both templates. The lower section shows sequence information for native BPTI, four homologous and three nonhomologous proteins. Sequence is provided only for those positions that differ from BPTI. Unbroken circles mark positions where the given sequence fails both templates. Dotted circles indicate failure with respect to only the full-chain template. In this illustration, all test sequences were tried only in the single alignment given by lining up the amino terminus of the test sequence with the amino terminus of BPTI. (Adapted from Ponder and Richards 1987.)

sequences by a factor of the order of 10^3–10^6. An additional option uses all atoms outside the packing unit as additional restricting atoms during the above checks. The implications of this option and its effects on results are discussed below.

(h) In the next step, all pairs of sites within the packing unit are surveyed, the *side-chain/side-chain check*. Starting with the restricted list from the main-chain check, all allowed rotamer pairs are determined and stored in a matrix. Possible side-chain/side-chain hydrogen bonds and potential disulfide bridges are noted as well. At this point, the time-consuming steric checks with all the required distance calculations are complete. In later testing for sequence acceptability for the packing unit, one only has to refer to this matrix for all pairs in the proposed sequence.

certain residues will not be found in any allowed sequence in the full template, and the appropriate element in the compositional template is blocked out. When complete, the clear positions in the two-dimensional template allow a rapid first estimate of the acceptability of a test sequence without computer intervention. Any sequence that will eventually pass the full template must also pass the compositional template. The reverse is not necessarily true. Many more sequences will pass the compositional test than will eventually pass the full template. Nonetheless, the compositional test may be useful and is easy to apply as a first screen.

Preliminary Results and Discussion

The rotamer library concept had to be tested first. Although the narrow distribution of χ values was encouraging, it was not clear how well the procedure would work for specific individual residues in the various structures. Individual interior residues in the native structures were removed, but all other atoms were left, and the full rotamer library was surveyed for replacements. In practically all cases in the most highly refined structures, and in more than 90% of the examples in the other structures, the native residue was found as the only acceptable residue, or among a small group considered acceptable, at each of the interior positions. The rotamer library approach thus appears to be a satisfactory approximation for this algorithm.

This observation by itself is of some interest. The mean χ angles were shown some time ago to correspond quite closely to the staggered conformations expected to represent energy minima. These positions are also those predicted on the basis of theoretical calculations on the isolated residues. There would thus appear to be no strain energy stored in the form of distorted torsional angles in the proteins of this basis set. Although an occasional residue may be forced into such a conformation, perhaps in the strong ligand fields found in metalloenzymes, for example, in general the residues will be in their most relaxed conformation in the native proteins. Since this is almost certainly true in the unfolded state, this observation may put substantial constraints on the paths for the folding reaction itself.

The next test was on three small proteins; crambin, rubredoxin, and scorpion neurotoxin. The packing units chosen for these proteins are shown in Figure 4. These proteins are so small, 46, 54, and 65 residues respectively, that they have very small "insides." However, there are some central residues in each protein, and the interior could be represented by a single packing unit. The tertiary templates were calculated for each protein and the statistics associated with these runs are shown in Table 1.

For all proteins the main-chain atoms plus CB represent about two-thirds of all the non-hydrogen atoms. Thus, the tremendous constraint on the allowed sequences produced simply by the main-chain overlap requirements is not unexpected. The increased restriction produced by the pairwise side-chain contacts is relatively small. This is due to the large number of small residue pairs where there will frequently be no side-chain contact at all. The packing constraint is again a very large factor, 10^2–10^4. The combined result of these constraints is an enormous reduction from the combinatorial maximum to the final number of allowed rotamer sequences, 100 to 300 in the examples chosen. There is a further reduction when these are reduced to the more conventional amino acid sequences. At this point, the only constraints are those of steric overlap and effective packing. If an additional constraint, such as absence of charged groups in the interior, is imposed, then the lists are further reduced.

The fact that a given amino acid sequence in many cases is represented by more than one rotamer sequence is interesting. This does not appear to correspond with the facts in known structures. The interior of most proteins is usually the clearest part of the X-ray structure with no evidence for multiple conformations of the side chains. In very high-resolution structures there are examples of multiple conformers, but these differ only slightly when found for interior residues (Smith et al. 1986). These observations show that even for the nonpolar residues, which make up the bulk of the tertiary templates, there are important energy terms not even implicitly accounted for in the present algorithm that select among the sterically acceptable rotamer sequences. An example of such a term would be the effect of the charge distribution in aromatic ring systems or carbonyl groups, as pointed out by Burley and Petsko (1985).

The enormous importance of the packing criterion in limiting the number of acceptable sequences is shown in Table 2. The first entry is the volume of the packing unit residues if they were all glycine. As the required volume for the packing unit is increased, there is at first very little effect, but soon there is a dramatic decrease in the number of allowed sequences. In the particular case of crambin, which is used for this example, the actual volume in the native structure is 659 Å^3. Note that there are no sequences that are capable of filling 700 Å^3 without steric overlap. There are possibly two sequences that might fill 690 Å^3. The difference between the native and the maximum packing is thus 30 Å^3. This volume is less than that of a single methyl group and only slightly larger than a methylene group. In this particular example, one cannot go from a sequence filling 660 Å^3 to one filling 690 Å^3 by simply changing one residue to another that is one carbon atom larger.

The rubredoxin case is interesting because of the large volume of the packing unit. Offhand, one might have thought that the larger volume would permit a much larger collection of acceptable sequences. This is not the case. The volume is so big that a large number of the largest residues are always required for proper filling, thus severely restricting the acceptable sequence list.

In recent computations, we have included in the

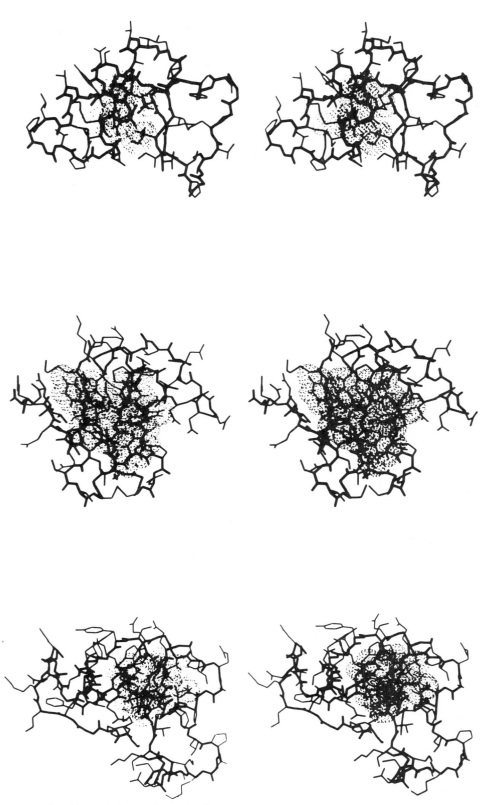

Figure 4. Stereo view of packing units in crambin, rubredoxin, and scorpion neurotoxin. Main-chain atoms are drawn in a heavy line. Hydrogen atoms are included only for residues contained in the packing unit. (*Upper*) Crambin with dot surface shown for residues 2, 13, 26, 30, and 32. (*Middle*) Rubredoxin with dot surface shown for residues 4, 11, 13, 30, 37, and 49. (*Lower*) Scorpion neurotoxin with dot surface shown for residues 5, 29, 34, 36, 48, 51, and 55. (Reprinted, with permission, from Ponder and Richards 1987.)

Table 1. Overall Results for Three Simple Tertiary Templates

	Number of sequences surviving sequential checks		
	crambin	rubredoxin	scorpion neurotoxin
Interior cavity:			
Number of residues	5	6	7
Volume in native	659	1256	897
Restricted by:			
None	1.4×10^9	9.1×10^{10}	6.1×10^{12}
Main chain only	85,652	152,915,040	4,717,440
Pairwise contacts	43,936	62,281,930	1,324,651
Packing constraint	95	236	284
Survivors as:			
Rotamer sequence	95	236	284
Amino acid sequence	34	44	70
Amino acid composition	18	20	58
Without charged residues:			
Amino acid sequence	34	30	14
Amino acid composition	18	14	13

(Reprinted, with permission, from Ponder and Richards 1987.)

rotamer library a tentative set of 13 Met structures. Interestingly, the sequence lists derived using the extended library often contain a large number of sequences with at least one Met residue. This observation is a direct result of the great flexibility of the Met side chain (i.e., three freely rotating χ angles). Conversely, a protein sequence containing a high proportion of Met sites might be able to arrange its side-chain conformations so as to fit several tyes of protein "fold." This could be one of many factors contributing to the relative rarity of the Met residue in known sequences.

Problems and Future Directions

If the template concept is to be useful, the sequence lists in the various templates must be mutually exclu-

Table 2. Impact of Packing Constraint

Minimum volume (Å^3)	Rotamer sequences	Amino acid sequences	Amino acid compositions
330	43936	8113	1494
350	43935	8112	1493
400	43768	8043	1483
450	41877	7590	1442
500	31715	5867	1286
550	15188	3177	894
560	11922	2624	788
570	9041	2049	671
580	6469	1637	559
590	4633	1201	437
600	3288	874	338
610	1976	575	241
620	1340	398	168
630	803	236	102
640	464	137	65
650	199	74	35
660	93	33	17
670	43	17	9
680	9	5	4
690	2	1	1
700	0	0	0

(Reprinted, with permission, from Ponder and Richards 1987.)

sive. As will be seen below, the present derivation is too restrictive to represent a class of structures rather than an individual structure. In addition, there will be errors in the reference structures and uncertainties in the proper allowed deviations. Thus, in checking a test sequence against a given template, it will be essential to derive a probability that the match is significant and not to demand that the match be perfect. Discrimination between templates will then be subject to the usual statistical tests. The appropriate weighting to set up such probabilities has yet to be worked out.

Cavity Distribution

The marked dependence of the size of the template on the volume criterion assumed for a given packing unit is shown in Table 2. Although proteins are, on average, well packed, cavities or packing defects do exist. They represent a small fraction of the total volume but are not necessarily uniformly distributed. As long as the entire core of the protein may be treated as a single packing unit, the cavity problem is adequately handled by adjustment of the volume criterion. However, for larger cores, where current computing capacity requires division into multiple packing units, the cavity problem is more severe. The use of a single criterion for all units implies a uniform cavity distribution. If the criterion is relaxed to allow for an occasional large cavity, then the total cavity volume summed over all packing units becomes unrealistically large. The seriousness of this problem has yet to be evaluated in detail.

Interior and Exterior Residues

There is clearly an "interaction" between the interior and exterior residues. The packing and overlap criteria must eventually be applied to the interface between these two groups as well as to the interior residues alone. Thus, the largest list of template sequences will be those developed solely with restriction by main-chain atoms. The allowed sets of exterior residues, eventually put in to complete the protein, will depend on which of the template sequences is used for the interior set. In this indirect sense, surface portions of the structure directly involved in biological function may be affected by the internal set. In the reverse case, if one wishes to maintain the external set so as to ensure function, the template sequences will be substantially more restricted than they would be by just the main chain. The more restricted template may be the most useful in the design of experimental tests.

Insertions and Deletions

To compare a sequence with a template for a given class, one must be prepared to handle the problem of possible insertions and deletions. Our assumption is that all such changes occur in the external residues, that the interior core does not suffer insertions or deletions, and that the template is independent of such sequence changes. For this to work, the core residues must be arranged on elements of secondary structure that have a defined length and that are inviolate for a particular structural class. The template must include two or more sites on each element in order that the position and orientation of that element be fixed. Changes made in regions of the sequence between the elements are then irrelevant, since these positions are not used in defining the template. The relative positions of the template sites are specified, and the order of the elements in the full chain is known. Algorithms for such a search are similar to recently developed "template" methods for sequence homology searches in protein and nucleic acid data bases (see e.g., Gribskov et al. 1987).

Structure Variations within a Class

Even reduced solely to the template cores, the individual structures within a recognized class are not identical. The most serious problem for the present approach is represented by the structure variations within each class. There is at this time no clear definition of a class. The human eye has a marvelous ability to detect similarities in form, but the decision as to whether two objects are the "same" or not has a strong subjective component that is difficult to quantify. Chothia and Lesk (1986) have recently reported a relation between structural and sequence homology in several protein families. Their results imply that rms deviations of roughly 2.5 Å in main-chain atoms of core regions will accommodate sequences with essentially no homology. The computer modeling experiments by Novotný et al. (1984) on "misfolded" protein structures seem to substantiate this view. If the tertiary structure is allowed to vary, then inevitably the number of sequences in the template will increase, possibly dramatically. A logical procedure for expanding the template has not yet been found, and the extent of the required expansion is not yet known. To be useful, the templates will still have to be mutually exclusive.

The globin family makes a good test case. The "globin fold" is generally regarded as the same in myoglobin, the hemoglobins, and the plant protein leghemoglobin, even though between the distant relatives there is no recognizable sequence homology. In an interesting recent study, Elber and Karplus (1987) performed an extensive molecular dynamics simulation on myoglobin followed by energy minimization of selected frames. As part of this work, they noted that the relative conformations of the helices during the simulation sampled essentially all of the structures found in the globin class. Comparison of different minimized structures from the simulation showed main-chain rms deviations between frame pairs of as much as 2.7 Å. With the help of the above authors, we have started a sampling of the templates computed from selected frames in this simulation. To date, only one packing unit has been investigated, and this may be misleading. The X-ray structure is represented by a template of about 1100 amino acid sequences. For eight time frames picked to represent the most extreme structures, the total list increases to 15,000. Obviously, not all of these sequences are compatible with all of the structures. In fact, only 12 are found in common among the eight frames. The dynamic simulation is just that, and at any instant in time there may be steric overlap or large cavities that will subsequently disappear. The current algorithm is based on equilibrium structures and thus may not be appropriate for analyzing the dynamic simulations in its present form. Dynamic structures are only relevant to the template analysis insofar as they accurately represent the variation in equilibrium main-chain structure for members of the studied protein's class.

Experimental Tests

Even at the present stage of development, the templates provide an interesting goal for mutagenesis experiments. It is not obvious that evolution will necessarily have tested the full range of options for the interior residues for a given class of structures. Once a convenient core has been obtained, there would seem to be little pressure to change, since function is relegated to the external residue set, and this set, by definition, can be easily changed without affecting the core. Permissible single-site changes appear to be rare in the template sequences so far examined. Required multiple mutations would thus render interior residue changes even less likely.

There seems to be an admirable opportunity to test both the template proposal and its possible evolutionary significance by setting out to make the full set of permissible changes for at least one packing unit. This will require random mutations simultaneously at several sequentially distant sites. A strong selection procedure would seem to be mandatory. The experimental difficulties are formidable, but perhaps worth a try if the proper system can be found. Regardless of the fate of the current proposal, the results should be very interesting and useful. Some collaborative efforts along these lines have been initiated.

Other more selective tests may also be very useful. Specific mutations, which would be predicted either to permit or to prevent successful folding, could be made. Making the DNA for such a test would be more straightforward than a peptide synthesis approach. However, the expression of the gene may present a problem because isolation of the nonfolding mutants would be as important as those that fold successfully. Here, as well, the experimental problems are not simple. If a small enough system can be found, hopefully excluding disulfide bonds, organic synthesis of the peptides may be quite practical and free from some of the biological difficulties.

ACKNOWLEDGMENTS

F.M.R. especially thanks Carl Pabo for discussions in the early stages of this study. The work was supported by a grant from the National Institute of General Medical Sciences, GM-22778. J.W.P. was supported in part by a postdoctoral fellowship from the National Institute of General Medical Sciences, GM-11537.

REFERENCES

Baker, E.N. and R.E. Hubbard. 1984. Hydrogen bonding in globular proteins. *Prog. Biophys. Mol. Biol.* **44:** 97.

Blundell, T. and M.J.E. Sternberg. 1985. Computer-aided design in protein engineering. *Trends Biotechnol.* **3:** 228.

Burley, S.K. and G.A. Petsko. 1985. Aromatic-aromatic interaction: A mechanism of protein structure stabilization. *Science* **229:** 23.

Chothia, C. 1975. Structural invariants in protein folding. *Nature* **254:** 304.

———.1976. The nature of the accessible and buried surfaces in proteins. *J. Mol. Biol.* **105:** 1.

Chothia, C. and A.M. Lesk. 1986. The relation between divergence of sequence and structure in proteins. *EMBO J.* **5:** 823.

Drexler, K.E. 1981. Molecular engineering: An approach to the development of general capabilities for molecular manipulation. *Proc. Natl. Acad. Sci.* **78:** 5275.

Elber, R. and M. Karplus. 1987. Multiple conformational states of proteins: A molecular dynamics analysis of myoglobin. *Science* **235:** 318.

Gribskov, M., A.D. McLachlan, and D. Eisenberg. 1987. Profile analysis: Detection of distantly related proteins. *Proc. Natl. Acad. Sci.* **84:** 4355.

Janin, J. 1979. Surface and inside volumes in globular proteins. *Nature* **277:** 491.

Janin, J., S. Wodak, M. Levitt, and B. Maigret. 1978. Conformation of amino acid side-chains in proteins. *J. Mol. Biol.* **125:** 357.

Levitt, M. and C. Chothia. 1976. Structural patterns in globular proteins. *Nature* **261:** 552.

Novotný, J., R. Bruccoleri, and M. Karplus. 1984. An analysis of incorrectly folded protein models. *J. Mol. Biol.* **177:** 787.

Pabo, C. 1983. Designing proteins and peptides. *Nature* **301:** 200.

Ponder, J.W. and F.M. Richards. 1987. Tertiary templates for proteins: Use of packing criteria in the enumeration of allowed sequences for different structural classes. *J. Mol. Biol.* **193:** 775.

Ramachandran, G.N. and V. Sasisekharan. 1968. Conformation of polypeptides and proteins. *Adv. Protein Chem.* **23:** 283.

Rashin, A.A. and B. Honig. 1984. On the environment of ionizable groups in globular proteins. *J. Mol. Biol.* **173:** 515.

Richards, F.M. 1974. The interpretation of protein structures: Total volume, group volume distributions and packing density. *J. Mol. Biol.* **82:** 1.

———.1977. Areas, volumes, packing, and protein structure. *Annu. Rev. Biophys. Bioeng.* **6:** 151.

Richardson, J.S. 1981. The anatomy and taxonomy of protein structure. *Adv. Protein Chem.* **34:** 167.

Schulz, G.E. and R.H. Schirmer. 1979. *Principles of protein structure.* Springer-Verlag, New York.

Smith, J.L., W.A. Hendrickson, R.B. Honzatko, and S. Sheriff. 1986. Structural heterogeneity in protein crystals. *Biochemistry* **25:** 5018.

Structural and Functional Relationships in the Adenylate Kinase Family

G.E. SCHULZ

Institut für Organische Chemie und Biochemie der Universität, 7800-Freiburg i.Br., Federal Republic of Germany

All cells make wide use of the adenine nucleotides AMP, ADP, and ATP to accept, store, and transfer chemical energy. The nucleotides are also essential as modulators of regulatory enzymes of glycolysis, of the citric acid cycle, and of oxidative phosphorylation. Consequently, all the factors affecting the concentrations of intracellular adenine nucleotides play important roles. One such factor is adenylate kinase (ATP: AMP phosphotransferase, EC 2.7.4.3, myokinase, AK), a ubiquitous small monomeric intracellular enzyme (M_r=20,000–26,000) that catalyzes the interconversion of the adenosine nucleotides according to $Mg^{++}ATP + AMP \rightleftharpoons Mg^{++}ADP + ADP$. The catalysis requires a divalent cation, preferentially Mg^{++} (Noda 1973).

The catalytic mechanism of adenylate kinase is an in-line displacement, as demonstrated by the observed inversion of chiral $ATP\gamma S\gamma^{18}O$ (Richard and Frey 1978). Thus, phosphoryl transfer takes place without the formation of an enzyme-phosphoryl complex of significant lifetime. NMR measurements indicate that the binding and/or release of substrates with concomitant conformational changes are the rate-limiting steps and not the breakage and formation of the anhydride bonds (Nageswara Rao et al. 1978).

The adenylate kinases are as ubiquitous as the adenine nucleotides. In mammals, three major isozymes, named AK1, AK2, and AK3, have been purified and studied in detail. AK1 is located in the cytosol and has been found in skeletal muscle, brain, and erythrocytes. AK2 is located in the intermembrane space of the mitochondria; it is the major isozyme of the liver and the kidney. AK3 is localized in the mitochondrial matrix and is a GTP:AMP phosphotransferase. All three isozymes are encoded in the nuclear genome, synthesized in the cytoplasm, and transported into the mitochondria. Yeast has at least one cytosolic and one mitochondrial adenylate kinase in the intermembrane space. Presumably, the roles of these two enzymes are similar to those of the mammalian AK1 and AK2.

Presently, a wide range of adenylate kinases have been characterized and are being structurally analyzed. A comparison of these data gives new information on the substrate binding sites and on the conformational changes of the enzyme during the catalytic cycle. The species-specific properties of the enzyme are not yet understood.

The glycine-rich loop of the adenylate kinases has attracted widespread interest, because it is likely to play a special role in phosphoryl transfer. It can bind tightly a divalent anion (Dreusicke and Schulz 1986), but it is also mobile (Sachsenheimer and Schulz 1977). Thus, one may speculate that this loop transports a phosphoryl group over a distance of a couple of angstroms during catalysis. The sequence of this glycine-rich loop has been found in a number of mononucleotide-binding proteins, among them the cancerogenic p21 proteins (Higgins et al. 1986).

MATERIALS AND METHODS

Thirty-five years ago, adenylate kinase was detected because of its interference with the hexokinase assay. Crystals of the enzyme were obtained rather early (Noda and Kuby 1957), but it took some time before crystals suitable for X-ray-diffraction analysis could be produced (Schirmer et al. 1970). Moreover, these crystals turned out to be rather fragile in correspondence with observations on other crystalline kinases (Shoham and Steitz 1980). During catalysis, this enzyme group has to undergo an induced fit, which usually involves a large conformational change that is detrimental to crystal stability. Thus, crystallization remained a severe problem in structure analyses, also after the first adenylate kinase structure had been solved (Schulz et al. 1974). In parallel with the X-ray analysis, the first amino acid sequence was established by Heil et al. (1974).

As listed in Table 1, the adenylate kinases of about two dozen species have been described. Presently, about one dozen sequences, one spatial structure at high, one at medium, and two at low resolution have been elucidated. Several structure analyses are running at various stages (Table 1). A family numbering scheme has been introduced by Schulz et al. (1986), which is here generally used. In order to find the positions of the substrates on the enzyme, which is a prerequisite for establishing the catalytic mechanism, several lines of analysis have been followed: In the crystalline enzyme, the substrate binding sites were investigated by soaking with substrates and using the difference-Fourier technique (Pai et al. 1977), as well as by cocrystallization with an inhibitor (Egner et al. 1987). NMR analyses of the enzyme have been pursued in several laboratories (McDonald et al. 1975; Rösch and Gross 1985; Fry et al. 1987), establishing the general region of the catalytic center. There are a number

Table 1. Established Sources and Running Structure Analyses of Members of the Adenylate Kinase Family

Species	Location	Year of first characterization	Sequence established	Crystals obtained	Structure analysis
Man	cytosol	1972	1976[a]	400 μm	—
Man	mitochondria	1982	—	—	—
Bovine	cytosol	1980	1984[b]	50 μm	—
Bovine	outer mitochondria	1966	1986[c]	50 μm	—
Bovine	inner mitochondria	1970	1986[d]	X-grade[+]	coming[e]
Porcine	cytosol	1970	1974[f]	X-grade	2.1 Å[g]
Porcine	outer mitochondria	1960	—	—	—
Porcine	inner mitochondria	1961	—	—	—
Rat	cytosol	1970	—	—	—
Rat	outer mitochondria	1968	—	—	—
Rabbit	cytosol	1957	1984[b]	400 μm	—
Chicken	cytosol	1986	1986[h]	—	—
Chicken	outer mitochondria	1982	—	—	—
Carp	cytosol	1975	1987[i]	X-grade	coming[i]
Cockroach	outer mitochondria	1966	—	—	—
Plant	outer chloroplast	1977	—	—	—
Yeast	cytosol	1967	1986[j]	X-grade	2.6 Å[k]
Yeast	mitochondria	1986	—	—	—
Yeast guanylate kinase		1985	coming[l]	400 μm	coming[l]
E. coli		1973	1985[m]	X-grade	coming[n]
Paracoccus denitrificans		1983	1987[o]	200 μm	—
Pseudomonas denitrificans		1974	—	—	—
B. subtilis		1969	—	—	—
B. stearothermophilus		1986	coming[p]	20 μm	—

[+] "X-grade" means that the crystals have sizes of the order of 500 μm and are well ordered so that an X-ray structure analysis can be done. [a]von Zabern et al. (1976). [b]Kuby et al. (1984). [c]Frank et al. (1986). [d]Tomasselli et al. (1986a). [e]K. Diederichs and G.E. Schulz (pers. comm.). [f]Heil et al. (1974). [g]D. Dreusicke et al. (in prep.). [h]Kishi et al. (1986). [i]C. Reuner et al. (in prep.). [j]Tomasselli et al. (1986b). [k]Egner et al. (1987). [l]A. Berger and G.E. Schulz, (pers. comm.). [m]Brune et al. (1985). [n]C. Mueller-Gronert and G.E. Schulz, (pers. comm.). [o]P. Spürgin et al. (in prep.). [p]J. Gogoll et al. (pers. comm.).

of experiments using chemical modification methods that also contribute to this endeavor (Yazawa and Noda 1976; Berghäuser and Schirmer 1978; Crivellone et al. 1985; Tagaya et al. 1987).

The importance of particular structural features in adenylate kinases can be worked out by overlaying the known sequences and three-dimensional structures. Sequences of five quite different species have been overlaid by Schulz et al. (1986) using a tailor-made alignment procedure. Assuming that substrate binding and catalysis are important and the participating residues therefore are conserved, such alignment yields data on substrate binding positions. An overlay of spatial structures was done by Egner et al. (1987), revealing appreciable conformational changes.

Recently, the genes of adenylate kinase of *Escherichia coli* (Brune et al. 1985; Saint-Girons et al. 1987) and yeast (K. Proba et al., in prep.) have been isolated and sequenced, so that site-directed mutagenesis becomes a methodological option. This opens a multitude of possibilities for experiments in the field of artificial evolution and in testing of chemical and structural hypotheses.

RESULTS AND DISCUSSION

The nine published adenylate kinase sequences are given in Figure 1. They can be subdivided into five sequences of cytosolic enzymes of vertebrates, which are rather similar and therefore easy to align, and four sequences of mitochondrial and microbial enzymes. An alignment with the mitochondrial and microbial enzymes has been done by Schulz et al. (1986), using the porcine adenylate kinase as a representative of the vertebrate cytosolic enzymes. This alignment was anchored at five highly homologous segments. For the regions between these anchors, the number of single-residue gaps was minimized and all possible alignments were evaluated using the natural exchange frequency matrix MDM78 (Dayhoff et al. 1983). The best fit of this rigorous search was taken as the result. In this procedure, a problem arose with the large insertion of 31 residues in the middle of the chain, because there emerged several solutions at quite different positions between the anchor segments having fit values not much below the best one. As shown below, this problem could only be solved with a further X-ray structure analysis. Figure 1 contains the corrected alignment of the 31-residue insertion, which had been placed incorrectly using the best fit on the basis of matrix MDM78.

For relating the members of the adenylate kinase family to each other, we take the percentage of identical amino acids as a suitable measure of sequence similarity. The results are given in Figure 2. A most obvious result of the sequence comparisons is the split of the family into two branches: the small variants, consisting of the cytosolic enzymes of vertebrates and the large variants, consisting of the mitochondrial and microbial adenylate kinases. Since the vertebrate cytosolic enzymes are rather closely related, we took the structurally best-known porcine enzyme as their repre-

```
(AK1 numbering)                                10        20        30        40        50        60        70        80        90       100

porcine cytosol           ac-MEEKLKKSKIIFVVGGPGSGKGTQCEKIVQKYGYTHLSTGDLLRAEVSSGSARGKMLSEIMEKGQLVPLETVLDMLRDAMVAKVDTSKGFLIDGYPREVKQGEEFE
human cytosol             ac-M......T..................Q................S.........K..................VN.................Q..........
rabbit cytosol            ac-M......A..................H................S.........K..................A..................Q.Q........
calf cytosol              ac-M......A..................Q................A.........M...................VN.................Q.Q........
chicken cytosol              MST...HH....................H................A.........A....E...D.........L.A................K.........
bovine outer mito.        APNVPAAEPVPESPKGVRAVLLGPPGAGKGTQAPKLAKNFCVHLATGDMLRAMVASGSELGKKLKATMDAGKLVSDEMVLELIEKNL-ETPPCKNGFLLDGFPRTVRQAEMLD
bovine inner mito.        GASARLLRAIMGAPGSGKGTVSSRITKHFELKHLSSGDLLRDNMLRGTEIGVLAKTFIDQGKLIPDDVMTRLVLHEL-KNLT-QYNWLLDGFPRTLPQA---E
yeast cytosol             ac-SSESIRMVLIGPPGAGKGTQAPNLQERFHAAHLATGDMLRSQIAKGTQLGLEAKKIMDQGGLVSDDIMVNMIKDELTNNPACKNGFLIDGFPRTIPQAEKLD
E.coli                    MRITILLGAPGAGKGTQAQFIMEKYGIPQISTGDMLRAAVKSGSELGKQAKDIMDAGKLVTDELVIALVKERI-AQEDCRNGFLLDGFPRTIPQA---D

a) p21 c-has/bas   (pos.5)    KLVVVGAGGVGKSA
b) F1-ATPase,beta  (pos.151)  KIGLFGGAGVGKTV
c) myosin,nematode (pos.172)  SMLITGESGAGKTE
d) G-protein       (pos.30)   KLLLLGAGESGKST

(family numbering)                   20        30        40        50        60        70        80        90       100       110


                                    110       120       130       140       150       160       170       180       190

RKIGQPTLLLYVDAGPETMTKRLLKR------------------------------GETS-GRVDDNEETIKKRLETYYKATEPVIAFVEKRGI-----VRKVNAEGSVDDVFSQVCTHLDTLK
.R.G......................R.....R....................................................E.........A..K
.R.A......Q...............................................................N.........A..K
.R.A......Q.................................................................N.........A..K
KK.AP......K...V...........................................................KG.............QL...T.E..Q..SY..K.
DLMEKRREKLDSVIEFSIPDSLLIRRITGRLIHPQSRSYHEEFNPPKEPMKDDITGEPLIRRSDDNKKALKIRLEAYHTQTTPLVEYYSKRGI-----HSAIDASQTPDVVFASILAAFSKATCKDLVM
AL--DRAYQIDTVINLNVPFEVIKQRLTARWIHPGSGRVYNIEFNPPKTMGIDDLTGEPIVQREDDRPETVVKRLKAYEAQTEPVLEYYRKGV-----LETFSGTET-NKIWPHVYAFLQTKLPQRSQETSVTP
QMLKEQGTPLEKAIELKVDDELLVARITGRLIHPASGRSYHKIFNPPKEDMKDDVTGEALVQRSDDNADALKKRLAAYHAQTEPIVDFYKKTGI----WAGVDASQPATVWADILNKLGKN
AM--KEAGINVDYVLEFDVPDELIVDRIVGRRVHAPSGRVYHVKFNPPKVEGKDDVTGEELTTRKDDQETVRKRIVEYHQMTAPLIGYSKEAEAGNTKYAKVDGTKPVAEVRADLEKILG

                      120       130       140       150       160       170       180       190       200       210       220       230       240       250
```

Figure 1. Sequences of nine adenylate kinases in the one-letter code. The group of vertebrate cytosolic enzymes (AK1) is so homologous that identical amino acid residues are indicated by dots in order to emphasize the differences. (For references, see Table 1.) The numbering on top corresponds to AK1, whereas the numbers beneath show the family numbering scheme used generally in this paper. References for the distantly related proteins are: a) Reddy et al. (1982); Tabin et al. (1982); b) Walker et al. (1982); c) Karn et al. (1983); d) Hurley et al. (1984).

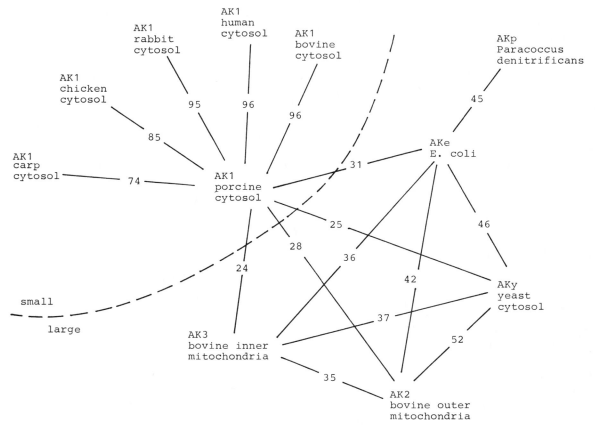

Figure 2. Percentages of identical amino acids in pairwise comparisons in the family of adenylate kinases. There is a clear separation between small and large variants of the enzyme.

sentative in the comparison with the other family members. As shown in Figure 2, the number of identical amino acids between small and large variants hovers around an average of 27%, whereas the internal averages of the groups of small and large variants are 89% and 41%, respectively.

The highest homology value within the large variants occurs between the bovine mitochondrial intermembrane adenylate kinase and the yeast cytosolic enzyme. Moreover, it has been shown that these enzyme species cross-react immunologically, whereas others do not (Watanabe et al. 1979). Since this relationship is rather peculiar, the localization of the sequenced enzyme from baker's yeast became a matter of discussion, in particular because yeast also harbors a mitochondrial adenylate kinase. However, the location has been confirmed by immunological tests (G. Schatz, pers. comm.), so that we are confronted with the fact that the eukaryotic yeast and vertebrate cytosolic enzymes differ much more from each other than do the vertebrate mitochondrial and the yeast cytosolic enzymes. This allows us to speculate that the vertebrate mitochondrial intermembrane adenylate kinase was a contribution of the invaded cell for the adaptation of the invading mitochondrion.

In each sequence comparison, in particular when more than two sequences are involved, a plot of the similarity as a function of residue position in the poly-

peptide chain may reveal interesting information. For the adenylate kinases, such a plot is given in Figure 3. The plot shows the highly homologous regions A, B, C, D, F, and G, which had been used an anchors for the alignment. These regions stand out as peaks higher than the 4-s.d. level above the average. The level of 3 s.d. above average indicated by a line in Figure 3 does not suffice for anchoring, because there are peaks above this level between regions D and F, where the small variant cannot be clearly aligned with the large variants from the sequence alone. These peaks are so high because there is strong conservation among the large variants.

Since we know the spatial structures of two adenylate kinases at medium and high resolution, respectively, the similarity plot (Fig. 3) can be depicted in three dimensions. For this purpose we used the high-resolution structure of the small variant from porcine muscle cytosol and marked the anchoring segments in Figure 4. Obviously, the most strongly conserved residues line the deep cleft of this enzyme, which is such a pronounced feature of the protein structure that one can barely imagine that the substrates Mg^{++}ATP and AMP can bind at a position outside this cleft. Therefore, the reason for the strong conservation in segments A, B, C, D, F, and G appears to be the maintenance of the catalytic function of the enzyme.

Although the general location of the active center is

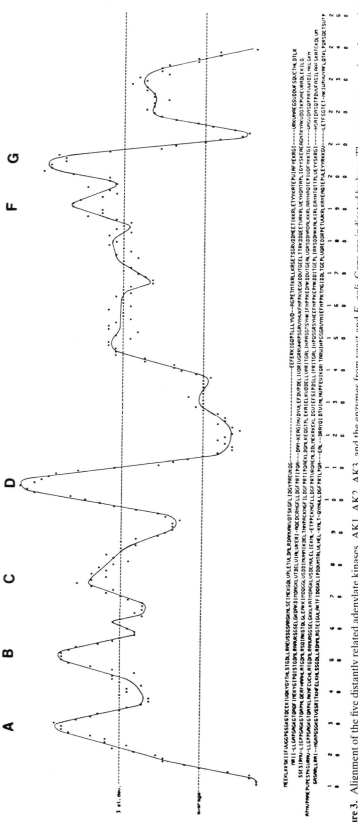

PEEFKLMFSKIIFUUGGPGSGKGTDCEKIUUKYGYIHLSTGDLLRPEUSGGSRRGKHLSEIMEKGQLUPLETULDMLRDMRUVRKUDTSKGFLIDGYPREUKQG------
MRII-LLGAPGAGKGTQAQFIMEKYGIPQISTGDMLRPAKASGSELGKQPWDIIMDRGKLVDELVIRLUKERI-RQEDCRNGFLLDGFPRTIPQN---DMY-KERGIMYDVULEFDUPDELIUDRIUGRRUMPSGROVMAKFMPXUEGKQDUTGEELTTRKQDDDETUXRKRLUEYHQMIAPLIGYYSKERAGMTKYRKUDGTKPUHEUARDLEKILG
SSFSIMTU-LIGYPCRKGGTQRPVLROEFMRMULRTGDMLRSQIMGTDLGLEMKKIMDGGGLUSDDITMRMTIKDELTTMMPRCKMGFILDGFPRTIPQEKLDQPLKEGGTPLEKRIELKUDDELUVRRITGRLIMPASGDSYMKIFMPMEDPMRDBUTGERLUQRSGDMRDKLKKPLRRYHRQIEPIUDFYKKTGI-----URGQDRSGPPRTUURDILMKLGRN
RPHJPRRKPUPKSPKGUMRU-ILGYPCRKGGTQRPVLRKMFCUCKLRTGDMLRMKRGKLVRTMDRGKLVSDEMLKLIEFKML-ETPPCKMGFLDGFPRTURGPMEFLDDLMEKRKEXLDSUIEFSIFPDSLLIPRTIGRLIMPQSGRSVMHEEFMPKEPMKQDITGEPLIRRSSDDMKKKRLKIRLEAYHTQITPLUEYYSKRGI-----HSRIDRSQTPDUFRSILMHISKRTCKDLUM
GASARRLLKMI-MGAPGSGKGTUSARITDHFELIKHLSSGDLLRDMRLRGTEIGULPKTFIDGGKLIPDDVMTRLVLHEL-KML-T-QYMALLDGFMRTLPQN-----ERL--DRRYGIDTUIMLMJPFEUIKGRITARUIHPGSGRUVMIETMPPKTMGIDDLTGEPLUQREDDRPETUXKRLKRYEMQTEPLJLEYYRKKGU------LETFSGTET-MKIUPKUYMFLQTKLPQRSQETSUTP

                        2   3   4   6   8   8   7   2   3   4   0   5   6   7   2   3   4   5   2
                        0   0   0   0   0   0   0   0   0   0   0   0   0   0   0   0   0   0   0

Figure 3. Alignment of the five distantly related adenylate kinases, AK1, AK2, AK3, and the enzymes from yeast and *E. coli*. Gaps are indicated by bars. The sequences are given in one-letter code. Family similarity, which is the average of the profiles of all ten pairwise comparisons between any two sequences, is plotted using a sampling length of seven residues in the alignment. Two guide lines are inserted; the lower one indicates the weighted mean of the natural exchange frequency matrix MDM78 (Dayhoff et al. 1983), whereas the upper one marks the level of 3 s.p. above this mean. Letters A, B, C, D, F, and G indicate segments of high homology.

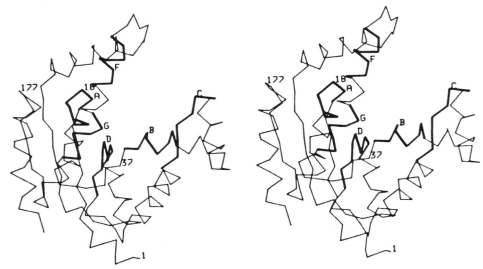

Figure 4. Stereo plot of the C_α atoms of porcine cytosolic adenylate kinase (AK1 numbering). Dark lines represent those stretches of amino acids that are at least 4 S.D. above the mean in Fig. 3.

most obvious from the structure, and although it was also corroborated by NMR measurements and chemical modification studies, a more detailed picture was very difficult to obtain. Early on, the crystals of the porcine cytosolic enzyme have been used for binding studies by soaking them with substrates and substrate analogs at high concentration (Pai et al. 1977). The main results of these studies are reported in Table 2 and Figure 5. In all experiments, the crystals became very fragile, so that none of them could be measured beyond 6 Å resolution. In many cases, which are not reported in Table 2, the crystals broke on soaking and could not be measured at all. The experiments were done in crystal forms A and B, which are the stable crystal forms of the native enzyme at high and low pH, respectively. The low-resolution results and their interpretation are depicted in Figure 5. As a conspicuous feature, they show the intercalation of one nucleotide between the parallel β sheet and one α helix, which could not be confirmed by other data yet.

With the help of the sequence comparison resulting in the similarity plot of Figure 4, the binding positions in Figure 5, which were reported (Pai et al. 1977) as a list of contacting residues, can be checked with respect to conservation. It turned out that the residues in con-

tact with the adenosines of the "AMP" and "ATP" sites are not much more strongly conserved than the average; only the residues in contact with the "phosphates" are strongly conserved (Schulz et al. 1986). Thus, one cannot expect that much more than the general area of the active center has been established with the soaking experiments.

For some time it has been known that Ap5A (see Table 2) is a potent inhibitor of adenylate kinases (Lienhard and Secemski 1973). Actually, it has been designed as such, because it mimics both substrates in a single compound. As a consequence, the cocrystallization of inhibitor and enzyme was an obvious task. Suitable crystals were obtained with the yeast enzyme. The Ap5A:adenylate kinase complex of this species has been elucidated at medium resolution (Egner et al. 1987). The result is shown in Figure 6.

The structure of this complex revealed a number of interesting features. First, it showed that the 31-residue insertion separating small and large variants is actually located at the deep cleft that accommodates the active center. The best fit of the sequence comparison had placed it far away from this cleft at the "lower" (Fig. 6) surface of the molecule. Although it is surprising that the largest change during evolution occurs at the active

Table 2. Binding Studies with Pig Muscle Adenylate Kinase Crystals

Compound	Concentration	pH	Crystal form	Binding position[a]
Ap5A	22 mM	6.4	A	"ATP" site[b]
Salicylate	saturated	6.2	A	"ATP" site
Decavanadate	10% saturated	7.7	A	region of phosphates
ATP and Mn[++]	30 mM each	6.1	B	"AMP" site
ANS[d]	saturated	5.8	B	"AMP" site

All measurements have been done at 6 Å resolution.
[a]The assignment of the binding positions of "AMP" and "ATP" followed chemical reasoning, placing His-45 and Asp-102 close to the transferred phosphoryl group.
[b]Ap5A, P^1,P^5-di(adenosine-5'-)pentaphosphate, was bound between symmetrically related positions of two neighboring molecules so that only one site at the enzyme was occupied.
[c]ANS, 1-anilino-8-naphthalenesulfonate.

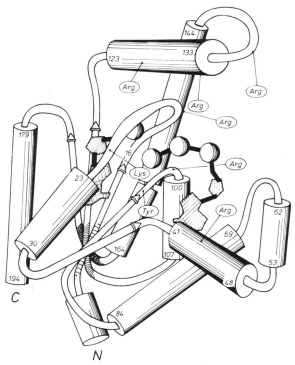

Figure 5. Assignment of Mg^{++}ATP- and AMP-binding sites of vertebrate cytosolic adenylate kinase as proposed by Pai et al. (1977) from crystallographic studies on the porcine enzyme. The positions have been obtained by soaking the crystals with substrate analogs and subsequent difference-Fourier analysis at 6 Å resolution (AK1 numbering).

center without changing the catalytic properties of the enzyme appreciably, the observation is corroborated by the fact that the inserted segment is highly conserved among the large variants, leading to high peaks between the anchoring segments D and F in the similarity plot of Figure 3.

Furthermore, the structure of the Ap$_5$A:enzyme complex showed parts of the inhibitor in a surprising

location. Although the ATP site and the phosphate region were actually occupied by adenosine B and the pentaphosphate within the very limited accuracy of the low-resolution studies of Pai et al. (1977), there occurred a clear-cut contradiction at adenosine A of Ap$_5$A, the location of which is quite different from the AMP site of the soaking experiments.

At first sight, one casually dispenses with the AMP site because it was found under rather extreme conditions, whereas Ap$_5$A cocrystallizes and is a good inhibitor designed for binding and expected to bind at both substrate sites. A closer inspection, as given in Table 3, however, shows that whereas adenosine B and the pentaphosphate of Ap$_5$A bind to strongly conserved residues, the same does not apply for adenosine A, which binds to no residue from any of the segments conserved in all species. Therefore, one has to conclude that adenosine A of the inhibitor does not bind to a substrate position. On the other hand, the AMP site of Pai et al. (1977) is probably also wrong, because none of the involved residues is well conserved. We conclude that the inhibitor designed for binding to both substrate positions, which in fact binds strongly to the enzyme, actually evades one of the substrate sites.

A comparison of the enzyme structure without substrates and the enzyme:inhibitor complex in Figure 7 shows appreciable differences. The chain segment 50–77 has moved over a rather long distance, closing the deep and spacious cleft observed in the enzyme without substrate (Fig. 4). Thus, Figure 7 seems to show an adenylate kinase before the induced fit overlaid with an adenylate kinase after the induced fit. Such a conformational change is necessary for all kinases (Jencks 1975). This change is much larger than a previously reported chain-fold difference occurring between two crystal forms of the porcine cytosolic enzyme (Sachsenheimer and Schulz 1977). Furthermore, the change is in a different region. A conformational change of similar magnitude has been observed with hexokinase on substrate binding (Shoham and Steitz 1980). The corres-

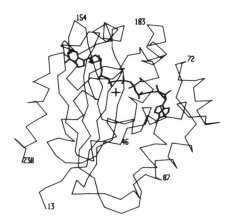 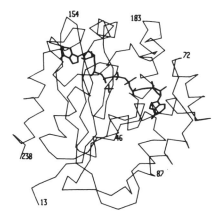

Figure 6. Stereo drawing of the C$_\alpha$ backbone model of yeast cytosolic adenylate kinase together with the bound inhibitor Ap$_5$A. Some residue positions are inserted. In the family numbering scheme, the 220 residues of the enzyme are placed from positions 13 to 238. The adenosines at the left- and right-hand sides are denoted A and B moieties, respectively; (+) indicates the Mg^{++} position.

Table 3. Residues Contacting Ap$_5$A in the Crystalline Complex between Ap$_5$A and Yeast Cytosolic Adenylate Kinase

Ap$_5$A moiety	Residue	Number of contacts	Generally conserved segments[a]	Earlier X-ray studies[b]
Adenosine site A[c]	Thr-32	1	—	—
	Leu-137	3	—	—
	Ala-150	1	—	—
	Ser-151	1	—	—
	Tyr-155	5	—	—
	Ala-220	1	—	—
	Gln-222	2/14	—	—
Pentaphosphate[c]	Pro-25	1	A	—
	Pro-26	8	A	—
	Gly-27	3	A	—
	Gly-29	7	A	AMP
	Lys-30	2	A	P
	Gly-31	2	A	—
	Thr-32	4	A	—
	Arg-53	1	B	P
	Arg-106	4	D	P
	Arg-141	8	—	—
	Arg-178	5/45	—	P
Adenosine site B[c]	Thr-48	9	B	—
	Gly-49	2	B	—
	Leu-52	1	B	—
	Arg-53	1	B	P
	Met-70	3	C	—
	Gly-74	2	C	—
	Leu-75	5	C	—
	Val-76	2	C	ATP
	Met-81	4	C	ATP
	Gly-103	5	D	—
	Phe-104	2	D	ATP
	Arg-106	3	D	P
	Gln-110	2	D	ATP
	Asp-180	1/42	—	—

Listed are all residues with at least one non-hydrogen atom at a distance of less than 3.5 Å from a non-hydrogen atom of the inhibitor (Egner et al. 1987).

[a]For nomenclature see Fig. 3.

[b]Pai et al. 1977.

[c]For definition see Egner et al. (1987) or Fig. 7.

pondence with hexokinase holds also with respect to the observation that the moving part is connected by two strands to the remaining chain fold. In contrast, one-stranded connections are generally observed be-tween domains that have been fused to each other during evolution (Schulz and Schirmer 1979).

The structure of porcine cytosolic adenylate kinase has been refined at a resolution high enough to deduce

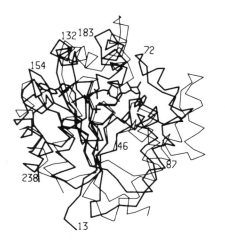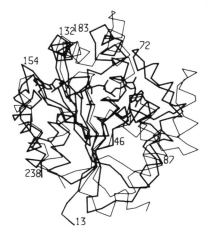

Figure 7. Chain-fold overlay of the porcine cytosolic (AK1, thin line) and the yeast cytosolic (thick line) adenylate kinases. Several residues are given. The chain overlay is based on the 24 residues of the central parallel β-pleated sheet and on α-helix residues 194–204. Ap$_5$A and Mg^{++} (+) as bound to the yeast enzyme are shown.

Table 4. The Strictly Conserved Residues in the Adenylate Kinase Family

Residue	Comment
Gly-24	no serious collision problem detectable
Gly-27, Gly-29, Gly-59 Gly-73, Gly-103	the backbone dihedral angles (φ, ψ) are in a forbidden region for non-glycines
Gly-31, Gly-49	a side chain is expected to collide with the substrate
Gly-63	a side chain would collide with helix 47-57
Arg-53	contacts phosphoryl group in the Ap$_5$A:yeast adenylate kinase complex
Arg-106	points into the deep cleft that harbors the active center
Arg-168	in porcine cytosolic AK the guanidinium group is close to sulfate ion-1, participates presumably in substrate binding
Arg-178, Arg-189	in porcine cytosolic AK the guanidinium groups contact sulfate ion-2
Asp-50	carboxyl is likely to bind to a substrate, possibly to a ribose
Asp-102	binds Mg^{++} in yeast adenylate kinase
Asp-180, Asp-181	in a highly mobile region of porcine cytosolic AK, conservation is peculiar
Pro-26	not clear, corresponds to position 12 of *ras*-protein p21, where an exchange causes cell transformation (Reddy et al. 1982; Tabin et al. 1982)
Pro-105	*cis*-peptide requires usually Pro
Pro-199	interrupts and bends the long α-helix at the surface
Lys-30, Thr-32, Leu-52, Leu-75, Gln-110	are likely to participate in substrate binding
Leu-190, Tyr-193, Thr-197, Tyr-204	are in the protein interior and may be important for protein stability

Note that about half of all glycines and arginines are strictly conserved.

structural details like hydrogen bonds, backbone dihedral angles, etc. (D. Dreusicke et al., in prep.). This allows us to draw some conclusions with respect to the conserved residues. The strictly conserved residues are listed in Table 4. For a number of them, the conservation can be explained. In particular, there are five glycines that are obviously conserved because their unusual dihedral angles do not allow side chains for steric reasons. Moreover, there is one *cis*-proline and several arginines and aspartates that participate in substrate binding. A most puzzling strict conservation occurs with Asp-180 and Asp-181, which are located in the most mobile segment of crystalline porcine cytosolic adenylate kinase. Presently, we think that these mobile residues play an important role in closing the deep cleft during the induced fit by electrostatic attraction to residues from the moving chain part. That the moving segment approaches these residues can be visualized in Figure 7. Altogether, we observe 30 strictly conserved residues, which amounts to 15%.

The glycine-rich loop of adenylate kinases, consisting of the segment Gly-Gly-Pro-Gly-Ser-Gly-Lys-Gly-Thr, has attracted widespread attention. The residues with single underlining are conserved in the adenylate kinase family, whereas the double-underlined residues are observed in quite a large range of mononucleotide-binding proteins (Higgins et al. 1986), a small part of which is shown in Figure 1. With the crystalline structures of porcine cytosolic adenylate kinase (Sachsenheimer and Schulz 1977; D. Dreusicke et al., in prep.), we see that this loop can bind a sulfate in the crystal, which presumably mimics a phosphoryl group of a substrate. Without a sulfate ion bound, this loop moves over a distance of about 5 Å. Moreover, the refinement at high resolution shows that the five peptide hydrogens of residues 27–31 point to the encircled sulfate, as shown in Figure 8. The orientation of the sulfate ion is unambiguous. The resulting distances between peptide nitrogens and sulfate oxygens range between 2.8 and 3.5 Å, so that hydrogen bonds can be

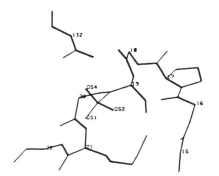 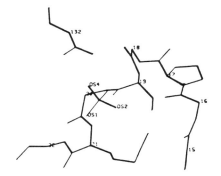

Figure 8. Stereo view of the segment -Gly-Gly-Pro-Gly-Ser-Gly-Lys-Gly- (residues 15–22 in the applied numbering of AK1; for family numbers, see Fig. 1) and Arg-132 (AK1 numbering) of porcine cytosolic AK1 in crystal form A together with a bound sulfate ion, which presumably occupies a phosphoryl binding site. The view is into the deep cleft of the enzyme toward the center of the molecule. The loop is not much exposed to solvent. The model is based on a refinement at 2.1 Å resolution (D. Dreusicke et al., in prep.). This segment appears to be conserved in a number of mononucleotide-binding proteins.

formed. Thus, the loop forms an anion hole for the sulfate or a phosphoryl group reminiscent of the anion hole of the serine proteases (Blow 1976). In contrast to the two involved peptide nitrogens in the serine proteases, adenylate kinase uses five peptide nitrogens, so that one may call this feature a giant anion hole for a divalent anion. We expect that this loop is intimately involved in the transfer of a phosphoryl group. It is conspicuous that the interactions in the giant anion hole are, for the most part, with the backbone, which is the basic structure of a polypeptide. Therefore, the anion hole in the adenylate kinases may reveal an archaic way of anion:protein interaction: The investigated kinase may allow us to visualize a primordial encounter between nucleotides and polypeptides.

ACKNOWLEDGMENTS

This paper comprises work done with a number of collaborators, whose contributions are gratefully appreciated. In particular, I thank Drs. R.H. Schirmer, E. Schiltz, A.G. Tomaselli, P.A. Karplus, and A. Wittinghofer for most interesting discussions.

REFERENCES

Berghäuser, J. and R.H. Schirmer. 1978. Properties of adenylate kinase after modification of Arg97 by phenylglyoxal. *Biochim. Biophys. Acta* **537:** 428.

Blow, D.M. 1976. Structure and mechanism of chymotrypsin. *Accts. Chem. Res.* **9:** 145.

Brune, M., R. Schumann, and A. Wittinghofer. 1985. Cloning and sequencing of the adenylate kinase gene (*adk*) of *Escherichia coli. Nucleic Acids Res.* **13:** 7139.

Crivellone, M.D., M. Hermodson, and B. Axelrod. 1985. Inactivation of muscle adenylate kinase by site-specific destruction of Tyr95 using potassium ferrate. *J. Biol. Chem.* **260:** 2657.

Dayhoff, M.O., W.C. Barker, and L.T. Hunt. 1983. Establishing homologies in protein sequences. *Methods Enzymol.* **91:** 524.

Dreusicke, D. and G.E. Schulz. 1986. The glycine-rich loop of adenylate kinase forms a giant anion hole. *FEBS Lett.* **208:** 301.

Egner, U., A.G. Tomaselli, and G.E. Schulz. 1987. Structure of the complex of yeast adenylate kinase with the inhibitor P^1,P^5-di(adenosine-5'-)pentaphosphate at 2.6 Å resolution. *J. Mol. Biol.* **195:** 649.

Frank, R., M. Trosin, A.G. Tomaselli, L. Noda, R.L. Krauth-Siegel, and R.H. Schirmer. 1986. Mitochondrial adenylate kinase (AK2) from bovine heart: The complete primary structure. *Eur. J. Biochem.* **154:** 205.

Fry, D.C., S.A. Kuby, and A.S. Mildvan. 1987. NMR studies of the AMP-binding site and mechanism of adenylate kinase. *Biochemistry* **26:** 1645.

Heil, A., G. Müller, L.H. Noda, T. Pinder, R.H. Schirmer, and I. von Zabern. 1974. The amino acid sequence of porcine adenylate kinase from skeletal muscle. *Eur. J. Biochem.* **43:** 131.

Higgins, C.F., I.D. Hiles, G.P. Salmond, D.R. Gill, J.A. Downie, I.J. Evans, I.B. Holland, L. Gray, S.D. Buckel, A.W. Bell, and M.A. Hermodson. 1986. A family of related ATP-binding subunits coupled to many distinct biological processes in bacteria. *Nature* **323:** 448.

Hurley, J.B., M.I. Simon, D.B. Teplow, J.D. Robishaw, and A.G. Gilman. 1984. Homologies between signal transducing G-proteins and *ras* gene products. *Science* **226:** 860.

Jencks, W.P. 1975. Binding energy, specificity, and enzymic catalysis: The circe effect. *Adv. Enzymol.* **43:** 219.

Karn, J., S. Brenner, and L. Barnett. 1983. Protein structural domains in the *Caenorhabditis elegans unc-54* myosin heavy chain gene are not separated by introns. *Proc. Natl. Acad. Sci.* **80:** 4253.

Kishi, F., M. Maruyama, Y. Tanizawa, and A. Nakazawa. 1986. Isolation and characterization of cDNA for chicken muscle adenylate kinase. *J. Biol. Chem.* **261:** 2942.

Kuby, S.A., R.H. Palmieri, A.H. Frischat, L.H. Wu, L. Maland, and M. Manship. 1984. Studies on adenosine triphosphate transphosphorylases. Amino acid sequence of rabbit muscle ATP-AMP transphosphorylase. *Biochemistry* **23:** 2393.

Lienhard, G.E. and I.I. Secemski. 1973. P^1,P^5-Di(adenosine-5'-)pentaphosphate, a potent multisubstrate inhibitor of adenylate kinase. *J. Biol. Chem.* **248:** 1121.

McDonald, G.G., M. Cohn, and L.H. Noda. 1975. Proton magnetic resonance spectra of porcine muscle adenylate kinase and substrate complexes. *J. Biol. Chem.* **250:** 6947.

Nageswara Rao, B.D., M. Cohn, and L.H. Noda. 1978. Differentiation of nucleotide binding sites and role of metal ion in the adenylate kinase reaction by ^{31}P NMR. *J. Biol. Chem.* **253:** 1149.

Noda, L.H. 1973. Adenylate kinase. In *The enzymes*, 3rd. edition (ed. P.D. Boyer), vol. 8, p. 279. Academic Press, New York.

Noda, L.H. and S.A. Kuby. 1957. Adenosine triphosphate-adenosine monophosphate transphosphorylase (myokinase). Isolation of the crystalline enzyme from rabbit skeletal muscle. *J. Biol. Chem.* **226:** 541.

Pai, E.F., W. Sachsenheimer, R.H. Schirmer, and G.E. Schulz. 1977. Substrate positions and induced-fit in crystalline adenylate kinase. *J. Mol. Biol.* **114:** 37.

Reddy, E.P., R.K. Reynolds, E. Santos, and M. Barbacid. 1982. A point mutation is responsible for the acquisition of transforming properties by the T24 human bladder carcinoma oncogene. *Nature* **300:** 149.

Richard, J.P. and P.A. Frey. 1978. Stereochemical course of thiophosphoryl group transfer catalyzed by adenylate kinase. *J. Am. Chem. Soc.* **100:** 7757.

Rösch, P. and K.-H. Gross. 1985. Assignment of aromatic spin systems in the ^{1}H nuclear magnetic resonance spectrum of adenylate kinase. *J. Mol. Biol.* **182:** 341.

Sachsenheimer, W. and G.E. Schulz. 1977. Two conformations of crystalline adenylate kinase. *J. Mol. Biol.* **114:** 23.

Saint-Girons, I., A.-M. Gilles, D. Margarita, S. Michelson, M. Monnot, S. Fermandjian, A. Danchin, and O. Bârzu. 1987. Structural and catalytic characteristics of *Escherichia coli* adenylate kinase. *J. Biol. Chem.* **262:** 622.

Schirmer, I., R.H. Schirmer, G.E. Schulz, and E. Thuma. 1970. Purification, characterization and crystallization of pork myokinase. *FEBS Lett.* **10:** 333.

Schulz, G.E. and R.H. Schirmer. 1979. *Principles of protein structure.* Springer-Verlag, New York.

Schulz, G.E., M. Elzinga, F. Marx, and R.H. Schirmer. 1974. Three-dimensional structure of adenylate kinase. *Nature* **250:** 120.

Schulz, G.E., E. Schiltz, A.G. Tomaselli, R. Frank, M. Brune, A. Wittinghofer, and R.H. Schirmer. 1986. Structural relationships in the adenylate kinase family. *Eur. J. Biochem.* **161:** 127.

Shoham, M. and T.A. Steitz. 1980. Crystallographic studies and model building of ATP at the active site of hexokinase. *J. Mol. Biol.* **140:** 1.

Tabin, C.J., S.M. Bradley, C.I. Bargmann, R.A. Weinberg, A.G. Papageorge, E.M. Scolnick, R. Dhar, D.R. Lowy, and E.H. Chang. 1982. Mechanism of activation of a human oncogene. *Nature* **300:** 143.

Tagaya, M., T. Yagami, and T. Fukui. 1987. Affinity labeling of adenylate kinase with adenosine diphosphopyridoxal. Presence of Lys21 in the ATP-binding site. *J. Biol. Chem.* **262:** 8257.

Tomasselli, A.G., R. Frank, and E. Schiltz. 1986a. The complete primary structure of GTP:AMP phosphotransferase from beef heart mitochondria. *FEBS Lett.* **202:** 303.

Tomasselli, A.G., E. Mast, W. Janes, and E. Schiltz. 1986b. The complete amino acid sequence of adenylate kinase from baker's yeast. *Eur. J. Biochem.* **155:** 111.

von Zabern, I., B. Wittmann-Liebold, R. Untucht-Grau, R.H. Schirmer, and E.F. Pai. 1976. Primary and tertiary structure of the principal human adenylate kinase. *Eur. J. Biochem.* **68:** 281.

Walker, J.E., M. Saraste, M.J. Runswick, and N.J. Gay. 1982. Distantly related sequences in the α- and β-subunits of ATP-synthase, myosin, kinases and other ATP-requiring enzymes and a common nucleotide binding fold. *EMBO J.* **1:** 945.

Watanabe, K., T. Itakura, and S. Kubo. 1979. Distribution of adenylate kinase isozymes in porcine tissues and their subcellular localization. *J. Biochem.* **85:** 799.

Yazawa, M. and L.H. Noda. 1976. Studies on tyrosine residues in porcine muscle adenylate kinase. *J. Biol. Chem.* **251:** 3021.

Facing up to Membranes: Structure/Function Relationships in Phospholipases

A. Achari, D. Scott, P. Barlow, J.C. Vidal, Z. Otwinowski,
S. Brunie,* and P.B. Sigler

Department of Biochemistry and Molecular Biology, University of Chicago, Chicago, Illinois 60637;
*Laboratoire de Biochimie, Ecole Polytechnique, 91128 Palaiseau, France

Phospholipases are unique enzymes in that they have evolved to attack aggregated substrates (e.g., phospholipids in a membrane). Only a trace of their full activity is exhibited against monomerically dispersed phospholipids. Moreover, phospholipase activity can be "tuned" by structural factors operating within the aggregate. These include steric influences on the head groups, hydration of the polar regions, chain-packing density, surface charge, and surface defects, all of which contribute to the physical state of the interfacial region (for review, see Israelachvili et al. 1980). Furthermore, perturbation of lamellar aggregates by insertion of amphipathic proteins may modulate phospholipase activity. For example, amphipathic peptides such as melittin from bee venom (Vogel 1981), cardiotoxins from some snake (*Elapidae*) venoms (Louw and Visser 1978), and polymixin B (bacterial), which are known to insert into phospholipid bilayers, increase the activity of extracellular phospholipases A_2 toward phospholipid vesicles, liposomes (Yunes et al. 1977), and cell membranes (Tönsing et al. 1983). They also increase the activity of endogenous phospholipases A_2 in bacterial and cultured cells (Shier 1979).

This responsiveness of phospholipases to the physical state of their substrate has generated considerable interest for two reasons. First, from an enzymological perspective, phospholipases represent a system in which biological macromolecules are specifically adapted to perform catalysis at the interface between two bulk phases. The ill-defined physical chemistry of this boundary between solvent and aggregated phospholipid may be further complicated by local inhomogeneities within the aggregate. Moreover, the asymmetry and anisotropy of the aggregated substrate undermine the assumptions of traditional kinetic treatments. For example: (1) Absorption of the enzyme to the aggregate may be a separate process from productive-mode binding at the active site, and (2) it is difficult to derive meaningful and useful definitions of enzyme and substrate concentrations at an interface. To make matters worse, no acylated or alkylated intermediates have been detected to help identify the critical functional groups of the catalytic machinery, nor has any source of nucleophile other than water been shown to participate in the solvolysis. To date, no structures have been convincingly solved by X-ray diffraction of a crystalline complex between a phospholipase A_2 and a substrate analog—although recent efforts have been

encouraging (Renetseder 1986). Indeed, despite the efforts of many groups over the last three decades (for reviews, see Verheij et al. 1981; Dennis 1983), there is still little consensus on how phospholipases work. This is true even of extracellular phospholipases A_2, for which four high-resolution crystal structures have been published (see below). Yet, to elucidate in chemical terms a wide range of important cellular events, it is essential that we understand the complexities of enzyme action in the unique physicochemical environment created by surfaces of membranes and other physiological phospholipid aggregates.

A second reason for interest in the mechanism of phospholipase action derives from the fact that phospholipases are being increasingly implicated in the web of biochemical events that underlie receptor-mediated transmembrane signaling and the inflammatory response. Phospholipase C (refer to Fig. 1 for nomenclature of phospholipases), a phosphodiesterase that hydrolyzes the glycerol-phosphate bond in phosphatidylinositols, releases the "second messengers" diacylglycerol (DAG) and 1,4,5-inositol trisphosphate ($InsP_3$) upon stimulation by agonist binding to over 25 different membrane receptors (for a recent review, see Sekar and Hokin 1986). Both DAG and $InsP_3$ apparently act synergistically to trigger cellular responses,

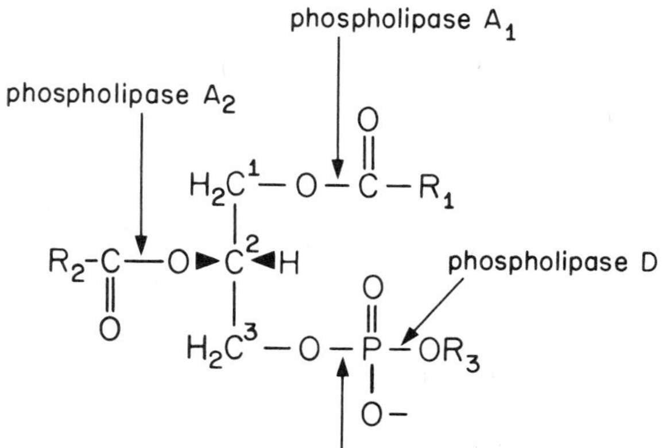

Figure 1. Nomenclature for phospholipases. R_1 and R_2 are fatty acyl chains, R_3 is commonly choline, ethanolamine, serine, glycerol, or inositol. The chiral specificity and numbering are the basis for the standard nomenclature (*sn*) for glycerides.

the former by activating protein kinase C and the latter by releasing calcium ion from internal stores. An intracellular phospholipase A_2 releases arachidonic acid, which serves as the starting material for the biosynthesis of the eicosanoids, such as prostaglandins, which are effectors of inflammation. It is likely that the production of these small molecular "messengers," i.e., DAG, $InsP_3$, and arachidonate, is controlled by regulating the activity of phospholipases. Since phospholipase activity can be influenced by local alterations of membrane structure, a fascinating possibility suggests itself for the mechanism of signal transduction. Specifically, small perturbations of membrane organization might be caused by ligand-induced conformational changes in a receptor molecule and/or ancillary integral membrane proteins. These perturbations could locally alter the susceptibility of the phospholipids in the cytosolic leaflet to hydrolysis by endogenous phospholipases. Thus, by modulating the phospholipase-mediated release of second messengers at the level of its substrate structure, the receptor system could switch on or off general metabolic events.

The Phospholipases A_2: A Model System

As part of our ongoing study of enzyme action at the membrane surface, we have employed the extracellular phospholipases A_2 as a model system. These calcium-requiring enzymes, which hydrolyze stereospecifically the acyl ester in position 2 of 3-*sn*-phosphoglycerides (Fig. 1), are particularly convenient to study, as they are abundantly available (from snake venom and mammalian pancreatic tissue), easily purified, stable under a great variety of experimental conditions, and readily crystallized. They are the best characterized of the phospholipases.

Vertebrate, extracellular phospholipases A_2 are composed of compact subunits (~ 14 kD) stabilized by seven disulfide bridges. Phospholipases A_2 may occur as monomers, homodimers, or—in the case of certain presynaptic neurotoxins—as the catalytic subunit of heterodimers or trimers. This large homologous family of enzymes may be divided into two structural classes based on the more than 30 complete amino acid sequences available in the literature (Heinrikson et al. 1977; Randolph et al. 1980; Dufton and Hider 1983). (The phospholipase A_2 from bee venom has only four disulfide bridges and a nonhomologous primary structure [Shipolini et al. 1974].) Group I enzymes, defined by a disulfide linkage between residues 11 and 69, include those from mammalian pancreas and the venoms of the snake families *Elapidae* and *Hydrophidae*. Group II enzymes, which possess a carboxy-terminal sequence extension linked by a disulfide to a cysteine near the presumed active site, consist of phospholipases A_2 from the venom of *Crotalidae* and *Viperidae* families.

In pancreatic tissue, a precursor (prophospholipase A_2) is produced. The active monomeric enzyme is formed after tryptic removal of the proenzyme's amino-terminal heptapeptide (de Haas et al. 1968) (Fig. 2a).

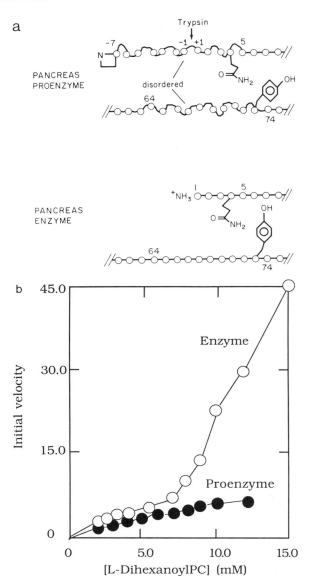

Figure 2. Tryptic activation of pancreas proenzyme. (*a*) Cleavage reaction. Residues 1–4 and 62–73 are converted from a disordered state in the proenzyme into a well-defined state in the enzyme (see text for more details and references). The amino terminus (−7) in the proenzyme is pyroglutamic acid. (*b*) Proenzyme- and enzyme-catalyzed hydrolysis of dihexanoyllecithin. Notice that the aggregation-induced enhancement of catalytic activity (above the critical micellar concentration, 10 mM) occurs only in the case of the enzyme.

This cleavage is accompanied by a conformational change in the newly generated amino-terminal segment (Abita et al. 1972) which, in turn, stabilizes the structure that confers on the enzyme the ability to bind specifically to aggregated phospholipids (Pieterson et al. 1974). Both precursor and enzyme are about equally active toward monomeric substrates; however, only the enzyme displays an enhanced catalytic activity toward aggregated phospholipids (Fig. 2b). The poor activity of the proenzyme toward aggregated substrates is apparently a direct consequence of its inability to bind to phospholipid-water interfaces (Pieterson et al. 1974).

Comparison of the crystal structures of the enzyme and its precursor should reveal a region of the protein that is involved in binding to aggregated substrate. This is discussed below. In contrast, no precursor of snake venom phospholipases A_2 has been identified. Some are stable dimers (Hachimori et al. 1971; Wells 1971) and act as such (Shen et al. 1975). Structural comparisons with the monomeric pancreas enzyme are discussed below.

What Makes *Aggregated* Phospholipids Better Substrates?

Almost all naturally occurring phospholipids reside and function in aggregates: either membranes, mixed micelles, vesicles, or lipoproteins. In a sense, phospholipids and their cognate enzymes have co-evolved to deal with the formation and turnover of micellar or lamellar aggregates. What then is the structural basis for the fact that aggregated phospholipids are much better substrates than monomers?

Three general theories for enhanced phospholipase A_2 activity against phospholipid aggregates. The enhanced phospholipase A_2 activity toward aggregated phospholipid compared with that for monomeric substrates has been regarded as either the result of a change in the enzyme molecule brought about by its interaction with the surface of the aggregated phospholipid, or a property pertaining to the substrate molecule within the aggregate that distinguishes it from the monomeric substrate molecule. (1) *Interfacial recognition site model.* From studies on mammalian pancreatic phospholipase A_2 (and its precursor) it has been postulated (Verheij et al. 1981) that a reversible interaction with the aggregated substrate occurs through a specific area on the enzyme, the so-called "interfacial recognition site." This induces a conformational change in the protein, leading to a reorientation of the active site residues and thereby an increased catalytic efficiency. The stereochemical details of the process have not been established, although an interfacial activation surface has been proposed for the crystal structure of the bovine pancreatic enzyme (Dijkstra et al. 1981a). The validity of this proposal is discussed below. (2) *The dual phospholipid model.* Another model that assumes a direct influence of phospholipid on the enzyme's architecture has been postulated for *Naja naja naja* phospholipase A_2 (Plückthun et al. 1986). An activating phospholipid is thought to induce the formation of an asymmetric enzyme dimer, with one subunit involved in the binding to the activator (a phosphorylcholine-containing molecule, either soluble or incorporated in the aggregate) and the other subunit involved in catalysis. Since two phospholipid molecules with different functions participate in one catalytic cycle, this scheme has been called the "dual phospholipid" model. (3) *The substrate model.* This model considers the enzyme structure to remain essentially constant and assumes that the enhancement of catalytic activity is due to the fact that phospholipid

aggregation restricts the distribution of conformations of the substrate to those resulting in a higher fraction of productive encounters with the enzyme (Wells 1974; Allgyer and Wells 1979).

There is scant evidence that the protein's conformation undergoes an interface-associated change that augments catalytic function (interfacial recognition-site model). The fact that binding of the pancreas enzyme to micelles causes a change in the protein's UV absorbance and fluorescence, which is different from the change observed for binding to monomers, has been ascribed to a perturbation in the environment of tryptophan at position 3 (van Dam-Mieras et al. 1975; Hillie et al. 1981). But this spectral change could be readily explained by direct interaction between the chromophore and the aggregated substrate (see discussion of the "activation network" below) without invoking a functionally significant change in the backbone conformation. Even if these spectral perturbations do reflect a genuine conformational change, it does not necessarily follow that the structural rearrangement causes a more catalytically efficient enzyme molecule.

The dual phospholipid model, which was suggested by Dennis and his colleagues for phospholipase A_2 from *N. n. naja* venom is supported by three lines of evidence. (1) To deal with the inhomogeneous character of the substrate, Dennis and colleagues have exploited "surface dilution kinetics." The decrease in the rate of hydrolysis that accompanies dilution of substrate by detergent in mixed micelles shows a concentration dependency consistent with a requirement by the enzyme for two phospholipid molecules (Deems et al. 1975; Roberts et al. 1977). This interpretation, however, depends heavily on the assumption that the Triton X-100 detergent has negligible influence on enzyme activity. (2) There exists a "helper effect," in which the rate of hydrolysis of a relatively poor substrate, phosphatidylethanolamine, is enhanced by the presence of phosphorylcholine-containing compounds (Adamich and Dennis 1978; Adamich et al. 1979; Roberts et al. 1979). This intriguing result clearly implies the simultaneous interaction of two different phospholipid molecules at distinct but "communicating" sites. It has been shown that the activator molecule can be either in the aggregate *or in solution* (Adamich et al. 1979). To elicit a similar response from both a soluble and aggregated helper molecule presents a puzzling stereochemical question, since we would not expect head groups of monomeric soluble substrates to interact with enzyme in the same way as the head groups from an aggregate. Although the dual phospholipid model is undoubtedly of importance to our understanding of *N. n. naja* phospholipase A_2 action, it may not be the primary element responsible for aggregation-induced activation common to all phospholipases A_2. (3) The enzyme from *N. n. naja* venom apparently must form dimers (or higher order aggregates) in order to exhibit enhanced catalysis of micellar substrates but dimerization is not necessary for hydrolysis of monomeric substrates (Lewis et al. 1977; Lombardo and Dennis 1985). This requirement is used to support the dual phospholipid model, as it conveniently provides a second binding site. However, dimerization cannot be regarded as a general mechanism for activity enhancement, since many phospholipases A_2 that are stable dimers *before* interacting with any phospholipid display the same increased activity toward micellar or vesicular substrates (Wells 1971). Moreover, the pancreas enzyme is thought to be fully active as a monomer (de Araujo et al. 1979).

Until recently there has been little evidence advanced for the modified substrate model originally derived from kinetic and thermodynamic arguments (Wells 1974; Allgyer and Wells 1979) using the enzyme from *Crotalus adamanteus* venom. The basic claim was that the enzyme that interacts with monomeric substrates is mechanistically indistinguishable from the enzyme that interacts with micelles. The default conclusion was that the *substrate* must undergo a change in conformation upon insertion into an aggregate that results in a more productive interaction with the active site. In experiments that are described more fully below, Barlow et al. (1988) have provided the first direct evidence in support of the modified substrate model. They showed that unless the phospholipid substrate is sufficiently flexible to undergo aggregation-induced deformation, it is *not* attacked at an accelerated rate when incorporated into a micelle.

Clearly the phospholipases represent a break from our conventional views of enzyme action. Understanding the unique catalytic task of these enzymes may warrant, indeed require, unorthodox approaches. For the past 6 years we have been addressing the following questions: (1) What structural features of the enzyme determine its ability to perform catalysis at a heterogenous interface? (2) What is special about the aggregated substrate that enhances its suceptibility to phospholipase and distinguishes it from the poorly hydrolyzed monomeric phospholipid?

Structural Studies of Phospholipases A_2: An Enzyme in Search of an Active Site

The crystallographic structures of three forms of phospholipase A_2 and one form of the proenzyme have been solved and refined to near-atomic resolution (Dijkstra et al. 1981b, 1982, 1983; Keith et al. 1981; Brunie et al. 1985). The calcium-containing monomeric bovine proenzyme (3.0 Å) and its activated form (1.7 Å), along with the porcine equivalent (2.6 Å) and the calcium-free form of the dimeric phospholipase A_2 from *Crotalus atrox* (2.5 Å), have provided the basis for our present understanding of the relationships between structure and mechanism.

The homologous family of phospholipase A_2 from vertebrates has a common "core" structure. Based on the analysis of amino acid sequences and crystal structures, a common numbering system has been proposed that accents the remarkable conformational homology among members of this family of proteins (Renetseder

et al. 1985). This numbering system takes advantage of a rigid core of three large α helices, as well as the highly conserved nature of three other sequence segments (Fig. 3). These structurally homologous sections range from 7 to 20 amino acids in length and together comprise 62% of the minimal sequence. When the homologous segments are combined and superimposed as a rigid structural unit, the Cα atoms in the bovine crystal structure deviated from their counterparts in the dimeric venom enzyme by a root mean square distance of less than 0.67 Å (Renetseder et al. 1985). Specific amino acids are invariantly conserved among phospholipases A_2; many of these residues appear to be involved in functional groupings. The evolutionary antecedent of this family is not clearly established. Phospholipase A_2 from insect venom—especially the honey bee—has been sequenced and its kinetics have been analyzed, but the three-dimensional structure is still unknown (Shipolini et al. 1974; Raykova and Blagoev 1986). Although there are segments that suggest sequence homology, the overall sequence does not suggest a clear path of molecular evolution. Since the function of bee venom phospholipase A_2 resembles that of vertebrate phospholipase A_2, the sequence/structure/function relationship is a rich one for evolutionary study.

The calcium-binding and catalytic residues are known. Phospholipases A_2 contain two well-established structural domains: a calcium-binding region and a catalytic network (Dijkstra et al. 1981a). A third site, one that recognizes and binds aggregated substrate, has been proposed by Brunie et al. (1985). Although distinct locales for each of these functions have been tentatively assigned, the biochemical and crystallographic evidence remains far from absolute, as we will describe.

Based on the crystallographic analysis of the pancreatic enzyme with Ba^{++} substituted for Ca^{++}, a calcium "cage" of five carbonyl oxygens was proposed as the calcium-binding site (Dijkstra et al. 1981b). This assignment has been substantiated by high-resolution refinements of the calcium-containing variants of the pancreatic protein (Dijkstra et al. 1981b, 1982, 1983). Three of the liganding carbonyls are contributed from a highly conserved "calcium-binding loop," and the remaining two are derived from the aspartate at sequence position 49. Chemical modification of Asp-49 with water-soluble carbodiimides abolishes phospholipasic activity (Fleer et al. 1981). Although this aspartate was originally believed to be invariant, it is replaced by lysine in at least one small subclass (K-49) of phospholipase A_2 (Maraganore et al. 1984). Replacing the carboxylate of Asp-49 with the side chain of the lysine clearly alters the Ca^{++}-binding capabilities of the K-49 variant and, consequently, the exact role of Ca^{++} in the enzyme's function. This unusual replacement has rendered the K-49 enzyme the object of crystallographic study both in our laboratory and elsewhere (Scott et al. 1986; H.M. Einspahr, pers. comm.).

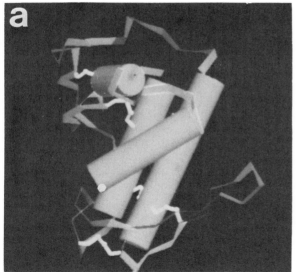
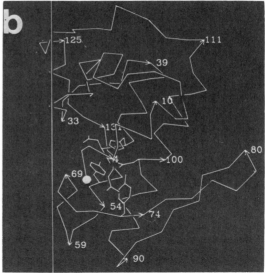
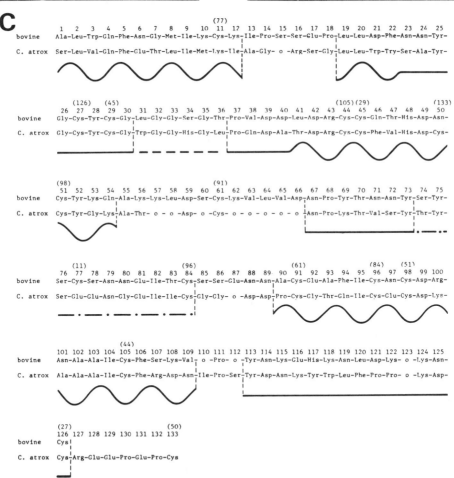

Figure 3. Structure of phospholipase A$_2$. Molecular structures shown here are the "right" subunit of the dimeric enzyme from *C. atrox* venom. (The complete dimer is shown in the same orientation in Figs. 4 and 5). (*a*) Schematic rendering of the polypeptide chain to emphasize helical components. (*b*) C$_\alpha$ trace with side chains involved in catalysis and activation (see text). In both *a* and *b* the position of the amino terminus is indicated by a white dot. (*c*) Homologous core of phospholipase A$_2$ taken from Renetseder et al. (1985). Sequences of bovine and *C. atrox* venom enzymes were aligned primarily on the basis of their conformational similarity and indicated here by a continuous heavy line (sinusoidal indicates helical structure). The broken lines indicate segments whose conformation deviates either locally (31–36) or globally (74–84) to make obvious functional or structural adjustments. Residues 59 and 61 of the *C. atrox* enzymes have been assigned their sequence numbers arbitrarily and deviate in position considerably from their bovine counterparts. The numbers in parentheses indicate the disulfide partner of the Cys residue below it. Position 123 contains an insertion in the equine phospholipase A$_2$.

445

446 ACHARI ET AL.

The putative catalytic network (Fig. 4), like the proposed calcium-binding region, is composed of highly conserved residues. Four absolutely conserved amino acids (His-48, Tyr-52, Tyr-73, and Asp-99) have been

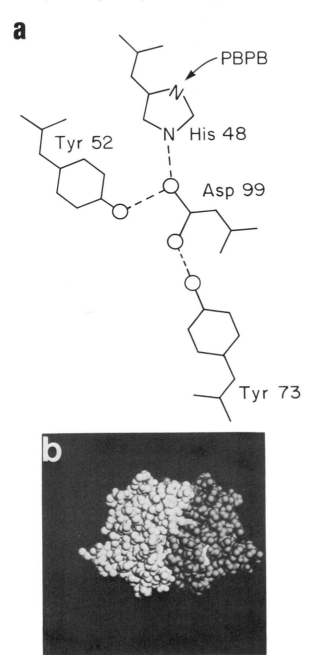

Figure 4. The catalytic network of *Crotalus atrox*. (*a*) A schematic representation of the four hydrogen-bonded conserved residues considered to be the catalytic system. PBPB is *para*-bromophenacyl bromide, which has been shown to specifically attack the N-1 of His-48. Alkylation of this residue abolishes catalytic activity and inhibits binding of both Ca++ and monomeric (but not aggregated) substrate. (*b*) Space-filling representation of the *C. atrox* dimer. The molecular dyad is vertical. The side chains of the catalytic network are highlighted in white (the ring of Tyr-73 is slightly exposed on the right and Tyr-52 can just be seen on the left).

shown by crystallographic study to form a tightly constructed hydrogen-bonded network whose three-dimensional structure is virtually identical in all cases. This constellation of residues has been referred to as the "catalytic network" (Brunie et al. 1985), since disruption of its electronic structure by chemical modification of His-48 or Tyr-73 destroys catalytic activity (Meyer et al. 1979; Verheij et al. 1980). Based on the presence of a water molecule hydrogen-bonded to the Nδ1 of His-48, Dijkstra et al. (1981a) originally proposed that the catalytic mechanism of phospholipase A$_2$ is analogous to that of the serine proteases. In the case of the phospholipases, a water molecule would be activated for nucleophilic attack on the ester substrate via a charge relay system involving the hydrogen bonds to His-48 and Asp-99 (Fig. 4). Although Brunie et al. (1985), noted that a corresponding water molecule was not present in the low-pH *C. atrox* crystal structure, there is density for a water molecule in the partially refined model of the *C. atrox* enzyme crystallized at neutral pH in the presence of calcium (D. Scott, unpubl.). Since the residues of the catalytic network of the mammalian and venom enzymes are all superimposable, one would expect a common mechanism. If a water molecule were an essential element, it is likely that it would be seen in all cases.

The binding site for aggregated substrate: Where is it? The structure of the *C. atrox* enzyme poses a challenge to the conventional understanding of phospholipase A$_2$ function. The dimer is a flat, oblate ellipsoid in which the two subunits are snugly interfaced across a molecular dyad (Fig. 3). With the possible exception of Tyr-73, however, the functional groups of the catalytic network face an internal cavity shielded from the solvent by the dyad-related subunit (Fig. 4b). This restriction of access to the proposed catalytic network is especially puzzling, since, as noted above, the optimal substrate for the enzyme is not the head group of a freely diffusible phospholipid molecule, but rather a phospholipid immersed in a bulky micelle or lamellar aggregate. An early proposal (Keith et al. 1981) suggested that the enzyme might dissociate upon binding calcium ion. This suggestion is contradicted by our crystallographic studies (A. Achari et al., in prep.) of the dimeric phospholipase A$_2$ from *C. atrox* at neutral pH, which establishes definitively that the basic dimeric architecture is preserved over a wide range of pH, both in the presence and absence of bound calcium ion. Moreover, kinetic studies (Shen et al. 1975) of the enzymes from *C. atrox*, *C. adamanteus* (Wells 1971; Smith and Wells 1981) and, more recently, *Agkistrodon piscivorus piscivorus* (F.J. Kézdy et al., unpubl.), further substantiate the concept of functional dimers with apparent dissociation constants ranging from 10^{-9} M (*C. adamanteus*) to 10^{-11} M (*C. atrox*). There is no evidence to suggest that these dimers must dissociate to function; indeed, the evidence is that the dimer is required for function against aggregated substrate.

Assuming the functional dimer has basically the same architecture as these crystal structures, several solutions are possible to the problem of a shielded catalytic site. First, productive interaction with aggregated substrate could cause a deshielding shift in conformation. A second and more likely possibility is a misassignment by Dijkstra et al. (1981a) of the so-called interfacial recognition surface, i.e., the site that recognizes and binds the aggregated substrate. A more plausible assignment for the part of the enzyme's surface that interacts with phospholipid aggregates is suggested by the observation that, whereas both the proenzyme and enzyme can bind and hydrolyze monomeric substrate, it is the presence of the nascent terminal amino group of the enzyme (created by tryptic digestion) that is required for binding to aggregated substrates and hence, for enhanced catalytic function (for review of evidence, see Verheij et al. 1981). When the refined

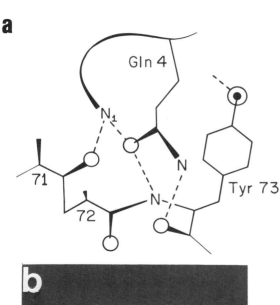

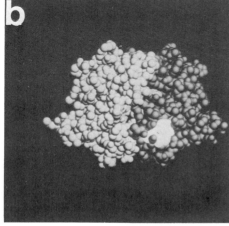

Figure 5. The "activation network." (*a*) A schematic representation oriented as it occurs in the "right" subunit of *C. atrox*. The network is a hydrogen-bonded system involving the amino-terminal amino group, the side chain of Gln-4, the backbone of Val-71, and all of Tyr-73. (*b*) Space-filling representation of the *C. atrox* dimer showing the elements of the activation network highlighted in white.

structure of the bovine pancreatic proenzyme is compared with that of the enzyme (Verheij et al. 1981; Dijkstra et al. 1982), the role of this terminal amino group can be clearly seen. It forms the heart of a hydrogen-bonded network that involves the nearly invariant Gln-4 and stabilizes the segment of the polypeptide carrying Tyr-73 (Fig. 2a), one of the four conserved catalytic residues. In the proenzyme, this network cannot exist and the segments −7 to 4 and 62 to 73 (see Fig. 2a) are consequently disordered. Thus, the amino terminus of the enzyme functions via a hydrogen-bonded "activation network" to shape an element of the enzyme's structure that (in contrast to the region assigned by Dijkstra et al. [1981a]) is on the surface of the dimer and quite accessible to aggregated substrate (see Fig. 5a). Brunie et al. (1985) gave detailed structural support to the previous suggestions of Verheij et al. (1981) that the amino terminus is likely to be an essential component of the interfacial binding apparatus. Unlike the "interfacial recognition surface" of Dijkstra et al. (1981a), which includes the active site His-48, the "activation network" is quite remote from His-48. The role of this activation network as the critical element in micellar or lamellar binding is consistent with alkylation studies using *p*-bromo-phenacyl bromide, which suggest that the binding site for monomeric substrate is physically distinct from the binding site for micelles (Volwerk et al. 1974).

This mode of activation proposed by Brunie et al. (1985) differs from that proposed by Dijkstra et al. (1981b), who suggested that the role of the enzyme's newly formed terminal amino group was to structure the active site through hydrogen-bonded interactions with catalytic functional groups. A part of this hydrogen-bonded system was a well-fixed water molecule. This explanation is not likely, since this water molecule is not part of the *C. atrox* enzyme's structure (134 fixed water molecules have been identified), yet the structure of the catalytic system is identical (Renetseder et al. 1985).

Functional Studies of Phospholipase A$_2$ Substrates: The Importance of Being Flexible

It was mentioned earlier that the most characteristic functional feature of phospholipases is the dependency of their catalytic activity on the physical state of their substrates. An especially striking example of this dependency, and an excellent model system for its study, is the spectacular burst of activity that occurs when short acyl chain phosphatidylcholines (PCs) form micelles, the so-called interfacial activation effect (Fig. 2b). It should be noted that the rate of hydrolysis of the aggregated substrate greatly exceeds the V_{max} extrapolated for an infinite monomeric concentration. This indicates that the aggregate does not serve just to increase the local concentration of substrate (Brockman et al. 1973), but rather that a different catalytic process is operating in the attack of phospholipases A$_2$ on aggregates as opposed to monomers. What are the features of the phospholipid aggregate that cause this enhancement in phospholipase A_2 activity?

We have discovered that one requirement for interfacial activation is that the substrate be flexible (Barlow et al. 1988). Figure 6 illustrates a semi-rigid PC analog specifically designed to test the importance of substrate deformability on phospholipase A_2 action. This short acyl chain analog has a built-in constraint that restricts the conformational flexibility of the glycerol-like backbone within the range determined by the puckering limits of an appropriately substituted all-*trans* cyclopentane-1,2,3-triol. The only other way in which it differs from the standard dihexanoyl PC is in the extra steric bulk of the "ethylene bridge." It is noteworthy that, in the case of long acyl chain analogs of this kind, only the phospholipid based on the all-*trans* cyclopentane-triol backbone was a substrate for phospholipase A_2 (A.J. Hancock and M.D. Lister, pers. comm.). Those based on the all-*cis* or the *cis-trans* cyclopentane-triols were not susceptible to catalytic hydrolysis. This was the reason for choosing an all-*trans* analog for our studies. Indeed, as can be seen from Table 1,

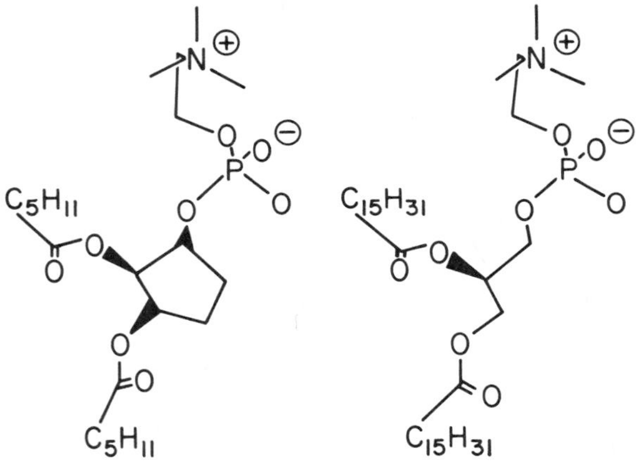

compound I is subject to catalytic attack by both snake venom and mammalian pancreas phospholipase A_2. Employing short acyl chains (six carbons) in the analog resulted in an experimentally accessible critical micellar concentration (CMC) of 11 mM (which is within 10% of that for the unconstrained equivalent—L-dihexanoyl PC) enabling us to conveniently study kinetics both above and below the CMC. The constrained analog appears to behave like its unconstrained counterpart when dispersed as a monomer. The kinetic mechanism for the hydrolysis of the constrained compound is similar to that observed for its unconstrained counterpart with all of the enzymes that we have examined; i.e., from porcine pancreas (proenzyme and enzyme), *C. atrox* venom (dimer), *A. p. piscivorus* venom (dimer), *A. p. piscivorus* venom (monomer, D-49), *A. p. piscivorus* venom (monomer, K-49). As a monomer, the constrained analog is slightly inferior to the L-dihexanoyl PC as a substrate for some enzymes, but it is a better substrate with others (refer to Table 1).

The constrained analogs, like naturally occurring lecithins, exhibit chiral specificity. Only the levorotatory enantiomer can be hydrolyzed. The (+) cyclopentanoid compound not only resists hydrolysis but, like its linear counterpart, serves as a competitive inhibitor for both the (−) enantiomer and the unconstrained reference compound. As a monomer, the K_i of the (+) compound approximates the K_m of its (−) enantiomorph.

The constrained substrate cannot be activated. The principal result of the work of Barlow et al. (1988) is that phospholipases A_2, when presented with the constrained substrate analog in aggregated form, have an observed rate of hydrolysis that does not exceed the V_{max} for the monomeric analog (Fig. 7). This is in striking contrast to the deformable linear analog whose hydrolysis is accelerated hundreds of times upon aggregation. In other words, the lack of flexibility in this analog prevents it from exhibiting the so-called interfacial activation effect.

It was important to establish that this difference in substrate behavior between the constrained and unconstrained compounds was primarily a consequence of their difference in conformational flexibility, as opposed to being a result of limited access of the substrate

Figure 6. The structure of the cyclopentanoid analog (I), fitted to the crystal structure for L-dipalmitoyl PC (II) (Hauser et al. 1981). The enantiomer of the cyclopentanoid analog illustrated here is the one which can be better fitted to the structure of the reference compound.

Table 1. Kinetic Parameters for Phospholipase A_2-catalyzed Hydrolysis of Monomeric L-Dihexanoyl PC (Unconstrained) and its (−)-Cyclopentanoid Analog (Constrained)

Phospholipase A_2	L-Dihexanoyl PC (CMC = 10 mM)		(−)-Cyclopentanoid analog (CMC = 11.2 mM)	
	K_m (mM)	V_{max} (units.mg^{-1})	K_m (mM)	V_{max} (units.mg^{-1})
Crotalus atrox	4.3(±0.6)	25(±2)	36(±9)	7(±1)
Porcine pancreas proenzyme	10 (±1)	9(±2)	13(±1)	17(±1)
Porcine pancreas enzyme	8.2(±0.6)	14(±3)	10(±1)	15(±2)

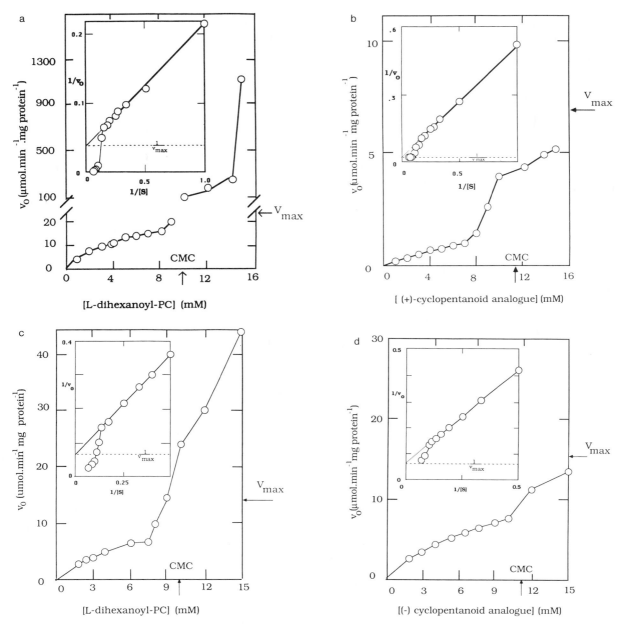

Figure 7. Hydrolysis of model substrates by phospholipase A_2. (*a*) *C. atrox* enzyme, L-dihexanoyl PC; (*b*) *C. atrox* enzyme, cyclopentanoid analog; (*c*) porcine pancreatic enzyme, L-dihexanoyl PC; (*d*) porcine pancreatic enzyme, cyclopentanoid analog. The experimental data were obtained with a spectrophotometric assay at 30°C. The reaction mixture contained 10 mM $CaCl_2$, 0.2 mM bromothymol blue:NaOH (pH 8), and 0.8–1.0 μg phospholipase A_2. (This "dye" assay was used rather than a "pH·stat" assay because it can be scaled down to save valuable substrate. However, as discussed in Barlow et al. (1988), the dye inhibits some phospholipases A_2.) V_{max} is the extrapolated rate of hydrolysis for the monomeric substrate at infinite concentration. Note that the enhanced rate for the micellar substrate (above the CMC) exceeds V_{max} only for the *un*constrained substrate. *Inset.* Same data plotted as double reciprocal plots of initial velocity as a function of substrate.

to the catalytic site created by the ethylene bridge or disparities in the physical chemistry of the respective aggregates. Since for pancreas enzyme, and at least one snake venom enzyme (the monomeric D-49 from *A. piscivorus*, data not shown), the constrained compound is a slightly better substrate than its counterpart, we are reasonably confident that the ethylene bridge is not a major obstacle to binding of the monomer to phospholipases A_2.

It could be argued that the constrained compounds produce aggregates having significantly different physical properties. There are three observations that suggest this is not the case. When compared to L-dihexanoyl PC, (1) the CMC for the cyclopentanoid analog occurs at an approximately similar concentration of phospholipid (11 mM compared to 10 mM for the L-dihexanoyl PC), (2) micelle formation is accompanied by the same typical changes in magnetic nonequivalence of the α-methylene protons (Plück-thun et al. 1986; Barlow et al. 1988), and (3) the constrained compound forms micelles of approximately similar size (the average aggregation number is about 50 monomers per micelle compared to 37 for the L-dihexanoyl PC [J.C. Vidal et al., unpubl. data]). The close correspondence of these parameters indicates that the physical properties of the aggregated constrained cyclopentanoid are not greatly perturbed by the constrained conformation of the polar group. It might still be argued that the enzyme does not associate with micelles of the analog because of an inappropriate polar surface. However, the enzyme does indeed "see" the analog micelles, as is evidenced by the discontinuity in the velocity versus substrate analog curve that occurs at the CMC (Fig. 7). Moreover, Figure 8 strongly suggests binding of enzyme to micelles of the analog. In this experiment, the addition of the nonhydrolyzable (+) enantiomer of the constrained analog is used to create mixed micelles containing the unconstrained L-dihexanoyl PC. Note that when the sum of the concentrations of inhibitor and substrate remains below the CMC, the addition of nonhydrolyzable constrained compound, as expected, progressively inhibits the enzymatic hydrolysis of L-dihexanoyl PC. However, when the total concentration of phospholipid reaches the CMC, the rate of hydrolysis of the L-dihexanoyl PC is markedly stimulated in the usual way. Not only does this result imply that the enzyme can bind to micelles consisting predominantly of the constrained analog, it also suggests that the enzyme is bound to the interface in an "active" form and in an appropriate orientation.

It might also be argued in terms of the dual phospholipid model that, although the constrained analog is

a substrate, it cannot fulfill the requirements of an "activator" or "helper." Barlow et al. (1988) have shown that monomeric nonhydrolyzable (+) cyclopentanoid analog stimulates hydrolysis of phosphatidyl-ethanolamine in mixed micelles with Triton X-100. The effect appears to be saturable and is completely analogous with the helper effect seen with other phosphorylcholine-containing compounds (Roberts et al. 1979). Therefore, the lack of a helper effect cannot be invoked to explain the failure to see enhanced hydrolysis in aggregates of the cyclopentanoid substrate.

It seems that the only hypothesis consistent with our result is one that proposes that aggregation restrains the range of conformations in normal flexible substrates to those that are favored by the enzyme's active site. These conformations presumably cannot be adopted by a nondeformable substrate analog. This is not to say that a conformational change of the enzyme at the interface and/or a neighboring headgroup helper effect does not occur—merely that alone they are insufficient to produce enhanced activity of phospholipase A_2 toward aggregated substrates.

Evolutionary Implications and Further Studies

From an evolutionary viewpoint, the phospholipases and aggregated phospholipids present a highly diversified enzyme/substrate system that developed to facilitate a variety of advanced functions typical of multicellular organisms. Phospholipases C and A_2 coordinate differentiated cellular activity by mediating transmembrane signaling. Venom phospholipases A_2 are enzymes that have evolved to paralyze or kill the prey by a variety of mechanisms involving highly targeted attacks on specific membranes (like those of myocardial cells or on the presynaptic membrane of the neuromuscular junction [Kini and Iwanaga 1986a,b]).

From a mechanistic viewpoint there are few precedents, either in structural biology or in enzymology, to help us understand even the most straightforward aspects of enzymatic attack on phospholipids in biological membranes and other phospholipid aggregates. There are even fewer precedents to suggest how certain phospholipases select specific membranes and are triggered to rapidly attack specific phospholipids in a designated location on the membrane surface. It is likely that protein/protein interactions play their usual regulatory role here as in most other processes; however, our structure/function studies of the extracellular phospholipases A_2 suggest an attractive and unifying hypothesis that we intend to explore further. We suggest that "shaping" or "conditioning" the substrate may modulate phospholipase activity. Just as the formation of aggregates converts a normal flexible phospholipid into a better substrate, we suggest that the modulation of phospholipase activity may be carried out to a great extent at the level of the substrate's structure. Perhaps in these late evolutionary events the flow of allosteric control has been reversed; integral membrane proteins may act as allosteric effectors of phospholipase sub-

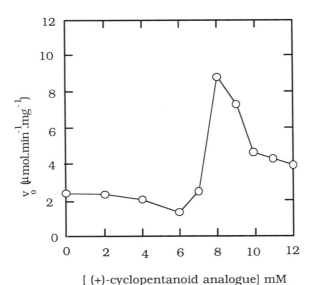

[(+)-cyclopentanoid analogue] mM

Figure 8. Enhanced activity of unconstrained substrate coaggregated with (+)-cyclopentanoid analog. The reaction mixtures contained 1.0 mM CaCl_2, 0.2 mM bromothymol blue:NaOH (pH 8), the concentrations of the (+)-cyclopentanoid analog indicated in the abscissa, 2.0 mM L-dihexanoyl PC and 0.6 μg of *C. atrox* phospholipase A_2.

strate conformation, making specific aggregated phospholipids in select regions of the membrane better or worse substrates.

It is clear that further structural and biochemical studies are required to understand the interaction between phospholipase A$_2$, a fairly rigid enzyme, and its true substrate, a very plastic assembly of flexible phospholipid molecules. Cloning of the phospholipase A$_2$ gene from mammalian pancreas (Ohara et al. 1986) and heterologous expression, coupled with site-directed mutagenesis, will provide an opportunity to directly explore the relationship between structure and function on the molecular level. However, the fact that the phospholipases A$_2$ seem to have a strict requirement for a specific aggregation-induced substrate conformation provides a challenge for future structural studies. The manner in which substrate binds to the enzyme remains very poorly understood. X-ray crystal structures of meaningful enzyme-substrate complexes are a compelling priority in the field. However, producing suitable cocrystals of phospholipase A$_2$ and aggregated substrate will be difficult, at best. Cocrystals with monomeric short-chain phospholipids may be misleading, since they are not necessarily the appropriate substrate analogs for understanding the effects at the membrane surface. On the other hand, our preliminary results with constrained phospholipids suggest that it might be possible to design compact and stable monomeric substrate analogs that conformationally mimic aggregated lipids and can be cocrystallized with phospholipases. This would appear to be a most fruitful avenue for future studies.

ACKNOWLEDGMENTS

Work was supported by grants from the United States Public Health Service (GM-22324) and the National Science Foundation (INT-8616103). We thank A.J. Hancock, Drs. M.D. Lister, E.A. Dennis, and H.Z. Sable for helpful discussions and Dr. Arthur Lesk for his computer graphics programs and help in their implementation.

REFERENCES

Abita, J.-P., M. Lazdunski, P.P.M. Bonsen, W.A. Pieterson, and G.H. de Haas. 1972. Zymogen-enzyme transformations: On the mechanism of activation of phospholipase A. Eur. J. Biochem. 30: 37.

Adamich, M. and E.A. Dennis. 1978. Specificity reversal in phospholipase A$_2$ hydrolysis of lipid mixtures. Biochem. Biophys. Res. Commun. 80: 424.

Adamich, M., M.F. Roberts, and E.A. Dennis. 1979. Phospholipid activation of cobra venom phospholipase A$_2$: Characterization of the phospholipid enzyme interaction. Biochemistry 18: 3308.

Allgyer, T.T. and M.A. Wells. 1979. Thermodynamic model for micelle formation by phosphatidylcholines containing short-chain fatty acids. Correlations with physical-chemical data and the effects of concentration on the activity of phospholipase A$_2$. Biochemistry 18: 4354.

Barlow, P.N., J.-C. Vidal, M.D. Lister, E.A. Dennis, and P.B. Sigler. 1988. Probing the role of substrate conformation in phospholipase A$_2$ action on aggregated phospholipids using constrained phosphatidylcholine analogues. J. Biol. Chem. (in press).

Brockman, H.L., J.H. Law, and F.J. Kézdy. 1973. Catalysis by adsorbed enzymes. The hydrolysis of tripropionin by pancreatic lipase adsorbed to siliconized glass beads. J. Biol. Chem. 248: 4965.

Brunie, S., J. Bolin, D. Gewirth, and P.B. Sigler. 1985. The refined crystal structure of dimeric phospholipase A$_2$ at 2.5 Å: Access to a shielded catalytic site. J. Biol. Chem. 260: 9742.

de Araujo, P.S., M.Y. Rosseneu, J.M.H. Kremer, E.J.J. van Zoelen, and G.H. de Haas. 1979. Structure and thermodynamic properties of the complexes between phospholipase A$_2$ and lipid micelles. Biochemistry 18: 580.

Deems, R.A., B.R. Eaton, and E.A. Dennis. 1975. Kinetic analysis of phospholipase A$_2$ activity towards mixed micelles and its implication for the study of lipolytic enzymes. J. Biol. Chem. 250: 9013.

de Haas, G.H., N.M. Postema, W. Nieuwenhuizen, and L.L.M. Van Deenen. 1968. Purification and properties of phospholipase A from porcine pancreas. Biochim. Biophys. Acta 159: 103.

Dennis, E.A. 1983. On phospholipases. In The enzymes, 3rd edition (ed. P.D. Boyer), vol. 16, p. 307. Academic Press, New York.

Dijkstra, B.W., J. Drenth, and K.H. Kalk. 1981a. Active site and catalytic mechanism of phospholipase A$_2$. Nature 289: 604.

Dijkstra, B.W., K.H. Kalk, W.G.J. Hol, and J. Drenth. 1981b. Structure of bovine pancreatic phospholipase A$_2$ at 1.7 Å resolution. J. Mol. Biol. 147: 97.

Dijkstra, B.W., G.J.H. van Nes, K.H. Kalk, N.P. Brandenburg, W.G.J. Hol, and J. Drenth. 1982. The structure of bovine pancreatic prophospholipase A$_2$ at 3.0 Å resolution. Acta Crystallogr. Sect. B Struct. Crystallogr. Cryst. Chem. B38: 793.

Dijkstra, B.W., R. Renetseder, K.H. Kalk, W.G.J. Hol, and J. Drenth. 1983. Structure of porcine pancreatic phospholipase A$_2$ at 2.6 Å resolution and comparison with bovine phospholipase A$_2$. J. Mol. Biol. 168: 163.

Dufton, M.J. and R.C. Hider. 1983. Classification of phospholipases A$_2$ according to sequences. Evolutionary and pharmacological implications. Eur. J. Biochem. 137: 545.

Fleer, E.A.M., H.M. Verheij, and G.H. de Haas. 1981. Modification of carboxylate groups in bovine pancreatic phospholipase A$_2$. Identification of aspartate-49 as Ca^{++}-binding ligand. Eur. J. Biochem. 113: 283.

Hachimori, Y., M.A. Wells, and D.J. Hanahan. 1971. Observations on the phospholipase A$_2$ of Crotalus atrox. Molecular weight and other properties. Biochemistry 10: 4084.

Hauser, H., I. Pascher, R.H. Pearson, and S. Sundell. 1981. Preferred conformation and molecular packing of phosphatidylethanolamine and phosphatidylcholine. Biochim. Biophys. Acta 650: 21.

Heinrikson, R.L., E.T. Krueger, and P.S. Keim. 1977. Amino acid sequence of phospholipase A$_2$-α from the venom of Crotalus adamanteus: A new classification of phospholipases A$_2$ based upon structural determinants. J. Biol. Chem. 252: 4913.

Hillie, J.D.R., G.M. Donné Op Den Kelder, P. Sauve, G.H. de Haas, and M.R. Egmond. 1981. Physico-chemical studies on the interaction of pancreatic phospholipase A$_2$ with a micellar substrate analogue. Biochemistry 20: 4068.

Israelachvili, J.N., S. Marcelja, and G. Horn. 1980. Physical principles of membrane organization. Q. Rev. Biophys. 73(2): 121.

Keith, C., D.S. Feldman, S. Deganello, J. Glick, K.B. Ward, E.O. Jones, and P.B. Sigler. 1981. The 2.5 Å crystal structure of a dimeric phospholipase A$_2$ from the venom of Crotalus atrox. J. Biol. Chem. 256: 8602.

Kini, R.M. and S. Iwanaga. 1986a. Structure-function relationships in phospholipases. I: Prediction of presynaptic neurotoxicity. Toxicon 24: 527.

———. 1986b. Structure-function relationships of phospholipases. II: Charge density distribution and the myotoxicity of presynaptically neurotoxic phospholipases. *Toxicon* **24:** 895.

Lewis, R.V., M.F. Roberts, E.A. Dennis, and W.S. Allison. 1977. Photoactivated heterobifunctional cross-linking reagents which demonstrate the aggregation state of phospholipase A$_2$. *Biochemistry* **16:** 5650.

Lombardo, D. and E.A. Dennis. 1985. Immobilized phospholipase A$_2$ from cobra venom. *J. Biol. Chem.* **260:** 16114.

Louw, A.I. and L. Visser. 1978. The synergism of cardiotoxin and phospholipase A$_2$ in hemolysis. *Biochim. Biophys. Acta* **512:** 163.

Maraganore, J.M., G. Merutka, W. Cho, W. Welches, F.J. Kézdy, and R.L. Heinrikson. 1984. A new class of phospholipases A$_2$ with lysine in place of aspartate 49. *J. Biol. Chem.* **259:** 13839.

Meyer, H., W.C. Puijk, R. Dijkman, M.M.E.L. Foda-van der Hoorn, F. Pattus, A.J. Slotboom, and G.H. de Haas. 1979. Comparative studies of tyrosine modification in pancreatic phospholipases. 2. Properties of the nitrotyrosyl, aminotyrosyl, and dansylaminotyrosyl derivatives of pig, horse, and ox phospholipases A$_2$ and their zymogens. *Biochemistry* **18:** 3589.

Ohara, O., M. Takami, E. Nakamura, Y. Tsuruta, Y. Fujii, M. Shin, H. Teraoka, and M. Okamata. 1986. Dog and rat pancreatic phospholipases A$_2$: Complete amino acid sequences deduced from complementary DNAs. *J. Biochem.* **99:** 733.

Pieterson, W.A., J.C. Vidal, J.J. Volwerk, and G.H. de Haas. 1974. Zymogen-catalyzed hydrolysis of monomeric substrates and the presence of a recognition site for lipid-water interfaces in phospholipase A$_2$. *Biochemistry* **13:** 1455.

Plückthun, A., J. DeBony, T. Fanni, and E.A. Dennis. 1986. Conformation of fatty acyl chains in α-phosphatidylcholine and β-phosphatidylcholine and phosphatidylethanolamine derivatives in sonicated vesicles. *Biochim. Biophys. Acta* **856:** 144.

Randolph, A., T.P. Sakmar, and R.L. Heinrikson. 1980. Phospholipase A$_2$: Structure, function and evolution. In *Frontiers in protein chemistry* (ed. A.B. Liu et al.), p. 297. Elsevier, Amsterdam.

Raykova, D. and B. Blagoev. 1986. Hydrolysis of short chain phosphatidylcholines by bee venom phospholipase A$_2$. *Toxicon* **24:** 791.

Renetseder, R. 1986. "X-ray crystallographic studies on structure and action of phospholipase A$_2$." Ph.D. thesis, University of Gröningen, The Netherlands.

Renetseder, R., S. Brunie, B.W. Dijkstra, J. Drenth, and P.B. Sigler. 1985. A comparison of the crystal structures of phospholipase A$_2$ from bovine pancreas and *Crotalus atrox* venom. *J. Biol. Chem.* **260:** 11627.

Roberts, M.F., R.A. Deems, and E.A. Dennis. 1977. Dual role of interfacial phospholipid in phospholipase A$_2$ catalysis. *Proc. Natl. Acad. Sci.* **74:** 1950.

Roberts, M.F., M. Adamich, R.J. Robson, and E.A. Dennis. 1979. Phospholipase activation of cobra venom phospholipase A$_2$: A lipid-lipid or lipid-enzyme interaction. *Biochemistry* **18:** 3301.

Scott, D.L., A. Achari, M. Zajac, and P.B. Sigler. 1986. Crystallization and preliminary diffraction studies of the Lys-49 phospholipase A$_2$ from *Agkistrodon piscivorus piscivorus*. *J. Biol. Chem.* **261:** 12337.

Sekar, M.C. and L.E. Hokin. 1986. The role of phosphoinositides in signal transduction. *J. Membr. Biol.* **89:** 193.

Shen, B.W., F.H.C. Tsoa, J.H. Law, and F.J. Kézdy. 1975. Kinetic study of the hydrolysis of lecithin monolayers by *Crotalus adamanteus* α-phospholipase A$_2$. Monomer-dimer equilibrium. *J. Am. Chem. Soc.* **97:** 1205.

Shier, W.T. 1979. Activation of high levels of endogenous phospholipase A$_2$ in cultured cells. *Proc. Natl. Acad. Sci.* **76:** 195.

Shipolini, R.A., G.L. Calewaert, R.C. Cottrell, and C.A. Vernon. 1974. The amino acid sequence and carbohydrate content of phospholipase A$_2$ from bee venom. *Eur. J. Biochem.* **48:** 447.

Smith, C.M. and M.A. Wells. 1981. A further examination of the active form of *Crotalus adamanteus* phospholipase A$_2$. *Biochim. Biophys. Acta* **289:** 147.

Tönsing, L., D.J.J. Potgeitrer, A. Louw, and L. Visser. 1983. The binding of snake venom cardiotoxin to heart cell membranes. *Biochim. Biophys. Acta.* **732:** 282.

van Dam-Mieras, M.C.E., A.J. Slotboom, W.A. Pieterson, and G.H. de Haas. 1975. The interaction of phospholipase A$_2$ with micellar interfaces. The role of the N-terminal region. *Biochemistry* **14:** 5387.

Verheij, H.M., A.J. Slotboom, and G.H. de Haas. 1981. Structure and function of phospholipase A$_2$. *Rev. Physiol. Biochem. Pharmacol.* **91:** 91.

Verheij, H.M., J.J. Volwerk, E.H.J.M. Janse, W.C. Puyk, B.E. Dijkstra, J. Drenth, and G.H. de Haas. 1980. Methylation of histidine-48 in pancreatic phospholipase A$_2$: Role of histidine and calcium ion in the catalytic mechanism. *Biochemistry* **19:** 743.

Vogel, H. 1981. Incorporation of melittin into phosphatidylcholine bilayers. Study of binding and conformational changes. *FEBS Lett.* **134:** 37.

Volwerk, J.J., W.A. Pieterson, and G.H. de Haas. 1974. Histidine at the active site of phospholipase A$_2$. *Biochemistry* **13:** 1446.

Wells, M.A. 1971. Evidence that the phospholipases A$_2$ of *Crotalus adamanteus* are dimers. *Biochemistry* **10:** 4074.

———. 1974. The mechanism of interfacial activation of phospholipase A$_2$. *Biochemistry* **13:** 2248.

Yunes, R., A.R. Goldhammer, W.K. Garner, and E.H. Cordon. 1977. Melittin facilitation of bee venom phospholipase A$_2$-catalyzed hydrolysis of unsonicated lecithin liposomes. *Arch. Biochem. Biophys.* **183:** 105.

Atomic Protein Structures Reveal Basic Features of Binding of Sugars and Ionic Substrates, and Calcium Cation

F.A. QUIOCHO, N.K. VYAS, J.S. SACK, AND M.N. VYAS

Howard Hughes Medical Institute and Departments of Biochemistry and of Physiology and Molecular Biophysics, Baylor College of Medicine, Houston, Texas 77030

Following the discovery of the sulfate-binding protein 20 years ago by Pardee and co-workers (1966), about two dozen single-chain, water-soluble proteins (collectively called "binding proteins") have been purified from osmotic-shock fluid of gram-negative bacteria (Wilson and Smith 1978; Ames 1986). The identification of these proteins as essential components of high-affinity active transport systems for a large variety of carbohydrates, amino acids, and ions, and the demonstration that a number of the sugar-binding proteins serve as initial receptors for the simple behavioral response of bacterial chemotaxis (Adler 1975) provided the impetus for our crystallographic study of the structure and function of these proteins.

Binding proteins, which are located in the periplasmic space, have molecular weights in the range of 25,000–45,000 and all contain one tight ligand-binding site with very similar dissociation constants (of about 0.1 μM), irrespective of the nature of the substrate. Protein components—confined in the cytoplasmic membrane and distinct for either transport or chemotaxis—are also required for both processes. It is believed that the binding of a substrate to the binding protein causes a conformational change, allowing it, rather than the unliganded protein, to form a productive complex with the membrane-bound protein components. The ensuing complex formation initiates active transport or flagella motion.

Seven binding proteins, each specific for L-arabinose, D-galactose/D-glucose, sulfate, leucine/isoleucine/valine, D-maltose, leucine, and phosphate are currently under investigation in our laboratory. The structures of the L-arabinose-binding protein and sulfate-binding protein have been extensively refined crystallographically at 1.7 Å resolution to R-factors of 14% (Quiocho and Vyas 1984; Pflugrath and Quiocho 1985; J.S. Sack and F.A. Quiocho, unpubl. data). Well-refined structures have been achieved for the D-galactose-binding protein (GBP) at 1.9 Å (Vyas et al. 1987), the Leu/Ile/Val-binding protein at 2.4 Å (J.S. Sack et al., in prep.), and the leucine-specific-binding protein at 2.5 Å (J.S. Sack et al., unpubl. data). The preliminary trace of the polypeptide backbone of the D-maltose-binding protein has recently been obtained, and a search for heavy-atom derivatives of the phosphate-binding protein is currently under way in our laboratory.

Apart from the knowledge of the tertiary structures, an important component of the structural analysis concerns the mode of binding of the various substrates. Indeed, we have discovered novel features that have led to new and fundamental understanding of the binding of sugars and of charged substrates (e.g., sulfate, aliphatic amino acids). We have also recently unraveled a novel calcium-binding site in the D-galactose-binding protein. These findings have far-reaching importance in the understanding of electrostatic interactions, the means whereby isolated buried ionic groups are stabilized, as well as the design, chemistry, and evolution of calcium-binding sites in proteins. A description of the structural features of the various binding protein-ligand interactions is the major thrust of this paper.

Tertiary Structures of Periplasmic Binding Proteins

There are remarkable similarities in both the tertiary structure and ligand-binding properties of the L-arabinose-, sulfate-, D-galactose-, Leu/Ile/Val-, and leucine-specific-binding proteins. All five proteins are ellipsoidal in shape (axial ratios = 2:1) and are composed of two similar yet distinct globular domains (Quiocho et al. 1987b). These structures have similar overall dimensions of approximately 40 × 35 × 70 Å. The two domains in all of the structures are connected by three separate peptide segments. Although these interdomain connecting segments are widely separated in the primary structure, they are spatially close together. Moreover, as these segments are located near the periphery of the protein molecules, they serve as the base or "boundary" of the deep cleft between the two domains. The cleft is where the substrate is bound and becomes almost totally engulfed (Newcomer et al. 1981; Quiocho and Vyas 1984; Pflugrath and Quiocho 1985; Vyas et al. 1987; J.S. Sack et al., unpubl. data).

The three-peptide-segment interdomain connectivity found in the binding proteins is very different from those commonly observed in many multidomain proteins in which each domain is formed from one continuous polypeptide segment with only one connection between any two domains (Schulz and Schirmer 1979). This type of connectivity in the binding proteins also complicates our understanding of protein folding.

In the binding-protein structures, the first third of the polypeptide chain constitutes the major part of the amino-terminal domain, and the second third forms the bulk of the carboxy-terminal domain. The final third of the chain follows a winding route by traversing both domains. Despite this complex folding pattern, the packing of the secondary structure in both domains is very similar. The domains have a central β sheet flanked by at least a pair of α helices. The interfaces between the sheet and helices are occupied predominantly by nonpolar residues. The α helices and β-sheet strands generally alternate along the chain, so that carboxyl termini of the strands and the amino termini of the helices point toward the binding-site cleft between the two domains.

Despite the similarity of the tertiary structures and mode of binding of the substrates, the binding proteins as a whole lack significant sequence homology.

Binding Protein-substrate Complexes

What is perhaps the most notable discovery emerging from the highly refined atomic structures of the liganded form of the periplasmic binding proteins is that substrates, although often unrelated and possessing completely different structures (e.g., saccharides, sulfate, and amino acids), are bound primarily by hydrogen bonds. This finding is fully consistent with the fact that these proteins bind their ligands with very similar tight affinity. Furthermore, this finding, together with the homology of the tertiary structures, suggests that the mechanisms by which these proteins undertake their function within transport or chemotaxis must be very similar.

Protein-sugar interactions. Protein-carbohydrate interactions play an important role in a wide range of biological and biochemical processes. Consequently, a detailed understanding of these interactions at the molecular level is of considerable importance. In terms of details and accuracy, the 1.7 Å resolution highly refined X-ray structure of the complex of L-arabinose-binding protein with its sugar substrate remains unsurpassed (Quiocho and Vyas 1984). We have also very recently completed extensive refinement of the 1.9 Å structure of the complex of D-galactose-binding protein with bound D-glucose (also a natural substrate) to an R factor of 14% (for preliminary account, see Vyas et al. 1987). We believe that these complexes not only exhibit essentially all the molecular features of protein-carbohydrate interactions, but also provide a useful framework to analyze other complexes and to formulate principles of such interactions. These features and principles are briefly presented herein. A more comprehensive review of the three-dimensional structures of proteins and enzymes with specificity for carbohydrates and sugar-protein interactions has recently appeared (Quiocho 1986). Based on the atomic structure of the complex of the binding protein with L-arabinose (Fig. 1), the salient features of protein-sugar interactions are as follows (Quiocho and Vyas 1984; Quiocho 1986).

Since hydroxyls are the basic functional groups of sugars, hydrogen bonds involving these groups are the major interactions conferring both the stereospecificity and stability of protein-sugar complexes. In the case of the binding protein-arabinose complex, ten excellent hydrogen bonds are formed (Quiocho and Vyas 1984). Although the anomeric hydroxyl groups participate almost exclusively as hydrogen-bond donors, all the other hydroxyls participate as donors and acceptors simultaneously. These patterns of hydrogen bonding of sugar-hydroxyl groups are consistent with the following concepts (Quiocho 1986): First the O-1 or anomeric hydroxyl, as a result of the "anomeric effect" is more acidic and thus a stronger-than-average hydrogen-bond donor. Second, because of cooperative or synergistic effect, the involvement of hydroxyl groups as hydrogen-bond donors and acceptors leads to stronger-

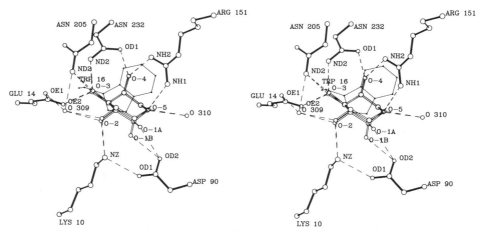

Figure 1. Stereoscopic view of the interaction between L-arabinose-binding protein and the bound α- or β- anomeric form of L-arabinose substrate. Both anomeric sugars (unfilled bonds) form ten hydrogen bonds (indicated by dashed lines) with the same binding site residues (solid lines) and water molecules. The α-anomeric hydroxyl is labeled O-1A and the β-anomeric hydroxyl, O-1B. Trp-16 (thinner lines) is partially stacked on the hydrophobic patch of the L-arabinose consisting of C-3, C-4, and C-5. See text for details.

than-average hydrogen bonds. And third, in the low dielectric constant environment of the sugar-binding site of proteins, hydrogen-bond formation should not leave "free" the hydrogen of the sugar hydroxyls. The last concept presupposes that the sugar hydroxyl in such an environment would be better as a hydrogen-bond donor or concurrently as a hydrogen-bond donor and acceptor rather than solely as an acceptor.

Nonanomeric hydroxyls serve simultaneously as hydrogen-bond donors and acceptors (Figs. 1 and 2). Remarkably, this "cooperative" hydrogen-bonding in the binding protein-arabinose complex can be described simply as

$$(NH)_n \rightarrow OH \rightarrow O \qquad (1)$$

where NH and O are hydrogen-bond donor and acceptor groups in the protein-binding site, respectively, OH is a nonanomeric sugar hydroxyl, and $n = 1$ or 2. The NH donor groups emanate from the side chains of Lys-10, Arg-151, Asn-205, and Asn-232, whereas the O acceptor groups come from Glu-14 and Asn-232 side chains and the isolated water molecule 309. This pattern of hydrogen-bonding may very well be a common feature of protein-sugar complexes (Quiocho 1986).

The bound arabinose is additionally hydrogen-bonded to the receptor via the sugar-ring oxygen (O-

5). In this case, the ring oxygen accepts two hydrogen bonds (Figs. 1 and 2).

The majority of the residues utilized in sugar binding have planar polar side chains with two or more functional groups that are engaged in multiple hydrogen bonds. These residues in the binding protein-arabinose complex are Asn, Glu, Asp, and Arg (Figs. 1 and 2). Two reasons account for these findings. First, two of the planar side chains (Arg-151 and Asn-232) make bidentate hydrogen bonds with the sugars. The geometry of these bidentate hydrogen bonds is such that the atoms OD1 and ND2 of Asn-232 and O-3 and O-4 of the sugar are coplanar, as are atoms NH1 and NH2 of Arg-151, and Ara O-5 and O-4. Second, all planar side chains, together with the sugar molecule, are involved in extensive networks of hydrogen bonds with other residues and water molecules in the binding-site region. At least three shells of residues around the sugar participate in these networks. Two of these shells are shown in Figure 2.

It is especially important to note that the formation of the hydrogen-bond networks leads to full utilization of all the functional groups of the essential side-chain residues and of *every one* of the potential hydrogen-bond donor groups of these residues (Arg-151, Asn-205, and Asn-232), arabinose, and the two bound water molecules (see Fig. 2). This finding is the principal basis

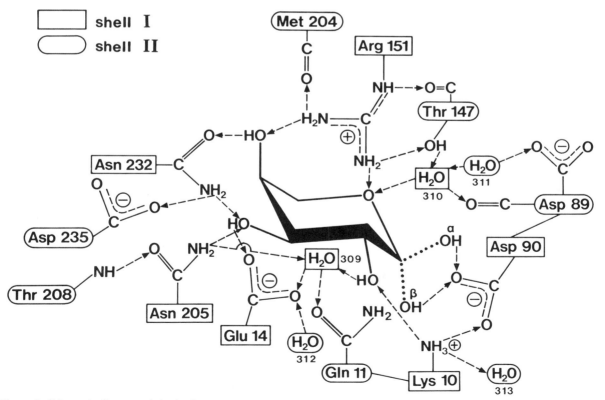

Figure 2. Schematic diagram of the intricate networks of hydrogen bonds formed in the complex of the L-arabinose-binding protein with the L-arabinose substrate. Shell I represents the essential residues hydrogen-bonded to the sugars and to adjacent second shell (shell II) of residues. Note especially that Arg-151 is not involved in salt linkages but is the source of five donor groups for five hydrogen bonds. (Adapted from Quiocho and Vyas 1984.)

of the third concept describing the patterns of hydrogen bonds expected for sugar hydroxyls (see above). Although Lys-10 differs from the rest of the essential residues, it is engaged in multiple interactions crucial to ligand binding. Its ammonium side chain is in an excellent position to donate a hydrogen bond to O-2 hydroxyl, to fix (via a salt link) an alignment of the essential Asp-90, and to make van der Waals' contacts with each of the anomeric hydroxyls.

The hydrogen-bonding scheme shown in Figure 2 (including the directions of the arrows) is dictated entirely by the result of the structural analysis of the complex. Remarkably, there is no ambiguity in the entire scheme. The structure of the binding protein-arabinose complex provides the first clear mapping of the hydrogen-bond networks in a protein-sugar complex.

The geometries of the cooperative hydrogen bonding shown in Equation (1) are those expected for maximal interactions (see Fig. 1). The O-3 hydroxyl is fully coordinated ($n = 2$) in an arrangement that is essentially tetrahedral, including the sugar C–O bond. The hydrogen-bonding geometry of O-4 hydroxyl simultaneously donating and accepting one hydrogen bond is such that the atoms C-4 and O-4 of the sugar, Arg-151 NH2, and Asn-232 OD1 are coplanar. Also, the H bond donated to or by O-4 hydroxyl is oriented so that both lone pairs of electrons on either acceptor group (the sugar-hydroxyl oxygen or the OD1 of Asn-232) are utilized in accepting the donor group. Similar analysis of the cooperative hydrogen bonding of O-2 hydroxyl leads to the same observations. As the sugar-ring oxygen accepts two hydrogen bonds in almost tetrahedral coordination, each of the lone pairs of electrons on the sugar-ring oxygen is directed at a hydrogen-bond donor group.

A novel stereospecificity has been revealed in the L-arabinose-binding protein: Both the α- and the β-anomeric forms of the sugar are substrates of the protein. The key to the ability of the binding protein to recognize both anomers—while using the same residues in hydrogen bonding—is the precise alignment of the atom OD2 of Asp-90, enabling the atom to accept a hydrogen bond from either the α (equatorial) or β (axial) anomeric hydroxyl (Figs. 1 and 2). This stereospecificity is fully consistent with the transport function of the binding protein: The open-chain aldehyde form, derived from both anomers of the translocated L-arabinose, is utilized by the cell in the biosynthesis of pentose phosphates (Engelsberg 1971). It is noteworthy that many of the enzymes of glucose metabolism (e.g., hexokinase, glucokinase, glucose-6-phosphatase) also act on both anomeric forms of their respective sugar substrates.

Protein-sugar complexes are further stabilized by van der Waals' forces (Quiocho 1986). About 45 van der Waals' contacts between non-hydrogen atoms in the range of 3.2–4.0 Å are formed between non-hydrogen atoms of the binding protein and arabinose. Of special significance is the observation that some of these contacts involve a cluster of nonpolar atoms within the L-arabinose (Quiocho and Vyas 1984). The disposition of both the equatorial O-3 and the axial O-4 hydroxyls to one side on the pyranose ring creates a hydrophobic patch composed of C-3, C-4, and C-5. As shown in Figure 1, Trp-16 is partially stacked with the hydrophobic patch. This specific type of interaction (i.e., stacking of aromatic residues with a sugar ring), which may prove more common than heretofore anticipated (Quiocho 1986), should confer substrate specificity by disallowing binding of sugar substrate epimers because of steric hindrance or polarity of the hydroxyls. It has been shown that the epimers of L-arabinose or D-galactose at positions C-3 and C-4 do not in fact bind to the L-arabinose-binding protein.

Finally, the arabinose bound to the binding protein and practically all of the hydrogen-bonding residues are buried and inaccessible to the bulk solvent (Quiocho and Vyas 1984). Based on the Lee and Richards (1971) criteria, the solvent-accessible area of the L-arabinose in the free state is reduced by 98% when bound in the L-arabinose-binding protein. An unusual finding is that the charged essential residue Arg-151 is not only completely sequestered, but uncompensated for; there are no anions, negatively charged residues, or water molecules close to the side chain of Arg-151. Nevertheless, each of the five hydrogen-bond donor groups of the guanidinium side chain is engaged in hydrogen bonding to the sugar and amino acid residues, notably via their peptide CO groups (Fig. 2). A general mechanism for stabilization of uncompensated buried ionic groups such as the Arg-151 will be presented below.

The complex between the D-galactose-binding protein and D-glucose is depicted in Figure 3. This complex also shows the same basic features discussed above for the mode of binding of L-arabinose to the arabinose-binding protein. One particular feature worth noting is that two aromatic residues are associated with the bound D-glucose—one on either side of the plane of the pyranose ring. The locations of the aromatic residues are consistent with there being two hydrophobic patches in D-glucose—one on either side of the pyranose ring.

Binding protein-ionic substrate interactions. Hydrogen bonding also constitutes the major interaction in the complex between the sulfate-binding protein and the sulfate dianion as shown in Figure 4. All the sulfate oxygens are engaged as acceptors for a total of seven excellent hydrogen bonds (Pflugrath and Quiocho 1985; J.S. Sack and F.A. Quiocho, unpubl. data). Five of the hydrogen bonds to the sulfate involve five main-chain peptide NH groups. Consequently, the final geometry of the sulfate-binding site greatly depends on the precise folding of the polypeptide backbone. We further note that all five peptide units are in turn coupled via their CO groups to arrays of hydrogen bonds.

Four unusual features also characterize the complex of the binding protein with sulfate. First and foremost,

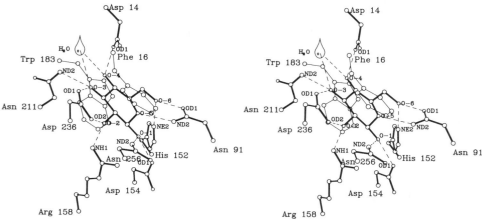

Figure 3. Stereoscopic view of the interactions in the complex of D-galactose-binding protein with D-glucose (also a natural substrate). Besides the hydrogen bonds involving all the sugar hydroxyls, the sugar substrate is sandwiched between two aromatic residues (Trp-183 and Phe-16) (N.K. Vyas et al., unpubl. data).

neither positively charged residues nor cations nor water molecules are within van der Waals' contact of the sulfate, thus precluding salt linkages to neutralize the sulfate charges. Second, the bound sulfate is buried about 7 Å below the protein surface and completely inaccessible to the bulk solvent. Third, as three of the five peptide NH groups hydrogen-bonded to the sulfate each constitute the first peptide unit of the first turn of a helix, the sulfate is in proximity to three α helices. However, the sulfate is not centered on any of the helix axes. Fourth, six of the seven hydrogen bonds donated to the sulfate are further involved (via peptide bonds) in hydrogen-bond arrays (see Fig. 4).

These arrays, starting with the sulfate oxygens, are as follows: (1) O-1 to peptide NH of 173; the CO group of the same peptide (from residue 172) in turn initiates a

continuous sequence of alternating peptide units and hydrogen bonds within an α helix. This left-handed "zigzag" line of hydrogen-bonded peptide units has the general form:

$$O \cdots NH_{i+4} \qquad (2)$$

where $i = m + 3(n - 1)$; m is the residue bearing the first peptide O, and $n = 1,2,3...$ indicates the extent of the hydrogen-bonded peptide units within the helix. (The helix array in this case has $m = 172$ and $n = 1$–3.) (2) O-1 to OG of Ser-130 to the peptide NH of residue 133, which is in turn part of an array in a helix with $m = 132$ and $n = 1$–5; (3) O-2 to peptide NH of residue 45, which is part of a helix array with $m = 44$ and $n = 1$–3; (4) O-2 to peptide NH of 131 and peptide CO

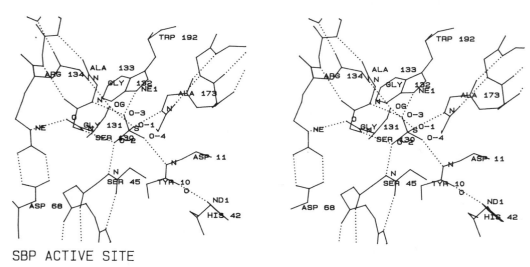

SBP ACTIVE SITE

Figure 4. The structure of the complex of the sulfate-binding protein with sulfate substrate as determined at 1.7 Å resolution. The seven hydrogen bonds formed in the complex are as follows. O-1 of the sulfate accepts two hydrogen bonds, one from the peptide NH of Ala-171 and the other from the OH of Ser-130. O-2 is the recipient of two NH hydrogen-bond donors from the peptide units of Gly-131 and Ser-45. O-3 forms two hydrogen bonds with NH groups: one from the peptide bond involving Gly-132 and the other from the side chain of Trp-192. O-4 is associated with only one hydrogen bond, that with the peptide NH of Asp-11. Only the first two turns of the three helices (44–54, 131–148, 172–181) close to the sulfate are shown.

of 130 to NE of Arg-134; (5) O-3 to peptide NH of Gly-132 which is part of a helix array with m = 131 and n = 1–5; and (6) O-4 to peptide NH of Asp-11 and peptide CO of residue 10 to His-42 ND1.

At least 41 van der Waals' contacts ranging from 3.2 to 4 Å are formed between non-hydrogen atoms of sulfate-binding protein and the sulfate (J.S. Sack and F.A. Quiocho, unpubl. data).

As there are no salt linkages nor cations in proximity to the sequestered sulfate dianion, the paramount question is "What is the mechanism for stabilizing the charges on the sulfate?"

The Leu/Ile/Val-binding protein structure—unlike the structures of L-arabinose-, D-galactose-, and sulfate-binding proteins—was determined without bound ligand (Saper and Quiocho 1983). In fact, it was necessary to remove the endogenous L-leucine bound to purified protein to obtain octahedral crystals that are suitable for high-resolution X-ray analysis; otherwise, crystals of the liganded form are thin needles. The Leu/Ile/Val-binding protein structure shows the two domains to be more separated than in the other binding-protein structures.

In a further experiment, Leu, Ile, or Val was soaked in crystals of Leu/Ile/Val-binding protein. Apparently due to crystal-packing forces, the presence of any one of these branched aliphatic amino acids did not cause the two domains to come close toward each other and totally enclose the substrate. However, each amino acid does bind isomorphously in a cavity located exclusively in the wall of the amino-terminal domain facing the cleft (Saper and Quiocho 1983).

Refinement at 2.8 Å resolution of the Leu/Ile/Val-binding protein structure with "diffused" leucine shows the amino acid substrate held in place primarily by seven hydrogen bonds: three to the ammonium group and four to the carboxylate group (see Fig. 5) (J.S. Sack and F.A. Quiocho, unpubl. data). It is noteworthy that four of these hydrogen bonds are formed with three peptide units. These peptide units are in turn part of hydrogen-bond arrays (Fig. 5). The bound leucine is only partially exposed to the bulk solvent; the solvent-

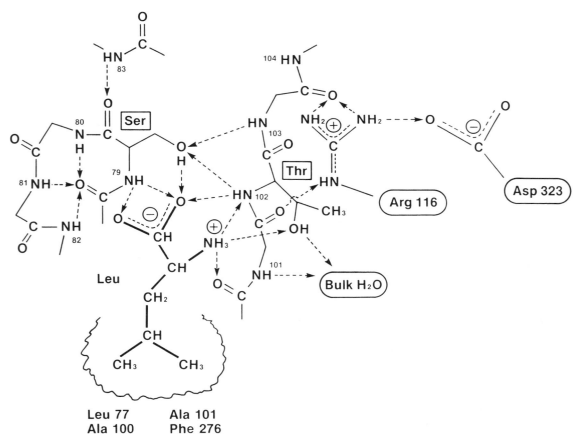

Figure 5. Schematic diagram of the complex between the Leu/Ile/Val-binding protein and L-leucine substrate. The hydrogen bonding is based on the structure refinement of the complex at 2.8 Å resolution. Thicker lines indicate the leucine substrate (Leu). The carboxylate group of Leu forms a total of four hydrogen bonds, whereas the ammonium group is involved in three hydrogen bonds. The main-chain peptide NH 79 forms a bidentate hydrogen bond with the two Leu carboxylate oxygens. It is possible for the peptide NH 102 to form a bidentate hydrogen bond and accept a hydrogen bond from the ammonium group of the bound Leu. The hydrogen-bond arrays mediated through the peptide bonds associated with the bound Leu are also indicated. (Adapted from Quiocho et al. 1987a.)

accessible area of the free leucine is reduced by 87% in the bound state. Furthermore, it is notable that neither countercharged residues nor ions are close to the ammonium and carboxylate groups of the bound leucine. How are the charges on the sequestered leucine zwitterion stabilized?

Charge Stabilization of Isolated Sequestered Ionic Groups

A discovery of fundamental importance resulting from our structural studies is that isolated ionic groups can be sequestered in proteins without formation of salt linkages or the presence of counterions. These groups include the ligand binding-site residue Arg-151 of the L-arabinose-binding protein (Fig. 2), the sulfate substrate bound to the sulfate-binding protein, and the leucine substrate bound to the Leu/Ile/Val-binding protein. Despite the differences in the nature and extent of the charges on the sulfate dianion, leucine zwitterion, and the positively charged arginine side chain, three key common features characterize the interactions of each of these buried ionic groups with the specific binding proteins (Quiocho et al. 1987a). First, the interactions are mediated primarily via hydrogen bonds with no obvious salt linkages or the presence of counterions. Second, the hydrogen bonds are formed chiefly with main-chain peptide units; the peptide CO groups being associated with the positively charged arginine residue, the NH moieties with the sulfate dianion, and both peptide groups with the leucine zwitterion. Third, the peptide units associated with the three charged groups are in turn coupled to a variety of hydrogen-bond arrays.

On the basis of the three common features outlined above, we have proposed a mechanism for stabilization of charges on isolated and sequestered ionic groups (Quiocho et al. 1987a). The mechanism also rests upon the facts that the peptide bond is a composite of a few canonical resonant structures—neutral and ionic resonant structures being the two predominant ones (Pauling 1960)—and that interactions (e.g., hydrogen bonding) involving the peptide bond influence the labile electronic structure of the peptide bond (Popov and Sheltova 1971; Llinás and Klein 1975). The mechanism simply considers the hydrogen bonds, particularly those involving the highly polarized main-chain peptide units, to be effective in stabilizing the sequestered charges on the positive Arg-151 residue, the bound sulfate dianion, and the leucine zwitterion substrates. The highly polarized peptide units are due to the hydrogen bonding of one end of the peptide units to the ionic groups and of the other end to arrays of hydrogen bonds or charged side-chain residues. In these situations, the dipole moment of each of the peptide units associated with the charged groups is likely to be somewhat greater than 5 Debye, the value obtained experimentally and theoretically for a peptide unit in α helix (Applequist and Mahr 1966; Wada 1976). Moreover, the ionic resonant form of the peptide unit ought to be stabilized, thus providing highly localized partial countercharges sufficient to neutralize the various ionic groups. The arrays of hydrogen bonds coupled to these charged groups could further disperse the buried charges. The importance of hydrogen bonds and associated arrays coupled via peptide bonds was originally proposed in the case of the binding protein-sulfate complex (Pflugrath and Quiocho 1985).

Although the binding proteins contain at least eight helices, the helix macrodipole does not appear to be of general importance in stabilization of the different charged groups described above. In fact, Arg-151 and the bound leucine substrate are nowhere near a helix terminus. There are three helix amino termini close to the sulfate molecule, but we believe that helix macrodipoles could play a major role in long-range attraction of the dianion. On the other hand, in the final complex formation, the more highly directional hydrogen bonds and peptide dipoles assume a more dominant role in not only conferring specificity upon the binding site and ensuring correctness of fit for the substrate but also in providing sufficient means for stablizing the buried isolated charges. Although hydrogen bonds are also important in the binding of neutral sugars to the sugar-binding protein and zwitterionic amino acids to the amino acid binding proteins, it is not obvious whether helix macrodipoles play a role in these protein-substrate complexes.

We have noted that the three basic features of the electrostatic interactions involving the three different charged groups described above, especially the peptide-bond-mediated hydrogen bonds, may be more common than heretofore anticipated (Quiocho et al. 1987a). Moreover, the proposed mechanism can readily be applied to processes requiring enhancement of reactive active site residues of enzymes and stabilization of enzyme reaction intermediates. Among the examples cited recently in support of these claims are flavodoxin, chymotrypsin, and related proteolytic enzymes, and rhodanese (Quiocho et al. 1987a). In chymotrypsin and other proteolytic enzymes, the tetrahedral anion intermediate in the catalyzed reaction is stabilized in the "oxyanion hole," primarily by hydrogen bonding with main-chain peptide units (Kraut 1977).

Protein-Calcium Interactions

In the course of refining the 1.9 Å resolution structure of the D-galactose-binding protein, we discovered a novel calcium-binding site (Vyas et al. 1987). This finding has important implications in understanding the designs, chemistry, and evolution of calcium-binding proteins.

Figure 6 shows the atomic structure around the Ca^{++} in the D-galactose-binding protein which is coordinated by seven ligands, all of which are protein oxygen atoms. The entire calcium-binding site is composed of a nine-residue loop (134–142) and a dipeptide segment (residues 204–205). The nine-residue segment loops around the calcium and deploys ligand atoms Asp-134

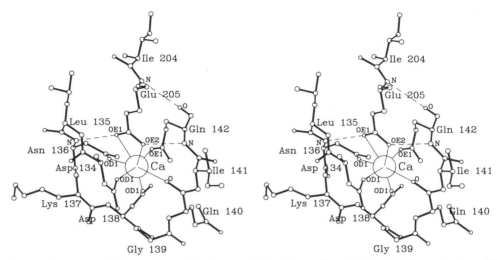

Figure 6. The atomic structure of the D-galactose-binding protein in the immediate vicinity of the bound calcium. The calcium is shown as a circle with the appropriate atomic radius, and coordinations are indicated by thinner lines. The calcium-binding site comprises a loop containing residues 134–142 and a dipeptide segment of residues 204–205. The nine-residue loop provides calcium ligand atoms Asp-134 OD1, Asn-36 OD1, Asp-138 OD1, Gln-140 peptide carbonyl O, and Gln-142 OE1. Glu-205 OE1 and OE2 atoms provide the remaining two ligands. The Ca⁺⁺ coordination geometry is a pentagonal bipyramid whose apices are occupied by oxygen atoms from Asp-134 OD1 and Gln-142 OE1. The hydrogen bonds involving Glu-205 are represented by dashed lines; other hydrogen bonds (not shown) that stabilize the conformation of the loop are discussed in the text.

OD1, Asn-136 OD1, Asp-138 OD1, Gln-140 O (peptide carbonyl oxygen), and Gln-142 OE1. Glu-205 OE1 and OE2 atoms provide the remaining two ligands. The Ca^{++} coordination geometry is an almost perfect pentagonal bipyramid whose apices are occupied by oxygen atoms from the side chains of the loop's first and ninth positions.

The Ca^{++} binding site is situated in the carboxy-terminal domain of the protein—at one end of the ellipsoidal, two-domain structure (Fig. 7). The nine-residue loop, the main component of the metal site, is immediately preceded by a reverse turn (type I) and followed by the first strand from the carboxy-terminal domain. The reverse turn itself is preceded by the first α helix in the domain. Residue Leu-204 is also considered structurally part of the entire calcium-binding site (see below), and this residue and Glu-205 lie near the beginning of the carboxy-terminal domain's third β strand.

The calcium-binding site in the D-galactose-binding protein is unique. Although the site is not immediately preceded and followed by helices, we find great structural and sequence similarities among the sites in the class of calcium-binding folds, better known as the EF hand and commonly found in calcium-modulated intracellular proteins (Kretsinger and Nockolds 1973; Herzberg and James 1985). In particular, the nine-residue loop of the extracellular galactose-binding protein adopts a conformation very similar to the first nine of the twelve-residue EF loop. Moreover, Glu-205, providing bidentate ligands to the metal, occupies a position equivalent to the invariant residue at coordinating position 12 of the EF loop. Additionally, the backbone atoms of residue 204 partly superimpose on those of the residue at position 11 of the EF loop.

Therefore, only the EF loop's position 10 is lacking any structural equivalence to the calcium-binding loop of the binding protein; but both this position and position 11 contain variable side chains, none appearing vital in binding the metal or maintaining structural integrity of the EF loop (Vyas et al. 1987). As further evidence of the similarity between the calcium-binding loop of the D-galactose-binding protein and the EF loop, we find that the root-mean-squares discrepancy between main-chain coordinates of the entire calcium-binding site in the binding protein superimposed on the parvalbumin EF loop is 0.60 Å (Vyas et al. 1987), which compares very well with those obtained from comparisons of several EF-hand proteins (Herzberg and James 1985).

Other notable similarities exist between the calcium-binding site of the D-galactose-binding protein and EF loop. The nine-residue loop in the binding protein–calcium-binding site contains residues resembling the highly conserved ones of many EF-hand loops (Table 1). They include some containing side-chain ligands at positions 1, 3, and 5, as well as others, located at positions 6 and 8, conferring structural constraint or stability on the calcium-binding site. In addition, the coordinating atom at position 7 is, in both the galactose-binding protein and EF loops, provided by the main-chain peptide carbonyl oxygen. Unlike residues with side chains, Gly-139 at position 6 is crucial, for it adopts a main-chain conformation with $\phi = 70°$, $\psi = 5°$), thereby ensuring that the chain direction changes to allow the peptide carbonyl oxygen of the residue in position 7 to coordinate the calcium. A hydrogen bond between Gly-139, peptide NH, and Asp-134 OD2 stabilizes the glycyl conformation. Conversely, the branched aliphatic side chain at position 8 is directed toward the interior of the domain and aids in stabilizing

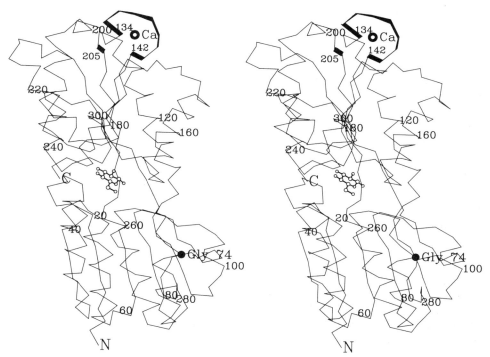

Figure 7. C$_\alpha$ backbone trace of galactose-binding protein (GBP) showing the locations of the binding sites for calcium, β-D-glucose, and the *trg* signal transducer. N represents the amino-terminal end and C the carboxyl end. Numbers are given for every 20 residues and for residues in the metal and transducer sites. The GBP structure is ellipsoid (axial ratio ≈ 2:1) and is composed of two very similar globular domains that are designated N and C domains, as the former contains the N(amino)-terminus and the latter the C(carboxyl)-terminus. The calcium (Ca, thick circle) is surrounded by residues highlighted by thicker lines between C$_\alpha$ atoms. The nine-residue metal-binding loop (134–142) is immediately preceded by a type I reverse turn (131–134) and followed by β strand (142–147). The reverse turn is preceded by the first helix (113–130) in the C domain. The dipeptide 204–205, also a part of the metal site, is located near the beginning of the third strand in the domain. Gly-74 (filled circle) is part of a site for interacting with the membrane-bound *trg* signal transducer (N.K. Vyas et al., unpubl. results). The sugar, which is located at the center of GBP, is 30 Å to the bound calcium and 18 Å to the *trg* site. (Adapted from Vyas et al. 1987.)

Table 1. Sequence Alignment of Ca^{++} Binding Sites in GBP and EF-hand Loops

		1 *	2	3 *	4	5 *	6	7 *	8	9 *	10	11	12 *	
GBP										142		204		
Site	134	Asp	Leu	Asn	Lys	Asp	Gly	Gln	Ile	Gln	—	Ile	Glu	205
Parv														
Loop CD	51	Asp	Gln	Asp	Lys	Ser	Gly	Phe	Ile	Glu	Glu	Asp	Glu	62
Loop EF	90	Asp	Ser	Asp	Gly	Asp	Gly	Lys	Ile	Gly	Val	Asp	Glu	101
TnC														
Loop I	30	Asp	Ala	Asp	Gly	Gly	Gly	Asp	Ile	Ser	Thr	Lys	Glu	41
Loop II	66	Asp	Glu	Asp	Gly	Ser	Gly	Thr	Ile	Asp	Phe	Glu	Glu	77
Loop III	106	Asp	Lys	Asn	Ala	Asp	Gly	Phe	Ile	Asp	Ile	Glu	Glu	117
Loop IV	142	Asp	Lys	Asn	Asn	Asp	Gly	Arg	Ile	Asp	Phe	Asp	Glu	153
ICaBP														
Loop III–IV	54	Asp	Lys	Asn	Gly	Asp	Gly	Glu	Val	Ser	Phe	Glu	Glu	65
CaM														
Loop I	20	Asp	Lys	Asp	Gly	Asn	Gly	Thr	Ile	Thr	Thr	Lys	Glu	31
Loop II	56	Asp	Ala	Asp	Gly	Asn	Gly	Thr	Ile	Asp	Phe	Pro	Glu	67
Loop III	93	Asp	Lys	Asp	Gly	Asn	Gly	Tyr	Ile	Ser	Ala	Ala	Glu	104
Loop IV	129	Asn	Ile	Asp	Gly	Asp	Gly	Glu	Val	Asn	Tyr	Glu	Glu	140

The sequence of the calcium-binding site in GBP (galactose-binding protein) (Vyas et al. 1987) is compared with EF loops of Parv (parvalbumin) (Coffee and Bradshaw 1973; Kretsinger and Nockolds 1973), TnC (troponin C) (Wilkinson 1976), ICaBP (vitamin-D-dependent intestinal calcium-binding protein) (Fullmer and Wasserman 1981), and CaM (calmodulin) (Watterson et al. 1980). A calcium ligand, determined crystallographically or predicted on the basis of sequence homology, is marked by an asterisk. As indicated by structure analysis, the ligand at position 7 is provided by the main peptide carbonyl oxygen of the main-chain peptide bond. The other ligands are provided by side-chain oxygens.

461

the loop. The invariant glutamate residue at position 12 has already been discussed.

Last, the calcium-binding loop in D-galactose-binding protein, as in the EF loop, is stabilized by hydrogen bonds. These hydrogen bonds in EF-hand proteins are in the form of reverse turns (one at the start and another at the end of the loop), "Asx turns", and a β sheet (Herzberg and James 1985). In the metal-binding loop of D-galactose-binding protein, a total of nine excellent hydrogen bonds are formed—three between main-chain atoms only, four between main-chain and side-chain atoms, and two between side chains. A reverse turn is located at the start of the nine-residue loop, which in turn is followed by an Asx turn, the only one in the binding protein–calcium-binding site. There is also only one Asx turn in the calcium-binding site of parvalbumin. A parallel β-sheet hydrogen bonding occurs between the residue 141 (position 8 residue) and residues 172 and 174 of an adjacent strand (Fig. 7). The other hydrogen bonds do not fall under any categories. For example, the carboxylate side chain of Glu-205 is held in place by hydrogen bonds (Fig. 6).

The preceding results suggest a variety of calcium-binding folds or units, containing very similar cation binding sites or loops. The binding sites or loops of these aforementioned units can be tethered to different types of secondary structure (i.e., helices, β strands, reverse turns). Thus, the conformational integrity of the metal site depends almost entirely on the hydrogen bonds, nonpolar interactions, and other structural features characteristic of the site itself (see above). The reverse turns at the start and at the end of the site are critical to achieving the requisite conformation. These turns can be part of the carboxyl and amino termini of helices, as in the EF loops, or they can be separate entities, as found at the beginning of the nine-residue calcium-binding loop of the galactose-binding protein. Interestingly, although the calcium-binding site in the binding protein is composed of a nine-residue loop (134–142) and a dipeptide segment (204–205), the main-chain CO group of the residue at position 9 (Gln-142) is hydrogen-bonded to the peptide NH group of the residue at position 12 (Glu-205), thus mimicking a reverse turn.

Despite the bacterial D-galactose-binding protein having no evolutionary relationship with the eukaryotic EF-hand proteins, our results indicate that the calcium-binding site found in both classes of proteins—especially the peptide loop—is designed to provide extremely tight and specific binding of the biologically important cation.

CONCLUSIONS

The study of the structure and function of the periplasmic binding protein, chiefly by X-ray crystallographic techniques, has resulted in a number of findings that provide new insight into a variety of protein-ligand interactions. The complexes of L-arabinose- and D-galactose-binding proteins with their respective

sugar substrates have revealed many, if not all, of the features of protein-saccharide interactions. The stereospecificity and affinity of carbohydrate binding are conferred principally by hydrogen bonds with primarily polar planar amino acid side chains and by partial stacking of the hydrophobic patches of the monopyranoside substrates with aromatic residues. The interactions involving the binding site residue Arg-151 of the L-arabinose-binding protein, the sulfate bound to the sulfate-binding protein, and the leucine substrate bound to the Leu/Ile/Val-binding protein indicate that isolated charges on ionic groups sequestered in proteins can be stabilized without salt linkages or counterions. These charged substrates and Arg-151 side-chain residue are held in place by several hydrogen bonds with primarily main-chain peptide units that in turn form part of hydrogen-bond arrays. A mechanism has been proposed whereby the highly polarized peptide bonds stabilize the buried charges on the various sequestered ionic groups. It is noteworthy that the ligand specificity and affinity of the L-arabinose- and D-galactose-binding protein depend on hydrogen bonding between the sugar substrates and binding site amino acid side chains, whereas the binding-protein-sulfate and binding-protein-leucine interactions rely heavily on main-chain peptide groups (Figs. 1–4). This reflects in part the necessity of the sulfate- and leucine-binding proteins not only to offset a much greater hydration energy of the ionic substrates, but also to provide a means to stabilize the charges on the substrates.

Apart from the similarity of the tertiary structures, the most notable discovery emerging from the highly refined structures of the binding proteins is that substrates, though having completely different structures (e.g., saccharides, sulfate, and amino acids) are held in place principally by hydrogen bonds. This finding is fully consistent with the fact that all binding proteins bind their ligands with very similar high affinity.

A novel calcium-binding site has been uncovered in the D-galactose-binding protein. Although the site has residues and adopts a conformation very similar to the site in the "helix-loop-helix" or EF-hand fold commonly found in intracellular calcium-binding protein, the site is not immediately preceded and followed by helices.

ACKNOWLEDGMENTS

This work was supported in part by the National Institutes of Health and the Welch Foundation.

REFERENCES

Adler, J. 1975. Chemotaxis in bacteria. *Annu. Rev. Biochem.* **44:** 341.
Ames, G.F.L. 1986. Bacterial periplasmic transport systems: Structure, mechanism, and evolution. *Annu. Rev. Biochem.* **55:** 397.
Applequist, J. and T.G. Mahr. 1966. The conformation of poly-L-tyrosine in quinoline from dielectric dispersion studies. *J. Am. Chem. Soc.* **82:** 23.

Coffee, C.J. and R.A. Bradshaw. 1973. Carp muscle calcium-binding protein. I. Characterization of the tryptic peptides and the complete amino acid sequence of component B. *J. Biol. Chem.* **248:** 3305.

Engelsberg, E. 1971. Regulation in the L-arabinose system. In *Metabolic pathways: Metabolic regulation* (ed. H.J. Vogel), p. 257. Academic Press, New York.

Fullmer, C.S. and R.H. Wasserman. 1981. The amino acid sequence of bovine intestinal calcium-binding protein. *J. Biol. Chem.* **256:** 5669.

Herzberg, O. and M.N.G. James. 1985. Common structural framework of the Ca^{++}/Mg^{++} binding loops of troponin C and other Ca^{++} binding proteins. *Biochemistry* **24:** 5298.

Kraut, J. 1977. Serine proteases: Structure and mechanism of catalysis. *Annu. Rev. Biochem.* **46:** 331.

Kretsinger, R.H. and C.E. Nockolds. 1973. Carp muscle calcium-binding protein. II. Structure determination and general description. *J. Biol. Chem.* **248:** 3313.

Lee, B.K. and F.M. Richards. 1971. The interpretation of protein structures: Estimation of static accessibility. *J. Mol. Biol.* **55:** 379.

Llinás, M. and M.P. Klein. 1975. Charge relay at the peptide bond. A proton magnetic resonance study of solvation effects on the amide electron density distribution. *J. Am. Chem. Soc.* **97:** 4731.

Newcomer, M.E., G.L. Gilliland, and F.A. Quiocho. 1981. L-Arabinose-binding protein-sugar complex at 2.4 Å resolution: Stereochemistry and evidence for a structural change. *J. Biol. Chem.* **256:** 13213.

Pardee, A.B., L.S. Prestidge, M.B. Whipple, and J. Dreyfuss. 1966. A binding site for sulfate and its relation to sulfate transport into *Salmonella typhimurium. J. Biol. Chem.* **241:** 3962.

Pauling, L. 1960. *Nature of the chemical bond.* 2nd edition. Cornell University, Ithaca, New York.

Pflugrath, J.W. and F.A. Quiocho. 1985. Sulphate sequestered in the sulphate-binding protein is bound solely by hydrogen bonds. *Nature* **314:** 257.

Popov, E.M. and V.N. Sheltova. 1971. Electronic structure and properties of peptides. *J. Mol. Struct.* **10:** 221.

Quiocho, F.A. 1986. Carbohydrate-binding proteins: Tertiary structures and protein-sugar interactions. *Annu. Rev. Biochem.* **55:** 287.

Quiocho, F.A. and N.K. Vyas. 1984. Novel stereochemistry of the L-arabinose-binding protein. *Nature* **310:** 381.

Quiocho, F.A., J.S. Sack, and N.K. Vyas. 1987a. Stabilization of charges on isolated ionic groups sequestered in proteins by polarized peptide units. *Nature* (in press).

Quiocho, F.A., N.K. Vyas, J.S. Sack, and M.A. Storey. 1987b. Periplasmic binding proteins: Structures and new understanding of protein-ligand interactions. In *Crystallography in molecular biology. NATO Adv. Study Inst. Ser. Ser. A Life Sci.* **126:** 385.

Saper, M.A. and F.A. Quiocho. 1983. Leucine, isoleucine, valine-binding protein from *Escherichia coli*: Structure at 3.0 Å resolution and location of the binding site. *J. Biol. Chem.* **258:** 11057.

Schulz, G.E. and R.H. Schirmer. 1979. *Principles of protein structure.* Springer-Verlag, New York.

Vyas, N.K., M.N. Vyas, and F.A. Quiocho. 1987. A novel calcium binding site in the galactose-binding protein of bacterial transport and chemotaxis. *Nature* **327:** 635.

Wada, A. 1976. The α-helix as an electric macro-dipole. *Adv. Biophys.* **9:** 1.

Watterson, D.M., F. Sharief, and T.C. Vanaman. 1980. The complete amino acid sequence of Ca^{2+}-dependent modular protein (calmodulin) of bovine brain. *J. Biol. Chem.* **255:** 962.

Wilkinson, J.M. 1976. The amino acid sequence of troponin C from chicken skeletal muscle. *FEBS Lett.* **70:** 254.

Wilson, D.B. and J.B. Smith. 1978. Bacterial transport proteins. In *Bacterial transport* (ed. B.P. Rosen), p. 495. Marcel Dekker, New York.

Structural Studies of Klenow Fragment: An Enzyme with Two Active Sites

T.A. STEITZ, L. BEESE, P.S. FREEMONT, J.M. FRIEDMAN, AND M.R. SANDERSON

Department of Molecular Biophysics and Biochemistry and The Howard Hughes Medical Institute,
Yale University, New Haven, Connecticut 06511

Among the catalytic activities that were presumably required very early in evolution is that of RNA and/or DNA polymerase. The ability to replicate the nucleic acid genome accurately is essential to the process of evolution. One might expect that the basic polymerase function of the present-day DNA polymerases evolved from a common ancestor, since an intermediate evolutionary state of switching from one polymerase to another is difficult to imagine. It may even turn out that RNA and DNA polymerases are evolutionarily and thus structurally related. A detailed understanding of the enzymatic mechanism of current DNA and RNA polymerases might or might not provide clues concerning the possible nature of earlier prebiotic RNA polymerases.

DNA polymerase I from *Escherichia coli* (Pol I) was the first DNA polymerase purified and is the best understood and perhaps the simplest of the known DNA polymerases (Kornberg 1980). Unlike many other replication enzymes, it is active as a single subunit. The molecule (molecular weight 103,000) has three enzymatic activities: a DNA polymerase, a 3′-5′ exonuclease thought to edit out mismatched terminal nucleotides, and a 5′-3′ exonuclease that removes DNA ahead of the growing point of a DNA chain. Deoxynucleoside monophosphate (dNMP) and deoxynucleoside triphosphate (dNTP) bind noncompetitively to the 3′-5′ exonuclease and polymerase active sites, respectively. The binding of both nucleotides as well as the enzymatic activities of Pol I require divalent metal ions.

A combination of structural, biochemical, and genetic studies have led to the conclusion that Pol I has three domains, each responsible for a separate enzymatic activity (Fig. 1). Limited proteolysis of Pol I removes the 35,000 dalton amino-terminal domain that contains the 5′-3′ exonuclease activity (Klenow and Henningsen 1970; Brutlag et al. 1980). The remaining 68,000 dalton large fragment (Klenow fragment) has the polymerization and editing 3′-5′ exonuclease activities.

The crystal structure of the Klenow fragment (Ollis et al. 1985b) shows that the 605-amino-acid polypeptide is folded into two distinct structural domains of approximately 200 and 400 amino acids (Fig. 2). The amino terminal one third of the Klenow fragment can bind two divalent metal ions and a molecule of dNMP. The larger carboxy-terminal domain forms a structure that

contains a deep cleft, about 20–24 Å wide and 25–35 Å deep. Above the cleft are 40 to 50 amino acid residues that are partially disordered in the crystal structure, indicating that this region is flexibly attached to the rest of the molecule.

Model building suggests that the cleft in the large domain can accommodate double-stranded B DNA. In this model the J and K α helices are placed partially into a major groove and may function like the thread of a nut to fix the exact position of a DNA major groove relative to the protein. This circumstance would require the polymerase to follow a spiral path along the DNA during DNA synthesis. Placing the duplex DNA into the cleft is consistent with (1) the observation that virtually all the positive electrostatic charge potential lies within the cleft (Warwicker et al. 1985), (2) the finding that mutants that weaken the enzyme's interaction with DNA lie within the cleft (Ollis et al. 1985b; Joyce et al. 1986a), and (3) the results of footprinting studies on the Klenow fragment bound to a primer terminus (Joyce et al. 1986b).

Extensive evidence has been obtained to establish that the 3′-5′ exonuclease active site resides on the small domain and the polymerase active site lies on the large domain. The carboxy-terminal domain (residues 515–928) has been overexpressed and purified as a

E. Coli DNA POLYMERASE I

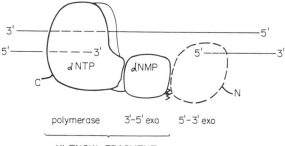

Figure 1. A schematic drawing of the apparent domain structure of *E. coli* DNA polymerase I. The solid lines represent the experimentally determined Klenow fragment structure; the dashed lines indicate a possible location for the small fragment produced by proteolytic cleavage of Pol I. The orientation of the nicked DNA substrate is such that the 5′-3′ exonuclease domain would be able to interact with the DNA 5′ end downstream from the primer terminus.

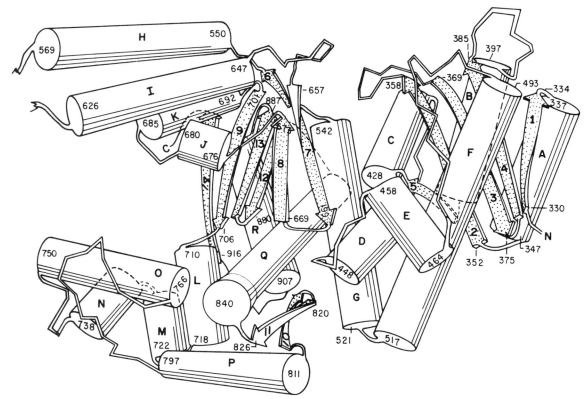

Figure 2. A schematic representation of the three-dimensional polypeptide fold of the Klenow fragment of *E. coli* DNA polymerase I. Regions of polypeptide that form α helix are represented by cylinders and those that form β sheet by arrows.

separate entity. Consistent with the hypothesis that the large domain of the Klenow fragment contains the polymerase active site, this purified domain has polymerase activity but no measurable exonuclease activity (Freemont et al. 1986). Furthermore, Rush and Konigsberg have cross-linked the dNTP analog, 8 azido-dATP, to Klenow fragment and have shown that it cross-links to Tyr-766, which is located at the end of helix O and whose side chain is pointing toward the proposed DNA-binding cleft (Joyce et al. 1986b). Finally, preliminary characterization of mutants within the proposed polymerase active site have reduced polymerase activity, but essentially unchanged exonuclease activity (A. Polesky and C. Joyce, pers. comm.).

That the small domain catalyzes the exonuclease reaction was suggested initially by its ability to bind dNMP, since dNMP was known (Que et al. 1978) to inhibit the 3'-5' exonuclease reaction. More recently, by site-directed mutagenesis of residues within the dNMP-binding region, two mutant proteins have been made that are completely devoid of 3'-5' exonuclease activity but retain the polymerase activity (V. Derbyshire, P.S. Freemont, M.R. Sanderson, T.A. Steitz, and C.M. Joyce, in prep.).

Refined Structure

The atomic coordinates of the Klenow fragment are being refined against the observed X-ray diffraction intensities extending to 2.75 Å resolution using restrained least-squares procedures (Hendrickson and Konnert 1980). The crystallographic R factor of the starting model after the coordinates were regularized was 0.42 at 3.3 Å resolution. Initial refinement was begun at 3.3 Å resolution and gradually extended to 2.75 Å resolution. Cycles of Konnert-Hendrickson least-squares refinement were alternated with rebuilding of the protein model into an electron density map. When the crystallographic R factor reached 0.24, individual temperature factors were used but were tightly restrained. In the later stages of the refinement, 35 water molecules have been added. Currently, the crystallographic R factor is 0.20 and the deviation of bond angles from ideality is 0.015. The rms shift in coordinates from the starting model is 1.1 Å.

The thermal parameters are largest in polypeptide regions that surround the deep cleft presumed to bind DNA. Two regions of polypeptide in the cleft region are particularly disordered and in stretches contain only a polyalanine backbone. Currently, 23 amino acids between residues 589 and 611 cannot be identified at all and are presumed to be disordered.

Exonuclease Active Site. Although the overall structure of the exonuclease active site is as previously published, a few important alterations and additions have been made in some details through the course of the refinement. As noted earlier (Ollis et al. 1985b), extra electron density accompanies the binding of the nucleoside monophosphate. Crystallographic studies of a mutant Klenow protein (V. Derbyshire et al., in prep.) and more recent crystallographic refinement are best explained if this extra density corresponds to the binding of a second metal ion that requires the binding of dNMP. The more tightly bound metal ion (site A) is a zinc atom in these crystals to which 1 mM $ZnSO_4$ has been added and is liganded to the side chains of Asp-501, Glu-355, and Asp-357 (Fig. 3). The chemical identity of the second metal ion has not been established, but it could be either a magnesium ion or a less-well-ordered Zn^{++} ion. Metal B is bound to the protein through Glu-355 and perhaps to Asp-424 via a layer of water molecules. The two metal atoms are 4.3 Å apart.

Pol I Homologies to Other Polymerases

Comparison of the amino acid sequence of Pol I with that of other DNA polymerases as well as with RNA polymerases shows only one protein that bears a strong sequence homology: T7 DNA polymerase (Ollis et al. 1985a). Numerous peptides located in the carboxy-terminal domain of the Klenow fragment show sequence homologies ranging between 30% and 50% identities. Those regions showing the strongest amino acid homology were found to line the large cleft thought to bind duplex DNA. Examination of the location of those side chains that are identical between T7 DNA polymerase and the Klenow fragment shows that they are clustered in the cleft and specifically around the region thought to contain the polymerase active site (around residues 880 and 786, Fig. 2). Thus, T7 DNA polymerase and Klenow fragment clearly evolved from a common ancestral polymerase.

Much weaker amino acid sequence homologies have been found between the ε subunit of DNA polymerase III (the subunit that contains the editing 3'-5' exo-

nuclease activity) and the small domain of the Klenow fragment (Joyce et al. 1986b). Among the residues that appear to be conserved are some of those that are essential for binding the metals and the nucleoside monophosphate product. In considering the mechanism of editing in these two polymerases, it is interesting to note that the editing exonuclease activity resides on a different subunit from the polymerase active site in Pol III and on a different structural domain in Pol I, suggesting that the polymerase and editing active sites are substantially separated in both Pol I and Pol III.

No convincing amino acid sequence homology has been observed between the Klenow fragment sequence and that of any eukaryotic DNA polymerases that have been sequenced to date (D.L. Ollis and T.A. Steitz, unpubl.). There are short stretches of amino acid sequence homology between and among various eukaryotic DNA polymerases. Interestingly, gene 43 from T4, the polymerase subunit, shows no amino acid sequence homology with the Klenow fragment but does show significant and strong sequence homology with those regions of the eukaryotic polymerases that are homologous among themselves (D.L. Ollis and T.A. Steitz, unpubl.). The lack of an identifiable sequence homology between Klenow and eukaryotic polymerases does not rule out a structural and functional homology, but it does mean that conclusions drawn from the Klenow fragment studies cannot be directly extrapolated to other polymerases at present.

Cocrystallization of Klenow Fragment with DNA Substrates

We have succeeded in obtaining crystallographically suitable crystals of three different complexes between the Klenow fragment and DNA. Two of these complexes we have solved at high resolution and the third is still under study. The two cocrystal structures examined at high resolution provide a wealth of detail concerning the interaction of single-stranded DNA with the exonuclease active site and suggest a model for how the 3 terminus of a growing DNA substrate shuttles between the polymerase and the exonuclease active sites.

The first cocrystal of Klenow fragment with DNA obtained was grown from solutions containing 38% saturated ammonium sulfate, 400 mM citrate (pH 5.6), EDTA to inhibit the exonuclease activity of the wild-type enzyme, and an 8-bp duplex DNA substrate with a 3 base, single-stranded 5' overhang:

$$5' \quad \text{A G A C C G G C C C G G} \quad 3'$$
$$\text{G G C C G G G C C}$$

High-performance liquid chromatography analysis of the resulting crystals establishes that the stoichiometry of duplex DNA to protein is one to one in the crystal and that equimolar amounts of both strands are present. Because these crystals have the same cell dimensions and space group as the structure that has been solved, it was possible to simply calculate a difference

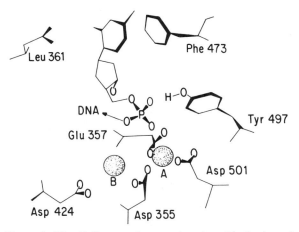

Figure 3. The 3'-5' exonuclease active site with the bound product molecule, dCMP. The side chains of residues interacting with the metal ions and dNMP are shown. The two binding sites for divalent metal ions, labeled A and B, are described in detail in the text.

electron density map using 3.5 Å X-ray diffraction data on a Hamlin-Xuong area detector kindly made available for our use by Dr. Sherin Abdel-Meguid at Monsanto research laboratories.

The difference electron density map between the DNA complex and the native Klenow fragment showed the presence of three single-stranded nucleotides bound at the exonuclease active site and a substantial degree of conformational change in the protein. One obvious structural change observed in the difference map was the movement of the two α helices I and H (Fig. 2) in toward the cleft. In this initial difference map there is little evidence for the remaining portion of the bound DNA. Refinement of this complex structure at 3.5 Å resolution has begun to show indication of additional DNA leading toward the cleft. The complementary strand of the duplex DNA is not yet visible.

Since this difference electron density map shows that the 3′ terminus of the DNA duplex used in the experiment is in the exonuclease active site, the enzyme appears to be melting the duplex and binding a partially denatured DNA. Possibly the high ionic strength in which the cocrystals were grown is favoring the binding of the DNA at the exonuclease active site rather than the polymerase active site, as normally occurs in solution at low ionic strength (Joyce et al. 1986b).

The observation that duplex DNA cocrystallized with Klenow fragment contained single-stranded DNA at the exonuclease active site suggested that short, single-stranded oligonucleotides might diffuse into the crystals and bind at the exo site, which indeed they appear to do. Crystals of the Asp→Ala-424 mutant of Klenow fragment that is devoid of exonuclease activity were soaked in ammonium sulfate solution containing 1 mM deoxythymidine tetranucleotide (dT_4), 1 mM zinc sulfate, and 5 mM magnesium sulfate for a week at room temperature. Data were measured to 2.8 Å resolution using the Hamlin-Xuong area detector at Yale; a difference electron density map calculated using multiple isomorphous replacement phases to 8 Å resolution and calculated refined phases between 8 and 2.8 Å resolution. A portion of this map is shown in Figure 4.

The binding of dT_4 produces few structural changes in the protein. Electron density corresponding to three of the four bases is very clear, and some indication of the presence of the fourth base is seen. The binding of a longer oligonucleotide did not appear to show additional electron density, suggesting that single-stranded

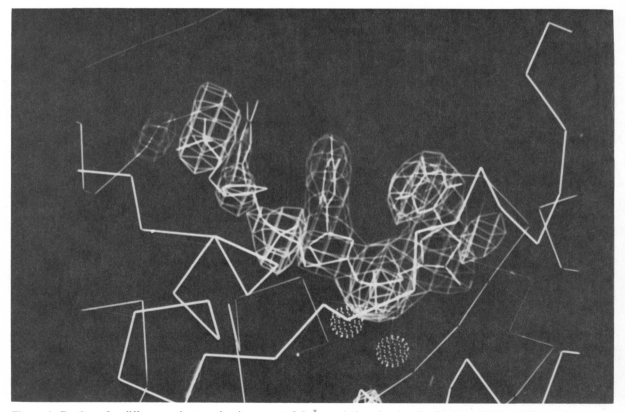

Figure 4. Portion of a difference electron density map at 2.8 Å resolution showing the binding of dT_4 to Klenow fragment. Coefficients in the Fourier calculation are $\{F_{424}(dT_4) - F_{wt}(Zn)\}$ exp α hybrid, where $F_{424}(dT_4)$ is the diffraction amplitude of the A424 mutant Klenow complexed with dT_4 and $F_{wt}(Zn)$ is the amplitude of the wild-type protein complexed with Zn and α hybrid corresponds to experimental phase angles in the 20–8 Å 2θ range and calculated phase angles in the 8–2.8 Å range. The positive electron density is contoured at a level of 4σ and a model of dT_3 is superimposed. The two metal positions are represented by a dotted surface.

DNA beyond three to four residues from the 3' terminus is partially or totally disordered.

The 3' terminal residue is binding in a fashion nearly identical with nucleoside monophosphate, except that the phosphate may lie in a slightly altered orientation (Fig. 5). The side chain of Leu-361 lies between the 3' terminal and penultimate bases and is interacting with both. The side chain of this residue, which is a methionine in the ϵ subunit of Pol III, may play an important role in stabilizing the denatured single-stranded 3' terminus in the exonuclease site. The penultimate phosphate is interacting with a glutamine side chain. No additional protein side chains appear to be moving into the region of the bond to be cleaved. Thus, only the two metal atoms and the hydroxyl of Tyr-497 are in contact with the phosphate and close enough to be directly involved in catalysis.

It may be of some interest to consider the relationship that might exist between the active site of the Klenow 3'-5' exonuclease and the active sites of RNA enzymes that catalyze RNA cleavage resulting in a 5' phosphate product (for example RNase P). Presently, it appears that two magnesium ions and possibly a hydroxyl (chemical entities present in RNA) may be sufficient to catalyze this nuclease reaction. Currently, we cannot, however, exclude the possibility that one or more of the carboxylates interacting with the metals plays an additional catalytic role.

Mutant Klenow fragment that is devoid of exonuclease activity has also been crystallized in the presence of the duplex DNA substrate, a dTTP analog, $MgSO_4$, and $ZnSO_4$ at low ionic strength and pH 7.0. These

crystals are currently small but have different unit cell dimensions from the crystal form already solved. It has not yet been determined whether these crystals contain DNA.

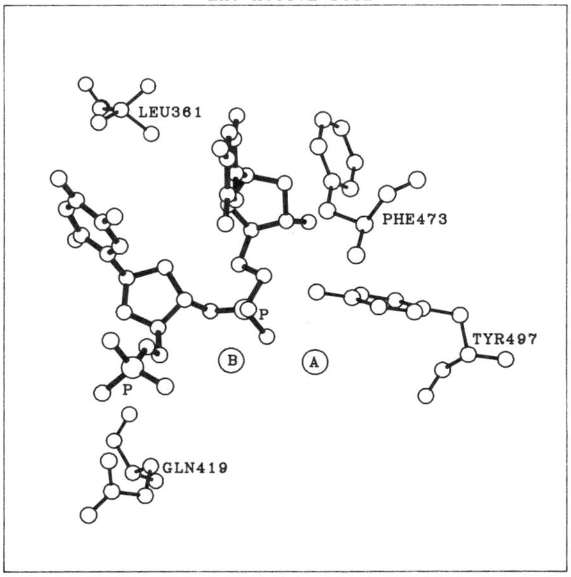

Relative Orientation of the Two Active Sites. The distance between the dNMP in the exonuclease active site and the proposed position of the 3' terminus in the polymerase active site is about 25–30 Å (Fig. 6). The single-stranded DNA that is observed in the cocrystals extends from the nucleoside-monophosphate-binding site toward the cleft anticipated to bind the duplex DNA. In fact, the 5' end of the experimentally observed single-stranded DNA intersects with the 3' end of the model built duplex. Thus, it is entirely plausible to assume that the 3' terminus of the primer strand goes from the polymerase active site to the exonuclease active site by sliding and unraveling several bases at its 3' terminus.

If the rate of sliding of the 3' terminus between the two active sites is significantly faster than the polymerase and exonuclease reactions, then the physical separation of these two active sites is of no consequence for the efficient coupling of the synthesis and editing reaction. The rate of sliding deduced for *lac* repressor (Berg et al. 1982) on DNA (10^6 bp/sec) is probably at least 4 orders of magnitude faster than would be required for Klenow fragment.

Competition Model for Editing

If the exonuclease active site lies 25–30 Å from the polymerase active site as it appears to do, how then are mismatched nucleotides that are misincorporated at the polymerase active site "recognized" and excised at the remote exonuclease active site? After an incorrect nucleotide is misincorporated at the polymerase active site, there are at least four possible subsequent steps. (1) The polymerase reaction can be reversed by pyrophosphorolysis, thus removing the incorrect base. (2) The 3' terminus can dissociate from the polymerase active site and slide to the exonuclease active site and

EXO ACTIVE SITE

Figure 5. The conformation of the 3' terminal two nucleotides of the dT$_4$ bound to the exonuclease active site along with those protein side chains and the two metals with which they interact. The dinucleotide coordinates were obtained by fitting them to the difference electron density of the dT$_4$ complex.

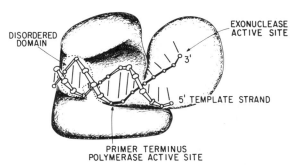

Figure 6. A schematic drawing showing the relationship between the binding sites for the 3' terminus of the primer strand when it is bound in the polymerase and exonuclease active sites. The extent of movement necessary to bring the primer terminus from the polymerase to the exonuclease active site is indicated by the darkened bonds.

be excised. (3) The 3' terminus can be translocated and the addition of the next nucleotide can proceed, thereby locking in a mismatched base pair. (4) The DNA can dissociate from the enzyme. The extent and nature of the editing that will occur depends on the competition among these four alternative reactions.

It is true for the Klenow fragment, as it is for other polymerases such as the one from phage T4, that correctly incorporated nucleotides are excised in addition to incorrectly incorporated nucleotides. About 10% of the correctly incorporated nucleotides are removed through exonuclease activity. However, to improve the fidelity of DNA synthesis, the enzyme must exert a significant bias in favor of excising mismatched base pairs over correctly matched base pairs. How is this achieved?

The excision of incorrectly matched base pairs could be enhanced either by the enzyme's possessing an increased rate of exonuclease activity for mismatched base pairs and/or by its showing a decreased rate of translocation. The former almost assuredly occurs since mismatched base pairs are thermally less stable as duplex and therefore melt out to form the single-stranded DNA required for binding to the exonuclease active site more readily than do correctly matched base pairs. Thus, the propensity for terminally mismatched base pairs to form single-stranded DNA would enhance the rate of exonuclease on mismatched base pairs (Kornberg 1980).

It is also possible that the polymerase active site is constructed in such a way as to prevent translocation of 3' termini containing mismatched base pairs. How might this be achieved? A steric blocking model (Steitz 1987) has been proposed that suggests that the polymerase may contain a "reading head" that lies in the minor groove and detects terminally mismatched base pairs. The crystal structures of duplex DNAs containing mismatched base pairs determined in the Kennard laboratory (Brown et al. 1985; Kennard 1985) establish that, at least with respect to the base pairs GT, AG, and AC, the sugar phosphate backbone can have the identical conformation as normal B DNA and thus, it is not likely to be the structural feature that the enzyme utilizes in detecting mismatched base pairs. Likewise, the enzyme is probably not detecting mismatched base pairs in the major groove since substitution of bulky groups at the 5 position of pyrimidines does not block activity of the enzyme (Dale et al. 1975). Since the pattern of hydrogen-bond acceptors in the minor groove is identical for all four base pair combinations (Seeman et al. 1976), and since the positioning of the minor groove hydrogen-bond acceptors differs in mismatched base pairs (Brown et al. 1985; Kennard 1985), it seems plausible that such an enzyme reading head could be detecting mismatched base pairs in the minor groove.

Thus, it is perhaps possible that a "reading head" on the polymerase "detects" in the minor groove the altered orientation of the hydrogen-bond acceptors of mismatched base pairs and either retards translocation or prevents formation of the enzyme conformation necessary for the polymerase reaction. The partially disordered regions of the Klenow fragment (residues 570–620 and 770–790) lie above the minor groove in the region of the proposed 3' terminus. Clearly, the crystal structure of a ternary complex with DNA and dNTP bound at the polymerase active site will directly address the issue of what role (if any) the polymerase active site plays in the detection of misincorporated bases.

ACKNOWLEDGMENTS

We thank Catherine Joyce, Nigel Grindley, Victoria Derbyshire, and Andrea Polesky for continuing discussion and collaboration on Pol I. This research was supported by American Cancer Society grant NP-421 and National Institutes of Health grant GM-22778 to Thomas A. Steitz, and by a Jane Coffin Childs Memorial Fund fellowship to Jonathan Friedman.

REFERENCES

Berg, O.G., R.B. Winter, and P.H. von Hippel. 1982. How do genome-regulatory proteins locate their DNA target sites? *Trends Biochem. Sci.* **7:** 52.

Brown, T., O. Kennard, G. Kneale, and D. Rabinovich. 1985. High resolution structure of a DNA helix containing mismatched base-pairs. *Nature* **315:** 604.

Brutlag, D., M.R. Atkinson, P. Setlow, and A. Kornberg. 1980. An active fragment of DNA polymerase produced by proteolytic cleavage. *Biochem. Biophys. Res. Commun.* **37:** 982.

Dale, R.M.K. and D.C. Ward. 1975. Mercurated polynucleotides: New probes for hybridization and selective polymer fractionation. *Biochemistry* **14:** 2458.

Freemont, P.S., D.L. Ollis, T.A. Steitz, and C.M. Joyce. 1986. A domain of the Klenow fragment of *Escherichia coli* DNA polymerase I has polymerase but no exonuclease activity. *Proteins* **1:** 66.

Hendrickson, W.A. and J.H. Konnert. 1980. Stereochemically restrained crystallographic least-squares refinement of macromolecule structures. In *Biomolecular structure, function, conformation and evolution* (ed. R. Srinevasan), p. 43. Pergamon Press, Oxford, England.

Joyce, C.M., D.N. Fujii, H.F. Laks, C.M. Hughes, and N.D.F. Grindley. 1986a. Genetic mapping and DNA sequence analysis of mutations in the *polA* gene of *E. coli*. *J. Mol. Biol.* **186:** 283.

Joyce, C.M., D.L. Ollis, J. Rush, T.A. Steitz, W.H. Konigsberg, and N.D.F. Grindley. 1985b. Relating structure to function for DNA polymerase I of *Escherichia coli*. *UCLA Symp. Mol. Cell. Biol.* **39:** 197.

Kennard, O. 1985. Structural studies of DNA fragments: The G·T wobble base pair in A, B and Z DNA; The G·A base pair in B-DNA. *J. Biomol. Struct. Dyn.* **3:** 205.

Klenow, H. and I. Henningson. 1970. Selective elimination of the exonuclease activity of the DNA polymerase from *E. coli* B by a limited proteolysis. *Proc. Natl. Acad. Sci.* **65:** 168.

Kornberg, A. 1980. *DNA replication*. W.H. Freeman, San Francisco, California.

Ollis, D.L., C. Kline, and T.A. Steitz. 1985a. Domain of *E. coli* DNA polymerase I showing sequence homology to T7 DNA polymerase. *Nature* **313:** 818.

Ollis, D.L., P. Brick, R. Hamlin, N.G. Xuong, and T.A. Steitz. 1985b. Structure of the large fragment of *E. coli* DNA polymerase I complexed with dTMP. *Nature* **313:** 762.

Que, B.G., K.M. Downey, and A. So. 1978. Mechanism of selective inhibition of 3′ to 5′ exonuclease activity of *E. coli* DNA polymerase I by nucleoside 5′-monophosphates. *Biochemistry* **17:** 1603.

Seeman, N.C., J.M. Rosenberg, and A. Rich. 1976. Sequence-specific recognition of double helical nucleic acids by proteins. *Proc. Natl. Acad. Sci.* **73:** 804.

Steitz, T.A. 1987. The Klenow fragment structure suggests mechanisms for fidelity and processivity of DNA polymerase I. In *Biological organization: Macromolecular interactions at high resolution* (ed. R. Burnett and H. Vogel), p. 45. Academic Press, New York.

Warwicker, J., D.L. Ollis, F.M. Richards, and T.A. Steitz. 1985. The electrostatic field of the large fragment of *E. coli* DNA polymerase. *J. Mol. Biol.* **186:** 645.

Zinc Fingers: A Novel Protein Fold for Nucleic Acid Recognition

A. KLUG AND D. RHODES

MRC Laboratory of Molecular Biology, Cambridge CB2 2QH, England

An essential part of gene expression and regulation is the binding of a regulatory protein to the recognition sequence of the gene on which it acts. Many such proteins have embedded in their structures a domain, or motif, that serves for binding to DNA. The best-understood protein structure used for DNA binding is the helix-turn-helix motif seen in the crystal structure of several bacterial regulatory proteins (for review, see Pabo and Sauer 1984; Anderson et al. 1987). Amino acid sequences that could form a similar structural motif are also present in the homeo box region of several eukaryotic proteins (Gehring 1985).

A few years ago, it was discovered in this laboratory (Miller et al. 1985) that the *Xenopus* transcription factor IIIA (TFIIIA) for the 5S RNA gene contains small sequence units repeated in tandem, and it was proposed that each unit is folded about a Zn atom to form separate structural domains. Similar units have subsequently been found to be present in the amino acid sequence of other transcription factors and more generally nucleic-acid-binding proteins. Thus a second and apparently more commonly used structural motif for DNA recognition has emerged: the "Zn finger."

Repetitive Zn-binding Domains in TFIIIA

TFIIIA is required for correct initiation of transcription of *Xenopus* 5S RNA genes by RNA polymerase III. This protein, of molecular weight 40,000, binds to a 50-bp region located within the coding sequence of 5S RNA genes (the internal control region) to form an initiation complex that is stabilized by the sequential addition of at least two more transcription factors (for review, see Brown 1984). TFIIIA is found in large quantities in the ovaries of immature frogs, stored as a 7S complex with its own gene product, 5S RNA (Picard and Wegnez 1979). TFIIIA therefore binds to both DNA and RNA. This presents an intriguing structural problem, as does the question of how such a small protein interacts with a long tract of DNA, and we began work on TFIIIA about 5 years ago.

In the course of trying to improve published purification methods, with the aim of producing the large quantities of protein necessary for structural studies, Jonathan Miller found that the stability of the 5S RNA/TFIIIA complex was greatly improved by excluding chelating agents such as dithiothreitol (DTT) and EDTA, suggesting that a metal was involved in the binding of the protein to RNA and DNA (Miller et al.

1985). Analysis by atomic absorption spectroscopy revealed that preparations of 7S-particle purified to homogeneity, in the absence of chelating agents, contained 7–11 atoms of Zn per mole of particle. This result was consistent with the fact that the protein contains a large number of histidine and cysteine residues (Picard and Wegnez 1979), the commonest ligands for Zn in enzymes and other proteins, and explained the finding by Hanas et al. (1983) that Zn is necessary for transcription of 5S genes.

Following on from earlier proteolytic studies on TFIIIA by Brown's group (Smith et al. 1984), which showed stable fragments at 30 kD and 20 kD, we found that on prolonged proteolysis the protein breaks down further, finally to a limit of about 3 kD. In the course of this, periodic intermediates differing in size by about 3 kD could be seen. The correspondence in size between these last two values suggested that the 30-kD domain of TFIIIA may contain a periodic arrangement of small, compact domains of size 3 kD. If each of such domains contained one Zn atom, that would account for the observed Zn content.

This novel idea of a small Zn-stabilized domain was strengthened by the timely publication of the sequence of TFIIIA derived from a cDNA clone (Ginsberg et al. 1984). By inspection, it could be seen that the large number of cysteines and histidines present in the protein appeared to occur in more or less regular patterns. A rigorous computer analysis showed that, of the 344 amino acids of the TFIIIA sequence, residues 13–276 form a continuous run of nine tandemly repeated, similar units of about 30 amino acids containing two invariant pairs of histidines and cysteines (Fig. 1). Repeating patterns in the sequence were also noticed by Brown et al. (1985) who, however, concluded that the whole protein was divided into twelve repeats, indexed on a 39-amino-acid unit.

From the three different lines of evidence described above, namely, (1) a 30-amino-acid repeat in the sequence that (2) corresponds in size to the observed periodic intermediates and limit digest product of 3 kD, and (3) the measured Zn content of 7–11 atoms, we proposed that most of the TFIIIA protein has a repeating structure in which each of the nine 30-amino-acid units folds around a Zn atom to form a small independent structural domain (Miller et al. 1985). Figure 2 shows a schematic representation of the proposed folding of a TFIIIA domain in which most 30-amino-acid residues are in the loop formed around the central Zn

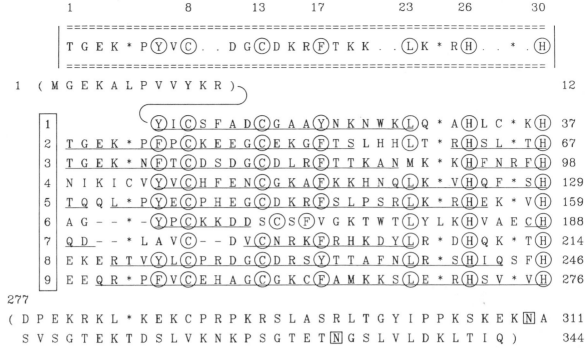

Figure 1. Amino acid sequence of transcription factor IIIA from *X. laevis* oocytes, aligned to show the repeated units. The repeat units are numbered 1–9 on the left side of the diagram. The boxed consensus sequence at the top shows the characteristic features of a typical repeat unit, numbered as for a length of 30 residues. (*) Positions where an insertion sometimes occurs in the normal pattern. (.) Variable positions in the sequence. In the main body of the repeats (—) indicates an alignment gap. The underlined regions are those that show clear evidence of a relationship with at least one other unit. (Reprinted, with permission, from Miller et al. 1985.)

atom, and a few amino acids provide the linkers between consecutive fingers. The Zn atom forms the basis of the folding by being tetrahedrally coordinated to the two invariant pairs of cysteines and histidines. Each repeat also contains, besides this unique conserved pattern of Cys-Cys....His-His, several other conserved amino acids, namely Tyr-6 (or Phe-6), Phe-17, and Leu-23, all of which are hydrophobic. The whole of the 30-amino-acid repeat is rich in basic and polar residues, but the largest number are found concentrated in the region between the second cysteine and first histidine (Fig. 2), implicating this region in particular in DNA binding.

The proposal that each 30-amino-acid unit is an independently folded, Zn-stabilized domain has gained support from two lines of research. First, in the gene for TFIIIA the positions of the intron-exon boundaries mark most of its proposed finger domains (Tso et al. 1986). Second, a study using EXAFS (extended X-ray absorption fine structure), described below, confirmed that the Zn ligands are two cysteines and two histidines (Diakun et al. 1986). In evolutionary terms, the multifingered TFIIIA may have arisen by gene duplication of an ancestral domain comprising about 30 amino acids. Because of the ability of one such self-contained small domain to bind to nucleic acid, we suggested that these domains might occur more widely than in just this case of TFIIIA (Miller et al. 1985). In the last few years, this prediction has been borne out.

Many Regulatory Proteins Contain TFIIIA-like DNA-binding Domains

The occurrence of protein sequences containing motifs homologous to the Zn finger of TFIIIA has already been the subject of two reviews (Berg 1986; Vincent 1986). In Table 1 we give a restricted list of proteins that contain amino acid units bearing some

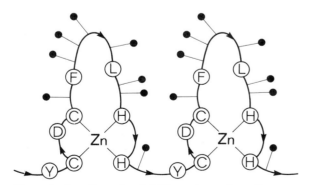

Figure 2. Two-dimensional folding scheme for a linear arrangement of repeated domains, each centered on a tetrahedral arrangement of Zn ligands. Circled residues are the conserved amino acids, which include the Cys and His zinc ligands, the negatively charged Asp-11, and the three hydrophobic groups that may form a structural core. (●) The most probable DNA-binding side chains. (Reprinted, with permission, from Miller et al. 1985.)

Table 1. A Partial List of Proteins (or cDNA Sequences) That Contain Sequences Homologous to the Zn-finger Motif of TFIIIA

	Name of sequence or protein	Type	Evidence for Zn- or DNA-binding	References
Xenopus	TFIIIA	CC–HH	Zn, DNA/RNA	Engelke et al. (1980); Ginsberg et al. (1984); Miller et al. (1985); Diakun et al. (1986)
	Xfin	CC–HH (one CC–HC)		
Drosophila	Serendipity	CC–HH		Ruiz i Altaba et al. (1987)
	Krüppel	CC–HH		Vincent et al. (1985)
	hunchback	CC–HH		Rosenberg et al. (1986)
	mk1, mk2	CC–HH		Tautz et al. (1987)
Mouse	Sp1	CC–HH	DNA	Chowdhury et al. (1987)
SV40	ADR1	CC–HH	DNA	R. Tjian (pers. comm.)
Yeast	SWI5	CC–HH	Zn, DNA	Hartshorne et al. (1986); Blumberg et al. (1987)
		(one CC–HC)		D. Stillman et al., (pers. comm.)
	PPR1	CC–CC	Zn, DNA	Johnston and Dover (1987); Keegan et al. (1986); Johnston (1987)
	ARGRII	CC–CC		Hartshorne et al. (1986)
		CC–CC		Messenguy et al. (1986)
Human	estrogen receptor	CC–CC	Zn?, DNA	Green et al. (1986); Bunce and Vessal (1987); Green and Chambon (1987)
	glucocorticoid receptor	CC–CC	DNA	Hollenberger et al. (1985); Giguere et al. (1986)
	c-erbA (thyroid hormone receptor)			
Rat	glucocorticoid receptor	CC–CC		Weinberger et al. (1986)
Chicken	estrogen receptor	CC–CC	DNA	Miesfeld et al. (1986, 1987)
	progesterone receptor	CC–CC		Krust et al. (1986)
E. Coli	Uvr A	CC–CC	Zn?, DNA	Conneely et al. (1986); Jeltsch et al. (1986)
Retroviruses	nucleic acid binding proteins	CC–HC	RNA	Doolittle et al. (1986)
				Covey (1986)
E. coli	Gene 32 protein	CH–CC	Zn, ss DNA, ss RNA	Giedroc et al. (1986)

Proteins are grouped in classes according to the type of proved or potential ligands to the Zn atom.

degree of sequence homology to the repeat of TFIIIA and might therefore be expected to form Zn-binding domains. The proteins for which a Zn requirement and/or DNA-binding has been demonstrated, or is strongly suggested, are indicated.

From the large number of published sequences, other subclasses of putative Zn-binding domains have started to emerge. In particular, instead of the classical arrangement of Cys-Cys....His-His of TFIIIA (and several other proteins) with a constant spacing of 12 or 13 amino acids between the inner ligands, a sequence unit having the same spacing but containing Cys-Cys....Cys-Cys is found. Such sequence units are seen in the first half of the two putative DNA-binding domains of several of the receptor proteins (Tables 1 and 2). The second half, which is encoded in a different exon, comprises a similar sequence unit but contains additional cysteines, allowing more than one possibility for theoretical folding, depending on which cysteines are used.

A similar situation is seen for the yeast regulatory proteins GAL4 and PPR1 in which there is a second pair of cysteines located at 13 and 16 residues away from the first pair of cysteines (Table 2). There is evidence that Zn is in this case also required for DNA binding (see below). A distinguishing character of these Cys-Cys....Cys-Cys domains is that they do not contain the conserved hydrophobic tyrosine, phenylalanine, and leucine, but instead contain acidic residues at invariant positions. It is possible that these amino acids form salt bridges with some of the basic residues, to substitute for the hydrophobic cluster we have postulated to be formed by the three hydrophobic groups found in the TFIIIA-type domain.

A third possible subclass showing combinations of histidine and cysteine is found in the nucleic-acid-binding proteins derived from the *gag* gene of retroviruses and T4 phage gene 32 protein. The spacing between the inner ligands is short (4 amino acids), but could coordinate Zn to form "stubbier" fingers (Table 1). Interestingly, a similar combination of cysteine and histidine is seen in the third putative finger of SWI5 (Table 2). However, it is very possible, by analogy with the structural Zn-binding site present in alcohol dehydrogenase (Eklund et al. 1976), that these shorter sequence units are not interacting directly with nucleic acids but are stabilizing the larger protein fold.

Besides the different families or classes of finger domains, there are differences in the sequences of the linkers that connect the finger loops. These are defined as the 5–8 amino acids that lie between the last histidine of one domain and the first cysteine of the next in the two-dimensional folding scheme (Fig. 2). In the three-dimensional structure these could, even within one protein, be folded differently or be all very similar. In TFIIIA all linkers have a different sequence except two having the sequence $\mathrm{TGEK_N^PT_T^P}$ (Fig. 1). This linker sequence TGEKPYX is highly conserved in Xfin from *Xenopus*, Krüppel from *Drosophila*, and mouse

mkr, suggesting some common evolutionary origin or perhaps some specific fold.

The conclusion from a number of deletion mutant studies of the hormone receptor proteins from humans and chicken (Giguere et al. 1986; Green and Chambon 1987) and the yeast transcriptional activators GAL4 (Keegan et al. 1986), SWI5 (K. Nagai et al., in prep.), and ADR1 (Blumberg et al. 1987), is that it is the region containing the putative Zn-binding domains that is responsible for binding to DNA (Table 1). The DNA-binding domain of these proteins alone, as is the case for TFIIIA, is not sufficient for the complete biological function. Other parts of the protein are needed, the so-called activation domains, presumably for making essential contacts with other components of the transcriptional machinery.

Do These Domains Bind Zn?

This is more difficult to show because many of the sequences listed in Table 1 derive from cDNA sequences or from proteins that cannot be purified in the amounts needed for measurements of Zn content. The abundance of TFIIIA made it possible for us to carry out EXAFS, an X-ray absorption technique that offers a means of characterizing the local environment of the metal sites. This study (Diakun et al. 1986) confirmed that there are approximately nine Zn atoms in the 7S particle and that all Zn atoms are in a similar environment. The Zn atom is coordinated by four ligands, two nitrogen atoms (from the histidines) at a distance of 2 Å and two sulfur atoms (from the cysteines) at 2.3 Å, in agreement with the tetrahedral coordination proposed by Miller et al. (1985).

More indirectly, there is physiological evidence on mutants consistent with Zn being an essential cofactor in the Cys-Cys....Cys-Cys-containing DNA-binding domain of the GAL4 protein (Johnston 1987). There had also been suggestions, as early as 1975, that the estrogen and progesterone receptors might be Zn-binding proteins (Lohmer and Toft 1975; Shymala and Yeh 1975). Certain zinc deficiency diseases that lead to a loss of estrogen or androgen sensitivity can be attributed to a failure of these hormones to fold their receptors properly in the absence of zinc (Bunce and Vessal 1987).

A strategy that allows one to study the metal requirement and DNA-binding properties of isolated Zn-binding domains is to express such sequences in *Escherichia coli*. Frankel et al. (1987), who have expressed a single finger of TFIIIA and show some evidence that Zn is necessary for folding of the synthetic amino acid chain, have not demonstrated specific DNA binding. This also applies to folding experiments in which Co has been used instead of Zn. In our laboratory we have, with our colleagues, been studying SWI5, which is an activator of HO gene transcription in yeast (Nasmyth et al. 1987). This protein contains three tandem, 30-amino-acid-long units bearing strong homology to the TFIIIA

Table 2. Comparison of the TFIIIA Consensus Sequence with the Putative Zn-binding Motif of Other Protein Sequences

TFIIIA consensus (9)	T	G	E	K	*	P	Ⓨ	V	Ⓒ	.	D	G	Ⓒ	D	K	R	Ⓕ	T	K	K	.	Ⓘ	K	*	R	Ⓗ	.	.	Ⓗ
Xfin consensus (37)	T	G	E	K	–	P	Ⓨ	.	Ⓒ	.	.	Ⓕ	.	.	.	s	.	Ⓘ	A	–	K	Ⓗ	.	R	–	T			Ⓗ
SW15	M	P	D	K	T	Ⓔ	L	F	P	G	Ⓒ	T	K	T	Ⓕ	K	R	R	Y	N	I	Q	–	T	Ⓗ				
	L	E	D	R	P	Ⓢ	D	H	P	G	Ⓒ	D	K	A	Ⓕ	V	R	N	H	D	R	–	K	–	s	Ⓗ			
	Q	O	E	K	A	Ⓐ	–	–	P	–	Ⓒ	G	K	K	Ⓕ	N	R	E	D	A	Ⓥ	–	R	S	R	M	I	Ⓒ	s G G
Estrogen receptor (human)	K	E	T	R	Y	Ⓒ	A	V	–	–	Ⓒ	N	D	Y	A	S	G	Y	H	Y	G	V	W	S	Ⓒ	E	G	–	– Ⓒ K A F
	K	R	S	I	O	G	H	N	D	Y	M	Ⓒ	P	A	T	N	Q	Ⓒ	T	I	D	K	N	R	R	K	S	Ⓒ	Q A Ⓒ R L R K Ⓒ Y E V G
GAL4	S	I	E	Q	A	Ⓒ	–	–	D	I	Ⓒ	R	L	K	K	L	K	C	S	K	E	K	P	K	Ⓒ	A	–	–	K Ⓒ L K N N

The sequences have been lined up to show their similarity to the 30-amino-acid repeat of TFIIIA. The same symbols as in Fig. 1 are used. The numbers above the sequence indicate the position of these DNA-binding domains in the sequence of the protein.

(Numbers above sequences: SW15 544; SW15 180; SW15 634; Estrogen receptor 249; GAL4 6; GAL4 35)

repeat (Table 2). This region, which is implicated in DNA binding (D. Stillman and K. Nasmyth, pers. comm.), has been expressed in *E. coli*, purified in its unfolded state and refolded in the presence of Zn, and shown to bind specifically to a region of about 15 bp of DNA (K. Nagai et al., in prep.). These experiments demonstrate that the isolated, three-finger motif of transcription factor SWI5 is sufficient for directing binding of the SWI5 protein to the promoter region of the HO gene and further, that Zn is a significant element in their structure.

Why Zinc?

The role of zinc in the DNA-binding finger appears to be purely structural. It might have an advantage over a disulfide bridge in bringing together two parts of a protein because it cannot be reduced in the reducing atmosphere inside the cell. A property particular to Zn, and not to Cu and Fe, is the absence of redox chemistry. Zn might be used in situations where the presence of redox reaction would lead to damaging radicals that could hydrolyze RNA or DNA and possibly even the protein chain (Williams 1984). The question of whether other metals, e.g., Co or Cd, can substitute for Zn has not been definitively settled, but in the experiments of Miller et al. (1985), in which various metals were tested for their ability to restore the partially dissociated 7S complex, only Zn was able to do so.

How Do Zn-binding Fingers Bind to DNA?

The nine small domains of TFIIIA interact with about 50 bp of the 5S RNA gene, so that each domain of the protein could, on the average, bind to about 5 bp of DNA (Fig. 3). Is there a pattern in the sequence of the internal control region of the 5S RNA gene that would match the repetitive structure of the protein that binds to it? There is no obvious repeat in the DNA sequence, but careful inspection of electrophoretic patterns of the naked 5S RNA gene cut with DNase I (and DNase II) revealed that within the internal control region there is a striking and fairly regular pattern of cuts occurring at about every five or six nucleotides. (Rhodes and Klug 1986). The origin of this periodic cutting is likely to be a periodicity in the DNA structure, and this in turn can be traced to the occurrence in the noncoding strand of short runs of guanines also at about every five or six nucleotides. It therefore appears that there is a framework for the recognition by each domain of TFIIIA of half a double-helical turn of DNA.

On examining the promoter regions of other closely related genes transcribed by RNA polymerase III, such as tRNA genes, we found that not only they, but also the transcription factor Sp1 binding site of the SV40 promoter show repeating G clusters, similar to those of the internal promoter of the 5S RNA gene. This suggested to us that the factors involved in the transcription of these genes might have Zn-binding fingers as

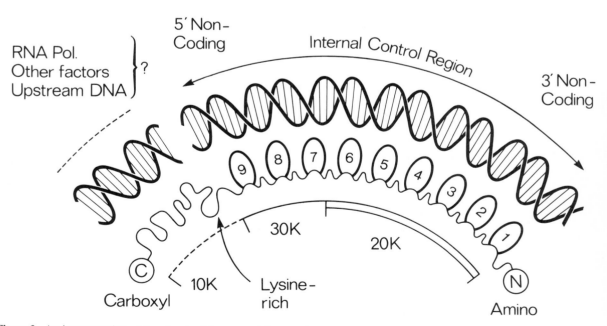

Figure 3. An interpretation of the structural features of the protein TFIIIA and its interactions with DNA. The DNA is drawn curved, as if resting on a long beaded surface of the protein. The internal control region of the 5S RNA gene (bases 40–100) is drawn as six turns of DNA, with the 5′ end of the noncoding strand at the left. The protein sequence runs from right to left. The amino end is followed by nine repeat units (residues 1–276) in contact with the control region. These units together form the 30-kD proteolytic fragment of TFIIIA. (Adapted from Miller et al. 1985.)

their DNA-binding domain (Rhodes and Klug 1986). Indeed the transcription factor Sp1 has since then been found to contain three sequence domains homologous to those of TFIIIA (R. Tjian, pers. comm.).

With our colleague Louise Fairall, we have investigated the contact points of TFIIIA with the internal control region of the 5S RNA gene by probing the accessibility of the DNA in the protein-DNA complex to dimethylsulfate and to micrococcal nuclease. The results of quantitative measurements, combined with those from our earlier DNase I and DNase II protection studies, are consistent with a series of multiple contacts about 5 bp apart, or half a double-helical turn, along the whole length of the internal control region. The nine patches of contact we have mapped could correspond to nine DNA-binding fingers in the protein (Rhodes 1985; Fairall et al. 1986).

Given the nature of repetitive structure of both protein and DNA, there are two possible simple models for the geometry of the interaction that produce contacts every half of a double-helical turn (Fig. 4). In model I, successive fingers follow the helical path of the major groove so that the protein might be said to snake around the DNA double helix (cf. Smith et al. 1984). On this model successive fingers make structurally

equivalent contact. In model II, the protein as a whole lies on one face of the DNA double helix, successive fingers pointing alternately on either side. In this model, only every other finger makes structurally equivalent contacts every 10 bp. The nuclease and methylation protection data is only consistent with TFIIIA making the type of interaction represented by model II. In brief, only one face of the DNA double helix is accessible, whereas the other is protected by the protein. Moreover, the methylation protection study shows that guanines located 10 nucleotides apart are protected, whereas the ones in between are not. This clearly is not the result one would expect if the protein spiraled around the double helix as in model I.

What Is the Tertiary Structure of a Zn Finger?

The answer will have to await the crystal or NMR structure of one of the many related complexes between Zn fingers and DNA. We have, however, already noted that in addition to the characteristic arrangements of cysteines and histidines coordinating the Zn, there are several other conserved amino acids (Table 2), of which three hydrophobic residues are likely to form a hydrophobic inner core of the folded

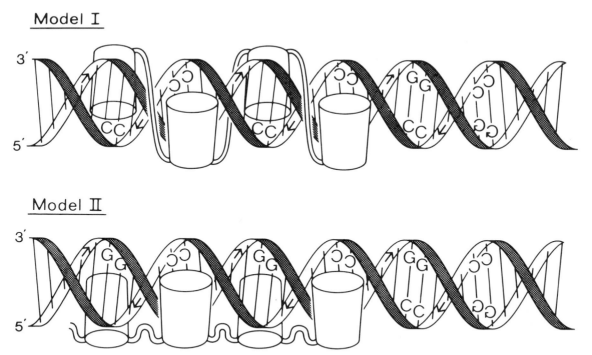

Figure 4. Schematic representation of two different models for the interaction of the TFIIIA domains with the double helix. For simplicity, the DNA-binding fingers of TFIIIA are represented by short cylinders, linked by thinner joints. In model I, TFIIIA follows the helical path of the major groove, each finger making contact from opposite faces of the DNA double helix at about every 5 bp. In this model, successive fingers make structurally equivalent contacts with guanine residues, which occur in the sequence of the internal control region of 5S RNA genes (noncoding strand) at about every 5 nucleotides. In model II, the protein lies on one face of the DNA helix, successive fingers pointing into the major groove alternately "in front" and "behind." Consequently, in this case, only every other finger makes structurally equivalent contacts located 10 bp apart, and the N-7 atoms of guanine residues 5 nucleotides apart are approached from different directions. The drawing is idealized, since the axis of the DNA helix need not be straight, nor the fingers arranged quite as regularly as shown. (Reprinted, with permission, from Fairall et al. 1986.)

structure (Fig. 1). In other words, the conserved amino acids provide the framework of tertiary folding, whereas the variable residues presumably determine the specificity of each domain. In the absence of a crystal structure, J. Berg (in prep. and this volume) has built on these original observations by fitting known structural motifs from other metalloproteins to a consensus sequence for Zn-binding fingers. The proposed three-dimensional model consists of an antiparallel β-sheet that contains the loop formed by the two cysteines and an α helix containing the His-His loop. The two structural units are held together by the Zn atom. Analogous to the way in which the helix-turn-helix motif binds DNA, DNA recognition is postulated to reside mostly in the helical region of the protein structure. A consequence of such a model is that the TFIIIA protein would have to spiral around the DNA helix as proposed in model I of Figure 4.

Conclusion: A Novel Motif for DNA or RNA Binding

We have listed in Table 1 many examples to show that the Zn-binding domains of TFIIIA are not some freak structure evolved for one particular gene or organism. In the case of TFIIIA we have suggested that a special multifingered design could have evolved to allow the polymerase to pass through the internal control region of the gene and yet remain bound through the internal promoter through the many rounds of transcription that are known to take place once the transcriptional complex is formed (Brown 1984). However, in RNA polymerase II transcription, it is likely that most factors bind upstream of the gene they regulate, so that two or three Zn fingers might suffice for specific DNA binding, as is shown experimentally for SWI5, GAL4, and several of the receptor proteins. On the other hand, primary sequences have now been found that are more TFIIIA-like (e.g., Krüppel) and indeed, in a sequence called Xfin from *Xenopus* (Ruiz i Altaba et al. 1987), may contain as many as 37 putative Zn-binding domains. In the latter case the finger motifs represent about 90% of the protein sequence. It is not yet clear what the role of these many-fingered proteins might be: one possibility, e.g., in the case of Krüppel and Xfin, could be in holding or carrying mRNA during developmental processes.

It thus appears that a novel protein motif for DNA binding has emerged for which TFIIIA is the type. It is an unusually small, self-folding domain in which Zn is a crucial component of its tertiary structure. This design for specific DNA recognition is distinctly different from the helix-turn-helix motif used for binding to DNA in several bacterial control proteins (for review, see Pabo and Sauer 1984). The latter has so far always been found embedded in a larger protein that binds to DNA as a dimer. The two-fold symmetry of the protein dimer corresponds to the palindromic nature of the DNA sequence to which it binds (Anderson et al. 1987). In contrast, the Zn-binding domain is a module that can be used singly without reference to DNA symmetry, and can be repeated in tandem to recognize DNA (or RNA) sequences of different lengths. Each domain is based on a similar framework that interacts with a small number of base pairs (about five in the case of TFIIIA and SWI5). Modulations in the amino acid sequence of each domain and sympathetic variations in the DNA sequence enable spatial registration of the interaction to be precise. The strength of the interaction and the number of Zn fingers can be varied, as can the spacing between them, thus achieving a high level of specificity in recognition. This modular design thus offers a large number of combinatorial possibilities for the specific recognition of DNA. It is not surprising that it is widespread throughout so many different types of organisms.

Some Remarks on Evolution

We have already mentioned that TFIIIA appears to be a highly evolved version of a small molecule of the size of one of the contemporary 3K domains stabilized by a metal ion. The primitive molecule could perhaps have assisted an early form of transcription. Evolution to the elaborate transcription apparatus found today could have taken place by gene duplication, with different repeats taking up extra functions. It is noteworthy, as remarked by Hanas et al. (1983), that RNA polymerase III contains zinc, and it could be that the initial activity of primitive TFIIIA promoted transcription in the absence of a polymerase molecule, which presumably only evolved later for greater efficiency.

Ginsberg et al. (1984) have noted a homology between a region of 5S DNA (or RNA) and the coding sequence of the TFIIIA gene and have suggested that TFIIIA could interact with its own gene or the derived RNA to autoregulate expression at the transcriptional or translational levels. The evolutionary origin of this contemporary property may be as follows. RNA is widely believed to have preceded DNA, so that a small primitive RNA could have coded for a small protein (the precursor of the 3K repeating unit) which bound back to the RNA and so stimulated its own production. These are the conditions for an Eigen-Schuster hypercycle (Eigen, this volume). Whatever the case, one would think that the zinc finger appeared rather early in evolution. What could be simpler than a relatively short (topological) loop of polypeptide folded back on itself with the aid of a metal ion, which is phenotypically stable and so could be passed on by exon shuffling? It is noteworthy that the finger, about 30 amino acids long, is of similar size to the elementary motif postulated to have been the origin of the α/β class of enzymes (Brändén 1987). It may therefore be that in the zinc finger we have another glimpse of the early history of protein evolution.

REFERENCES

Anderson, J.F., M. Ptashne, and S.C. Harrison. 1987. Structure of the bacteriophage 434 repressor-operator complex. *Nature* **326**: 846.

Berg, J.M. 1986. Potential metal-binding domains in nucleic acid binding proteins. *Science* **232:** 485.

Blumberg, H., A. Eisen, A. Sledziewski, D. Bader, and E.T. Young. 1987. Two zinc fingers of a yeast regulatory protein shown by genetic evidence to be essential for its function. *Nature* **328:** 443.

Bränden, C.I. 1987. Relation between functional loop regions and intron positions in α/β domains. In *Crystallography in molecular biology* (ed. D. Moras et al.), p. 359. Plenum Press, New York.

Brown, D.D. 1982. How a simple animal gene works. *Harvey Lect.* **76:** 27.

———. 1984. The role of stable complexes that repress and activate eucaryotic genes. *Cell* **37:** 359.

Brown, R.S., C. Sander, and P. Argos. 1985. The primary structure of transcription factor TFIIIA has 12 conserved repeats. *FEBS Lett.* **186:** 271.

Bunce, G.E. and M. Vessal. 1987. Effect of zinc and/or pyridoxine deficiency upon oestrogen retention and oestrogen receptor distribution in the rat uterus. *J. Steroid Biochem.* **26:** 303.

Chowdhury, K., V. Deutch, and P. Gruss. 1987. A multigene family encoding several "finger" structures is present and differentially active in mammalian genomes. *Cell* **48:** 771.

Conneely, O.M., W.P. Sullivan, D.O. Toft, M. Birnbaumer, R.G. Cook, B.L. Maxwell, T. Zarucki-Schulz, G.L. Greene, W.T. Schrader, and B.W. O'Mally. 1986. Molecular cloning of the chicken progesterone receptor. *Science* **233:** 767.

Covey, S.N. 1986. Amino acid sequence homology in gag region of reverse transcribing elements and the coat protein gene of cauliflower mosaic virus. *Nucleic Acids Res.* **2:** 623.

Diakun, G.P., L. Fairall, and A. Klug. 1986. EXAFS study of the zinc-binding sites in the protein transcription factor IIIA. *Nature* **324:** 689.

Doolittle, R.F., M.S. Johnson, I. Husain, B. VanHouten, D.C. Thomas, and A. Sancar. 1986. Domainal evolution of a prokaryotic DNA repair protein and its relationship to active-transport proteins. *Nature* **323:** 451.

Eklund, H., B. Nordström, E. Zeppezauer, G. Söderlund, I. Ohlsson, T. Boiwe, B.O. Söderberg, O. Tapia, and C.-I. Bränden. 1976. Three-dimensional structure of horse liver alcohol dehydrogenase at 2.4 Å resolution. *J. Mol. Biol.* **102:** 27.

Engelke, D.R., S.-Y. Ng, D.S. Shastry, and R.G. Roeder. 1980. Specific interaction of a purified transcription factor with an internal control region of 5S RNA genes. *Cell* **19:** 717.

Fairall, L., D. Rhodes, and A. Klug. 1986. Mapping of the sites of protection on a 5S RNA gene by the *Xenopus* transcription factor IIIA: A model for the interaction. *J. Mol. Biol.* **192:** 577.

Frankel, A.D., J.M. Berg, and C.O. Pabo. 1987. Metal-dependent folding of a single zinc finger from transcription factor IIIA. *Proc. Natl. Acad. Sci.* **84:** 4841.

Gehring, W.J. 1985. Homeotic genes, the homeo box and the genetic control of development. *Cold Spring Harbor Symp. Quant. Biol.* **50:** 243.

Giedroc, D.P., K.M. Keating, K.R. Williams, W.H. Koningsberg, and J.E. Coleman. 1986. Gene 32 protein, the single-stranded DNA binding protein from bacteriophage T4, is a zinc metallo protein. *Proc. Natl. Acad. Sci.* **83:** 8452.

Giguere, V., S.M. Hollenberg, M.G. Rosenfeld, and R.M. Evans. 1986. Functional domains of the glucocorticoid receptor. *Cell* **48:** 645.

Ginsberg, A.M., B.O. King, and R.G. Roder. 1984. *Xenopus* 5S gene transcription factor, TFIIIA: Characterization of a cDNA clone and measurement of RNA levels throughout development. *Cell* **39:** 479.

Green, S. and P. Chambon. 1987. Oestradiol induction of a glucocorticoid-responsive gene by chimeric receptor. *Nature* **325:** 75.

Green, S., P. Walter, V. Kumar, A. Krust, J.-M. Bornert, P. Argos, and P. Chambon. 1986. Human oestrogen receptor cDNA: Sequence, expression and homology to v-erb-A. *Nature* **320:** 134.

Hanas, J.S., D.J. Hazuda, D.F. Bogenhagen, F.Y.H. Wu, and C.W. Wu. 1983. *Xenopus* transcription factor A requires zinc for binding to the 5S RNA gene. *J. Biol. Chem.* **258:** 14120.

Hartshorne, T.A., H. Blumberg, and E.T. Young. 1986. Sequence homology of the yeast regulatory protein ADR1 with *Xenopus* transcription factor TFIIIA. *Nature* **320:** 283.

Hollenberg, S.M., C. Weinberger, E.S. Ong, G. Cerelli, A. Oro, R. Lebo, E.B. Thompson, M.G. Rosenfeld, and R.M. Evans. 1985. Primary structure and expression of a functional human glucocorticoid receptor DNA. *Nature* **318:** 635.

Jeltsch, J.M., Z. Krozowski, S. Quirin-Stricker, H. Gronemeyer, R.J. Simpson, J.M. Garnier, A. Krust, E. Jacob, and P. Chambon. 1986. Cloning of the chicken progesterone receptor. *Proc. Natl. Acad. Sci.* **83:** 5424.

Johnston, M. 1987. Genetic evidence that zinc is an essential co-factor in the DNA binding domain of GAL4 protein. *Nature* **328:** 353.

Johnston, M. and J. Dover. 1987. Mutations that inactivate a yeast transcriptional regulatory protein cluster in an evolutionary conserved binding domain. *Proc. Natl. Acad. Sci.* **84:** 2041.

Keegan, L., G. Gill, and M. Ptashne. 1986. Separation of DNA binding from the transcription-activating function of a eukaryotic regulatory protein. *Science* **231:** 699.

Krust, A., S. Green, P. Argos, V. Kumar, P. Walter, J.-M. Bornert, and P. Chambon. 1986. The chicken oestrogen receptor sequence: Homology with v-erb A and human oestrogen and glucocorticoid receptors. *EMBO J.* **5:** 891.

Lohmar, P.H. and D.O. Toft. 1975. Inhibition of the binding of progesterone receptor to nuclei: Effects of o-phenanthrobine and rifamycin AF/103. *Biochem. Biophys. Res. Commun.* **67:** 8.

Messenguy, F., E. Dubois, and F. Descamps. 1986. Nucleotide sequence of the ARGRII regulatory gene and amino acid sequence homologies between ARGRII, PPRI and GAL4 regulatory proteins. *Eur. J. Biochem.* **157:** 77.

Miesfeld, R., P.J. Godowski, B.A. Maler, and K.R. Yamamoto. 1987. Glucocorticoid receptor mutants that define a small region sufficient for enhancer activation. *Science* **236:** 423.

Miesfeld, R., S. Rusconi, P.J. Gadowski, B.A. Maler, S. Okret, A.-C. Wikström, J.-A. Gustavsson, and K.R. Yamamoto. 1986. Genetic complementation of a glucocorticoid receptor deficiency by express of cloned receptor DNA. *Cell* **48:** 389.

Miller, J., A.D. McLachlan, and A. Klug. 1985. Repetitive zinc-binding domains in the protein transcription factor IIIA from *Xenopus* oocytes. *EMBO J.* **4:** 1609.

Nasmyth, K., A. Seddon, and G. Ammerer. 1987. Cell cycle regulation of SW15 is required for mother-cell-specific HO transcription in yeast. *Cell* **49:** 549.

Pabo, C.O. and R.T. Sauer. 1984. Protein-DNA recognition. *Annu. Rev. Biochem.* **53:** 293.

Pelham, H.R.B. and D.D. Brown. 1980. A specific transcription factor can bind either the 5S RNA gene or the 5S RNA. *Proc. Natl. Acad. Sci.* **77:** 4170.

Picard, B. and M. Wegnez. 1979. Isolation of a 7S-particle from *Xenopus laevis* oocytes: A 5S RNA protein complex. *Proc. Natl. Acad. Sci.* **76:** 241.

Rhodes, D. 1985. Structural analysis of a triple complex between the histone octamer, a *Xenopus* gene for 5S RNA and transcription factor IIIA. *EMBO J.* **4:** 3473.

Rhodes, D. and A. Klug. 1986. An underlying repeat in some transcriptional control sequences corresponding to half a double helical turn of DNA. *Cell* **46:** 123.

Rosenberg, U.B., C. Schröder, A. Priess, A. Kienlin, S. Cote, I. Riede, and H. Jäckle. 1986. Structural homology

of the product of the *Drosophila* Krüppel gene with
Xenopus transcription factor IIIA. *Nature* **319**: 336.

Ruiz i Altaba, A., H. Perry-O'Keefe, and D.A. Melton. 1987.
Xfin: An embryonic gene encoding a multifingered protein
in *Xenopus*. *EMBO J.* (in press).

Shyamala, G. and Y.-F. Yeh. 1975. Is the estrogen receptor of
mammary glands a metallo-protein? *Biochem. Biophys.
Res. Commun.* **64**: 408.

Smith, D.R., I.J. Jackson, and D.D. Brown. 1984. Domains
of the positive transcription factor specific for the *Xenopus*
5S RNA gene. *Cell* **37**: 645.

Tautz, D., R. Lehmann, H. Schnürch, R. Schuh, E. Seifert,
A. Kienlin, K. Jones, and H. Jäckle. 1987. Finger protein
of novel structure encoded by hunchback, a second member of the gap class of *Drosophila* segmentation genes.
Nature **327**: 383.

Tso, J.Y., D.J. Van Den Berg, and L.J. Korn. 1986. Structure
of the gene for *Xenopus* transcription factor TFIIIA. *Nucleic Acids Res.* **14**: 2187.

Vincent, A. 1986. TFIIIA and homologous genes. The finger
proteins. *Nucleic Acids Res.* **14**: 4385.

Vincent, A., H.V. Colot, and M. Rosbash. 1985. Sequence
and structure of the Serendipity locus of *Drosophila
melanogaster*. A densely transcribed region including a
blastoderm-specific gene. *J. Mol. Biol.* **186**: 146.

Weinberger, C., C.C. Thompson, E.S. Ong, R. Lebo, D.J.
Gruol, and R.M. Evans. 1986. The c-erb-A gene encodes a
thyroid hormone receptor. *Nature* **324**: 641.

Williams, R.J.P. 1984. Zinc: What is its role in biology?
Endeavour New Ser. **8**: 65.

Some Evolutionary Relationships of the Primary Biological Catalysts Glutamine Synthetase and RuBisCO

D. EISENBERG, R.J. ALMASSY, C.A. JANSON, M.S. CHAPMAN, S.W. SUH, D. CASCIO, AND W.W. SMITH
*Molecular Biology Institute and the Department of Chemistry and Biochemistry,
University of California, Los Angeles, California 90024*

The polypeptide folds of two primary biological catalysts have been determined by X-ray crystallography. One is glutamine synthetase (GS) from *Salmonella typhimurium*, which catalyzes the entry of nitrogen into metabolism, and the other is ribulose bisphosphate carboxylase/oxygenase (RuBisCO) from tobacco, which catalyzes the entry of carbon into metabolism. Both are oligomeric structures having complicated patterns of interdomain and intersubunit contacts.

In this paper we consider three questions: (1) What are the patterns of folding of polypeptide chains in GS and RuBisCO, and how do the folded domains interact in the oligomeric enzyme? (2) Which features of the folding patterns are conserved in distantly related species and which are changed? and (3) What do the patterns of conservation and change tell us about the evolution of these catalytic functions?

Both GS and RuBisCO are primary biological catalysts in the sense that they catalyze the first steps at which nitrogen and carbon, respectively, are brought into cellular metabolism. GS (Ginsburg 1972; Ginsburg and Stadtman 1973) brings nitrogen into metabolism by condensing ammonia with glutamate, with the aid of ATP, to form glutamine:

$$\text{L-Glutamate} + \text{NH}_4^+ + \text{ATP} \longrightarrow$$
$$\text{L-Glutamine} + \text{ADP} + \text{P}_i$$

Glutamine is in turn a source of nitrogen in the biosynthesis of numerous nitrogen-containing metabolites, including amino acids, nucleotides, and amino sugars. Some nine of these end products of glutamine metabolism are feedback inhibitors of bacterial GS. GS in enteric bacteria is also regulated by covalent modification of a tyrosine residue by adenylylation (Shapiro et al. 1967). GS is adenylylated by a multienzyme cascade system in response to high levels of glutamine, and this modified GS has heightened sensitivity to the feedback inhibitors. In higher cells, GS also plays a central metabolic role. In plants, for example, GS assimilates ammonia produced by nitrogen fixation in roots and also assimilates ammonia released by photorespiration in leaves.

The three-dimensional structure of the 12-subunit GS from *S. typhimurium* has been determined at 3.5 Å (Almassy et al. 1986) and is described briefly below. A remarkable feature of the enzyme structure is that the

catalytic site is formed from portions of two polypeptide chains, at the subunit interface. This finding in itself suggests that bacterial GS is not a "primitive" enzyme, in that primitive GS enzymes presumably contained a catalytic site completely within one polypeptide chain.

The question of how the GS function evolved deepens when we consider that plant and animal GS molecules contain 8 identical subunits (Meister 1974), rather than 12 as in bacteria. In this paper, we present a speculative hypothesis on the relationship of the structure of the plant GS with 8 subunits to the bacterial molecule with 12 subunits. It is based in part on the observation that some segments of the amino acid sequences of plant and bacterial GS molecules are more strongly conserved than others. The stronger conservation tends to be in segments that form features of the active site. We show that features of the active sites can be conserved in an octameric GS molecule, provided that the symmetry of the octamer is lower than that of an ideally symmetric molecule. A lower symmetry octamer is consistent with some measurements on stoichiometry of binding.

RuBisCO catalyzes the first step of the Calvin cycle of photosynthesis (Miziorko and Lorimer 1983; Ellis and Gray 1986), in which carbon is brought into cellular metabolism in the form of carbon dioxide:

$$\text{CO}_2 + \text{Ribulose-1,5-bisphosphate} + \text{H}_2\text{O} \longrightarrow$$
$$\text{2 3-Phosphoglycerate}$$

RuBisCO also catalyzes the oxidation of ribulose bisphosphate in the first step of photorespiration.

The RuBisCO in plants has the subunit stoichiometry L_8S_8 (Baker et al. 1975), in which L is the large polypeptide chain (M_r 53,000) containing the catalytic residues and S is the small subunit (M_r 15,000). Recently, we have determined a moderate resolution structure for RuBisCO from tobacco (Chapman et al. 1987). It reveals that the catalytic site, like that of GS, is at the interface of two polypeptide chains. A portion of the molecule, containing just two L chains, resembles the structure of the L_2 RuBisCO from the photosynthetic bacterium *Rhodospirillum rubrum* (Schneider et al. 1986). Thus the tertiary structures of *R. rubrum* and plant RuBisCOs are similar for the large subunit polypeptide common to both enzymes, although the quaternary structures are different.

METHODS

X-ray crystallographic methods were used to determine the three-dimensional structures of GS to 3.5 Å resolution and of RuBisCO to 3.0 Å resolution. Some details have been reported by Almassy et al. (1986) and Chapman et al. (1987); additional information on structure determination will be presented elsewhere. Atomic models for both have been built and refined partially to crystallographic R factors of about 0.35. Refinement is continuing for both models, and it is anticipated that the preliminary structures reported here will change in details.

Alignment of the GS amino acid sequence from *S. typhimurium* (Janson et al. 1986) to that of GS from alfalfa (Tischer et al. 1986) was achieved with the University of Wisconsin Genetics Computer Group software package, mainly with the program BESTFIT, using a gap weight of 3.0 and a length weight of 0.1.

RESULTS

Structure of GS from *S. typhimurium*

In bacterial GS, the 12 subunits are arranged with 622 symmetry, just as the carbon atoms of two face-to-face benzene rings. Each subunit contains 468 amino acid residues and two metal ions at the active site. In Figure 1, one layer of 6 subunits is viewed down the 6-fold molecular axis; for clarity the layer below is omitted. In this paper, we are concerned mainly with the interaction of adjacent subunits within one such layer.

Each subunit has two folding domains (Fig. 1). The N domain is formed from the 103 amino-terminal residues, and is mainly a five-strand β sheet. However, this domain contains two α helices: it starts with a 12-residue helix and also contains a short 6-residue helix starting at amino acid 40. The C domain is much larger (residues 104–468). It contains 11 major α helices, and a β sheet with six antiparallel strands. This β sheet forms part of a cylindrical active site at the interface of two subunits within a ring. The rest of the cylinder is formed by two β strands from the neighboring subunit. These two strands are in the N domain; they are residues 44–52 and 59–70, bracketing a loop that contains Trp-57. This antiparallel, eight-strand cylinder is identified in the electron density as the active site both from the two metal ions it contains, and from a difference Fourier map showing that the transition-state analog binds within.

The polypeptide fold of a single GS subunit is shown in Figure 2. The two metal ions are depicted as circles in the active site at the top of the figure. Surrounding these ions are six heavy arrows, representing the six prominent β strands of the C domain. The other two β strands forming the active-site cylinder are at the bottom of the figure, with the position of Trp-57 marked at the bottom of the two strands. This two-strand segment of the structure is called the Trp-57 loop.

In summary, the six active sites within one ring of the GS molecule are between adjacent subunits. The major

portion of the active site, including six antiparallel extended strands and eight metal ligands, is donated by the C domain of one subunit; the minor portion, including two β strands, is donated by the N domain of the neighboring subunit.

Relationship between Bacterial and Plant GS Amino Acid Sequences

Amino acid sequences have been inferred from gene sequences for GS from alfalfa (Tischer et al. 1986) and Chinese hamster (Hayward et al. 1986), as well as from *Anabaena* (Tumer et al. 1983), *S. typhimurium* (Janson et al. 1986), and *E. coli* (Colombo and Villafranca 1986). The sequences from alfalfa and Chinese hamster can be readily aligned with over 50% of paired residues being identical (Tischer et al. 1986), a level of similarity that suggests very similar protein folds (Sweet and Eisenberg 1983). Similarly, the sequences from *Anabaena*, *S. typhimurium*, and *E. coli* can be readily aligned (Janson et al. 1986). In contrast, the similarity between the GS amino acid sequences of *S. typhimurium* (or the other bacterial GS) and of higher cells is much smaller, but not insignificant, as is shown in Figure 3. There are four segments in the paired sequences that show strong similarity.

Where in the known three-dimensional structure of bacterial GS do the segments of strong similarity fall? One of these segments includes residues 49–67 in *S. typhimurium*. This segment is the loop containing Trp-57, which can be seen at the bottom of Figure 2. By comparison with Figure 1, it is possible to see that this loop is part of the active site of the adjacent subunit. The second strongly conserved segment extends from

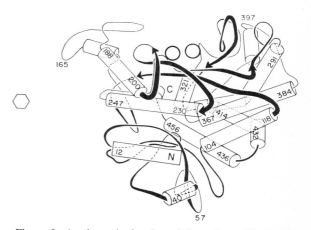

Figure 2. A schematic drawing of the polypeptide chain of one subunit of GS from *S. typhimurium*. (Reprinted, with permission from Almassy et al. 1986.) This subunit corresponds to the one on the right center of Fig. 1. The metal ions are indicated by two circles in the upper center, and the 6-fold axis by the hexagon on the left. Cylinders represent α helices; 6 heavy arrows, prominent β strands surrounding the metals. The amino-terminal folding domain (residues 1–103) is at the bottom. The central loop is at the upper left. The β loop is the U just below the helical end marked 247. (Reprinted, with permission, from Almassy et al. 1986.)

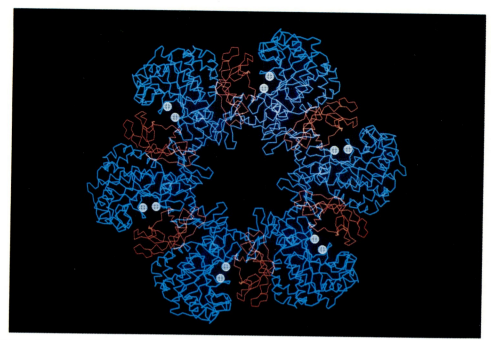

Figure 1. GS from *S. typhimurium* projected down the 6-fold molecular axis. The six subunits of the upper ring are shown as lines connecting sequential α carbon atoms. The N domains (residues 1–103) are shown in red and the C domains (residues 104–468) in blue. The central cavity, 40 Å in diameter, is filled with solvent, except for the central loops from each subunit, which protrude in about 15 Å. The active sites are cylindrical channels, each holding two Mn^{++} ions, shown as white circles. The N and C domains that meet at each active site are on *different* subunits. The molecule, including side chains, is 143 Å in diameter.

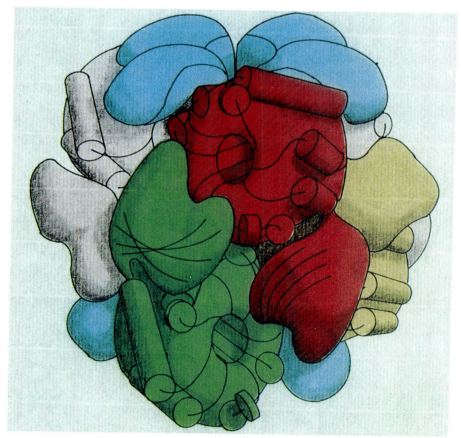

Figure 4. The spatial arrangement of subunits and domains in tobacco RuBisCO. (Reprinted, with permission, from Chapman et al. 1987.) S subunits are in blue, and each L subunit is in a different color. Notice that the amino-terminal domain of the green L subunit sits close to the mouth of the α/β barrel of the red barrel domain. Small helical carboxy-terminal domains of the L subunits are omitted for clarity.

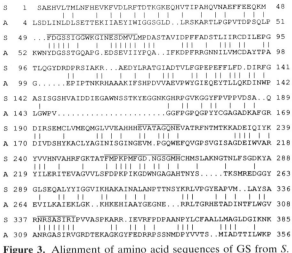

```
S    1  SAEHVLTMLNFHEVKFVDLRFTDTKGKEQHVTIPAHQVNAEFFEEQKM  48
        |  | | | | | | | | | | |   | |  | | | | | |
A    4  LSDLINLDLSETTEKIIAEYIWIGGSGLD..LRSKARTLPGPVTDPSQLP  51

S   49  ...FDGSSIGGWKGINESDMVLMPDASTAVIDPFFADSTLIIRCDILEPG  95
           |||||  |   |  |||||| |||    |||  | |||  || | ||
A   52  KWNYDGSSTGQAPG.EDSEVIIYPQA..IFKDPFRRGNNILVMCDAYTPA  98

S   96  TLQGYDRDPRSIAKR...AEDYLRATGIADTVLFGPEPEFFLFD.DIRFG  141
           ||  ||  | |    ||  |  |   |||  ||  || || |
A   99  G......EPIPTNKRHAAAKIFSHPDVVAEVPWYGIEQEYTLLQKDINWP  142

S  142  ASISGSHVAIDDIEGAWNSSTKYEGGNKGHRPGVKGGYFPVPPVDSA..Q  189
        |                                   |
A  143  LGWPV.....................GGFPGPQGPYYCGAGADKAFGR  169

S  190  DIRSEMCLVMEQMGLVVEAHHHEVATAGQNEVATRFNTMTKKADEIQIYK  239
        ||  |  |   | |||||| |||  |||   |  |   |   | |||
A  170  DIVDSHYKACLYAGINISGINGEVM.PGQWEFQVGPSVGISAGDEIWVAR  218

S  240  YVVHNVAHRFGKTATFMPKPMFGD.NGSGMHCHMSLAKNGTNLFSGDKYA  288
        |||   |  |   ||  | |     ||
A  219  YILERITEVAGVVLSFDPKPIKGDWNGAGAHTNYS.....TKSMREDGGY  263

S  289  GLSEQALYYIGGVIKHAKAINALANPTTNSYKRLVPGYEAPVM..LAYSA  336
        | ||  ||  ||  ||  | |  ||        |||   | | ||
A  264  EVILKAIEKLGK..KHKEHIAAYGEGNE...RRLTGRHETADINTFLWGV  308

S  337  RNRSASIRIPVVASPKARR.IEVRFPDPAANPYLCFAALLMAGLDGIKNK  385
        |||||||||          ||  || ||     ||||      |||
A  309  ANRGASIRVGRDTEKAGKGYFEDRRPSSNMDPYVVTS..MIADTTILWKP  356
```

Figure 3. Alignment of amino acid sequences of GS from *S. typhimurium*, labeled S, and from alfalfa, labeled A. Identical or similar residues in the two sequences are indicated by vertical lines. Four strongly conserved segments discussed in the text are indicated by overbars.

residue 212 to 220 in the sequence. In Figure 2 this is a turn and β strand that pass next to the metal ions in the active site. The third conserved segment comprises residues 255–270, another turn and β strand in the active site. A turn and β strand in the active-site cylinder comprise the fourth conserved segment, residues 338-345. In short, all of the strongly conserved segments of sequence between bacterial and alfalfa GS are known in *S. typhimurium* GS to line the active-site cylinder. This suggests that the polypeptide geometries of the active sites of the alfalfa and bacterial enzymes are similar.

In the alignment of Figure 3, a large gap appears in the alfalfa sequence between residues 147 and 148. The segment of the bacterial sequence that aligns in this gap corresponds to two extended loops in the known GS structure. The first of these is the "β loop", which makes contact with the lower layer of 6 subunits. The β loop is visible in Figure 2 as the U-shaped loop just under the end of the helix marked by residue 247. The second loop is the "central loop", which protrudes into the central aqueous cavity of the dodecameric enzyme. This loop is marked by residue 165 in Figure 2. The sequence alignment of Figure 3 suggests that these two loops may be absent in the GS of higher cells.

Structure of RuBisCO from Tobacco

At low resolution, RuBisCO resembles a keg with the axis of the keg being the 4-fold axis of the 16-subunit molecule. The keg is 105 Å along the 4-fold axis and about 132 Å in diameter at its widest point. Along the 4-fold axis there is an open channel, 28 Å wide at the center of the molecule and 6 Å at its narrowest constriction (Chapman et al. 1986).

The arrangement of subunits in tobacco RuBisCO is depicted schematically in Figure 4, where the 4-fold keg

axis runs vertically. Clustered around the 4-fold axis at both the top and bottom of the molecule are tetramers of S subunits, shown in blue. Bridging between the two tetramers of S subunits are elongated L subunits, each one a different color in Figure 4. The L subunits have two main folding domains. The amino-terminal (N) domain of about 150 residues is a β-sheet structure with two α helices on the inside, toward the 4-fold axis. The larger domain is an α/β barrel (B) domain, with dimensions and topology very similar to the α/β barrel of triosephosphate isomerase (Banner et al. 1975).

The active site of RuBisCO is at the opening of the α/β barrel onto the solution, as surmised by analogy to other α/β barrel enzymes, and from our preliminary fitting of segments of the amino acid sequence into the electron density. From Figure 4 it can be seen that the active-site region is near the N domain of the adjacent L subunit. Thus RuBisCO, like GS, has its active site at the junction of two domains, which are on different polypeptide chains.

Relationship of Tobacco RuBisCO to *R. rubrum* RuBisCO

In earlier work, we compared the amino acid sequence of the L subunit of tobacco (477 residues) to that of *R. rubrum* (466 residues) (Janson et al. 1984). The method of hydrophobicity correlation was used to assess the probability that the two polypeptide chains are folded in a similar manner. It was found that there is a reasonably high correlation in the hydrophobicities of the pairs of residues in the aligned sequences, suggesting that the two polypeptide chains are folded in the same general way.

This inference, based on comparison of amino acid sequences, has now been confirmed by X-ray diffraction studies of structure. The structure of *R. rubrum* RuBisCO at 3 Å resolution has been reported by Schneider et al. (1986). The polypeptide chain is folded into two main domains, and the L_2 molecule has the same general fold and dimensions as that for one of the four L_2 dimers in the plant L_8S_8 form. The red and green L subunits of Figure 4 contribute one such dimer. Moreover, a 2-fold axis of symmetry relates the two subunits of the *R. rubrum* dimer in nearly the same way that one of the 2-fold axes of the tobacco RuBisCO relates the green and red *L* chains in Figure 4. The S subunits in the L_8S_8 tobacco RuBisCO are not present in *R. rubrum*. It is possible that the tetramers of S subunits in the plant enzyme may function as a scaffold for tetramerizing L_2 dimers of the type found both in *R. rubrum* and tobacco.

DISCUSSION

Possible Relationship of Bacterial and Higher GS Structures

It may be possible to infer some aspects of the structure of GS from higher cells. In this section we argue that the active sites found at the junction of subunits in bacterial GS are present also in higher GS molecules. This speculation is based in part on the comparison of amino acid sequences made in Figure 3 above, and in part on a comparison of the catalytic and ligand-binding behavior of the two classes of GS.

GS molecules from liver, brain, and plant tissues are somewhat smaller in subunit mass than bacterial GS (M_r = 39,000–50,000 versus 52,000) and have 8 subunits rather than 12 (Tate and Meister 1973). Many of the catalytic and regulatory properties of GS from higher cells are like those from bacteria, but some differ. GS from liver, brain, pea, and *E. coli* all require divalent cations for activity, act on D- as well as L-glutamate, and are inhibited by L-methionine-S-sulfoximine, glycine, alanine, and carbamyl phosphate (Tate et al. 1972). On the other hand, tryptophan, histidine, and glucosamine-6-phosphate inhibit GS from *E. coli* and slightly inhibit GS from pea but do not inhibit GS from liver or brain. GSs from enteric bacteria are regulated by adenylylation, but GSs from *Bacillus subtilis* and higher cells are not. Tate and Meister (1971) summarize the situation as follows: "...the active catalytic sites of these enzymes (and the mechanisms of the reactions catalyzed) are probably quite similar."

Three similarities between the bacterial and higher GSs argue that the protein fold of the higher GS resembles that of the bacterial molecule. The first is the similarity in subunit size. The second is the strong similarity of four segments of the amino acid sequence, discussed above. The third is the similarity in catalytic and regulatory function described in the preceding paragraph. However, with the active site at the interface between two subunits, how can identical subunits be positioned to form both 12mers (bacteria) and octamers (higher cells) and in both cases maintain the active conformation at the subunit interfaces?

In fact, an octamer can be formed from subunit pairs that preserve the intersubunit geometry of the active sites of bacterial GS. However, this packing reduces the symmetry of the octamer to one with half its active-site peptide segments not actually forming active sites. This packing is illustrated by Figure 5, where the top layer of the octamer is depicted as four GS subunits of the bacterial type. Two subunit pairs of the bacterial type are preserved, so that the four subunits form two potent active sites and four impotent half active sites. In this model, a lower layer of four GS subunits is related to the upper layer by two 2-fold axes in the plane of the paper. Thus the symmetry of the octamer is 222, rather than the maximum possible 422.

A consequence of this model is that higher cell GS would be expected to exhibit "half-of-the-sites" activity. In fact, half-of-the-sites binding has been reported for several substrates and effectors. Tate and Meister (1971) found that four moles of methionine sulfoximine bind to octameric rat liver GS and completely inactivate the enzyme. Wedler et al. (1982) found that octameric sheep brain GS binds four moles of Mn^{++} tightly and then four moles more somewhat less tightly. Thus higher GS may demonstrate the half-

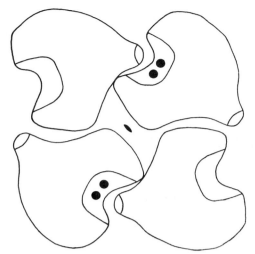

Figure 5. A hypothetical subunit arrangement for GS from higher cells. The enzyme is an octamer, with only the upper layer of four subunits shown. Subunits are arranged in an upper pair and a lower pair, with the two members of each pair having the same spatial relationship as a pair of subunits from bacterial GS (as in Fig. 1). However, the four pairs are arranged with 222 symmetry, rather than 622 symmetry of the six pairs in Fig. 1. The result is that one complete active site is present at the interface of each subunit pair. These complete active sites are indicated by two circles, representing the catalytic metal ions. Each pair also has two vestigial half active sites which could conceivably act as regulatory sites.

of-the-sites activity that must be observed in a symmetry 222 octamer that preserves subunit pairs of the type observed in bacterial GS. It should be noted, however, that there could be reasons for half-of-the-sites function other than the diminished symmetry oligomer proposed here. A recent study of the binding of Mn to brain GS is in conflict with earlier work (Maurizi et al. 1986).

The subunit-level model for higher cell GS shown in Figure 5 is also consistent with the loss of the central loop in higher GS suggested by Figure 3. This curious structural feature of *S. typhimurium* GS protrudes into the central solvent channel. It interacts with the active site (see Almassy et al. 1986), but could conceivably interfere with tight association of two subunit pairs. Finally, there is one feature of the model of Figure 5 that is inconsistent with the sequence alignment of Figure 3. It is that lack of any strong homology between the carboxy-terminal amino acid sequences of bacterial and higher cell GS. The carboxyl termini are important for holding together the two layers of bacterial GS, and these interlayer contacts might be expected to be preserved in higher GS, constructed as in the model of Figure 5. Given this lack of homology in the carboxyl termini, as well as the ongoing discussion about binding data mentioned above, the model of Figure 5 must be regarded as highly speculative.

Complexity of the primary biological catalysts. GS and RuBisCO catalyze the primary steps in the assimilation of nitrogen and carbon, respectively. In bacterial systems they might have been expected to have primitive structures. In fact, the structures are very complex: Both structures involve multiple subunits, two main domains in both GS and RuBisCO subunits, and active sites formed from two domains at the junction of subunits. Clearly these primary catalysts have evolved from simpler enzymatic units.

One intriguing question regards the pathway of development from single-domain, single-subunit precursors of these multiple-subunit enzymes containing multiple-domain subunits. The first step might have been multiple-domain formation (i.e., evolution of protomeric chains resembling the GS subunit or the RuBisCO L subunit). Then, the second step would have been oligomerization of these subunits. Alternatively, oligomers of single-domain subunits could have been formed first, followed by development of folding domains within the subunits. From our present knowledge of the structures, neither possibility can be ruled out.

Patterns of evolutionary change and conservation in GS and RuBisCO. In comparing structures of bacterial and higher cell primary catalysts, which features are preserved and which are changed? Quaternary structures are not conserved from one kingdom to another. Bacterial GS contains 12 identical subunits, whereas higher cell GS contains 8. Similarly RuBisCO from the photosynthetic bacterium *R. rubrum* has 2 identical L chains with symmetry 2, and RuBisCO from plants has 8 L and 8 S subunits with symmetry 422. However, within the octamer of L subunits, there are 4 L_2 pairs, each resembling the dimensions of the *R. rubrum* pair (Schneider et al. 1986; Chapman et al. 1987). The variation among species of quaternary structures of enzymes has been noted often before, and a detailed description of comparative RuBisCO quaternary structures has been given by McFadden et al. (1986).

There are indications that tertiary folds of RuBisCO and GS are conserved among kingdoms. The pattern of folding of the L subunit within the tobacco L_8S_8 RuBisCO (Chapman et al., 1987) is at least qualitatively similar to that of *R. rubrum* RuBisCO (Schneider et al. 1986). Both chains have two domains, each domain is similar to its counterpart in the other protein, and the geometry of connection of the two domains is similar in the two molecules.

In GS there are also indications that the tertiary folds of bacterial and higher cell GS are at least partially conserved. This indication is from the conservation of residues in active-site peptides. The observation that one of these conserved regions lies in the N domain of bacterial GS and the other three lie in the C domain suggests that higher cell GS, like bacterial GS, has a two-domain structure.

In short, at our present state of knowledge it appears that the tertiary structures and domain structure of GS and RuBisCO are conserved among kingdoms more strongly than are primary or quaternary structures.

What advantage might there be to an organism of an altered quaternary structure in an enzyme that preserves its tertiary fold? The most obvious answer is that a preserved tertiary structure maintains a useful catalytic function, whereas an altered quaternary structure presents new opportunities for regulation. In RuBisCO, the tetramerized L_2 structure of the plant enzyme permits interaction of the four L_2 pairs, perhaps mediated by the S subunits that appear to act as a scaffold for the L_2 pairs. In the hypothetical higher GS structure of Figure 5, the 8 open "half-active sites" could conceivably function in the octamer as regulatory sites. Each putative regulatory half site belongs to the same subunit as part of a full active site; consequently, the binding of an effector could be communicated to the catalytic center through the subunit.

Testing of these speculative notions must await more detailed comparison of RuBisCO structures, as well as the determination of the structure of higher cell GS.

ACKNOWLEDGMENTS

The authors gratefully acknowledge support from the National Institutes of Health research (United States Public Health Service GM-31299).

REFERENCES

Almassy, R.J., C.A. Janson, R. Hamlin, N.-H. Xuong, and D. Eisenberg. 1986. Novel subunit-subunit interactions in the structure of glutamine synthetase. *Nature* 323: 304.

Baker, T.S., D. Eisenberg, F.A. Eiserling, and L. Weissman. 1975. The structure of form I crystals of D-ribulose-1,5-diphosphate carboxylase. *J. Mol. Biol.* 91: 391.

Banner, D.W., A.C. Bloomer, G.A. Petsko, D.C. Phillips, C.I. Pogson, and I.A. Wilson. 1975. Structure of chicken muscle triose phosphate isomerase determined crystallographically. *Nature* 255: 609.

Chapman, M.S., S.W. Suh, D. Cascio, W.W. Smith, and D. Eisenberg. 1987. The quaternary structure of plant RuBisCO limits sliding-layer conformational change. *Nature* (in press).

Chapman, M.S., W.W. Smith, S.W. Suh, D. Cascio, A. Howard, R. Hamlin, N.-H. Xuong, and D. Eisenberg. 1986. Structural studies of RuBisCO from tobacco. *Philos. Trans. R. Soc. Lond. B Biol. Sci.* 313: 367.

Colombo, G. and J.J. Villafranca. 1986. Amino acid sequence of *Escherichia coli* glutamine synthetase deduced from the DNA nucleotide sequence. *J. Biol. Chem.* 261: 10587.

Ellis, R.J. and J.C. Gray, eds. 1986. *Ribulose bisphosphate carboxylase-oxygenase.* The Royal Society, London.

Ginsburg, A. 1972. Glutamine synthetase of *Escherichia coli*: Some physical and chemical properties. *Adv. Protein Chem.* 26: 1.

Ginsburg, A. and E.R. Stadtman. 1973. Regulation of glutamine synthetase in *Escherichia coli*. In *The enzymes of glutamine metabolism* (ed. S. Prusiner and E.R. Stadtman), p. 92. Academic Press, New York.

Hayward, B.E., A. Hussain, R.H. Wilson, A. Lyons, V. Woodcock, B. McIntosh, and T.J.R. Harris. 1986. The cloning and nucleotide sequence of cDNA for an amplified glutamine synthetase gene from the Chinese hamster. *Nucleic Acids Res.* 14: 999.

Janson, C.A., W.W. Smith, and D. Eisenberg. 1984. Preliminary structural studies of ribulose-1,5-bisphosphate carboxylase/oxygenase from *Rhodospirillum rubrum*. *J. Biol. Chem.* 259: 11594.

Janson, C.A., P.S. Kayne, R.J. Almassy, M. Grunstein, and D. Eisenberg. 1986. DNA-encoded sequence of glutamine synthetase from *Salmonella typhimurium*: Implications for the protein structure. *Gene* 46: 297.

Maurizi, M.R., H.B. Pinkofsky, P.J. McFarland, and A. Ginsburg. 1986. Mg^{2+} is bound to glutamine synthetase extracted from bovine or ovine brain in the presence of L-
methionine-S-sulfoximine phosphate. *Arch Biochem.
Biophys.* **246:** 494.

McFadden, B.A., J. Torres-Ruiz, H. Daniell, and G. Sarojini.
1986. Interaction, functional relations and evolution of
large and small subunits in RuBisCO from prokaryota and
eukaryota. *Philos. Trans. R. Soc. Lond. B Biol. Sci.*
313: 347.

Meister, A. 1974. Glutamine synthetase of mammals. In *The
enzymes*, 3rd. edition (ed. P.D. Boyer), vol. 10, p.10.
Academic Press, New York.

Miziorko, H.M. and G.H. Lorimer. 1983. Ribulose-1,5-
bisphosphate carboxylase/oxygenase. *Annu. Rev. Biochem.* **52:** 507.

Schneider, G., Y. Lindqvist, C.-I. Branden, and G. Lorimer.
1986. Three-dimensional structure of ribulose-1,5-bisphos-
phate carboxylase/oxygenase from *Rhodospirillum rubrum* at 2.9 Å resolution. *EMBO J.* **5:** 3409.

Shapiro, B.M., H.S. Kingdon, and E.R. Stadtman. 1967.
Adenylylglutamine synthetase: A new form of the enzyme
with altered regulatory and kinetic properties. *Proc. Natl.
Acad. Sci.* **58:** 642.

Sweet, R.M. and D. Eisenberg. 1983. Correlation of sequence
hydrophobicities measures similarity in three-dimensional
protein structure. *J. Mol. Biol.* **171:** 479.

Tate, S.S. and A. Meister. 1971. Regulation of rat liver
glutamine synthetase: Activation by α-ketoglutarate and
inhibition by glycine, alanine, and carbamyl phosphate.
Proc. Natl. Acad. Sci. **68:** 781.

————.1973. Glutamine synthetases of mammalian liver and
brain. In *The enzymes of glutamine metabolism* (ed. S.
Prusiner and E.R. Stadtman), p. 77. Academic Press, New
York.

Tate, S.S., L. Fang-Yun and A. Meister. 1972. Rat liver
glutamine synthetase. *J. Biol. Chem.* **247:** 5312.

Tischer, E., S. DasSarma, and H.M. Goodman. 1986. Nucleotide sequence of an alfalfa glutamine synthetase gene.
Mol. Gen. Genet. **203:** 221.

Tumer, N.E., S.J. Robinson, and R. Haselkorn. 1983. Different promoters for *Anabaena* glutamine synthetase gene
during growth using molecular or fixed nitrogen. *Nature*
306: 337.

Wedler, F.C., R.B. Denman, and W.G. Roby. 1982. Glutamine synthetase from ovine brain is a manganese(II)
enzyme. *Biochemistry* **21:** 6389.

Structural and Evolutionary Aspects of the Key Enzymes in Photorespiration; RuBisCO and Glycolate Oxidase

C.-I. Brändén, G. Schneider, Y. Lindqvist, I. Andersson, S. Knight, and G. Lorimer*

*Department of Molecular Biology, Swedish University of Agricultural Sciences, Biomedical Center, S-75124 Uppsala, Sweden; *Central Research and Development Department, E.I. du Pont de Nemours and Company, Wilmington, Delaware 19898*

Photorespiration, which occurs in most photosynthetic organisms, involves an oxidation of reduced carbon in the form of sugar molecules to carbon dioxide. The energy released in this process is dissipated as heat. No net ATP or NADH is produced in this series of enzymatic reactions. Photorespiration is a major process in the carbon metabolism of plants; up to 50% of the solar energy that is absorbed, converted, and stored as reduced carbon is released again by this process with no apparent benefit for the plant.

The process is initiated by one of the key enzymes in the Calvin cycle of carbon dioxide fixation, ribulose bisphosphate carboxylase/oxygenase (RuBisCO), due to its dual enzymatic function (Miziorko and Lorimer 1983). RuBisCO can add either carbon dioxide or oxygen to the key metabolite of the cycle, ribulose bisphosphate. The first reaction is part of the Calvin cycle, the second leads to the formation of glycolate and to photorespiration through the glycolate shunt. Glycolate oxidase is the first enzyme in this shunt that is present in most organisms with an oxidative metabolism.

There are a number of evolutionary questions that can be asked about photorespiration. The first and most often discussed is why this process has evolved and why it has stayed in the photosynthetic system until the present time. This is, in our opinion, more a teleological question than a scientific one, and for our purposes it is sufficient to know that the process can be reduced by artificial means or by changed physiology of the plant leaves with no apparent harmful effects on the plant but with a considerable increase in plant productivity.

The second question, whether it is possible to compete with evolution and change the ratio of oxygenation/carboxylation of the enzyme RuBisCO by genetic engineering, is more interesting scientifically and is the aim of the study we have undertaken on RuBisCO by a combination of X-ray crystallography and site-directed mutagenesis.

Third, recent X-ray studies (Xia et al. 1987) have shown that there is in yeast an enzyme that is evolutionarily related to glycolate oxidase and that traps the energy released in this oxidation and channels it to reduced cytochrome *c*. We predict that in algae that have learned how to live with an energy crisis a similar mechanism has evolved and that the enzyme that oxidizes glycolate, glycolate dehydrogenase, is evolutionarily related to yeast flavocytochrome b2.

We have determined the X-ray structures of glycolate oxidase from spinach (Lindqvist and Brändén 1985) and of RuBisCO from a photosynthetic bacterium, *Rhodospirillum rubrum* (Schneider et al. 1986b). We have also recently obtained a high-resolution electron density map of the more complex RuBisCO from spinach and have related this map to the RuBisCO structure from *Rh. rubrum*. These structures will be described and discussed.

METHODS

Glycolate Oxidase

The structure determination of glycolate oxidase to 2.2 Å resolution has been described (Lindqvist and Brändén 1980, 1985). We have compared this structure and that of yeast flavocytochrome b2 (Xia et al. 1987) in collaboration with Scott Mathews by superposition of α-carbon atoms from both structures using a program kindly provided by M. Rossmann.

RuBisCO from *Rhodospirillum rubrum*

Crystallization procedures, methods for data collection, and the structure to 2.9 Å resolution have been published (Brändén et al. 1986; Schneider et al. 1986a,b). Recombinant RuBisCO from *Rh. rubrum*, expressed in *Escherichia coli* (Somerville and Somerville 1984), was used for all X-ray work.

Phase angles were initially determined from two heavy-atom derivatives and refined (Bricogne 1976) using the local noncrystallographic two-fold symmetry of our crystals. An initial model was built from the averaged electron density map. Crystallographic refinement to higher resolution is now in progress. The model described here has an R factor of 26.5% at 2.9 Å resolution.

RuBisCO from Spinach

Crystallization conditions and preliminary X-ray studies on RuBisCO from spinach have been reported

(Andersson and Brändén 1984; Brändén et al. 1986). X-ray data to 2.4 Å resolution were collected at the Daresbury synchrotron radiation source using the wiggler beam line for native enzyme, two heavy-atom derivatives, and a Co-substituted enzyme. The native crystals were of a quaternary complex with carbon dioxide, Mg, and a six-carbon sugar molecule that is believed to function as an analog for one of the transition states. Data were collected on film using the rotation method with 1° oscillation. These data were processed using a program package kindly provided by J. Remington (Eugene University, Oregon) and modified by A. Jones (University of Uppsala). To search for heavy-atom positions in Pattersson space, a program was written that utilizes the noncrystallographic symmetry. The space group of our crystals is C222₁ and there is a pseudo-four-fold axis almost parallel to the c axis. The position of this pseudo-four-fold axis is such that it gives a pseudo-F-centered pattern in the diffraction to low resolution.

From this pseudosymmetry it is easy to deduce that the molecular center of the molecule must be close to either (0,0.25,0.25) or (0.25,0,0) in this space group. This was confirmed by R-value searches using the transform of a hollow sphere with an outer radius of 50 Å and an inner radius of 8 Å. It was not possible, however, to distinguish between the two alternative positions from this search. The distinction was made on the basis of the heavy-atom difference Pattersson vector search that was initially carried out for both alternatives. It was then found that the cross vectors between different sites made the best fit if the molecular center was placed at position (0,0.25,0.25). From the position of the big peak in the low-resolution native Pattersson due to the pseudo-F-centering, it was then obvious that the two halves of the molecule are related by separate four-fold axes, the positions of which differ by about 2 Å in the a direction. These two four-fold axes are related by the crystallographic two-fold axis parallel to the b axis. The subunit arrangement that we have deduced in this way is very different from that recently suggested to occur in the RuBisCO molecules from *Alcaligenes eutrophis* (Holzenburg et al. 1987). There, the two four-fold axes were suggested to be 36 Å apart in the two halves of the molecule. We have confirmed our arrangement by an electron density map to high resolution in which we could identify the orientation of the large subunits from the structure of the *Rh. rubrum* molecule.

Our vector search program first searches through the Harker sections and provides a ranking list of possible heavy-atom sites. These positions were then expanded using the noncrystallographic symmetry, and all possible combinations of these sites were tested against the difference Pattersson maps. This procedure was repeated until one consistent set of sites remained. For the mercury derivative we obtained 16 sites and for the gold derivative 12 sites that gave good agreement with the maps to low resolution, but we noticed that many vectors were slightly offset from the peaks in the high-resolution maps. After considerable confusion, we finally realized that there was a small translation component in the c direction associated with the pseudo-four-fold axes. By incorporating this translation into our pseudosymmetry we obtained very good agreement between calculated vector positions and observed Pattersson peaks and a considerable improvement in the averaged electron density maps. From cross-difference Fourier maps we included some additional minor sites. Electron density maps were initially plotted on sheets and later adjusted to a model of the *Rh. rubrum* RuBisCO molecule on the display using FRODO (Jones 1985).

RESULTS AND DISCUSSION

Glycolate Oxidase

The glycolate oxidase molecule is octameric with strict 422 symmetry. Figure 1 shows a view of the octameric molecule down the four-fold axis illustrating the large solvent-filled hole through the middle of the molecule. Each subunit has about 370 amino acid residues. The most striking feature of the subunit structure is an α/β barrel of eight parallel β strands surrounded by eight helices. This domain comprises about 250 residues and binds the coenzyme FMN. The remaining residues form a number of helices scattered outside one half of the barrel. Figure 2 shows a schematic diagram of the subunit structure. A stereo diagram of the barrel with bound FMN is given in Figure 3.

The barrel is a structural motif that has been found in a variety of structures with different functions and usually completely different amino acid sequences. So far, the motif has only been found in enzymes, and the active sites of these enzymes are always at the carboxyl

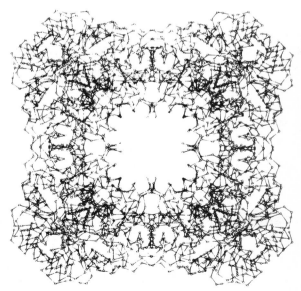

Figure 1. Diagram of the α carbon atoms of the octameric glycolate oxidase molecule viewed down the four-fold symmetry axis.

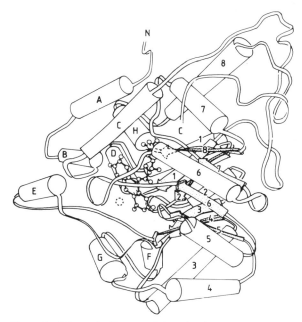

Figure 2. Schematic diagram of the subunit structure of glycolate oxidase seen from a side perpendicular to the barrel axis. Cylinders represent helices and arrows represent β strands. FMN bound at the carboxyl end of the barrel is shown as a ball and stick model.

This structural motif has now been described for the following enzymes in addition to glycolate oxidase: triosephosphate isomerase (Banner et al. 1975), pyruvate kinase (Stuart et al. 1979), taka-amylase (Matsuura et al. 1980), phosphogluconate aldolase (Mavridis et al. 1982), xylose isomerase (Carrell et al. 1984), trimethylamine dehydrogenase (Lim et al. 1986), RuBisCO (Schneider et al. 1986b), muconolactone isomerase (Goldman et al. 1987), flavocytochrome b2 (Xia et al. 1987), and the bifunctional enzyme phosphoribosylanthranilate isomerase : indoleglycerol phosphate synthase (Priestle et al. 1987). The last enzyme has two barrels in one polypeptide chain catalyzing different reactions. All these barrels have very similar geometry. The common core of eight β strands and eight helices comprises around 160 residues, the α carbon atoms of which superpose with a root-mean-square deviation of around 2.6 Å in any pairwise comparison. An exception is glycolate oxidase and flavocytochrome b2, which show a much higher degree of similarity. For all the remaining comparisons there is no significant amino acid sequence homology, not even for the superposed residues. Corresponding loop regions have, in general, different lengths in these barrels, but there is a consistent trend that loop regions at the amino end of the strands are shorter than those at the carboxyl end.

We thus have here a common structural motif in many enzymes of different amino acid sequences and different functions. Since neither sequence nor function is conserved, it seems most probable that these barrels have not evolved from a common ancestral barrel structure, but have a different evolutionary history. They might have evolved in a strictly convergent fashion quite independently of each other, but a case can be made for a different history. An analysis of intron positions in the genes for some of these barrels has shown (C.-I. Brändén, pers. comm.) that these positions are concentrated in regions either within or close to the loops at the carboxyl end of the β strands and very few are at the other end of the barrel. It has been

edge of the parallel β strands. The carboxyl ends of these strands and the beginning of the loop regions that connect these β strands with the following α helices form a funnel-shaped active site. Most residues that participate in binding and catalysis are located in these regions of the polypeptide chain. The remaining residues from the β strands and the helices form the hydrophobic cores that stabilize the barrel structure. Thus, residues that participate in the specific function of these barrel structures are clearly separated from residues that are responsible for the structural stability of the barrels.

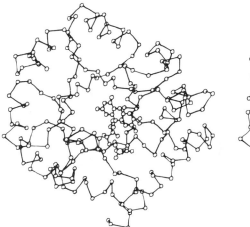
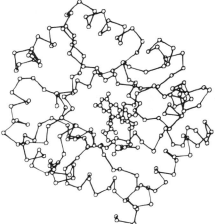

Figure 3. Stereo view of the α carbon skeleton of the barrel domain in glycolate oxidase with bound FMN viewed from the carboxyl end of the β sheet along the barrel axis.

suggested that this reflects an evolutionary history where these barrels have been constructed by joining small exons coding for simple α-β units. If such units are joined into an α/β barrel, all splice regions will occur in the loops at the carboxyl ends of the β strands. This is consistent with the greater variability in lengths of these loop regions and with the position of the active sites at this end in all the barrels. The probability of evolving enzymes with different catalytic sites around the intron positions is much higher than from random changes around the surface of the molecule or from random point mutations at the other end of the barrel.

Two of these enzymes, glycolate oxidase and flavocytochrome b2, show some similarities in their catalytic reactions. They both utilize FMN to oxidize small α-hydroxy acids, glycolate and lactate, respectively, in a two-step process. In the first step, the substrate is oxidized and FMN is reduced in a reaction that would be expected to have similarities in the mechanism since the only difference is a small change in the size of the substrate. In the second step, FMN is reoxidized by quite different mechanisms. In flavocytochrome b2, the electron is transferred to a cytochrome that is present as a second domain of the enzyme. This cytochrome then transfers the electron to the pool of cytochrome c in the yeast cell. In glycolate oxidase, the electron is transferred to oxygen and hydrogen peroxide is formed.

Xia et al. (1987) noticed that the FMN-binding domain of flavocytochrome b2 showed larger similarities to glycolate oxidase than to other barrel structures. In particular, the two large loop regions outside the barrel had a similar arrangement of helices. In a comparison we have made of these structures in collaboration with Scott Mathews, we find that around 320 residues superpose with a root-mean-square error of 1.6 Å, which is far greater structural homology than is found for any other barrel comparison. Unfortunately, the amino acid sequence of glycolate oxidase has not been described so we cannot make a comparison at the sequence level of these two enzymes. However, by comparing this result with that of other structures that have homologous sequences (Chothia and Lesk 1986), we can estimate that glycolate oxidase and the FMN-binding domain of flavocytochrome b2 have a sequence homology in the region of 30–50%.

The comparison of these two structures has thus revealed an interesting example of functional adaptation by evolutionary gene transfer. Flavocytochrome b2 might have evolved by gene fusion of separate ancestral flavin-binding and cytochrome b2 domains, whereas glycolate oxidase evolved from the flavin-binding domain alone. Alternatively and less likely, the ancestral gene coded for one protein carrying both domains from which glycolate oxidase evolved by deletion of the cytochrome domain. Cytochrome b2, which is homologous to the cytochrome domain in flavocytochrome b2, would then have evolved by deletion of the flavin-binding domain.

RuBisCO in algae has an oxygenase activity quite similar to that in green plants. The fate of glycolate that results from this activity is, however, different. Here there is a different enzyme glycolate dehydrogenase that starts the degradation of glycolate. This enzyme has not been characterized biochemically, except to show that it is quite different from glycolate oxidase. On the basis of our comparison between glycolate oxidase and flavocytochrome b2, we predict that glycolate dehydrogenase is related to flavocytochrome b2. Water absorbs a considerable amount of light energy, so algae have been under severe selection pressure to conserve energy, in contrast to green plants. It would be quite advantageous for algae to preserve the large amounts of energy released in glycolate oxidation by channeling it to cytochrome c instead of oxygen.

RuBisCO from *Rhodospirillum rubrum*

RuBisCO from higher plants, algae, and most photosynthetic microorganisms is a complex multisubunit protein. The enzyme molecule consists of eight large (MW 56,000) and eight small (MW 15,000) subunits. The catalytic function resides on the large subunit; the function of the small subunits is unknown. Primary structures for the large subunits of higher plant and algal carboxylases are very similar. The amino acid sequence homologies among these carboxylases are in the range of 70–80%.

In contrast to these carboxylases, the enzyme from the photosynthetic bacterium *Rh. rubrum* differs considerably in amino acid and subunit composition. This carboxylase is a dimer of large subunits and lacks small subunits. The overall amino acid homology to higher plant large subunits is 25% (Nargang et al. 1984). However, despite this low overall sequence homology, some peptide regions are highly conserved. Three of these peptide regions have been identified as parts of the active site by chemical methods (Lorimer 1981; Fraij and Hartman 1982; Herndon et al. 1982). A number of mutagenesis experiments on residues in these peptide regions have been carried out prior to our determination of the three-dimensional structure of the enzyme (Gutteridge et al. 1984; Estelle et al. 1985; Niyogi et al. 1986; Terzaghi et al. 1986; Hartman et al. 1987).

The structure of the dimeric molecule is shown in Figure 4. The dimensions are approximately $50 \times 72 \times 105$ Å. Each subunit consists of two domains, as is seen in the schematic diagram of Figure 5. The amino-terminal domain comprises amino acid residues 1–137 and the larger carboxy-terminal domain is built up from residues 138–466. The amino-terminal domain is centered around a central, mixed five-stranded β sheet. Two α helices are found on one side and one α helix on the other side of the β sheet. The connection to the carboxy-terminal domain is a short α helix, followed by a piece of extended chain.

The carboxy-terminal domain has an α/β barrel structure, as was found for glycolate oxidase. This domain starts with an α helix, which does not belong to

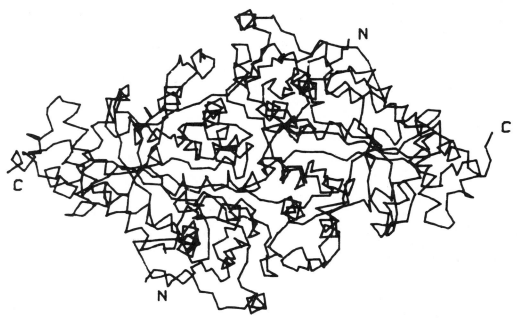

Figure 4. Stereo diagram of the α carbon atoms in the dimer molecule of RuBisCO from *Rh. rubrum*.

the α/β barrel motif. This helix is located at the amino-terminal end of the β strands of the barrel and closes off the barrel from this side. After this helix, the chain enters the first strand of the barrel. There are also other

additional secondary structural elements outside the barrel motif in this domain. After helix 6, the polypeptide chain forms two antiparallel β strands before going back into the barrel. These two antiparallel β

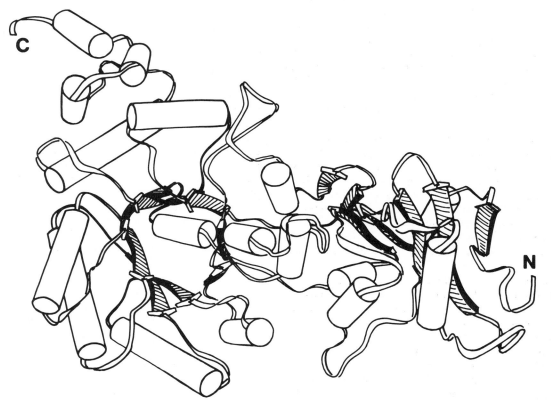

Figure 5. Schematic diagram of the structure of one subunit of RuBisCO from *Rh. rubrum*. Cylinders represent α helices and arrows represent β strands. (Drawing by Ulla Uhlin.)

strands are involved in domain-domain interactions (Fig. 5). A small additional α helix is found in the loop between strand 8 and helix 8 of the α/β barrel. At the carboxy-terminal end of the polypeptide chain, we find three consecutive α helices.

Our gene product contains 24 extra amino acids from β-galactosidase at the amino-terminal end. We do not observe electron density for these additional 24 amino acid residues. These residues are probably disordered in our crystals.

The subunit-subunit interactions are tight and extensive, as can be seen in Figure 4. Two main interface areas are found. One such area is between the carboxy-terminal domains of the two subunits, which build up the core of the molecule. The second contact area is between the carboxy-terminal domain of one subunit and the amino-terminal domain of the second subunit. Amino acid residues from loops 1, 2, and 3 at the carboxyl end of the β strands of the barrel in one subunit interact with the amino-terminal domain of the second subunit. Loops 1 and 2 exhibit extensive amino acid sequence homology between the bacterial and higher plant enzymes. Parts of these conserved peptide regions are involved in these subunit-subunit interactions. This is in agreement with our recent finding that not only the subunit structures, but also the dimer interactions of the *Rh. rubrum* dimer are essentially preserved in the spinach molecule.

The active site of RuBisCO is found at the carboxyl end of the eight parallel β strands of the carboxy-terminal domain. Active site residues are, as expected, located at the carboxyl end of the β strands and in the loops between the strands and the helices of the barrel. This side of the barrel is close to the amino-terminal domain of the second subunit. Glu-48, which is part of a highly conserved region in the amino-terminal domain, is close to the active site.

Three conserved lysine residues, 166, 191, and 329, have been suggested to be involved in either catalysis or the activation process (Lorimer 1981; Herndon et al. 1982; Herndon and Hartman 1984). Lys-191 is involved in the activation of the enzyme, and it has been suggested that Lys-166 is the base that initiates catalysis by abstracting the C-3 proton from the substrate (Nargang et al. 1984; Hartman et al. 1987). This reaction is analogous to the enolization in the mechanism of triosephosphate isomerase (Straus et al. 1985). Lys-329 has been identified as an active site residue by chemical modification.

All three lysine residues are found at the carboxyl end of β strands or in loops between these strands and the helices of the α/β barrel. Lys-166 is located in the loop after strand 1, Lys-191 is the last residue in strand 2, and Lys-329 is found in loop 6. The function of Lys-191 is best understood. This residue is involved in the activation process of the enzyme, a process common to all carboxylases. During activation, a carbamate is formed between the amino group of Lys-191 and an activator carbon dioxide molecule. This carbamate is stabilized by Mg. Figure 6 shows the surround-

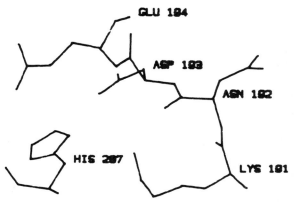

Figure 6. A picture of protein atoms in the vicinity of Lys-191 in the active site of RuBisCO from *Rh. rubrum*.

ings of Lys-191 in our crystal structure that are from the nonactivated enzyme. Two acidic residues, Asp-193 and Glu-194, are found in close proximity to Lys-191. These two residues are conserved in all carboxylases. It is very likely that these two residues are part of the Mg-binding site in the activated ternary complex. In close proximity to this site is the side chain of His-287. From our present model, it is possible that this side chain is also involved in binding the metal ion in the ternary complex. This would be in agreement with EPR measurements of the activated ternary complex, where Mg has been replaced by Cu (Brändén et al. 1984; Styring and Brändén 1985). From these studies, a nitrogen ligand has been proposed to be part of the coordination sphere of the metal ion. Upon formation of the quaternary complex, this nitrogen ligand is displaced, presumably by oxygen atoms from the substrate.

Lys-191 has been replaced by Glu in a site-directed mutagenesis experiment (Estelle et al. 1985). The negative charge of the activated carbamylated form of this residue is preserved by the mutation, but the mutant is inactive, presumably because it is unable to bind Mg. We have done model-building experiments of a ternary complex where we assumed that Mg is coordinated to Asp-193, Glu-194, and the carbamate on residue 191. In this model it is obvious that the replacement of the carbamylated lysine side chain by the shorter Glu side chain does not give a proper metal-binding site. The oxygen atoms of the carboxyl group of Glu-191 are too far away from the metal for direct coordination. Consequently, the proper surrounding of the Mg-binding site is not maintained and the enzyme can no longer bind Mg in its proper place.

Lys-166 has been replaced with a number of other residue types; Gly, Ala, Ser, Glu, Arg, Cys, and His. All seven mutants are severely deficient in carboxylase activity (Hartman et al. 1987). The glycine mutant is completely inactive, but it can be carbamylated, as demonstrated by its ability to tightly bind a transition state analog. On the basis of these experiments, it has been suggested that Lys-166 does not participate directly in activation or substrate binding but catalyzes enolization of the substrate. Our X-ray structure is not incompatible with these suggestions, although other explanations for the kinetic properties of these mutants are not excluded.

RuBisCO from Spinach

The crystals of spinach RuBisCO contain half a molecule, four large subunits and four small subunits, in the asymmetric unit. These are related by noncrystallographic pseudo-four-fold axes parallel to the c axis with translation components of about 2 Å along c. In our improved electron density map to low resolution we could identify a number of α helices. From the amino acid sequence homology between the enzymes from spinach and from *Rh. rubrum* we expected that the large subunit of the spinach enzyme would have domain structures similar to the *Rh. rubrum* subunit. We could very quickly identify the typical eight-helix motif of the α/β barrel due to the specific geometric arrangement of these helices. From the arrangement of the four barrel motifs in the asymmetric unit coupled with the crystallographic symmetry, it was then obvious that they were arranged pairwise in a way similar to the dimer arrangement in the *Rh. rubrum* molecule. A high-resolution electron density map was then calculated, and we have started building the *Rh. rubrum* molecule into this map. It is obvious from this map that details of both the subunit and the domain arrangements are different. Characterization of these differences as well as the structure of the small subunit for which we see well-defined electron density is now in progress.

ACKNOWLEDGMENTS

This work was supported by grants from the Swedish Natural Science Research Council and from the Swedish Agricultural Research Council.

REFERENCES

Andersson, I., and C.-I. Brändén. 1984. Large single crystals of spinach ribulose-1,5-bisphosphate carboxylase/oxygenase suitable for X-ray studies. *J. Mol. Biol.* 172: 363.

Banner, D.W., A.C. Bloomer, G.A. Petsko, D.C. Phillips, C.I. Pogson, I.A. Wilson, P.H. Corran, A.J. Furth, J.D. Milman, R.E. Offord, J.D. Priddle, and S.G. Waley. 1975. Structure of chicken muscle triose phosphate isomerase determined crystallographically at 2.5 Å resolution using amino acid sequence data. *Nature* 255: 609.

Brändén, R., T. Nilsson, and S. Styring. 1984. Ribulose-1,5-bisphosphate carboxylase/oxygenase incubated with Cu(II) and studied by electron paramagnetic resonance spectroscopy. *Biochemistry* 23: 4373.

Brändén, C.-I., G. Schneider, Y. Lindqvist, I. Andersson, S. Knight, and G.H. Lorimer. 1986. X-ray structural studies of Rubisco from *Rhodospirillum rubrum* and spinach. *Philos. Trans. R. Soc. Lond. B Biol. Sci.* 313: 359.

Bricogne, G. 1976. Methods and programs for direct-space exploitation of geometric redundancies. *Acta Crystallogr. Sect. A.* 32: 832.

Carrell, H.L., B.H. Rubin, T.J. Hurley, and J.P. Glusker. 1984. X-ray crystal structure of D-xylose isomerase at 4-Å resolution. *J. Biol. Chem.* 259: 3230.

Chothia, C. and A.M. Lesk. 1986. The relation between the divergence of sequence and structure in proteins. *EMBO J.* 5: 823.

Estelle, M., J. Hanks, L. McIntosh, and C.R. Somerville. 1985. Site-specific mutagenesis of ribulose-1,5-bisphosphate carboxylase/oxygenase. *J. Biol. Chem.* 260: 9523.

Fraij, B. and F.C. Hartman. 1982. 2-Bromoacetylaminopentitol 1,5-bisphosphate as an affinity label for ribulose bisphosphate carboxylase/oxygenase from *Rhodospirillum rubrum*. *J. Biol. Chem.* 257: 3501.

Goldman, A., D.L. Ollis, and T.A. Steitz. 1987. Crystal structure of muconate lactonizing enzyme at 3 Å resolution. *J. Mol. Biol.* 194: 143.

Gutteridge, S., I. Sigal, B. Thomas, R. Arntzen, A. Cordova, and G. Lorimer. 1984. A site-specific mutation within the active site of ribulose-1,5-bisphosphate carboxylase of *Rhodospirillum rubrum*. *EMBO J.* 3: 2737.

Hartman, F.C., T.S. Soper, S.K. Niyogi, R.J. Mural, R.S. Foote, S. Mitra, E.H. Lee, R. Machanoff, and W.F. Larimer. 1987. Function of Lys-166 of *Rhodospirillum rubrum* ribulosebisphosphate carboxylase/oxygenase as examined by site-directed mutagenesis. *J. Biol. Chem.* 262: 3496.

Herndon, C.S. and F.C. Hartman. 1984. 2-(4-bromacetamido)-anilino-2-deoxypentitol 1,5-bisphosphate, a new affinity label for ribulose bisphosphate carboxylase/oxygenase from *Rhodospirillum rubrum*. *J. Biol. Chem.* 259: 3102.

Herndon, C.S., I.C. Norton, and F.C. Hartman. 1982. Reexamination of the binding site for pyridoxal 5'-phosphate in ribulosebisphosphate carboxylase/oxygenase from *Rhodospirillum rubrum*. *Biochemistry* 21: 1380.

Holzenburg, A., F. Mayer, G. Harauz, M. van Heel, R. Tokuoka, T. Ishida, K. Harata, G.P. Pal, and W. Saenger. 1987. Structure of D-ribulose-1,5-bisphosphate carboxylase/oxygenase from *Alcaligenes eutrophus* H16. *Nature* 325: 730.

Jones, A. 1985. Interactive computer graphics: FRODO. *Methods Enzymol.* 115: 157.

Lim, L.W., N. Shamala, F.S. Mathews, D.J. Steenkamp, R. Hamlin, and N.H. Xuong. 1986. Three-dimensional structure of the iron-sulfur flavoprotein trimethylamine dehydrogenase at 2.4-Å resolution. *J. Biol. Chem.* 261: 15140.

Lindqvist, Y. and C.-I. Brändén. 1980. Structure of glycolate oxidase from spinach at a resolution of 5.5 Å. *J. Mol. Biol.* 143: 201.

———. 1985. Structure of glycolate oxidase from spinach. *Proc. Natl. Acad. Sci.* 82: 6855.

Lorimer, G. 1981. Ribulosebisphosphate carboxylase: Amino acid sequence of a peptide bearing the activator carbon dioxide. *Biochemistry* 20: 1236.

Matsuura, Y., M. Kusunoki, W. Harada, N. Tanaka, Y. Iga, N. Yasuoka, H. Toda, K. Narita, and M. Kakudo. 1980. Molecular structure of takaamylase A. Backbone chain folding at 3 Å resolution. *J. Biochem.* 87: 1555.

Mavridis, I.M., H.M. Hatada, A. Tulinsky, and L. Lebioda. 1982. Structure of 2-keto-3-deoxy-6-phosphogluconate aldolase at 2.8 Å resolution. *J. Mol. Biol.* 162: 419.

Miziorko, H.M. and G. Lorimer. 1983. Ribulose-1,5-bisphosphate carboxylase-oxygenase. *Annu. Rev. Biochem.* 52: 507.

Nargang, F., L. McIntosh, and C.R. Somerville. 1984. Nucleotide sequence of the ribulosebisphosphate carboxylase gene from *Rhodospirillum rubrum*. *Mol. Gen. Genet.* 193: 220.

Niyogi, S.K., R.S. Foote, R.J. Mural, F.W. Larimer, S. Mitra, T.S. Soper, R. Machanoff, and F.C. Hartman. 1986. Nonessentiality of histidine 291 of *Rhodospirillum rubrum* ribulose-bisphosphate carboxylase/oxygenase as determined by site-directed mutagenesis. *J. Biol. Chem.* 261: 10087.

Priestle, J.P., M.G. Grutter, J.L. White, M.G. Vincent, M. Kania, E. Wilson, T.S. Jardetzky, K. Kirschner, and J.N.

Jansonius. 1987. Three-dimensional structure of the bifunctional enzyme N-(5'-phosphoribosyl) anthranilate isomerase-indole-3-glycerol-phosphate synthase from *Escherichia coli*. *Proc. Natl. Acad. Sci.* **84**: 5690.

Schneider, G., C.-I. Brändén, and G. Lorimer. 1986a. New crystal forms of ribulose-1,5-bisphosphate carboxylase/oxygenase from *Rhodospirillum rubrum*. *J. Mol. Biol.* **187**: 141.

Schneider, G., Y. Lindqvist, C.-I. Brändén, and G. Lorimer. 1986b. Three-dimensional structure of ribulose-1,5-bisphosphate carboxylase/oxygenase from *Rhodospirillum rubrum* at 2.9 Å resolution. *EMBO J.* **5**: 3409.

Somerville, C.R. and S.C. Somerville. 1984. Cloning and expression of the *Rhodospirillum rubrum* ribulosebisphosphate carboxylase gene in *E. coli*. *Mol. Gen. Genet.* **193**: 214.

Straus, D., R. Raines, E. Kawashima, J.R. Knowles, and W. Gilbert. 1985. Active site of triosephosphate isomerase: In vitro mutagenesis and characterization of an altered enzyme. *Proc. Natl. Acad. Sci.* **82**: 2272.

Stuart, D.I., M. Levine, H. Muirhead, and D.K. Stammers. 1979. Crystal structure of cat muscle pyruvate kinase at a resolution of 2.6 Å. *J. Mol. Biol.* **134**: 109.

Styring, S. and R. Brändén. 1985. Identification of ligands to the metal ion in Cu(II) activated ribulose-1,5-bisphosphate carboxylase/oxygenase by the use of electron paramagnetic resonance spectroscopy and ^{17}O-labeled ligands. *Biochemistry* **24**: 6011.

Terzaghi, B.E., W.A. Laing, J.T. Christeller, G.B. Petersen, and D.F. Hill. 1986. Ribulose 1,5-bisphosphate carboxylase—Effect on the catalytic properties of changing methionine-330 to leucine in the *Rhodospirillum rubrum* enzyme. *Biochem. J.* **235**: 839.

Xia, Z.-X., N. Shamala, P.H. Bethge, L.W. Lim, H.D. Bellamy, N.H. Xuong, F. Lederer, and S. Mathews. 1987. Three-dimensional structure of flavocytochrome b2 from baker's yeast at 3.0 Å resolution. *Proc. Natl. Acad. Sci.* **84**: 2629.

Calcium Coordination and the Calmodulin Fold: Divergent versus Convergent Evolution

R.H. KRETSINGER

Department of Biology, University of Virginia, Charlottesville, Virginia 22901

In 1975 I presented "Hypothesis: Calcium-modulated proteins contain EF-hands" as part of a general summary of the function of calcium within the cytosol. In brief review, the general theory consists of five summary ideas or hypotheses.

1. The concentration of Ca^{++} ion within the cytosols of all quiescent cells, eukaryotic or prokaryotic, is very low, about 10^{-7} M or pCa 7. This generalization has been amply confirmed for numerous plants, animals, fungi, and protocists. It is probably valid for bacteria as well.

2. The sole function of calcium in the cytosol is to transmit information, or to function as a messenger. There may be a few exceptions in which calcium at 10^{-7} M confers structural stability. However, because free Mg^{++} is present at $10^{-2.5}$ M, the binding molecule requires very high affinity and selectivity for calcium. The concentration of free Ca^{++} ion rises to pCa ~ 5.5 during stimulation, thereby reducing the Mg^{++}/Ca^{++} ratio from $10^{4.5}$ to $10^{3.0}$.

3. The target of calcium functioning as a second messenger is a protein in the cytosol, by definition a calcium-modulated protein. Phospholipids, although strongly affected by millimolar concentrations of calcium, do not have the selectivity to bind $10^{-5.5}$ M Ca^{++} ions in the presence of $10^{-2.5}$ M Mg^{++}. The change in potential due to the flux of Ca^{++} across membranes may be detected by membrane proteins in some neurons, as are voltage changes caused by Na^+ fluxes.

4. Calcium-modulated proteins contain EF-hands. This 29-amino-acid domain consisting of helix, loop, helix is now more properly called the calmodulin fold. It seemed reasonable that the common function of transducing the information inherent in a pulse of Ca^{++} ions into a change in conformation of an enzyme or structural protein might be performed by members of a single homolog family.

5. Calcium was initially extruded by early cells because calcium salts are highly insoluble; only later in evolution was the resulting gradient ($[Ca^{++}]_{out}$ $10^{-2.8}$ M, $[Ca^{++}]_{cytosol}$ $10^{-7.0}$ M) exploited to transmit information. This hypothesis is admittedly somewhat more speculative. However, it is now well established that introducing millimolar calcium into the cytosol is toxic. Many extracellular fluids are near saturation in calcium phosphate or other counteranions. The proteins, frequently glycosylated, that regulate nucleation and biomineralization were proposed not to be homologs of the calmodulin fold.

In this paper I will summarize a few characteristics of the 27 proteins that contain two to six copies of the calmodulin fold (Table 1). Interestingly, functions for only 10 of these have been established. Numerous noncytosolic proteins bind calcium and are not homologs of calmodulin. Given this background, I will address 8 proteins not considered to be calcium modulated, 6 of which function in extracellular environments having millimolar calcium concentrations. Their proposed calcium-binding sites resemble those of the EF-hand. Does this represent convergent or divergent evolution?

CALMODULIN SUPERFAMILY

General Description

Over 20 distinct "families" of proteins are included in the "superfamily" of EF-hand proteins. Family refers to a cluster of proteins with distinguishable structural or functional characteristics. Homology among all families of the superfamily is inferred from primary sequence or from tertiary structure.

The families listed in Table 1 share various characteristics and are certainly homologous with one another. Yet, they do display variations that are relevant to the subsequent question of divergent versus convergent evolution. Although it is inappropriate to list some 300 sequences of two to six domains of multiple isotypes of over 20 families, the selected sequences in Tables 2, 3, and 4 illustrate the "canonical" EF-hand and several of its more important variations.

The general characteristics of the EF-hand have been reviewed on numerous occasions. Helix E consists of nine residues with side chains at positions 2, 5, 6, and 9 facing the inside of the molecule. The calcium-binding loop coordinates calcium with side-chain oxygens of Ser, Thr, Asx, or Glx. These can be assigned to the vertices of an octahedron: X (position 10); Y 12; Z 14; $-X$ 18; $-Z$ 21. One of the carboxylates may coordinate calcium with two oxygen atoms, i.e., the calcium is seven coordinate with six amino acids involved. The oxygen at $-Y$ 16 comes from the carbonyl group of the main chain; the side chain is exposed to the solvent and variable. Helix F extends from residues 22 through 29, with 22, 25, 26, and 29 facing inward. Usually EF-hands occur in pairs with the two hands having numerous hydrophobic contacts and being related by an approximate twofold axis.

Table 1. Domain Structures of the Calmodulin Superfamily

	1	2	3	4	seq	cDNA	gDNA	3D
Calmodulin	Ca	Ca	Ca	Ca	+	+	+	+
cal-1	Ca*	Ca*	Ca*	Ca*			+	
CM1	Ca*	Ca*	Ca*	Ca*			+	
Spec 1 (*S. purpuratus*)	Ca*	Ca*	Ca*	Ca*		+	+	
Calcineurin	Ca	Ca	Ca	Ca	+	+		
CDC31 (yeast)	Ca*	O	O	Ca*		+		
TNC (skeletal)	Ca	Ca	Ca	Ca	+	+	+	+
TNC (cardiac)	O	Ca	Ca	Ca	+	+		
TNC (*Halocynthia*)	O	Ca*	O	Ca*	+			
Essential LC	O	O	O/?	O	+	+	+	
Calpain, heavy	Enz–Ca	Ca	O	O	+	+		
Calpain, light	(G)n–Ca	Ca	O	O		+		
Aequorin	Ca	Enz	Ca	Ca	+	+		
Regulatory LC	Ca	O	O	O	+	+	+	
Ca vector protein	O	O	Ca	Ca	+			
SCBP (shrimp)	Ca	Ca	Ca	??	+			
SCBP (*Amphioxus*)	Ca	Ca	Ca	??	+			
SCBP (sandworm)	Ca	??	Ca	Ca	+			
SCBP (scallop)	Ca	??	Ca	??	+			
Calbindin 28kD	Ca*	O	Ca*		+			
(six domains)	Ca*		Ca*	O				
Parvalbumin		O	Ca	Ca	+	+		+
Oncomodulin		O	Ca	Ca	+			
ICBP 9kD	Ca'	Ca			+	+		+
S-100	Ca'	Ca			+			
CF antigen	Ca'	Ca				+		
2A9	Ca'*	Ca*				+		
p10	Ca'*	Ca*				+		

Domains are numbered 1, 2, 3, and 4, based on an interpretation of gene duplication and reduplication. Parvalbumin and oncomodulin have lost domain 1; ICBP 9kD and its near relatives are inferred to have lost domains 3 and 4. Calbindin (Hunziker 1986) is inferred to have evolved from an eight-domain precursor with domains 4 and 6 being deleted. In the heavy (Emori et al. 1986b) and light (Emori et al. 1986a) chains of calpain four domains are spliced to the carboxyl terminus of another region. Ca indicates that domain binds calcium based on crystallographic or binding studies; Ca* implies calcium binding based primarily on amino acid sequence; Ca' implies an ICBP-1-type domain; O implies loss of calcium binding. Amino acid sequences were determined directly (seq) or from cDNA or genomic, gDNA sequences. 3D means that the crystal structure is available. More recent references are: cal-1 from *C. elegans* (Salvato et al. 1986), CM1 expressed calmodulin pseudogene from chick (Stein et al. 1983), Spec 1 (Hardin et al. 1985), calcineurin (Aitken et al. 1984), CDC31 (Baum et al. 1986), troponin C (TNC) from *H. roretzi* (Takagi and Konishi 1983), essential light chain of myosin (Collins et al. 1986), aequorin (Charbonneau et al. 1985), calcium vector protein from *Amphioxus* (Kobayashi et al. 1987), SCBP from *Amphioxus* (Takagi et al. 1986), cystic fibrosis (CF) antigen (Dorin et al. 1987), 2A9 (Calabretta et al. 1986), p10 (Gerke and Weber 1985; Glenney and Tack 1985). Similar abbeviations are used in Tables 2–6.

Table 2. Sequences of Intestinal Calcium-binding Protein (9kD) Domain 1 and Homologs

		2 2 2 2 2 2 2	
	1 2 3 4 5 6 7 8 9	2 3 4 5 6 7 8 9	

	-8 -5 -3 0 $+5$
Common	* n * * n F * * n * * * E G D * * * L * K * E L K * L n * * E
	X Y Z $-$Y $-$Z
	=O =O =O =O
ICBP 9kD	E E L K G I F E K Y A A K E G D P N Q L S K E E L K L L L Q T E F
	A S Q I A
S-100α	E T L I N V F H A H S G K E G D K Y K L S K K E L K E L L Q T E L
S-100β	V A L I D V F H Q Y S G R E G D K H K L K K S E L K E L I N N E L
CF Ag	N S I I D V Y H K Y S L I K G N F H A V Y R D D L K K L L E T E C
2A9	G L L V A I F H K Y S G R E G D K H T L S K K E L K E L I Q K E L
P10	E T M M F T F H K F A – – – G D K G Y L T K E D L R V L M E K E F

ICBP domain 1 is two residues longer than the canonical EF-hand. Positions in helix E, 1–9, and in helix F, 22–29 are numbered as in the canonical EF-hand. Positions within the calcium-binding loop are numbered relative to the residue coordination calcium at vertex $-$Y. =O indicates coordination with the carbonyl oxygen atom of the main chain.

Table 3. Helices E and F of Calmodulin Homologs

Position markers (helix E and helix F):
Block 1: `E n * * n n * * n X Y Z̄ Y X Z n * * n`
Block 2 (right of number): `E n * * n n * * n X Y Z̄ Y X Z n * * n n * * n`

Domains		Seq 1	Seq 2	N	Seq 3	Seq 4
CaM	1 and 2	EFKEAFSLFD A	ELGTVMRSL	7	ELQDMINEVD VG	EFLTMMARK SL K N
	3 and 4	EIREAFRVFD LI K	ELRHVMTNL I SI	7	EVDEMIREAD K V	EFVQMMTAK KV MSR T IEG R V A
TNC	1 and 2	EFKAAFDMFD	ELGTVMRML	7	ELDAIIEEVD	EFLVMMVRQ
	3 and 4	ELAECFRIFD SDL M	ELAEIFRAS KIMLQST G	7	EIESLMKDGD D EI D	EFLKMMEGV ET K
Parv	3 and 4	DVKKAFAIID ELAEV GAL TAEAI HVA QI L KF D E Y	ELKLFLQNF GFV KG ENI IS C A V	10	ETKTFLKAGD EALMADA SN A	EFTALVKA- WSNMASGS ET IDET VK HKA GS MW Q K
cal-1	1 and 2	EFREAFMMFD	ELGIAMRSL	7	EILEMINEVD	EFCVMMKRM
	3 and 4	MIREAFRVFD	EFRYFMVHM	7	EVDEMIKEVD	EFVKMMSNQ
CM1	1 and 2	EFKEAFSLFD	ELGTVMRSL	7	ELQDMVGEVD	EFLSLMARK
	3 and 4	EIREAFRVFD	ELRHVMTNL	7	EVDEMIKEAD	EFVRMMTEK
Spec	1 and 2	EFKRRFKNKD	ELGEFFKST	7	QIDKMISDVD	EMLMGIAEQ
	3 and 4	HYTKAFDDMD	ELEALSAS	7	KIKAIIQKAD	EFMKLIKSC
CN	1 and 2	KLRFAFRIYD	ELFQVLKMM	12	IVDKTIINAD	EFSAVVGGL
	3 and 4	EILRAFKVFD	EFKFIMQKV	8	EVEEAMKEAD	EFMDLIKSK
Vect	3 and 4	WGDALFDIVD	EWKAYTKAA	7	DCEETFRVCD	EMTRQHLGF
Aeq	3 and 4	QVKDIFRFID	ELKYFLQKF	10	ETKSLMDAAD	EFQEMVHS -
Onc	3 and 4	VKYIVRYMYD	DFECLVARV	23	LWNEIAELAD	EFKQAVQKN
SCBPsh	1 and 2	QKDTFDFFLD	DFEEMIKRY	22	EWRDLKGRAD	EYLAMWEKT
SCBPAm1 and 2		SCRSMVNLMD	EFNILWNRI	1	NYLAIFRKFD	EMRMAIESA)
(CalpH[1 and 2]		T KI DML	YV TK		K QK Y EI	E KL ESA)
(CalpL[1 and 2]		TCRSMVAVMD	EFKYLWNNI	1	KWQAIYKQFD	ELPGAFEAA)

The first sequence indicated for calmodulin is from mammal; all known variants are listed beneath without species designation. The first sequence listed for troponin C is from rabbit skeletal muscle; other variants from cardiac, domains 3 and 4 only, are listed below. The first sequence listed for parvalbumin is from carp, isotype pI 4.25; others listed below. Other sequences are indicated only if the domain is a member of a pair in which both are inferred to bind calcium and in which neither appears to have suffered a deletion or insertion. The dashed line indicates that tertiary structures of the lower molecules are not known. The number between domain 1 (or 3) and 2 (or 4) indicates the number of intervening amino acids.

Table 4. Calcium-binding Loops of Calmodulin Homologs

	1					2														
	X	Y	Z	−X	−Z	X	Y	Z	−X	−Z	X	Y	Z	−X	−Z	X	Y	Z	−X	−Z
CaM	D	D	NG	IT	E	D	D	NG	ID	PE	D	D	NG	IS	E	D	D	DG	VN	E
		D					D					D		T		N		I		
cal-1	D	D	NG	IS	E	D	D	NG	IE	E	D	D	NG	IT	E	D	D	DG	ID	E
CM1	D	D	DG	IT	E	D	D	SG	ID	PE	D	D	NG	IS	E	D	N	DG	VN	E
Spec1	(D	D	SK	IT	E	D	D	SG	ID	E	D	D	NG	LRP	E	D	N	DG	ID	E)
CN	D	D	SG	LS	E	D	D	NG	VD	E	D	D	DG	IS	E	D	D	DG	IS	E
CDC31	(D	N	DG	LD	E											D	D	DG	IN	E)
TNC sk	D	D	GG	IS	E	D	D	SG	ID	E	D	N	DG	ID	PE	D	N	DG	ID	E
cd									V											
TNC HR						D	D	SG	ID	E						D	N	DS	ID	E
Calp H	(D	D	NG	LG	E	D	D	SG	MS	E)										
		T							N											
Calp L	(D	D	TG	LG	E	D	D	SG	IC	E)										
Aeq	D	N	NG	IS	E						D	D	NG	IT	E	D	D	SG	LD	E
RLC	D	N	DG	ID	D															
		D		VS																
				N																
CaVP											(D	N	DG	ID	E	D	D	NG	ID	PE)
SCBP sh	D	D	DG	LD	D	D	N	DG	VT	E	D	D	DG	VG	E					
SCBP Am	D	N	DG	IQ	D	D	N	DD	VS	E	D	S	DG	VD	E					
SCBP sw	D	D	DG	IT	D						D	N	DN	IS	E	D	N	DG	LS	E
SCBP sc	D	N	DG	IS	N						D	D	DR	ID	E					
CALB 28	(D	D	NG	MD	E						D	D	SG	ID	E					
	D	N	DG	LE	E						D	D	NG	ID	E)					
Parv											D	D	SG	IE	E	D	D	DG	IG	E
											E	D		V					D	
																			H	
Onco											D	D	SG	LD	E	D	D	DG	IG	E
ICBP 9kD						D	N	DG	VS	E										
						D	N													
S-100 α						D	D	DG	VD	E										
β									C											
2A9						(D	N	DG	VN	E)										
CF Ag						(D	N	DG	VN	E)										
p10						(D	C	DG	VG	S)										

The amino acid sequences, and variants, for all domains that (are inferred to) bind calcium are listed for positions 10(X), 12(Y), 14(Z), 15, 17, 18(−X), and 21(−Z). Occurrences of Pro at positions 19 and 20 are also indicated.

In the following sections, I will examine in detail variations on this basic theme in light of recently published sequence and structural information. In general, only those amino acid or DNA sequences published during the past year are referenced; previous sequences are available in the Los Alamos data bank.

Loss of Calcium Binding

There are numerous examples of loops having lost the ability to coordinate calcium either by change of residue, deletion, or insertion. Loss of calcium coordination by point mutation is inferred to have occurred in domain 3 of the alkaline light chain of myosin and domain 4 of sarcoplasm calcium-binding protein (SCBP) of shrimp. Loss by deletion is exemplified by domain 2 of parvalbumin or domain 2 SCBP of scallop. Insertions are seen in domain 2 of alkaline light chain.

The inability to bind calcium does not reduce the functional significance of that domain to its protein. However, it does appear that this is a departure from the dominant evolutionary theme. Such domains will not be included in this evaluation. As indicated in Table 1, the ability to bind calcium is often inferred from the amino acid sequence. Admittedly, the argument here is cyclic and could easily lead one to overlook new variations, such as the first domain of the 9-kD intestinal calcium-binding protein (ICBP 9kD) (Szebenyi and Moffat 1986).

Loss of Helices

In several instances, alignment of sequences by homology indicates the loss of all or part of either helix E or helix F, for instance, as seen in domain 3 of the essential light chain. One would be reluctant to speculate as to its tertiary structure; its recognition as a homolog was aided by its association with other domains more easily recognized as EF-hands. One cannot say what effect such a loss would have on a seemingly canonical calcium-binding loop.

Domain Pairing

Turning to the association of individual domains with other EF-hands or with other types of domains or with other proteins, we again see a standard motif and variations. As seen in calmodulin, troponin C, parvalbumin, and ICBP 9kD, pairs of domains fit together with the inner aspects of their four helices and the Ilu, Leu, or Val at position 17 to form a hydrophobic core somewhat exposed to the solvent on the side opposite from the two calcium ions. In calmodulin and troponin C, these partially exposed surfaces probably interact with their target proteins.

In parvalbumin, the AB domain, now called domain 2 since the first domain is inferred to have been deleted, is unpaired. Its hydrophobic aspect covers the otherwise exposed hydrophobic region of the 3,4 pair.

In the monomeric aequorin there are three EF-hand domains and an intervening fourth region of probably different evolutionary origin. The hydrophobic surface of the third EF-hand may interact with a complementary hydrophobic region on the inferred catalytic domain.

The 28-kD calcium-binding protein from chicken is now called calbindin. It consists of six domains, called I, Ia, II, III, IV, and IVa by Hunziker (1986); none resemble the unique first domain of ICBP 9kD. From our preliminary analysis we infer that domains I, II, III, and IV more closely resemble the 1 and 3 type, whereas Ia and IVa resemble 2 and 4. We cannot infer their pairing or lack thereof.

Consistent with the original prediction, all of the homologs listed in Table 1 are found in the cytosol. None have been identified in prokaryotes. Although we refer to them as calcium modulated, functions are known for only ten. Calmodulin, calcineurin, skeletal and cardiac troponin C, and the regulatory light chain activate their associated enzyme or structural protein upon binding calcium. The alkali or essential light chain is required for myosin function, although none of its four domains still bind calcium. The three calcium-binding domains of aequorin and four of both heavy and light chains of calpain impart calcium activation to the catalytic domains to which they are fused. Parvalbumins have been suggested to function as a capacitor or temporal buffer (Gillis et al. 1982) and ICBP 9kD to facilitate transport of calcium (Kretsinger et al. 1982). The remaining 14 homologs have not been demonstrated to be involved in the function of calcium as a cytosolic messenger.

Gene Splicing

EF-hands have been observed in multiples of 2, 3, 4, and 6 in monomeric proteins that have evolved by duplication(s) of a single precursor domain. This interpretation is reinforced by the closer similarity of domains 1–3 and of domains 2–4 (Baba et al. 1984). This precursor four-domain molecule, presumably resembling today's calmodulins, existed in the precursor of protocists, fungi, animals, and plants. In at least three instances—aequorin, heavy and light chains of calpain—a protein has obviously evolved by fusion of several EF-hands with catalytic domains of other evolu-

tionary origin. The full EF-hand is found in these cases. However, when evaluating possible homologs, one should appreciate that only portions of domains might be found in the fusion protein. Perhaps relevant, introns in this superfamily seem distributed throughout the domain and are not clustered in interdomain regions (P. Maisonpierre and C. Emerson, in prep.).

Intestinal Calcium-binding Protein Variation

Domain 1 of ICBP 9kD (ICBP-1) differs significantly from the canonical EF-hand. As Szebenyi and Moffat (1986) discuss in detail, the loop about the calcium ion is two residues longer but follows the same general course. They introduce a valuable notation. The ligand at the −Y vertex, a carbonyl oxygen in both canonical and ICBP-1 domains, is numbered 0 and the glu at −Z is +5 in both types of domains. X, Y, and Z in the ICBP-1 domains are numbered −8, −5, and −3 (Table 2). Certainly the α and β subunits of S-100 bind calcium in ICBP-1-type loops as do probably the cystic fibrosis antigen (Dorin et al. 1987) and the A29 gene product (Calabretta et al. 1986). The light chain of calpactin, or p10, may not bind two equivalents of calcium, at least when not complexed with the heavy chain. The second of its two domains appears to be canonical; however, the first shows general similarity to the ICBP-1 domain but has suffered a three-amino-acid deletion (Gerke and Weber 1985; Glenney and Tack 1985). With these recently available sequences, one can refine the consensus proposed by Szebenyi and Moffat (1986) as shown in Table 2. The "n**nn**n" pattern is retained in helix E; however, position 1 is variable, Glu is not preferred. The second helix (F) changes from the "n**nn**n" pattern to "LK*Ln**E." Why the exposed Lys is conserved is not obvious, nor are the conservations of the Leus as the unique hydrophobics. The terminal Glu is exposed to the solvent. Often this position is exposed as well in the canonical EF-hand.

In the calcium-binding loop, Glu is consistently found at Y and Asp at Z, even though both coordinate with carbonyl oxygens. Glu at −Z is the only residue to coordinate with its side chain. The side chain of Leu at +1 contributes to the core of the molecule, in an analogous function but different position to the "Ilu" of the canonical hand. Why Lys is conserved at +3 is not obvious. CFAg appears to have diverged earliest from this branch and has Lys at Y, Asn at Z, Asp at −Z, Val at +1, and Arg at +3. All sequences, including p10, conserve Gly at −1. If one searches a new sequence for EF-hands, one should include an ICBP-1 probe.

Canonical Helices

Even a cursory examination of all of the amino acid sequences of all of the domains of all of the isotypes of all 27 families convinces one of their wide variability. Many individual domains would not appear to be related to another given member. Yet nearly all have been recognized by the

"En**nn**nD*D*DG*ID**En**nn**n"

search pattern. Given the large data base of several hundred domains, one can suggest more discriminating consensuses. Very frequently a search of the entire data base reveals one of the stronger alignments being with a calmodulin domain. This probably reflects the fact that calmodulin has changed little over time. Furthermore, we will assume that it reflects a precursor in which there were two paired canonical domains, both of which bind calcium. Table 3 lists the sequence variations of helices E and F for calmodulin, troponin C, and parvalbumin, the three for which crystal structures are available. The ICBP 9kD variant has been treated separately. The others are inferred to have at least one pair near isostructural with these three. Domains 1 and 2 of both heavy and light chains of calpain are enclosed in parentheses because there is only one residue between the last residue of domain 1 (1–29) and the first of domain 2 (2–1). The same close spacing obtains between domains 3 and 4, which are inferred not to bind calcium. Most canonical pairs, 1 and 2 or 3 and 4, of domains are separated by seven to ten residues.

One can infer from Table 3 a more accurate, but also more cumbersome, test sequence for helices E and F of domains 1 and 3 and with slight variation of domains 2 and 4. After an evaluation of the calcium-binding loops (Table 4), the summary consensus is presented in Table 5.

Calcium-binding Loops

The essential features of the normal calcium-binding loops can be evaluated from the precedents summarized in Table 4. Parentheses enclose sequences whose structures and calcium affinities are not well established. More weight is given to those of known crystal structure. Register is maintained; there are no insertions or deletions. There seems to be little systematic variation between domains 1 and 3 and domains 2 and 4 or between loops in canonical domains whose mate is missing or aberrant. When considered one residue at a time, the consensus of Table 5, very similar to that proposed by Szebenyi and Moffat (1986), seems the most reasonable revision of that originally proposed by Tufty and Kretsinger (1975). Asp is invariant at vertex X. Asp or Asn are found at Y. Calcium binding has not been established for protein p10, which has Cys at Y. The Z ligand is variable with Asp, Asn, Ser, or Thr present. Note that Ser and Thr have one carbon between the main-chain α-carbon and the oxygen atom; Asp and Asn have two; Glu and Gln three. In most parvalbumins, domain 3, Ser reaches the Ca^{++} ion without an intervening water. In troponin C, domain 1, Gly is found at Z. In the crystal structure, domains 1 and 2 are apo; water is inferred to be the Z ligand in $TNC*Ca_4$. The −Y ligand is the main-chain carbonyl oxygen; the side chain is highly variable. The −X ligand is the most variable with several examples of all

six residues. The distance from the main chain accommodates the two carbons of Glu as seen in parvalbumin. In TNC domains 3 and 4, calcium is coordinated by water, which in turn is hydrogen bonded to Asp. Correspondingly, in ICBP 9kD, domain 2, water bridges Ser to calcium. Our crystallographic studies of calmodulin (Kretsinger et al. 1986), whose refinement is not yet complete, indicate a similar water coordination at the four −X vertices. When Gly is at −X as in parvalbumin, domain 4, water coordinates calcium but is not part of a defined bridge. At −Z one finds Glu in the four proteins of known crystal structure, but in domain I of the regulatory light chain and the four SCBPs, there is Asp or Asn. In the light chain of calpain the Cys may hydrogen bond to a water that in turn coordinates calcium. A similar situation may obtain for the Cys at +X, domain 2 of p10.

The Gly following the Z ligand permits a sharp turn ($\phi = 90°$, $\psi = 0°$) not available to other amino acids. Four possible exceptions occur: Lys in domain 1 of Spec1, Asp in 2 of SCBP of *Amphioxus*, Asn in 3 of SCBP sandworm and Arg of SCBP scallop, and fourth, Ser in 4 of TNC *Halocynthia*. Calcium binding in these domains is probable but not established. Three interesting exceptions occur in parvalbumins, assumed very similar in tertiary structure to that of carp; Asp in 3 of hake isotype pI 4.36 and His in 4 of ray 4.45 and Asp in 4 of *Coelocanth* 5.40.

At the position preceding −X there is always a hydrophobic residue, usually Ilu, Val, or Leu; Met is seen twice. Possibly of functional significance, Cys is at −X in domain II of the β subunit of S100.

The remaining four positions in the loop appear to be highly variable; however, an evaluation of pairs of positions or triplets may reveal additional correlations. Several of the (inferred) calcium-binding loops contain Pro at positions 19 and 20; as will be discussed, ϕ values are near the −60° obliged for Pro.

Various authors, perhaps most thoroughly Reid (1985), have searched for correlations between calcium affinity and carboxylate number or relative disposition. Given our available data, I find no such correlation.

As evaluated in detail by Herzberg and James (1985), residues 10(X), 11, 12(Y), and 13 form a type I β bend, and residues 18(−X), 19, 20, and 21(−Z) form a type III β bend. They evaluated crystal structures of parvalbumin, ICBP, and troponin C. We see no exceptions to their summary in calmodulin. The ϕ and ψ angles that characterize these bends at residues 11 and 12 and at residues 19 and 20 are listed in Table 5. Furthermore, there are consistently seen four Asx turns in which the amine nitrogen of residue n + 2 forms a hydrogen bond with the side-chain oxygen of Asp, Asn, Ser, or Thr at residue n. These are of type 3 (12[Y] to 10[X], and 20 to 18[−X]), type 3′ (14[Z] to 12[Y]), and type 1′ (16[−Y] to 14[Z]), see Table 5 for ϕ, ψ values. Only Gly (15) can assume $\phi = 90$, $\psi = 0$ for an Asx 1′ type loop. Gly is often found at position 13, $\phi = 60°$, $\psi = 30°$, but with small change in angle other

Table 5. Consensus Summary for EF-hand Domains: ICBP, 1 and 3 and 2 and 4

```
ICBP   *  n  *  *  n  F  *  *  *  n  *  *  *  E  G  D  *  *  *  E  L  K  *  L  n  *  *  E
                      -8                                             +5
                      =O                -5    -3        0
                                        =O    =O        =O
               1  2  3  4  5  6  7  8  9
                      X              Y     Z        -Y        -X           -Z


1 and 3  E  n  *  *  n  F  *  n  n  D  *  D  G  *  I  G  *  E  L  *  *  *  n  n  *  *  *  *
                            A           D  N     L  S                            2 2 2 2 2 2 2 2
                               F        N  S     V  T                            2 3 4 5 6 7 8 9
                                        S        D                               2 2
                                                 N                               2 9
                                                 E


2 and 4  E  n  *  *  n  n  *  *  *  *  F  *  *  n  n  *  *  *  *


         ///3\\\///3\\\///1'\\\              ///3\\\
         X  *  Y  *  Z  *  -Y               -X  *  *   -Z
         D (P) D (G) D  G                    D (P)(P)  E
         !- - - -I- - - -!                   !- - -III- - -!

   φ    -60  -90   60   90                  -60  -60
   ψ    -30   -0   30    0                  -30  -30
```

ICBP refers to the first domain of the 9-kD intestinal calcium-binding protein. There are 29 residues in the canonical calcium-binding domain. The ICBP-type domain is two residues longer. Residues that coordinate calcium are referred to the vertices of an octahedron in linear sequence: X, Y, Z, -Y, -X, -Z. Within the calcium-binding loop, residues can be counted from -Y at zero which in both domains coordinates calcium with carbonyl oxygen as indicated by =O. Asterisks refer to highly variable positions, n to the hydrophobic residues, Val, Leu, Ilu, Met, and Phe. The calcium-binding loop is expanded in the lower portion of the table. In Asx turns of types 3, 3', and 1', indicated by ///\\\, the main-chain nitrogen of residue $n + 2$ forms a hydrogen bond to the side-chain oxygen of Asx or Ser. In β bends of types I and III, indicated by !------!, the main-chain nitrogen of residue $n + 3$ forms a hydrogen bond with the carbonyl oxygen of residue n. φ and ψ values are listed beneath the residues involved in these bends. At position -Y - 1 the values 0, -90 are accessible to only Gly. At -Y - 3 Gly is often found; however, only an acceptably small change in φ, ψ accommodates other residues. Pro, whose φ value is fixed at -60 is often found at positions -Y + 3 and -Y + 4.

residues can assume this conformation, as seen in the left-hand α helix. At positions 11, 19, and 20, ϕ is $-60°$. There are several examples of Pro occurring at position 19, where it would not interfere with the hydrogen bond of the Asx. The Pro in calmodulin domain 2, position 20 does not significantly change the course of the loop, but cannot donate a hydrogen bond.

An interesting observation concerns the course of the main chain around the calcium. If the first ligand defines the X and the second the Y vertex, and if one recognizes that adjacent ligands do not span the diameter, $+X$ to $-X$, then there are only ten traces about the four remaining vertices: Z, $-X$, $-Y$, $-Z$; Z, $-X$, $-Z$, $-Y$; Z, $-Y$, $-X$, $-Z$; Z, $-Y$, $-Z$, $-X$; $-Z$, $-X$, $-Y$, Z; $-Z$, $-X$, Z, $-Y$; $-Z$, $-Y$, $-X$, Z; $-Z$, $-Y$, Z, $-X$; $-X$, Z, $-Y$, $-Z$; and $-X$, $-Z$, $-Y$, Z. The twelve EF-hands of known crystal structures all observe X, Y, Z, $-Y$, $-X$, $-Z$; one might suspect a putative homolog having a different course.

The two β-bends and four Asx turns plus the constraints of six calcium ligands and one residue contributing to the hydrophobic core seem to necessitate this X, Y, Z, $-Y$, $-X$, $-Z$ trace. However, the necessity of these bends and turns is contradicted by the existence of calcium-binding proteins having quite different conformations. The counterargument that the important point is the difference between the apo and the calcium form has not been resolved by knowing the structure of troponin C, which in that crystal form has domains 1 and 2 apo (Herzberg and James 1985; Sundaralingam et al. 1985).

Consensus Domains

In Table 5, I summarize the conclusions from an examination of the data in Tables 2, 3, and 4. Inevitably this process resembles a self-fulfilling prophecy in that one tends to find what one looks for. Even so, given the past success of En**nn, etc., the results of Table 5 should provide more discriminating references in three senses. First, the 1 and 3 and 2 and 4 consensuses are weighted toward domains that (probably) bind calcium. As noted, there are many domains, equally loved by Nature, that do not bind calcium. A computerized search of the data base of individual sequences for similarities to a putative domain will frequently show higher overall scores to non-EF-hands than to identified homologs. These consensus sequences provide a filter or weighting scheme to evaluate such results. Second, numerous homologs that do not bind calcium have been identified. Attention to the characteristics of the loop should help determine whether they do bind calcium. Unfortunately, we have not found correlates of affinity. Third, the major variant, the ICBP-1 domain, differs significantly from the EF-hand domain. Possible homologs should be identified when evaluated relative to the unique characteristics of the ICBP-hand.

Obviously, an uncritical application of these consensuses can lead one to overlook new conformations. Their use is hardly a substitute for experimental results.

Linker Connecting Domains 2 and 3

Many aspects of the structures of troponin C and calmodulin had been anticipated (Kretsinger and Barry 1975) based on the homology of troponin C and parvalbumin (Collins et al. 1973). Both the 1,2 and 3,4 pairs of domains were correctly predicted to have exposed hydrophobic surfaces on the sides opposite the two calcium-binding sites. The linker connecting helix F2 to helix E3 would supposedly bend to permit apposition of the two hydrophobic surfaces. Aitken et al. (1984) calculated the helix-forming tendency of the linker region of calmodulin and of calcineurin using the Chou and Fasman algorithm, as did Sundaralingam et al. (1985) for troponin C, and as did Kobayashi et al. (1987) for calmodulin, TNC, and the calcium vector protein. For all four proteins a nonhelical region was predicted in the middle of the linker. Certainly the greatest surprise to come from the crystal structures of troponin C (Herzberg and James 1985; Sundaralingam et al. 1985) and of calmodulin (Babu et al. 1985; Kretsinger et al. 1986) was the extended helix comprising helix F2, linker, and helix E3, quite straight for seven turns in calmodulin, slightly bent in the middle of eight turns in troponin C. In Table 6 are listed the amino acid sequences of the linkers between domains 2 and 3 of proteins in which both domains 2 and 3 are anticipated to be competent to bind calcium. Since our ability to predict helices has already been found wanting, one would be reluctant to speculate on the helicity of the $2 \rightarrow 3$ linker in other homologs. This seems a highly variable region with little similarity between one family and another. The linkers of the heavy and the light chains of calpain are only six residues long, that of calmodulin eight, and that of the SCBP of *Amphioxus* sixteen. Most of the linkers are rich in hydrophilic groups and have a net negative charge. Calmodulin has four Glus or Asps and one Lys; however, shrimp SCBP has three Lys and no Glu or Asp. In contrast, the linker of CDC31 of yeast has three of eight and that of Spec1 has four of nine hydrophobic residues. Five of the listed linkers have Pro and hence cannot be unbent helices. At this time, one must reserve judgment as to the generality of precedent of a helical linker provided by troponin C and by calmodulin. In any case, the helix may well be bent when, or if, the calcium-modulated protein is coupled to a target; part of the target specificity may reside in this bend.

CALCIUM-BINDING PROTEINS LACKING EF-HANDS

At least five extracellular proteins of known crystal structure bind calcium, as recently summarized by Szebenyi and Moffat (1986). None of these five (trypsin, thermolysin, concanavalin A, phospholipase A, or *Staphylococcus* nuclease) are homologous to one another or to the 27 EF-hand homologs of Table 1 or to the eight analogs to be discussed, see Table 7. Most of the coordinating amino acids come from a stretch of 20

Table 6. Linker (2→3) of Calmodulin and Homologs

	En n n n		En n n nD
	-Z		X
Calp H	E M R M A I E S A	G F K L N K	K L Y E L I I T R Y
Calp L	E L P G A F E A A	G F H L N E	H L Y N M I I R R Y
CaVP	E W L T L C S K W	V R Q D D E E	E I L R A F K V F D
cal-1	E F C V M M K R M	M K E T D S E	M I R E A N F V F D
CaM	E F L T M M A R K	M K D T D S E E	E I R E A F R V F D
CM1	E F L S L M A R K	M R D S D S E E	E I R E A F R V F D
CN	E F I E G V S Q F	S V K G D K E Q	K L R F A F R I Y D
CDC31	D F Y I V M G E K	I L K R D P L D	E I K R A F Q L F D
RLC	V F L T M F G E K	L K G A D P E D	V I T G A F K V L D
	M S I S D S	S T T E	T L R N A M F
Spec1	E M L M G I A E Q	M V K W T W K E E	H Y T K A F D D M D
ELC	Q F L P M L Q A I	S N N K D Q G T Y E	D F V E G L R V F D
TNC sk	E F L V M M V R Q	M K E D A K G K S E E	E L A D C F R I F D
cd	C	D S	S L M
TNC Hr	E F C L M M T R Q	M Q A Q E E A K I P E R E E K	E L S E A F R L F D
SCBP sh	E F K Q A V Q K N	C K G K A F A N F P N A F K V	F I G N Q F K T I D
SCBP Am	E Y L A M W E K T	I A T C K S V A D L P A W C Q N	R I P F L F K G M D

amino acids. However, thermolysin uses two aspartate carboxylates separated by 51 residues. The number of carboxylates ranges from one to four with little correlation with calcium affinity. Nature has many ways of wrapping a protein around a Ca^{++} ion.

DOMAINS RESEMBLING THE CALMODULIN FOLD

We have described a score of proteins judged to be homologs of calmodulin and five other calcium-binding proteins that appear quite unrelated, to one another or to this superfamily. Proteins have many oxygen atoms and can obviously employ a variety of conformations to point five to seven oxygen atoms at a 0.99-Å radius sphere. Yet if it is so easy to coordinate calcium, why has the EF-hand been retained and modified so many

times in the course of evolution? Hopefully an evaluation of several closer analogs will provide an answer or, better yet, pose a more insightful question.

Lysozyme

In (1975) Tufty and Kretsinger scanned the then-meager data base of protein sequences and found a bimodal distribution of alignment scores. The vast majority of sequences that were not homologous to the EF-hand showed a Poisson distribution of alignment scores. The parvalbumin and troponin C that were used to construct the test as well as the essential light chain of myosin scored with high significance. The next highest score came from T4 lysozyme residues 42–70 (Table 7). The initial results of the crystal structure determination of T4 lysozyme were just available (Matthews

Table 7. Amino Acid Sequences of Proteins with Domains Resembling the Calmodulin Fold

				1 1 1 1 1 1 1 1 1 1 2 2 2 2 2 2 2 2 2 2
				1 2 3 4 5 6 7 8 9 0 1 2 3 4 5 6 7 8 9 0 1 2 3 4 5 6 7 8 9
				X Y Z −Y−X −Z
Protein	Ca	Location	3-D Structure	E n * * n n * * n D * D * D G * I D * * E n * * n n * * n
T4 Lysozyme	no	extracellular	helix-loop-helix	A K S E L D K A I G R N C N G V I T K D E A E K L F N Q D
				42 70
α-Lactalbumin	yes	extracellular	helix-loop-helix	N I C D I S C D K F L D D D I T D D I M C A K K I L D I K
				61 89
Galactose-binding protein	yes	bacteria membrane	"helix"-loop-β-strand	K H W A A N Q G W D L N K D G Q I Q F V L L K G E P G H P
				121 153
Uteroglobin	no	extracellular	helix-loop-helix	S Y E T S L K E F E P D D T M K D A G M Q M K K V L D S L
				20 48
Sodium channel rat I	?	transmembrane		M F Y E V W E L F D P D A T Q F I E F C K L S D F A A A L
				1797 1825
rat II				M F Y E V W E K F D P D A T Q F M E F E K L S Q F A A A L
				1807 1835,
Electrophorus				R I H C L D I L F A F T K R V L G E S G E M D A L R I Q M
				1861 1889
Osteonectin	yes	extracellular matrix		C T T R F F E T C D L D N D K Y I A L E E W A G C F G I K
				264 292
Thrombospondin	yes	extracellular		N G E G D A C A A D I D G D G I L N E R D N C Q Y V Y N V
				773 801
Protein kinase C	?	cytosol		G E Y Y N V P I P E G D E E G N V E L R Q K F E K A K L G
				283 311

References: T4 Lysozyme (Tufty and Kretsinger 1975); α-Lactalbumin (Stuart et al. 1986); Galactose binding (Vyas et al. 1987); Uteroglobin (Baker 1985); Sodium channel (Babitch and Anthony 1987); Osteonectin (Engel et al. 1987); Thrombospondin (Lawler and Hynes 1986); Protein kinase C (Parker et al. 1986).

and Remington 1974). We noted, "It may be simply a thermodynamically preferred conformation which has been arrived at by an alternate evolutionary route." As we learned of the refinement of the structure (final description) we added "in proof" that, "The revised lysozyme loop fits less well to the EF-hand than does the structure used in their original publications. This revision seems to strengthen the interpretation of convergent evolution and to weaken the prediction of calcium binding and homology."

α-Lactalbumin

Weaver et al. (1985) compared the primary and tertiary structures of goose, chicken, and phage lysozymes and concluded, "that all three classes of lysozyme diverged from a common evolutionary precursor, even though their amino acid sequences appear to be unrelated." The loop of T4 lysozyme, 51–62, was aligned with a loop 77–90 of hen egg-white lysozyme (HEWL) two residues longer. In turn, α-lactalbumin has long been known to be homologous to c-type lysozymes, such as found in the chicken egg white (Brew et al. 1967; Qasba and Safaya 1984). The 77–90 loop of HEWL aligns with residues 74–87 of human (or baboon) α-lactalbumin. Stuart et al. (1986) recently completed the crystal structure refinement of baboon α-lactalbumin and found "...a Ca^{++}-binding fold that resembles an EF hand only superficially and presumably has no evolutionary relationship with it." Calcium is coordinated by carboxylate groups of Asp-82, Asp-87, and Asp-88, and by carbonyl oxygens of Lys-79 and Asp-84; two water molecules complete a pentagonal bipyramide. Ile-85 (similar to Ile EF-17) appears to stabilize the loop and form part of the hydrophobic core of α-lactalbumin. Stuart et al. convincingly argue that this calcium-binding ability is a recent acquisition and represents convergent evolution.

Galactose-binding Protein

Vyas et al. (1987) and Quiocho et al. (this volume) recently determined the crystal structure of the periplasmic D-galactose-binding protein of *Escherichia coli*. A Ca^{++} ion is coordinated by five ligands from every second residue of a nine-residue loop, 134–142 (see Fig. 6 Quiocho et al., this volume). The carboxylate group of Glu-205 coordinates calcium with two oxygen atoms. The galactose-binding site is 45 Å from the calcium-binding site. The main-chain coordinates of the nine residues, 134–142, plus those from residues 204 and 205, superimpose on the EF-loop of parvalbumin (domain 4, 10–18 and 20–21) with rms deviation of 0.60 Å. The Gly analogous to domain 4, residue 15 "adopts a main-chain conformation ($\phi = 70°$, $\psi = 5°$) that assures that the chain direction changes appropriately to allow the peptide carbonyl oxygen of the residue in 4–16 "to coordinate the calcium." Compare this to the $\phi = 90°$, $\psi = 0°$ listed in Table 5. Ilu-141 (analogous to EF-17) contributes its side chain to a hydropho-

bic region. The residues immediately preceding residue 134 form a β bend; however, they extend the immediately preceding helix in such a way that the general direction of the preceding "helix" as designated in Table 7 is similar to helix E of the EF-hand. Similarly, the direction of the following extended strand points in a direction similar to that assumed by helix F.

Uteroglobin

Uteroglobin is found in uterine fluid. It is a homodimer; each monomer is 70 amino acids long. Baker (1985) found that it shows some similarity to the essential light chain of myosin with a comparison score of 7.2 standard deviations ($P \sim 10^{-12}$) but cautioned "these analyses do not determine whether these proteins are derived from a common ancestor or whether the similarities...are the result of convergent evolution." They note that the loop region lacks Gly-15 and Ilu-17 and would not be expected to bind calcium. In the crystal structure (Morize et al. 1987) refined with data measured to 1.3 Å resolution, there is quite clearly an α helix from residues 18–27 (analogous to EF-hand $2 \rightarrow 8$) and from 32–47 (EF $13 \rightarrow 28$) but definitely no Ca^{++} ion. These two helices are nearly parallel, as opposed to being perpendicular as found in the EF-hand.

Sodium Channel

The amino acid sequences of the sodium channel proteins from rat brain (I and II) and from *Electrophorus electricus* were deduced by Noda et al. (1986) from their cDNA sequences. They suggested four transmembrane helices with the carboxyl terminus in the cytosol. Babitch and Anthony (1987) identified near the carboxyl terminus several sites that resemble EF-hands (Table 7). They reviewed the literature on the possible calcium modulation and concluded that "the possibility that sodium channel proteins may bind calcium at an internal site appears to remain an open question, though they clearly bind Ca^{++} at an external site." In all three proteins (rat I and II and eel) there are two putative EF-hand domains. The amino terminus of the second is 26 residues from the carboxyl terminus of the first; whether the domains interact is not known. In each protein the first of the two has greater similarity to the canonical EF-hand than does the second. The most significant departures from precedent are the lack of Gly at EF-15 and a Lys at −Z (EF-21) that usually has Glu.

Osteonectin

Osteonectin, apparently the same as SPARC and BM-40, is an abundant extracellular glycoprotein whose function remains unknown. Engel et al. (1987) inferred an increase in content of α helix of about 35% from circular dichroic spectra associated with binding calcium. From the amino acid sequence they inferred two calcium-binding regions, one near the amino terminus rich in glutamic acid and the second resembling an EF-hand near the carboxyl terminus (Table 7). One especially intriguing aspect of their EF-hand model is the postulate that Cys-272 (EF-9) and Cys-288 (EF-25) form a disulfide bond. This they could readily do without distorting the standard structure.

Thrombospondin

Thrombospondin is a trimeric glycoprotein of molecular weight 420,000; it probably mediates cell-to-cell interaction. Lawler and Hynes (1986) identified a continuous, eightfold repeat of about 38 residues (Table 2). The consensus sequence of the central regions (D*D*DG*LD**D) is very similar to the EF-hand; however, there is no indication of a flanking helix E. Each monomer of thrombospondin binds several equivalents of calcium with $pk_d(Ca) \sim 7$. Removal of calcium causes an elongation of the narrow waist of the molecule. Lawler and Hynes suggest that these Ca^{++} ions, probably 24 per trimer, bind at the identified loops.

Protein Kinase C

Protein kinase C is serine- and threonine-specific and is the major phorbol ester receptor. It requires calcium, phospholipid, and diacylglycerol for activity. Whether the Ca^{++} ion(s) is coordinated entirely by the protein or partially by either the phospholipid or diacylglycerol has yet to be determined. Parker et al. (1986) determined the amino acid sequence of the α form and proposed a glutamic-acid-rich region as the probable calcium-binding site. They note that the putative calcium ligands would be in register with the EF-loop and there would appear to be a second helix F; two Pros preclude the possibility of a preceding helix E. In the companion paper, Coussens et al. (1986) present the DNA sequences of the β and γ forms and note the similarity of all three. The putative calcium-binding regions of β and γ show even less resemblance to the EF-hand than does the α isotype.

CONCLUSIONS

Quite certainly Nature has evolved for the extracellular proteins a wide variety of calcium-binding proteins. Some, like α-lactalbumin and the galactose-binding protein, have domains that closely resemble the calmodulin fold yet surely are not homologous. To distinguish homology and divergent evolution from analogy and convergence requires both structure and sequence data. However, even with this information, one may have to withhold judgment until one has a better idea of the protein's function and recent evolutionary history. There are now numerous examples of proteins not homologous to calmodulin that bind calcium, of proteins with related sequences that do not bind calcium, and of proteins with related structures that are

not homologous. Yet the generalization that "calcium-modulated proteins contain EF-hands and that proteins containing EF-hands are involved in calcium-modulated processes" still seems valid. Why?

REFERENCES

Aitken, A., C.B. Klee, and P. Cohen. 1984. The structure of the B subunit of calcineurin. *Eur. J. Biochem.* **139:** 663.

Baba, M., M. Goodman, J. Berger-Cohn, J. Demaille, and G. Matsuda. 1984. The early adaptive evolution of calmodulin. *Mol. Biol. Evol.* **1:** 442.

Babitch, J.A. and F.A. Anthony. 1987. Grasping for calcium-binding sites in the *Electrophorus electricus* sodium channel with an EF hand. *J. Theor. Biol.* **127:** 451.

Babu, Y.S., J.S. Sack, T.J. Greenhough, C.E. Bugg, A.R. Means, and W.J. Cook. 1985. Three-dimensional structure of calmodulin. *Nature* **315:** 37.

Baker, M.E. 1985. Evidence that progesterone binding uteroglobin is similar to myosin alkali light chain. *FEBS Lett.* **189:** 188.

Baum, P., C. Furlong, and B. Byers. 1986. Yeast gene required for spindle pole body duplications: Homology of its product with Ca^{2+}-binding proteins. *Proc. Natl. Acad. Sci.* **83:** 5512.

Brew, K., T.C. Vanaman, and R.L. Hill. 1967. Comparison of the amino acid sequence of bovine α-lactalbumin and hens egg white lysozyme. *J. Biol. Chem.* **242:** 3747.

Calabretta, B., R. Battini, L. Kaczmarek, J.K. de Riel, and R. Baserga. 1986. Molecular cloning of the cDNA for a growth factor-inducible gene with strong homology to S-100, a calcium-binding protein. *J. Biol. Chem.* **261:** 12628.

Charbonneau, H., K.A. Walsh, R.O. McCann, F.G. Prendergast, M.J. Cormier, and T.C. Vanaman. 1985. Amino acid sequence of the calcium-dependent photoprotein aequorin. *Biochemistry* **24:** 6762.

Collins, J.H., J.D. Potter, M.J. Horn, G. Wilshire, and N. Jackman. 1973. The amino acid sequence of rabbit skeletal muscle troponin C: Gene replication and homology with calcium-binding proteins from carp and hake muscle. *FEBS Lett.* **36:** 268.

Collins, J.H., R. Jakes, J. Kendrick-Jones, J. Leszyk, W. Barouch, J.L. Theibert, J. Spiegel, and A.G. Szent-Györgyi. 1986. Amino acid sequence of myosin essential light chain from the scallop *Aquipecten irradians. Biochemistry* **25:** 7651.

Coussens, L., P.J. Parker, L. Rhee, T.L. Yang-Feng, E. Chen, M.D. Waterfield, U. Francke, and A. Ullrich. 1986. Multiple, distinct forms of bovine and human protein kinase C suggest diversity in cellular signaling pathways. *Science* **233:** 859.

Dorin, J.R., M. Novak, R.E. Hill, D.J.H. Brock, D.S. Secher, and V. van Heyningen. 1987. A clue to the basic defect in cystic fibrosis from cloning the CF antigen gene. *Nature* **326:** 614.

Emori, Y., H. Kawasaki, S. Imajoh, S. Kawashima, and K. Suzuki. 1986a. Isolation and sequence analysis of cDNA clones for the small subunit of rabbit calcium-dependent protease. *J. Biol. Chem.* **261:** 9472.

Emori, Y., H. Kawasaki, H. Sugihara, S. Imajoh, S. Kawashima, and K. Suzuki. 1986b. Isolation and sequence analysis of cDNA clones for the large subunits of two isozymes of rabbit calcium-dependent protease. *J. Biol. Chem.* **261:** 9465.

Engel, J., W. Taylor, M. Paulsson, H. Sago, and B. Hogan. 1987. Calcium binding domains and calcium induced conformational transition of SPARC (osteonectin, BM-40), an extracellular glycoprotein expressed in mineralized non mineralized tissues. *Biochemistry* **26:** 6958.

Gerke, V. and K. Weber. 1985. The regulatory chain in the p36-kd substrate complex of viral tyrosine-specific protein kinase is related in sequence to the S-100 protein of glial cells. *EMBO J.* **4:** 2917.

Gillies, J.M., D.B. Thomason, J. LeFevre, and R.H. Kretsinger. 1982. Parvalbumin and muscle relaxation: A computer simulation study. *J. Muscle Res. Cell Motil.* **3:** 377.

Glenney, J.R., Jr., and B.F. Tack. 1985. Amino-terminal sequence of p36 and associated p10: Identification of the site of tyrosine phosphorylation and homology with S-100. *Proc. Natl. Acad. Sci.* **82:** 7884.

Hardin, S.H., C.D. Carpenter, P.E. Hardin, A.M. Bruskin, and W.H. Klein. 1985. Structure of the Spec1 gene encoding a major calcium-binding protein in the embryonic ectoderm of the sea urchin, *Strongylocentrotus purpuratus. J. Mol. Biol.* **186:** 243.

Herzberg, O. and M.N.G. James. 1985. Common structural framework of the two Ca^{2+}/Mg^{2+} binding loops of troponin C and other Ca^{2+} binding proteins. *Biochemistry* **24:** 5298.

Hunziker, W. 1986. The 28-kDa vitamin D-dependent calcium-binding protein has a six-domain structure. *Proc. Natl. Acad. Sci.* **83:** 7578.

Kobayashi, T., T. Takagi, K. Konishi, and J.A. Cox. 1987. The primary structure of a new M_r 18,000 calcium vector protein from *Amphioxus. J. Biol. Chem.* **262:** 2613.

Kretsinger, R.H. 1975. Hypothesis: Calcium modulated proteins contain EF-hands. In *Calcium transport in contraction and secretion* (ed. E. Carafoli et al.), p. 469. North-Holland Publishing, Amsterdam.

Kretsinger, R.H. and C.D. Barry. 1975. The predicted structure of the calcium-binding component of troponin. *Biochim. Biophys. Acta* **405:** 40.

Kretsinger, R.H., J.E. Mann, and J.G. Simmons. 1982. Model of the calcium-binding component of troponin. *Biochim. Biophys. Acta* **405:** 40.

Kretsinger, R.H., J.E. Mann, and J.G. Simmons. 1982. Model of facilitated diffusion of calcium by the intestinal calcium binding protein. In *Proceedings of the Fifth Workshop on Vitamin D* (ed. A.W. Norman), p. 233. de Gruyter, New York.

Kretsinger, R.H., S.E. Rudnick, and L.J. Weissman. 1986. Crystal structure of calmodulin. *J. Inorg. Biochem.* **28:** 289.

Lawler, J. and R.O. Hynes. 1986. The structure of human thrombospondin, an adhesive glycoprotein with multiple calcium-binding sites and homologies with several different proteins. *J. Cell Biol.* **103:** 1635.

Matthews, B.W. and S.J. Remington. 1974. The three dimensional structure of the lysozyme from bacteriophage T4. *Proc. Natl. Acad. Sci.* **71:** 4178.

Morize, I., E. Surcouf, M.C. Vaney, Y. Epelboin, M. Buehner, F. Fridlansky, E. Milgrom, and J.P. Mornon. 1987. Refinement of the $C222_1$ crystal form of oxidized uteroglobin at 1.34 Å resolution. *J. Mol. Biol.* **194:** 725.

Noda, M., T. Idedka, T. Kayano, H. Suzuki, H. Takeshima, M. Kurasaki, H. Takahaski, and S. Numa. 1986. Existence of distinct sodium channel messenger RNAs in rat brain. *Nature* **320:** 188.

Parker, P.J., L. Coussens, N. Totty, L. Rhee, S. Young. E. Chen, S. Stabel, M.D. Waterfield, and A. Ullrich. 1986. The complete primary structure of protein kinase C—the major phorbol ester receptor. *Science* **233:** 853.

Qasba, P.K. and S. Afaya. 1984. Similarity of the nucleotide sequences of rat α-lactalbumin and chicken lysozyme genes. *Nature* **308:** 377.

Reid, R.E. 1985. The functional nature of calcium binding loops in calmodulin, troponin C and parvalbumin. *J. Theor. Biol.* **44:** 353.

Salvato, M., J. Sulston, D. Albertson, and S. Brenner. 1986. A novel calmodulin-like gene from the nematode *Caenorhabditis elegans. J. Mol. Biol.* **190:** 281.

Stein, J.P., R.P. Munzaal, L. Lagace, E.C. Lai, B.W. O'Malley, and A.R. Means. 1983. Tissue-specific expression of a chicken calmodulin pseudogene lacking intervening sequences. *Proc. Natl. Acad. Sci.* **80:** 6485.

Stuart, D.I., K.R. Acharya, N.P.C. Walker, S.G. Smith, M. Lewis, and D.C. Phillips. 1986. α-Lactalbumin possesses a novel calcium binding loop. *Nature* **324:** 84.

Sundaralingam, M., R. Bergstrom, G. Strasburg, S.T. Rao, P. Roychowdhury, M. Greaser, and B.C. Wang. 1985. Molecular structure of troponin C from chicken skeletal muscle at 3-angstrom resolution. *Science* **227:** 945.

Szebenyi, D.M.E. and K. Moffat. 1986. The refined structure of vitamin D-dependent calcium-binding protein from bovine intestine. Molecular details, ion binding, and implications for the structure of other calcium-binding proteins. *J. Biol. Chem.* **261:** 8761.

Takagi, T. and K. Konishi. 1983. Amino acid sequence of troponin C obtained from ascidian (*Halocynthia roretzi*) body wall muscle. *J. Biochem.* **94:** 1753.

Takagi, T., K. Konishi, and J.A. Cox. 1986. Amino acid sequence of two sarcoplasmic calcium binding proteins from the photochordate *Amphioxus. Biochemistry* **25:** 3585.

Tufty, R.M. and R.H. Kretsinger. 1975. Troponin and parvalbumin calcium binding regions predicted in myosin light chain and T7 lysozyme. *Science* **187:** 167.

Vyas, N.K., M.N. Vyas, and F.A. Quiocho. 1987. A novel calcium binding site in the galactase-binding protein of bacterial transport and chemotaxis. *Nature* **329:** 635.

Weaver, L.H., M.G. Grütter, S.J. Remington, T.M. Gray, N.W. Isaacs, and B.W. Matthews. 1985. Comparison of goose-type, chicken-type, and phage-type lysozymes illustrates the changes that occur in both amino acid sequence and three-dimensional structure during evolution. *J. Mol. Evol.* **21:** 97.

Biosynthesis, Processing, and Evolution of Bovine Pancreatic Trypsin Inhibitor

T.E. Creighton and I.G. Charles

Medical Research Council, Laboratory of Molecular Biology, Cambridge CB2 2QH, England

Functional products of gene expression are generally obtained only after the initial linear polypeptide chain has folded to its native three-dimensional conformation (Creighton 1984). Unfolded proteins are usually inactive biologically. Folding is believed to be a spontaneous self-assembly process, directed solely by the amino acid sequence of the polypeptide chain under the appropriate physiological conditions, and occurs shortly after assembly of the polypeptide chain on the ribosome.

Most studies of protein folding have been carried out in vitro, using the intact polypeptide chain. Even under such well-controlled conditions, elucidating the nature of the folding transition has been hampered by its cooperativity: Partially folded intermediates are unstable relative to the fully folded and fully unfolded states and hence can be observed, at best, as transient kinetic intermediates (Creighton 1985). The most detailed folding pathway known is that of bovine pancreatic trypsin inhibitor (BPTI), which was elucidated using disulfide bonds between its six Cys residues to trap, isolate, and characterize the inherently unstable intermediates that define the pathway.

The relevance of such a folding pathway to in vivo conditions remains to be demonstrated. Experimental studies of in vivo protein folding have primarily demonstrated that individual structural domains of a nascent polypeptide chain tend to fold as they are completed (Bergmann and Kuehl 1979; Peters and Davidson 1982). There are reasons for believing that an individual protein domain should not fold productively until after completion of its polypeptide chain on the ribosome, when folding could occur by the same pathway as in vitro. Experimental determination of folding of the nascent chain in vivo should be possible using techniques like those used with BPTI in vitro, to determine which, if any, disulfide bonds are formed between Cys residues.

To carry out such in vivo studies of biosynthetic folding, the gene for BPTI has been isolated and characterized. These studies also produced the gene for a similar protein found in bovine spleen (Fioretti et al. 1983, 1985), designated the spleen inhibitor (SI).

EXPERIMENTAL PROCEDURES

The original clones of bovine genome fragments encoding the primary structures of BPTI and SI were isolated with a unique sequence DNA probe of 86 nucleotides synthesized according to the amino acid sequence of BPTI (Anderson and Kingston 1983; Kingston and Anderson 1986). Using the BPTI genomic segment as probe, clones were isolated that encode cDNA copies of the mRNA molecules of BPTI and SI. The remainders of the two genomic segments were then isolated, sequenced, and characterized (Creighton and Charles 1987).

RESULTS

The two genes encoding BPTI and SI, depicted in Figure 1, are homologous over their length, except for the upstream promoter regions. Probably as a result of these differences, the two genes tend to be transcribed into mRNA at two different start sites, with that for SI being 90 bp upstream. Otherwise, the two genes have the same sites for splicing out the two introns, for translation initiation and termination, and for addition of poly(A) tails.

Both genes encode polypeptide products of 98 or 100 amino acid residues, depending on which of the two AUG codons is used for initiation of translation; the first is the more probable. The sequences encoding the two mature proteins are uninterrupted by introns, but are flanked by two homologous introns. Intron A is at least 2700 bp long in each case, and the two versions differ in having at least one nonhomologous segment. Intron B is 450 bp in the BPTI gene; that of SI is one shorter.

Each primary polypeptide product is predicted to consist of a 35- or 33-residue amino extension, the mature protein of 58 residues, and a carboxyl extension of 7 residues. The amino-terminal extensions contain a segment with all the characteristics of signal peptides that result in translocation of the nascent chain through the membrane of the endoplasmic reticulum. The signal peptides of BPTI and SI are unlikely to comprise the entire amino extensions, but their virtually identical sequences indicate that the signal peptide of each is most likely to extend to residue -16, -14, or -8 (von Heijne 1986).

DISCUSSION

Biosynthesis of BPTI and SI

The finding that BPTI is synthesized as a larger precursor was surprising, for there were few indications of its existence. Consequently, it is necessary to establish the biological significance of this precursor, which would presumably apply also to SI.

The least interesting possibility is that the precursor is necessary simply to provide a minimum polypeptide length that might be required for insertion of the nascent chain through a membrane, as has been proposed for the precursor forms of other small proteins (Steiner et al. 1985). However, the mature forms of these other proteins are longer than the precursors of BPTI and SI. Other possible functions of the extensions are that they are involved in folding or cellular targeting of the proteins.

Processing of the BPTI and SI Precursors

Proteolytic processing of the BPTI and SI precursors, to yield the mature proteins of 58 amino acid residues, must occur in several steps. The first is likely to be removal of the putative signal peptide, which usually occurs on the nascent chain. The site of this cleavage must be determined experimentally, as no unique site is predicted from the amino acid sequence. Nevertheless, this site is most unlikely to coincide with the amino terminus of the mature protein, but is predicted to leave an amino extension of 7, 13, or 15 residues.

Removal of the amino and carboxyl extensions could occur by a variety of mechanisms, for there are few indications of intermediates accumulating. Siekmann et al. (1986) have reported the natural occurrence of small quantities of BPTI with an additional pyroglutamic acid residue at the amino terminus, which presumably arose from having the Gln-1 residue at the amino terminus. D. Barra et al. (in prep.) have isolated two alternative forms of SI, both retaining residues −1 and −2 of the amino extension and either the first 5 or 6 residues of the carboxyl extension. Other minor variant forms of BPTI (Siekmann et al. 1986) and SI (Fioretti et al. 1983) may also be relevant to the processing of the two precursors.

The terminal residues of mature BPTI are very resistant to proteolytic removal, and they normally interact in the final folded conformation to form a salt bridge (Brown et al. 1978) and to confer additional stability on the folded conformation (Goldenberg and Creighton 1984). Consequently, it is possible that the amino and carboxyl extensions are removed by nonspecific proteolysis until the stable and resistant mature protein is generated. A minor natural variant lacking residue 58 (Siekmann et al. 1986), the normal mature carboxyl terminus, may represent an aberrant pathway or simply molecules that have undergone loss of one additional residue. The Pro-2 residue might be important for stopping proteolysis at the amino terminus (Schwartz 1986). Otherwise, the amino acid sequences of the amino- and carboxy-terminal regions of the precursors or the mature proteins have none of the characteristics of other specific cleavage sites in other proteins.

Folding of the BPTI and SI Precursors

The extensions of the BPTI and SI precursors could conceivably play a role in folding and formation of the three disulfide bonds of the two proteins. On the other hand, there are few indications that such a phenomenon should be significant. Mature BPTI is able to refold readily, and the in vitro pathway for formation of its three disulfide bonds has been elucidated in detail (Creighton 1985). Folding and disulfide formation can occur within less than a minute, and the process is increased in rate by the enzyme protein-disulfide isomerase, which is likely to be involved in folding in vivo (Creighton et al. 1980). The extensions could have unforeseen consequences for the folding of the protein, and it is possible that the presence of any such extensions could increase the rate of folding of BPTI. Mature BPTI folds most readily through rearrangements of the two-disulfide intermediates, apparently due to the necessity of going through a high-energy distorted form of the native conformation (Goldenberg and Creighton 1985). The chain termini of mature BPTI are on the surface of the folded native protein and interact favorably in a salt bridge (Brown et al. 1978). By cross-linking them with a peptide bond (Goldenberg and Creighton 1984), it was found that they seem to have no particular role in folding except to stabilize the fully folded protein. Peptide extensions in the BPTI precursor would not be expected to interfere with the final folded conformation, but might destabilize it slightly by disrupting the final salt bridge. This would be the case if the extensions were involved in no other interactions, since they could then not form a comparable salt bridge. Such a destabilizing effect could diminish the energetic barrier to folding, so the precursor might fold more rapidly by sequentially forming the three disulfide bonds without undergoing the disulfide rearrangements.

The SI protein is likely to fold by a pathway very similar to that of BPTI, since the seven amino acid replacements seem unlikely to have any substantial structural effects. Much less similar homologs of BPTI fold by similar pathways, and it is likely that protein-folding pathways, as well as folded conformations, have been conserved during evolutionary divergence (Hollecker and Creighton 1983).

Folding in vivo is likely to take place within a precursor retaining at least part of the amino and carboxyl extensions, so folding of the appropriate precursors, after removal of the signal peptide, will be determined experimentally in vitro.

Cellular Targeting of BPTI and SI

Mature BPTI is found histochemically to be localized within mast cells (Fritz et al. 1979; Shikimi and Kobayashi 1980; Businaro et al. 1987), whereas mature SI is found in smooth muscle cells of numerous bovine organs (Businaro et al. 1987). The different cellular

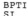

```
BPTI        CTGTAAGGAGATTACAGACTGTTCAAGCCTGACCCCAGA
SI             GGT CATTACTGA   CT GTCCG GAATAACGAGTG
                                                    ↑


TCTTGCCTTTCCT--CTCCCCTCCTTATCTCCTGCTCCCACCCTTCACCTGGGGTATGAA
      C    G   CA


                          ↓                            -35
                                                       MetLysMetSer
AAGCACAGTCAACCCCCAGCTTTCCCCAGGAGCCCTCCTTGCAAGGCCATGAAGATGAGC


   -30           -25          -20          -15
ArgLeuCysLeuSerValAlaLeuLeuValLeuLeuGlyThrLeuAlaAlaSerThrPro
CGGCTCTGCCTCTCCGTAGCCCTTCTGGTCCTCCTGGGCACCCTGGCGGCCAGCACTCCA
                A
                Ile

   -10          -5
GlyCysAspThrSerAsnGlnAlaLysA
GGGTGTGACACCAGCAACCAGGCCAAAG/GUAAGU...Intron.A....AUCCCUGCAG
                        A


   -1 +1         5           10          15
laGlnArgProAspPheCysLeuGluProProTyrThrGlyProCysLysAlaArgIle
/CCCAGCGGCCTGACTTCTGCCTAGAGCCTCCATATACGGGTCCCTGCAAGGCCAGAATT
                                                        A   G
                                                        LysMet

   20          25          30          35
IleArgTyrPheTyrAsnAlaLysAlaGlyLeuCysGlnThrPheValTyrGlyGlyCys
ATCAGATACTTCTACAACGCCAAGGCTGGGCTCTGCCAGACCTTTGTATATGGCGGCTGC
                              T       G                   T
                              Phe     Glu

   40          45          50          55
ArgAlaLysArgAsnAsnPheLysSerAlaGluAspCysMetArgThrCysGlyGlyAla
AGAGCTAAAAGAAACAATTTCAAGAGCGCAGAGGACTGCATGAGGACCTGTGGTGGTGCT
A       G   C           G
Lys     Ser             Arg

   60                                      65
IleGlyProTrpG                              luAsnLeu
ATTGGGCCCTGGG/GUAAGA...Intron.B....CUUUUUACAG/AGAACCTGTGAACT
     C
     Arg


GTGCTCCCCTGAGATGCTGAAGTATGAGGAGGACCCACCCAAGGCTGGCCTCTATCTGCT

TCTGAAAAATTTCAGCCTCCTTTTATTTCTTCTCAACCCTCCCCTCCTCAGCAGAAATCT

GTCTCTTTCCTTCCTCCACAGGTCCACTTACTTTAGCCCTATCTCATCCAGTTTGCTCTA

AGCACCATGAAAGCAAATCTTCCCTTTGTCCCTCACACTTCCCACAATTTCTGGCACAAA

GGAGAAGGTCCAGAAATATTGGAGGAAGGAAGGAATGAAGTTCCCCATGACTGGAGCATC

TGTAGAGTCTGAGATTTAAATCTGGATTCTTGTCCTAATCTTCCTCCTCACGGCATCCTT

ACCTTCATCCTCCACCCCACCATCACTGCTCTCCCTCTACTGGCGAAAGTAGAATTTCCA

TCATCGAGTTTTCAGCTCAGTGGTGGGAGAGGTCTTTTCATGAACGAAACCTCCTCCTCA
                                            -       G

CATTGATTTGAAGGTCTGTGGCTTCAAAGAGTCTGGCCTTATCTTTAAATAAATTCATAT

TTTAATTAAACTAACTGGAGTGGATTGTGTTGTT
      ∨∨
      poly A
```

Figure 1. Sequences of the genes for BPTI and SI and of their putative polypeptide products. The BPTI gene sequence is shown in its entirety, except for the bulk of the two introns, with the predicted amino acid sequence of the polypeptide product above it. The gene and polypeptide sequences for SI are indicated below those for BPTI only where they differ. The sequences of the mature proteins are shown in bold face. The transcription initiation sites are indicated by the arrows. That for BPTI is 33 bp downstream from a TATA-like sequence, TATG, whereas that for SI has a similar sequence ATTA in the same relative position. Poly(A) addition in both genes occurs somewhere within the sequence TAAA; this site is preceded and followed by the usual sequences AATAAA and GTGTT, respectively. Intron splice sites are indicated by /.

513

locations of the two proteins presumably reflect the cell-specific expression of their two genes, controlled by their different promoters (Fig. 1). The organ distribution of mature BPTI protein is similar to that of its mRNA (Kingston and Anderson 1986), so the protein is probably retained in the organ where it is synthesized. Comparable information is not available for SI, but cDNA copies of its mRNA were cloned from lung mRNA, an organ where the mature SI protein is found in only very small amounts (Fioretti et al. 1983).

Despite its name, mature BPTI is found in virtually all tissues of the cow, parallel with the distribution of mast cells. It is found in tissues, not in extracellular fluids, and appears to be an intracellular protein (Fritz and Wunderer 1983). Consequently, finding a putative signal sequence at the amino terminus of its precursor was unexpected. If the protein is not secreted after entering the endoplasmic reticulum, it is most likely to be retained within an intracellular organelle, of which mast cells have many. Most proteins destined for the endoplasmic reticulum, the Golgi, and lysosomes are synthesized with signal peptides, but those destined for mitochondria, peroxisomes, and other microbodies are not (Borst 1986).

A major question of cell biology is how these proteins are targeted to the proper intracellular targets (Kelly 1985). Proteins destined for lysosomes are tagged with mannose-6-phosphate groups, but this is unlikely to be the sole mechanism (Owada and Neufeld 1982; Waheed et al. 1982; Hoflack and Kornfeld 1985). At least some lysosomal proteins are processed proteolytically to remove carboxyl extensions (Erickson and Blobel 1983), similar to BPTI and SI.

There are similarities between the BPTI and SI carboxyl extensions and the carboxy-terminal sequences of most of the proteins found in intracellular organelles (Creighton and Charles 1987); an updated compilation of carboxy-terminal sequences of the primary gene product, before any proteolytic processing, is presented in Table 1. The terminal residue (Z) is nearly always hydrophobic, and residue Z-1 is almost always either basic, or small and polar. Residue Z-2 is almost always small or acidic. Residue Z-3 is usually basic if residue Z-1 was not, or Gly, Ala, or Trp. Of the four proteins listed in Table 1 that clearly do not have such a consensus sequence, three are from yeast, and the fourth, lysosomal hexosaminidase, is discussed later. Comparable sequences are not found at the termini of secreted proteins, although it is not clear where proteins in granules used as storage before secretion should be included. The similarities in the sequences of Table 1 raised the possibility that such sequences were involved in targeting to intracellular organelles (Creighton and Charles 1987).

The apparently similar sequence -Lys-Asp-Glu-Leu has been independently noted to be present at the carboxyl termini of three soluble endoplasmic reticulum proteins and shown to stop the usual secretion of hen egg-white lysozyme when added to its carboxyl terminus (Munro and Pelham 1987). We added five of the other seemingly similar sequences from Table 1 to lysozyme, but the extended proteins were largely secreted when the modified lysozyme gene was expressed in Cos cells (Munro and Pelham 1987). Therefore, these sequences may not be sufficient to target a protein, or the Cos cells may not have the appropriate cellular machinery.

There may not be a single mechanism for targeting proteins to organelles, as the phenomenon is likely to be cell specific. With the lysosomal proteins, the mannose-6-phosphate label appears not to be the sole mechanism, for in certain cells some of the proteins are directed to lysosomes even in the absence of this targeting system (Owada and Neufeld 1982; Waheed et al. 1982). An exception is hexosaminidase, which is secreted in the absence of the mannose phosphate system (Waheed et al. 1982); it may be pertinent that its carboxy-terminal sequence also differs from the general consensus (Table 1). This is consistent with the proposal that the consensus carboxy-terminal sequence, in addition to the mannose-6-phosphate system, is involved in targeting proteins to lysosomes and other organelles.

Other evidence indicates a role for amino-terminal sequences (Bankaitis et al. 1986), but the amino extensions of BPTI and SI do not seem to be homologous to other such sequences.

Positive Selection in the Evolutionary Divergence of BPTI and SI

The two genes for BPTI and SI undoubtedly arose by gene duplication and have undergone only limited evolutionary divergence. However, the nature of the divergence that has occurred is very different from that observed in most other gene families, where the rate of divergence of each nucleotide of the gene is usually inversely proportional to its apparent functional importance. Just the opposite is observed with the BPTI and SI genes. Their most conserved regions are the identical 5′ untranslated regions of the mRNA molecules and the very long 3′ untranslated regions, which differ in only 2 of the 554 nucleotides (0.4% different). The most variable regions are those coding for protein (5.2% different), especially the mature protein; they are more variable than even the introns (2.9% and 3.1% different). Moreover, within the coding regions, 9 of the 11 nucleotide differences produce amino acid differences, whereas silent mutations occur more frequently in most other genes. Of the 9 amino acid differences, 7 occur within the mature proteins, and 3 of these occur within those segments of the proteins, residues 11–19 and 34–39, that are observed crystallographically to be in direct physical contact with the proteases to which they bind and inhibit (Ruhlmann et al. 1973; Chen and Bode 1983).

Greater than average variability of some positions in the active-site regions is apparent in the 27 other known protein sequences that clearly are homologous with

Table 1. Carboxy-terminal Sequences of Proteins Found in Intracellular Organelles

Organelle Protein		Z-3 Z	Reference
Lysosomes			
Procathepsin B	human, mouse	-Trp-Glu-Lys-Ile	a
	rat	-Trp-Gly-Arg-Phe	a
Procathepsin D	human	-Ala-Ala-Arg-Leu	b
α-Galactosidase A	human	-Lys-Asp-Leu-Leu	c
β-Glucuronidase	rat	-Pro-Phe-Thr-Phe	d
Hexosaminidase α	human	-Phe-Glu-Gln-Thr	e, v
Hexosaminidase β	human	-His-Glu-Asn-Met	v
Peroxisomes			
Catalase	human	-Lys-Ala-Asn-Leu	f
	bovine, rat	-Lys-Ala-Asn-Leu	g
Bifunctional enzyme	rat	-Gly-Ser-Lys-Leu	h
Dihydroxyacetone synthase	yeast	-Glu-Gly-Lys-Ala	i
Methanol oxidase	yeast	-Leu-Ala-Arg-Phe	j
Uricase II	soybean	-Trp-Ser-Lys-Leu	k
AcylCoA Oxidase I	yeast	-Ile-Leu-Ser-Ser	l
II	yeast	-Ile-Leu-Ser-Lys	l
D-Amino acid oxidase	pig	-Pro-Ser-His-Leu	m
Endoplasmic reticulum			
Protein disulfide isomerase	bovine	-Lys-Asp-Glu-Leu	n
Grp 78	rat	-Lys-Asp-Glu-Leu	o
Grp 94	hamster	-Lys-Asp-Glu-Leu	p
Trypanosomal glycosomes			
P-Glycerate kinase		-Trp-Ser-Ser-Leu	q
Aldolase		-Gly-Asn-Thr-Tyr	r
Triose-P isomerase		-Lys-Ala-Thr-Gln	s
Glyceraldehyde-P dehydrogenase		-Ala-Ala-Lys-Leu	t
Melanosomes			
Tyrosinase	Mouse	-His-Ser-Met-Val	u

References: [a]Chan et al. (1986); [b]Faust et al. (1985); [c]Bishop et al. (1986); [d]Nishimura et al. (1986); [e]Myerowitz et al. (1985); [f]Quan et al. (1986); [g]Furuta et al. (1986); [h]Osumi et al. (1985); [i]Janowicz et al. (1985); [j]Ledeboer et al. (1985); [k]Nguyen et al. (1985); [l]Okazaki et al. (1986); [m]Ronchi et al. (1982); [n]Edman et al. (1985); [o]Munro and Pelham (1986); [p]Sorger and Pelham (1987); [q]Osinga et al. (1985); [q]Osinga et al. (1985); [r] Clayton (1985); [s]Swinkels et al. (1986); [t]Michels et al. (1986); [u]Shibahara et al. (1986); [v]Korneluk et al. (1986).

BPTI and SI (Table 2). Most of these proteins have demonstrable protease inhibitor activity, although of varying specificity, and all the amino acid residues believed to be important for the three-dimensional structure of BPTI (Wlodawer et al. 1987) have been conserved (Creighton 1975). Alignment of the sequences is also straightforward, due to the virtual absence of insertions and deletions. A single insertion apparently occurred in the silkworm inhibitor, and a single deletion in the two homologous β-bungarotoxin B chains; the alignments of these three proteins are uncertain in the corresponding regions of the polypeptide chain, but all other alignments are unambiguous. In Figure 2, the variability of each position is expressed as the number of different amino acids observed at that position, divided by the frequency of the most common amino acid (Wu and Kabat 1970).

The most variable position is residue 17, within the active-site region of BPTI (Fig. 2). Other markedly variable active-site positions are 34 and 39. BPTI and SI differ at two of these three positions. Other positions within the active-site regions are very conserved, apparently for functional and structural reasons; examples are the Cys residues 14 and 38 that form a disulfide

bond, the Gly residues at positions 12, 36, and 37, Pro residues at 13, and aromatic residues at 35 (Creighton 1975). These structural constraints probably limited the divergence of the active-site regions of this family of inhibitors.

The most plausible explanation for these observations is that the evolutionary divergence of this gene family has been accelerated by positive selective pressure. This would also account for the difficulty in constructing phylogenetic trees from the sequences of Table 2, due to the need to invoke numerous parallel and reverse mutations. Other explanations for the differences between BPTI and SI genes are possible, such as that their introns and untranslated regions may play unexpected functional roles, for example, in thus far unobserved alternative modes of expression of these genes. The phenomenon of gene conversion may also complicate the divergence of closely similar duplicated genes, such as those of BPTI and SI. These alternative explanations are made less likely by the observation of a similar, but less dramatic, hypervariability of active-site regions in other members of this protease inhibitor family (Fig. 2) and in other inhibitor families (Hill and Hastie 1987; Laskowski et al. 1987).

Table 2. Protein Sequences Homologous to BPTI

Protein		Reference	Sequence (positions 1–60)
BPTI			RPDFCLEPP-YTGPCKARIIRYFYNAKAGLCQTFVYGGCRAKRNNFKSAEDCMRTCGGA
SI			RPDFCLEPP-YTGPCKAKMIRYFYNAKAGFCETFVYGGCKAKSNNFRSAEDCMRTCGGA
Bovine colostrum inhibitor		a	FQTPPDLCQLPQ-ARGPCKAALLRYFYNSTSNACEPFTYGGCQGNNNNFETTEMCLRICEPPTDKS
Turtle egg-white inhibitor		b	QFDKRDICRLPP-EQGPCKGRIPRYFYNPASRMCESFIYGGCKGNKNNFKTKAECVRACRPPERPGVCPKT-
Snail inhibitor K		c	EGRPSFCNLPA-ETGPCKASFRQYYYNSKSFFCQQFIYGGCRGNQNRFDTTQQCQGVCV
Sea anemone inhibitor		d	INGDCELPK-VVGPCRARFPRYYYNSSSKRC　　)KVCGVRS
Russell's viper inhibitor		e	HDRPTFCNLAP-ESGRCRGHLRRIYYNLESNKCKVFFYGGCGGNANNFETRDECRETCGGK
Ringhal's cobra inhibitor		f	RPDFCELPA-ETGLCKAYIRSFHYNLAAQQCLQFIYGGCGGNANRFKTIDECRRTCVG
Cape cobra inhibitor		f	RPRFCELPA-ETGLCKARIRSFHYNRAAQQCLEFIYGGCGGNANRFKTIEECRRTCVV
Toxin B, black mamba		g	RPYACELIV-AAGPCMFFISAFYYSKGANKCYPFTYSGCRGNANRFKTIEECRRTCVV
Toxin E, black mamba		h	LQHRTFCKLPA-EPGPCKASIPAFYYNWAAKKCQLFHYGGCKGNANRFSTIEKCRHACVG
Toxin I, black mamba		i	QPLRKLCILHR-NPGRCYQKIPAFYYNQKKKQCEGFTWSGCGGNSNRFKTIEECRRTCIRK
green mamba		i	QPRRKLCILHR-NPGRCYDKIPAFYYNQKKKQCEGFTWSGCGGNANRFKTIEECRRTCVG
Toxin K, black mamba		j	AAKYCKLPL-RIGPCKRKIPSFYYKWKAKQCLPFDYSGCGGNANRFKTIEECRRTCVG
green mamba		j	AAKYCKLPV-RYGPCKKKIPSFYYKWKAKQCLPFDYSGCGGNANRFKTIEECRRTCVG
Banded krait inhibitor		k	KNRPTFCNLLP-ETGRCNALIPAFYYNSHLHKCQKFNYGGCGGNANNFKTIDECERTCAAKYGRSS
Long-nosed viper chymotrypsin inhibitor		l	RDRPKFCYLPA-DPGRCLAYMPRFYYNPASNKCEKFIYGGCRGNANNFKTWDECRHTCVASEIQPR
Long-nosed viper trypsin inhibitor		m	QDHPKFCYLPA-DPGRCKAHIPRFYYDSASNKCNKFIYGGCPGNANNFKTWDECRQTCGASA
Silkworm chymotrypsin inhibitor		n	TTDLPICEQAFGDAGLCFGYMKLYSYNQETKNCEEFIYGGCQGNDNRFSTLAECEQKCIN
β1-bungarotoxin B chain		o	RQRHRDCDKPP-DKGNCGP-VRAFYYDTRLKTCKAFQYRGCDGNHGNFKTETLCRCECLVYP
B2-bungarotoxin B chain		p	RKRHPDCDKPP-DTKICQT-VRAFYYKPSAKRCVQFRYGGCDGDHGNFKSDHLCRCECELYR
Inter-α-trypsin inhibitor, Domain 1	bovine	q	KADSCQLDY-SQGPCLGLFKRYFYNGTSMACETFLYGGCMGNLNNFLSQKECLQTCR-
	human	r	KEDSCQLGY-SAFPCMGMTSRYFYNGTSMACETFQYGGCMGNGNNFVTQKECLQTCR-
	equine	q	KEDSCQLDH-AQGPCLGMISRYFYNGTSMACETFQYGGCLGNGNNFASQKECLETCR-
	porcine	q	KEDSCELGY-SQGPCLGMIKRYFYNGSSMACETFHYGGCMGNGNNFVSQKECLQTCR-
Domain 2	bovine	q	TVEACNLPI-VQGPCRAFIQLWAFDAVKGKCVRFSYGGCKGNGNKFYSQKECKEYCGIPGEADERLLR
	human	r	TVAACNLPI-VRGPCRAFIQLWAFDAVKGKCVLFPYGGCQGNGNKFYSQKECREYCGVPGDGDEELLRF
	equine	q	TVAACNLPI-VQGPCRAFIRLWAFDAAQGKCVLFTYGGCRGNGNKFYSQKECKEYCGIPGDGDEELLR
	porcine	q	TVSACSLPI-VQGPCRAFIRLWAFDAAQGKCVLFNYGGCQGNGNKFYSQKECKEYCGVPGEEDELLR

References: [a]Cechova et al. (1976); [b]Kato and Tominaga (1979); [c]Tschesche and Dietl (1975); [d]Wunderer et al. (1976); [e]Takahashi et al. (1974); [f]Hokama et al. (1976); [g]Strydom and Joubert (1981); [h]Joubert and Strydom (1978); [i]Strydom (1973); [j]Joubert and Taljaard (1980); [k]Liu et al. (1983); [l]Ritonja et al. (1983a); [m]Ritonja et al. (1983b); [n]Sasaki (1984); [o]Kondo et al. (1982); [p]Kondo et al. (1982); [q]Hochstrasser et al. (1985); [r]Kaumeyer et al. (1986).

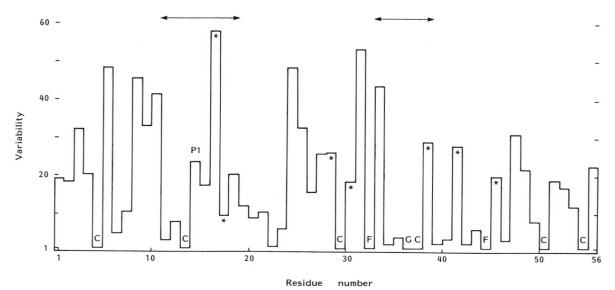

Figure 2. Variability of the amino acid residue positions in proteins homologous to BPTI. The variability of each position is defined as the number of amino acids observed to occur at that position, divided by the frequency of the most prevalent amino acid (Wu and Kabat 1970), using the alignment of Table 2. The active-site regions of the protease inhibitors are indicated by the arrows; the residue most responsible for determining protease specificity is labeled P1. Positions at which BPTI and SI differ are marked with asterisks. Positions that are invariant (variability = 1.0) are indicated with the one-letter code for the conserved amino acid residue.

The phenomenon of positive selection may be so apparent with protease inhibitors, in contrast to proteins with other biological functions, because of their evolutionary competition with a variety of target proteases. Accordingly, the protease specificities of the members of the various protease inhibitor families would be expected to vary, as has generally been observed. Interestingly, the residue at position 15 of the BPTI family, which is given the designation P1 and is generally considered to be the prime determinant of protease specificity, is variable, but not remarkably so (Fig. 2). The most variable positions are those at the fringe of the area of contact between protease and inhibitor (Ruhlmann et al. 1973; Chen and Bode 1983). The three active-site differences between BPTI and SI involve chemically similar amino acid side chains, implying only subtle differences in protease specificity. Only small differences in the affinities of BPTI and SI for porcine kallikrein have been reported, with indistinguishable affinities for three other proteases of the trypsin family (Fioretti et al. 1985). Clearly, the functional basis of the evolutionary divergence of these families of proteases and their inhibitors needs to be studied further.

The small number of differences between the SI and BPTI genes is therefore likely to indicate that the two genes arose only recently by gene duplication, or at least only recently escaped the constraint of gene conversion. In contrast, the wide variety of species in which members of the BPTI family are found, from mammals to snails, silkworms, and sea anemones, presumably reflects the ancient origin of this family.

It is remarkable that the apparent role of positive selection is so very obvious in the closely related pairs,

especially BPTI and SI (Fig. 1), whereas it is not so striking in the distantly related proteins (Fig. 2). This may indicate that positive selection acted to accelerate the evolutionary divergence primarily at the early stages after each gene duplication. Presumably, selection would be for a new protease specificity that happened to be beneficial. Once the new specificity had evolved, the gene would be subject to negative selection to maintain this new specificity. In contrast, selection against change at crucial structural positions and neutral evolutionary divergence at nonfunctional positions would continue so that the initial positive divergence would become less apparent with increasing time (Fig. 2).

REFERENCES

Anderson, S. and I.B. Kingston. 1983. Isolation of a genomic clone for bovine pancreatic trypsin inhibitor by using a unique-sequence synthetic DNA probe. *Proc. Natl. Acad. Sci.* **80:** 6838.

Bankaitis, V.A., L.M. Johnson, and S.D. Emr. 1986. Isolation of yeast mutants defective in protein targeting to the vacuole. *Proc. Natl. Acad. Sci.* **83:** 9075.

Bergmann, L.W. and W.M. Kuehl. 1979. Formation of an interchain disulfide bond on nascent immunoglobulin light chains. *J. Biol. Chem.* **254:** 8869.

Bishop, D.F., D.H. Calhoun, H.S. Bernstein, P. Hantzopoulos, M. Quinn, and R.J. Desnick. 1986. Human α-galactosidase A: Nucleotide sequence of a cDNA clone encoding the mature enzyme. *Proc. Natl. Acad. Sci.* **83:** 4859.

Borst, P. 1986. How proteins get into microbodies (peroxisomes, glyoxysomes, glycosomes). *Biochim. Biophys. Acta* **866:** 179.

Brown, L.R., A. De Marco, R. Richarz, G. Wagner, and K. Wüthrich. 1978. The influence of a single salt bridge on static and dynamic features of the globular solution conformation of the basic pancreatic trypsin inhibitor. [1]H and ^{13}C nuclear-magnetic-resonance studies of the native and the transaminated inhibitor. *Eur. J. Biochem.* **88:** 87.

Businaro, R., E. Fioretti, L. Fumagalli, G. Citro, G. de Renzis, and F. Ascoli. 1987. Vascular localization of bovine pancreatic trypsin inhibitor-related molecular forms in bovine spleen. *Eur. J. Biochem.* **165:** 79.

Cechova, D. 1976. Trypsin inhibitor from cow colostrum. *Methods Enzymol.* **45:** 806.

Chan, S.J., B. San Segundo, M.B. McCormick, and D.F. Steiner. 1986. Nucleotide and predicted amino acid sequences of cloned human and mouse preprocathepsin B cDNAs. *Proc. Natl. Acad. Sci.* **83:** 7721.

Chen, Z. and W. Bode. 1983. Refined 2.5 Å X-ray crystal structure of the complex formed by porcine kallikrein A and the bovine pancreatic trypsin inhibitor. *J. Mol. Biol.* **164:** 283.

Clayton, C.E. 1985. Structure and regulated expression of genes encoding fructose biphosphate aldolase in *Trypanosoma brucei. EMBO J.* **4:** 2997.

Creighton, T.E. 1975. Homology of protein structures: Proteinase inhibitors. *Nature* **255:** 743.

———. 1984. *Proteins: Structures and molecular properties.* W.H. Freeman, New York.

———. 1985. The problem of how and why proteins adopt folded conformations. *J. Phys. Chem.* **89:** 2452.

Creighton, T.E. and I.G. Charles. 1987. Sequences of the genes and polypeptide precursors for two bovine protease inhibitors. *J. Mol. Biol.* **194:** 11.

Creighton, T.E., D.A. Hillson, and R.B. Freedman. 1980. Catalysis by protein-disulphide isomerase of the unfolding and refolding of proteins with disulphide bonds. *J. Mol. Biol.* **142:** 43.

Edman, J.C., L. Ellis, R.W. Blacher, R.A. Roth, and W.J. Rutter. 1985. Sequence of protein disulphide isomerase and implications of its relationship to thioredoxin. *Nature* **317:** 267.

Erickson, A.H. and G. Blobel. 1983. Carboxyl-terminal proteolytic processing during biosynthesis of the lysosomal enzymes β-glucuronidase and cathepsin D. *Biochemistry* **22:** 5201.

Faust, P.L., S. Kornfeld, and J.M. Chirgwin. 1985. Cloning and sequence analysis of cDNA for human cathepsin D. *Proc. Natl. Acad. Sci.* **82:** 4910.

Fioretti, E., I. Binotti, D. Barra, G. Citro, F. Ascoli, and E. Antonini. 1983. Heterogeneity of the basic pancreatic inhibitor (Kunitz) in various bovine organs. *Eur. J. Biochem.* **130:** 13.

Fioretti, E., G. Iacopino, M. Angeletti, D. Barra, F. Bossa, and F. Ascoli. 1985. Primary structure and antiproteolytic activity of a Kunitz-type inhibitor from bovine spleen. *J. Biol. Chem.* **260:** 11451.

Fritz, H. and G. Wunderer. 1983. Biochemistry and applications of aprotinin, the kallikrein inhibitor from bovine organs. *Arzneim.-Forsch.* **33:** 479.

Fritz, H., J. Krucki, I. Russe, and H.G. Riebich. 1979. Immunofluorescence studies indicate that the basic trypsin-kallikrein-inhibitor of bovine organs (Trasylol) originates from mast cells. *Hoppe-Seyler's Z. Physiol. Chem.* **360:** 437.

Furuta, S., H. Hayashi, M. Hijikata, S. Miyazawa, T. Osumi, and T. Hashimoto. 1986. Complete nucleotide sequence of cDNA and deduced amino acid sequence of rat liver catalase. *Proc. Natl. Acad. Sci.* **83:** 313.

Goldenberg, D.P. and T.E. Creighton. 1984. Folding pathway of a circular form of bovine pancreatic trypsin inhibitor. *J. Mol. Biol.* **179:** 527.

———. 1985. Energetics of protein structure and folding. *Biopolymers* **24:** 167.

Hill, R.E. and N.D. Hastie. 1987. Accelerated evolution in the reactive centre regions of serine protease inhibitors. *Nature* **326:** 96.

Hochstrasser, K., E. Wachter, G.J. Albrecht, and P. Reisinger. 1985. Kunitz-type proteinase inhibitors derived by limited proteolysis of the inter-α-trypsin inhibitor, X. The amino acid sequences of the trypsin-released inhibitors from horse and pig inter-α-trypsin inhibitors. *Biol. Chem. Hoppe-Seyler* **366:** 473.

Hoflack, B. and S. Kornfeld. 1985. Lysosomal enzyme binding to mouse P388D[1] macrophage membranes lacking the 215-kDa mannose 6-phosphate receptor: Evidence for the existence of a second mannose 6-phosphate receptor. *Proc. Natl. Acad. Sci.* **82:** 4428.

Hokama, Y., S. Iwanaga, T. Tatsuki, and T. Suzuki. 1976. Snake venom proteinase inhibitors. III. Isolation of five polypeptide inhibitors from the venoms of *Hemachatus haemachatus* (Ringhal's cobra) and *Naja nivea* (Cape cobra) and the complete amino acid sequences of two of them. *J. Biochem.* **79:** 559.

Hollecker, M. and T.E. Creighton. 1983. Evolutionary conservation and variation of protein folding pathways. *J. Mol. Biol.* **168:** 409.

Janowicz, Z.A., M.R. Eckart, C. Drewke, R.O. Roggenkamp, C.P. Hollenberg, J. Maat, A.M. Ledeboer, C. Visser, and C.T. Verrips. 1985. Cloning and characterization of the *DAS* gene encoding the major methanol assimilatory enzyme from the methylotrophic yeast *Hansenula polymorpha. Nucleic Acids Res.* **13:** 3043.

Joubert, F.J. and D.J. Strydom. 1978. Snake venoms. The amino-acid sequence of trypsin inhibitor E of *Dendroaspis polylepis polylepis* (black mamba) venom. *Eur. J. Biochem.* **87:** 191.

Joubert, F.J. and N. Taljaard. 1980. Snake venoms. The amino acid sequences of two proteinase inhibitor homologues from *Dendroaspis augusticeps* venom. *Hoppe-Seyler's Z. Physiol. Chem.* **361:** 661.

Kato, I. and N. Tominaga. 1979. Trypsin-subtilisin inhibitor from red sea turtle eggwhite consists of two tandem domains—one Kunitz—one of a new family. *Fed. Proc.* **38:** 832.

Kaumeyer, J.F., J.O. Polazzi, and M.P. Kotick. 1986. The mRNA for a proteinase inhibitor related to the HI-30 domain of inter-α-trypsin inhibitor also encodes α-1-microglobulin (protein HC). *Nucleic Acids Res.* **14:** 7839.

Kelly, R.B. 1985. Pathways of protein secretion in eukaryotes. *Science* **230:** 25.

Kingston, I.B. and S. Anderson. 1986. Sequences encoding two trypsin inhibitors occur in strikingly similar environments. *Biochem. J.* **233:** 443.

Kondo, K., K. Narita, and C.-Y. Lee. 1978. Amino acid sequences of the two polypeptide chains in β[1]-bungarotoxin from the venom of *Bungarus multicinctus. J. Biochem.* **83:** 101.

Kondo, K., H. Toda, K. Narita, and C.-Y. Lee. 1982. Amino acid sequence of β[2]-bungarotoxin from *Bungarus multicinctus* venom. The amino acid substitutions in the B chains. *J. Biochem.* **91:** 1519.

Korneluk, R.G., D.J. Mahuran, K. Neote, M.H. Klavins, B.F. O'Dowd, M. Tropak, H.F. Willard, M.-J. Anderson, J.A. Lowden, and R.A. Gravel. 1986. Isolation of cDNA clones coding for the α-subunit of human β-hexosaminidase. Extensive homology between the α- and β-subunits and studies on Tay-Sachs disease. *J. Biol. Chem.* **261:** 8407.

Laskowski, M., Jr., I. Kato, W. Ardelt, J. Cook, A. Denton, M.W. Empie, W.J. Kohr, S.J. Park, K. Parks, B.L. Schatzley, O.L. Schoenberger, M. Tashiro, G. Vichot, H.E. Whatley, A. Wieczorek, and M. Wieczorek. 1987. Ovomucoid third domains from 100 avian species: Isolation, sequences, and hypervariability of enzyme-inhibitor contact residues. *Biochemistry* **26:** 202.

Ledeboer, A.M., L. Edens, J. Maat, C. Visser, J.W. Bos, and C.T. Verrips. 1985. Molecular cloning and characterization of a gene coding for methanol oxidase in *Hansenula polymorpha. Nucleic Acids Res.* **13:** 3063.

Liu, C.-S., T.-C. Wu, and T.-B. Lo. 1983. Complete amino acid sequences of two protease inhibitors in the venom of *Bungarus fasciatus*. *Int. J. Pept. Protein Res.* **21:** 209.

Michels, P.A.M., A. Poliszczak, K.A. Osinga, O. Misset, J. Van Beeumen, R.K. Wierenga, P. Borst, and F.R. Opperdoes. 1986. Two tandemly linked identical genes code for the glycosomal glyceraldehyde-phosphate dehydrogenase in *Trypanosoma brucei*. *EMBO J.* **5:** 1049.

Munro, S. and H.R.B. Pelham. 1986. An hsp70-like protein in the ER: Identity with the 78 kd glucose-regulated protein and immunoglobulin heavy chain binding protein. *Cell* **46:** 291.

———. 1987. A C-terminal signal prevents secretion of luminal ER proteins. *Cell* **48:** 899.

Myerowitz, R., R. Piekarz, E.F. Neufeld, T.B. Shows, and K. Suzuki. 1985. Human β-hexosaminidase α chain: Coding sequence and homology with the β chain. *Proc. Natl. Acad. Sci.* **82:** 7830.

Nguyen, T., M. Zelechowska, V. Foster, H. Bergmann, and D.P.S. Verma. 1985. Primary structure of the soybean nodulin-35 gene encoding uricase II localized in the peroxisomes of uninfected cells of nodules. *Proc. Natl. Acad. Sci.* **82:** 5040.

Nishimura, Y., M.G. Rosenfeld, G. Kreibich, U. Gubler, D.D. Sabatini, M. Adesnik, and R. Andy. 1986. Nucleotide sequence of rat preputial gland β-glycuronidase cDNA and *in vitro* insertion of its encoded polypeptide into microsomal membranes. *Proc. Natl. Acad. Sci.* **83:** 7292.

Okazaki, K., T. Takechi, N. Kambara, S. Fukui, I. Kubota, and T. Kamiryo. 1986. Two acyl-coenzyme A oxidases in peroxisomes of the yeast *Candida tropicalis*: Primary structures deduced from genomic DNA sequence. *Proc. Natl. Acad. Sci.* **83:** 1232.

Osinga, K.A., B.W. Swinkels, W.C. Gibson, P. Borst, G.H. Veeneman, J.H. Van Boom, P.A.M. Michels, and F.R. Opperdoes. 1985. Topogenesis of microbody enzymes: A sequence comparison of the genes for the glycosomal (microbody) and cytosolic phosphoglycerate kinases of *Trypanosoma brucei*. *EMBO J.* **4:** 3811.

Osumi, T., N. Ishii, M. Hijikata, K. Kamijo, H. Ozasa, S. Furuta, S. Miyazawa, K. Kondo, K. Inoue, H. Kagamiyama, and T. Hashimoto. 1985. Molecular cloning and nucleotide sequence of the cDNA for rat peroxisomal enoyl-CoA: hydratase-3-hydroxyacyl-CoA dehydrogenase bifunctional enzyme. *J. Biol. Chem.* **260:** 8905.

Owada, M. and E.F. Neufeld. 1982. Is there a mechanism for introducing acid hydrolases into liver lysosomes that is independent of mannose 6-phosphate recognition? Evidence from I-cell disease. *Biochem. Biophys. Res. Commun.* **105:** 814.

Peters, T., Jr. and L.K. Davidson. 1982. The biosynthesis of rat serum albumin. *In vivo* studies on the formation of the disulfide bonds. *J. Biol. Chem.* **257:** 8847.

Quan, F., R.G. Korneluk, M.B. Tropak, and R.A. Gravel. 1986. Isolation and characterization of the human catalase gene. *Nucleic Acids Res.* **14:** 5321.

Ritonja, A., B. Meloun, and F. Gubensek. 1983a. The primary structure of *Vipera ammodytes* venom chymotrypsin inhibitor. *Biochim. Biophys. Acta* **746:** 138.

———. 1983b. The primary structure of *Vipera ammodytes* venom trypsin inhibitor I. *Biochim. Biophys. Acta* **748:** 429.

Ronchi, S., L. Minchiotti, M. Galliano, B. Curti, R.P. Swenson, C.H. Williams, Jr., and V. Massey. 1982. Primary structure of D-amino acid oxidase from pig kidney. II. Isolation and sequence of overlap peptides and the complete sequence. *J. Biol. Chem.* **257:** 8824.

Ruhlmann, A., D. Kukla, P. Schwager, K. Bartels, and R. Huber. 1973. Structure of the complex formed by bovine trypsin and bovine pancreatic trypsin inhibitor. *J. Mol. Biol.* **77:** 417.

Sasaki, T. 1984. Amino acid sequence of a novel Kunitz-type chymotrypsin inhibitor from hemolymph of silkworm larvae, *Bombyx mori*. *FEBS Lett.* **168:** 227.

Schwartz, T.W. 1986. The processing of peptide precursors. Proline-directed arginyl cleavage and other monobasic processing mechanisms. *FEBS Lett.* **200:** 1.

Shibahara, S., Y. Tomita, T. Sakakura, C. Nager, B. Chaudhuri, and R. Muller. 1986. Cloning and expression of cDNA encoding mouse tyrosinase. *Nucleic Acids Res.* **14:** 2413.

Shikimi, T. and T. Kobayashi. 1980. Production of antibody to aprotinin and location of this compound in bovine tissue. *J. Pharmacobio-Dyn.* **3:** 400.

Siekmann, J., H. Tschesche, H.R. Wenzel, E. Rauenbusch, W. Schröder, H. Schutt, and E. Truscheit. 1986. Naturally occurring isoinhibitors and chemically or enzymatically modified derivatives of bovine trypsin inhibitor (Kunitz)—Separation and characterization by high performance ion-exchange chromatography. *Biol. Chem. Hoppe-Seyler* **367:** 92.

Sorger, P.K. and H.R.B. Pelham. 1987. The glucose-regulated protein grp94 is related to heat shock protein hsp90. *J. Mol. Biol.* **194:** 341.

Steiner, D.F., S.J. Chan, J.M. Welsh, and S.C.M. Kwok. 1985. Structure and evolution of the insulin gene. *Annu. Rev. Genet.* **19:** 463.

Strydom, D.J. 1973. Protease inhibitors as snake venom toxins. *Nat. New Biol.* **243:** 88.

Strydom, D.J. and F.J. Joubert. 1981. The amino acid sequence of a weak trypsin inhibitor B from *Dendroaspis polylepis polylepis* (black mamba) venom. *Hoppe-Seyler's Z. Physiol. Chem.* **362:** 1377.

Swinkels, B.W., W.C. Gibson, K.A. Osinga, R. Kramer, G.H. Veeneman, J.H. Van Boom, and P. Borst. 1986. Characterization of the gene for the microbody (glycosomal) triosephosphate isomerase of *Trypanosoma brucei*. *EMBO J.* **5:** 1291.

Takahashi, H., S. Iwanaga, T. Kitagawa, Y. Hokama, and T. Suzuki. 1974. Snake venom proteinase inhibitors. II. Chemical structure of inhibitor II isolated from the venom of Russell's viper (*Vipera russelli*). *J. Biochem.* **76:** 721.

Tschesche, H. and T. Dietl. 1975. The amino-acid sequence of isoinhibitor K from snails (*Helix pomatia*). *Eur. J. Biochem.* **58:** 439.

von Heijne, G. 1986. A new method for predicting signal sequence cleavage sites. *Nucleic Acids Res.* **14:** 4683.

Waheed, A., R. Pohlmann, A. Hasilik, K. von Figura, A. van Elsen, and J.G. Leroy. 1982. Deficiency of UDP-N-acetylglucosamine:lysosomal enzyme N-acetylglucosamine-1-phosphotransferase in organs of I-cell patients. *Biochem. Biophys. Res. Commun.* **105:** 1052.

Wlodawer, A., J. Deisenhofer, and R. Huber. 1987. Comparison of two highly refined structures of bovine pancreatic trypsin inhibitor. *J. Mol. Biol.* **193:** 145.

Wu, T.T. and E.A. Kabat. 1970. An analysis of the sequences of the variable regions of Bence-Jones proteins and myeloma light chains and their implications for antibody complementarity. *J. Exp. Med.* **132:** 211.

Wunderer, G., L. Beress, W. Machleidt, and H. Fritz. 1976. Broad-specificity inhibitors from sea anemones. *Methods Enzymol.* **45:** 881.

The Design of a Four-helix Bundle Protein

W.F. DeGrado, L. Regan, and S.P. Ho

E.I. du Pont de Nemours and Company, Central Research and Development Department, Wilmington, Delaware 19898

The design of proteins with predetermined structural properties is a necessary first step in the de novo design of novel enzymes and receptors. A major problem associated with the design of proteins is the high flexibility inherent in polypeptide chains. It has been estimated that a protein of 100 residues can adopt up to 10^{100} different conformations, a number that is as large as the number of atoms in the universe (Creighton 1984)! The mechanism by which a protein adopts a relatively well-defined set of conformations out of such a large number of possibilities is only beginning to be understood, and it is not possible to predict the three-dimensional structure of a protein from its amino acid sequence.

Recently, the protein folding problem has been rephrased in light of the ease with which one can now prepare proteins of virtually any amino acid sequence (Drexler 1981; Pabo 1983). If it is not possible to predict the three-dimensional structure of a protein from its sequence, might it not be possible to do just the inverse? Could one begin with a reasonable three-dimensional structure and then design a peptide sequence that would fold into this structure? We think that this should be possible if a design is chosen that is relatively simple and rich in secondary structural elements. The design of protein secondary structures has become fairly straightforward. It has long been known that certain amino acids have clear-cut preferences for adopting a given secondary structure (Chou and Fasman 1978), and more recent studies with synthetic peptides have shown the importance of hydrophobic periodicity (Eisenberg et al. 1984; DeGrado and Lear 1985) and electrostatic interactions (Shoemaker et al. 1987) in determining the stability of α helices and β sheets. Thus, it is now routinely possible to design peptides that incorporate single secondary structural units (Kaiser and Kezdy 1984; O'Neil et al. 1987). A logical next step would be to design secondary structures that can pack together to form a globular protein with a predetermined three-dimensional structure. In this paper, we will describe our progress along these lines toward the design of a synthetic four-helix bundle protein.

Our designed protein (Eisenberg et al. 1986; Ho and DeGrado 1987) is an idealized version (Fig. 1) of a class of proteins that includes myohemerythrin, apoferritin, tobacco mosaic virus coat protein, and cytochrome c' (Weber and Salemme 1980). These proteins contain a common four-helix bundle structural motif that is comprised of four helices connected by three loops. The helices in the bundle are nearly an-

tiparallel to one another with a slight tilt of about 20°. As a result of this tilt, the helices diverge from a point of closest approach, forming a cavity that can ac-

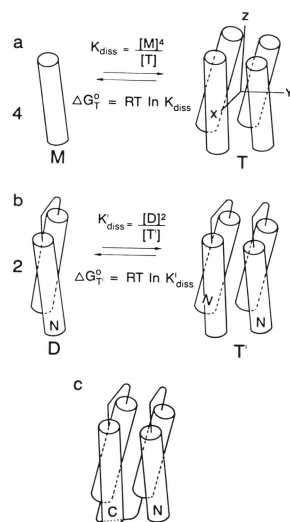

Figure 1. An incremental approach to the design of a four-helix bundle protein. (*a*) The sequence of an amphiphilic helix is designed with the aim of obtaining stable tetrameric aggregates in solution. (*b*) Once the sequence of the helix has been optimized, sequences for the loops are evaluated. Using the best helix sequence obtained in step *a*, various designed loop sequences are evaluated on the basis of the stability of the resulting dimer of helical hairpins. (*c*) The ultimate four-helix bundle is constructed from four optimized helices and three optimized loops. Dissociation constants and free energies are experimentally determined as a measure of the stability of the tetramers and dimers.

commodate binuclear iron in myohemerythrin or a heme in cytochrome c'. The formation of cavities near the end of the bundles appears to be quite a general attribute of this folding pattern (Weber and Salemme 1980), making this motif an attractive target for understanding protein folding as well as for the eventual design of synthetic binding sites. In our approach to the design of a four-helix bundle, we decided to first make a fairly short bundle in which the helices were too short to diverge very far from one another. At a later date we intend to extend the helices from one side of the bundle to form a cavity that could be lined with appropriate side chains for binding and catalysis.

Chothia and co-workers (Chothia et al. 1977; Chothia 1984) have proposed a very simple hypothesis to account for the observed geometry of the helical packing in four-helix bundles as well as the stability of these structures. They observed a regularity in the packing of the side chains that comprise the solvent inaccessible core of four-helix bundles. Residues at positions $i - 4$, i, and $i + 4$ appear to form a ridge that packs against residues at positions $k - 3$, k, and $k + 3$ on a neighboring helix. This defines the packing angle between neighboring helices and allows tight packing of the apolar side chains, thereby driving the folding process. Electrostatic interactions between helical macrodipoles (Sheridan et al. 1982) are also thought to contribute to the stability of the structure. Finally, the loops between the helices probably serve to stabilize the structure.

In our design of a four-helix bundle protein (Eisenberg et al. 1986; Ho and DeGrado 1987), we idealized the pseudo 2,2,2 symmetry that is found in the structures of natural four-helix bundle proteins (Weber and Salemme 1980). This provided two distinct advantages over other approaches to protein design (Moser et al. 1983; B.W. Erickson et al., pers. comm.). First, the modeling was significantly simplified; rather than designing an entire protein, it was only necessary to design a single helix, which, upon application of a 2,2,2 symmetry operator, would adopt a structure with a tightly packed interior. Second, the design of the protein could be approached in the iterative, experimental manner described in Figure 1. The first step of this approach involved the evaluation of single helices that self-assemble into homotetramers. The free energy for the self-assembly process could be conveniently monitored from the monomer-to-tetramer equilibrium constant. Evaluation of several different designs allowed optimization of the helical sequence. In the next step of the project, loops were inserted between two identical helical sequences in an attempt to prepare a helical hairpin that would assemble into a four-helix bundle, as shown in Figure 1b. Finally, the entire sequence for the four-helix bundle was prepared by connecting four identical helices with three identical loops.

Methods and Experimental Procedures

The synthesis and characterization of peptides 1–4 were reported previously (Eisenberg et al. 1986; Ho and DeGrado 1987).

DNA oligonucleotides were synthesized on an Applied Biosystems DNA synthesizer and on a Coder 300 (du Pont) DNA synthesizer. The oligonucleotides were purified by excision and elution from denaturing polyacrylamide gels (Maniatis et al. 1982) followed by C18 (Sep-Pac, Waters) chromatography. Restriction enzymes and DNA-modifying enzymes were purchased from New England Biolabs, Bethesda Research Laboratories, and Pharmacia. They were used according to the manufacturers' specifications. *Escherichia coli* protein extraction and Western blot analyses were performed as described previously (Burnette 1981; Regan et al. 1986).

Results

Design of the helical sequence. The design of the helical sequence was first accomplished using physical models (Eisenberg et al. 1986; Ho and DeGrado 1987). Models of four 16-residue helices were arranged so that their side chains could interact in a manner similar to that described by Chothia (1984) for a four-helix bundle. Leu side chains were placed at positions that project into the interior of the structure, and Glu and Lys side chains were placed at positions projecting toward the exterior of the structure. All three of these residues are known to strongly favor helix formation (Chou and Fasman 1978). In addition, glycine residues were placed at the amino and carboxyl termini of the structure to help break the helix and also to help induce the formation of a turn when the loops were added at a later stage. The resulting structure, peptide 1, was synthesized by the Merrifield solid phase method. A fragment comprising the 12 carboxy-terminal residues of peptide 1 was also isolated during the purification. This peptide (1a) was found to form tetramers in aqueous solution (Eisenberg et al. 1986). A subsequent analysis (Ho and DeGrado 1987) of a model of peptide 1 suggested that its sequence could be improved. In models, the Leu residue at position 11 appeared to be excessively exposed to solvent, and the Glu residue at position 13 was partially buried. Consequently, Leu was changed to Lys at position 11 and Glu was changed to Leu at position 13. In addition, it appeared likely that the Lys at position 2 of peptide 1 and the α-carboxylate at the carboxyl terminus might interact unfavorably with the helical macrodipole. Therefore, these were converted to a Glu and an α-carboxamide, respectively. The resulting peptide (2) should form a more stable tetramer if the model is correct.

The assembly of the above peptides into tetramers could be assessed by circular dichroism (CD) spectroscopy. In very dilute aqueous solution the peptides are monomers and show low helicity. In concentrated solutions, they form tetramers in which the peptides form helices that are stabilized by long-range interactions between the apolar side chains. These conformational changes are reflected in the CD spectra of the peptides. The concentration dependence of the spectra are extremely well described by a simple monomer-to-tetramer equilibrium (Fig. 2). Analysis of these curves

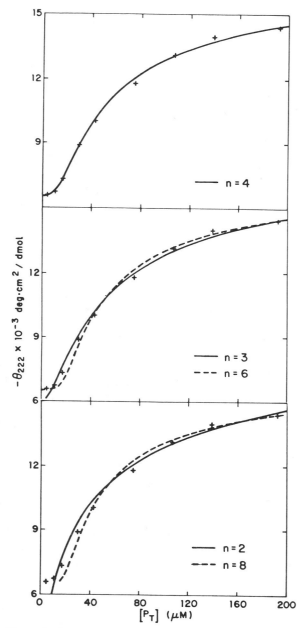

Figure 2. Concentration dependence of the ellipticity of $\alpha_1 A$ at 222 nm. The lines are computer-generated, theoretical curves describing various monomer-n-mer equilibria. (*Top*) Monomer-tetramer equilibrium, (*middle*) monomer-trimer and monomer-hexamer equilibria, and (*bottom*) monomer-dimer and monomer-octamer equilibria. The data are optimally fit by a cooperative monomer-to-tetramer equilibrium.

provides three useful parameters: the stability of the tetramers ($RT \ln K_{diss}$) and the approximate helical contents of the monomeric and tetrameric forms of the peptides (Table 1). Peptide 2 was found to form such stable tetramers that it was necessary to measure the monomer-to-tetramer equilibrium at various guanidine hydrochloride concentrations and then extrapolate the values of these parameters to zero guanidine concentration.

The helical content of the monomeric form depended markedly on the peptide chain length; the 12-residue peptide 1a was approximately 15% helical as a monomer, whereas the 16-residue peptides 1 and 2 were approximately 30% helical. The helical content for the tetrameric form of all three of these peptides was approximately 70%. The stabilities of the tetramers depended both on chain length and sequence and were in accord with the predictions based on computer modeling; peptide 1a was the least stable, followed by peptide 1, with peptide 2 being the most stable. The tetramer of peptide 2 was stabilized by approximately 20 kcal/mol. This large value shows that the sequence of peptide 2 is well designed for forming helical tetramers.

The design of a helical hairpin. We next attempted to design a hairpin loop that would connect two molecules of peptide 2 in a head-to-tail manner. Examination of models of tetramers of peptide 2 suggested that the ends could be joined by a single Pro if the helices were slightly unwound. Thus, peptide 3, which contains two copies of peptide 2 connected by a single Pro residue, was synthesized. Size exclusion chromatography of this peptide indicated that it was forming trimers rather than the desired dimer of helical hairpins. Operating under the assumption that the trimer formed by peptide 3 had a conformation similar to that illustrated in Figure 3, we proceeded to introduce substitutions that should destabilize the trimeric conformer with respect to the desired dimeric conformer. Two Arg residues were therefore inserted directly after the Pro with the expectation that this should electrostatically destabilize the trimer. Now, if a trimer were to form, the Arg residues from neighboring peptides would be buried together near the center of the trimer structure, thus resulting in unfavorable electrostatic interactions. Indeed, peptide 4 (Table 1) appeared to form dimers rather than trimers, as assessed by size exclusion chromatography. In addition, the concentration dependence of the CD spectra for this peptide indicated that peptide 4 was in a monomer-to-dimer equilibrium.

Peptide 4 has been substantially stabilized toward guanidine hydrochloride denaturation as compared to peptide 2. At approximately equal peptide concentrations, about twice as much guanidine hydrochloride is required to unfold peptide 4 as is required to unfold peptide 2 (Fig. 4). This success notwithstanding, a detailed analysis of the thermodynamic data for peptide 4 suggests that it might be possible to further optimize the loop sequence to provide an even more stable protein. The dimers of peptide 4 are stabilized with respect to their unfolded monomers by approximately 13 kcal/mol. Comparison of this number with that for the tetramers of peptide 2 indicates that the loop sequence could be substantially improved (Ho and De-Grado 1987).

Design of a gene encoding peptide 5. The gene for peptide 5 was constructed from eight synthetic DNA oligonucleotides. It was cloned into the vector pTM201/NS3-3 (K. Knight and R.T. Sauer, in prep.)

Table 1. Amino Acid Sequences and Free Energies of Tetramerization or Dimerization of Synthetic Peptides

Peptide	Sequence	$RT \ln K_{diss}$ (kcal/mol)
1[1]	Ac-GluLeuLeuLysLysLeuLeuGluGluLeuLysGly-COOH	−11.4
2[1]	Ac-GlyLysLeuGluGluLeuLeuLysLysLeuLeuGluGluLeuLysGly-COOH	−19
3[1]	Ac-GlyGluLeuGluGluGluLeuLeuLysLysLeuLys GluLeuLeuLysGly-CONH₂	−22
4[2]	Ac-GlyGluLeuGluGluGluLeuLeuLysLysLeuLys GluLeuLeuLysGlyProArgArg	
	GlyGluLeuGluGluGluLeuLeuLysLysLeuLys GluLeuLeuLysGly-CONH₂	−13

Data taken from Ho and DeGrado (1987).
[1]Monomer-tetramer equilibria.
[2]Monomer-dimer equilibrium.

at the *NcoI* and *NruI* sites, using standard techniques (Maniatis et al. 1982). This resulted in plasmid pα_4-1 in which peptide 5 is expressed from the inducible *tac* promoter (De Boer et al. 1983). (See Fig. 5.) The gene was designed such that unique restriction sites were introduced at conveniently spaced locations near the end of the helices. This should facilitate the introduction of future changes into peptide 5 by "cassette" mutagenesis (Richards 1986). Restriction analysis confirmed that all sites were indeed present in the synthetic gene.

Expression of peptide 5 in *E. coli* was detected using polyclonal antibodies generated against peptide 4. Western blot analysis (Burnette 1981) of protein extracts from strains containing the synthetic gene showed that peptide 5 was produced in *E. coli* and that its expression was inducible by the addition of isopropyl β-D-thiogalactopyranoside (Fig. 6). Further analysis revealed that the majority of peptide 5 is present in a soluble form within the bacteria. This facilitates protein purification, which is currently in progress.

Discussion

The folding of a protein is a complex process that includes helix formation, helix termination, helix packing, and loop formation. Few of these processes are very well understood, so that it seemed unlikely that a sequence that fulfilled each of these functions could be designed in a single step. Instead, it seemed more prudent to devise an incremental experimental approach, which would allow each aspect of folding to be dissected and optimized separately.

First, consider helix formation as evaluated by the helical contents of the monomeric forms of peptides 1, 1a, and 2. Helix formation by the 12-residue peptide, 1a, is quite unfavorable at room temperature, as it contains about 15% helix in dilute solution. Clearly, it is energetically unfavorable to fold this peptide into a helix, and this decreases the overall stability of the helical tetramers formed by this peptide. In contrast, peptides 1 and 2 show unusually high helical contents (approximately 30%) as monomers in water at room temperature. Few other peptides show this high a degree of monomolecular helix formation at room temperature (Shoemaker et al. 1987). Stabilizing interactions that might account for this high degree of helicity include salt bridges between Glu to Lys side chains (Eisenberg et al. 1986; Ho and DeGrado 1987) and partial dehydration of the apolar side chains in the helical conformation. Also, peptides 1 and 2 both have their amino termini blocked by an acetyl group, which

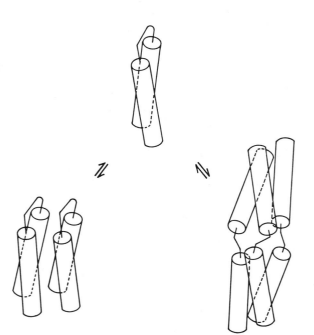

Figure 3. Diagrammatic representation of trimer formation instead of the desired dimer of helical hairpins.

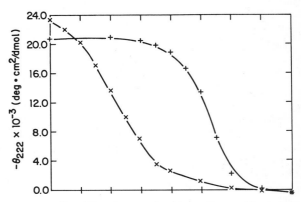

Figure 4. Guanidine denaturation curves for peptides 3 (×) and 4 (+).

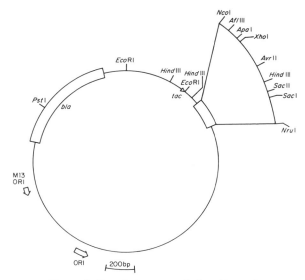

Figure 5. Restriction map of plasmid pα_4-1.

stabilizes helix formation (Shoemaker et al. 1987). If one assumes that helix formation is an all-or-nothing process, then it can be calculated that helix formation by peptides 1 and 2 is only slightly unfavorable and on the order of a single kcal/mol. In any case, it appears that the sequences of peptides 1 and 2 have been well designed from the point of view of allowing helix formation to occur at a low energetic cost.

Peptide 2 forms more stable tetramers than peptide 1, which indicates that the packing interactions must be more favorable for peptide 2. (Both peptides have equal helicities as monomers, which suggests that helix formation is approximately energetically equivalent for both peptides.) This is in agreement with our computer modeling, which suggests that peptide 2 should form a more stable tetramer than peptide 1. The observed free energy of tetramerization of peptide 2 is consistent with dehydration of the apolar side chains being the driving force for folding. The observed free energy corresponds to −0.8 to −0.9 kcal/(mol of Leu side chains) in reasonable agreement with the value of −1.2 estimated for the transfer of a Leu side chain from water to the interior of a protein (Guy 1985).

Helix formation and loop formation appeared to be a problem in the design of peptide 3. Based on hydrodynamic measurements, it seemed likely that this peptide was forming trimers of extended rods rather than dimers of folded helical hairpins. The ease with which this problem was isolated and remedied clearly demonstrates the value of approaching the design of proteins in an iterative, experimental manner. It also illustrates an important point that must be considered in the design of new proteins. *Natural proteins have evolved not only to stabilize a given, desired fold, but also to destabilize all other possible alternatives.* A would-be designer of proteins must do no less if he or she is to succeed. One must try to consider all alternatives to the desired, designed fold and selectively destabilize the alternative folding pathways.

The hydrodynamic and thermodynamic data described herein provide excellent evidence to suggest that we have succeeded in designing proteins that are composed of four α helices. However, we cannot presently conclude that the helices are arranged into a four-helix bundle as illustrated in Figure 1. An elucidation of the helical packing geometry must await the solution of the crystal structures of peptides 1–5. Crystals of peptide 1a have been grown and diffract to high resolution (Eisenberg et al. 1986).

In the near future, we hope to purify and examine the properties of the single-chain four-helix peptide 5. If it can be shown to form a four-helix bundle, we will next try to convert it to a ligand-binding protein. By extending the helices one to two turns it should be possible to create a cavity capable of binding small, apolar compounds. The loops between the helices provide a natural location for adding catalytic groupings, including metal-binding sites. The locations of the restriction sites in the gene encoding peptide 5 should facilitate these manipulations.

ACKNOWLEDGMENTS

We thank Professor David Eisenberg for his collaboration and for many helpful discussions. We thank K. Knight and R. Sauer for a gift of plasmid pTM201/NS3-3. We thank Dan Oprian and Zelda Wasserman for helpful advice on various aspects of this work. We also thank K. Smithyman for his technical assistance throughout this work, and Carol Farber for preparing the manuscript.

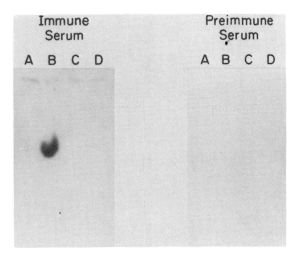

Figure 6. Western blot analysis of *E. coli* protein extracts. (Lane *A*) Extract from strain X-90 with plasmid pα_4-1 grown in uninduced conditions. (Lane *B*) Extract from strain X-90 with plasmid pα_4-1 grown with 5 mM isopropyl-β-D-thio-galactopyranoside. (Lane *C*) Extract from strain X-90 with the vector pTM201/NS3-3 grown in uninduced conditions. (Lane *D*) Extract from strain X-90 with the vector pTM201/NS3-3 in induced conditions. Left panel shows the filter probed with antipeptide 4 immune serum. Right panel shows the filter probed with preimmune serum.

REFERENCES

Burnette, W.W. 1981. Western blotting: Electrophoretic transfer of proteins from sodium dodecyl sulphate-polyacrylamide gels to unmodified nitrocellulose and radiographic detection with antibody and radioiodinated protein A. *Anal. Biochem.* **112**: 195.

Chothia, C. 1984. Principles that determine the structure of proteins. *Annu. Rev. Biochem.* **53**: 537.

Chothia, C., M. Levitt, and D. Richardson. 1977. Structure of proteins: Packing of α-helices and β-pleated sheets. *Proc. Natl. Acad. Sci.* **74**: 4130.

Chou, P.Y. and G.D. Fasman. 1978. Prediction of the secondary structure of proteins from their amino acid sequence. *Adv. Enzymol.* **47**: 45.

Creighton, T.E. 1984. *Proteins,* p. 161. W.H. Freeman, New York.

DeBoer, H.A., L.J. Comstock, and M. Vasser. 1983. The *tac* promoter: A functional hybrid derived from the *trp* and *lac* promoters. *Proc. Natl. Acad. Sci.* **80**: 21.

DeGrado, W.F. and J.D. Lear. 1985. Induction of peptide conformation at apolar/water interfaces: A study with peptides of defined hydrophobic periodicity. *J. Am. Chem. Soc.* **107**: 7684.

Drexler, K.E. 1981. Molecular engineering: An approach to the development of general capabilities for molecular manipulation. *Proc. Natl. Acad. Sci.* **78**: 5275.

Eisenberg, D., R.M. Weiss, and T.C. Terwilliger. 1984. The hydrophobic moment detects periodicity in protein hydrophobicity. *Proc. Natl. Acad. Sci.* **81**: 140.

Eisenberg, D., W. Wilcox, S.M. Eshita, P.M. Pryciak, S.P. Ho, and W.F. DeGrado. 1986. Design, synthesis and crystallization of a helical peptide. *Proteins Struct. Funct. Genet.* **1**: 16.

Guy, H.R. 1985. Amino acid side-chain partition energies and distribution of residues in solution. *Biophys. J.* **47**: 61.

Ho, S.P. and W.F. DeGrado. 1987. Design of a four-helix bundle: Synthesis of peptides which self-associate into a helical protein. *J. Am. Chem. Soc.* (in press).

Kaiser, E.T. and F.J. Kézdy. 1984. Amphiphilic secondary structure: Design of peptide hormones. *Science* **24**: 639.

Maniatis, T., E.F. Fritsch, and J. Sambrook. 1982. *Molecular cloning: A laboratory manual.* Cold Spring Harbor Laboratory, Cold Spring Harbor, New York.

Moser, R., R.M. Thomas, and B. Gutte. 1983. An artifical crystalline DDT-binding polypeptide. *FEBS Lett.* **157**: 247.

O'Neil, K.T., H.R. Wolfe, Jr., S. Erickson-Viitanen, and W.F. DeGrado. 1987. Alpha-helical periodicity reflected in the fluorescence properties of calmodulin-binding peptides. *Science* **236**: 1454.

Pabo, C.O. 1983. Molecular technology: Designing peptides and proteins. *Nature* **301**: 200.

Regan, L., J.D. Dignam, and P. Schimmel. 1986. A bacterial and silkworm enzyme share a common epitope which maps to the catalytic domain of each. *J. Biol. Chem.* **261**: 5241.

Richards, J.H. 1986. Cassette mutagenesis shows its strength. *Nature* **323**: 187.

Sheridan, R.P., R.M. Levy, and F.R. Salemme. 1982. α-Helix dipole model and electrostatic stabilization of 4-α-helical proteins. *Proc. Natl. Acad. Sci.* **79**: 4545.

Shoemaker, K.R., P.S. Kim, E.V. York, J.M. Stewart, and R.L. Baldwin. 1987. Tests for the helix dipole model for stabilization of α-helices. *Nature* **326**: 563.

Weber, P.C. and F.R. Salemme. 1980. Structural and functional diversity in 4-α-helical proteins. *Nature* **287**: 82.

The Serpins: Evolution and Adaptation in a Family of Protease Inhibitors

R.W. Carrell,* P.A. Pemberton,[†] and D.R. Boswell*

*Department of Haematological Medicine and [†]Medical Research Council, M.I.T.I. Unit,
University of Cambridge, Cambridge, CB2 2QL, United Kingdom

The serpins are a superfamily of serine protease inhibitors that have undergone divergent evolution over a period of some 600 million years (Hunt and Dayhoff 1980; Carrell and Boswell 1986). The best-studied member of the family is the human plasma protein α_1-antitrypsin (Carrell et al. 1982), which is now known to function primarily as an inhibitor of leucocyte elastase and for this reason is alternatively named α_1-proteinase inhibitor (Travis and Salvesen 1983). Here we will retain the historical name abbreviated to antitrypsin.

Antitrypsin is a characteristic member of the serpins in that it is a single-chain glycoprotein of near 400 residues that functions by forming a tight 1:1 complex with its cognate protease, neutrophil (leucocyte) elastase. This complex slowly dissociates to yield active enzyme and inactive cleaved inhibitor. The crystallographic structure of post-complex antitrypsin has been determined by Loebermann et al. (1984) and shown to be a highly ordered globular molecule with 40% as pleated sheets and 30% as α helices. The reactive center of the serpins is typically formed by an X-Ser that acts as a substrate for the target protease, hence antitrypsin has a Met-Ser reactive center with the methionine providing a putative cleavage site for neutrophil elastase.

An unexpected finding in the crystallographic structure of the postcomplex antitrypsin is the separation of its reactive center methionine and serine to opposite poles of the molecule at a distance of 70 Å. To reconstruct the native inhibitor by rejoining the Met-Ser, it is necessary to withdraw a central strand from the major pleated sheet of the molecule to form a stretched loop of some 16 residues. This exposed and stretched loop (Fig. 1) places the reactive center in an accessible position with probable distortion of the Met-Ser bond. It is likely that in this way the neutrophil elastase is presented with an ideal substrate that fits precisely into its active center to give stable complex formation between enzyme and inhibitor.

A consequence of the strain imposed by the stretched loop is that the native molecule is in a stressed, somewhat unstable (S) form. Cleavage of the reactive center loop of the native serpins will predictably give a stable conformation as the strain is relieved and the molecule takes up a relaxed (R) form (Carrell and Owen 1985). Thus the crystallization of antitrypsin by Loebermann and colleagues required conversion to the R form, a recapitulation of the much earlier experience of the Carlsberg group (Linderstrom-Lang 1952) who found that another serpin, ovalbumin, could only be crystallized after similar cleavage to the stable plakalbumin.

In this paper we provide evidence from alignments that all of the 19 serpins whose sequences are currently known share the same overall tertiary structure. However, even closely related members of the family share little more than 30% common sequence, so the question arises as to why evolution has resulted in such diversity of composition. The answer does not appear to be just the need to provide specialized inhibitory activity. This point will be considered in greater detail in the discussion but can be illustrated here by the example shown in Figure 2 of the single mutation of the methionine at the reactive center of antitrypsin to an arginine, to give a complete switch in inhibitory activity from inhibition of elastase to inhibition of thrombin (Owen et al. 1983). This primary dependence of inhibitory activity on the reactive center P_1 residue, or more correctly on the P_1-P_2 residues, has been repeatedly confirmed by subsequent site-specific recombinant mutants of antitrypsin (Table 1) (Rosenberg et al. 1984; Jallat et al. 1986). Thus, the need for inhibitory specificity explains only a proportion of the sequence diversity of the serpins, and a significant contribution appears to arise from subsidiary functions of the molecule. This is true of the unstructured amino terminus of the serpins, which shows an almost complete loss of

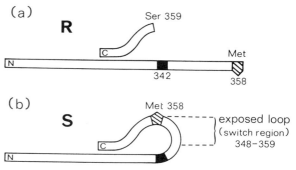

Figure 1. The structure of the serpins is based on the relaxed (R) form of antitrypsin shown diagrammatically (*a*). The native stressed (S) form has to be reconstituted by a deduced exposed loop that hinges near residue 342 (*b*). This loop is accessible to proteases and acts as an irreversible switch, as well as a putative substrate for the target protease.

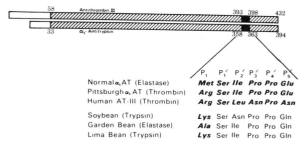

	P_1	P_1'	P_2'	P_3'	P_4'	P_5'
Normal α₁AT (Elastase)	**Met**	**Ser**	**Ile**	**Pro**	**Pro**	**Glu**
Pittsburgh α₁AT (Thrombin)	**Arg**	**Ser**	**Ile**	**Pro**	**Pro**	**Glu**
Human AT-III (Thrombin)	**Arg**	**Ser**	**Leu**	**Asn**	**Pro**	**Asn**
Soybean (Trypsin)	**Lys**	Ser	Asn	Pro	Pro	Gln
Garden Bean (Elastase)	**Ala**	Ser	Ile	Pro	Pro	Gln
Lima Bean (Trypsin)	**Lys**	Ser	Ile	Pro	Pro	Gln

Figure 2. Amino acid sequences of antitrypsin with 394 residues and antithrombin with 432 residues. The sequences can be aligned to give a 30% identity in structure over most of their length (hatched area). This brings in alignment the reactive centers of both molecules (solid area). These centers are compared with the known reactive centers of plant proteinase inhibitors. The P_1 residue acts as a bait that determines the specificity of enzyme inhibition as indicated. The change in this P_1 position from a methionine to an arginine in antitrypsin Pittsburgh explains the change in inhibitory specificity from elastase to thrombin.

homology reflecting its varied roles; for example, as a peptide donor in angiotensinogen (Kageyama et al. 1984) and as an allosteric binding site in antithrombin (Owen et al. 1987). Another subsidiary domain we will consider in more detail here is the exposed loop sequence flanking the amino-terminal aspect of the reactive center. In particular, evidence will be given of the way that evolution has modified the sequence to provide a proteolytic switch for the S–R transition. In the case of the plasma serpins this allows the leucocyte to control inhibitory activity at foci of inflammation.

This ability to undergo a profound molecular transition during inflammation may explain why the tertiary structure of the serpin molecule has been faithfully retained during evolution, even in those members of the family that have lost their inhibitory activity and have evolved seemingly more trivial (in a biochemical sense) functions. Examples are angiotensinogen, which has almost certainly no inhibitory activity but functions as a donor of the octapeptide angiotensin, and thyroxine-binding globulin, which acts as a carrier of the small di-tyrosyl derivative, thyroxine (Flink et al. 1986).

METHODS

Sequence alignment. Alignment of the serpins was carried out using the Needleman-Wunsch algorithm with modification to penalize insertion of gaps in regions of defined secondary structure (Lesk et al. 1986). References to sequence data of members of the superfamily are given in the legend of Figure 3.

Enzymes and reagents. Benzoyl-arginyl-ethyl ester, cytocholasin *b*, *N*-formyl-methionyl-leucyl-phenylalanine (fMLP), antitrypsin antisera, porcine pancreatic trypsin, and the snake venom from *Bitis arietan* were supplied by Sigma. C1-inhibitor antiserum was supplied by Atlantic antibodies and antithrombin antiserum by Dakopatts.

Purified human neutrophil elastase (HNE) was a gift from P. George (Pathology Department, Christchurch Clinical School, University of Otago, Christchurch, New Zealand), *Pseudomonas aeruginosa* elastase was a gift from Kaziyuki Morihara (Kyoto Research Laboratories, Tokyo, Japan).

The plasma used for all protein purifications was freshly drawn, made 10 mM in EDTA/benzamidine and frozen at −70°C. For all other assays plasma was either freshly drawn into 10 mM EDTA/benzamidine or had been stored at −70°C for 18 months.

Preparation of serpins. These were isolated from human plasma by chromatography: C1-inhibitor by the method of Harrison (1983), antitrypsin as described by Jeppsson et al. (1985), and antithrombin by the method of McKay (1981). Thyroxine-binding globulin was kindly provided by Dr. M.B. Pepys, Royal Postgraduate Medical School, London.

Protease cleavage of serpins. Cleavage of antithrombin by human neutrophil elastase was carried out as described by Carrell and Owen (1985) at an enzyme:inhibitor ratio of 1:100, in the presence of heparin. Other cleavages, including those by snake venoms, followed the general method of Kress et al. (1983) with enzyme:inhibitor ratios of 1:50 or less.

Human neutrophil isolation and incubation. Human neutrophils were isolated on the day of use from whole blood by Ficoll-Hypaque fractionation and used at 5 × 10⁶ cells/ml in phosphate-buffered saline containing 1 mM MgCl₂, 1 mM CaCl₂, and 5 mM glucose. To a 1-ml aliquot of isolated human neutrophils was added 1 μl of cytocholasin *b*, and the cells were incubated at 37°C for 2 minutes. The tripeptide fMLP (1 μl) was then added and the cells incubated for a further 10 minutes. The cells were spun down and the supernatant removed. C1-inhibitor was diluted with this supernatant to 1 mg/ml and incubated at 37°C for 2 hours. Samples were taken at 15-minute intervals up to 2 hours and assayed for plasmin inhibitory activity, for cleavage products, and for heat stability.

Antithrombin was mixed with a 2:5 times dilution of the stimulated neutrophil supernatant and incubated as for the C1-inhibitor cleavage. Samples were taken and monitored for inactivation by trypsin inhibition, by SDS-PAGE, and by heat stability assays.

Heat stability assays. Native or enzyme-inactivated inhibitors were diluted to 0.2 mg/ml in 75 mM sodium phosphate, 75 mM glycine, and 75 mM Tris (pH 7.5) and heated at 40, 50, 60, 70, 80, 90, and 100°C for 2 hours in screwcap tubes. These samples were centrifuged, filtered, and 3 μl aliquots assayed by rocket immunoelectrophoresis. Similar samples were then heated at 60°C for 2 hours, aliquots taken every 20 minutes and treated as above. The same procedure was carried out with the protease and neutrophil cleaved inhibitor preparations.

Purification of low M_r cleavage fragments. Fragments from the neutrophil enzyme and snake venom digests were separated by reverse-phase high-perfor-

Table 1. Protease-Inhibitor Association Constants: Mutants Compared to Normal Serpins

Serpin $P_2 - P_1 - P_1'$ Protease	Plasma antitrypsin Pro-MET-Ser	Pittsburgh antitrypsin Pro-Arg-Ser	Valine recombinant Pro-Val-Ser	Antithrombin Gly-ARG-Ser	C1-inhibitor Ala-ARG-Thr
Human neutrophil elastase	7×10^7	2×10^3	2×10^7	nil	—
Porcine pancreatic elastase	1×10^5	nil	1×10^6	nil	—
Porcine pancreatic trypsin	4×10^4	7×10^6	nil	2×10^6	—
Human thrombin	5×10^1	3×10^5	nil	1×10^{6} [a]	—
Human kallikrein	7×10^1	1×10^5	—	3×10^6	2×10^4
Human Xa	2×10^2	2×10^4	nil	—	—
Human XIa	7×10^1	1×10^5	—	2×10^2	2×10^2
Human XIIf	nil	8×10^2	—	5×10^1	3×10^4
Human plasmin	2×10^2	2×10^5	nil	1×10^4	1×10^4
Human cathepsin G	4×10^5	2×10^4	7×10^2	nil	—

[a] With heparin.

```
                                    1         2         3         4         5         6         7         8         9         1
                                    0         0         0         0         0         0         0         0         0         0
0
Sequence Number
Secondary Structure
Antitrypsin Human                                                                              mpssvswqilllaqlcclvpvslaEDPQGDAAQKTDTS-
Antitrypsin Baboon                                                                                   lllaglccllpqslaEDPQGDAAQKTDTP-
Antitrypsin Mouse
Heparin Cofactor II       GSKGPLDQLEKGGETAQSADPQWEQLNNKNLSMPLLPADFHKENTVTNDWIPEGEEDDDYLDLEKIFSEDDDYIDIVDSLSVSPTDSDVSAGNIL-
Antithrombin                               mysnvigtvtsgkrkvyllslllligfwdcvtcHGSPVDICTAKPRDIPMNPMCIYRSPEKKATEDEGSEQK-
C1-Inhibitor              NPNATSSSSQDPESLQDRGEGKVATTVISKMLFVEPILEVSSLPTTNSTTNSATKITANTTDEPTTQPTTEPTTQPTIQPTQPTTQLPTDSPTQPTTGS-
Rabbit O R F
Endothelial P A I                                                                            mqmspaltclvlglalvf
Thyroxine B G                                                                     mspflylvllvlglhatihcASPEGKVTA
Antichymo Mouse
Antichymo Human                                                                  mermlpllalgllaagfcpavlchpNSPLDEENLTQE-
Antiplasmin                                                                            NQEQVSPLTLLKLGNQEPGGQTALKSPPGV
Ovalbumin
Gene Y Protein
Placental P A I
Angiotens Rat             mtptgaglkatifciltwvsltagDRVYIHPFHLLYYSKSTCAQLENPSVETLPEPTFEPVPIQAKTSPVDEKTLRDKLVLATEK-
Angiotens Human           mrkrapqsemapagvslratilcllawaglaagDRVYIHPFHLVIHNESTCEQLAKANAGKPKDPTFIPAPIQAKTSPVDEKALQDQLVLVAAK-
Barley Z Protein


                                    1         2         3         4         5         6         7         8         9         2
                                    0         0         0         0         0         0         0         0         0         0
0
Sequence Number
Secondary Structure       !°°°°°°°°°°A°°°°°°°!   !==B6==!°°°°°°°B°°°°°°!  !°°°°°C°°°°°!
Antitrypsin Human         -HHDQDHPTFNKITPNLAEFAFSLYRQLAHQSNS-TNI-FFSPVSIATAFAMLSLGTKADTHDEILEGLNFN-LTEI------------------------
Antitrypsin Baboon        -PHDQNHPTLNKITPSLAEFAFSLYRQLAHQSNS-TNI-FFSPVSIATAFAMLSLGTKADTHSEILEGLNFN-LTEI------------------------
Antitrypsin Mouse
Heparin Cofactor II       -QLFHGKSRIQRLNILNAKFAFNLYRVLKDQVNTFDNI-FIAPVGISTAMGMISLGLKGETHEQVHSILHFKDVFNA-----------------------
Antithrombin              -IPEATNRRVWELSKANSRFATTFYQHLADSKNDNDNI-FLSPLSISTAFAMTKLGACNDTLQQLMEVFKFDTISEK-----------------------
C1-Inhibitor              -FCPGPVTLCSDLESHSTEAVLGDALVDFSLKLY--HA-FSAMKKVETNMAFSPFSIASLLTQVLLGAGQNT-KTNL------------------------
Rabbit O R F                                      MFNVVRVRDIGLWTFRYVYNESDNVVFSPYGLTSALSVL-----------------------
Endothelial P A I         gegsaVHHPPSYVAHLASDFGVRVFQQVAQASKD-RNV-VFSPYGVASVLAMLQLTTGGETQQQIQAAMGFK-----------------------
Thyroxine B G             CHSSQPNATLYKMSSINADFAFNLYRRFTVETPD-KNI-FFSPVSISAALVMLSFGACCSTQTEIVGTLGFN-LTDT------------------------
Antichymo Mouse
Antichymo Human           -NQDRGTHVDLGLASANVDFAFSLYKQLVLKALD-KNV-IFSPLSISTALAFLSLGAHNTTLTEILKASSSP-HGDL------------------------
Antiplasmin               CSRDPTPEQTHRLARAMMAFTADLFSLVAQTS-TCSNL-ILSPLSVALALSHLALGAQNHTLQRLQQVLH-----------------------
Ovalbumin                             mGSIGAASMEFCFDVFKELKVHHAN-ENI-FYCPIAIMSALAMVYLGAKDSTRTQINKVVRFDKLPGF-----------------------
Gene Y Protein            MDSISVTNAKFCFDVFNEMKVHHVN-ENI-LYCPLSILTALAMVYLGARGNTESQMKKVLHFDSITGA-----------------------
Placental P A I           MEDLCVANTLFALNLFKHLAKASPT-QNL-FLSPWSISSTMAMVYMGSRGSTEDQMAKVLQF-NEVGANAVTPMTPENFTSCGFMQQIQKG
Angiotens Rat             -LEAEDRQRAAQVAMIANFMGFRMYKMLSEARGVASGA-VLSPPALFGTLVSFYLGSLDPTASQLQVLLGVPVKEGD-----------------------
Angiotens Human           -LDTEDKLRAAMVGMLANFLGFRIYGMHSELWGVVHGATVLSPTAVFGTLASLYLGALDHTADRLQAILGVPWKDKN
Barley Z Protein


                                    1         2         3         4         5         6         7         8         9         3
                                    0         0         0         0         0         0         0         0         0         0
0
Sequence Number
Secondary Structure       !°°°°°°°D°°°°°°!    !====A2=====!   !°°°°°E°°°°°!===A1==!  !°°°°°°°F°°°°°°!
Antitrypsin Human         ----------PEAQIHEGFQELLRTLNQPDSQ--LQLTTGNGLFLSEGLKLVDKFLEDVKKLYHSE-AFTVNFGD-TEEAKKQINDYVEKGTQGKIVDLV
Antitrypsin Baboon        ----------PEAQVHEGFQELLRTLNKPDSQ--LQLTTGNGLFLNKSLKVVDKFLEDVKNLYHSE-AFSVNFED-TEEAKKQINNYVEKGTQGKVVDLV
Antitrypsin Mouse
Heparin Cofactor II       ------SSKYEITTIHNLFRKLTHRLFRRNFG--YTLRSVNDLYIQKQFPILLDFKTKVREYYFAE-AQIADFSD--PAFISKTNNHIMKLTKGLIKDAL
Antithrombin              ----------TSDQIHFFFAKLNCRLYRKANK--SSKLVSANRLFGDKSLTFNETYQDISELVGYAK-LQPLDFKENAEQSRAAINKWVSNKTEGRITDVI
C1-Inhibitor              ---------ESILSYPKDFTCVHQALKGFTTK----GVTSVSQIFHSPDLAIRDTFVNASRTLYSSS-PRVLSNN--SDANLELINTWVAKNTNNKISRLL
Rabbit O R F              ----------RIAAGGNTKREIDVPESVVEDS--DAFLALRELFVDASVPLRPEFTAEFSSRFNTS-VQRVTFN--SENVKDVINSYVKDKTGGDVPRVL
Endothelial P A I         ----------IDDKGMAPALRHLYKELMGPWNK--DEISTTDAIFVQRDLKLVQGFMPHFFRLRST-VKQVDFSE-VERARFIINDWVKTHTKGMISNLL
Thyroxine B G             ----------PMVEIQHGFQHLICSLNFPKKE--LELQIGNALFIGKHLKPLAKFLNDVKTLYETE-VFSTDFSN-ISAAKQEINSHVEMQTKGKVVGLI
Antichymo Mouse
Antichymo Human           ----------LRQKFTQSFQHLRAPSISSSDE--LQLSMGNAMFVKEQLSLLDRFTEDAKRLYGSE-AFATDFQD-SAAAKKLINDYVKNGTRGKITDLI
Antiplasmin               --------AGSGPCLPHLLSRLCQDLG-PG------AFRLAARMYLQKGFPIKEDFLEQSEQLFGAK-PVSLT--GKQEDDLANINQWVKEATEGKIQEFL
Ovalbumin                 -GDSIEAQCGTSVNVHSSLRDILNQITKPND--VYSFSLASRLYAEERYPILPEYLQCVKELYRGG-LEPINFQTAADQARELINSWVESQTNGIIRNVL
Gene Y Protein            -GSTTDSQCGSSEYVHNLFKELLSEITRPNA--TYSLEIADKLYVDKTFSVLPEYLSCARKFYTGG-VEEVNFKTAAEEARQLINSWVEKETNGQIKDLL
Placental P A I           SYPDAILQAQAADKIHSSFRSLSSAINASTGD--YLLESVNKLFGEKSASFREEYIRLCQKYYSSE-PQAVDFLECAEEARKKINSWVKTQTKGKIPNLL
Angiotens Rat             -CTSRLDGH-KVLTALQAVQGLLVTQGGSSSQTPLLQSTVVGLFTAPGLRLKQPFVESLGPFTPAIFPRSLDLSTDPVLAAQKINRFVQAVTGWKMNLPL
Angiotens Human           -CTSRLDAH-KVLSALQAVQGLLVAQGRADSQAQLLLSTVVGVFTAPGLHLKQPFVQGLALYTPVVLPRSLDF-TELDVAAEKIDRFMQAVTGWKTGCSL
Barley Z Protein


                                    1         2         3         4         5         6         7         8         9         4
                                    0         0         0         0         0         0         0         0         0         0
0
Sequence Number
Secondary Structure       !=====A3====!             !====C3====! !=B1=!  !===B2===!  !==B3==!       !°°°
Antitrypsin Human         KELDRD--TVFALVNYIFFKGKWERPFEVKDTEE-EDFHVDQVTTVKVPMMKRLGMF--NIQHCKK-LSSWVLLMKYL-GNATAIFFLPD-----EGKLQ
Antitrypsin Baboon        KELDRD--TVFALVNYIFFKGKWERPFEVEATEE-EDFHVDQATTVKVPMMRRLGMF--NIYHCEK-LSSWVLLMKYL-GNATAIFFLPD-----EGKLQ
Antitrypsin Mouse                 SPANYILFKGKWKKPFDPENTEE-AEFHVDESTTVKVPMMTLSGML--DVHHCST-LSSWVLLMDYA-GNATAVFLLPD-----DGKMQ
Heparin Cofactor II       ENIDPA--TQMMILNCIYFKGSWVNKFPVEMTHN-HNFRLNEREVVKVSMMQTKGNF--LAANDQE-LDCDILQLEYV-GGISMLIVVPHK----MSGMK
Antithrombin              PSEAINELTVLVLVNTIYFKGLWKSKFSPENTRK-ELFYKADGESCSASMMYQEGKF--RYRRVAE--GTQVLELPFKGDDITMVLILPKP----EKSLA
C1-Inhibitor              DSLPSD--TRLVLLNAIYLSAKWKTTFDPKKTRM-EPPHFKNSV-IKVPMMNSKKYP-VAHFIDQT-LKAKVGQLQLSHNLSLVILVPQNL----KHRLE
Rabbit O R F              DASLDRD-TKMLLLSSVRMKTSWRHVFDPSFTTD-QPFYSGNV-TYKVRMMNKIDTL-KTETFTLRNVGYSVTELPYKRRQTAMLLVVP-----DDLGE
Endothelial P A I         GKGAVDQLTRLVLVNALYFNGQWKTPFPDSSTHR-RLFHKSDGSTVSVPMMAQTNKFNYTEFTTPDGHYYDILELPYHGDTLSMFIAAPYE-KEVPLSA
Thyroxine B G             QDLKPN--TIMVLVNYIHFKAQWANPFPDSKTEDSSSFLIDKTTTVQVPMMHQMEQY--YHLVDME-LNCTVLQMDYS-KNALALFVLPK-----EGQME
Antichymo Mouse                   VVLVNYIYFKGKWISFDPQDTFE-SEFYLDEKRSVKVPMMKMKLL--TTRHFRDEE-LSCSVLELKYT-GNASALLILPD-----QGRMQ
Antichymo Human           KDP--DSQTMMVLVNYIFFKAKWEMPFDPQDTHQ-SRFYLSKKKWVMVPMMSLHHL-TIPYFRDEE-LSCTVVELKYT-GNASALFILPD-----QDKME
Antiplasmin               SGLPED--TVLLLLNAIHFQGFWRNKFDPSLTQR-DSFHLDEQFTVPVEMMQARTYP-LRWFLLEQ-PEIQVAHFPFK-NNMSFVVLVPTH--FEWNVS
Ovalbumin                 QPSSVDSQTAMVLVNAIVFKGLWEKAFKDEDTQA-MPFRVTEQESKPVQMMYQIGLF--RVASMAS-EKMKILELPFASGTMSMLVLLPDE----VSGLE
Gene Y Protein            VSSSIDFGTTMVFINTIYFKGIWKIAFNTEDTRE-MPFSMTKEESKPVQMMCMNNSF--NVATLPA-EKMKILELPYASGDLSMLVLLPDE----VSGLE
Placental P A I           PEGSVDGDTRMVLVNAVYFKGKWKTPFEKKLNGL-YPFRVNSAQRTPVQMMYLREKL--NIGYIED-LKAQILEIPYA-GDVSMFLLLPDEIADVSTGLE
Angiotens Rat             EGVSTDS--TLFFNTYVHFQGKM-RGFSQ-LTGL-HEFWVDNSTSVSVPMLSGTGNF--QHWSDAQ-NNFSVTRVPL--GESVTLLLIQPQ----CASDL
Angiotens Human           MGASVDS--TLAFNTYVHFQGKM-KGFSL-LAEP-QEFWVDNSTSVSVPMLSGMGTF--QHWSDIQ-DNFSVTQVPF--TESACLLLIQPH----YASDL
Barley Z Protein          YISSSDNLK-VLKLPYAKGHDKRQFSMYILLPG--AQDGL
```

Figure 3. (*Continued on facing page.*)

```
                                                                                                            5
                          1          2          3          4          5          6          7          8          9          0
Sequence Number           0          0          0          0          0          0          0          0          0          0
Secondary Structure       °G°°°!!°°H°°°!            !==C2==!!====A6====!  !°°I°°!                   !======A5======!!======A4====
Antitrypsin Human         HLENELTHDIITKFLENEDR--RSASLHLPKLSITGTYDLK-SVLGQLGITKVFSNGAD-LSGVTEEA--PLKLSKAVHKAVLTIDEKGTEAAGAMFLEA
Antitrypsin Baboon        HLENELTHDIITKFLENENR--RSANLHLPKLAITGTYDLK-TVLGHLGITKVFSNGAD-LSGVTEDA--PLKLSKAVHKAVLTIDEKGTEAAGAMFLEA
Antitrypsin Mouse         HLEQTLSKELISKFLLNRRR--RLAQIHFPRLSISGEYNLK-TLMSPLGITRIFNNGAD-LSGITEENA-PLKLSQAVHKAVLTIDETGTEAAAVTVLLA
Heparin Cofactor II       TLEAQLTPRVVERWQKSMTN--RTREVLLPKFKLEKNYNLV-ESLKLMGIRMLFDKNGN-MAGISDQR---IAIDLFKHQGTIITVNEEGTQATTVTTVGF
Antithrombin              KVEKELTPEVLQEWLDELEE--MMLVVHMPRFRIEDGFSLK-EQLQDMGLVDLFSPEKSKLPGIVAEGRDDLYVSDAFHKAFLEVNEEGSEAAASTAVVI
C1-Inhibitor              DMEQALSPSVFKAIMEKLEMSKFQPTLLTLPRIKVTTSQDMLSIMEKLEFFD-FSYDLN-LCGLTEDP--DLQVSAMQHQTVLELTETGVEAAAASAISV
Rabbit O R F              IVRALDLSLVRFWIRNMRK---DVCQVVMPKFSVESVLDLR-DALQRLGVRDAFDPSRADFGQASPSN--DLYVTKVLQTSKIEADERGTTASSDTAITL
Endothelial P A I         LTNILSAQLISHWKGNMTR---LPRLLVLPKFSLETEVDLR-KPLENLGMTDMFRQFQADFTSLSDQE--PLHVAQALQKVKIEVNESGTVASSSTAVIV
Thyroxine B G             SVEAAMSSKTLKKWNRLLQK--GWVDLFVPKFSISATYDLG-ATLLKMGIQHAYSENAD-FSGLTEDN--GLKLSNAAHKAVLHIGEKGTEAAAVPEVEL
Antichymo Mouse           QVEASLQPETLRKWRKTLFPS-QIEELNLPKFSIASNYRLEEDVLPEMGIKEVFTEQAD-LSGIIETK--KLSVSQVVHKAVLDVAETGTEAAAATGVIG
Antichymo Human           EVEAMLLPETLKRWRDSLEFR-EIGELYLPKFSISRDYNLN-DILLQLGIEEAFTSKAD-LSGITGAR--NLAVSQVVHKVVSDVFEEGTEASAATAVKI
Antiplasmin               QVLANLSWDTLHPPLVWE----RPTKVRLPKLYLKHQMDLV-ATLSQLGLQELF-QAPD-LRGISEQ---SLVVSGVQHQSTLELSEVGVEAAAATSIAM
Ovalbumin                 QLESIINFEKLTEWTSSNVMEERKIKVYLPRMKMEEKYNLT-SVLMAMGITDVFSSSAN-LSGISSAE--SLKISQAVHAAHAEINEAGREVVGSAEAGV
Gene Y Protein            RIEKTINFDKLREWTSTNAMAKKSMKVYLPRMKIEEKYNLT-SILMALGMTDLFSRSAN-LTGISSVD--NLMISDAVHGVFMEVNEEGTEATGSTGAIG
Placental P A I           LLESEITYDKLNKWTSKDKMAEDEVEVYIPQFKLEEHYELR-SILRSMGMEDAFNKGRANFSGMSERN--DLFLSEVFHQAMVDVNEEGTEAAAGTGGVM
Angiotens Rat             DRVEVLVFQHDFLTWIKNPPP-RAIRLTLPQLEIRGSYNLQ-DLLAQAKLSTLLGAEAN-LGKMGDTN--PRVGEVLNSILLELQAGEEEQPTESAQQPG
Angiotens Human           DKVEGLTFQQNSLNWMKKLSP-RTIHLTMPQLVLQGSYDLQ-DLLAQAELPAILHTELN-LQKLSNDR--IRVGEVLNSIFFELEA-DEREPTESTQQLN
Barley Z Protein          WSLAKRLSTEPEFIENHIPKQTVEVGRFQLPKFKISYQFEASSLLRALGLQLPFSEEAD-LSEMVDSS-QGLEISHVFHKSFVEVNEEGTEAGAATVAMG
```

```
                                                                                                            6
                          1          2          3          4          5          6          7          8          9          0
Sequence Number           0          0          0          0          0          0          0          0          0          0
Secondary Structure       ===!!=====C1=====!  !===B4===!!===B5====!
Antitrypsin Human         IP-MSIPPE-----VKFNKPFVFLMIEQNTKSPLFMGKVVNPTQK
Antitrypsin Baboon        IP-MSIPPE-----VKFNKPFVFLMIEQNTKSPLFIGKVVNPTQK
Antitrypsin Mouse         VP-YSMPPI-----LRFDHPFLFIIFEEHTQSPLFVGKVVDPTHK
Heparin Cofactor II       MP-LSTQVR-----FTVDRPFLFLIYEHRTSCLLFMGRVANPSRS
Antithrombin              AG-RSLNPN-----RVTFKANRPFLVFIREVPLNTIIFMGRVANPCVK
C1-Inhibitor              A--RTLLV------FEVQQPFLFVLWDQQHKFPVFMGRVYDPRA
Rabbit O R F              IP-RNALTA-----IVANKPFMFLIYHKPTTTVLFMGTIITKGEKVIYDTEGRDDVVSSV
Endothelial P A I         SA-RMAPEE-----IIMDRPFLFVVRHNPTGTVLFMGQVMEP
Thyroxine B G             SD-QPENTFLHPI-IQIDRSFMLLILERSTRSILFLGKVVNPTEA
Antichymo Mouse           GIRKAILPA-----VHFNRPFLFVIYHTSAQSILFMAKVNNPK
Antichymo Human           TL-LSALVETRTI-VRFNRPFLMIIVPTDTQNIFFMSKVTNPSKPRACIKQWGSQ
Antiplasmin               S--RMSLSS-----FSVNRPFLFFIFEDTTGLPLFVGSVRNPNPSAPRELKEQQDSPGNKDFLQSLKGFPRGDKLFGPDLKLVPPMEEDYPQFGSPK
Ovalbumin                 DA-ASVS-EE----FRADHPFLFCIKHIATNAVLFFGRCVSP
Gene Y Protein            NIKHSLELEE----FRADHPFLFFIRYNPNTNAILFFGRYWSP
Placental P A I           TG-RTGHGG-----PQFVADHPFLFLIMHKITKCILFFGRFCSP
Angiotens Rat             SP--------EVLDVTLSSPFLFAIYERDSGALHFLGRVDNPQNVV
Angiotens Human           KP--------EVLEVTLNRPFLFAVYDQSATALHFLGRVANPLSTA
Barley Z Protein          VA-MSNPLKVDLVDFVANHPFLFLIREDIAGVVVFVGHVTNPLISA
```

Figure 3. Alignment of the serpins with secondary structure notation; α helix (○○○), β sheet (= = =). Lower case letters indicate leader sequence. Proposed exposed loop formed by strand A4 with P_1-P_1' at A4-C1 interstrand position. Sequences: antitrypsin human (Carrell et al. 1982); antitrypsin baboon (Kurachi et al. 1981); antitrypsin mouse (Hill et al. 1984); heparin cofactor human (Ragg 1986); antithrombin human (Chandra et al. 1983a); C1-inhibitor human (Bock et al. 1985); rabbit ORF (Upton et al. 1986); endothelial plasminogen activator inhibitor human (Pannekoek et al. 1986); thyroxine-binding globulin human (Flink et al. 1986); antichymotrypsin mouse (Hill et al. 1984); antichymotrypsin human (Chandra et al. 1983b); antiplasmin human (Holmes et al. 1987); ovalbumin chicken (McReynolds et al. 1978); ovalbumin gene Y chicken (Heilig et al. 1982); placental plasminogen activator inhibitor human (Ye et al. 1987); angiotensinogen rat (Ohkuba et al. 1983); angiotensinogen human (Kageyama et al. 1984); and barley Z protein (Hejgaard et al. 1985).

mance liquid chromatography using an acetonitrile/trifluoroacetic acid gradient. Peaks were monitored at 214 nm, and aliquots from each were dried down under vacuum and subjected to 5–20% SDS-PAGE and amino acid analysis. Both low and high molecular weight fragments purified in this fashion were sequenced by the gas phase method (Applied Biosystems).

RESULTS

The homologous alignment of serpins, with secondary structure annotations, is shown in Figure 3. A tabulation of identity fractions and evolutionary distances in PAMs (accepted point mutations percent) is shown in Figure 4.

The results of the digestion of the four serpins with a range of proteases and the results of subsequent sequence and other studies will be reported in detail in separate publications by the authors (P.A. Pemberton et al., in prep.) with P.J. Lachmann and R.A. Harrison regarding C1-inhibitor, with M.B. Pepys and others regarding thyroxine-binding globulin, and with P. Christey regarding antithrombin. The results can be readily summarized as follows. Most of the proteases cut at two sites, the first being near the amino terminus of the molecule, prior to the commencement of ordered structure at helix A and the second being in the peptide loop containing the reactive center. Cleavage of the reactive center loop did occur with all the reported proteases, the position of cleavage being confirmed by sequence studies of the released carboxy-terminal fragment. The newly determined sites of loop cleavage are shown in Figure 5, arrowed 7, 8, 9, 10, 12, and 13. Figure 5 also includes cleavage sites determined independently by other workers as referenced in the legend. In particular, neutrophil leucocyte elastase rapidly cleaved and inactivated antithrombin (in the presence of heparin) and C1-inhibitor but not (or only slowly) antitrypsin. Both C1-inhibitor and antithrom-

		1	2	3	4	5	6	7	8	9	10	11	12	13	14	15	16	17	18
1	Antitrypsin Human	*	8	51	173	166	218	267	182	104	98	116	176	157	160	153	236	238	221
2	Antitrypsin Baboon	92	*	51	173	167	231	275	193	102	103	123	175	159	158	156	242	247	228
3	Antitrypsin Mouse	61	61	*	172	158	190	247	203	110	101	116	172	140	152	155	221	231	215
4	Heparin Cofactor II	28	28	28	*	170	299	257	204	172	136	165	198	165	145	152	302	323	233
5	Antithrombin	29	29	30	28	*	233	240	174	179	122	157	177	151	132	137	321	315	194
6	C1-Inhibitor	23	21	26	16	21	*	273	250	237	165	219	219	275	257	210	350	317	285
7	Rabbit O R F	18	18	20	19	21	18	*	171	239	187	222	245	248	249	204	>350	>350	211
8	Endothelial P A I	27	25	24	24	28	20	28	*	198	175	174	181	183	170	165	269	268	249
9	Thyroxine B G	42	43	41	28	27	21	21	25	*	101	114	194	188	193	169	293	301	240
10	Antichymo Mouse	44	42	43	34	37	29	26	28	43	*	55	137	145	140	144	210	224	212
11	Antichymo Human	39	37	39	29	30	22	22	28	39	59	*	184	165	166	157	260	290	214
12	Antiplasmin	27	28	28	25	27	22	20	27	25	34	26	*	180	188	186	257	256	180
13	Ovalbumin	30	30	34	29	31	18	20	27	26	33	29	27	*	59	119	265	275	215
14	Gene Y Protein	30	30	31	33	35	19	20	28	25	34	29	26	58	*	107	273	320	181
15	Placental P A I	31	30	31	31	34	23	24	29	28	33	30	26	38	41	*	278	300	185
16	Angiotens Rat	21	20	22	16	15	14	13	18	17	23	19	19	19	18	18	*	46	315
17	Angiotens Human	21	20	21	15	16	16	13	18	16	22	17	19	18	15	16	64	*	>350
18	Barley Z Protein	22	22	23	21	25	17	23	20	20	23	23	27	23	27	26	16	14	*

Figure 4. Serpin identity percentage (lower left triangle) and evolution distances in PAM, accepted point mutations per 100 residues (upper right triangle).

bin were similarly rapidly inactivated by direct incubation with stimulated neutrophils.

All the enzymes causing cleavage and inactivation reported in Figure 5 gave a concomitant and striking change in the heat stability of the serpin substrate. The four serpins prior to cleavage (ovalbumin not tested here) were all denatured by heating for 40 minutes at 60°C. However, following cleavage the inactivated inhibitors remained stable in solution even after prolonged heating at 90°C.

As predicted, thyroxine-binding globulin, even though it has no recognizable inhibitory activity, underwent the same increase in stability after cleavage by neutrophil elastase.

DISCUSSION

The serpins provide an intriguing model of the way in which evolution can provide a range of functions within the one superfamily. The alignments (Fig. 3) show shared features of sequence indicating a common tertiary structure and evolutionary origin (Fig. 6). Additional support for a common structure is provided here by the demonstration that members of the family undergo the same conformational change on cleavage of the reactive center loop sequence.

Exposed Loop and S–R Transition

As shown in Figure 5, the serpins are susceptible to proteolytic cleavage of the peptide loop extending to each side (P_{10}–P_4) of the reactive center (P_1–P_1). In each case, this cleavage is accompanied by a profound change in thermal stability. To confirm the general nature of this S–R transformation, a new member of the family, thyroxine-binding globulin, which has no apparent inhibitory activity, was tested. Rapid catalytic cleavage by neutrophil elastase occurred, accompanied by a change in denaturation temperature from 60°C in

the native protein to greater than 80°C in the cleaved form.

The sites of cleavage within the serpin family, shown in Figure 5, provide useful information for the reconstruction of the reactive center loop. In the crystallographic R structure of Loebermann (Loebermann et al. 1984), the 15 residues amino-terminal to the reactive center, P_2–P_{16}, form the central strand (A4) of the large six-membered A β sheet. Consequently, these residues are inaccessible to proteolytic attack in the cleaved postcomplex molecule. We do not know the conformation of the intact loop in the native (S) form. However, the cleavage sites shown in Figure 5 indicate that residues P_{10}–P_4' must be accessible in the intact molecule; i.e., the reactive center loop must be predominantly formed by withdrawal of the A4 strand from the β sheet (Fig. 1). This conclusion carries with it the prediction, confirmed here, that cleavage of the reactive center loop will result in a conformational change to a more stable relaxed structure. Inferential support for this is given by the observation in Huber's laboratory (Loebermann et al. 1984) that cleaved antitrypsin crystallized more readily than the native protein, and also by the earlier experience in the Carlsberg laboratory where cleaved ovalbumin (plakalbumin) was seen to crystallize spontaneously on storage in the refrigerator. This has been confirmed by Wright (1984), who has obtained good, X-ray-diffractible plakalbumin crystals. It is only recently that the first report has been made of crystallization of an intact serpin, antithrombin, by Samama et al. (1987).

Functional and Pathological Significance of the S–R Transition

The evidence supports the presence of a stressed loop as a general feature of the serpin superfamily. Why has nature preserved this tense native structure, and why has there been the preservation of a stable

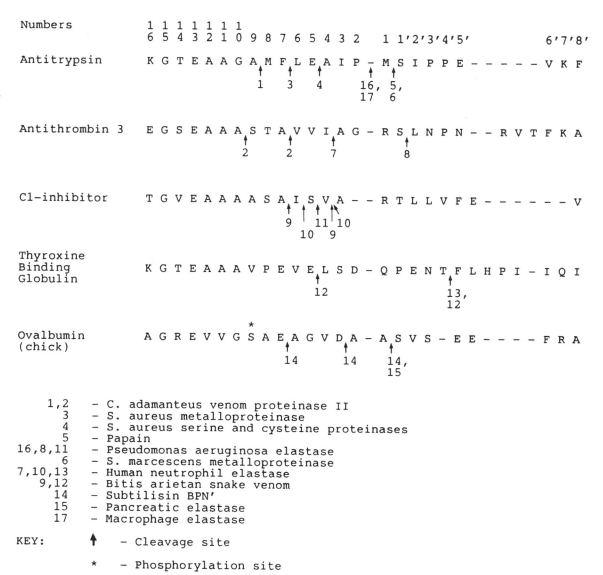

Figure 5. Serpin reactive center loop cleavage sites. Numbering is related to P_1–P_1' reactive center; the invariant glycine at P_{15} acts as a hinge for strand A4, which extends from it to the P_1 reactive center. Reference: Cleavage site 1 (Kress et al. 1979); 2 (Kress and Catanese 1981); 3, 4 (Potempa et al. 1986); 5 (Johnson and Travis 1977); 6 (Virca et al. 1982); 7 (Carrell and Owen 1985); 8 (P. Christey, unpubl.); 9, 10 (P.A. Pemberton et al., unpubl.); 11 (Salvesen et al. 1985); 12, 13 (P.A. Pemberton, unpubl.); 14, 15 (Linderstrom-Lang 1952; Wright 1984); 16 (Morihara et al. 1984); 17 (Banda et al. 1987).

postcleavage structure? The best suggestion in response to the first part of the question is that the stressed loop provides a strained conformation at the P_1–P_1' bond that is favorable to formation of a stable, intermediate state complex with the target protease. However, this is speculative, and there is no supporting experimental evidence.

In answer to the second part: There are advantages in the maintenance of a stable postcleavage conformation, as this provides what is in effect a switch; i.e., an effective means for the inactivation and subsequent removal of inhibitors. Both neutrophil leucocytes and

macrophages secrete enzymes, including elastases and collagenases, that catalytically cleave and inactivate the plasma serpins (Carrell and Owen 1985; Banda et al. 1987). This proteolytic inactivation of the serpins by leucocytes along with reversible inactivation of antitrypsin by oxidation of its reactive center methionine (Fig. 7) allows the localized modification of proteolysis that occurs around an inflammatory focus.

It is not difficult to see how evolution can advantageously adapt this S–R transition in those members of the family that have a prime function other than protease inhibition. Thus, as is shown here, the hormone-

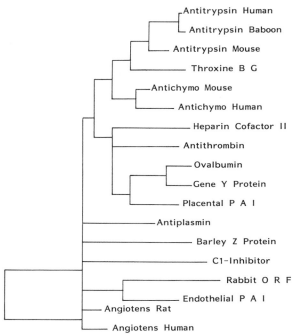

Figure 6. Evolution of the serpins. Tree drawn to scale in accepted point mutations per hundred residues.

carrier thyroxine-binding globulin undergoes a conformational change on cleavage by neutrophil elastase that provides the potential for localized modification of its function at sites of inflammation.

Reactive Center Variation

The inhibitory specificity of the serpins is primarily determined by the reactive center P_1 residue. The natural mutant illustrated in Figure 2 shows how a single P_1 mutation can result in a complete change in inhibitory profile (Table 1). This is confirmed by subsequent genetically engineered variants (Carrell 1986; Jallat et al. 1986). Thus, a single mutation could provide the initial response needed to meet a new proteolytic challenge. Such an event must have occurred in mouse antitrypsin subsequent to primate and rodent

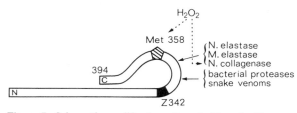

Figure 7. Schematic modification sites. Antitrypsin, like several other plasma serpins, can be inactivated by oxidation of methionine, at (or near) the reactive center, by neutrophil leucocyte oxidants. This together with cleavage of loop sites by leucocyte enzymes provides an advantage in allowing the localized inactivation of serpins at sites of inflammation. The last mechanism has been utilized by invading organisms that have evolved enzymes to pathologically inactivate the plasma serpins. (N) Neutrophil; (M) macrophage. See Fig. 5 for details.

divergence, since mouse antitrypsin (Fig. 3) has a reactive center tyrosine, in contrast to the methionine of humans, with a consequently changed inhibitory specificity (Hill et al. 1984).

Hill and Hastie (1987) have proposed that the variability of reactive center regions provides evidence for positive Darwinian selection. Their proposal that this sequence variation is based on selection of precise inhibitory activities is supported by the independent findings with the ovomucoid inhibitors by Laskowski et al. (this volume). Our conclusions are in keeping with this but broaden the proposal as follows. The reactive center of substratelike inhibitors, by definition, must be accessible and hence, exteriorly placed on the molecule. In the serpins, the reactive center is on a peptide loop that, because of its external position, will be relatively free from the conformational constraints that conserve internally placed residues. This relative freedom from constraint allows a wide range of acceptable variation, with positive selection taking place on the basis of two functional roles. The first is selection based on modification of inhibitory activity, as proposed by Hill and Hastie; the other is selection based on modified cleavage susceptibility. There will be functional advantages in the evolution of sequences on the exposed loop that allow local cleavage and inactivation as a physiological process, demonstrated here by neutrophil elastase modification of thyroxine-binding globulin. From a survival point of view, there will be even greater pressure for conservation of mutational changes that provide resistance to loop cleavage by pathogenic proteases. An example of this is seen with the rattlesnake protease that rapidly cleaves the reactive center loop of mammalian antitrypsins. The notable exception is that of the antitrypsin of a mammal most exposed to rattlesnakes, the opossum, which has apparently evolved a loop sequence resistant to cleavage by rattlesnake protease (Kress et al. 1986).

ACKNOWLEDGMENTS

This work was supported by the Medical Research Councils of the United Kingdom and New Zealand.

REFERENCES

Banda, M.J., E.J. Clark, S. Sinha, and J. Travis. 1987. Interaction of mouse macrophage elastase with native and oxidized human α_1 proteinase inhibitor. *J. Clin. Invest.* **79:** 1314.

Bock, S.C., K. Skriver, E. Nielson, H.C. Thogersen, B. Wiman, V.H. Donaldson, R.L. Eddy, J. Marriana, E. Radziejewska, R. Huber, T.B. Shows, and S. Magnusson. 1985. Human C1 inhibitor: Primary structure, cDNA cloning, and chromosomal localisation. *Biochemistry* **25:** 4292.

Carrell, R.W. 1986. Reactive centre variants of alpha-1-antitrypsin. A range of anti-inflammatory agents. *Biotechnol. Genet. Eng. Rev.* **4:** 291.

Carrell, R.W. and D.R. Boswell. 1986. Serpins: A family of serine protease inhibitors. In *Protease inhibitors* (ed. A. Barrett and G. Salvesen), p. 403. Elsevier, Amsterdam.

Carrell, R.W. and M.C. Owen. 1985. Plakalbumin, alpha-1-antitrypsin, antithrombin and the mechanism of inflammatory thrombosis. *Nature* **317:** 730.

Carrell, R.W., J.-O. Jeppsson, C.-B. Laurell, S.O. Brennan, M.C. Owen, L. Vaughan, and D.R. Boswell. 1982. Structure and variation of human alpha-1-antitrypsin. *Nature* **298**: 329.

Chandra, T., R. Stackhouse, V.J. Kidd, and S.L.C. Woo. 1983a. Isolation and sequence characterization of a cDNA clone of human antithrombin III. *Proc. Natl. Acad. Sci.* **80**: 1845.

Chandra, T., R. Stackhouse, V.J. Kidd, K.J.H. Robson, and S.L.C. Woo. 1983b. Sequence homology between human alpha-1-antichymotrypsin, alpha-1-antitrypsin and antithrombin III. *Biochemistry* **22**: 5055.

Flink, F., T.J. Bailey, T.A. Gustafson, B.E. Markham, and E. Morkin. 1986. Complete amino acid sequence of human thyroxin-binding globulin deduced from cloned DNA: Close homology to the serine antiprotease. *Proc. Natl. Acad. Sci.* **83**: 7708.

Harrison, R.A. 1983. Human C1-inhibitor: Improved isolation and preliminary structural characterisation. *Biochemistry* **22**: 5001.

Heilig, R., R. Muraskowsky, C. Kloepfer, and J.L. Mandle. 1982. The ovalbumin gene family: Complete sequence and structure of the Y gene. *Nucleic Acids Res.* **10**: 4363.

Hejgaard, J., S.K. Rasmussen, A. Brandt, and I. Svendsen. 1985. Sequence homology between barley endosperm protein Z and protease inhibitors of the alpha-1-antitrypsin family. *FEBS Lett.* **180**: 89.

Hill, N.D. and R.E. Hastie. 1987. Accelerated evolution in the reactive centre regions of serine protease inhibitors. *Nature* **326**: 96.

Hill, R.E., P.H. Shaw, P.A. Bovd, H. Baumann, and N.D. Hastie. 1984. Plasma protease inhibitors in mouse and man: Divergence within the reactive centre regions. *Nature* **311**: 175.

Holmes, W.E., L. Nelles, H.R. Lijnen, and D. Collen. 1987. Primary structure of human alpha-2-antiplasmin, a serine protease inhibitor (serpin). *J. Biol. Chem.* **262**: 1659.

Hunt, L.T. and M.O. Dayhoff. 1980. A surprising new protein superfamily containing ovalbumin, antithrombin III and alpha-1-proteinase inhibitor. *Biochem. Biophys. Res. Commun.* **95**: 864.

Jallat, S., D. Carvallo, L.H. Tessier, D. Roecklin, C. Roitsch, F. Ogushi, R.G. Crystal, and M. Courtney. 1986. Altered specificities of genetically engineered alpha₁-antitrypsin variants. *Protein Eng.* **1**: 29.

Jeppsson, J.-O., H. Lillja, and M. Johansson. 1985. Isolation and characterization of two minor fractions of alpha-1-antitrypsin by high-performance liquid chromatographic chromatofocusing. *J. Chromatog.* **327**: 173.

Johnson, D. and J. Travis. 1977. Inactivation of human alpha-1-proteinase inhibitor by Thiol proteinases. *Biochem. J.* **163**: 639.

Kageyama, R., H. Ohkubo, and S. Nakanisi. 1984. Primary structure of human preangiotensinogen deduced from the cloned cDNA sequence. *Biochemistry* **23**: 3603.

Kress, L.F. and J.J. Catanese. 1981. Identification of the cleavage sites resulting from enzymatic inactivation of human antithrombin III by *Crotalus adamanteus* proteinase II in the presence and absence of heparin. *Biochemistry* **20**: 7432.

Kress, L.F., J.J. Catanese, and T. Hirayama. 1983. Analysis of the effects of snake venom proteinases on the activity of human plasma C1-esterase inhibitor, α₁-antichymotrypsin and α₂-antiplasmin. *Biochim. Biophys. Acta* **745**: 113.

Kress, L.F., J.J. Catanese, and L.G. Sheflin. 1986. Regulation of rattlesnake venom proteolytic and haemorrhagic activity by inhibitors isolated from opossum serum. *J. Cell Biochem.* (suppl.) **10a**: 264 (Abstr.).

Kress, L.F., T. Kurachi, S.-K. Chan, and M. Lasowski. 1979. Characterization of the inactive fragment resulting from limited proteolysis of human alpha-1-proteinase inhibitor by *Crotalus adamanteus* proteinase II. *J. Biol. Chem.* **254**: 5317.

Kurachi, K., T. Chandra, S.J. Friezneo Degen, T.T. White, T.L. Marchioro, S.L.C. Woo, and E.W. Davie. 1981. Cloning and sequence of cDNA coding for alpha-1-antitrypsin. *Proc. Natl. Acad. Sci.* **78**: 6826.

Lesk, A.M., M. Levitt, and C. Chothia. 1986. Alignment of distantly related proteins using variable gap penalties. *Protein Eng.* **1**: 77.

Linderstrom-Lang, K.U. 1952. The enzymatic breakdown of ovalbumin. *Med. Sci.* **6**: 73.

Loebermann, H., R. Tokuoka, J. Deisenhofer, and R. Hiber. 1984. Human alpha-1-proteinase inhibitor: Crystal structure analysis of two crystal modifications, molecular model and preliminary analysis of the implications for function. *J. Mol. Biol.* **177**: 531.

McKay, E.J. 1981. A simple two step procedure for the isolation of antithrombin III from biological fluids. *Thromb. Res.* **21**: 375.

McReynolds, L., B.W. O'Malley, A.D. Nisbett, J.E. Fothergill, D. Givol, S. Fields, M. Robertson, and G.G. Brownlee. 1978. Sequence of chicken ovalbumin mRNA. *Nature* **273**: 723.

Morihara, K., H. Tsusuki, M. Harada, and T. Iwato. 1984. Purification of human plasma alpha-1-proteinase inhibitor and its inactivation by *Pseudomonas aeruginosa* elastase. *J. Biochem.* **95**: 795.

Ohkubo, H., R. Kageyama, M. Ujihara, T. Hirose, S. Inayama, and S. Nakanishi. 1983. Cloning and sequence analysis of cDNA for rat angiotensinogen. *Proc. Natl. Acad. Sci.* **80**: 2196.

Owen, M.C., S.O. Brennan, J.H. Lewis, and R.W. Carrell. 1983. Mutation of antithrombin to antitrypsin. Antitrypsin Pittsburgh (358 Met–Arg), a fatal bleeding disorder. *N. Engl. J. Med.* **309**: 694.

Owen, M.C., J.Y. Borg, C. Soria, J. Soria, J. Caen, and R.W. Carrell. 1987. Heparin binding defect in a new antithrombin III variant. Rouen, 47 Arg to His. *Blood* **5**: 1275.

Pannekoek, H., H. Veerman, H. Lambers, P. Diergaarde, C.L. Verweij, A.-J. van Zonneveld, and J.A. van Mourik. 1986. Endothelial plasminogen activator inhibitor (PAIO: A new member of the serpin gene family). *EMBO J.* **5**: 2542.

Potempa, J., W. Watorek, and J. Travis. 1986. The inactivation of human plasma alpha-1-proteinase inhibitor by proteinases from *Staphylococcus aureus*. *J. Biol. Chem.* **261**: 14330.

Ragg, H. 1986. A new member of the plasma protease inhibitor gene family. *Nucleic Acids Res.* **14**: 1073.

Rosenberg, S., P.J. Barr, R.C. Najarian, and R.A. Hallewell. 1984. Synthesis in yeast of a functional oxidation-resistant mutant of human alpha 1-antitrypsin. *Nature* **312**: 77.

Salvesen, G.S., J.J. Catanese, L.F. Kress, and J. Travis. 1985. Primary structure of the reactive site of human C1-inhibitor. *J. Biol. Chem.* **260**: 2432.

Samama, J.P., M. Delarue, D. Moras, M. Petitou, J.G. Lormean, and J. Choay. 1987. Crystallographic investigation of antithrombin III. *Thromb. Haemostasis.* **58**: 264 (Abstr.).

Travis, J. and G.S. Salvesen. 1983. Human plasma proteinase inhibitors. *Annu. Rev. Biochem. Chem.* **52**: 655.

Upton, C., R.W. Carrell, and G. McFadden. 1986. A novel member of the serpin superfamily is encoded on a circular plasmid-like DNA specimen isolated from rabbit cells. *FEBS Lett.* **207**: 115.

Virca, G.D., D. Lyerly, A. Kreger, and J. Travis. 1982. Inactivation of human plasma alpha-1-proteinase inhibitor by a metalloproteinase from *Serratia marcescens*. *Biochim. Biophys. Acta* **704**: 267.

Wright, H.T. 1984. Ovalbumin is an elastase substrate. *J. Biol. Chem.* **259**: 14335.

Ye, R.D., T.C. Wun, and J.E. Sadler. 1987. cDNA cloning and expression in *Escherichia coli* of a plasminogen activator inhibitor from human placenta. *J. Biol. Chem.* **262**: 3718.

The Role of Protein Folding in the Evolution of Protein Sequences

T. STACKHOUSE,* J.J. ONUFFER,* C.R. MATTHEWS,* S.A. AHMED,[†] AND E.W. MILES[†]

Department of Chemistry, Pennsylvania State University, University Park, Pennsylvania 16802;
[†]Laboratory of Biochemical Pharmacology, NIADDKD, National Institutes of Health, Bethesda, Maryland 20205

The concept that protein folding proceeds through intermediate, partially folded forms has been gaining acceptance since Levinthal first proposed that the folding mechanism is not likely to be a random search of all possible conformations (Levinthal 1968). Although the early stages of folding may involve relatively large numbers of partially folded forms, recent data on several globular proteins suggest that only a few intermediates may be present at later stages (Beasty et al. 1986; Touchette et al. 1986).

The idea that folding pathways and discrete intermediates exist implies that certain amino acids play key roles in folding and others play lesser roles. Studies on the α subunit of tryptophan synthase and dihydrofolate reductase from *Escherichia coli* have shown that single amino acid replacements can be used to identify amino acids whose replacement alters a rate-limiting step in folding, near the native conformation (Beasty et al. 1986; Touchette et al. 1986). These results have begun to provide an understanding of the structural basis of rate-limiting steps in the folding of both proteins.

Another way of viewing the essential nature of individual amino acids in folding is to ask whether the folding mechanisms of homologous proteins are conserved during evolution. Changes at critical amino acids would, by definition, significantly alter the stability or perhaps the rate-limiting steps in folding. Presumably, changes that decrease the yield of final, folded product would be selected against during evolution.

Previous comparisons of a series of pancreatic ribonucleases showed that the same folding mechanism was operative (Krebs et al. 1983), including the presence of a highly populated, nativelike intermediate (Krebs et al. 1986). Differences in amplitudes and relaxation times for the slow folding phases in porcine ribonuclease were attributed to a unique Pro 114-Pro 115 sequence in the porcine protein (Grafl et al. 1986). Other features of the folding model are rather similar to that for bovine ribonuclease. Studies on three homologous protease inhibitors showed that the same disulfide intermediates appear, suggesting that the folding mechanism is conserved in this system as well (Hollecker and Creighton 1983).

To test the generality of these conclusions, we have examined the folding and stability of the α subunit of tryptophan synthase from *E. coli* (EC α subunit), *Salmonella typhimurium* (ST α subunit) and a series of hybrids produced by random combination of the structural genes for the parent proteins. The 85% homology between EC α subunit and ST α subunit permits a test of the roles of the 40 replacements in the 268-residue polypeptide. The hybrids provide a more refined view of the effect of the replacements on folding and stability and, in addition, an interesting alternative to the construction of mutant proteins.

EXPERIMENTAL PROCEDURES

Protein purification. The EC α subunit (E.C.4.2.1.20) was purified from *E. coli* containing plasmid pBN 55 (a gift from Brian Nichols, University of Illinois at Chicago), the ST α subunit either from *S. typhimurium* or from *E. coli* containing plasmid pSTP 26 which carries the ST α subunit gene (a gift from Ronald Bauerle, University of Virginia) and the 6–34, 8–32, 12–28, 14–26, and 15–25 hybrid α subunit proteins from *E. coli* containing the appropriate plasmid (Schneider et al. 1981). The procedure used in purification has been described elsewhere (Matthews et al. 1983; T. Stackhouse et al., in prep.).

Protein purity and concentration determination. The purity of each protein was shown by the appearance of a single band on Coomassie-blue-stained native and sodium dodecylsulfate polyacrylamide gel electrophoresis. The protein concentration was determined by absorbance measurements at 278 nm using a molar extinction coefficient of 12,600 M^{-1} cm^{-1} (Matthews and Crisanti 1981) for all the proteins in this study. The seven Tyr residues are strictly conserved, as is the absence of Trp residues. The reversibility was determined by the recovery of the absorbance spectrum and always exceeded 90%.

Chemicals. Ultrapure urea was purchased from Schwarz/Mann; all other chemicals were reagent grade. The buffer used in all folding experiments was 10 mM potassium phosphate (pH 7.8), 0.2 mM Na_2EDTA, and 1 mM 2-mercaptoethanol.

Spectroscopic methods. Equilibrium and kinetic measurements of the denaturant-induced unfolding and refolding reactions were performed with UV difference spectroscopy at 25°C on a Cary 118 C spectrophotometer. Equilibrium and kinetic methods for monitoring the unfolding reactions have been described previously (Crisanti and Matthews 1981).

Data analysis. The equilibrium unfolding data was fit to a three-state model and has been described in detail elsewhere (Beasty et al. 1986). The free energy difference between a pair of stable conformations was assumed to depend linearly on the denaturant concentration (Schellman 1978).

The transient responses in absorbance at 286 nm to changes in urea concentration were fit to one or a sum of exponentials by a nonlinear least-squares fitting program and the amplitudes and relaxation times for each kinetic phase obtained (Beasty et al. 1986).

RESULTS

The α Subunit System

The amino acid sequences of the EC and ST α subunits are shown in Figure 1. The 40 amino acid replacements are generally conservative, although there are a few notable exceptions, e.g., Glu-113 (EC) → Ala (ST), Ala-198 (EC) → Glu (ST), Asp-225 (EC) → Arg (ST), Glu-249 (EC) → Lys (ST), and Ala-254 (EC) → Glu. Note also that the degree of conservation is not uniform along the sequence, with only 15 changes in the region 1–188 and 25 changes in the region 189–268. These differences may be related to the observation that these two regions behave as independent folding domains (Miles et al. 1982; Beasty and Matthews 1985).

The hybrid α subunits were constructed such that the amino terminus is derived from *S. typhimurium* and the carboxyl terminus from *E. coli* (Schneider et al. 1981); the regions in which the recombination occurred are also shown in Figure 1. The nomenclature used to denote a particular hybrid is to list the number of replacements in the amino terminus that originate from the ST α subunit, followed by the number in the carboxyl terminus that originate from the EC α subunit. For example, 6–34 is the hybrid that contains the *S. typhimurium* sequence in the region from 1 to 58 (6 replacements in *E. coli*) and the *E. coli* sequence from 59 to 268 (34 replacements in *S. typhimurium*).

The validity of a comparison of the folding kinetics and stability depends critically on the assumption that the three-dimensional structures of this set of α subunits are the same. This assumption is supported by three observations: (1) The far UV circular dichroism spectra of this set of proteins is identical within experimental error (T. Stackhouse, unpubl. results). (2) The ST α subunit and the five hybrids can all activate the β_2 subunit from *E. coli* (Schneider et al. 1981). (3) Antisera to EC α subunit recognizes ST α subunit and the five hybrids (Schneider et al. 1981). Therefore, the secondary and tertiary structures of the entire set of α subunit proteins must be very similar.

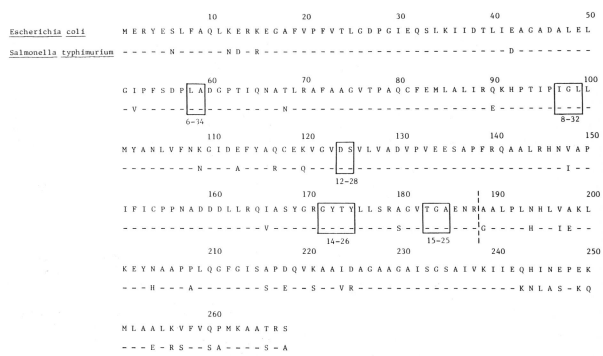

Figure 1. The amino acid sequences of EC α subunit and ST α subunit (Schneider et al. 1981). Dashes indicate identical amino acids in both sequences. Boxes indicate the regions where recombination has occurred for the respective hybrid α subunits. The vertical dashed line indicates the proposed junction between the amino and carboxyl domains (Miles et al. 1982). This figure has been taken from T. Stackhouse et al. (in prep.).

Equilibrium Folding Studies

The equilibrium unfolding of the EC α subunit by urea (Matthews and Crisanti 1981) and guanidine hydrochloride (Yutani et al. 1979) has been shown to proceed by a three-state mechanism that involves a stable, partially folded intermediate. The intermediate has a folded amino domain, residues 1–188, and an unfolded carboxyl domain, residues 189–268 (Miles et al. 1982). This multistate behavior is apparent both in difference UV spectroscopy at 286 nm (Matthews and Crisanti 1981) and in circular dichroism at 222 nm (Yutani et al. 1979).

The dependence of the apparent fraction of unfolded EC α subunit, F_{app}, on the urea concentration is shown in Figure 2.[1] The native form, N, is stable up to approximately 2 M urea. The increase in F_{app} between 2 and 3 M urea corresponds to the transition from N to the stable intermediate, I. The break in the F_{app} curve at ~3 M urea and the subsequent unfolding transition of lower cooperativity corresponds to the transition from I to the unfolded form, U.

---

[1]F_{app} was calculated from the difference UV spectrum at 286 nm from the equation $F_{app} = (\epsilon_{OBS} - \epsilon_{NAT})/(\epsilon_{UNF} - \epsilon_{NAT})$ where ϵ_{OBS} is the observed extinction coefficient and ϵ_{NAT} and ϵ_{UNF} are the extinction coefficient of the native and unfolded forms, all at the same urea concentration. The values for ϵ_{NAT} and ϵ_{UNF} in the transition region were obtained by linear extrapolation from the baseline regions.

The equilibrium unfolding reaction for the ST α subunit detected by difference UV spectroscopy at 286 nm also follows a three-state model; however, the difference between the two transitions is less apparent (Fig. 2). The N $\leftrightarrow$ I transition for ST α subunit occurs at higher urea concentrations than that for the EC α subunit, whereas the I $\leftrightarrow$ U transition occurs at a lower urea concentration than that for EC α subunit. By fitting both data sets to a three-state model and assuming a linear dependence of the free energy change on the urea concentration, the effects of stability can be quantified. In the absence of denaturant, the difference in free energy between N and I, ΔG_{NI}, for the ST α subunit is 0.4 ± 0.1 kcal mol^{-1} greater than that for EC α subunit. The free energy difference between I and U, ΔG_{IU}, is 0.4 ± 0.1 kcal mol^{-1} less for ST α subunit than for EC α subunit (T. Stackhouse et al., in prep.). Under these conditions, ΔG_{NI} and ΔG_{IU} for the EC α subunit are 5.7 ± 0.4 and 5.0 ± 0.6 kcal mol^{-1}, respectively. Thus, the effects of the 40 amino acid replacements in the EC and ST α subunits on the relative stabilities of N, I, and U are rather small.

To determine if the hybrid α subunits also have a stable folding intermediate, the equilibrium unfolding reactions for the 6–34, 8–32, 12–28, 14–26, and 15–25 hybrids were monitored by difference UV spectroscopy (Fig. 3). An adequate fit of all five hybrids again required a three-state model in which a more cooperative

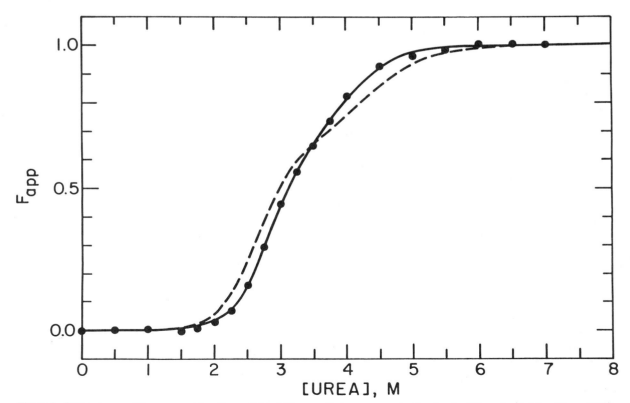

Figure 2. Dependence of the apparent fraction unfolded, F_{app}, on the urea concentration for the ST α subunit ($\bullet$—$\bullet$) at pH 7.8, 25°C. The line indicates a fit to a three-state model. The transition curve for the EC α subunit (−−) under the same conditions is shown for comparison. This figure has been taken from T. Stackhouse et al. (in prep.).

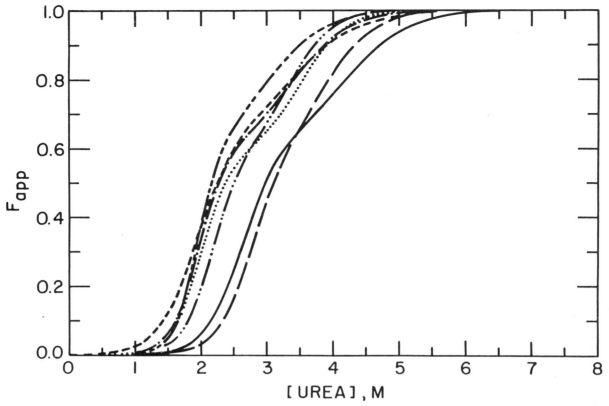

Figure 3. Dependence of the apparent fraction unfolded, F_{app}, on the urea concentration for the EC α subunit (—), the ST α subunit (– –), and the 6–34 (– · –), 8–32 (– · · –), 12–28 (— · · —), 14–26 (· · · ·), and 15–25 (----) hybrid α subunits at pH 7.8, 25°C. The lines indicate results of the nonlinear least-squares fit of the data to a three-state model. To simplify the figure, the data points have not been included; however, the computer fits to the actual data are comparable to that shown in Fig. 2 for the ST α subunit. This figure has been taken from T. Stackhouse et al. (in prep.).

$N \leftrightarrow I$ transition is followed by a less cooperative $I \leftrightarrow U$ transition. Although there are small differences between the hybrids, the general behavior is that both the $N \leftrightarrow I$ and $I \leftrightarrow U$ transitions for all five hybrids are destabilized with respect to both the EC and ST α subunits. Compared to EC α subunit, the decreases in ΔG_{NI} range from 1.1 to 2.2 Kcal mol^{-1} and the decreases in ΔG_{IU} range from 0.9 to 1.6 kcal mol^{-1}, (T. Stackhouse et al., in prep.). Thus, although all of the hybrid proteins are less stable than either parent, the effects of combining the EC and ST α subunits at a variety of sites on the relative stabilities of N, I, and U are again rather small.

Kinetic Folding Studies

The proposed kinetic folding mechanism for the EC α subunit involves a series of native, intermediate, and unfolded forms (Beasty et al. 1986; Hurle et al. 1987; T. Stackhouse et al., in prep.). As shown in Figure 4, there are proposed to be three unfolded forms U_1, U_2, and U_3 that interconvert by slow reactions that may be *cis/trans* isomerizations at X-Pro peptide bonds (Brandts et al. 1975; Crisanti and Matthews 1981; Hurle et al. 1987). These unfolded forms rapidly fold or condense ($\tau < 10$ msec) to their respective intermediate

forms, I_1, I_2, and I_3. These three species then fold to N by a series of slow reactions. The $I_1 \rightarrow I_2$ and $I_2 \rightarrow I_3$ reactions are thought to reflect isomerization reactions, whereas the $I_3 \rightarrow N$ reaction has been shown to be a domain association reaction between the amino domain, 1–188, and the carboxyl domain, 189–268 (Beasty et al. 1986). Unfolding is rate limited by the $N \rightarrow I_3$ reaction.

The urea dependence of the relaxation times that are observed in the unfolding and refolding reactions for EC α subunit are shown in Figure 5. Note that the fast folding reactions that link unfolding and intermediate forms cannot be directly detected because of transient aggregation effects. Consequently, only the relaxation times for the slower ($\tau > 10$ sec) folding reactions are shown. The unfolding reaction is completely accounted for by a single exponential change in absorbance whose relaxation time decreases as the final urea concentration is increased; on a semilogarithmic plot, the decrease is linear with increasing urea concentrations. This reaction corresponds to the $N \rightarrow I_3$ step in the above mechanism (Fig. 4).

Refolding is more complex, showing two relaxation times that have quite different dependences on the urea concentration (Fig. 5). The relaxation time for the slower reaction is independent of the urea concentra-

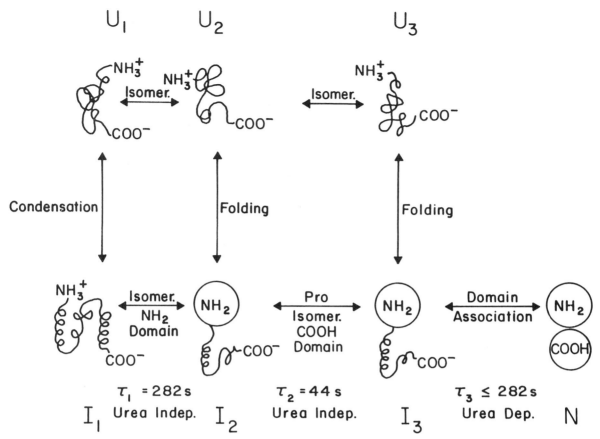

Figure 4. Kinetic model for the folding of EC α subunit at pH 7.8, 25°C. Proposed structures of intermediates and the relaxation times for individual steps are indicated. This figure has been taken from T. Stackhouse et al. (in prep.).

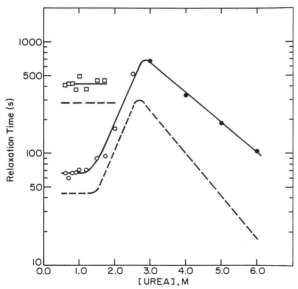

Figure 5. Semilog plot of the urea dependence of the relaxation times for single phase in unfolding ($\bullet$), and the fast ($\bigcirc$) and slow ($\square$) phases in refolding for the ST α subunit at pH 7.8, 25°C. The dependence for the EC α subunit (----) is shown for comparison. This figure has been taken from T. Stackhouse et al. (in prep.).

tion and has an average value of 282 seconds at pH 7.8, 25°C. This reaction is proposed to correspond to the $I_1 \rightarrow I_2$ reaction in the folding model. The relaxation time for the faster reaction decreases as the urea concentration decreases down to 1.5 M urea. Below 1.5 M urea, this relaxation time also becomes independent of the final urea concentration; the average value is 44 seconds below 1.5 M urea. This process is first limited by the $I_3 \rightarrow N$ reaction and depends on the final urea concentration because it involves an actual folding reaction. As this process accelerates at low urea concentration, the $I_2 \rightarrow I_3$ step, which is independent of the urea concentration, becomes rate limiting.

Intermediates I_2 and I_3 are likely to correspond to the single stable intermediate detected in the equilibrium experiment. The I_1 species has an extinction coefficient at 286 nm that is similar to that for the unfolded forms. It would therefore contribute to the observed spectrum as another unfolded form.

Examination of the number of kinetic phases, and magnitudes of the relaxation times, and the urea dependence of these relaxation times for the ST α subunit shows that although there are quantitative differences from the EC α subunit, the slow folding reactions must be quite similar. Unfolding is again well described by a single exponential whose relaxation time is four- to fivefold larger than for EC α subunit. Refolding involves one or more fast reactions that are not directly detected but presumed to exist because the amplitudes of the observed phases do not account for the absorbance change expected from the equilibrium studies. Two slower folding reactions that show the same type of urea dependence as the two phases detected in the EC α subunit were directly observed. The relaxation time for the urea-dependent $I_3 \rightarrow N$ reaction is twice as large as that from EC α subunit. The $I_1 \rightarrow I_2$ and $I_2 \rightarrow I_3$ have average relaxation times of 420 and 67 seconds, respectively. In addition, the relative amplitudes of these two slow phases in the folding of ST α subunit are nearly identical to those from the EC α subunit (T. Stackhouse et al., in prep.). Therefore, the same rate-limiting steps appear in the folding of both EC and ST α subunits.

The urea dependence of the relaxation times for unfolding and refolding of the five EC/ST hybrid α subunits were measured to determine whether the same slow steps limit the folding of these species as well. The slower phase in refolding for all the hybrids except 14–26 is urea independent and falls in the range between the EC and ST α subunits (T. Stackhouse et al., in prep.). The slow refolding phase for the 14–26 hybrid has a significantly longer relaxation time ($1500 < \tau < 3000$ sec), which depends on the final urea concentration. The probable explanation for this apparent change in mechanism will be discussed below.

The urea dependences of the single phase in unfolding and the faster of the two observed phases in refolding of all five hybrid proteins are shown in Figure 6. Although there are small differences between the unfolding relaxation times for all five hybrids, the relaxation times are very similar to that for the EC α subunit. In contrast, the refolding relaxation times for all five hybrids are significantly longer than that for the EC α subunit. Also, the refolding relaxation times for the hybrids do not become independent of the urea concentration at low urea concentrations.

To determine if these changes in the faster observed folding reaction for all five hybrids and the slower folding reaction for the 14–26 hybrid correspond to a change in the folding mechanism, the refolding studies were repeated in the presence of 20% sucrose (w/v). Sucrose is known to stabilize folded forms of proteins over unfolded forms, and a thermodynamic explanation has been provided (Lee and Timasheff 1981). The significance of increasing the stability of folded forms is that the refolding reactions can be accelerated (Hurle et al. 1987). One explanation for the absence of the urea-independent portion of the faster folding phase is that the $I_3 \rightarrow N$ reaction is rate limiting even at 0.6 M urea, the lowest urea concentration studied. If this reaction can be accelerated by sucrose, the urea-independent $I_2 \rightarrow I_3$ reaction may again become rate limiting at sufficiently low urea concentrations.

The effect of 20% sucrose on the refolding reactions of the 8–32, 12–28, 14–26, and 15–25 hybrid α subunits

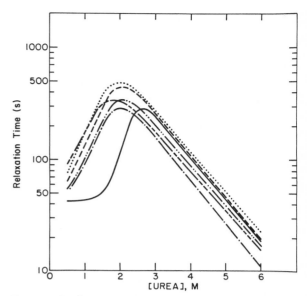

Figure 6. Semilog plot of the urea dependence of the relaxation time for the single phase in unfolding and the faster phase in refolding of the EC α subunit (—) and the 6–34 (– · –), 8–32 (– · · –), 12–28 (———), 14–26 (· · · ·), and 15–25 (- - - -) hybrid α subunits at pH 7.8, 25°C. The data points have not been included to simplify the figure. The scatter of the data about the lines is comparable to that shown for the ST α subunit in Fig. 5. This figure has been taken from T. Stackhouse et al. (in prep.).

is shown in Figure 7. The results for EC α subunit in 20% sucrose are also shown for comparison. As expected, the refolding relaxation times for the EC α subunit

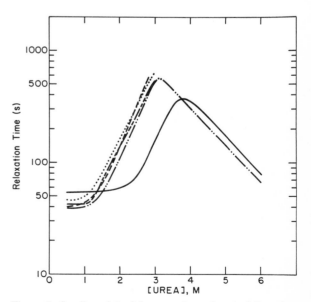

Figure 7. Semilog plot of the urea dependence of the relaxation time for the single phase in unfolding and the faster phase in refolding in the presence of 20% (w/v) sucrose for the EC α subunit (—) and the 8–32 (– · ·), hybrid α subunit at pH 7.8, 25°C. Refolding data only is shown for the 12–28 (———), 14–26 (· · · ·), and 15–25 (- - - -) hybrid α subunits. This figure has been taken from T. Stackhouse et al. (in prep.).

and the four hybrids decrease relative to their values in the absence of sucrose (Fig. 6). Also apparent for the hybrids below 1 M urea is the urea-independent behavior of this relaxation time observed for both EC and ST α subunits. Therefore, the $I_2 \rightarrow I_3$ folding reaction also occurs for the hybrid α subunits.

The presence of sucrose also accelerated the slower folding phase for the 14–26 hybrid so that the relaxation time is independent of the urea concentration and very close in magnitude to that for the EC α subunit (T. Stackhouse et al., in prep.). Presumably, this change reflects a shift in the $U_1 \rightarrow I_1$ equilibrium to favor the more folded I_1 species. This shift would remove the contribution of a prior, rapid equilibrium between U_1 and I_1 on the relaxation time for the $I_1 \rightarrow I_2$ step. Thus, the kinetic folding model for the EC α subunit adequately describes the slow folding steps in the hybrid α subunits as well.

DISCUSSION

Detailed equilibrium and kinetic studies on the folding of the α subunit from tryptophan synthase from *E. coli*, *S. typhimurium*, and five interspecies hybrids show that all fold via the same rate-limiting steps and that all involve one or more stable intermediates. Thus, it seems very likely that the folding mechanism has been conserved *throughout* the process by which the EC and ST α subunits have diverged from a common ancestor (Nichols et al. 1981).

This conclusion is supported by a previous equilibrium study of the guanidine-hydrochloride-induced unfolding of the EC, ST, and 14–26 hybrid α subunits (Yutani et al. 1984). These workers concluded that all three proteins fold via a three-state mechanism that involves a stable intermediate with a folded amino domain.

The similar equilibrium transition curves and refolding relaxation times for all five hybrids suggest that the nine replacements that occur between residues 58 and 184 have little effect on stability or the rate-limiting steps in folding. This conclusion must be drawn with caution because the pairwise comparison of these hybrid proteins involves more than one amino acid replacement, with the exception of the 14–26 and 15–25 hybrids. Site-directed mutagenesis is required to determine definitively the role of an individual amino acid in stability and folding.

The abrupt change in stability and kinetics of folding when the 6–34 hybrid and the EC α subunit are compared shows that one or more of the six replacements in the region from 1 to 58 do play an important role in stability. The observation that the relaxation time for refolding is selectively affected means that the difference in free energies between I_3 and the transition state between I_3 and N increases, whereas that between N and the transition state is not altered. A reaction coordinate diagram that summarizes these observations and others is shown in Figure 8.

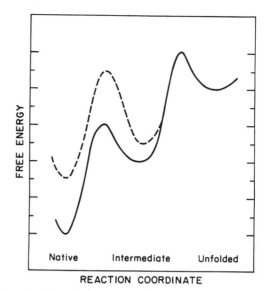

Figure 8. Hypothetical reaction coordinate diagrams for the EC α subunit (—) and the 6–34 hybrid α subunit (----). The diagrams have been arbitrarily aligned by equating the free energies of the unfolded forms and exaggerated to emphasize the selective effects of the hybrid on the I → N refolding reaction; the rate of the N → I unfolding reaction for the 6–34 hybrid is the same as for EC α subunit. This figure has been taken from T. Stackhouse at al. (in prep.).

The decreased stabilities of both the N ↔ I and I ↔ U transitions for the hybrid dictate an increase in the free energy of N and I, relative to their counterparts in EC α subunit. The kinetic consequence of this decrease in stability, a selective effect on the relaxation time for refolding between I and N, implies that the change in the transition state energy must follow that of the native conformation. The effects on the energy of the transition state between U and I are not known.

The structural implications of these results are twofold: (1) At least some part of the amino terminus (1–58) must change its association with the remainder of the protein between I and N. Because the amino domain (1–188) appears to be folded in a rather nativelike fashion in the intermediate (Higgins et al. 1979; Beasty and Matthews 1985), it is possible that the amino terminus interacts with the carboxyl domain in the final, folded protein. (2) This interaction between the amino terminus and the remainder of the protein is established in the transition state.

The selective effect of one or more of the six replacements in the region from 1 to 58 on the relaxation time for refolding suggests that the replacements at positions 6, 12, 13, 15, 42, and 52 may act as equilibrium mutants (Beasty et al. 1986). Such mutants alter the stability but do not *selectively* affect the energy of the transition state.

In contrast, kinetic mutants and mixed equilibrium-kinetic mutants alter selectively the energy of the transition state and, by definition, display changes in the relaxation times for both unfolding and refolding. This type of behavior is apparent when the relaxation times for EC and ST α subunit are compared (Fig. 5). Both unfolding and refolding relaxation times for the urea-dependent reaction are larger for ST α subunit. Because the hybrids, which are various fusions of the EC and ST amino domains, are all equilibrium mutants, it is reasonable to presume that the mixed equilibrium-kinetic effect apparent in the comparison of EC and ST α subunits arises in the carboxyl domain (189–268). Again, site-directed mutagenesis is required to pinpoint those amino acids that play key roles in this domain association reaction.

The conclusions drawn from this study regarding the conservation of the folding mechanism of the α subunit of tryptophan synthase are in agreement with those from earlier studies on ribonuclease A (Krebs et al. 1983) and protease inhibitors (Hollecker and Creighton 1983). Therefore, it seems very likely that the conservation of the folding mechanism is indeed an important evolutionary constraint.

The use of hybrid proteins to examine this question is particularly interesting because it permits an artificial "acceleration" of the evolutionary process along what must be non-natural pathways. The observation that the folding mechanism is conserved in these proteins as well suggests that each individual amino acid replacement has an independent effect on stability and folding and that those effects are rather small. Thus, the total effect of multiple replacements is also small.

ACKNOWLEDGMENTS

The authors are pleased to acknowledge the support of the National Institutes of Health through grant GM-23303 (C.R.M.) and a Research Career Development Award 1 KO4 AG 00153 (C.R.M.). The authors also thank Mark Hurle and Neil Tweedy for critical discussions and Gail Feldman for typing the manuscript.

REFERENCES

Beasty, A.M. and C.R. Matthews. 1985. Characterization of an early intermediate in the folding of the α subunit of tryptophan synthase by hydrogen exchange measurement. *Biochemistry* **24**: 3547.

Beasty, A.M., M.R. Hurle, J.T. Manz, T. Stackhouse, J.J. Onuffer, and C.R. Matthews. 1986. Effects of the Phe 22→Leu, Glu 49→Met, Gly 234→Asp and Gly 234→Lys mutations on the folding and stability of the α subunit of tryptophan synthase from *Escherichia coli*. *Biochemistry* **25**: 2965.

Brandts, J.R., H.R. Halverson, and M. Brennan. 1975. Consideration of the possibility that the slow step in protein denaturation reactions is due to *cis-trans* isomerism of proline residues. *Biochemistry* **14**: 4953.

Crisanti, M.M. and C.R. Matthews. 1981. Characterization of the slow steps in the folding of the α subunit of tryptophan synthase. *Biochemistry* **20**: 2700.

Grafl, R., K. Lang, A. Wrba, and F.X. Schmid. 1986. Folding mechanism of porcine ribonuclease. *J. Mol. Biol.* **191**: 281.

Higgins, W., T. Fairwell, and E.W. Miles. 1979. An active proteolytic derivative of the α subunit of tryptophan synthase. Identification of the site of cleavage and characterization of the fragments. *Biochemistry* **18**: 4827.

Hollecker, M. and T.E. Creighton. 1983. Evolutionary conservation and variation of protein folding pathway. Two protease inhibitor homologues from black mamba venom. *J. Mol. Biol.* **168**: 409.

Hurle, M.R., G.A. Michelotti, M.M. Crisanti, and C.R. Matthews. 1987. Characterization of a slow folding reaction for the α subunit of tryptophan synthase. *Proteins* **2**: 54.

Krebs, H., F.X. Schmid, and J. Jaenicke. 1983. Folding of homologous proteins: The refolding of different ribonucleases is independent of sequence variations, proline content and glycosylation. *J. Mol. Biol.* **169**: 619.

———. 1986. Native-like folding intermediates of homologous ribonucleases. *Biochemistry* **24**: 3846.

Lee, J.C. and S.N. Timasheff. 1981. The stabilization of proteins by sucrose. *J. Biol. Chem.* **256**: 7193.

Levinthal, C. 1968. Are there pathways for protein folding? *J. Chim. Phys.* **69**: 44.

Matthews, C.R. and M.M. Crisanti. 1981. Urea-induced unfolding of the α subunit of tryptophan synthase: Evidence for a multistate process. *Biochemistry* **20**: 784.

Matthews, C.R., M.M. Crisanti, J.T. Manz, and G.L. Gepner. 1983. Effect of a single amino acid substitution on the folding of the α subunit of tryptophan synthase. *Biochemistry* **22**: 1445.

Miles, E.W., K. Yutani, and K. Ogasahara. 1982. Guanidine hydrochloride induced unfolding of the α subunit of tryptophan synthase and of the two α proteolytic fragments: Evidence for stepwise unfolding of the two α domains. *Biochemistry* **21**: 2586.

Nichols, B.P., M. Blumenberg, and C. Yanofsky. 1981. Comparison of the nucleotide sequence of trpA and sequences immediately beyond operon of *Klebsiella aerogenes*, *Salmonella typhimurium* and *Escherichia coli*. *Nucleic Acids Res.* **9**: 1743.

Schellman, J.A. 1978. Solvent denaturation. *Biopolymers* **17**: 1305.

Schneider, W.P., B.P. Nichols, and C. Yanofsky. 1981. Procedure for production of hybrid genes and proteins and its use in assessing significance of amino acid differences in homologous tryptophan synthase α polypeptides. *Proc. Natl. Acad. Sci.* **78**: 2169.

Touchette, N.A, K.M. Perry, and C.R. Matthews. 1986. The folding of dihydrofolate reductase from *Escherichia coli*. *Biochemistry* **25**: 5445.

Yutani, K., K. Ogasahara, M. Suzuki, and Y. Sugino. 1979. Comparison of denaturation by guanidine hydrochloride of the wild type tryptophan synthase α subunit of *E. coli* and two mutant proteins. *J. Biochem.* **85**: 915.

Yutani, K., T. Sato, K. Ogashara, and E.W. Miles. 1984. Comparison of denaturation of tryptophan synthase α-subunits from *Escherichia coli*, *Salmonella typhimurium*, and an interspecies hybrid. *Arch. Biochem. Biophys.* **229**: 448.

Positive Darwinian Selection in Evolution of Protein Inhibitors of Serine Proteinases

M. Laskowski, Jr., I. Kato, W.J. Kohr, S.J. Park, M. Tashiro, and H.E. Whatley

Department of Chemistry, Purdue University, West Lafayette, Indiana 47907

The Neutral Theory of Molecular Evolution by M. Kimura (1983) deservedly stands as a statement of consensus among molecular evolutionists. It asserts that the overwhelming majority of fixations of mutations are selectively neutral. Selection (negative Darwinian selection) relentlessly weeds out the strongly deleterious mutations. Positive Darwinian selection is rare. We agree with this theory, but we note that it deals with what happens most of the time. We believe that a minority of proteins are species specific and frequently exhibit positive Darwinian selection. The purpose of this paper is to present some evidence that protein inhibitors of serine proteinases exhibit in their evolution characteristics associated with positive Darwinian selection. Although the "neutral theory" is now widely believed, there are still many "selectionists" who oppose it. However, the theory is based on or supported by five phenomenological generalizations, which are almost universally believed and which are explicitly or implicitly stated in most elementary biochemistry texts. As we point out later, the belief in these is so strong that it may in fact serve to thwart investigations that may challenge that belief. The five phenomenological generalizations are based on Kimura (1983), but they are not direct quotes, in order to make them as "theory free" as possible. We first acquaint the reader briefly with protein inhibitors of serine proteinases and then show cases where their evolution seems to conflict with the generalization of the neutral theory.

PROTEIN INHIBITORS OF SERINE PROTEINASES

Target Enzymes Are Not Clearly Known

Proteinases are ubiquitous. As is now well known, they have a cradle-to-grave association with all proteins; for many they also exercise important control functions (prepeptide and propeptide removal, zymogen activation, etc.). Although controlled proteolysis is essential to life, rampant proteolysis is fatal. As we do not wish to have all of our blood clot at once, or to eat our own pancreas, or, if we are an intestinal parasite, to be eaten by our host, we must have proteinase inhibitors. Stated in this way, the general function of protein proteinase inhibitors is obvious. Yet one of

the major difficulties of this field of study is that the detailed target enzymes against which the inhibitors are aimed are seldom known. This is in part because many of the inhibitors are not highly specific and can inhibit many different proteinases reasonably well, in part because there are many proteinases, and in part because it is now clear that for some inhibitors the target enzymes are endogenous but for others they are exogenous, thus making the search for the true target even wider.

Because of lack of knowledge of true target enzymes, the study of inhibitors has proceeded with "off the shelf" enzymes such as bovine trypsin and bovine chymotrypsin A, porcine elastase, etc. Despite this limitation, the interaction of serine proteinases with their cognate inhibitors is now one of the best understood of protein-protein associations (Laskowski and Sealock 1971; Laskowski and Kato 1980).

Classification of protein inhibitors of proteinase is given in Table 1. The macroglobulins are not true inhibitors. Instead, they are proteinase traps, which upon cleavage of their "bait regions," wrap themselves around the enzymes to block the access of large substrates. The enzymatic active site remains open in complex, and small substrates are readily turned over (Barrett and Starkey 1973; Harpel 1973; Sottrup-Jensen et al. 1984). Macroglobulins "inhibit" most, but not all, enzymes against which they were tested. They are present both in blood plasma and in eggs.

In contrast, other inhibitory proteins combine with active sites of enzymes and block all of the activities. Such inhibitors are seldom (never) promiscuous enough to interact with proteinases of more than one mechanistic class. Therefore, they can be grouped into four classes corresponding to the four classes of proteinases.

Of the four classes of inhibitors, those of serine proteinases are by far the most extensively studied. In particular, it is the only class for which the position of the reactive sites has been determined and where three-dimensional structures of enzyme-inhibitor complexes

Table 1. Protein Proteinase Inhibitors

Macroglobulins
Inhibitors of Single Mechanistic Classes
1. Serine proteinase inhibitors
2. Cysteine proteinase inhibitors
3. Aspartic acid proteinase inhibitors
4. Metallo proteinase inhibitors

Taken from Laskowski (1986).

An article with a title similar to that of this paper was recently published (Brown 1987).

(Read and James 1986) have been determined, thus allowing for the assignment of contact residues. Thus, this discussion must be restricted to serine proteinase inhibitors. However, it is anticipated that similar analyses will be possible for other inhibitors in the near future, especially the intensively studied inhibitors of cysteine proteinases—the cystatins (Mueller-Esterl et al. 1985; Barrett 1987).

Most protein inhibitors of serine proteinase share a common mechanism of inhibition, the reactive site mechanism, and show considerable similarity in the conformation of their contact regions (Laskowski and Kato 1980; Read and James 1986). However, many pairs of protein inhibitors of serine proteinases show little similarity in overall three-dimensional structure. Consequently, we believe that there are many inhibitor families that are related to one another by convergent rather than divergent evolution. The presently well-established families are listed in Table 2. New families are now found less frequently than before and it is likely that their ultimate number will be no greater than 20–30. Within the families, the evolution is divergent, and it is this divergent evolution that is our topic here.

The Reactive Site Model

Moses Kunitz and co-workers (Kunitz and Northrop 1936; Kunitz 1947a,b) have firmly established that serine proteinase inhibition (at that time simply trypsin inhibition) was a result of a reversible, protein-protein association between the enzyme and inhibitor to form an inactive complex. In the 1960s and 1970s it was shown (for reviews, see Laskowski and Sealock 1971; Laskowski and Kato 1980) that inhibitors are substrates for the proteinases they inhibit. Each inhibitor domain contains a single peptide bond, called the reactive-site peptide bond, which combines with the enzyme in a substrate-like manner. This complex can then dissociate reversibly to either the enzyme and the virgin reactive-site intact inhibitor, I, or to the enzyme and the reactive-site hydrolyzed modified inhibitor, I*, as shown by the relation

$$E + I \underset{k_{off}}{\overset{k_{on}}{\rightleftharpoons}} C \underset{k_{on}^*}{\overset{k_{off}^*}{\rightleftharpoons}} E + I^*$$

The formation of I* and especially the formation of the complex C from I* and E allows for facile determination of the reactive-site peptide bond by chemical studies. The reactive-site peptide bond can also be readily identified from three-dimensional structures of enzyme-inhibitor complexes, where the catalytic serine of the enzyme approaches the carbon of the reactive site of the peptide bond inhibitor somewhat closer than van der Waals distance. In such structures we can also identify the contact residues between the enzyme and the inhibitor. There are typically 11–15 of them. Both chemical evidence (e.g., Ardelt and Laskowski 1985) and X-ray crystallography (Read and James 1986) agree on the reactive-site assignments and show that within a single inhibitory domain all enzymes that are inhibited are inhibited on the same reactive site. Furthermore, in most cases the reactive site can be assigned to all new members of an established family by homology. Difficulties arise only when there are deletions and insertions near the reactive site, such as is the case among serpins. Not quite all protein inhibitors of serine proteinases obey the reactive-site model exactly in all of its details. In most inhibitors, modified inhibitor can still combine with enzyme to form C. This implies reversibility of the reactive-site peptide bond hydrolysis. This is aided by the reactive site's being within one or more disulfide-bridged rings in most, but not all inhibitors. The exceptions are eglin (potato I family) and the serpins. In the case of the serpins, reversal of proteolysis is in fact highly unlikely and the detailed mechanism of interaction differs.

Table 2. Families of Protein Inhibitors of Serine Proteinases

Animals
Bovine pancreatic trypsin inhibitor (Kunitz) family[a]
Pancreatic secretory trypsin inhibitor (Kazal) family[b]
Ascaris inhibitor family[c]
Chelonianin family[d]
Serpin family (mechanistically distinct)[e]
Hirudin family[f]

Plants
Soybean trypsin inhibitor (Kunitz) family[g]
Soybean proteinase inhibitor (Bowman-Birk) family[h]
Potato 1 family[i]
Potato 2 family[j]
Barley trypsin inhibitor family[k]
Squash inhibitor family[l]

Microbial
Streptomyces subtilisin inhibitor (SSI) family[m]

Other families

Expanded from Laskowski (1986).
[a]Gebhard et al. (1986); Gebhard and Hochstrasser (1986). [b]Laskowski et al. (1980, 1987); a list of all known Kazal sequences is maintained at Purdue. Currently, it contains about 300 domain sequences. [c]Babin et al. (1984). [d]Kato and Tominaga (1979) reported on chelonianin, which consists of one Kunitz and one chelonianin domain. Antileukoproteinase (Seemüller et al. 1986b) consists of two chelonian-type domains. [e]Carrell and Travis (1985). [f]Seemüller et al. (1986a). [g]Hejgaard et al. (1983). [h]Ikenaka and Norioka (1986). [i]Graham et al. (1985a). [j]Graham et al. (1985b). [k]Campos and Richardson (1983); Odani et al. (1983); Mahoney et al. (1984). [l]Joubert (1984); Wieczorek et al. (1985). [m]Hiromi et al. (1985).

FIVE GENERALIZATIONS THAT THE INHIBITORS DEFY

First Generalization

Orthologous proteins from closely related species are functionally identical or closely similar.

The oldest of the five generalizations we propose precedes both the neutral theory of Kimura (1968) and that of King and Jukes (1969) and even macromolecular sequencing. It was based on the unity of life notion and has served as a mainstay of biochemistry during this century.

It is the belief in this generalization that allows us to talk about "the specificity of trypsin" or "the allosteric behavior of hemoglobin" without specifying the species. It is this belief that leads us to isolate myoglobin from whales or acetylcholinesterase from electric eels solely because these proteins are very abundant in those species, and to study these proteins without excessive worry that they will be *very* different from their human counterpart. We regret the use of the splendid but much newer word orthologous (Fitch and Margoliash 1970) in this generalization, but this word adds a good bit of clarity.

Ovomucoids are one of the more abundant (10% of total protein, about 10 g/L, thus 3×10^{-4} M) proteins in avian egg white. Their primary function is undoubtedly that of a storage protein, but it was known since the turn of the century that chicken ovomucoid is the major component reponsible for trypsin inhibition (Delezenne and Pozerski 1903) by egg white. As chicken ovomucoid was most accessible, it was the only one to be studied until Rhodes et al. (1960) (see also Feeney and Allison 1969) isolated ovomucoids from about a dozen avian species and tested them for inhibitory activity against trypsin and chymotrypsin. They found that some of them inhibited only one enzyme molecule per mole (single headed), others two (double headed), and yet others three (triple headed). Almost as a corollary, they also found that ovomucoids from closely related species have very different inhibitory specificities; e.g., chicken (*Gallus gallus*), turkey (*Meleagris gallopavo*), and ring-necked pheasant (*Phasianus colchicus*) ovomucoids are strong inhibitors of trypsin, but golden pheasant (*Chrysolophus pictus*) ovomucoid is very weak. In contrast, turkey, ring-necked pheasant, and golden pheasant ovomucoids are strong inhibitors of chymotrypsin, whereas chicken ovomucoid is ineffective. We believe that the paper of Rhodes et al. was ahead of its time and did not receive the attention it deserved.

The above observations were easier to understand when we sequenced several ovomucoids and located their reactive sites (Fig. 1). It is seen there that chicken ovomucoid (and all avian ovomucoids we have studied) consists of three tandem, homologous domains. The domains are closely homologous to pancreatic secretory trypsin inhibitor (Kazal), and thus, ovomucoids belong to the Kazal family of inhibitors (Table 2). Each domain has a single, actual or putative reactive site. After the sequence of ovomucoid became known, it was clear that the study of inhibitory activity of entire ovomucoid is rather complex. It is better to study the individual domains. It is possible to isolate ovomucoid second and third domains (generally without internal nicking) by hydrolysis with proteinase V8 from *Staphylococcus aureus* or with some other proteinase (Laskowski et al. 1987). Of these, the third domains are easiest to get and we have isolated and sequenced them from ovomucoids from 112 species of birds. We have also measured equilibrium constants, K_a^{obs}, for the interaction of most of these with five enzymes: bovine chymotrypsin, porcine pancreatic elastase, sub-

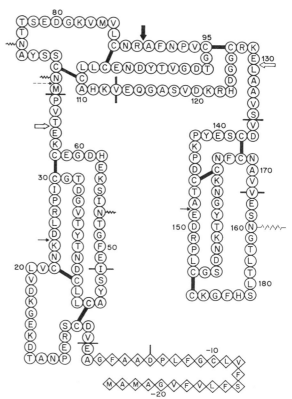

Figure 1. Amino acid sequence of ovomucoid based on Kato et al. (1987). Letters in diamonds indicate the prepeptide; letters in circles indicate the mature protein. Heavy black lines are disulfide bridges, zigzag lines are carbohydrate attachment sites, and the broken line indicates partial glycosylation. A heavy black arrow indicates the well-known trypsin reactive site located in the second domain. Regular arrows are the less-studied reactive sites of the first and third domains. Open arrows are the points of specific hydrolysis by *Staphylococcus aureus* proteinase V8 used to obtain second and third domains. The dashed arrow is the point of CNBr cleavage used to obtain the first domain. Lines are positions of exon/intron junctions in the ovomucoid gene (Stein et al. 1980).

tilisin Carlsberg and *Streptomyces griseus* proteinases A and B. We are currently adding data on human leukocyte elastase. In contrast to the first generalization, the Rhodes et al. (1960) qualitative conclusion on entire ovomucoids was dramatically confirmed by quantitative measurements on isolated third domains. For the inhibition of chymotrypsin, K_a^{obs} is 1.8×10^{10} M^{-1} for turkey ovomucoid third domains and only 1.9×10^3 for chicken. Similar large variations are seen for inhibition of other enzymes and for other closely related pairs of bird species.

Avian ovomucoids are almost certainly products of single-copy genes and orthologous. Stein et al. (1980) and Scott et al. (1987) found only a single chicken ovomucoid gene. Bogard et al. (1980) found that Japanese quail that are heterozygous for Ser-32 and Gly-32 ovomucoid third domains have a precise 50% Ser-32 and 50% Gly-32 distribution in their eggs. The ovomucoids were isolated from eggs of various species by physical techniques, and in each case a single protein was found, except for polymorphisms, which are discussed above and more extensively below.

Second Generalization

In closely related proteins residues at structurally *and* functionally *important positions are nearly unvaried, whereas there are relatively many changes (fixations of mutations) at structurally and functionally neutral positions.*

This generalization is so widely believed by practicing biochemists that whenever several sequences of related proteins are presented, the unvaried residues are almost always pointed out as the important ones and the varied ones as trivial. Due to this belief, it is held that sequencing of closely related proteins is useless because it is expected to produce only a few more trivial positions.

When the sequences of ovomucoid third domains from 112 species are compared (Fig. 2) we note that some positions are unvaried and others are highly varied (at position 18 there are nine alternatives). This is what is expected from similar comparisons for any large set of homologous protein sequences. For further interpretation we utilize three-dimensional structural data that are available on two free ovomucoid third domains: Japanese quail (Weber et al. 1981; Papamokos et al. 1982) and silver pheasant (Bode et al. 1985), and for three complexes of turkey ovomucoid third domain with *Streptomyces griseus* proteinase B (Fujinaga et al. 1982; Read et al. 1983), human leukocyte elastase (Bode et al. 1986), and with bovine chymotrypsin (Fujinaga et al. 1987).

The unvaried or slightly varied positions all can be rationalized (Laskowski et al. 1987) on the basis of their importance to the three-dimensional structure of the molecule. Ovomucoid third domains in particular, and serine proteinase inhibitors in general, do not differ from the majority of proteins in this regard. *Structurally* important positions are conserved.

Figure 2, aside from providing the alternatives at each position, also indicates those positions that are in contact with the enzyme in enzyme-inhibitor complexes. It has been shown repeatedly (e.g., Ardelt and Laskowski 1985) that all enzymes that are inhibited by the same inhibitory domain are inhibited at the same reactive site. The markings in Figure 2 indicate that essentially the same residues of turkey ovomucoid third domain are in contact with all the studied cognate enzymes. We take the 12 positions, 13–21, 32, 33, and 36, where two of the three studied enzymes make contact as the consensus contact residues, all others as consensus noncontact residues. As is seen in Figure 2, this is an approximation; however, all the additional contacts seen in Figure 2 are only glancing interactions. Probably an even greater approximation is the use of turkey ovomucoid data for all avian ovomucoid third domains. Small residues at a given position are less likely to make contact than large ones. As an example,

6	Val Ile	
7	Asp Asn	
8	Cys	
9	Ser	
10	Glu Asp Gly	
11	Tyr His	
12	Pro	
13	Lys Arg Thr Met Gln	◆ ■ ●
14	Pro His Ser	◆ ■ ●
15	Ala Val Asp Ser Gly Glu Thr	◆ ■ ●
16	Cys	◆ ■ ●
17	Thr Pro Ser Arg Leu Met	◆ ■ ●
18	Leu Pro Met Val Gln Ser Ala Thr Lys Gly	◆ ■ ●
19	Glu Asp Leu	◆ ■ ●
20	Tyr Phe Asn Asp Leu Gln Glu His Arg	◆ ■ ●
21	Arg Met Phe Lys Val Thr Leu	◆ ■ ●
22	Pro	
23	Leu Val Ile Phe	
24	Cys	
25	Gly	
26	Ser	
27	Asp Asn	
28	Asn Ser	
29	Lys Gln Ile Glu	◆
30	Thr Ser Ile	◆
31	Tyr	
32	Gly Ser Asn Ala Asp Val Arg His	◆ ■ ●
33	Asn Ser Asp	◆ ■
34	Lys Arg Glu	
35	Cys	
36	Asn Asp Ala Ser Gly Tyr	◆ ■ ●
37	Phe	
38	Cys	
39	Asn Ser	■
40	Ala	
41	Val Ala Phe	
42	Val Ala Leu Met	
43	Glu Asp Gln Lys His	
44	Ser Lys	
45	Asn Ser	
46	Gly Val	
47	Thr -	
48	Leu -	
49	Thr Ile Asn Ser	
50	Leu Val Phe	
51	Ser Arg Gly Asn	
52	His Arg Asn	
53	Phe Leu Ile	
54	Gly Glu	
55	Lys Glu Thr Gln	■
56	Cys	

Figure 2. The amino acid sequence of turkey ovomucoid third domains (shown vertically) and alternatives based on sequences of 111 additional avian species (shown horizontally). 101 species are from Laskowski et al. (1987); the remaining 11 species are results from our laboratory (H. Whatley et al., unpubl.). The numbering is based on connecting peptide extended third domain fragment, first introduced by Weber et al. (1981). The horizontal line divides the sequence at the reactive-site peptide bond. Residues in contact with human leukocyte elastase (◆) (Bode et al. 1986; W. Bode, pers. comm.), bovine chymotrypsin A (■) (Fujinaga et al. 1987) and *Streptomyces griseus* proteinase B (●) (Read et al. 1983) are indicated. Contact is said to occur if any C, N, O, or S atom of the inhibitor residue is within 4.0 Å of a C, N, O, or S atom of the enzyme.

Gly-32 in turkey is not in contact with chymotrypsin, but computer modeling shows that all seven alternatives that we show at this position are. Extensive computer modeling of this type suggests that the division into contact and noncontact residues is sound.

Turning now to Figure 2, we note that there is an astonishing correlation between the number of alternatives and being in contact. The seven most varied positions are all in contact.

The question now arises: Are these positions functional? If the function is defined as inhibition of any of the six enzymes we have studied, the answer is clearly yes. Table 3 is a compilation of data on effects of *natural* substitutions in contact and in noncontact positions based on observations by Park (1985). It is clear

Table 3. Changes in Contact Matter a Lot; Changes not in Contact Matter Little

K_a^{obs} ratios	In contact	Not in contact
$1.0 \rightarrow 2.5$	29%	92%
$2.5 \rightarrow 10.0$	23%	7%
$10.0 \rightarrow 100$	29%	1%
$100 \rightarrow 10^7$	19%	0%
Number of comparisons	265	96
Positions involved	10/12	18/39

Based on interactions with five proteinases: four from trypsin superfamily (bovine chymotrypsin Aα, porcine elastase, and *Streptomyces griseus* proteinases A and B) and one from subtilisin family (subtilisin Carlsberg). Of these, two are vertebrate and three microbial.

that *all* contact positions matter a great deal to K_a^{obs} and *noncontact* positions matter relatively little. Thus, the functionally most important positions are the ones that vary most.

Since "off the shelf" cognate enzymes rather than biological target enzymes were used for the K_a^{obs} determination, an objection might be raised that all of the observed changes in contact positions might be synonymous for the true target enzyme. We regard this possibility as highly unlikely on the basis of what we know about serine proteinases, on the basis of computer modeling, and on the basis of simple inspection of the various residues listed in Figure 2.

We also have determined about 130 sequences of ovomucoid first domains and 15 sequences of ovomucoid second domains. Unfortunately, for these we do not have three-dimensional structures. Therefore, we assume that residues homologous to the contact residues in the third domain are in contact. Subject to this assumption, the contact residues in first and second domains show a hypervariability comparable to that of ovomucoid third domains. The presumed physiological role of pancreatic secretory trypsin inhibitors (Kazal) is to prevent excessive autolytic activation of trypsinogen in the pancreas and in pancreatic juice. Therefore, they all are inhibitors of trypsin. However, the comparison of the eight known complete and fragmentary vertebrate inhibitors shows both Lys and Arg at P_1, both Pro and Thr at P_2, both Ile and Asn at P_1', both Asn and Asp at P_3'. The notion that contact residues vary in inhibitor evolution underlies all of the inhibitor literature, but in most cases we are looking at paralogous rather than at orthologous proteins.

The Third Generalization

In cases where two allelic proteins both have a large frequency (polymorphic locus), both are functionally equivalent.

This generalization is really a corollary of Kimura's theory (Kimura 1983). Protein polymorphisms represent new mutants in the process of fixation. Since it is the neutral changes that are fixed, the two allelic proteins should be equivalent.

In the process of sequencing the ovomucoid third domains from 112 species, we have come across five

polymorphisms. Since we came across these by accident, we assume that both forms are present at high frequencies (in the case of Japanese quail the frequency is 30% of the ancestral Gly-32 and 70% of the new Ser-32; Bogard et al. 1980; Laskowski et al. 1987). Of these five cases, one involves a noncontact residue, four are contact; of these, two are at the major specificity position P_1. Probably the least conservative change is in Montezuma quail (*Cyrtonyx montezumae*) where the change is indicated below.

	P_4	P_3	P_2	P_1	↓	P_1'	P_2'	P_3'	
OMMNQ3L	Ala	Cys	Thr	<u>Leu</u>		Glu	Tyr	Val	....
OMMNQ3S	Ala	Cys	Thr	<u>Ser</u>		Glu	Tyr	Val	....

The K_a^{obs} values of both forms were determined and they are

	Chymotrypsin	Elastase	Subtilisin	SGPA	SGPB
OMMNQ3L	4.9×10^9	8.7×10^9	3.5×10^{10}	3.2×10^{11}	4.2×10^{10}
OMMNQ3S	9.6×10^5	2.8×10^8	1.4×10^9	2.2×10^8	2.9×10^7

A riposte to all of the observations summarized above is an assertion that inhibition of serine proteinases is not a function of ovomucoid third domains. Then especially rapid evolution is not a paradigm break but just what would be expected of pseudogenes, fibrinopeptides, and insulin C peptides. An immediate answer is that the exposed residues on the opposite side of the molecule fix mutations less rapidly, but it only remains to postulate that those on the slowly evolving side do have a function.

A possible approach to resolving this problem is to show that the fixation of mutations in contact positions is faster than the neutral mutation rate. Such a calculation requires both reliable phylogenetic trees for intraordinal divergence of the bird species we have studied and divergence times. Since the bird fossil record is sparse, neither is highly reliable. However, the same goal can be accomplished by internal comparison of pairs of long stretches of contiguous DNA. If the fixation of mutations is faster for nonsynonymous changes in the contact region than for synonymous changes or changes in introns and in pseudogenes, the point is made without need for divergence times and for trees. Unfortunately, all of our sequences are protein sequences, because our main objective was to obtain variants for detailed sequence to reactivity studies. Protein sequencing served us not only to determine the sequence, but to characterize the preparations we used. However, it is clear that to complete the ovomucoid argument, gene sequences of ovomucoids from many species and not just chicken (Stein et al. 1980) should be known. Fortunately for us, however, sets of gene sequences of closely related proteinase inhibitors other than ovomucoids have recently appeared in the literature. As the authors argue that the differences observed are due to selection and we agree, we continue the discussion with their data.

Fourth and Fifth Generalizations

In the DNA sequences of genes, the coding parts fix mutations less frequently than the noncoding parts (introns, pseudogenes, 3' noncoding regions).

Within the coding portions of genes, synonymous changes are appreciably more common than nonsynonymous changes.

These generalizations, albeit recent, are widely supported and widely accepted. In closely related sequences the rate of change of noncoding regions serves as a measure of neutral mutation rate, as does the rate of change in synonymous codons.

Recently Fioretti et al. (1985) isolated from bovine spleen and found in many bovine tissues a close homolog of bovine pancreatic trypsin inhibitor (BPTI) (Kunitz) and named it spleen inhibitor II (SI). The two differ at 7 of the 58 residues. Of these 7, 3 are among the 12 residues in enzyme inhibitor contact as determined by X-ray crystallography. The gene sequences of BPTI and of SI as well as cDNA sequences of their mRNAs were determined by Kingston and Anderson (1986) and by Creighton and Charles (1987). The two mRNAs differ in length, but 874 nucleotides are common. Of these, 12 differ, but of these 12 differences, 9 are in the 174 nucleotide region coding for the mature proteins. Of these 9 differences, only 2 are synonymous and, as already stated, 3 are not only nonsynonymous but in contact. The data clearly suggest selection. However, the two inhibitors are clearly paralogous.

Recently Hill and Hastie (1987) and Yoon et al. (1987) obtained nucleotide sequences of two pairs of rat serpins. These rat serpins are especially closely related to mouse contrapsin and to human α_1-antichymotrypsin. Within each pair the long amino-terminal region 1 is quite closely homologous ($\sim 80-90\%$). This is followed by region 2, consisting of 45 nucleotides, where there is little similarity between the two sequences. It is this region that surrounds the reactive-site peptide bond. In the carboxy-terminal region the homology resumes (albeit less strongly). The surprising fact about the two pairs is that they have one common member so there are three rat serpin genes, all with the striking region 2 hypervariability. Hill and Hastie (1987) show that the rate of nonsynonymous replacements in region 2 is far greater than the rate of

synonymous replacements for regions 1 and 3. Furthermore, they estimate that the rate of divergence of the reactive-site region between rat spi-2.1 gene and mouse contrapsin (assumed orthologous) is 6–8 times greater than the expected neutral mutation rate. These data are in contradiction to the fourth and fifth generalizations. Numerous other tests all suggest selection as the most obvious explanation of the extremely rapid divergence in the reactive-site region. A caveat might be added as the reactive-site region for serpins is defined solely as the hypervariable region surrounding the reactive site, since thus far no one has succeeded in crystallizing a serpin-proteinase complex. This was not for lack of trying.

The data specifically discussed here are particularly strong examples suggesting positive Darwinian selection of enzyme-inhibitor contact residues. However, a look at aligned sequences of the various proteinase inhibitor families (e.g., Fig. 2) indicates a relatively large number of changes among contact residues, when these can be identified from X-ray crystallography, and of the residues surrounding the reactive site in those families where X-ray structures of complexes are not yet available. The notion of hypervariability of these residues is an old one (Kato et al. 1978; Laskowski and Kato 1980), but until recently we lacked the courage to definitively state that we believe protein inhibitors of serine proteinases are frequently subject to positive Darwinian selection.

Why Do Inhibitors Evolve Differently?

We are asserting positive Darwinian selection for serine proteinase inhibitors that belong to several different families. What do they have in common that makes them evolve differently? We should say at the outset that we are puzzled and not at all sure of the answer.

A. Chemical tolerance of radical replacements without necessary loss of activity. We believe that the major reason for the correctness of neutral mutation theory is the great intolerance of proteins to mutations of structurally or functionally important residues. Generally, such mutations simply impair function. On the other hand, in inhibitors, functional residue replacements often lead to a change in specificity and not to a loss of function. To rephrase in everyday jargon, positive Darwinian selection of inhibitors is technologically possible.

B. An important reason why many orthologous proteins do not undergo significant positive Darwinian selection is that the gain of a new desirable specificity may be accompanied by complete loss of the old desirable specificity. Thus, gene duplication and separate evolution of the descendant paralogous genes is the main mechanism for acquisition of new specificity. Proteinase inhibitors of serine proteinases have two characteristics that may make the loss of initial specificity somewhat more tolerable. Many of them are products of tandem gene duplication and elongation, such as is seen in avian ovomucoids with three domains (Fig. 1). The current champion is ovoinhibitor with seven tandem domains (Scott et al. 1987). Since all domains are (at least potentially) inhibitory, the loss of the original specificity may sometimes be compensated by overlapping specificity of another domain. The other related compensation for the loss of initial specificity stems from the fact that in many rich sources of inhibitors (e.g., blood, egg white, plant seeds), many different inhibitors tend to occur together, all at relatively high levels. Among these inhibitors there is often at least one that is not very specific (e.g., macroglobulin) both in blood and in egg white. Again to translate this to common language, not only is it technologically possible, but we can afford it.

C. One anticipates that proteins that evolve to interact with other proteins in the producing organism will evolve rather slowly as the mutual need to adjust to each other will slow the process down. Such is not the case if the target protein is exogenous to the producing organism. Many inhibitors clearly have exogenous target enzymes (e.g., the thrombin inhibitor from leeches, hirudin; the trypsin and chymotrypsin inhibitors from the intestinal parasite *Ascaris lumbricoides;* and Kunitz-type inhibitors in snake venoms). Green and Ryan (1972) have presented convincing evidence that the role of many plant inhibitors is defense against invading insects. It is quite plausible, as discussed by Laskowski et al. (1987), that the role of inhibitors in avian egg white is the inhibition of proteinases of invading microorganisms. The postulated role of human serpins is the inhibition of human enzymes (Travis and Salvesen 1983), but Hill and Hastie (1987) raise the possibility of an additional role in defense against parasitic proteinases. If the frequent role of inhibitors is the inhibition of foreign enzymes, then rapid evolution has a purpose. To go on with the common language translation: not only is it technologically possible and affordable, but there may even be some reason for it.

After listing these possible causes of positive Darwinian selection among inhibitors, we were struck by the fact that these resembled those frequently listed to explain the truly great diversity of antibodies. As we have already pointed out (Laskowski et al. 1987), the mechanisms for achieving this diversity among antibodies and inhibitors are quite different, as is the time scale on which they are achieved. Yet analogies between inhibitors and antibodies are also of interest.

The obvious fault of this paper is that neither we nor our colleagues provide a clear demonstration of the specific advantage gained for the organism by rapid evolution of the enzyme-inhibitor contact residues. We are looking for such examples, but as we are not biologists, our hopes are slim. We hope that many others will join us in this quest.

In summary, we believe, along with Kimura (1983), that the evolution of most proteins is predominantly neutral and that the five consensus generalizations apply to most proteins. In the natural history of most proteins there may be episodes where positive Darwinian selection takes over, but its contribution to overall evolution is modest. In contrast with Kimura (1983), we believe that there are a few groups of proteins where, for a number of reasons, positive Darwinian selection is a major (although clearly not the only) cause of evolutionary change. We assert that protein inhibitors of serine proteinases are such a group. It is of interest to ask whether there are other such groups and if so, why they were not found as yet. The following list of reasons occurs to us.

1. There may be very few of them.
2. Acquisition of a set of related proteins usually involves a functional assay. It is therefore likely that members of the set will be functionally similar. This point often arises in inhibitor research. Many investigators simply "fish" for trypsin inhibitors and thus restrict their set to inhibitors with Lys and Arg P_1 residues. In contrast, ovomucoids are isolated on the basis of their physical properties without a functional assay, and the great variety of P_1 residues is apparent.
3. Journals, granting agencies, and the scientific ethos are against determining sequences of closely related genes and proteins, but it is only such sequencing that can find exceptions to the neutral evolution.

ACKNOWLEDGMENTS

Isolation sequencing and characterization of inhibitors was a huge task. We are grateful to the following members of our group at Purdue for help in this effort: W. Ardelt, W.C. Bogard, C.-W. Chi, J. Cook, A. Denton, M.W. Empie, D.A. Estell, W. Finkenstadt, C.A. Kelly, T.R. Leary, T.-Y. Lin, J. Otlewski, K. Parks, B.L. Schatzley, Oe. Schoenberger, J. Schrode, R.W. Sealock, M. Tashiro, G. Vichot, N. Warne, A. Wieczorek, M. Wieczorek, K.A. Wilson, and R. Wynn. We were fortunate to get help from some of the best practitioners of the art of X-ray crystallography: M. Fujinaga, M.N.G. James, R.J. Read, A. Sielecki, W. Bode, O. Epp, R. Huber, E. Papamokos, and E. Weber. M.L. benefited greatly by studying molecular evolution with W.M. Fitch (now at the University of California) at the University of Wisconsin at Madison. We thank the National Institutes of Health for grant GM-10831.

REFERENCES

Ardelt, W. and M. Laskowski, Jr. 1985. Turkey ovomucoid third domain inhibits eight different serine proteinases of varied specificity on the same...Leu[18]-Glu[19]...reactive site. *Biochemistry* **24:** 5313.

Babin, D.R., R.J. Peanasky, and S.M. Goos. 1984. The isoinhibitors of chymotrypsin/elastase from *Ascaris lumbricoides:* The primary structure. *Arch. Biochem. Biophys.* **232:** 143.

Barrett, A.J. 1987. The cystatins: A new class of peptidase inhibitors. *Trends Biochem. Sci.* **12:** 193.

Barrett, A.J. and P.M. Starkey. 1973. The interaction of α_2-macroglobulin with proteinases. Characteristics and specificity of the reaction, and a hypothesis concerning its molecular mechanism. *Biochem. J.* **133:** 709.

Bode, W., O. Epp, R. Huber, M. Laskowski, Jr., and W. Ardelt. 1985. The crystal and molecular structure of the third domain of silver pheasant ovomucoid (OMSVP3). *Eur. J. Biochem.* **147:** 387.

Bode, W., A.-Z. Wei, R. Huber, E. Meyer, J. Travis, and S. Neumann. 1986. X-ray crystal structure of the complex of human leukocyte elastase (PMN elastase) and the third domain of the turkey ovomucoid inhibitor. *EMBO J.* **5:** 2453.

Bogard, W.C., Jr., I. Kato, and M. Laskowski, Jr. 1980. A Ser^{162}/Gly^{162} polymorphism in Japanese quail ovomucoid. *J. Biol. Chem.* **255:** 6569.

Brown, A.L. 1987. Positively darwinian molecules? *Nature* **326:** 12.

Campos, F.A.P. and M. Richardson. 1983. The complete amino acid sequence of the bifunctional α-amylase/trypsin inhibitor from seeds of ragi (Indian finger millet, *Eleusine coracana* Gaertn.). *FEBS. Lett.* **152:** 300.

Carrell, R. and J. Travis. 1985. α_1-Antitrypsin and the serpins: Variation and countervariation. *Trends. Biochem. Sci.* **10:** 20.

Creighton, T.E. and I.G. Charles. 1987. Sequences of the genes and polypeptide precursors for two bovine protease inhibitors. *J. Mol. Biol.* **194:** 11.

Delezenne, C. and E. Pozerski. 1903. Inhibitory action of the native ovalbumin on the tryptic digestion of heat denatured ovalbumin. *C.R. Seances Soc. Biol. Fil.* **55:** 935.

Feeney, R.E. and R.G. Allison. 1969. *Evolutionary biochemistry of proteins.* Wiley-Interscience, New York.

Fioretti, E., G. Iacopino, M. Angeletti, D. Barra, F. Bossa, and F. Ascoli. 1985. Primary structure and antiproteolytic activity of a Kunitz-type inhibitor from bovine spleen. *J. Biol. Chem.* **260:** 11451.

Fitch, W.M. and E. Margoliash. 1970. The usefulness of amino acid and nucleotide sequences in evolutionary studies. *Evol. Biol.* **4:** 67.

Fujinaga, M., R.J. Read, A. Sielecki, W. Ardelt, M. Laskowski, Jr., and M.N.G. James. 1982. The refined crystal structure of the molecular complex of SGPB, a serine protease, with the third domain of the ovomucoid inhibitor from turkey. *Proc. Natl. Acad. Sci.* **79:** 4868.

Fujinaga, M., A.R. Sielecki, R.J. Read, W. Ardelt, M. Laskowski, Jr., and M.N.G. James. 1987. Crystal and molecular structures of the complex of α-chymotrypsin with its inhibitor turkey ovomucoid third domain at 1.8 Å resolution. *J. Mol. Biol.* **195:** 397.

Gebhard, W. and K. Höchstrasser. 1986. Inter-α-trypsin inhibitor and its close relatives. In *Proteinase inhibitors* (ed. A.J. Barrett and G. Salvesen), p. 389. Elsevier, Amsterdam.

Gebhard, W., H. Tschesche, and H. Fritz. 1986. Biochemistry of aprotinin and aprotinin-like inhibitors. In *Proteinase inhibitors* (ed. A.J. Barrett and G. Salvesen), p. 375. Elsevier, Amsterdam.

Graham, J.S., G. Pearce, J. Merryweather, K. Titani, L. Ericsson, and C.A. Ryan. 1985a. Wound-induced proteinase inhibitors from tomato leaves. I. The cDNA-deduced primary structure of pre-inhibitor I and its post-translational processing. *J. Biol. Chem.* **260:** 6555.

———. 1985b. Wound-induced proteinase inhibitors from tomato leaves. II. The cDNA-deduced primary structure of pre-inhibitor II. *J. Biol. Chem.* **260:** 6561.

Green, T.R. and C.A. Ryan. 1972. Wound-induced proteinase inhibitor in plant leaves. Possible defense mechanism against insects. *Science* **175:** 776.

Harpel, P.C. 1973. Human plasma α_2-macroglobulin-enzyme interactions. Evidence for proteolytic modification of the subunit chain structure. *J. Exp. Med.* **138:** 508.

Hejgaard, J., I. Svendsen, and J. Mundy. 1983. Barley α-amylase/subtilisin inhibitor. II. N-terminal amino acid sequence and homology with inhibitors of the soybean trypsin inhibitor (Kunitz) family. *Carlsberg Res. Commun.* **48:** 91.

Hill, N.D. and R.E. Hastie. 1987. Accelerated evolution in the reactive center regions of serine protease inhibitors. *Nature* **326:** 96.

Hiromi, K., K. Akasaka, Y. Mitsui, B. Tonomura, and S. Murao. 1985. *Protein protease inhibitor—The case of Streptomyces subtilisin inhibitor (SSI).* Elsevier, New York.

Ikenaka, T. and S. Norioka. 1986. Bowman-Birk family serine proteinase inhibitors. In *Proteinase inhibitors* (ed. A.J. Barrett and G. Salvesen), p. 361. Elsevier, Amsterdam.

Joubert, F.J. 1984. Proteinase inhibitors from *Lonchocarpus capassa* (apple-leaf seed). *Phytochemistry* **23:** 1401.

Kato, I. and N. Tominaga. 1979. Trypsin-subtilisin inhibitor from red sea turtle eggwhite consists of two tandem domains—one Kunitz—one of a new family. *Fed. Proc.* **38:** 832 (Abstr.).

Kato, I., W.J. Kohr, and M. Laskowski, Jr. 1978. Evolution of avian ovomucoids. In *Regulatory proteolytic enzymes and their inhibitors* (ed. S. Magnusson et al.), vol. 47, p. 197. Federation of European Biochemical Societies, Copenhagen.

Kato, I., J. Schrode, W.J. Kohr, and M. Laskowski, Jr. 1987. Chicken ovomucoid. Determination of its amino acid sequence, of the trypsin reactive site and preparation of all three of its domains. *Biochemistry* **26:** 193.

Kimura, M. 1968. Evolutionary rate at the molecular level. *Nature* **217:** 624.

———. 1983. *The neutral theory of molecular evolution.* Cambridge University Press, Cambridge.

King, J.L. and T.H. Jukes. 1969. Non-Darwinian evolution. *Science* **164:** 788.

Kingston, I.B. and S. Anderson. 1986. Sequences encoding two trypsin inhibitors occur in strikingly similar genomic environments. *Biochem. J.* **233:** 443.

Kunitz, M. 1947a. Crystalline soybean trypsin inhibitor. II. General properties. *J. Gen. Physiol.* **30:** 291.

———. 1947b. Isolation of a crystalline protein compound of trypsin and soybean trypsin inhibitor. *J. Gen. Physiol.* **30:** 311.

Kunitz, M. and J.H. Northrop. 1936. Isolation from beef pancreas of crystalline trypsinogen, trypsin, a trypsin inhibitor and an inhibitor-trypsin compound. *J. Gen. Physiol.* **19:** 991.

Laskowski, M., Jr. 1986. Protein inhibitors of serine proteinase—Mechanism and classification. In *Nutritional and toxicological significance of enzyme inhibitors in foods* (ed. M. Friedman), p. 1. Plenum Publishing, New York.

Laskowski, M., Jr. and I. Kato. 1980. Protein inhibitors of proteinases. *Annu. Rev. Biochem.* **49:** 593.

Laskowski, M., Jr. and R.W. Sealock. 1971. Protein proteinase inhibitors—Molecular aspects. In *The enzymes,* 3rd edition (ed. P.D. Boyer), vol. 3, p. 375. Academic Press, New York.

Laskowski, M., Jr., I. Kato, W.J. Kohr, C.J. March, and W.C. Bogard. 1980. Evolution of the family of serine proteinase inhibitors homologous to pancreatic secretory trypsin inhibitor (Kazal). *Protides Biol. Fluids Proc. Colloq.* **28:** 123.

Laskowski, M., Jr., I. Kato, W. Ardelt, J. Cook, A. Denton, M.W. Empie, W.J. Kohr, S.J. Park, K. Parks, B.L. Schatzley, O.L. Schoenberger, M. Tashiro, G. Vichot, H.E. Whatley, A. Wieczorek, and M. Wieczorek. 1987. Ovomucoid third domains from 100 avian species. Isolation, sequence and hypervariability of enzyme-inhibitor contact residues. *Biochemistry* **26:** 202.

Mahoney, W.C., M.A. Hermodson, B. Jones, D.D. Powers, R.S. Corfman, and G.R. Reeck. 1984. Amino acid sequence and secondary structural analysis of the corn inhibitor of trypsin and activated Hageman factor. *J. Biol. Chem.* **259:** 8412.

Mueller-Esterl, W., H. Fritz, J. Kellermann, F. Lottspeich, W.

Machleidt, and V. Turk. 1985. Genealogy of mammalian cysteine proteinase inhibitors. Common evolutionary origin of stefins, cystatins and kininogens. *FEBS. Lett.* **191:** 221.

Odani, S., T. Koide, T. Ono, and K. Ohnishi. 1983. Structural relationship between barley (*Hordeum vulgare*) trypsin inhibitor and castor-bean (*Ricinus communis*) storage protein. *Biochem. J.* **213:** 543.

Papamokos, E., E. Weber, W. Bode, R. Huber, M.W. Empie, I. Kato, and M. Laskowski, Jr. 1982. Crystallographic refinement of Japanese quail ovomucoid, a Kazal-type inhibitor, and model building studies of complexes with serine proteases. *J. Mol. Biol.* **158:** 515.

Park, S.J. 1985. "Effect of amino acid replacements in ovomucoid third domains upon their association with serine proteinases." Ph.D. thesis, Purdue University, West Lafayette, Indiana.

Read, R.J. and M.N.G. James. 1986. Introduction to the protein inhibitors: X-ray crystallography. In *Proteinase inhibitors* (ed. A.J. Barrett and G. Salvesen), p. 301. Elsevier, Amsterdam.

Read, R.J., M. Fujinaga, A.R. Sielecki, and M.N.G. James. 1983. Structure of the complex of *Streptomyces griseus* protease B and the third domain of the turkey ovomucoid inhibitor at 1.8 Å resolution. *Biochemistry* **22:** 4420.

Rhodes, M.B., N. Bennett, and R.E. Feeney. 1960. The trypsin and chymotrypsin inhibitors from avian egg whites. *J. Biol. Chem.* **235:** 1686.

Scott, M.J., C.S. Huckaby, I. Kato, W.J. Kohr, M. Laskowski, Jr., M.-J. Tsai, and B.W. O'Malley. 1987. Ovoinhibitor introns specify functional domains as in the related and linked ovomucoid gene. *J. Biol. Chem.* **262:** 5899.

Seemüller, U., J. Dodt, E. Fink, and H. Fritz. 1986a. Protein-ase inhibitors of the leech *Hirudo medicinalis* (hirudins, bdellins, eglins). In *Proteinase inhibitors* (ed. A.J. Barrett and G. Salvesen), p. 337. Elsevier, Amsterdam.

Seemüller, U., M. Arnhold, H. Fritz, K. Wiedenmann, W. Machleidt, R. Heinzel, H. Appelhans, H.-G. Gassen, and F. Lottspeich. 1986b. The acid-stable proteinase inhibitor of human mucous secretions (HUSI-I, antileukoprotease). *FEBS Lett.* **199:** 43.

Sottrup-Jensen, L., T.M. Stepanik, T. Kristensen, D. Wierz-bicki, C.M. Jones, P.B. Lonblad, S. Magnusson, and T.E. Peterson. 1984. Primary structure of human α_2-macro-globulin. V. The complete structure. *J. Biol. Chem.* **259:** 8318.

Stein, J.P., J.F. Catterall, P. Kristo, A.R. Means, and B.W. O'Malley. 1980. Ovomucoid intervening sequences specify functional domains and generate protein polymorphism. *Cell* **21:** 681.

Travis, J. and G.S. Salvesen. 1983. Human plasma proteinase inhibitors. *Annu. Rev. Biochem.* **52:** 655.

Weber, E., E. Papamokos, W. Bode, R. Huber, I. Kato, and M. Laskowski, Jr. 1981. Crystallization, crystal structure analysis and molecular model of Japanese quail ovomucoid third domain, a Kazal-type inhibitor. *J. Mol. Biol.* **149:** 109.

Wieczorek, M., J. Otlewski, J. Cook, K. Parks, J. Leluk, A. Wilimowska-Pelc, A. Polanowski, T. Wilusz, and M. Laskowski, Jr. 1985. The squash family of serine proteinase inhibitors. Amino acid sequences and association equilibrium constants of inhibitors from squash, summer squash, zucchini, and cucumber seeds. *Biochem. Biophys. Res. Commun.* **126:** 646.

Yoon, J.-B., H.C. Towle, and S. Seelig. 1987. Growth hormone induces two mRNA species of the serine protease inhibitor gene family in rat liver. *J. Biol. Chem.* **262:** 4284.

Stereochemistry of Cooperative Mechanisms in Hemoglobin

M.F. Perutz,* G. Fermi,* B. Luisi,* B. Shaanan,† and R.C. Liddington‡
*MRC Laboratory of Molecular Biology, Cambridge, CB2 2QH, England; †Department of Structural Chemistry, Weizmann Institute, Rehovot 76100, Israel; ‡Department of Chemistry, York University, York YO1 5DD, England

Hemoglobin (Hb) is the respiratory protein of the red blood cells that carries O_2 from the lungs to the tissues and facilitates the return transport of CO_2 from the tissues to the lungs. The physicist J.J. Hopfield has called it the hydrogen atom of biochemistry because understanding of its functions is so fundamental to proteins generally. One of these functions is allostery, the switching of proteins between active and inactive structures in response to chemical stimuli. Another is the formation of coordination complexes with transition metals for a great variety of catalytic and other actions. Hemoglobin may be unique in exploiting changes in Fe–N bond lengths accompanying the transition from high-spin to low-spin ferrous iron for the purpose of efficient oxygen transport: without use of that spin transition, fast-moving animals could not have evolved. The isolation of the iron atoms in separate pockets of the globin prevents collisions between them, which means that their reactions with ligands can be studied without any of the elaborate apparatus of matrix isolation needed for investigating the reaction mechanisms of simpler metal complexes. Finally, hemoglobin shows how nature uses conjugated bases with pK values in the physiological pH range to sensitize proteins to small pH changes in their environment.

Hemoglobin has a molecular weight of 64,500 and is a tetramer made up of two α chains, each containing 141 amino acid residues, and two β chains, each containing 146 amino acid residues. Each chain carries one heme. The α chains contain seven helical segments and the β chains eight, interrupted by nonhelical segments. Each chain also carries short nonhelical segments at the amino and carboxyl termini. Myoglobin (Mb) is a similar protein consisting of a single chain of 153 amino acid residues and one heme. It is found in muscle, where it stores the O_2 transferred to it from hemoglobin and liberates the O_2 to the mitochondria for oxidative phosphorylation of adenosine diphosphate. The hemes in Mb and Hb are held in pockets formed by several helical and nonhelical segments; their Fes are 5-coordinated to N_ϵ of histidines F8, also known as proximal, and to the four porphyrin nitrogens (N_{porph}); the porphyrin is in van der Waals contact with another histidine on the distal side (E7) and also makes contact with 18 other amino acid side chains, most of which are nonpolar. The propionate side chains of the porphyrin protrude into the solvent and form hydrogen bonds with basic side chains of the globin (HisCD3[45]α and

LysE10[66]β) (Fermi and Perutz 1981; Dickerson and Geis 1983) (Figs. 1 and 2).

The heme irons in Hb and Mb combine reversibly with O_2 to form dioxygen complexes and, in the process, change from high-spin FeII to low-spin FeII. The reaction of O_2 with Mb is a simple bimolecular one, but the reaction with Hb is cooperative, with a free energy of cooperativity, under conditions that mimic physiological ones, of 3.6 kcal mol^{-1} (15 kJ mol^{-1})$heme^{-1}$. The oxygen affinity of Mb is independent of pH and ionic strength, but that of mammalian Hb is lowered by H^+, Cl^-, CO_2, and 2,3-D-diphosphoglycerate (DPG), all of which are present in the red cell. They are known collectively as the heterotropic ligands, and ligands that combine with the heme iron are called homotropic. The interactions between the various ligands reacting with Hb are known as the cooperative effects. They are needed to ensure efficient respiratory transport.

The cooperative binding of O_2 is manifested by its sigmoid equilibrium curve and ensures uptake and release of O_2 over the comparatively narrow range of partial O_2 pressures that distinguishes the lungs ($pO_2 \sim 100$ mm Hg) from the tissues ($pO_2 \sim 30$–40 mm Hg). Hb binds one H^+ for every two O_2 molecules released; this uptake biases the equilibrium of the reaction between CO_2 and H_2O in the direction of HCO_3^-, thus promoting the transport of CO_2 by the blood serum. Conversely, the protons released by the metabolic products, lactic and carbonic acids, facilitate the release of O_2 to the tissues.

In the hemoglobins of bony vertebrates, the cooperative effects arise from an equilibrium between two alternative Hb structures, the oxy or relaxed (R) and deoxy or tense (T) structure. The O_2 affinity of the R structure is slightly larger than the average of free α and β subunits; that of the T structure is lower by the equivalent of the free energy of cooperativity. The O_2 equilibrium of Hb can be described by the O_2 association constants K_T and K_R, usually expressed in (mm Hg)$^{-1}$, and by the equilibrium constant $L_o = [T]/[R]$ in the absence of O_2. Imai has shown empirically that log $K_T/K_R = A - 0.25$ log L_o, where A is a constant, which leaves K_R and K_T as the only independent variables. K_T varies over a wide range as a function of $[H^+]$, $[Cl^-]$, $[CO_2]$, and [DPG]; K_R varies as a function of $[H^+]$ below pH 7, but is little affected by the other ligands (Baldwin 1975; Imai 1982).

The T and R structures differ in the arrangement of

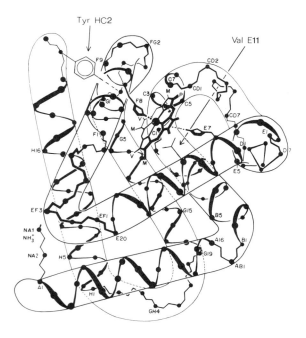

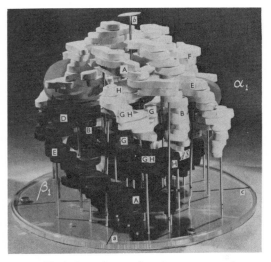

Figure 1. (*Top*) Secondary and tertiary structure characteristic of the hemoglobins. Starting from the amino terminus the helical segments are denoted A to H, and the nonhelical ones NA, AB, BC, etc., to HC, which denotes a segment of 3 nonhelical residues at the carboxyl terminus. Residues within each segment are numbered from the amino end, A1 to A16, etc. We label each residue by its structural position followed by its position in the sequence, e.g., GluA3(6)β. The tetramer has pseudotetrahedral symmetry. (*Bottom*) Model of oxyhemoglobin. The α chains are white, the β chains black; the gray disks represent the hemes, the sign at the top the dyad axis, HS the reactive CysF9(93)β. The FG and C segments at the $\alpha_1\beta_2$ contact are marked. On transition to the deoxy structure, the $\alpha_1\beta_1$ dimer on the left turns relative to the $\alpha_2\beta_2$ dimer on the right, so that FGβ_2 moves toward and Cα_1 away from the observer; the gap between β_1 and β_2 widens. A true dyad relating the chains α_1 to α_2 and β_1 to β_2 runs along a 50-Å long and ~10-Å wide water-filled central cavity. Pseudodyads at right angles to the true dyad and to each other relate α_1 to β_1 and α_1 to β_2. The diagram shows the helical and nonhelical segments, the heme, the proximal HisF8, the distal HisE7, and the distal ValE11.

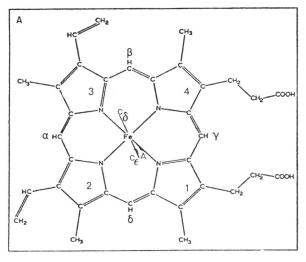

Figure 2. (*A*) Heme with imidazole of HisF8 projected into its plane. (*B*) Interatomic distances around Fe in 2-MeIm-(TpivPP)FeII. The diagrams illustrate the meanings of angles A and B in Table 1.

the four subunits, referred to as the quaternary structure, and the conformation of the subunits, referred to as the tertiary structure. The quaternary R $\rightleftharpoons$ T transition consists of a rotation of the dimer $\alpha_1\beta_1$ relative to the dimer $\alpha_2\beta_2$ by 12–15° and a translation of one dimer relative to the other by 0.8 Å. The $\alpha\beta$ dimers move relative to each other at the symmetry-related contacts $\alpha_1\beta_2$ and $\alpha_2\beta_1$ and at the contacts $\alpha_1\alpha_2$ and $\beta_1\beta_2$; the contacts $\alpha_1\beta_1$ and $\alpha_2\beta_2$ remain rigid.

At the $\alpha_1\beta_2$ interface the nonhelical segment FGα_1 is in contact with helix Cβ_2 and helix Cα_1 with FGβ_2. During the R $\rightleftharpoons$ T transition, the contact FGα_1–Cβ_2 acts as a ball and socket joint, whereas the contact Cα_1–FGβ_2 acts as a two-way switch that shifts Cα_1 relative to FGβ_2 by about 6 Å, like the knuckles of one hand moving over those of the other. Intermediate positions of the switch are blocked by steric hindrance. The gaps along the central cavity between α_1 and α_2 and between β_1 and β_2 narrow on transition from T to R. The shape of the $\alpha_1\beta_1$ and $\alpha_2\beta_2$ dimers is altered by changes in tertiary structure: for example, on oxygenation, the distance between the α carbons of residues FG1α_1 and β_1 shrinks from 45.6 to 41.3 Å. These changes make an $\alpha_1\beta_1$ dimer that has the tertiary oxy structure a misfit in the quaternary T structure, and an $\alpha_1\beta_1$ dimer that has the tertiary deoxy structure a misfit in the quaternary R structure (Baldwin and Chothia 1979; A. Lesk and M.F. Perutz, unpubl.).

The key questions for the understanding of Hb function are these: How does the reaction with O_2 affect the stereochemistry at and around the heme so as to trigger the transition from the T to the R structure? What are the constraints of the T structure and how do they lower the O_2 affinity? By what mechanisms do the heterotropic ligands influence the O_2 affinity? Single-crystal X-ray analyses of deoxy and oxyhemoglobin, and of analogs of intermediates in the reactions with O_2 or CO, together with chemical, spectroscopic, and magnetic studies, have furnished some of the answers. Table 1 lists the structures on which our analysis of the cooperative mechanism rests. We shall now review these in turn.

The Structures of Deoxy and Oxyhemoglobin

Changes on oxygenation in stereochemistry of the hemes. Table 1 and Figures 3 and 4 summarize the stereochemistry of the hemes in deoxyhemoglobin (DHb) and oxyhemoglobin (HbO$_2$) (Shaanan 1983; Fermi et al. 1984). In DHb, the Fes are displaced from the planes of the porphyrin nitrogens, and the porphyrins are domed, as predicted by Gelin et al. (1983). On oxygenation, the porphyrins flatten and the Fe–N$_{Porph}$ bond lengths contract, thus moving the Fes toward the porphyrin planes. In consequence, the proximal histidines come 0.5–0.6 Å closer to the porphyrin planes in HbO$_2$ than in DHb. A water molecule that is hydrogen bonded to the distal histidines (E7) of the α subunits in DHb dissociates in HbO$_2$.

Are these stereochemical changes at the hemes intrinsic or are they influenced by the globin or the crystal lattice? The Fe–N$_{porph}$ distances and the displacements of the Fes from the planes of the N$_{porph}$s in DHb and DMb are the same as in two synthetic 5-coordinated FeII-porphyrins (Table 1) (Hoard 1975; Jameson et al. 1980). The average Fe–N$_{porph}$ distances measured in crystals of DHb and HbO$_2$ also agree with those measured in solution by extended X-ray fluorescence spectroscopy (EXAFS) (Eisenberger et al. 1978; Perutz et al. 1982; Fermi et al. 1987). The conformation of the hemes in human DHb is the same within error in crystals of space group P2$_1$ grown in (NH$_4$)$_2$SO$_4$ solutions and in crystals of space group P2$_1$2$_1$2 grown in polyethylene glycol (PEG) solutions. The degree of doming of the porphyrin, on the other hand, appears to be influenced by the constraints of the globin and by those of the crystal lattices in the synthetic iron porphyrins.

Hb, Mb, and the model complexes bind O_2 to the Fes in the bent, terminal η^1 mode (Fig. 4). The Fe–O–O angle varies over a wide range, depending on the shape

and chemical constitution of the heme pocket, but its influence on the strength of the Fe–O_2 bond is unknown. Single-crystal neutron diffraction of MbO$_2$ has proved that N$_\epsilon$H of the distal histidine (E7) donates a hydrogen bond to the bound O_2 (Phillips and Schoenborn 1981). N$_\epsilon$H–O distances in the α subunits are similar to those in MbO$_2$; in the β subunits they are longer, indicative of weaker bonds, which may be related to the lower oxygen affinity of the β subunits (Table 1). Other interatomic distances in the heme complexes of HbO$_2$, MbO$_2$, and the two synthetic Fe-porphyrins are very similar, but the displacements of the Fes from the plane of the N$_{porph}$ values vary, apparently due to steric factors on the proximal side. In HbO$_2$ and MbO$_2$ these take the form of variations that the angle of the imidazole plane of HisF8 makes with the plane normal to the heme that contains N(1)$_{porph}$, Fe, and N(3)$_{porph}$ (A in Fig. 2A). The smaller that angle the greater the displacement of the Fe, apparently due to repulsion of C$_\epsilon$ and C$_\delta$ of the proximal histidine by the two porphyrin nitrogens (Gelin and Karplus 1977; Gelin et al. 1983).

Changes on oxygenation in tertiary structure of the globin: The α subunits. Since the $\alpha_1\beta_1$ contact undergoes no significant changes during the R → T transition, the atoms at this contact can serve as a reference frame for changes in tertiary structure elsewhere; except for residues G1–4 and H18–21, the B, G, and H helices were also found to be static (Baldwin and Chothia 1979). The largest movements relative to either of these frames occur in helix F, in segment FG, and in residues G1–4, H18–21, and HC1–3. We shall use the BGH reference frame because it gives the smallest rms deviation for all the other atoms (0.29 Å in the α subunits). Figure 3A shows the heme environment of DHb superimposed on that of HbO$_2$. It can be seen that on oxygenation, helix Fα shifts toward the heme and to the right and carries the FG segment with it. In DHb the imidazole of HisF8 is tilted relative to the heme normal; in HbO$_2$ the shift of helix F relative to DHb aligns it with the heme normal. Relative to the BGH frame, the heme turns clockwise by 1° on going from DHb to HbO$_2$. Taking as a reference frame residues F1–8 to which the heme is attached, the heme flattens and turns clockwise by 10°; the motion of its right-hand edge pushes down LeuFG3(91)α and ValFG5(93)α, which form part of the $\alpha_1\beta_2$ contact where the quaternary switch occurs (Figs. 3 and 4). In the T structure, the amino and carboxyl termini form the hydrogen bonds shown in Figure 5A. In the R structure, these hydrogen bonds are broken, and the terminal residues are seen only at the low level of electron density (0.25–0.5 e/Å^3), implying that they are disordered. The map shows indications that the guanidinium of the carboxy-terminal arginine is hydrogen bonded to a phosphate or sulfate ion that lies on the dyad symmetry axis in the central cavity, but that ion would be absent in the red cell, where the guanidinium groups would be free.

Table 1. Heme Stereochemistry in Hemoglobin, Myoglobin, and Synthetic Iron Porphyrins

Species, derivative, and medium	Quaternary structure	Resolution (Å)	Subunit	Bond length (Å) $Fe\text{-}N_{porph}$ crystal	$Fe\text{-}N_{porph}$ EXAFS[21]	$Fe\text{-}N_\varepsilon$	Distances to/between planes (Å) $Fe\text{-}P_{heme}$	$Fe\text{-}P_N$	$N_\varepsilon\text{-}P_{heme}$	$P_N\text{-}P_C$	Angles (°) A	B	$Fe\text{-}O$ (Å)	$Fe\text{-}O\text{-}O$ (°)	$N_\varepsilon\text{-}O_2$ (Å)	$N_\varepsilon\text{-}O_1$ (Å)	Ref.[a]
Human DHb: $(NH_4)_2SO_4$	T	1.74	α mean	2.08(3)		2.16(6)	0.58(3)	0.40(5)	2.72(6)	0.16(6)	18	78					8
			β mean	2.05(3)		2.09(6)	0.50(3)	0.36(5)	2.58(6)	0.10(6)	23	79					
Human DHb: (PEG)	T	2.1	α mean	2.03(4)	2.06(1)	2.16(8)	0.56(4)	0.34(4)	2.72(8)	0.21(8)	15	80					7, 9
			β mean	2.03(4)		2.21(8)	0.48(6)	0.42(8)	2.69(10)	0.05(19)	21	76					
Horse BME-DHb: $(NH_4)_2SO_4$	R	1.8	α	2.02(3)		1.99(8)	0.41	0.26	2.39		14	86					10
			β	2.07(3)		2.14(14)	0.45	0.27	2.58		16	84					
Sperm whale Mb: $(NH_4)_2SO_4$		2.0		2.03(10)		2.22( )	0.47	0.42	2.67		12	87					2
2-MeIm(TpivPP)FeII				2.072(5)	2.08(4)	2.095(5)	0.43	0.40	2.52	0.12							4
Human HbO_2: $NaKHPO_4$	R	2.1	α	1.99(5)	1.98(1)	1.94(9)	0.16(8)	0.12(8)	2.1(1)	0.04	11	84	1.66(8)	153.0(7)	2.6(1)	3.0(1)	6
			β	1.96(6)		2.07(9)	0.00(8)	−0.11(8)	2.1(1)	0.06	27	91	1.87(13)	159.0(12)	3.5(2)	3.2(2)	
Human $(\alpha FeII\text{-}O_2)_2(\beta FeII)$ in PEG	T	2.1	α1	2.04(4)		2.14(10)	0.41(4)	0.17(5)	2.55(8)	0.20(8)	6	79	1.82(4)	153 (4)	2.8(1)	2.9(2)	7, 9
			α2	2.03(4)		2.34(12)	0.31(4)	0.20(5)	2.66(8)	0.19(8)	16	80					
Sperm whale MbO_2: $(NH_4)_2SO_4$		1.6		1.95(6)	1.98(1)	2.07(6)	0.45	0.18	2.28(6)		1	90	1.83(6)	115.0(5)	2.9(2)	3.3(2)	5
2-MeIm(TpivPP)FeII-O_2				1.996(4)	1.98(1)	2.017(4)	0.11	0.086	2.217	0.07			1.898(7)	129.0			4
Horse Hb^+ H_2O; $(NH_4)_2SO_4$	R	2.0	α	2.03(5)		2.08(9)	0.13	0.07	2.17		14	84					1, 10
			β	2.04(3)		2.14(10)	0.19	0.10	2.32		18	84					
bis H_2O-TPP FeII				2.045(8)				0									3

$Fe\text{-}P_{heme}$: Displacement of Fe from mean plane of porphyrin Ns and Cs, including the first atom of each side chain.

$Fe\text{-}P_N$: Displacement of Fe from mean plane of porphyrin Ns.

$P_N\text{-}P_C$: Displacement of plane of porphyrin Ns from plane of porphyrin Cs. This is the doming parameter.

A: Angle between plane of imidazole of HisF8 projected onto the heme and line N_1–N_3 (Fig. 2A).

B: Angle between line C_ε – C_δ of HisF8 and heme normal (Fig. 2B).

2-MeIm(TpivPP)FeII: (2-methylimidazole)-meso-tetra(1,1,1,1,-o-pivalamidophenyl)porphyrinatoiron(II).

2-MeIm(TPP): (2-methylimidazole)tetraphenylporphyrinatoiron(II).

[a] 1. Ladner et al. 1977; 2. Takano 1977; 3. Kastner et al. 1978; 4. Jameson et al. 1980; 5. Phillips 1980; 6. Shaanan 1983; 7. Brzozowski et al. 1984; 8. Fermi et al. 1984; 9. Liddington 1988; 10. Luisi 1986.

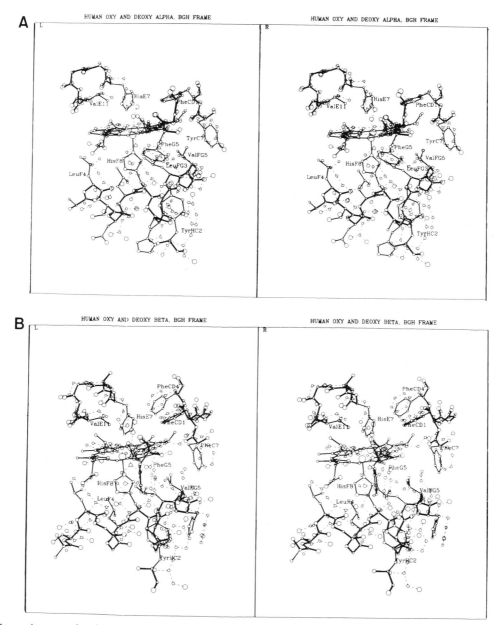

Figure 3. Change in stereochemistry of the hemes and the surrounding globin after superposition of the B, G, and H helices of (A) the α and (B) the β chains of human deoxyhemoglobin (solid lines) and oxyhemoglobin (broken lines). Note the flattening of the hemes and the movements of HisF8 toward the hemes on oxygenation; also the rotation of the heme and the large movements of HisE7 and ValE11 in β (Shaanan 1983; Fermi et al. 1984). The view in this and subsequent stereo pictures is approximately from the central dyad and perpendicular to it, looking toward the surface of the molecule.

The β subunits. Figure 3B shows that on oxygenation, helix F moves toward the heme and in the direction of the FG segment, carrying that segment with it and aligning HisF8 with the heme normal. The movement of F and FG is transmitted to residue G1 and dissipated beyond G5. The center of the heme moves further into its pocket along a line linking porphyrin N_1 to N_3, and the heme rotates about an axis close to the line linking N_2 to N_4. Referred to residues F1 to F6, the iron stays still and the porphyrin becomes coplanar with it, as shown at the bottom of Figure 4. In the T structure, $C_\gamma H_3$ of ValE11(67) obstructs the ligand site at the iron; in the oxygenated R structure that obstruction is cleared by a concerted shift of helices D and E and the CD segment, together with the beginning of helix B, away from and across the heme.

The carboxy-terminal histidines form different sets of hydrogen bonds in the T and R structures, as a result of which their pK_a values drop on oxygenation from 8.0 to 6.5, and protons are released. The conformation of the reactive sulfhydryl groups of CysF9(93)β also changes (Fig. 5B).

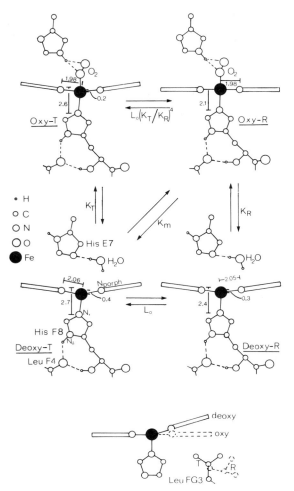

Figure 4. Schematic diagram of changes in heme stereochemistry on binding of O_2 by the α subunits in the R and T structures. On uptake of oxygen by the T structure, the heme remains domed and the iron remains displaced from the porphyrin plane, due to the constraints by the tightly packed side chains of the globin around the heme; on the other hand, the porphyrin becomes domed on dissociation of oxygen from the R structure, which does not constrain it to the flat conformation. The bottom diagram shows the change in conformation of the heme, seen when residues F1–F6 of DHb and HbO_2 are superimposed. The heme flattens and in so doing, pushes down the side chains of LeuFG3 and ValFG5 (hidden behind FG3 in the diagram). This may be one of the ways the change in conformation of the heme is transmitted to the $\alpha_1\beta_2$ contact, thus triggering the T→R transition. L = [T]/[R]. At the ith step of oxygenation $L_i = L_o(K_R/K_T)^i$. The numbers in the diagram indicate the distances in angstroms of N_ϵ from the mean plane of the porphyrin carbons and nitrogens, including the pyrrols and the first carbon of the side chains (N_ϵ–P_{porph}); the mean distance between the iron and the porphyrin nitrogens (Fe–N_{porph}); and the displacement of the iron from the mean plane of the porphyrin nitrogens and carbons (Fe–P_N). In deoxy-R, Fe–N_{porph} is the mean of α and β.

Partially liganded hemoglobins in the quaternary T structure: From deoxyhemoglobin to $(\alpha FeII\text{-}O_2)_2$ $(\beta FeII)_2$. This derivative was obtained by exposure to air of orthorhombic crystals of DHb grown in PEG (Table 1 and Fig. 6). The molecules lie in general positions in the unit cell, so that subunits α_1 and α_2

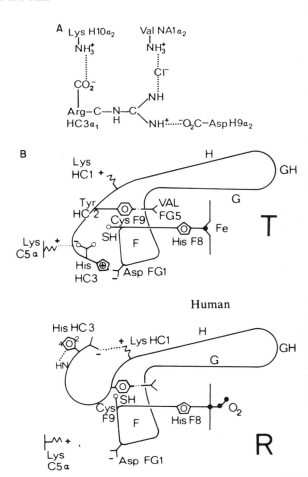

Figure 5. (*A*) Hydrogen bonds made by ionized groups between subunit α_1 and α_2 in deoxyhemoglobin. (*B*) Hydrogen bonds made by HisHC3(146)β in deoxy- (T) and oxyhemoglobin (R). Note also the changing orientations of the side chain of CysF9(93)β. The orientation in T is found in high-spin, and the one shown in R is found in low-spin derivatives; in mixed-spin derivatives the two orientations are in equilibrium. The salt bridges made by DPG are shown in Fig. 10 of Fermi and Perutz (1981).

make different lattice contacts; their coordinates were refined separately. The refined structure shows full occupancy by O_2 at the α hemes and no evidence of O_2 bound to the β hemes, but up to 30% of the β hemes may have become oxidized to methemoglobin (Hb^+H_2O). In both α subunits the reaction with O_2 causes the Fes to move by 0.15 Å toward the porphyrin that remains domed as in DHb, but the tilt of the proximal histidine is slightly reduced. The distal residues remain unperturbed; only the water molecule that is hydrogen bonded to HisE7(58)α in DHb is displaced by the heme-linked O_2. In one of the α subunits, the motion of the Fe produces a small concerted shift of residues F5–9, of the main chain of FG4, and of the side chains of FG4 and FG5; in the other α subunit, the motion of the Fe stretches the Fe–N_ϵ bond by ~0.2 Å, with hardly detectable shifts of F or FG (Figs. 4 and 6) (Brzozowski et al. 1984; Liddington 1986). These differences are due, presumably, to the

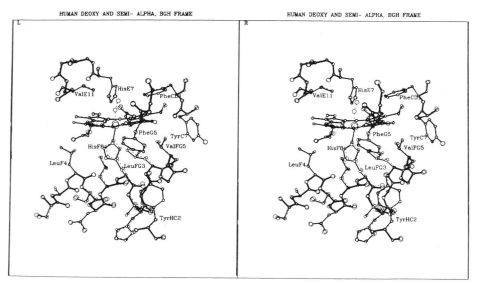

Figure 6. Change in stereochemistry of the heme and the surrounding globin seen after superposition of the B, G, and H helices in one of the α chains of human deoxyhemoglobin (solid lines) and in $(\alpha FeII\text{-}O_2)_2(\beta FeII)_2$ (broken lines). Symbols as in Fig. 3 (Brzozowski et al. 1984; Liddington 1986).

different lattice contacts of the two α subunits. However, the important features that are common to both subunits are the doming of the hemes as in DHb and localization of strain to the immediate neighborhood of the Fes and proximal histidines.

From deoxyhemoglobin to $(\alpha NiII)_2(\beta FeIICO)_2$ in the T structure.

This derivative crystallizes with unit cell dimensions similar to those of the ligand-free T structure, but the molecular packing is so different that the structure had to be solved by molecular replacement (B. Luisi et al., unpubl.). The electron density map shows Ni-porphyrin to be planar and the Ni to be 4-coordinated with a Ni-N_ϵ(His) distance of 3.2 Å; this

large distance biases the allosteric equilibrium strongly toward the T structure, just as in the abnormal human Hb Boston, where the replacement HisE7 $\rightarrow$ Tyr causes the iron atom to be linked to the distal tyrosine instead of the proximal histidine. These structures behave as if the metal atoms were displaced from the porphyrin plane by over 1 Å instead of the normal 0.55 Å, and had pushed the proximal histidines away with them. Figure 7 shows the marked changes in tertiary structure around the liganded β hemes after superposition of the B, G, and H helices on those of the ligand-free T structure. CO is seen to be accommodated by a change in tilt of the heme and its attached helix F, combined with shifts in the distal residues. The map clearly shows the shift of the distal histidine and valine. The heme

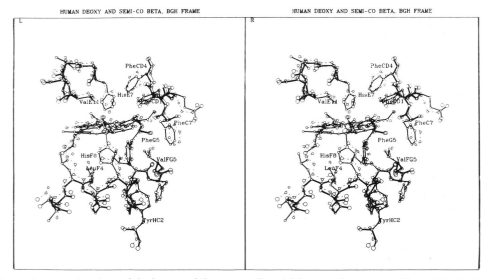

Figure 7. Change in stereochemistry of the heme and the surrounding globin seen after superposition of the B, G, and H helices in one of the β chains of human deoxyhemoglobin (solid lines) and in $(\alpha NiII)_2(\beta FeIICO)_2$ (broken lines). Symbols as in Fig. 3.

pocket is closed as in the ligand-free T structure. The CO occupancy is different in the two β subunits, apparently due to different lattice constraints. The packing of the residues at the $\alpha_1\beta_2$ interface is the same as in normal, fully deoxy, T structure. We shall call t_β the tertiary structure of the β chains in $(\alpha\text{FeII})_2(\beta\text{FeII})_2$, where the ligand site is blocked by ValE11, the t'_β in $(\alpha\text{NiIII})_2(\beta\text{FeIICO})_2$, where the site is occupied by a ligand. The ligand-binding properties of this hybrid Hb have been determined by Shibayama et al. (1986).

From deoxyhemoglobin to $(\alpha\text{FeII-CO})_2(\beta\text{MnII})_2$ and to $(\alpha\text{FeII-CO})_2(\beta\text{CoII})_2$ in the T structure.

Crystalline hybrid Hbs carrying iron porphyrin in the α chains and a metalloporphyrin that fails to combine with O_2 or CO in the β chain are isomorphous with those of normal DHb. A difference electron density map of the hybrid $(\alpha\text{FeII-CO})_2(\beta_2\text{MnII})$ minus DHb at 3.0 Å resolution showed no significant density in the β subunits, as 5-coordinated MnII and FeII porphyrins are isomorphous. In the α subunits the map has pairs of positive and negative peaks indicative of a movement of the ligated Fes and of residues F6(85) to FG1(89) toward the porphyrin. Restrained least-squares refinement leads to tentative estimates of 0.3 Å for the movements of the Fe and the imidazole of HisF8(87)α and of 0.2 Å for some of the main-chain atoms (Arnone et al. 1986).

The Co–N_{porph} bond is 0.1 Å shorter than the Fe–N_{porph} bond; consequently the displacement of the metal from the plane of the N_{porph} in CoII(TPP)(1,2-diMeIm) is only 0.15 Å (Lauher and Ibers 1974), compared to 0.42 Å in FeII(TPP)(2-MeIm). In deoxy$(\alpha\text{CoII})_2(\beta\text{CoII})_2$ the displacement of Co from the mean plane of the porphyrin nitrogens and carbons is 0.25 Å less than that of the iron in FeII DHb, but this closer approach of the Co to the porphyrin is compensated by a stretching of the Co–N_ϵ bond, so that the distance of N_ϵ from the porphyrin plane remains the same as in ferrous deoxyhb and the substitution of Co from Fe causes no perceptible changes in the structure of the globin (Fermi et al. 1982). The difference electron density map of $(\alpha\text{FeII-CO})_2(\beta\text{Co})_2$ minus DHbA at 2.9 Å resolution shows the Co atoms in the β subunits to be flanked by pairs of positive and negative peaks, due to the smaller displacement Co from the porphyrin planes compared to Fe, but again there is no change in the structure of the globin. Difference peaks appear near both the ligated α hemes: a large positive peak on the distal side represents the CO; a negative peak next to it is due to the removal of the H_2O bound to HisE7(58)α in DHb; a negative peak on the proximal side of the iron shows that it has moved closer to the porphyrin, and pairs of positive and negative peaks flanking helix F show that residues F5 to FG1 have also moved closer to the porphyrin. In one of the α subunits these movements are transmitted to the FG segments, but in the other they are not. No refinement of this structure has yet been done (Luisi 1986).

From met to deoxyhemoglobin in the R structure.

When crystals of HbO_2 or methemoglobin (Hb^+H_2O) are reduced to DHb with $Na_2S_2O_4$, they break up and their diffraction pattern is lost, but crystals of horse Hb^+H_2O that have been reacted with bis(N-maleimidomethyl) ether (BME) remain intact even when fully reduced (Simon et al. 1967). The structure of BME DHb was determined at 1.8 Å resolution and compared with the structure of horse Hb^+H_2O at 2.0 Å resolution (Ladner et al. 1977) after both structures had been subjected to combined least-squares and energy refinement. With helices B, G, and the first 11 residues of H as a reference frame, rms differences between main-chain atoms were found to be greatest for helices E and Fα and for D, E, and Fβ. The α hemes stay put, and the β hemes tilt very slightly in the same direction as on transition from R to T. The Fes move away from the plane of the N_{porph}s by 0.2 Å and from the mean plane of the porphyrin by 0.3 Å; the porphyrins become domed as in DHb in the T structure (Figs. 4 and 8). Table 1 shows the Fe–N distances to be the same within error as in human DHb in the T structure, whereas the displacement of the Fes from the plane of the N_{porph}s is less by about 0.1 Å. The close similarity between the 5-coordinated hemes in the T and R structures found in crystals has been corroborated by studies of the X-ray absorption near edge structures (XANES) of solution of carp DHb in the two quaternary structures. Their XANES curves were identical, implying that the Fe–N distances remain the same with 0.01 Å displacement, and that the displacements of the Fes from the plane of the N_{porph}s differ by no more than 0.1 Å (Bianconi et al. 1986). There is a concerted movement of the two subunits relative to each other at the $\alpha_1\beta_2$ contact, as if the molecule were trying to make the R→T switch, but could not muster enough energy to go more than a small part of the way. For example, during the R→T switch, the distance between the Cβs of ThrC3(38)α_1 and HisFG4(97)β_2 increases by 6.5 Å, whereas on going from met (R) to deoxy (R) that distance increases by only 0.5 Å. There is no significant difference density at the carboxyl termini of the four chains (Luisi 1986).

$(\alpha\text{FeIIIH}_2O)_2(\beta\text{FeIIIH}_2O)_2$ and $(\alpha\text{FeIIIF}^-)_2(\beta\text{FeIIIF}^-)_2$ in the T structure.

These two liganded T structures are isomorphous with the unliganded T structure and exhibit smaller changes in tertiary structure around the β hemes than $(\alpha\text{NiII})_2(\beta\text{FeCO})_2$, because the smaller heme ligands experience less steric hindrance by the distal residues than CO or O_2 (Fermi and Perutz 1977; Liddington 1986).

The Heterotropic Ligands

All the heterotropic ligands lower oxygen affinity by forming hydrogen bonds that specifically stabilize and

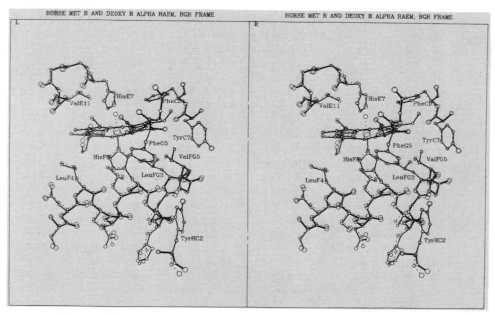

HORSE MET R AND DEOXY R ALPHA HAEM, BGH FRAME

HORSE MET R AND DEOXY R ALPHA HAEM, BGH FRAME

Figure 8. Same as Fig. 6, but the derivatives superimposed are horse methemoglobin (broken lines) and BME deoxyhemoglobin (solid lines) (Luisi 1986). (Reprinted with permission, from Perutz et al. 1987.)

constrain the T structure. For each mole of O_2 taken up at pH 7.4 and 25°C, human Hb liberates 0.2 mole H^+ in a deionized solution, 0.5 mole H^+ in 0.1 M Cl^-, and 0.7 mole H^+ in the presence of a molar excess of DPG (Kilmartin 1974; Perutz et al. 1980). This is known as the alkaline Bohr effect. In deionized solutions all the protons come from HisHC3(146)β, which donates a hydrogen bond to AspF61(94)β in the T structure and accepts a hydrogen bond from its own main-chain NH in the R structure (Fig. 5B) (Kilmartin et al. 1980; Shih and Perutz 1987). In consequence, its pK_a drops from 8.0 in DHb to 6.5 or less in HbO_2 (Matsukawa et al. 1984). The binding of Cl^- by the T structure raises the pK_a values of ValNA1(1)α and LysEF6(82)β, which contribute an additional 0.28 mole H^+ to the Bohr effect. DPG enters a cleft flanked by the amino termini and helices H of the β chains and forms hydrogen bonds with ValNA1(1), HisNA2(2), LysEF6(82), and HisH21(143) (Fig. 10 in Brzozowski et al. 1984). The rise in pK_a values of their cationic groups contributes 0.33 mole H^+ to the Bohr effect (Kilmartin 1974). CO_2 forms carbamino groups with ValNA1(1)α and β, and these in turn make hydrogen bonds with cationic groups of the globin.

In 0.1 M Tris-HCl + 0.1 M NaCl at pH 7.4 and 21.5 °C, the first mole of O_2 taken up releases 0.64(7) mole H^+, the second and third mole of O_2 combined release 1.62(27), and the fourth mole of O_2 releases only 0.05(6) mole H^+ (Chu et al. 1984). How is their release related to the allosteric transition from T to R? Allosteric theory allows the equilibrium constant $L_j = [T]/[R]$ at the ith step of oxygenation to be calculated from $L_i = L_o(K_R/K_T)^i$. Under the above nonphysiological conditions $L_1 = 8.7 \times 10^4 \times 0.0073 = 633$

(Baldwin 1975; Imai 1982). Thus, more than a quarter of the Bohr protons are discharged before 1/600 of the Hb molecules have switched from T to R, which implies that the hydrogen bonds responsible for H^+ discharge must break in the T structure. On the other hand, $(\alpha NiII)_2(\beta FeIICO)$ and $(\alpha FeIIO_2)_2(\beta FeII)$ in the T structure offer no evidence in favor of combination of O_2 with the hemes causing rupture of the salt bridges. The bulk of the protons are released in the $T \rightarrow R$ transition, which takes place mostly at the second and third oxygenation steps. After the third oxygenation step $L_3 = 0.034$, leaving a little more than 1/30 of the Hb molecules in the T structure, which is roughly equivalent to the fraction of 1/20 of the protons to be discharged at the fourth oxygenation step.

Stereochemical Mechanism

In 1970, Perutz proposed that "the oxygenation of hemoglobin is accompanied by structural changes in the subunits triggered by shifts of the iron atoms relative to the porphyrin and, in the β subunits, also by the steric effect of oxygen itself. The oxygen-free form is constrained by salt bridges (hydrogen bonds between oppositely charged ions), which are broken by the energy of heme-heme interaction with the release of H^+. 2,3-Diphosphoglycerate may add to the constraints by being stereochemically complementary to a site between the β chains; this complementarity is lost on oxygenation" (Perutz 1970).

Role of the hemes. In 1970 the resolution of the best electron density maps was 2.8 Å, which was insufficient to resolve the atoms of the porphyrin; methods for refining atomic coordinates in protein structures did not yet exist. Bolton and Perutz measured the displacements of the Fes from the porphyrins, assumed to be planar, with a ruler in a Richards box and obtained values of 0.75 Å for horse DHb and 0.3 Å for horse Hb^+H_2O, the only derivatives then available (Bolton and Perutz 1970). The uncertainties of these measurements aroused much controversy about the proposal that the T → R equilibrium is governed by the displacement of the Fes from the plane of the porphyrin. Recent X-ray analyses at high resolution have confirmed that the iron atoms do shift and show that the conformation of the porphyrins also changes. As a result, the N_ϵs of the proximal histidines move relative to the mean porphyrin plane by 0.6 Å in the α and 0.5 Å in the β subunits (Fig. 4). Do those movements trigger the allosteric transitions between the R and T structures, and if so, how are these transitions initiated?

Our semi-liganded derivatives in the T structure show that on combination of O_2 or CO with the α hemes, the Fes move by 0.15 Å toward the plane of the N_{porph}s and the doming of the pyrroles is preserved. The movements of the Fes are transmitted to the proximal histidines and their adjoining residues, leaving the bulk of the protein unperturbed. Thus, perturbations are confined to what Gelin et al. have called the "allosteric core" (Gelin et al. 1983). On loss of Fe-linked H_2O and reduction of the Fes in BME-Hb in the R structure, the Fes move away from the plane of the N_{porph}s by 0.2 Å; the movements are transmitted not just to the proximal histidines and their adjoining residues, but also to the $\alpha_1\beta_2$ and $\alpha_2\beta_1$ contacts that shift a short way toward their positions in the T structure.

There have been suggestions that the hydrogen bonds between N_δ of HisF8 and the carbonyl of LeuF4 play a part in the allosteric mechanism (Valentine et al. 1979; Stein et al. 1980). The length of these bonds may change in transition states, but it remains the same in DHb and HbO_2 (Shaanan 1983). There has also been a suggestion that changes in charge transfer interactions between the porphyrin and PheCD1 contribute to the free energy of cooperativity (Shelnutt et al. 1979), but the distance between the phenylalanine side chain and the porphyrin is too large (3.8–4.1 Å) for such interactions to occur. *We are thus left with the distances of the Fes and the proximal histidines from the porphyrin as the only determinants of the allosteric equilibrium visible in the α subunits.*

CONCLUSIONS

Changes in quaternary structure are initiated by changes in the allosteric core of the protein (Gelin et al. 1983). In deoxyhemoglobin the porphyrins are domed and the iron atoms are displaced by 0.4 Å from the plane of the porphyrin nitrogens, regardless of the quaternary structure of the globin. On binding O_2 or CO, the iron atoms move toward the porphyrin. These remain domed in the T structure, but flatten on transition to the R structure. As a result, on transition from deoxyhemoglobin in the quaternary T structure of oxyhemoglobin in the quaternary R structure, the iron atoms and the proximal histidines move toward the mean planes of the porphyrins by 0.5–0.6 Å. In deoxyhemoglobin in the quaternary T structure, combination of the β hemes with O_2 or CO is blocked by the distal valine; in the R structure this block is removed by a shift of the β hemes relative to helix E.

In reaction intermediates, combination with O_2 or CO of the α hemes in the T structure causes the iron atoms, the proximal histidines, and their adjoining residues to move *toward* the porphyrin by 0.15–0.3 Å, and the porphyrins to remain domed, showing that their conformation is constrained by the globin. On combination with CO of the β hemes, a transition in tertiary structure from t_β to t'_β changes the tilt of the heme, shifts the iron and proximal histidine toward the porphyrin, and moves the distal residues away from the ligand site. On loss of heme ligands from the R structure, the transition from R to T is initiated by movements of the iron, the proximal histidines, and their adjoining residues *away* from the porphyrin by 0.3 Å, and by doming of the porphyrins (Fig. 4). *The doming and undoming of the porphyrins, the movements of the irons and of the proximal histidines, and, in the β subunits, the movement of the distal residues relative to the heme, are seen as the only perturbations that could set the changes in quaternary structure in motion.*

There is uncertainty concerning the location of the strain responsible for the low oxygen affinity of the T structure. Existing evidence indicates that the location of the strain varies from derivative to derivative and in hemoglobins of different species, depending on the relative strength of the restraints of the globin and of the Fe–N bonds (Nagai 1983), but this does not imply, as is sometimes claimed, that the mechanism of cooperativity differs in different species. The majority of the residues in contact with the hemes and those essential for the allosteric switch between the R and T structures are the same in all bony vertebrates. If the components of the machine have remained the same, its mechanism cannot have changed. Only the response to heterotropic ligands has evolved differently in different phyla (Perutz 1984).

ACKNOWLEDGMENTS

A longer version of this article was published in September 1987 in *Accounts in Chemical Research* (Perutz et al. 1987). We thank the American Chemical Society for permission to reproduce it here. The work of M.F.P. and B.L. was supported by National Institutes of Health grant BBCB 2 ROI HL31461-04 and National Science Foundation grant DMB-8609842. B.L. held a Peterhouse Research Studentship, B.S. held a European Molecular Biology Organisation Fellowship, and R.C.L. held a Science and Engineering Research Council Studentship, followed by a Medical Research Council Postdoctoral Fellowship. G.F. is on the scientific staff of the Medical Research Council.

REFERENCES

Arnone, A., P. Rogers, N.V. Blough, J.L. McGourty, and B.M. Hoffman. 1986. X-ray diffraction studies of a partially liganded hemoglobin [α(FeII-CO)β(MnII)]₂. *J. Mol. Biol.* **188**: 693.

Baldwin, J.M. 1975. Structure and function of haemoglobin. *Prog. Biophys. Mol. Biol.* **29**: 225.

Baldwin, J.M. and C. Chothia. 1979. Haemoglobin: The structural changes related to ligand binding and its allosteric mechanism. *J. Mol. Biol.* **129**: 175.

Bianconi, A., A. Congiu-Castellano, M. Dell'Aricia, A. Giovanelli, S. Morante, E. Burattini, and P.J. Durham. 1986. Local Fe site structure in the tense-to-relaxed transition in carp deoxyhemoglobin: A XANES (X-ray absorption near edge structure) study. *Proc. Natl. Acad. Sci.* **83**: 7736.

Bolton, W. and M.F. Perutz. 1970. Three-dimensional Fourier synthesis of horse deoxyhaemoglobin at 2.8 Å resolution. *Nature* **228**: 551.

Brzozowski, A., Z. Derewenda, E. Dodson, G. Dodson, M. Grabowski, R. Liddington, T. Skarzynski, and D. Vallely. 1984. Bonding of molecular oxygen to T-state human haemoglobin. *Nature* **307**: 74.

Chu, A.H., B.W. Turner, and G.K. Ackers. 1984. Effects of protons on the oxygenation-linked subunit assembly in human hemoglobin. *Biochemistry* **23**: 604.

Dickerson, R.E. and I. Geis. 1983. *Hemoglobin. Benjamin Cummings,* Menlo Park, California.

Eisenberger, P., R.G. Shulman, B.M. Kincaid, G.S. Brown, and S. Ogawa. 1978. Extended X-ray absorption fine structure determination of iron nitrogen distances in haemoglobin. *Nature* **274**: 30.

Fermi, G. and M.F. Perutz. 1977. Structure of human fluoromethaemoglobin with inositol hexaphosphate. *J. Mol. Biol.* **114**: 421.

―――. 1981. Haemoglobin and myoglobin. In *Atlas of biological structures* (ed. D.C. Phillips and F.M. Richards). Clarendon Press, Oxford, England.

Fermi, G., M.F. Perutz, and R.G. Shulman. 1987. Iron distances in hemoglobin: Comparison of X-ray crystallographic and extended X-ray absorption fine structure studies. *Proc. Natl. Acad. Sci.* **84**: 6167.

Fermi, G., M.F. Perutz, L.C. Dickinson, and J.C.W. Chien. 1982. Structure of human deoxy cobalt haemoglobin. *J. Mol. Biol.* **55**: 495.

Fermi, G., M.F. Perutz, B. Shaanan, and R. Fourme. 1984. The crystal structure of human deoxyhaemoglobin at 1.7 Å resolution. *J. Mol. Biol.* **175**: 159.

Gelin, B. and M. Karplus. 1977. Mechanism of tertiary structural change in hemoglobin. *Proc. Natl. Acad. Sci.* **74**: 801.

Gelin, B.R., A.W.-M. Lee, and M. Karplus. 1983. Hemoglobin tertiary structural change on ligand binding. Its role in the co-operative mechanism. *J. Mol. Biol.* **171**: 489.

Hoard, J. 1975. Stereochemistry of porphyrins and metalloporphyrins. In *Porphyrins and metalloporphyrins.* (ed. K.M. Smith), p. 317. Elsevier, Amsterdam.

Imai, K. 1982. *Allosteric effects in haemoglobin.* Cambridge University Press, England.

Jameson, G.B., F.S. Molinaro, J.A. Ibers, J.P. Collman, J.I. Brauman, E. Rose, and K.S. Suslick. 1980. Models for the active site of oxygen-binding hemoproteins. Dioxygen binding properties and the structures of (2-methylimidazole)-meso-tetra (α,α,α,α-o-pivalamidophenyl)porphyrinato-iron(II)-ethanol and its dioxygen adduct. *J. Am. Chem. Soc.* **102**: 3224.

Kastner, M.E., W.E. Scheidt, T. Mashiko, and C.A. Reed. 1978. Size coordination in high spin ferric porphyrins. A structural type and model for aquomet hemoglobin. *J. Am. Chem. Soc.* **100**: 6354.

Kilmartin, J.V. 1974. Influence of DPG on the Bohr effect on human hemoglobin. *FEBS. Lett.* **38**: 147.

Kilmartin, J.C., J.H. Fogg, and M.F. Perutz. 1980. Role of C-terminal histidine in the alkaline Bohr effect of human hemoglobin. *Biochemistry* **19**: 3189.

Ladner, R.C., E.J. Heidner, and M.F. Perutz. 1977. The structure of horse methaemoglobin at 2.0 Å resolution. *J. Mol. Biol.* **114**: 385.

Lauher, J.W. and J.A. Ibers. 1974. Stereochemistry of cobalt porphyrins. II. The characterization and structure of meso-tetraphenylporphinatobis(imidazole) cobalt (III) acetate monohydrate monochloroformate, [Co(Im)₂(TPP)]-[OAc]·H₂O·CHCl₃. *J. Am. Chem. Soc.* **96**: 4447.

Liddington, R.C. 1986. "The origins of co-operativity in hemoglobin: An X-ray analysis of the liganded T state." Ph.D. thesis, York University, England.

Luisi, B. 1986. "Studies of intermediate states of hemoglobin." Ph.D. thesis, University of Cambridge, England.

Matsukawa, S., Y. Itatani, K. Mawatari, Y. Shimokawa, and Y. Yoneyama. 1984. Quantitative evaluation for the role of β146His and β142His residues in the Bohr effect of human hemoglobin in the presence of 0.1 M chloride ion. *J. Biol. Chem.* **259**: 11479.

Nagai, K. 1983. The nature of the Fe-His bond in haemoglobin. In *Brussels hemoglobin symposium* (ed. E.G. Schenk and C. Paul). Editions de l'Universite de Bruxelles, Brussels.

Perutz, M.F. 1970. Stereochemistry of cooperative effects in haemoglobin. *Nature* **228**: 726.

―――. 1984. Species adaptation in a protein molecule. *Adv. Protein Chem.* **36**: 213.

Perutz, M.F., G. Fermi, B. Luisi, and R.C. Liddington. 1987. Stereochemistry of cooperative effects in hemoglobin. *Accts. Chem. Res.* **20**: 309.

Perutz, M.F., S.S. Hasnain, P.J. Duke, J.S. Sessler, and J.E. Hahn. 1982. Stereochemistry of iron in deoxyhemoglobin. *Nature* **295**: 535.

Perutz, M.F., J.V. Kilmartin, K. Nishikura, J.H. Fogg, P.J.G. Butler, and H.S. Rollema. 1980. Identification of residues contributing to the Bohr effect of human haemoglobin. *J. Mol. Biol.* **138**: 649.

Phillips, S.E.V. 1980. Structure and refinement of oxymyoglobin at 1.6 Å resolution. *J. Mol. Biol.* **142**: 531.

Phillips, S.E.V. and B.P. Schoenborn. 1981. Neutron diffraction reveals oxygen-histidine hydrogen bond in oxymyoglobin. *Nature* **292**: 81.

Shaanan, B. 1983. Structure of human oxyhaemoglobin at 2.1 Å resolution. *J. Mol. Biol.* **171**: 31.

Shelnutt, J.A., D.O. Rousseau, J.L. Friedman, and S.R. Simon. 1979. Protein-heme interaction in hemoglobin: Evidence from Raman difference spectroscopy. *Proc. Natl. Acad. Sci.* **76**: 4409.

Shibayama, N., H. Morimoto, and T. Kitagawa. 1986. Properties of chemically modified Ni(II)-Fe(II) hybrid hemoglobins: Ni(II) protoporphyrin IX as a model for a permanent deoxy-heme. *J. Mol. Biol.* **192**: 331.

Shih, D.T.-B. and M.F. Perutz. 1987. Influence of anions and protons on the adair constants of haemoglobins A and cowtown (His HC3(146)β → Leu). *J. Mol. Biol.* **195**: 419.

Simon, S.R., W.H. Konigsberg, W. Bolton, and M.F. Perutz. 1967. Identity of structure of horse deoxy- and oxyhaemoglobin after reaction with bis(N-maleidomethyl) ether. *J. Mol. Biol.* **28**: 451.

Stein, P., M. Mitchell, and T.G. Spiro. 1980. H-bond and deprotonation effects on the resonance Raman iron-imidazole mode in deoxyhemoglobin models: Implications for hemoglobin cooperativity. *J. Am. Chem. Soc.* **102**: 7795.

Valentine, J.S., R.P. Sheridan, L.C. Allen, and P.C. Kahn. 1979. Coupling between oxidation state and hydrogen bond conformation in heme proteins. *Proc. Natl. Acad. Sci.* **76**: 1009.

Porphyrin Iron(III) Mixed Function Oxidases: An Evolutionary Endpoint for Transition Metal(III) Reactions with Oxygen Donors

T.C. BRUICE

Department of Chemistry, University of California at Santa Barbara, Santa Barbara, California 93106

Peroxidases, catalases, and cytochrome P-450 enzymes have in common iron(III) protoporphyrin-IX as a cofactor. The reactions catalyzed by these enzymes can be, for the most part, duplicated by use of transition metal(III) porphyrins. Porphyrins serve admirably well as conjugated and rigidly planar ligands that prevent other than transformations of the ligated metal moiety at axial positions. The adjacent and distal axial positions serve to separate the enzyme-bound (distal) ligand from the reactive face (adjacent) of the iron(III). These features are not required, however, to mimic the chemical conversions that are catalyzed by peroxidases, catalases, and cytochrome P-450 enzymes. Indeed, other simple ligands may be used with a number of transition metals (cf. Samsel et al. 1985). Porphyrins were selected as components of living organisms at an early time, as attested to by the observation that petroleum is a rich source of porphyrins.

In the oxidation reactions catalyzed by peroxidases, catalases, and cytochrome P-450, an oxidant is initially formed that might be described as a "porphyrin-iron-oxene" compound. The formation of the porphyrin-iron-oxene compound occurs by reaction of the iron(III) porphyrin with a reagent that may be symbolically represented as Z-OH. With horseradish (HR) peroxidase (distal axial ligand a histidine imidazole) and catalase (distal axial ligand a tyrosine hydroxyl function), Z-OH represents HO-OH (for both enzymes) and, in addition, alkyl-O-OH (for the peroxidase). The porphyrin-iron-oxene compound formed in these reactions is known as compound I. Much evidence exists to support the structure of compound I as being an iron(IV)-oxo porphyrin π-cation radical (Eq. 1, where X is imidazole or tyrosine-O^-, cf. Moss et al. 1969; Dolphin et al. 1971; Schultz et al. 1979; Roberts et al. 1981).

$$(\text{Porph})\text{Fe}^{\text{III}}(X) + Z\text{-OH} \rightarrow (^{+}\cdot\text{Porph})(X)\text{Fe}^{\text{IV}}(O) + ZH \quad (1)$$

With cytochrome P-450 enzymes (distal axial ligand a thiolate of cysteine) Z-OH may represent a host of oxidants (such as HO-OH, alkyl-O-OH, RC(O)O-OH, arene-IO, aniline N-oxides), but under physiological circumstances it represents $2e^- + O_2 +$ one or two protons (building blocks for peroxide). Nothing is known about the structure of the porphyrin-iron-oxene intermediate formed with cytochrome P-450 because its formation (1) requires the presence of the substrate bound

at the active site and (2) is rate-limiting in the oxidation of the substrate. When $R\text{-}S^-$ species are ligated to metal ions of higher oxidation states (M^{n+1}), they undergo $1e^-$ oxidation, and a covalent bond is formed between $RS\cdot$ and M^n (Sawyer et al. 1986). It is safe to assume that the structure of the porphyrin-iron-oxene species of cytochrome P-450 reflects this feature so that the second $1e^-$ deficiency resides with the thiolate ligand rather than in the porphyrin ring system as a porphyrin π-cation radical (Eq. 2). Chemical systems that incorporate such features have not been prepared.

$$(\text{Porph})(\text{CysS}^-)\text{Fe}^{\text{III}} + Z\text{-OH} \rightarrow (\text{Porph})(\text{CysS}\cdot)\text{Fe}^{\text{IV}}(O) + ZH \quad (2)$$

Aside from the structures of the porphyrin-iron-oxene species of HR peroxidase, catalase, and cytochrome P-450, a complete description of these systems requires a knowledge of the mechanisms of formation of the porphyrin-iron-oxene species and a description of their reactions with substrates. The electrochemical stepwise oxidation of iron(III)-hydroxy porphyrins to iron(IV)-oxo porphyrins (compound II oxidation level) and iron(IV)-oxo porphyrin π-cation radicals (compound I oxidation level) have been investigated (Calderwood et al. 1985; Lee et al. 1985; Calderwood and Bruice 1986). Also, the second-order rate constants have been determined for "oxene" equivalent transfer from a series of percarboxylic acids and alkyl hydroperoxides (YOOH) to meso-tetrakis(phenyl)porphinato transition metal(III) chlorides ([TPP]Cr^{III}[Cl], [TPP]Fe^{III}[Cl], [TPP]Mn^{III}[Cl], [TPP]Co^{III}[Cl]) (Lee and Bruice 1985, 1986; Yuan and Bruice 1985a,b, 1986; Balasubramanian and Bruice 1987). All reactions involving oxene equivalent transfer from percarboxylic acids were shown to involve heterolytic O–O bond scission (Eq. 3), and the logs of the second-order rate constants k_{YOOH} were determined to be linearly related to the pK_a of the leaving carboxylic acid (YOH).

$$R\text{-C(O)-O-O-H} + ([\text{TPP}]M^{\text{III}}[\text{Cl}]) \xrightarrow{k_{\text{YOOH}}} R\text{-C(O)-O-H} + ([\text{TPP}]M^{\text{V}}[\text{Cl}][O])$$
$$(3)$$

The slopes of plots (β_{1g}) of log k_{YOOH} versus pK_a of YOH were found to be markedly negative (-0.35 to -1.25), which is expected for such a polar reaction. When k_{YOOH} values for alkyl hydroperoxides were determined and included in the plots of log k_{YOOH} versus pK_a of YOH for percarboxylic acids, it was found that a single linear free-energy line was obtained with

(TPP)Cr^{III}(Cl). Thus, alkyl hydroperoxides most likely react with (TPP)Cr^{III}(Cl) to provide (TPP)Cr^V(O)(Cl) by heterolytic O–O bond scission. With imidazole-ligated meso-tetrakis(phenyl)porphinato manganese(III) chloride ([TPP][ImH]Mn^{III}[Cl]) as well as (TPP)Fe^{III}(Cl) and (TPP)Co^{III}(Cl), there was found to be a break in the slope of the linear free-energy plots with the most electron-rich alkyl peroxides residing on a line of very small negative slope. This has been interpreted as a change of mechanism from heterolytic to homolytic O–O bond scission (Eq. 4).

$$Alkyl\text{-}O\text{-}OH + ([TPP]Fe^{III}[Cl]) \xrightarrow{K_{YOOH}} ([TPP]Fe^{IV}[Cl][OH]Alkyl\text{-}O\cdot)$$
$$([TPP]Fe^{IV}[Cl][OH]Alkyl\text{-}O\cdot) \xrightarrow{fast} ([^+\cdot TPP]Fe^{IV}[O][Cl]) + Alkyl\text{-}OH$$
$$([TPP]Fe^{IV}[Cl][OH]Alkyl\text{-}O\cdot) \xrightarrow{fast} (TPP)Fe^{III}(Cl) + Alkyl\text{-}O^+ + HO^-$$
$$([TPP]Fe^{IV}[Cl][OH]Alkyl\text{-}O\cdot) \xrightarrow{fast} ([TPP]Fe^{IV}[Cl][OH]) + Alkyl\text{-}O\cdot$$

$$(4)$$

Studies have been initiated to determine the role of general catalysis in the transfer of an oxene equivalent from Z-OH species to iron(III) and manganese(III) porphyrins (Bruice et al. 1986; Zipplies et al. 1986; Balasubramanian et al. 1987). These and the investigations that will follow are predicated on the proposed role of an imidazolyl group of a histidine residue as a general base at the active site of peroxidases. These investigations are being carried out in water using water-soluble metalloporphyrins that do not form μ-oxo dimer. In the reaction of the manganese(III) porphyrin with H_2O_2 (Eq. 5, where X=H_2O, HO$^-$, or imidazole) the rate-controlling oxene equivalent transfer is not subject to general catalysis (by any of the oxygen-centered or nitrogen-centered bases and acids investigated) at any pH.

$$(Porph)Mn^{III}(X) + H_2O_2 \rightarrow (Porph)Mn^V(O)(X) + H_2O$$
$$(Porph)Mn^V(O)(X) + H_2O_2 \rightarrow (Porph)Mn^{III}(X) + O_2 + H_2O$$

$$(5)$$

When an iron(III) porphyrin is used as catalyst, the single nitrogen base buffer employed (collidine/collidine·H$^+$) is a catalyst, but a number of oxygen bases and acids are not. Much remains to be done to gain an understanding of the role of general catalysis in these systems.

A question that begs an answer concerns the rates of oxygen transfer from porphyrin-iron-oxene and porphyrin-manganese-oxene species to organic substrates. The two reactions of interest are oxygen insertion (Eq. 6) and epoxidation (Eq. 7). These are the most interesting reactions catalyzed by cytochrome P-450.

$$(^+\cdot Porph)Fe^{IV}(O)(X) + RCH_3 \rightarrow (Porph)Fe^{III}(X) + RCH_2OH \qquad (6)$$

$$(^+\cdot Porph)Fe^{IV}(O)(X) + \;\rangle C = C\langle\; \rightarrow (Porph)Fe^{III}(X) + -\overset{O}{\overset{\diagup\diagdown}{\underset{|}{C}} - \underset{|}{C}} -$$

$$(7)$$

The dynamics of the reactions of Equations 6 and 7

cannot be explored with the enzyme, since the formation of the porphyrin-iron-oxene compound is rate-determining. Until the present, the same may be said of chemical systems. Meunier and co-workers (1984) introduced the use of ClO$^-$ as an oxene equivalent transfer agent and studied the epoxidation of alkenes by using a rapidly stirred biphasic system consisting of an organic phase containing manganese(III) porphyrin plus nitrogen base ligand, a phase transfer agent, and a basic aqueous phase containing LiOCl. Epoxides were obtained in high yield. Collman and co-workers (1983, 1984, 1985a,b) subsequently carried out a number of kinetic studies with the Meunier machine. From these studies they proposed that the rates of epoxidation, rather than oxene equivalent transfer to manganese(III) porphyrin, are rate-determining and that intermediate to epoxide formation there arises a metallaoxetane. Though the evidence for formation of a stable metallaoxetane intermediate has been questioned (Nakagaki et al. 1987), the facility of the oxene equivalent transfer to the metal center has not (Eq. 8a: where ImR represents a N-substituted imidazole).

$$([P]Mn^{III}[ImR])^+ + ClO^- \rightarrow (P)Mn^V(O)(ImR) + Cl^- \qquad (8a)$$

$$(P)Mn^{III}(OH)(ImR) + (P)Mn^V(O)(ImR) \rightarrow 2(P)Mn^{IV}(O)(ImR) + H^+$$

$$(8b)$$

$$(P)Mn^V(O)(ImR) + \;\rangle C = C\langle\; \rightarrow ([P]Mn^{III}[ImR])^+ + -\overset{O}{\overset{\diagup\diagdown}{\underset{|}{C}} - \underset{|}{C}} -$$

$$(8c)$$

We find (Nakagaki et al. 1987) that we can prepare homogeneous solutions of rather high ClO$^-$ concentration by simply shaking an organic solvent containing a high concentration of phase transfer agent with an aqueous solution of LiOCl. The organic solvent containing the ClO$^-$ may then be mixed on a stopped-flow bench with a like solution containing metalloporphyrin plus nitrogen base ligand and alkene substrate. Without substrate, the manganese(IV)-oxo species is formed due to the reactions of Equations 8a and 8b (Fig. 1), and at high substrate concentration there is scarcely any accumulation of manganese(IV)-oxo species due to the trapping of the manganese(V)-oxo porphyrin by alkene (Eq. 8c). By monitoring the rate of formation of manganese(IV)-oxo species (and its yield) as a function of alkene concentration, the second-order rate constants associated with Equations 8a and 8c may be determined. Thus, when employing meso-tetrakis-(2,4,6-trimethylphenyl)porphinato manganese(III) hydroxide with norbornene, the rate constant for Equation 8a is $\sim 6 \times 10^5$ M^{-1} sec^{-1} and the epoxidation rate of Equation 8c is $\sim 1.2 \times 10^4$ M^{-1} sec^{-1}. This procedure is being extended to include other metalloporphyrins and other alkenes.

There is presently much interest in the mechanism of alkene epoxidation by hypervalent metallo-oxo porphyrin species. In the epoxidation of an alkene, a number of other products are generally obtained. The yields

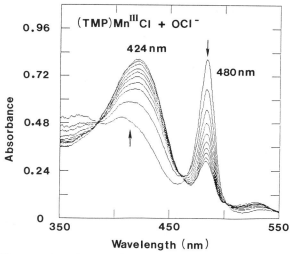

Figure 1. Repetitive spectral scans (10 msec between scans) using a homogeneous solution (wet CH_2Cl_2) showing the conversion of meso-tetrakis-(2,4,6-tetraphenyl)porphinato manganese(III) chloride (478 nm) to a manganese(IV)-oxo porphyrin species (426 nm) on reaction with ClO^-.

of these other products are dependent on conditions, the nature of the oxene equivalent transfer reagent, the alkene, and the metalloporphyrin. The question arises as to whether these additional products are derived from intermediates that are formed along the reaction path to epoxide. Does epoxide formation represent a multistep mechanism, or is it concerted? In Figure 2 are represented three pathways that can account for the products obtained in the epoxidation of *cis*-stilbene by C_6F_5IO when catalyzed by a number of iron(III) tetraphenylporphyrins (A. Castellino and T. Bruice, in prep.). Pathway a involves the intermediacy of a por-

phinato iron(III)-oxo carbocation (2) that partitions between epoxide and the rearrangement products diphenylacetaldehyde (by phenyl migration), deoxybenzoin (by hydrogen migration), *trans*-stilbene oxide (by rotation about the C–C bond and ring closure), etc. In pathway b, the first step involves the formation of a caged pair consisting of a carbocation radical (1) and $(Porph)M^{IV}(O)$. The reaction involves an outer sphere $1e^-$ transfer from the alkene to the hypervalent metallo-oxo porphyrin. Pathway c is consistent with the proposed radical character of the hypervalent metallo-oxo bond (Traylor et al. 1986). One could construct an alternate reaction scheme by having a concerted epoxidation mechanism and all other products arise as a result of competing reaction paths.

To assess the likelihood of formation of intermediate radical species, we have synthesized Z-1,2-bis($2^t,3^t$-diphenylcyclopropyl)ethene and examined its epoxidation (Eq. 9) by C_6F_5IO with meso-tetrakis(pentafluorophenyl)porphinato iron(III) chloride catalyst (A.J. Castellino and T.C. Bruice, work in progress).

$$\text{(9)}$$

The *cis*-epoxide was formed in 80% yield based on the concentration of C_6F_5IO oxene equivalent transfer reagent employed. The rate constant for the cyclopropylcarbinyl radical → allyl carbinyl radical rearrangement of Equation 10 has been clocked as 10^9 sec^{-1} (Mathew and Warkentin 1986).

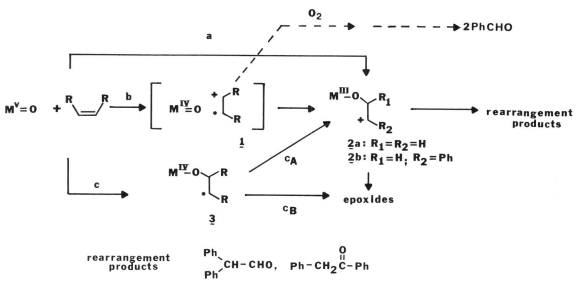

Figure 2. Plausible stepwise mechanisms for oxygen insertion into alkenes. $M^V=O$ symbolically represents the formal state of the metalloporphyrin catalyst after oxene equivalent transfer. No structural inference is to be made from this representation.

$$(10)$$

Though not verified experimentally, it is our anticipation that the rearrangement of Equation 11 should have a clocked time of about 10^{10} sec^{-1}.

$$(11)$$

If this proves to be so, then the theoretical yield of *cis*-epoxide obtained for the reaction of Equation 9 would require that any radical intermediate present would have a half-life of about 10^{11} sec^{-1}. Such a result would make questionable the radical cation (1) and iron-oxo carbinyl (3) intermediates of Figure 2.

ACKNOWLEDGMENTS

The studies referred to herein have been supported by the National Institutes of Health and the American Cancer Society.

REFERENCES

Balasubramanian, P.N. and T.C. Bruice. 1987. Oxygen transfer involving non heme iron. II. The influence of leaving group ability on the rate constant for oxygen transfer to (EDTA)Fe^{III} from percarboxylic acids and hydroperoxides. *Proc. Natl. Acad. Sci.* **84**: 1734.

Balasubramanian, P.N., E.S. Schmidt, and T.C. Bruice. 1987. Catalase modeling. II. The dynamics of reaction of a water-soluble and non-μ-oxo dimer forming manganese(III) porphyrin with hydrogen peroxide. *J. Am. Chem. Soc.* (in press).

Bruice, T.C., M.F. Zipplies, and W.A. Lee. 1986. The pH dependence of the mechanism of reaction of hydrogen peroxide with a non-aggregating non-μ-oxo dimer forming iron(III) porphyrin in water. *Proc. Natl. Acad. Sci.* **83**: 4646.

Calderwood, T.S. and T.C. Bruice. 1986. Electrochemical generation of iron(IV)-oxo porphyrins and iron(IV)-oxo porphyrin π-cation radicals. *Inorg. Chem.* **25**: 3722.

Calderwood, T.S., W.A. Lee, and T.C. Bruice. 1985. Spectral and electrochemical identification of iron(IV)-oxo porphyrin and iron(IV)-oxo porphyrin π-cation species. *J. Am. Chem. Soc.* **107**: 8272.

Collman, J.P., T. Kodadek, S.A. Raybuck, and B. Meunier. 1983. Oxygenation of hydrocarbons by cytochrome P-450 model compounds: Modification of reactivity by axial ligands. *Proc. Natl. Acad. Sci.* **80**: 7039.

Collman, J.P., J.I. Brauman, B. Meunier, S.A. Raybuck, and T. Kodadek. 1984. Epoxidation of olefins by cytochrome P-450 model compounds: Mechanism of oxygen atom transfer. *Proc. Natl. Acad. Sci.* **81**: 3245.

Collman, J.P., T. Kodadek, S.A. Raybuck, J.I. Brauman, and L.M. Papazian. 1985a. Mechanism of oxygen atom transfer from high valent iron porphyrins to olefins: Implications to the biological epoxidation of olefins by cytochrome P-450. *J. Am. Chem. Soc.* **108**: 4343.

Collman, J.P., J.I. Brauman, B. Meunier, T. Hayashi, T. Kodadek, and S.A. Raybuck. 1985b. Epoxidation of olefins by cytochrome P-450 model compounds: Kinetics

and stereochemistry of oxygen atom transfer and origin of shape selectivity. *J. Am. Chem. Soc.* **107**: 2000.

Dolphin, D., A. Forman, D.C. Borg, J. Fajer, and R.H. Felton. 1971. Compounds I of catalase and horseradish peroxidase: π-Cation radicals. *Proc. Natl. Acad. Sci.* **68**: 614.

Lee, W.A. and T.C. Bruice. 1985. Homolytic and heterolytic oxygen-oxygen bond scissions accompanying oxygen transfer to iron(III) porphyrins by percarboxylic acids and hydroperoxides. A mechanistic criterion for peroxidase and cytochrome P-450. *J. Am. Chem. Soc.* **107**: 513.

———. 1986. The transfer of oxygen from percarboxylic acids and alkyl hydroperoxides to (meso-tetraphenyl-porphinato) cobalt(III) chloride. *Inorg. Chem.* **25**: 131.

Lee, W.A., T.S. Calderwood, and T.C. Bruice. 1985. Stabilization of higher states of iron porphyrins by hydroxide and methoxide ligands. Electrochemical generation of iron-(IV)-oxo porphyrins. *Proc. Natl. Acad. Sci.* **82**: 4301.

Mathew, L. and J. Warkentin. 1986. The cyclopropylmethyl free radical clock. Calibration for the range 30-89° C. *J. Am. Chem. Soc.* **108**: 7981.

Meunier, B., E. Guilmet, M.E. De Carvalho, and R. Poilblanc. 1984. Sodium hypochlorite: A convenient source for olefin epoxidation catalyzed by (porphyrinato)manganese complexes. *J. Am. Chem. Soc.* **106**: 6668.

Moss, T.H., A. Erenbert, and A.J. Beardon. 1969. Mössbauer spectroscopic evidence for the electronic configuration of iron in horseradish peroxidase and its peroxide derivatives. *Biochemistry* **8**: 4159.

Nakagaki, P.C., R.W. Lee, P.N. Balasubramanian, and T.C. Bruice. 1987. Observations and comments on the mechanism of epoxidation of alkenes by manganese(III) porphyrins with hypochlorite. *Proc. Natl. Acad. Sci.* (in press).

Roberts, J.E., B.M. Hoffman, R. Rutter, and L.P Hager. 1981. Electro-nuclear double resonance of horseradish peroxidase compound I. *J. Biol. Chem.* **256**: 2118.

Samsel, E.G., K. Srinivasan, and J.K. Kochi. 1985. Mechanism of the chromium-catalyzed epoxidation of olefins. Role of oxochromium(V) cations. *J. Am. Chem. Soc.* **107**: 7606.

Sawyer, D.T., G.S. Srivatsa, M.E. Bodini, and W.P. Schaefer. 1986. Redox chemistry and spectroscopy of toluene-3,4-dithio (TDTH$_2$) and of its M(TDT)$_2^{2-/-}$ complexes with zinc(II), copper(II), nickel(II), cobalt(II), iron(II), and manganese(II). Formation of a stable d^n-($\cdot$SR) bond upon oxidation by one electron. *J. Am. Chem. Soc.* **108**: 936.

Schultz, C.E., P.W. Devaney, H. Winkler, P.G. Debrunner, N. Doan, R. Chiang, R. Runtler, and L.P. Hager. 1979. Horseradish peroxidase compound I: Evidence for spin coupling between the heme iron and a "free" radical. *FEBS Lett.* **103**: 102.

Traylor, T.G., T. Wakano, B.E. Dunlap, P.S. Traylor, and D. Dolphin. 1986. Mechanisms of hemin-catalyzed alkene epoxidation. The effect of catalyst on the regiochemistry of epoxidation. *J. Am. Chem. Soc.* **108**: 2782.

Yuan, L.-C., and T.C. Bruice. 1985a. The mechanisms of "oxygen atom" transfer to tetraphenylporphinato chromic chloride. *J. Am. Chem. Soc.* **107**: 512.

———. 1985b. Oxygen donation to manganese(III) tetraphenylporphyrin chloride. Low reactivity of hydroperoxides as oxygen donors to manganese(III) porphyrins. *Inorg. Chem.* **24**: 986.

———. 1986. The influence of nitrogen base ligation and hydrogen bonding on the rate constants for oxygen transfer from percarboxylic acids and alkyl hydroperoxides to *meso*-tetraphenyl-porphinato manganese(III) chloride. *J. Am. Chem. Soc.* **108**: 1643.

Zipplies, M.F., W.A. Lee, and T.C. Bruice. 1986. Influence of hydrogen ion activity and general acid-base catalysis on the rate of decomposition of hydrogen peroxide by a novel non-aggregating water-soluble iron(III) tetraphenylporphyrin derivative. *J. Am. Chem. Soc.* **108**: 4433.

S-Adenosylmethionine and the Mechanism of Hydrogen Transfer in the Lysine 2,3-Aminomutase Reaction

P.A. Frey AND M.L. Moss

Institute for Enzyme Research, Graduate School, and Department of Biochemistry,
College of Agricultural and Life Sciences, University of Wisconsin-Madison, Madison, Wisconsin 53705

Many enzymatic reactions involve chemical transformations that cannot be brought about by the catalytic actions of the functional groups in amino acids. The enzymes catalyzing these reactions exhibit extended catalytic capabilities by virtue of the actions of coenzymes or other cofactors, which lend specific and, in many cases, reasonably well-understood physicochemical properties to the catalytic process.

Enough is known about the mechanism of action of most coenzymes that the reactions in which they are involved can be recognized by their chemical types. However, certain reactions that should, on this basis, require the assistance of a particular coenzyme turn out not to involve that coenzyme. In these cases, some new, formerly unrecognized coenzyme must be present to provide the required catalytic properties. This appears to be the case with lysine 2,3-aminomutase.

Clostridium SB_4 can grow on lysine as its sole source of carbon and nitrogen. Lysine catabolism in this organism is an interesting process outlined in Figure 1, in which the six carbons are transformed into three molecules of acetyl-CoA, and the amino groups are converted to ammonia (Stadtman 1973). Lysine breakdown begins with the rearrangement of amino groups in the molecule, the 2-amino group being shifted to carbon 3 and the 6-amino group to carbon 5. After conversion of the 3- and 5-amines to ketones and activation of the carboxylate as the CoA ester, the molecule is properly functionalized for a series of β-ketothiolase reactions leading to the formation of three moles of acetyl-CoA.

The most difficult steps in lysine catabolism are the first two, the lysine 2,3-aminomutase and β-lysine 5,6-aminomutase reactions. These rearrangements are coenzyme B_{12}-type reactions. Indeed, the β-lysine 5,6-aminomutase is adenosylcobalamin-dependent (Stadtman 1972). Adenosylcobalamin-dependent rearrangements proceed by cross-migration of a hydrogen and another group ($-X$ in Eq. 1) between adjacent carbons. The 5′-deoxyadenosyl moiety of adenosylcobalamin plays a crucial mechanistic role by mediating hydrogen transfer (Abeles, 1972; Barker 1972).

$$-\underset{X}{\overset{|}{C}}_\beta - \underset{H}{\overset{|}{C}}_\alpha - \;\rightleftarrows\; -\underset{H}{\overset{|}{C}}_\beta - \underset{X}{\overset{|}{C}}_\alpha - \tag{1}$$

The lysine aminomutase reactions follow this pattern

with $-X = NH_3^+$. Another lysine aminomutase in *Clostridium sticklandii*, lysine 5,6-aminomutase, is also an adenosylcobalamin-dependent enzyme (Stadtman 1972). Both of the lysine 5,6-aminomutases are pyridoxal phosphate-dependent as well.

Lysine 2,3-aminomutase catalyzes Equation 2, the

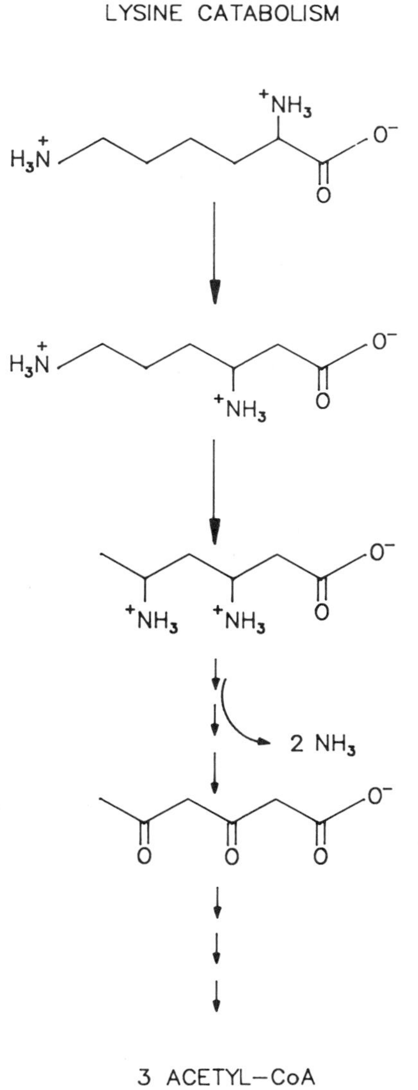

LYSINE CATABOLISM

Figure 1. Lysine metabolism in *Clostridia.*

interconversion of L-lysine and L-β-lysine (L-3,6-diaminohexanoate).

$$^+H_3N—CH_2CH_2CH_2CH_2—\underset{\underset{^+NH_3}{|}}{CH}—CO_2^- \Longrightarrow$$

$$^+H_3N—CH_2CH_2CH_2—\underset{\underset{^+NH_3}{|}}{CH}—CH_2—CO_2^- \quad (2)$$

Although the reaction follows the pattern of Equation 1, its cofactor requirements differ from those for the 5,6-aminomutases in that adenosylcobalamin is not involved, and the enzyme is activated by iron, a reducing system, and S-adenosylmethionine. The lysine 2,3-aminomutase described by Barker and his associates has a molecular weight estimated at 285,000 and a subunit M_r of 48,000 (Chirpich et al. 1970; Zappia and Barker 1970). It is a pyridoxal phosphate enzyme that contains approximately 2.8 moles of iron per mole of enzyme. The activity is stimulated three- to fourfold by added iron, 20% by added pyridoxal phosphate and 2.5-fold by S-adenosylmethionine (Chirpich et al. 1970).

The mechanistic functions of S-adenosylmethionine, pyridoxal phosphate, and iron in this reaction are not obvious. The known properties of pyridoxal phosphate do not suggest a means by which it could promote the reaction by a pathway involving low-energy intermediates. S-Adenosylmethionine is usually a methyl-donor substrate in metabolism, but methyl transfer has no obvious significance for this rearrangement. Although iron is thought to be essential, its function, too, is mysterious. The rearrangement itself is a chemically difficult reaction of a type that is expected to require a vitamin B_{12} coenzyme.

We have recently undertaken to investigate the mechanism of the lysine 2,3-aminomutase reaction, with special reference to the mechanism by which hydrogen transfer proceeds and the role of pyridoxal phosphate. We have observed the involvement of S-adenosylmethionine in hydrogen transfer in a manner reminiscent of that of adenosylcobalamin in coenzyme B_{12}-dependent rearrangements.

MATERIALS AND METHODS

Materials. Uniformly labeled L-[^{14}C]lysine · HCl, S-adenosyl[*methyl*-^{3}H]methionine, [2,8,5'-^{3}H]ATP, and [2,8-^{3}H]ATP were obtained from Amersham. S-[2,8,5'-^{3}H]adenosylmethionine and S-[2,8-^{3}H]adenosylmethionine were synthesized enzymatically from methionine and [2,8,5'-^{3}H]ATP or [2,8-^{3}H]ATP using S-adenosylmethionine synthase generously provided by Dr. Douglas Markham of the Institute for Cancer Research, Fox Chase Cancer Center, Philadelphia, PA. L-β-Lysine was synthesized as described by Van Tamelen and Smissman (1953).

Lysine 2,3-aminomutase was purified from cells of *Clostridium* SB$_4$ grown on lysine as the source of carbon and nitrogen essentially as described by Chirpich et al. (1970) through the acetone fractionation step with minor modifications. The enzyme was further purified by gel permeation chromatography through an Ultro-Pac TSK-G 3000 SWG column (21.5 × 500 mm) guarded by an Ultro-Pac TSK-G SWGPG column (21.5 × 75 mm) from LKB, Bromma, Sweden, using 30 mM Tris · acetate at pH 7.3 as the buffer. It was further purified by chromatography through DEAE-Sephadex A-50 eluted with a gradient of NaCl in 30 mM Tris · HCl. The best preparations exhibited a specific activity of 12 units/mg · protein.

Methods. Lysine 2,3-aminomutase was assayed as described (Chirpich et al. 1970). This assay procedure involved activation of the enzyme by preliminary incubation with sodium dithionite, dihydrolipoate, ferric ammonium citrate, and pyridoxal phosphate under Ar, essentially as described by Chirpich et al. (1970), substituting ferric ammonium citrate and dihydrolipoate for ferrous ammonium sulfate and glutathione and extending the preliminary incubation from 1 hour to 6 hours. The activated enzyme was then assayed exactly as described by Chirpich et al. (1970) by incubation with S-adenosylmethionine and L-[^{14}C]lysine. At the conclusion of the incubation period, the L-[^{14}C]lysine and L-β-[^{14}C]lysine were isolated and separated by paper electrophoresis and L-β-[^{14}C]lysine measured by radiochemical analysis using liquid scintillation counting. One unit of activity corresponded to the amount of enzyme required to convert one micromole of L-lysine to L-β-lysine in 1 minute under the standard assay conditions (Chirpich et al. 1970).

In the tritium transfer experiments, 3–18 units of lysine 2,3-aminomutase were first activated by incubation under Ar with 0.04 mM pyridoxal phosphate, 18 mM dihydrolipoate, 1.1 mM ferric ammonium citrate, 1.1 mM sodium dithionite, and 40 mM Tris · HCl buffer at pH 8.0 in a total volume of 0.44 ml for 6 hours at 37°C. A 0.4-ml aliquot of the activated enzyme was combined with a solution consisting of 0.5 M K-phosphate buffer at pH 7.9, 0.4 ml; 24 mM Na-dithionite, 0.4 ml; 0.12 M L-lysine · HCl, 0.04 ml; tritium-labeled S-adenosylmethionine diluted with carrier to give a final concentration of 0.02 mM; and H$_2$O to give a final volume of 4.94 ml. The reaction vessel, a 15-ml ampoule, was sealed under Ar after the addition of lysine 2,3-aminomutase. After 1 hour at 30°C, the ampoule was opened and 0.05 ml of 90% TCA added to stop the reaction. Activated charcoal (7 mg) was added to 3.94 ml of the supernatant fluid from the TCA precipitation, and after centrifugation the supernatant fluid was applied to a 0.6 × 5.5 cm column of Dowex 50W X4 ion exchange resin in the H$^+$ form. The column was washed with 10 ml of water and eluted with 36 ml of 1 M HCl. Fractions containing L-lysine and L-β-lysine, which were eluted together, were identified by colorimetric assay using ninhydrin; selected fractions throughout the elution were subjected to radiochemical assay by liquid scintillation counting. Tritium-labeled L-lysine and L-β-lysine were separated by paper electrophoresis at 5000 V for 10 minutes on Whatman no. 1 filter paper using 0.2 M formic acid as the electrolyte. Areas corresponding to L-lysine and L β-lysine were identified by electrophoresis of standards used as markers beside the radioactive samples. The markers were located by spraying with 3% ninhydrin in ethanol, and the corresponding areas from the radio-electrophoretogram were cut out and assayed radiochemically by liquid scintillation counting.

RESULTS

Purification of Lysine 2,3-aminomutase

Barker and his co-workers first described the purification and properties of lysine 2,3-aminomutase from *Clostridium* SB$_4$ in 1970 (Chirpich et al. 1970). Their purification procedure was typical in that it involved sonic disruption of bacteria grown on L-lysine as the sole source of carbon and nitrogen, streptomycin sulfate precipitation of nucleic acids, ammonium sulfate fractionation, heat denaturation of labile proteins, acetone fractionation at low temperature, and ion exchange chromatography through a column of DEAE-Sephadex. The purified enzyme appeared to be nearly homogeneous.

We have repeated the purification described by Chirpich et al. (1970) through the acetone fractionation step. We confirmed the reported results in general, with slight variations attributable to differences in extracts obtained in the two laboratories. The DEAE-Sephadex chromatography described in the earlier work involved an unusual protocol that was difficult to reproduce, the reasons for which became clear to us as our work progressed. In our first attempts to apply very high resolution chromatographic methods in place of the previously described DEAE-Sephadex procedure, we observed that chromatography of this enzyme through a Pharmacia Mono Q column or a large Ultro-Pac TSK-G 3000 gel permeation column resulted in good resolution of proteins but led to major or even complete activity losses, even though the traverse times through the columns were 30 minutes or less. In other experiments, it became clear that lysine was carried along with the enzyme through the early purification steps, and that added [^{14}C]lysine became associated with the enzyme sufficiently intimately to survive gel filtration through Sephadex G-25. We hypothesized that the enzyme might be stabilized by lysine and that high-resolution chromatographic procedures led to inactivation by virtue of the removal of lysine. Therefore, we carried out gel permeation chromatography through the Ultro-Pac TSK-G 3000 high-performance liquid chromatography (HPLC) column in a buffer supplemented with 0.1 mM L-lysine. The enzyme appeared in the effluent in a highly purified and active state in a reasonably well-isolated band.

Purification of lysine 2,3-aminomutase is now being perfected in this laboratory. The procedure we currently use is similar to that reported by Chirpich et al. (1970) through the acetone fractionation step, except that we include 0.1 mM L-lysine and 5 mM phenylmethylsulfonyl fluoride in all buffers and carry out the heat denaturation of labile proteins at a lower temperature (50°C rather than 60°C). We complete the purification with gel permeation chromatography through the Ultro-Pac TSK-G 3000 HPLC column and a conventional DEAE-Sephadex chromatography, all in the presence of 0.1 mM L-lysine. Our best preparations exhibit a specific activity of 12 units/mg · protein, about twice the activity reported by Chirpich et al. (1970). We attribute the higher specific activity mainly to stabilization by lysine during purification and to an improved procedure described in the next section.

Chirpich et al. (1970) originally characterized this enzyme as a protein with an overall M_r of 285,000. Zappia and Barker (1970) reported a subunit M_r of 48,000, as determined by polyacrylamide gel electrophoresis in 0.1 M sodium dodecyl sulfate (SDS), and suggested a hexameric quaternary structure. We have been unable to obtain an active preparation that failed to show a multiband pattern upon SDS-polyacrylamide gel electrophoresis. In addition to the major band, we have observed two smaller proteins in apparently reproducible ratios in our most active preparations. Zappia and Barker (1970) also observed a smaller protein in addition to the major component in ultracentrifugation experiments carried out in the presence of 50 mM SDS.

Activation of Lysine 2,3-aminomutase

Lysine 2,3-aminomutase is purified in an inactive state and must be activated by incubation with a reducing system. Maximum activity is obtained when ferrous ammonium sulfate and pyridoxal phosphate are included in the activation system. In the activation procedure utilized by Chirpich et al. (1970), sodium dithionite and glutathione in addition to enzyme, ferrous ammonium sulfate, and pyridoxal phosphate are incubated 1 hour under anaerobic conditions. We utilize a similar procedure, except that we substitute dihyrolipoate for glutathione and extend the incubation time to 6 hours under anaerobic conditions. In our hands, dihydrolipoate leads to higher activities than glutathione.

S-Adenosylmethionine and the Hydrogen Transfer Mechanism

To determine whether S-adenosylmethionine participates directly in hydrogen transfer, we carried out the reaction using enzyme that had been activated with S-adenosylmethionine labeled with tritium in various positions. We then isolated L-lysine and L-β-lysine as a mixture and analyzed them for tritium. These experiments implicated S-adenosylmethionine in the hydrogen transfer process of the reaction.

In our first experiments, we used lysine 2,3-aminomutase purified to a specific activity of 3 units/mg·protein and obtained the results in Table 1. In the experiment in which we activated lysine 2,3-aminomutase with S-[2,8,5'-³H]adenosylmethionine, 16.3% of the radioactivity appeared in L-lysine and L-β-lysine. No significant tritium appeared in lysine either when enzyme was omitted or when the enzyme had not been subjected to the preliminary activation described above. Furthermore, no significant radioactivity could be detected in lysine when either S-[2,8-³H]adenosylmethionine or S-adenosyl[methyl-³H]methionine was used to activate the enzyme.

Separation of the mixture of tritium-labeled L-lysine and L-β-lysine in Table 1 by paper electrophoresis, under the conditions used to separate them in the assay procedure, enabled us to measure the relative amounts of tritium in each isomer. The tritium content of L-lysine in Table 1 was found to be 0.29×10^5 cpm and that of L-β-lysine was 1.3×10^5 cpm, showing that all of the tritium isolated with the mixture was associated with L-lysine or L-β-lysine. Five repetitions of this experiment gave similar results corresponding to a K_{eq} of 5.3 ± 0.3 favoring L-β-lysine at pH 7.7 and 30°C. This was similar to the published value of the K_{eq}, which has been reported to be 5.7 or 6.7 at 37°C (Costilow et al. 1966; Chirpich et al. 1970). The close correspondence between K_{eq} and the relative tritium contents of L-lysine and L-β-lysine further supported their identification as the radioactive products.

The amount of S-[2,8,5'-³H]adenosylmethionine used in Table 1 exceeded the amount of lysine 2,3-aminomutase on a molar basis, as estimated from the amount of enzyme activity in the reaction mixture and the molecular weight of the enzyme. The transfer experiment in the first line of Table 1, i.e., using S-[2,8,5'-³H]adenosylmethionine as the coenzyme, was repeated with larger and smaller amounts of enzyme, with the results shown in Table 2. The amounts of radioactivity in L-lysine and L-β-lysine were clearly dependent on the amount of enzyme used, although not directly pro-

Table 2. Effect of Enzyme Concentration on Tritium Transfer

Lysine 2,3-aminomutase[a] (units)	% ³H in lysines[b] (cpm)
18	26
9	16
3	6

[a]The reaction mixtures were identical to the complete reaction in Table 1 except that the amount of enzyme was varied as indicated.

[b]The values tabulated are the % of the total ³H in S-[2,8,5'-³H]adenosylmethionine isolated in L-lysine and L-β-lysine.

portional. Since the reaction times were quite long, we concluded that the interaction of S-adenosylmethionine with lysine 2,3-aminomutase is not freely reversible since, if it were reversible, the amount of tritium mobilized should have been maximal and the same in all of the experiments. A double reciprocal plot of the data in Table 2 was linear, and extrapolaton to infinite [enzyme] indicated that the maximum amount of tritium that could be incorporated into lysine from S-[2,8,5'-³H]adenosylmethionine corresponded to between 60% and 80% of the tritium in the coenzyme. According to the manufacturer's specifications, 66% of the tritium was in the 5' position and the balance in the 2 and 8 positions. Therefore, if both 5' hydrogens were labeled, that is, if the labeling was nonstereospecific, both 5' hydrogens were mobilized in the hydrogen transfer process. This could happen only if the bond between the 5' carbon and the sulfur in methionine were broken in the course of the hydrogen transfer process.

The experiments in Tables 1 and 2 were carried out with enzyme at a specific activity of 3 units/mg·protein that was highly purified but not homogeneous. The key experiment, that utilizing S-[2,8,5'-³H]adenosylmethionine as the coenzyme, has been repeated with identical results using essentially homogeneous enzyme displaying a specific activity of 12 units/mg·protein. Inasmuch as no tritium from either S-[2,8,³H]adenosylmethionine or S-adenosyl[methyl-³H]methionine was transferred to L-lysine or L-β-lysine, the 5' hydrogens must be involved in a hydrogen transfer pool with substrate-derived hydrogens, whereas the methyl and 2 and 8 hydrogens cannot participate. We cannot as yet exclude the other methionyl and ribosyl hydrogens from this pool, although we have no reason to expect them to be involved.

Table 1. Transfer of Tritium from S-Adenosylmethionine to Lysine

Reaction mixture	³H in lysine (cpm)
Complete[a]	1.59×10^5
−enzyme	0.006×10^5
unactivated enzyme[b]	0.006×10^5
S-adenosyl[methyl-³H]methionine[c]	0.003×10^5
S-[2,8-³H]adenosylmethionine[c]	0.010×10^5

[a]The complete reaction mixture is described in the methods section and contained 9.74×10^5 cpm of S-[2,8,5'-³H]adenosylmethionine (4.9 mCi/m·mol).

[b]The reaction mixture was complete in all respects except that the enzyme was not activated by preliminary incubation with dihydrolipoate, ferric ammonium citrate, dithionite, and pyridoxal phosphate prior to initiating the reaction.

[c]In place of S-[2,8,5'-³H]adenosylmethionine.

DISCUSSION

Proteins have diverse three-dimensional structures that give them the potential to catalyze a broad range of biochemical reactions. The catalytic mechanisms involving protein function in enzymatic reactions are reasonably well understood. A crucially important catalytic force is the binding process itself, which involves hydrophobic, electrostatic, hydrogen bonding, and dipolar forces between the active site and the substrate (Jencks 1975). The binding process overcomes much of the entropy barrier to reaction. Binding interactions also stabilize transition states by immobilizing substrates in conformations that resemble the structures of transition states. Such conformations often lie at energies higher than those of the ground states of free substrates; therefore, catalysis by binding often entails raising the structural energy levels of substrates by interactions in the Michaelis complexes that simultaneously lower the transition state energies. Other crucially important enzymatic mechanisms support the interconversions of Michaelis complexes by providing low-energy transition states. These include general acid-base catalysis and nucleophilic catalysis, which are provided for by the functional groups of amino acid residues.

The principal limitation of proteins as catalysts is that the range of chemical reaction types that can be catalyzed is bounded by the chemical properties of the amino acid functional groups. Residues such as histidine, lysine, glutamate, aspartate, and cysteine can support general acid-base and nucleophilic catalysis and binding interactions, but they cannot provide electrophilic catalysis or support the formation of intrinsically unstable free radicals or carbanions. The mechanisms of many enzymatic reactions must involve such unstable intermediates; in these cases a cofactor such as a metal ion or coenzyme is always found to play a crucial catalytic role.

The mechanisms by which most of the coenzymes act in supporting enzymatic reactions are reasonably well understood. Thiamin pyrophosphate and pyridoxal phosphate, for example, provide access to catalytic pathways that avoid the formation of highly unstable carbanions, that is, by stabilizing requisite carbanions. Adenosylcobalamin is thought to promote rearrangements by initiating substrate free-radical formation through abstraction of a hydrogen by the 5' free radical of the 5'-deoxyadenosyl moiety, as illustrated in Figure 2. The substrate-derived free radical then rearranges to a product-derived free radical, which is converted to the product by abstraction of a hydrogen and regeneration of the 5'-deoxyadenosyl free radical (Abeles 1971; Barker 1972).

The lysine 2,3-aminomutase reaction is analogous to the adenosylcobalamin-dependent rearrangements and to the β-lysine 5,6-aminomutase reaction in particular. However, adenosylcobalamin is not involved. The role of S-adenosylmethionine as a cofactor is clarified by our experiments, which implicate the 5'-deoxyadenosyl group of S-adenosylmethionine in mediating hydrogen transfer in a manner that appears to be similar to the function of the 5'-deoxyadenosyl moiety of adenosylcobalamin in coenzyme B_{12}-dependent reactions. Our results allow us to conclude that the lysine 2,3-aminomutase reaction mechanism involves the generation of a hydrogen transfer pool that includes one substrate-derived hydrogen and the 5' hydrogens of the nucleoside moiety in S-adenosylmethionine. The function of this pool involves the cleavage of the nucleoside from methionine, since both 5' hydrogens, which are sterically important, are involved. If the function of the 5'-deoxyadenosyl moiety is similar to that of adenosylcobalamin in the B_{12}-dependent reactions, the reaction mechanism probably involves free radicals and a rearrangement similar to that illustrated in Figure 3.

The question of the mechanistic involvement by pyridoxal phosphate in the lysine 2,3-aminomutase and the β-lysine 5,6-aminomutase reactions is interesting

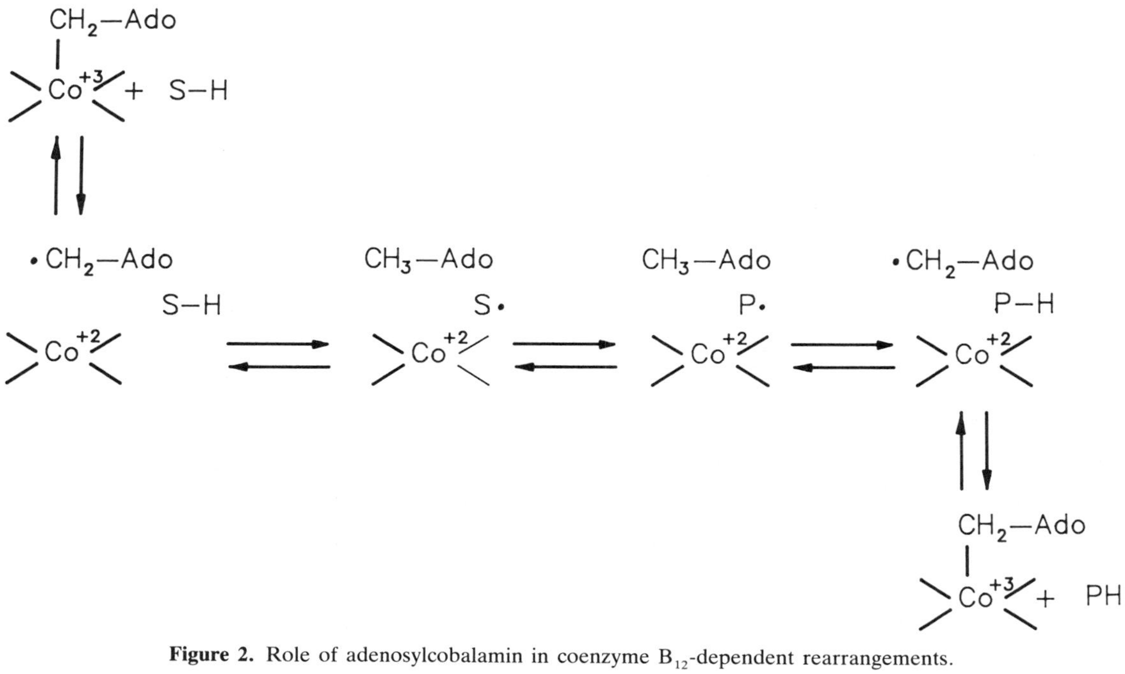

Figure 2. Role of adenosylcobalamin in coenzyme B_{12}-dependent rearrangements.

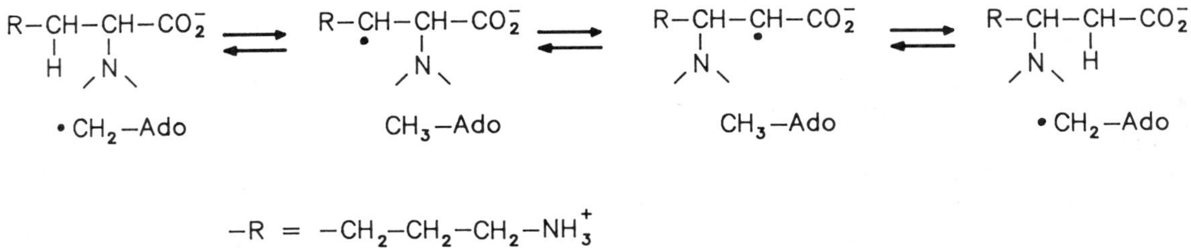

Figure 3. A hypothetical free-radical mechanism for lysine aminomutase reactions.

and not clearly defined. Although pyridoxal phosphate plays a central role in many reactions of amino acid metabolism, its function is generally to potentiate bond cleavages by stabilizing carbanions. This capability of pyridoxal phosphate does not offer a satisfying mechanistic rationale for its involvement in the lysine aminomutases. It is not known in the case of lysine 2,3-aminomutase whether pyridoxal phosphate reacts with the 2-amino group to form an aldimine; however, there is evidence in the β-lysine 5,6-aminomutase reaction that pyridoxal phosphate forms an aldimine with the transferred amino group (Stadtman 1973).

Aldimine formation between the transferred amino group and pyridoxal phosphate can promote the rearrangement mechanism shown in Figure 3 by providing a driving force for the migration of nitrogen and stabilizing a rearrangement intermediate. This mechanism, illustrated in Figure 4, explains the rearrangement on the basis that the free radical generated in the first step can form an aziridine free radical, in which the unpaired electron is stabilized by delocalization throughout the pyridine ring of pyridoxal phosphate. The aziridine free radical is electronically symmetrical with respect to the rearrangement and can reopen to either the substrate or product-related free radical. Hydrogen transfer from 5'-deoxyadenosine to either of these species leads to substrate or product formation. This is a very attractive and novel role for pyridoxal phosphate.

Aberhart and Gould and their co-workers carried out a stereochemical study of hydrogen transfer in the lysine 2,3-aminomutase reaction and obtained results fully in accord with those reported here. They found that the reaction proceeds with transfer of the 3-pro-R hydrogen of L-lysine to the 2-pro-R position of L-β-lysine (Aberhart et al. 1983). They also mixed L-[3-^{2}H$_2$]lysine with L-lysine in a molar ratio of 1:10 and carried out a mass spectral analysis of the L-β-lysine

produced. They observed only monodeutero-species and concluded that hydrogen transfer was largely intermolecular under their conditions. They could not exclude a degree of intramolecular transfer with the limited information from their experiment. Their data indicated that the mechanism involves either a compulsory intermolecular hydrogen transfer between substrate molecules or a hydrogen transfer pool such as that proposed in Figures 2 and 3 above. They were also able to show that the amino group migration is an intramolecular process, consistent with the mechanism in Figures 3 and 4.

Our experiments implicate the 5'-deoxyadenosyl group of S-adenosylmethionine as part of the hydrogen transfer pool in the lysine 2,3-aminomutase reaction mechanism. They imply that the function of S-adenosylmethionine is to supply this nucleoside in such a way as to support its action by a mechanism similar to that of the 5'-deoxyadenosyl moiety of adenosylcobalamin in coenzyme B$_{12}$-dependent rearrangements. Many questions are raised by our results, including whether the involvement of the deoxyadenosyl 5'-hydrogens is kinetically competent, whether S-adenosylmethionine reversibly or irreversibly donates the 5'-deoxyadenosyl moiety to some entity on the enzyme, whether free radicals are actually intermediates, whether pyridoxal phosphate stabilizes a free-radical intermediate, and whether iron interacts chemically with S-adenosylmethionine or with the 5'-deoxyadenosyl moiety of the coenzyme. The question of whether the enzyme consists of more than one type of subunit also remains. Finally, the mechanistic relationship of this reaction with the adenosylcobalamin-dependent reactions, when unmasked, may clarify both reaction mechanisms. The nature of the hydrogen transfer cofactor in lysine 2,3-aminomutase may also shed light on the evolutionary origin of coenzymes that potentiate free-radical formation.

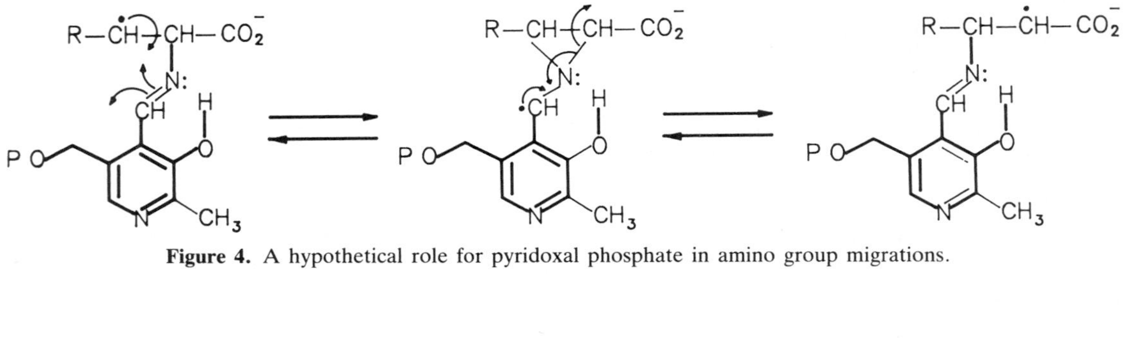

Figure 4. A hypothetical role for pyridoxal phosphate in amino group migrations.

ACKNOWLEDGMENTS

This research was supported by grant AM-28607 from the National Institute of Arthritis, Metabolism and Digestive and Kidney Diseases. Robert Petrovich assisted us with the purification of 2,3-aminomutase, especially with the development of high-performance gel permeation chromatography as a purification step. We are grateful to Dr. Douglas Markham for a gift of S-adenosylmethionine synthase.

REFERENCES

Abeles, R.H. 1971. Dehydrations requiring vitamin B_{12} coenzyme. In *The enzymes* 3rd edition (ed. P.D. Boyer), vol. 5, p. 481. Academic Press, New York.

Aberhart, D.J., S.J. Gould, H.-J. Lin, T.K. Thiruvengadam, and B.H. Weiller. 1983. Stereochemistry of lysine 2,3-aminomutase isolated from *Clostridium subterminale* SB4. *J. Am. Chem. Soc.* **105**: 5461.

Barker, H.A. 1972. Coenzyme B_{12}-dependent mutases causing carbon chain rearrangements. In *The enzymes* 3rd edition (ed. P.D. Boyer), vol. 6, p. 509. Academic Press, New York.

Chirpich, T.P., V. Zappia, R.N. Costilow, and H.A. Barker. 1970. Lysine 2,3-aminomutase. Purification and properties of a pyridoxal phosphate and S-adenosylmethionine-activated enzyme. *J. Biol. Chem.* **245**: 1778.

Costilow, R.N., O.M. Rochovansky, and H.A. Barker. 1966. Isolation and identification of β-lysine as an intermediate in lysine fermentation. *J. Biol. Chem.* **241**: 1573.

Jencks, W.P. 1975. Binding energy, specificity, and enzymatic catalysis. The Circe effect. *Adv. Enzymol.* **43**: 210.

Stadtman, T.C. 1972. B_{12} coenzyme-dependent amino group migrations. In *The enzymes* 3rd edition (ed. P.D. Boyer), vol. 6, p. 539. Academic Press, New York.

―――. 1973. Lysine metabolism by *Clostridia. Adv. Enzymol.* **38**: 413.

Van Tamelen, E.E. and E.E. Smissman. 1953. Streptolin. The structure and synthesis of isolysine. *J. Am. Chem. Soc.* **75**: 2031.

Zappia, V. and H.A. Barker. 1970. Studies on lysine 2,3-aminomutase. Subunit structure and sulfhydryl groups. *Biochim. Biophys. Acta* **207**: 505.

Metal Ions in Proteins: Structural and Functional Roles

J.M. BERG

Department of Chemistry, The Johns Hopkins University, Baltimore, Maryland 21218

Metal ions play important roles in many biological systems. In particular, metal ions are required for the activity of a large number of enzymes and proteins. Metal ions are well suited for these functions because of the following properties: (1) Metal ions are almost always positively charged and, hence, electrophilic. They can act as Lewis acids for binding and activating substrates. (2) Many metals can exist stably in a number of different oxidation states differing by one or by several units. This allows these metals to participate in various types of oxidation-reduction processes. (3) Metal ions generally bind four or more ligands. By binding several protein side chains, metals can act as multidentate cross-linking agents.

In some metalloproteins, the coordination sphere around the metal ion is relatively static in that the coordination number and gross coordination geometry do not change as the protein executes its function. In others, the coordination environment is quite dynamic with changes in geometry, including changes in the ligands bound, playing an essential role in protein function. Furthermore, as noted above, some proteins contain metal ions that undergo changes in oxidation level, whereas others have ions that remain in a single oxidation state. Consideration of the static versus dynamic natures of the coordination spheres and oxidation states of various metal ions in proteins can be used to develop the classification scheme shown in Figure 1.

Metal Ions In Proteins

Coordination Sphere

		Static	Dynamic
Oxidation State	Static	**Binding Proteins** Aspartate Transcarbamylase Regulatory Subunit (Zn) Calmodulin (Ca)	**Hydrolases** Carboxypeptidase A (Zn) Urease (Ni)
	Dynamic	**Electron Carriers** Cytochrome c (Fe) Plastocyanin (Cu)	**Oxidoreductases and Oxygen Carriers** Cytochrome P-450 (Fe) Hemocyanin (Cu)

Figure 1. Classification scheme for the functions of metal ions in proteins according to the static versus dynamic natures of their coordination spheres and oxidation levels.

The first class includes proteins for which both the coordination sphere and the oxidation state change during the course of function. The most obvious members of this class are oxidoreductases, enzymes that execute oxidation-reduction reactions of substrates. A specific example is cytochrome P-450. In the cytochromes P-450, an iron atom is bound to the four nitrogens of a porphyrin ring and to a thiolate group from a protein cysteine residue with the sixth position in an octahedral structure available for substrate binding (Poulos et al. 1985). During the catalytic cycle the iron undergoes the following changes: $Fe^{+++} \rightarrow Fe^{++} \rightarrow (Fe^{++}[O_2] \leftrightarrow Fe^{+++}[O_2^-]) \rightarrow (Fe=O)^{+++} \rightarrow Fe^{+++}$ (Coon and White 1980). Thus, the dynamic nature of the coordination sphere is required for dioxygen binding, and changes in oxidation state are required for dioxygen binding and activation. Another less obvious group of proteins in this class are the oxygen carriers. Although changes in the coordination sphere are clearly required for dioxygen binding, the necessity for changes in oxidation state is not as apparent. However, for the three well-characterized types of oxygen carriers, dioxygen is not bound as O_2^0 but as a more reduced form (O_2^-, O_2^{--}, or HO_2^-), indicating that an internal oxidation-reduction process has occurred. In hemocyanin, for example, the deoxy form has two Cu(I) ions, whereas the oxy form contains two Cu(II) ions bridged by a peroxide ligand (Eickman et al. 1979).

The second class consists of proteins in which the coordination sphere is dynamic, but the oxidation state of the metal ion remains constant. The prototypical examples of such proteins are the zinc(II)-containing peptidases such as carboxypeptidase A (Vallee et al. 1983). In these proteins, the zinc ions act as Lewis acids to bind and polarize substrate carbonyl groups and/or to bind and activate water/hydroxide. Since zinc has only one stable oxidation level, no oxidation-reduction process can be involved. Another example is provided by urease, which has an active site that appears to contain two Ni(II) ions (Blakeley and Zerner 1984). Although oxidation-reduction processes are possible with nickel, a mechanism has been proposed in which one Ni(II) ion acts to bind and activate urea and the other activates a bound hydroxide ion for attack (Blakeley and Zerner 1984).

The third class includes those proteins in which the coordination sphere remains relatively static while the metal ion is involved in an oxidation-reduction process. These proteins are generally electron carriers involved in transferring single electrons. Examples include cytochrome c and plastocyanin. The coordination spheres of the metal ion in these proteins are changed only very slightly as the metal ions changes oxidation state. Indeed, this small structural change is certainly important in facilitating fast electron transfer by minimizing the reorganizational energy component to the activation energy.

The final class of protein is that in which both the coordination sphere and the oxidation state are fixed. In these proteins, the metal ions act to cross-link several amino acid side chains and hence to stabilize a particular protein structure. Thus, the metal ions play a purely structural role, but since three-dimensional structure and function are intimately connected, they have dramatic effects on protein function as well. Examples of such proteins include calcium-binding proteins such as calmodulin, and zinc proteins such as the regulatory subunit of aspartate transcarbamylase. In the calcium-binding proteins, the Ca^{++} ions are bound in an α helix-loop–α helix structure termed the EF-hand with the ligands all from a short stretch (about 12 residues) of sequence (Seamon and Kretsinger 1983). These proteins respond to changes in calcium concentration in a manner that is fundamental to the function of Ca^{++} as a second messenger. In aspartate transcarbamylase, the Zn^{++} is bound by four cysteinate residues from a single protein domain that is involved in interactions between the regulatory and catalytic subunits (Honzatko et al. 1982); removal of the Zn^{++} causes dissociation of the holoenzyme (Nelbach et al. 1972).

Recognition of the importance of "structural zinc" has been greatly increased recently by the discovery that zinc appears to play such a role in several classes of proteins involved in nucleic acid binding and gene regulation. This development has been made possible largely by the observation that these proteins contain characteristic patterns of cysteine and histidine residues within relatively short segments of amino acid sequence, suggesting the presence of small structural domains organized around bound metal ions. The remainder of this paper will discuss the structural and functional roles of such metal-binding domains.

RESULTS AND DISCUSSION

Transcription Factor IIIA and the "Zinc Finger" Proteins

The occurrence of metal-binding domains in nucleic-acid-binding proteins was first hypothesized based on analysis of the sequence of the protein transcription factor IIIA from *Xenopus* (TFIIIA). This protein binds both the approximately 50-bp internal control region of the 5S RNA genes to activate transcription and the 5S RNA molecule itself in a 1:1 complex that acts as a storage particle (Pelham and Brown 1980). The protein sequence was determined from a cDNA clone (Ginsberg et al. 1984), and two groups reported that the sequence contained nine tandem imperfect repeats of an approximately 30-amino-acid sequence with two con-

served cysteine residues and two conserved histidine residues with some hydrophobic residues conserved as well (Brown et al. 1985; Miller et al. 1985). The consensus sequence of these repeats is (Phe,Tyr)-X - Cys - $(X)_4$ - Cys - $(X)_3$ - Phe - $(X)_5$ - Leu - $(X)_2$ - His - $(X)_3$ -His-$(X)_5$. Furthermore, it was shown that the storage particle contains 7–11 zinc ions if it was isolated under conditions that avoided the use of chelating agents (Miller et al. 1985), extending an earlier report that the particle and protein contained 2–3 zinc ions (Hanas et al. 1983). Based on these observations, it was proposed that each repeat bound a zinc ion tetrahedrally through the cysteine and histidine residues to form an independent structural domain that was termed a "zinc finger" (Miller et al. 1985).

A variety of evidence supports the existence of these domains. First, the protein was known to have a highly asymmetrical shape, based on sedimentation studies (Bieker and Roeder 1984) and on the fact that a single protein molecule protected about 50 bp of DNA from digestion (Bieker and Roeder 1984; Smith et al. 1984). The hypothesis that three-quarters of the protein are built of nine relatively independent structural units fits nicely with these observations. Second, limited proteolysis of the storage particle yielded fragments with sizes consistent with the existence of domains of approximately 3–3.5 kD (Miller et al. 1985). Third, the structure of the TFIIIA gene has been determined, and it was found that introns occur between repeats 1–2,2–3,3–4,4–5,5–6, and 6–7, strongly suggesting that these units have structural significance (Tso et al. 1986). Fourth, a 30-amino-acid peptide corresponding to one repeat has been prepared, and it has been shown to fold into a stable structure in the presence of Zn^{++} or similar divalent metal ions, but not in their absence (Frankel et al. 1987). Finally, spectroscopic studies of the metal-binding site are consistent with the hypothesis. X-ray absorption studies of the storage particle suggest that each zinc has two nitrogen ligands at 2.0 Å and two sulfur ligands at 2.3 Å (Diakun et al. 1986). Furthermore, the spectroscopic properties of the Co^{++} complex of the single-repeat peptide suggest a tetrahedral site and are entirely consistent with the proposed structure (Frankel et al. 1987).

Subsequently, several other proteins have been discovered to contain quite similar sequences. The consensus sequences are essentially identical, except that two residues are present between the cysteine residues rather than four as observed in TFIIIA. Four of these were discovered in a manner entirely independent of the knowledge of the zinc finger sequence. These include the product of the *Drosophila* segmentation gene *Krüppel* (Rosenberg et al. 1986), the β and δ open reading frames from the *Drosophila serendipity* locus (Vincent et al. 1985), and the yeast positive control protein ADR1 (Hartshorne et al. 1986). More recently, several open reading frames have been isolated using nucleic acid probes derived from the *Krüppel* gene. These include one from *Drosophila* (Kr h) (Schuh et al. 1986) and two from mouse (MKR1 and

MKR2) (Chowdhury et al. 1987). In addition, hybridization studies using *Krüppel*-derived probes and studies using antisera against a 12-amino-acid peptide derived from *Krüppel* indicate that a wide variety of eukaryotes have nuclear proteins that contain the zinc finger motif (Schuh et al. 1986).

Other Potential Metal-binding Domains

The widespread occurrence of TFIIIA-like metal-binding sequences raised the question of whether other classes of metal-binding domains also occur in other nucleic-acid-binding proteins. Such domains would be similar to the TFIIIA-like structures in that they would have four metal-binding residues within a short stretch of amino acid sequence, but they would not be homologous to the TFIIIA-like sequences in a formal sense. To address this question, a systematic search procedure was devised (Berg 1986). A search template of the form $Cys-(X)_{2-4}-Cys-(X)_{2-15}-a-(X)_{2-4}-b$ or $a-(X)_{2-4}-b-(X)_{2-15}-Cys-(X)_{2-4}-Cys$, where a and b can be either Cys or His, was developed. The form of this template was loosely based on the TFIIIA-like sequences, and the spacing of two to four residues between the outer sets of metal-binding ligands was chosen based on an analysis of structurally characterized metalloproteins. It should be noted that such a procedure cannot (and is not intended to) find all potential binding sites since many such sites involve amino acids that are widely separated in the amino acid sequence. The involvement of all metal-binding residues within a short stretch of sequence provides a definition of a metal-binding domain. Furthermore, the goal of the search was to identify *potential* metal-binding domains. Once identified, the actual role of metal ions in these systems (if any) must be investigated experimentally.

The template was used to search a computer-based protein sequence library. Five classes of proteins involved in nucleic-acid-binding or gene regulation were identified (Berg 1986). Of these, I shall discuss two in detail. The first group consists of the low-molecular-weight nucleic-acid-binding proteins from retroviruses. The proteins are encoded within the *gag* gene, expressed as part of a polyprotein, and freed by proteolysis. The final products have less than 100 amino acids and contain either one or two sequences of the form $Cys-(X)_2-Cys-(X)_4-His-(X)_4-Cys$. Although no direct evidence is yet available concerning the involvement of metal ions in these proteins, several observations support this hypothesis. First, some proteins contain one such sequence, whereas others contain two, with the spacing between the two varying from 5 to 22 residues. These facts suggest that each sequence forms an independent structural unit. Second, Gly residues occur frequently in positions 5 and, especially, 8. These are analogous to the Gly residues in the metal-binding sequences of rubredoxins ($Cys-[X]_2-Cys-Gly$) and azurins ($Cys-[X]_3-Gly-His$), where they allow type II β turns and, concomitantly, additional hydrogen bonds to

form. Finally, these sequences are quite similar to the sequence $Cys-(X)_3-His-(X)_5-Cys-(X)_2-Cys$ from the bacteriophage T4 helix-destabilizing (gene 32) protein, which was also identified as a potential metal-binding domain by the search procedure (Berg 1986). This protein has recently been shown to contain one zinc ion per molecule, and spectroscopic studies of the Co^{++}-substituted protein are consistent with this binding site (Giedroc et al. 1986).

The function of these proteins is not completely understood. In vitro studies of the isolated proteins indicated that they are nonspecific nucleic-acid-binding proteins with a preference for single-stranded substrates (Davis et al. 1976; Schulein et al. 1978; Smith and Bailey 1979). In vivo photo-cross-linking studies, however, indicated the presence of specific binding sites on the viral RNA (Darlix and Spahr 1982; Méric et al. 1984). More recent studies of mutants have strongly suggested that the proteins play a role in RNA packaging (Méric and Spahr 1986). A 2-amino-acid insertion within one of the two potential metal-binding domains of the Rous sarcoma virus protein p12 caused a marked decrease in the amount of dimeric viral RNA present in the virion, whereas more dramatic mutations led to little RNA incorporation whatsoever. These results suggest that the proteins may recognize a site (sequence or structure) on the viral RNA that is required for packaging. One possible explanation for the differences between the in vitro and in vivo studies is that the proteins have been isolated in the presence of EDTA and other potential chelating agents. Interestingly, treatment of free TFIIIA with low concentrations of EDTA causes loss of zinc with concomitant abolition of site-specific DNA-binding activity, although the protein still binds nucleic acids (particularly single stranded) nonspecifically (Hanas et al. 1983). TFIIIA is normally isolated as a complex with 5S RNA, which is substantially less sensitive to chelating agents.

The second class of proteins consists of one class of products of the adenovirus E1A genes (Berk 1986). These proteins contain a sequence of the form $Cys-(X)_2-Cys-(X)_{13}-Cys-(X)_2-Cys$ (Berg 1986). Two overlapping mRNAs are transcribed from the E1A genes. These differ by a small internal sequence (93–138 nucleotides) that is removed by splicing from one of the messages but not the other. The messages remain in the same reading frame, however, so that the two protein products have identical amino- and carboxy-terminal ends and differ only by the presence of an internal sequence of 31–46 amino acids. Importantly, the potential metal-binding domain sequences occur in this region, which is unique to the larger protein product.

The E1A gene products have several activities (Berk 1986). They increase the efficiency of transcription of other early viral genes and some endogenous cellular genes, they play a role in cell transformation, and they repress the effect of certain enhancer elements. Studies of mutant genes have revealed that only the larger protein is active in transcriptional activation, whereas both proteins have repression and transformation activities (Lillie et al. 1986). A variety of studies have indicated that the larger E1A protein is not itself a DNA-binding protein but instead interacts with cellular transcription factors to increase the efficiency of transcription of certain genes (Berk 1986). In particular, a TATA-box-binding transcription factor has been implicated in studies of E1A protein *trans*-activation of the adenovirus E1B promoter (Wu et al. 1987).

These results suggest that the potential metal-binding domain in the larger E1A protein may be involved in a protein-protein contact. As noted in the introduction, such a role for a metal-binding domain has a precedent in the regulatory subunit of aspartate transcarbamylase (Honzatko et al. 1982). This protein is a dimer of a polypeptide that has two structural domains called the allosteric effector domain and the zinc domain. The dimer is held together by interactions between β sheets of the allosteric effector domains, and the zinc domain mediates interactions between the regulatory dimer and the catalytic subunits. The zinc domain consists of residues 101–153 and contains the metal-binding sequence Cys-109–$(X)_4$–Cys-114–$(X)_{25}$–Cys-138–$(X)_2$–Cys-141. The interactions with the catalytic subunits involve residues close to the zinc-binding residues, namely, residues Asp-111, Lys-139, Tyr-140, and Glu-142. Thus, the bound zinc stabilizes a structure that is essential for this protein-protein interaction.

A Predicted Structure for the Zinc Finger Domain

A question arises from the observations of the TFIIIA-like and other potential metal-binding sequences: Can these sequences be used to predict more detailed three-dimensional structures for the metal-binding domains? Recent analysis of the TFIIIA-like zinc finger sequences suggests that the answer may be "yes" for certain cases (Berg 1987).

As noted above, the TFIIIA-like repeats have the consensus sequence ([Phe,Tyr]-X-Cys-$[X]_{2or4}$-Cys-$[X]_3$-Phe)-($[X]_4$)-(X-Leu-$[X]_2$-His-$[X]_3$-His)-($[X]_5$). The sequence has been divided into four parts that will be discussed below. The first part of the sequence contains the two cysteines and two conserved aromatic residues. Two structurally characterized proteins have sequences of the isolated sequences of the form Cys-$(X)_{2or4}$-Cys that are involved in binding single metal ions: rubredoxin (Fe) (Watenpaugh et al. 1979) and aspartate transcarbamylase regulatory subunit (Zn) (Honzatko et al. 1982). Each of these proteins contains two such sites. Analysis of the structures of these metal-binding sequences revealed that the structures are quite conserved from one protein to another. The regions with sequences shown below are of particular interest:

Rubredoxin:
Tyr-4-Thr-Cys-Thr-Val-Cys-Gly-Tyr-Ile-**Tyr**

Aspartate transcarbamylase:
Leu-136-Lys-Cys-Lys-Tyr-Cys-Glu-Lys-Glu-**Phe**

In addition to the two cysteine residues, these sequences also have hydrophobic amino acids in the positions corresponding to the conserved hydrophobic residues from the TFIIIA-like sequences. Importantly, structures of these two regions are extremely similar. The α carbon atoms for these stretches of 10 residues may be superimposed with a rms deviation of 0.72 Å. The structures are antiparallel β sheets with two hydrogen bonds between the first and last residues and an additional hydrogen bond between the NH group of the first cysteine and the carbonyl group of the second residue past the second cysteine. A major factor contributing to the similarity of the Cys-$(X)_{2\ or\ 4}$-Cys structures is the presence of NH to cysteine sulfur hydrogen bonds (Adman et al. 1975). Bonds are formed between the cysteine sulfur of residue n and the NH group of residue $n + 2$. These bonds orient the peptide units in a way that places large constraints on the total conformation.

The histidine residues occur in regions with the form X-Leu-$(X)_2$-His-$(X)_3$-His. Three structurally characterized proteins have two metal-binding histidine residues separated by three residues: thermolysin (Zn) (Matthews et al. 1972), hemerythrin (Fe) (Stenkamp et al. 1982), and hemocyanin (Cu) (Gaykema et al. 1985). In each case, the region is α helical with the metal bound to the ϵ-nitrogens of the two histidines. The presence of an α helix in the zinc finger structure is supported by two additional observations. First, the conserved Leu residue is positioned such that it would lie on the same face of an α helix as the histidines. Second, secondary structure prediction methods averaged over 39 of the zinc finger sequences have been used to predict that the region X-Leu-$(X)_2$-His-$(X)_2$ is helical (Brown and Argos 1986).

The two substructures (the β sheet containing the cysteine residues and the α helix containing the histidines) can be combined around a tetrahedral metal ion and connected via a bend consisting of the four residues that lie between them. Only one arrangement (corresponding to one absolute configuration around the tetrahedral zinc ion) is possible due to the length of the bend region. This structure places the conserved leucine residue in position to neatly pack against the two conserved aromatic residues to form a small hydrophobic core. Two schematic views of the predicted structure are shown in Figure 2. Pairs of these structures would be connected by the remaining linker sequence. This sequence generally contains five residues with the sequence Thr-Gly-Glu-Lys-Pro occurring frequently. This region is predicted to be in a relatively extended conformation.

Fairall, Rhodes, and Klug proposed two models for the interaction between TFIIIA and the 5S RNA gene based on nuclease digestion and chemical protection experiments (Fairall et al. 1986). In model I TFIIIA wraps around the DNA following the major groove, whereas in model II the protein lies on one face of the DNA with alternate fingers lying in two different planes at an angle to one another. The two models differ in their structural requirements for the individual metal-

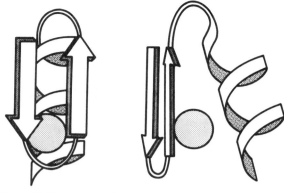

Figure 2. Two views of a proposed structure for the metal-binding domains from TFIIIA and related proteins (zinc finger domains). The structure has the form β-β-α with a zinc ion tetrahedrally coordinated by two cysteine and two histidine residues.

binding domains. In model II, the true repeat is two domains so that alternate domains contact the DNA through different faces, suggesting a symmetrical structure for the domain. In addition, this model suggests that the amino terminus and carboxyl terminus of the domain should exit from the same end of the finger. In contrast, each domain in model I interacts with the DNA in the same manner, and the amino and carboxyl termini should exit from opposite ends of the finger. The structure for the zinc finger domain developed clearly favors model I, with the protein lying largely in the major groove of the DNA (Berg 1987). A schematic view for the proposed protein-DNA complex is shown in Figure 3. It must be noted that the derived structure is based on the consensus sequence; variations from the consensus do occur and are probably crucial for the process of protein-nucleic acid recognition.

Structural and Potential Regulatory Roles of Metal-binding Domains

A final question remains about the occurrence of metal-binding domains in these nucleic-acid-binding

and gene-regulatory proteins: Why are metal ions involved at all? A structural role is evident but the particular characteristics of metal ion stabilization of a small domain need further elaboration. Consider the hypothetical folding pathway shown in Figure 4 using a TFIIIA-like peptide as an example. In the absence of metal ion the peptide exists as a random coil. There are insufficient stabilizing interactions in the folded state (hydrogen bonds, hydrophobic interactions, van der Waals interactions) to overcome the factors stabilizing the unfolded state (conformational entropy, interactions with solvent). Upon reaction with one equivalent of metal ion in aqueous solution, the metal-binding residues (in this case two cysteinates and two histidines) displace the six water molecules from the metal ion to form a peptide-metal ion complex, but it is assumed that no additional "folding" occurs. A major contribution driving this reaction is the entropy of release of the six water molecules from the metal ion. The enthalpy of the metal-binding process may be positive in that six metal-ligand bonds are broken and only four are formed (albeit with more tightly binding ligands). Finally, the peptide folds to assume its final conformation. This process will be driven by the stabilizing interactions noted above with the conformational entropy of the "unfolded" peptide-metal ion complex being significantly reduced by the cross-links involving the bound metal ion. Thus, metal ion stabilization of small domains (which are not expected to be folded in the absence of bound metal ion) is founded on two entropic contributions: the entropy of water molecules released from the aquo complex of the "free" metal ion and the reduced conformational entropy of the peptide with a metal ion bound to four side chains.

Do metal ions play any other roles in these proteins? One feature that many of the zinc finger proteins such as TFIIIA and *Krüppel* appear to have in common is

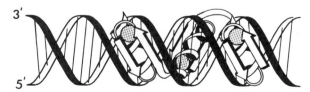

Figure 3. A model proposed for the interaction of a protein consisting of TFIIIA-like metal-binding domains and DNA based on the predicted structure for the individual domains. The α helix from each domain lies in the major groove of the DNA and makes sequence-specific contacts, whereas the β sheet lies further away from the DNA helical axis and makes contacts with the sugar-phosphate backbone. The linker region also lies in the major groove. This model is related to model I proposed by Fairall, Rhodes, and Klug (Fairall et al. 1986).

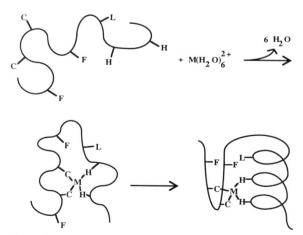

Figure 4. A hypothetical folding pathway for a TFIIIA-like peptide. The metal-free peptide exists as a random coil. This species binds a metal ion to form a relatively unfolded metal-peptide complex that then folds into its final conformation. This scheme is not intended to represent a real folding process but rather to illustrate some of the thermodynamic contributions to the stability of the final structure.

that they are involved in control of development. This suggests the possibility that zinc may be involved in developmental control in some manner. No direct information is yet available to support this hypothesis, but several additional observations allow the construction of one speculative scenario: (1) Free TFIIIA is quite sensitive to chelating agents (such as EDTA), losing its site-specific DNA-binding activity upon removal of zinc (Hanas et al. 1983); (2) TFIIIA bound to nucleic acids (at least 5S RNA) is less sensitive to such treatment (Hanas et al. 1983); and (3) metallothioneins, very cysteine-rich proteins involved in binding metal ions such as zinc and cadmium, are tightly regulated developmentally, with their expression being sensitive to the presence of steroid hormones and of certain metal ions. This tight regulation has suggested that these proteins have functions other than heavy-metal detoxification (Karin 1985). Early in development, metallothionein concentration is relatively low and free zinc concentration is expected to be relatively high. Thus, if free zinc finger proteins are produced, they bind zinc and are activated to bind their DNA target sites. Later, as metallothionein expression is elevated, the free zinc concentration should fall so that newly synthesized zinc finger proteins may not be activated, but existing zinc finger protein-nucleic acid complexes would be stable. Thus, the initial relatively high zinc concentration is reflected in the genome even after the free zinc concentration is reduced by increases in metallothionein concentration. Clearly, further chemical and biological studies are required to more completely elucidate the structural and functional roles of zinc in nucleic-acid-binding and gene-regulatory proteins.

ACKNOWLEDGMENTS

I thank the Camille and Henry Dreyfus Foundation and the National Institutes of Health for support of this work.

REFERENCES

Adman, E., K.D. Watenpaugh, and L.H. Jensen. 1975. NH—S hydrogen bonds in *Peptococcus aerogenes* ferredoxin, *Clostridium pasteurianum* rubredoxin, and *Chromatium* high potential iron protein. *Proc. Natl. Acad. Sci.* **72:** 4854.

Berg, J.M. 1986. Potential metal binding domains in nucleic acid binding proteins. *Science* **232:** 485.

———. 1987. A proposed structure for the zinc binding domains from transcription factor IIIA and related proteins. *Proc. Natl. Acad. Sci.* (in press).

Berk, A.J. 1986. Adenovirus promoters and E1A transactivation. *Annu. Rev. Genet.* **20:** 45.

Bieker, J.J. and R.G. Roeder. 1984. Physical properties and DNA-binding stoichiometry of a 5S gene-specific transcription factor. *J. Biol. Chem.* **259:** 6158.

Blakeley, R.L. and B. Zerner. 1984. Jack bean urease: The first nickel enzyme. *J. Mol. Catal.* **23:** 263.

Brown, R.S. and P. Argos. 1986. Fingers and helices. *Nature* **324:** 215.

Brown, R.S., C. Sander, and P. Argos. 1985. The primary structure of transcription factor TFIIIA has 12 consecutive repeats. *FEBS Lett.* **186:** 271.

Chowdhury, K., U. Deutsch, and P. Gruss. 1987. A multigene family encoding several "finger" structures is present and differentially active in mammalian genomes. *Cell* **48:** 771.

Coon, M.J. and R.E. White. 1980. Cytochrome P-450, a versatile catalyst in monooxygenation reactions. In *Metal ion activation of dioxygen* (ed. T.G. Spiro), p. 73. Wiley-Interscience, New York.

Darlix, J.-L.and P.-F. Spahr. 1982. Binding sites of viral protein P19 onto Rous sarcoma virus RNA and possible controls of viral functions. *J. Mol. Biol.* **160:** 147.

Davis, J., M. Scherer, W.P. Tsai, and C. Long. 1976. Low-molecular-weight, Rauscher leukemia virus protein with preferential binding for single-stranded RNA and DNA. *J. Virol.* **18:** 709.

Diakun, G.P., L. Fairall, and A. Klug. 1986. EXAFS study of the zinc-binding sites in the protein transcription factor IIIA. *Nature* **324:** 698.

Eickman, N.C., R.S. Himmelwright, and E.I. Solomon. 1979. Geometric and electronic structure of oxyhemocyanin: Spectral and chemical correlations to met apo., half met, met, and dimer active sites. *Proc. Natl. Acad. Sci.* **76:** 2094.

Fairall, L., D. Rhodes, and A. Klug. 1986. Mapping of the sites of protection on a 5S RNA gene by the *Xenopus* transcription factor IIIA: A model for the interaction. *J. Mol. Biol.* **192:** 577.

Frankel, A.D., J.M. Berg, and C.O. Pabo. 1987. Metal-dependent folding of a single zinc finger from transcription factor IIIA. *Proc. Natl. Acad. Sci.* **84:** 4841.

Gaykema, W.P.J., A. Volbeda, and W.G.J. Hol. 1985. Structure determination of *Panulirus interruptus* haemocyanin at 3.2 Å resolution. Successful phase extension by sixfold density averaging. *J. Mol. Biol.* **187:** 255.

Giedroc, D.P., K.M. Keating, K.R. Williams, W.H. Konigsberg, and J.E. Coleman. 1986. Gene *32* protein, the single-stranded DNA binding protein from bacteriophage T4, is a zinc metalloprotein. *Proc. Natl. Acad. Sci.* **83:** 8452.

Ginsberg, A.M., B.O. King, and R.G. Roeder. 1984. *Xenopus* 5S gene transcription factor, TFIIIA: Characterization of a cDNA clone and measurement of RNA levels throughout development. *Cell* **39:** 479.

Hanas, J.S., D.J. Hazuda, D.F. Bogenhagen, F.Y.-H. Wu, and C.-W. Wu. 1983. *Xenopus* transcription factor A requires zinc for binding to the 5S RNA gene. *J. Biol. Chem.* **258:** 14120.

Hartshorne, T.A., H. Blumberg, and E.T. Young. 1986. Sequence homology of the yeast regulatory protein ADR1 with *Xenopus* transcription factor IIIA. *Nature* **320:** 283.

Honzatko, R.B., J.L. Crawford, H.L. Monaco, J.E. Ladner, B.F.P. Edwards, D.R. Evans, S.G. Warren, D.C. Wiley, R.C. Ladner, and W.N. Lipscomb. 1982. Crystal and molecular structures of native and CTP-liganded aspartate carbamyltransferase from *Escherichia coli*. *J. Biol. Chem.* **160:** 219.

Karin, M. 1985. Metallothioneins: Proteins in search of function. *Cell* **41:** 9.

Lillie, J.W., M. Green, and M.R. Green. 1986. An adenovirus E1a protein region required for transformation and transcriptional repression. *Cell* **46:** 1043.

Matthews, B.W., J.N. Jansonius, P.M. Colman, B.P. Schoenborn, and D. Dupourque. 1972. Three-dimensional structure of thermolysin. *Nature* **238:** 37.

Méric, C. and P.-F. Spahr. 1986. Rous sarcoma virus nucleic acid-binding protein p12 is necessary for viral 70S RNA dimer formation and packaging. *J. Virol.* **60:** 450.

Méric, C., J.-L. Darlix, and P.-F. Spahr. 1984. It is Rous sarcoma virus protein P12 and not P19 that binds to Rous sarcoma virus RNA. *J. Mol. Biol.* **173:** 531.

Miller, J., A.D. McLachlan, and A. Klug. 1985. Repetitive zinc-binding domains in the protein transcription factor IIIA from *Xenopus* oocytes. *EMBO J.* **4:** 1609.

Nelbach, M.E., V.P. Pigiet, Jr., J.C. Gerhart, and H.K.

Schachman. 1972. A role for zinc in the quaternary structure of aspartate transcarbamylase from *Escherichia coli*. *Biochemistry* **11**: 315.

Pelham, H.R.B. and D.D. Brown. 1980. A specific transcription factor that can bind either the 5S RNA gene or 5S RNA. *Proc. Natl. Acad. Sci.* **77**: 4170.

Poulos, T.L., B.C. Finzel, I.C. Gunsalus, G.C. Wagner, and J. Kraut. 1985. The 2.6-Å crystal structure of *Pseudomonas putida* cytochrome P-450. *J. Biol. Chem.* **260**: 16122.

Rosenberg, U.B., S. Schröder, A. Preiss, A. Kienlin, S. Côté, I. Riede, and H. Jäckle. 1986. Structural homology of the product of the *Drosophila Krüppel* gene with *Xenopus* transcription factor IIIA. *Nature* **319**: 336.

Schuh, R., W. Aicher, U. Gaul, S. Côté, A. Preiss, D. Maier, E. Seifert, U. Nauber, C. Schröder, R. Kemler, and H. Jäckle. 1986. A conserved family of nuclear proteins containing structural elements of the finger protein encoded by *Krüppel,* a *Drosophila* segmentation gene. *Cell* **47**: 1025.

Schulein, M., W.N. Burnette, and J.T. August. 1978. Stoichiometry and specificity of binding of Rauscher oncovirus 10,000-dalton (p10) structural protein to nucleic acids. *J. Virol.* **26**: 54.

Seamon, K.B. and R.H. Kretsinger. 1983. Calcium-modulated proteins. In *Calcium in biology* (ed. T.G. Spiro), p. 1. Wiley-Interscience, New York.

Smith, B.J. and J.M. Bailey. 1979. The binding of an avian myeloblastosis virus basic 12,000 dalton protein to nucleic acids. *Nucleic Acids Res.* **7**: 2055.

Smith, D.R., I.J. Jackson, and D.D. Brown. 1984. Domains of the positive transcription factor specific for the *Xenopus* 5S RNA gene. *Cell* **37**: 645.

Stenkamp, R.E., L.C. Sieker, and L.H. Jensen. 1982. Restrained least-squares refinement of *Themiste dyscritum* methydroxohemerythrin at 2.0 angstroms resolution. *Acta Crystallogr. Sect. B Struct. Crystallogr. Cryst. Chem.* **38**: 784.

Tso, J.Y., D.J. Van Den Berg, and L.J. Korn. 1986. Structure of the gene for *Xenopus* transcription factor TFIIIA. *Nucleic Acids Res.* **14**: 2187.

Vallee, B.L., A. Galdes, D.S. Auld, and J.F. Riordan. 1983. Carboxypeptidase A. In *Zinc enzymes* (ed. T.G. Spiro), p. 25. Wiley-Interscience, New York.

Vincent, A., H.V. Colot, and M. Rosbash. 1985. Sequence and structure of the *serendipity* locus of *Drosophila melanogaster*: A densely transcribed region including a blastoderm-specific gene. *J. Mol. Biol.* **186**: 149.

Watenpaugh, K.D., L.C. Sieker, and L.H. Jensen. 1979. The structure of rubredoxin at 1.2 angstroms resolution. *J. Mol. Biol.* **131**: 509.

Wu, L., D.S.E. Rosser, M.C. Schmidt, and A.J. Berk. 1987. A TATA box implicated in E1A transcriptional activation of a simple adenovirus 2 promoter. *Nature* **326**: 512.

Lactobacillus leichmannii and Escherichia coli Ribonucleotide Reductases: Chemical and Structural Similarities

A.I. LIN, G.W. ASHLEY, AND J. STUBBE

Department of Biochemistry, University of Wisconsin, Madison, Wisconsin 53706

Ribonucleotide reductases are proteins required for de novo DNA biosynthesis that catalyze the conversion of nucleotides to deoxynucleotides (Eq. 1) (Reichard and Ehrenberg 1983).

The reductases isolated from *E. coli* (ribonucleoside diphosphate reductase, RDPR) and *L. leichmannii* (ribonucleoside triphosphate reductase, RTPR), the most intensely studied systems from a mechanistic point of view, share a number of common features (Ashley and Stubbe 1987). Substrate reduction (NDP, NTP) is accompanied by thiol oxidation. Replacement of the C–OH bond of substrate with the C–H bond of product occurs with retention of configuration, with the H being derived from solvent. In addition, there is a large solvent isotope effect on this reduction: 3.5 for RDPR, and 4.0 for the RTPR. Thioredoxin from *E. coli* is capable of reducing the protein disulfide of both RDPR and RTPR (Lammers and Follmann 1983).

Although the features described above suggest chemical similarities between these reductases, physical data indicate that these proteins are remarkably distinct. Structural studies of Thelander (1973) and the recent gene sequence (Carlson et al. 1984) show that the RDPR is composed of two nonequivalent subunits. Subunit B_1, $M_r = 175$ kD, is composed of two very similar polypeptides, and binds the NDP substrates and contains the redox active thiols. Subunit B_2, $M_r = 87$ kD, is composed of two equivalent polypeptides and contains one binuclear iron center (Fig. 1A, proposed structure) and one stable tyrosyl radical. The active site has been proposed to be at the interface of the two subunits, and a half site reactivity model has been proposed to accommodate the signal tyrosyl radical (Thelander and Reichard 1979).

On the other hand, RTPR uses NTPs as substrates. Blakley (1978) has shown that the protein is a single polypeptide chain, $M_r = 76$ kD, and that its cofactor is

coenzyme B_{12}, adenosylcobalamin (AdoCbl) (Fig. 1B). The AdoCbl · RTPR complex can undergo homolytic cleavage of the C–Co bond to produce Co(II), and presumably 5′-deoxyadenosyl radical, in a kinetically competent fashion (Tamao and Blakley 1973).

Our hypothesis for investigating the mechanism of both reduction reactions is that even though the proteins and their cofactors are structurally unique, the chemical aspects of the reduction might be quite similar. Both proteins contain a metal center stabilizing an organic radical, and hence radical involvement in these reduction reactions has been proposed.

A chemical model system has provided an excellent starting point for the investigation of radical mediated cleavage of a carbon hydroxyl bond and subsequent reduction (Eq. 2).

Studies of Walling and Johnson (1975) and Gilbert et al. (1972) indicate that to cleave the C–OH bond of ethylene glycol (analogous to the 2′,3′-*cis* diol of the nucleotide), a species resembling HO · mediates a hydrogen atom abstraction from the carbon adjacent to the bond being cleaved. When ethylene glycol is the substrate, cleavage of the C–OH bond requires acid catalysis to produce the cation radical intermediate. When chloroethanol is the substrate, loss of Cl⁻ requires no acid catalysis. In both cases, the radical cations undergo a number of subsequent reactions, one of which is a one-electron reduction and protonation to produce acetaldehyde.

This chemical model has served as the basis for thinking about the enzyme-catalyzed reduction reactions (Fig. 2). This mechanism proposes that a protein radical mediates hydrogen atom abstraction from the 3′ position of the nucleotide to produce **1**. The thiols proposed to be involved in the redox chemistry then might serve as a general acid catalyst to facilitate cleavage of a C–OH bond, producing a cation radical intermediate **2**. Subsequent reduction of this intermediate

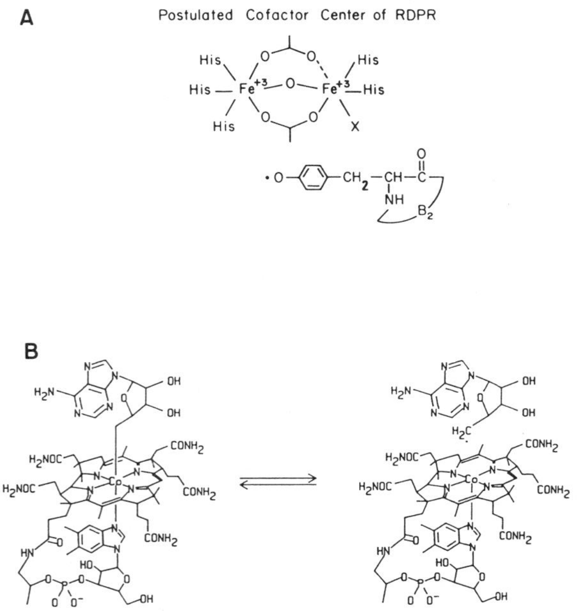

A

Postulated Cofactor Center of RDPR

B

Figure 1. (*A*) Proposed structure for the binuclear iron center and tyrosyl radical, the cofactor of *E. coli* ribonucleotide reductase. (*B*) Adenosylcobalamin, the cofactor of *L. leich-mannii* ribonucleotide reductase.

and return of the hydrogen atom from the protein residue to the 3' carbon would lead to product.

This proposal makes predictions that have been examined experimentally using both the RDPR and RTPR proteins. Using [3'-³H] and [3'-²H] nucleotides, primary isotope effects on both reductase reactions have been demonstrated. In addition, studies using [3'-²H] ribonucleotides and NMR spectroscopy have demonstrated that the hydrogen abstracted from the 3' position in the starting material is returned to the 3' position in the product. Even more intriguing is our recent demonstration with RTPR that the 5'-deoxyadenosyl radical, presumably produced from the observed homolytic cleavage of the C–Co bond of AdoCbl, is not the X· in Figure 2 (Ashley et al. 1986).

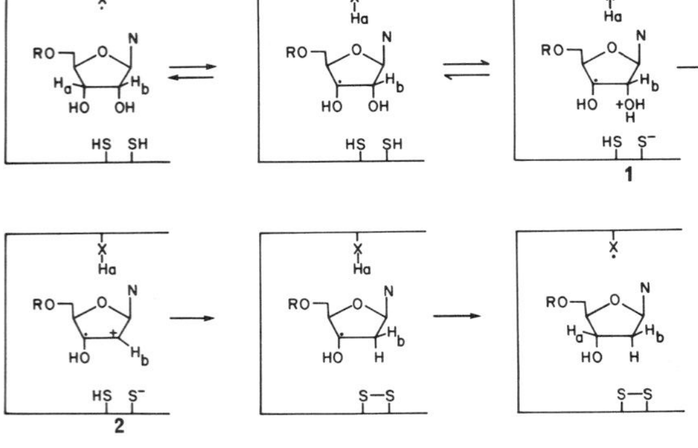

Figure 2. Proposed mechanism for reduction of nucleotides to deoxynucleotides catalyzed by ribonucleotide reductases. X· is an amino acid radical proposed to be involved in catalysis.

Instead, we propose that the 5'-deoxyadenosyl radical abstracts a hydrogen atom from a protein residue XH to produce protein radical X·, which mediates the chemistry. These studies with the normal substrate emphasize the amazing similarities in the catalytic capabilities of the *E. coli* and *L. leichmannii* reductases (Ashley and Stubbe 1987).

Finally, the interaction of both reductases with 2'-chloro-2'-deoxynucleotides (2'-chloro-2'-deoxynucleoside 5'-diphosphate, ClNDP; and 2'-chloro-2'-deoxynucleoside 5'-triphosphate, ClNTP) has been investigated in some detail. The 2'-chloro-2'-deoxynucleotides are potent inactivators of both enzymes. The similarities between the two systems are indicated in Equation 3.

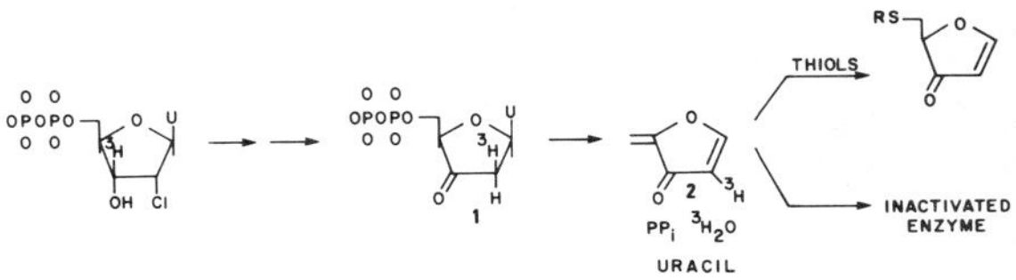

Both proteins catalyze cleavage of the 3' C–H bond as the initial step in the production of a 3'-keto-2'-deoxynucleotide. This unstable compound decomposes, probably nonenzymatically, to produce uracil, $PP_i(PPP_i)$ and 2-methylene-3(2H)-furanone; this furanone is responsible for enzyme inactivation. These results again emphasize the similar chemical capabilities of these structurally diverse proteins (Ashley and Stubbe 1987).

The present paper extends the initial studies with 2'-chloro-2'-nucleotides in an attempt to determine if the AdoCbl reductase mediates a stereospecific hydrogen shift from the 3' position of chloronucleotide to the 2' position of the 3'-keto-2'-deoxynucleotide, as has been recently shown with the *E. coli* reductase. In addition, an attempt has been made to identify the peptide sequence containing the redox active thiols involved in the *E. coli* reductase and the peptide modified by inactivation of *L. leichmannii* reductase by 2-methylene-3(2H)-furanone. Results from these studies again support the original hypothesis, that the enzymes are capable of similar catalytic transformations, and raise the intriguing possibility that there may be some structural similarities as well.

EXPERIMENTAL PROCEDURES

[3'-³H]ClUTP to [2'(proS)-³H]-3'-keto-dUTP catalyzed by RTPR. Details of these studies will be presented elsewhere (G.W. Ashley et al., in prep.).

Preparation of NaBH₄-reduced ClUTP-inactivated RTPR. Prereduced RTPR (116 nmol, 1.35 U/mg) was treated with [2'-³H]ClUTP (1500 nmol, 4.0×10^6 cpm/μmol) and AdoCbl (1500 nmol) in 1.5 ml of 0.3 M Tris-HCl, pH 7.4, 1 mM EDTA at 37°C. Reaction was initiated by addition of AdoCbl, and 50 μl aliquots of a 2.0 M solution of NaBH₄ in 10 mM NaOH were added at 0, 2, and 5 minutes. After an additional 10 minutes, the protein was isolated by gel filtration on a 1.4×20 cm column of Sephadex G-50 (0.3 M Tris-HCl, pH 8.3) and concentrated by centrifugal ultrafiltration (Centricon-30). The protein had a specific activity of 2.7×10^6 cpm/μmol, indicating binding of 0.65 ^{3}H per RTPR. RTPR activity assays indicated that the enzyme had lost 63% of its activity; thus, there was approximately 1.0 alkylation per RTPR molecule inactivated.

Trypsin digestion. The modified protein (106 nmol) was dissolved in 1.0 ml of 0.3 M Tris-HCl, pH 8.3, containing 4 mM EDTA, 30 mM dithiothreitol (DTT), and 6 M guanidine-HCl. After 30 minutes at 37°C, iodoacetamide (50 mg, 270 μmol) was added and the mixture was kept for 30 minutes in the dark. After addition of 30 μl of 2-mercaptoethanol, the solution was dialyzed against H_2O (2×500 ml) in the dark. Analysis of the dialysis fluid indicated a maximum loss of 5% of the radiolabel. The precipitated protein was collected by suspension in H_2O and lyophilized. The protein was redissolved in 300 μl of 0.10 M NH_4HCO_3, pH 8.2. A 0.40 mg portion of TPCK-Trypsin (1:20 w/w) was added and the mixture was kept at 37°C for 5 hours. The resulting peptide mixture was separated by high-performance liquid chromatography (HPLC) (Vydac C18 reversed-phase peptide column, H_2O/ CH_3CN [0–45% CH_3CN over 90 min] containing 0.1% CF_3COOH, flow rate 1.0 ml/min, detection at 220 nm). Fractions were collected manually every 1.0 minute, and 100 μl aliquots were analyzed for radioactivity by addition to 8 ml of scintillation cocktail (Eco-Scint) followed by liquid scintillation counting. The sole region of radioactivity (eluting between 21% and 23% CH_3CN) was pooled and evaporated. This region was rechromatographed on HPLC using a 10 mM NH_4OAc, pH 6.8/CH_3CN gradient (0–35% CH_3CN over 90 min). Again, a single region of radioactivity was observed, eluting between 14% and 17% CH_3CN. As several UV-absorbing peaks were observed in this region, however, the radioactive region was pooled, evaporated, and rechromatographed in the same system using a shallower gradient (10–13% CH_3CN over 30 min). This resulted in resolution of three closely migrating radiolabeled regions. The peptide corresponding to the first radioactive area could be purified by rechromatography using H_2O/CH_3CN, 0.1% CF_3COOH (10–20% CH_3CN over 30 min), which removed some contaminating peptides. The second and third radioactive regions have not been sufficiently purified to allow sequencing.

Sequencing of the peptide from the first radioactive region by automated Edman degradation gave the sequence: D-L-E-L-V-D-Q-T-D-*-E-G-G-A-*-P-I-K. Analysis of the cycles from the Edman degradation by liquid scintillation counting indicated radioactivity only in cycle 10.

Preparation of redox active thiol radioalkylated RDPR. Prereduced B_1 (40 nmol) was added to a reaction mixture containing 50 mM HEPES (pH 7.6), 15 mM $MgSO_4$, 1 mM EDTA, 0.25 mM dTTP, 4 nmol B_2 in a volume of 0.64 ml, which was degassed and equilibrated with argon. CDP (256 nmol) was added and the reaction mixture was incubated for 10 minutes. The protein was denatured in 6 M guanidine-HCl, 0.1 M Tris-HCl (pH 8.5), 15 mM $MgSO_4$, 1 mM EDTA, and alkylated with ICH_2CONH_2 (120 μmol) in a final volume of 3.2 ml for 3 hours in the dark. The protein was isolated by gel filtration on a 1.5×16 cm Sephadex G-50 column equilibrated in 0.1 M Tris-HCl (pH 8.0), 2 M guanidine-HCl and concentrated to 0.8 ml by centrifugal ultrafiltration (Centricon 30). The protein solution containing 37 nmol B_1 was treated with 610 μl of 0.1 M Tris (pH 8.0), 8.3 M guanidine-HCl. The mixture was evacuated and equilibrated with argon. DTT (592 nmol) was added and the reaction mixture was incubated for 30 minutes at room temperature. [1-^{14}C]ICH_2- $CONH_2$ (18.5 μmol [185 μl], specific activity = 1.93×10^6 cpm/μmol) was then added and the mixture was incubated for an additional 3 hours at room temperature in the dark. The protein was isolated by gel filtration (1.5×16 cm) and had a specific activity of 1.01×10^7 μmol (5.4 labels/B_1). Typical overall recovery of B_1 was 60%. A control experiment was run using an identical protocol to that described above except that the CDP was omitted. The protein isolated from the control experiment had a specific activity of 2.33×10^6 cpm/μmol (1.2 labels/B_1).

Trypsin digestion. The protein (15 nmol) was dialyzed against 4 l H_2O in the dark overnight. The precipitated protein was collected and lyophilized. After suspension in 1 ml of 0.1 M NH_4HCO_3, pH 8.0, TPCK-Trypsin (87.5 μg, 1:30 [w/w]) was added and the mixture was kept at 37°C for 24 hours. After several hours the solution became clear. The resulting peptide mixture was separated by HPLC (Vydac C18 reverse-phase peptide column, H_2O/CH_3CN [0–50% CH_3CN over 75 min] containing 0.1% CF_3COOH [solvent system A], flow rate 1.0 ml/min, detection at 220 nm). Fractions (1 ml) were collected manually, and 100 μl aliquots of each fraction were analyzed for radioactivity. Four regions of radioactivity (I, II[A], II[B], III) were pooled separately and evaporated.

Regions II(A) and II(B) were rechromatographed on HPLC using a 20 mM KPi (pH 7.2)/CH_3CN gradient (0–30% CH_3CN over 45 min) (solvent system B). In each case a single peak of radioactivity comigrated with a well-defined peak ($A_{220\ nm}$) and eluted at 13.5% CH_3CN for II(A) and 14.5% CH_3CN for II(B).

The peptides in region III were dissolved in 0.15 ml of 0.1 M NH_4HCO_3, pH 7.8, containing 2 mM EDTA. A 0.9 μg portion of *Staphylococcus aureus* V8 protease (1:30 [w/w]) was added and the mixture was kept at 37°C for 5 hours. The resulting peptide mixture was chromatographed using solvent system A. Four regions of radioactivity (eluting between 23% and 32% CH_3CN) were observed and pooled separately and evaporated. Regions III(A), III(B), and III(C) (containing 21%, 41%, and 24% of the total label, respectively) were rechromatographed separately by using solvent system B. In the case of III(A) and III(C), a single peak of radioactivity was observed, eluting at 19.5% CH_3CN (III[A]) and 21.5% CH_3CN (III[C]). A broad region of radioactivity was observed on rechromatography of III(B) (eluting between 20% and 21% CH_3CN).

Purified II(A), II(B), III(A), III(C), and the front region of III(B) (78% of III[B]) peptides were reinjected separately on HPLC using solvent system A and then sequenced.

RESULTS

RTPR can mediate a 3' to 2' hydrogen shift in the conversion of ClUTP to 3'-keto-dUTP.

Recent efforts by Ator and Stubbe (1985) have shown that E. coli RDPR catalyzes the stereospecific conversion of [3'-^{3}H]ClUDP to [2'(proS)-^{3}H]3'-keto-dUDP. A similar experiment is reported with RTPR using the protocol outlined in Figure 3. These studies are more complex than the studies with the E. coli reductase for two reasons. The first is that in approximately 1 out of every 200 turnovers, RTPR catalyzes the conversion of ClUTP to dUTP. Hence, dUTP can be produced by the normal enzymatic reduction process as well as by the $NaBH_4$ trapping of 3'-keto-dUTP. The second is that the E. coli RDPR is extensively protected by $NaBH_4$ from ClUDP inactivation, whereas the L. leichmannii reductase can only be protected for 12 turnovers prior to inactivation.

Incubation of ClUTP (specific activity 6.0×10^6 cpm/μmol) with RTPR in the presence of $NaBH_4$ results in the production of both xylo-dUTP and dUTP (specific activity 9.2×10^5 cpm/μmol). Both of these nucleotides have been subjected to chemical and enzymatic degradation processes to locate the ^{3}H label (G.W. Ashley et al., in prep.). Only the xylo-dUTP, whose sole mode of production is by $NaBH_4$ trapping, will be discussed. Location of the label was established using the protocol in Figure 3. The xylo-dUTP was treated with alkaline phosphatase and converted to 3'-xylo-2'-deoxyuridine. The 3' hydroxyl of xylo-2'-deoxyuridine was inverted using diethylazodicarboxylate/triphenylphosphine and benzoic acid, followed by hydrolysis of the benzoate esters. All of the ^{3}H was retained during this procedure. The [^{3}H]deoxyuridine was then treated with deoxyuridine hydroxylase to produce uridine, which retained 98.6% of its radiolabel. The 3'- and 5'-hydroxyls of the uridine were blocked and the 2'-OH oxidized to produce 3',5'O-(1,1,3,3-tetraisopropyldisiloxyl)2'-keto-uridine, which contained no radiolabel. Therefore, of the ^{3}H that is not exchanged with the media (15%) during the RTPR-catalyzed conversion of [3'-^{3}H]ClUTP to 3'-keto-dUTP, 98.6% is located in the 2'-proS position and 1.4% in the 2'-proR position of [2'-^{3}H]3'-keto-dUTP. Although the L. leichmannii reductase is clearly different from the E. coli reductase, both proteins are able to mediate stereospecific hydrogen shifts in the production of 3'-keto-2'-deoxynucleotides.

Isolation of a peptide radiolabeled by interaction of [2'-^{3}H]ClUTP with RTPR.

Inactivation of 116 nmol of RTPR with 1500 nmol of [2'-^{3}H]ClUTP in the presence of 65 mM $NaBH_4$ results in 63% inactivation and 0.65 equivalents of ^{3}H covalently bound per equivalent of RTPR. The $NaBH_4$ is essential to stabilize the radiolabel on the peptide(s). The inactive protein is denatured and alkylated with iodoacetamide, digested with trypsin, and analyzed by HPLC (Fig. 4A,B). Region I in Figure 4B, which accounts for ~30% of the labeled material, has been sequenced and analyzed by fast-atom bombardment-mass spectroscopy. The molecular weight of the peptide is 2010 and the sequence is D-L-E-L-V-D-Q-T-D-*-E-G-G-A-*-P-I-K, where * represents an unidentified amino acid residue. Recently, in an experiment to identify the redox active thiols analogous to that described subsequently with E. coli protein, both *s have been identified as cysteines.

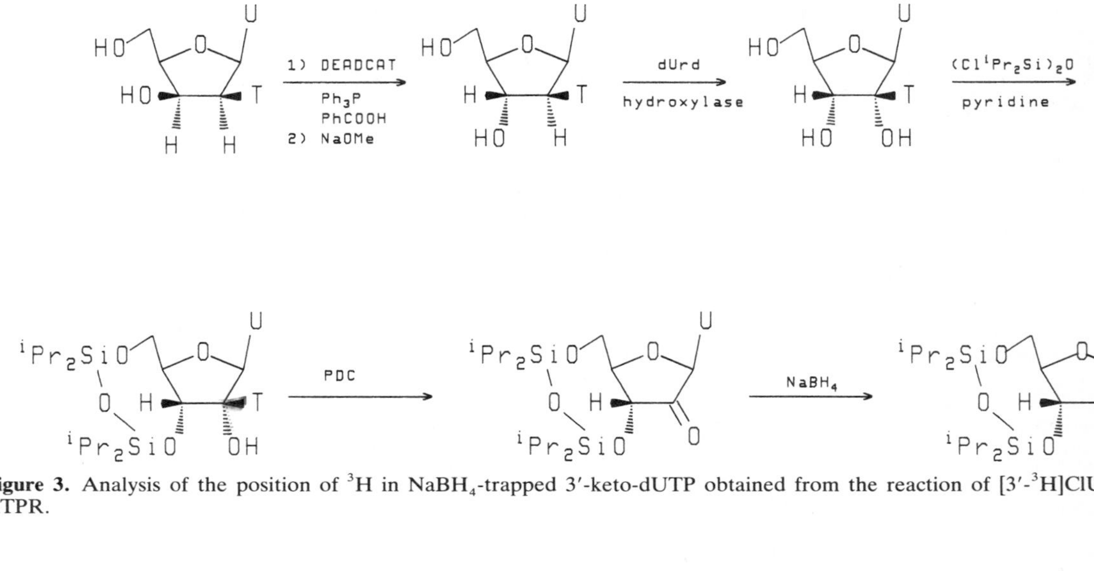

Figure 3. Analysis of the position of ^{3}H in $NaBH_4$-trapped 3'-keto-dUTP obtained from the reaction of [3'-^{3}H]ClUTP with RTPR.

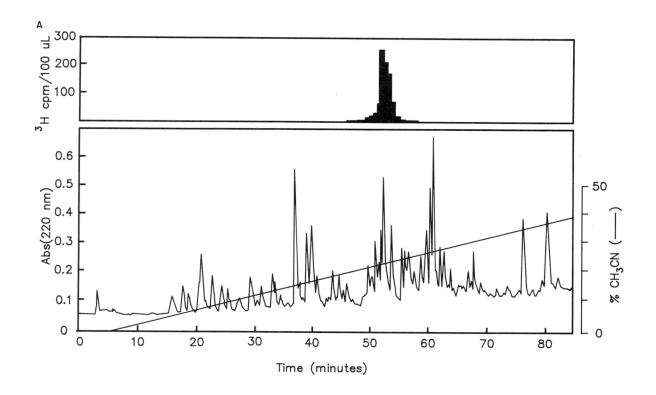

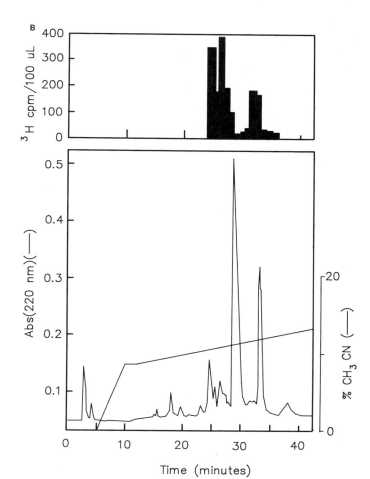

Figure 4. HPLC trace of the trypsin digest of radiolabeled RTPR. (*A*) Initial chromatography of digest using H_2O/CH_3CN containing 0.1% CF_3-CO_2H. Vertical bars represent ^3H cpm measured in 100 μl aliquots of fractions. (*B*) Rechromatography of radioactive region of initial digest using 10 mM NH_4OAc, pH 6.8/CH_3CN.

The observed molecular weight of the peptide is consistent with one cysteine being modified by a reduced 2-methylene-3(2H)-furanone derivative.

Identification of peptide(s) containing the redox active thiols of the B_1 subunit of E. coli RDPR.

The recently corrected gene sequence of the B_1 subunit of RDPR (J. Fuchs, pers. comm.) indicates that it contains 24 cysteine residues. The protocol used to isolate the thiols postulated to be involved in CDP reduction is indicated in Figure 5. RDPR was prereduced with 10–20 mM DTT for 20 minutes to 1 hour, and the reductant was then removed by Penefsky column. The RDPR was incubated with variable amounts of CDP for 10 minutes, and the protein was denatured in 6 M guanidine · HCl and alkylated with ICH_2CONH_2 in the dark under argon for 3 hours. A control experiment was run using an identical protocol except that the CDP was omitted. The ICH_2CONH_2 was removed by Sephadex G-50 chromatography and the protein was reduced with DTT and then alkylated with $[^{14}C]ICH_2$-$CONH_2$. The alkylated protein was then separated from the small molecules by gel filtration. The amount of radiolabeled B_1 in the experiment and control was determined, as was the amount of dCDP produced at the beginning and the end of the incubation of RDPR with CDP. The change in the amount of dCDP should reflect one-half the number of equivalents of thiols oxidized during this incubation period, and hence one-half the expected number of equivalents of iodoacetamide labels bound per B_1. The results of several experiments using catalytic amounts of B_2 are indicated in Table 1.

The number of dCDPs produced in a number of experiments using excess CDP varied from 2.5 to 3.6 depending on the ratio of $B_1:B_2$ and the concentration of RDPR. The amount of $[^{14}C]ICH_2CONH_2$ alkylation in the same experiments varied from 5 to 6 equivalents/equivalent of B_1. In the corresponding controls, however, 1.2–1.5 equivalent ICH_2CONH_2 labeling/equivalent of B_1 was always observed even though no spontaneous thiol oxidation occurred (Table 1).

To analyze the distribution of radiolabel on B_1, the alkylated protein was treated with trypsin and the resulting peptides analyzed by HPLC (Fig. 6A,B). Three broad regions of radioactivity are observed and have been designated I, II, and III in Figure 6A. The control experiment (Fig. 6B) has also been analyzed in a simi-

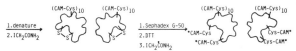

Figure 5. Analysis used to identify the redox active thiols of E. coli RDPR.

lar fashion and indicates distribution of label in the same three regions (Table 2). The amount of radioactivity in region I has always been almost identical in both experiment and controls, and therefore is not considered further. The distribution of label between regions II and III varies depending on the amount of CDP used to oxidize the redox active thiols (Table 2). With 0.5 equivalent of CDP the predominant radiolabeling is in region II, whereas with excess CDP a distribution of 53%:37% in II to III is routinely observed. Results from a number of additional experiments suggest that region II is labeled prior to region III.

Regions II and III have been pooled separately and subjected to further purification in an attempt to define the peptide(s) modified. Region II was subdivided into regions A and B (Fig. 6A), and in each case a single modified peptide has been isolated and sequenced:

Region II
A D_{734}-G-A-E-D-A-Q-D-D-L-V-P-S-I-Q-D-D-G-C-E-S-G-A-C-K$_{758}$
B D_{734}-G-A-E-D-A-Q-D-D-L-V-P-S-I-Q-D-D-G-C-E-S-G-A-C-K-I$_{759}$

Thus ~53% of alkylated peptides reside at the carboxy-terminal end of the B_1 gene.

Region III was less tractable, but when the entire region was pooled and retreated with SV-8 protease, ~70% of the label also can be accounted for in a single region of the protein:

Q_{218}-F-S-S-C-V-L-I-E-C-G-D-S-L-D-S-I-N-A-T-S-S-A-I-V-K$_{243}$

Table 1. Stoichiometry of ICH_2CONH_2 Alkylation and dCDP Production

		Equivalents dCDP/B_1			
Equivalents CDP[a]/B_1		0 min	10 min	diff.	Equivalents ICH_2CONH_2/B_1
Experiment	6.0	3.2	0.1	3.1	5.0
Control	6.0	3.1	3.1	0	1.5
Experiment	2.0	3.0	1.3	1.7	5.0
Control	2.0	2.9	2.9	0	1.5
Experiment	0.5	2.7	2.3	0.4	2.0
Control	0.5	2.8	2.8	0	1.4

[a]All experiments contained 20 nmol B_1 and 2 nmol B_2.

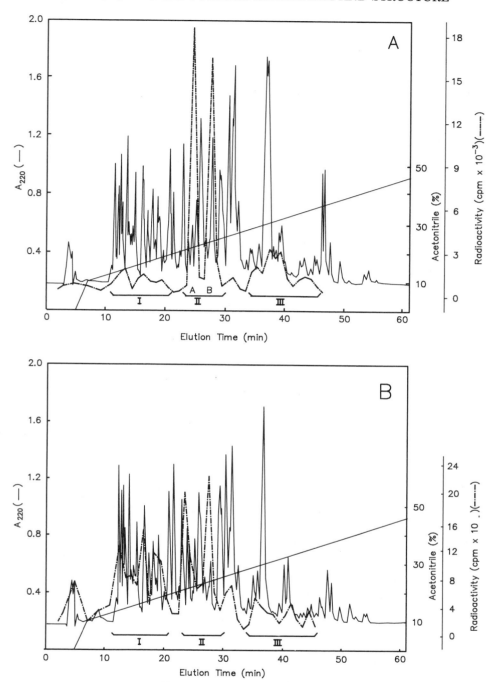

Figure 6. HPLC trace of the trypsin digest of [^{14}C]carboxamidomethylated RDPR prepared by the protocol outlined in Fig. 5: (A) Experiment. (B) Control in the absence of CDP as described in experimental procedures. Chromatography of digest using H$_2$O/CH$_3$CN containing 0.1% CF$_3$CO$_2$H.

The remaining 30% of the label in this region we have not yet been able to purify well enough to sequence. Intriguingly, region II of *E. coli* RDPR has a sequence that is remarkably similar to the peptide modified by 2-methylene-3(2H)-furanone in RTPR inactivation by ClUTP.

E. coli (region II) G-C-E-S-G-A-C-K-I
L. leichmannii D-C-E-G-G-A-C-P-I-K

DISCUSSION

Previous studies from our laboratory have demonstrated the amazing similarities in the catalytic capabilities of the *E. coli* and *L. leichmannii* reductases. Recently, detailed studies on the interaction of *E. coli* RDPR with [3'-^{3}H]ClUDP have revealed that 33% of the time the enzyme catalyzes transfer of its 3'-^{3}H stereospecifically to the 2'-proS position to produce 3'-keto-dUDP (Ator and Stubbe 1985), whereas 67%

Table 2. Distribution of Equivalents of $[^{14}C]ICH_2CONH_2$ in Regions I, II, and III from Figure 6, A and B

| | Equivalents ICH_2CONH_2 (% total labeling) Region | | |
	I	II	III
Excess $CDP/B_1{}^a$			
Experiment	0.55 (10)	2.84 (53)	2.0 (37)
Control	0.44 (34)	0.57 (45)	0.27 (21)
0.5 CDP/B_1			
Experiment	0.54 (28)	1.1 (55)	0.32 (17)
Control	0.54 (42)	0.53 (41)	0.22 (17)

^{a}Average of three different experiments.

of the time the $3'\text{-}^3H$ is transferred to solvent. Although similar studies with the $[3'\text{-}^3H]ClUTP$ and RTPR are more complex than those with RDPR, a similarity between the two systems has again been observed. The analysis shown in Figure 3 indicates that 1 out of 6.5 times the tritium from $[3'\text{-}^3H]ClUTP$ is transferred to the 2'-proS position of the resulting 3'-keto-dUTP.

In addition, since 1 equivalent of ClUTP appeared to cause extensive inactivation of RTPR, an attempt was made to isolate and sequence the radiolabeled peptide(s). Although it is tempting to speculate based on this stoichiometry that the modified peptide(s) may be at the active site of RTPR, no evidence exists supporting this premise. In fact, preliminary studies using $ICH_2\text{-}CONH_2$ in amounts stoichiometric with RTPR suggest that there are several groups on the protein that are activated toward nucleophilic attack and result in protein inactivation. However, the results obtained thus far are still suggestive. Thirty percent of the radiolabel is found attached to a peptide whose sequence is quite similar to the carboxy-terminal end of the RDPR B_1 subunit. As indicated below, we believe that this carboxy-terminal end contains thiols at the enzyme's active site and is involved in substrate reduction. Thus far we have been unable to purify the remaining 70% of the labeled RTPR peptide(s). In a variety of systems these peptide(s) have very similar chromatographic behavior. We believe that difficulties in purification may be related to heterogeneity of alkylation with $ICH_2\text{-}CONH_2$, incomplete trypsin digest, or diastereomeric mixtures of the furanone alkylated peptides. Since the sequence of *L. leichmannii* reductase is presently unknown, further purification of peptide(s) is required prior to sequence analysis.

An additional similarity between the *E. coli* RDPR and *L. leichmannii* RTPR is that subsequent to their inactivation by 2-methylene-3(2H)-furanone, a slow increase in absorbance on both proteins is observed at 320 nm. Extensive model studies (G.W. Ashley, unpubl.) indicate that a reasonable explanation for this absorption change is indicated in Equation 4.

PROPOSED STRUCTURE FOR 320 nm ABSORBANCE ON RTPR

Both the carboxy-terminal peptide of the *E. coli* B_1 subunit and peptide modified by 2-methylene-3(2H)-furanone of the *L. leichmannii* RTPR contain a lysine residue near the reactive cysteines. The significance of these observations awaits further investigation.

Attempts to identify the thiols involved in CDP reduction of *E. coli* RDPR met with a number of unexpected results. The first surprise, foreshadowed by early studies of Thelander in 1973, indicates that more than the expected one or two dCDPs are produced. (Only one dCDP would be expected if this protein exhibits half site reactivity. DTT was used to prereduce RDPR and was removed subsequent to the experiment by use of a Penefsky column. Although control experiments indicated no DTT remaining by this protocol, the appropriate control with B_1 and DTT cannot be done, due to the high concentration of thiols in B_1. If any DTT remains, the amount of dCDP produced would be greater than predicted from one turnover.) The second surprise is that more than one set of thiols are modified.

Although the results indicated in Table 1 and Figure 6, A and B, are reproducible, we also caution that they are still preliminary. The experiments are difficult and the observed heterogeneity could result from a number of considerations. First, the requirements for "total" prereduction of RDPR are not clear. Second, since B_1 contains 24 cysteines, quantitative alkylation with unlabeled iodoacetamide is difficult and perhaps accounts for radiolabeled B_1 in the control. All attempts to remove or decrease the 1.3 equivalents of radiolabel associated with B_1 from the control experiment have thus far failed. Third, incomplete trypsin digestion, as evidenced by studies with region IIA and IIB, can also result in heterogeneity.

With these problems in mind, we have developed the following model to account for these results (Fig. 7). This model indicates that there are two sets of redox active thiols per protomer. Previous reports of Thelander indicate no disulfides in B_1, hence, based on this model, prereduced B_1 should be able to accept 8 e⁻s in going from a fully oxidized to a fully reduced state. We postulate that the thiols located at the carboxy-terminal end of the gene are those directly involved in CDP reduction. This hypothesis is based on the observation that when prereduced B_1 is incubated with 0.5 equivalents of CDP, the carboxy-terminal region is alkylated first. In addition, the sequences of the B_1 gene from four different organisms have been reported (Sjöberg et al. 1985). All contain two cysteines in the carboxy-terminal region.

We postulate that the other set of thiols in the middle of the gene, Cys-222 and Cys-227, are involved in shuttling e⁻s between thioredoxin and the active site of RDPR. To account for the more than two dCDPs produced per B_1 subunit, one could invoke the possibility that two dCDPs are produced readily from one prereduced protomer, consistent with a half site's reactivity model, but that additional dCDPs could be produced subsequent to reorganization of the B_1 and B_2 subunits to reform active protein.

The variability in the number of equivalents of label on acetamide-modified B_1, the observation of one equivalent of label on the control, and the lack of 1:2 correspondence between the measured number of dCDPs produced with the alkylated cysteines make this interpretation tentative. (The possibility cannot be ruled out that the active site is composed of one cysteine from the carboxy-terminal end and one from the 222–227 region.) However, recent cloning and over-

expression of the B_1 subunit of reductase makes this hypothesis (Fig. 7) testable using site-directed mutagenesis. The function of both sets of thiols is amenable to biochemical assay.

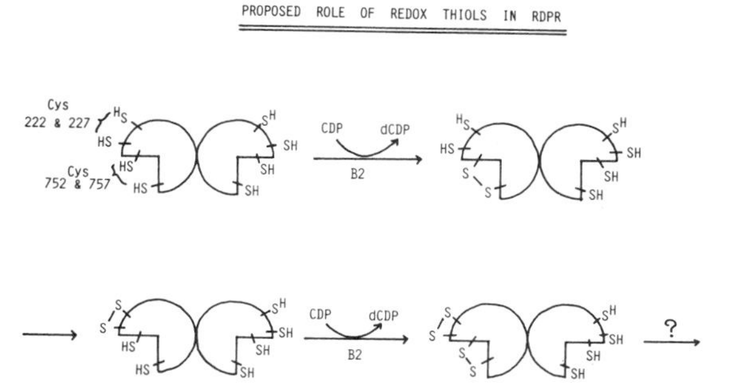

The unexpected result from the peptide studies discussed above is that a similar peptide has been obtained from both reductases. Whether this observation is coincidental or is implicating similar active site structures requires further experimentation. (Analogous experiments to those described with *E. coli* reductase to identify the redox with *L. leichmannii* reductase have recently been completed. The same peptide has been isolated as the one from the ClUTP inactivation experiment.) However, regardless of the conclusions from the peptide mapping, the ribonucleotide reductases from *E. coli* and *L. leichmannii* have been shown to be remarkably similar in a number of their catalytic capabilities.

ACKNOWLEDGMENTS

This research was supported by grant GM-29595 from the United States Public Health Service. G.W.A. is a National Institutes of Health postdoctoral fellow. We thank M. Ator and G. Harris, who provided the foundation on which these studies were built.

REFERENCES

Ashley, G.W. and J. Stubbe. 1987. Current ideas on the chemical mechanism of ribonucleotide reductases. *Pharmacol. Ther.* **30**: 301.

Ashley, G.W., G. Harris, and J. Stubbe. 1986. The mechanism of *Lactobacillus leichmannii* ribonucleotide reductase: Evidence for 3′-carbon-hydrogen bond cleavage and a unique role for coenzyme B_{12}. *J. Biol. Chem.* **261**: 3958.

Ator, M. and J. Stubbe. 1985. Mechanism of inactivation of *Escherichia coli* ribonucleotide reductase by 2′-chloro-2′-deoxyuridine 5′-diphosphate: Evidence for generation of a 2′-deoxy-3′-ketonucleotide via a net 1,2 hydrogen shift. *Biochemistry* **24**: 7214.

Blakley, R.L. 1978. Ribonucleotide triphosphate reductase from *Lactobacillus leichmannii*. *Methods Enzymol.* **L1**: 246.

Carlson, J., J.A. Fuchs, and J. Messing. 1984. Primary structure of the *Escherichia coli* ribonucleoside diphosphate reductase operon. *Proc. Natl. Acad. Sci.* **81**: 4294.

Gilbert, B.C., J.P. Larkin, and R.O.C. Norman. 1972. Electron spin resonance studies. Part XXXIII. Evidence for heterolytic and homolytic transformations of radicals from 1,2-diols and related compounds. *J. Chem. Soc. Perkin Trans.* **II**: 794.

Lammers, M. and H. Follmann. 1983. The ribonucleotide reductase—A unique group of metalloenzymes essential for cell proliferation. *Struct. Bonding* **54**: 27.

Reichard, P. and A. Ehrenberg. 1983. Ribonucleotide reductase—A radical enzyme. *Science* **221**: 514.

Sjöberg, B.M., H. Eklund, J.A. Fuchs, J. Carlson, N.W. Standart, J.V. Ruderman, S.J. Bray, and T. Hunt. 1985. Identification of the stable free tyrosine residue in ribonucleotide reductase. *FEBS Lett.* **183**: 99.

Tamao, Y. and R.L. Blakley. 1973. Direct spectrophotometric observation of an intermediate formed from deoxyadenosylcobalamin in ribonucleotide reduction. *Biochemistry* **12**: 24.

Thelander, L. 1973. Physicochemical characterization of

PROPOSED ROLE OF REDOX THIOLS IN RDPR

Figure 7. Proposed role for two sets of redox active thiols in RDPR: e⁻ acceptors from thioredoxin and direct participants in substrate reduction.

ribonucleotide diphosphate reductase from *Escherichia coli*. *J. Biol. Chem.* **248:** 4591.

Thelander, L. and P. Reichard. 1979. Reduction of ribonucleotides. *Annu. Rev. Biochem.* **48:** 133.

Walling, C. and R.A. Johnson. 1975. Fenton's reagent VI. Rearrangements during glycol oxidations. *J. Am. Chem. Soc.* **97:** 2405.

The Development of Enzyme Catalytic Efficiency: An Experimental Approach

J.D. HERMES, S.C. BLACKLOW, AND J.R. KNOWLES

Department of Chemistry, Harvard University, Cambridge, Massachusetts 02138

Enzymes are formidably efficient catalysts that mediate specific chemical transformations at rates rarely approached by even the best of man-made catalytic assemblies. From one angle, the challenge for the physical-organic chemist is to try to delineate the reaction mechanism and to understand the chemical and physical origins of the large rate enhancements that we observe. From a more biological viewpoint, however, the problem is to understand how, over evolutionary time, enzymes have become so effective. These two questions are related, of course, and if we could trace the development of catalytic efficiency, we should be better able to understand the nature of enzyme catalysis as we find it today. In this paper, we outline the first steps of an attempt to monitor the improvement in catalytic efficiency of an enzyme as its gene is mutagenized at random and more efficient catalysts are selected for.

Some years ago, following the determination of all the rate constants for the reaction catalyzed by triosephosphate isomerase, we suggested that this enzyme has reached the end of its development as a catalyst (Albery and Knowles 1976). When the rate data are presented together as a free-energy profile (Fig. 1), two features stand out. First, the transition state of highest free energy is that for the binding of the less stable substrate (i.e., the "on" rate for R-glyceraldehyde 3-phosphate), which has a rate constant of 4×10^8 M^{-1} s^{-1}. We suggested at that time (and have since confirmed by viscosity variation experiments) that the reaction is encounter-controlled. That is, the reaction in the thermodynamically downhill direction cannot be any faster (presuming only that the substrate and the enzyme are freely diffusing species). (The fact that substrate encounter rates for different enzymes vary over one or two orders of magnitude may reflect the differ-

ing contributions to the overall encounter rate of active-site size and shape, desolvation phenomena, and, for charged substrates, electric field effects. The latter have been nicely scrutinized for the case of superoxide dismutase by Klapper et al. [1986]. In any case, the dependence of the reaction rate on the encounter frequency is what is at issue here.) Second, when a standard state is chosen equal to the in vivo concentration of triosephosphates (a concentration must, of course, be specified, so that second-order and first-order rate constants can be represented in the same profile), the most stable ground state is that of free enzyme plus the more stable substrate (i.e., isomerase plus dihydroxyacetone phosphate [DHAP]). Any enzymic reaction having these two features cannot become a more efficient catalyst, provided that the reacting species diffuse freely and provided that the ambient substrate levels do not alter significantly. Neither destabilization of the intermediate states of the reaction nor stabilization of the reaction transition states (as distinct from those for substrate binding) can increase the overall rate of a reaction such as that illustrated in Figure 1: these states are already kinetically insignificant.

The Evolution to Catalytic Perfection

The characteristics of the free-energy profile for triosephosphate isomerase illustrated in Figure 1 led us to speculate on the sequence of events that could have produced, over evolutionary time, the energetics for a perfect catalyst. We suggested that an enzyme could show three different levels of discrimination in binding its substrates (Albery and Knowles 1976). At the lowest level, the enzyme could bind all bound species more or less tightly. In terms of Figure 2, the least sophisticated (and, we argued, the most facile) change in the enzyme could lead to the tighter binding of *all* the bound states (the substrate *s*, the transition state *ts*, and the product *p*) as a whole. If Figure 2A represents the primordial catalyst, the free-energy barrier could be lowered by such "uniform binding" of all the internal states. In the case of triosephosphate isomerase, for example, an improvement in the phosphate-binding site would result in the uniformly tighter binding of all bound species (substrate, intermediate, product, and reaction transition states). Such binding can, of course, be overdone, since if the internal states are bound *too* tightly, the enzyme becomes stuck in a free-energy well from which escape for another turnover is slow. The optimum condition (for an enzyme that maintains its substrates and

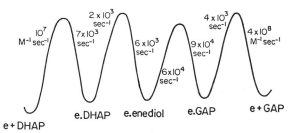

Figure 1. The free energy profile for wild-type triosephosphate isomerase from chicken muscle. (e) Enzyme; (DHAP) dihydroxyacetone phosphate; (GAP) R-glyceraldehyde 3-phosphate.

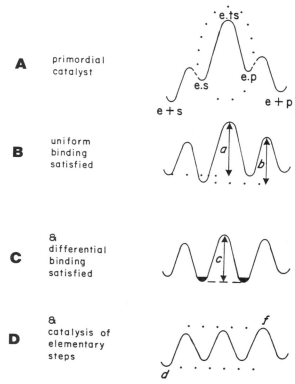

Figure 2. Free energy profiles illustrating the three types of binding energy. Uniform binding does not discriminate among *s*, *ts*, and *p*, and all the internal states (enclosed in the dotted oval) are bound more or less tightly to the enzyme. At the optimum, (*a*) = (*b*). Differential binding discriminates between *s* and *p*, and equalizes the internal thermodynamics so that the free energies of *e.s* and *e.p* are equal, resulting in a lower energy barrier (*c*). Finally, the enzyme discriminates between *s* and *ts*, and reduces the barrier (*c*). The lowest free-energy profile is that for a "perfect" enzyme, where in the downhill direction (right to left) the diffusive transition state (*f*) is the highest barrier, and in the uphill direction (left to right) no intermediate accumulates because at the ambient concentration of *s*, (*d*) has the lowest free energy.

products at equilibrium in vivo: i.e., for an enzyme that is not at a metabolic control point) will be as illustrated in Figure 2B, when the two free energies *a* and *b* are equal. Any movement of the internal states, by stronger or looser uniform binding, would be kinetically damaging, by increasing barrier *b* or barrier *a*, respectively.

Having satisfied the uniform binding condition, the enzyme could effect a more discriminating change that allows the differential binding of *p* rather than *s*. The optimum here, for reversible systems, occurs when the free energies of the two bound states *es* and *ep* are equal, as shown in Figure 2C. This optimum is derived from the presumption that elementary steps of enzyme-catalyzed reactions behave like single-step organic reactions, in that there exists a free-energy relationship between the overall free-energy change for a reaction, ΔG_o, and its activation free energy, $\Delta G^{\ddagger}$. Quantitative expressions of this relationship are found in the Brønsted and Hammett equations, and, qualitatively, in

Hammond's postulate. We argued that such differential binding, for which the enzyme must recognize the difference between *s* and *p*, would be less easy to achieve than uniform binding, and would normally follow the optimization of uniform binding. This idea, that the equilibrium constant for the *es* ⇌ *ep* equilibrium will be close to unity (and certainly nearer to one than the overall *s* ⇌ *p* equilibrium), has been supported by measurements on a number of enzyme systems that operate under reversible conditions in vivo (see Table 1). (We should emphasize that, as has been pointed out by others [Chin 1983; Ellington and Benner 1987], enzymes that are "off equilibrium" in vivo, e.g., the regulatory enzymes referred to above, are expected not to show equalized internal thermodynamics. In this paper, we are concerned with the majority of enzymes, which are simply the catalytic mediators of metabolic flux.) It is evident from the data in Table 1 that the free energies of such enzyme-bound substrates and products are matched, whether the overall equilibrium constant is very far from unity (as for the reactions catalyzed by myosin ATPase or tyrosyl-tRNA synthetase) or whether the overall equilibrium constant is quite close to unity anyway (as for the reaction catalyzed by enolase). Whether or not our explanation for the origins of differential binding is correct, the tendency for the equilibrium constant between enzyme-bound substrates and products to be close to one for reversible systems seems inescapable.

Having satisfied the differential binding condition illustrated in Figure 2C, what more can the enzyme achieve? The most discriminating binding interaction is one in which the enzyme preferentially interacts with a transition state rather than with the intermediate states that flank it. In terms of Figure 2C, the enzyme can

Table 1. Equilibrium Constants for Free (K_{eq}) and Enzyme-bound (K_{int}) Substrates[a]

Enzyme	K_{eq}	K_{int}	Reference
Tyrosyl-tRNA synthetase	3×10^{-7}	2.3	b
Methionyl-tRNA synthetase	3×10^{-7}	1.7	b, c
Isoleucyl-tRNA synthetase	3×10^{-7}	0.2	b, d
Phosphoglycerate kinase	3×10^{-4}	0.8	e
Creatine kinase	0.025	0.4	e, f
Arginine kinase	0.1	1.2	g, h
Adenylate kinase	0.4	1.6	i
Enolase	4.3	1.1	f, j
Phosphoglucomutase	17	2.5	k
Lactate dehydrogenase	3×10^4	4	l
Myosin ATPase	3×10^5	9	l

[a]This compilation only contains data for those enzymes (for which K_{int} has been studied) that are believed to operate in vivo under reversible conditions (i.e., to maintain their substrates at equilibrium). Not listed, therefore, are hexokinase,[m] pyruvate kinase,[n] fructose 1,6-bisphosphate,[o] and dihydrofolate reductase.[p]
[b]Wells and Fersht (1986). [c]Fayat et al. (1980). [d]Holler and Calvin (1972). [e]Nageswara Rao et al. (1978b). [f]J. Burbaum (unpubl. quench experiments). [g]Nageswara Rao et al. (1976). [h]Nageswara Rao and Cohn (1977). [i]Nageswara Rao et al. (1978a). [j]Brewer and Ellis (1983). [k]Ray and Long (1976). [l]Gutfreund and Trentham (1975). [m]Wilkinson and Rose (1979). [n]Nageswara Rao et al. (1979); Stackhouse et al. (1985). [o]Benkovic and deMaine (1982). [p]Fierke et al. (1987).

effect a further rate acceleration by binding *ts* in preference to *s* or *p*. This process results in the acceleration of an elementary step, and such preferential binding is what Haldane and Pauling proposed many decades ago (Haldane 1930; Pauling 1946). Within the formalism of Figure 2, this catalysis of an elementary step will take us from the situation illustrated in Figure 2C to the "perfect" enzyme shown in Figure 2D.

The sequence of events from Figure 2A to Figure 2D is, of course, entirely conjectural, and is based on a simple view of the statistical probabilities of the consequences of random changes in the amino acid sequence of an enzyme. The three kinds of binding interaction proposed do, however, embrace all possible effects on the relative free energies of intermediates and transition states in an enzyme-catalyzed reaction, and one of the purposes of this paper is to examine whether the existence of such a hierarchy of binding interactions is susceptible to experimental test. One approach would be to look for enzyme fossils, and to see if there exist today, in different ecological niches, examples of both more and less highly evolved enzymes. Thus, in the case of triosephosphate isomerase, for which we know that the enzyme from chicken breast muscle is perfect (Figs. 1, 2D), can we find sources of less highly evolved enzymes that have energetics that are in the class of systems illustrated by Figure 2C or Figure 2B? The answer to this question is "no." When one looks at the specific catalytic activity of the triosephosphate isomerases from cows, chickens, human erythrocytes, *Bacilli*, algae, coelancanth, *Dissostichus* (an ice fish), and (even) archebacteria, they are all the same within experimental error (Hermes et al. 1987). That is, any isomerase that we now isolate from a natural source appears to be perfect, and there are no functioning fossils. We can, however, make what might be called a pseudo-fossil.

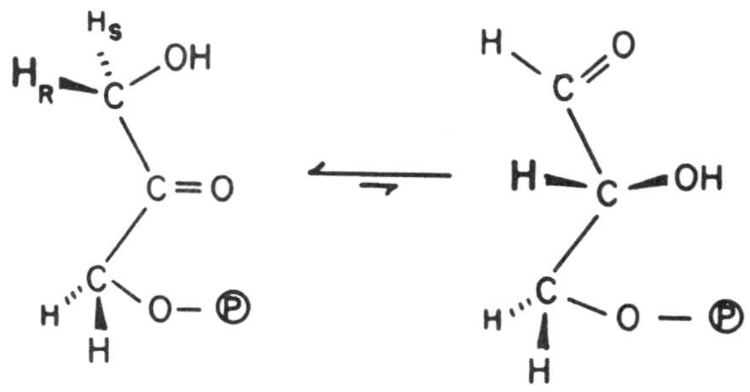

The Generation of Sluggish Isomerases by Site-directed Mutagenesis

Any structural alteration that one makes in a perfect catalyst must, by definition, either have no catalytic effect or have an adverse consequence. As part of an investigation of the structure : function relationships in triosephosphate isomerase, we have changed several of the amino acid residues that are in the active site of the enzyme and that are believed to participate directly in the catalyzed reaction (Fig. 3). For example, Glu-165, the residue that is believed to act as the catalytic base that abstracts either the pro-*R* proton from C-1 of dihydroxyacetone phosphate or the C-2 proton of *R*-glyceraldehyde 3-phosphate, has been changed to Asp (Straus et al. 1985). The mutant enzyme (a mutant of the chicken enzyme expressed in a strain of *Escherichia coli* from which the endogenous isomerase gene has been excised) is about 500 times less active than the wild type (see Table 2) (Raines et al. 1986). Analogously, a mutant in which His-95, a residue that is well positioned to act as a general acid catalyst in the enoli-

Figure 3. The reaction catalyzed by triosephosphate isomerase.

zation, has been changed to Asn, is about 1500 times less active than the wild-type enzyme. These two sluggish mutants are clearly imperfect catalysts, and as such should be susceptible to evolutionary improvement. We do not for a moment suggest that either of them was an actual intermediate state in primordial time in the development of the perfect isomerase that now exists, but each of them can be used as a starting point in a study of the improvement in enzyme efficiency brought about by random mutagenesis of the gene. This effort to trace the forward evolution of an enzyme is being made as described below.

Forward Evolution by Random Mutagenesis

First, the gene for a slow isomerase mutant is subjected to random mutagenesis using several of the chemical reagents (e.g., nitrous acid, formic acid, and hydrazine) evaluated by Myers et al. (1985). Each DNA strand is mutagenized independently, and the product DNA is inserted back into a plasmid vector such that only changes in the isomerase structural gene will be found. (In the search for more efficient isomerases, we want to avoid selecting for "promoter-up" mutants or other genetic alterations that result in a higher level of expression of the starting enzyme.) Transformants that produce the same levels of a more efficient isomerase are now selected for. Fortunately, a powerful selection can be devised. The host strain of *E. coli* used in our experiments is DF502, which is isomerase-minus. This strain grows on glucose (which, as illustrated in Fig. 4, provides both of the triosephosphates) or on a mixture of glycerol (which is two metabolic steps from dihydroxyacetone phosphate) *plus* lac-

Table 2. Catalytic Activity of Triosephosphate Isomerases

Enzyme	Amino acid at position			Relative catalytic activity
	165	95	96	
Wild type	Glu	His	Ser	100
Mutant E165D	Asp	His	Ser	0.23
Pseudorevertant from E165D	Asp	His	Pro	5.4
Mutant H95N	Glu	Asn	Ser	0.070
Pseudorevertant from H95N	Glu	Asn	Pro	3.8
Mutant S96P	Glu	His	Pro	9.3

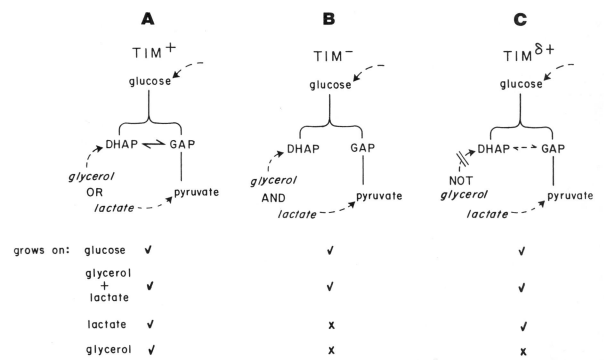

Figure 4. Growth patterns of: (*A*) a wild-type *E. coli* strain that produces normal levels of triosephosphate isomerase; (*B*) DF502, a strain of *E. coli* from which the endogenous isomerase gene has been excised; (*C*) DF502 transformed with a plasmid encoding a sluggish isomerase (that produces less than 75 pico-units/cell).

tate (which is six metabolic steps from *R*-glyceral-dehyde 3-phosphate). The host strain will *not* grow on either glycerol alone or lactate alone, since in the absence of triosephosphate isomerase only one of the two triosephosphates can be produced. Now, in a transformant where the plasmid carries the gene for a sluggish mutant isomerase (e.g., either E165D or H95N: see Table 2), we found that slow growth on lactate alone occurred, but *no* growth on glycerol alone could be seen. Herein lies the selection, since a transformant containing a sluggish isomerase (that drives the production of less than 75 pico-units of enzyme per cell) will not survive on glycerol alone, whereas a transformant containing wild-type isomerase (that produces about 85,000 pico-units of enzyme per cell) grows well. We therefore selected the transformants that derive from random mutagenesis of the isomerase gene for growth on glycerol alone. In passing, one may be curious about the biochemical basis of this selection. In the absence of any experimental results that bear on the issue, we speculate that a transformant containing only low amounts of isomerase activity will, when grown on glycerol alone, accumulate unusual amounts of di-hydroxyacetone phosphate. This metabolite can decompose nonenzymatically to the toxic material methylglyoxal, which kills the cell (Cooper 1984). The longer (and thermodynamically more uphill) route from lactate to glyceraldehyde phosphate (which also decomposes to methylglyoxal) would be expected to result in a much lower accumulation of this triosephosphate in cells grown on lactate alone. Whatever the molecular basis for the selection, however, its existence allows the

search for second-site suppressor mutants of the two isomerases E165D and H95N to be conducted.

As is evident from Table 2, a second-site suppressor mutant has been found from each of the sluggish isomerases. In the case of mutant E165D, a second-site change of Ser-96 to Pro yielded a pseudorevertant that is 25 times more active. Curiously, from the other sluggish mutant H95N, the *same* second-site change of Ser-96 to Pro was found to increase the catalytic activity 50-fold. At first sight it is remarkable that two such different changes at the active site of triosephosphate isomerase, one (E165D) that moved the carboxylate base and one (H95N) that altered a putative general acid, should *each* be compensated for by the same (S96P) second-site mutation. A relatively trivial explanation for this finding would be that the chemical mutagens used have found a "hot spot" in the gene. This would suggest that there are many ways to suppress the E165D and H95N mutations by changes at second sites, and that we have simply found the one that is most accessible to chemical mutagens. To test this possibility, we have reembarked on the search for second-site suppressors using the "impure oligonucleotide primer" approach, which should allow a search for pseudorevertants that is more nearly random. A second possibility to explain the fact that S96P partially suppresses both of the initially deleterious mutations, E165D and H95N, is that the S96P change always makes a better catalyst and is independent of other alterations, and the only reason that it is not already part of the wild-type enzyme is because the chemical steps of the wild-type isomerase are no longer under selective pressure (see Fig. 1). This argument has, however, no validity: when the S96P change is effected in the wild type, catalytic efficiency is lost, down to a level comparable with that of the two pseudorevertants (see Table 2). It is clear, then, that the two pseudorevertants represent different cooperative changes that in each case partially compensate for the initial reduction in catalytic power. Although in the absence of high-resolution structural information on these mutant isomerases it is unwise to attempt to understand their catalytic properties in structural terms, a glance at the structure of the native enzyme (Fig. 5) shows the proximity of Ser-96 both to Glu-165 and to His-95. We should not be surprised by the existence of nonadditive catalytic effects when neighboring active-site residues are changed.

Whatever the detailed relationships between structure and function turn out to be, we can start to define the nature of the catalytic changes that are evident in the two pseudorevertants described in Table 2. If the catalyzed reaction is conflated into three steps—substrate binding, catalytic conversion to product, and product release—the reaction energetics of the wild type, the E165D mutant, and the E165D, S96P pseudorevertant can all be presented as shown in Figure 6. First, we see that the E165D mutation has had but little effect on substrate or product binding (i.e., on the free energies of e · DHAP and e · GAP: see Fig. 6); the main consequence is a decreased transition-state stability that results in the mutant being some 500-fold less effective than the wild type. In the pseudorevertant, catalytic efficiency has improved primarily by virtue of a change in uniform binding. That is, all the bound states (substrate, transition state, and product) interact with the enzyme somewhat more strongly, resulting in a catalyst with an almost unchanged k_{cat}, but with a second-order rate constant (k_{cat}/K_m) that is some 25-fold higher than the mutant from which it

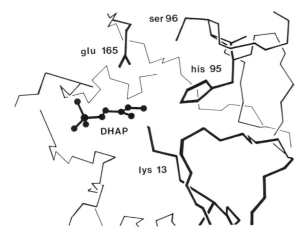

Figure 5. The active site of triosephosphate isomerase. The model is built from the coordinates of the native chicken enzyme (Banner et al. 1975), and the substrate dihydroxyacetone phosphate (DHAP) has been positioned on the basis of the sulfate (phosphate) binding site and a *cis*-enediol intermediate, minimizing nonbonding contacts with the protein.

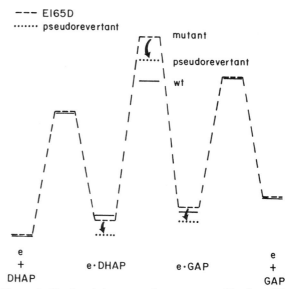

Figure 6. Conflated three-step free-energy profiles for wild-type triosephosphate isomerase (—), the mutant E165D enzyme (– – –), and the derived pseudorevertant E65D, S96P (· · · ·).

derives. Tempting as it might be to suggest that this first pseudorevertant proves that uniform binding is indeed (as our theory suggests) the most facile and most probable functional improvement in catalytic efficiency, the pseudorevertant from the other sluggish isomerase mutant, H95N, shows that this conclusion is premature, if not unwarranted. In Figure 7, the energetic changes for this second case are illustrated. Once again, the chosen mutation (H95N) barely affects the free energies of the enzyme-bound intermediates, and essentially all the 1500-fold reduction in catalytic rate lies in a higher transition-state free energy. In this case, however, the pseudorevertant *only* involves the transition state, and both k_{cat} and k_{cat}/K_m rise together (see Fig. 7).

It is clear from the aforementioned that we have only taken the first, tentative steps toward an understanding of the development of the catalytic efficiency of an enzyme. Before any claims can be made about the relative probability of different interactions between the enzyme and substrate, transition state, and product, a reasonable variety of pseudorevertants will have to be generated and evaluated. Before we can have any real understanding of the relationships between different amino acid changes and their catalytic consequences, a precise knowledge of the detailed three-dimensional structure of the mutants and of their pseudorevertants will be required. Finally, before any estimate can be made of the structural uniqueness of the enzymes that we find around us, and before we can begin to assess how many different constellations of active-site amino acids would lead to catalysts of an effectiveness equal to wild type, more artificial evolutionary "steps" will have to be taken. We hope, however, that these approaches may lead to some illumination of the path that has produced, in Nature, enzymes of such formidable catalytic power.

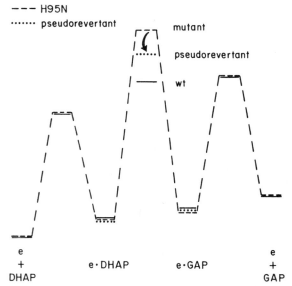

Figure 7. Conflated three-step free-energy profiles for wild-type triosephosphate isomerase (—), the mutant H95N enzyme (– – –), and the derived pseudorevertant H95N, S96P (· · · ·).

ACKNOWLEDGMENTS

This work was supported by the National Institutes of Health and by Merck, Sharp and Dohme.

REFERENCES

Albery, W.J. and J.R. Knowles. 1976. Evolution of enzyme function and the development of catalytic efficiency. *Biochemistry* 15: 5631.

Banner, D.W., A.C. Bloomer, G.A. Petsko, D.C. Phillips, C.I. Pogson, I.A. Wilson, P.H. Corran, A.J. Furth, J.D. Milman, R.E. Offord, J.D. Priddle, and S.G. Waley. 1975. Structure of chicken triosephosphate isomerase determined crystallographically at 2.5 Å resolution using amino acid sequence data. *Nature* 255: 609.

Benkovic, S.J. and M.M. deMaine. 1982. Mechanism of action of fructose 1,6-bisphosphatase. *Adv. Enzymol.* 53: 45.

Brewer, J.M. and P.D. Ellis. 1983. ^{31}P NMR studies of the effect of various metals on substrate binding to yeast enolase. *J. Inorg. Biochem.* 18: 71.

Chin, J. 1983. Perfect enzymes: Is the equilibrium constant between the enzyme's bound species unity? *J. Am. Chem. Soc.* 105: 6502.

Cooper, R.A. 1984. Metabolism of methylglyoxal in microorganisms. *Annu. Rev. Microbiol.* 38: 49.

Ellington, A.D. and S.A. Benner. 1987. The thermodynamic details of enzyme catalysis. *J. Theor. Biol.* 127: 491.

Fayat, G., S. Blanquet, B.D. Nageswara Rao, and M. Cohn. 1980. ^{31}P NMR of the reversible methionine activation reaction catalyzed by methionyl-tRNA synthetase of *Escherichia coli. J. Biol. Chem.* 255: 8164.

Fierke, C.A., K.A. Johnson, and S.J. Benkovic. 1987. Construction and evaluation of the kinetic scheme associated with dihydrofolate reductase from *Escherichia coli. Biochemistry* 26: 4085.

Gutfreund, H. and D.R. Trentham. 1975. Energy changes during the formation and interconversion of enzyme-substrate complexes. *Ciba Found. Symp.* 31: 69.

Haldane, J.B.S. 1930. *Enzymes.* Longmans, Green and Co., London.

Hermes, J.D., S.C. Blacklow, K.A. Gallo, A.J. Bauer, and J.R. Knowles. 1987. The evolution of enzyme function. *UCLA Symp. Mol. Cell. Biol.* 69: (in press).

Holler, E. and M. Calvin. 1972. Isoleucyl transfer ribonucleic acid synthetase of *Escherichia coli* B. A rapid kinetic investigation of the L-isoleucine activating reaction. *Biochemistry* 20: 3741.

Klapper, I., R. Hagstrom, R. Fine, K. Sharp, and B. Honig. 1986. Focussing of electric fields in the active site of Cu-Zn superoxide dismutase: Effects of ionic strength and amino-acid modification. *Proteins* 1: 47.

Myers, R.M., L.S. Lerman, and T. Maniatis. 1985. A general method for saturation mutagenesis of cloned DNA fragments. *Science* 229: 242.

Nageswara Rao, B.D. and M. Cohn. 1977. ^{31}P Nuclear magnetic resonance of bound substrates of arginine kinase reaction. *J. Biol. Chem.* 252: 3344.

Nageswara Rao, B.D., D.H. Buttlaire, and M. Cohn. 1976. ^{31}P NMR studies of the arginine kinase reaction. *J. Biol. Chem.* 251: 6981.

Nageswara Rao, B.D., M. Cohn, and L. Noda. 1978a. Differentiation of nucleotide binding sites and role of metal ion in the adenylate kinase reaction by ^{31}P NMR. *J. Biol. Chem.* 253: 1149.

Nageswara Rao, B.D., M. Cohn, and R.K. Scopes. 1978b. ^{31}P NMR study of bound reactants and products of yeast 3-phosphoglycerate kinase at equilibrium and the effect of sulfate ion. *J. Biol. Chem.* 235: 8056.

Nageswara Rao, B.D., F.J. Kayne, and M. Cohn. 1979. ^{31}P NMR studies of enzyme-bound substrates of rabbit muscle pyruvate kinase. *J. Biol. Chem.* 254: 2689.

Pauling, L. 1946. Molecular architecture and biological reactions. *Chem. Eng. News* 24: 1375.

Raines, R.T., E.L. Sutton, D.R. Straus, W. Gilbert, and J.R. Knowles. 1986. Reaction energetics of a mutant triosephosphate isomerase in which the active-site glutamate has been changed to aspartate. *Biochemistry* 25: 7142.

Ray, W.J. and J.W. Long. 1976. Thermodynamics and mechanism of the PO$_3$ transfer process in the phosphoglucomutase reaction. *Biochemistry* 15: 3993.

Stackhouse, J., K.P. Nambiar, J.J. Burbaum, D.M. Stauffer, and S.A. Benner. 1985. Dynamic transduction of energy and internal equilibria in enzymes: A reexamination of pyruvate kinase. *J. Am. Chem. Soc.* 107: 2757.

Straus, D., R. Raines, E. Kawashima, J.R. Knowles, and W. Gilbert. 1985. Active site of triosephosphate isomerase: *In vitro* mutagenesis and characterization of an altered enzyme. *Proc. Natl. Acad. Sci.* 82: 2772.

Wells, T.N.C. and A.R. Fersht. 1986. Use of binding energy in catalysis analyzed by mutagenesis of the tyrosyl-tRNA synthetase. *Biochemistry* 25: 1881.

Wilkinson, K.D. and I.A. Rose. 1979. Isotope trapping studies of yeast hexokinase during steady-state catalysis. *J. Biol. Chem.* 254: 12567.

Crystallography and Site-directed Mutagenesis of Yeast Triosephosphate Isomerase: What Can We Learn about Catalysis from a "Simple" Enzyme?

T.C. ALBER,* R.C. DAVENPORT, JR.,[†] D.A. GIAMMONA,[‡]
E. LOLIS, G.A. PETSKO, AND D. RINGE
Department of Chemistry, Massachusetts Institute of Technology, Cambridge, Massachusetts 02139

If there is any hope of completely understanding the catalytic action of any enzyme, surely the best candidate for the protein is triosephosphate isomerase (TIM). (Following a convention initially established by Knowles's and Phillips's groups at Oxford, we use TIM as an abbreviation for the enzyme and TPI to represent its gene.) This enzyme catalyzes the simplest reaction in all of metabolic biochemistry, the interconversion of the 3-carbon triosephosphates dihydroxyacetone phosphate (DHAP) and D-glyceraldehyde-3-phosphate (D-GAP). The reaction is just the transfer of a proton, the pro-R hydrogen from carbon 1 of DHAP, stereospecifically to carbon 2 to form the D-isomer of GAP (Fig. 1). Isomerization of these two sugar phosphates, which are the products of the aldolase-catalyzed degradation of fructose 1-6 biphosphate, provides the net gain of ATP that makes glycolysis an efficient energy-producing pathway. Since only D-GAP is utilized by glycolysis, TIM ensures that those carbon atoms from glucose that end up in DHAP are converted to GAP and funneled down to pyruvate, with concomitant production of ATP.

Although the equilibrium constant on the enzyme is not known, K_{eq} for the overall reaction is 300 to 1 in favor of DHAP. The large magnitude of this number arises from the combination of an apparent K_{eq} of 22 with a hydration equilibrium of 29 for the hydrated and unhydrated forms of D-GAP (Trentham et al. 1969); only the unhydrated forms of the triosephosphates are substrates for or even bind to the isomerase (Webb et al. 1977). The enzyme is highly specific. Free triose sugars do not bind to the enzyme; a phosphate group is required. Dihydroxyacetone sulfate is not a substrate, and α-glycerol phosphate is a competitive inhibitor (Wolfenden 1969).

The simplicity of the TIM reaction allowed Albery and Knowles and their co-workers to determine, by means of an elegant series of isotopic labeling experiments, the complete free energy profile of the catalytic process (summarized in Albery and Knowles 1976a).

These data showed that the highest free energy transition state was that for the diffusion-limited bimolecular association of GAP with the enzyme. Looked at in reverse, if DHAP is given as substrate, the rate-limiting step is product release.

Albery and Knowles further argued, on the basis of the free energy profile, that TIM had reached evolutionary perfection as a catalyst (for details, see Albery and Knowles 1976b, and the article by Hermes et al., this volume). For our purposes, the availability of the complete free energy profile for the TIM-catalyzed reaction meant that the mechanism could be understood in great detail. In particular, if a mutant was made by site-directed mutagenesis that produced an interesting effect on catalysis, the free energy profile of that mutant could be determined, and the specific microscopic step(s) that were altered by the mutation could be identified (for an example, see Hermes et al., this volume).

TIM is a very good catalyst. Richard (1984) has determined that the enzyme accelerates the rate of GAP to DHAP isomerization by almost 10 orders of magnitude over the rate enhancement provided by a simple base catalyst such as the acetate ion. Moreover,

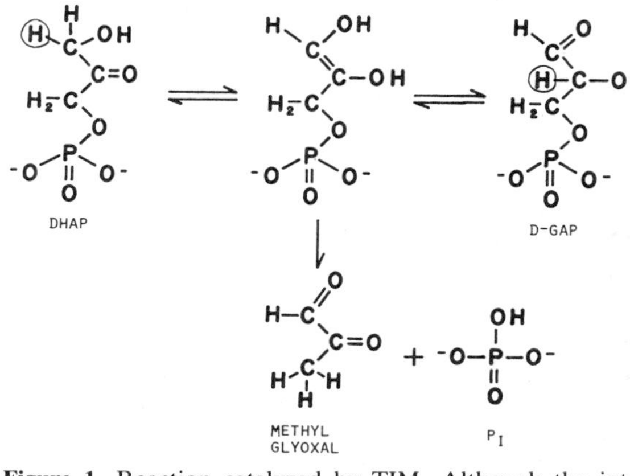

Figure 1. Reaction catalyzed by TIM. Although the intermediate is depicted as a *cis* enediol, it is possible that there really are symmetrical *cis*-enediolates. The pro-R hydrogen abstracted from DHAP by the enzyme is circled, as is the hydrogen abstracted from D-GAP.

Present addresses: *Departments of Biochemistry and Chemistry, University of Utah, Salt Lake City, Utah 84112; [†]Department of Biology, Massachusetts Institute of Technology, Cambridge, Massachusetts 02139; [‡]Bolt, Beranek and Newman, Cambridge, Massachusetts 02139.

as indicated by the free energy profile, the enzymatic reaction rate is very fast in physical-chemical terms. k_{cat}/K_m (the pseudo first-order rate constant for the reaction of enzyme with substrate) in the thermodynamically favorable direction GAP to DHAP is 4×10^8 M^{-1} s^{-1}, which is close to the expected diffusion-controlled limit (see above). TIM has been isolated, purified, and sequenced from a number of organisms. The enzyme from all sources is a dimer of two identical subunits, each of molecular weight 28,000, and contains no cofactors, metal ions, or prosthetic groups. The challenge of understanding catalysis by TIM is the challenge of determining how such tremendous catalytic potency is achieved with only the structural features and chemical reactivity provided by water and the 20 naturally occurring amino acid side chains.

An Organic Chemist's Look at the TIM Reaction

Elegant isotope labeling studies by I.A. Rose and his co-workers (Rieder and Rose 1959; Rose 1962) established the general mechanistic features of the TIM reaction. Proton transfer is mediated by a single enzymatic base, and the reaction proceeds via an intermediate that is either a *cis* enediol phosphate (Fig. 1) or one of the two possible symmetrical enediolates. Chemical labeling by Offord, Waley, Knowles, and Hartman (e.g., Waley et al. 1970) has identified the base as the side-chain carboxylate of Glu-165.

Immediately a mechanistic problem appears. The normal side-chain pKa of glutamic acid is 4.5. There is evidence that in the protein this is raised to between 6 and 7 (Hartman and Ratrie 1977), but even if the pKa were higher, it would appear that glutamate is too weak a base to remove a proton from carbon. The pKa of the pro-R hydrogen of free DHAP has not been determined, but it is unlikely to be lower than 15. The enzyme must therefore solve two problems: increase the basicity of the essential carboxylate and make the hydrogen to be transferred more acidic. This is the essential feature of enzymatic catalysis: the enhancement of intrinsic chemical reactivity by protein structure.

Knowles has pointed out that the pKa of the transferred hydrogen could be lowered by polarization of the adjacent carbonyl group (Webb and Knowles 1974). Electron withdrawal to the oxygen atom would weaken the carbon–hydrogen bond and promote enolization. Two possible polarization mechanisms suggest themselves: hydrogen bonding to the carbonyl oxygen by a neutral donor and electrostatic interaction by a cation, which may or may not also directly hydrogen-bond. The latter has the advantage of providing electrostatic stabilization for incipient negative charge development on the carbonyl oxygen, which is expected to occur in the enediolate-like transition state. These considerations apply whichever direction the reaction runs. There is direct evidence for polarization of the substrate carbonyl from infrared spectroscopy (Belasco and Knowles 1980).

Thus, before the structure of TIM had been solved, one had a very good idea of what its active site probably looked like. In addition to Glu-165, there should be some mechanism for recognition of the phosphate group and one or two electrophilic groups (possibly His, Lys, or Arg). The most likely scenario would be one electrophile for each carbonyl, but a centrally positioned, single electrophile might suffice.

The problem with this seemingly straightforward treatment is that *cis* enediol phosphates are prone to undergo elimination reactions, and the TIM reaction intermediate is no exception. It will readily eliminate to form methyl glyoxal and inorganic phosphate (Campbell et al. 1979) (Fig. 1). Since the enzyme accelerates the isomerization reaction, and therefore the production of intermediate, one would expect rate enhancement of the elimination reaction as well. Astonishingly, this is not the case. Somehow, TIM is able to speed up isomerization by nearly 10 orders of magnitude (relative to a simple base catalyst—the rate enhancement over the uncatalyzed reaction is much greater) while disfavoring elimination by 4 orders of magnitude (Rose 1981). Any structural explanation for catalysis must account for this selectivity.

The Crystal Structure of TIM

The three-dimensional structure of TIM from chicken muscle was determined in the early 1970s in Phillips's laboratory at Oxford (Banner et al. 1975). Chicken TIM crystals do not tolerate the addition of substrates or inhibitors, so we turned our attention to the enzyme from yeast. This article will concentrate on the results from our lab on yeast TIM, but all of these data depend in some fashion on the pioneering work by Phillips and co-workers on chicken TIM. Yeast and chicken TIM have essentially identical crystal structures and kinetic properties, so the results of studies on one enzyme transfer to the other. We will discuss here the crystal structure of yeast TIM, solved at 3 Å resolution (Alber et al. 1981) and currently under refinement at 1.9 Å resolution (E. Lolis, pers. comm.).

TIM is a homodimer with an extensive, mostly hydrophobic subunit interface. Monomers have a strikingly symmetrical β/α folding pattern that has come to be termed the "TIM barrel." The core of the monomer consists of eight strands of parallel twisted β-pleated sheet wrapped around the surface of an imaginary cylinder. Each strand is connected to the next in the expected right-handed crossover manner (Richardson 1981), by one (or occasionally two) α-helical segment. To a first approximation, the structure can be represented as (β, α) (Fig. 2). The connections between sheet and helix are not smooth, and short segments of polypeptide normally bridge the two regular secondary structure elements. In some cases, these segments are classic β turns, but often they are irregular in conformation and are simply termed "loops." Two of them are quite long (> 7 residues) and deserve special attention. Residues 72–79 protrude from the surface of the mono-

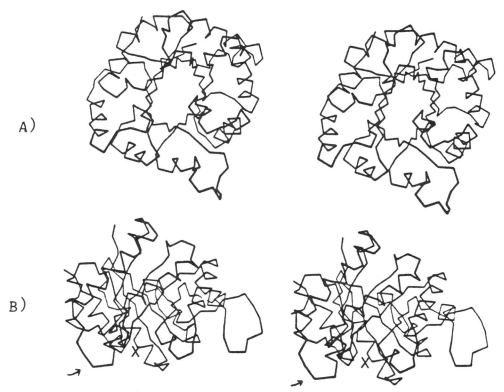

Figure 2. Two orthogonal stereoviews of the α-carbon backbone of one monomer of TIM. In *(A)*, the orientation of viewing is looking directly down the eight-stranded parallel β barrel, with the carboxy-terminal end of the barrel (the location of the active site) nearest the observer. In *(B)*, the active site is indicated by an $\times$, and the ten-residue loop that undergoes a conformational change on substrate binding is denoted by an arrow.

mer but are completely buried in the dimer; they form an interdigitating loop that leaves one monomer, forms extensive contacts with a pocket on the other monomer, and then returns (Fig. 3). Although this loop does not generate all of the intersubunit contacts, it does form most of them. The pocket into which the loop penetrates is one wall of the active site cleft on that monomer, and it appears that hydrogen bonding from the loop is essential for integrity of the active site. Thus, the active sites lie, in part, at the subunit interface, and the integrity of the active site would seem, on purely structural grounds, to depend on dimerization.

The other long loop comprises residues 168–177. This loop sticks out into the solvent. Curiously, the amino acid sequence of this loop is highly conserved throughout the evolutionary history of the enzyme, from bacteria to people. Yet, the apex of the loop is about 14 Å from the active site Glu-165 and is even farther from the subunit interface, the only other two regions of high amino acid sequence conservation in TIM (Alber and Kawasaki 1982). This fact presents another critical question: Why has nature preserved, through several billion years of evolution, the amino acid sequence of a portion of the protein that is 14 Å away from where the action is?

The active site of TIM is a pocket containing Glu-165. This pocket is located near the center of the cir-

cular-like structure shown in Figure 2, at the carboxy-terminal end of the β-sheet cylinder, the end where all of the α-helical segments begin. Hol et al. (1978) have pointed out that the dipole moment of the peptide bond gives rise to an appreciable macrodipole for an α helix, owing to the alignment of the peptide dipoles by the helical hydrogen bonding. The positive end of the helix dipole is the amino-terminal end, so the TIM active site is at the focus of the positive electrostatic potential produced by the helices. Since TIM binds dianionic sugar phosphates and needs to stabilize anionic character in the transition state, the α-helix dipoles may be important for both substrate binding and catalysis.

More than ten enzymes have now been found to have domains that possess the characteristic TIM barrel. Some of the others are pyruvate kinase, KDPG aldolase, glycolate oxidase, Taka amylase, muconate lactonizing enzyme, ribulose bis-phosphate carboxylase oxygenase, tryptophan synthase α subunit (C. Hyde, pers. comm.), glucose isomerase (Farber et al. 1987), and the two components of the bifunctional enzyme phosphoribosyl-anthranilate isomerase/indole-3-glycerolphosphate synthase. Structural comparisons of the TIM domain in these enzymes have been attempted by us as well as others. Frequently, the best overlap is achieved when the barrels are superimposed with the strands out of numerical register. The number and orientation of the helical segments and loops vary

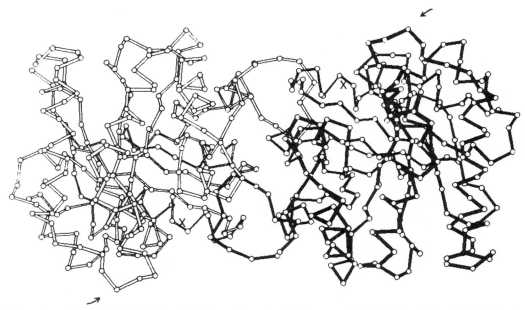

Figure 3. View down the twofold axis of the TIM dimer. One subunit is drawn with filled-in bonds for clarity. This view shows how the two subunits interact via the interdigitating loop. In each subunit, the active site is marked with an ×, and the ten-residue loop that undergoes a conformational change on substrate binding is denoted by an arrow.

enormously within this set of structures. Structural data of this type have been used to postulate convergent evolution or that the TIM barrel is a particularly stable protein structural framework onto which many different active sites can be grafted. Arguments about evolution are ad hoc, and we do not wish to debate the relative merits of various methods of structure superposition. Rather, we simply point out three interesting common facts: (1) All of these enzymes have their active sites in a homologous location at the carboxy-terminal end of the β barrel, even though many of them do not use anionic substrates and some even require a bound cation in the active site. (2) As originally pointed out by Rose (1982), it is possible to write reaction mechanisms for all of these enzymes in which one of the intermediates or substrates has two *cis* oxygen atoms on adjacent carbons. Moreover, for all of them, an enediol or diolate, in which the carbons are doubly bonded, is a possible intermediate, although it is true that these enediol mechanisms are not always the simplest ones to write. (3) We have noted that TIM-barrel enzymes seem to occur in pairs in metabolic pathways, catalyzing consecutive transformations. In view of these observations, which represent structure/function relationships rather than semiautomatic comparison of atomic coordinates, we think that it would be premature to conclude that no evolutionary relationship exists among these proteins until possible functional commonality has been investigated more carefully.

The crystal structure of TIM, combined with the earlier mechanistic studies, allowed a set of precise questions to be formulated. These are: (1) What are the catalytic electrophiles? (2) What is the function of the flexible loop (168–177)? (3) How does the enzyme prevent the elimination reaction? (4) How does TIM achieve its great catalytic potency?

The Structure of the Enzyme–Substrate Complex

Answers for some of these questions emerged from the crystal structure of the Michaelis complex of TIM with its physiological substrate DHAP. Direct observation of this structure is possible because TIM catalyzes a single-substrate/single-product reaction. For a hydrolase, an attempt to do the crystal structure of a Michaelis complex at room temperature by conventional crystallography would be futile: Substrate could be diffused into the solvent-filled channels in the crystal, but it would rapidly be hydrolyzed to products that would diffuse away (unless product binding was tight). Averaged over the time required for data collection (days to a week or more), the occupancy of the enzyme–substrate complex would be negligible. However, TIM catalyzes a simple single-substrate/single-product equilibration: If substrate is soaked into the crystal, it will be converted to product, but product is just the substrate for the back reaction. So the crystalline enzyme system will settle to equilibrium, and as long as the substrate concentration in the mother liquor around the crystal is kept in excess of K_m, the thermodynamically favored complex will dominate what is observed in the crystal. The free energy profile of Albery and Knowles (1976a) indicates that, for TIM, the predominant form will be the enzyme–DHAP complex.

We prepared this complex (TIM–DHAP) by diffusing 10 mM DHAP into a crystal of TIM mounted in a flow cell (Petsko 1985) on the diffractometer at −15°C. The low temperature was used to reduce the rate of methyl glyoxal production by the elimination reaction, which has a much bigger temperature coefficient than the isomerization (Campbell et al. 1979). Substrate binding was followed by monitoring the intensities of a set of medium-resolution strong reflections (for an example, see Alber et al. 1976).

As soon as the wave of substrate reached the crystal, there were large changes in intensity and small changes in the unit cell parameters. The intensity profiles also became broad (2°), limiting data collection to 3.5 Å resolution. These changes were complete in less than 10 minutes.

Data were collected to 3.5 Å resolution and a difference electron density map was calculated using native amplitudes and phases (Alber et al. 1981). The map showed the substrate bound in the pocket containing Glu-165. The phosphate group, clearly identified by its high electron density, lay nearest the solvent. However, most dramatic was a large difference density feature indicating a conformational change in the loop, residues 168–177. This loop had moved over 6 Å through space to fold down like a giant flap or lid onto the phosphate end of the substrate, thus closing off the active site (Fig. 4).

This conformational change following substrate binding is consistent with the fact that product release is rate-limiting for TIM: The loop must move back out of the way to allow GAP to escape from the active site pocket. If there is a disorder-to-order transition as well, it may also contribute directly to catalysis by raising the free energy of the enzyme–substrate complex (Alber 1981). What is especially interesting is that the loop movement provides a rationale for the disfavoring of the unwanted elimination reaction. For this reaction to occur, methyl glyoxal and inorganic phosphate must separate. They cannot do this because the intermediate is held in the active site by the loop. Elimination reactions are also solvent- and buffer-catalyzed, and the closing of the loop protects the bridging oxygen from contact with bulk solvent. This same loop movement has also been observed, at low resolution, in crystals of chicken TIM complexed with an inhibitor (Phillips et al. 1977), making it unlikely that our observations are due to crystal artifacts.

We have tested this assumed role for the flexible loop by site-directed mutagenesis. The yeast TPI gene was cloned and sequenced by Alber and Kawasaki (1982) and has been expressed in *Escherichia coli* (Petsko et al. 1984; Davenport 1985). Site-directed mutagenesis was carried out by the two-primer oligonucleotide method of Zoller and Smith (1983) using single-stranded bacteriophage M13 as a vector. We elected to change Thr-172, which is the residue in the loop that directly makes contact with the phosphate group of the substrate, to aspartic acid on the assumption that charge repulsion between the Asp carboxylate and substrate phosphate would prevent closure of the loop. We predicted that the mutant of TIM would still catalyze isomerization but show increased methyl glyoxal production.

The mutant has been made, sequenced, expressed in *E. coli*, and purified by antibody affinity chromatography (for details of the procedure, see Casal et al. 1987). Characterization of the protein is not yet complete, but preliminary kinetic analysis shows that k_{cat}/K_m for the direction GAP to DHAP is reduced by approximately tenfold over that for the wild-type enzyme, with a substantial portion of the reduction being in k_{cat}. Assuming that closure has indeed been prevented, the loop would appear to play a role in orienting as well as binding the substrate.

Methyl glyoxal production has not yet been quantitated for this mutant; there is an endogenous methyl glyoxal synthase in *E. coli* (Cooper 1984), and the mutant TIM must be proven to be free from this activity before proper measurements are made. The existence of an enzyme that converts DHAP to methyl glyoxal has caused us to speculate that methyl glyoxal synthase may be a "loopless TIM." Possible evolutionary relationship between these two enzymes must remain fanciful until methyl glyoxal synthase is sequenced and studied structurally. This is work we plan to do.

The Structure of the Enzyme–Transition State Analog Complex

The disorder in the crystal lattice caused by DHAP binding limits the structure of the Michaelis complex to 3.5 Å resolution. Slow degradation of substrate to methyl glyoxal by the enzyme prevents direct cocrystallization of this complex. Consequently, we cocrystallized yeast TIM in the presence of saturating concentrations of the competitive inhibitor phosphoglycolohydroxamate (PGH). PGH has a stereochemistry and charge configuration that resemble the putative enediolate transition state, and inhibits yeast TIM with a K_i of 15 μM, indicating substantially tighter binding than either substrate or the substrate–analog inhibitor α-glycerol phosphate (Collins 1974). The enzyme–transition state analog complex (TIM–PGH) crystallizes in a different crystal from native yeast TIM. This structure was solved by a combination of single isomorphous replacement and molecular replacement methods (D. Ringe et al., in prep.) and is now being refined at 1.9 Å resolution (Davenport 1985). The structure shows the flexible loop in the "closed" position, as expected, with PGH bound in the active site in a manner identical to that deduced, at lower resolution, for the substrate DHAP. From this high-resolution crystal structure we have formulated hypotheses about the roles of the various active site residues and have begun to test these hypotheses by site-directed mutagenesis.

The Active Site of TIM

Both DHAP and PGH are bound in an extended conformation. No positively charged residues make contact with the phosphate; it is held in place by hydrogen bonds from several glycine-containing loops, particularly 209–212 and 232–234. Main-chain hydrogen bonding to phosphate is a common mode of binding in proteins, especially those that do not carry out chemis-

A)

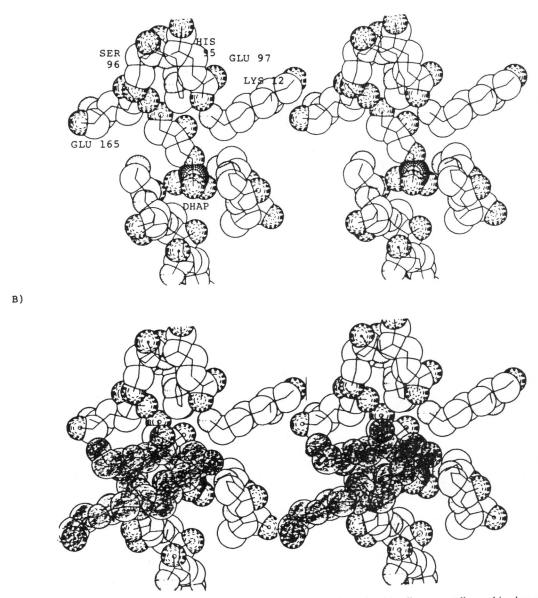

B)

Figure 4. (*A*) Stereodrawing of the active site of the TIM-DHAP complex, as determined by direct crystallographic observation at 3.5 Å resolution. All atoms are indicated by spheres of their appropriate van der Waals radii. The substrate is in the center, with the phosphate atom having a dark circle. Carbon atoms are clear, oxygens are dashed, and nitrogens are dotted. In this picture, the ten-residue loop from 168 to 177 has been omitted for clarity. This may be imagined as the hypothetical structure of the Michaelis complex immediately after substrate has entered the active site but before the loop has closed. (*B*) Full structure of the TIM-DHAP complex, including the 168–177 loop (in dark atoms). It is clear that the conformational change in this loop has sealed off the active site from direct contact with bulk solvent.

try on the phosphate group (for an example, see Smith et al. 1983). Cationic side chains are used to bind phosphate oxygens when phosphate is transferred or hydrolyzed (probably because charge stabilization is needed for the anionic pentacoordinate transition state in phosphate ester chemistry). Main-chain hydrogen bonds and helix dipoles solvate phosphate groups when the phosphate is only needed for specificity of binding.

There are some exceptions to these generalizations about phosphate-binding sites, but the rules are generally obeyed. In TIM, the absence of cationic side chains bound to the sugar phosphate is consistent with the enzymatic function of sugar isomerization rather than phosphate cleavage. We presume that the negative charge on the phosphate is compensated by the positive helix dipoles that are oriented toward the active site.

The long carboxy-terminal helix (235–246) appears to be particularly important in this regard. Since there are only main-chain hydrogen bonds to the phosphate, mutagenesis cannot be used to probe the phosphate-binding site. Although replacement of glycine by proline is a theoretical possibility, a proline side chain would interfere sterically with phosphate binding. There are few other hydrogen bonds between the enzyme and DHAP or PGH, supporting the observation from analog studies that a phosphate group is required for tight binding to TIM. TIM thus resembles most other enzymes in having a specificity-determining binding site that is distinct from the site where chemistry is carried out. This general design principle of enzymatic catalysis is sensible, since chemical transformations involve changes in charge and geometry, which would disrupt the interactions needed for the tight binding that ensures specificity. We thus speak of TIM as having a specificity subsite (the phosphate-binding site) and a catalytic subsite.

The catalytic subsite consists of Glu-165, Cys-126, His-95, Ser-96, Glu-97, Asn-10, and Lys-12. Only Glu-165 and Cys-126 are on the side of the substrate where proton transfer occurs. The remainder of the residues interact with the substrate (or each other) on the carbonyl side of the sugar. Glu-165 and Cys-126 are thus on the side where proton abstraction occurs, whereas the other side chains contain the putative electrophilic components.

The Nucleophilic Side

Glu-165 — The catalytic base. In the TIM–PGH and TIM–DHAP structures, the carboxylate group of Glu-165 is perfectly positioned for nucleophilic abstraction of the pro-R proton from C1 of DHAP and direct transfer to C2. To test the importance of the position of this residue, Straus et al. (1985) have carried out site-directed mutagenesis of the cloned gene for chicken TIM and changed Glu-165 to Asp. This mutation is discussed in detail elsewhere in this volume, but, for convenience, we note that the intention was to keep the chemistry the same but to move the base about 1 Å farther from the substrate. The fundamental kinetic parameters k_{cat} and K_m have been determined in both directions for this mutant, as has the complete free energy profile (Raines et al. 1986). K_m is only slightly affected, but k_{cat} is reduced by several orders of magnitude in both the forward and reverse directions. The free energy profile for the mutant shows that only the transition-state free energies have been seriously altered. Glu-165 → Asp mutation has slowed each of the enolization steps by a factor of about 1000. (This reduction is probably due to a slowing of the actual proton transfer process, rather than an alteration in the geometry of the bound substrate that could affect interactions with the electrophilic side of the active site. Support for this view comes from the observation that the K_i for PGH binding to the mutant is only slightly altered from its value for the wild-type enzyme.) In an attempt to explain these observations, Alagona et al. (1986) carried out ab initio self-consistent field calculations on a model system, the abstraction of a proton from hydroxyacetone by formate. They concluded that a longer oxygen-to-carbon distance in the transition state, as expected from the change of Glu to Asp, could explain the observed rate reduction.

On request from Knowles and associates, we undertook to calculate the structure of the mutant enzyme in its complex with DHAP. Our starting point was the coordinate set for wild-type yeast TIM with substrate bound. The method of structure prediction was the minimum perturbation approach developed by Karplus and co-workers (Shih et al. 1985). We replaced Glu-165 by Asp in the enzyme–substrate complex coordinate set, using computer graphics to position the aspartate side chain. We then cranked the two side-chain torsion angles of Asp-165 through all possible values in 10° increments, keeping the rest of the protein fixed. At each point in the torsion angle scan, the interaction potential energy between Asp-165 and the surrounding protein atoms was computed. The resulting energy map, which resembles a Ramachandran diagram, was inspected for low energy regions (i.e., side-chain torsion angle combinations that yielded energies similar to those in the wild-type protein structure). Each of these low energy structures was then subjected to full energy minimization, with all atoms in a 7 Å sphere about the α carbon of the mutant residue allowed to move freely, while atoms outside this sphere were under harmonic restraints. An adapted-basis Newton Raphson minimizer was used. A variation of this procedure has been used with success by Snow and Amzel (1986) to model immunoglobulin variable regions.

The minimum perturbation approach yielded two minima separated by large energy barriers. One minimum energy structure places the side-chain carboxylate oxygens of Asp-165 over 5 Å from the nearest substrate atom, an impossible position for catalysis. The other structure, which is the lowest energy structure found in the calculation, has one carboxylate oxygen 2.9 Å from C1 of DHAP, just as observed in the wild-type TIM–DHAP crystal structure (Fig. 5). Although the distance from Asp-165 to the substrate in this model is the same as the distance from the oxygen of Glu-165 to DHAP in the wild-type enzyme–substrate complex, the orientation of the carboxylate group is quite different in the mutant. Replacement of Glu by Asp is not a structurally conservative mutation: It moves the bulky carboxylate group closer to the surface of the protein. In the TIM active site, this movement causes the carboxylate to collide with the backbone of the protein around Gly-209. To relieve this steric crowding, the carboxylate must rotate (this is the minimum energy position found), and when it does, it can only reach the substrate in a conformation in which the outer (anti) orbital of the oxygen atom acts as the proton acceptor (Figs. 5 and 6). In the wild-type TIM–DHAP structure, where the longer side chain of glutamate pushes the carboxylate beyond the 209 loop,

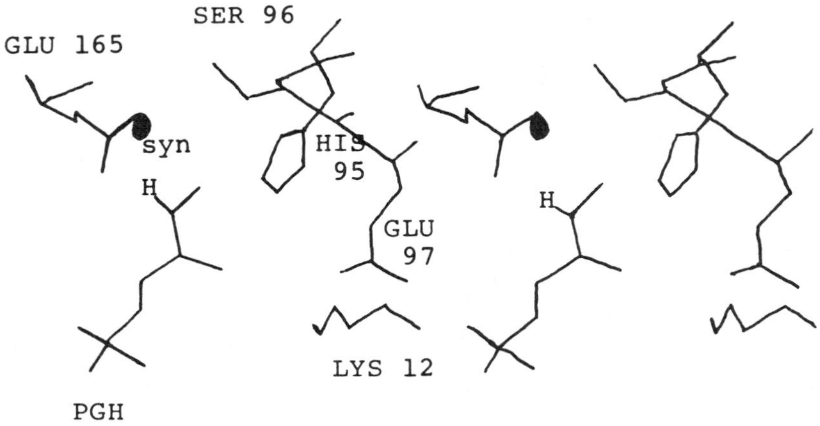

GLU 165

SER 96

syn

H

HIS 95

GLU 97

LYS 12

PGH

Figure 5. Stereo line drawing of the active site of the TIM-PGH complex, as determined by direct crystallographic observation at 1.9 Å resolution, our most highly refined view of a TIM complex to date. Substrate binds in a manner analogous to that of PGH, as is clear from comparison of this figure with Fig. 4. Every covalent bond is denoted by a line segment. Only some of the catalyic residues are shown, and once again the 168–177 loop has been omitted for clarity. Note that the carboxylate side chain of Glu 165 is oriented so that the inner or syn orbital (indicated on the figure) is positioned for proton abstraction.

the syn orbital (the orbital on the same side of the C–O bond as the C = O bond) is the proton acceptor. Gandour (1981) has pointed out that the anti orbital is 10,000-fold less basic than the syn orbital. If that equilibrium difference is used in the Bronsted formula together with a β of about 0.7, a rate reduction of 1,000-fold for proton transfer is calculated for the mutant enzyme. This is the same value as observed experimentally.

Although these calculations do not establish that the difference in orbital usage is responsible for the reduced activity of the Asp-165 mutant, they do provide a testable hypothesis. The three-dimensional structure of the mutant enzyme, complexed to PGH, will indicate

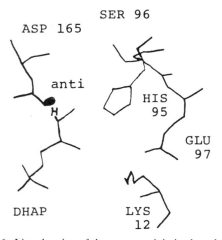

Figure 6. Line drawing of the energy-minimized model structure of the complex of the E165D mutant of TIM with DHAP. In this lowest-energy model, the replacement of Glu-165 by Asp has caused a rotation of the carboxylate (to avoid a steric clash with a backbone loop nearby, as the side chain of Asp is shorter), so that now only the outer or anti orbital of the oxygen is available for proton abstraction. The anti oribital is believed to be at least 10,000-fold less basic than the syn oribital.

whether the anti orbital is in fact the only one available for proton transfer.

Cys-126—The anchor. The calculated structure for the Asp mutant raises the question of whether the observed structure for the wild-type Glu-165, where the more basic syn orbital is used for proton transfer, is in fact the minimum energy conformation of this residue. Calculations using the minimum perturbation approach indicate that it is. There is an interesting structural reason for this. The longer side chain of glutamate is able to make contact with the –SH group of Cys-126. The sulfhydryl possibly hydrogen-bonds to one of the carboxylate oxygens. That hydrogen bond holds Glu-165 in the position where the syn orbital is available for proton donation. In fact, the cysteine sulfur donates its hydrogen to the anti orbital of the carboxylate, leaving the syn orbital free.

Hydrogen bonding to a carboxylate normally reduces the basicity of the oxygen atoms, unless the hydrogen-bond donor atom is much less electronegative than oxygen. Sulfur is the only hydrogen-bond donor commonly found in proteins that meets this criterion. We suggest that the requirement for anchoring Glu-165 without diminishing its base strength is the reason for the invariance of cysteine at position 126 in all TIMs sequenced to date. An interesting experiment would be to change the cysteine to serine, making the donor atom oxygen. This mutation is currently being made.

The Electrophilic Side

His-95, Lys-12, and Asn-10—The electrophiles. In both the TIM–DHAP and TIM–PGH structures there are three residues that are in contact with the carbonyl and hydroxyl oxygen atoms of the triosephosphates. One of these, which is uncharged and may be purely involved in substrate binding, is Asn-10. Mutation of this residue to valine or alanine would be of interest.

The other two residues may have more complex roles. Lys-12 is positively charged at neutral pH and is close to the C2 oxygen of the substrate. We speculate that its role may be to stabilize the transition state by charge–charge interaction. A mutant TIM with glutamine replacing the lysine has been made but not yet characterized: In crude cell extract it shows little or no TIM activity. The positive charge on Lys-12 will also affect the oxygen at C1, since electrostatic interactions remain strong at reasonably long distances, and the dielectric of the active site will be very low when the flexible loop is in the closed position, so there should be little screening. We conclude that a single amino acid may have an effect on more than one substrate atom. Simple notions of one-side-chain/one-interaction would seem inappropriate for TIM, and possibly for many other enzymes as well.

His-95 is the most complex of the putative electrophiles. It is hydrogen-bonded to the C1 substrate oxygen through its ϵ NH. If it has the normal histidine pKa of about 6, it could function as an acid, protonating the substrate carbonyl to form the *cis*-enediol intermediate. (If His-95 does not do this, the proton needed to form the enediol may come from water, or the intermediate may be the charged enediolate.) The crystal structure is ambiguous on this point. Protein crystallography cannot ordinarily detect protons, so the ionization state of the histidine must be inferred from its environment and interactions. In the refined native structures of yeast and chicken TIM, His-95 appears to be hydrogen-bonded through its δ nitrogen to the main-chain –NH of Ser-96 at the beginning of a short, irregular α helix. Since the backbone amide must be protonated, the structure suggests that the δ nitrogen of the histidine is unprotonated. The ϵ nitrogen must carry the proton, and the histidine, by this analysis, is neutral. If it is, its two possible roles are as an acid (although this is unlikely as on deprotonation the histidine would become anionic) or, more likely, as an electrophile. Electrophilic catalysis could be accomplished solely by the neutral histidine hydrogen-bonding to the substrate oxygen at C1, but it is also possible that the histidine could act as a relay for the positive dipole of the short, irregular helix. In that case, it would also have an electrostatic role.

If we ignore the implications of the hydrogen bonding of His-95 and assume it has the normal proton distribution (δ nitrogen protonated at pH 7, ϵ nitrogen able to be in either state; see Bachovchin and Roberts 1978), then its two possible roles are electrostatic or as an acid. No matter which protonation state we favor, the logical test of the function of this residue is to replace it with a side chain that is uncharged and incapable of functioning as an acid. We have mutated His-95 to glutamine (Davenport 1985). Glutamine is a better choice than asparagine because it retains hydrogen bonding at a position comparable to that of the ϵ nitrogen. If only hydrogen bonding to the substrate were important, the glutamine mutant should be fully active. If acid behavior were essential for catalysis, Gln-95

would inactivate the enzyme. If an electrostatic effect is important at this position, the mutant TIM might have reduced activity.

His-95 to Gln TIM is an active enzyme. Kinetic measurements indicate that K_m is unchanged, but k_{cat} in both directions is reduced by a factor of about 200. This observation is in keeping with the hypothesis that His-95 is not essential as an acid but does act to stabilize the transition state electrostatically. Support for this view comes from inhibition studies of the mutant enzyme: Simple competitive inhibitors are bound equally tightly by wild-type TIM and the H95Q mutant, but the transition-state analog inhibitor PGH binds to the mutant over 50-fold less well than to the wild-type enzyme.

To see if Gln-95 still hydrogen-bonded to the substrate, we cocrystallized the mutant enzyme with PGH and determined the structure of the complex at 3 Å resolution. This structure determination is not complete, but even at its current low resolution we can see that the mutation has caused a rearrangement in the groups on the electrophilic side of the active site. Whereas His-95 did not interact with any of the other electrophiles, Gln-95 moves away from the His position in order to make contact with Glu-97 and, possibly, Lys-12. Lys-12, in turn, moves to a position midway between the C1 and C2 oxygens of the substrate. These structural changes make a simple interpretation of the kinetic results of the mutation problematic, to say the least. Nevertheless, it is interesting to note that acidity is certainly not required for catalysis, at least at position 95, and that the active site of TIM has sufficient electrostatic redundancy, probably due to the helix dipoles as well as Lys-12, to survive loss of one electrophile without losing all catalytic power.

Glu-97—The other anchor. Lys-12 is normally held in place near the C2 oxygen of the substrate by a salt bridge to the side-chain carboxylate of Glu-97. This residue is buried at the hydrophobic subunit interface, so its protonation state is also open to question, but its invariance combined with the presence of the lysine makes the assumption of deprotonation reasonable. Mutation of this residue to glutamine would shed light on this question.

Ser-96—The mystery. The only other conserved residue in the vicinity of the substrate sugar atoms is the side-chain hydroxyl of Ser-96. This residue is conserved in all TIMs. Unfortunately, in all of our crystal structures, its side chain points away from the substrate and is not involved in any interaction with either triose or protein atoms! Its proximity to His-95 and Glu-165 suggested a possible "charge relay" analogous to that found in the serine proteases. Experiments designed to test this possibility by reacting the serine with serine-protease inhibitor reagents have thus far proved negative. The role of Ser-96 is thus a mystery. (The recent observation by Knowles and co-workers of a pseudo-revertant in which Ser-96 has been changed to Pro along with the Glu-165 to Asp mutation only deepens the mystery. See Hermes et al., this volume, for details.) We therefore must keep in mind the possibility that all of our mechanistic deductions about TIM are completely incorrect, since they provide no role for Ser-96. Mutation of this residue into all 19 other amino acids would seem warranted.

CONCLUSIONS

Although our combined crystallographic and mutagenesis studies have raised many new questions, they have provided some answers to the set of questions with which we began this work. Our major findings are summarized briefly:

1. TIM is able to prevent the unwanted elimination reaction by means of a flexible loop that sterically desolvates the substrate and disfavors elimination by mass action.
2. Desolvation of the active site maximizes all electrostatic effects by reducing the effective dielectric.
3. Glu-165 acts as the catalytic base. It is held in optimal position for proton transfer by a hydrogen bond from Cys-126. Steric desolvation of the active site increases the pKa of Glu-165 when substrate binds.
4. The likely catalytic electrophiles are Asn-10, Lys-12, and His-95.
5. Acid catalysis by His-95 is not essential for isomerization.
6. Rather than a unique electrophile for each substrate oxygen, the enzyme seems to provide a positive electrostatic potential by means of a combination of side chains and α-helix dipoles. Thus, it is more accurate to speak of a catalytic surface than a specific site for electrophilic catalysis.
7. Substrate specificity is chiefly provided by helical dipole and backbone hydrogen bonding to the phosphate group.
8. The active site of TIM is complementary, in both stereochemistry and charge configuration, to the transition state of the reaction it catalyzes.
9. There is no such thing as a "simple" enzyme.

There are a number of questions that remain unanswered. Some of the most pressing are: What are the pKa values of the various catalytic groups? How fast does the loop move, and is there a trigger for its movement? What is the role of Ser-96? Where does the proton needed to form the enediol come from? It should be obvious that neither X-ray crystallography nor site-directed mutagenesis is the most appropriate technique to address many of these questions.

Finally, we offer some comments about the evolution of catalytic efficiency. Our studies show that the active site of TIM contains a great deal of "fail-safe" structural character. Mutation in any one catalytic residue still leaves a number of features that can function, albeit at a reduced rate. In view of the possibility of adventitious mutations, such overdesigning of catalytic groups seems a sensible safety feature. Our studies also show that the enzyme has both simple and sophisticated rate enhancement methods. It uses the simple tools of base

catalysis, solvent exclusion, and proximity, but it also is set up to bind the charged transition state more tightly than either substrate. Stabilization of charged transition states would seem to be a general, important feature of enzymatic catalysis. But above all, our studies show that the simple notions of functional group organic chemistry are inadequate for treatment of even a "simple" enzyme. TIM uses both backbone and side-chain groups to interact with the substrate. Positive charges that it needs for binding and catalysis are provided by helical dipoles as well as by charged side chains. There is no easily identifiable "cationic group;" the cation is the whole enzyme, the structure of the protein provides a cationic region. Here we have a rationale for the large size of enzymes. Here also we have a suggestion that heterogenous surface catalysts may be better analogs for the structural principles of enzymatic catalysis than previously suspected.

ACKNOWLEDGMENTS

The authors thank Professor Sir David C. Phillips, F.R.S., for his continued interest and encouragement. We are also grateful to J.R. Knowles, F.C. Hartman, R.G. Wolfenden, I.A. Rose, S.G. Waley, R.E. Offord, A.C. Bloomer, D.W. Banner, I.A. Wilson, P.S. Rivers, G.K. Farber, E. Nickbarg, R.T. Raines, and D. Tsernoglou for advice and many useful discussions. This work was supported by National Institutes of Health grant GM-26788 to G.A.P. and D.R.

REFERENCES

Alagona, G., C. Ghio, and P.A. Kollman. 1986. Simple model for the effect of glu 165 and asp 165 mutation on the rate of catalysis in triose phosphate isomerase. *J. Mol. Biol.* **191:** 23.

Alber, T. 1981. "Structural origins of the catalytic power of triose phosphate isomerase." Ph.D. thesis, Massachusetts Institute of Technology, Cambridge.

Alber, T. and G. Kawasaki. 1982. Nucleotide sequence of the triose phosphate isomerase gene of *Saccharomyces cerevisiae. J. Mol. Appl. Genet.* **1:** 419.

Alber, T., G.A. Petsko, and D. Tsernoglou. 1976. Crystal structure of an elastase-substrate complex at −55°C. *Nature* **263:** 297.

Alber, T., D.W. Banner, A.C. Bloomer, G.A. Petsko, D.C. Phillips, P.S. Rivers, and I.A. Wilson. 1981. On the three-dimensional structure and catalytic mechanism of triosephosphate isomerase. *Philos. Trans. R. Soc. Lond. B* **293:** 159.

Albery, W.J. and J.R. Knowles. 1976a. Free-energy profile for the reaction catalyzed by triosephosphate isomerase. *Biochemistry* **15:** 5627.

———. 1976b. Evolution of enzyme function and the development of catalytic efficiency. *Biochemistry* **15:** 5631.

Bachovchin, W.W. and J.D. Roberts. 1978. Nitrogen-15 nuclear magnetic resonance spectroscopy. The state of histidine in the catalytic triad of alpha-lytic protease. Implications for the charge-relay mechanism of peptide-bond cleavage by serine protease. *J. Am. Chem. Soc.* **100:** 8041.

Banner, D.W., A.C. Bloomer, G.A. Petsko, D.C. Phillips, C.I. Pogson, and I.A. Wilson. 1975. Structure of chicken triosephosphate isomerase determined crystallographically at 2.5 Å resolution. *Nature* **255:** 609.

Belasco, J.G. and J.R. Knowles. 1980. Direct observation of substrate distortion by triosephosphate isomerase using

Fourier transform infrared spectroscopy. *Biochemistry* **19:** 472.

Campbell, I.D., R.B. Jones, P.A. Kiener, and S.G. Waley. 1979. Enzyme-substrate and enzyme-inhibitor complexes of triose phosphate isomerase studied by 31-P nuclear magnetic resonance. *Biochem. J.* **179:** 607.

Casal, J.I., T.J. Ahern, R.C. Davenport, G.A. Petsko, and A.M. Klibanov. 1987. Subunit interface of triosephosphate isomerase: Site-directed mutagenesis and characterization of the altered enzyme. *Biochemistry* **26:** 1258.

Collins, K.D. 1974. An activated intermediate analog. *J. Biol. Chem.* **249:** 136.

Cooper, R.A. 1984. Metabolism of methylglyoxal in microorganisms. *Annu. Rev. Microbiol.* **38:** 49.

Davenport, R.C. 1985. "Yeast triose phosphate isomerase: Studies by X-ray crystallography and site-directed mutagenesis." Ph.D. thesis, Massachusetts Institute of Technology, Cambridge.

Farber, G.K., G.A. Petsko, and D. Ringe. 1987. The crystal structure of xylose isomerase from *Streptomyces* olivochromogenes at 3 Å resolution. *Protein Eng.* (in press).

Gandour, R.D. 1981. On the importance of orientation in general base catalysis by carboxylate. *Bioorganic Chem.* **10:** 169.

Hartman, F.C. and H. Ratrie III. 1977. Apparent equivalence of the active-site glutamyl residue and the essential group with pKa 6.0 in triosephosphate isomerase. *Biochem. Biophys. Res. Commun.* **77:** 746.

Hol, W.J.G., P.T. Van Duijnen, and H.J. Berendsen. 1978. The alpha-helix dipole and the properties of proteins. *Nature* **273:** 443.

Petsko, G.A. 1985. Flow cell construction and use. *Methods Enzymol.* **114:** 141.

Petsko, G.A., R.C. Davenport, Jr., D. Frankel, and U.L. RajBhandary. 1984. Probing the catalytic mechanism of yeast triose phosphate isomerase by site-specific mutagenesis. *Biochem. Soc. Trans.* **12:** 229.

Phillips, D.C., M.J.E. Sternberg, J.M. Thornton, and I.A. Wilson. 1977. An analysis of the three-dimensional structure of chicken triosephosphate isomerase. *Biochem. Soc. Trans.* **5:** 642.

Raines, R.T., D.R. Straus, W. Gilbert, and J.R. Knowles. 1986. The kinetic consequences of altering the catalytic residues of triosephosphate isomerase. *Philos. Trans. R. Soc. Lond. A* **317:** 371.

Richard, J.P. 1984. Acid-base catalysis of the elimination and isomerization reactions of triose phosphates. *J. Am. Chem. Soc.* **106:** 4926.

Richardson, J.S. 1981. The anatomy and taxonomy of protein structure. *Adv. Protein Chem.* **34:** 168.

Rieder, S.V. and I.A. Rose. 1959. The mechanism of the triosephosphate isomerase reaction. *J. Biol. Chem.* **234:** 1007.

Rose, I.A. 1962. Mechanisms of C–H bond cleavage in aldolase and isomerase reactions. *Brookhaven Symp. Biol.* **15:** 293.

———. 1981. Chemistry of proton abstraction by glycolytic enzymes (aldolase, isomerases and pyruvate kinase). *Philos. Trans. R. Soc. Lond. B* **293:** 131.

———. 1982. Enzymology of enol intermediates. *Methods Enzymol.* **87:** 84.

Shih, H.H.-L., J. Brady, and M. Karplus. 1985. Structure of proteins with single-site mutations: A minimum perturbation approach. *Proc. Natl. Acad. Sci.* **82:** 1697.

Smith, W.W., K.A. Pattridge, M.L. Ludwig, G.A. Petsko, D. Tsernoglou, M. Tanaka, and K.T. Yasunobu. 1983. Structure of oxidized flavodoxin from *Anacystis nidulans*. *J. Mol. Biol.* **165:** 737.

Snow, M.E. and L.M. Amzel. 1986. Calculating three-dimensional changes in protein structure due to amino-acid substitutions: The variable region of immunoglobulins. *Proteins* **1:** 267.

Straus, D., R.T. Raines E. Kawashima, J.R. Knowles, and W. Gilbert. 1985. Active site of triosephosphate isomerase: In vitro mutagenesis and characterization of an altered enzyme. *Proc. Natl. Acad. Sci.* **82:** 2272.

Trentham, D.R., C.H. McMurray, and C.I. Pogson. 1969. The active chemical state of D-glyceraldehyde 3-phosphate in its reactions with D-glyceraldehyde 3-phosphate dehydrogenase, aldolase, and triose phosphate isomerase. *Biochem. J.* **114:** 19.

Waley, S.G., J.C. Miller, I.A. Rose, and E.L. O'Connell. 1970. Identification of the site in triosephosphate isomerase labelled by glycidol phosphate. *Nature* **227:** 181.

Webb, M.R. and J.R. Knowles. 1974. The existence of an electrophilic component in the reaction catalysed by triosephosphate isomerase. *Biochem. J.* **141:** 589.

Webb, M.R., D.N. Standring, and J.R. Knowles. 1977. Phosphorus-31 nuclear magnetic resonance of dihydroxyacetone phosphate in the presence of triose phosphate isomerase. *Biochemistry* **16:** 2738.

Wolfenden, R.G. 1969. Transition state analogs for enzyme catalysis. *Nature* **223:** 704.

Zoller, M.J. and M. Smith. 1983. Oligonucleotide-directed mutagenesis of DNA fragments cloned into M13 vectors. *Methods Enzymol.* **100:** 468.

Evolution of Catalysis in the Serine Proteases

J.N. HIGAKI,* B.W. GIBSON,* AND C.S. CRAIK*[†]

*Department of Pharmaceutical Chemistry, [†]Department of Biochemistry and Biophysics,
University of California, San Francisco, California 94143

The hydrolytic cleavage of peptide bonds by proteases is an ancient biochemical reaction prevalent in
all forms of living organisms. Hydrolysis of a peptide
substrate by a protease requires specificity in binding
and catalytic efficiency. Certain constellations of amino
acid residues comprise the substrate binding pocket,
which in turn confers the unique substrate specificity of
each enzyme. Productive binding of the substrate in
this pocket positions the scissile bond next to a characteristic set of functional amino acid residues arranged in
a particular conformation to form the active site. The
active-site residues polarize the peptide bond by nucleophilic attack on the carbon–oxygen bond assisted
by the donation of a proton to the peptide amide
nitrogen. The evolution of this highly sophisticated
protein "machine" has been the topic of previous
studies involving protein sequencing, crystallography,
and enzyme kinetics (Neurath 1984). A prototypic hydrolytic enzyme that has been the subject of many of
these studies is the serine protease trypsin (Kraut
1977). We have applied the techniques of recombinant
DNA technology to this enzyme to address questions
on the evolution of catalysis.

Although the primary sequences of serine proteases
are diverse, with the exception of subtilisin, the three-
dimensional structure of this family of enzymes is highly conserved. *All* serine proteases have virtually identical active sites, an important feature of which is the
catalytic triad composed of His-57, Asp-102, and Ser-
195. The Ser oxygen serves as a nucleophile to attack
the carbonyl carbon of the substrate. The His imidazole
acts as a base, assisting in the transfer of a proton from
the Ser hydroxyl to the substrate-leaving group. Our
previous kinetic and structural characterization of a
variant trypsin in which Asp-102 was changed to an Asn
suggests that the role of the Asp is to maintain the
conformation and tautomeric form of His-57 that is
required for catalysis (Craik et al. 1987; Sprang et al.
1987). Superposition of the atoms of the amino acid
residues composing the active sites of trypsin and subtilisin shows virtual identity, less than 1.0 Å root-mean-
square difference (Kraut 1977). The similarity of the
active centers of these two serine proteases that have
otherwise disparate three-dimensional structures is a
prime example of evolutionary convergence of active
center geometries in enzymes. What about other enzymes that are specific for a substrate with a carbonyl
group that undergoes a trigonal to tetrahedral carbon
transition during catalysis?

A functionally related family of enzymes to the

serine proteases are the thiol proteases, papain being
the most extensively studied member of the family.
Papain contains three residues in the catalytic site that
may serve analogous functions to those of His-57, Asp-
102, and Ser-195 (Fig. 1). The active center nucleophile
in papain is Cys-25 with its essential thiol group within
hydrogen-bonding distance to the N-1 nitrogen of His-
159. The N-3 nitrogen of the imidazole ring is hydrogen-bonded to the side chain of the Asn-175
(Husain and Lowe 1968; Kamphuis et al. 1984). Superposition of the atoms of these amino acid residues in
the active centers of trypsin and papain shows a root-
mean-square difference of only 1.0 Å, suggesting that
convergence of active-site geometry is a common occurrence (Garavito et al. 1977). We have tested this
hypothesis by replacing the active site Ser-195 in rat
trypsin with a Cys and the active site Asp-102 with an
Asn to mimic the active site of papain.

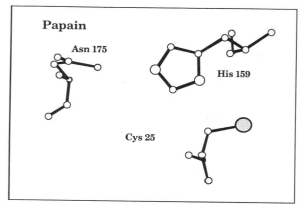

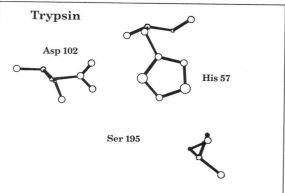

Figure 1. Comparison of the active-site geometries for papain
and trypsin.

EXPERIMENTAL PROCEDURES

Prokaryotic Expression of Trypsinogen

To construct the full length coding sequence for rat anionic trypsinogen, the 5′ portion of the trypsinogen II gene was ligated to the 3′ portion of the rat trypsinogen cDNA via a unique *Eco*RI restriction endonuclease site (Craik et al. 1985). This resulted in a full length copy of the trypsinogen coding sequence including the trypsinogen signal peptide, which was not included in the cDNA. Since this "minigene" contained the first intervening sequence of the trypsin gene starting at the codon for amino acid − 2, the intron was removed via site-directed mutagenesis to yield the full length coding sequence for rat anionic trypsinogen.

The prokaryotic expression vector for rat anionic trypsinogen was constructed from a pBR322 plasmid containing the DNA sequence encoding the signal peptide and regulatory regions of bacterial alkaline phosphatase (*pho*A). A *Bam*HI–*Sal*I fragment encoding rat anionic trypsinogen was ligated in frame with the *pho*A signal peptide. The resulting plasmid conferred ampicillin resistance to *Escherichia coli* and was called pTRAP.

E. coli transformed with pTRAP was induced to express high levels of trypsinogen (∼1 mg/l) by depleting phosphate from the growth media. Alternatively, since constitutive production of trypsinogen was not deleterious to *E. coli*, a strain, SM138, lacking a functional alkaline phosphatase repressor (*E. coli* K12, F⁻, ara D139, Δ [lac] U169, rps1 150, B1⁻, rel A1, *pho*R⁻) was transformed with the vector resulting in the high level constitutive production of trypsinogen. The major portion (>95%) of the expressed trypsinogen was localized in the periplasmic space; thus substitution of the natural signal peptide of trypsinogen with the alkaline phosphatase signal peptide allowed trypsinogen to be secreted into the periplasmic space. This was accompanied by proteolytic processing of the alkaline phosphatase signal peptide and subsequent folding of trypsinogen into the native conformation.

Site-directed Mutagenesis

Replacement of Ser-195 with a Cys to make trypsinogen S195C was accomplished using a 26 base synthetic oligonucleotide synthesized by solid phase phosphoramidite chemistry on a 380B DNA synthesizer (Applied Biosystems, Inc., Foster City). The oligonucleotide, 5′-TCCTGCCAAGGAGAT*TGT*GGTG-GCCC-3′ was used to prime the synthesis of a single-stranded DNA sequence encoding trypsinogen containing a Cys (TGT) in place of a Ser (TCT) at position 195 (S195C). Mutagenesis, transformation of JM101, screening, and sequencing were carried out as described previously (Craik et al. 1985). To introduce the S195C mutation into the pTRAP expression vector, mutant M13 RF DNA containing the S195C mutation was isolated and subsequently digested with the restriction endonucleases *Xho*I and *Sst*I in order to remove a

380-bp fragment containing the mutated sequence. This fragment was then ligated into *Xho*I-*Sst*I digested pTRAP and the ligated product was used to transform *E. coli* (MH-1). Transformed cells were selected by ampicillin resistance. The colonies were transferred to nitrocellulose filters and the filters were probed with radiolabeled S195C oligonucleotide. The filters were then washed at successively higher temperatures to discriminate between mutant and wild-type clones.

To construct the double mutant trypsinogen D102N, S195C, plasmid DNA containing the trypsinogen S195C substitution was digested with the restriction endonucleases *Xho*I and *Sst*I, to isolate a 380-bp fragment encoding the Ser-195 to Cys mutation. This fragment was ligated into the pTRAP vector already containing a trypsinogen D102N substitution, thereby introducing the S195C mutation into the trypsinogen D102N sequence. Positive transformants were screened as described above for the single S195C mutation. The resulting plasmid contained both the D102N and the S195C substitutions and was used to transform competent SM138 cells for constitutive expression in these cells.

Protein Purification

Two hundred liters of *E. coli* expressing trypsinogen D102N, S195C were grown in a New Brunswick fermentor for 12 hours. Cells were harvested using a Sharples continuous flow centrifuge, typically yielding a 1.5-kg cell pellet. The cell pellet was resuspended in 6 liters of 25% sucrose in 10 mM Tris-HCl, pH 8.0. To release the contents of the periplasmic space, a 600-ml aliquot of a 5 mg/ml lysozyme solution in 20 mM EDTA, pH 8.0, was then added to the suspension and the mixture was incubated at room temperature for 4 hours. The lysis solution was centrifuged at $10,000 \times g$ for 40 minutes and the supernatant, consisting of the periplasmic fraction, was diluted with an equal volume of water. The mixture was then brought to 70% (w/v) with ammonium sulfate and the slurry was stirred at 4°C for 12 hours. This solution was then centrifuged at $12,000 \times g$ for 30 minutes and the supernatant discarded. The pellet was redissolved in 250 ml 10 mM MES, pH 6.0, and dialyzed exhaustively against 10 mM MES, pH 6.0, at 4°C.

After dialysis, the solution was centrifuged at $23,300 \times g$ for 30 minutes at 4°C and the supernatant was then loaded onto a 5×27 cm DEAE-cellulose column and eluted with a gradient from 0 to 0.5 M NaCl in 10 mM MES, pH 6.0. Fractions were monitored by SDS-PAGE and Western blotting. Trypsinogen S195C and trypsinogen D102N,S195C eluted at approximately 0.2 M NaCl. These fractions were pooled and dialyzed against 10 mM sodium citrate, pH 4.0. After dialysis the samples were loaded onto a 2.7×29 cm CM-cellulose column equilibrated in 10 mM sodium citrate, pH 4.0, and eluted with a linear gradient from 0 to 0.5 M NaCl. Fractions containing trypsinogen were again pooled and dialyzed against 10 mM MES, pH 6.0, with 2 mM

CaCl$_2$ and the dialyzed sample was then activated by adding porcine enterokinase to a 50:1 final (w/w) ratio of trypsinogen to enterokinase. The activation proceeded for 6 hours at 37°C. The activated sample was then loaded onto a 10-ml immobilized p-aminobenzamidine column and washed with a 50-ml volume of 10 mM MES, pH 6.0, followed by a second 50-ml wash of 10 mM MES, pH 6.0, containing 0.5 M NaCl. Bound trypsin was eluted with three 10-ml volumes of 0.1 M formic acid. The pH of the eluted samples was then adjusted to pH 4.0 with 0.5 M sodium citrate, pH 4.0, and the samples were concentrated to a final concentration of approximately 0.5 mg/ml by ultrafiltration using Centricon-10 microcentrifuge tubes (Amicon).

Characterization of Trypsin S195C and Trypsin D102N,S195C

Quantitative determination of the free sulfhydryl groups of the mutant trypsins was performed using 5,5'-dithiobis(2-nitrobenzoic acid) (DTNB). A buffer solution consisting of 0.1 M Tris-HCl, pH 8.0, with 0.02 M CaCl$_2$ and 0.05–0.1 mM dithiothreitol (DTT) was degassed and saturated with N$_2$. A 0.5-mg sample of the appropriate trypsin mutant was added to this buffer to a final concentration of 0.2 mg/ml. The solution was maintained under N$_2$ at 4°C for 1 hour or more. After reduction, the sample was concentrated by ultrafiltration to a final volume of approximately 0.2 ml. Excess DTT was removed by gel filtration on a 6-ml Sephadex G25F column equilibrated in degassed and N$_2$-saturated 0.1 M Tris-HCl, pH 8.0, containing 0.02 M CaCl$_2$. A 1.0-ml protein fraction was collected, and the protein concentration in this sample was determined by absorbance at 280 nm. A 10-μl aliquot of 0.01 M DTNB in dimethylformamide was added to the protein sample and allowed to react at room temperature for 5 minutes. The absorbance of the solution was measured at 412 nm and the sulfhydryl concentration was calculated from the concentration of the thionitrobenzoate anion using a molar extinction coefficient of 13,600 M^{-1}cm^{-1}. The sulfhydryl/protein molar ratios for reduced and nonreduced protein are listed in Table 1.

Tryptic Digestion of Trypsin D102N,S195C

Efficient and complete proteolysis of trypsin requires reduction of the six disulfide bridges in the enzyme and alkylation of the resultant free sulfhydryls. This was accomplished by dissolving 3.8 mg of trypsin D102N, S195C in 1.0 ml of 0.01 M DTT, 6 M guanidine hydrochloride. The sample was allowed to denature at room

temperature for 10 minutes before increasing the pH to 8.5 with the addition of 30 μl of 2 M Tris ([hydroxymethyl]aminomethane). The reduction was allowed to proceed under N$_2$ for 2 hours at room temperature.

After reduction was complete, a 1.0-ml aliquot of 50 mM Tris-HCl, pH 8.5, containing 6 M guanidine hydrochloride and 0.5 M iodoacetic acid was added to the reduced protein solution. The alkylation was allowed to proceed for 30 minutes in the dark at room temperature under N$_2$. The sample was then dialyzed exhaustively against 1 mM HCl. During the dialysis, the denatured and alkylated protein precipitated out of solution. The entire sample was then lyophilized to dryness.

A 1-mg sample of the denatured and alkylated trypsin D102N,S195C was resuspended in 0.10 ml of 0.05 M Tris-HCl, pH 8.0, containing 0.02 M CaCl$_2$. TPCK-treated trypsin (1.35 mg/ml) was added to the resuspended protein for a final ratio of trypsin D102N, S195C to trypsin of 50:1. The digestion was incubated at 37°C for 3 hours and stopped by decreasing the pH with a 1:1 (v/v) addition of 15% acetic acid.

Trypsin Assays

Since preliminary assays of trypsin S195C and trypsin D102N,S195C indicated that the tryptic activity of these mutants was severely compromised, a sensitive fluorometric assay was used to more accurately assess the relative levels of activity in these mutants. Highly purified samples of trypsin S195C and trypsin D102N, S195C were concentrated to a final concentration of 1–2 mg/ml. Tryptic activity was monitored fluorometrically by following the release of free aminofluorocoumarin (AFC) from benzyloxycarbonyl-Arg-AFC (Z-Arg-AFC) or from the tripeptide D-Val-Leu-Arg-AFC. A typical assay consisted of 10–20 μg of enzyme in degassed and N$_2$-saturated 0.01 M Tris-HCl, pH 8.0, containing 0.02 M CaCl$_2$ and 20 μM substrate. The excitation wavelength was adjusted to 400 nm and the emission wavelength was set at 505 nm.

HPLC Analysis

The tryptic digest of carboxymethyl-trypsin D102N, S195C was chromatographed by reverse phase high performance liquid chromatography (HPLC) on a Vydac C$_{18}$ column (4.5 mm × 25 cm). Approximately 7.6 nmoles of the tryptic hydrolyzate was injected onto the column that was equilibrated with 0.1% trifluoroacetic acid (TFA) in H$_2$0 (solvent A). The peptides were eluted with a linear gradient of 0.1% TFA in acetonitrile (solvent B). The gradient was developed at 1% B/min and taken to a final concentration of 60% B at a flow rate of 1.0 ml/min. Peptides were detected at 215 nm with a Beckman 163 UV detector and fractions were collected in 1.5-ml polypropylene tubes. Samples were then dried using a Savant liquid concentrator and resuspended in 20–50 μl of 5% acetic acid or 0.1% TFA prior to mass spectrometric analysis.

Table 1. Sulfhydryl Content of Thiol Trypsins

Protein	Sulfhydryl/Protein	
	non-reduced	reduced
Trypsin S195C	negligible	1.6
Trypsin D102N,S195C	negligible	1.1

Mass Spectrometry

Tryptic peptides were analyzed directly by liquid secondary ion mass spectrometry (LSIMS) (for review, see Burlingame et al. 1986) after HPLC fractionation. In all cases, samples were dissolved in 20–30 μl of 0.1 TFA and 1–5 μl aliquots were transferred to the LSIMS probe and dried in vacuo. A 0.5-μl mixture of thioglycerol:glycerol (1:1) was added to the probe tip to dissolve the sample, and approximately 0.1 μl of 0.1 N HCl was added to acidify the solution. A prototype Wien EXB mass spectrometer equipped with a Cs^+ ion gun (Antek, Palo Alto, CA) (Aberth 1986a) was used to determine the molecular weights of the various tryptic peptides at high mass ($m/z > 2000$). A 10-keV primary beam was used to sputter off secondary sample ions, which were then accelerated at 40 keV. Mass spectra were taken in the static mode with a mass resolution of 800, which produced a mass range of ±200 daltons at m/z 4000. In this mode, ions were simultaneously detected over a 3–5-minute period on a channel electron multiplier array (CEMA) detector. Typically, 10–100 pmol of polypeptide were used for each analysis on the Wien instrument to obtain the corresponding molecular weight centroids to within ±2 daltons at m/z 4000. Mass calibrations were made from a monoisotopic CsI-RbI spectrum run under identical conditions (Aberth 1986b). Peptides of lower mass ($m/z < 2000$) were analyzed on a Kratos MS 50F double-focusing mass spectrometer operating at a mass resolution of 2000. The peptide samples were prepared as described previously, except that approximately 0.5 nmol was used for each experiment. A Cs^+ ion LSIMS ion source (Falick et al. 1986) was used with a primary beam energy of about 8 keV and a secondary accelerating voltage of 8 keV.

For the analysis of the HPLC fraction containing tryptic peptide with MH^+ 1173, a VG ZAB-SE 4F tandem mass spectrometer fitted with a fast atom bombardment source was used to obtain a MS/MS daughter ion spectrum as described previously (Crabb et al. 1986).

RESULTS AND DISCUSSION

To test whether the active site amino acid residues of papain could function as an efficient catalytic unit in the three-dimensional environment of the trypsin polypeptide chain, Asp-102 and Ser-195 of trypsin were changed to Asn and Cys, respectively. The modification of Ser-195 to a Cys has been accomplished chemically in the prokaryotic serine protease, subtilisin (Neet et al. 1969; Polgar and Bender 1969), and *Streptomyces griseus* trypsin (Yokosawa et al. 1977). However, to date there have been no eukaryotic serine proteases modified to thiol enzymes. The reshuffling of the six disulfides that occurs upon chemical modification of the active site Ser to a Cys precludes any subsequent analysis of the mutant enzyme. The S195C and D102N, S195C mutations were thus introduced

genetically via oligonucleotide site-specific mutagenesis. The resulting enzymes were heterologously expressed in *E. coli* under control of the alkaline phosphatase promoter. The mutant trypsins were efficiently secreted into the periplasm at high levels (~1 mg/l) and subsequently purified to homogeneity. Tight binding of the thiol trypsins to an affinity column of *p*-aminobenzamidine suggested that the presence of the additional Cys did not affect native folding of the mutant enzymes. Both trypsin S195C and trypsin D102N, S195C reacted with DTNB to near stoichiometric levels after mild treatment with DTT, indicating that a reversibly oxidized thiol group was present. In the absence of DTT, the active site sulfhydryl was prone to oxidation and presumably formed the sulfenic acid derivative. The sulfhydryl content of greater than unity for trypsin S195C is presumably due to partial reduction of other readily reducible disulfides in the enzyme. In particular, the disulfide at position 191–220 in bovine trypsinogen has been shown to be more highly susceptible to reduction than the other disulfides (Sondack and Light 1971).

The need to confirm the mutational changes in the DNA at the protein level was essential since secondary chemical reactions, e.g., oxidation of Cys and deamination of Asn, could give rise to erroneous interpretations of the effect of the amino acid substitution on the enzyme function. To verify the two separate amino acid substitutions, mass spectrometry was used for the mass analysis of several large peptides ($M_r > 2000$) and for MS/MS analysis in the case of multiple co-eluting peptides. Tryptic digestions of reduced and alkylated mutant trypsins followed by HPLC separation permitted facile isolation of the peptide fragments of interest for mass spectrometric analysis (Gibson and Biemann 1984) (Fig. 2).

In the case of the Ser-195 to Cys substitution, the Cys residue was expected to be located within a large peptide eluting late in the HPLC chromatogram. This peptide was also expected to have a calculated molecular weight for the protonated molecular ion (MH^+) of m/z

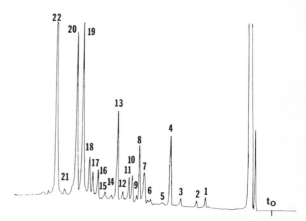

Figure 2. Tryptic digest of 7.6 nmole of carboxymethylated rat trypsinogen separated by reverse-phase HPLC.

4093.4 consisting of the sequence Asp-Ser-Cys-Gln-Gly-Asp-Cys-Gly-Gly-Pro-Val-Val-Cys-Asn-Gly-Gly-Leu-Gln-Gly-Ile-Val-Ser-Trp-Gly-Tyr-Gly-Cys-Ala-Leu-Pro-Asp-Asn-Pro-Gly-Val-Tyr-Thr-Lys, spanning residues 189–230. Furthermore, three Cys residues in their carboxymethylated form should be present in this peptide. However, if the active-site sulfhydryl was irreversibly oxidized to the sulfinic acid derivative, no reaction of Cys-195 with iodoacetic acid would be expected. This would result in a calculated molecular weight difference of 10, 26, or 42 mass units lower than detected, depending on the oxidation state of the thiol group. The mass analysis of various peptides that eluted late in the chromatogram (Fig. 2) required the use of a Wien mass spectrometer capable of efficient high mass detection. The LSIMS spectrum of peak 19 gave a centroid for the unresolved MH$^+$ at 4093.7 (Fig. 3), confirming that Ser-195 had indeed been converted to carboxymethyl Cys-195. The carboxymethylated form of Cys-195 indicated that the active-site thiol was present in the sulfhydryl form following reduction with DTT and could thus react with iodoacetic acid.

The conversion of Asp-102 to Asn was confirmed at the protein level in a similar experiment. Since the peptide that contained this substitution was expected to have a mass below 2000, a Kratos MS 50F mass spectrometer was used, which is capable of nominal mass resolution in this range. In the spectrum of HPLC peak 11, three separate MH$^+$ were observed at m/z 1125, 1173, and 1231 (Fig. 4). The second MH$^+$ at 1173 agreed with the predicted tryptic peptide inclusive of residues 98–107 with an Asn in place of Asp at position 102. A mass of 1174 is expected if Asp is present at position 102. The mass of the neighboring peak at 1174 was consistent with the natural isotopic abundance for the isotopically pure peptide at m/z 1173. The ratio of peaks with m/z 1173 and 1174 required that less than 4% of the deaminated product from the peptide was present in this mixture. Similarly, no other peptides in the chromatogram were detected with m/z 1174, verifying the quantitative conversion of Asp to Asn at position 102.

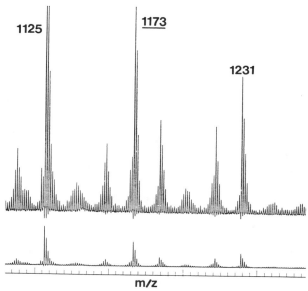

Figure 4. Partial LSIMS spectrum of HPLC peak 11, showing tryptic peptide containing Asn-102 with MH$^+$ 1173, in addition to two other coeluting peptides with MH$^+$ 1125 and 1231.

To further confirm that MH$^+$ 1173 was indeed the peptide containing Asn-102, analysis of its fragment ions was necessary. Since this peptide coeluted with two other peptides, interpretation of the lower mass fragment ions was not possible. To circumvent this problem, an MS/MS experiment was carried out where the MH$^+$ 1173 ion was selected in the first mass spectrometer, collisionally activated with helium in the field free region, and the resulting fragments (daughter ions) separated in the second mass spectrometer. The MS/MS spectrum of this MH$^+$ 1173 ion (data not shown) easily confirmed that this peptide was the tryptic fragment spanning residues 98–107 with an Asn in position 102 (Fig. 5).

The specific activities of trypsin D102N, S195C and trypsin S195C were determined using the fluorogenic substrates Z-Arg-AFC and D-Val-Leu-Arg-AFC (Table 2). No detectable activity was observed for either mu-

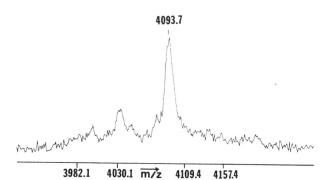

Figure 3. Wien LSIMS spectrum of HPLC peak 19 with an average of MH$^+$ 4093.7. Mass calibration was carried out with CsI-RbI standard, whose exact masses correspond to the numbers listed on the bottom mass scale.

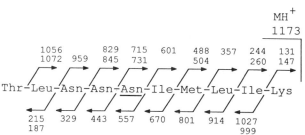

Figure 5. Fragmentation of the tryptic peptide with MH$^+$ 1173 under MS/MS conditions confirming the identity of the tryptic peptide from amino acids 98–107, including the Asp-102 to Asn substitution. Arrows represent the bonds cleaved during the MS/MS experiment with charge retention on either the amino terminus (←) or carboxyl terminus (→). The numbers placed above or below these arrows represent the masses of the fragment ions observed.

Table 2. Peptidase Activities of Thiol Trypsins

Enzyme	Z-Arg-AFC	D-Val-Leu-Arg-AFC
Trypsin	4.2×10^{-3}	3.5
Trypsin S195C	$<1 \times 10^{-6}$	1.8×10^{-5}
Trypsin D102N,S195C	$<1 \times 10^{-6}$	$<1 \times 10^{-6}$

Numbers are specific activities (μ mole min^{-1} mg^{-1}).

tant using Z-Arg-AFC as substrate; however, trypsin S195C showed a low level of activity approximately 2×10^5 times less than trypsin toward the tripeptide-AFC substrate. Presumably, both trypsin and trypsin S195C were able to form more substrate interactions with the tripeptide substrate than with the single residue substrate, resulting in the increased activity observed with D-Val-Leu-Arg-AFC.

The loss of activity resulting from the replacement of the active-site residues in trypsin with those of papain might be explained by secondary chemical events. However, since we have confirmed the presence of Asn at position 102, the deamination of Asn to Asp did not occur. Furthermore, the presence of Cys at position 195 indicated that the conditions used in this study maintained Cys-195 in the free sulfhydryl form. The loss of activity observed in these mutant forms of trypsin might alternatively be explained by gross structural anomalies. The Asn-102, His-57, Cys-195 triad of amino acid residues, although available, might not have adopted the appropriate three-dimensional conformation in the mutant enzyme. The different hydrogen-bonding pattern of an Asp at position 102 might result in a distorted active-site geometry. Similarly, the larger van der Waals radius of the sulfur atom (1.7 Å) compared to the oxygen atom (1.35 Å) at position 195 could affect the arrangement of atoms at the active site. However, since the refined structure of the single mutant trypsin D102N, which is 10^4 times less reactive than trypsin at neutral pH (Craik et al. 1987), shows that the loss of activity was not due to an altered active-site conformation or any gross structural changes, it is likely that the active sites of trypsin S195C and trypsin D102N,S195C are also maintained. Furthermore, the tight binding properties of the thiol trypsins to an affinity resin during the purification scheme suggested that positioning of the free sulfhydryl at the active site did not induce significant conformational changes in the enzyme.

The reduced activity observed for trypsin S195C was consistent with the expected activity based on the chemical modification studies of subtilisin and *Streptomyces griseus* trypsin (Neet et al. 1969; Polgar and Bender 1969; Yokosawa et al. 1977). The further reduction in activity observed for trypsin D102N, S195C suggested that positioning the catalytic triad of papain in the active site of trypsin was not sufficient for catalyzing the hydrolysis of peptide bonds. Although it was noted previously that the chirality of the tetrahedral intermediate in the thiol protease papain is of opposite hand to that found in the serine protease trypsin

(Garavito et al. 1977), it is unlikely that this difference would result in the observed abolishment of activity. The peptide substrate should still be able to adopt the appropriate conformation such that the correct hand of the tetrahedral intermediate is maintained for the given enzyme. It is more likely that other residues in or near the active sites of the serine and cysteine enzymes account for the loss of activity. These experiments thus underscore the requirements for conservation of the amino acid residues in and around the active sites of the serine and cysteine proteases. Furthermore, they show that the convergent geometry of the active-site residues, although essential, is not sufficient for the formidable rate observed in the proteolytic enzymes.

ACKNOWLEDGMENTS

We thank R.J. Fletterick for helpful discussions and W. Aberth for the Wien filter mass spectrometer analysis. Support by National Science Foundation grant DMB-8608086 (C.S.C.) and the National Institutes of Health Division of Research Resources grant RR-01614 (A.L. Burlingame) is gratefully acknowledged. J.H. is the recipient of a National Institutes of Health postdoctoral fellowship (GM-11598).

REFERENCES

Aberth, W. 1986a. Instrumental conditions of secondary ion mass spectrometry that affect sensitivity for observation of very high masses. *Anal. Chem.* **58:** 165R.
———. 1986b. High mass analysis capability of a Wien spectrometer. *Int. J. Mass Spectrom. Ion Phys.* **68:** 204.
Burlingame, A.L., T.A. Baillie, and P.J. Derrick. 1986. Mass spectrometry. *Anal. Chem.* **58:** 165R.
Crabb, J.W., L.G. Armes, S.A. Carr, C.M. Johnson, G.D. Roberts, R.S. Bordoli, and W.L. McKeerhan. 1986. Complete primary structure of prostatropin, a prostrate epithelial cell growth factor. *Biochemistry* **25:** 4988.
Craik, C.S., S. Roczniak, C. Largman, and W.J. Rutter. 1987. The catalytic role of the active site aspartic acid in serine proteases. *Science* **237:** 909.
Craik, C.S., C. Largman, T. Fletcher, S. Roczniak, P.J. Barr, R.J. Fletterick, and W.J. Rutter. 1985. Redesigning trypsin: Alteration of substrate specificity. *Science* **228:** 291.
Falick, A.M., G.H. Wang, and F.C. Walls. 1986. Ion source for liquid matrix secondary ionization mass spectrometry. *Anal. Chem.* **58:** 1308.
Garavito, R.M., M.G. Rossman, P. Argos, and W. Eventoff. 1977. Convergence of active center geometries. *Biochemistry* **16:** 5065.
Gibson, B.W. and K. Biemann. 1984. Strategy for the mass spectrometric verification and correction of the primary structures of proteins deduced from their DNA sequences. *Proc. Natl. Acad. Sci.* **81:** 1956.
Husain, S.S. and G. Lowe. 1968. Evidence for histidine in the active site of papain. *J. Biochem.* **82:** 869.
Kamphuis, I.G., K.H. Kalk, M.B.A. Swarte, and J. Drenth. 1984. Structure of papain refined at 165 Å resolution. *J. Mol. Biol.* **179:** 233.
Kraut, J. 1977. Serine proteases; structure and mechanism of catalysis. *Annu. Rev. Biochem.* **46:** 331.
Neet, K.E., A. Nanci, and D.E. Koshland, Jr. 1969. Properties of thiolsubtilisin. *J. Biol. Chem.* **243:** 6392.
Neurath, H. 1984. Evolution of proteolytic enzymes. *Science* **224:** 350.

Polgar, L. and M.L. Bender. 1969. Chromatography and activity of thiolsubtilisin. *Biochemistry* **8:** 136.

Sondack, D.L. and A. Light. 1971. Comparative studies on the modification of specific disulfide bonds of trypsinogen and chymotrypsinogen. *J. Biol. Chem.* **246:** 1630.

Sprang, S., T. Standing, R.J. Fetterick, R.M. Stroud, J.

Finer-Moore, N.-H. Xuong, R. Hamlin, W.J. Rutter, and C.S. Craik. 1987. The three-dimensional structure of Asn102 mutant of trypsin: Role of Asp102 in serine protease catalysis. *Science* **237:** 905.

Yokosawa, H., S. Ojima, and S. Ishii. 1977. Thioltrypsin. *J. Biochem.* **82:** 869.

Transmission of Regulatory Conformational Changes through Proteins

P.E. Thorsness, S.L. Mowbray, and D.E. Koshland, Jr.
Department of Biochemistry, University of California, Berkeley, California 94720

Response to the external environment and to the changing internal needs of the cell is an essential feature of catalysts operating in a living system. Enzymes cannot always be turned on at full speed, since there are different needs for pathway products at various times.

Two aspects of the control of catalysis are under investigation in our laboratory. Each reveals interesting features about the evolution of regulatory control. The first system deals with the regulation at a metabolic branchpoint that is essential for the growth of the organism. The second deals with the manner in which a receptor transmits information across a membrane barrier and integrates the response to more than one stimulus.

REGULATION OF A METABOLIC BRANCHPOINT

Kinetics of the Branchpoint

A critical branchpoint in *Escherichia coli* occurs during growth on acetate where the two enzymes, isocitrate dehydrogenase (IDH) and isocitrate lyase, work on the common substrate isocitrate (Kornberg 1966). One path through IDH leads to the Krebs cycle and produces energy but burns both carbons of acetate, the nutrient source. Hence, no net carbon would be available for cell growth or repair if all the nutrient went through this pathway. The organism avoids this dilemma by shunting approximately 30% of the acetate through isocitrate lyase of the glyoxylate bypass (Fig. 1). These carbons then go to build the cell constituents that are essential to the survival of the organism. In the normal wild-type cell, isocitrate lyase has a relatively high K_m (600 μm) for isocitrate, and isocitrate dehydrogenase has a very low K_m (8 μm). The intracellular isocitrate concentration is approximately 100 μM (LaPorte et al. 1984). Isocitrate lyase is therefore extremely sensitive to changing concentrations of isocitrate, whereas IDH is almost always saturated with substrate. Since IDH is very active, its activity must be reduced to a level that allows sufficient flux through the glyoxylate bypass. That is done by converting the IDH to the inactive, phosphorylated form during growth on acetate (Bennett and Holms 1975; Garnak and Reeves 1979; LaPorte and Koshland 1983; Nimmo and Nimmo 1984). The dependence of the flux through the glyoxylate bypass on the V_{max} of IDH is shown in Figure 2. This curve was generated using the kinetic parameters determined for IDH and isocitrate lyase in vitro (LaPorte et al. 1984).

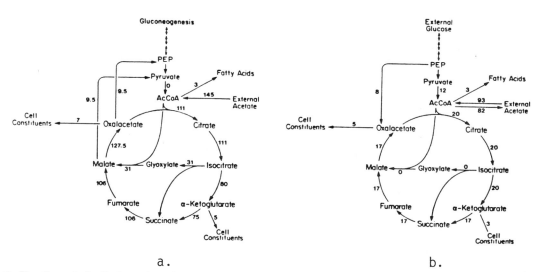

a.   b.

Figure 1. Flux through the Krebs cycle and glyoxylate bypass. (*a*) Flux (expressed in mM/min) through pathways during growth on acetate. (*b*) Flux after addition of glucose to cells adapted to growth on acetate. Note that the flux through the glyoxylate bypass goes to zero after addition of glucose. Data is from Walsh and Koshland (1985).

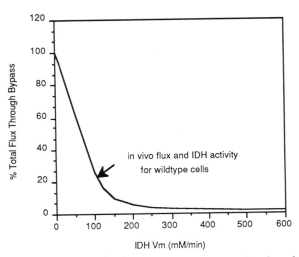

Figure 2. Flux through the glyoxylate bypass as a function of the isocitrate dehydrogenase activity. This relationship was calculated based on the kinetic constants determined from preparations of purified isocitrate lyase and isocitrate dehydrogenase (Laporte et al. 1984).

The inactivation of IDH by phosphorylation is a tightly regulated process. The enzymes that modify IDH are encoded by a single gene and are associated with the same polypeptide chain (LaPorte and Koshland 1982). The addition of a single phosphate from ATP, catalyzed by the IDH kinase, to a serine residue on IDH causes complete inactivation. The reverse reaction is catalyzed by the IDH phosphatase. The metabolites implicated in regulating the activities of the kinase and phosphatase are isocitrate and 3-phosphoglycerate (LaPorte and Koshland 1983). The phosphorylation of IDH has been shown to be ultrasensitive (Goldbetter and Koshland 1981; LaPorte and Koshland 1983) to the concentration of these molecules. The ultrasensitivity stems in large part from the zero-order kinetics displayed by the modifying enzymes. The intracellular concentration of IDH ($\sim$40 μm) is such that it saturates the modifying enzymes, the IDH kinase/phosphatase. The kinetic constraints of the kinase/phosphatase are in turn controlled by the effector concentrations.

An interesting feature of this regulatory system is the location of the competing modifying activities on the same polypeptide chain. Although this may be simply a step in the physical evolution of the phosphatase activity (the kinase having to evolve first), it also provides some convenient kinetic features. The ultrasensitive response of the phosphorylation system to effector molecules depends not on the absolute activity of the kinase or phosphatase but on the ratio of their activities. By keeping the modifying enzymes on the same polypeptide chain, the ratio of activities will remain constant no matter what the extent of gene expression. The ultrasensitive response is also dependent on metabolic effectors acting at more than one step of the regulatory system. This type of ultrasensitivity is termed "multistep ultrasensitivity" (Goldbetter and Koshland

1984). Isocitrate and 3-phosphoglycerate both activate the phosphatase and inhibit the kinase. This tight regulation of the futile cycle is the consequence of natural selection. It has been proposed that the energy expended in regulation of cellular processes by covalent modification is of sufficient dimensions as to mandate that the system must be highly regulated for survival in a competitive environment (Goldbetter and Koshland 1987).

Our in vitro and theoretical analyses (LaPorte et al. 1984) allowed us to make some predictions about the distribution of carbon flux at the branchpoint under various conditions. Specifically, a strain that did not have an IDH V_{max} in the range indicated in Figure 2 as that of a wild-type cell on acetate would have difficulty diverting the correct amount of carbon flux through the glyoxylate bypass necessary for efficient growth. Most IDH kinase/phosphatase mutants are unable to grow on acetate (LaPorte et al. 1985). Using a ^{14}C-acetate labeling technique (Walsh and Koshland 1984), it was shown that an IDH kinase/phosphatase mutant that grew very poorly on acetate and had only dephosphorylated IDH diverted only a few percent of the total flux through the bypass, in contrast to the wild-type diversion of about one-third of the total flux (Fig. 3a,b).

Pseudorevertant Analysis of Branchpoint Regulation

Our analysis of the branchpoint indicated that a strain that could not phosphorylate IDH, but had lower total IDH activity so that correct distribution of flux at the branchpoint could occur, would be viable. It is possible to isolate such strains as pseudorevertants from kinase/phosphatase mutants that normally do not grow on acetate (LaPorte et al. 1985). These pseudorevertant isolates were found to have altered their IDH V_{max} by mutating the IDH structural gene, *icd*. When the carbon flux was measured in vivo, the distribution and rate of carbon flux were found to be identical to the related wild-type strain (Fig. 3c,d). The growth rate of these pseudorevertants is identical to that of wild-type cells.

To a first approximation the pseudorevertants are as viable as wild-type cells when it comes to growth on acetate under these restricted conditions. However, the flexible covalent modification system of a wild-type cell allows adaptation to different intracellular concentrations of isocitrate dehydrogenase. When a cell contains a multicopy plasmid that overproduces IDH 15-fold, the cell adapts by phosphorylating 98% of the protein, leaving the amount of IDH in the active form that is necessary for the correct dispersion of carbon at the branchpoint (LaPorte et al. 1985). The pseudorevertants lacking the kinase can work at one concentration but are inherently unable to adapt to changes in their IDH concentration.

The flexibility of the wild-type cell with respect to varied concentrations of IDH stems from the same features of the covalent modification that give rise to

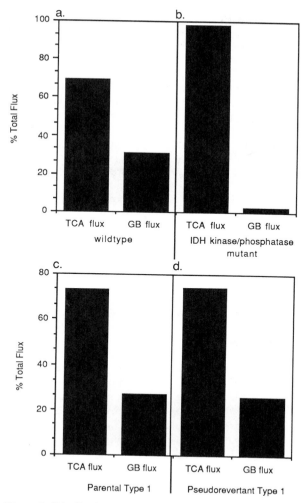

the ultrasensitive regulation of the phosphorylation state. Because one of the modifying enzymes is saturated with its substrate, in this case the phosphatase, the variation of the substrate, phospho-IDH, over a wide range of concentration has little effect on the activity of the phosphatase. The kinase remains responsive to the concentration of its substrate, IDH, and at steady state the concentration of active IDH will remain independent of the total IDH present. Depending on the carbon source the cell is using to grow, IDH concentrations can range from 30 to 80 μM in vivo.

Mechanism of Inactivation by Covalent Modification

How is the inactivation by covalent modification achieved? Because the IDH protein has been cloned and sequenced, it was possible to replace the serine that is phosphorylated by other amino acids, which are shown in Table 1 (Thorsness and Koshland 1987). It is seen that replacements of this serine by alanine, tyrosine, threonine, and cysteine alter the kinetic properties of the protein, but do not shut it off entirely. The fact that residues both smaller than serine and larger than serine still allow active protein indicates that the size of the phosphate group added will not turn off activity per se. On the other hand, the substitution of aspartate for serine completely inactivates the protein. Aspartate is not larger than tyrosine and is approximately the same size as threonine, yet inactivates the protein. The difference is the presence of a negative charge similar to that of the phosphate when the serine is phosphorylated. The strong implication, therefore, is that it is the negative charge of the serine phosphate that inactivates the protein. These results also suggest that it would be relatively easy to select a form of IDH that has reduced activity and can thus divert flux through the glyoxylate bypass. However, it would not allow the glyoxylate bypass to be turned off under conditions when the bypass becomes unnecessary, such as during growth on glucose. The answer that apparently was achieved over evolution was to use phosphorylation to obtain the inactive protein in a reversible manner, which could regenerate the initial, highly active enzyme.

Figure 3. Distribution of isocitrate flux at the branchpoint in vivo during growth on acetate. Flux at the branchpoint is measured using ^{14}C-acetate, as described by Walsh and Koshland (1984). The percentage of flux passing through IDH is labeled as "TCA flux" and the flux passing through the glyoxylate bypass is labeled as "GB flux". (*a*) Distribution of flux for cells with IDH kinase/phosphatase (wild-type). (*b*) Distribution of flux for an IDH kinase/phosphatase mutant. (*c*) Distribution of flux for Parental type 1, which has IDH kinase/phosphatase activity. (*d*) Distribution of flux for Pseudorevertant type 1, which does not have a functional IDH kinase/phosphatase.

Table 1. Kinetic Constants of Normal and Altered IDH Proteins

Residue 113	V_{max} [a]	K_m NADP (μM)	K_m Isocitrate (μM)
Serine	100	7	8
Threonine	66	68	26
Tyrosine	12	72	124
Cysteine	8	65	71
Alanine	40	31	18
Aspartate	0[b]	—	—

Residue 113 of the wild-type protein is the serine that is phosphorylated.

[a]The specific activities of the proteins have been normalized to the wild-type (serine at residue 113) protein.

[b]The aspartate-113 mutant had activity no greater than the background level, which was less than 1% of wild type. (Reprinted, with permission, from Thorsness and Koshland 1987.)

These results indicate that other mutations could lead to viable cells, and this indeed has been found. For example, a mutant lacking kinase but with fully active IDH has also been found to be viable. What may have happened in this case is that selection for an allosteric effector in larger amounts essentially decreases the rate of IDH, providing another way of regulating the flux through that pathway. It is equally possible that mutants that lower the K_m of isocitrate lyase would have the effect of compensating for higher IDH activity, but such mutants have not as yet been found.

THE MECHANISM OF TRANSMEMBRANE SIGNALING

Structure of the Receptor

Another area in which we can learn something about conformational changes resulting from covalent modification is represented by receptors. Most of the work in our laboratory has concentrated on the receptor that allows chemotaxis to aspartate in gram-negative bacteria (Clarke and Koshland 1979; Springer et al. 1979; Wang and Koshland 1980). The available evidence suggests that the aspartate receptor has the general structure shown in Figure 4 (Krikos et al. 1983; Russo and Koshland 1983; Krikos et al. 1985; Mowbray et al. 1985). In this model the amino terminus of the protein lies on the cytoplasmic side of the bacterial inner membrane. A short hydrophobic sequence then goes through the membrane to the periplasm, where a soluble domain of roughly 150 amino acids serves as the site of ligand recognition. Another hydrophobic segment then recrosses to the cytoplasm, where the remainder of the protein (about 350 amino acids) forms a second soluble unit associated with signaling and containing the sites of methylation involved in adaptation. This model, based on sequence information initially, was supported by the finding that limited cleavage with protease after residue 259 produced two distinct fragments of the receptor (Mowbray et al. 1985). The amino-terminal fragment, which contained both proposed membrane-spanning elements, was indeed membrane-bound, and able to bind aspartate with unaltered affinity ($K_d \sim 10^{-6}$ M). The carboxy-terminal fragment was soluble in the absence of detergent, and contained the sites of covalent modification.

When aspartate binds on the external domain of the receptor, that information is transmitted into the cell by a conformational change that alters the signaling regions in the cytoplasm and also causes a change at the methylation sites. The resulting slow methylation eventually turns off the signal sent initially. The sequence homologies of this protein to the other membrane receptors for chemotaxis, the serine receptor, the dipeptide receptor, and the transducer for ribose and galactose, indicate that the receptors are highly similar (Boyd et al. 1983; Krikos et al. 1983; Russo and Koshland 1983; Bollinger et al. 1984). The carboxy-terminal domain is in each case quite highly conserved, with the highest regions of homology being near the methylation sites and the region between. One region of 45 amino acids is 87% conserved among the four receptors. The amino-terminal end, where the specificity for the ligand molecules is determined, has much more variability. Some pairs of receptors exhibit no statistically significant homology in this region. Thus, like the antibodies, the chemotaxis receptors may be said to have certain constant and variable domains. The process operating here appears to be gene duplication followed by selection rather than domain recombination in each generation as in antibody expression.

The chemotaxis receptors are structurally similar to other receptors, such as the EGF receptor (Ullrich et al. 1984), the insulin receptor (Ullrich et al. 1985), and others, in which a very small transmembrane region appears to connect two large domains with the sequence characteristics of a soluble protein. How signaling information can be transmitted across a membrane barrier using only two small transmembrane segments is a fundamental question in the study of these systems.

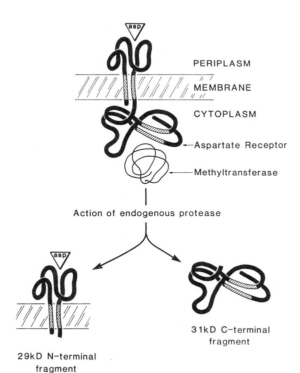

Figure 4. Model of receptor structure. Soluble domain in the periplasm is the determinant of ligand specificity. This is linked through a small transmembrane region to a cytoplasmic domain that is the site of adaptation and signaling functions. Cleavage with an endogenous protease produces two fragments. A membrane-bound fragment includes the amino-terminal half of the receptor and binds aspartate with unaltered affinity. A carboxy-terminal soluble fragment contains the sites of covalent modification.

Covalent Modification of the Receptor

The chemotaxis proteins provide an interesting contrast to the isocitrate dehydrogenase described above, since instead of a single phosphorylation site, binding of the ligand at one site induces changes at several specific glutamic acid residues that serve as methylation sites (Kehry et al. 1983; Terwilliger and Koshland 1984). The question arises as to why the receptors have *multiple* sites of modification, when it is possible in other systems to turn off an activity with only *one* covalent modification.

One clue to the value of multiple modification comes from the basic nature of the methylation-response system. Increases in the concentration of attractants are reflected by increases in the methylation of receptors, and increases in repellents cause decreases in the methylation state (Springer et al. 1979). Although we will talk in the following discussion of units of methylation added to receptor in response to attractants as though no methyl groups were initially present, in reality some methyl groups (an average of 0.5 methyl group per receptor) are always present, even in completely unstimulated receptor (Terwilliger and Koshland 1984). Thus, the receptor is poised to respond either way; methyl groups may be added in response to attractants, or removed when a repellent is introduced.

Behavioral Responses

Another clue to the purpose of multiple methylation has been found in recent studies (Mowbray and Koshland 1987). The aspartate receptor of chemotaxis has been identified as the protein product of the *tar* gene (Clarke and Koshland 1979; Wang and Koshland 1980). This gene had previously been implicated in signaling for aspartate, as well as maltose and some repellents (Silverman and Simon 1977; Springer et al. 1977). Although aspartate can bind directly to the Tar protein, maltose must first bind to the maltose-binding protein from the maltose transport system, which then in turn can bind to the Tar protein (Koiwai and Hayashi 1979; Richarme 1982; Manson et al. 1985). The net effect is similar in the two cases, differing only in that the response to aspartate is roughly three times that to maltose. The finding that both maltose and aspartate work through the same gene was not itself so surprising, since alternate allosteric sites on the same protein have been revealed for many enzymes. However, it was unexpected when behavioral studies revealed that the two responses were additive and independent (Mowbray and Koshland 1987). Responses to maltose occurred whether or not the cells had been adapted to aspartate, and vice versa. Binding of either effector thus could induce a change in the receptor even after the response to a previous stimulus has been nullified by adaptation.

Further studies showed that the methylation had much the same additivity and independence as the behavioral responses. The zero state of the receptor is defined as the adapted state that occurs when the receptor is covalently modified to match the strength of the attractant added. Roughly one unit of methyl groups (~ 0.5/receptor) are added as a result of

saturating maltose stimulation, whether or not pre-adaptation to aspartate has occurred. Approximately three units of methylation (1.5/receptor) result from saturating aspartate stimulation, regardless of pre-stimulus with maltose. Binding of both attractants simultaneously causes four units of methyls to be added.

In the case in which a single protein carried both signals, one would expect the conformational change induced by one stimulus to modify or eliminate the response to a second stimulus through that same protein. The actual observations to additivity and independence were similar to those obtained with separate receptors, like the serine receptor and the aspartate receptor, rather than the results to be expected for a single protein product. The immediate suspicion was then that two separate receptor proteins were involved, generated from the same gene, perhaps by different reading frames, by different transcriptional or translational processing, or by posttranslational modification. These alternatives were eliminated by demonstration that a single protein produced responses to the two separate effectors (Mowbray and Koshland 1987). Thus, the two hydrophobic segments of the sequences were not only transmitting information across the membrane, but were capable of doing so in increments that reflected the strength of the effector, whether or not its complementary ligand was present.

Molecular Mechanism

We shall explain in molecular terms how the receptor is capable of integrating two types of conformational changes in such a sophisticated way. Our basic premise of receptor action is that ligand binding on the external domain causes a relative movement through the transmembrane sections, resulting in distortion of the intracellular signaling and methylation domains, and that methylation acts as a balancing force. One model through which additivity might be introduced into the system is shown in Figure 5. Binding of aspartate causes a twisting of the protein, generating a signal that is transmitted to the flagella. Methylation of the receptor is also stimulated, which exerts a force on the protein in the opposite direction. A neutralization of the aspartate signal results when three units of methylation have been added. Thus, the "push" of the aspartate binding causes one change in conformation and the "pull" of the methylation causes the reverse conformational change; their equalization leads to adaptation. When maltose binds through its maltose-binding protein, a similar but less extensive response occurs that requires only one unit of methylation to counterbalance it. When both aspartate and maltose are added together, it is necessary to add four units of methylation to the receptor to return to the zero state. The type of conformational change described in Figure 5 is such that it can be added to incrementally even after the receptor has preadapted to another stimulus. Response also does not depend on whether saturating or subsaturating

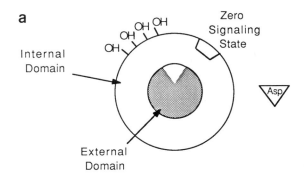

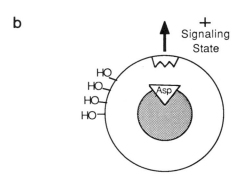

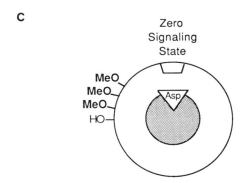

Figure 5. Twist model for receptor signaling and adaptation. The receptor is shown from a top view, with the external, ligand-binding domain shown shaded, and the internal, signaling and adaptation domains shown unshaded behind it. (*a*) The zero state of the receptor is shown with no ligand bound, little methylation, and no signal being sent. (*b*) Binding of the ligand aspartate causes a relative twisting motion between the two domains through the membrane-spanning region. This stress deforms the internal portion of the receptor and results in a signal being sent. (*c*) Methylation releases the stress caused by the twisting motion. Three units of methylation are necessary to counteract the aspartate effect. Maltose would act by a similar, but smaller, twist, and the addition of both ligands simultaneously would result in the largest twist and methylation response.

concentrations of the stimuli are added. Roughly speaking, one-third saturation by aspartate or complete saturation by maltose both lead to one unit of methylation, and to the same behavioral response.

We have described other possible mechanisms by which transmembrane signaling can occur, making use

of the same principles (Mowbray and Koshland 1987). An evolutionary selection has thus allowed multiple covalent modification to provide an integrating device for stimuli, allowing the receptor to be reset to zero as necessary for adaptation. The overall effects of the integration-signaling-adaptation system are illustrated further in Figure 6.

Evolution of the Additive Response

A comparison of the *E. coli* and *Salmonella* aspartate receptors may illustrate how the maltose function arose. *Salmonella typhimurium* also has an aspartate receptor and a maltose-binding protein involved in transport, but this organism does not chemotax to maltose. The aspartate receptor from *Salmonella* is very similar to that from *E. coli* and has been replaced by it in genetic engineering experiments. The hybrid strain is perfectly normal with respect to aspartate chemotaxis, but is defective in maltose chemotaxis (Mizuno et al. 1986). The reverse experiment has also been done, i.e., the *Salmonella* maltose-binding protein has been put into *E. coli*. It was found that maltose taxis could take place normally in this strain (Dahl and Manson 1985). Therefore, it is clear that certain properties of the sequence of the *E. coli* receptor determined the cell's ability to chemotax to maltose. One can postulate the evolutionary development of the maltose response from these facts. After induction, the maltose-binding protein concentration in the periplasm of each organism is roughly 1 mM, high enough to be effective even when binding to the Tar protein is relatively weak.

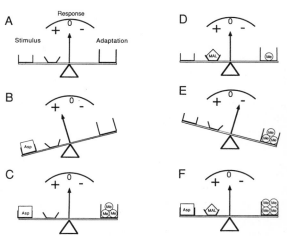

Figure 6. Balance between ligand binding and covalent modification. (*A*) The unstimulated receptor is shown in its zero state without methylation. (*B*) The binding of aspartate temporarily brings the system to a positively signaling position that can then subsequently be restored to balance by three units of methylation (*C*). (*D*) The binding of maltose at a different site requires only one unit of methylation to counteract its effect. (*E*) The removal of stimulus without corresponding removal of the methyl groups will induce a negative signal. (*F*) The binding of both maltose and aspartate simultaneously can be counterbalanced by the addition of further methyl groups.

Apparently, at some time after the divergence of *Salmonella* and *E. coli*, maltose-binding protein of the latter species must have interacted with a mutated aspartate receptor in such a way as to alter its conformation. Since that allowed the organism to respond to maltose as well as to aspartate, it gave it an added advantage that was selected for over evolutionary time and remained a feature of the *E. coli* strain. That selection ultimately led to a sophisticated integration of signals in a single protein and probably carries valuable lessons for the mechanism of transmembrane signaling in receptors of similar structure.

As stated above, the aspartate receptor is one of a small family of transmembrane chemotaxis receptors of varying function. As the first gene in an operon that contains other proteins involved in methylation and chemotaxis, the aspartate receptor is a good candidate for the "oldest" chemotaxis receptor. Another, similar receptor (that for dipeptides; Manson et al. 1986) that immediately follows it is probably the result of a tandem gene duplication and subsequent divergence (Wang et al. 1982). The serine receptor (Boyd et al. 1983), located elsewhere in the genome, is probably more or less directly evolved from the aspartate receptor, due to its similar function as an amino acid receptor, and relationship in its sequence. Another binding-protein-dependent receptor (the ribose-galactose receptor; Bollinger et al. 1984) occupies yet another location, and may have been derived less directly through the dipeptide receptor.

CONCLUSION

Two systems involving covalent modification indicate how intricate and sophisticated conformational changes can provide feedback that allows cells to respond to changing conditions. In one case, a single phosphate can inactivate a protein at a critical branchpoint in response to changes in nutrients. In the other, methylation at four sites provides for the integration of multiple signals in sensory transduction. Both suggest evolutionary selection to provide a physiologically optimized system.

ACKNOWLEDGMENTS

This work was supported by grants from the National Institutes of Health and the National Science Foundation.

REFERENCES

Bennett, P.M. and W.H. Holms. 1975. Reversible inactivation of the isocitrate dehydrogenase of *Escherichia coli* ML308 during growth on acetate. *J. Gen. Microbiol.* **87:** 37.

Bollinger, J., C. Park, S. Harayama, and G. Hazelbauer. 1984. Structure of the Trg protein: Homologies with and differences from the other sensory transducers of *Escherichia coli*. *Proc. Natl. Acad. Sci.* **87:** 3287.

Boyd, A., K. Kendall, and M.I. Simon. 1983. Structure of the serine chemoreceptor in *Escherichia coli*. *Nature* **301:** 623.

Clarke, S. and D.E. Koshland, Jr. 1979. Membrane receptors for aspartate and serine in bacterial chemotaxis. *J. Biol. Chem.* **254:** 9695.

Dahl, M.K. and M.D. Manson. 1985. Interspecific reconstitution of maltose transport and chemotaxis in *Escherichia coli* with maltose-binding protein from various enteric bacteria. *J. Bacteriol.* **164:** 1057.

Garnak, M. and H.C. Reeves. 1979. Phosphorylation of isocitrate dehydrogenase of *Escherichia coli*. *Science* **203:** 1111.

Goldbetter, A. and D.E. Koshland, Jr. 1981. An amplified sensitivity arising from covalent modification in biological systems. *Proc. Natl. Acad. Sci.* **78:** 6840.

———. 1984. Ultrasensitivity in biochemical systems controlled by covalent modification: Interplay between zero-order and multistep effects. *J. Biol. Chem.* **259:** 14441.

———. 1987. Energy expenditure in the control of biochemical systems by covalent modification. *J. Biol. Chem.* **262:** 4460.

Kehry, M.R., M.W. Bond, W.W. Hunkapiller, and F.W. Dahlquist. 1983. Enzymatic deamidation of methyl-accepting chemotaxis proteins in *Escherichia coli* catalyzed by the *cheB* gene product. *Proc. Natl. Acad. Sci.* **80:** 3599.

Koiwai, O. and H. Hayashi. 1979. Studies on bacterial chemotaxis, IV. Interaction of maltose receptor with a membrane-bound chemosensing component. *J. Biochem.* **86:** 27.

Kornberg, H.L. 1966. The role and control of the glyoxylate cycle in *Escherichia coli*. *Biochem. J.* **99:** 1.

Krikos, A., N. Mutoh, A. Boyd, and M.I. Simon. 1983. Sensory transducers of *E. coli* are composed of discrete structural and functional domains. *Cell* **33:** 615.

Krikos, A., M.P. Conley, A. Boyd, H. Berg, and M.I. Simon. 1985. Chimeric sensory transducers of *Escherichia coli*. *Proc. Natl. Acad. Sci.* **82:** 1326.

LaPorte, D.C. and D.E. Koshland, Jr. 1982. A protein with kinase and phosphatase activities involved in regulation of the tricarboxylic acid cycle. *Nature* **300:** 458.

———. 1983. Phosphorylation of isocitrate dehydrogenase as a demonstration of enhanced sensitivity in covalent regulation. *Nature* **305:** 286.

LaPorte, D.C., P.E. Thorsness, and D.E. Koshland, Jr. 1985. Compensatory phosphorylation of isocitrate dehydrogenase: A mechanism for adaptation to the intracellular environment. *J. Biol. Chem.* **260:** 10563.

LaPorte, D.C., K. Walsh, and D.E. Koshland, Jr. 1984. The branchpoint effect: Ultrasensitivity and subsensitivity to metabolic control. *J. Biol. Chem.* **259:** 14068.

Manson, M.D., V. Blank, G. Brade, and C.F. Higgins. 1986. Peptide chemotaxis in *E. coli* involves the Tap signal transducer and the dipeptide permease. *Nature* **321:** 253.

Manson, M.D., W. Boos, P.J. Bassford, Jr., and B.A. Rasmussen. 1985. Dependence of maltose transport and chemotaxis on the amount of maltose binding protein. *J. Biol. Chem.* **260:** 9727.

Mizuno, T., N. Mutoh, S.M. Panasenke, and Y. Imae. 1986. Acquisition of maltose chemotaxis in *Salmonella typhimurium* by the introduction of the *Escherichia coli* chemosensory transducer gene. *J. Bacteriol.* **165:** 890.

Mowbray, S.L. and D.E. Koshland, Jr. 1987. Additive and independent responses in a single receptor: Aspartate and maltose stimuli on the Tar protein. *Cell* **50:** 171.

Mowbray, S.L., D.L. Foster, and D.E. Koshland, Jr. 1985. Proteolytic fragments identified with functional domains of the aspartate chemoreceptor. *J. Biol. Chem.* **260:** 11711.

Nimmo, G.A. and H.G. Nimmo. 1984. The regulatory properties of isocitrate dehydrogenase kinase and isocitrate dehydrogenase phosphatase from *Escherichia coli* ML308 and the roles of these activities in the control of isocitrate dehydrogenase. *Eur. J. Biochem.* **141:** 409.

Richarme, G. 1982. Interaction of the maltose-binding protein with membrane vesicles of *Escherichia coli*. *J. Bacteriol.* **149:** 662.

Russo, A.F. and D.E. Koshland, Jr. 1983. Separation of signal transducer and adaptation functions of the aspartate receptor in bacterial sensing. *Science* **220:** 1016.

Silverman, M. and M. Simon. 1977. Chemotaxis in *Escherichia coli:* Methylation of the *che* gene products. *Proc. Natl. Acad. Sci.* **74:** 3317.

Springer, M.S., M.F. Goy, and J. Adler. 1977. Sensory transduction in *Escherichia coli:* Two complementary pathways in information processing that involve methylated proteins. *Proc. Natl. Acad. Sci.* **74:** 3312.

———. 1979. Protein methylation in behavioral control mechanisms and in signal transduction. *Nature* **280:** 279.

Terwilliger, T. and D.E. Koshland, Jr. 1984. Sites of methyl esterification and deamidation on the aspartate receptor involved in bacterial chemotaxis. *J. Biol. Chem.* **259:** 7719.

Thorsness, P.E. and D.E. Koshland, Jr. 1987. The inactivation of isocitrate dehydrogenase by phosphorylation is mediated by the negative charge of the phosphate. *J. Biol. Chem.* **262:** 10422.

Ullrich, A., J.R. Bell, E.Y. Chen, R. Herrera, L.M. Petruzelli, T.J. Dull, A. Gray, L. Coussens, Y.-C. Liao, M. Tsubokawa, A. Mason, P.H. Seeburg, C. Grunfeld, O.M. Rosen, and J. Ramachandran. 1985. Human insulin receptor and its relationship to the tyrosine kinase family of oncogenes. *Nature* **313:** 756.

Ullrich, A., L. Coussens, J.S. Hayflick, T.J. Dull, A. Gray, A.W. Tam, J. Lee, Y. Yarden, T.A. Libermann, J. Schlessinger, J. Downward, E. Mayes, N. Whittle, M.D. Waterfield, and P.H. Seeburg. 1984. Human epidermal growth factor receptor cDNA sequence and aberrant expression of the amplified gene in A431 epidermoid carcinoma cells. *Nature* **309:** 418.

Walsh, K. and D.E. Koshland, Jr. 1984. Determination of flux through the branchpoint of two metabolic cycles: The tricarboxylic acid cycle and the glyoxylate shunt. *J. Biol. Chem.* **259:** 9646.

———. 1985. Branchpoint control by the phosphorylation of isocitrate dehydrogenase: A quantitative examination of fluxes during a regulatory transition. *J. Biol. Chem.* **260:** 8430.

Wang, E.A. And D.E. Koshland, Jr. 1980. Receptor structure in the bacterial sensing system. *Proc. Natl. Acad. Sci.* **77:** 7157.

Wang, E.A., K.L. Mowry, D.O. Clegg, and D.E. Koshland, Jr. 1982. Tandem duplication and multiple functions of a receptor gene in bacterial chemotaxis. *J. Biol. Chem.* **257:** 4673.

Implications for Enzymic Catalysis from Free-energy Reaction Coordinate Profiles

C.A. Fierke,* R.D. Kuchta,* K.A. Johnson,[†] and S.J. Benkovic*

*Department of Chemistry and [†]Department of Molecular and Cell Biology,
Pennsylvania State University, University Park, Pennsylvania 16802

The power of pre-steady-state techniques employing stopped-flow and rapid-quench methods or of steady-state measurements combining isotope-effect techniques has provided a number of examples of free-energy reaction profiles for differing enzymes; dihydrofolate reductase (Fierke et al. 1987), DNA polymerase I (Kuchta et al. 1987), mechanochemical ATPases (Johnson 1985), and triosephosphate isomerase (Albery and Knowles 1976a). Such detailed descriptions have provided impressive, valuable insights into the coupling between the overall thermodynamic free-energy change for the given reaction and specific steps in the kinetic sequence for enzyme turnover (Jencks 1986) and have furnished predictions about the relationship between the ground- and transition-state levels for enzyme-ligand complexes for enzymes operating at high catalytic efficiency as a consequence of evolution (Albery and Knowles 1976b, 1977; Chin 1983; Stackhouse et al. 1985). In this paper, we describe the free-energy reaction rate profiles for these enzymes; *Escherichia coli* dihydrofolate reductase (DHFR), the Klenow fragment of DNA polymerase I, and the mechanochemical enzymes, myosin and dynein. The analysis highlights the relationship of the free-energy profiles for each enzyme to specific functions of these enzymes to optimize catalytic efficiency, nucleic acid base selectivity, or work.

Dihydrofolate Reductase

The complete kinetic sequence (Scheme 1) for the reduction of dihydrofolate (H_2F) by NADPH (NH) to tetrahydrofolate (H_4F) and $NADP^+$ (N) catalyzed by *E. coli* DHFR has been determined using a variety of transient state kinetic methods (Fierke et al. 1987). Two key features of Scheme 1 are: (1) The rate-limiting step under V_{max} conditions is H_4F dissociation at a rate that is more than tenfold slower than the chemical reduction step at pH 7, and (2) the dissociation of H_4F is increased sixfold by NADPH binding to the binary $E.H_4F$ product complex, creating a preferred pathway for product dissociation and interlocking successive catalytic cycles.

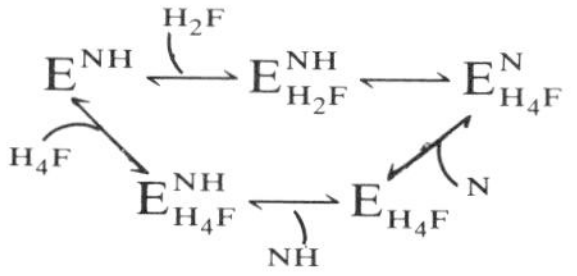

Figure 1 depicts a reaction coordinate diagram for this scheme under conditions approximating those of the *E. coli* cell, namely 1.0 mM NADPH, 1.5 mM $NADP^+$ (Lilius et al. 1979), 0.3 μM H_2F and 13 μM H_4F (D. Duch, pers. comm.), 0.1 M NaCl, pH 7.0, 25°C. It is apparent that under these conditions two nonchemical steps are partially rate limiting: H_2F binding and H_4F dissociation. Although the reaction is highly irreversible, the presence of H_4F causes accumulation of $E.NH.H_4F$ and $E.N.H_4F$ that is manifested in the stability of the enzyme-bound H_4F complexes.

Given the definition of the kinetic sequence under physiological conditions, one can calculate the steady-state turnover velocity and its reciprocal, the reaction flux. A maximum catalytic flux is set by the observed rate of H_2F binding to the enzyme because the higher concentration of NADPH maintains the reductase in the E.NH form. We have chosen to calculate the maximum flux, $1/\nu^0$, employing a measured association rate constant of 4×10^7 M^{-1} s^{-1} for H_2F binding to E.NH as a diffusion-controlled process (Fierke et al. 1987; M. Penner and C. Frieden, pers. comm.). Thus, at the above conditions, $1/\nu^0 = 0.083$ s. Under the same conditions, the observed flux is $1/\nu = 0.56$ s so that the enzyme is operating at 15% of its maximal flux, where $E_f = \nu/\nu^0$. (This efficiency could be less if, under cellular conditions, channeling of H_2F to the enzyme were occurring [Young et al. 1985].)

Consequently, the division of the free-energy change of the chemical reaction into the steps exhibited in Figure 1 is a very satisfactory solution to the problem of catalyzing the given reactions and approaches that observed for triosephosphate isomerase ($E_f = 0.6$) (Albery and Knowles 1976b), even though the chemistry carried out by DHFR is more complex. In the absence of H_4F, the efficiency of DHFR increases to 0.37. It is not known if this product inhibition is a cellular control mechanism.

We now ask what changes would be necessary to further optimize this efficiency. It is reasonable to simplify Scheme 1 to Scheme 2 by collapsing the interconversion of $E.N.H_4F \rightleftharpoons E.NH.H_4F$ to a single step because the measured association rate constants involving N and NH are nearly identical and diffusion limited. The designated rate coefficients are also included.

Scheme 1

$$E^{NH} \xrightleftharpoons{H_2F} E^{NH}_{H_2F} \rightleftharpoons E^{N}_{H_4F}$$
$$E^{NH}_{H_4F} \rightleftharpoons E^{N}_{H_4F}$$

Scheme 2

$$E^{NH} \underset{k_2}{\overset{k_1[H_2F]}{\rightleftharpoons}} E^{NH}_{H_2F} \underset{k_4}{\overset{k_3}{\rightleftharpoons}} E^{N}_{H_4F} \underset{k_6}{\overset{k_5}{\rightleftharpoons}} E^{NH}_{H_4F} \underset{k_8[H_4F]}{\overset{k_7}{\rightleftharpoons}} E^{NH}$$

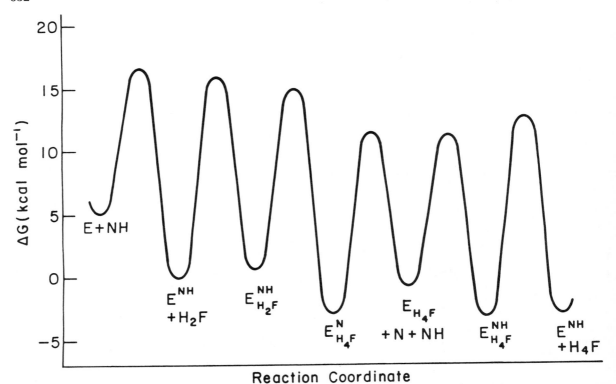

Figure 1. Gibbs free-energy reaction coordinate diagram for *E. coli* dihydrofolate reductase calculated for conditions approximating those of an *E. coli* cell: 1.0 mM NADPH, 1.5 mM NADP, 0.3 µM H$_2$F, 13 µM H$_4$F, and 0.1 M NaCl, pH 7.0, 25°C.

Albery and Knowles (1976b) have described three theoretical means to improve enzymic catalysis: (1) uniform binding in which all internal intermediate ground and transition states are bound with equal affinity; (2) differential binding in which the stabilities of the internal intermediates and associated transition states are varied relative to one another; and (3) catalysis of individual steps in which further improvement is achieved by fine tuning the energetics of elementary steps. It is clear from an examination of Figure 1 that ground-state destabilization of E.NH.H$_4$F might represent a means for further improving E_f.

Uniform binding criteria. The flux calculated for Scheme 2 is given by the reciprocal of the steady-state velocity where

$$v = (k_1[S]k_3k_5k_7 - k_2k_4k_6k_8[P])/\{k_6(k_3 + k_4)$$
$$\times (k_1[S] + k_8[P]) + k_5(k_7 + k_8[P])(k_2 + k_3)$$
$$+ k_2k_4(k_6 + k_7 + k_8[P])$$
$$+ k_1[S](k_7(k_3 + k_4) + k_5(k_3 + k_7))\} \qquad (1)$$

The flux is then maximized after substitution for

$$k_7 = K_e k_2 k_4 k_6 k_8 [P]/(k_1[S]k_3k_5) \qquad (2)$$

by differentiation of Equation 1 with respect to k_2 holding both $K_2 = k_3/k_4$ and $K_3 = k_5/k_6$ constant. (The

rate steps designated by k_1 and k_8 are diffusion limited.) This result is given in Equation 3.

$$\frac{k_2}{k_1k_3[S]} = \left(\frac{k_8[P]}{k_1[S]} + 1\right)\left(\frac{1}{K_2K_3} + \frac{1}{K_3} + 1\right)\left(\frac{k_4 + k_5}{k_5k_7}\right) \qquad (3)$$

When the actual rate coefficients for the reductase are inserted, the free energy of activation calculated from the left-hand side of Equation 3 is greater than that from the right-hand side by 1.6 kcal mol^{-1}, so that the uniform binding criteria are nearly satisfied. It also can be demonstrated that for these values of k_i, Equation 3 reduces to

$$k_2/(k_1k_3[S]) \simeq 3/k_7 \qquad (4)$$

Consequently, the most efficient situation arises when the free-energy difference between the most stable reactant ground state (E.NH) and the transition state for the chemical step approximates the free-energy difference between the most stable reaction product ground state (E.NH.H$_4$F) and the transition state for product loss as suggested earlier (Albery and Knowles 1976b). A unique solution for the uniform binding criteria then is found by solving simultaneously Equations 2 and 3 with the results illustrated in Figure 2A. It is obvious that an increased E_f (0.3) is achieved by destabilizing the central intermediates and associated transition states by about 0.8 kcal mol^{-1}.

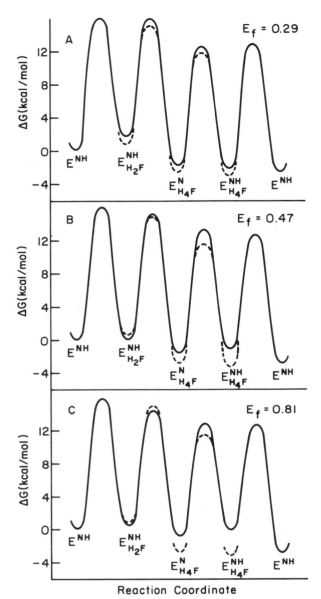

Figure 2. Optimization of the efficiency of dihydrofolate reductase: (*A*) with respect to uniform binding as described by Eq. 3 varying k_2 and k_7 but keeping K_2 and K_3 constant; (*B*) with respect to both uniform binding (Eq. 3) and differential binding allowing both K_2 and K_3 to vary assuming $k_f = C_{eq}K_{eq}^\beta$, where $C_2 = 11.7$, $C_3 = 126$ (taken from wild-type data), and $\beta = 0.5$, giving final values of $K_2 = 16$ and $K_3 = 0.3$; (*C*) by transition-state stabilization as the rate constants, k_3, k_4, k_5, and k_6 were all increased tenfold, and then the efficiency was maximized as described for B, assuming $\beta = 0.5$, $C_2 = 117$, and $C_3 = 1260$, giving final values of $K_2 = 9$ and $K_3 = 0.4$.

Differential binding. One striking feature of the free-energy reaction coordinate diagram for this enzyme is the marked departure from unity of the internal chemical equilibrium linking E.NH.H_2F and E.N.H_4F. We explored the potential to maximize E_f by systematically varying K_2 and K_3 and calculating the flux. Two constraints were imposed: (1) that uniform binding remain optimized according to Equation 3 and (2) that

the effect of changing the relative positions of the internal ground states on the position of their respective transition states follow a linear free-energy relationship where $k_f = CK^{\beta_i}$ (Moore and Pearson 1981). (The scaling C term was evaluated from the experimental kinetic data.) For $\beta = 0.5$, the optimized free-energy profile is shown in Figure 2B; this scheme features an increased stability for E.NH.H_2F but decreased stability for E.N.H_4F and E.NH.H_4F and the latter intervening transition state. For optimal efficiency, the values of K_2 and K_3 change from 380 to 16 and 2.4 to 0.3, respectively. Although these decreases are approximately tenfold, the change in E_f is less than twofold (0.47).

To investigate further the dependency of the flux on K_2 and β, we varied both K_2 and β while maintaining the optimal uniform binding constraint and holding $K_3 = 2.4$. The results (Fig. 3) show a dramatic insensitivity of E_f to the value of K_2; for example, K_2 varies by 10^3, whereas E_f changes less than twofold ($\beta = 0.5$). This plot also shows that when $\beta = 1$, the observed internal equilibrium constant ($K_2 = 380$) is in the region of maximal efficiency under these conditions. An analogous experimental situation actually occurs because the rate constant for the conversion of E.NH.H_2F $\rightarrow$ E.N.H_4F is pH dependent and controlled by the carboxyl of Asp-27 ($pK_a = 6.5$) (Fierke et al. 1987), where

$$k_3 = 950/(1 + K_a/[H^+]) \tag{5}$$

Here an increase in pH is equivalent to decreasing the ground-state levels of E.NH and E.NH.H_2F relative to the other internal ground states until the chemical reduction step is primarily rate limiting. This change does not improve E_f (k_7 remains unchanged), so that when $K_2 \rightarrow 1$, $E_f \rightarrow 0.02$. Thus, the intermediates for the chemical step need not be at equal free energy for high catalytic efficiency.

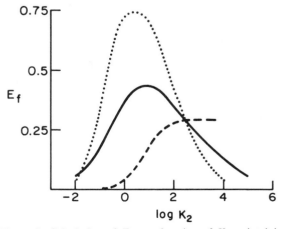

Figure 3. Calculation of E_f as a function of K_2 maintaining uniform binding (Eq. 3) and assuming ($k_f = C_{eq}K_{eq}^\beta$) at three values of β: 0 (...); 0.5 (—); and 1.0 (---).

Catalysis of individual steps. A final fine tuning of the free-energy reaction profile was achieved by stabilizing the two internal transition states by 0.5 and 0.8 kcal mol^{-1}, respectively, when the uniform binding criterion and $\beta = 0.5$ were retained. The resulting free-energy profile is shown in Figure 2C with E_f increased to 0.81. It should be emphasized that this profile represents only one of a number of adequate solutions, i.e., other combinations of β, K_2, and K_3 are satisfactory in which the internal ground states are far less balanced (Fig. 3), provided that none of the ground states for the bound intermediates are more stable than the most stable bound reactant or product or none of the intermediate transition states are less stable than the least stable transition state for reactant or product combination with the enzyme (Jencks 1982).

Given the high efficiency of native dihydrofolate reductase, it is likely that specific amino acid substitutions will generally decrease rather than increase the efficiency of the enzyme. Table 1 lists the efficiency of various site-specific mutations in which the change was localized to the folate-binding site. In all cases, the efficiency of the mutant is less than the wild type, owing primarily to an unfavorable compensation between an increased product dissociation rate constant, k_7, and a decreased rate constant for binding of H$_2$F, k_1, or hydride transfer, k_3.

DNA Polymerase I

The Klenow fragment of DNA polymerase I from *E. coli* catalyzes the addition of dNTP to the 3' end of the primer strand in the template-primer duplex with the concomitant release of PP$_i$ (Kornberg 1980). The enzyme also possesses a $3' \rightarrow 5'$ exonuclease activity that has been postulated to perform an editing role through hydrolytic excision of an improperly paired nucleotide (Brutlag and Kornberg 1972). Recently, we have been able to establish and evaluate, employing rapid-quench kinetic techniques, the minimal kinetic sequence for the polymerization process that is illustrated as a free-energy reaction coordinate diagram in Figure 4 (Kuchta et al. 1987). The profile was constructed assuming a standard state of 5 nM DNA, 20 μM PP$_i$, and 5 μM dNTP. There are several noteworthy features: (1) Dis-

sociation of the polymerase from the duplex is the slow step under nonprocessive conditions; (2) the conversion of E.D$_n$ to E.D$_{n+1}$ is limited by a nonchemical step involving the ternary complexes E.D$_n$.dNTP and E'.D$_n$.dNTP that accounts for 2.7 kcal mol^{-1} of the overall free-energy change of 3.7 kcal mol^{-1}; and (3) the chemical polymerization step is estimated as greater than 1000 s^{-1} with a free-energy difference of 0.5 kcal mol^{-1} between the E'.D$_n$.dNTP and E.D$_{n+1}$.PP$_i$ complexes.

A necessary aspect of polymerase catalysis is to accomplish rapid replication with high fidelity. Various estimates of the error frequency in vivo vary from 10^{-8} to 10^{-12} misincorporations per nucleotide added (Englisch et al. 1985). There are numerous models for proofreading (Hopfield 1974, 1980; Ninio 1975; Loeb and Kunkel 1982), but let it suffice for our discussion that such systems have in common at least two or more steps that each express a selectivity for a correctly versus an incorrectly base-paired nucleotide so that the selection may be amplified. For example, proposed selection steps include the binding of dNTP to E.D$_n$ and the hydrolytic excision of dNMP from the 3' terminus of the primer. This selectivity may be viewed as either thermodynamic (ground-state) or kinetic (transition-state) discrimination and is independent of the locus of the step in question in the turnover sequence.

We have recently presented evidence that the step interconverting E.D$_n$.dNTP and E'.D$_n$.dNTP probably represents an important selectivity step (Kuchta et al. 1987). The rate of the misincorporation of dATP into the sequence

    T C G C A G C C G
    A G C G T C G G C A G G T T C C C A A A

compared to dTTP is disfavored by 6.4 kcal mol^{-1}, the product of a 2.6-fold discrimination in forming E.D$_n$.dNTP and a decrease in V_{max} (for E.D$_n$.dNTP $\rightarrow$ E'.D$_n$.dNTP) of 2.9×10^4 (Fig. 5). On the other hand, the catalytic efficiency with the correct nucleotide as calculated for DHFR from flux measurements was only 4%.

We then ask whether the optimal balance between nucleotide selectivity and catalytic efficiency had been achieved by the polymerase. The kinetic sequence in Figure 4 was condensed by combining the polymerization and pyrophosphate release steps into a single irreversible step. (There is no detectable selectivity in the chemical polymerization step [Mizrahi et al. 1985; R.D. Kuchta, unpubl. results].)

Table 1. Efficiency of DHFR Mutants

	% Efficiency
Wild-type	15
Phe-31 $\rightarrow$ Tyr	3.9[a]
Phe-31 $\rightarrow$ Val	1.1[a]
Thr-113 $\rightarrow$ Val	3.1
Leu-54 $\rightarrow$ Gly	0.016[b,c]
Asp-27 $\rightarrow$ Ser	0.008[b,d]
Asp-27 $\rightarrow$ Asn	0.006[b,d]
Phe-31, Leu-54 $\rightarrow$ Val-31, Gly-54	0.00011[b,c]

[a]Taken from Chen et al. (1987).
[b]The flux for these mutants was calculated as $1/\nu = (K_m + [S])/(V_{max}[S])$.
[c]Taken from Mayer et al. (1986).
[d]Taken from Howell et al. (1986).

Scheme 3

$$\text{E.D}_n + \text{dNTP} \underset{k_2}{\overset{k_1}{\rightleftharpoons}} \text{E.D}_n.\text{dNTP} \underset{k_4}{\overset{k_3}{\rightleftharpoons}} \text{E'.D}_n\text{dNTP}$$

$$\overset{k_5}{\longrightarrow} \text{E.D}_{n+1} + \text{PP}_i$$

For purposes of this discussion, the discrimination between correct and incorrect nucleotides was limited

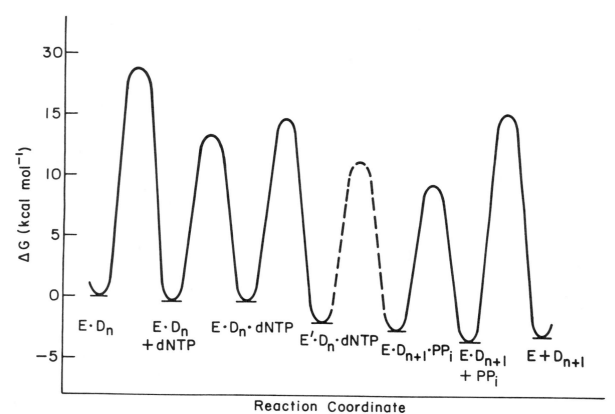

Figure 4. Gibbs free-energy profile for DNA polymerase I with a standard state of 5 nM DNA (D_n and D_{n+1}), 5 μM dNTP, and 20 μM PP_i.

to two initial steps so that the overall maximum selectivity (S_M) available is defined as

$$S_M = (k_1/k_1')(k_2'/k_2)(k_3/k_3') \qquad (6)$$

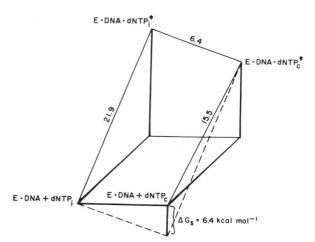

Free Energy Diagram for Polymerization of Correct vs. Incorrect dNTPs.

Figure 5. Gibbs free-energy diagram of the ground and transition states for polymerization of a correct ($dNTP_c$, 5 μM) and incorrect ($dNTP_i$, 5 μM) dNTP.

where k_1, k_2, k_3, and k_1', k_2', k_3' refer to incorporation of the correct and incorrect nucleotides, respectively (Hopfield 1974). The selectivity, S, of the polymerase is then the ratio of the steady-state velocities for correct and incorrect nucleotide incorporation given for Scheme 3 by Equation 7.

$$S \equiv \frac{\nu_c}{\nu_i} = \frac{\dfrac{k_1 k_3 k_5 [dNTP_c]}{k_2 k_4 + k_2 k_5 + k_3 k_5 + k_1 [dNTP_c](k_3 + k_4 + k_5)}}{\dfrac{k_1' k_3' k_5' [dNTP_i]}{k_2' k_4' + k_2' k_5' + k_3' k_5' + k_1' [dNTP_i](k_3' + k_4' + k_5')}} \qquad (7)$$

The selective efficiency, E_s, equals S/S_M.

To examine selectivity under various conditions, we set $[dNTP_c] = [dNTP_i]$; $k_1' = k_1$; and $k_3 > k_4$ (Eq. 7). Four limiting selectivity conditions occur as illustrated in Table 2, where $k_2 > k_3$ (column I) and $k_3 > k_2$ (column II) both subdivided into low and high dNTP concentrations. In this model, the maximal selectivity (compare to Eq. 6) occurs for the case of low dNTP when $k_2 > k_3$, a situation that is intermediate to the conditions under which the polymerase is operative. At high dNTP levels when $k_2 > k_3$ the selectivity is reduced by the factor k_2'/k_2 as the polymerase becomes saturated. At the other limit of $k_5 < k_3 > k_2$ all selec-

Table 2. Selectivity as a Function of the Rate Constants

[dNTP]	Case I $k_2 > k_3$	Case II $k_3 > k_2$
High	$\dfrac{k_3}{k'_3}$	$\dfrac{k_3}{k'_3}$ (1, if $k_3 > k_5$)
Low	$\dfrac{k_3}{k'_3} \cdot \dfrac{k'_2}{k_2}$ $(k_5 > k_3,\ k_3 > k_4)$	1

tivity is lost since $E.D_n.dNTP$ is irreversibly committed to product regardless of dNTP level.

It is apparent that the catalytic efficiency of the polymerase can be improved by lowering the transition state for the interconversion of $E.D_n.dNTP$ and $E'.D_n.dNTP$; indeed increasing k_3 to $10^5\ s^{-1}$ increased E_f to 0.53. This, of course, is at the expense of S, which decreases to unity. The relationship between selective efficiency and catalytic efficiency was further examined by varying the free energy of the transition state for k_3 and the concentration of dNTP (Fig. 6). Selectivity factors of $k'_2/k_2 = 3$ and $k_3/k'_3 = 1000$ were chosen based on experimental data (R.D. Kuchta, unpubl. results). The dashed line demarcates region I ($k_2 > k_3$) and region II ($k_3 > k_2$) with the predictions for a given dNTP level extrapolating to the limits in Table 2. The polymerase operates at the designated positions favoring E_s over E_f. Two features are noteworthy: (1) E_s is improved to the extent that the k_3 step is rate limiting and (2) this simple model is incapable of having $E_f + E_s > 1$, i.e., no relationship is found above the 45° diagonal in Figure 6.

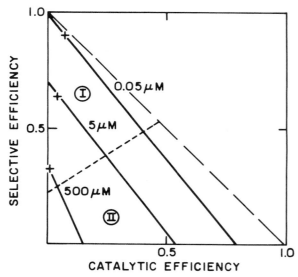

Figure 6. Varying k_3 affects selective and catalytic efficiency. The effect of varying k_3 (and hence k_4) of Scheme 3 while keeping k_3/k_4 constant upon the rate of incorporation of a correct and incorrect dNTP was evaluated using the computer program SIMUL (Barshop et al. 1983) at various dNTP levels and the kinetic parameters of Fig. 4.

One solution to the dilemma of high nucleotide selectivity but low catalytic efficiency is to introduce alternative methods for maintaining fidelity. DNA polymerase I, like other prokaryotic polymerases, possesses a $3' \rightarrow 5'$ exonuclease activity capable of mismatch repair (Kornberg 1980; Fersht et al. 1982). Also, by combining the selectivity and catalytic functions into a single step, a small improvement in this ratio (up to the 45° diagonal in Fig. 6) may be achieved. It is curious that a two-step rather than a one-step kinetic sequence was chosen to execute selectivity and polymerization. Perhaps it is a problem of active-site design. Finally, the near balance between the levels of $E'.D_n.dNTP$ and $E.D_{n+1}.PP_i$ may be more a consequence of the large free-energy utilization in the previous step rather than specific pressure to improve the chemical step.

Myosin and Dynein

Mechanochemical ATPases, myosin and dynein, catalyze the hydrolysis of ATP to ADP and P_i, in a process that is linked to filament movement (Taylor 1979; Eisenberg and Hill 1985; Johnson 1985). Figure 7 shows the free-energy profile for myosin and actomyosin, based on a slightly abbreviated scheme. Recent work (Trybus and Taylor 1982; Rosenfeld and Taylor 1984) has shown that the binding of ADP and ATP occurs in three steps, involving two first-order transitions following the collision complex; we have simplified the scheme to a single step following the collision complex as shown in Figure 7. The dashed line shows the corresponding free-energy profile for actomyosin based on best estimates for the rate constants with myosin bound to actin (White and Taylor 1976; Johnson and Taylor 1978; Taylor 1979; Stein et al. 1981; Johnson 1985). In addition, we have set the ground states for myosin and actomyosin to be equal, thus ignoring the large change in free energy that occurs with the formation of the actomyosin complex in order to focus on the comparison of the free-energy profiles. Although the dissociation and reassociation of actomyosin are crucial to the coupling of ATP hydrolysis to movement, one can more readily see the effect of actin on the free-energy profile by overlapping the ground states.

The mechanochemical ATPases have evolved to maximize the efficiency of energy coupling to perform work, and accordingly one would not expect them to be efficient in the Albery and Knowles sense (1976b). In fact, estimates of enzymatic efficiency at 1 mM physiological ATP concentration are in the range of 10^{-7} for myosin and 10^{-5} for actomyosin. This low turnover is a necessary consequence of the requirements for high efficiency to perform work and the rapid turnover of ATP being very wasteful. The basis for this low enzymatic efficiency can be understood by inspection of the free-energy profile. The ATP concentration is three orders of magnitude greater than the K_m and the rate-limiting step is an extremely slow product release. In the free-energy profile, it can be seen quite clearly that

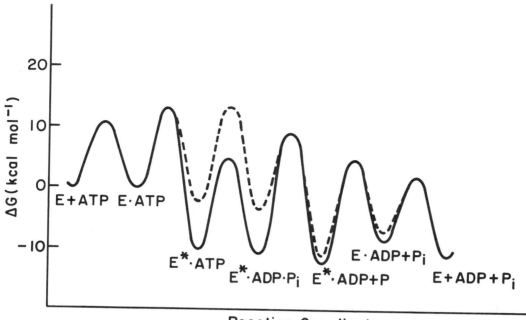

Figure 7. Gibbs free-energy profile for myosin (—) and actomyosin (---) calculated for conditions approximating those in muscle: 1.0 mM ATP, 1 mM P_i, and 0.01 mM ADP. The ground-state free energies of myosin and actomyosin have been set to zero to make a direct comparison between the two.

the bound substrate and products (E.ATP and E. $ADP.P_i$) are in a deep well. The data approximate a case of extreme uniform binding that leads to lowered enzymatic efficiency. The effect of the actin is to bring the bound products and substrate out of the well and to increase catalytic efficiency by a factor of 200, but the enzyme is still extremely inefficient if one only considers the rate of turnover. On the other hand, the efficiency of coupling to perform work has been estimated to be 60%. It is interesting to note that the equilibrium constant at the active site is near unity. Clearly, an internal equilibrium of unity is not sufficient to insure efficient catalysis, but in this case is a necessary component of the coupling mechanism to insure optimal efficiency to do work.

The mechanochemical ATPase, dynein, that couples microtubule-dependent sliding forces in cilia and flagella, exhibits a free-energy profile similar to that described for myosin (Johnson 1985). Dynein is somewhat more efficient as an enzyme catalyst because the turnover number is two orders of magnitude faster. Nonetheless, dynein is efficient in mechanochemical coupling because it has optimized the free-energy change for the chemical reaction to perform a work function, not to simply carry out catalysis.

SUMMARY

The constraints on the internal ground and transition states of enzyme-bound intermediates are mandated by the overall free-energy change in the direction of flux (Chin 1983; Stackhouse et al. 1985; Raines 1986) and the barrier for combination with reagent. Within these confines there are many solutions to transit the reaction coordinate. The path taken may reflect the function of the enzyme in question; particularly, whether in addition to catalysis there is a need to optimize reaction accuracy (Cramer and Freist 1987), to perform mechanochemical coupling (Jencks 1980), or to create metabolic control (Newsholme and Crabtree 1981; Koshland 1984).

REFERENCES

Albery, W.J. and J.R. Knowles. 1976a. Free-energy profile for reaction catalyzed by triosephosphate isomerase. *Biochemistry* **15**: 5627.

———. 1976b. Evolution of enzyme function and the development of catalytic efficiency. *Biochemistry* **15**: 5631.

———. 1977. Efficiency and evolution of enzyme catalysis. *Angew. Chem. Int. Ed. Engl.* **16**: 285.

Barshop, B.A., R.F. Wrenn, and C. Frieden. 1983. Analysis of numerical methods for computer simulation of kinetic processes: Development of KINSIM—A flexible, portable system. *Anal. Biochem.* **130**: 137.

Brutlag, D. and A. Kornberg. 1972. Enzymatic synthesis of deoxyribonucleic acid. *J. Biol. Chem.* **241**: 241.

Chen, J.-T., K. Taira, C.-P. Tu, and S.J. Benkovic. 1987. Probing the functional role of Phe-31 of *E. coli* dihydrofolate reductase by site-directed mutagenesis. *Biochemistry* **26**: 4093.

Chin, J. 1983. Perfect enzymes: Is the equilibrium constant between the enzyme's bound species unity? *J. Am. Chem. Soc.* **105**: 6502.

Cramer, F. and W. Freist. 1987. Molecular recognition by energy dissipation, a new enzymatic principle: The example isoleucine-valine. *Accts. Chem. Res.* **20**: 79.

Eisenberg, E. and T.L. Hill. 1985. Muscle contraction and free energy transduction in biological systems. *Science* **227**: 999.

Englisch, V., D. Gauss, W. Freist, S. Englisch, H. Sternbach, and F. von der Haar. 1985. Error rates of the replication and expression of genetic information. *Angew. Chem. Int. Ed. Engl.* **24:** 1015.

Fersht, A.R., J.W. Knill-Jones, and W.-C. Tsui. 1982. Kinetic basis of spontaneous mutation. *J. Mol. Biol.* **156:** 37.

Fierke, C.A., K.A. Johnson, and S.J. Benkovic. 1987. Construction and evaluation of the kinetic scheme associated with dihydrofolate reductase from *E. coli. Biochemistry* **26:** 4085.

Hopfield, J.J. 1974. Kinetic proofreading: A new mechanism for reducing errors in biosynthetic processes requiring high specificity. *Proc. Natl. Acad. Sci.* **71:** 4135.

———. 1980. The energy relay: A proofreading scheme based on dynamic cooperativity and lacking all characteristic symptoms of kinetic proofreading in DNA replication and protein synthesis. *Proc. Natl. Acad. Sci.* **77:** 5248.

Howell, E.E., J.E. Villafranca, M.S. Warren, S.J. Oatley, and J. Kraut. 1986. Functional role of aspartic acid-27 in dihydrofolate reductase revealed by mutagenesis. *Science* **231:** 1123.

Jencks, W.P. 1980. The utilization of binding energy in coupled vectorial processes. *Adv. Enzymol. Relat. Areas Mol. Biol.* **51:** 75.

———. 1982. Intrinsic binding energy, enzymatic catalysis and coupled vectorial processes. In *Cyclotrons to cytochromes. Essays in molecular biology and chemistry* (ed. N.O. Kaplan), p. 485. Academic Press, New York.

———. 1986. On the economics of binding energies. In *Proceedings of the XVIII Solday Conference on Chemistry: Design and synthesis of organic molecules based on molecular recognition* (ed. G. van Binst), p. 59. Springer-Verlag, Berlin.

Johnson, K.A. 1985. Pathway of the microtubule-dynein ATPase and the structure of dynein: A comparison with actomyosin. *Annu. Rev. Biophys. Biophys. Chem.* **14:** 161.

Johnson, K.A. and E.W. Taylor. 1978. Intermediate states of subfragment 1 and actosubfragment 1 ATPase: Reevaluation of the mechanism. *Biochemistry* **17:** 3432.

Kornberg, A. 1980. *DNA replication.* Freeman Publications, San Francisco.

Koshland, D.E., Jr. 1984. Control of enzyme activity and metabolic pathways. *Trends Biochem. Sci.* **9:** 155.

Kuchta, R.D., V. Mizrahi, P.A. Benkovic, K.A. Johnson, and S.J. Benkovic. 1987. The kinetic mechanism of DNA polymerase I. *Biochemistry* (in press).

Lilius, E.-M., V.-M. Multanen, and V. Toivonen. 1979. Quantitative extraction and estimation of intracellular nicotin-amide nucleotides of *Escherichia coli. Anal. Biochem.* **99:** 22.

Loeb, L.A. And T.A. Kunkel. 1982. Fidelity of DNA synthesis. *Annu. Rev. Biochem.* **52:** 429.

Mayer, R.J., J.-T. Chen, K. Taira, C.A. Fierke, and S.J. Benkovic. 1986. Importance of a hydrophobic residue in binding and catalysis by dihydrofolate reductase. *Proc. Natl. Acad. Sci.* **83:** 7718.

Mizrahi, V., R.N. Henrie, J.F. Marlier, K.A. Johnson, and S.J. Benkovic. 1985. Rate-limiting steps in the DNA polymerase I reaction pathway. *Biochemistry* **24:** 4010.

Moore, J.W. and R.G. Pearson. 1981. *Kinetics and mechanism.* Wiley-Interscience, New York.

Newsholme, E.A. and B. Crabtree. 1981. Flux-generating and regulatory steps in metabolic control. *Trends Biochem. Sci.* **6:** 53.

Ninio, J. 1975. Kinetic amplification of enzyme discrimination. *Biochimie* **57:** 587.

Raines, R. 1986. "Perfection in enzymatic catalysis: The energetic consequences of maximizing *in vivo* flux." Ph.D. thesis, Harvard University, Cambridge, Massachusetts.

Rosenfeld, S.S. and E.W. Taylor. 1984. Reactions of 1-N^6-ethenoadenosine nucleotides with myosin subfragment 1 and acto-subfragment 1 of skeletal and smooth muscle. *J. Biol. Chem.* **259:** 11920.

Stackhouse, J., K.P. Nambiar, J.J. Burbaum, D.M. Stauffer, and S.A. Benner. 1985. Dynamic transduction of energy and equilibria in enzymes. A reexamination of pyruvate kinase. *J. Am. Chem. Soc.* **107:** 2757.

Stein, L.A., P.B. Chock, and E. Eisenberg. 1981. Mechanism of the actomyosin ATPase: Effect of actin on the ATP hydrolysis step. *Proc. Natl. Acad. Sci.* **78:** 1346.

Taylor, E.W. 1979. Mechanism of actomyosin ATPase and the problem of muscle contraction. *Crit. Rev. Biochem.* **8:** 103.

Trybus, K.M. and E.W. Taylor. 1982. Transient kinetics of adenosine 5'-diphosphate and adenosine 5'-(β,γ-imidotriphosphate) binding to subfragment 1 and actosubfragment 1. *Biochemistry* **21:** 1284.

White, H.D. and E.W. Taylor. 1976. Energetics and mechanism of actomyosin adenosine triphosphatase. *Biochemistry* **15:** 5818.

Young, M., G. Wasserman, P. Benkovic, and S. Benkovic. 1985. Kinetic investigations of potential channelling between enzymes involved in de novo purine biosynthesis. In *Proceedings of the Second Workshop on Folyl and Antifolyl Polyglutamates* (ed. I.D. Goldman), p. 76. Praeger, New York.

Kinetic Devices in Protein Synthesis, DNA Replication, and Mismatch Repair

J. NINIO

Institut Jacques Monod du C.N.R.S., 75251 Paris Cedex 05, France

Enzymes are reputed to accomplish highly specialized tasks, thanks to an active site whose shape matches closely that of the substrate. The cell also needs general practitioner enzymes, just so for the tasks requiring the highest accuracy. Thus, a single macromolecular assembly, the ribosome, must select a correct tRNA in response to 61 different codons. A polymerase must insert the correct nucleotide in response to each of the four nucleotides of the template. For such situations, designing a clever binding site is not enough. The greatest attention must be paid to the "wiring diagram" of the reaction mechanism and to the time window allocated to each step. The following intuitive example illustrates the importance of appropriate timing. After a DNA replication error is made, mismatch binding proteins detect the error, which is ultimately excised from the newly synthesized patch of DNA carrying it. In *Escherichia coli*, the repair system distinguishes the daughter strand of DNA, on which lies the error, from the parental strand by the fact that it is undermethylated (Radman et al. 1980). After a while, when both strands are methylated, it is too late. Repair requires a methylating enzyme to label the strands, but when this enzyme is overproduced, the time window for repair is too narrow, and the strain becomes hypermutable (Herman and Modrich 1981).

In this spirit, the kinetic theory of accuracy relates the error rates in complex processes to the kinetics of substrate processing. It teaches how to read an enzyme reaction scheme and interpret it in terms of choice strategies. It successfully predicted a number of now well-established effects like the influence on replication errors at one site, of the concentration of nucleotide to be incorporated next, or the stoichiometry of GTP consumption to amino acid incorporation in protein synthesis in response to a given codon, according to whether cognate or noncognate tRNAs are used. The most publicized aspect of this theory is the concept of kinetic proofreading or kinetic amplification (Hopfield 1974; Ninio 1975). I shall concentrate here on more elementary principles, which are at work in almost every experimental situation, and whose manifestations continue to mystify many biologists. A broad coverage of the field, including the required mathematics, can be found in Kirkwood et al. (1986).

Kinetic Modulation

Take a black and white photograph of a white, a grey, and a black ball, over a white background. De-pending on the exposure time and the contrast grade of the paper print, the darkness of the balls will appear in various ratios. Similarly, by changing in a nonspecific way the rate constant for a step in an enzyme reaction, the apparent specificity of the enzyme may change. This is the effect we will now explore.

Consider an enzyme acting on two substrates, correct and incorrect, that differ by their sticking times to the enzyme, θ^C and θ^I. Assume this is the only property by which the substrates are distinguished, and assume the enzyme takes, on average, a time τ to convert S into P. Then, the probability of transforming a bound substrate into product is, for a Michaelis enzyme (Ninio 1974),

$$p(\theta, \tau) = \theta/(\theta + \tau) \tag{1}$$

so that the discrimination—the ratio of correct to incorrect products at equal collision frequencies of the substrates—is

$$D = \frac{\theta^C}{\theta^I} \times \frac{\theta^I + \tau}{\theta^C + \tau} \tag{2}$$

By changing τ, which is a characteristic of the enzyme mechanics independent of substrate binding, one changes the discriminative power of the enzyme. If the enzyme is an extremely active one, τ will be small compared to the θs, both substrates are transformed into product with a probability of one, and there is no discrimination. If τ is large compared to the θs, the probability of converting a substrate into product will be proportional to θ, and discrimination given by the ratio θ^C/θ^I. Moderate changes in either θ or τ will have little effect on p if θ/τ is large, and almost proportional effects if θ/τ is small. Thus, sensitivity to context is a distinctive property of weak interactions, as observed repeatedly (e.g., Bouadloun et al. 1986).

Mutants of *E. coli* with high-fidelity or low-fidelity ribosomes are well known (Gorini 1971). Their effects on various types of protein synthesis errors can be analyzed in terms of general changes in the kinetic parameters of protein synthesis, the τs or the θs (Ninio 1974; Schwartz and Lysikov 1974; Blomberg 1977). Actually, if the kinetic interpretation is correct, one can calculate some kinetic parameters of translation in vivo. Thus, from the analysis of the data in Gorini (1971), the following proposals were made (Ninio 1974): On a wild-type ribosome, the efficiency of reading $p(\theta,\tau)$ of a codon by a cognate tRNA is about

90–99%. For nonsense suppressors su2, su3, and su7, it ranges from 30% to 90%. For the high-fidelity mutant *strA1* the efficiency would fall to about 50% for a cognate codon (two trials would be needed, on average, for each successful incorporation) and to 0.5–5% for the above suppressors.

There was formerly an alternative interpretation (Woese 1970; Gorini 1971). Depending upon the codon, the ribosome adopts a peculiar configuration that allows it to probe some part of the tRNA structure outside the anticodon, and determine whether or not the "tRNA type" matches the "codon type." Such ideas are still alive, in various amended forms. For Yarus (1982), a high-fidelity ribosome "is presumed to have a more tightly fitting template with which to compare the entire extended anticodon-message complex." If cognate tRNAs were tightly bound on high-fidelity ribosomes, their binding would be rarely abortive, and no extra GTP should be wasted to make a peptide bond. The opposite is observed. A high-fidelity ribosome does reject cognate tRNAs, so that the GTP consumed per amino acid incorporated may be twice as high as in wild-type ribosomes (Ruusala et al. 1984). A 50% drop in efficiency is just what was predicted 10 years before, using the kinetic ideas (Ninio 1974).

Similar kinetic modulation effects apply to DNA polymerases. Let us call k_2 the kinetic constant for excision, and k_1 the kinetic constant for nucleotide incorporation. Taking the simplest kinetic model, with just these two constants, the probability for a misincorporated nucleotide to escape from the editing function is

$$p = k_1[\text{dNTP}]/(k_2 + k_1[\text{dNTP}]) \qquad (3)$$

where the dNTP here is that to be incorporated after the error. From Equation 3, which is analogous to Equation 1, two effects are predicted (Ninio 1975; Bernardi and Ninio 1978; Galas and Branscomb 1978). First, the errors at one position must grow with the concentration of the nucleotide to be incorporated next. This "next nucleotide effect" has been established quite carefully in various systems (Fersht 1979; Kunkel et al. 1981). Second, by playing with the global nucleotide concentration one should be able to transform the phenotype of a polymerase mutant from low- to high- or high- to low-fidelity. This again has been confirmed with T4 polymerases (Clayton et al. 1979).

Choice Strategies and Memory

To optimize their choices, humans examine all possibilities, retain the most interesting ones, compare these, eventually reconsider the case, etc. The quality of the final decision depends on the capacity to compare in memory all competing offers. There is another choice strategy used by humans that requires little memory and may be applied to enzymes. It operates as follows: Examine a first offer, reject it, and raising accordingly one's acceptance threshold, look for a bet-

ter offer. If there is one, still raise the threshold. If after a certain time no valuable offer is made, lower the threshold. *E. coli* DNA polymerase I follows this logic: the more it polymerizes, the more active its editing function (Papanicolaou et al. 1986). Stringency increases with the availability of substrate.

An inverse strategy may apply to ribosomes. When a cell is starved for an amino acid, and a codon for this amino acid must be read, there is a deficit in cognate-acylated tRNA and errors are expected to increase in proportion to this deficit. This is not usually the case. Wild-type *E. coli* has a means to make up for substrate imbalance. The chosen strategy restores the accuracy at starved codons without changing the accuracy at other codons. Assume the ribosome is able to switch between a laxist state (small τ) and the stringent one (high τ). Just after making a peptide bond, it is in the laxist state. While it waits for the next tRNA, it has a given probability per unit time to fall into the stringent state. As the "offers" drop, it becomes more demanding. This scheme achieves effective but not complete error damping (Ninio 1986a).

Such a device might operate in mnemonic enzymes. These enzymes may switch between two states of high and low catalytic efficiency. The probability of being in one state rather than the other is influenced by the concentration of substrate (Ricard et al. 1986; Cornish-Bowden and Cárdenas 1987). The switch is perhaps a device to buffer metabolic errors against sudden substrate depletion.

There are some indications that ribosomes start synthesis inefficiently and progressively warm up: Synthesis often aborts after a few peptide bonds are made (Tanaka and Teraoka 1968). In parallel, the peptidyl-transferase center becomes more resistant to virginiamycin M (Chinali et al. 1987). Thus, independently of the "accuracy tuner," ribosomes would start synthesis in a stringent state, then proceed in the laxist state. Thus, the accuracy tuning effect could be difficult to demonstrate on the first peptide bonds. This may explain the discrepancy between the tenfold effect of ppGpp (which unlocks the accuracy tuner) in an in vitro protein synthesis system (Wagner et al. 1982), and the twofold effect observed in a dipeptide synthesis system (Dix and Thompson 1986).

An objection to the accuracy tuner, as formulated initially, was raised by Gallant (1986). Consider a nonsense codon. Since the concentration of release factor is very small, a nonsense codon is starved. Thus, the reading of these codons by nonsense suppressors should be sensitive to amino acid starvation (I gloss over the genetic technicalities), which is not the case (Weiss et al. 1984). Therefore, another element, which Gallant identifies as the binding of deacylated tRNA, must come into the picture. It would be during this binding that the ribosome would switch between the two states (Gallant 1986). This would make the accuracy tuner more effective. Furthermore, Gallant speculates that uncharged tRNA may be acylated on the ribosome, while bound to the A site. This proposal is less credible, for then, why would the ribosome need an active mechanism to expel deacylated tRNA (Richter 1976)? The question whether or not ribosomes stall at nonsense codons is an interesting one. Tate et al. (1983) suggest that the release factors may bind to the nonsense codon before reaching the A site. By the time the codon is presented by the ribosome, the local concentration in release factors may have increased significantly.

Whether or not some enzymes (or ribosomes) use duplicate binding sites to concentrate substrates in the vicinity of their active sites, and whether or not such a device might work efficiently is not known at present.

Proofreading and Amplification

Most DNA polymerases and aminoacyl tRNA ligases manufacture substantial amounts of incorrect products, then destroy these using associated editing (proofreading) activities. These activities are tuned to the elimination of the most prominent errors made in the synthetic step (Fersht and Dingwall 1979). Similarly, mismatch repair is most efficient on the errors made by the DNA polymerases and which escaped from immediate excision (Jones et al. 1987).

Tautomeries, considered to be a most likely source of replication errors, do not contribute significantly to the error spectrum. I speculate that the polymerases, in order to get rid of errors due to tautomeries, could use a mechanism involving a disruption of the last base pair as an obligate step. Replication would occur in two stages, at two different sites on the polymerase. First, the incoming dNTP would pair to the nucleotide to be replicated, unstacked, in a site 1. Then, the polymerase would open up this base pair and transfer the dNTP to a site 2, where it would come close to the free 3′ terminus of the primer. While the bond is synthesized, the replicated nucleotide would flip back, and the editing activity would then check the last base pair. If the first binding event is due to a tautomery, the transfer of the dNTP from site 1 to site 2, in the unpaired state, allows the nucleotide to return to its natural tautomeric form. Such a mechanism, suggested to me by the results of Lecomte et al. (1986) would explain why the dNTP- and dNMP-binding sites are wide apart in the crystal structure of E. coli Pol I large fragment (Ollis et al. 1985). The site identified as the proofreading site may also be the actual site for synthesis. However, this would not agree with the separation of polymerizing and proofreading activities on two different subunits of E. coli Pol III (Scheuermann and Echols 1984). If opening of the base pair is a mandatory step in the polymerase reaction, this also explains why DNA polymerases make only short fragments at low temperature, when base pairs are the most stable (McClure and Jovin 1975).

It is hard to see how the ribosome might probe the correctness of the product it just manufactured. Thus, other means of enhancing accuracy must be used. Returning to the analogy of the photographic picture of clear and dark objects over a clear background, what is needed is a high-contrast paper print that would provide a dark image of a dark object, and would be practically insensitive to a clear object, below a certain threshold of luminance. Ribosome discrimination was described above in terms of sticking time parameters, the θs, and characteristic times for making the peptide bond, the τs. The limiting discrimination, for the most usual mechanisms of reactions is given by θ^C/θ^I. How to go beyond that limit? By introducing a time delay T such that now, the ribosome discriminates according to $\theta^C - T$ and $\theta^I - T$. One clearly sees, on paper, that a ratio $(x - T)/(y - T)$ may be much larger than x/y when $x > y$. The difficulty, solved independently by Hopfield (1974) and Ninio (1975), was to construct a scheme that achieved this trick while obeying the classical constraints of enzyme kinetics. Let us see first the features the two schemes have in common, when applied to the ribosome.

In both cases, when tRNA binds to the ribosome it stays there according to a sticking time θ, and leaves the ribosome with a uniform probability per unit time. However, the presence of tRNA (eventually complexed with Tu and GTP) is not enough to allow efficient peptide bond formation. For this, a second event must occur, which requires GTP hydrolysis. The time delay T is the time that elapses from the instant of tRNA binding to the instant of GTP hydrolysis. During this time, the tRNA may leave as usual, but the peptide bond cannot be formed. Applied to ribosomes, Hopfield's scheme assumes that tRNA binds as an EF-Tu-GTP complex, which seems to be the general case, under normal conditions, in E. coli. The delayed reaction scheme of Ninio (1975) would require independent binding of tRNA and EF-Tu-GTP. A specific prediction of the scheme is that if EF-Tu-GTP binds in the absence of tRNA, there must be an efficient hydrolysis of GTP, which is in fact observed but rarely discussed (e.g., Thompson et al. 1986). In modern in vitro systems for studying protein synthesis (Ruusala et al. 1984; Dix and Thompson 1986), there is a large excess of tRNA–EF-Tu-GTP ternary complex. These systems confirm the validity of Hopfield's scheme but, by design, they do not probe the possible parallel pathway of independent tRNA and EF-Tu-GTP binding. The study of EF-Tu mutants (Vijgenboom et al. 1985) will perhaps clarify this point.

Although the kinetic amplification schemes may be difficult to understand, their implementation is particularly easy. For instance, in the scheme of independent binding of main substrate and energy donor, the amplification of specificity merely requires an activity of nonspecific hydrolysis of ATP or GTP in the absence of the other substrate.

There is another kinetic amplification scheme that uses memory (Hopfield 1980). Discrimination is also based on the θs. The enzyme may accomplish a catalytic act, from which it derives some free energy. The free energy is then used to enhance the accuracy of the reaction carried out with the next substrate.

In the case of an enzyme having an editing function, the discrimination of this function can be amplified by a kinetic trick (Ninio 1975; Hopfield 1978). What matters here is the time during which proofreading is exerted, between product formation and product departure. It is essential that the probability distribution of these times be skewed, with respect to the exponential decay, with a deficit of short time intervals. For instance, there must be a delay to the departure of the product.

On the other hand, there seems to be no way to amplify the discrimination of a forward step (Ninio 1977). For instance, if discrimination is based on different k_{cat}s with respect to correct and incorrect substrates, it is impossible to form products in ratios greater than the correct/incorrect k_{cat} ratios, assuming equal substrate concentrations.

Diffusional Proofreading and Mismatch Repair

Mismatch repair in bacteria corrects all polymerization errors but one in a hundred or one in a thousand (for reviews, see Claverys and Lacks 1986; Radman and Wagner 1986). A detecting enzyme or enzyme complex binds to a site of mismatch in double-stranded DNA. After that, other proteins open the DNA on both sides, on a section of a few hundred nucleotides, cut out the DNA strand containing the error, thus leaving a wide gap, which is then refilled by a DNA polymerase.

Let us compare the error levels before and after mismatch correction. Consider a chromosome of length L and assume the DNA polymerase makes E errors on average. Its error rate per incorporated nucleotide is E/L. Consider now that a mismatch has a probability p of being detected, and let l be the length of the excision track. On average, a DNA length of $(pE)l$ will be subject to resynthesis. Now mismatch detection is itself subject to errors, so let q be the probability of an illegitimate detection, leading to removal of an entirely correct DNA section. A further $(qL)l$ stretch of DNA will have to be resynthesized for this reason. Let f be the error rate of the polymerase responsible for resynthesis. After mismatch repair there are still some errors originating from two sources: the original replication errors that escaped detection, amounting to $E(1-p)$ and the errors generated by resynthesis. The average number F of errors after repair is thus:

$$F = E(1-p) + (pE + qL)lf \qquad (4)$$

If a factor of 10^3 must be gained in accuracy, $F/E = 10^{-3}$ by definition, and two conditions must be satisfied separately:

$$1 - p < 10^{-3} \qquad (5)$$

$$(pE + qL)lf < 10^{-3}E \qquad (6)$$

Condition 5 is obvious and says that the detecting enzyme may not leave more than one mismatch in a

thousand undetected. In the previous sections we discussed enzyme accuracy in terms of the probability of abortion of reactions involving the incorrect substrate. The price for accuracy was a reduced efficiency toward the correct substrate. Here, the cognate substrate of the detecting protein must be processed with almost absolute efficiency. Let us examine the requirements toward the noncognate substrate. Equation 4 gives some indications, but since it contains too many variables, we shall eliminate one by assuming that the two sources of errors contribute about equally to the final error level, thus

$$E(1-p) = (pE + qL)lf \qquad (7)$$

$$\frac{1}{f} = \frac{L}{E}\left(\frac{ql}{1-p}\right) + \frac{pl}{1-p} \qquad (8)$$

Take the case where the error rate of the major polymerase is $e = E/L = 10^{-6}$, and assume an accuracy gain by mismatch repair of 10^3, thus $1 - p = 10^{-3} = (1-p)/p$ and, rearranging Equation 8,

$$f = \frac{10^{-3}}{l} \times \frac{1}{1 + \dfrac{q}{e}} \qquad (9)$$

Consider an average repair patch of length $l = 1000$ and a situation where the probability of excising a patch without mismatch is 10^{-5}. For one legitimate excision, there would be ten illegitimate ones. f would be equal to 10^{-7}, which means that the repair polymerase must be ten times more accurate than the major polymerase. In *E. coli* long-patch resynthesis is under the responsibility of Pol III, so that we may assume equal fidelities of replication and repair synthesis: $f = e = 10^{-6}$. This is realistic if the size of repair patches is about 300 instead of 1000, and the accuracy gain by repair is also 300 rather than 1000.

The major unsolved problem is how to achieve a high efficiency of detection. One may think of just raising the production of detecting proteins. To switch from a 0.99 binding probability to the desired 0.999 probability, one would need to multiply by ten the concentration of proteins, thus multiplying by ten the number of illegitimate detections. We would lose on one side what we gained on the other. Note, by the way, that an overproducer of detecting proteins would have a mutator phenotype.

What is needed is a device by which a mismatch would have the effect of raising the concentration of detecting enzymes in its vicinity. Imagine the detecting protein accomplishing a random walk on the DNA and passing through the mismatch. We would like the mismatch to modify the parameters of the random walk in such a way as to increase significantly the probability of subsequent return of the protein, within a defined interval of time. This model implies that the detecting enzyme moves in both directions with equal probability (otherwise, the chances of return would be too small).

I thus imagine that there are three modes of binding of the detecting protein. The protein would have the capacity to collapse over a DNA section, but normally it would be locked in a noncollapsible state. At the beginning, the protein performs a random walk on the DNA. An encounter with the mismatch unlocks the enzyme, making it capable of collapsing, and also alters the parameters of the random walk (by changing the frictional properties of the protein). Of course, neither of these two events needs to be absolutely specific. Our understanding of diffusional processes within the cell is too poor yet to allow us to make a precise treatment of the scheme. However, the model of unlocking and collapse leads to a broad prediction. A protein may be used only once (unless there is another protein to energize it) and this property may in principle be demonstrated in vitro. Note that kamikaze enzymes are involved in the repair of some chemical lesions (Lindahl et al. 1982). In vivo, the cell may repair only a limited number of mismatches, not greater than the number of detecting proteins. Beyond that number, there should be a neat saturation of the capacity for repair. This is observed in several cases (e.g., Rydberg 1977). Beyond a certain level of errors, cells behave as though they were completely deficient for mismatch repair.

Ambiguity Displacements and Codon-anticodon Recognition

The wobble hypothesis (Crick 1966) is a historical accident. It would perhaps not have seen the light of day, had the first sequenced tRNA been a tRNA$_f^{Val}$ from *E. coli* rather than a tRNA^{Ala} from yeast. The tRNA$_f^{Val}$ anticodon VAC where V is uridine 5-oxyacetic acid probably reads the codons GUU, GUA, GUG, whereas the wobble hypothesis would have suggested an anticodon IAC reading the codons GUU, GUC, and GUA.

The present results, taken together (for review, see Buckingham and Grosjean 1986), give an impression of great disorder, and the temptation is great to be satisfied with the doctrine that everything matters—the ribosome structure, the nucleotides adjacent to the anticodon, the elongation factors, etc. There are many in vitro results suggesting more flexible reading rules than predicted by the wobble. Most codons may be read through unorthodox third-position pairings (Samuelson et al. 1983) or even first- or second-position mispairings (Hornig et al. 1984; Nègre et al. 1986). In vivo, in yeast, the amber codon UAG is read by a normal tRNA^{Gln} through first-position mispairing (Weiss and Friedberg 1986). On the other side, third-position reading may be stricter than predicted by the wobble hypothesis. Thus, in *Schizosaccharomyces pombe*, the serine codon UCA *is not* read by the anticodon IGA (Munz et al. 1981). Furthermore, there is nowhere evidence that inosine in the wobble position has a wider reading spectrum than guanine.

The most disquieting case is the glycine codon GGA. It is normally read in *E. coli* by a glycine tRNA with anticodon U*CC, U* being an unknown derivative of U (Murgola and Pagel 1980). The single-copy gene for this tRNA may be mutated in the anticodon region, thus generating a mixed missense/nonsense suppressor for codons UGA and UGG, the anticodon being U*CA. *E. coli* still grows, under these circumstances, although not in all usual media. By which tRNA is the glycine codon now read? Most specialists would have suspected one of the other two remaining glycine tRNAs, through an extended third-position wobble. Actually, the codon is read by its mutated tRNA, through first-position mispairing (Prather et al. 1981). Observations of this kind become intelligible by making use of a principle which is both crude and subtle (Ninio 1971). I assume that (1) the physical ambiguity of codon-anticodon recognition is "less unsymmetrical with respect to the three positions of the codon-anticodon association than assumed by the wobble hypothesis," (2) by suppressing some anticodons, or by modifying nucleotides in the anticodons so as to decrease by the same amount the interactions with cognate and noncognate codons, translation can become, on the whole, more accurate. A third-position wobble may be a camouflage for a first-position ambiguity!

Let us take, as in Table 1, a tRNA for glycine with an anticodon 3'CCG5', which would read the glycine codon GGC by Watson-Crick base pairs, the glycine codon GGU by wobble in position 3, the serine codon AGC by C·A mispair in the first position, and the serine codon AGU by first-position mispairing and third-position wobble. Sticking times are as in Table 1. In the initial situation, the tRNA sticks as well to the cognate codon GGU as to the noncognate codon AGC. The rule of the game is to improve specificity without ever acting specifically on the first position. In column 2 of Table 1, we perform the essential trick, which is to equalize G·C and G·U pairing in position 3. Then, we use the subsidiary tricks discussed in the previous sections: We decrease all sticking times by the same factor (column 3) and we take proofreading into account (column 4). If formerly, the codon GGU was read by another, error-prone tRNA, and there was no way to make it work more accurately, this tRNA may now be eliminated.

It is widely believed that tRNA structure is optimized for efficient reading (Yarus 1982; Yarus et al. 1986). However, if we analyze the post-transcriptional modifications in the anticodon loops, it becomes clear that most of them either increase binding and decrease accuracy, or decrease binding and increase accuracy. Here are a few examples. The A → ms^{2}i^{6}A modification belongs to the first type. Strains deficient for this modification make fewer errors than wild type (e.g., Janner et al. 1980; Bouadloun et al. 1986). The decrease in binding strength can be demonstrated both in vitro (Houssier and Grosjean 1985) and in vivo by the frequent release of unfinished peptides (Petrullo and Elseviers 1986). The C → N^4-acetyl cytidine modification belongs to the second type. In *E. coli*, initiator tRNA$_f^{Met}$ reads several codons besides AUG, using

Table 1. Conversion of a First-position Ambiguity into a Third-position Degeneracy

Anticodon: 3' CCG 5'		Initial situation		Equalize G.C and G.U in wobble position		Divide all θs by 10		Amplify p^2
		θ	p	θ	p	θ	p	p^2
Glycine codons	GGU	1000	0.9	5000	0.98	500	0.84	0.7
	GGC	25000	0.99	5000	0.98	500	0.84	0.7
	GGA	100	0.5	100	0.5	10	0.09	0.08
	GGG	100	0.5	100	0.5	10	0.09	0.08
Serine codons	AGU	40	0.29	200	0.66	20	0.165	0.028
	AGC	1000	0.9	200	0.66	20	0.165	0.028

The elongation probabilities, given by p, are calculated according to Eq. 1, assuming $\tau = 100$. Starting with a situation in which first-position are not less stable than third-position mismatches, we end up with a clear discrimination between legitimate and illegitimate interactions. The essential trick is to act upon the G in the wobble position, so as to weaken G.C pairing and equalize it with G.U pairing.

first-position mismatches. It has a normal C in the wobble position, whereas the elongator $tRNA_m^{Met}$ has an N^4-acetyl cytidine. If this nucleotide is chemically converted to C, there is an increase in binding efficiency, and a widening of the reading spectrum of the tRNA (Stern and Schulman 1978), just as predicted (Ninio 1971).

I suggest that most modifications of U in the wobble position of eubacterial or eukaryotic tRNAs increase both orthodox binding and misreadings (e.g., Colby et al. 1976; Grossenbacher et al. 1986), whereas modification of C (Comer et al. 1975; Stern and Schulman 1978) or G (Bienz and Kubli 1981; Beier et al. 1984) decrease normal binding and increase accuracy.

Implicit in Table 1 is the idea that the difference between the first and third positions does not lie in the basic ambiguity of base pairings here and there. It lies in the fact that the pairing properties may be more easily manipulated in the third than in the first position. This is consistent with our representation of the anticodon loop (e.g., Fuller and Hodgson 1967; Westhof et al. 1983). There is a paradoxical result going in this direction. The $A \rightarrow ms^2i^6A$ modification affects the (remote) third-position errors, but is without influence on the (adjacent) first-position errors (Bouadloun et al. 1986). If general, this result would be of crucial importance to our understanding of the code.

There are a few points in my original hypothesis (Ninio 1971) that need revision. Discrimination was discussed in terms of free-energy differences between cognate and noncognate interactions, whereas we would rather speak now of elongation probabilities (Eq. 2). In analyzing possible mismatches, the $U \cdot C$ pair was given excessive weight. Modern estimates make it the least stable one and highlight instead the $G \cdot G$ pair (Papanicolaou et al. 1984; Aboul-ela et al. 1985). The variety of resources the cell can mobilize to enhance accuracy was not fully appreciated, and the discussion focused too narrowly on anticodon sequences.

The evolution of tRNA was then viewed as always moving in the direction of lower efficiencies. I see it now as a zigzag motion. From a state 1 of efficiency e_1 and accuracy a_1, a first change leads to a state 2 of

efficiency $e_2 < e_1$ and accuracy $a_2 > a_1$. Then a second change, in the opposite direction, would lead to $e_3 > e_2$ and $a_3 < a_2$, the overall effect of the two changes being a slight gain either in accuracy or in efficiency, for instance: $e_3 = e_1$ and a_3 slightly superior to a_1. The central thesis that an ambiguity somewhere can be converted into a degeneracy elsewhere must be reemphasized. One of the most general predictions that can be derived from this framework concerns the heterologous systems.

Consider two translation apparatuses taken from phylogenetically distant organisms. Translation is accurate in both systems. What happens if one adds to one system a tRNA species extracted from the other? If we follow Yarus (1982) and believe that every tRNA is fully optimized to bind to its cognate ribosome, and the ribosome checks an extended portion of the tRNA, ribosomes are expected to ignore or reject the heterologous tRNAs. If, on the contrary, tRNA design is a result of a large number of compromises on strength and accuracy, and mutual adjustments with the other tRNAs of the same cell, then mixing the components of two translation apparatuses must lead to high error levels. A tRNA from one species may read both cognate and noncognate codons on ribosomes of another species (Ninio 1971). This feature is repeatedly observed in heterologous translation systems (Bergquist et al. 1968; Richer 1978; Grosjean et al. 1980).

Let us push this idea to its ultimate consequence. Consider an in vivo situation where there is some mixing of the components of two translation apparatuses due to endosymbiosis (the mitochondria), predation (the protozoan ciliates), or infection (the mycoplasms). Then, the translation of one particular codon may be so ambiguous that the assignment of this codon could evolve. This might be the key to the observed divergence in the genetic code (Ninio 1983, 1986b).

REFERENCES

Aboul-ela, F., D. Koh, and I. Tinoco, Jr. 1985. Base-base mismatches. Thermodynamics of double helix formation for $dCA_3XA_3G + dCT_3YT_3G$ (X, Y = A,C,G,T). *Nucleic Acids Res.* **13:** 4811.

Beier, H., M. Barciszewska, and H.-D. Sickinger. 1984. The molecular basis for the differential translation of TMV RNA in tobacco protoplasts and wheat germ extracts. *EMBO J.* **3**: 1091.

Bergquist, P.L., D.W.J. Burns, and C.A. Plinston. 1968. Participation of redundant transfer ribonucleic acids from yeast in protein synthesis. *Biochemistry* **7**: 1751.

Bernardi, F. and J. Ninio. 1978. The accuracy of DNA replication. *Biochimie* **60**: 1083.

Bienz, M. and E. Kubli. 1981. Wild-type tRNA$_G^{Tyr}$ reads the TMV-RNA stop codon, but Q base-modified tRNA$_Q^{Tyr}$ does not. *Nature* **294**: 188.

Blomberg, C. 1977. The kinetic recognition process for tRNA at the ribosome. *J. Theor. Biol.* **66**: 307.

Bouadloun, F., T. Srichaiyo, L.A. Isaksson, and G.R. Björk. 1986. Influence of modification next to the anticodon in tRNA on codon context sensitivity of translational suppression and accuracy. *J. Bacteriol.* **166**: 1022.

Buckingham, R.H. and H. Grosjean. 1986. The accuracy of mRNA-tRNA recognition. In *Accuracy in molecular processes. Its control and relevance to living systems* (ed. T.B.L. Kirkwood et al.), p. 83. Chapman and Hall, London.

Chinali, G., M. Di Giambattista, and C. Cocito. 1987. Ribosome protection by tRNA derivatives against inactivation by virginiamycin M: Evidence for two types of interaction of tRNA with the donor site of peptidyl transferase. *Biochemistry* **26**: 1592.

Claverys, J.-P. and S.A. Lacks. 1986. Heteroduplex deoxyribonucleic acid base mismatch repair in bacteria. *Microbiol. Rev.* **50**: 133.

Clayton, L.K., M.F. Goodman, E.W. Branscomb, and D.J. Galas. 1979. Error induction and correction by mutant and wild type T4 DNA polymerases. Kinetic error discrimination mechanisms. *J. Biol. Chem.* **254**: 1902.

Colby, D.S., P. Schedl, and C. Guthrie. 1976. A functional requirement for modification of the wobble nucleotide in the anticodon of a T4 suppressor tRNA. *Cell* **9**: 449.

Comer, M.M., K. Foss, and W.H. McClain. 1975. A mutation of the wobble nucleotide of a bacteriophage T4 transfer RNA. *J. Mol. Biol.* **99**: 283.

Cornish-Bowden, A. and M.L. Cárdenas. 1987. Co-operativity in monomeric enzymes. *J. Theor. Biol.* **124**: 1.

Crick, F.H.C. 1966. Codon-anticodon pairing: The wobble hypothesis. *J. Mol. Biol.* **19**: 548.

Dix, D.B. and R.C. Thompson. 1986. Elongation factor Tu-guanosine 3'-diphosphate 5'-diphosphate complex increases the fidelity of proofreading in protein biosynthesis: Mechanism for reducing translational errors introduced by amino acid starvation. *Proc. Natl. Acad. Sci.* **83**: 2027.

Fersht, A.R. 1979. Fidelity of replication of phage φX174 DNA by DNA polymerase III holoenzyme: Spontaneous mutation by misincorporation. *Proc. Natl. Acad. Sci.* **76**: 4946.

Fersht, A.R. and C. Dingwall. 1979. Evidence for the double-sieve editing mechanism for selection of amino acids in protein synthesis: Steric exclusion of isoleucine by valyl-tRNA synthetases. *Biochemistry* **18**: 2627.

Fuller, W. and A. Hodgson. 1967. Conformation of the anticodon loop in tRNA. *Nature* **215**: 817.

Galas, D.J. and E.W. Branscomb. 1978. Enzymatic determinants of DNA polymerase accuracy. Theory of coliphage T4 polymerase mechanisms. *J. Mol. Biol.* **124**: 653.

Gallant, J.A. 1986. Uncharged tRNA error damping model. *FEBS Lett.* **206**: 185.

Gorini, L. 1971. Ribosomal discrimination of tRNAs. *Nature* **234**: 261.

Grosjean, H., S. de Henau, C. Houssier, and R.H. Buckingham. 1980. Wild-type *E. coli* tRNA^{Trp} efficiently suppresses UGA opal codon in an eukaryotic cell-free protein synthesis: Evolutionary implications. *Arch. Int. Physiol. Biochim.* **88**: 168.

Grossenbacher, A.-M., B. Stadelmann, W.-D. Heyer, P. Thuriaux, J. Kohli, C. Smith, P.F. Agris, K.C. Kuo, and C. Gehrke. 1986. Antisuppressor mutations and sulfur-carrying nucleosides in transfer RNAs of *Schizosaccharomyces pombe*. *J. Biol. Chem.* **261**: 16351.

Herman, G.E. and P. Modrich. 1981. *Escherichia coli* K12 clones that overproduce *dam* methylase are hypermutable. *J. Bacteriol.* **145**: 644.

Hopfield, J.J. 1974. Kinetic proofreading: A new mechanism for reducing errors in biosynthetic processes requiring high specificity. *Proc. Natl. Acad. Sci.* **71**: 4135.

———. 1978. Origin of the genetic code: A testable hypothesis based on tRNA structure, sequence, and kinetic proofreading. *Proc. Natl. Acad. Sci.* **75**: 4334.

———. 1980. The energy relay: A proofreading scheme based on dynamic cooperativity and lacking all characteristic symptoms of kinetic proofreading in DNA replication and protein synthesis. *Proc. Natl. Acad. Sci.* **77**: 5248.

Hornig, H., P. Woolley, and R. Lührmann. 1984. Decoding at the ribosomal A site. The effect of a defined codon-anticodon mismatch upon the behaviour of bound aminoacyl transfer RNA. *J. Biol. Chem.* **259**: 5632.

Houssier, C. and H. Grosjean. 1985. Temperature jump relaxation studies on the interactions between transfer RNAs with complementary anticodons: The effect of modified bases adjacent to the anticodon triplet. *J. Biomol. Struct. Dyn.* **3**: 387.

Janner, F., G. Vögeli, and R. Fluri. 1980. The antisuppressor strain *sin1* of *Schizosaccharomyces pombe* lacks the modification isopentenyladenosine in transfer RNA. *J. Mol. Biol.* **139**: 207.

Jones, M., R. Wagner, and M. Radman. 1987. Repair of a mismatch is influenced by the base composition of the surrounding nucleotide sequence. *Genetics* **115**: 605.

Kirkwood, T.B.L., R.F. Rosenberger, and D.J. Galas, eds. 1986. *Accuracy in molecular processes. Its control and relevance to living systems.* Chapman and Hall, London.

Kunkel, T.A., R.M. Schaaper, R.A. Beckman, and L.A. Loeb. 1981. On the fidelity of DNA replication. Effect of the next nucleotide on proofreading. *J. Biol. Chem.* **256**: 9883.

Lecomte, P., O.P. Doubleday, and M. Radman. 1986. Evidence for an intermediate in DNA synthesis involving pyrophosphate exchange. A possible role in fidelity. *J. Mol. Biol.* **189**: 643.

Lindahl, T., B. Demple, and P. Robins. 1982. Suicide inactivation of the *E. coli* O^6-methylguanine-DNA methyltransferase. *EMBO J.* **1**: 1359.

McClure, W.R. and T.M. Jovin. 1975. The steady state kinetic parameters and non-processivity of *Escherichia coli* deoxyribonucleic acid polymerase I. *J. Biol. Chem.* **250**: 4073.

Munz, P., U. Leupold, P. Agris, and J. Kohli. 1981. *In vivo* decoding rules in *Schizosaccharomyces pombe* are at variance with in vitro data. *Nature* **294**: 187.

Murgola, E.J. and F.T. Pagel. 1980. Codon recognition by glycine transfer RNAs of *Escherichia coli* in vivo. *J. Mol. Biol.* **138**: 833.

Nègre, D., A.J. Cozzone, and Y. Cenatiempo. 1986. Accuracy of natural messenger translation: Analysis of codon-anticodon recognition in a simplified cell-free system. *Biochemistry* **25**: 6391.

Ninio, J. 1971. Codon-anticodon recognition: The missing triplet hypothesis. *J. Mol. Biol.* **56**: 63.

———. 1974. A semi-quantitative treatment of missense and nonsense suppression in the *strA* and *ram* ribosomal mutants of *Escherichia coli*. Evaluation of some molecular parameters of translation in vivo. *J. Mol. Biol.* **84**: 297.

———. 1975. Kinetic amplification of enzyme discrimination. *Biochimie* **57**: 587.

———. 1977. Are further kinetic amplification schemes possible? *Biochimie* **59**: 759.

———. 1983. *Molecular approaches to evolution.* Princeton University Press, Princeton.

————. 1986a. Fine tuning of ribosomal accuracy. *FEBS Lett.* **196**: 1.

————. 1986b. Divergence in the genetic code. *Biochem. Syst. Ecol.* **14**: 455.

Ollis, D.L., P. Brick, R. Hamlin, N.G. Xuong, and T.A. Steitz. 1985. Structure of large fragment of *Escherichia coli* DNA polymerase I complexed with dTMP. *Nature* **313**: 762.

Papanicolaou, C., M. Gouy, and J. Ninio. 1984. An energy model that predicts the correct folding of both the tRNA and the 5S RNA molecules. *Nucleic Acids Res.* **12**: 31.

Papanicolaou, C., P. Lecomte, and J. Ninio. 1986. Mnemonic aspects of *E. coli* DNA Polymerase I. Interaction with one template influences the next interaction with another template. *J. Mol. Biol.* **189**: 435.

Petrullo, L.A. and D. Elseviers. 1986. Effect of a 2-methyl-thio-N6-isopentenyladenosine deficiency on peptidyl-tRNA release in *Escherichia coli*. *J. Bacteriol.* **165**: 608.

Prather, N.E., E.J. Murgola, and B.H. Mims. 1981. Primary structure of an unusual glycine tRNA UGA suppressor. *Nucleic Acids Res.* **9**: 6421.

Radman, M. and R. Wagner. 1986. Mismatch repair in *Escherichia coli*. *Annu. Rev. Genet.* **20**: 523.

Radman, M., R.E. Wagner, B.W. Glickman, and M. Meselson. 1980. DNA methylation, mismatch correction and genetic stability. In *Progress in environmental mutagenesis* (ed. M. Alacevic), p. 121. Elsevier, Amsterdam.

Ricard, J., J.-M. Soulié, J. Buc, and M. Bidaud. 1986. Kinetic implications of the occurrence of several relaxations in the conformational transition of mnemonical enzymes. *Eur. J. Biochem.* **159**: 247.

Richer, L.L. 1978. The efficiency of methionine incorporation from isoaccepting species of tRNA^{Met} into rabbit globin in an homologous reticulocyte lysate system. *Biochim. Biophys. Acta* **517**: 76.

Richter, D. 1976. Stringent factor from *Escherichia coli* directs ribosomal binding and release of uncharged tRNA. *Proc. Natl. Acad. Sci.* **73**: 707.

Ruusala, T., D. Andersson, M. Ehrenberg, and C.G. Kurland. 1984. Hyper-accurate ribosomes inhibit growth. *EMBO J.* **3**: 2575.

Rydberg, B. 1977. Bromouracil mutagenesis in *Escherichia coli*. Evidence for involvement of mismatch repair. *Mol. Gen. Genet.* **152**: 19.

Samuelson, T., T. Axberg, T. Boren, and U. Lagerkvist. 1983. Unconventional reading of the glycine codons. *J. Biol. Chem.* **258**: 13178.

Scheuermann, R.H. and H. Echols. 1984. A separate editing exonuclease for DNA replication: The ε subunit of *Escherichia coli* DNA polymerase III holoenzyme. *Proc. Natl. Acad. Sci.* **81**: 7747.

Schwartz, V.S. and V.N. Lysikov. 1974. Physical mechanisms of ribosomal screen. (In Russian). *Dokl. Akad. Nauk SSR* **217**: 1446.

Stern, L. and L.H. Schulman. 1978. The role of the minor base N^4-acetylcytidine in the function of the *Escherichia coli* noninitiator methionine transfer RNA. *J. Biol. Chem.* **253**: 6132.

Tanaka, K. and H. Teraoka. 1968. Effect of erythromycin on polylysine synthesis directed by polyadenylic acid in an *Escherichia coli* cell-free system. *J. Biochem.* **64**: 635.

Tate, W.P., H. Hornig, and R. Lührmann. 1983. Recognition of termination codon by release factor in the presence of a tRNA-occupied A site. Evidence for flexibility in accommodation of the release factor on the ribosome. *J. Biol. Chem.* **258**: 10360.

Thompson, R.C., D.B. Dix, and A.M. Karim. 1986. The reaction of ribosomes with elongation factor Tu · GTP complexes. Aminoacyl-tRNA independent reactions in the elongation cycle determine the accuracy of protein synthesis. *J. Biol. Chem.* **261**: 4868.

Vijgenboom, E., T. Vink, B. Kraal, and L. Bosch. 1985. Mutants of the elongation factor EF-Tu, a new class of nonsense suppressors. *EMBO J.* **4**: 1049.

Wagner, E.G.H., M. Ehrenberg, and C.G. Kurland. 1982. Kinetic suppresssion of translational errors by (p)ppGpp. *Mol. Gen. Genet.* **185**: 269.

Weiss, R., J. Murphy, G. Wagner, and J. Gallant. 1984. The ribosome's frame of mind. *Proc. Alfred Benz. Symp.* **19**: 208.

Weiss, W.A. and E.C. Friedberg. 1986. Normal yeast tRNA$_{CAG}^{Gln}$ can suppress amber codons and is encoded by an essential gene. *J. Mol. Biol.* **192**: 725.

Westhof, E., P. Dumas, and D. Moras. 1983. Loop stereochemistry and dynamics in transfer RNA. *J. Biomol. Struct. Dyn.* **1**: 337.

Woese, C.R. 1970. Codon recognition: The allosteric ribosome hypothesis. *J. Theor. Biol.* **26**: 83.

Yarus, M. 1982. Translational efficiency of transfer RNA's: Uses of an extended anticodon. *Science* **218**: 646.

Yarus, M., S.W. Cline, P. Wier, L. Breeden, and R.C. Thompson. 1986. Actions of the anticodon arm in translation on the phenotypes of RNA mutants. *J. Mol. Biol.* **192**: 235.

On the Evolution of Specificity and Catalysis in Subtilisin

J.A. WELLS,* B.C. CUNNINGHAM,* T.P. GRAYCAR,[†] D.A. ESTELL,[†] AND P. CARTER*
*Department of Biomolecular Chemistry, Genentech Incorporated, South San Francisco, California 94080;
[†]Research Department, Genencor, Incorporated, South San Francisco, California 94080

Serine proteases are present in almost all organisms and exhibit a wide range of substrate specificities (for reviews, see Stroud 1974; Kraut 1977). The enzymes are characterized by a set of three catalytic residues consisting of a serine, a histidine, and an aspartic acid (the catalytic triad). Nature has apparently evolved the catalytic triad structure and the resulting serine protease mechanism at least twice. In particular, subtilisin (from species of bacillus) and chymotrypsin (from mammalian pancreas) are genetically unrelated and their corresponding tertiary structures are entirely different. However, it is possible to virtually superimpose the catalytic triad and some features of the substrate-binding site from these convergently related enzymes (Kraut et al. 1971).

We and others have chosen the subtilisin ($M_r \cong$ 27,500) from *Bacillus amyloliquefaciens* as a model system for protein engineering (for review, see Wells et al. 1987c). The X-ray structure of the wild-type enzyme has been determined at high resolution (Wright et al. 1969; Drenth et al. 1972; R.R. Bott et al., in prep.). Sequences from a number of different subtilisins have been determined (Markland and Smith 1971) and kinetic properties of some of these enzymes extensively studied (Philipp and Bender 1983).

The subtilisin gene from *B. amyloliquefaciens* has been cloned and the enzyme expressed in a secreted form in *B. subtilis* (Wells et al. 1983; Vasantha et al. 1984). Protein engineering of subtilisin has been used to introduce disulfide bonds (Katz and Kossiakoff 1986; Wells and Powers 1986; Pantoliano et al. 1987), to improve the oxidative (Estell et al. 1985) and alkaline stability (Cunningham and Wells 1987), to alter the pH profile of the enzyme (Thomas et al. 1985; Russell et al. 1987), and to probe the importance of a residue involved in transition-state stabilization (Wells et al. 1986; Bryan et al. 1986). These studies demonstrate the potential for functional modifications of subtilisin that may have been exploited during its evolution.

Here, we review two strategies for altering the substrate specificity of subtilisin (Fig. 1). Previously, the substrate specificity of subtilisin has been altered by changing enzyme residues capable of making direct contact with a bound substrate. By appropriate amino acid substitutions it has been possible to sterically exclude binding of large substrates, promote binding of hydrophobic substrates (Estell et al. 1986), or enhance binding of charged substrates (Wells et al. 1987b).

Extending this approach, we show here the degree to which the specificity properties of two functionally and evolutionarily divergent subtilisins can be switched by exchange of substrate contact residues (Wells et al. 1987a). These key substitutions represent less than 4% of the sequence differences between the two natural variant enzymes studied. Thus, mutation of substrate contact residues provides a powerful mechanism for divergence of substrate specificity within this homologous enzyme family.

In the second approach that we call "substrate-assisted catalysis," the catalytic His is removed and its catalytic function is restored partially by a His side chain from a bound substrate (Carter and Wells 1987). In this case, substrates are distinguished at the level of catalysis by virtue of their ability to supply the missing catalytic function. We propose substrate-assisted catalysis as a possible evolutionary mechanism for installing

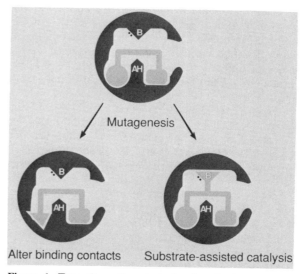

Figure 1. Two alternative strategies for altering substrate specificity by site-directed mutagenesis of an enzyme. In the first approach (*left*), binding site contact residues of the enzyme (darkly shaded) are changed to alter the chemical and structural complementarity of the binding site for the substrate (lightly shaded). In the second approach (*right*) called substrate-assisted catalysis, one of the catalytic groups (AH or :B representing a catalytic acid or base, for example) is removed such that it may be replaced by a similar functional group from a bound substrate.

the His in the catalytic triad to help explain the convergent evolution of the two serine protease families.

MATERIALS AND METHODS

Mutations in the cloned *B. amyloliquefaciens* gene were constructed by mismatched oligonucleotide site-directed mutagenesis (Zoller and Smith 1982), as modified by Carter et al. (1985), or cassette mutagenesis (Wells et al. 1985). We have described previously the construction of Glu156Ser,[1] Tyr217Leu, and Gly169Ala mutations as well as combined multiple mutations at these sites (Wells et al. 1987a,b). Construction of the His64Ala mutant and the double mutant Ser24Cys:His64Ala has been described previously (Carter and Wells 1987). Mutant and wild-type subtilisin genes were expressed and secreted from a protease-deficient strain of *B. subtilis*, BG2036 (Yang et al. 1984). Enzymes were purified from culture supernatants as reported previously (Estell et al. 1985). In the case of the Ser24Cys:Ala64His enzyme, substantial modifications to fermentation and protein purification were made to produce high yields and to ensure the purity of this catalytic site mutant (Carter and Wells 1987).

RESULTS

Recruitment of the Specificity Properties of *B. licheniformis* Subtilisin into the *B. amyloliquefaciens* Enzyme by Alteration of Substrate Contact Residues

The protein sequences of the *B. licheniformis* and *B. amyloliquefaciens* subtilisins differ at 86 out of 275 residues, including a single amino acid deletion (Wells et al. 1983; Jacobs et al. 1985). Furthermore, these two enzymes differ by factors of up to 60 in catalytic efficiency (k_{cat}/K_m) toward particular substrates (Wells et al. 1987a).

Despite large changes in sequence ($\sim 31\%$) and substrate specificity, the X-ray structures of these two enzymes containing bound protease inhibitors (Hirono et al. 1984; McPhalen et al. 1985; Bode et al. 1986), substrate analogs (Robertus et al. 1972b; Matthews et al. 1975; Poulos et al. 1976), and product complexes (Robertus 1972a; R. Bott and M. Ultsch, unpubl.) show virtually identical features for substrate binding. However, these enzymes differ at two positions that can make direct contact with a bound substrate. Position 156, which is Glu in the *B. amyloliquefaciens* subtilisin and Ser in the *B. licheniformis* enzyme, is within 4 Å (van der Waals distance) of the P1-binding site.[2] This charge difference probably contributes to the fact that the *B. amyloliquefaciens* enzyme is better on

Lys P1 substrates and worse on Glu P1 substrates compared to the *B. licheniformis* subtilisin (Fig. 2). This view is supported by an X-ray structure of a bound Lys P1 substrate affinity label showing that the Lys substrate side chain can form a salt bridge with Glu-156 in *B. amyloliquefaciens* subtilisin (Poulos et al. 1976).

A second potential difference in substrate contact is at position 217 (located in the P1'-binding site), which is a Tyr in *B. amyloliquefaciens* and a Leu in *B. licheniformis*. Model building indicates the *p*-nitroanilide group in synthetic substrates can make van der Waals contact with residue 217 (Wells et al. 1987a). A third substitution near the P1-binding site, but further than 3 Å from making direct contact with a large P1 substrate, is at position 169, which is Gly in *B. amyloliquefaciens* and Ala in *B. licheniformis*. The Ala substitution may have indirect effects on substrate binding by making van der Waals contact with the carbonyl at position 152. This affects the position of Ala-152, which makes direct contact with the P1 substrate side chain.

To test the extent to which substitutions at these three sites account for the large differences in substrate specificity between the two natural variant subtilisins, the three *B. licheniformis* substitutions (Glu156Ser, Gly169Ala, and Tyr217Leu) were introduced together into the *B. amyloliquefaciens* gene. The triple mutant and both natural variant wild-type subtilisins were analyzed for substrate specificity by kinetic analysis of seven

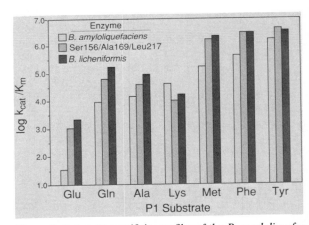

Figure 2. Substrate specificity profiles of the *B. amyloliquefaciens* wild-type (lightly shaded), the *B. amyloliquefaciens* triple mutant, Glu156Ser/Gly169Ala/Tyr217Leu (medium shaded), and the *B. licheniformis* wild-type (darkly shaded) subtilisins. Bars represent the logarithm of the k_{cat}/K_m ratios ($s^{-1} M^{-1}$) for each enzyme toward substrates containing different P1 amino acids (shown below each set of bars). Substrates have the form *N*-succinyl-L-Ala-L-Ala-L-Pro-L-[X]-*p*-nitroanilide (where X is the P1 amino acid). Data is taken from Wells et al. (1987a).

---

[1]This notation describes mutations by giving first the wild-type amino acid, the sequence position, and then the mutant amino acid. Multiply mutated enzymes are indicated by combined single mutations separated by colons.

[2]The protease substrate nomenclature of Schechter and Berger (1967) is used here and can be represented as:

$$\text{NH}_2\text{—Pn}\ldots\text{P2—P1—}\overset{\overset{\displaystyle O}{\|}}{\text{C}}\text{—}\overset{\overset{\displaystyle H}{|}}{\text{N}}\text{—P1'—P2'}\ldots\text{Pn'—COOH},$$

where the scissile peptide bond is between the P1 and P1' residues.

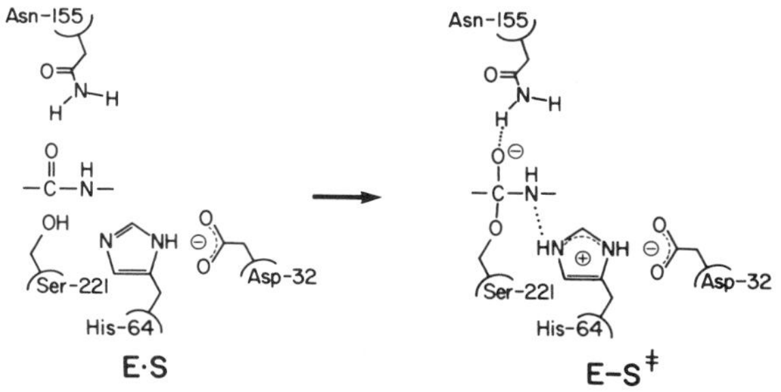

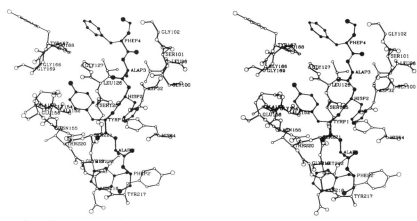

Figure 3. Diagram of important catalytic residues involved in the enzyme mechanism of subtilisin. In the enzyme substrate complex (E·S) the scissile amide bond of the substrate is positioned over the catalytic Ser-221. In proceeding to the first tetrahedral transition-state complex, the proton on Ser-221 is transferred to the NE2 nitrogen of His-64. This permits attack by the Ser-221 OG on the scissile carbonyl producing a tetrahedral oxyanion that is further stabilized by a hydrogen bond to Asn-155 and Ser-221 backbone NH (not shown).

homologous P1 substrates that vary in size and charge (Fig. 2). The catalytic efficiencies (k_{cat}/K_m) of the triple mutant nearly match those of the *B. licheniformis* enzyme. Although the specificity of the triple mutant is very close to the *B. licheniformis* enzyme, there are significant differences toward small hydrophilic or charged P1 substrates (Ala, Gln, Glu, or Lys). Thus, other amino acid changes that are not directly involved in making substrate contacts must account for these differences. Further analysis of the Glu156Ser, Gly169Ala, and Tyr217Leu single mutants and combined mutants at these sites is presented elsewhere (Wells et al. 1987a).

Alteration of Specificity by "Substrate-assisted Catalysis"

The catalytic His-64 plays a crucial role in the hydrolytic mechanism of subtilisin (Fig. 3). In the rate-limiting acylation step for amide hydrolysis, the im-

idazole acts as a catalytic base by accepting the proton from the hydroxyl of Ser-221, permitting attack on the carbonyl carbon of the scissile peptide (for review, see Kraut 1977). Subsequently, the protonated His-64 acts as an acid by donating the proton to the amine-leaving group. In deacylation the His-64 functions as a general base to permit a water molecule to attack the acyl–enzyme bond, and next as an acid to transfer the proton to the catalytic serine that completes the catalytic cycle.

Molecular modeling of a substrate bound to the active site of subtilisin revealed that a His P2 side chain can occupy a position where the imidazole nitrogens can be virtually superimposed on the corresponding nitrogens of the catalytic His-64 (Fig. 4). The dihedral bond angles and distances to the catalytic Ser and Asp are reasonable for a His P2 side chain. The hydrogen bond angle to the Ser-221 hydroxyl is similar for the His P2 substrate and His-64 side chains, although the hydrogen bond angle to the Asp-32 carboxylate is less favorable. This model has been described more extensively elsewhere (Carter and Wells 1987).

To provide space for the His P2 substrate side chain, the catalytic His was replaced by an Ala. In addition, a Ser24Cys mutation was introduced into subtilisin, which is normally cysteine-free. This free thiol has no substantial effect on catalytic properties, but it permits reversible attachment to an activated thiol sepharose column that is an essential purification step.

To evaluate the effect of the His64Ala mutation on enzyme specificity and catalysis, kinetic parameters were determined for the Ser24Cys (wild-type analog) and Ser24Cys:His64Ala enzymes (Table 1) toward substrates containing either Ala or His P2 side chains. The His64Ala mutation causes a large drop in k_{cat}/K_m ($\sim 10^6$) toward the Ala P2 substrate. Almost all of this can be accounted for by a decreased k_{cat} term. In contrast, the His64Ala mutation causes a much smaller decrease in k_{cat}/K_m toward the His P2 substrate. Much of this effect results from an increased K_m as well as a decreased k_{cat} term.

Figure 4. Stereo view of a substrate model (filled atoms) L-Phe-L-Ala-L-His-L-Tyr-L-Ala-L-Phe representing residues P4 to P2′ bound to the active site of *B. amyloliquefaciens* subtilisin (open atoms). This model shows the superposition of the His P2 side chain with His-64. The dihedral angles for the His P2 side chain have been adjusted to optimize the hydrogen bond distances and angles between the imidazoyl nitrogens and the OG of Ser-221 and OD of Asp-32.

Table 1. Kinetic Parameters for Ser24Cys and the Double Mutant Ser24Cys:His64Ala

Substrate P2 residue	Ser24Cys			Ser24Cys:His64Ala		
	k_{cat}	K_m	k_{cat}/K_m	k_{cat}	K_m	k_{cat}/K_m
	s^{-1}	μM	$s^{-1} M^{-1}$	s^{-1}	μM	$s^{-1} M^{-1}$
Ala	8.1	10	8.0×10^5	8.1×10^{-6}	32	0.25
His	4.6	23	2.0×10^5	1.6×10^{-2}	380	42

Substrates have the form N-succinyl-L-Phe-L-Ala-L-[X]-L-Phe-p-nitroanilide when X (the P2 amino acid) is either Ala or His. Reactions were run in 0.10 M Tris-HCl (pH 8.6) at 25°C as described previously (Carter and Wells 1987).

Comparisons of catalytic efficiencies (k_{cat}/K_m) toward different substrates show that the Ser24Cys enzyme prefers the Ala P2 substrate by a factor of four over the His P2 substrate. In contrast, the Ser24Cys:His64Ala mutant enzyme prefers the His P2 substrate to the Ala P2 substrate by a factor of 170. Additional lines of evidence from pH profiles and specific cleavage of peptide substrates further demonstrate the extreme substrate preference for the His64Ala mutant (Carter and Wells 1987).

DISCUSSION

We have presented two strategies for engineering the substrate specificity of subtilisin (Fig. 1) that may have been utilized in evolution. In the first approach, differences in direct binding contacts between two natural variant subtilisins (that result from 3 substitutions out of 86) are found to account for most of the differences in substrate specificity. These mutations do not simply alter substrate binding (K_s)[3]; in fact, most of the changes in k_{cat}/K_m for the Tyr217Leu mutation result from alterations in the k_{cat} term (Wells et al. 1987a). Generally, these mutations act independently and therefore have an additive effect on the energy available for transition-state binding.

The mutations involving direct contact residues (such as Glu156Ser and Tyr217Leu) generally have greater effects on substrate specificity than mutations that act indirectly to alter the conformation of binding site (such as Gly169Ala). Thus, the modification of residues that directly or indirectly affect substrate binding provides a mechanism for the diversification of substrate specificity from an ancestral enzyme.

In the second approach, called substrate-assisted catalysis, substrates are distinguished by their participation in the enzyme mechanism (Carter and Wells 1987). Presumably, His P2 substrates are hydrolyzed by a serine protease-like mechanism using their own His side chain in place of the missing catalytic His. Substrates lacking a His P2 side chain may depend on hydroxide ion to deprotonate the catalytic serine (a

much slower process at pH 8.0) or direct attack by hydroxide. This strategy produces large changes in substrate preference to give enzymes with exquisite substrate specificity. This approach is applicable in situations where catalytic groups (such as general acids and bases, nucleophiles, etc.) may be precisely replaced by similar functional groups from a bound substrate. A possible example where nature has apparently employed a derivative of substrate-assisted catalysis is in the maturation of human rhinovirus (Rossman et al. 1985; Arnold et al. 1987), where the protein VP0 is processed to VP2 and VP4. Rossman proposed that in the final stages of capsid assembly, an RNA base inserts between a serine residue and the carboxyl terminus in VP0 to permit the Ser OG to attack the scissile peptide bond producing VP2 and VP4.

It is highly unlikely that the catalytic triad in subtilisin evolved in one step, but more likely that it was installed in separate events. The following is one of many possible scenarios whereby substrate-assisted catalysis may have facilitated establishment of the catalytic triad (Fig. 5). If the genetic ancestor of subtilisin were capable of binding peptide substrates containing a His residue, then introducing a Ser residue nearby may have imparted a further catalytic advantage to His P2 substrates. This putative evolutionary intermediate in the catalytic triad (Fig. 5, middle) may have had functional significance. For example, high catalytic efficiency toward His P2 substrates may have imparted a selective advantage for cellular defense, specific proteolytic processing, or protein scavenging, among others. Such properties may have been especially important in the context of other primordial proteases that may have been poor catalysts by comparison. In subsequent mutational events, a His side chain in the enzyme could be fixed by selection and so relax substrate specificity toward His P2 side chains (Fig. 5, bottom). Thus, by substrate-assisted catalysis, the substrate may have acted as a catalytic "crutch" and "space-saver" until the enzyme could acquire the catalytic His by mutation.

In summary, modification of substrate binding contact residues provides a mechanism for the evolution of diverse substrate specificities. In addition, substrate-assisted catalysis is a potential means for ancestral subtilisin to have introduced the catalytic histidine and may help to account for the convergent evolution of serine proteases.

---

[3]For the two-step reaction mechanism for serine proteases, if acylation is rate-limiting, then $K_m \cong K_s$ (Gutfreund and Sturtevant 1956). This is the case for hydrolysis of N-succinyl-L-Ala-L-Ala-L-Pro-L-Phe-p-nitroanilide by wild-type subtilisin (Wells et al. 1986).

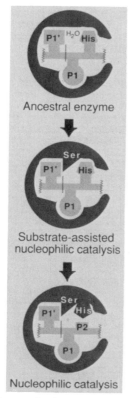

Figure 5. Possible use of substrate-assisted catalysis to facilitate installation of the catalytic triad in serine proteases. The ancestors to serine proteases (*top*, darkly shaded) may have bound His P2 substrates (lightly shaded), among others. If a Ser were fixed next to the His P2 side chain (*center*) a large rate acceleration may have resulted on His P2 substrates from substrate-assisted nucleophilic catalysis. Finally, the enzyme could have fixed a His relaxing the requirement for a His side chain at the P2 position (*bottom*). This is only one of many possible scenarios in which substrate-assisted catalysis could have been utilized in the evolution of intermediate enzyme forms and does not speculate on the timing for introduction of the catalytic Asp. The dotted line shows the position of the hydrolyzed peptide bond and the jagged lines represent the continuation of the substrate.

ACKNOWLEDGMENTS

We are grateful to Dr. Rick Bott for making unpublished crystallographic data available prior to publication, to colleagues at Genentech and Genencor for their support and encouragement, and to Wayne Anstine for preparation of drawings and manuscript.

REFERENCES

Arnold, E., M. Luo, G. Vriend, M.G. Rossman, A.C. Palmenberg, G.D. Parks, M.J.H. Nicklin, and E. Wimmer. 1987. Implications of the picornavirus capsid structure for polypeptide processing. *Proc. Natl. Acad. Sci.* **84:** 21.

Bode, W., E. Papamokos, D. Musil, U. Seemueller, and H. Fritz. 1986. Refined 1.2 Å crystal structure of the complex formed between subtilisin Carlsberg and the inhibitor eglin C. Molecular structure of eglin and its detailed interaction with subtilisin. *EMBO J.* **5:** 813.

Bryan, P., M.W. Pantoliano, S.G. Quill, H.Y. Hsiao, and T. Poulos. 1986. Site-directed mutagenesis and the role of the oxyanion hole in subtilisin. *Proc. Natl. Acad. Sci.* **83:** 3743.

Carter, P. and J.A. Wells. 1987. Engineering enzyme specificity by "substrate-assisted catalysis." *Science* **237:** 394.

Carter, P., H. Bedouelle, and G. Winter. 1985. Improved oligonucleotide site-directed mutagenesis using M13 vectors. *Nucleic Acids Res.* **13:** 4431.

Cunningham, B.C. and J.A. Wells. 1987. Improvement in the alkaline stability of subtilisin using an efficient random mutagenesis and screening procedure. *Protein Eng.* **1:** 319.

Drenth, J., W.A.J. Hol, J.N. Jansonius, and R. Koekoek. 1972. A comparison of the three-dimensional structures of subtilisin BPN' and subtilisin Novo. *Eur. J. Biochem.* **26:** 107.

Estell, D.A., T.P. Graycar, and J.A. Wells. 1985. Engineering an enzyme by site-directed mutagenesis to be resistant to chemical oxidation. *J. Biol. Chem.* **260:** 6518.

Estell, D.A., T.P. Graycar, J.V. Miller, D.B. Powers, J.P. Burnier, P.G. Ng, and J.A. Wells. 1986. Probing steric and hydrophobic effects on enzyme-substrate interactions by protein engineering. *Science* **233:** 659.

Gutfreund, H. and J.M. Sturtevant. 1956. The mechanism of the reaction of chymotrypsin with *p*-nitrophenyl acetate. *Biochem. J.* **63:** 656.

Hirono, S., H. Akagawa, Y. Mitsui, and Y. Iitaka. 1984. Crystal structure at 2.6 Å resolution of the complex of subtilisin BPN' with *Streptomyces* subtilisin inhibitor. *J. Mol. Biol.* **178:** 389.

Jacobs, M., M. Eliasson, M. Uhlen, and J. Flock. 1985. Cloning, sequencing and expression of subtilisin Carlsberg from *Bacillus licheniformis*. *Nucleic Acids Res.* **13:** 8913.

Katz, B.A. and A. Kossiakoff. 1986. The crystallographically determined structures of atypical strained disulfides engineered into subtilisin. *J. Biol. Chem.* **261:** 15480.

Kraut, J. 1977. Serine proteases: Structure and mechanism of catalysis. *Annu. Rev. Biochem.* **46:** 331.

Kraut, J., J.D. Robertus, J.J. Birktoft, R.A. Alden, P.E. Wilcox, and J.C. Powers. 1972. The aromatic substrate binding site in subtilisin BPN' and its resemblance to chymotrypsin. *Cold Spring Harbor Symp. Quant. Biol.* **36:** 117.

Markland, F.S. and E.L. Smith. 1971. Subtilisins: Primary structure, chemical and physical properties. In *The enzymes*, 3rd. edition (ed. P.D. Boyer), vol. 5, p. 561. Academic Press, New York.

Matthews, D.A., R.A. Alden, J.J. Birktoft, S.T. Freer, and J. Kraut. 1975. X-ray crystallographic study of boronic acid adducts with subtilisin BPN' (NOVO). *J. Biol. Chem.* **250:** 7120.

McPhalen, C.A., I. Svendsen, I. Jonassen, and M.N.G. James. 1985. Crystal and molecular structure of chymotrypsin inhibitor 2 from barley seeds in complex with subtilisin Novo. *Proc. Natl. Acad. Sci.* **82:** 7242.

Pantoliano, M.W., R.C. Ladner, P.N. Bryan, M.L. Rollence, J.F. Wood, and T.L. Poulos. 1987. Protein engineering of subtilisin BPN': Enhanced stabilization through the introduction of two cysteines to form a disulfide bond. *Biochemistry* **26:** 2077.

Philipp, M. and M.L. Bender. 1983. Kinetics of subtilisin and thiolsubtilisin. *Mol. Cell. Biochem.* **51:** 5.

Poulos, T.L., R.A. Alden, S.T. Freer, J.J. Birktoft, and J. Kraut. 1976. Polypeptide halomethyl ketones bind to serine proteases as analogs of the tetrahedral intermediate. *J. Biol. Chem.* **251:** 1097.

Robertus, J.D., J. Kraut, R.A. Alden, and J.J. Birktoft. 1972a. Subtilisin: A stereochemical mechanism involving transition-state stabilization. *Biochemistry* **11:** 4293.

Robertus, J.D., R.A. Alden, J.J. Birktoft, J. Kraut, J.C. Powers, and P.E. Wilcox. 1972b. An X-ray crystallographic study of the binding of peptide chloromethyl ketones to subtilisin BPN'. *Biochemistry* **11:** 2439.

Rossman, M.G., E. Arnold, J.W. Erickson, E.A. Franken-berger, J.P. Griffith, H.J. Hecht, J.E. Johnson, G. Kramer, M. Luo, A.G. Mosser, R.R. Rueckert, B. Sherry, and G. Vriend. 1985. Structure of a human common cold virus and functional relationship to other picornaviruses. *Nature* **317:** 145.

Russell, A.J., P.G. Thomas, and A.R. Fersht. 1987. Electrostatic effects on modification of charged groups in the active site cleft of subtilisin by protein engineering. *J. Mol. Biol.* **193:** 803.

Schechter, I. and A. Berger. 1967. On the size of the active site in proteins. *Biochem. Biophys. Res. Commun.* **27:** 157.

Stroud, R.M. 1974. A family of protein-cutting proteins. *Sci. Am.* **131:** 74.

Thomas, P.G., A.J. Russell, and A.R. Fersht. 1985. Tailoring the pH dependence of enzyme catalysis using protein engineering. *Nature* **318:** 375.

Vasantha, N., L.D. Thompson, C. Rhodes, C. Banner, J. Nagle, and D. Filpula. 1984. Genes for alkaline protease and neutral protease from *Bacillus amyloliquefaciens* contain a large open reading frame between regions coding for signal sequence and mature protein. *J. Bacteriol.* **159:** 811.

Wells, J.A. and D.B. Powers. 1986. *In vivo* formation and stability of engineered disulfide bonds in subtilisin. *J. Biol. Chem.* **266:** 6564.

Wells, J.A., M. Vasser, and D.B. Powers. 1985. Cassette mutagenesis: An efficient method for generation of multiple mutations at defined sites. *Gene* **34:** 315.

Wells, J.A., B.C. Cunningham, T.P. Graycar, and D.A. Estell. 1986. Importance of hydrogen-bond formation in stabilizing the transition state of subtilisin. *Philos. Trans. R. Soc. Lond. A Math. Phys. Sci.* **317:** 415.

———. 1987a. Recruitment of substrate-specificity properties from one enzyme into a related one by protein engineering. *Proc. Natl. Acad. Sci.* **84:** 5167.

Wells, J.A., E. Ferrari, D.J. Henner, D.A. Estell, and E.Y. Chen. 1983. Cloning, sequencing, and secretion of *Bacillus amyloliquefaciens* subtilisin from *Bacillus subtilis*. *Nucleic Acids Res.* **11:** 7911.

Wells, J.A., D.B. Powers, R.R. Bott, T.P. Graycar, and D.A. Estell. 1987b. Designing substrate specificity by protein engineering of electrostatic interactions. *Proc. Natl. Acad. Sci.* **84:** 1219.

Wells, J.A., D.B. Powers, R.R. Bott, B.A. Katz, M.H. Ultsch, A.A. Kossiakoff, S.D. Power, R.M. Adams, H.H. Heyneker, B.C. Cunningham, J.V. Miller, T.P. Graycar, and D.A. Estell. 1987c. Protein engineering of subtilisin. In *Protein engineering* (ed. D.L. Oxender and C.F. Fox), p. 279. Alan R. Liss, New York..

Wright, C.S., R.A. Alden, and J. Kraut. 1969. Structure of subtilisin BPN' at 2.5 Å resolution. *Nature* **221:** 235.

Yang, M., E. Ferrai, and D.J. Henner. 1984. Cloning of the neutral protease gene of *Bacillus subtilis* and the use of the cloned gene to generate an *in vitro* deletion mutation. *J. Bacteriol.* **160:** 15.

Zoller, M.J. and M. Smith. 1982. Oligonucleotide-directed mutagenesis using M13-derived vectors: An efficient and general procedure for production of point mutations in any fragment of DNA. *Nucleic Acids Res.* **10:** 6487.

The Role of RNA and Protein in Ribosome Function: A Review of Early Reconstitution Studies and Prospects for Future Studies

M. NOMURA

Department of Biological Chemistry, University of California, Irvine, California 92717

Although the major research effort of our laboratory during recent years has been on the genes for ribosomal components and the regulation of their expression, I have agreed to write an article reviewing the earlier work related to ribosome structure and function, based mostly on our own research on ribosome reconstitution from the late 1960s to the early 1970s, as well as studies on ribosome mutations in general.

The emphasis in current research on ribosome structure and function is on rRNA as the probable component directly involved in ribosome function, in contrast to the earlier studies that appeared to concentrate on ribosomal proteins (r-proteins). However, it should be noted that the earlier workers did not ignore possible roles of rRNAs. In fact, not only was the importance of rRNAs recognized, but some strong evidence existed supporting the idea that RNA played a functional role. However, because there are many proteins in the ribosomes and it was easier technically to dissect the proteins in those early days, most studies concentrated on the proteins. Although there was abundant evidence to indicate that r-proteins are important for assembly, functional roles of r-proteins in the finished ribosomes were clearly established only for a few proteins in these earlier studies. Since the main theme of this volume is the origin of catalytic function, reviewing the old reconstitution studies at this time may still be pertinent to this volume; it may be useful in assessing the relative roles of r-proteins and rRNAs in the present-day ribosomes, allowing speculation on the nature of the primitive ribosomes and their evolution to the present-day ribosomes.

In addition to discussing ribosome structure and function, I have also decided to describe, in the addendum to this article, some recent observations related to the evolution of r-protein genes, which came from our studies on the regulation of ribosome synthesis.

The Function of 16S rRNA Studied by In Vitro Reconstitution

Since as much as two thirds of the total mass of ribosomes are RNA, the possible role of rRNAs in ribosome function was an obvious question from the very beginning of ribosome research. Even leaving aside the suggestion that the primitive ribosome could have been made entirely of RNA (Crick 1968; Orgel

1968), it was reasonable to think about direct interactions between mRNA (or tRNA) and rRNA by mechanisms such as base pairing or base-phosphate interactions. This possibility was first suggested by Watson as early as 1964 (Watson 1964). However, experimental approaches to study this question were not technically easy.

Although the first 30S ribosome reconstitution demonstrated an absolute requirement for the presence of 16S rRNA for functional reconstitution (Traub and Nomura 1968a), 16S rRNA is also required for physical assembly and therefore, it was difficult to prove direct involvement of RNA in translation. In contrast to the protein fraction that was known to consist of many (later nominally shown to be 21) different molecules, the RNA portion of the 30S subunit is a single, large molecule, and it was technically difficult to dissect it into various parts at that time. Thus, the approaches taken were to modify rRNA, then test the activity by reconstitution, using (a) substitution of 16S rRNA by heterologous RNA (Nomura et al. 1968; Held et al. 1974a); (b) chemical modification of 16S rRNA (Nomura et al. 1968; Noller and Chaires 1972); and (c) specific alterations of 16S rRNA by mutation or some other physiological means (Bowman et al. 1971; Helser et al. 1971; Lai et al. 1973). In this third approach, the presence of seven copies of rRNA genes made the isolation of rRNA mutants with functional alterations difficult. Exceptions were those mutations affecting base modification. Despite these limitations, the first indication of the importance of 16S rRNA in the ribosome function came from some of those earlier reconstitution experiments.

The first strong indication of the importance of 16S rRNA in ribosome function came from research, including that carried out in our laboratory, on the mode of action of colicins, including colicin E3. We had discovered that E3 specifically inhibits protein synthesis in sensitive *Escherichia coli* cells (Nomura 1964) and that ribosomes, specifically 30S subunits, isolated from E3-treated cells were almost completely inactive in in vitro protein synthesis (Konisky and Nomura 1967). Such inactive ribosomes were apparently physically intact as judged by techniques such as sedimentation analysis of the ribosome particle and rRNA, as well as gel electrophoretic analysis of protein components. Thus, the basis for colicin-mediated inactivation was initially a mystery. Subsequent reconstitution analysis of the inactive 30S subunits convincingly demonstrated that it is the RNA that is inactive and that the protein fraction is fully functional (Bowman et al. 1971). Ultimately, the presence of a single nucleolytic cleavage at a position about 50 nucleotides from the 3' end was demonstrated (Bowman et al. 1971; Senior and Holland 1971). Although the particles reconstituted with the "E3-16S rRNA" (with the 3' end cleaved) lacked one protein (S21) (Bowman et al. 1971), the functionally important role played by the 3'-end portion of 16S rRNA was strongly indicated by two observations obtained through reconstitution experiments. First, all of the proteins, including S21, were present in the original E3-inactivated ribosomes as functionally active proteins. Second, the omission of S21 in reconstitution (with the intact 16S rRNA) caused only a partial (40–60%) decrease in activity (Nomura et al. 1970; Held et al. 1974b) and could not account for the near-complete inactivation caused by E3-catalyzed cleavage. Therefore, the near-complete inactivation caused by cleavage of the 3'-end fragment (which represents only about 3% of the entire molecule) was difficult to explain as a result of a hypothetical effect of cleavage on some protein components.

As is now well known, the 3'-end fragment includes the region complementary to the Shine-Dalgarno sequence of mRNA and is important for the initiation of protein synthesis (Shine and Dalgarno 1974; Steitz and Jakes 1975). In addition, the region deleted by E3 may also function together with the region around 1400 as the decoding site in codon-anticodon interaction (Noller et al. 1986).

The second type of reconstitution experiment that suggested the importance of rRNA was analysis of drug-resistant ribosomes. For example, kasugamycin inhibits initiation. Ribosomes from E. coli mutants resistant to kasugamycin were found to be deficient in methylation of 16S rRNA, and reconstitution experiments demonstrated that this alteration is responsible for resistance (Helser et al. 1971). Similarly, erythromycin-induced resistance to lincomycin in Staphylococcus aureus involves methylation of 23S rRNA, and reconstitution experiments showed that this alteration is responsible for resistance (Lai et al. 1973). These experiments suggested that these antibiotics act directly on rRNAs that were functionally important. However, resistance to many other antibiotics acting on E. coli ribosomes was shown to involve alterations in r-proteins, as in the case of streptomycin resistance (see below). Therefore, one could not exclude an alternative interpretation that the rRNA modifications in these mutant ribosomes prevent antibiotics from reaching functionally important target sites consisting of proteins.

Another reconstitution experiment that led to the suggestion of the importance of 16S rRNA was heterologous reconstitution using components from E. coli and Bacillus stearothermophilus. It was demonstrated that substitution of B. stearothermophilus 16S

rRNA for E. coli 16S rRNA in reconstitution with purified components causes about a twofold decrease in translational activity of R17 RNA, whereas activity in poly(U)-dependent polyphenylalanine synthesis or AUG-dependent formylmethionyl tRNA binding remained the same (Held et al. 1974a). It was also observed that the substitution of both Bacillus 16S RNA and Bacillus protein S12 for E. coli 16S rRNA and S12 caused a drastic decrease in R17 RNA translation without decreasing poly(U) translational activity. The decrease was much stronger than when S12 alone was substituted. In these experiments, the effects of the substitution were clearly not on assembly, but on a specific aspect of ribosomal function. Thus, the suggestion was made that direct interaction of some parts of 16S RNA with mRNA is involved in recognition of initiation signals on natural mRNA (Held et al. 1974a). Of course, as is well known, the more specific proposal made by Shine and Dalgarno (1974), followed by extensive sequence analysis of translation initiation sites, as well as experimental tests of the model (Steitz and Jakes 1975; Steitz 1980), has established the interaction of 16S rRNA with mRNA. However, the role of rRNA demonstrated in the original heterologous reconstitution cannot be explained by sequence differences in the 3' end of 16S rRNA between the two bacterial species, since the essential regions complementary to the Shine-Dalgarno sequence in these two species were found to be identical (Sprague et al. 1977). Thus, additional rRNA sequences, together with certain other r-proteins such as S12 (see above) or S1 (Isono and Isono 1975), must contribute to the initiation reaction (discussed by Sprague et al. 1977).

The Function of r-Proteins Studied by In Vitro Reconstitution of 30S Subunits

The existence of many different proteins in the ribosomes was already known in the 1960s (Waller 1964). Thus, after initial success in reconstituting active 30S subunits from 16S rRNA and unfractionated proteins, we (and others) carried out purification of all the 30S r-proteins in order to perform reconstitution experiments using purified components. It was then natural to define the components of the system (i.e., 16S rRNA and each of the 21 r-proteins) and to analyze their role in ribosome assembly, structure, and function. Many reconstitution experiments, such as single-component omission experiments, were carried out, not because we believed that proteins and not RNA were responsible for ribosome function, but because the question was well defined and the analysis was technically feasible. We expected that these different protein molecules each played unique roles, and this expectation was confirmed with respect to their roles in assembly (Mizushima and Nomura 1970; Held et al. 1974c). In addition, reconstitution experiments with the unfractionated 30S protein mixture and 16S rRNA had already indicated that the alteration caused by an interesting mutation, streptomycin resistance (Str-R), affects a protein and not 16S rRNA (Traub and Nomura 1968b). In fact, because of the effects of streptomycin and Str-R mutations on translational fidelity, identification of the protein controlled by the *str* locus (S12) and its functional characterization were the first major reconstitution experiments to suggest that at least one r-protein, S12, is either directly or indirectly involved in translation (Ozaki et al. 1969).

The analysis of the role of S12 through reconstitution also gave interesting results. Particles lacking S12, but containing all other proteins, were almost as active as the control particle containing S12 when translation was carried out with synthetic mRNA in the presence of high concentrations of Mg^{++}. However, the particle lacking S12 showed a great reduction in misreading, induced not only by streptomycin but also by a variety of other agents, such as ethanol. In addition, the particle showed greatly reduced activity in the initiation reaction and in the translation of phage f2 RNA. These results suggest that S12 is directly or indirectly involved in ribosome function, perhaps interacting with the initiator tRNA or initiation factors, thus helping the initiator tRNA to bind in the correct position (Ozaki et al. 1969; Nomura et al. 1970).

However, results obtained with S12 turned out to be an exception, rather than the rule. With many other proteins, single-component omission affected assembly, as judged by the sedimentation pattern of the assembled particles. Specifically, the particles produced after incubation did not have the same compact structure as the intact 30S ribosomal subunits (Nomura et al. 1970). In addition, in many instances, the omission of a single protein led to the formation of particles that were deficient not only in the protein omitted, but also in certain other proteins (Mizushima and Nomura 1970). In these instances, it was difficult to decide whether the large decrease observed in the activity of the reconstituted particles was caused by the absence of the protein omitted or by the observed defects in assembly. Only with a few proteins (S2, S6, S12, S13, S20, and S21) did omission affect function without causing measurable effects on physical assembly or on the physical properties of the assembled particles. Furthermore, the decrease in activity in these instances was only partial or insignificant (except for S12, which was mentioned above) (Nomura et al. 1970; Held et al. 1973). I should add that more recent experiments have suggested that S21 is primarily required for initiation (Van Duin and Wijnands 1981), which is somewhat different from the earlier results we obtained in which functions in both initiation and elongation were suggested (Held et al. 1974b). In addition, S1 is a protein primarily required for initiation function and not for assembly (Van Dieijen et al. 1976). However, S1 is only loosely associated with ribosomes, and could almost be considered an initiation factor.

In fact, one important conclusion that came from the reconstitution studies was that some r-proteins are clearly required for facilitating the assembly reaction or for maintaining the stability of the assembled particles

but are not involved directly in protein synthesis. For example, under the standard reconstitution conditions but in the absence of protein S16, particles containing all of the other proteins were assembled slowly, but once assembled, had physical and functional properties (as judged by many available techniques) almost identical to control particles with all of the r-proteins. The particles missing S16 could be isolated and were stable once assembled. Hence, the sole function of S16 appears to be in facilitating assembly (Held and Nomura 1975). In the case of the omission of S18 or S9, particles with nearly full activity (as assayed by poly(U)-dependent polyphenylalanine synthesis) were also gradually formed, but the particles lost activity upon isolation and purification. This loss of activity was shown to be due to the loss of other r-proteins (Held and Nomura 1975). Thus, the function of these proteins appears to be related to assembly and/or maintenance of the assembled structure. (Similar observations were later made in connection with *E. coli* 50S ribosome reconstitution [Spillmann and Nierhaus 1978; Nowotny and Nierhaus 1980].) Therefore, the results of early reconstitution studies on the 30S subunits do favor the concept that most r-proteins are perhaps required for assembly and maintenance of the correct ribosome structure, whereas the main function of 30S subunits, that is, binding of mRNA and the initiator tRNA (and other tRNAs when acting in concert with the 50S subunit), is probably carried out by 16S rRNA.

The role of some r-proteins such as S12 (encoded by the *str* locus), which were originally thought to be more directly involved in ribosome function, might actually act more indirectly. An example might be the maintenance of a local RNA structure (an "active center") that is perhaps directly involved in the interaction with mRNA or tRNA. This view is still consistent with the observations that omission of a single protein in the in vitro reconstitution system or mutational alterations affecting that protein give more drastic and/or specific effects on ribosome function without affecting the assembly or global conformation of rRNA. Similar arguments apply not only to S12 but also to other proteins, such as S3, S10, S11, and S14, which were strongly required for 30S ribosomal functions, but whose omission gave only small effects on the structure of the assembled particles (Traub et al. 1967; Mizushima and Nomura 1970; Nomura et al. 1970; Held et al. 1973).

Regarding the possibility of a functionally important interaction of S12 with 16S rRNA, it should be noted that streptomycin probably binds to 16S rRNA (Biswas and Gorini 1972). Even though S12 was identified as the determinant of streptomycin sensitivity, S12 (from sensitive *E. coli*) itself did not show any streptomycin-binding activity (Ozaki et al. 1969). In addition, reconstituted S12-deficient particles always showed a weak but definite sensitivity to streptomycin. The addition of wild-type S12 increased sensitivity, and addition of the mutant S12 (from the *str*^{r} cells) decreased sensitivity (Ozaki et al. 1969). Although mutants selected for Str-R always carried mutations in the gene-encoding protein S12 in *E. coli*, Str-R mutations in *Euglena gracilis* chloroplasts were found to be due to an alteration in 16S rRNA (Montandon et al. 1985). By introducing the same base substitution at the equivalent position in *E. coli* 16S rRNA (C912 to U) by in vitro mutagenesis, Montandon and co-workers (1986) recently demonstrated that this RNA alteration *in fact* renders *E. coli* cells (and ribosomes) streptomycin-resistant. These observations support the suggestion mentioned above, namely, that S12 interacts with a specific region of 16S rRNA and influences its conformation.

Reconstitution Studies of the 50S Subunit

Although the first reconstitution of 50S subunits was achieved in our laboratory using components from *B. stearothermophilus* 50S subunits (Nomura and Erdmann 1970), and some analyses of the component molecules, including 5S RNA, required for 50S functions were carried out with this system (Erdmann et al. 1971; Fahnestock and Nomura 1972; Cohlberg and Nomura 1976; Auron and Fahnestock 1981), more detailed and extensive studies were carried out by Nierhaus and his co-workers using an *E. coli* 50S reconstitution system that they had developed (Nierhaus and Dohme 1974; for reviews, see Nierhaus 1980, 1982). Since the 50S subunits carry out peptide bond formation, the tacit assumption at that time was that this catalytic function was carried out by a protein(s) and not by RNA. Also, it was assumed that the functions of 5S and 23S rRNAs were probably related to the binding of substrates, peptidyl-tRNA and incoming aminoacyl-tRNA at the correct positions, and/or the maintenance of the correct structure so that the presumed "peptidyltransferase protein(s)" could function in a proper way. Thus, after much effort to identify the peptidyltransferase proteins, Nierhaus and his co-workers concluded that L2, L3, L4, L15, and L16, together with 23S rRNA, constitute the peptidyltransferase center (Nierhaus 1980; Hampl et al. 1981; Schulze and Nierhaus 1982). However, many other proteins were also found to be strongly stimulatory, and it was not obvious why so many proteins must participate in the catalysis of a single biochemical reaction. In addition, subsequent genetic studies have demonstrated that one of these essential proteins, L15, is completely dispensable for cell growth (Lotti et al. 1983; Ito et al. 1984). Additionally, reconstitution studies on *B. stearothermophilus* 50S subunits by Auron and Fahnestock (1981) led to identification of seven r-proteins most directly involved in the peptidyltransferase reaction. They were homologs of *E. coli* L2, L3(or L6), L4, L5, L14, L16, and L20, and did not include L15.

Of course, since the discovery of the ability of RNA to function as a catalyst (Kruger et al. 1982; Guerrier-Takada et al. 1983), our thoughts on the peptidyltransferase activity have been greatly altered, and the possibility that 23S rRNA itself might be the catalytic component now seems likely. (Earlier reconstitution experiments indicated that 5S RNA does not play a major role in peptidyltransferase activity [see Fahnestock and Nomura 1972; Schulze and Nierhaus 1982].) From the sites of affinity labeling with peptidyl-tRNA analogs (Barta et al. 1984) and mutations conferring resistance to antibiotics inhibitory to peptidyltransferase (obtained using multicopy plasmids, see a later section), Noller and his co-workers have suggested a model for the functional organization of the peptidyltransferase site that involves interaction between two widely separated domains of 23S rRNA (Barta et al. 1984; Douthwaite et al. 1985; Noller et al. 1986). If 23S rRNA is in fact the peptidyltransferase, the function of the various proteins required for reconstitution of activity in vitro might be to fold 23S rRNA in the proper way so that these separate domains of the rRNA molecule are brought together to form the catalytic center. Such a model provides an elegant explanation for the requirement for so many different r-proteins to generate a single catalytic activity.

Ribosomal Protein Mutations Affecting Ribosomal Functions

If r-proteins are involved in some essential ribosomal functions, one would predict the existence of r-protein mutants that show defects in function both in vivo and in vitro. Surprisingly, despite isolation of many temperature-sensitive or cold-sensitive mutants with altered r-proteins, we have only a very few well-studied examples of defined functional defects. For instance, if the r-proteins implicated in peptidyltransferase function participate directly in the reaction, one would expect to find conditionally lethal mutations with alterations in these proteins accompanied by defects in peptidyltransferase activity assayed in vitro. No such mutants have yet been isolated. Several well-characterized temperature-sensitive and cold-sensitive mutants were shown to be mostly defective in assembly based on in vivo analysis of protein synthesis and ribosome assembly. These include temperature-sensitive mutations with alterations in S2 (Bollen et al. 1979), S4 (Olsson et al. 1974; Hayes and Schmitt 1980), S12 (Nashimoto et al. 1985), S17 (Herzog et al. 1979), and L24 (Cabezón et al. 1977), as well as cold-sensitive mutations with alterations in S5 (Nashimoto and Nomura 1970; Wittman et al. 1974), S8 (Geyl et al. 1977), S20 (Wittman et al. 1974), L3 (Lhoest and Colson 1981), and L30 (Geyl et al. 1977). The very frequent occurrence of r-protein mutations with assembly-defective phenotypes (see above and Guthrie et al. 1969; Tai et al. 1969) appears to support the general thesis that many r-proteins are important in the assembly of the ribosomes, but probably play only minor functional roles in the assembled ribosomes.

In addition, Dabbs has isolated many mutants lacking individual r-proteins as "suppressors" of drug-dependent *E. coli* mutants. Proteins missing in these mutants include S1, S6, S9, S13, S17, S20, L1, L11, L15, L19, L24, L27, L28, L29, L30, and L33 (for a summary review, see Dabbs 1986). Although most of these mutants grow poorly, the fact that they do grow indicates that none of these r-proteins is absolutely required for protein synthesis. As mentioned above, the dispensability of L15 for protein synthesis under normal growth conditions was also clearly demonstrated using a strain carrying a well-characterized amber mutation in the L15 gene and a temperature-sensitive amber suppressor (Ito et al. 1984). These observations again appear to support the notion that rRNAs, and not r-proteins, are the key components directly participating in ribosomal functions.

Even if rRNAs are directly responsible for ribosome function, the results of in vitro reconstitution studies suggest that certain r-proteins are not required for assembly or maintenance of subunit structure and stability, but are required more directly for ribosomal functions. These functions might include maintaining or modulating some local RNA structures at the active centers of the rRNAs. Therefore, one should expect to encounter r-protein mutations affecting such functions.

In fact, there are reports of temperature-sensitive mutants whose ribosomes showed temperature sensitivity when assayed in vitro (e.g., Kang 1970a,b; Kushner et al. 1977: Champney 1980; Armstrong-Major and Champney 1985). In some instances, the altered r-proteins in these mutants were identified (S10, S15, and L22; Champney 1980). Of course, the best-studied r-protein mutations in this regard are str^r mutations. As already mentioned above, ribosomes isolated from str^r mutants show reduced misreading in vitro, as well as resistance to the inhibitory action of streptomycin. In addition, the ribosomes isolated from a str^r mutant showed restricted read-through of UGA termination codons and restricted suppression of amber mutations by a tRNA suppressor in vitro, restrictions similar to those observed in vivo (Yates et al. 1977). This str^r mutant was also shown to have a reduced rate of protein chain elongation and a reduced growth rate in the absence of streptomycin (Zengel et al. 1977). Analysis of in vitro translation using ribosomes from this mutant by Kurland, Ehrenberg, and their co-workers showed that ribosomes from this mutant have a twofold increase in K_m for the AA-tRNA-EF-Tu-GTP ternary complex as measured in vitro (Ruusala et al. 1984). This result and their previous analyses of the mechanism of proofreading led these workers to attribute the observed increase in proofreading and the reduction in elongation rate and growth rate to this alteration in K_m (Ehrenberg et al. 1986).

In the course of studies on the regulation of ribosome synthesis, we have recently discovered that a cold-sensitive, spectinomycin-resistant mutant actually has a primary defect in the initiation of protein synthesis, and that the mutation is in the gene coding for S5 (*spc*). The mutant cells grow at 42°C almost as fast as the parental strain. Upon shift to 20°C, the rate of total protein synthesis in the mutant cells relative to that of the parent cells decreases almost immediately by a factor of 3–5. Ribosomes isolated from the mutant cells grown at

40°C showed a strongly reduced activity in the initiation reaction assayed at 20°C, but not at 40°C, relative to the parent ribosomes. In contrast, no significant difference was observed between the mutant and the parent ribosomes when an elongation assay was carried out at 20°C (G. Threadgill et al., unpubl. experiments). Thus, S5 is clearly essential for initiation (at least at 20°C). If S5 functions by altering a local structure of 16S rRNA, such a structural alteration might be uniquely recognizable at 20°C with the isolated mutant ribosomes. Isolation of such ribosomal mutants with a clear defect in a ribosome function that can be measured in vitro will certainly help define the roles played by the individual r-proteins in ribosomal functions.

rRNA Mutations

In contrast to r-protein genes that occur in single copy, the rRNA genes exist in seven copies in the *E. coli* genome. For this reason, it was previously difficult to isolate discrete rRNA mutations (other than those affecting base modifications). However, after isolation of rRNA genes on plasmids combined with advances in techniques for genetic manipulation, it has now become possible using multicopy plasmids carrying rRNA genes to isolate mutations either by selection (Sigmund and Morgan 1982; Mark et al. 1983; Douthwaite et al. 1985) or by in vitro mutagenesis (see Dahlberg 1986). Since conditional expression systems are now available in which the entire rRNA operon is fused to an inducible promoter such as λ P_L or a phage T7 promoter (de Boer et al. 1985; Gourse et al. 1985; Dahlberg 1986), almost any desired alterations in the nucleotide sequence can be introduced without worrying about lethality to cells carrying the altered genes. Using this approach, the importance of complementarity between the 3'-end region of 16S rRNA and the Shine-Dalgarno sequence of mRNA has been convincingly demonstrated (de Boer et al. 1985; Dahlberg 1986). As mentioned above, multicopy plasmids have been used to demonstrate that a single base substitution in 16S rRNA renders ribosomes Str-R (Montandon et al. 1986). Clearly, these approaches provide powerful means for examining the rRNA regions suspected to be important in ribosomal functions.

CONCLUDING REMARKS

In reviewing the results of earlier reconstitution studies and mutant analyses, it is evident that they are consistent with the current thought of ribosomes as an RNA enzyme as originally emphasized by Woese (1980); i.e., rRNAs are directly involved in ribosomal functions. Research on ribosome structure and function should then have two major goals. One is to prove (or disprove) convincingly the direct functions of rRNAs, especially the presumed catalytic function of 23S rRNA in peptide bond formation. Except for the direct role of 16S rRNA in mRNA recognition, experimental evidence for direct function of rRNA is still circumstantial, at best. The success obtained with RNase P in demonstrating the catalytic activity of an RNA component (Guerrier-Takada et al. 1983) suggests that a search for experimental conditions to demonstrate ribosomal functions with protein-free RNA deserves serious effort.

The second goal is to define the roles of r-proteins in ribosome function. A role in ribosome assembly has been amply demonstrated and studied in detail for many of the individual r-proteins (see above and Nomura and Held 1974; Röhl and Nierhaus 1982). In addition to functioning in assembly, r-proteins in present-day ribosomes may contribute to both efficiency and flexibility (e.g., regulation) in translation, even if rRNAs were the only functional components of primitive ribosomes. Precise functional roles of r-proteins should be defined and molecular mechanisms elucidated, as discussed above, for example, in connection with S12. Elucidation of three-dimensional arrangements of 30S r-proteins by Moore, Engelman, and their co-workers (Moore et al. 1986; Moore, this volume), and the current attempts to elucidate three-dimensional structure of 16S rRNA in relation to the positions of 30S r-proteins (see e.g., Noller and Lake 1984; Brimacombe et al. 1986; Noller et al., this volume) will certainly be very useful in this endeavor. Although the pendulum in ribosome research has now swung toward RNA both technically and conceptually, the reason for evolving the present-day ribosomes with so many protein molecules should also be explained.

ACKNOWLEDGMENTS

The author thanks Dr. Christopher L. Greer for his useful comments on the manuscript. The work from the author's laboratory described in this article has been supported by grants from the National Institutes of Health (currently GM-35949) and the National Science Foundation (currently DMB-85 43776).

ADDENDUM

Heterogeneity of GC Content within a Single Bacterial Genome and Its Implication for Evolution

M. NOMURA, F. SOR,* M. YAMAGISHI, AND M. LAWSON

Departments of Biological Chemistry and Microbiology and Molecular Genetics, University of California, Irvine, California 92717

It is known that the base composition of genomic DNA varies widely, between 25% and 75% guanine-cytosine (GC) content, among various different bac-

teria, and that heterogeneity within a single bacterial species is relatively small (Rolfe and Meselson 1959; Sueoka et al. 1959). In contrast, compositional heterogeneity of mammalian DNA is larger than that of bacterial DNA (Sueoka 1961). However, the conclusion about the heterogeneity within a single species was originally obtained from the analysis of the buoyant density of large DNA fragments in a CsCl gradient, and the variation of GC content among smaller regions of the genome has only recently become a subject of analysis, thanks mostly to the accumulation of nucleotide sequence data on various isolated genes from a single bacterial species. In connection with our studies on the regulation of L11 ribosomal protein (r-protein) operon expression, we have recently isolated and sequenced L11 r-protein operons from *Serratia marcescens* and *Proteus vulgaris* (Sor and Nomura 1987). (The purpose of the research was to study the possible conservation of the structures of sites involved in the interaction between mRNA and L1 repressor, and we have demonstrated that both *Serratia* L1 and *Proteus* L1 can function as a repressor to regulate *Escherichia coli* L11 operon in vivo [Sor and Nomura 1987].) The sequence data have allowed us to compare the sequence divergence of these r-protein genes between *S. Marcescens* and *E. coli* with that of some other genes, such as $trp(G)D$ (Nichols et al. 1980), studied previously. The results of preliminary analyses suggest that the directional mutation pressure affecting GC content of genomes (Sueoka 1962 and in prep.; Jukes 1985; Muto and Osawa 1987) may have operated differently in different regions of a single bacterial genome, although the range of diversity may not be as great as that seen in vertebrates. Here, we limit our discussion only to the comparison between *E. coli* genome and *S. marcescens* genome.

The L11 operon consists of the genes for L11 (*rplK*) and L1 (*rplA*). The nucleotide sequence of the *S. marcescens rplKA* region determined covers the coding regions (1128 nucleotides) for the two genes together with their 5'- and 3'-flanking regions (231 nucleotides and 122 nucleotides, respectively) (Sor and Nomura 1987). The GC content of the coding regions and the noncoding regions (the upstream and downstream regions plus 3 nucleotides in the intercistronic region) were found to be 51% and 47%, respectively. These values are similar to the values (52%, 45%) in the corresponding regions in *E. coli* (Table 1). Thus, the GC content of the *rplKA* coding region (as well as the surrounding noncoding region) in *S. marcescens* does not reflect the GC content of the entire genome (See Table 1). This situation is in sharp contrast to the $trp(G)D$ gene studied thoroughly by Yanofsky and his co-workers (Nichols et al. 1980). The *trpG* gene from *S. marcescens* has a higher GC content (65%) than the corresponding region (*trp[G]D*) from *E. coli* (55%), and therefore, the divergence in this gene reflects the GC contents of the two genomes (Nichols et al. 1980; Table 1). By comparing the $trp(G)D$ sequences from the two organisms, Nichols et al. (1980) have noted

*Institut Curie, batiment 110, Centre Universitaire, Orsay, F91405 France.

Table 1. GC Contents of the *rplKA* Region, *trp(G)D*, *ompA*, and *lpp* Genes

	Chromosomal location (min)	Number of nucleotides analyzed	%GC	
			E. Coli	*S. marcescens*
rplKA	90			
Noncoding regions		356	45	47
Coding regions		1128	52	51
First and second positions			52	51
Third position			52	50
trp(G)D	28			
Coding region		579	<u>55</u>	<u>65</u>
First and second positions			52	56
Third position			<u>61</u>	<u>82</u>
lpp	36			
Coding region		234	51	50
First and second positions			50	51
Third position			49	50
ompA	22			
Coding region		1038	54	55
First and second positions			52	54
Third position			56	56
Entire genome			51	59

The GC contents of the coding region and the third codon position of *trp(G)D* are underlined to indicate large differences between *E. coli* and *S. marcescens*. The GC contents of genomes are from Sober (1970). Other references are given in the text.

that most of the nucleotide substitutions that result in an increase of GC content (from *E. coli* to *S. marcescens*) are neutral mutations in the third position of codons that do not alter the amino acid, i.e., synonymous substitutions at the third position. The numbers of these synonymous substitutions are given in Table 2, together with the corresponding values found for the *rplKA* genes. It is evident that the frequency of occurrence of synonymous substitutions at the third position of codons in the *rplKA* genes is quite high (18%), although not as high as that in the *trp(G)D* system (33%). Yet, in contrast to the synonymous substitutions in the *trp* system that are mostly AT→GC, substitutions in both directions are equally frequent in the *rplKA* genes. This difference is reflected in the GC content of the third codon position as listed in Table 1; no increase in the case of *rplKA* (52% to 50%) and a large increase in the case of *trp(G)D* (61% to 82%) from *E. coli* to *S. marcescens*.

There are two other genes that were isolated and sequenced both from *E. coli* and *S. marcescens* present in the GenBank sequence data base. They are the *lpp* gene (Nakamura and Inouye 1980) and the *ompA* gene (Braun and Cole 1984). The GC contents of the coding regions and the GC contents of the third position of the

codons of these genes are given in Table 1. No difference exists in the GC contents of these two genes between *S. marcescens* and *E. coli*, as in the case of *rplKA*. In fact, Nakamura and Inouye (1980) have already noticed this feature. Although the *lpp* gene is a small gene and the number of the neutral substitutions are rather small to make a statistically strong case, the synonymous substitutions at the third codon position are biased to GC→AT rather than AT→GC (from *E. coli* to *S. marcescens*). In addition, Nakamura and Inouye (1980) have found that an (incomplete) open-reading frame that exists upstream of the *lpp* gene shows synonymous base substitutions representing mostly AT to GC (from *E. coli* to *S. marcescens*), as in the case of the *trp(G)D*. Therefore, the remarkable differences observed in the direction of synonymous base substitutions between *rplKA* and *trp(G)D* do not appear to be exceptional.

There are two possible ways to explain the observed differences in the GC content (and in the direction of synonymous base substitutions) among chromosomal regions within a single bacterial species. One possibility is that variation in GC content is simply a reflection of past recombinational events (e.g., transfer of the *rplKA* region from an ancestor of *E. coli* to an ancestor

Table 2. Synonymous Substitutions (at the Third Codon Position) in *rplKA* and *trp(G)D* from *E. coli* to *S. marcescens*

Genes	Total number of codons	Synonymous substitutions		
		AT→GC	GC→AT	Total (%)
rplKA	376	30	36	66 (18)
trp(G)D	193	48	15	63 (33)

of *S. marcescens*). Although this is a formal possibility, we do not think it very likely, since several independent recombinational events have to be invoked to explain unique GC contents of several (and probably many) separate regions. In addition, studies on the genetic structure of natural populations of bacteria indicate recombinational events to be very limited (e.g., see Selander 1985). The second possibility is that mutational pressures are different in different chromosomal regions, and we shall examine this possibility below.

To explain the wide variation of DNA base composition among different bacteria and its relatively small heterogeneity within individual species, Sueoka has proposed a theory of directional mutation pressure (Sueoka 1962 and in prep.). He has suggested that the overall mutation rate of individual bacteria has a directional effect toward higher or lower GC content of DNA, and that this mutational pressure generates greater directional change in the neutral part of the genome than in the functionally significant part. Since a mutation at the third codon position to GC or AT usually leads to another synonymous codon without amino acid alteration, the effect of the proposed directional mutation pressure (also called "AT/GC pressure"; see Muto and Osawa 1987) is more evident in the GC content of the third codon position than the average GC content of the genome of an organism (Muto and Osawa 1987; N. Sueoka, in prep.). Muto and Osawa (1987) have also pointed out that the GC content of rRNA and tRNA genes has a positive linear correlation with the GC content of the genomic DNA, but the correlation is much less striking than with the protein genes. They have suggested that these RNA genes are more resistant to the directional mutation pressure, since the rRNA and tRNA genes are not translated and most of their sequences are under functional constraints. Thus, an important question is whether the apparent absence of the directional base substitution between *E. coli* and *S. marcescens* observed with the *rplKA* genes is a reflection of a strong functional constraint on their mRNA sequences. We think that the explanation on the basis of functional constraint probably does not apply here. First, the homology of the upstream noncoding region between *E. coli* and *S. marcescens* is less than that in the coding regions. The upstream region (about 230 nucleotides sequenced) showed only 73% homology (compared to 89% in the coding regions), suggesting less functional constraint than the coding regions. The downstream region (covering 122 nucleotides sequenced) immediately following the *rplA* gene does not show any noticeable homology, suggesting perhaps no functional constraint in this region (Sor and Nomura 1987). Yet, the GC content of these regions is about the same in the two organisms analyzed as is found in the coding regions (Table 1). Second, the synonymous codon changes observed are significant in numbers, as much as 18% of the total codons, and appear to be distributed randomly throughout the coding regions. In addition, approximately half of the synonymous codon changes in each gene are balanced by the corresponding opposite changes so that the pattern of codon usage in the *rplKA* genes is very similar between *E. coli* and *S. marcescens*, as was found in the comparative analysis of *trp* operon genes of *E. coli* and *Salmonella typhimurium* (Nichols and Yanofsky 1979; Crawford et al. 1980; Yanofsky and vanCleemput 1982). In addition, the expression of a hybrid operon consisting of *E. coli rplK* and *S. marcescens rplA* in *E. coli* cells appears to be as efficient as the intact *E. coli rplKA* operon (Sor and Nomura 1987), indicating that the alteration of the *rplA* mRNA sequence to the *S. marcescens* sequence (as well as the alteration of the *rplA* gene product, L1 protein, from the *E. coli* form to the *S. marcescens* form) is probably functionally neutral. Therefore, as argued by Yanofksy and his co-workers for the *trp* operon genes (Nichols et al. 1980; Yanofsky and vanCleemput 1982), we think that the many observed synonymous codon changes do not reflect selective values in evolution.

It is known that, in vertebrates, different genes have widely different GC contents. It has been discovered recently that the genomes of vertebrates consist of domains with different GC content, and each domain probably contains several genes (Bernardi et al. 1985; Aota and Ikemura 1986). Sueoka has suggested that several different mutational pressures may operate on different locations of the genome, and the cause for this difference may reside in local structural elements of the chromatin that may influence, for example, substitution errors in DNA replication or repair systems (N. Sueoka, in prep.). A similar suggestion has also been made by Cox (1972), based on a somewhat different reasoning. Although the presence of domains within a chromosome in higher eukaryote genomes has been well known, as exemplified by the presence of many replicons or the presence of cytologically observable bands and loops, bacterial chromosomes have usually been considered not to have such comparable domains. Although we do not know the size of each of the GC-rich regions or AT-rich regions in a bacterial chromosome, bacterial chromosomes do show a regional heterogeneity in GC content. Although we cannot exclude the possibility of past recombinational events as the cause of the present-day heterogeneity, it appears more likely that different regions of a bacterial chromosome are subject to dissimilar mutational pressures. Although it may not be as extreme as in vertebrates, the difference in mutational pressures might be a reflection of differences in structural features of different regions of the chromosome, as has been suggested by N. Sueoka (in prep.) for vertebrate chromosomes. Such nonuniformity in the structural features, if it does exist, may have significance in the regulation of gene expression.

ACKNOWLEDGMENTS

We thank Drs. Noboru Sueoka and Richard E. Lenski for discussion and comments on the manuscript. This work was supported by National Institutes of Health grant GM-35949 and National Science Foundation grant DMB-8543776.

REFERENCES

Aota, S. and T. Ikemura. 1986. Diversity in G + C content at the third position of codons in vertebrate genes and its cause. *Nucleic Acids Res.* **14:** 6345.

Armstrong-Major, J. and W.S. Champney. 1985. Temperature-sensitive translation of MS2 bacteriophage RNA. *Biochim. Biophys. Acta* **824:** 140.

Auron, P.E. and S.R. Fahnestock. 1981. Functional organization of the large ribosomal subunit of *Bacillus stearothermophilus. J. Biol. Chem.* **256:** 10105.

Barta, A., G. Steiner, J. Brosius, H.F. Noller, and E. Kuechler. 1984. Identification of a site on 23S ribosomal RNA located at the peptidyl transferase center. *Proc. Natl. Acad. Sci.* **81:** 3607.

Bernardi, G., B. Olofsson, J. Filipski, M. Zerial, J. Salinas, G. Cuny, M. Meunier-Rotival, and F. Rodier. 1985. The mosaic genome of warm-blooded vertebrates. *Science* **228:** 953.

Biswas, D.K. and L. Gorini. 1972. The attachment site of streptomycin to the 30S ribosomal subunit. *Proc. Natl. Acad. Sci.* **69:** 2141.

Bollen, A., R. Lathe, A. Herzog, D. Denicourt, J.P. Lecocq, L. Desmarez, and R. Levalle. 1979. A conditionally lethal mutation of *Escherichia coli* affecting the gene coding for ribosomal protein S2 (*rpsB*). *J. Mol. Biol.* **132:** 219.

Bowman, C.M., J.E. Dahlberg, T. Ikemura, J. Konisky, and M. Nomura. 1971. Specific inactivation of 16S ribosomal RNA induced by colicin E3 *in vivo. Proc. Natl. Acad. Sci.* **68:** 964.

Braun, G. and S.T. Cole. 1984. DNA sequence analysis of the *Serratia marcescens ompA* gene: Implications for the organization of an enterobacterial outer membrane protein. *Mol. Gen. Genet.* **195:** 321.

Brimacombe, R., J. Atmadja, A. Kyriatsoulis, and W. Stiege. 1986. RNA structure and RNA-protein neighborhoods in the ribosome. In *Structure, function, and genetics of ribosomes* (ed. B. Hardesty and G. Kramer), p. 184. Springer-Verlag, New York.

Cabezón, T., A. Herzog, J. Petre, M. Yaguchi, and A. Bollen. 1977. Ribosomal assembly deficiency in an *Escherichia coli* thermosensitive mutant having an altered L24 ribosomal protein. *J. Mol. Biol.* **116:** 361.

Champney, W.S. 1980. Protein synthesis defects in temperature-sensitive mutants of *Escherichia coli* with altered ribosomal proteins. *Biochim. Biophys. Acta* **609:** 464.

Cohlberg, J.A. and M. Nomura. 1976. Reconstitution of *Bacillus stearothermophilus* 50S ribosomal subunits from purified molecular components. *J. Biol. Chem.* **251:** 209.

Cox, E.C. 1972. On the organization of higher chromosomes. *Nature* **239:** 133.

Crawford, I.P., B.P. Nichols, and C. Yanofsky. 1980. Nucleotide sequence of the *trpB* gene in *Escherichia coli* and *Salmonella typhimurium. J. Mol. Biol.* **142:** 489.

Crick, F.H.C. 1968. The origin of the genetic code. *J. Mol. Biol.* **38:** 367.

Dabbs, E.R. 1986. Mutant studies on the prokaryotic ribosome. In *Structure, function, and genetics of ribosomes* (ed. B. Hardesty and G. Kramer), p. 733. Springer-Verlag, New York.

Dahlberg, A.E. 1986. Site-directed mutagenesis of *Escherichia coli* ribosomal RNA. In *Structure, function, and genetics of ribosomes* (ed. B. Hardesty and G. Kramer), p. 686. Springer-Verlag, New York.

de Boer, H., P. Ng, and A. Hui. 1985. Synthesis of specialized ribosomes in *Escherichia coli*. In *Sequence specificity in transcription and translation* (ed. R. Calendar and L. Gold), p. 419. Alan R. Liss, New York.

Douthwaite, S., J.B. Prince, and H.F. Noller. 1985. Evidence for functional interaction between domains II and V of 23S ribosomal RNA from an erythromycin-resistant mutant. *Proc. Natl. Acad. Sci.* **82:** 8330.

Ehrenberg, M., D. Andersson, K. Bohman, P. Jelenc, T. Ruusala, and C.G. Kurland. 1986. Ribosomal proteins tune rate and accuracy in translation. In *Structure, function, and genetics of ribosomes* (ed. B. Hardesty and G. Kramer), p. 573. Springer-Verlag, New York.

Erdmann, V.A., S. Fahnestock, K. Higo, and M. Nomura. 1971. Role of 5S RNA in the functions of 50S ribosomal subunits. *Proc. Natl. Acad. Sci.* **68:** 2932.

Fahnestock, S.R. and M. Nomura. 1972. Activity of ribosomes containing 5S RNA with a chemically modified 3'-terminus. *Proc. Natl. Acad. Sci.* **69:** 363.

Geyl, D., A. Böck, and H.G. Wittman. 1977. Cold-sensitive growth of a mutant of *Escherichia coli* with an altered ribosomal protein S8: Analysis of revertants. *Mol. Gen. Genet.* **152:** 332.

Gourse, R.L., Y. Takebe, R.A. Sharrock, and M. Nomura. 1985. Feedback regulation of rRNA and tRNA synthesis and accumulation of free ribosomes after conditional expression of rRNA genes. *Proc. Natl. Acad. Sci.* **82:** 1069.

Guerrier-Takada, C., K. Gardiner, T. Marsh, N. Pace, and S. Altman. 1983. The RNA moiety of ribonuclease P is the catalytic subunit of the enzyme. *Cell* **35:** 849.

Guthrie, C., H. Nashimoto, and M. Nomura. 1969. Structure and function of *E. coli* ribosomes. VIII. Cold-sensitive mutants defective in ribosome assembly. *Proc. Natl. Acad. Sci.* **63:** 384.

Hampl, H., H. Schulz, and K.H. Nierhaus. 1981. Ribosomal components from *Escherichia coli* 50S subunits involved in the reconstitution of peptidyltransferase activity. *J. Biol. Chem.* **256:** 2284.

Hayes, F. and S. Schmitt. 1980. Defective assembly of the small ribosomal subunit in temperature-sensitive mutant of *Escherichia coli. Eur. J. Biochem.* **107:** 95.

Held, W.A. and M. Nomura. 1975. *Escherichia coli* 30S ribosomal proteins uniquely required for assembly. *J. Biol. Chem.* **250:** 3179.

Held, W.A., W.R. Gette, and M. Nomura. 1974a. Role of 16S ribosomal ribonucleic acid and the 30S ribosomal protein S12 in the initiation of natural messenger ribonucleic acid translation. *Biochemistry* **13:** 2115.

Held, W.A., S. Mizushima, and M. Nomura. 1973. Reconstitution of *Escherichia coli* 30S ribosomal subunits from purified molecular components. *J. Biol. Chem.* **248:** 5720.

Held, W.A., M. Nomura, and J.W.B. Hershey. 1974b. Ribosomal protein S21 is required for full activity in the initiation of protein synthesis. *Mol. Gen. Genet.* **128:** 11.

Held, W.A., B. Ballou, S. Mizushima, and M. Nomura. 1974c. Assembly mapping of 30S ribosomal proteins from *Escherichia coli*: Further studies. *J. Biol. Chem.* **249:** 3103.

Helser, T.L., J.E. Davies, and J.E. Dahlberg. 1971. Change in methylation of 16S ribosomal RNA associated with mutation of kasugamycin resistance in *Escherichia coli. Nature* **233:** 12.

Herzog, A., M. Yaguchi, T. Cabezón, M.-C. Corchuelo, J. Petre, and A. Bollen. 1979. A missense mutation in the gene coding for ribosomal protein S17 (*rpsQ*) leading to ribosomal assembly defectivity in *Escherichia coli. Mol. Gen. Genet.* **171:** 15.

Isono, S. and K. Isono. 1975. Role of ribosomal protein S1 in protein synthesis: Effects of its addition to *Bacillus stearothermophilus* cell-free system. *Eur. J. Biochem.* **56:** 15.

Ito, K., D.P. Cerretti, H. Nashimoto, and M. Nomura. 1984. Characterization of an amber mutation in the structural gene for ribosomal protein L15, which impairs the expression of the protein export gene, *secY*, in *Escherichia coli. EMBO J.* **3:** 2319.

Jukes, T.H. 1985. A change in the genetic code in *Mycoplasma capricolum. J. Mol. Evol.* **22:** 361.

Kang, S.-S. 1970a. A mutant of *Escherichia coli* with temperature-sensitive streptomycin protein. *Proc. Natl. Acad. Sci.* **65:** 544.

———. 1970b. Temperature sensitive alteration of 30S subunits demonstrated by *in vitro* reassociation of functional ribosomes. *Nature* **225:** 1132.

Konisky, J. and M. Nomura. 1967. Interaction of colicins with bacterial cells. II. Specific alteration of *Escherichia coli* ribosomes induced by colicin E3 *in vivo*. *J. Mol. Biol.* **26:** 181.

Kruger, K., P.J. Grabowski, A.J. Zaug, J. Sands, D.E. Gottschling, and T.R. Cech. 1982. Self-splicing RNA: Autoexcision and autocyclization of the ribosomal RNA intervening sequence of tetrahymena. *Cell* **31:** 147.

Kushner, S.R., V.F. Maples, and W.S. Champney. 1977. Conditionally lethal ribosomal protein mutants: Characterization of a locus required for modification of 50S subunit proteins. *Proc. Natl. Acad. Sci.* **74:** 467.

Lai, C.-J., B. Weisblum, S.R. Fahnestock, and M. Nomura. 1973. Alteration of 23S ribosomal RNA and erythromycin-induced resistance to lincomycin and spiramycin in *Staphylococcus aureus*. *J. Mol. Biol.* **74:** 67.

Lhoest, J. and C. Colson. 1981. Cold-sensitive ribosome assembly in an *Escherichia coli* mutant lacking a single group in ribosomal protein L3. *Eur. J. Biochem.* **121:** 33.

Lotti, M., E.R. Dabbs, R. Hasenbank, M. Stöffler-Meilicke, and G. Stöffler. 1983. Characterisation of a mutant from *Escherichia coli* lacking protein L15 and localisation of protein L15 by immuno-electron microscopy. *Mol. Gen. Genet.* **192:** 295.

Mark, L.G., C.D. Sigmund, and E.A. Morgan. 1983. Spectinomycin resistance due to a mutation in an rRNA operon of *Escherichia coli*. *J. Bacteriol.* **155:** 989.

Mizushima, S. and M. Nomura. 1970. Assembly mapping of 30S ribosomal proteins from *E. coli*. *Nature* **226:** 1214.

Montandon, P.-E., R. Wagner, and E. Stutz. 1986. *E. coli* ribosomes with a C912 to U base change in the 16S rRNA are streptomycin resistant. *EMBO J.* **5:** 3705.

Montandon, P.-E., P. Nicolas, P. Schürmann, and E. Stutz. 1985. Streptomycin-resistance of *Euglena gracilis* chloroplasts: Identification of a point mutation in the 16S rRNA gene in an invariant position. *Nucleic Acids Res.* **13:** 4299.

Moore, P.B., M. Capel, M. Kjeldgaard, and D.M. Engelman. 1986. A 19 protein map of the 30S ribosomal subunit of *Escherichia coli*. In *Structure, function, and genetics of ribosomes* (ed. B. Hardesty and G. Kramer), p. 87. Springer-Verlag, New York.

Nashimoto, H. and M. Nomura. 1970. Structure and function of bacterial ribosomes. XI. Dependence of 50S ribosomal assembly on simultaneous assembly of 30S subunits. *Proc. Natl. Acad. Sci.* **67:** 1440.

Nashimoto, H., A. Miura, H. Saito, and H. Uchida. 1985. Suppressors of temperature-sensitive mutations in a ribosomal protein gene, *rpsL*, of *Escherichia coli* K12. *Mol. Gen. Genet.* **199:** 381.

Nichols, B.P. and C. Yanofsky. 1979. Nucleotide sequences of *trpA* of *Salmonella typhimurium* and *Escherichia coli*: An evolutionary comparison. *Proc. Natl. Acad. Sci.* **76:** 5244.

Nichols, B.P., G.F. Miozzari, M. vanCleemput, G.N. Bennett, and C. Yanofsky. 1980. Nucleotide sequences of the *trpG* regions of *Escherichia coli*. *Shigella dysenteriae*, *Salmonella typhimurium* and *Serratia marcescens*. *J. Mol. Biol.* **142:** 503.

Nierhaus, K.H. 1980. Analysis of the assembly and function of the 50S subunit from *Escherichia coli* ribosomes by reconstitution. In *Ribosomes: Structure, function, and genetics* (ed. G. Chambliss et al.), p. 267. University Park Press, Baltimore.

———.1982. Structure, assembly, and function of ribosomes. *Curr. Top. Microbiol. Immunol.* **97:** 81.

Nierhaus, K.H. and F. Dohme. 1974. Total reconstitution of functionally active 50S ribosomal subunits from *Escherichia coli*. *Proc. Natl. Acad. Sci.* **71:** 4713.

Noller, H.F. and J.B. Chaires. 1972. Functional modification of 16S ribosomal RNA by kethoxal. *Proc. Natl. Acad. Sci.* **69:** 3115.

Noller, H.F. and J.A. Lake. 1984. Ribosome structure and function: Localization of rRNA. *Membr. Struct. Funct.* **6:** 217.

Noller, H.F., M. Asire, A. Barta, S. Douthwaite, T. Gold-

stein, R.R. Gutell, D. Moazed, J. Normanly, J.B. Prince, S. Stern, K. Triman, S. Turner, B. Van Stolk, V. Wheaton, B. Weiser, and C.R. Woese. 1986. Studies on the structure and function of ribosomal RNA. In *Structure, function, and genetics of ribosomes* (ed. B. Hardesty and G. Kramer), p. 143. Springer-Verlag, New York.

Nomura, M. 1964. Mode of action of colicines. *Cold Spring Harbor Symp. Quant. Biol.* **28:** 315.

Nomura, M. and V.A. Erdmann. 1970. Reconstitution of 50S ribosomal subunits from dissociated molecular components. *Nature* **228:** 744.

Nomura, M. and W.A. Held. 1974. Reconstitution of ribosomes: Studies of ribosome structure, function and assembly. In *Ribosomes* (ed. M. Nomura et al.), p. 193. Cold Spring Harbor Laboratory, Cold Spring Harbor, New York.

Nomura, M., P. Traub, and H. Bechmann. 1968. Hybrid 30S ribosomal particles reconstituted from components of different bacterial origins. *Nature* **219:** 793.

Nomura, M., S. Mizushima, M. Ozaki, P. Traub, and C.V. Lowry. 1970. Structure and function of ribosomes and their molecular components. *Cold Spring Harbor Symp. Quant. Biol.* **34:** 49.

Nowotny, V. and K.H. Nierhaus. 1980. Protein L20 from the large subunit of *Escherichia coli* ribosomes is an assembly protein. *J. Mol. Biol.* **137:** 391.

Olsson, M., L. Isaksson, and C.G. Kurland. 1974. Pleiotropic effects of ribosomal protein S4 studied in *Escherichia coli* mutants. *Mol. Gen. Genet.* **135:** 191.

Orgel, L.E. 1968. Evolution of the genetic apparatus. *J. Mol. Biol.* **38:** 381.

Ozaki, M., S. Mizushima, and M. Nomura. 1969. Identification and functional characterization of the protein controlled by the streptomycin-resistant locus in *E. coli*. *Nature* **222:** 333.

Röhl, R. and K.H. Nierhaus. 1982. Assembly map of the large subunit (50S) of *Escherichia coli* ribosomes. *Proc. Natl. Acad. Sci.* **79:** 729.

Rolfe, R. and M. Meselson. 1959. The relative homogeneity of microbial DNA. *Proc. Natl. Acad. Sci.* **45:** 1039.

Ruusala, T., D. Andersson, M. Ehrenberg, and C.G. Kurland. 1984. Hyper-accurate ribosomes inhibit growth. *EMBO J.* **3:** 2575.

Schulze, H. and K.H. Nierhaus. 1982. Minimal set of ribosomal components for reconstitution of the peptidyltransferase activity. *EMBO J.* **5:** 609.

Selander, R.K. 1985. Protein polymorphism and the genetic structure of natural populations of bacteria. In *Population genetics and molecular evolution* (ed. T. Ohta and K. Aoki), p. 85. Springer-Verlag, Berlin.

Senior, B.W. and I.B. Holland. 1971. Effect of colicin E3 upon the 30S ribosomal subunits of *Escherichia coli*. *Proc. Natl. Acad. Sci.* **68:** 959.

Shine, J. and L. Dalgarno. 1974. The 3′-terminal sequence of *E. coli* 16S ribosomal RNA: Complementarity to nonsense triplets and ribosome binding sites. *Proc. Natl. Acad. Sci.* **71:** 1342.

Sigmund, C.D. and E.A. Morgan. 1982. Erythromycin resistance due to a mutation in a ribosomal RNA operon of *Escherichia coli*. *Proc. Natl. Acad. Sci.* **79:** 5602.

Sober, H.A., ed. 1970. *Handbook of biochemistry: Selected data for molecular biology* 2nd edition, p. H83. CRC Press, Boca Raton, Florida.

Sor, F. and M. Nomura. 1987. Cloning and DNA sequence determination of the L11 ribosomal protein operon of *Serratia marcescens* and *Proteus vulgaris*: Translational feedback regulation of the *Escherichia coli* L11 operon by heterologous L1 proteins. *Mol. Gen. Genet.* (in press).

Spillmann, S. and K.H. Nierhaus. 1978. The ribosomal protein L24 of *Escherichia coli* is an assembly protein. *J. Biol. Chem.* **253:** 7047.

Sprague, K.U., J.A. Steitz, R.M. Grenley, and C.E. Stocking. 1977. 3′ Terminal sequences of 16S rRNA do not explain translational specificity differences between *E. coli* and *B. stearothermophilus* ribosomes. *Nature* **267:** 462.

Steitz, J.A. 1980. RNA·RNA interactions during polypeptide chain initiation. In *Ribosomes: Structure, function, and genetics* (ed. G. Chambliss et al.), p. 479. University Park Press, Baltimore.

Steitz, J.A. and K. Jakes. 1975. How ribosomes select initiator regions in mRNA: Base pair formation between the 3′ terminus of 16S rRNA and the mRNA during initiation of protein synthesis in *Escherichia coli. Proc. Natl. Acad. Sci.* **72:** 4734.

Sueoka, N. 1961. Variation and heterogeneity of base composition of deoxyribonucleic acids: A compilation of old and new data. *J. Mol. Biol.* **3:** 31.

———. 1962. On the genetic basis of variation and heterogeneity of DNA base composition. *Proc. Natl. Acad. Sci.* **48:** 582.

Sueoka, N., J. Marmur, and P. Doty. 1959. Dependence of the density of deoxyribonucleic acids on guanine-cytosine. *Nature* **183:** 1432.

Tai, P.-C., D.P. Kessler, and J. Ingraham. 1969. Cold-sensitive mutations in *Salmonella typhimurium* which affect ribosome synthesis. *J. Bacteriol.* **97:** 1298.

Traub, P. and M. Nomura. 1968a. Structure and function of *E. coli* ribosomes. V. Reconstitution of functionally active 30S ribosomal particles from RNA and proteins. *Proc. Natl. Acad. Sci.* **59:** 777.

———. 1968b. Streptomycin resistance mutation in *Escherichia coli*: Altered ribosomal protein. *Science* **160:** 198.

Traub, P., K. Hosokawa, G.R. Craven, and M. Nomura. 1967. Structure and function of *Escherichia coli* ribosomes. IV. Isolation and characterization of functionally active ribosomal proteins. *Proc. Natl. Acad. Sci.* **58:** 2430.

Van Dieijen, G., P.H. Van Knippenberg, and J. Van Duin. 1976. The specific role of ribosomal protein S1 in the recognition of native phage RNA. *Eur. J. Biochem.* **64:** 511.

Van Duin, J. and R. Wijnands. 1981. The function of ribosomal protein S21 in protein synthesis. *Eur. J. Biochem.* **118:** 615.

Waller, J.P. 1964. Fractionation of the ribosomal protein from *Escherichia coli. J. Mol. Biol.* **10:** 319.

Watson, J.D. 1964. The synthesis of proteins from ribosomes. *Bull. Soc. Chim. Biol.* **46:** 1399.

Wittman, H.G., G. Stöffler, W. Piepersberg, P. Buckel, D. Ruffler, and A. Böck. 1974. Altered S5 and S20 ribosomal proteins in revertants of an alanyl-tRNA synthetase mutant of *Escherichia coli. Mol. Gen. Genet.* **134:** 225.

Woese, C.R. 1980. Just so stories and Rube Goldberg machines: Speculations on the origin of the protein synthetic machinery. In *Ribosomes: Structure, function, and genetics* (ed. G. Chambliss et al.), p. 357. University Park Press, Baltimore.

Yanofsky, C. and M. vanCleemput. 1982. Nucleotide sequence of *trpE* of *Salmonella typhimurium* and its homology with the corresponding sequence of *Escherichia coli. J. Mol. Biol.* **155:** 235.

Yates, Y.L., W.R. Gette, M.E. Furth, and M. Nomura. 1977. Effects of ribosomal mutations on the read-through of a chain termination signal: Studies on the synthesis of bacteriophage λ 0 gene protein *in vitro. Proc. Natl. Acad. Sci.* **74:** 689.

Zengel, J.M., R. Young, P.P. Dennis, and M. Nomura. 1977. Role of ribosomal protein S12 in peptide chain elongation: Analysis of pleiotropic streptomycin-resistant mutants of *Escherichia coli. J. Bacteriol.* **129:** 1320.

New Aspects of Structure, Assembly, Evolution, and Function of Ribosomes

K.H. Nierhaus, R. Brimacombe, V. Nowotny, C.L. Pon, H. J. Rheinberger, B. Wittmann-Liebold, and H.-G. Wittmann

Max-Planck-Institut für Molekulare Genetik, D-1000 Berlin 33, Federal Republic of Germany

Bacterial ribosomes consist of 50–60 proteins and three (5S, 16S, and 23S) rRNA molecules. Now that the determination of the primary structure of all the ribosomal components from *Escherichia coli* is complete (for reviews, see Noller 1980; Giri et al. 1984), current research is concentrating on regulation of the biosynthesis of ribosomal components, the architecture of the ribosome, principles of the ribosomal assembly and functions, and the evolutionary relatedness between components of the translational apparatus derived from various organisms. In this paper, we survey some of our recent contributions, with particular emphasis on the ribosomal elongation cycle.

The Three-dimensional Arrangement of 16S rRNA in situ in the 30S Ribosomal Subunit

The secondary structure of the 16S rRNA from *E. coli* is now well established by both experimental and phylogenetic methods (e.g., Brimacombe et al. 1983; Huysmans and De Wachter 1986), and a large body of intra-RNA and RNA-protein cross-linking data obtained in this laboratory has been used to fold this secondary structure into a three-dimensional model (R. Brimacombe et al., in prep.). All the cross-links were induced in intact 30S subunits (or in some cases in growing *E. coli* cells) and the sites of cross-linking were precisely localized on the RNA by oligonucleotide analysis. The RNA-protein cross-linking data (including 28 sites, and involving 13 of the 21 proteins of the 30S ribosomal subunit) were used to relate the RNA structure to the distribution of the proteins as determined by neutron scattering (Moore et al. 1986) or immunoelectron microscopy (e.g., Stöffler and Stöffler-Meilicke 1986).

The three-dimensional model of the 16S RNA has overall dimensions of 220 Å × 140 Å × 90 Å, in good agreement with electron microscopic estimates for the 30S subunit. The shape of the model is also recognizably the same as that seen in electron micrographs, and the positions in the model of bases localized on the surface of the 30S subunit by immunoelectron microscopy (the 5′ and 3′ termini, the m⁷G and m⁶A residues, and C-1400) correspond closely to their experimentally observed positions. A view of the model is shown in Figure 1, in which several of these features, as well as the "cleft" in the subunit, can clearly be seen.

The distances between the RNA-protein cross-link

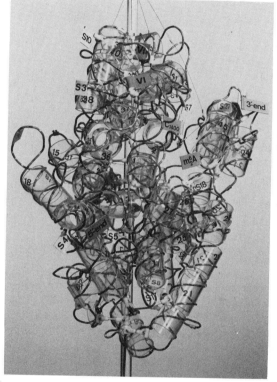

Figure 1. View of the three-dimensional model of 16S RNA (R. Brimacombe et al., in prep.). The wire represents the phosphate backbone of the RNA, and the Perspex tubes define the double-helical elements. Features such as RNA-protein cross-link sites, intra-RNA cross-link sites, or immunoelectron microscopically located bases are indicated by "flags" (see R. Brimacombe et al., in prep., for details).

sites in the model correlate well with the distances between protein centers of mass obtained by neutron scattering (Moore et al. 1986), only 2 out of 66 distances falling outside the expected tolerance limits. The model fits well with previously published data on RNA-protein binding sites and tertiary interactions in the RNA. Mutation sites on the RNA causing resistance to antibiotics lie close to the positions of the corresponding proteins. Mutations which also cause resistance to the respective antibiotics and the sequences proposed to be involved in a secondary structural "switch" are also close neighbors in the model.

All nine of the modified bases in the *E. coli* 16S RNA

show a remarkable distribution, in that they lie roughly in a plane, forming a "collar" around the "neck" of the 30S subunit between the head and body regions. These modified bases are all in exposed positions in the model. Similarly, 87% of the sites on 16S RNA found to be accessible to chemical modification in the 30S subunit are at exposed sites in the model, whereas, in contrast, 70% of the sites corresponding to positions that have ribose 2'-O-methylations in the 18S RNA from *Xenopus laevis* are at nonexposed (i.e., internal) positions. Insertions in eukaryotic 18S RNA and corresponding deletions in chloroplast or mammalian mitochondrial rRNA relative to the *E. coli* 16S RNA (see Brimacombe et al. 1983) represent distinct topographical "subdomains" in the structure. Some, but by no means all, of the RNA helices proposed to be coaxial in the 16S RNA can be brought into coaxial positions, but it is clearly premature to try to formulate rules governing this property of multihelical RNA molecules. All these features are discussed in detail by R. Brimacombe et al. (in prep.), together with the appropriate literature references. Cross-linking data from other authors, in particular intra-RNA cross-links formed using isolated 16S RNA as the substrate for the cross-linking reactions, are generally not compatible with our model, the model being radically different from that proposed by Expert-Bezançon and Wollenzien (1985) on the basis of the latter type of data.

Neutron-scattering Analysis of the 50S Ribosomal Subunit

Neutron scattering has been applied to the elucidation of the quaternary structure of the 30S subunit. By integrating two deuterated proteins into a protonated ribosomal matrix, the distance between the mass centers of the corresponding proteins can be assessed. The distances obtained in this way have been used to reconstruct the spatial arrangement of 19 of the 21 S proteins (Moore et al. 1986). We are applying a modified strategy for analysis of the 50S structure, in which protonated components are integrated into a "homogenized" (see below) deuterated ribosome. With this strategy, not only distances but also shape parameters of single protonated components or ligands can be determined directly in situ (Nierhaus et al. 1983).

Protons (^{1}H) scatter neutrons in a manner remarkably different from the other elements most frequently found in biological samples (C, N, O, P, and S), whereas the heavy hydrogen isotope deuterium (^{2}H or D) scatters neutrons in a manner similar to the other elements. Thus, the scattering densities of biological molecules are predominantly determined by their relative proton content, which is different for nucleic acids and proteins (51% and 37%, respectively). In consequence, all complexes consisting of these two molecular classes are heterogeneous for the neutron beam.

We have homogenized the ribosome by reconstitut-ing the 50S subunit from differentially deuterated rRNA and protein fractions, both of which have a scattering density equivalent to that of 90% D_2O. The deuterated components are derived from two different cell batches, one of which is grown at a D_2O concentration such that all nucleic acids of the bacteria match at 90% D_2O, the other one being grown at a D_2O concentration where all the proteins achieve that scattering density. A reconstituted deuterated ribosome, which has been transferred to a buffer containing 90% D_2O, thus exhibits the advantage of becoming "invisible" for the neutron beam (the "glassy ribosome"). A second advantage of this strategy lies in the fact that the measured sample is dominated by deuterons. Of the neutrons scattered by deuterons, 75% show interference phenomena ("coherently" scattered neutrons, the other 25% being incoherently scattered), as compared with only 2% of the neutrons scattered by protons. Both factors, i.e., homogenization and deuteron dominance, are responsible for the improved signal-to-noise ratio observed with this experimental design (for a detailed description, see Nowotny et al. 1986).

When one protonated protein is incorporated in the deuterated ribosome, the radius of gyration of the respective component in situ can be measured directly (for a recent compilation, see Nowotny et al. 1986). When two protonated proteins are incorporated, the distance between the mass centers of gravity of the respective proteins can be determined. These pair distances can be used for triangulation of the mass centers of the proteins, and the current model, comprising eleven proteins, is depicted in Figure 2. The model can be oriented within the 50S subunit in such a manner that an excellent correlation is found with the epitopes

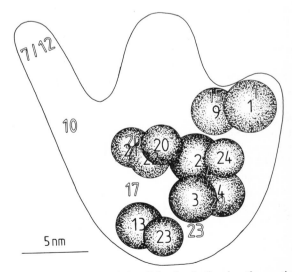

Figure 2. Rear view of the 50S subunit showing the spatial arrangement of 11 L proteins. Epitopes of 5 of these proteins (L1, L4, L9, L20, and L23) have been located on the surface of the 50S subunit by means of immunoelectron microscopy (Stöffler and Stöffler-Meilicke 1986), and the neutron-scattering model has been arranged to achieve an optimal overlap with the epitopes of the 5 proteins.

of those five proteins whose positions have also been determined by means of immunoelectron microscopy (Stöffler and Stöffler-Meilicke 1986).

Reconstitution Analysis of the 50S Assembly

Despite the complicated structure of the *E. coli* ribosome with its 55 different components, fully active subunits can be reconstructed in vitro from the separated proteins and rRNA (total reconstitution). The total reconstitution of the small subunit is a one-step procedure (20 mM Mg^{++}, 40°C), and the analysis of the 30S assembly by means of this technique has been reviewed by Nomura and Held (1974).

The total reconstitution of the large subunit from *E. coli* ribosomes requires a two-step procedure (4 mM Mg^{++}, 44°C → 20 mM Mg^{++}, 50°C; Dohme and Nierhaus 1976). The 50°C incubation lasts for 90 minutes, whereas in vivo the 50S assembly takes only a few minutes at 37°C (Schlessinger 1974). This enormous difference raises the question of the physiological significance of the results obtained by total reconstitution in vitro, and this point will be given particular consideration in this survey of the 50S assembly (Table 1).

The three reconstitution intermediates sequentially formed in the course of 50S assembly in vitro are termed $RI_{50}(1)$, $RI_{50}^*(1)$, and $RI_{50}(2)$, (Table 1). They are very similar to the corresponding precursor particles found in vivo, as far as their S values (Table 1) and protein content (Herold and Nierhaus 1987) are concerned. The rate-limiting steps are very similar, if not identical, both in vivo and in vitro.

Table 1. Features of the 50S Assembly

1. In vitro:3 intermediates $RI_{50}(1) \rightarrow RI_{50}^*(1) \rightarrow RI_{50}(2) \rightarrow$ 50S
   (33S)(42S)(48S)

   In vivo:3 precursors $p_1 50S \rightarrow p_2 50S \rightarrow p_3 50S \rightarrow$ 50S
   (32S)(43S)(~50S)
2. The assembly starts with only two proteins (assembly initiator proteins): L24 and L3.
3. The early assembly reactions depend on only five proteins: L4, L13, L20, L22, and L24 (early assembly proteins). L3 stimulates.
4. The five early assembly proteins bind exclusively to the 5' end of the 23S rRNA: assembly gradient.
5. At least two of the early assembly proteins, L20 and L24 are mere assembly proteins. They are not involved in both late assembly and function of the 50S subunit.

Interestingly, the $RI_{50}(1)$ and $RI_{50}^*(1)$ particles contain an identical set of ribosomal components, despite the drastic difference between their respective S values (33S and 42S). Likewise, the $RI_{50}(2)$ particle contains a complete set of 50S components but is totally inactive. The conformational changes involved ($RI_{50}[1] \rightarrow RI_{50}^*[1]$ and $RI_{50}[2] \rightarrow 50S$, respectively) require different ionic milieus and incubation temperatures (Dohme and Nierhaus 1976), which explains the need for a two-step procedure.

A step-by-step analysis of the 50S reconstitution process has led to the assembly map, the latest version of which contains all of the 50S components (Fig. 3; Herold and Nierhaus 1987). The bar at the top represents the three fragments into which the 23S rRNA can

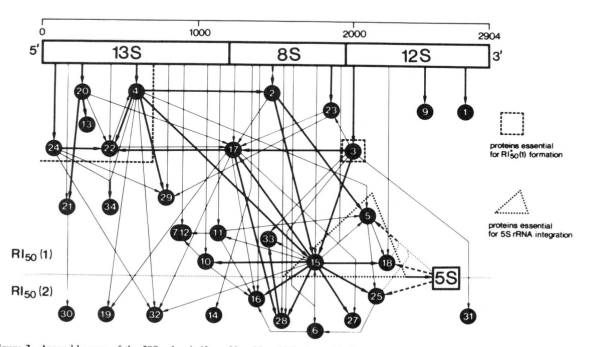

Figure 3. Assembly map of the 50S subunit (from Herold and Nierhaus 1987). Lx→ (→) Ly, binding of Ly is strongly (weakly) dependent on Lx. Dotted lines indicate the encircled proteins are essential for mediating the binding of 5S rRNA to 23S rRNA. Proteins enclosed by dashed lines are important or essential for the conformational change from $RI_{50}^*(1)$ to $RI_{50}(1)$ (for review, see Nierhaus 1980). Components below the finely dotted line are not present on the $RI_{50}(1)$ particle.

be easily split. An arrow from L20 to L13, for example, indicates that L13 can only be assembled after L20 has been incorporated. A line separates the proteins found in the $RI_{50}^*(1)$ particle (above) from those present in addition in the $RI_{50}(2)$ particle (below).

Although the 50S subunit contains 20 proteins which can bind to "naked" 23S rRNA in vitro (23S rRNA-binding proteins, as indicated by arrows from the 23S rRNA to a protein in Fig. 3), only two of these, namely L24 and L3, are able to act as assembly-initiator proteins. It is likely that the existence of just two initiator proteins represents an optimum (for further details, see Nowotny and Nierhaus 1982).

Proteins essential for the early assembly (Table 1) bind near the 5' end of the 23S rRNA (for review, see Nierhaus 1980). Clearly, in vivo the early assembly reactions occur between the few early assembly proteins and a short 5' region of the nascent 23S rRNA, whereas in vitro we are dealing with the mature 23S rRNA and all of the ribosomal proteins at the same time. Therefore, the early assembly in vivo has an enormous entropic advantage over that in vitro. This advantage is a feature of the "assembly gradient" (Nierhaus 1980), which means that the progress of the rRNA synthesis dictates the progress of assembly. The entropic advantage of the assembly gradient is probably one important reason why ribosomes can assemble within a few minutes at 37°C in the cell, in contrast to the 90 minutes at 50°C required for the in vitro assembly. Furthermore, a maintenance of the assembly gradient principle in eukaryotic cells is the only explanation that can be offered for the complicated and circumstantial mode of ribosome assembly in vivo. Eukaryotic ribosomal proteins are imported from the cytosol into the nucleoli, thus enabling rRNA synthesis and ribosomal assembly to be coupled.

Two of the early assembly proteins, L20 and L24, have been identified as mere "assembly proteins," which are essential for the early assembly but play no role in the late assembly or the functions of the 50S subunits (for review, see Nierhaus 1980).

With the help of the reconstitution technique, it has been possible to analyze the peptidyltransferase center. Six components have been identified as being essential for its reconstitution, namely 23S rRNA, L2, L3, L4, L15, and L16 (Schulze and Nierhaus 1982), all of which are interconnected via strong assembly dependencies (see Fig. 3). The same set (except L15) has been identified in a similar analysis of 50S subunits from *Bacillus stearothermophilus* (Auron and Fahnestock 1981). If there is a catalytically active component in the 50S subunit, then it must necessarily be one of these components; if it is a protein, L2 is a likely candidate (for further discussion, see Herold and Nierhaus 1987).

Evolution

Because of their occurrence in all organisms, ribosomes and their constituents are ideal subjects for phylogenetic investigations. The extensive studies that have been made on the structure of ribosomal proteins and RNAs from many organisms have already yielded interesting information, not only concerning the evolution of ribosomes but also concerning the relatedness of eubacteria, archaebacteria, and eukaryotes to each other and hence their relative positions within the phylogenetic tree.

Among the various approaches used for evolutionary studies on ribosomal proteins, e.g., two-dimensional polyacrylamide gel electrophoresis and immunological methods, the determination and comparison of the amino acid sequences is the most informative. The results that we have so far obtained by this approach can be summarized as follows (for more details, see Wittmann-Liebold 1986).

(1) When the amino acid sequences of the 52 proteins present in the *E. coli* ribosome were compared with one another by the computer program RELATE, only 4% of all possible combinations were found to show some homology, and in these cases the homologous regions were rather short, i.e., no extensive homology among the numerous *E. coli* ribosomal proteins could be detected by comparison of their amino acid sequences.

(2) There are several internal repeats within the primary structure of the largest protein of the *E. coli* ribosome, demonstrating that the gene of this protein has evolved from smaller units by multiple gene duplications.

(3) A comparison of ribosomal proteins from the gram-positive *Bacillus stearothermophilus* with those from the gram-negative *E. coli* showed a wide range of homology, depending on the protein pair concerned. The most conserved protein is S12, where 76% of the amino acids are identical in both species, whereas only 25% of the amino acids are identical in protein L32 from the two organisms. Interestingly, those proteins that are important for ribosomal functions, for example, in the poly(U) or the peptidyltransferase tests, are more conserved than those that have been found to be functionally less important.

(4) The extent of homology between ribosomal proteins from chloroplasts of higher plants and those from *E. coli* is approximately the same as that between gram-positive and gram-negative eubacteria.

(5) Since the phylogeny of the archaebacteria is still a subject of controversy, the comparison of ribosomal proteins from these bacteria with those from other organisms is of particular interest. The 16 ribosomal proteins from *Halobacterium marismortui*, whose complete primary structures have been elucidated by M. Kimura and his co-workers (Arndt et al. 1986), can be divided as follows. Several of these proteins are homologous to ribosomal proteins either from eubacteria or from eukaryotes. On the other hand, some proteins show a significant homology with both those from eubacteria and those from eukaryotes, whereas a few proteins reveal no homology at all. It is possible that in the latter case a homology with eukaryotes will be detected when the structures of more proteins from

eukaryotic ribosomes are known. Interestingly, one halobacterial protein is homologous in its amino-terminal part to the eubacterial protein S8 and in its carboxy-terminal part to the eubacterial protein S15. Since this halobacterial protein is approximately as long as both eubacterial proteins combined, this phenomenon could be explained by gene fusion or gene splitting during evolution.

(6) The ribosomal proteins from lower and higher eukaryotes (yeast and rat, respectively) are strongly homologous to each other, whereas homology between proteins from eubacterial and eukaryotic ribosomes is rare. It is likely that the determination of the tertiary structure of the proteins by X-ray structure analysis will show a higher degree of homology than is apparent from the primary structure.

In the case of rRNA, the sequences have been highly conserved throughout evolution, and it is this high level of conservation that has enabled the secondary structure models already mentioned above (Brimacombe et al. 1983; Huysmans and De Wachter 1986) to be developed. The extent of homology between, for example, the 16S RNA from *E. coli* and that from *Zea mays* chloroplast ribosomes is of the order of 75%. Differences in length between the RNA molecules from the different classes of ribosomes (eukaryotes, prokaryotes, and mitochondria) are accommodated by deletion or insertion of discrete domains, rather than by a general contraction or expansion of the structure. A number of short sequence regions appear to be virtually universally conserved in all the sequences studied. In the case of the small subunit RNA, an up-to-date list of the complete sequences available has been compiled by Huysmans and De Wachter (1986).

Mechanism of Initiation of Prokaryotic Protein Synthesis

Translational initiation requires the formation of a complex consisting of the 30S ribosomal subunit, fMet-tRNA$_f^{Met}$, and the mRNA region containing the ribosomal binding site (RBS) that includes the initiation triplet. Formation of this complex requires three initiation factors (IF1, IF2, and IF3) and one molecule of GTP, which binds to IF2, changing its conformation and increasing its activity (Pon et al. 1985). Through the joining of a 50S subunit to the 30S initiation complex, a 70S initiation complex is formed in which fMet-tRNA is located in the ribosomal P site, whereas the A site is available to accept the aminoacyl-tRNA corresponding to the second mRNA codon (Gualerzi et al. 1986).

The structural properties of the initiation factors, their molecular interactions, and their topographical localization on the ribosome have been extensively studied by a number of techniques, including bifunctional cross-linking, selective chemical modifications, and ^{1}H-NMR spectroscopy; these results have recently been reviewed (Gualerzi et al. 1986).

Formation of the 30S initiation complex has been investigated primarily using model systems in which either fMet-tRNA, its analog NAcPhe-tRNA, or a fluorescent derivative of the latter was bound to the 30S subunit in response to synthetic oligo- or polynucleotides (e.g., AUG, poly[AUG], poly[U]). Based on the available data, a model illustrating the likely mechanism of translational initiation is presented in Figure 4. This entails a random binding mechanism in which the native 30S subunit, two binary complexes (30S-mRNA and 30S-fMet-tRNA), and a preternary complex in which the 30S-bound mRNA and fMet-tRNA are not yet interacting, are in rapid equilibrium. A rate-limiting ribosomal conformational transition (C in Fig. 4), probably consisting of several steps, leads to the formation of the actual 30S initiation complex in which mRNA and fMet-tRNA are mutually interacting, presumably through codon-anticodon base pairing (Gualerzi et al. 1986).

Recent data indicate that IF2 does not function as an fMet-tRNA carrier (Canonaco et al. 1986; Gualerzi and Wintermeyer 1986); accordingly, ribosomal binding of the initiator tRNA is shown in Figure 4 as occurring without the direct participation of IF2, which is depicted as being bound to the 30S subunit in a complex with GTP (Pon et al. 1985) and in the presence of the other two factors. Ejection of the initiation factors from the ribosome occurs upon binding of the 50S ribosomal subunit, which yields a 70S initiation complex (Pon and Gualerzi 1986). Prior to its ejection from the ribosome, IF2 triggers a ribosome-dependent GTPase. The formation of a 70S initiation complex, which probably entails a ribosomal conformational change, is virtually irreversible. The possibility that the IF2-dependent GTP hydrolysis may play a role in a proofreading mechanism is presently under investigation. Steady-state and pre-steady-state kinetic analyses of the formation of 30S initiation complexes in which the individual factors were omitted showed that the three factors affect on and off rates of the transition from preternary complex to 30S initiation complex (Gualerzi et al. 1986). Thus, by influencing the half-life of the 30S initiation complex, the factors may determine the kinetic selection of the correct complexes, which enter elongation via their fixation in the 70S initiation complex.

More recently, synthetic genes encoding model mRNAs have been assembled and expressed to obtain mRNAs of minimal size and coding capacity, but endowed with the relevant characteristics (e.g., a canonical RBS) of natural mRNAs. These mRNAs interact with *E. coli* ribosomes even in the absence of initiation factors, but depend completely on their presence to promote the ribosomal binding of fMet-tRNA and to direct protein synthesis. Both initiation and termination occur faithfully in this system at the AUG and UAA codons, respectively (Gualerzi et al. 1987). The activity of the mRNA containing a consensus RBS was compared with that from which the Shine-Dalgarno sequence had been completely deleted. It was found that initiation begins in the correct frame from the

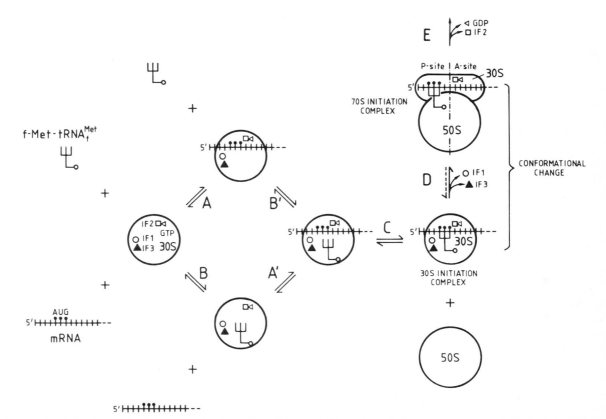

Figure 4. Mechanism of initiation complex formation. Schematic illustration of the proposed random-order mechanism of initiation complex formation. Steps A, B, B', and A' are in rapid equilibrium. Step C is rate limiting and probably consists of at least two first-order rearrangements of the preternary complex. (Reprinted, with permission, from Gualerzi et al. 1986.)

single AUG triplet even in the absence of this sequence; furthermore, at least in vitro, the Shine-Dalgarno sequence provides a modest advantage (four- to fivefold stimulation of translation) only at low inputs of mRNA and fMet-tRNA. Taken together, the results obtained with these mRNAs are consistent with the model discussed above (Fig. 4). Furthermore, the data indicate that in addition to being neither necessary nor sufficient for initiation, the Shine-Dalgarno sequence is not required for the selection of the correct reading frame. Instead, it is suggested that the Shine-Dalgarno sequence, whose interaction with the 30S subunit is completely unaffected by the initiation factors (Gualerzi et al. 1987), is useful in increasing the local (i.e., around the P-site decoding area) concentration of a more or less relevant initiation triplet; selection of the more relevant triplet is achieved kinetically by the combined action of the initiation factors which control on and off rates of the decoding process.

Mechanism of the Ribosomal Elongation Cycle

Saturation experiments with poly(U)-programmed ribosomes from *E. coli* and three kinds of tRNA, namely, deacylated tRNA^{Phe}, Phe-tRNA^{Phe}, and AcPhe-tRNA^{Phe} (as a simple analog of peptidyl-tRNA) yielded different results for each tRNA species (Rheinberger et al. 1981):

(1) Three deacylated tRNA^{Phe} molecules could be bound per ribosome. The P site was occupied first, followed by a new site, the E site, and finally the A site was filled. E stands for "exit", according to a proposal of Wettstein and Noll (1965). In the absence of poly(U), or in the presence of miscognate poly(A), one deacylated tRNA was bound to the P site. This indicates that the two additional binding sites bind deacylated tRNA via codon-anticodon interaction.

(2) Phe-tRNA binding leveled off at 1.5 molecules per ribosome as a result of a 30% contamination with deacylated tRNA. It is, however, clear that one ribosome can carry two Phe-tRNAs simultaneously at the A and P sites, as indicated by the formation of Phe$_2$.

(3) In contrast, only one AcPhe-tRNA molecule could be bound per 70S, although the AcPhe-tRNA preparation contained the same percentage (and not more) of deacylated tRNA. Since the AcPhe-tRNA can be present at either the A or the P site, the binding of AcPhe-tRNA seems to be governed by an exclusion principle, namely, if the P site is occupied by AcPhe-tRNA, then the A site cannot bind a second AcPhe-tRNA molecule. A recent thorough analysis confirmed this exclusion principle and demonstrated by means of a quantitative puromycin reaction that 80% to 100% of our ribosomes participate in tRNA binding (Geigenmüller et al. 1986).

These unexpected binding properties could be repro-

duced with ribosomes from the extreme halophilic archaebacterium *Halobacterium halobium* (Saruyama
and Nierhaus 1986), which diverged from the *E. coli*
line at least 1.6 billion years ago (Osawa and Hori
1980).

With regard to the functional importance of the E
site, the first assumption was that after peptide bond
formation the deacylated tRNA is not released from
the P site but is instead translocated to the E site. In
fact, a cotranslocation of peptidyl-tRNA and deacylated tRNA from A to P and P to E sites, respectively,
could be demonstrated, and the lack of coupling between translocation and tRNA release is now a well-
documented fact in poly(U)- and poly(A)-dependent
systems (feature 1 in Table 2; Rheinberger and Nierhaus 1983, 1986a,b; Rheinberger et al. 1986; Saruyama
and Nierhaus 1986).

After translocation, the occupation of the A site by a
ternary complex, Phe-tRNA * EF-Tu * GTP, triggers
the release of deacylated tRNA from the E site (Rheinberger and Nierhaus 1986a). Thus, occupation of the A
site results in an affinity drop at the E site, causing the
release of deacylated tRNA. In the experiment described below, we test whether the reverse is also true,
i.e., whether occupation of the E site reduces the A-site
affinity.

A poly(U)-programmed ribosome is increasingly
filled with deacylated tRNA^{Phe} (Fig. 5C). Next, various
amounts of Ac[^{3}H]Phe-tRNA are added, and the binding is measured at 0°C (Fig. 5A). Increasing the number of bound deacylated tRNA molecules from $\nu = 1$ to
$\nu = 2$ abolishes the binding of AcPhe-tRNA at 0°C. In
sharp contrast, at 37°C the binding of AcPhe-tRNA is
not affected in this ν range (Fig. 5B). This finding
indicates that the second deacylated tRNA does not
compete with the A-site ligand AcPhe-tRNA for one
and the same binding site, particularly since the second

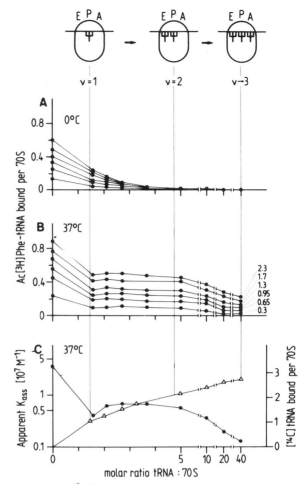

Figure 5. Ac[^{3}H]Phe-tRNA binding to poly(U)-programmed
70S ribosomes prefilled with various amounts of nonlabeled
deacylated tRNA^{Phe}. The level of prefilling was assessed in a
control experiment with deacylated [^{14}C]tRNA^{Phe} (triangles in
C). The binding of various amounts of Ac[^{3}H]Phe-tRNA was
determined at 0°C (*A*) and 37°C (*B*). The applied amounts of
AcPhe-tRNA (molar ratios of AcPhe-tRNA to 70S) are given
in *B* at the right edge. The figure has been adapted from
Rheinberger and Nierhaus (1986a).

Table 2. Features of the Allosteric Three-site Model

1. A ribosome contains three tRNA binding sites A, P, and
   E. In the course of elongation a tRNA occupies successively the sites in the order A → P → E. The E site exclusively binds deacylated tRNA.
2. A and E sites are allosterically linked via negative
   cooperativity, i.e., occupation of one site decreases the
   affinity of the other and vice versa.
   Consequences:
      An elongating ribosome can adopt two states:
         The pretranslocational state, where A and P sites
         have high affinities for tRNA.
         The posttranslocational state, where P and E sites
         have high affinities.
      Deacylated tRNA is released upon A-site occupation
      and not during translocation.
3. Both tRNAs present on the ribosome before and after
   translocation undergo codon-anticodon interaction simultaneously.
4. Both elongation factors EF-Tu and EF-G promote the
   transition from one state to the other: EF-Tu that of the
   post- to the pretranslocational, and EF-G that of the pre-
   to the posttranslocational transition.

deacylated tRNA binds to the ribosome with about the
same affinity as does AcPhe-tRNA to the A site (0.4 ×
10^7 to 0.6×10^7 M^{-1} at 15 mM Mg^{++}). It follows that the
second deacylated tRNA binds to the E site, which
must be physically distinct from the A site. Furthermore, the occupation of the E site reduces the A-site
affinity, whereas if only the P site is occupied by deacylated tRNA and the E site is free (i.e., $\nu = 1$), AcPhe-
tRNA can bind to the A site at 0°C (see Fig. 5A).

Clearly, the A and E sites are allosterically linked via
negative cooperativity, i.e., occupation of one site reduces the affinity of the other and vice versa. This
important feature can be illustrated by a simple experiment where we make use of the fact that the second
deacylated tRNA binds to the E site.

Ac[^{3}H]Phe-tRNA is added to a poly(U)-pro-
grammed ribosome that carries two deacylated
[^{14}C]tRNA molecules at the P and E sites (Fig. 6). At

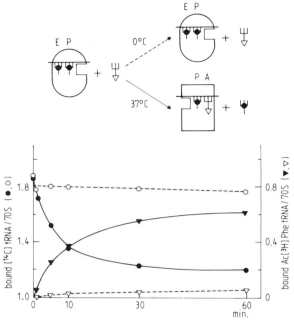

Figure 6. Binding of Ac[³H]Phe-tRNA at 0°C and 37°C to poly(U)-programmed ribosomes carrying two deacylated [¹⁴C]tRNA^Phe molecules at E and P sites (adapted from Rheinberger and Nierhaus 1986a).

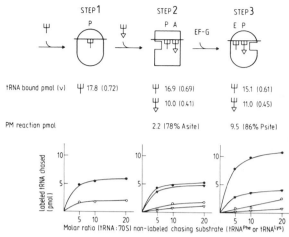

Figure 7. Poly(A)-programmed 70S ribosomes are prepared carrying [¹⁴C]tRNA^Lys and Ac[³H]Lys-tRNA^Lys. The labeled tRNAs are chased by increasing amounts of nonlabeled tRNA^Lys (cognate chasing substrate; ●, ▼) or tRNA^Phe (noncognate chasing substrate; ○, ▽). ○ and ●, amount of chased [¹⁴C]tRNA. ▽ and ▼, amount of chased Ac[³H]Lys-tRNA. ν is the occupation number (e.g., 0.72 means that each ribosome carries 0.72 molecules of [¹⁴C]tRNA^Lys statistically). For experimental details, see Rheinberger and Nierhaus (1986b).

0°C, no AcPhe-tRNA is bound during a period of 60 minutes, indicating the low binding affinity of the A site induced by the occupied E site. However, at 37°C, Ac[³H]Phe-tRNA is bound to the A site, and for every molecule bound, one deacylated tRNA is released from the E site. This experiment clearly demonstrates the mutually negative cooperativity between the A and E sites. Furthermore, three deacylated tRNAs are found on the ribosome only at a nonphysiologically high excess of tRNA over ribosomes. If an acylated tRNA is present, two tRNAs are preferentially found on the ribosome.

The negative cooperativity between the A and E sites has the important consequence that two high-affinity sites always exist on the ribosome. In the pretranslocational state, these are the A and P sites, and in the postranslocational state, the P and E sites (feature 2 in Table 2). In the following experiment, we investigate whether or not both tRNAs present on the ribosome simultaneously undergo codon-anticodon interaction.

It has already been shown that the second deacylated tRNA binds only in the presence of the cognate mRNA (Rheinberger et al. 1986). A deacylated [¹⁴C]tRNA^Lys is bound to the P site of poly(A)-programmed ribosomes (Fig. 7, step 1), and in step 2 Ac[³H]Lys-tRNA is bound to the A site. Then, the Ac[³H]Lys-tRNA is translocated from the A to the P site, and the [¹⁴C]tRNA^Lys from the P to the E site, respectively (step 3). At all three steps the chasing effects of increasing amounts of added nonlabeled tRNA^Lys (cognate) or tRNA^Phe (noncognate) are studied. If a tRNA molecule were bound via codon-anticodon interaction, the cog-

nate chasing substrate would be expected to be more effective than the noncognate one. At all three steps and for both tRNA species ([¹⁴C]tRNA^Lys and Ac[³H]Lys-tRNA), the cognate chasing substrate is 3–12 times more efficient than the noncognate one. The most pronounced effect is found at the E site. This experiment clearly shows that a tRNA can undergo codon-anticodon interaction at all three sites (A, P, and E), and it provides striking evidence that both tRNAs present at the A and P or P and E sites, respectively, simultaneously undergo codon-anticodon interaction (feature 3 in Table 2).

According to the allosteric three-site model, the ribosome adopts two functionally different states in the course of elongation, namely, the pre- and postranslocational states. The elongation factors facilitate the transitions between these states, namely EF-Tu, the post- to pretranslocational transition (concomitant with A-site binding), and EF-G, the pre- to posttranslocational transition (translocation). Both elongation factors accelerate the elongation cycle by reducing the activation energies involved (A. Bartetzko and K.H. Nierhaus, unpubl. observation; feature 4 in Table 2).

Figure 8 depicts the elongation cycle in the frame of the allosteric three-site model. The interference points of some antibiotics are indicated and will be discussed elsewhere (T.-P. Hausner et al., in prep.).

The main features of the allosteric three-site model were elucidated at 15 mM Mg⁺⁺. A point made in critiques of these experiments was that at Mg⁺⁺ concentrations below 10 mM the E site becomes more and more nonfunctional. Since the effective Mg⁺⁺ concentration in vivo lies in the range of 1–3 mM, it was

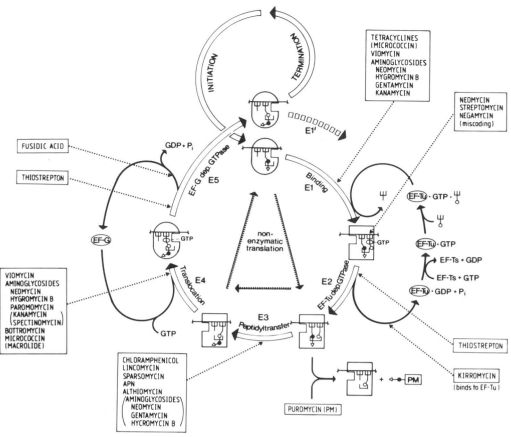

Figure 8. The elongation cycle of the ribosome: The pretranslational state is symbolized by a "rectangular" ribosome, the posttranslational state by a "rounded" ribosome. The interference points of some antibiotics are indicated. For further details, see T.-P. Hausner et al. (in prep.) and Nierhaus and Wittmann (1980).

concluded that the E site plays no important role in vivo (Robertson et al. 1984).

However, we demonstrated that all three sites become inactivated in a coordinated and parallel fashion at decreasing Mg^{++} concentrations below 10 mM in standard Mg^{++}/NH_4^+ systems. The inactivation at low Mg^{++} can be prevented by the addition of polyamines (0.6 mM spermine and 0.4 mM spermidine). Under these conditions, tRNA binding is still quantitative at 6 mM Mg^{++}. Furthermore, the E site is fully functional, and the features of the allosteric three-site model apply even at 3 mM Mg^{++} (Rheinberger and Nierhaus 1987). Model-building studies revealed the feasibility of three deacylated tRNAs being bound simultaneously by a single ribosome via codon-anticodon interaction. However, if one tRNA is acylated, only two tRNAs are allowed (Nagano and Harel 1987), in full agreement with the allosteric three-site model.

The significance of the allosteric three-site model is seen in the existence of two adjacent codon-anticodon interactions before and after translation. This constraint, together with the necessity to make contact at the peptidyltransferase center, has evidently been a factor in the evolution of the universal L-shape of all tRNAs. It should be noted that eukaryotic tRNA[Phe]

from yeast can be used efficiently in poly(Phe) synthesis systems with ribosomes from archaebacterial *H. halobium* as well as from eubacterial *E. coli*. No other component of the translational apparatus shows this universal property (for further discussion, see Nierhaus et al. 1986).

REFERENCES

Arndt, E., G. Breithaupt, and M. Kimura. 1986. The complete amino acid sequence of ribosomal protein H-S11 from the archaebacterium *Halobacterium marismortui*. *FEBS Lett.* **194:** 227.

Auron, P.E. and S.R. Fahnestock. 1981. Functional organization of the large ribosomal subunit of *Bacillus stearothermophilus*. *J. Biol. Chem.* **256:** 10105.

Brimacombe, R., P. Maly, and C. Zwieb. 1983. The structure of ribosomal RNA and its organization relative to ribosomal protein. *Prog. Nucleic Acids Res.* **28:** 1.

Canonaco, M.A., R.A. Calogero, and C.O. Gualerzi. 1986. Mechanism of translational initiation in prokaryotes. Evidence for a direct effect of IF2 on the activity of the 30S ribosomal subunit. *FEBS Lett.* **207:** 198.

Dohme, F. and K.H. Nierhaus. 1976. Total reconstitution and assembly of 50S subunits from *Escherichia coli* ribosomes *in vitro*. *J. Mol. Biol.* **107:** 585.

Expert-Bezançon, A. and P. Wollenzien. 1985. Three-dimensional arrangement of the *E. coli* 16S ribosomal RNA. *J. Mol. Biol.* **184:** 53.

Geigenmüller, U., T.P. Hausner, and K.H. Nierhaus. 1986. Analysis of the puromycin reaction: The ribosomal exclusion principle for AcPhe-tRNA binding re-examined. *Eur. J. Biochem.* **161:** 715.

Giri, L., W.E. Hill, H.G. Wittmann, and B. Wittmann-Liebold. 1984. Ribosomal proteins: Their structural and spatial arrangement in prokaryotic ribosomes. *Adv. Protein Chem.* **36:** 56.

Gualerzi, C.O. and W. Wintermeyer. 1986. Prokaryotic initiation factor 2 acts at the level of the 30S ribosomal subunit. A fluorescence stopped-flow study. *FEBS Lett.* **202:** 1.

Gualerzi, C.O., R.A. Calogero, M.A. Canonaco, M. Brombach, and C.L. Pon. 1987. Selection of mRNA by ribosomes during prokaryotic translational initiation. In *Genetics of translation* (ed. M.F. Tuite et al.). Springer-Verlag, Heidelberg. (In press.)

Gualerzi, C.O., C.L. Pon, R.T. Pawlik, M.A. Canonaco, M. Paci, and W. Wintermeyer. 1986. Role of the initiation factors in *E. coli* translational initiation. In *Structure, function, and genetics of ribosomes* (ed. B. Hardesty and G. Kramer), p. 621. Springer-Verlag, New York.

Herold, M. and K.H. Nierhaus. 1987. Incorporation of six additional proteins, to complete the assembly map of the 50S subunit from *Escherichia coli* ribosomes. *J. Biol. Chem.* **262:** 8826.

Huysmans, E. and R. De Wachter. 1986. Compilation of small ribosomal subunit RNA sequences. *Nucleic Acids Res.* (suppl.) **14:** r73.

Moore, P.B., M. Capel, M. Kjeldgaard, and D.M. Engelman. 1986. A 19 protein map of the 30S ribosomal subunit of *Escherichia coli*. In *Structure, function, and genetics of ribosomes* (ed. B. Hardesty and G. Kramer), p. 87. Springer-Verlag, New York.

Nagano, K. and M. Harel. 1987. Approaches to a three-dimensional model of *E. coli* ribosome. *Prog. Biophys. Mol. Biol.* **48:** 67.

Nierhaus, K.H. 1980. Analysis of the assembly and function of the 50S subunit from *Escherichia coli* ribosomes by reconstitution. In *Ribosomes: Structure, function, and genetics* (ed. G. Chambliss et al.), p. 267. University Park Press, Baltimore.

Nierhaus, K.H. and H.G. Wittmann. 1980. Ribosome function and its inhibition by antibiotics in prokaryotes. *Naturwissenschaften* **67:** 234.

Nierhaus, K.H., H.-J. Rheinberger, U. Geigenmüller, A. Gnirke, H. Saruyama, S. Schilling, and P. Wurmbach. 1986. Three tRNA binding sites involved in the ribosomal elongation cycle. In *Structure, function, and genetics of ribosomes* (ed. B. Hardesty and G. Kramer), p. 454. Springer-Verlag, New York.

Nierhaus, K.H., R. Lietzke, R.P. May, V. Nowotny, H. Schulze, K. Simpson, P. Wurmbach, and H. Stuhrmann. 1983. Shape determinations of ribosomal proteins *in situ*. *Proc. Natl. Acad. Sci.* **80:** 2889.

Noller, H.F. 1980. Structure and topography of ribosomal RNA. In *Ribosomes: Structure, function, and genetics* (ed. G. Chambliss et al.), p. 3. University Park Press, Baltimore.

Nomura, M. and W.A. Held. 1974. Reconstitution of ribosomes: Studies of ribosome structure, function and assembly. In *Ribosomes* (ed. M. Nomura et al.), p. 193. Cold Spring Harbor Laboratory, Cold Spring Harbor, New York.

Nowotny, V. and K.H. Nierhaus. 1982. Initiation proteins for the assembly of the 50S subunit from *Escherichia coli* ribosomes. *Proc. Natl. Acad. Sci.* **79:** 7238.

Nowotny, V., R.P. May, and K.H. Nierhaus. 1986. Neutron-scattering analysis of structural and functional aspects of the ribosome: The strategy of the glassy ribosome. In *Structure, function, and genetics of ribosomes* (ed. B. Hardesty and G. Kramer), p. 101. Springer-Verlag, New York.

Osawa, S. and H. Hori. 1980. Molecular evolution of ribosomal components. In *Ribosomes: Structure, function, and genetics* (ed. G. Chambliss et al.), p. 333. University Park Press, Baltimore.

Pon, C.L. and C.O. Gualerzi. 1986. Mechanism of translational initiation in prokaryotes. IF3 is released from ribosomes during and not before 70S initiation complex formation. *FEBS Lett.* **195:** 215.

Pon, C.L., M. Paci, R.T. Pawlik, and C. Gualerzi. 1985. Biochemical and biophysical characterization of the interaction between IF2 and guanosine nucleotides. *J. Biol. Chem.* **260:** 8918.

Rheinberger, H.-J. and K.H. Nierhaus. 1983. Testing an alternative model for the ribosomal peptide elongation cycle. *Proc. Natl. Acad. Sci.* **80:** 4213.

———. 1986a. Allosteric interactions between the ribosomal transfer RNA-binding sites A and E. *J. Biol. Chem.* **261:** 9133.

———. 1986b. Adjacent codon-anticodon interactions of both tRNAs present at the ribosomal A and P or P and E sites. *FEBS Lett.* **204:** 97.

———. 1987. The ribosome E site at low Mg^{2+}: Coordinate inactivation of ribosomal functions at Mg^{2+} concentrations below 10 mM and its prevention by polyamines. *J. Biomol. Struct. Dyn.* (in press).

Rheinberger, H.-J., H. Sternbach, and K.H. Nierhaus. 1981. Three tRNA binding sites on Escherichia coli ribosomes. *Proc. Natl. Acad. Sci.* **78:** 5310.

———. 1986. Codon-anticodon interaction at the ribosomal E site. *J. Biol. Chem.* **261:** 9140.

Robertson, J.M., R. Lill, and W. Wintermeyer. 1984. Elongation factor G-induced release of tRNA during ribosomal translocation. In *Proceedings of the 5th Symposium* (ed. J. Zelinka and J. Balan), p. 307. Slovak Academy of Sciences, Bratislava.

Saruyama, H. and K.H. Nierhaus. 1986. Evidence that the three-site model for the ribosomal elongation cycle is also valid in the archaebacterium *Halobacterium halobium*. *Mol. Gen. Genet.* **204:** 221.

Schlessinger, D. 1974. Ribosome formation in *Escherichia coli*. In *Ribosomes* (ed. M. Nomura et al.), p. 393. Cold Spring Harbor Laboratory, Cold Spring Harbor, New York.

Schulze, H. and K.H. Nierhaus. 1982. Minimal set of ribosomal components for reconstitution of the peptidyltransferase activity. *EMBO J.* **1:** 609.

Stöffler, G. and M. Stöffler-Meilicke. 1986. Immuno electron microscopy on *Escherichia coli* ribosomes. In *Structure, function, and genetics of ribosomes* (ed. B. Hardesty and G. Kramer), p. 28. Springer-Verlag, New York.

Wettstein, F.O. and H. Noll. 1965. Binding of transfer ribonucleic acid to ribosomes engaged in protein synthesis: Number and properties of ribosomal binding sites. *J. Mol. Biol.* **11:** 35.

Wittmann-Liebold, B. 1986. Ribosomal proteins: Their structure and evolution. In *Structure, function, and genetics of ribosomes* (ed. B. Hardesty and G. Kramer), p. 326. Springer-Verlag, New York.

Evolving Ribosome Structure and Function: rRNA and the Translation Mechanism

M. OAKES, A. SCHEINMAN, M. RIVERA, D. SOUFER,
G. SHANKWEILER, AND J. LAKE

Molecular Biology Institute and Department of Biology, University of California, Los Angeles, California 90024

Major advances have been made in recent years in our understanding of the structure, function, and evolution of ribosomes. Among these advances one notes that the overall three-dimensional structures of ribosomes and ribosomal subunits are known; the primary and secondary structures of the rRNAs are known for diverse organisms; the approximate locations of many ribosomal proteins (r-proteins) and of some sequences of the rRNAs are known; many aspects of ribosome function have been related to ribosome structure; and finally, comparative studies of ribosomes have revealed some of the early steps in the evolution of ribosomes and of the cells that contain them.

In this chapter, we will focus on the structure and evolution of rRNA and the molecular mechanisms of protein synthesis. In light of the recent experimental emphasis on RNA (for review, see e.g., Noller 1984), this chapter emphasizes the role and the functioning of RNA in the mechanism.

Three-dimensional Ribosome Structure

Homologous structures are found in ribosomes from all known organisms, including eukaryotes, halobacteria, methanogens, eubacteria, and eocytes (Lake 1985). There is now general agreement concerning the overall structure and morphology of the *Escherichia coli* ribosome. The asymmetric model for the ribosome and its subunits (Lake 1976) is accepted. Details of the structure are provided elsewhere (for reviews, see e.g., Lake 1981a), but the outlines are given below. The *E. coli* structures shown in Figure 1 serve to illustrate the related features are found in ribosomes from all organisms.

The smaller subunit, at the left, is divided into two unequal parts by an indentation and a region of accumulated negative stain. These parts are the head, or the upper third, and the base, or lower two thirds. A region of the small subunit, called the platform, extends from the base of the small subunit and forms a cleft between it and the head.

The structure of the large subunit, like that of the small, is asymmetric. It consists of a central protuberance, or head, and protrusions inclined approximately 50° to either side of the central protuberance (lower central panel of Fig. 1). One of these, the "L7/L12 stalk," is at the right and contains the only multiple-copy proteins present in the *E. coli* ribosome. In a projection approximately orthogonal to this (shown in the upper central panel of Fig. 1), the large subunit is characterized by a notch on the upper surface.

In the monomeric ribosome, the small subunit is positioned asymmetrically on the large subunit, as shown at the right of Figure 1. This allows the platform of the small subunit to contact the large subunit, so that the partition between the head and body of the small subunit is approximately aligned with the notch of the large subunit.

Ribosomal Domains

Ribosomes from all organisms are divided into two general functional regions. They are the translational domain and the exit, or secretory, domain (Bernabeu and Lake 1982). These two domains are found at opposite ends of the ribosome (see Fig. 2). The translational domain includes the head and the platform of the small subunit and the L7/L12 stalk, the central protuberance, and the L1 ridge of the large subunit.

In general, almost all of the proteins of the *E. coli* small ribosomal subunit that have been mapped by immunoelectron microscopy are located in the translational domain (see Fig. 3). In the large subunit, many ribosomal proteins are found in the translational domain, although at least one, L17, is located in the exit domain (see Fig. 3). Within the translational domain itself, several functional regions are found. These regions are all important in understanding the functioning of ribosomes during protein synthesis and will be discussed in the following sections.

RESULTS

Mapping rRNA Regions in the Translational Domain Using DNA Hybridization Electron Microscopy

rRNAs from all extant organisms have homologous primary sequences and secondary structures. Many regions from distantly related organisms are extremely conserved, whereas other regions are highly diverged (for review, see Gutell et al. 1985). The conserved regions are of considerable interest, since the conservation is thought to imply their functional importance. In addition, a number of conserved regions are single stranded and hence, are amenable to study by DNA hybridization microscopy (Oakes et al. 1986). In this section, we discuss the locations of three regions of the

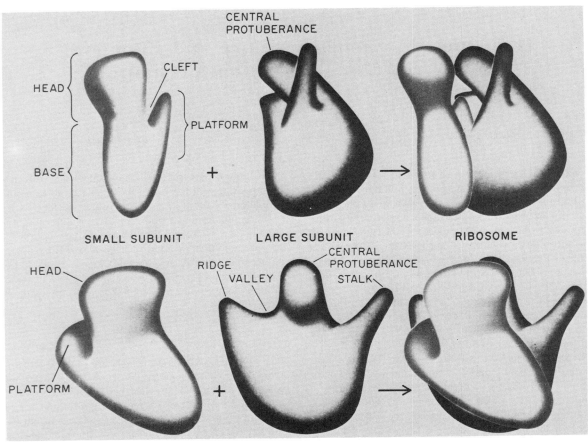

Figure 1. The three-dimensional asymmetric model of the ribosome (Lake 1976, 1981a). This model gives an asymmetric shape to the two subunits of which a ribosome consists. The small subunit (*left*) includes a head, a base, and a platform. The large subunit (*center*) includes a central protuberance, flanked by a ridge on one side and a stalk on the other. Two orientations of the model are shown. The length of a ribosome is about 250 Å.

small subunit rRNA. These are the 1400 region, the 787 region, and the Shine-Dalgarno messenger-binding site (Shine and Dalgarno 1974).

DNA hybridization electron microscopy is a technique used to map specific rRNA sequences in three dimensions. In this technique, a synthetic oligonucleotide probe, complementary to a specific rRNA sequence and carrying an attached biotin, is hybridized to ribosomal subunits. The locations of biotins on subunits can then be mapped by electron microscopy to determine the probe's three-dimensional site of attachment.

Complementary DNA probes have been employed previously to study the base-pairing potential of regions of the 16S rRNA including the 3′ terminus and have also been used in conjunction with RNase H, an enzyme that digests RNA-DNA hybrids (Kopylov et al. 1975; Taniguchi and Weissmann 1978; Eckhardt and Lührmann 1979; Backendorf et al. 1981; Mankin et al. 1981; Van Duin et al. 1984; Oakes et al. 1986; Tapprich and Hill 1986). These studies have confirmed that many regions of 16S rRNA are able to bind oligonucleotide probes. Information suggesting which regions of 16S rRNA might be accessible to DNA probes has been

gained by chemical modification and nuclease digestion techniques. Some examples are kethoxal modification of guanines, dimethyl sulfate modification of adenine, and carbodiimide modification of uracil and guanine (Noller and Chaires 1972; Peattie and Gilbert 1980; Moazed et al. 1986).

We have chosen DNA probes complementary to sequences that may be on or near the platform of the 30S subunit. The platform has a unique structure when compared with the rest of the 30S subunit. It has a thickness of approximately 25–30 Å, which places constraints on how helices of 16S rRNA can be positioned within the platform structure. Helices longer than one repeat cannot run perpendicular to the plane of the platform; therefore, the long axes of rRNA helices must run parallel to the plane of the platform as shown in the model in Figure 4 (Noller and Lake 1984).

The three-dimensional locations of several 16S rRNA sequences have been determined. In the initial searches for useful probes, we assayed for the ability of complementary DNA to bind to ribosomes by sucrose-density centrifugation and/or by Penefsky columns. DNA probes were ^{32}P-labeled with T$_4$ polynucleotide kinase and incubated with at least a fivefold molar

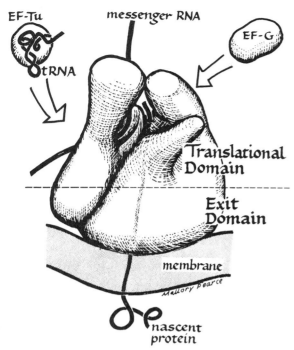

Figure 2. Diagrammatic representation of the exit and translational domains of the ribosome and their orientations with respect to the membrane-binding site. (Adapted from Bernabeu and Lake 1982).

excess of subunits. The ability of the DNA probe to bind subunits is reflected by the radioactivity comigrating with subunits during centrifugation (Fig. 5). Probes capable of binding to 30S subunits were biotinylated with bio-dUTP or bio-dCTP and terminal transferase

(Bollum 1974). The strong binding of avidin to biotin and the ability to visualize avidin directly by electron microscopy make biotin a useful label. For each mapping, the subunits were first heat-activated, then incubated with biotinylated DNA probe, and, finally, avidin DN was added for a shorter incubation time (Oakes et al. 1986). Unbound avidin was removed by centrifugational chromatography and the eluant stained using the double-layer carbon technique (Lake 1979b). Micrographs were obtained with a Philips 400 electron microscope. In the following sections, we examine the small subunit RNA sequences in *E. coli* and in the yeast *Saccharomyces cerevisiae*.

The 1400 Region Is Exposed in the Cleft of the Small Subunit

The ribosomal sequence coresponding to *E. coli* 16S rRNA nucleotides 1392–1407, the "1400 region," is highly conserved phylogenetically and has functional significance. This sequence probably is exposed in active small subunits, since within this region, nucleotide 1405 can be modified by kethoxal and the region is accessible to cobra venom ribonuclease (Noller 1974; Chapman and Noller 1977; Vassilenko et al. 1981). The region also appears to be adjacent to an anticodon-binding site, since C_{1400} can be cross-linked to the "wobble" nucleotide of a modified tRNA bound to the peptidyl-tRNA-binding (P) site (Ofengand et al. 1979; Prince et al. 1982). Other evidence that the 1400 region is near the anticodon-binding site comes from tRNA protection of 16S bases (Meier and Wagner 1984; Moazed and Noller 1986) from attack by a combination of structure-specific chemical probes. It was shown that

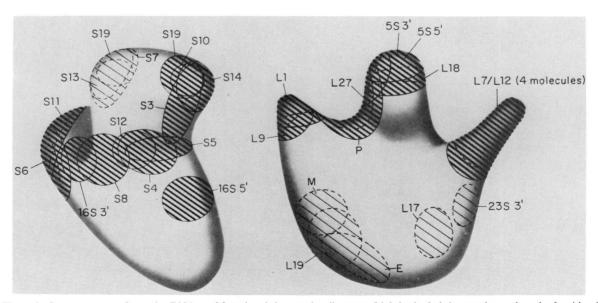

Figure 3. Summary map of protein, RNA, and functional sites on the ribosome. Lightly shaded sites are located on the far side of the subunits. The letters P, M, and E represent the peptidyltransferase site, the membrane-binding site, and the nascent protein exit site. The letters S and L refer to small and large subunit protein and 16S 5′, 23S 3′, etc., refer to the 5′ and 3′ ends, respectively, of the rRNAs.

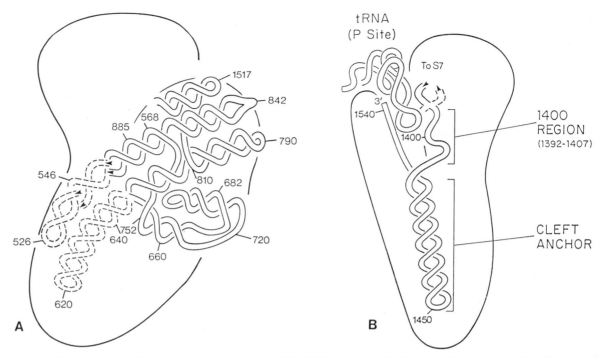

Figure 4. (*A*) Schematic model of the hypothetical path of 16S rRNA in the small subunit platform (adapted from Noller and Lake 1984). Chains in dashed lines are on the far side of the subunit. Although the details of the RNA locations are hypothetical, the platform region contains several of the sequences described in this paper. (*B*) Diagrammatic representation of the location of *E. coli* rRNA sequence 1392–1407. The locations inferred for the penultimate helix, the cleft anchor, and for the P site are shown together with the 1400 site (adapted from Oakes et al. 1986).

G_{1401} is protected from DMS by poly(U)-directed binding of $tRNA_{yeast}^{Phe}$ and that C_{1399} and G_{1401} are also protected by $tRNA^{Phe}$ alone. In yeast 18S rRNA the identical sequence is found at positions 1618–1633. The yeast 18S rRNA exhibits primary and secondary struc-

tural homology with *E. coli* 16S rRNA and has a similar reactivity with kethoxal (Chapman and Noller 1979). This suggests that the 1400-region-like rRNA sequences in both these subunits could be located at similar three-dimensional sites.

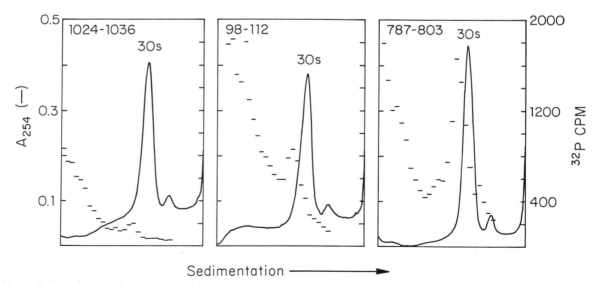

Figure 5. The ability of DNA probes to bind subunits measured by radioactivity migrating with the subunits during centrifugation, as described in the text. In this figure, three 16S nucleotide sequences were analyzed, 98–112, 787–803, and 1024–1036. Complementary DNA probes to these sequences bound to 30S subunits in varying degrees. The greatest binding was observed with 787–803, lesser binding with the probe complementary to 98–112, and very little binding with 1024–1036. The 787 sequence is readily mapped; sequence 98 is harder, but is being mapped, and 1024 is probably not possible.

In the *E. coli* ribosome, the 1400 region (1392–1407) is located at the level of the neck near the cleft (Fig. 6). This sequence is highly conserved, and therefore, the same probe was used with yeast 40S subunits. As shown in Figure 6, the sequence in yeast 18S rRNA (1618–1633) is located in a site topologically equivalent to the *E. coli* site. The 1400 site, as mapped, is shown schematically in Figure 4B.

The significance of the 1400 mapping site is that it identifies the site of the anticodon-codon interaction. Other studies had previously identified this site through the mapping of proteins or other ligands. The 1400 region mapping is more direct, however. Some of these studies are described below.

One special group of small subunit proteins is found on the platform. Proteins S6, S11, S15, and S18 are in this group (see Fig. 3). Because of the thinness (~ 30 Å) of the platform, it is possible for a protein to be exposed on both the exterior and the interface surfaces of the platform. Several lines of experimentation have linked these proteins to mRNA binding. Single-component omission experiments (Nomura et al. 1970; discussed in Lake 1979a) have suggested that S11 may be participating directly in the selection of the correct tRNA, i.e., in the codon-anticodon interaction. Protein S18 has been cross-linked to mRNA using a variety of affinity-labeling analogs (for review, see Cooperman 1978). Also, the platform has been implicated as the decoding site by affinity immunoelectron microscopy of the 3′ end of a cross-linked tRNA (Keren-Zur et al. 1979).

Important rRNA markers are found on the platform. The 3′ end of 16S RNA has been localized there (Olson and Glitz 1979; Shatsky et al. 1979) and the two N^6-dimethyladenosine nucleosides at positions 1518 and 1519 have also been placed there by immunoelectron microscopy (Politz and Glitz 1977). Recently, the initiation codon of a Shine-Dalgarno-containing message has been mapped on the platform (Oakes et al. 1984). In addition, proteins S6, S15, and S18, also located on the platform, represent one of the best-mapped and best-understood regions of the ribosome (Lake 1981b; Noller and Lake 1984).

Finally, the cleft is strongly implicated as being a tRNA-binding site, during the initiation step of protein synthesis. The locations of proteins S13 and S19, the locations of the platform proteins, and the locations of S12 taken together suggest the binding site for initiation factors, IF-1, IF-2, and IF-3 (Lake and Kahan 1975). Consideration of the results of both cross-linking (Bollen et al. 1975; Van Duin et al. 1975; Heimark et al. 1976; Langberg et al. 1977; Schwartz and L. Kahan, pers. comm.) and protein localization by immunoelectron microscopy had suggested that IF-3, IF-2, and IF-1 were positioned across the cleft between S13, S19-II, and S12 on the head of the small subunit and S11 on the platform. In eukaryotic small subunits, eIF3 was shown to bind in a similar region on the platform (Emanuilov et al. 1978).

All of these experiments point out the importance of the cleft in mRNA-tRNA interaction. Because of these data, we were interested in studying the arrangement of rRNA in this vicinity even more closely through DNA hybridization microscopy. As a result, we have mapped region 787 in preliminary studies.

Another highly conserved sequence in *E. coli* 16S rRNA is 787–803. This sequence is an excellent candidate for mapping, since it was previously shown to be exposed by RNase-H cleavage (Tapprich and Hill 1986). We have localized this sequence by DNA hybridization electron microscopy on the platform of the 30S subunit (Fig. 7A). It is near the site where the Shine-Dalgarno sequence was also mapped (Fig. 7B) by us. DNA probes have previously been used to study the base-pairing potential of the 3′ terminus of 16S rRNA and have been found to inhibit initiation complex formation (Taniguchi and Weissmann 1978; Eckhardt and Lührmann 1979; Backendorf et al. 1981; Van Duin et al. 1984). In our experiments, shown in Figure

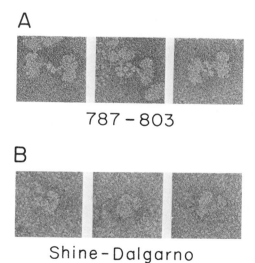

A

787 – 803

B

Shine–Dalgarno

Figure 7. DNA hybridization electron microscopy of the 16S rRNA regions in the *E. coli* sequence. (*A*) Mapping the 787–803 site using 30S pairs. (*B*) Mapping the Shine-Dalgarno complementary site using 30S monomers. Both sites are on the platform.

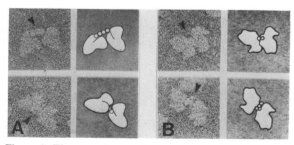

Figure 6. Electron micrographs of eubacterial (*E. coli*) small subunits after hybridization with the 1400-region probe and labeling with avidin. Electron micrographs of eukayrotic (*S. cervisiae*) small subunits and their reaction with the 1400-region probe. Pairs of subunits are shown. The column of each row is a schematic diagram of the adjacent micrograph. (Magnification × 212,500.)

7B, we also localized the Shine-Dalgarno region on the platform of the 30S subunit. This is in agreement with the localization of the 3' terminus by immunoelectron microscopy (Olson and Glitz 1979; Shatsky et al. 1979).

DNA hybridization electron microscopy offers an exciting technique to probe the three-dimensional structure of 16S rRNA. Furthermore, reliable control experiments make it possible to directly monitor the site of DNA-probe binding. These controls use RNase H, an enzyme that can cleave an RNA molecule at the site of DNA-RNA hybrid formation, such as is found at the probe-binding sites. In these controls, 30S subunits are heat activated and incubated with DNA probe and RNase H (Tapprich and Hill 1986). The resulting 5' and 3' sequences can be observed by polyacrylamide gel electrophoresis and the site of scission determined (Fig. 8). Control experiments used with the 787 probe and the 1400 probe are shown in lanes 1–5. A pattern of smaller sequences, as seen in all the controls, reveals the routine endogenous nuclease activity that is normally encountered during subunit preparation, but shows no unusual bands. Lanes 8 and 9 are experiments with 1400 and 787 probes, respectively. Lane 9 shows an enhancement of the bands Q2 and Q3, corresponding to lengths of approximately 800 and 745, produced

upon incubation with the 787 probe. The bands Q2 and Q3 are doublets, since the site of RNase-H cleavage is slightly different from the endogenous nick. Lane 8 (which has been incubated with the 1400 probe) has a new band at about 1400, resulting from RNase-H activity. As described in Figure 8, the double cutting experiment in lane 7 shows that the 790 fragment is from the 3' end of the 16S and confirms that the cut is near 787. Furthermore, this has been demonstrated directly by sequencing the 790 and 1400 bands. These RNase-H experiments have added confidence to DNA hybridization electron microscopy and established it as an important tool for mapping the locations of specific RNA sequences.

Thus, we hope that we will be able to work out, at moderate resolution, the packing of rRNA helices within the platform. Figure 4A shows a very preliminary model proposed by Noller and Lake (1984) for the positioning of helices in this region, based on the knowledge of the locations of ribosomal proteins and the protective functions of these proteins. It is already obvious from the experiments described above that the model, shown in Figure 4A, will need to be modified, but it illustrates the level of resolution at which we hope to understand the packing of rRNA in subunits.

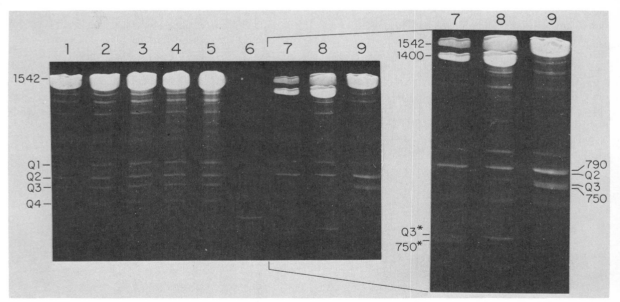

Figure 8. RNase-H control experiments demonstrate the binding sites of the 1400 and 787 probes. The controls in lanes 1–5 show the effects of digestion using incomplete reaction mixtures. (Lane 1) 30S subunits; (lane 2) 30S + DNA 787 + DNA 1400; (lane 4) 30S + DNA 787; (lane 5) 30S + DNA 1400. In these controls, the pattern is constant and independent of probe or RNase H. A characteristic pattern of rRNA nicking is present in which a series of four bands, referred to as the "quartet," is prominent. These bands are indicated as Q1, Q2, Q3, and Q4. RNA size standards are run in lane 6. Lanes 7–9 contain experimental results and all reaction components are present. Lane 9 contains DNA probe 787, lane 8 contains DNA probe 1400, and lane 7 contains both the DNA probes, 1400 and 787. The effect of the 1400-dependent RNase-H cut (lane 8) is to make a 1400 fragment at the top of the lane migrate just below the 16S band (corresponding to a loss of about 150 nucleotides). The Q3 band of the quartet is also removed (reappearing as a new band) from the 3' end of the molecule. The effect of the 787-dependent scission (in lane 9) is to generate two additional bands near the middle two bands of the quartet. The upper band, marked 790, corresponds to the 5' end of the RNA and the lower band, marked 750, corresponds to the 3' end. This is shown in the double digestion experiment of lane 7, in which the lower band of the pair (but not the upper) is digested. It can also be seen (lane 7) that a new fragment marked 750* is created (just below Q3*). These results have been confirmed by direct sequencing of the 1400 and 790 bands.

DISCUSSION

Evolution of Ribosome Function and Structure

A rational discussion of the evolution of ribosome function and structure must be based on a comparison of ribosomal mechanisms in diverse organisms and a knowledge of the evolutionary relationships among them. For this, one needs to know the evolutionary tree that connects all organisms. Whether the origins of translation, the origins of introns, or those of any other molecular process are being discussed, the variations of mechanisms among organisms can be rigorously analyzed only in the context of the evolutionary tree.

During the last five years, our understanding of the phylogeny of all organisms has undergone a significant change. It now appears, from analysis both of 16S rRNA sequences and of ribosomal structures (Lake 1986), that the eukaryotes evolved from a sulfur-metabolizing group of prokaryotes, the eocytes. A

new class of tree-construction algorithms for nucleic acid sequence analysis, evolutionary parsimony (Lake 1987), has ruled out the archaebacterial tree (Woese 1981) and explains it as an artifact caused by the unequal rate treeing paradox (see Lake, this volume). This algorithm is not affected by unequal rates of nucleotide substitution.

The eocyte tree on which our analysis is based is shown in Figure 9. Its most important features are the early bifurcation (not a trifurcation) that separates organisms into two groups. These groups are a protobacterial group on the left, consisting of the eubacteria, halobacteria, and methanogens (including Thermoplasma) and a proto-eukaryotic group on the right that includes the sulfur-metabolizing eocytes and the eukaryotes.

In addition to understanding the distribution of properties (i.e., character states), one must have a method of extrapolating these properties of extant organisms to

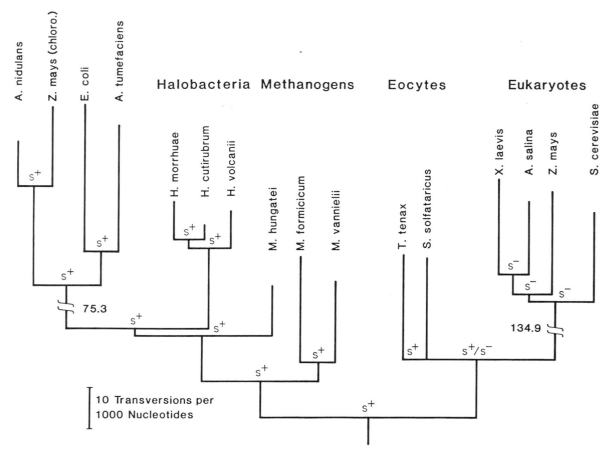

Figure 9. The sequence-derived, rooted evolutionary tree that relates extant organisms. The five groups are the eubacteria, halobacteria, methanogens, eocytes, and eukaryotes. The presence of a Shine-Dalgarno complementary sequence is indicated by an S + and its absence by an S − . The assignment of these character states to the ancestral nodes represents the first stage in parsimony analysis to determine the ancestral distribution of this mechanism. (In the next iteration, of the Fitch [1977] procedure, the S + /S − at the eocyte/eukaryote node would be replaced by an S + .) The most parsimonious assignment of character states indicates the last common ancestor of extant organisms had a Shine-Dalgarno-like mechanism.

the predicted properties of the nodes. For this, we use parsimony analysis (Fitch 1977). It is applied in the following example to the Shine-Dalgarno sequence as an example of this type of analysis (Shine and Dalgarno 1974).

The Last Common Ancestor of Extant Organisms Probably Used a Shine-Dalgarno-like Method of Messenger Selection

Parsimony analysis (Fitch 1977) is one of the most generally accepted techniques for assigning character states to the nodes of a tree. We have used this method to extrapolate our results from extant organisms to these ancestral ones. The Shine-Dalgarno sequence is a good example of how this analysis can be applied. Messenger-binding sequences are present on the small subunit rRNAs of eubacteria, halobacteria, methanogens, and eocytes, but are absent from eukaryotic small subunit RNA. Parsimony analysis applied to this distribution of character states then predicts that the eubacterial-halobacterial ancestor also had a Shine-Dalgarno region, since both of its descendants have the sequence. By repeatedly applying this analysis, one can proceed successively to nodes deeper within the tree. At the conclusion, one predicts that those nodes marked with an "S + " in Figure 7 correspond to ribosomes with the Shine-Dalgarno complementary region, and an "S − " indicates the ancestor lacked this function. This present-day distribution of character states thus implies that this mechanism of message selection was lost on the line leading to the eukaryotic cell. Most importantly, it indicates that the last common ancestor of extant organisms probably used a Shine-Dalgarno-like mechanism of message selection.

The Translation Mechanism of the Last Common Ancestor of All Extant Organisms

Given the evolutionary tree, one can predict some additional properties of the primitive protein synthesis mechanism of the last common ancestor. Fortunately, the two groups for which the most information is available on the mechanisms of protein synthesis are the eukaryotes and the eubacteria. Because these two groups are on opposite sides of the tree in Figure 7, features found in *both* eubacteria and eukaryotes (in the absence of dissenting information on the function of the halobacterial, methanogenic, and eocytic ribosomes) are most parsimoniously assigned to the common ancestor. (This would not necessarily hold had the archaebacterial tree been found valid.) In the following paragraphs we view the mechanism of protein synthesis in the light of parsimony analysis and in the light of DNA hybridization microscopy mappings of rRNA and other studies.

During protein synthesis, amino acids are added to the growing polypeptide chain in a series of reactions known as the elongation cycle. One of the accomplish-ments of studies of ribosome structure has been to learn what structural changes correspond to this cycle of additions. The biochemistry of the elongation cycle is quite well understood, whereas the structural correlates of this process are just starting to become understood. The biochemical process is as follows in both eubacteria and eukaryotes. Each iteration of the elongation cycle requires the participation of molecules called elongation factors (EFs) and also two molecules of GTP. At the beginning of each microcycle, the peptidyl-tRNA bearing the nascent chain is bound to the ribosome at the P-tRNA-binding site. Next an incoming aminoacyl-tRNA bearing the amino acid specified by the next unread codon on the mRNA binds to the recognition, or R, site (Lake 1977). It binds in complex with EF-Tu (EF-1 in eukaryotes) and GTP. The binding is controlled by the initial recognition of a codon on the mRNA by the anticodon of the tRNA. Following the initial recognition, the aminoacyl-tRNA is transferred to the A site, where, following a second checking of the mRNA-tRNA pairing, its amino acid accepts the nascent chain. Finally, in the second GTP-requiring step of the elongation microcycle, EF-G (EF-2) ejects the P-site tRNA and inserts the peptidyl-tRNA from the A site into the P site. The cycle is then repeated as subsequent codons are read.

The data available on the locations of functional sites in the ribosome have previously been integrated into the model for the functioning of the elongation cycle that is illustrated in Figure 10. The proposed mechanism has been discussed widely (Lake 1981a, 1985) and the experimental support for its features will not be repeated here, except to note that recently direct support for this model has come from structural studies in which the EF-Tu-binding site has been mapped in three dimensions (Girshovich et al. 1986; Langer and Lake 1986).

Four functional sites on the ribosomal surface now seem to have been determined by so many experiments in so many different laboratories that their locations can be considered known with new certainty. These regions are (1) the site of the codon-anticodon interaction is in the cleft; (2) the cleft is also a cradle for the A- and P-site-bound tRNAs; (3) the peptidyltransferase site is located on the side of the large subunit central protuberance; and (4) the site of the EF-Tu binding is on the neck of the small subunit and faces the cytoplasm, rather than the subunit interface. The first two of these conclusions have been described in the Results section and the last two will be discussed here. We note that the first conclusions would seem to be valid for both eubacteria and eukaryotes, since the DNA hybridization electron microscopy mappings of the 1400 region in *Escherichia coli* and in yeast (Oakes et al. 1986), in conjunction with cross-linking studies (Prince et al. 1982), locate the codon-anticodon interaction in both eubacteria and eukaryotes. Similarly, the platform and cleft structures are extremely conserved in ribosomes from eubacteria, halobacteria, methanogens, eocytes, and eukaryotes. Thus, the locations of the A

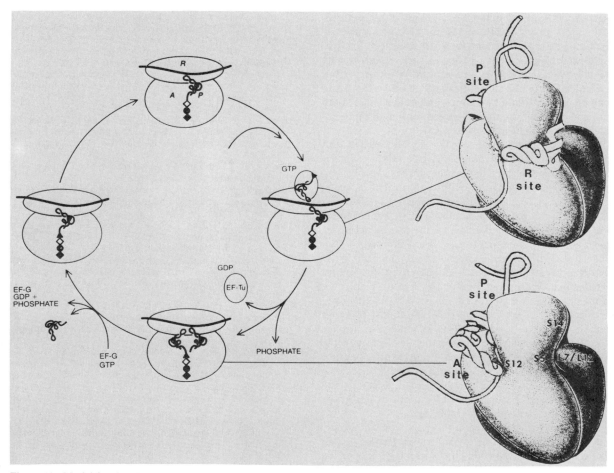

Figure 10. Model for the elongation cycle of protein synthesis in the last common ancestor of extant organisms. At the right are shown the likely locations of the tRNA-binding sites during specific stages of the cycle.

and P sites seem unlikely to vary in the different organisms.

The first evidence suggesting that the central protuberance was the site of the peptidyltransferase center was provided by immunoelectron microscopy. In particular, this was inferred from the location of the codon-anticodon site on the platform of the small subunit (Lake 1976). More direct evidence was provided by a mapping of protein L27 on the side of the central protuberance opposite the L7/L12 stalk (Lake 1980; Lake and Strycharz 1981), since L27 is consistently found among the proteins labeled by modified aminoacyl-tRNAs when they are bound to either the peptidyl site or to the aminoacyl site (for discussions, see Traut et al. 1974; Cooperman 1978). Most recently, the binding site of an analog of puromycin has been directly mapped on the central protuberance (Olson et al. 1982). Hence, evidence for this site is quite strong and, together with the location of the A and P sites in the cleft, is quite strongly supported in eubacteria and supported, but less strongly, in eukaryotes.

For a decade, much evidence has suggested that the EF-Tu-binding site was at a site distinct from the A and P sites. Recently, this has been shown to be the case in

experiments conducted in two different laboratories. These experiments have mapped the recognition site on the small subunit at a site that is distant from the A site (Girshovich et al. 1986; Langer and Lake 1986). Both groups concluded that the EF-Tu site is on the exterior surface of the small subunit, i.e., on the ribosomal surface that faces away from the interface between small and large subunits and is exposed to the cytoplasm. Although the R site has not yet been mapped in eukaryotic ribosomes, the extensive homology between EF-Tu and EF-1 and the conservation of ribosomal structure in the vicinity of the R site both suggest that the location of the R site is conserved.

The R-site Switch Mechanism May Be the Primitive Mechanism

If we attempt to incorporate the data presented in this chapter on the locations of functional sites into the elongation cycle of all ribosomes, then the model at the right of Figure 10 seems the most reasonable. The codon-anticodon site should almost certainly be placed on the platform near the cleft, and the bulk of data now suggest that the recognition site is on the external surface of the small subunit, as illustrated in Figure 10. The most likely locations for the A- and P-tRNA-binding sites would seem to be in the cleft. The locations in Figure 10 have been proposed previously (Lake 1981a), and they are especially attractive because switching of a tRNA from the R site to the A site can be accomplished by a conformational change of the anticodon loop from the 5′ stacked configuration to the 3′ stacked configuration (Lake 1976).

Since this mechanism is indicated in both left and right branches of the evolutionary tree (and much of it has been demonstrated in the other three branches), we argue that one can most simply interpret it as being used by the last common ancestor. The most parsimonious interpretation of these data is that this mechanism corresponds to that possessed by the last common ancestor of all extant organisms. Furthermore, it is a mechanism in which conformational changes in an RNA molecule (the tRNA anticodon loop) are central to the machinery, and thus it has a certain intrinsic appeal in light of the recent emphasis on possible primitive roles for RNA. At the time of the last common ancestor, both of the elongation factors were present, the Shine-Dalgarno mechanism was in place, and the peptidyltransferase center on the central protuberance of the large subunit was established. Furthermore, the essential rRNA architecture was formed, as is reflected by the extreme conservation of locations of sequences such as the small subunit "1400 region."

The proposals presented in this paper are admittedly speculative. In the spirit of this volume, however, we hope that they will provide others with a glimpse of the questions that can be approached using a combination of techniques from molecular biology and evolutionary analysis.

ACKNOWLEDGMENTS

We thank J. Washizaki for electron microscopy and photography. This work was supported by research grants from the National Science Foundation (PCM-83-16926) and the National Institute of General Medical Science (GM-24034) to J.A.L.

REFERENCES

Backendorf, C., C.J.C. Ravensbergen, J. Van der Plas, J.H. van Boom, G. Veeneman, and J. Van Duin. 1981. Basepairing potential of the 3′ terminus of 16S RNA: Dependence on the functional state of the 30S subunit and the presence of protein S21. *Nucleic Acids Res.* 9: 1425.

Berabeu, C. and J.A. Lake. 1982. Nascent polypeptide chains emerge from the exit domain of the ribosomal subunit: Immune mapping of the nascent chain. *Proc. Natl. Acad. Sci.* 79: 3111.

Bollen, A., R.L. Heimark, A. Cozzone, R.R. Traut, J.W.B. Hershey, and L. Kahan. 1975. Cross-linking of initiation factor IF-2 to *Escherichia coli* 30S ribosomal proteins with dimethylsuberimidate. *J. Biol. Chem.* 250: 4310.

Bollum, F.J. 1974. Terminal deoxynucleotidyl transferase. In *The Enzymes*, 3rd. edition (ed. P.D. Boyer), vol. 10, p. 145. Academic Press, New York.

Chapman, N.M. and H.F. Noller. 1977. Protection of specific sites in 16S RNA from chemical modification by association of 30S and 50S ribosomes. *J. Mol. Biol.* 109: 131.

Cooperman, B.S. 1978. Affinity labeling studies on *Escherichia coli* ribosomes. *Bioorg. Chem.* (suppl.) 4: 81.

Eckhardt, H. and R. Lührmann. 1979. Blocking of the initiation of protein biosynthesis by a pentanucleotide complementary to the 3′ end of *Escherichia coli* 16S rRNA. *J. Biol. Chem.* 254: 11185.

Emanuilov, I., D.D. Sabatini, J.A. Lake, and C. Freienstein. 1978. Localization of eukaryotic initiation factor 3 on native small ribosomal subunits. *Proc. Natl. Acad. Sci.* 75: 1389.

Fitch, W. 1977. On the problem of generating the most parsimonious tree. *Am. Nat.* 111: 223.

Girshovich, A.S., E.S. Bochkareva, and V.D. Vasiliev. 1986. Localization of elongation factor Tu on the ribosome. *FEBS Lett.* 197: 192.

Gutell, R.R., B. Weiser, C.R. Woese, and H.F. Noller. 1985. Comparative anatomy of 16S-like ribosomal RNA. *Prog. Nucleic Acid Res. Mol. Biol.* 32: 155.

Heimark, R.L., L. Kahan, K. Johnston, J.W.B. Hershey, and R.R. Traut. 1976. Cross-linking of initiation factor IF3 to proteins of the *Escherichia coli* 30S ribosomal subunit. *J. Mol. Biol.* 105: 219.

Keren-Zur, M., M. Boublik, and J. Ofengand. 1979. Localization of the decoding region on the 30S *Escherichia coli* ribosomal subunit by affinity immunoelectron microscopy. *Proc. Natl. Acad. Sci.* 76: 1054.

Kopylov, A.M., N.V. Chichkova, A.A. Bogdanov, and S.K. Vasilenko. 1975. Complementary binding of oligonucleotide with 16S RNA and ribosomal ribonucleoprotein. *Mol. Biol. Rep.* 2: 95.

Lake, J.A. 1976. Ribosome structure determined by electron microscopy of *Escherichia coli* small subunits, large subunits and monomeric ribosomes. *J. Mol. Biol.* 105: 131.

———. 1977. Aminoacyl-tRNA binding at the recognition site is the first step of the elongation cycle of protein synthesis. *Proc. Natl. Acad. Sci.* 74: 1903.

———. 1979a. Ribosome structure and tRNA binding sites. In *Transfer RNA: Structure, properties, and recognition* (ed. P.R. Schimmel et al.), p. 393. Cold Spring Harbor Laboratory, Cold Spring Harbor, New York.

———. 1979b. Practical aspects of immune electron microscopy. *Methods Enzymol.* 61: 250.

———. 1980. Ribosome structure and functional sites. In *Ribosomes: Structure, function and genetics* (ed. G. Chambliss et al.), p. 207. University Park Press, Baltimore.

———. 1981a. The ribosome. *Sci. Am.* 245: 84.

———. 1981b. Protein synthesis in prokaryotes and eukaryotes: The structural bases. In *Electron microscopy of proteins* (ed. R. Harris), vol. 1, p. 617. Academic Press, London.

———. 1985. Evolving ribosome structure: Domains in archaebacteria, eubacteria, eocytes and eukaryotes. *Annu. Rev. Biochem.* 54: 507.

———. 1986. In defence of bacterial phylogeny. *Nature* 321: 657.

———. 1987. A rate-independent technique for analysis of nucleic acid sequence: Evolutionary parsimony. *Mol. Biol. Evol.* 4: 167.

Lake, J.A. and L. Kahan. 1975. Ribosomal proteins S5, S11, S13 and S19 localized by electron microscopy of antibody-labeled subunits. *J. Mol. Biol.* 99: 631.

Lake, J.A. and W.A. Strycharz. 1981. Ribosomal proteins L1, L17, and L27 from *Escherichia coli* localized at single sites on the large subunit by immune electron microscopy. *J. Mol. Biol.* 153: 979.

Langberg, S., L. Kahan, R.R. Traut, and J.W.B. Hershey. 1977. Binding of protein synthesis initiation factor IF1 to 30S ribosomal subunits: Effects of other initiation factors and identification of proteins near the binding site. *J. Mol. Biol.* 117: 307.

Langer, J.A. and J.A. Lake. 1986. Elongation factor Tu localized on the exterior surface of the ribosomal subunit. *J. Mol. Biol.* **187**: 617.

Mankin, A.S., E.A. Skripkin, N.V. Chichkova, A.M. Kopylov, and A.A. Bogdanov. 1981. An enzymatic approach for localization of oligodeoxyribonucleotide binding sites on RNA. *FEBS Lett.* **131**: 253.

Meier, N. and R. Wagner. 1984. Binding of tRNA alters the chemical accessibility of nucleotides within the large ribosomal RNAs of *E. coli* ribosomes. *Nucleic Acids Res.* **12**: 1473.

Moazed, D. and H.F. Noller. 1986. Transfer RNA shields specific nucleotides in 16S ribosomal RNA from attack by chemical probes. *Cell* **47**: 985.

Moazed, D., S. Stern, and H.F. Noller. 1986. Rapid chemical probing of confirmation in 16S ribosomal RNA and 30S ribosomal subunits using primer extension. *J. Mol. Biol.* **187**: 399.

Noller, H.F. 1974. Topography of 16S RNA in 30S ribosomal subunits. Nucleotide sequences and location of sites of reaction with kethoxal. *Biochemistry* **13**: 4694.

―――. 1984. Structure of ribosomal RNA. *Annu. Rev. Biochem.* **53**: 119.

Noller, H.F. and J.B. Chaires. 1972. Functional modification of 16S ribosomal RNA by kethoxal. *Proc. Natl. Acad. Sci.* **69**: 3115.

Noller, H.F. and J.A. Lake. 1984. Ribosome structure and function: Localization of rRNA. *Membr. Struct. Funct.* **6**: 217.

Nomura, M., S. Mizushima, M. Ozaki, P. Traub, and C.V. Lowry. 1970. Structure and function of ribosomes and their molecular components. *Cold Spring Harbor Symp. Quant. Biol.* **34**: 49.

Oakes, M.I., M.W. Clark, E. Henderson, and J.A. Lake. 1984. 16S Ribosomal RNA mapped by electron microscopy complementary DNA probes. *J. Cell Biol.* **99**(4): 13a (Abstr.)

―――. 1986. DNA hybridization electron microscopy: Ribosomal RNA nucleotides 1392–1407 are exposed in the cleft of the small subunit. *Proc. Natl. Acad. Sci.* **83**: 275.

Ofengand, J., R. Liou, J. Kohut III, I. Schwartz, and R.A. Zimmermann. 1979. Covalent cross-linking of transfer ribonucleic acid to the ribosomal P site. Mechanism and site of reaction in transfer ribonucleic acid. *Biochemistry* **18**: 4322.

Olson, H.M. and D.G. Glitz. 1979. Ribosome structure: Localization of 3′ end of RNA in small subunit by immunoelectronmicroscopy. *Proc. Natl. Acad. Sci.* **76**: 3769.

Olson, H.M., P.G. Grant, B.S. Cooperman, and D.G. Glitz.

1982. Immunoelectron microscopic localization of puromycin binding on the large subunit of the *Escherichia coli* ribosome. *J. Biol. Chem.* **257**: 2649.

Peattie, D.A. and W. Gilbert. 1980. Chemical probes for higher-order structure in RNA. *Proc. Natl. Acad. Sci.* **77**: 4679.

Politz, S.M. and D.G. Glitz. 1977. Ribosome structure: Localization of N^6, N^6-dimethyladenosine by electron microscopy of a ribosome-antibody complex. *Proc. Natl. Acad. Sci.* **74**: 1468.

Prince, J.B., B.H. Taylor, D.L. Thurlow, J. Ofengand, and R.A. Zimmermann. 1982. Covalent crosslinking of $tRNA_1^{Val}$ to 16S RNA at the ribosomal P site: Identification of crosslinked residues. *Proc. Natl. Acad. Sci.* **79**: 5450.

Shatsky, I.N., L.V. Mochalova, M.S. Kojouharova, a.A. Bogdanov, and V.D. Vasiliev. 1979. Localization of the 3′ end of *Escherichia coli* 16 S RNA by electron microscopy of antibody-labelled subunits. *J. Mol. Biol.* **133**: 501.

Shine, J. and L. Dalgarno. 1974. The 3′-terminal sequence of *Escherichia coli* 16S ribosomal RNA: Complementarity to nonsense triplets and ribosome binding sites. *Proc. Natl. Acad. Sci.* **71**: 1342.

Taniguchi, T. and C. Weissmann. 1978. Inhibition of Qβ RNA 70S ribosome initiation complex formation by an oligonucleotide complementary to the 3′ terminal region of *E. coli* 16S ribosomal RNA. *Nature* **275**: 770.

Tapprich, W.E. and W.E. Hill. 1986. The involvement of bases 787–794 of *Escherichia coli* 16S ribosomal RNA in ribosomal subunit association. *Proc. Natl. Acad. Sci.* **83**: 556.

Traut, R.R., R.L. Heimark, T.-T. Sun, J.W.B. Hershey, and A. Bollen. 1974. Protein topography of ribosomal subunit from *Escherichia coli*. In *Ribosomes* (ed. M. Nomura et al.), p. 271. Cold Spring Harbor Laboratory, Cold Spring Harbor, New York.

Van Duin, J., C.J.C. Ravensbergen, and J. Doornbos. 1984. Basepairing of oligonucleotides to the 3′ end of 16S ribosomal RNA is not stabilized by ribosomal proteins. *Nucleic Acids Res.* **12**: 5079.

Van Duin, J., C.G. Kurland, J. Dondon, and M. Grunberg-Manago. 1975 Near neighbors of IF3 bound to 30S ribosomal subunits. *FEBS Lett.* **59**: 287.

Vassilenko, S.K., P. Carbon, J.P. Ebel, and C. Ehresmann. 1981. Topography of 16S RNA in 30S subunits of 70S ribosomes, accessibility to cobra venom ribonuclease. *J. Mol. Biol.* **152**: 699.

Woese, C.R. 1981. Archaebacteria. *Sci. Am.* **244**: 98.

Slippery Runs, Shifty Stops, Backward Steps, and Forward Hops: −2, −1, +1, +2, +5, and +6 Ribosomal Frameshifting

R.B. Weiss,* D.M. Dunn,* J.F. Atkins,*† and R.F. Gesteland*
*Department of Human Genetics and Howard Hughes Medical Institute, University of Utah Medical Center, Salt Lake City, Utah 84132; †Department of Biochemistry, University College, Cork, Ireland

Frameshift mutations frequently express residual levels of gene activity; that is, they are often leaky. This leakiness can be used as a tool to define the functional components that affect the reading frame during gene expression (Atkins et al. 1972; Fox and Weiss-Brummer 1980; Weiss and Gallant 1983). Recent technological advances in the capability to efficiently build synthetic DNA sequences have facilitated the construction of small, defined "frameshift windows." These windows are regions where frameshift events can be detected and measured. The cloned synthetic window is fused onto the 5' coding region of an active β-galactosidase gene that provides a sensitive monitor for the frameshift events. Fusions onto the *lacZ* gene have the advantages of simple colorimetric assays for β-galactosidase activity and little or no effect of the fused sequence on the specific activity or stability of the enzyme (Miller and Albertini 1983). A frameshift event also leaves a clue to its character in the protein sequence translated from the window's mRNA sequence. Recovery of the frameshift-containing β-galactosidase in sufficient yield and purity for determining its amino-terminal sequence provides hard evidence for the occurrence of a frameshift, and this sequence may be used to infer the kind of event generating the loss of reading frame.

Frameshift windows are defined at their 3' border by a stop codon in the zero frame relative to the translation start and at their 5' border by a stop codon in the monitored outgoing frame. Ribosomes can only enter the window by translating in the zero frame, and they can only exit by shifting to the −1 or +1 frame, only one of which results in the production of active β-galactosidase. A 2p, 3p, or 4p designation is given to windows that monitor the −1, 0, or +1 frame. Frameshift windows also have as a formal property the ability to determine the level (replication or transcription versus translation) at which the shift occurs. This property involves "reframing" the window's sequence so that the sequence remains the same but the frames in which the ribosome translates through it have both been shifted. Translational frameshifts should be sensitive to such reframing since ribosomes read frame, but the levels of transcriptional shifts or genetic reversion of the frameshift should not be altered by reframing, since the enzymatic machinery involved in these processes is not known to detect the reading frame.

This paper is confined to several key results from a construction project initiated several years ago, in which many *lacZ* frameshift windows have been built in and partially characterized. We focus on high-level translational shifts (> 0.1% of in-frame levels) here for two reasons: (1) They occur quite frequently and unexpectedly during construction of specific sequences and (2) interest in the mechanisms responsible for high-level shifts has recently been augmented by several cases of high-level ribosomal shifts that are necessary for proper gene expression and whose efficiency appears to be programmed in the mRNA (Dunn and Studier 1983; Craigen et al. 1985; Clare and Farabaugh 1985; Jacks and Varmus 1985; Mellor et al. 1985; Shimotohno et al. 1985; Jacks et al. 1987; Moore et al. 1987). The synthetic *lacZ* high-level shifts described here all occur within strings of repeated nucleotides (henceforth called strings) or between overlapping or nonoverlapping homologous codons. These strings and variably spaced homologous codons share the potential for correct decoding in the zero frame followed by a shift to a new frame that can be stabilized by good codon:anticodon pairing. This investigation has confirmed the location of several of these shifts and has begun to reveal a variety of events ranging from −2 to +6 nucleotides shifted relative to the zero frame. In all cases, good codon:anticodon pairing is available to the alleged shifting tRNA in both the incoming and outgoing frames, giving the paramount definition of the reading frame to the tRNA:mRNA interaction. However, mRNA sequence contexts can enhance the frequency of certain types of shifts, and the consequences of two mRNA contexts on these types of shifts are described.

EXPERIMENTAL PROCEDURES

Construction of *lacZ* Frameshifts

Oligonucleotides were synthesized by an Applied Biosystems 380A or B DNA synthesizer, and the crude material was cloned into a uniquely restricted pBR322 vector containing an engineered derivative of the *lacZ* gene. This places the synthetic sequence two codons downstream from the Z translation start, within in a region nonessential for β-galactosidase function. Inserts were verified by dideoxy sequencing of the plasmid DNA (Chen and Seeburg 1985). The primary *lacZ* vector has *lac* operon sequence from codon 5 of *Z* through codon 66 of *Y*, replacing the *Eco*RI-*Ava*I section of pBR322. The *Hin*dIII/*Apa*I cloning sites and the ribosome-binding site (based on the sequence of *Escherichia coli* lipoprotein ribosome-binding site) were constructed synthetically. A 269-bp *Bam*HI fragment from plasmid containing a *Tac* promoter was inserted just upstream of the synthetic ribosome-binding site, and an 800-bp fragment containing a T7 promoter was inserted between the *Eco*RI site of the pBR backbone and the upstream *Bam*HI site bordering the *Tac* promoter. The bacterial strain used is *E. coli* K-12 SU1675 del- *prolac*, *recA56*/F'I^Q (rec$^-$ derivative of CSH26; Miller 1972).

Purification and Amino-terminal Sequencing of Frameshifted β-Galactosidase

Cell extracts of saturated cultures of *E. coli* SU1675 *prolac*, *recA56* grown in superbroth (Davis et al. 1980) were prepared by sonication or freeze-thawing in 50 mM KPO$_4$ (pH 7.4), 150 mM NaCl, 0.1% Tween-20, and 10 mM β-mercaptoethanol. β-Galactosidase was purified by either passage through an anti-β-galactosidase affinity column (Protosorb, Promega Biotech) or by precipitation with anti-β-galactosidase antibody (Cooper Biomedical) and protein-A-Sepharose CL-4B beads. When necessary, the sample was further purified by high-pH electroblotting from a 7.5% SDS-acrylamide gel onto an aminopropyl-glass fiber filter (Aebersold et al. 1986). The GF-C filters were prepared by heating in neat trifluoroacetic acid (TFA) (Pierce, Sequanal grade) on a heating block at 68–70°C for 45 minutes. They were air-dried in a hood on Whatman No. 1 sheets for 2 hours, and then treated with a freshly prepared solution of γ-aminopropyltriethoxysilane (Pierce, 5% in 95% aqueous acetonitrile) at room temperature for 5 minutes with agitation. The filters were then taken through three washes of acetonitrile (each filter being handled separately), blotted, and cured at 105–110°C for 1 hour; this procedure is based on that of Aebersold et al. (1986). The electroblotted filter was stained with 3,3-dipentyloxacarbocyanine iodide (Aebersold et al. 1986); the β-galactosidase band was excised from the filter and placed in the cartridge of an ABI 470a gas-phase protein sequencer equipped with an on-line ABI 120a high-performance liquid chromatography (HPLC) analyzer. The program 03RPTH was utilized, cartridge temperature set at 45°C, and 40% of the phenylthiohydantoin (PTH) amino acids from each cycle were chromatographed by the on-line HPLC.

β-Galactosidase Activity Measurements

Whole-cell assays were based on the procedure according to Miller (1972). Stationary phase cultures were diluted 1/40 into Luria broth (LB) + 2 mM isopropyl-β-D-thiogalactoside (IPTG), grown at 37°C with rapid shaking, and chilled to 0°C at an OD$_{600}$ of 0.7–0.8. Whole-cell assays were done in a final volume of 1.0 ml Z-buffer, the assays were started with the addition of 0.2 ml of 4 mg/ml *O*-nitrophenyl-β-D-galactopyranoside and stopped with the addition of 0.5 ml of 1 M Na$_2$CO$_3$ (pH 11). All reactions were run at 28°C. The assay tubes were centrifuged before reading the OD$_{420}$.

RESULTS

Shifty Stops

Constructing frameshift mutations within the dispensable amino-terminal region of β-galactosidase takes advantage of the simple enzymatic assay for β-galactosidase activity (the range of in vivo detection spans at least five orders of magnitude); this permits easy measurement of the leakiness. Even low levels of frameshifted β-galactosidase produced from these constructs can be purified in one step by immunoaffinity chromatography, or in two steps using immunoprecipitation followed by SDS-acrylamide gel electrophoresis and electroblotting onto activated glass fiber filters. These techniques yield material suitable for amino-terminal sequencing, and the confinement of the frameshift window near the translation start puts this region within reach.

In an initial series of constructions, it was noted that placement of a string of repetitive nucleotides next to the 3′ stop codon border sometimes resulted in a sharp increase in the window's leakiness. This observation is shown in Table 1. When a GGG glycine codon is located 5′ to a stop codon (construct 4p101 CGG-GGG-UAA, Table 1) the reading frame shifts at the zero frame GGG by −2 nucleotides. This occurs at a level of approximately 2% relative to a similar in-frame construct (p900 series, Table 1). Comparison of the mRNA sequence of 4p101 with its protein sequence (Fig. 1a) leads to the inference that the glycine tRNA decoding the zero frame GGG shifts backwards by two nucleotides onto the 5′ overlapping GGG. This inference is strengthened by the decrease in the level of shifting observed when the first G in the 5′ overlapping GGG is altered (4p101 C̲GG-GGG-UAA:140 units versus 4p102 CA̲G-GGG-UAA:40 units and 4p103 CC̲G-GGG-UAA:12 units, Table 1). When the zero frame GGG is changed to a GGA glycine or GAA glutamate codon, −2 shifting is still observed at appreciable levels, and in the latter case, glutamate is incorporated at the shift site (data not shown), implying that a glutamate decoding tRNA reads the zero frame GAA glutamate codon and then shifts −2 onto the 5′ overlapping GGG glycine codon. Also, a sharp decrease in the level of shifting can be seen when the 3′ stop is changed to a sense codon in the 4p1100 series. Stop codons, especially UGA and UAA, elevate the level of this type of shift.

Enhancement of −1 frameshifting on 4 base G strings by a bordering 3′ stop codon is also seen (Table 1) by comparing 2p302 G-GGG-UAA:140 units with

Table 1. Frameshifting on Strings of Repetitive Nucleotides is Enhanced by a 3′ Stop Codon Border

Series	Sequence	β-Galactosidase activity (whole-cell units)
	Met- Lys- Ser- Leu- Asp- Arg- Gly- [−2 shift]	
	Gly- Lys- Gly-	
4p101	A U G-A A A-A G C-U U A-G A U-C G G-G G G-U A A-G G G-C	170
102	A	40
103	C	12
4p1103	A U G-A A A-A G C-U U A-G A C-C G G-G G G-U G A-C U G-U A A-G	230
1108	U A A	135
1122	U A G-G U G	40
1132	U G G-C U G-U A A	10
4p801	A U G-A A A-A G C-U U A-G A U-C G C-G C G-U G A-G G G-C	1
	Met- Lys- Ser- Phe- Asn- Leu- Gly- [−1 shift]	
	Val-Lys-Gly-	
2p302	A U G-A A A-A G C-U U U-A A U-C U G-G G G-U A A-A G G-G C	140
2p2613	A U G-A A A-A G C-U U U-A A U-C U G-G G G-C U U-C A C-U A A-C G G-G C	8
2p403	A U G-A A A-A G C-U U U-A A U-C U U-G G G-U A A-A G G-G C	5
2p3901	A U G-A A A-A G C-U U U-A A C-U U A-A U C-U G G-G G C-U U C-A C U-A C C-U A A-	1
3p901	A U G-A A A-A G C-U U A-G A U-U G G-A A U-A A G-G G C-	10100
902	U C	10000
903	G G	4600

The ribosome-binding site, AUG start, and frameshift windows were derived from synthetic DNA inserts cloned into a plasmid-borne *lacZ* gene. The host is *E. coli* SU1675 F′I^Q. Cultures were grown in LB at 37°C with aeration from a 1:40 dilution of a fresh saturated culture until an OD_{600} of ~0.7; whole cell β-galactosidase assay conditions are described in Miller (1972), except assays were centrifuged to remove cell debris before measuring the OD_{420}. The amino acid sequences superimposed above certain constructs were determined by amino-terminal sequencing of the purified frameshift β-galactosidase from those constructs. The 5′ stop codon border is overlined and the 3′ stop codon border is underlined.

2p2613 G-GGG-CUU:8 units. In 2p301, the reading frame slips −1 at the zero frame GGG glycine codon (Fig. 1b). Construct 4p403 U-GGG-UAA:5 units suggests the importance of good base-pairing potential in the outgoing frame when compared with 2p302 G-GGG-UAA:140 units (Table 1). The influence of the zero frame 3′ stop codon in enhancing the rate of −2

and −1 shifting on G strings indicates that the shift is occurring during translation. However, the origin of a comparatively low level of activity of 2p2613 is unclear. To test whether the signal is produced mainly from translational shifting, the window is reframed in construct 2p3901. The same sequence from the 2p2613 window is contained in 2p3901 (plus extra nucleotides necessary for reframing) but the ribosome translates into the window in another frame, a frame in which G-GGG Gly codons are not encountered; amino-terminal sequence analysis indicates that the G-GGG sequence in 2p2613 is the shift site (data not shown). If the activity of 2p2613 results from the addition of a single G residue into the G-GGG sequence, then 2p2613 and 2p3901 should have equal levels of activity; however, if it results from a translational slip on the G-GGG sequence, then the activity of 2p3901 should be lower than 2p2613. The decreased activity of 2p3901 (1 unit, Table 1) confirms the translational component of the shift emanating from 2p2613 (8 units).

If a GGG or GGA-decoding glycine tRNA can shift back −2 onto an overlapping GGG codon, and a GAA-decoding glutamate tRNA can shift back −2 onto an overlapping GGG, it might be expected that a GCG-decoding alanine tRNA would shift back −2 onto an overlapping GCG. 4p801 CGC-GCG-UGA (Table 1) demonstrates that this event is two orders of magnitude less frequent than the shift in 4p1103 CGG-GGG-UGA. One explanation is that the ability to backshift is tRNA-specific, whereas another view might require intermediate pairing, that is, a tRNA must step −1 with correct pairing before stepping −2, or an equivalent view would hold that purines may not pass purines on the opposite strand.

Inspection of sequences naturally occurring 5′ to ter-

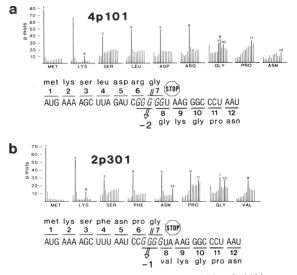

Figure 1. Amino-terminal sequence analysis of shifting on strings of repetitive nucleotides. Each panel shows the yield in pmols of PTH amino acids analyzed during each sequencing cycle; the data are not corrected for injection or base line. A number over a vertical line represents the major PTH amino acid recovered from that cycle. Underneath the panels are interpretations of the shifts seen by superimposing the protein sequence and the mRNA sequence.

mination codons of *E. coli* genes (from NIH GenBank and EMBL data libraries, January 1987) reveals that shifty stops of the type shown in Table 1 are rather prevalent, raising the prospect that in some cases they may be there for a purpose. Some potential uses for shifty stops might be required functional heterogeneity at the carboxyl terminus and translational coupling to downstream mRNA signals, for instance, translation start signals or mRNA degradation signals; such hypothetical uses of shifty stops remain to be tested. Why 3′ stop codon borders should enhance the rate of shifting on strings relative to sense codon borders is not known, but it may be a consequence of release factor action at stop codons, or the enhancement may occur prior to release factor binding.

tRNA Hopping

Can tRNAs move from their zero-frame codon to nearby similar codons, and do such tRNA "hops" occur? Construct 4p801 CGC-GCG-UGA suggests that tRNAs are not able to hop backward from their zero frame codon to a nearby similar codon at a high rate. However, in other constructs, several cases of forward hops appear to occur at high rates, in contrast to the attempted backward hop in 4p801. Table 2 lists the β-galactosidase activity, mRNA sequence, and protein sequence derived from three synthetic constructs in *lacZ* that are capable of testing sequences for tRNA hopping. One interpretation of the evidence is that in construct 2p4001 (GUG-UG) the valine tRNA decoding at GUG codon 7 hops onto the GUG overlapping codons 7 and 8, in construct 2p4101 (AAC-UCA-AU) the asparagine tRNA decoding at AAC codon 4 hops onto the AAU codon overlapping codons 5 and 6, and in construct 3p4201 (CUU-UAG-CUA) the leucine tRNA decoding the CUU at codon 7 hops over codon 8 and onto the CUA at codon 9, leading to shifts in the reading frame by +2, +5, and +6 nucleotides. The β-galactosidase levels produced from these constructs (ranging from 0.4 to 1.0% of average in-frame levels) implies that hopping occurs quite frequently. Another interpretation of the pattern of activities and protein

sequences displayed by these constructs is that during expression, the mRNA is altered in some manner as to be translated into the observed protein sequence; reversion of the frameshift lesion cannot explain these hops, since genetic variation is not observed at the required level. The translational basis of the observed +2 and +5 hops is testable by reframing the windows. Construct 2p4001 is also a synthetic analog of the *trpE91* frameshift window (Atkins et al. 1983) first isolated in *Salmonella typhimurium* and for which many external −1 frameshift suppressors exist. Recently, one of these suppressors, *E. coli hopR*, has been shown to suppress via hopping at the GUG-UG (B. Falahee and J. Atkins, unpubl.).

The precise sequence requirements and generality of tRNA hopping remain uncharacterized; however, potential examples for utilizing a programmed hop during gene expression may be found among the plant RNA viruses. Tobacco mosaic virus (TMV) encodes a 183-kD read-through polypeptide synthesized by leaky termination at the TMV 126-kD polypeptide amber stop (Pelham 1978; Goelet et al. 1982), beet necrotic yellow vein virus RNA (Bouzoubaa et al. 1986), and turnip yellow mosaic virus RNA (Haenni et al. 1987) encode similar amber read-through polypeptides. In these three cases, the leaky amber terminator is flanked by CAA glutamine codons (CAA-UAG-CAA). It is possible these amber stops leak because of stop-hopping, similar to the leucine tRNA stop-hop seen in construct 4p4201 CUU-UAG-CUA.

Programmed Ribosomal Frameshifts

Two cases of programmed high-level frameshifting, *E. coli* peptide chain release factor 2 (RF2) and Rous sarcoma virus *gag-pol* polyprotein and related retroviral shifts, display similar motifs of shifting that appear related to the synthetic *lacZ* high-level shifts; however, the rates of 30% shifting and above indicate that they are doing something extra. The known retroviral shifts are −1 on pyrimidine or purine strings and their levels range from 3 to 30%; this high level requires mRNA sequences 3′ to the string, which may form stem-loop

Table 2. tRNA Hopping

Series	β-Galactosidase activity (whole-cell assays, % in-frame level)
A. [+2 hop] Met-Lys-Ser-Phe-Asp-Gly-Val . . . Arg-Leu 2p4001- A U G-A A A-A G C-U U U-G A U-G G A-<u>G U G-U G</u>A-G G U-U A A-	0.5
B. [+5 hop] Met-Glu-Ile-Asn- . . . Leu-Glu-Gly 2p4101- A U G-G A G-A U U-<u>A A C</u>-U C <u>A-A U</u>C-U A G-A G G-G U A-	0.4
C. [+6 hop] Met-Lys-Ser-Leu-Gly-Tyr-Leu- . . . Arg-Arg 3p4201- A U G-A A A-A G C-U U A-G G G-U A U-<u>C U U</u>-U A G-<u>C U A</u>-C G A-C G G-	1.0

The first AUG in each construct is the translation start codon, and the amino-terminal sequence determined for each construct is superimposed above the mRNA sequence. The β-galactosidase activity is given as a percentage of in-frame levels (in-frame level = average of 3p900 series, Table 1). The similar codons inferred to be involved in the hops are underlined.

structures (Jacks et al. 1987; Moore et al. 1987). The reading frame in RF2 mRNA shifts +1 on a CUU-U pyrimidine string (Craigen et al. 1985), and the rate of shifting is approximately 30% (Craigen and Caskey 1986). A mutational analysis of synthetic RF2 frameshift window (see below) suggests that both upstream and downstream elements flanking the CUU-U string enhance the rate of shifting. One possible recipe for programming high-level frameshifts derived from these examples is to begin with a codon:anticodon pair embedded within a string of repetitive mRNA nucleotides, and then perturb this inherently ambiguous pairing potential with outlying mRNA:ribosome interplay of various kinds.

The RF2 shift has been analyzed by synthetically reconstructing a 30-nucleotide mRNA sequence sufficient for high-level shifting near the 5' end of the *lacZ* gene; Table 3 displays some of the variants of this sequence that define the components of the site. The 25% ratio of β-galactosidase produced from out-of-frame versus in-frame synthetic RF2-*lacZ* constructs (4p2101 versus 3p1201, Table 3) demonstrates that the high rate of shifting has been recreated within *lacZ*. The protein sequences (Fig. 2) of two synthetic derivatives, 4p2101, an analog of the RF2 window, and 4p2203, which changes the UGA stop to a UGG tryptophan codon, both suggest that a leucine tRNA decoding at the CUU-UGA/G sequence slips +1 at the string of pyrimidines.

The requirement for a string at the shift site is seen

Table 3. Variants of the Synthetic RF2-*lacZ* Frameshift Window

Series		β-Galactosidase activity (whole-cell units)
	Val-Leu-Arg-Gly-Tyr-Leu-Asp-Tyr-Glu	
3p1201	-G U U-C U U-A G G-G G G-U A U-C U U-G A C-U A C-G A G-	24600
	Val-Leu-Arg-Gly-Tyr-Leu -Asp-Tyr-Glu	
4p2101	-G U U-C U U-A G G-G G G-U A U-C U U-U G A-C U A-C G A-G	6600
4p1601	-G U U-C U U-A <u>G-A</u> G G-U A U-C U U-U G A-C U A-C G A-G	1400
1602-	U-G	660
1603-	G-U	280
4p1701	-G U U-C U U-A G G-G <u>G G-C</u> A U-C U U-U G A-C U A-C G A-G	2500
1706-	G C-G	260
1716-	C G-A	50
4p1801	G -U U C-U U A-G G G-G G U-<u>U</u> A U-C U U-U G A-C U A-C G A-G	390
1802-	G	35
4p1901	-G U U-C U U-A G G-G G G-U <u>U A</u>-C U U-U G A-C U A-C G A-G	9300
1905-	C G	5400
	Val-Leu-Arg-Gly-Tyr-Val -Asp-Tyr-Glu	
4p2001	-G U U-C U U-A G G-G G G-U A U-<u>G U U</u>-U G A-C U A-C G A-G	1900
2003-	U U A	60
2004-	C U A	35
2005-	G U A	25
2006-	G U G	25
2007-	A U A	15
4p2100	-G U U-C U U-A G G-G G G-U A U-C U U-<u>U G A</u>-C U A-C G A-G	6600
2201-	U A G	3800
2102-	U A A	3600
2203-	U G G	830
2103-	U U A	560
2204-	U U G	530
4p2301	-G U U-C U U-A G <u>A</u>-G G G-U A U-C U U-<u>U U G</u>-C U A-C G A-G	45
	Val-Leu-Arg-Gly-Tyr-Gly -Asp-Tyr-Glu	
4p2501	-G U U-C U U-A <u>G</u> G-G G G-U A U-<u>G G G</u>-U G A-C U A-C G A-G	1500
2502-	U	260
4p1302	-<u>U G</u> U-C U U-A G G-G G G-U A U-C U U-U G A-C U A-C G A-G	5400
4p1403	-G U <u>G-G</u> U U-A G G-G G G-U A U-C U U-U G A-C U A-C G A-G	4100
4p1501	-G U U-C <u>U A</u>-A G G-G G G-U A U-C U U-U G A-C U A-C G A-G	3700
1504-	G G	220
4p4301	-U <u>G G-U G G</u>-C U U-A G G-G G G-U A U-C U U-U G A-C U A-C	5400
4302	G G-C G G	4200
4303	G G-G G G	170
4304	G G-A G G	140

The codon demarcating the 5' border of these series is located 6 codons in from the AUG start codon. The host is *E. coli* SU1675 F'I^{O}, cultures were grown in LB at 37°C with aeration from a 1:40 dilution of a fresh saturated culture until an OD$_{600}$ of ~0.7; whole cell β-galactosidase assay conditions are described in Table 1. The amino acid sequences shown above certain constructs were determined by amino-terminal sequencing of the purified frameshift β-galactosidase. Critical residues in each series are underlined.

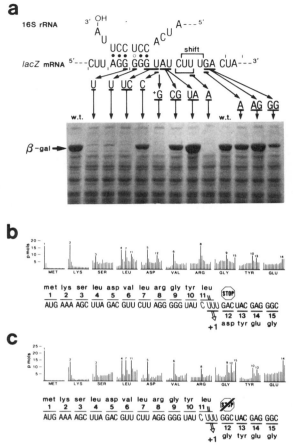

Figure 2. Variants of the synthetic RF2 frameshift window and amino-terminal sequencing of 4p2101 and 4p2203. The Coomassie-stained 7.5% SDS-PAGE gel (*a*) of whole cell lysates shows the amount of β-galactosidase produced from each construct in LB at 37°C; the w.t. designation refers to 4p2101. From left to right, the constructs shown are: 4p2101, 4p1602, 4p1603, 4p1707, 4p1701, 4p1802, 4p1905, 4p1901, 4p2004, 4p2101, 4p2102, 4p2201, and 4p2203 (see Table 3). Amino-terminal sequence analysis and interpretation (*b*) for 4p2101 and (*c*) for 4p2203.

with the constructs that disrupt the string (4p2003 UUA, 4p2004 CUA, 4p2005 GUA, 4p2006 GUG, and 4p2007 AUA; Table 1) and eliminate high-level shifting. It is also possible to substitute one string for another and still maintain high-level shifting (4p2001 GUU-UGA shifts a valine tRNA +1 at this position, and 4p2501 GGG-UGA shifts a glycine tRNA +1, Table 3). A decrease similar to that seen in Table 1 for stop to sense substitutions is seen in the 4p2100 and 4p2200 series (Table 3). This suggests that the CUU-UGA sequence is a shifty stop.

Decreases in the rate of shifting caused by changes upstream of the shifty stop are shown in series 4p1600-1900. Severe decreases are seen when single or multiple changes are introduced 3–7 nucleotides upstream of the CUU-UGA (4p1600 and 4p1700 series, Table 3). Changes within the UAU sequence located between this upstream element and the shifty stop do not grossly affect the level of shifting (4p1901 UUA and 4p1905

UCG, Table 3), but single nucleotide insertions within this region do have severe effects (4p1801 U-UAU and 4p1802 U-GAU, Table 3).

Substitutions further upstream of sequence only slightly alter the level of shifting (4p1300–1500 series, Table 3), except for the change in 4p1504, which decreases shifting by approximately 20-fold (Table 3). One explanation for this decrease is that this substitution creates an overlapping duplication of the region inferred to be critical in the 4p1600 and 1700 series. This region resembles the Shine-Dalgarno (SD) nucleotides of ribosome-binding sites, a region known to function via base pairing with nucleotides near the 3' end of 16S rRNA (Shine and Dalgarno 1974; Steitz and Jakes 1975). In 4p1504, an SD-like sequence (GGAGG) overlaps the SD-like sequence inferred to be necessary for high-level shifting, implying perhaps that if the 16S rRNA pairs with this upstream GGAGG sequence it is then unavailable for pairing with the AGGGGG sequence necessary for shifting. Interference by upstream core SD-like sequences is tested explicitly in series 4p4300 (Table 3). When the sequences GGGGG or GGAGG are placed three nucleotides upstream of the AGGGGG, interference is evident (4p4303 GGGGG-170 units and 4p4304 GGAGG-140 units, Table 3), but when GGUGG or GGCGG is substituted here, only slight effects are observed (4p4301 GGUGG-5400 units and 4p4302 GGCGG-4200 units, Table 3). This pattern of SD-like effects on shifting implies that pairing between the mRNA and 16S rRNA may occur close to the decoding sites within elongating ribosomes and this pairing can enhance the rate of +1 shifting on properly spaced shifty stops. A comparison of 4p2204 UUG-530 units, a stop to a sense codon change, with 4p2301 AGAG-GG...UUG-45 units, a change of both the SD-like element and the stop codon, demonstrate that the enhanced level of shifting caused by the SD-like element is not confined to shifty stops but works on sense strings as well (see amino-terminal sequence of 4p2202, Fig. 2). Critical changes in the synthetic RF2 window are summarized in Figure 2, which displays the β-galactosidase levels produced by these mutants as seen by Coomassie-blue staining of an SDS-acrylamide gel of whole-cell lysates. The postulated pairing between the mRNA and 16S rRNA is also shown in Figure 2.

CONCLUSIONS

Application of technical improvements in the array of experimental approaches currently available has provided a fresh look at the basis of frameshift leakiness. The novel events observed include the stop codon effect upon shifting on strings, tRNAs that appear to hop forward on the mRNA from their zero-frame codon to a similar codon, and a postulated SD-like interaction within elongating ribosomes. Some of these events have evidently become grist for evolution's mill, having been turned into sophisticated control points for particular genes. The rationale for nature having constructed the RF2 shift site and bordering it with a UGA codon is to provide an efficient autoregulatory loop for RF2 expression (Craigen and Caskey 1986), since RF2 is involved in termination at UGA and UAA codons. In doing so, both the SD-like and stop codon effect on enhancing shifts on pyrimidine or purine strings have been used to advantage. Retroviruses have also taken advantage of enhanced shifting on strings by using 3′ sequence elements to elevate the level of shifting (Jacks et al. 1987, Moore et al. 1987). The rationale there appears designed for producing nested proteins in a defined ratio from a single translation start. How many more examples of these types of controls exist remains to be seen, but they contain the prospect of illuminating the design of the ribosome's translocation mechanism.

ACKNOWLEDGMENTS

Regina Zeikus and Bernadette Falahee provided excellent assistance in protein sequencing. We thank Al Dahlberg, Larry Gold, Tyler Jacks, Shalha Thompson, R.J. Goldberg, Bill Craigen, and Jon Gallant for helpful conversations. This research was supported by the Howard Hughes Medical Institute and National Science Foundation grant DMB-8408649. R. Weiss is a fellow of the Helen Hay Whitney Foundation.

REFERENCES

Aebersold, R.H., D.B. Teplow, L.E. Hood, and S.B.H. Kent. 1986. Electroblotting onto activated glass: High efficiency preparation of proteins from analytical SDS-PAGE for direct sequence analysis. *J. Biol. Chem.* **261:** 4229.

Atkins, J.F., D. Elseviers, and L. Gorini. 1972. Low activity of β-galactosidase in frameshift mutants of *Escherichia coli*. *Proc. Natl. Acad. Sci.* **69:** 1192.

Atkins, J.F., B.P. Nichols, and S. Thompson. 1983. The nucleotide sequence of the first externally suppressible −1 frameshift mutant, and of some nearby leaky frameshift mutants. *EMBO J.* **2:** 1345.

Bouzoubaa, S., V. Ziegler, D. Beck, H. Guilley, K. Richards, and G. Jonard. 1986. Nucleotide sequence of beet necrotic yellow vein virus RNA-2. *J. Gen. Virol.* **67:** 1689.

Chen, E.Y. and P.H. Seeburg. 1985. Supercoil sequencing: A fast and simple method for sequencing plasmid DNA. *DNA* **4:** 165.

Clare, J. and P. Farabaugh. 1985. Nucleotide sequence of a yeast Ty element: Evidence for an unusual mechanism of gene expression. *Proc. Natl. Acad. Sci.* **82:** 2829.

Craigen, W.J. and C.T. Caskey. 1986. Expression of peptide chain release factor 2 requires high-efficiency frameshift. *Nature* **322:** 273.

Craigen, W.J., R.G. Cook, W.P. Tate, and C.T. Caskey. 1985. Bacterial peptide chain release factors: Conserved primary structure and possible frameshift regulation of release factor 2. *Proc. Natl. Acad. Sci.* **82:** 3616.

Davis, R.W., D. Botstein, and J.R. Roth. 1980. *Advanced bacterial genetics: A manual for genetic engineering.* Cold Spring Harbor Laboratory, Cold Spring Harbor, New York.

Dunn, J.J. and F.W. Studier. 1983. Complete nucleotide sequence of bacteriophage T7 DNA and the locations of T7 genetic elements. *J. Mol. Biol.* **166:** 477.

Fox, T.D. and B. Weiss-Brummer. 1980. Leaky +1 and −1 frameshift mutations at the same site in a yeast mitochondrial gene. *Nature* **288:** 60.

Goelet, P., G.P. Lomonosoff, P.J.G. Butler, M.E. Akam, M.J. Gait, and J. Karn. 1982. Nucleotide sequence of tobacco mosaic virus. *Proc. Natl. Acad. Sci.* **79:** 5818.

Haenii, A.L., M.D. Morch, G. Drugeon, R. Valle, R. Joshi, and T.M. Denial. 1987. Gene expression in turnip yellow mosaic virus. *UCLA Symp. Mol. Cell. Biol.* **54:** 149.

Jacks, T. and H.E. Varmus. 1985. Expression of Rous sarcoma virus *pol* gene by ribosomal frameshifting. *Science* **230:** 1237.

Jacks, T., K. Townsley, H.E. Varmus, and J. Majors. 1987. Two efficient ribosomal frameshifting events are required for synthesis of mouse mammary tumor virus *gag*-related polyproteins. *Proc. Natl. Acad. Sci.* **84:** 4298.

Mellor, J., S.M. Fulton, M.J. Dobson, W. Wilson, S.M. Kingsman, and A.J. Kingsman. 1985. A retrovirus-like strategy for expression of a fusion protein encoded by yeast transposon Ty1. *Nature* **313:** 243.

Miller, J. 1972. *Experiments in molecular genetics.* Cold Spring Harbor Laboratory, Cold Spring Harbor, New York.

Miller, J.H. and A.M. Albertini. 1983. Effects of surrounding sequence on the suppression of nonsense codons. *J. Mol. Biol.* **164:** 59.

Moore, R., M. Dixon, R. Smith, G. Peters, and C. Dickson. 1987. Complete nucleotide sequence of a milk-transmitted mouse mammary tumor virus: Two frameshift suppression events are required for translation of *gag* and *pol*. *J. Virol.* **61(2):** 480.

Pelham, H.R.B. 1978. Leaky UAG termination codon in tobacco mosaic virus RNA. *Nature* **272:** 469.

Shimotohno, K., Y. Takahashi, N. Shimizu, T. Gojobori, D.W. Golde, I.S.Y. Chen, M. Miwa, and T. Sugimura. 1985. Complete nucleotide sequence of an infectious clone of human T-cell leukemia virus type II: An open reading frame for the protease gene. *Proc. Natl. Acad. Sci.* **82:** 3101.

Shine, J. and L. Dalgarno. 1974. The 3′ terminal sequence of *Escherichia coli* 16S ribosomal rRNA: Complementarity to nonsense triplets and ribosome binding sites. *Proc. Natl. Acad. Sci.* **71:** 1342.

Steitz, J.A. and K. Jakes. 1975. How ribosomes select initiator regions in mRNA: Base pair formation between the 3′ terminus of 16S rRNA and the mRNA during initiation of protein synthesis in *Escherichia coli*. *Proc. Natl. Acad. Sci.* **72:** 4734.

Weiss, R.B. and J.A. Gallant. 1983. Mechanism of ribosome frameshifting during translation of the genetic code. *Nature* **302:** 389.

Studies on the Architecture and Function of 16S rRNA

H.F. Noller,* S. Stern,* D. Moazed,* T. Powers,* P. Svensson,* and L.-M. Changchien[†]

*Thimann Laboratories, University of California at Santa Cruz, Santa Cruz, California 95064;
[†]Laboratory of Molecular Biology, University of Wisconsin, Madison, Wisconsin 53706

Ribosomes are responsible for translation of the genetic code. Since the process of translation serves to link genotype with phenotype, as emphasized by Woese (1980), ribosomes occupy a unique and central position in the functioning of biological systems. The extraordinarily high conservation of primary and secondary structure of rRNA (Gutell et al. 1985) implies that ribosomes are very ancient macromolecular structures, perhaps the most ancient that exist, along with tRNA. This high degree of conservation also suggests that the three-dimensional structure of ribosomes is conserved, presumably because their proper functioning is dependent on maintaining many crucial structural elements in correct geometrical relationship with each other. Presently available information (see Hardesty and Kramer 1986) is consistent with the view that ribosomes are intricately designed molecular machines, rather than passive surfaces on which translation takes place.

Our understanding of ribosome structure has progressed without benefit of X-ray crystallography, although recent results with crystalline *Halobacterium* 50S subunits (Makowski et al. 1987) provide hope that this situation will change. A sense of the morphology of ribosomes and their subunits has come from electron microscopy (see Oakes et al., this volume). The most detailed quantitative information concerning the three-dimensional structure of the ribosome is a map of the positions of the 21 *Escherichia coli* 30S ribosomal proteins, obtained from neutron diffraction studies by Moore et al. (this volume). This information can be correlated with electron microscopy models via placement of ribosomal proteins by immuno-electron microscopy (IEM) (Oakes et al. 1986; Stöffler and Stöffler-Meilicke 1986). Finally, indications of the folding of rRNA within the ribosome may be inferred from protein-RNA and RNA-RNA cross-linking (Brimacombe et al. 1986), identification of protein binding sites on rRNA (Zimmermann 1980), IEM studies using antibodies directed toward certain features of rRNA (e.g., Politz and Glitz 1977), and the secondary structures of the rRNAs, deduced from comparative sequence analysis and supported by extensive experimental evidence (for a review, see Woese et al. 1983; Noller 1984; Gutell et al. 1985).

Early structure-function studies were concerned with the assignment of specific translational functions (e.g., tRNA and mRNA binding, peptidyltransferase, translocation, etc.) to various soluble protein factors, as opposed to the ribosome itself. By now it is clear, however, that under the appropriate solvent conditions, virtually all such functions can be executed by purified ribosomes or ribosomal subunits in the absence of factors (albeit at reduced efficiency, in many cases). More recently, similar questions have been raised concerning the role of ribosomal proteins. It has been argued from an evolutionary standpoint that the primitive ribosome must have been a functional RNA molecule (Crick 1968; Woese 1980; Noller and Woese 1981). This view has gained considerable support since the discovery of catalytic RNA (Cech and Bass 1986). Apart from the Shine-Dalgarno mechanism for mRNA selection (reviewed by Steitz 1980), there is now extensive experimental evidence in support of the view that ribosomal RNA participates directly in many, if not all, of the steps of the translation process (for a review, see Noller 1984; Noller et al. 1986). Taken together with the findings that many ribosomal proteins can be eliminated from cells without loss of viability (Dabbs 1986), one is led to ask, what purpose(s) do the ribosomal proteins serve? This amounts to a complete reversal of the paradigm that defined the conventional point of view in this field until relatively recently.

In this paper, we summarize some recent efforts aimed toward (1) understanding the molecular mechanism of assembly of 30S ribosomal subunits, (2) predicting the three-dimensional folding of the main features of the 16S rRNA structure, (3) identification of sites of interaction of 16S rRNA with tRNA, and (4) the use of antibiotics to distinguish between possible functional roles for these sites. Our approach exploits the use of chemical and enzymatic probing in conjunction with primer extension to monitor the higher order structure of rRNA and its interaction with specific functional ligands (Moazed et al. 1986a; Stern et al. 1987). We find evidence for interaction of twenty 30S ribosomal proteins with specific sites in 16S rRNA, and use this and other information, together with the neutron diffraction map of the locations of the corresponding proteins (Moore et al., this volume) to construct a preliminary model for the three-dimensional folding of 16S rRNA in the 30S subunit. In addition, tRNA shields specific sites in 16S rRNA from our probes. These sites fall into three experimentally distinguishable classes; we discuss the possible mechanistic roles of these sites, and evidence for functionally relevant conformational changes in 16S rRNA. Finally, we discuss the assembly and function of the 30S subunit in the context of our preliminary structural model for 16S rRNA.

METHODS

To localize the sites of interaction of ligands with 16S rRNA, we used a recently developed "footprinting" method (Moazed et al. 1986a; Stern et al. 1987). The various complexes containing 16S rRNA are treated with chemical or enzymatic probes, which attack exposed nucleotides in the RNA according to their respective base and structure specificities (Table 1). The precise sites of attack are identified by primer extension with avian myeloblastosis virus reverse transcriptase, which pauses or stops at modified bases or sites of strand cleavage. A set of synthetic DNA oligomers is used to prime at ~200-nucleotide intervals along the 16S rRNA chain. In this way, the availability of virtually every nucleotide in the RNA may be monitored; in purines, the N1 and N7 positions can be monitored independently (Table 1). Interaction of a ligand with a base is manifested as a decrease in the intensity of the cDNA band corresponding to the stop or pause generated by the modification (see Fig. 1). It is important to note that such decreases in intensity can be the result of either direct contact or indirect (allosteric) interaction between the RNA and its ligand. Enhanced reactivities are also observed; these are almost certainly attributable to ligand-induced conformational changes in the RNA.

Three-dimensional modeling of the folding of 16S rRNA was done using an Evans and Sutherland PS 330/VAX 11-750 computer graphics system. Each double-stranded segment of the secondary structure (Fig. 2) was converted to a set of three-dimensional RNA A helical coordinates, in which each nucleotide is represented by a point centered at its phosphorus atom. Single-stranded regions are displayed simply as straight lines joining consecutive base-paired segments. This structure is displayed, superimposed on a map of the positions of the 30S ribosomal proteins (see Moore et al., this volume), and individual helical elements are disconnected, moved, and rejoined using a modification of the interactive molecular modeling program FRODO (Jones 1982).

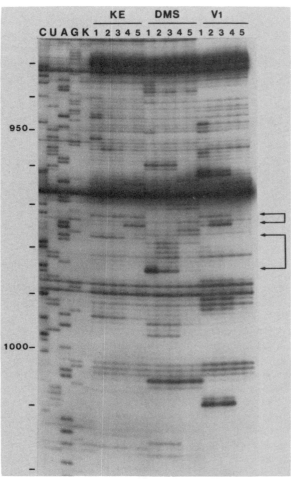

Figure 1. An example of the application of chemical and enzymatic footprinting, using primer extension, to 16S rRNA-protein interactions. Naked 16S rRNA (lane *1*), or its RNP complexes with ribosomal proteins S7 (lane *2*), S7 + S9 (lane *3*), S7 + S19 (lane *4*), or S7 + S9 + S19 (lane *5*) were probed with kethoxal (KE), dimethyl sulfate (DMS), or cobra venom nuclease (V_1). Dideoxy sequencing lanes are shown at left, and nucleotide positions in the 16S rRNA sequence are indicated. The brackets shown at right indicate regions of the RNA whose susceptibility to the probes is enhanced by protein S7, and subsequently protected by S19 (T. Powers, unpubl. results). Protein S19 has no effect in the absence of S7 (not shown). Details of the method are described in Stern et al. (1987).

Table 1. Chemical and Enzymatic RNA Structural Probes

	Base specificity			
Probes	G	A	C	U
Kethoxal	N1, N2			
Dimethyl sulfate	N7	N1	N3	
CMCT	N1			N3
Diethyl pyrocarbonate	N7	N7		
RNase T_1	+			
RNase A			+	+
RNase V_1	helical structures			

All of the listed probes are believed to be single-strand-specific, except for RNase V_1, and the reaction of dimethyl sulfate with guanine at N7. See Stern et al. (1987) and Van Stolk and Noller (1987) for details.

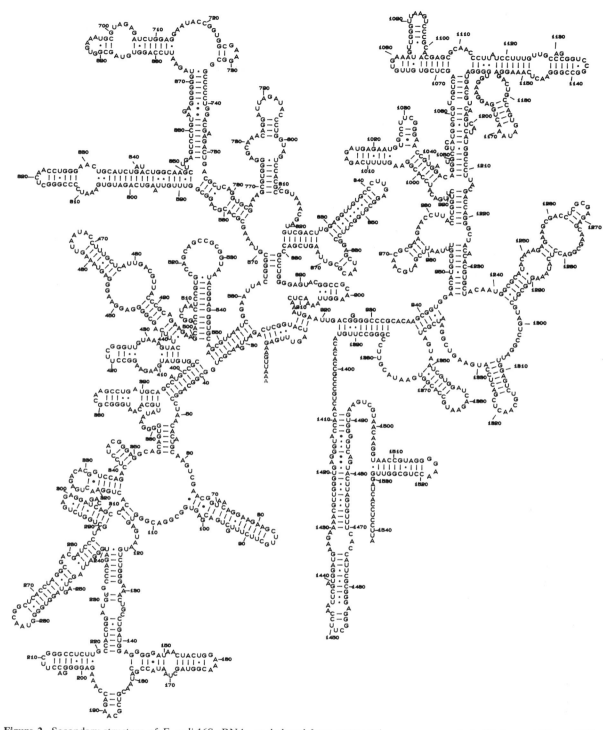

Figure 2. Secondary structure of *E. coli* 16S rRNA, as deduced from comparative sequence analysis (Noller and Woese 1981; Woese et al. 1983; Gutell et al. 1985).

Sites of Interaction between Ribosomal Proteins and 16S rRNA

The *E. coli* 30S ribosomal subunit is composed of 16S rRNA and 21 different ribosomal proteins, held together by noncovalent interactions. Nomura and his colleagues showed by in vitro reconstitution of active 30S subunits that these macromolecules have the capacity for self-assembly, suggesting an intricate system of interacting molecular recognition mechanisms (Traub and Nomura 1968). Step-wise reconstitution from 16S rRNA and purified ribosomal proteins provided a picture of the assembly interdependencies of the different macromolecular components, known as the 30S assembly map (Mizushima and Nomura 1970; Held et al. 1974). Several proteins, including S4, S7, S8, S15, S17, and S20, are able to bind to 16S rRNA independently. These proteins, which we call the primary binding proteins, have been the subject of most of the published studies on rRNA-protein interaction (for a review, see Zimmermann 1980). For the most part, they have been localized relatively imprecisely to large regions of 16S rRNA, with some notable exceptions. Little has been learned about the possible interaction of the secondary binding proteins (which we define as requiring one or more primary binders for assembly) with 16S rRNA. Chemical and UV cross-linking experiments have provided information regarding proximity of specific proteins to sites in 16S rRNA, but do not necessarily imply that interaction between the cross-linked sites occurs naturally (for a review, see Brimacombe et al. 1986).

Among the important questions concerning ribosome assembly are: Do the secondary and tertiary binding proteins interact, directly or indirectly, with rRNA? Which features of 16S rRNA interact with specific ribosomal proteins? Do the proteins induce conformational changes in the RNA during assembly? What is the mechanism of cooperativity of assembly that is implicit in the assembly map? And, what can we infer concerning the biological role of the ribosomal proteins? Finally, an important motivation for localization of protein binding sites is that it enables us to begin to understand the three-dimensional folding of 16S rRNA in the 30S subunit, based on the positions of the 21 proteins obtained by neutron diffraction (Moore et al., this volume). In the following, we briefly summarize our progress toward an understanding of protein-RNA interactions during assembly of the 30S subunit.

Our general approach has been to construct protein-RNA complexes in vitro, and subject them to the various chemical and enzymatic probes listed in Table 1. The effect of each individual protein is taken to be the difference beween the modification patterns observed with and without a given protein. This footprinting approach has several advantages over some other methods. Most importantly, it is a very gentle method; on the average, each RNA molecule is modified only at a few residues, minimizing disruption of higher order structure in the RNP complexes. It can be used with a wide variety of chemical and enzymatic probes, yielding information about each base in the RNA chain; a significant feature is that one can also know positively whether a base is *un*reactive, which is often an important piece of negative information. The mechanisms and stereochemistry of the chemical probing reactions are well understood, and the atoms that are attacked by probes are known precisely. One may distinguish between reactivity at N1 versus N7 in the same base, for example (Moazed et al. 1986b). Finally, only microgram amounts of nonradioactive RNA are required, and even large RNA chains can be probed at every base

in a matter of days. The first application of this approach was to localize the interactions between the primary binding protein S4 and 16S rRNA (Stern et al. 1986). All of the strong protections caused by S4 are found to be clustered around the junction of five helices near position 500 in the upper part of the 5' domain, as indicated in Figure 3. The nucleotides protected by S4 are contained within a much more compact region of the secondary structure than one might have anticipated on the basis of nuclease protection studies, in which the S4-associated RNA was found to comprise most of the 5' domain (for a review, see Zimmermann 1980).

The effects of the other primary binding proteins S7, S8, S15, S17, and S20 have been localized by a similar approach (T. Powers et al.; S. Stern et al.; P. Svensson et al.; all in prep.); their locations are also indicated in Figure 3. Most of these locations are in good agreement with the results of earlier studies. The effects of protein S7 are localized to the 3' major domain and surround the sites where this protein has been cross-linked to 16S rRNA by Brimacombe and co-workers, at positions 1240 and 1377–1378 (Wower and Brimacombe 1983). Protein S15 protects nucleotides in the central domain in and around the stem at position 740, in agreement with previous studies (Müller et al. 1979; Gregory et al. 1984).

Some surprises were found, also. Besides protecting nucleotides in the stem at position 600, its "classical" binding site (Zimmermann et al. 1980), S8 shows extensive effects elsewhere in the central domain, with numerous protections in the 570–590, 810–830, and 850–870 regions. These results suggest that S8 makes widespread contacts and/or has a major effect on the conformation of the central domain, in keeping with its important role in assembly (Mizushima and Nomura 1970; Held et al. 1974). Protein S17 has been localized previously only to the 5' domain. Our studies show that it strongly protects nucleotides in the stem region within positions 245–280, a region previously thought to bind S20. We also observe protection of nucleotides in this same region by S20, but weaker than that found for S17. Furthermore, S20 affects many positions outside of the 245–280 stem, including G108, nucleotides in the 180–200 region, the loop around position 330, and nucleotides in the penultimate stem between positions 1430 and 1470. These results suggest that protection of the 245–280 stem by S20 may be nonspecific, and that this region interacts instead primarily with S17. Finally, we failed to detect any effects from protein S13 in the absence of other proteins, in support of the conclusions reached by other groups who have questioned whether S13 in fact behaves as a primary binding protein (for a review, see Zimmermann 1980).

To assess the effects of the secondary binding proteins (S6, S9, S16, S18, and S19), we constructed RNP complexes from 16S rRNA and mixtures of ribosomal proteins, based on the assembly map of Held et al. (1974). Thus, proteins S4, S8, and S20 are required to bind S16; accordingly, the effects of assembly of S16,

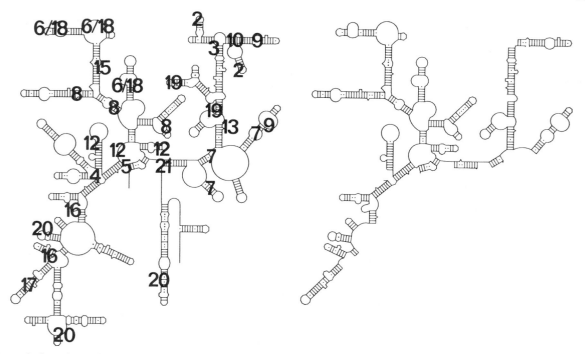

Figure 3. Locations of regions of 16S rRNA that are protected from chemical and enzymatic probes by assembly of specific ribosomal proteins (Stern et al. 1986 and in prep.; T. Powers et al.; P. Svensson et al.; both in prep.; L.-M. Changchien and H.F. Noller, unpubl.). The number of each protein is centered on regions where significant protein-dependent protections are observed. The diagram at the *right* indicates the actual regions of 16S rRNA presented in our 3-dimensional model (Fig. 4, A–C).

for example, were determined by comparison of the results of probing RNP complexes made with S4 + S8 + S20 + S16 versus S4 + S8 + S20. The RNP complexes used in these experiments are listed in Table 2. In every case, new effects are observed that are specifically dependent on the presence of the secondary binding proteins. In every case, the nucleotides affected by assembly of the secondary binding proteins are in the same domain as those affected by the corresponding primary binding proteins. At least some of the

Table 2. Mixtures of 30S Ribosomal Proteins Used in Assembly Experiments

Target protein	Mixture of other proteins used to probe assembly of target protein
S2	ΣI, ΣII, S3, S10, S13, S14
S3	ΣI, ΣII, S10, S13, S14
S4	none
S5	ΣI, S2, S3, S6, S9, S10, S11, S12, S13, S14, S18, S19, S21
S6	S15, S18
S7	none
S8	none
S9	S7
S10	ΣI, ΣII, S13, S14
S11	ΣI, S5, S6, S12, S18
S12	ΣI
S13	ΣI, ΣII
S14	ΣI, ΣII, S13
S15	none
S16	S4, S8, S20
S17	none
S18	S6, S15
S19	S7
S20	none; S4, S8
S21	ΣI, S5, S6, S11, S12, S18

Complexes were formed using the above mixtures, with or without the target protein, and 16S rRNA. Effects of the target protein were deduced by the results of probing the complexes containing or lacking the target protein. ΣI contains S4, S8, S7, S15, S16, S17, and S20. ΣII contains S5, S6, S9, S11, S12, S18, S19, and S21. Protein S20 was probed on its own, or in combination with S4 and S8.

effects of each secondary binding protein are in locations directly adjacent to regions affected by the corresponding primary binding protein. Thus, nucleotides affected by S16 are near those affected by S4 and S20, nucleotides affected by S6 and S18 are near those affected by S15, and some of the effects dependent on S9 and S19 are adjacent to those produced by protein S7 (see Fig. 3).

An important point that can be raised here is whether our probing results bear on the observed cooperativity of assembly of the ribosomal components. In several cases, primary binding proteins induce enhanced reactivity of certain nucleotides. Many of these enhanced nucleotides then become protected upon assembly of the corresponding secondary binding protein. This suggests a possible mechanism for a sequential assembly pathway, in which the primary binding protein induces a local conformational change in 16S rRNA; the altered RNA conformation is then recognized by the secondary binding protein. This represents an extreme kind of model; the corresponding opposite extreme would be that direct protein-protein contact between the primary and secondary binding proteins accounts for the cooperativity. Our findings suggest that both kinds of mechanisms play a role in assembly. Some proteins, such as S7 and S9, may use a combination of these two mechanisms. Yet another possibility is that protein-protein interaction could induce conformational changes in a protein, activating its RNA-binding capabilities.

An example which supports the first kind of mechanism is the dependence of S19 on S7 (T. Powers et al., in prep.). Nucleotides in the 975–980 region are enhanced by S7, but become strongly protected upon addition of S19 (Fig. 1; the region of interest is indicated by brackets). A particularly striking example suggesting RNA-mediating cooperativity is the S4→S16→S12 assembly pathway (Held et al. 1974). The primary binding protein S4 induces enhanced reactivity of nucleotides 361–364 (Stern et al. 1986). Addition of the secondary binding protein S16 (which is bound in the presence of S4, S8, and S20) protects these same nucleotides (S. Stern et al., in prep.). In turn, we observe S16-dependent enhancement of nucleotides 21, 524, 887, and 894, whose subsequent protection depends on the tertiary binding protein S12 (S. Stern et al., in prep.; S. Stern, unpubl.). These findings are highly suggestive of the involvement of protein-induced RNA conformational rearrangements in the cooperativity of protein assembly.

We have tested each of the 30S subunit proteins, except S1, for possible effects on 16S rRNA during assembly; all 20 proteins reproducibly affect the reactivity of specific nucleotides to our probes. Our current view of the approximate regions of 16S rRNA affected by each protein is summarized in Figure 3; a detailed description of these results will be presented elsewhere. We do not know yet whether any or all of the secondary and tertiary binding proteins actually make contact with 16S rRNA. For the present, it can be said that they all interact, either directly or indirectly, with the RNA.

Molecular Modeling Studies on the Folding of 16S rRNA in the 30S Ribosomal Subunit

We anticipated that the foregoing studies on protein-RNA interaction might provide information that would help to understand the three-dimensional folding of 16S rRNA. By far the most accurate and complete data on the three-dimensional solution structure of the ribosome is the set of coordinates for the placement of the centers of mass of the twenty-one 30S subunit proteins, as determined by Moore and his colleagues (see Moore et al., this volume). If we make the plausible, but largely untested, assumption that the main footprints associated with assembly of specific proteins represent regions of the 16S rRNA that are in contact with, or proximal to, the corresponding proteins, then the probing data provide a wealth of detailed constraints on the folding of the RNA. This important assumption has been put to test in several specific cases. For example, many of the protein contacts inferred in this way are consistent with protein-RNA cross-linking data (Brimacombe et al. 1986), or are contained within RNA fragments that are capable of specific binding to their cognate proteins (Zimmermann 1980). Our assumption is unlikely to be correct in every case, and so wherever possible should be supported by independent evidence. Two previous folding schemes for 16S rRNA have been proposed (Expert-Besançon and Wollenzien 1985; Nagano and Harel 1987); our model differs significantly from each of them. Several of the features of a partial model for 16S rRNA (Noller and Lake 1984) are supported by our present studies.

Our strategy in this model-building exercise is based on the following constraints: (1) the secondary structure of 16S rRNA (Fig. 2), whose accuracy has been extensively documented by comparative sequence analysis (Woese et al. 1983; Gutell et al. 1985) and tested experimentally (for a review, see Noller 1984; Moazed et al. 1986a); (2) placement of the 30S subunit proteins by neutron diffraction (Moore et al., this volume); (3) our protein footprinting results (Fig. 3), which (based on the foregoing assumption) place strongly protected regions of the RNA in contact with the corresponding protein; (4) certain RNA-RNA cross-links reported by Stiege and coworkers (Stiege et al. 1986); and (5) stereochemical rules based on crystal structures of tRNA and other RNA derivatives (Saenger 1984). Other information was used to test the self-consistency of the model that was developed using the above constraints. Modeling was carried out using the interactive molecular modeling program FRODO, as described in Methods.

Our initial questions were: Is it possible to satisfy all of the above constraints simultaneously? If so, are there a large or small (or even unique) number of possible models which do so? It was difficult to anticipate the importance of potential constraints imposed by the dimensions and geometry of the RNA helices themselves, which are comparatively large, rigid structures, and constraints imposed by the connectivity relationships between helices in conjunction with the known limits of internucleotide distances. Both of these factors significantly constrain the possible choices available at each stage of the modeling procedure.

A preliminary version of our model is shown in Figure 4A. The ribosomal proteins are displayed as dotted spheres whose volumes are calculated from their anhydrous molecular weights, with their centers of mass positioned as determined by neutron diffraction studies (Moore et al., this volume). The RNA chain is represented by lines connecting the positions of helical phosphate residues; nonhelical regions, including loops, are thus shown only as straight lines connecting helical phosphates. We display only that portion of the RNA chain that we consider to be relatively well constrained by the presently available data. Figure 3 shows the corresponding regions of the secondary structure that appear in the model. In the following, we summarize some of the main conclusions of this study.

(1) The pseudoknot helix. The length of the extended chain between the centers of the regions protected by S4 and S7 is close to the measured distance between S4 and S7, as pointed out previously (Noller and Lake 1984). We have arranged three of the connected helices, 27–37/547–566, 9–13/21–25, and 17–19/916–918, as a continuous, coaxially stacked pseudoknot structure (Fig. 4B). This structure seems to form a central core around which the 30S subunit is built; all three major domains emerge from it. We place the 37/547 end of this structure in the sphere of protein S4, and its 17/918 end oriented so that the connection can eventually be made to S7. The rotation of the pseudoknot helix about its own helical axis, as well as the solid angle by which it pivots with respect to S4 are fixed mainly by three constraints. Protection of A26 by S5 and G558 by S12 are consistent with the location of these two proteins on opposite sides of the pseudoknot helix, facing their respective protected nucleotides. This axial orientation places A918 at the uppermost position of the end of the pseudoknot, which directs the chain naturally up toward S7. Placement of the 510 and 530 regions on S12, following our footprinting results, is made possible by orienting the 500–517/534–545 helix orthogonally to the pseudoknot helix, making a sharp turn around position 546. This placement is achieved optimally with the pseudoknot oriented as shown in Figure 4B.

(2) The 5′ domain. The rest of the 5′ domain emerges from the S4-proximal end of the pseudoknot. We assume that the 39–47/394–403 and 368–379/384–383 helices stack coaxially. The lower part of the 5′ domain thus exits from their junction, and the cluster of S16-dependent protections in this region controls the placement of this coaxial helix, following our rules. Trial and error show that this can be realized in two different ways; one scheme pivots the coaxial 380 stem around position 38 to place it above the pseudoknot helix, and the other scheme places it below. Here, we display the latter version and the arrangement of features in the 290–360 region that follows from this choice. This arrangement is strongly supported by in

vivo UV-induced cross-links between positions 31 and 48, and between positions 366–369 and 398–400 (Stiege et al. 1986). Orientation of the 240–259/267–286 stem is fixed by S17 at the bottom and S16 and S20 at the top. The remainder of the 5′ domain is insufficiently constrained by our criteria to suggest how it might be structured.

(3) The central domain. This domain exits from the middle of the pseudoknot helix at position 556, which is oriented toward protein S12, as described. The location of S8-protected nucleotides in the central domain (Fig. 3) places the 570 region near protein S8, which is on the S5-proximal side of the pseudoknot helix. Thus, nucleotides 557–567, which connect the central domain to the pseudoknot helix, must cross from the S12 side to the S5 side. The choice of whether this strand crosses over or under the pseudoknot helix was determined initially by modeling trials; the best solution was to cross under, as shown in Figure 4B. This was subsequently supported by protection of nucleotides in the 557–567 linker by S12, which can only be satisfied by crossing under. The orientation of the structures in the 576–765 region is dictated by the positions of proteins S8, S15, S16, and S18. The result involves a sharp turn centered on the internal loop at positions 580/760, so that the 588–606/632–651 stem folds back to make contact with S8; this also places the 630 loop toward the bottom of the subunit, proximal to S17, to which it has been cross-linked (Brimacombe et al. 1986). The two stems formed by residues 655–751 then reach from S15 (near position 745) across to S6 (near position 720) and S18 (near position 690). The cross-link between the 690 and 790 regions (Atmadja et al. 1986) then establishes the orientation of the 790 stem toward protein S18. Footprinting results position the 860 region near S8. Orientation of the 840 stem is not well defined; enzymatic footprinting dependent on S6 + S18 near the end of the stem suggests that it points toward these two proteins. The phylogenetic variability of the 840 stem argues for placement below the conserved 690 and 790 regions, where stems of greater length would avoid interfering with the phylogenetically constant part of the structure. Finally, the 900 region emerges from the closure of the three-base-pair 567–569/881–883 helix and connects to position 916 at the S7-proximal end of the pseudoknot. Its placement is determined solely by its S12-dependent protections.

(4) The 3′ major domain. The 923–933/1384–1393 helix connects the pseudoknot to the region protected by protein S7, in the 3′ major domain. The remainder of the helical backbone of the domain follows a closed spiral path dictated by the footprinting results. Following the secondary structure diagram (Fig. 2), progressing upwards from position 940 (centered on S7), the 946–955/1225–1235 helix spans the gap between S7 and S19. After making a 90° turn, the compound helix comprising residues 1046–1067/1189–1211 joins S19 to S3 and S10. The final segment of the domain backbone, ending in the loop near position 1140, is folded back to form an acute angle with the preceding section,

bringing S9 into contact with the 1124/1145 internal loop, where it protects several bases. The other S9-protected region, around position 1280, constrains the 1240–1290 compound structure; it reaches directly from S7 toward S9, lying above the 1120–1150 region stem, which approaches S9 from the opposite direction. This arrangement is constrained by the observation that both the 1280 and the 1125/1145 regions are protected by S9.

This model is admittedly a preliminary one and, at best, can approach an overall precision on the order of ±10–15 Å. The main reasons for this limitation are the uncertainty of the placements of the proteins, our ignorance of the detailed structures of the individual proteins and how they interact with the RNA, and the absence of useful constraints in some regions of the structure. Of considerable importance is the extent to which the key assumption (that footprint sites indicate regions of contact with the corresponding proteins) will turn out to be correct. In this respect, our model represents a series of specific predictions, which we expect will be tested extensively in future experiments.

Based on our chosen criteria, the paths of most of the main features of the 16S rRNA chain are well constrained, within the limits of the attainable precision. Protected regions of the RNA are placed in proximity to the positions of their respective proteins, while obeying known stereochemical rules in folding the RNA chain. An important finding is that nearly all of the imposed criteria can be satisfied, and that, in our experience, it is difficult to see how this could be accomplished by a folding scheme which differs fundamentally from this one. We view our model as a useful framework for discussions of ribosome structure and function (see below) and hope that it will be of use in the design of critical experiments in this area.

Localization of Functional Sites in 16S rRNA

If the ribosome (or, at least, the primitive ribosome) is viewed as an RNA enzyme, or "ribozyme," then it is reasonable to think of tRNA as its "substrate." There is an appreciable body of experimental evidence to support the possibility that tRNA makes direct contacts with rRNA when it is bound to the ribosome (Noller and Chaires 1972; Prince et al. 1982; Brow et al. 1983; Barta et al. 1984; Moazed and Noller 1986). Here, we summarize recent studies aimed toward identification

of nucleotides in 16S rRNA that interact with, or are otherwise perturbed by, binding of tRNA to ribosomes. A second series of experiments identifies bases that are involved in the interaction of several antibiotics with 30S subunits. Together, the results of these two studies provide a basis for assignment of specific sites in 16S rRNA to three distinct functional classes and for predicting their possible relationships to the translational process.

In earlier experiments, we showed that chemical modification of a few nucleotides in 30S subunits causes loss of their ability to bind tRNA (Noller and Chaires 1972). If tRNA is bound prior to modification, it protects ribosomes against inactivation. We therefore reasoned that sites protected by tRNA from chemical attack should include nucleotides that are somehow important for tRNA binding. Our approach was to bind tRNA^{Phe} to ribosomes in vitro in the presence of poly (U), and to probe the resulting complexes in comparison with vacant ribosomes. Identification of tRNA-protected sites was carried out using the same primer extension approach described above. tRNA shields a set of highly conserved nucleotides from our probes (Moazed and Noller 1986; summarized in Fig. 5). The protected bases can be classified according to whether their protection is strictly mRNA-dependent (class I); mRNA-independent at high Mg^{++} concentrations (class II); or protected also by 50S subunits (class III). Several of these sites were also identified in earlier experiments as protected in tRNA-occupied polysomes, but not in vacant ribosomes (Brow and Noller 1983). A striking result is that all of the sites are similarly protected by a 15-nucleotide tRNA fragment consisting of only the anticodon stem and loop. On the basis of their observed protection behavior, we suggested that class I nucleotides are protected by A-site-bound tRNA, and class II nucleotides by P-site-bound tRNA. We suggested that class III protections could be the result of tRNA-induced and/or 50S subunit-induced conformational changes, since if they were caused by direct interaction, one would expect tRNA and 50S subunits to compete for binding to 30S subunits, which they do not.

Many of the tRNA-protected nucleotides occur in universally conserved sequences that were predicted to be important functional regions (Noller and Woese 1981; Woese et al. 1983). The conserved sequence around C1400 has been placed in the decoding region,

Figure 4. (A) Stereo computer graphics display of a preliminary 3-dimensional folding scheme for 16S rRNA, as described in the text. Ribosomal proteins are positioned according to Moore et al. (this volume) and are shown as dotted spheres with volumes based on their anhydrous molecular weights. The RNA is displayed as a series of vectors connecting the positions of phosphorus atoms in helical parts of the structure (see Fig. 2). Only the regions shown in the right side of Fig. 3 are displayed (~60% of the 16S rRNA chain). Single-stranded regions are shown as straight lines connecting helical elements. The three major domains are shown in *red* (5' domain), *yellow* (central domain), and *blue* (3' major domain). The view is from the 50S-distal (cytoplasmic) side of the 30S subunit. The platform (*left*) is formed by the central domain, the head (*top*) by the 3' major domain, and the remainder by the 5' domain. (B) A view of the pseudoknot helix from the S4 end of the 30S subunit. Rudimentary parts of the domains are colored as in A, except for the pseudoknot helix, which is shown in *orange*. (See text for discussion.) (C) A view of the 16S rRNA model from the 50S-proximal side, showing the clustering of class II sites around positions 690, 790, 926, and 960. The class I sites around position 530, in contrast, are remote (65–85 Å) from the class II sites, and are constrained by the positions of proteins S4 and S12 (see Fig. 3).

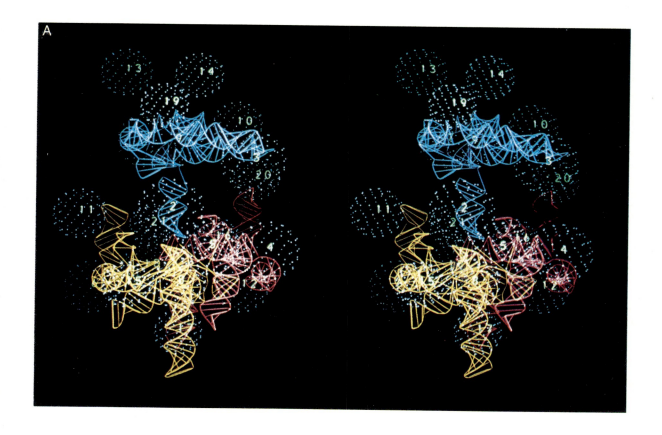

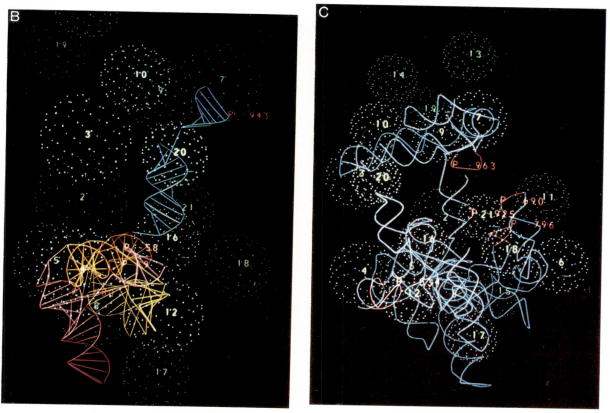

Figure 4. (*See facing page for legend.*)

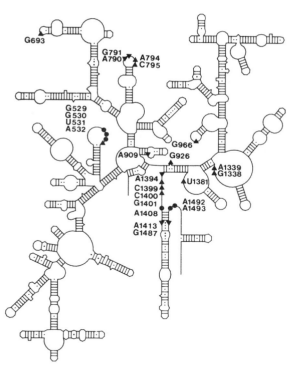

Figure 5. Sites protected from chemical probes by tRNA (Moazed and Noller 1986). (●) Class I sites; (▲) class II sites; (▼) class III sites.

from studies in which C1400 was cross-linked directly to the wobble base of tRNA by UV-induced photochemical attack (Prince et al. 1982), and so it should not be surprising to note tRNA-dependent protection of positions 1399–1401 (Fig. 5). Interestingly, strongly protected sites are distributed widely in the secondary structure, among all three major domains. This observation suggests that extensive three-dimensional folding must occur in order to bring these sites within

proximity of one another in the 30S subunit (see below). At least one result, however, seems difficult to explain in this way. Three of the class I nucleotides occur in the 530 loop of the 5′ domain, at positions 529, 530, and 531, whereas the other three are at the base of the penultimate stem near the decoding region, at positions 1408, 1492, and 1493. These two regions of the RNA have been localized in the 30S subunit by several approaches; there is general agreement that they are 65–85 Å apart, whereas the maximum dimension of the anticodon stem-loop fragment that protects these bases has a maximum dimension on the order of 25 Å. Thus, the effects seen in the 530 loop may be the result of an induced conformational change, rather than direct protection. Given the uncertainties involved in estimating the relevant distances, we cannot be sure of this at present. In any case, tRNA-dependent changes in reactivity in the 530 loop are likely to be indicative of some crucial translational event, because of universal conservation of sequence in the loop region. In the 18-nucleotide segment between positions 515 and 533, only two nucleotides show any variation among the dozens of sequenced eubacterial, archaebacterial, and eukaryotic 16S-like rRNAs (Woese et al. 1983; Gutell et al. 1985).

Many antibiotics interfere with protein synthesis by blocking specific steps of the translational cycle (reviewed by Cundliffe 1980). We have probed the interaction of several well-known antibiotics with ribosomes, in an effort to correlate their known modes of action with specific structural features of 16S rRNA (Moazed and Noller 1987). Interestingly, each antibiotic that we have tested produces a corresponding footprint in the RNA modification pattern; our findings are summarized in Table 3.

Of particular interest, in the context of our discussion of tRNA-protected sites, are the effects of antibiotics that are known to perturb events at the A and P sites.

Table 3. Protection of Specific Bases in *E. coli* 16S rRNA by Antibiotics

| Antiobiotic | Binding to 70S ribosome | | Binding to 30S subunits | |
	strong	weak	strong	weak
Streptomycin	A913, A914, A915	U911, C912	A912, A914, A915	U911, C912, A909, A1413, G1487, G1494
Tetracycline	A892	U1052↑, C1054↑	A892	U1052,↑, C1054↑
Spectinomycin	C1063, G1064	G973↑	C1063, G1064	G973↑
Hygromycin	G1494	A1408↑	—	G1494, A1408↑
Neomycin Paromomycin Gentamycin Kanamycin	A1408, G1494	C525↑	A1408, G1494	C525↑ A790, G791, A909, A1394, A1413, G1497
Edeine	G693, G926 A794, C795	—	G693, G926 A794, C785	A790, G791, A1394

Data from chemical footprinting experiments with 70S ribosomes and 30S subunits for the different antibiotics, according to whether they show strong or weak protection (from Moazed and Noller 1987). The chemical reaction specificities of U911, U1052, and C1063 are unusual, and not presently understood. Neomycin also shows weak enhancement of A65 and weak protection at N7 of G833, G836, G849, and G851 in 30S subunits. Gentamycin and kanamycin also give weak protection at N7 of G832, G833, G836, and G849 in both 30S subunits and 70S ribosomes. In addition, kanamycin weakly protects G851 and G852, and weakly enhances G973.

Edeine, which interferes with P-site tRNA binding, protects G693, A794, C795, and G926. All four of these nucleotides are class II sites (Table 4), supporting our assignment of this class to P-site tRNA protection. Hygromycin and the neomycin-related group of aminoglycosides (neomycin, kanamycin, gentamycin, and paromomycin) protect G1494; A1408 is enhanced by hygromycin, but protected by the neomycins, which also cause enhancement of C525. These drugs are all known to induce miscoding, which is presumably due to perturbation of A-site binding of tRNA. Their effects are all in or proximal to class I nucleotides (Table 4), supporting assignment of this class of sites to A-site binding. The effects of streptomycin and tetracycline are more mysterious. Streptomycin is believed to induce miscoding by interfering with proofreading in the A site, whereas tetracycline appears to interfere with aminoacyl-tRNA binding (reviewed by Cundliffe 1980). Both drugs might therefore be expected to affect class I sites. Instead, protection by streptomycin is focused at position 915, and that by tetracycline at A892, in the vicinity of the class III site at A909. In addition, position 915 shows weak mRNA-dependent protection by tRNA that might be construed as class I behavior (see, for example, Fig. 2c of Moazed and Noller 1986). We conclude that there is an important, but poorly understood, relationship between the 890–915 and 1400/1500 regions. This is further illustrated by the fact that tetracycline and streptomycin inhibit the action of colicin E3, which makes a phosphodiester bond scission at position 1493 (Nomura et al. 1974).

Our findings closely corroborate the results of genetic studies, in which point mutations conferring drug resistance have been localized in 16S rRNA (reviewed in Moazed and Noller 1987). In each case where such a mutation has been characterized, protection by the corresponding drug is found at or close to the site of mutation. This is well illustrated by spectinomycin, which is believed to affect the translocation step. A C→U change at position 1192 of 16S rRNA confers spectinomycin resistance (Sigmund et al. 1984). Our probing studies show that C1063 and G1064, which are on the opposite helical strand (G1064 forms a base pair with C1192; see Fig. 2), are protected by spectinomycin, at once suggesting a relationship between the target site of this drug and the site of mutation, and confirming the phylogenetically derived secondary structure involving this region of the RNA.

Streptomycin, edeine, and the neomycin group antibiotics affect the class III sites, when probed in complex with 30S subunits. Three of the class III sites are protected by streptomycin, the other three by edeine, and all six by the neomycin group (Table 4). This seems to imply the existence of two subclasses of class III sites, both of which are protected by 50S subunits or tRNA (Moazed and Noller 1986). The lack of competition between streptomycin and the neomycin group antibiotics lends additional support to our assignment of class III protections to conformational changes induced by ligand binding. It is intriguing that similar effects are produced either by tRNA, 50S subunits, or certain antibiotics, suggesting that the behavior of the class III sites may provide important clues to the functional interrelationships between these three kinds of ligands. The properties of the class I, II, and III sites are summarized in Table 4.

Structure and Function

What implications can be drawn from our preliminary structural model for the assembly and mechanism of action of ribosomes? First, can one rationalize the roles of the ribosomal proteins in 30S subunit assembly? We note some general, but not absolute,

Table 4. Sites of Protection of 16S rRNA from Chemical Probes by tRNA

	Positions	Strict mRNA dependence	Antibiotic protection		Functional correlate
Class I sites	G529, G530, U531 A1408, A1492, A1493	yes	neomycin paromomycin kanamycin gentamycin	A1408 G1494	A-site binding
			hygromycin (enhances A1408)	G1494	
Class II sites	(A532), G693, A794 C795, G926, $_m^2$G966, C1338 A1339, U1381, C1399, C1400, G1401(N7)	no	edeine	G693, A794, C795, G926	P-site binding
Class III sites	A790, G791, A909, A1394, A1413, G1487	protected by tRNA or 50S subunits	streptomycin	A909, A1413, G1487	conformational changes involving specific translational events
			edeine	A790, G791 A1394	
			neomycin group	A790, G791, A909, A1394, A1413, G1487	

Reprinted, with permission, from Moazed and Noller (1986).

relationships between the assembly map and our inferred structure. Primary binding proteins often (S4, S7, S8, and S20), but not always (S15 and S17), seem to be positioned at the junctions of multiple helical elements, as if to control or adjust their relative directions. The secondary binding proteins often seem to be positioned so as to influence major bends in the 16S rRNA structure. At least two of the tertiary binding proteins, S12 and S21, both of which have been strongly implicated in ribosome function, appear to affect functional sites in the RNA. In both cases, they appear to convert the local conformation from a non-native one into a structure that more closely resembles the active one. S12 influences the 530 loop, the site of the aforementioned class I protections, and the 890–915 region, which contains a class III site (A909) and the sites of protection by tetracycline and streptomycin. Protein S21 affects the 923–933/1384–1393 stem and the adjacent 1394–1400 region. Among other effects, S21 appears to be involved in the assembly-dependent enhancement of G926 (Moazed et al. 1986a), an important class II site. These observations suggest that some late-assembling ribosomal proteins may have what might be termed a regulatory role, converting the virtually assembled ribosome into a biologically active structure at the final stage of assembly.

Second, to what extent can one begin to draw connections between the functional sites described above and the structural model? The clearest example is the set of class II sites that are protected by edeine (G693, A794, C795, and G926). Although they appear to be widely distributed in the secondary structure (Fig. 2), they are clustered near one another in the three-dimensional model (Fig. 4C). Their location clearly corresponds to the cleft seen in electron micrographs of the 30S subunit, based on the locations of features identified by IEM studies. G926 would be located on the side of the head facing the cleft, whereas G693, A794, and C795 would all be located on the platform. In addition, the $^2_mG966$ would reach down from the head into the same general region. It is not difficult to imagine that the anticodon stem-loop could make simultaneous contact with all four of these bases. This location is in remarkable agreement with the placement of P-site-bound tRNA by electron microscopy (Gornicki et al. 1984).

Based on the constraints used in our modeling studies, it is difficult to see how the two sets of class I sites (around positions 530 and 1408/1492, respectively) could be proximal to each other. It should be noted, however, that the base of the penultimate stem (around position 1408) is not well constrained; it is conceivable that it could reach the 530 region by maximally extending the single-stranded 1400 region sequence (although probing data indicate that the latter region is highly structured in some way). Even if this were feasible, it would then place the anticodon stem-loop regions of A- and P-site tRNAs far from each other (~65–85 Å, in our model); their interaction with adjacent codons makes this impossible.

The class III sites are located in and around the cleft region, with the apparent exception of the interesting site at A909. It is premature to speculate on the nature of this intriguing class of nucleotides. Clearly, they are deserving of further study.

From the studies described above, and from the results of many other laboratories, it is apparent that we are currently in a stage of rapid expansion of our knowledge of the structure and function of ribosome. The view that rRNA is the fundamental functional component of the ribosome seems to have gained wide experimental support, and presently serves as a central paradigm in studies of the molecular biology of ribosomes. A true understanding of the mechanism of translation continues to elude us; application of novel approaches, combined with a deeper understanding of the capabilities of RNA, will be essential in realizing this goal.

ACKNOWLEDGMENTS

We thank Professor Peter B. Moore for providing unpublished coordinates for the positions of ribosomal proteins, and for helpful discussions; Professor R.R. Traut and Dr. B. Nag for supplying purified ribosomal proteins for preliminary studies; Professor Olke Uhlenbeck for providing the yeast tRNA^{Phe} anticodon stem-loop fragment; Dr. Gisela Kramer for a gift of edeine; Professor Elizabeth Blackburn for paromomycin, and Dr. J. Sack and Dr. F. Quiocho for providing FRODO. This work was supported by grant GM-17129 from the National Institutes of Health. Computer modeling was carried out in the University of California at Santa Cruz Molecular Graphics Laboratory, supported in part by grant DMB-8521802 from the National Science Foundation Biological Instrumentation Program. We thank Bryn Weiser and Tim Bullock for writing computer programs used in these studies. P.S. was supported by a fellowship from the Royal Swedish Academy of Sciences.

REFERENCES

Atmadja, J., W. Stiege, M. Zobawa, B. Greuer, M. Osswald, and R. Brimacombe. 1986. The tertiary folding of *Escherichia coli* 16S RNA , as studied by *in situ* intra-RNA cross-linking of 30S ribosomal subunits with bis-(2-chloroethyl)-methylamine. *Nucleic Acids Res.* **14:** 659.

Barta, A., G. Steiner, J. Brosius, H.F. Noller, and E. Kuechler. 1984. Identification of a site on 23S ribosomal RNA located at the peptidyl transferase center. *Proc. Natl. Acad. Sci.* **81:** 3607.

Brimacombe, R., J. Atmadja, A. Kyriatsoulis, and W. Stiege. 1986. RNA structure and RNA-protein neighborhoods in the ribosome. In *Structure, function, and genetics of ribosomes* (ed. B. Hardesty and G. Kramer), p. 184. Springer Verlag, New York.

Brow, D.A. and H.F. Noller. 1983. Protection of ribosomal RNA from kethoxal in polyribosomes. Implication of specific sites in ribosome function. *J. Mol. Biol.* **163:** 27.

Cech, T.R. and B.L. Bass. 1986. Biological catalysis by RNA. *Annu. Rev. Biochem.* **55:** 599.

Crick, F.H.C. 1968. On the origins of translation. *J. Mol. Biol.* **38:** 367.

Cundliffe, E. 1980. Antibiotics and prokaryote ribosomes: Action, interaction and resistance. In *Ribosomes* (ed. G. Chambliss et al.), p. 555. University Park Press, Baltimore.

Dabbs, E. 1986. Mutant studies on the prokaryotic ribosome. In *Structure, function, and genetics of ribosomes* (ed. B. Hardesty and G. Kramer), p. 733. Springer Verlag, New York.

Expert-Besançon, A. and P. Wollenzien. 1985. Three-dimensional arrangement of the *Escherichia coli* 16S ribosomal RNA. *J. Mol. Biol.* **184:** 53.

Gornicki, P., K. Nurse, W. Hellmann, M. Boublik, and J. Ofengand. 1984. High resolution localization of the tRNA anticodon interaction site on the *Escherichia coli* 30S ribosomal subunit. *J. Biol. Chem.* **259:** 10493.

Gregory, R.J., M.L.O. Zeller, D.L. Thurlow, R.L. Gourse, M.J.R. Stark, A.E. Dahlberg, and R.A. Zimmermann. 1984. Interaction of ribosomal proteins S6, S8, S15 and S18 with the central domain of 16S ribosomal RNA from *Escherichia coli*. *J. Mol. Biol.* **178:** 287.

Gutell, R.R., B. Weiser, C.R. Woese, and H.F. Noller. 1985. Comparative anatomy of 16S-like ribosomal RNA. *Prog. Nucleic Acids Res. Mol. Biol.* **32:** 155.

Hardesty, B. and G. Kramer, eds. 1986. *Structure, function, and genetics of ribosomes*. Springer Verlag, New York.

Held, W., B. Ballou, S. Mizushima, and M. Nomura. 1974. Assembly mapping of 30S ribosomal proteins from *Escherichia coli*: Further studies. *J. Biol. Chem.* **249:** 3103.

Jones, T.A. 1982. A graphics fitting program for macromolecules. In *Computational crystallography* (ed. D. Sayre), p. 303. Clarendon Press, Oxford.

Makowski, I., F. Frolow, M.A. Saper, M. Shoham, H.G. Wittmann, and A. Yonath. 1987. Single crystals of large ribosomal particles from *Halobacterium marismortui* diffract to 6 Å. *J. Mol. Biol.* **193:** 819.

Mizushima, S. and M. Nomura. 1970. Assembly mapping of 30S ribosomal proteins from *E. coli*. *Nature* **226:** 1214.

Moazed, D. and H.F. Noller. 1986. Transfer RNA shields specific nucleotides in 16S ribosomal RNA from attack by chemical probes. *Cell* **47:** 985.

———. 1987. Interaction of antibiotics with functional sites in 16S ribosomal RNA. *Nature* **327:** 389.

Moazed, D., S. Stern, and H.F. Noller. 1986a. Rapid chemical probing of conformation in 16S ribosomal RNA and 30S ribosomal subunits using primer extension. *J. Mol. Biol.* **187:** 399.

Moazed, D., B. Van Stolk, S. Douthwaite, and H.F. Noller. 1986b. Interconversion of active and inactive 30S ribosomal subunits is accompanied by a conformational change in the decoding region of 16S rRNA. *J. Mol. Biol.* **191:** 483.

Müller, R., R.A. Garrett, and H.F. Noller. 1979. The structure of the RNA binding site of ribosomal proteins S8 and S15. *J. Biol. Chem.* **254:** 3873.

Nagano, K. and M. Harel. 1987. Approaches to a three-dimensional model of *E. coli* ribosome. *Prog. Biophys. Mol. Biol.* **48:** 67.

Noller, H.F. 1984. Structure of ribosomal RNA. *Annu. Rev. Biochem.* **53:** 119.

Noller, H.F. and J.B. Chaires. 1972. Functional modification of 16S ribosomal RNA by kethoxal. *Proc. Natl. Acad. Sci.* **69:** 3115.

Noller, H.F. and J.A. Lake. 1984. Ribosome structure and function: Localization of rRNA. In *Membrane structure and function* (ed. E.E. Bittar), vol.6, p. 217. John Wiley, New York.

Noller, H.F. and C.R. Woese. 1981. Secondary structure of 16S ribosomal RNA. *Science* **212:** 403.

Noller H.F., M. Asire, A. Barta, S. Douthwaite, T. Goldstein, R.R. Gutell, D. Moazed, J. Normanly, J.B. Prince, S. Stern, K. Triman, S. Turner, B. Van Stolk, V. Wheaton, B. Weiser, and C.R. Woese. 1986. Studies on the structure

and function of ribosomal RNA. In *Structure, function, and genetics of ribosomes* (ed. B. Hardesty and G. Kramer), p. 143. Springer Verlag, New York.

Nomura, M., J. Sidikaro, K. Jakes, and N. Zinder. 1974. Effects of colicin E3 on bacterial ribosomes. In *Ribosomes* (ed. M. Nomura et al.), p. 805. Cold Spring Harbor Laboratory, Cold Spring Harbor, New York.

Oakes, M., E. Henderson, A. Scheinman, M. Clark, and J.A. Lake. 1986. Ribosome structure, function and evolution: Mapping ribosomal RNA, proteins and functional sites in three dimensions. In *Structure, function, and genetics of ribosomes* (ed. B. Hardesty and G. Kramer), p. 47. Springer Verlag, New York.

Politz, S.M. and D.G. Glitz. 1977. Ribosome structure: Localization of N6,N6-dimethyladenosine by electron microscopy of a ribosome-antibody complex. *Proc. Natl. Acad. Sci.* **74:** 1468.

Prince, J.B., B.H. Taylor, D.L. Thurlow, J. Ofengand, and R.A. Zimmermann. 1982. Covalent crosslinking of tRNA$_1^{Val}$ to 16S RNA at the ribosomal P site: Identification of crosslinked residues. *Proc. Natl. Acad. Sci.* **79:** 5450.

Saenger, W. 1984. *Principles of nucleic acid structure*. Springer-Verlag, New York.

Sigmund, C.D., M. Ettayebi, and E.A. Morgan. 1984. Antibiotic resistance mutations in 16S and 23S ribosomal RNA genes of *Escherichia coli*. *Nucleic Acids Res.* **12:** 4653.

Steitz, J.A. 1980. RNA-RNA interactions during polypeptide chain initiation. In *Ribosomes* (ed. G. Chambliss et al.), p. 479. University Park Press, Baltimore.

Stern, S., D. Moazed, and H.F. Noller. 1987. Analysis of RNA structure using chemical and enzymatic probing monitored by primer extension. *Methods Enzymol.* (in press).

Stern, S., R.C. Wilson, and H.F. Noller. 1986. Localization of the bonding site for protein S4 on 16S ribosomal RNA by chemical and enzymatic probing and primer extension. *J. Mol. Biol.* **192:** 101.

Stiege, W., J. Atmadja, M. Zobawa, and R. Brimacombe. 1986. Investigation of the tertiary folding of *Escherichia coli* ribosomal RNA by intra-RNA cross-linking in vivo. *J. Mol. Biol.* **191:** 135.

Stöffler, G. and M. Stöffler-Meilicke. 1986. Immuno electron microscopy on *Escherichia coli* ribosomes. In *Structure, function, and genetics of ribosomes* (ed. B. Hardesty and G. Kramer), p. 28. Springer Verlag, New York.

Traub, P. and M. Nomura. 1968. Structure and function of *E. coli* ribosomes. V. Reconstitution of functionally active 30S ribosomal particles from RNA and protein. *Proc. Natl. Acad. Sci.* **59:** 777.

Van Stolk, B.J. and H.F. Noller. 1987. Use of RNA-DNA hybridization to facilitate chemical probing of large RNA molecules. *Methods Enzymol.* (in press).

Woese, C.R. 1980. Just-so stories and Rube Goldberg machines: Speculations on the origin of the protein synthetic machinery. In *Ribosomes* (ed. G. Chambliss et al.), p. 357. University Park Press, Baltimore.

Woese, C.R., R.R. Gutell, R. Gupta, and H.F. Noller. 1983. Detailed analysis of higher-order structure of 16S-like ribosomal RNAs. *Microbiol. Rev.* **47:** 621.

Wower, I. and R. Brimacombe. 1983. The localization of multiple sites on 16S RNA which are cross-linked to proteins S7 and S8 in *Escherichia coli* 30S ribosomal subunits by treatment with 2-iminothiolane. *Nucleic Acids Res.* **11:** 1419.

Zimmermann, R.A. 1980. Interactions among protein and RNA components of the ribosome. In *Ribosomes* (ed. G. Chambliss et al.), p. 135. University Park Press, Baltimore.

Evolution of Eukaryotic rRNA: Constraints Imposed by RNA Interactions

S.A. Gerbi,* C. Jeppesen,* B. Stebbins-Boaz,* and M. Ares, Jr.[†‡]
*Division of Biology and Medicine, Brown University, Providence, Rhode Island 02912; †Department of Molecular Biophysics and Biochemistry, Yale University School of Medicine, New Haven, Connecticut 06510

In this chapter we will discuss the effects of alterations within the ribosomal DNA (rDNA) genes. RNA interactions that are important for regions within rRNA impose selective constraints upon propagation of mutations within the gene. As a consequence, there are functionally important regions in rRNA that are highly conserved in primary sequence, even between different kingdoms. rRNA also has an evolutionarily conserved core secondary structure. Finally, in this chapter we will examine U3 small nuclear RNA (snRNA), and discuss whether its structure can support models of its putative interaction with the rRNA precursor.

Structure of *Xenopus* rDNA Transcription Unit

The rDNA of *Xenopus laevis*, the South African clawed toad, was the first eukaryotic gene to be cloned (Morrow et al. 1974), and we have used this model system to study its evolution. Figure 1 depicts a typical repeat unit of *X. laevis* rDNA; there are about 450 tandem copies of this rDNA repeat in the nucleolus organizer region (Brown and Weber 1968a,b). The stretch coding for the 40S RNA precursor alternates with the so-called nontranscribed spacer (NTS). Recent evidence suggests that the NTS is, in fact, also transcribed as part of a larger precursor that must be

rapidly processed (DeWinter and Moss 1986; Labhart and Reeder 1986, 1987). Further processing events remove RNA from the external transcribed spacer (ETS) and internal transcribed spacers (ITS) to yield the mature molecules of 5.8S, 18S, and 28S rRNA. The sequence for the 11,580 nucleotides of *X. laevis* rDNA has been determined (Table 1).

Selection Superimposed on Molecular Drive

Mutations occur at essentially random positions within the rDNA, but the evolutionary consequences of each mutation depends on its position. For example, when the rDNA of *X. borealis* (Brown et al. 1977) was compared to *X. laevis* rDNA, it was found that the spacers differed greatly, whereas the rDNA coding regions were extremely similar (Brown et al. 1972; Furlong and Maden 1983; Furlong et al. 1983). Within any given individual, all repeated rDNA copies are virtually identical with one another. The coupling of intraspecific homogeneity with interspecific heterogeneity for sequences of a tandemly repeated gene family is called horizontal, coincidental, or concerted evolution (Brown et al. 1972; Brown and Sugimoto 1974). The constant turnover in rDNA sequence can be gradually corrected by "molecular drive," which includes the processes of unequal crossing-over, gene conversion, and transposition (Dover 1982; Dover and Flavell 1984). Molecular drive can spread variants through the multiple copies of rDNA, and could fix these changes within all individuals of a species under certain circumstances (discussed by Walsh 1985).

---

‡Present address: Biology Department, Thimann Laboratories, University of California-Santa Cruz, Santa Cruz, California 95064

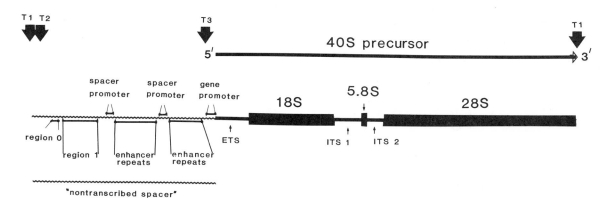

Figure 1. Structure of a typical repeat unit of rDNA from *X. laevis*, which has been sequenced in its entirety (see Table 1).

Table 1. Sequence of *Xenopus laevis* rDNA

Region	Length (nucleotides)	Reference
ETS	712	Maden et al. (1982)
18S	1825	Salim and Maden (1981)
ITS 1	557	Hall and Maden (1980)
5.8S	162	Hall and Maden (1980)
ITS 2	262	Hall and Maden (1980)
28S	4110	Ware et al. (1983)
NTS	3952	Sollner-Webb and Reeder (1979); Moss et al. (1980); Labhart and Reeder (1986 and pers. comm.)
Total:	11,580	

If molecular drive were the only force acting on rDNA to homogenize the multiple copies after random changes, then the variation between species should be uniform throughout the whole rDNA gene. In fact, this is not the case. Not only do spacers vary more than the rRNA coding regions, but even within the coding regions some sequences are more highly conserved than others. This suggests that selection pressures are superimposed on the products of molecular drive. Negative selection will drive downward the number of rDNA copies with a deleterious alteration, and positive selection will result in the spread of useful changes. In rDNA, much selection is influenced by RNA interactions necessary for ribosome biogenesis and ribosome function. Examples of such RNA interactions will be reviewed in the following sections.

CONSERVED PRIMARY SEQUENCE WITHIN rRNA

Heterologous hybridization experiments have demonstrated that portions of rRNA sequence have been highly conserved between different eukaryotic species (Sinclair and Brown 1971; Birnstiel and Grunstein 1972; Gerbi 1976). Southern blot hybridization showed that the evolutionarily conserved regions are scattered throughout 18S and 28S rRNA at distinct locations (Cox and Thompson 1980; Gourse and Gerbi 1980a). With the accumulation of rDNA sequences for many different species (see Tables II and III in Gerbi 1985; Gutell et al. 1985; Huysmans and DeWachter 1986), it has became possible to align sequences to determine regions of conservation at the nucleotide level (for early examples, see Olsen et al. 1983 for 16S–18S rRNA and Ware et al. 1983 for 23S–28S rRNA alignments). When used judiciously, rRNA sequence comparisons between different taxa can provide a powerful molecular approach for phylogenetics (Lane et al. 1985; Pace et al. 1986; Rothschild et al. 1986).

Certain regions within rRNA are conserved even between kingdoms. Selection must be very strong at these areas to prevent changes from being perpetuated. We will now describe the functions attributed to some of these highly conserved areas in rRNA.

Intermolecular Interactions: RNA-protein

rRNA interacts with proteins in ribosome biogenesis and also for ribosome function. Initially it was thought that perhaps the main function of rRNA was to act as a scaffold on which the early binding ribosomal proteins were laid during ribosome biogenesis. Although this is certainly one function for rRNA, we know now that rRNA has several other roles as well for ribosome function during protein synthesis.

L1 ribosomal protein provides a good example of the scaffold function for rRNA. We found that *Escherichia coli* ribosomal protein L1 can bind to *Dictyostelium discoideum* 26S rRNA (Gourse et al. 1981). The L1 protected regions in *E. coli* 23S, *D. discoideum* 26S, and the counterpart region in *X. laevis* 28S rRNA all share similarities in secondary structure and also share two stretches of conserved primary sequence (Gourse et al. 1981). These similarities also extend to other bacteria (Branlant et al. 1981; P. Cahill et al., pers. comm.). Presumably these are features that must be maintained in the rRNA in order for it to be able to bind ribosomal protein L1. The L11-L1 polycistronic mRNA of *E. coli* lacks the majority of the two conserved stretches found in rRNA but retains some of the same secondary structure features (Gourse et al. 1981; Baughman and Nomura 1983, 1984), and this may explain why L1 protein binds to its own message less well than to rRNA for L1 autoregulation.

Another area containing evolutionarily conserved sequence is the GTPase center located one third of the way in from the 5' end of 23S rRNA. This region associates with the protein EF-G, as demonstrated by cross-linking (Sköld 1983). The antibiotic thiostrepton blocks the interaction of EF-G with the ribosome, thereby stopping EF-G-dependent GTPase activity and inhibiting translocation (Thompson et al. 1982). The bacterium that makes thiostrepton is *Streptomyces azureus;* it may be resistant itself to thiostrepton because it methylates an A residue in the putative GTPase center (Thompson et al. 1982). *Xenopus* and other eukaryotes have a G instead of an A at this position, but site-directed mutagenesis shows that this cannot be the sole explanation for the decreased sensitivity of eukaryotes to thiostrepton (J. Thompson et al., pers. comm.).

A third example of an evolutionarily conserved region that is possibly important for rRNA-protein interactions is the peptidyltransferase center, located one quarter of the way inward from the 3′ end of 23S–28S rRNA. Peptidyl-tRNA and aminoacyl-tRNA must be positioned appropriately in the ribosome so that transpeptidation can occur. Note that a protein with peptidyltransferase activity has not yet been purified, and it is conceivable that this activity is not protein based. The peptidyltransferase center includes the sites of base mutation rendering mitochondrial ribosomes resistant to erythromycin (Sor and Fukuhara 1982, 1984) and chloramphenicol (Dujon 1980; Blanc et al. 1981a,b; Kearsay and Craig 1981; Slott et al. 1983); the same is true for eubacterial ribosomes (Skinner et al. 1983; Sigmund et al. 1984; Ettayebi et al. 1985). Also in archaebacterial ribosomes the sites of anisomycin resistance help to define the peptidyltransferase center (Hummel and Böck 1987). These studies suggest that this area of rRNA has been conserved to maintain a conformational pocket that holds the 3′ ends of the aminoacyl- and peptidyl-tRNAs in appropriate orientation to allow transpeptidation to occur. Cross-linking experiments demonstrate directly that tRNA is associated with this region of rRNA (Barta et al. 1984; Hall et al. 1985).

Intermolecular Interactions: RNA-RNA

Some conserved regions within rRNA interact with other RNA molecules during translation. The first example of such an RNA-RNA interaction was the finding of Shine and Dalgarno (1974) that the sequence CUCC adjacent to the 3′ end of prokaryotic 16S rRNA has a complementary region upstream of the AUG initiation codon in mRNA. The reality of this mRNA-rRNA interaction has been supported by several studies (Steitz and Jakes 1975; reviewed in Kozak 1983; Hui and deBoer 1987; Jacob et al. 1987). Although the Shine-Dalgarno sequence is found in the 16S rRNAs of eubacteria, archaebacteria, and chloroplasts, it is missing in mitochondria and in the cytoplasmic ribosomes of eukaryotes (Hagenbüchle et al. 1978). Even though the Shine-Dalgarno sequence is not present in eukaryotes, psoralen cross-linking has implicated association of mRNA with the 3′ end of 18S rRNA (Nakashima et al. 1980). An additional 18S mRNA-rRNA interaction has been hypothesized by Thompson and Hearst (1983), whereby the hypermodified base amψ found one third of the way in from the 3′ end of 18S rRNA may be base-paired with the 3′ end of 18S rRNA, allowing it to interact specifically with the m^{7}G cap found at the 5′ end of eukaryotic mRNAs.

During translation, tRNAs also come into close association with rRNA. A conserved 17-mer is found slightly inward from the 3′ end of 16S–18S rRNA in all known cases. This 17-mer includes C_{1400} in *E. coli* 16S rRNA and the equivalent in other species, which have been cross-linked to tRNA (Ofengand et al. 1982; Prince et al. 1982; Ehresmann and Ofengand 1984;

Gornicki et al. 1984; Ciesiolka et al. 1985). Mutation to paromomycin resistance maps to this region of rRNA, supporting the view that it is part of the decoding site (Li et al. 1982; Spangler and Blackburn 1985), as do site-directed mutagenesis studies (Krzyzosiak et al. 1987). It should be noted that no base pairing seems to be involved for the association of tRNA to the conserved 17-mer area of 16S–18S rRNA. Furthermore, DNA hybridization electron microscopy has shown that this region of 16S–18S rRNA that interacts with tRNA is exposed in the cleft of the small ribosomal subunit (Keren-Zur et al. 1979; Oakes et al. 1986). tRNA spans the interface between the two ribosomal subunits, and also associates with the peptidyltransferase center in 23S–28S rRNA as described in the preceding section (Barta et al. 1984; Hall et al. 1985).

Intramolecular Interactions: RNA Switches

It is conceivable that a stretch of sequence within rRNA might have more than one possible pairing partner within rRNA. At different stages of translation, one stem might open up and a new stem might be formed with an alternate stretch of complementary sequence. It has been speculated that such an RNA switch mechanism may be central to the process of translation (reviewed by Brimacombe et al. 1983); a chain of RNA switches that could cycle the conformation of the ribosome back to its ground state has been formulated for *E. coli* 16S rRNA (Thompson and Hearst 1983). RNA pairing interactions important for switching could be intramolecular (between two stretches of the same molecule) or intermolecular (e.g., between rRNA and a small RNA pairing partner such as 5S RNA, tRNA, or 5.8S RNA). In either case, when more than one pairing partner is involved, mutation at one position would favor compensatory mutations at the complementary nucleotides of both of its alternate pairing partners. Since such simultaneous multiple compensatory mutations are unlikely to occur, there would be negative selection against mutation of just one of the three interacting partners. The net effect would be evolutionary conservation of sequences utilized for RNA switches. It remains to be seen if data support the hypothesis of RNA switches. Instead of breaking and remaking stems, an alternate model is that changes in coaxial alignments of helices might drive functionally important changes in tertiary conformation of rRNA.

NONCONSERVED PRIMARY SEQUENCE WITHIN rRNA

Co-evolution to Retain a Core Secondary Structure of rRNA

As discussed above, functional constraints may preserve certain sequences within rDNA, since alteration of these sequences would be deleterious for rRNA function. Other regions within rRNA do not seem to have the same requirement for preservation of the actual nucleotide sequence, but may still be subject to other structural constraints.

Co-evolution can occur when RNA-RNA interactions are at stake. For instance, if it is important to retain a base-paired stem as part of the rRNA secondary structure, then mutation of a base on just one side of the stem would be selected against; only when a compensatory mutation occurs for its complementary base-pairing partner would selection permit fixation of the mutations. There is an increasing body of experimental data on the secondary structure of rRNAs; compensatory base changes are taken as additional evolutionary support for the existence of specific stems in rRNA. Covariation may also be found to maintain the tertiary structure of rRNA (Gutell et al. 1986).

Interruptions within the Core Secondary Structure of rRNA

Compensatory base changes suggest that the experimentally derived secondary structures for *E. coli* 16S and 23S rRNAs also are conserved as core structures in ribosomes from all bacteria, plants, animals, and organelles (summarized in Tables IV and V of Gerbi 1985; see also Brimacombe et al. 1983; Woese et al. 1983; Noller 1984). Can mutations occur that do not disrupt the core secondary structure of rRNA? Introns are one such example. These intervening sequences interrupt highly conserved sequences of some rDNAs (summarized in Gerbi et al. 1982), the most striking of which are the 87 bases in a row with no mismatch that are conserved beween *Xenopus* 28S rDNA (which lacks an intron) and the region surrounding the intron of *Tetrahymena* rDNA (Gourse and Gerbi 1980b). This conserved region doubtless represents an area of important function for rRNA, and disruption of this region would be harmful. *Tetrahymena* copes with such interruptions by removing introns via self-splicing so that the mature rRNA is no longer interrupted (Kruger et al. 1982). In other cases (such as *Drosophila*), where there are both intron-plus and intron-minus copies of rDNA in the genome, only the intron-minus copies of rDNA seem to be transcribed (reviewed by Beckingham 1982). Introns have not yet been found in the rDNA of vertebrates.

Eukaryotes carry additional sequences ("expansion segments"; Clark et al. 1984) that are not present in the core structure of *E. coli* rRNA, and are not usually removed by RNA processing. The location of expansion segments within regions of rRNA of little primary sequence conservation supports the idea that they can be tolerated in the mature rRNA molecules because they do not disrupt a region of functional importance. Since the length and sequence of expansion segments is quite variable between species (though some secondary structure features are preserved within but not between kingdoms; Michot and Bachellerie 1987), it seems plausible that they may not have any role in the ribosome. Indeed, it appears that if an expansion segment is too large and might create a steric hindrance to the

ribosome, it can be removed during rRNA maturation. One example of such RNA processing is the excision of the 3'-most expansion segment in higher plant chloroplast 23S rRNA. Unlike intron removal, subsequent splicing does not occur, so a separate 4.5S RNA molecule results that corresponds to the 3' end of *E. coli* 23S rRNA (Edwards et al. 1981; Machatt et al. 1981; Mackay 1981; Clark and Gerbi 1982).

A second example of removal of an expansion segment is found during rRNA processing in insects and many lower eukaryotes, thereby subdividing 28S rRNA into 28S α and 28S β halves (Delanversin and Jacq 1983; Ware et al. 1985; Fujiwara and Ishikawa 1986). In yeast 26S rRNA the counterpart expansion segment is not removed; it is smaller and apparently does not interfere with binding of yeast ribosomal protein L25 to this area (El-Baradi et al. 1985). Interestingly, yeast ribosomal protein L25 binds even tighter to the homologous region of *E. coli* 23S rRNA, which lacks an expansion segment altogether (El-Baradi et al. 1985).

In contrast to the expanded structure of eukaryotic rRNA, the rRNA of mammalian mitochondria appears to be decreased in size relative to *E. coli* rRNA, due to several "amputations" of blocks of sequence. Sometimes these amputations coincide with positions at which eukaryotic expansion segments are found inserted into the core structure (e.g., Mankin and Kopylov 1981).

DOES U3 snRNA INTERACT WITH rRNA PRECURSOR?

As described above, some regions within rRNA are highly conserved in primary sequence because they represent areas of functional importance for RNA-protein or RNA-RNA interactions. Other regions within rRNA are not conserved in primary sequence, but co-evolve by compensatory base changes to retain base-paired stems necessary for the conserved core secondary structure of rRNA. Let us now see whether these rules of RNA evolution can give information about another case of intermolecular RNA-RNA interaction, namely the postulated association of U3 snRNA with rRNA precursor.

Previous Work on U3 snRNA

snRNAs are present in eukaryotic nuclei and have been highly conserved in size and sequence throughout evolution. These RNAs are U-rich, and so were initially named U1–U6 snRNA; they exist associated with proteins in ribonucleoprotein particles (snRNPs). snRNAs are transcribed by RNA polymerase II (Gram Jensen et al. 1979; Reddy and Busch 1981), and lack a poly(A) tail at their 3' end. A unique trimethylguanosine cap occurs at the 5' end of all snRNAs except U6 (Reddy et al. 1972; Reddy and Busch 1981).

Several different snRNA molecules are utilized during mRNA splicing. The function of U3 snRNA is less clear. U3 snRNA is localized in the nucleolus, where it has been shown to be associated with nucleolar RNA sedimenting at 28S–32S (Prestayko et al. 1970; Zieve and Penman 1976; Reddy et al. 1981). In addition to U3 snRNA-rRNA interaction by hydrogen bonding, much U3 snRNP is bound to preribosomal RNP by protein interactions (Epstein et al. 1984). The observations above led to the belief that U3 snRNP plays a role in the processing removal of ITS 2 to convert 32S pre-rRNA into 28S rRNA.

How might U3 snRNP function in rRNA processing? It has been noticed that there is extensive primary sequence and secondary structure conservation between eukaryotic 5.8S RNA and the 5′ end of prokaryotic 23S rRNA (Nazar 1980; Jacq 1981; Clark and Gerbi 1982), suggesting that the 5.8S gene has become separated from the main body of the 28S gene by the insertion of the ITS 2 sequence (Fig. 1). The ITS 2 resembles the introns found in mRNA genes, since the ITS 2 is a sequence inserted into what was once probably a contiguous gene for the large rRNA. However, unlike intron splicing, the processing of the ITS 2 transcript does not entail religation of the 5.8S and 28S RNA products. Instead of being spliced together, 5.8S and 28S RNA are joined together by hydrogen bonds (Pene et al. 1968; Weinberg and Penman 1968; Prestayko et al. 1970), involving both termini of 5.8S RNA (Pace et al. 1977; Sitz et al. 1981; Peters et al. 1982; Walker et al. 1982; for review, see Walker and Pace 1983). The analogy between ITS 2 and introns prompted the hypothesis that U3 snRNA plays a role in the excision of the ITS 2 transcript (Bachellerie et al. 1983; Crouch et al. 1983; Tague and Gerbi 1984). As shown in Figure 2, we speculated that U3 snRNA base-pairs with a sequence found at the 5′ end of ITS 2, which is conserved in those vertebrates studied thus far (Tague and Gerbi 1984). However, this U3-ITS 2 interaction does not appear in nonvertebrates (Tague and Gerbi 1984).

Primary Sequence of *Xenopus* U3 snRNA

We used comparative sequence analysis to test the hypothesized interaction of U3 snRNA with ITS 2. We chose *X. laevis* and *X. borealis* as model systems be-cause previously Furlong and Maden (1983) had compared the ITS 2 sequences from these two species. Figure 3 summarizes their results, which show that conserved tracts are interspersed between divergent sequences. We predicted that if any of the conserved tracts in ITS 2 base-pair with U3 snRNA, then both *X. laevis* and *X. borealis* U3 snRNA should have an identical sequence that is complementary to the conserved tract of ITS 2. Alternatively, if co-evolution has occurred, then compensatory base changes should be found between a nonconserved stretch of ITS 2 sequence and the complementary region of U3 snRNA.

We prepared cDNA clones of U3 snRNA from both *X. laevis* and *X. borealis*, using a synthetic oligonucleotide complementary to the 3′ end of the molecule to prime first strand synthesis. The DNA sequence of both strands of these two cDNA clones was determined by the method of Maxam and Gilbert (1980), and subsequently confirmed by dideoxy primer extension off U3 snRNA templates. The very 3′ end was deduced from RNA sequencing of *X. laevis* U3 snRNA. As can be seen in Figure 4, the primary sequence of U3 snRNA is almost identical between these two species of *Xenopus*; both have a U3 snRNA sequence of 219 nucleotides with only a few positions differing between the two. With these data we can rule out compensatory base changes between nonconserved sequences in ITS 2 and U3 snRNA. Therefore, if U3 snRNA hydrogen bonds to ITS 2, such an association must be with one or more of the conserved tracts in ITS 2 (Fig. 3). When we compared the sequence of the conserved tracts in ITS 2 to that of *Xenopus* U3 snRNA (Fig. 4), only tract 0 of ITS 2 showed any appreciable complementarity to the U3 sequence.

How widely conserved are U3 snRNA sequences? We have aligned the U3 snRNA sequences of both species of *Xenopus* with the complete U3 snRNA sequences now available from rat (Reddy et al. 1979; Stroke and Weiner 1985), human (Suh et al. 1986), *Dictyostelium* (Wise and Weiner 1980), and the yeast *Saccharomyces cerevisiae* (Hughes et al. 1987). Regions of evolutionary conservation between these species for U3 snRNA are shown by enclosed boxes in Figure 4. Note that the last box contains much of the stretch of U3 snRNA hypothesized to base pair with tract 0 of ITS 2 (Fig. 2).

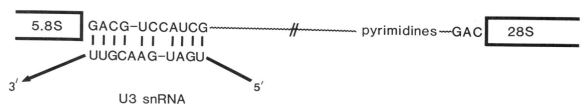

Figure 2. A hypothetical model for pairing vertebrate U3 snRNA to ITS 2 (Bachellerie et al. 1983; Tague and Gerbi 1984) is depicted here for *X. laevis*.

internal transcribed spacer 2

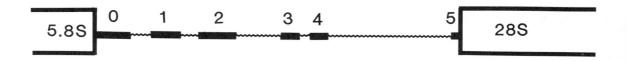

ITS 2 tracts conserved between X.laevis and X.borealis

Figure 3. ITS 2 tracts that are conserved between *X. laevis* and *X. borealis* are depicted by blackened boxes (modified from Furlong and Maden 1983).

Secondary Structure of U3 snRNA

We used chemical modification (Inoue and Cech 1985; Lempereur et al. 1985; Moazed et al. 1986) to determine if nucleotides within the conserved boxes of U3 snRNA are single stranded and therefore available for hydrogen bonding to rRNA precursor. Nuclei were isolated from *X. laevis* livers and U3 snRNP was modified in situ; only those accessible nucleotides that are not base paired will be reactive with the chemical reagent. Subsequently, the modified unbound U3 snRNA was purified and used as a template for synthetic oligonucleotide-directed primer extension (variation of

method of Qu et al. 1983). Reverse transcriptase pauses or stops one nucleotide before the modified residue (Hagenbüchle et al. 1978; Youvan and Hearst 1979); therefore, positions of chemical modification can be read from a sequencing gel.

Figure 5 shows our secondary structure model for *X. laevis* U3 snRNA. Base pairing is indicated by bars only if phylogenetic comparisons yield two or more compensatory base changes per stem. No nucleotides that are susceptible to strong modification by chemicals are located in base-paired stems of this model. The evolutionarily conserved sequences in U3 snRNA indicated by boxes in Figure 4 are depicted by wavy line brackets

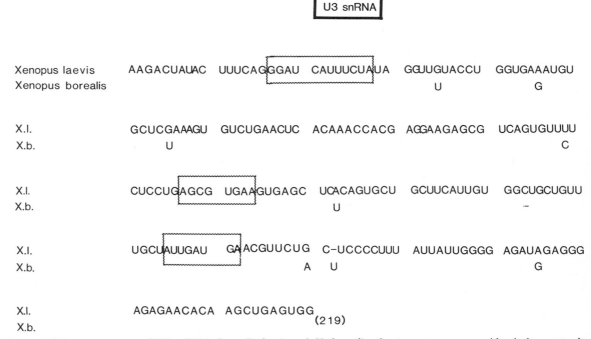

Figure 4. Primary sequence of U3 snRNA from *X. laevis* and *X. borealis*; the two sequences are identical except where differences are indicated. There seems to be population polymorphism for residue 99 in *X. laevis*: some frogs have a U at this position (as indicated in the figure), and other frogs have a C (identical to the *X. borealis* sequence at this region). RNA sequencing ambiguities occurred for residues A_{210} and U_{213}. The wavy lines enclose boxes 1, 2, and 3 that are conserved in sequence in all organisms studied so far (see text).

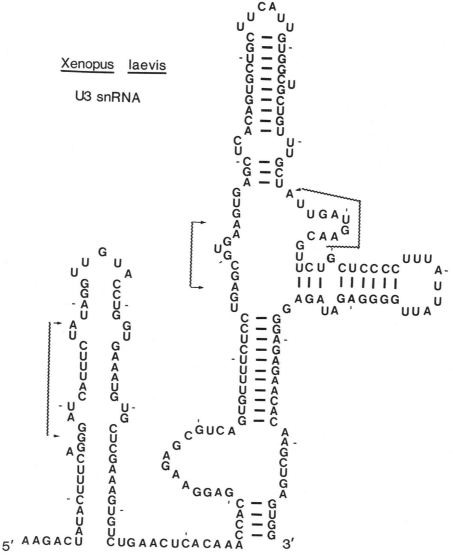

Figure 5. Secondary structure model of *X. laevis* U3 snRNA, supported by chemical modification data and by compensatory base changes in various organisms. Base-pairing bars are not drawn in for the 5′-most stem because phylogenetic comparisons and chemical modification data do not support their existence.

in Figure 5. There is no evidence for base pairing for any of these three conserved boxes. Chemical modification can be found at residues within all three conserved boxes of U3 snRNP. Their accessibility for chemical reaction suggests that these nucleotides in U3 snRNA could be available for base pairing with precursor rRNA.

Do any of the conserved boxes in U3 snRNA interact with rRNA precursor? It has been proposed that a region near box 1 of U3 snRNA might interact with the ETS of rRNA precursor (I.L. Stroke and A.M. Weiner, pers. comm.), that box 2 might base-pair with a termination processing region of rRNA precursor (Parker and Steitz 1987) and that box 3 includes much of a region that might base-pair with ITS 2 (Fig. 2). It is possible that U3 snRNA is used for some or all of these

roles. However, arguments can be raised against each of the three proposed interactions, as will be discussed more fully elsewhere. None of the models for base pairing of U3 snRNA to rRNA precursor fare well when phylogenetic comparisions are made. Proteins of the U3 snRNP particle have already been shown to play a major role for U3 snRNP binding in the nucleolus (Epstein et al. 1984), and perhaps proteins are sufficient for U3 snRNP binding. Alternatively, there may be other forces needed for RNA-RNA association besides hydrogen bond base pairing, as suggested earlier in this chapter by the conserved sequence at the end of 16S–18S rRNA that closely associates with tRNA despite a lack of sequence complementarity in the latter. Finally, U3 snRNP might play a structural role for nucleolar organization rather than have an enzymatic function for cleavage events in rRNA processing. The role of U3 snRNP in the nucleolus still awaits further investigation for its elucidation.

ACKNOWLEDGMENTS

We thank John Hughes and Kathy Parker for sharing their unpublished data with us; Bob Zimmerman and also Al Dahlberg's lab group for referral to recent references; and Carol King and Jessie Kerr for typing assistance. M.A. thanks Alan M. Weiner for laboratory space, supplies, and encouragement. This work was supported by United States Public Health Service grant GM-20261 to S.A.G.; B.S.-B. was a United States Public Health Service trainee supported by GM-07601.

REFERENCES

Bachellerie, J.-P., B. Michot, and F. Raynal. 1983. Recognition signals for mouse pre-rRNA processing. *Mol. Biol. Rep.* **9:** 79.

Barta, A., G. Steiner, J. Brosius, H.F. Noller, and E. Kuechler. 1984. Identification of a site on 23S ribosomal RNA located at the peptidyl transferase center. *Proc. Natl. Acad. Sci.* **81:** 3607.

Baughman, G. and M. Nomura. 1983. Localization of the target site for translational regulation of the L11 operon and direct evidence for translational coupling in *Escherichia coli. Cell* **34:** 979.

———. 1984. Translational regulation of the L11 ribosomal protein operon of *Escherichia coli*: Analysis of the mRNA target site using oligonucleotide-directed mutagenesis. *Proc. Natl. Acad. Sci.* **81:** 5389.

Beckingham, K. 1982. Insect rDNA. In *The cell nucleus: rDNA* (ed. H. Busch and L. Rothblum), vol. 10, p. 205. Academic Press, New York.

Birnstiel, M.L. and M. Grunstein. 1972. The ribosomal cistrons of eukaryotes—A model system for the study of evolution of serially repeated genes. *FEBS Symp.* **23:** 349.

Blanc, H., C.A. Adams, and D.C. Wallace. 1981a. Different nucleotide changes in the large rRNA gene of the mitochondrial DNA confer chloramphenicol resistance on two human cell lines. *Nucleic Acids Res.* **9:** 5785.

Blanc, H., C.T. Wright, M.J. Bibb, D.C. Wallace, and D.A. Clayton. 1981b. Mitochondrial DNA of chloramphenicol-resistant mouse cells contains a single nucleotide change in the region encoding the 3' end of the large ribosomal RNA. *Proc. Natl. Acad. Sci.* **78:** 3789.

Branlant, C., A. Krol, A. Machatt, and J.-P. Ebel. 1981. The secondary structure of the protein L1 binding region of ribosomal 23S RNA. Homologies with putative secondary structures of the L11 mRNA and of a region of mitochondrial 16S rRNA. *Nucleic Acids Res.* **9:** 293.

Brimacombe, R., P. Maly, and C. Zweib. 1983. The structure of ribosomal RNA and its organization relative to ribosomal protein. *Prog. Nucleic Acid Res. Mol. Biol.* **28:** 1.

Brown, D.D. and K. Sugimoto. 1974. The structure and evolution of ribosomal and 5 S DNAs in *Xenopus laevis* and *Xenopus mulleri. Cold Spring Harbor Symp. Quant. Biol.* **38:** 501.

Brown, D.D. and C.S. Weber. 1968a. Gene linkage by RNA-DNA hybridization. I. Unique DNA sequences homologous to 4S RNA, 5S RNA and ribosomal RNA. *J. Mol. Biol.* **34:** 661.

———. 1968b. Gene linkage by RNA-DNA hybridization. II. Arrangement of the redundant gene sequences for 28S and 18S ribosomal RNA. *J. Mol. Biol.* **34:** 681.

Brown, D.D., I.B. Dawid, and R.H. Reeder. 1977. *Xenopus borealis* misidentified as *Xenopus mulleri. Dev. Biol.* **59:** 266.

Brown, D.D., P.C. Wensink, and E. Jordan. 1972. A comparison of the ribosomal DNA's of *Xenopus laevis* and *Xenopus mulleri*: The evolution of tandem genes. *J. Mol. Biol.* **63:** 57.

Ciesiolka, J., P. Gornicki, and J. Ofengand. 1985. Identification of the site of cross-linking in 16S rRNA of an aromatic azide photoaffinity probe attached to the 5' anticodon base of A site bound tRNA. *Biochemistry* **24:** 4931.

Clark, C.G. and S.A. Gerbi. 1982. Ribosomal RNA evolution by fragmentation of the 23S progenitor: Maturation pathway parallels evolutionary emergence. *J. Mol. Evol.* **18:** 329.

Clark, C.G., B.W. Tague, V.C. Ware, and S.A. Gerbi. 1984. *Xenopus laevis* 28S ribosomal RNA: A secondary structure model and its evolutionary and functional implications. *Nucleic Acids Res.* **12:** 6197.

Cox, R.A. and R.D. Thompson. 1980. Distribution of sequences common to the 25–28S-ribonucleic acid genes of *Xenopus laevis* and *Neurospora crassa. Biochem. J.* **187:** 75.

Crouch, R.J., S. Kanaya, and P.L. Earl. 1983. A model for the involvement of the small nucleolar RNA (U3) in processing eukaryotic ribosomal RNA. *Mol. Biol. Rep.* **9:** 75.

Delanversin, G. and B. Jacq. 1983. Séquence de la région de la coupure centrale du précurseur de l'ARN ribosomique 26S de *Drosophile. C.R. Seances Acad. Sci. Ser. III Sci. Vie* **296:** 1041.

DeWinter, R.F.J. and T. Moss. 1986. The ribosomal spacer in *Xenopus laevis* is transcribed as part of the primary ribosomal RNA. *Nucleic Acids Res.* **14:** 6041.

Dover, G. 1982. Molecular drive: A cohesive mode of species evolution. *Nature* **299:** 111.

Dover, G. and R.B. Flavell. 1984. Molecular co-evolution: rDNA divergence and the maintenance of function. *Cell* **38:** 622.

Dujon, B. 1980. Sequence of the intron and flanking exons of the mitochondrial 21S rRNA gene of yeast strains having different alleles at the ω and *rib-1* loci. *Cell* **20:** 185.

Edwards, K., J. Bedbrook, T.A. Dyer, and H. Kössel. 1981. 4.5S rRNA from *Zea mays* chloroplasts shows structural homology with the 3' end of prokaryotic 23S rRNA. *Biochem. Int.* **2:** 533.

Ehresmann, C. and J. Ofengand. 1984. Two-dimensional gel electrophoresis technique for determination of the cross-linked nucleotides in cleavable covalent RNA-RNA complexes. Application to *Escherichia coli* and *Bacillus subtilis* acetyl valyl-tRNA covalently linked to *E. coli* 16S and yeast 18S ribosomal RNA. *Biochemistry* **23:** 438.

El-Baradi, T.T.A.L., H.A. Raué, V.C.H.F. de Regt, E.C. Verbree, and R.J. Planta. 1985. Yeast ribosomal protein L25 binds to an evolutionary conserved site on yeast 26S and *E. coli* 23S rRNA. *EMBO J.* **4:** 2101.

Epstein, P., R. Reddy, and H. Busch. 1984. Multiple states of U3 RNA in Novikoff hepatoma nucleoli. *Biochemistry* **23:** 5421.

Ettayebi, M., S.M. Prasad, and E.A. Morgan. 1985. Chloramphenicol-erythromycin resistance mutations in a 23S rRNA gene of *Escherichia coli. J. Bacteriol.* **162:** 551.

Fujiwara, H. and H. Ishikawa. 1986. Molecular mechanism of introduction of the hidden break into the 28S rRNA of insects: Implication based on structural studies. *Nucleic Acids Res.* **14:** 6393.

Furlong, J.C. and B.E.H. Maden. 1983. Patterns of major divergence between the internal transcribed spacers of ribosomal DNA in *Xenopus borealis* and *Xenopus laevis*, and of minimal divergence within ribosomal coding regions. *EMBO J.* **2:** 443.

Furlong, J.C., J. Forbes, M. Robertson, and B.E.H. Maden. 1983. The external transcribed spacer and preceding region of *Xenopus borealis* rDNA: Comparison with the corresponding region of *Xenopus laevis* rDNA. *Nucleic Acids Res.* **11**: 8183.

Gerbi, S.A. 1976. Fine structure of ribosomal RNA. I. Conservation of homologous regions within ribosomal RNA of eukaryotes. *J. Mol. Biol.* **106**: 791.

———. 1985. Evolution of ribosomal DNA. *Molecular evolutionary genetics*, (ed. R.J. MacIntyre), p. 419. Plenum Publishing, New York.

Gerbi, S.A., R.L. Gourse, and C.G. Clark. 1982. Conserved regions within ribosomal DNA: Locations and some possible functions. In *The cell nucleus: rDNA* (ed. H. Busch and L. Rothblum), vol. 10, p. 351. Academic Press, New York.

Gornicki, P., K. Nurse, W. Hellmann, M. Boublik, and J. Ofengand. 1984. High resolution localization of the tRNA anticodon interaction sites on the *Escherichia coli* 30S ribosomal subunit. *J. Biol. Chem.* **259**: 10493.

Gourse, R.L. and S.A. Gerbi. 1980a. Fine structure of ribosomal RNA. III. Location of evolutionarily conserved regions within ribosomal DNA. *J. Mol. Biol.* **140**: 321.

———. 1980b. Fine structure of ribosomal RNA. IV. Extraordinary evolutionary conservation in sequences that flank introns in rDNA. *Nucleic Acids Res.* **8**: 3623.

Gourse, R.L., D.L. Thurlow, S.A. Gerbi, and R.A. Zimmermann. 1981. Specific binding of a prokaryotic ribosomal protein to a eukaryotic ribosomal RNA: Implications for evolution and autoregulation. *Proc. Natl. Acad. Sci.* **78**: 2722.

Gram Jensen, E., P. Hellung-Larsen, and S. Frederiksen. 1979. Synthesis of low molecular weight RNA components A, C and D by polymerase II in α-amanitin-resistant hamster cells. *Nucleic Acids Res.* **6**: 321.

Gutell, R.R., H.F. Noller, and C.R. Woese. 1986. Higher order structure in ribosomal RNA. *EMBO J.* **5**: 1111.

Gutell, R.R., B. Weiser, C.R. Woese, and H.F. Noller. 1985. Comparative anatomy of 16S-like ribosomal RNA. *Prog. Nucleic Acid Res. Mol. Biol.* **32**: 156.

Hagenbüchle, O., M. Santer, J.A. Steitz, and R.J. Mans. 1978. Conservation of the primary structure at the 3′ end of 18S rRNA from eukaryotic cells. *Cell* **13**: 551.

Hall, C.C., J.E. Smith, and B.S. Cooperman. 1985. Mapping labeled sites in *Escherichia coli* ribosomal RNA: Distribution of methyl groups and identification of a photoaffinity-labeled RNA region putatively at the peptidyltransferase center. *Biochemistry* **24**: 5702.

Hall, L.M.C. and B.E.H. Maden. 1980. Nucleotide sequence through the 18S-28S intergene region of a vertebrate ribosomal transcription unit. *Nucleic Acids Res.* **8**: 5993.

Hui, A. and H.A. de Boer. 1987. The specialized ribosome system: Preferential translation of a single mRNA species in a subpopulation of mutated ribosomes. *Proc. Natl. Acad. Sci.* **84**: 4762.

Hughes, J.M.X., D.A.M. Konings, and G. Cesareni. 1987. The yeast homologue of U3 snRNA. *EMBO J.* **6**: 2145.

Hummel, H. and A. Böck. 1987. 23S Ribosomal RNA mutations in halobacteria conferring resistance to the anti-80S ribosome targeted antibiotic anisomycin. *Nucleic Acids Res.* **15**: 2431.

Huysmans, E. and R. DeWachter. 1986. Compilation of small ribosomal subunit RNA sequences. *Nucleic Acids Res.* (suppl.) **14**: r73.

Inoue, T. and T.R. Cech. 1985. Secondary structure of the circular form of the *Tetrahymena* rRNA intervening sequence: A technique for RNA structure analysis using chemical probes and reverse transcriptase. *Proc. Natl. Acad. Sci.* **82**: 648.

Jacob, W.F., M. Santer, and A.E. Dahlberg. 1987. A single base change in the Shine-Dalgarno region of 16S rRNA of *E. coli* affects translation of many proteins. *Proc. Natl. Acad. Sci.* **84**: 4757.

Jacq, B. 1981. Sequence homologies between eukaryotic 5.8S rRNA and the 5′ end of prokaryotic 23S rRNA: Evidences for a common evolutionary origin. *Nucleic Acids Res.* **9**: 2913.

Kearsay, S.E. and I.W. Craig. 1981. Altered ribosomal RNA genes in mitochondria from mammalian cells with chloramphenicol resistance. *Nature* **290**: 607.

Keren-Zur, M., M. Boublik, and J. Ofengand. 1979. Localization of the decoding region on the 30S *Escherichia coli* ribosomal subunit by affinity immunoelectron microscopy. *Proc. Natl. Acad. Sci.* **76**: 1054.

Kozak, M. 1983. Comparison of initiation of protein synthesis in procaryotes, eucaryotes and organelles. *Microbiol. Rev.* **47**: 1.

Kruger, K., P.J. Grabowski, A.J. Zaug, J. Sands, D.E. Gottschling, and T.R. Cech. 1982. Self-splicing RNA: Autoexcision and autocyclization of the ribosomal RNA intervening sequence of *Tetrahymena*. *Cell* **31**: 147.

Krzyzosiak, W., R. Denman, K. Nurse, W. Hellmann, M. Boublik, C.W. Gehrke, P.F. Agris, and J. Ofengand. 1987. *In vitro* synthesis of 16S ribosomal RNA containing single base changes and assembly into a functional 30S ribosome. *Biochemistry* **26**: 2353.

Labhart, P. and R.H. Reeder. 1986. Characterization of three sites of RNA 3′ end formation in the *Xenopus* ribosomal gene spacer. *Cell* **45**: 431.

———. 1987. Heat shock stabilizes highly unstable transcripts of the *Xenopus* ribosomal gene spacer. *Proc. Natl. Acad. Sci.* **84**: 56.

Lane, D.J., B. Pace, G.J. Olsen, D.A. Stahl, M.L. Sogin, and N.R. Pace. 1985. Rapid determination of 16S ribosomal RNA sequences for phylogenetic analyses. *Proc. Natl. Acad. Sci.* **82**: 6955.

Lempereur, L., M. Nicoloso, N. Riehl, C. Ehresmann, B. Ehresmann, and J.-P. Bachellerie. 1985. Conformation of yeast 18S rRNA. Direct chemical probing of the 5′ domain in ribosomal subunits and in deproteinized RNA by reverse transcriptase mapping of dimethyl sulfate-accessible sites. *Nucleic Acids Res.* **13**: 8339.

Li, M., A. Tzagoloff, K. Underbrink-Lyon, and N.C. Martin. 1982. Identification of the paromomycin-resistance mutation in the 15S rRNA gene of yeast mitochondria. *J. Biol. Chem.* **257**: 5921.

Machatt, M.A., J.-P. Ebel, and C. Branlant. 1981. The 3′-terminal region of bacterial 23S ribosomal RNA: Structure and homology with the 3′-terminal region of eukaryotic 28S rRNA and with chloroplast 4.5S rRNA. *Nucleic Acids Res.* **9**: 1533.

Mackay, R.M. 1981. The origin of plant chloroplast 4.5S ribosomal RNA. *FEBS Lett.* **123**: 17.

Maden, B.E.H., M. Moss, and M. Salim. 1982. Nucleotide sequence of an external transcribed spacer in *Xenopus laevis* DNA: Sequences flanking the 5′ and 3′ ends of 18S rRNA are non-complementary. *Nucleic Acids Res.* **10**: 2387.

Mankin, A.S. and A.M. Kopylov. 1981. A secondary structure model for mitochondrial 12S rRNA: An example of economy in rRNA structure. *Biochem. Int.* **3**: 587.

Maxam, A.M. and W. Gilbert. 1980. Sequencing end-labeled DNA with base-specific chemical cleavages. *Methods Enzymol.* **65**: 499.

Michot, B. and J.-P. Bachellerie. 1987. Comparisons of large subunit rRNAs reveal some eukaryote-specific elements of secondary structure. *Biochimie* **69**: 11.

Moazed, D., S. Stern, and N.F. Noller. 1986. Rapid chemical probing of conformation in 16S ribosomal RNA and 30S ribosomal subunits using primer extension. *J. Mol. Biol.* **187**: 399.

Morrow, J.F., S.N. Cohen, A.C.Y. Chang, H.W. Boyer, H.M. Goodman, and R.B. Helling. 1974. Replication and transcription of eukaryotic DNA in *Escherichia coli*. *Proc. Natl. Acad. Sci.* **71**: 1743.

Moss, T., P.G. Boseley, and M.L. Birnstiel. 1980. More ribosomal spacer sequences from *Xenopus laevis*. *Nucleic Acids Res.* **8**: 467.

Nakashima, K., E. Daryzynkiewicz, and A.J. Shatkin. 1980. Proximity of mRNA 5'-region and 18S rRNA in eukaryotic initiation complexes. *Nature* **286:** 226.

Nazar, R.N. 1980. A 5.8S rRNA-like sequence in prokaryotic 23S rRNA. *FEBS Lett.* **119:** 212.

Noller, H.F. 1984. Structure of ribosomal RNA. *Annu. Rev. Biochem.* **53:** 119.

Oakes, M.I., M.W. Clark, E. Henderson, and J.A. Lake. 1986. DNA hybridization electron microscopy: Ribosomal RNA nucleotides 1392–1407 are exposed in the cleft of the small subunit. *Proc. Natl. Acad. Sci.* **83:** 275.

Ofengand, J., P. Gornicki, K. Chakraburtty, and K. Nurse. 1982. Functional conservation near the 3' end of eukaryotic small subunit RNA: Photochemical crosslinking of P site-bound acetylvalyl-tRNA to 18S RNA of yeast ribosomes. *Proc. Natl. Acad. Sci.* **79:** 2817.

Olsen, G.J., R. McCarroll, and M.L. Sogin. 1983. Secondary structure of the *Dictyostelium discoideum* small subunit ribosomal RNA. *Nucleic Acids Res.* **11:** 8037.

Pace, N.R., G.J. Olsen, and C.R. Woese. 1986. Ribosomal RNA phylogeny and the primary lines of evolutionary descent. *Cell* **45:** 325.

Pace, N.R., T.A. Walker, and E. Schroeder. 1977. Structure of the 5.8S RNA component of the 5.8S-28S ribosomal RNA junction complex. *Biochemistry* **16:** 5321.

Parker, K.A. and J.A. Steitz. 1987. Structural analyses of the human U3 ribonucleoprotein particle reveal a conserved sequence available for base pairing with pre-rRNA. *Mol. Cell. Biol.* **7:** 2899.

Pene, J.J., E. Knight, and J.E. Darnell. 1968. Characterization of a new low molecular weight RNA in HeLa cell ribosomes. *J. Mol. Biol.* **33:** 609.

Peters, M.A., T.A. Walker, and N.R. Pace. 1982. Independent binding sites in mouse 5.8S ribosomal ribonucleic acid for 28S ribosomal ribonucleic acid. *Biochemistry* **21:** 2329.

Prestayko, A.W., M. Tonato, and H. Busch. 1970. Low molecular weight RNA associated with 28S nucleolar RNA. *J. Mol. Biol.* **47:** 505.

Prince, J.B., B.H. Taylor, D.L. Thurlow, J. Ofengand, and R.A. Zimmermann. 1982. Covalent crosslinking of tRNA$_1^{val}$ to 16S RNA at the ribosomal P site: Identification of crosslinked residues. *Proc. Natl. Acad. Sci.* **79:** 5450.

Qu, L.H., B. Michot, and J.-P. Bachellerie. 1983. Improved methods for structure probing in large RNAs: A rapid "heterologous" sequencing approach is coupled to the direct mapping of nuclease accessible sites. Application to the 5' terminal domain of eukaryotic 28S rRNA. *Nucleic Acids Res.* **11:** 5903.

Reddy, R. and H. Busch. 1981. U snRNA's of nuclear snRNP's. In *The cell nucleus: Nuclear particles* (ed. H. Busch), vol. 8, p. 261. Academic Press, New York.

Reddy, R., D. Henning, and H. Busch. 1979. Nucleotide sequence of nucleolar U3B RNA. *J. Biol. Chem.* **254:** 11097.

Reddy, R., W.-Y. Li, D. Henning, Y.C. Choi, K. Nohga, and H. Busch. 1981. Characterization of subcellular localization of 7–8 S RNAs of Novikoff hepatoma. *J. Biol. Chem.* **256:** 8452.

Reddy, R., T.S. Ro-Choi, D. Henning, H. Shibata, Y.C. Choi, and H. Busch. 1972. Modified nucleosides of nuclear and nucleolar low molecular weight ribonucleic acid. *J. Biol. Chem.* **247:** 7245.

Rothschild, L.J., M.A. Ragan, A.W. Coleman, P. Heywood, and S.A. Gerbi. 1986. Are rRNA sequence comparisons the Rosetta stone of phylogenetics? *Cell* **47:** 640.

Salim, M. and B.E.H. Maden. 1981. Nucleotide sequence of *Xenopus laevis* 18S ribosomal RNA inferred from gene sequence. *Nature* **291:** 205.

Shine, J. and L. Dalgarno. 1974. The 3'-terminal sequence of *E. coli* 16S ribosomal RNA: Complementarity to nonsense triplets and ribosome binding sites. *Proc. Natl. Acad. Sci.* **71:** 1342.

Sigmund, C.D., M. Ettayebi, and E.A. Morgan. 1984. Antibiotic resistance mutations of 16S and 23S ribosomal RNA genes of *Escherichia coli*. *Nucleic Acids Res.* **12:** 4653.

Sinclair, J. and D.D. Brown. 1971. Retention of common nucleotide sequences in the ribosomal deoxyribonucleic acid of eukaryotes and some of their physical characteristics. *Biochemistry* **10:** 2761.

Sitz, T.O., M. Banjeree, and R.N. Nazar. 1981. Effect of point mutations on 5.8S ribosomal ribonucleic acid secondary structure and the 5.8S-28S ribosomal ribonucleic acid junction. *Biochemistry* **20:** 4029.

Skinner, R., E. Cundliffe, and F.J. Schmidt. 1983. Site of action of a ribosomal RNA methylase responsible for resistance to erythromycin and other antibiotics. *J. Biol. Chem.* **258:** 12701.

Sköld, S.-E. 1983. Chemical crosslinking of elongation factor G to the 23S RNA in 70S ribosomes from *Escherichia coli*. *Nucleic Acids Res.* **11:** 4923.

Slott, E.F., R.O. Shade, and R.A. Lansman. 1983. Sequence analysis of mitochondrial DNA in a mouse cell line resistant to chloramphenicol and oligomycin. *Mol. Cell. Biol.* **3:** 1694.

Sollner-Webb, B. and R.H. Reeder. 1979. The nucleotide sequence of the initiation and termination sites for ribosomal RNA transcription in *Xenopus laevis*. *Cell* **18:** 485.

Sor, F. and H. Fukuhara. 1982. Identification of two erythromycin resistance mutations in the mitochondrial gene coding for the large ribosomal RNA in yeast. *Nucleic Acids Res.* **10:** 6571.

———. 1984. Erythromycin and spiramycin resistance mutations of yeast mitochondria: Nature of the *rib2* locus in the large ribosomal RNA gene. *Nucleic Acids Res.* **12:** 8313.

Spangler, E.A. and E.H. Blackburn. 1985. The nucleotide sequence of the 17S ribosomal RNA gene of *Tetrahymena thermophila* and the identification of point mutations resulting in resistance to the antibiotics paromomycin and hygromycin. *J. Biol. Chem.* **260:** 6334.

Steitz, J.A. and K. Jakes. 1975. How ribosomes select initiator formation between the 3' terminus of 16S rRNA and the mRNA during initiation of protein synthesis in *Escherichia coli*. *Proc. Natl. Acad. Sci.* **72:** 4734.

Stroke, I.L. and A.M. Weiner. 1985. Genes and pseudogenes for rat U3A and U3B small nuclear RNA. *J. Mol. Biol.* **184:** 183.

Suh, D., H. Busch, and R. Reddy. 1986. Isolation and characterization of a human U3 small nucleolar RNA gene. *Biochem. Biophys. Res. Commun.* **137:** 1133.

Tague, B.W. and S.A. Gerbi. 1984. Processing of the large rRNA precursor: Two proposed categories of RNA-RNA interactions in eukaryotes. *J. Mol. Evol.* **20:** 362.

Thompson, J., F. Schmidt, and E. Cundliffe. 1982. Site of action of a ribosomal RNA methylase conferring resistance to thiostrepton. *J. Biol. Chem.* **257:** 7915.

Thompson, J.F. and J.E. Hearst. 1983. Structure-function relations in *E. coli* 16S RNA. *Cell* **33:** 19.

Walker, T.A. and N.R. Pace. 1983. 5.8S ribosomal RNA. *Cell* **33:** 320.

Walker, T.A., K.D. Johnson, G.J. Olsen, M.A. Peters, and N.R. Pace. 1982. Enzymatic and chemical structure mapping of mouse 28S ribosomal ribonucleic acid contacts in 5.8S ribosomal ribonucleic acid. *Biochemistry* **21:** 2320.

Walsh, J.B. 1985. Interaction of selection and biased gene conversion in a multigene family. *Proc. Natl. Acad. Sci.* **82:** 153.

Ware, V.C., R. Renkawitz, and S.A. Gerbi. 1985. rRNA processing: Removal of only nineteen bases at the gap between 28Sα and 28Sβ rRNAs in *Sciara coprophila*. *Nucleic Acids Res.* **13:** 3581.

Ware, V.C., B.W. Tague, C.G. Clark, R.L. Gourse, R.C. Brand, and S.A. Gerbi. 1983. Sequence analysis of 28S ribosomal DNA from the amphibian *Xenopus laevis*. *Nucleic Acids Res.* **11:** 7795.

Weinberg, R.A. and S. Penman. 1968. Small molecular weight monodisperse nuclear RNA. *J. Mol. Biol.* **39:** 289.

Wise, J.A. and A.M. Weiner. 1980. *Dictyostelium* small nuclear RNA D2 is homologous to rat nucleolar RNA U3 and is encoded by a dispersed multigene family. *Cell* **22:** 109.

Woese, C.P., R.R. Gutell, R. Gupta, and H.F. Noller. 1983. A detailed analysis of the higher-order structure of 16S-like ribosomal RNAs. *Microbiol. Rev.* **47:** 621.

Youvan, D.C. and J.E. Hearst. 1979. Reverse transcriptase pauses at N^2-methylguanine during *in vitro* transcription of *Escherichia coli* 16S ribosomal RNA. *Proc. Natl. Acad. Sci.* **76:** 3751.

Zieve, G. and S. Penman. 1976. Small RNA species of the HeLa cell: Metabolism and subcellular localization. *Cell* **8:** 19.

On the Modus Operandi of the Ribosome

P.B. Moore

Department of Chemistry and Department of Molecular Biophysics and Biochemistry
Yale University, New Haven, Connecticut 06511

There are many reasons for discussing the ribosome at a symposium on the evolution of catalytic function. It is the polymerase-like enzyme that catalyzes peptide bond formation during protein synthesis. The ancestral ribosome had to have been in existence very early in evolution, at the time the genome was "invented." Furthermore, ribosome action is required so that the phenotypic effect of genetic changes in an organism may be acted upon by selective forces. Thus, its properties influence the feedback that the genome gets from the environment, and hence the manner in which organisms evolve. Ribosomes are also interesting evolutionarily because their catalytic activity almost certainly depends heavily on RNA chemistry (see Woese 1980; Moore 1986), and RNA-dependent enzymes are generally regarded as primitive.

Ribosomes are large; the prokaryotic version has a molecular weight near 2.3×10^6, and this mass supports just one active site. In the ribosome from *Escherichia coli*, 52 different proteins and three RNAs are found. A single particle contains one copy each of 54 of these components. The fifty-fifth is present in four copies (see Wittmann-Liebold 1986). Protein accounts for about 35% of the total mass; the rest is RNA. In general design, prokaryotic ribosomes are similar to their larger, protein-rich, eukaryotic homologs (see Wool 1986).

As protein synthesis proceeds, the prokaryotic ribosome associates transiently with (at least) seven different protein factors, as well as with its aminoacyl tRNA substrates and its mRNA template. In addition, some of these macromolecules move across the surface of the ribosome as the peptide chain elongates. (The eukaryotic version of the same events is similar to the prokaryotic one, but even more complicated, as usual.)

We do not have a clear understanding of where the macromolecular ligands of the ribosome bind to the ribosome during protein synthesis, let alone how they move around. Were these matters understood, even at low resolution, the answers to some long-standing, fundamental questions about ribosomal function would probably emerge, e.g., why ribosomes are invariably two-subunit enzymes. Thus, an analysis of the quaternary structure of the ribosomal complex at different stages of protein synthesis would advance our understanding of that process significantly.

Several years ago, D.M. Engelman and I developed a method for determining the quaternary structure of objects like the ribosome and its complexes with ligands and substrates (Engelman and Moore 1972).

The method involves neutron scattering measurements on solutions of ribosomes whose components have been selectively labeled with deuterium. Our initial goal, which was to use the method to map the protein structure of the small ribosomal subunit from *E. coli* in three dimensions, was reached just a few months ago (M.S. Capel et al.; P.B. Moore and M.S. Capel; both in prep.). The map of the quaternary structure of the small subunit that has emerged from this work is described briefly below.

The neutron map has no information in it about active site placements as such; the positions of none of the ligands of the subunit have yet been measured by neutron scattering. There is a considerable literature on the relationship of the ribosome's chemical structure to its function, however, and this literature has been under scrutiny to see if the data it contains can be merged with the neutron map to tell us something useful about the "macromolecular choreography" of protein synthesis.

Despite the fact that experiments have been done that identify protein components near virtually all the binding sites of the 30S ribosomal subunit, disappointingly few of these sites can be localized accurately with respect to the neutron map. Moreover, some of the data can be interpreted to mean that the reason precise localizations have not been obtained is because they do not exist in some cases. It is conceivable that there may be some fundamental differences between the way this RNA-based enzyme works and the modus operandi of more conventional protein enzymes. The case supporting this point of view will be made below.

METHODS

The ribosomal proteins and RNAs of *E. coli* can be prepared in deuterated form because the organism grows in media that contain only ^2H. By taking advantage of the fact that ribosomes can be reconstituted from their macromolecular constituents in vitro (Traub and Nomura 1968), particles can be constructed having any pattern of deuterium labeling whatever at the quaternary level.

Neutrons having wavelengths in the angstrom range are scattered differently by ^1H and ^2H (see Bacon 1975). This isotope effect is so large that the scattering profile given by a solution of ribosomes is measurably altered when just one protonated protein constituent is replaced by its deuterated counterpart. When two deuterated proteins are present in the particle, the incremental scatter they produce contains information not only about the size and shape of the two proteins individually, but also about their relative positions in the particle. The latter can be measured independently of the former.

Four reconstitutions are made: (1) a reconstitution in which both of the proteins of interest are deuterium labeled, (2) a preparation in which neither is labeled, and (3) and (4) the two possible preparations where only one of the two is labeled. It is easy to show that the portion of the scattering that carries information about their relative positions, $I_x(s)$, can be obtained by summing and differencing the scattering profiles of the four samples, suitably normalized, point by point:

$$I_x(s) = (I_1[s] + I_2[s]) - (I_3[s] + I_4[s]) \qquad (1)$$

s is the equivalent Bragg angle: $s = 2 \sin(\theta)/\lambda$, where θ is half the scattering angle and λ is the neutron wavelength.

For spherical proteins, $I_x(s)$ will approximate a damped $\sin(2\pi sd)/(2\pi sd)$ curve, where d is the distance between the centers of the two labeled proteins. Where the curve first crosses zero, $s = 1/2d$. The Fourier transform of $I_x(s)$ corresponds to the distribution of lengths of all vectors joining a deuterium in one of the labeled proteins with a deuterium in the other. The second moment of that length distribution, M, is related to several quantities of structural interest:

$$M = R_i^2 + R_j^2 + d_{ij}^2 \qquad (2)$$

where R_i is the radius of gyration of the deuterium distribution of the ith protein in situ, and d_{ij} is the distance between the centroids of the two deuterium distributions (May 1978; Moore et al. 1978; Stoekel et al. 1979). (It is assumed that the distribution of hydrogens in a protein satisfactorily approximates its distribution of mass.)

In any structure having more than eight components, more pairwise second moments can be measured than there are independent coordinates and radii of gyration to be determined. If an appropriate set of measurements is made, therefore, a model of the structure can be computed that specifies the positions of component centers and their radii of gyration. The theoretical and the practical aspects of this experiment have been described in detail elsewhere (Engelman 1979; Moore 1979; Moore and Engelman 1979; Ramakrishnan and Moore 1981; Capel and Ramakrishnan 1987; M.S. Capel et al., in prep.).

RESULTS

The Placement of Proteins in the 30S Ribosomal Subunit

The small ribosomal subunit from *E. coli* contains 21 protein molecules and a single molecule of RNA; 78 pairwise relationships are required to map its proteins.

Over the past 12 years, 105 $I_x(s)$ functions have been measured for 93 different protein pairs, enough to overspecify the map of the small subunit by a small amount (M.S. Capel et al., in prep.).

Figure 1 shows two views of the model of the distribution of proteins within the 30S subunit that results from the analysis of these data. The two views are rotated by 180° with respect to each other. The left-hand view will be referred to as the "front" view, and the right-hand one as the "back" view. The front view corresponds to the appearance of the particle from the side that is exposed to the cytoplasm in the 70S couple. The back view is the side the 50S subunit "sees." The centers of the spheres are at the locations calculated for the centroids of the proteins whose number they carry. The volume of each sphere represents the anhydrous volume of the corresponding protein drawn to the scale of the figure.

The protein array is about 190 Å in its longest dimension, from the "top" of S13 to the "bottom" of S17. It is thinnest in the direction of the line of sight in Figure 1. In that direction it is about 80 Å thick. The standard errors of the coordinates of the centroids run from 4 to 15 Å. (15 Å is the radius of an average protein in this map.)

Neutron mapping produces estimates for the radii of gyration of the ribosomal proteins in situ. Unfortunately, the errors associated with most of the radius gyration estimates obtained are quite large. All that can be said at this point is that protein S1 has a highly elongated conformation in the ribosome, and that S4 and possibly S2 may be moderately elongated as well. For the remaining proteins the data are not well enough determined to permit definitive conclusions to be drawn.

DISCUSSION

Comparisons of the Neutron Map with Other Structural Data

Those working on ribosomes have not been idle since 1972, waiting for us to provide them with a map of protein positions, but have explored many alternative approaches, of which the most effective by far has been electron microscopy. Electron microscopists have localized the positions of the antigenic determinants of many ribosomal proteins with respect to the overall shape of the subunits using protein-specific antibodies as stains. The technique is known as immunoelectron microscopy (IEM).

Figure 2 compares the IEM map produced by Lake and his colleagues at UCLA (Oakes et al. 1986) with the neutron map. Both images are drawn to roughly the same scale, and the neutron map has been rotated to make the correlation between protein positions in the two images obvious. The correspondence is excellent (P.B. Moore and M.S. Capel, in prep.). A satisfactory correlation also exists between the neutron map and the IEM map generated by Stoeffler and his coworkers

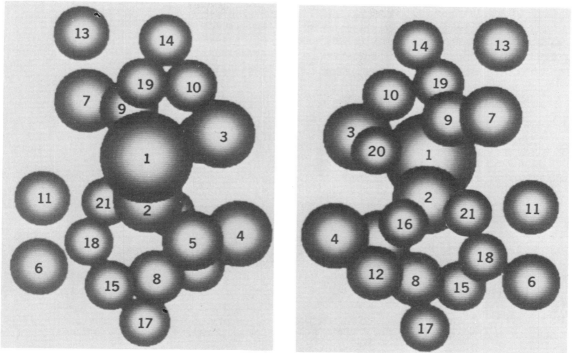

Figure 1. Two views of the neutron map of the 30S ribosomal subunit from *E. coli.* Proteins are depicted as spheres whose volumes represent the volume actually occupied by the protein in question to the scale of the figure. Proteins are designated by the usual numbering system, S1, ..., S21. (*Left*) the particle from the side accessible to the cytoplasm in the 70S ribosomal couple; (*right*) the subunit rotated 180° around a vertical axis in the plane of the figure, as it would be "seen" from the 50S subunit in the 70S couple. From the "top" of S13 to the "bottom" of S17 is about 190 Å.

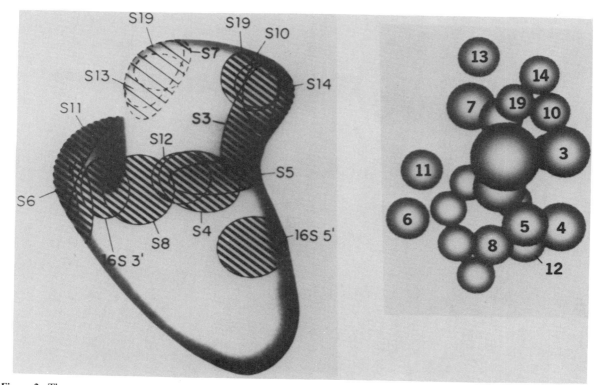

Figure 2. The neutron map compared with the immunoelectron microscopic map of Oakes et al. (1986). (*Left*) IEM image of the Lake group (reprinted, with permission, from Lake 1985.); (*right*) the cytoplasmic view of the neutron map. The two images are drawn to approximately the same scale.

(Stoeffler and Stoeffler-Meilicke 1986; M.S. Capel et al., in prep.). The fact that the two IEM maps and the neutron map agree in large measure gives us confidence that we have a reasonably accurate understanding of where the proteins are in the small subunit.

Self-assembly in Three Dimensions

Shortly after ribosomal reconstitution was discovered, the Nomura group analyzed the nucleoproteins produced when small subunit reconstitutions were done in the absence of each of the 21 proteins. This study elucidated the protein-protein interactions involved in the assembly process (Mizushima and Nomura 1970; Held et al. 1974). Figure 3 shows the strongest of these dependencies plotted on the neutron map. A protein at the head of an arrow will not add to a reassembling particle unless the protein at the butt of the arrow is already present.

Nomura's "assembly map" describes functional relationships between proteins in the ribosome, and it makes sense in terms of the protein structure of the particle (see P.B. Moore and M.S. Capel, in prep.). Proteins that interact strongly during assembly are neighbors in the completed particle. Furthermore, the trend of the arrows suggests that assembly is a process that nucleates in two different parts of the particle. One nucleation point is near S7 in the head of the subunit, and the second one is near S8.

Mapping Functional Sites in the Ribosome

Many of the experiments that have been done to localize ribosomal active sites with respect to their RNA have produced results as pleasing as the geometric mapping of the assembly just described.

For example, Ofengand and co-workers have discovered that the anticodons of some tRNAs bound to ribosomes in the P site photocross-link to 16S RNA at C1400 in high yield, and that similar cross-links can be made to the same residue using A-site-bound tRNAs, appropriately derivatized at their anticodons (see Ofengand et al. 1986). The controls done establish that the tRNAs in question are properly positioned on the ribosome *after cross-linking*. There is no doubt that C1400 is very close to the site where tRNAs interact with mRNA triplets.

It happens that C1400 is in the middle of a highly conserved sequence toward the 3' end of the 16S RNA, not far from a second, well-defined, RNA functional site, the Shine-Dalgarno sequence at the 3' end of 16S RNA. The Shine-Dalgarno sequence is responsible for aligning mRNAs on the small subunit during initiation (Shine and Dalgarno 1974; see Steitz 1980).

The 50S subunit supplies a third example of an RNA localization. Several residues in 23S RNA, which are well separated in its sequence, have been implicated in the peptidyltransferase function by a variety of methods, including affinity labeling using tRNAs carrying derivatized amino acids. When 23S RNA is folded into its canonical secondary structure, all these residues are brought together (Barta et al. 1984). Thus, the decoding function, the peptidyltransferase function, and the alignment function all map to discrete locations in the RNA primary or secondary structure.

When experiments are done to map functions with respect to ribosomal proteins, on the other hand, the

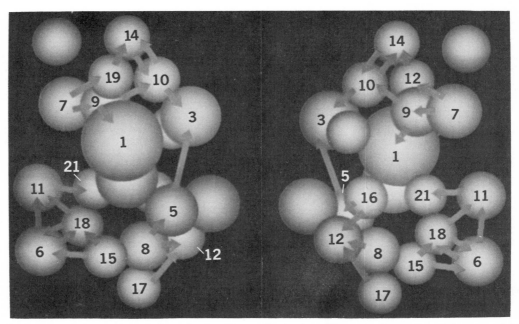

Figure 3. Protein-protein interactions during subunit self-assembly in vitro. The strong interactions between proteins during self-assembly (Mizuchima and Nomura 1970; Held et al. 1974) are shown superimposed on the neutron map of the 30S subunit. Proteins at the head of arrows require the presence of proteins at the butts of arrows in order to join the 30S assembly during reconstitution. Both the cytoplasmic and the interface views of the subunit are shown.

result is often messy. For example, Figure 4 shows the spatial distribution of all the proteins that have been reported as cross-linking to initiation factor 3 (IF-3). There are eight of them, spread all over the structure, and it is obvious that IF-3 cannot cross-link to all of them simultaneously. Where is the IF-3 binding site? The IF-3-ribosomal protein affinity labeling data do not answer this question, and the IF-3 data by no means constitute a worst case. The contrast between the vagueness of these protein-related results and the definiteness of the RNA localizations mentioned above is striking.

Why Have So Many Proteins Been Identified with the Binding Site of IF-3?

It is natural to attribute data like these to experimental fault. Affinity labeling is a demanding technique, and there is absolutely no doubt that unresolved technical difficulties have contributed to the confusion about active site locations (see P.B. Moore and M.S. Capel, in prep.).

Before ascribing all the problems in interpretation of protein localization data to poor experimental technique, however, it might be wise to examine the prejudices one brings to their interpretation. Everyone "knows" what the active sites of enzymes are like. They have well-defined geometries that ensure that when substrates bind they will be aligned accurately with

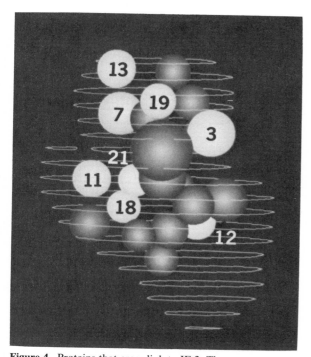

Figure 4. Proteins that cross-link to IF-3. The neutron map is shown superimposed on the electron microscopic image of Stoeffler and Stoeffler-Meilicke (1986). The numbered, light-colored proteins have been identified as cross-linkable to IF-3. References to the original cross-linking data may be found in Lambert et al. (1983).

critical, catalytically important protein residues and/or cofactors. "Accurate" in this context implies tolerances of an angstrom or less. The geometric accurateness of enzymes is , of course, the basis of the "lock and key" metaphor for the interaction of substrates with protein enzymes. If ribosomes were like other enzymes, proper affinity data should identify no more than one or two ribosomal components at each active site, not eight, as in the case of IF-3.

Are There Nonlocalized Sites on the Ribosome?

Some of the existing affinity data hint at the possibility that ribosomes may not work in a lock and key fashion. The most striking data in this regard that I am aware of were produced by Cantor's group in the early 1970s (see Pellegrini and Cantor 1977). They carried out a series of affinity labeling experiments using aminoacyl tRNAs derivatized at the α amino group to identify components at the peptidyltransferase site. In some cases, the affinity labeling was done with derivatized aminoacyl tRNAs that were nonradioactive, and the ribosomal components that had reacted with these compounds were made radioactive in a second step so they could be identified. The second step involved transfer of the amino acids covalently bound to the ribosome to radioactive aminoacyl tRNAs added to the system after the cross-linking reaction. The only way a protein could become radiolabeled under these circumstances was if the amino acid moiety of the affinity adduct could be transferred to the radioactive aminoacyl tRNA, presumably by the peptidyltransferase of the ribosome. This criterion for the validity of the affinity labeling identifications is a very strong one, and is the same one used by Barta et al. (1984) to identify the peptidyltransferase site in 23S RNA.

Four proteins were identified with the peptidyltransferase site by the two-step strategy: L2, L11, L18, and L27. Figure 5 shows where those proteins map on the 50S subunit, something that was not known in the mid-1970s. L11 is at the base of the L7/L12 stalk. L18 binds to 5S RNA in vitro, and is found near the top of the "central protuberance" where both the 3' and 5' ends of 5S RNA map by IEM. L27 maps to the region below the base of the central protuberance (see Oakes et al. 1986; Stoeffler and Stoeffler-Meilicke 1986), and the position of L2 can be established from cross-linking results (see Traut et al. 1986). The proteins in question spread over 80–100 Å of the subunit's surface.

It is conceivable that these proteins have long processes that converge at a point in the 50S subunit close to the U2585 region on 23S RNA (Barta et al. 1984), but this seems improbable. It is just as plausible to conclude that there are many places the amino acid on a P-site-bound tRNA can reside on the ribosome that are acceptable to the peptidyltransferase, even though that conclusion is completely at odds with our understanding of how conventional enzymes work.

It is possible to evade the conclusion that ribosomes are "sloppy" enzymes in this case. Aminoacyl tRNAs are high-energy compounds; the formation of peptide

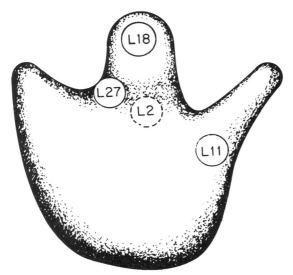

Figure 5. The location of 50S subunit proteins identified in peptidyltransferase affinity labeling experiments. The electron microscopic appearance of the 50S subunit is shown redrawn from Oakes et al. (1986). The locations given for L11, L18, and L27 are consensus locations from IEM experiments (see Oakes et al. 1986; Stoeffler and Stoeffler-Meilicke 1986). The position assigned L2 is inferred from cross-linking data (see Traut et al. 1986).

bonds from aminoacyl tRNAs is an exothermic process. Moreover, aminoacyl tRNAs are not very stable. Maybe the peptide transfer reaction requires no "help" from the ribosome once two aminoacyl tRNAs have become bound to its surface. This "escape route" is tantamount to saying that there is no peptidyltransferase on the ribosome. This thesis is not without its difficulties, however. How can chloramphenicol inhibit the peptidyltransferase activity, as it is known to do, if there is no peptidyltransferase? Furthermore, this line of argument leaves one puzzled by the results of Barta et al. (1984), which seem to identify a specific RNA site with that activity. The peptidyltransferase can be "saved," however, by postulating that the reactions that led to the labeling seen by Cantor and his colleagues were side reactions of protein synthesis.

There are other lines of evidence that support the view that ribosomal flexibility is the source of the Pellegrini-Cantor result. The Shine-Dalgarno mechanism for aligning mRNAs on ribosomes is an example. The number of nucleotides that separate the Shine-Dalgarno alignment point on a bacterial mRNA from its initiator AUG ranges from 3 to 13 bases (Gren 1984). Allowing 3 Å per base, this variation corresponds to 30 Å, a distance larger than the diameter of many enzymes! One can argue that mRNAs are flexible, and that loops form which accommodate these inconveniences within a constant geometric framework, etc., but it is unusual for a protein enzyme-substrate combination to loop out anything in order to accommodate variation in substrate size.

A third example comes from another experiment of Ofengand and colleagues (Ofengand et al. 1984). They

have shown that tRNA covalently bonded to the small subunit at its elbow region when it is in the A site can translocate without breaking the bond, already a startling observation. The criterion for translocation is that in the presence of EF-G, and only in the presence of EF-G, the amino acid on its 3' end becomes available for transfer by peptidyltransferase to puromycin. The same tRNA derivative bound in the normal manner to the P site is a perfectly acceptable tRNA, but it labels nothing. Clearly, there are two different geometries possible for the central region of tRNA relative to the ribosome that are compatible with P-site function.

Are Ribosomes Flexible?

I have provided arguments that preserve the notion of a fixed geometry ribosome against the pressure exerted by the peptidyltransferase affinity labeling experiments and the Shine-Dalgarno puzzle. Presumably, one can generate similar explanations for the tRNA result, but I am not sure how to do it at this point. The alternative is to accept the fact that all three can be explained by a single hypothesis, namely, that ribosomal sites are far more delocalized and flexible than those on conventional all-protein enzymes.

One can think of reasons why flexibility might be advantageous. First, the tRNAs the ribosome must accommodate are not identical, and their differences cannot be allowed to impede their function at the ribosomal level. Second, tRNAs are very large. If they have to bind to the ribosome so that both their 3' ends and their anticodon ends are simultaneously held in rigidly fixed locations on the ribosome, the geometric constraints that must be met so that a ribosome-tRNA collision is productive become quite severe. Geometric tolerance should permit ribosomes to operate faster.

The Role of RNA

If the particle really is as tolerant of geometric variability as the results just cited indicate it may be, one is left with the problem of understanding how functions like the decoding interaction and proofreading can be carried out with the accuracy required by a system that is unable to call upon well-defined geometries to help it. The answer to this question may be that the ribosome "runs on" RNA.

Specificity in interactions between nucleic acids is guaranteed by base pairing. Base pairing, in turn, is a local, secondary interaction that can take place whenever the appropriate sequences come within reach of each other. Specificity in protein interactions usually involves the assembly of groups of residues, which are well-separated in the protein's sequence, into a special, three-dimensional arrangement that requires nonlocal, tertiary interactions within the protein. It could be that the ribosome does not "care" what happens spatially between the anticodon and the CCA end of the molecule, as long as the proper rRNA sequences have a reasonably high probability of encountering the critical aligning sequences on the tRNA (e.g., its anticodon and the CCA sequence at its 3′ end). Protein enzymes cannot be so "laid back," since they depend on long-range, internal interactions that will not tolerate much deviation from the prescribed geometry.

Is There Evidence for Structural Flexibility in the Neutron Data?

The data we collect on the 30S subunit by neutron scattering is affected by motion within the structure. Each data set reports the distribution of distances between protons in two different proteins, averaged over all particles in a population and over long periods of time. A number of years ago, D.G. Schindler (pers. comm.) noticed that the variances of the length distributions obtained by Fourier inverting the $I_x(s)$ functions we measure should always be less than the sum of the squares of the radii of gyration of the two proteins to which they refer. Schindler's inequality is true for single objects whose structures do not vary with time. It can be violated if there is motion or variation from particle to particle.

The neutron map provides estimates for radii of gyration and distances between proteins that can be compared to the measured variances to find out whether the Schindler inequality is violated or not. Most of the data sets we measured have been tested. If there is motion within the particle, its magnitude is small compared to the errors in the data.

CONCLUSIONS

The considerations outlined above leave a number of puzzles. First, site-labeling experiments directed at RNA seem to give clean results, whereas similar experiments directed at protein give vague, delocalized results. Given the fact that the positions of proteins in the ribosome are determined by their interactions with rRNA, one would expect to get either definite results with both or indefinite results with both. Why are we seeing mixed results? Second, the functional plasticity of the ribosome that is hinted at by the examples cited above makes it difficult to understand how the ribosome achieves the specificity it must have in anticodon-codon interactions. Furthermore, the structural flexibility that would appear to be a necessary property of the particle if it is to be functionally flexible has not been detected by the neutron scattering experiments on which the model presented above is based. It is clear that the hypothesis that ribosomes are flexible helps explain some of the data we have, but does not provide satisfactory explanations for all the facts in hand at this point.

The information we have today describing how the ribosomal particle functions is obviously inadequate to either prove or disprove the hypothesis that the ribosome is a flexible enzyme. What is clear, however, is that the data we are getting on the relationship between ribosomal structure and function are not the data expected of an ordinary enzyme, and it is important that we understand why this is so. However the flexibility hypothesis fares in the end, it is possible that ancient RNA-driven enzymes may not follow the same rules as the modern all-protein enzymes with which we are more familiar.

ACKNOWLEDGMENTS

The neutron map shown above is the product of the work of many. I acknowledge with gratitude the contributions made by the following: Drs. M.S. Capel, M. Kjeldgaard, J.A. Langer, V. Ramakrishnan, D.G. Schindler, D.K. Schneider, I.-Y. Sillers, and S. Yabuki. Professor Donald M. Engleman has been a valued collaborator for many years on this project. From its inception, the project depended on his imagination and enthusiasm. Dr. Benno Schoenborn designed and constructed the data-gathering equipment necessary for this work; our debt to him is large. I also acknowledge the technical assistance of Mrs. Betty Freeborn throughout. These individuals deserve credit for the map shown here. I thank Drs. D.M. Crothers, H.F. Noller, and J. Ofengand for discussing with me matters related to ribosome function. However, neither they nor any of the individuals mentioned above are responsible for the speculations this paper contains. This work is supported by a grant from the National Institutes of Health (AI-09167). The neutron data on which the map depends were collected at Brookhaven National Laboratory under the auspices of the Department of Energy.

REFERENCES

Bacon, G.E. 1975. *Neutron diffraction*. Oxford University Press, London.

Barta, A., G. Steiner, J. Brosius, H.F. Noller, and E. Kuechler. 1984. Identification of a site on the 23S ribosomal RNA located at the peptidyl transferase center. *Proc. Natl. Acad. Sci.* **81:** 3607.

Capel, M.S. and V. Ramakrishnan. 1987. Neutron-scattering topography of the proteins of the small ribosomal subunit. *Methods Enzymol.* (in press).

Engelman, D.M. 1979. Neutron scattering measurement of protein pair scattering functions from ribosomes containing deuterated proteins. *Methods Enzymol.* **59:** 656.

Engelman, D.M. and P.B. Moore. 1972. A new method for the determination of biological quaternary structure by neutron scattering. *Proc. Natl. Acad. Sci.* **69:** 1997.

Gren, E.J. 1984. Recognition of messenger RNA during translational initiation in *Escherichia coli*. *Biochimie* **66:** 1.

Held, W.A., B. Ballou, S. Mizushima, and M. Nomura. 1974. Assembly mapping of 30S ribosomal proteins from *Escherichia coli*. *J. Biol. Chem.* **249:** 3103.

Lake, J.A. 1985. Evolving ribosome structure: Domains in archaebacteria, eubacteria, eocytes, and eukaryotes. *Annu. Rev. Biochem.* **54:** 507.

Lambert, J.M., G. Boileau, J.A. Cover, and R.R. Traut. 1983. Crosslinks between ribosomal proteins of 30S subunits in 70S tight couples and in 30S subunits. *Biochemistry* **22:** 3913.

May, R. 1978. Ph.D. thesis, Technical University, München.

Mizushima, S. and M. Nomura. 1970. Assembly mapping of 30S ribosomal proteins from *E. coli*. *Nature* **226:** 1214.

Moore, P.B. 1979. The preparation of deuterated ribosomal materials for neutron scattering. *Methods Enzymol.* **59:** 639.

———. 1986. Polypeptide polymerase: The structure and function of the ribosome in 1985. In *Proceedings of the Robert A. Welch Conferences on Chemical Research XXIX. Genetic Chemistry: The Molecular Basis of Heredity*, p. 185. Robert A. Welch Foundation, Houston, Texas.

Moore, P.B. and D.M. Engelman. 1979. On the feasibility and interpretation of intersubunit distance measurements using neutron scattering. *Methods Enzymol.* **59:** 629.

Moore, P.B., J.A. Langer, and D.M. Engelman. 1978. The measurement of the locations and radii of gyration of proteins in the 30S ribosomal subunit of *E. coli* by neutron scattering. *J. Appl. Crystallogr.* **11:** 479.

Oakes, M., E. Henderson, A. Scheinman, M. Clark, and J.A. Lake. 1986. Ribosomes structure, function, and evolution: Mapping ribosomal RNA, proteins, and functional sites in three dimensions. In *Structure, function, and genetics of ribosomes* (ed. B. Hardesty and G. Kramer), p. 47. Springer-Verlag, New York.

Ofengand, J., J. Ciesiolka, R. Denman, and K. Nurse. 1986. Structural and functional interactions of the tRNA-ribosome complex. In *Structure, function, and genetics of ribosomes* (ed. B. Hardesty and G. Kramer), p. 473. Springer-Verlag, New York.

Ofengand, J., P. Gornicki, K. Nurse, and M. Boublik. 1984. On the structural organization of the tRNA-ribosome complex. *Proc. Alfred Benz. Symp.* **19:** 293.

Pellegrini, M. and C.R. Cantor. 1977. Affinity labeling of ribosomes. In *Molecular mechanism of protein synthesis* (ed. H. Weissbach and S. Pestka), p. 203. Academic Press, New York.

Ramakrishnan, V.R. and P.B. Moore. 1981. Analysis of neutron distance data. *J. Mol. Biol.* **153:** 719.

Shine, J. and L. Dalgarno. 1974. The 3'-terminal sequence of *Escherichia coli* 16S ribosomal RNA: Complementarity to nonsense triplets and ribosome binding sites. *Proc. Natl. Acad. Sci.* **71:** 1342.

Steitz, J.A. 1980. RNA-RNA interactions during polypeptide chain initiation. In *Ribosomes: Structure, function and genetics* (ed. G. Chambliss et al.), p. 479. University Park Press, Baltimore.

Stoeffler, G. and M. Stoeffler-Meilicke. 1986. Immuno electron microscopy on *Escherichia coli* ribosomes. In *Structure, function, and genetics of ribosomes* (ed. B. Hardesty and G. Kramer), p. 28. Springer-Verlag, New York.

Stoekel, P., R. May, I. Strell, Z. Geha, W. Hoppe, H. Heumann, W. Zillig, and H.L. Crespi. 1979. Determination of intersubunit distances and subunit shape parameters in DNA-dependent RNA polymerase by neutron scattering. *J. Appl. Crystallogr.* **12:** 176.

Traub, P. and M. Nomura. 1968. Structure and function of *E. coli* ribosomes V. Reconstitution of functionally active 30S ribosomal particles from RNA and proteins. *Proc. Natl. Acad. Sci.* **59:** 777.

Traut, R.R., D.S. Tewari, A. Sommer, G.R. Gavino, H.M. Olson, and D.G. Glitz. 1986. Protein topography of ribosomal functional domains: Effects of monoclonal antibodies to different epitopes in *Escherichia coli* protein L7/L12 on ribosome function and structure. In *Structure, function, and genetics of ribosomes* (ed. B. Hardesty and G. Kramer), p. 286. Springer-Verlag, New York.

Wittmann-Liebold, B. 1986. Ribosomal proteins: Their structure and evolution. In *Structure, function, and genetics of ribosomes* (ed. B. Hardesty and G. Kramer), p. 326. Springer-Verlag, New York.

Woese, C.R. 1980. Just so stories and Rube Goldberg machines: Speculations on the origin of the protein synthetic machinery. In *Ribosomes: Structure, function, and genetics* (ed. G. Chambliss et al.), p. 357. University Park Press, Baltimore.

Wool, I.G. 1986. Studies of the structure of eukaryotic (mammalian) ribosomes. In *Structure, function, and genetics of ribosomes* (ed. B. Hardesty and G. Kramer), p. 391. Springer-Verlag, New York.

Approaches to the Determination of the Three-dimensional Architecture of Ribosomal Particles

A. YONATH,[*][†] K.R. LEONARD,[‡] S. WEINSTEIN,[*][§] AND H.G. WITTMANN[§]

[*]Department of Structural Chemistry, Weizmann Institute of Science, Rehovot, Israel;
[†]Max-Planck Research Unit for Structural Molecular Biology, Hamburg, Federal Republic of Germany;
[‡]European Molecular Biology Laboratory, Heidelberg, Federal Republic of Germany;
[§]Max-Planck Institute for Molecular Genetics, West Berlin (Dahlem)

The intricate and accurate process of biosynthesis of protein molecules occurs in a similar manner on ribosomes of all organisms. Ribosomes consist of two subunits that associate upon initiation of protein biosynthesis. Each subunit is a structurally defined assembly of proteins and RNA chains with a characteristic sedimentation coefficient (e.g., 30S and 50S for the small and the large ribosomal subunits from bacteria). During the last two decades a vast amount of information has been accumulated about the function and the chemical, biological, and genetic properties of ribosomes (for review, see Chambliss et al. 1979; Wittmann 1982, 1983; Hardesty and Kramer 1986). This knowledge has shed light on the entire process of protein biosynthesis, although the understanding of the detailed mechanism of this process is still severely limited by the lack of a molecular model.

As objects for crystallographic studies, ribosomal particles are of enormous size, with no internal symmetry. Furthermore, they are unstable and flexible. Therefore, even the first necessary step of these studies, namely crystallization, seemed, until recently, to be a formidable task. Despite that, a systematic exploration of crystallization conditions supported by development of innovative experimental techniques for fine control of the volume of the crystallization drops, as well as for sophisticated seeding (Yonath et al. 1982a; Yonath and Wittmann 1987a,b), led to reproducible production of crystals of intact ribosomal particles.

Bacterial ribosomes were chosen because they are well characterized biochemically, they can be prepared in high purity and large amounts, and they provide a system that is independent of in vivo events. Thus, the natural capacity of eukaryotic ribosomes to form two-dimensional sheets, stuck to cell membranes (e.g., Milligan and Unwin 1986), has been extended by us to a higher degree of organization, expressed in vitro. As a result, three-dimensional crystals and two-dimensional sheets of intact ribosomal particles from *Escherichia coli*, *Bacillus stearothermophilus*, *Thermus thermophilus,* and *Halobacterium marismortui* have been obtained (Table 1 and Yonath et al. 1980, 1982b, 1983a,b, 1984, 1986a,b,c, 1987; Wittmann et al. 1982; Yonath 1984; Shevack et al. 1985; Wittmann and

Yonath 1985; Piefke et al. 1986; Shoham et al. 1986; Makowski et al. 1987; Yonath and Wittmann 1987a,b,c). Currently, crystals grow from virtually every preparation of large ribosomal particles from *B. stearothermophilus* and *H. marismortui*, but, because of the intricate nature of the particles, the exact conditions for the growth of well-ordered and large crystals must still be slightly varied for each ribosomal preparation. Moreover, the quality of the crystals depends, in a manner not yet fully characterized, on the procedure used in preparing the particles and on the bacterial strain. There is a strong correlation between crystallizability and biological activity of all our crystallization systems. So far, inactive ribosomal particles could not be crystallized. Moreover, in spite of the natural tendency of ribosomes to disintegrate, all crystallized particles retain their biological activity, even for several months, in contrast to the short lifetime of isolated ribosomes in solution. This property accords well with the hypothesis that when external conditions (e.g., hibernation) demand prolonged storage of potentially active ribosomes in living organisms, temporary periodic organization occurs in vivo.

Synchrotron radiation provides the most intense, well-collimated X-ray beam. It is essential for crystallographic data collection from crystals of ribosomal particles due to their large unit cell dimensions (Table 1), their fragility, and their sensitivity. Until recently, all our crystallographic studies, including the assessment of the quality of the crystals and the determination of the resolution limits and the unit-cell parameters, had to be carried out solely with synchrotron radiation. The newly developed method of crystallographic data collection at cryotemperature (Hope 1985) paved the way for conducting preliminary experiments with less powerful X-ray sources, such as rotating anodes.

Phase information is essential for maturation of crystallographic studies. We are currently attempting to determine phases by both conventional and novel heavy-atom techniques. A great advantage for the production of heavy-atom derivatives is the large variety of ribosomal components and the wide spectrum of materials that interact specifically with these components (e.g., antibiotics; for review, see Nierhaus and Witt-

Table 1. Packing Parameters of Two- and Three-dimensional Crystals of Ribosomal Particles

| Source | Crystal form | Cell Dimensions, (Å) determined by | |
		electron microscopy	X-ray crystallography
70S *E. coli*	A[a]	340 × 340 × 590; 120°; P6	
70S *Bacillus stearothermophilus*	2D[b], AS[a]	200 × 440; 93°	
50S *Halobacterium marismortui*	1, P[a]	310 × 350; 105°	
	2, P	148 × 186; 95°	147 × 181; 97°
	3, P	170 × 180; 75°	214 × 300 × 590; C222₁
50S *Bacillus stearothermophilus*	1, A	130 × 254; 95°	
	2, A	156 × 288; 97°	
	3, A	260 × 288; 105°	
	4, A	405 × 405 × 256; 120°	
	5, A	213 × 235 × 315; 120°	
	6[c], A	330 × 670 × 850; 90°	360 × 680 × 920; P2₁2₁2₁
	2D, A	145 × 311; 108°; P2	
	2D, AS[a]	148 × 360; 109°; P1	

[a]Crystals are grown by vapor diffusion from alcohols or their mixtures (A), polyethylene glycol (P), or by mixing with ammonium sulfate (AS).
[b]All forms, unless marked 2D, are three-dimensional crystals. 2D = two-dimensional sheets.
[c]Same form and parameters for crystals of the large ribosomal subunits of – L11 mutant of the same source.

mann 1980). In favorable cases, derivatives can be used for an unambiguous localization of specific ribosomal components. Results of electron microscopy may also contribute toward phase determination. The model of the particle under study, obtained at medium resolution by three-dimensional image reconstruction of two-dimensional sheets, could be placed in the crystallographic unit cell using crystal-packing information derived from the electron micrographs of thin sections of the investigated crystal (Leonard et al. 1982). This, together with information obtained from crystallographic studies of isolated individual ribosomal components at high resolution (Leijonmarck et al. 1980; Appelt et al. 1981; Wilson et al. 1986), can be used for iterative phase determination by molecular replacement methods, assuming that the conformations of crystallized isolated components are similar to their conformations within the ribosome.

EXPERIMENTAL PROCEDURES

Ribosomes and their subunits were prepared and their integrity and activity were checked as described (Arad et al. 1987b; Yonath and Wittmann 1987a). Procedures for the production of three-dimensional crystals and two-dimensional sheets, the crystallographic data collection, and the three-dimensional image reconstruction are described in detail (Yonath et al. 1982a, 1986c; Arad et al. 1984, 1987b; Piefke et al. 1986; Makowski et al. 1987; Yonath and Wittmann 1987a,b,c). All crystallographic studies reported here have been performed using synchrotron radiation, at 4°C and −180°C (Hope 1985).

Radioactive *N*-ethylmaleimide was reacted with ribosomal particles to determine the accessibility of

sulfhydryl groups of ribosomal proteins of the 50S subunits from *B. stearothermophilus* and *H. marismortui*. For the latter, this procedure was also used to locate these groups, since the sequence of only a few proteins from this source is known.

A gold cluster and its radioactive derivative were prepared following basically a known procedure (Bartlett et al. 1978). Functional groups were attached to the gold clusters for covalent binding to ribosomal particles through accessible sulfhydryl groups (S. Weinstein and W. Jahn, in prep.). The extent of binding of the gold cluster was determined by measuring the radioactivity associated with the 50S particles, as well as by neutron activation (performed at Soreq Nuclear Research Laboratories, Israel). The proteins that bind *N*-ethylmaleimide were identified by locating the radioactivity on a two-dimensional gel electropherogram of the ribosomal proteins.

RESULTS AND DISCUSSION

Three-dimensional Image Reconstruction

The large size of ribosomal particles, which is an obstacle for crystallographic studies, permits their direct investigation by electron microscopy. Thus, in the case of intact ribosomal particles, a combination of X-ray crystallography with electron microscopy and three-dimensional image reconstruction should be possible and is expected to provide a powerful tool for our studies. Using electron microscopy, the initial steps of crystallization can be detected and the tendency of crystallization of native and modified particles can be followed rather quickly, in contrast to the long time needed for the growth of large three-dimensional crystals. Results from electron microscopy can also be used to locate and orient the particles within the crystallographic unit cells, and models obtained by three-dimensional image reconstruction may facilitate extraction of phase information. Thus, structure determination by three-dimensional image reconstruction from two-dimensional sheets is justified not only in its own right, but also because of its expected contribution to the determination of phases needed for crystallographic analysis. Therefore, we have pursued, side by side, X-ray crystallography using three-dimensional crystals and three-dimensional image reconstruction from two-dimensional sheets.

We have developed two procedures for the growth of two-dimensional sheets of ribosomal particles: (1) in hanging drops from alcohols (AL) (Arad et al. 1984); and (2) on flat surfaces using mixtures of salts and alcohols (ST) (Piefke et al. 1986; Arad et al. 1987 and in prep.; Yonath et al. 1987). These sheets were negatively stained with either gold-thioglucose or uranyl acetate and used for three-dimensional image reconstruction studies.

Gold-thioglucose is an inert stain and is expected to reveal the outer contour of the particles. Additional information may be obtained from sheets stained with uranyl acetate. This stain is chemically reactive; thus along with its ability to elucidate the external contour of the particle, it may interact with the negatively charged components of the ribosomal particles (most likely the rRNA). The extent of this interaction is somewhat irregular, since it depends on the accessibility of the appropriate components and may be influenced by irregularities of the electron microscopy grid. In general, the resolution and the quality of sheets that have been negatively stained by uranyl acetate are lower than those of sheets stained by gold-thioglucose. In favorable cases the influence of the staining procedure is minimal. An example may be the tunnel of the large ribosomal subunits (see below). It is resolved in all reconstructions of the two-dimensional sheets of 50S subunits from *B. stearothermophilus*, independent of the staining material (Yonath et al. 1987), as well as in the reconstructed model of the unstained sheets from chick embryos (Milligan and Unwin 1986).

The two-dimensional sheets of 70S particles from B. stearothermophilus. These are built of dimers, packed in relatively small unit cells: $190 \pm 15 \times 420 \pm 15$ Å, $\gamma = 107° \pm 3°$ (Fig. 1). Optical diffraction patterns of electron micrographs of negatively stained specimens with uranyl acetate and of cross-linked sheets stained with gold-thioglucose extend to 40 Å and 47 Å, respectively.

Eleven reconstructions of sheets from three different preparations have been performed. The resulting model of the ribosomal particle (Fig. 1) has average dimensions similar to those determined by other physical methods (Wittmann 1983). On the basis of the known molecular weight of the 70S particle (2.3×10^6)

and of the volume obtained from the three-dimensional image reconstruction, the calculated density of the particle is 1.3–1.4 g/cm^3, and the V_m for a hypothetical crystal of the thickness of the sheets (about 200 Å) is 2.6–2.7 Å^3/dalton.

Several features were revealed by the analysis (Fig. 1) of models derived from the gold-thioglucose-stained sheets. The two ribosomal subunits are arranged around an empty space of a volume of $4 \times 10^5 \pm 2 \times 10^5$ Å^3. This space is large enough to accommodate most of the components of protein biosynthesis. There are variations in the size of this space as revealed in different reconstructions. This may result from sheets, built of ribosomes that may carry some components of protein biosynthesis, such as tRNA or fractions of mRNA.

Because only a small fraction of the particles in the drop actually consists of two-dimensional sheets, they could not be separated from the rest of the drop. Therefore, we tested the migration profile on sucrose gradients of the ribosomal particles in the crystallizing drops. It was found that particles subjected to crystallization conditions comigrate with standard particles.

The two ribosomal subunits are fairly separated. Only the two ends of the small subunit are in contact with the large subunit. The sum of the contact areas is 400–800 Å^2. The overall shapes of both subunits have been compared with models that have previously been suggested for these particles. There is a similarity between the model of the small subunit obtained by visualization of single particles (Wittmann 1983) and that revealed by our studies. Isolated 30S particles seem to be wider than the reconstructed ones within the 70S particles. This may be a consequence of the contact of the isolated particles with the flat electron microscope grid. In contrast, particles within the crystalline sheets are held together by their interactions with the 50S particles as well as by interparticle crystalline forces. These construct a network that may stabilize the conformation of the particles and decrease, or even eliminate, the influence of the flatness of the grids. The portion of the reconstructed 70S particle that we assigned as the large subunit may be correlated to the image of this subunit as revealed in our previous studies (Fig. 2 and Yonath et al. 1987), both at 28 Å (the actual resolution of the studies) and at 55 Å.

Reconstruction of models of 70S ribosomes from sheets stained with uranyl acetate led to a model that shows the features described above, as well as regions where uranyl acetate, acting as a positive stain, was incorporated into the particle. This may indicate that in these regions the RNA is concentrated and/or easily exposed to the stain. Such regions could be located on the surface of the large subunit where it faces the internal empty space. Penetration of uranyl acetate to the region assigned as "collar's ridge" on the small subunits was also detected. In both cases, the staining of these areas with uranyl acetate may stem either from the existence of exposed rRNA regions, as previously found (Milligan and Unwin 1986), or from the presence of mRNA and tRNA in these locations.

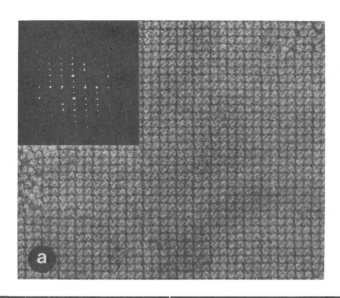

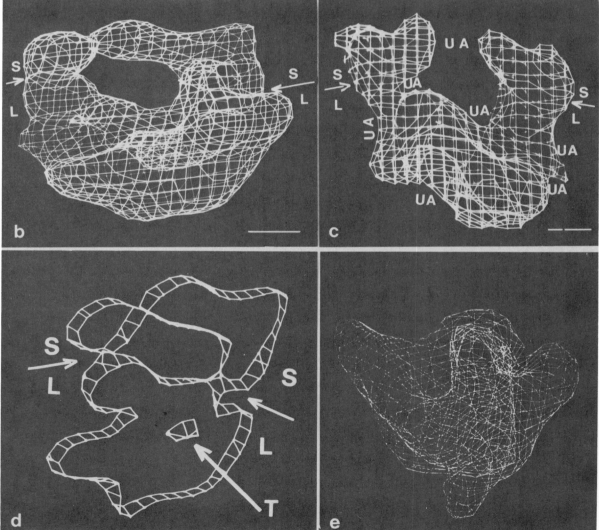

Figure 1. (*See facing page for legend.*)

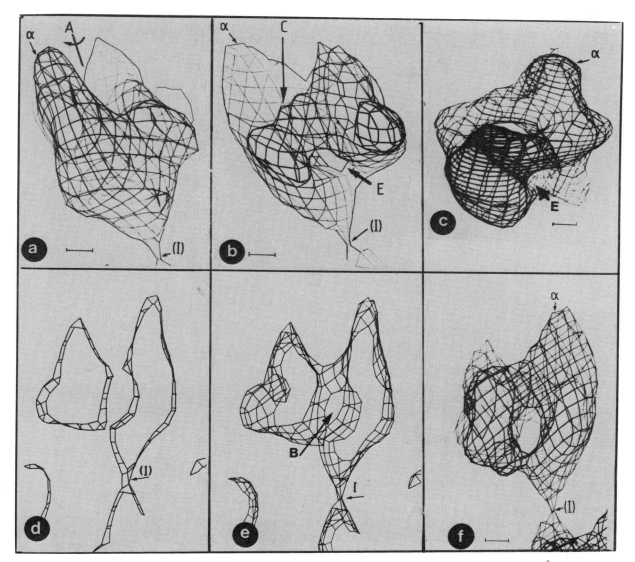

Figure 2. Computer graphic display of the outline of the reconstructed model of the 50S ribosomal subunit at 30 Å resolution. α marks the longest arm. E is the exit site. (*a*) A side view of the model. The entire particle and part of a second one are shown. The arrow (I) points at the crystal contact between the two particles. A marks the approximate axis around which the model was turned to obtain the view shown in *b*. Bar length=20 Å. (*b*) The model shown in *a* rotated about the A axis. C points at the cleft between the projecting arms, at the site it turns into the tunnel. (*c*) A view into the tunnel from the cleft. (*d*) The outline of a 20-Å-thick section in the middle of the reconstructed model, showing that the tunnel spans the particle. (*e*) The outline of a 40-Å-thick section in the middle of the reconstructed model. The branching of the tunnel is seen (B). (*f*) The model viewed into the branch of the tunnel from the exit point.

Figure 1. Computer graphic display of the outline of the reconstructed model of the 70S ribosome at 47 Å resolution. (*a*) Image of a two-dimensional sheet (× 28,000) of 70S particles from *B. stearothermophilus*, stained by gold-thioglucose, and an optical diffraction pattern from an area containing about 20 × 15 unit cells. (*b*) Computer graphic display of the outline of the reconstructed model of the 70S ribosome at 47 Å resolution, stained with gold-thioglucose. L and S indicate the 50S and the 30S subunits, respectively. The arrows point at the interface between the two subunits. Bar length=20 Å. (*c*) Computer graphic display of the outline of the reconstructed model of the 70S ribosome at 42 Å resolution stained with uranyl acetate, at a similar orientation to that shown in *b*. UA shows the regions to which uranyl acetate binds. L and S indicate the 50S and the 30S subunits. The arrows point at the interface between the two subunits. Bar length=20 Å. (*d*) The outline of a 20-Å-thick section in the middle of the reconstructed model of the 70S ribosome. T indicates part of the tunnel. (*e*) The 30 Å resolution reconstructed model of the 50S subunit, obtained as in Fig. 2, viewed in a projection which resembles models derived from electron microscopy studies of single particles.

733

The model for the 50S subunits. This was reconstructed at 30 Å resolution. Two-dimensional sheets of these particles from *B. stearothermophilus* have been obtained from three different preparations using both above mentioned procedures. In all cases the sheets consist of small unit cells (e.g., $145 \pm 10 \times 311 \pm 20$ Å, $\gamma = 108 \pm 3°$ for the AL sheets). These cell dimensions are close to those of forms 1 and 2 of three-dimensional crystals of the same particles (Table 1 and Yonath 1984). Both AL and ST are well ordered, and optical diffraction patterns of electron micrographs of negatively stained specimens extend to 30 Å and 28 Å, respectively. In both cases each unit cell contains two particles with dimensions similar to those obtained by other methods (for reviews, see Chambliss et al. 1979; Wittmann 1982, 1983; Hardesty and Kramer 1986). Based on the known molecular weight of this particle (1.6×10^6 daltons), and on the thickness of the sheets (160–170 Å), as determined by the three-dimensional image reconstruction studies, the calculated density of a 50S particle is 1.3–1.4 g/cm^3, and the V_m for a hypothetical crystal is 2.6–2.7 Å^3/dalton. Both are in good agreement with values tabulated by Matthews (1968) and calculated for three-dimensional crystals of 50S subunits from *H. marismortui* (Makowski et al. 1987), as well as for other large nucleoprotein structures (Hogle 1982; Richmond et al. 1984).

Interparticle contacts within the sheets are clearly revealed in our three-dimensional map (Fig. 2). The best-defined contact area is 5–12 Å in diameter, compatible with the regular intermolecular interactions found in crystals of proteins or nucleic acids. As these dimensions are beyond the resolution of our studies, the nature of these contacts cannot be identified.

The main features revealed by our analysis are shown in Figure 2. The particle has a concave surface that consists of several protrusions 25–30 Å in diameter, the approximate size of globular proteins of molecular weights typical of many ribosomal proteins. A long arm is located on one side of the particle (bottom of the particle shown in Fig. 2). Several projecting arms, two of which are longer than the others, are arranged radially around the other edge (upper side of the particle shown in Fig. 2), near the presumed interface with the 30S subunit (Fig. 1). A narrow elongated cleft is formed between the projecting arms and turns into a tunnel of a diameter of up to 25 Å and a length of 100–120 Å. This tunnel is present in all reconstructions of the ST sheets, independent of the staining material, as well as in reconstructed 80S ribosomes from chick embryos (Milligan and Unwin 1986). In every reconstructed particle there is a region of low density that branches off the tunnel to form a Y (or V) shape, and terminates on the other side of the particle (Fig. 2). As yet, we cannot determine the exact nature of this region. It may be a loosely packed protein region, but in some reconstructed models the density of the branch is so low that it appears as a branch of the main tunnel.

The functional significance of the tunnel is still to be determined. Originating at the presumed site for actual protein biosynthesis and terminating on the other end of the particle, and being of a diameter large enough to accommodate even the largest amino acids, this tunnel appears to provide the path taken by the nascent polypeptide chain. Furthermore, this tunnel is of a length that could accommodate and protect from proteolytic enzymes a peptide of about 40 amino acids in an extended conformation (Malkin and Rich 1967; Blobel and Sabatini 1970; Smith et al. 1978). It remains to be seen whether the tunnel terminates at a location compatible with that assigned by immunoelectron microscopy as the exit site for the growing polypeptide chain (Bernabeau and Lake 1982).

We have also reconstructed a model using a selected subset of diffraction data at lower resolution (55 Å). At this resolution the particle is almost spherical and shows only two thick and short arms instead of the elongated arms resolved in the 30 Å resolution studies. This accords well with the shape of the portion of the reconstructed model (at 47 Å) of the 70S particle assigned as the 50S subunit (Fig. 1), as well as with models derived from electron microscopy studies of single particles. It should be mentioned that the tunnel is clearly resolved in the low-resolution reconstructed model of the 50S particle, whereas in the 70S reconstructed particle there are only some indications for its existence. Thus, a portion of the tunnel could be detected in a section through the particle (Fig. 1). As mentioned above, the 70S particles were harvested while active, and it is feasible that nascent protein chains are still attached to a part of them. It is conceivable that the tunnel is only partially resolved due to this and/or to the intrinsic low resolution of this reconstruction.

Several models for 50S ribosomal subunits were suggested previously, based on electron microscopic visualization and averaging of single particles. Our model is more similar to those that have no flat surfaces and to those in which the projecting arms are arranged radially. It can be positioned so that its projected view resembles the usual image seen when single particles are investigated by electron microscopy (Fig. 1e). In addition, there are a few filtered images of two-dimensional sheets tilted by certain angles, which show the same shape and include the characteristic features that have been visualized by electron microscopy of single particles (Fig. 3). At the same time, there are some discrepancies in the nature of the gross structural features between our model and the others, which, as in the case of the 70S particles, probably stem from the basic differences between visualization of isolated particles in projection and the inherently more objective character of structure analysis by diffraction methods.

As mentioned above, the resolution of the sheets stained with uranyl acetate is somewhat lower (32–35 Å) than that of the sheets stained with gold-thioglucose. Consequently, the reconstructed model shows less detail. However, the essential features—the concave shape, the tunnel, and the projecting arms—are resolved. Comparison of this model with that obtained

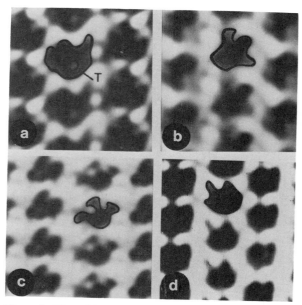

Figure 3. Filtered images of electron micrographs of sheets of 50S subunits from *B. stearothermophilus* in which the depicted view resembles that derived from electron microscopy of single particles. (*a*) AL sheets stained with uranyl acetate. The tunnel T can be detected. Tilt of 25°. (*b–d*) ST sheets stained with gold thioglucose. Tilts of 35°, 20° and 30°, respectively.

from the same sheets stained with gold-thioglucose shows regions (on one of the long arms, on the body of the particle, and near the interface with the 30S) where uranyl acetate, acting as a positive stain, is incorporated into the particle. This may indicate that in these regions the rRNA is concentrated and/or easily exposed to the stain.

There is a significant shortening of the long projecting arms in models reconstructed from sheets grown from alcohols. This may indicate that the arms are positioned firmly in an environment of salts, but may flex when exposed to alcohols. Inherent flexibility of the long arms has been observed also in reconstruction of rotated single particles (Verschoor et al. 1985).

Assignment of the known functional domains of 70S particles and of 50S subunits to the various structural features still awaits further investigations. In view of the recent progress of our crystallographic studies and of our ability to reproducibly produce two-dimensional sheets of native as well as modified ribosomal particles, we are hopeful that we shall be able to locate specific sites on a detailed model in the foreseeable future.

Crystallographic Studies

The process of crystal growth is initiated by nucleation. Although many biological molecules and complexes have been crystallized, little is known about the mechanism of nucleation. Most of the data currently available concerning the process of nucleation of crystals of biological systems are based on rather indirect evidence, such as monitoring aggregation under crys-

tallization conditions by scattering techniques. Crystals of ribosomal particles provided an excellent system for direct investigation of nucleation. In our experimental setup, the crystallization process was interrupted before the formation of mature crystals, and the crystallization medium was examined by electron microscopy. It was found that the first step in crystal growth is unspecific aggregation and that nucleation starts by a rearrangement within the aggregates (Yonath et al. 1982b).

Crystallographic studies are currently being performed on crystals from the large ribosomal subunits from *B. stearothermophilus* and *H. marismortui*. Two crystal forms of 50S subunits from *B. stearothermophilus* have been grown. The first are obtained directly in X-ray capillaries at 4°C by vapor diffusion from mixtures of methanol and ethylene glycol as long pointed needles that may reach the size of $1.5 \times 0.3 \times 0.2$ mm (Fig. 4). Since most of them grow with one of their faces adhering to the walls of the capillaries, it was possible to irradiate them without removing the original growth solution. This is essential since any handling of these crystals is virtually impossible. Although most of the crystals grow with their long axes parallel to the capillary axis, a fair number grow in different directions. Thus, using synchrotron radiation, it was possible to determine the unit cell constants ($360 \times 680 \times 920$ Å) of an orthorhombic form ($P2_12_12_1$) and to obtain diffraction patterns from all the zones (Fig. 4) without manipulating the crystals (Yonath et al. 1984, 1986c). A fair amount of crystallographic data to 18 Å resolution has been collected from these crystals.

Several diffraction patterns of single crystals as well as those of samples containing large numbers of microcrystals of this form include oriented arcs and distinct spots, with spacings similar to those measured from diffuse diffraction patterns of ribosome gels and extracted rRNA (Klug et al. 1961; Langridge and Holmes 1962) and extending to 3.5 Å. For aligned crystals the average arc length is 60°. Such patterns may arise from partial orientation of the nucleic acid component within the particle.

Recently, a second form of crystals from this source has been obtained. Here the growth solution contains polyethylene glycol, magnesium chloride, and ammonium sulfate. Crystals of this form grow within 10–14 days at 4°C, appear as polygons, and reach a maximum size of $0.1 \times 0.1 \times 0.1$ mm. Extensive attempts to increase their size by seeding have been, so far, unsuccessful.

Crystals of the 50S subunits from *H. marismortui* grow as thin plates at 19°C by vapor diffusion from polyethylene glycol in the presence of salts that mimic, to some extent, the composition of the natural environment of these bacteria, the Dead Sea. Although fragile, these crystals can be manipulated. Thus, seeding was used for obtaining larger (maximum size $0.6 \times 0.6 \times 0.2$ mm) as well as more ordered crystals (Fig. 5). We have taken advantage of the major role played by the Mg^{++} concentration in crystallization of ribosomal particles.

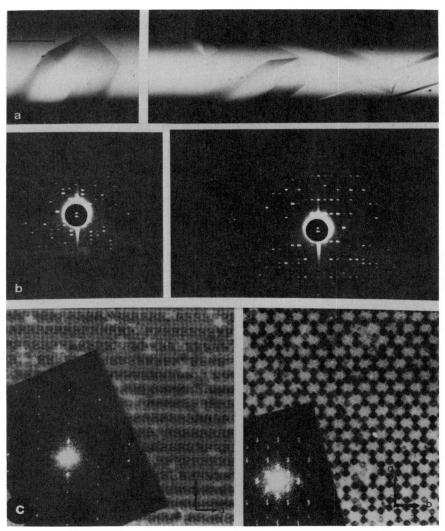

Figure 4. (*a*) Crystals of the 50S ribosomal subunits from *B. stearothermophilus* grown in 0.5-mm X-ray capillaries by vapor diffusion at 4°C. Crystallization mixture of 20 μl 50S ribosomal subunits (10–20 mg/ml) in H-I buffer (Yonath et al. 1980), 0.01 M spermine, 1% methanol, and 10 mM HEPES or glycine buffer (pH 8.4) was equilibrated with a reservoir of 12% methanol, 12% ethylene diol, and 0.5 M $NaCl_2$, pH 8.4. (*b*) X-ray diffraction patterns from crystals similar to those shown in *a*, obtained at −4°C with synchrotron radiation (A1 station at CHESS/CORNELL Univ. operating at 5 GeV, current 30–40 mA) with 0.3 mm collimated X-ray beam with wavelength of 1.55 Å, on a HUBER precession camera equipped with a He path. Exposure time 3 min, crystal to film distance 200 mm. (*Left*) 1° rotation photograph of Ok1 zone, 680 × 920 Å. (*Right*) 0.4° rotation photograph of hk0 zone, 360 × 680 Å. (*c*) Electron micrographs of positively stained (2% uranyl acetate) thin sections of crystals similar to those shown in *a* that have been fixed in 0.2% glutaraldehyde and embedded in resin ERL 4206. Optical diffraction patterns are inserted. (*Left*) Section approximately perpendicular to that shown on the right. Repeat distances measured from optical diffraction: 330 × 1050 Å. This corresponds to the h01 zone (360 × 920 Å) in the X-ray patterns. (*Right*) Micrograph showing the characteristic open packing of this crystal form. The orthogonal choice of axes corresponds to the 680 × 920 Å zone observed in the X-ray diffraction patterns. Lattice spacing calculated from optical diffraction: 670 × 850 Å.

It was found that three-dimensional crystals of 50S ribosomal subunits from *B. stearothermophilus* grow in relatively low Mg^{++} concentration, whereas the production of two-dimensional sheets requires a high Mg^{++} concentration, at which growth of three-dimensional crystals is prohibited. Similarly, for spontaneous crystal growth of 50S subunits from *H. marismortui*, the lower the Mg^{++} concentration is, the thicker the crystals are. With these points in mind, a variation of the standard seeding procedure has been developed. Thin

crystals of the 50S subunits from *H. marismortui* grown spontaneously under the lowest possible Mg^{++} concentration are transferred to mixtures in which the Mg^{++} concentration is so low that the transferred crystals almost dissolve, but after several days new microcrystals can be observed. These reach their maximum size after 3–4 weeks, are 10–30-fold thicker than the original seeds, are very well ordered, and diffract to a resolution of 5.5 Å (Fig. 6). They have relatively small unit cells of 214 × 300 × 584 Å ($C222_1$), which are compactly packed, in contrast to the open structure of the large crystals of *B. stearothermophilus* (Fig. 4).

Between −2°C and 4°C, these crystals are rather stable in the synchrotron beam. However, their higher resolution diffraction terms decay within the first few minutes. Thus only 1–3 rotation patterns could be taken from an individual crystal, and more than 260 crystals were needed to collect an entire data set. Recently, we have shown that at −180°C, irradiated crystals hardly show radiation damage for days. Thus, for the first time, a full data set could be collected from a single crystal. Moreover, under these conditions, the life expectation of the crystals is long enough to allow X-ray diffraction experiments using rotating anodes as X-ray generators. Thus, initial parameters such as quality of crystals, their resolution, unit cell constants, and isomorphism may be determined at conventional X-ray diffraction laboratories, and the progress of the struc-

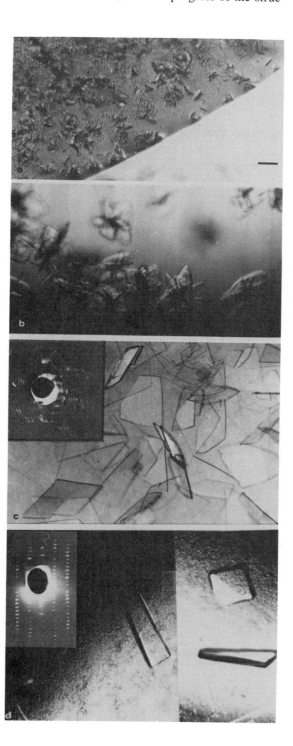

Figure 5. Growth of large, ordered three-dimensional crystals of the 50S ribosomal subunits from *H. marismortui* by vapor diffusion at 19°C (Bar length=0.2 mm). (*a*) Microcrystals obtained within 1–2 days. Droplets of 7–8% polyethylene glycol (PEG), 2.5 M KCl, 0.5 M NH$_4$Cl, 0.15–0.20 M MgCl$_2$, and 10 mM spermidine (pH 5.0–5.2) were equilibrated with 3.0 M KCl, 9% PEG, 0.5 M NH$_4$Cl, and 0.20 M MgCl$_2$. (*b*) Crystals obtained within 2–3 days in droplets containing lower KCl concentration than used in *a*. Droplet of 4–5% PEG, 1.2–1.7 M KCl, 0.5 M NH$_4$Cl, 0.10 M MgCl$_2$, and 10 mM spermidine were equilibrated with reservoirs as in *a*. (*c*) Crystals obtained within 3–5 days from droplets similar to those used for *b*, equilibrated with reservoirs of lower KCl concentrations. Droplet of 4–5% PEG, 1.2 M KCl, 0.5 M NH$_4$Cl, 0.05–0.10 M MgCl$_2$, and 10 mM spermidine (pH 5.0–5.6) were equilibrated with 1.7 M KCl, 9% PEG, 0.5 M NH$_4$Cl, and 0.10 M MgCl$_2$. An X-ray diffraction pattern taken perpendicular to the thin axis of the crystals, obtained under conditions similar to those described in Fig. 6, is inserted. (*d*) Crystals obtained by seeding of crystals from *c* in a crystallization drop containing 5% PEG, 1.2 M KCl, 0.5 M NH$_4$Cl, 0.03 M MgCl$_2$ (pH 5.6), which was equilibrated with 7% PEG, 1.7 M KCl, 0.5 M NH$_4$Cl, and 0.03 M MgCl$_2$ (pH 5.6). Seeds were small, well-shaped crystals, transferred into a stabilization solution of 7% PEG in 1.7 M KCl, 0.5 M NH$_4$Cl, and 0.05 M MgCl$_2$ (pH 5.6). An X-ray diffraction pattern taken perpendicular to the thin axis of the crystals, obtained under conditions described in Fig. 6, is inserted.

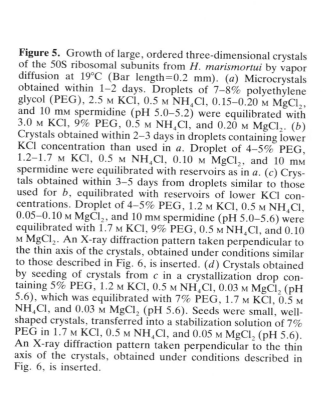

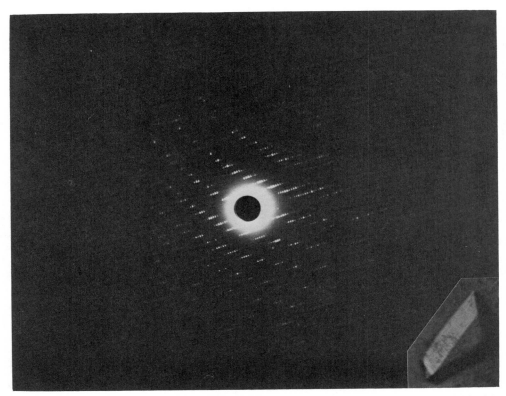

Figure 6. A 1° rotation pattern of a crystal similar to the inserted one. The pattern was obtained at −180°C with synchrotron radiation (7.1 station at SSRL). Wavelength, 1.54 Å; exposure time, 2 min; crystal to film distance, 135 mm. (*Insert*) A crystal of the 50S ribosomal subunits of *H. marismortui* obtained under similar conditions to Fig. 5 (*d*).

ture determination is hoped to be less dependent on the availability of synchrotron radiation.

Most recently we were able to obtain three-dimensional crystals from small (30S) ribosomal subunits from *Thermus thermophilus*. These have been grown at 4°C in X-ray capillaries, as described in Yonath et al. (1982b), using a mixture of ethylbutanol and ethanol at pH 8.3. Characterization of the crystal is currently underway.

Heavy-atom Derivatives

The most common method in protein crystallography to derive phases is multiple isomorphous replacement (MIR). For an object as large, asymmetric, and complex as the 50S ribosomal subunit, it is necessary to use extremely dense and compact compounds. Heavy-atom clusters are most suitable for this purpose.

An example of a suitable candidate for this purpose is a gold cluster, $Au_{11}(CN)_3(P[C_6H_4\text{-}p\text{-}CH_2NR]_3)_7$, of a molecular weight of about 5200 and in which the gold core has a diameter of 8.5 Å. Several variations of this cluster, prepared with phosphine ligands in which NR is a combination of NH_2, $NHCOCH_3$, and $N(COCH_3)\text{-}CH_2CH_2OH$ (Fig. 7) have been prepared (S. Weinstein and W. Jahn, in prep.). The variants in which NR is either NH_2 or $N(COCH_3)CH_2CH_2OH$ or a mixture of these are soluble in the crystallization solution of 50S

subunits from *H. marismortui*. One of these variants, with all $NR=NH_2$, was used for the formation of a heavy-atom derivative by soaking of native crystals in its solution. Crystallographic data (to 18 Å resolution) show isomorphous unit cell constants with observable differences in the intensities.

Because the surface of the ribosomal subunits is a composite of a variety of potential interaction sites, soaking in solutions of a heavy-atom cluster may give rise to multiple binding and complicate phase determination or make it impossible. Thus, in order to obtain usable heavy-atom derivatives, these clusters should preferably be covalently bound to one or a few specific sites on the ribosomal particles. This may be achieved by covalent binding of a suitable heavy-atom cluster with exposed chemically active groups of ribosomal proteins (e.g., —SH) or ends of rRNA on the intact particles prior to crystallization. Another possibility is to attach a heavy-atom cluster to tailor-made carriers that bind to specific sites on ribosomes or on ribosomal components that can then be reconstituted into the particles. To this end the following approaches were taken: First, free sulfhydryls on the surface of the 50S subunit have been located by reacting with radioactive *N*-ethylmaleimide. The binding sites were analyzed by locating radioactivity in two-dimensional gels of the ribosomal proteins. It was found that in the case of 50S subunits from *B. stearothermophilus* there are two proteins (L11 and L13) that definitely bind *N*-ethyl-

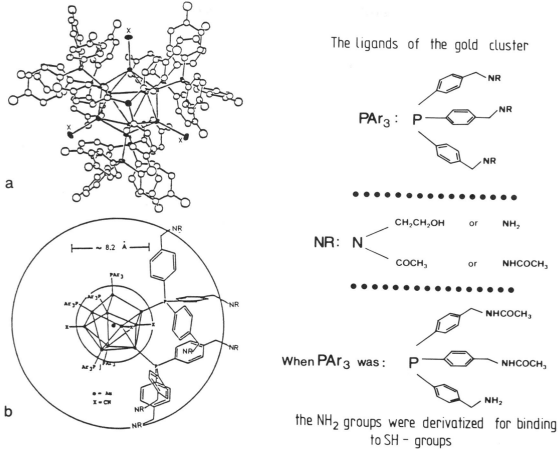

Figure 7. (*a*) Postulated molecular structure of $Au_{11}(CN)_3(P[C_6H_4\text{-}p\text{-}CH_2NR]_3)_7$ based on the crystal structure of $Au_{11}I_3(P[p\text{-}FC_6H_4]_3)_7$ (Bellon et al. 1972). (*b*) Semi-schematic presentation of $Au_{11}(CN)_3(P[C_6H_4\text{-}p\text{-}CH_2NR]_3)_7$ depicting the gold core of 8.2 Å diameter and the arrangement of the ligands around it (Wall et al. 1982).

maleimide. For *H. marismortui* most of the radioactivity was associated with one protein. Second, the gold cluster described above was prepared such that it could be bound to accessible —SH groups. Since this cluster is rather bulky, its accessibility was increased by the insertion of spacers, differing in length, to the cluster as well as to the free —SH groups on the ribosomal particles. Radioactive ^{14}C-labeling of this cluster as well as neutron activation analysis enabled us to determine the extent of the association of the cluster with the particles. The results of both analytical methods show that a spacer of minimum length of about 10 Å between the —SH group of a ribosomal protein and the N atom on the cluster is needed for significant binding. Furthermore, the extent of binding depends also on the structure of the spacer (S. Weinstein and W. Jahn, in prep.). Preliminary experiments indicate that the products of the derivatization reaction with 50S particles could be crystallized.

In parallel, a mutant of *B. stearothermophilus* that lacks protein L11 was obtained by growing cells in the presence of thiostrepton at 60°C. The 50S mutated ribosomal subunits crystallize in two and three dimensions under the same conditions as, and are isomor-

phous to, those obtained from the 50S ribosomal subunits of the wild type (Yonath et al. 1986a). This shows that L11, the missing protein, is not involved in crystal forces in the native crystals (in contrast, removal of protein L12 prevents crystallization). As mentioned above, *N*-ethylmaleimide binds to the —SH group of protein L11 on the ribosome particle. Furthermore, this binding does not reduce the activity and does not interfere with the crystallizability of the modified particles. Thus, modifying L11 with heavy-atom clusters is not expected to interfere with crystal packing and isomorphism. These observations open a new route for the preparation of specifically bound heavy atoms, by attaching clusters to the isolated protein, followed by reconstitution of the modified compound into the mutated particles.

Since protein L11 is believed to be nearly globular (Giri et al. 1984), its location may be determined in a Patterson electron density map with coefficients of |F(wild)|-|F(mutant)|, and may serve, by itself, as a super large heavy-atom derivative. At preliminary stages of structure determination, this approach may provide phase information and reveal the location of the missing protein.

CONCLUDING REMARKS

We have demonstrated here that diffraction methods can be employed for the determination of the three-dimensional structure of intact ribosomal particles. We expect that our studies, supported by biophysical, biochemical, and genetic knowledge, will yield a reliable model for the ribosome and lead to the understanding of the molecular mechanism of protein biosynthesis.

ACKNOWLEDGMENTS

We would like to thank Dr. H. Hope for introducing cryotemperature crystallography; Dr. W. Jahn for his involvement in the studies on the gold cluster; Drs. M.A. Saper, K.S. Bartels, F. Frolow, C. Kratky, and G. Weber for their efforts in data collection; Dr. F.L. Hirshfeld for his critical comments; Drs. J. Sussman and B. Shaanan for assisting us with computing and display problems; Dr. M. Shoham for his contribution to the crystallization process; Drs. K. Wilson, H.D. Bartunik, J. Helliwell, M. Papiz, K. Moffat, W. Schildcamp, P. Pizackerley, and E. Merrit for providing us with synchrotron radiation facilities; and I. Makowski, T. Arad, P. Webster, H.S. Gewitz, J. Piefke, J. Müssig, J. Halfon, C. Glotz, B. Romberg, G. Idan, and H. Danz for technical assistance. This work was supported by Bundesministerium für Forschung und Technologie (05 180 MP B0), National Institutes of Health (GM-34360), and Minerva research grants.

REFERENCES

Appelt, K., J. Dijk, R. Reinhardt, S. Sanhuesa, S.W. White, K.S. Wilson, and Y. Yonath. 1981. The crystallization of ribosomal proteins from the 50S subunit of the *Escherichia coli* and *Bacillus stearothermophilus* ribosome. *J. Biol. Chem.* **256**: 11787.

Arad, T., K.R. Leonard, H.G. Wittmann, and A. Yonath. 1984. Two-dimensional crystalline sheets of *Bacillus stearothermophilus* 50S ribosomal particles. *EMBO J.* **3**: 127.

Arad, T., J. Piefke, S. Weinstein, H.S. Gewitz, A. Yonath, and H.G. Wittmann. 1987a. Three-dimensional image reconstruction from ordered arrays of 70S ribosomes. *Biochimie* (in press).

Arad, T., J. Piefke, H.S. Gewitz, B. Romberg, C. Glotz, J. Müssig, A. Yonath, and H.G. Wittmann. 1987b. The growth of ordered two-dimensional sheets of ribosomal particles from salt-alcohol mixtures. *Anal. Biochem.* (in press).

Bartlett, P.A., B. Bauer, and S.J. Singer. 1978. Synthesis of water soluble undecagold cluster compounds of potential importance in electron microscopy and other studies of biological systems. *J. Amer. Chem. Soc.* **100**: 5085.

Bellon, P., M. Manassero, and M. Sansoni. 1972. Crystal and molecular structure of tri-iodoheptakis(tri-fluorophenylphosphine)undecagold. *J. Chem. Soc. (Dalton Trans.)* 1481.

Bernabeau, C. and J.A. Lake. 1982. Nascent polypeptide chains emerge from the exit domain of the large ribosomal subunit: Immune mapping of the nascent chain. *Proc. Natl. Acad. Sci.* **79**: 3111.

Blobel, G. and D.D. Sabatini. 1970. Controlled proteolysis of nascent polypeptides in rat liver cell fractions. *J. Cell Biol.* **45**: 130.

Chambliss, G., G.R. Craven, J. Davies, K. Davies, L. Kahan, and M. Nomura, eds. 1979. *Ribosomes: Structure, function, and genetics*. University Park Press, Baltimore.

Giri, L., W.E. Hill, H.G. Wittmann, and B. Wittmann-Liebold. 1984. Ribosomal proteins: Their structure and spatial arrangements in prokaryotic ribosomes. *Adv. Protein Chem.* **36**: 1.

Hardesty, B. and G. Kramer, eds.. 1986. *Structure, function, and genetics of ribosomes*. Springer-Verlag, Heidelberg.

Hogle, J.M. 1982. Preliminary studies of crystals of poliovirus type I. *J. Mol. Biol.* **160**: 663.

Hope, H. 1985. New techniques for handling of air-sensitive crystals. In *American Crystal Association Abstracts*, Ser. 2, vol. 13, abstract PA3.

Klug, A., K.C. Holmes, and J.T. Finch. 1961. X-ray diffraction studies on ribosomes from various sources. *J. Mol. Biol.* **3**: 87.

Langridge, R. and K.C. Holmes. 1962. X-ray diffraction studies of concentrated gels of ribosomes from *E. coli*. *J. Mol. Biol.* **5**: 611.

Leijonmarck, M., S. Eriksson, and A. Liljas. 1980. Crystal structure of a ribosomal component at 2.6 Å resolution. *Nature* **286**: 824.

Leonard, K.R., T. Arad, B. Tesche, V.A. Erdmann, H.G. Wittmann, and A. Yonath. 1982. Crystallization, electron microscopy and three-dimensional reconstruction studies of ribosomal subunits. In *Electron microscopy 1982*, vol. 3, p. 9. Offizin Paul Hartung, Hamburg.

Makowski, I., F. Frolow, M.A. Saper, M. Shoham, H.G. Wittmann, and A. Yonath. 1987. Single crystals of large ribosomal particles from *Halobacterium marismortui* diffract to 6 Å. *J. Mol. Biol.* **193**: 819.

Malkin, L.I. and A. Rich. 1967. Partial resistance of nascent polypeptide chains to proteolytic digestion due to ribosomal shielding. *J. Mol. Biol.* **26**: 329.

Matthews, B.W. 1968. Solvent content of protein crystals. *J. Mol. Biol.* **33**: 491.

Milligan, R.A. and P.N.T. Unwin. 1986. Location of exit channel for nascent protein in 80S ribosomes. *Nature* **319**: 693.

Nierhaus, K.H. and H.G. Wittmann. 1980. Ribosomal function and its inhibition by antibiotics in prokaryotes. *Naturwissenschaften* **67**: 234.

Piefke, J., T. Arad, H.S. Gewitz, A. Yonath, and H.G. Wittmann. 1986. The growth of ordered two-dimensional sheets of 70S ribosomes from *Bacillus stearothermophilus*. *FEBS Lett.* **209**: 104.

Richmond, T., J.T. Finch, B. Rushton, D. Rhodes, and A. Klug. 1984. Structure of the nucleosome core particle at 7 Å resolution. *Nature* **311**: 533.

Shevack, A., H.S. Gewitz, B. Hennemann, A. Yonath, and H.G. Wittmann. 1985. Characterization and crystallization of ribosomal particles from *Halobacterium marismortui*. *FEBS Lett.* **184**: 68.

Shoham, M., J. Müssig, A. Shevack, T. Arad, H.G. Wittmann, and A. Yonath. 1986. A new crystal form of the large ribosomal subunits from *Halobacterium marismortui*. *FEBS Lett.* **208**: 321.

Smith, W.P., P.C. Tai, and B.D. Davis. 1978. Interaction of secreted nascent chains with surrounding membrane in *Bacillus subtilis*. *Proc. Natl. Acad. Sci.* **75**: 5922.

Verschoor, A., J. Frank, and M. Boublik. 1985. Investigation of the 50S ribosomal subunit by electron microscopy and image analysis. *J. Ultrastruct. Res.* **92**: 180.

Wall, J.S., J.F. Hainfeld, P.A. Bartlett, and S.J. Singer. 1982. Observation of an undecagold cluster compound in the scanning transmission electron microscope. *Ultramicroscopy* **8**: 397.

Wilson, K.S., K. Appelt, J. Badger, I. Tanaka, and S.W. White. 1986. Crystal structure of a prokaryotic ribosomal protein. *Proc. Natl. Acad. Sci.* **83**: 7251.

Wittmann, H.G. 1982. Components of bacterial ribosomes. *Annu. Rev. Biochem.* **51:** 155.

———. 1983. Architecture of prokaryotic ribosomes. *Annu. Rev. Biochem.* **52:** 35.

Wittmann, H.G. and A. Yonath. 1985. Diffraction studies on crystals of ribosomal particles. In *The structure and function of the genetic apparatus* (ed. C. Nicolini and P.O.P. Ts'o), p. 177. Plenum Press, New York.

Wittmann, H.G., J. Müssig, H.S. Gewitz, J. Piefke, H.J. Rheinberger, and A. Yonath. 1982. Crystallization of *Escherichia coli* ribosomes. *FEBS Lett.* **146:** 217.

Yonath, A. 1984. Three-dimensional crystals of ribosomal particles. *Trends Biochem. Sci.* **9:** 227.

Yonath, A. and H.G. Wittmann. 1987a. Crystallographic and image reconstruction studies on ribosomal particles from bacterial sources. *Methods Enzymol.* (in press).

———. 1987b. Crystallographic and image reconstruction studies on ribosomes. In *Modern methods in protein chemistry* (ed. H. Tschesche). W. de Gruyter-Verlag, Berlin. (In press.)

———. 1987c. Towards a molecular model for the large ribosomal particle. In *Molecular structures, biological activity and chemical reactivity* (ed. J. Stezowski). Oxford Press, England. (In press.)

Yonath, A., K.R. Leonard, and H.G. Wittmann. 1987. A tunnel in the large ribosomal subunit revealed by three-dimensional image reconstruction. *Science* **236:** 813.

Yonath, A., J. Müssig, and H.G. Wittmann. 1982a. Parameters of crystal growth of ribosomal subunits. *J. Cell. Biochem.* **19:** 145.

Yonath, A., M.A. Saper, and H.G. Wittmann. 1986a. Studies on crystals of intact ribosomal particles. In *Structure, func-*tion, and genetics of ribosomes* (ed. B. Hardesty and G. Kramer), p. 112. Springer-Verlag, Heidelberg.

Yonath, A., H.D. Bartunik, K.S. Bartels, and H.G. Wittmann. 1984. Some X-ray diffraction pattern from single crystals of the large ribosomal subunit from *Bacillus stearothermophilus. J. Mol. Biol.* **177:** 201.

Yonath, A., J. Piefke, J. Müssig, H.S. Gewitz, and H.G. Wittmann. 1983a. A compact three-dimensional crystal form of the large ribosomal subunit from *Bacillus stearothermophilus. FEBS Lett.* **163:** 69.

Yonath, A., M.A. Saper, F. Frolow, I. Makowski, and H.G. Wittmann. 1986b. Characterization of single crystals of the large ribosomal particles from a mutant of *Bacillus stearothermophilus. J. Mol. Biol.* **192:** 161.

Yonath, A., J. Müssig, B. Tesche, S. Lorenz, V.A. Erdmann, and H.G. Wittmann. 1980. Crystallization of the large ribosomal subunits from *Bacillus stearothermophilus. Biochem. Int.* **1:** 428.

Yonath, A., B. Tesche, S. Lorenz, J. Müssig, V.A. Erdmann, and H.G. Wittmann. 1983b. Several crystal forms of the *Bacillus stearothermophilus* 50S ribosomal particles. *FEBS Lett.* **154:** 15.

Yonath, A., G. Khavitch, B. Tesche, J. Müssig, S. Lorenz, V.A. Erdmann, and H.G. Wittmann. 1982b. The nucleation of crystals of the large ribosomal subunit from *Bacillus stearothermophilus. Biochem. Int.* **5:** 629.

Yonath, A., M.A. Saper, I. Makowski, J. Müssig, J. Piefke, H.D. Bartunik, K.S. Bartels, and H.G. Wittmann. 1986c. Characterization of single crystals of the large ribosomal particles from *Bacillus stearothermophilus. J. Mol. Biol.* **187:** 633.

Peptide-specific Ribosomes, Genomic Tags, and the Origin of the Genetic Code

N. MAIZELS AND A.M. WEINER

Department of Molecular Biophysics and Biochemistry, Yale University School of Medicine, New Haven, Connecticut 06510

Contemporary protein synthesis requires more than 100 components. The ribosome itself consists of two large RNAs, one or two small RNAs, and over 50 polypeptides. In addition, active translation requires an mRNA template, numerous initiation, elongation, and termination factors, several dozen specifically charged tRNAs, the cognate tRNA synthetases, and a continuing source of ATP and GTP. To reconstruct the origin of protein synthesis, it is necessary to conceive of a scenario in which one of these interdependent components had a role in the absence of the others. Most previous models have focused on the emergence of the ribosome and the genetic code, and have simply assumed the prior existence of tRNAs, tRNA synthetases, and suitable mRNAs.

We have suggested that tRNA-like structures first evolved as tags at the 3' ends of RNA genomes to mark these genomes for replication in the ancient RNA world (Weiner and Maizels 1987). We showed that this genomic tag model can account for the existence of a population of relatively homogeneous tRNAs, as well as for their specific aminoacylation via a series of reactions completely analogous to contemporary tRNA charging. If this scenario is correct, the first tRNAs and tRNA synthetases predate the other major components of the translation apparatus. Early ribosomes then most likely evolved to facilitate the use of this population of charged tRNAs in polypeptide synthesis. In this paper, we outline arguments for believing that a rudimentary genetic code evolved *before* mRNA. This would imply that the principal components of the translation apparatus evolved in this order: tRNAs, tRNA synthetases, the ribosome, the genetic code, and finally mRNA.

Here we argue that the driving force for the evolution of protein synthesis was the ability of early ribosomes to synthesize useful proteins, which were not random polypeptides but essentially homopolymers. We revive the notion of the peptide-specific ribosome (Brenner et al. 1961; Brenner 1962; Gros et al. 1961) and propose that during a brief period in the early evolution of protein synthesis, each ribosome did in fact carry its own template. Base pairing between this *internal template* and a region on the tRNA defined both the location and sequence of the anticodon within the tRNA structure, thereby establishing the rudiments of the genetic code. Although a peptide-specific ribosome would not have been as versatile as a modern template-dependent ribosome, it would have had two striking virtues as a precursor of the modern protein-synthesizing apparatus: Peptide-specific ribosomes provide a pathway for the evolution of a rudimentary genetic code, as well as a plausible genetic origin for the first external templates or mRNAs.

Spontaneous Peptide Bond Formation

Peptide bond formation requires a source of activated amino acids. Once a tRNA synthetase activity had evolved, the earliest oligopeptides were probably synthesized by spontaneous peptide bond formation between activated aminoacyl-tRNAs. The first primitive ribosome would then have evolved to accelerate peptide synthesis by positioning the charged tRNAs adjacent to each other. In fact, in light of the many unsuccessful attempts to isolate a ribosomal protein with peptidyltransferase activity, the suspicion is beginning to emerge that modern ribosomes accelerate spontaneous peptide bond formation primarily by aligning the charged tRNAs (Moore 1985; Moore; Noller et al.; and Nomura et al.; all this volume). In addition, the facility with which the translation apparatus catalyzes formation of unnatural bonds such as esters, thioesters, thioamides, and phosphinoamides further supports the notion that the peptidyltransferase center does not participate directly in peptide bond formation. Its primary functions are probably to align the reacting groups and to promote general acid/base catalysis, deprotonating the α-amino group of the aminoacyl-tRNA, and possibly protonating the carbonyl group of the peptidyl-tRNA (for review, see Spirin and Lim 1986).

We wish to emphasize here, as we have previously (Weiner and Maizels 1987), that a primitive ribosome with only two equivalent tRNA-binding sites need not have been restricted to the synthesis of dipeptides. After such a ribosome had catalyzed formation of the first peptide bond, the discharged tRNA might dissociate and be replaced by another charged tRNA *before* the newly made dipeptidyl-tRNA dissociated from the ribosome. In this case, a second round of peptide bond formation could produce a tripeptidyl-tRNA, and so forth. Eventually, spontaneous hydrolysis of the peptidyl-tRNA bond would release the free polypeptide.

Early Ribosomes May Have Produced Homopolymers

The synthesis of random polypeptides is unlikely to have been sufficiently useful to drive the evolution of the protein-synthesizing apparatus. Instead, the first *useful* oligopeptides were probably homopolymers containing amino acids with chemically similar side chains—basic, hydrophobic, perhaps even acidic. We therefore suggest that each stage in the early evolution of protein synthesis was optimized for the synthesis of homopolymers. Initially, such synthesis may have reflected the existence of only a single class of tRNA synthetases, capable of charging tRNAs with amino acids carrying only a single class of side chain. At this stage, homopolymers would necessarily have been the sole polypeptide products of both spontaneous and ribosome-accelerated polymerization.

Basic amino acids may have participated most readily in both tRNA charging and spontaneous peptide bond formation, because the positively charged amino acid side chains could form ionic bonds with the negatively charged phosphate backbone of the RNAs (Weiner and Maizels 1987). Also, the resulting basic peptides would have been especially useful in an RNA world, because they could increase both the rate and variety of RNA-catalyzed reactions by efficiently neutralizing the backbone charge. Thus, the first biologically synthesized polypeptides may have functioned much like the modern polyamines, spermine and spermidine.

In addition, interaction of basic (but not neutral) polypeptides with a nucleic acid has been shown to facilitate inclusion of the resulting nucleoprotein complex within a lipid vesicle, suggesting an important role for basic polypeptides in early compartmentation (Jay and Gilbert 1987). Compartmentation must have been a *very* early event in evolution: A genome and its products must have remained together as a unit, since extensive mixing of molecular components would otherwise preclude evolution by natural selection.

Variant tRNA Synthetases Posed Both a Danger and a Challenge

Although at first there may have been only one kind of tRNA synthetase and one kind of peptide-specific ribosome, natural variation would inevitably have led to the emergence of variant tRNA synthetases with novel charging specificities, posing both a danger and a challenge to the primitive protein-synthesizing apparatus. A ribosome that directed indiscriminate polymerization of several different amino acids would have produced random polypeptides, conferring little, if any, selective advantage. Thus, there was strong selective pressure for the emergence of new classes of peptide-specific ribosomes that could recognize the new species of charged tRNA and polymerize them into *homo*polymers.

The Early Evolution of the Genetic Code

As Crick first pointed out, nucleic acids are not chemically suited to forming a three-dimensional template with cavities or pockets that can arrange specific amino acids for polymerization (Crick 1957). Instead,

he postulated the existence of *bifunctional* "adapter molecules" which could simultaneously or sequentially recognize *both* a nucleic acid sequence *and* the specific amino acid it encoded. The discovery of the role of tRNA in protein synthesis dramatically confirmed the adapter hypothesis and also suggested that the adapter molecules recognize the mRNA template through base pairing. Since molecular evolution tends to be conservative, this would imply that very early tRNAs also recognized their template through base pairing.

The adapter hypothesis provided no clues about the mechanism responsible for specific aminoacylation of different primitive tRNAs. One possible explanation was that each of the primitive amino acids may have interacted chemically with its cognate anticodon (see Hopfield 1978). In this view, it was chemistry that dictated the primitive genetic code, and the code itself was in some respects inevitable, given the available nucleic acid bases and amino acids. However, experiments designed to demonstrate such an interaction (for review, see Lacey and Mullins 1983) are not compelling.

In contrast, if the specificity of aminoacylation is determined by the interaction of the tRNA synthetase with its tRNA (Weiner and Maizels 1987), there will be no chemical interaction between the amino acid and the anticodon. The interaction of the *synthetase* with the tRNA would determine the specificity of aminoacylation. A code that developed in this fashion would be an historical accident: Any combination of bases could have encoded a particular amino acid, and the broad outlines of the code we know would have been fixed by those codons that happened to be immortalized first.

The Role of the Anticodon Loop

We argued above that the synthesis of random polypeptides would not have been advantageous, and thus that it was essential for primitive ribosomes to discriminate between charged tRNAs bearing different aminoacyl groups. How might this have occurred? One possibility is that the primitive ribosome recognized the aminoacyl group of the charged tRNA. This would, however, condemn the ribosome to be *terminally* peptide-specific. No such ribosome, even if it existed, could have been a precursor of the modern ribosome. We suggest instead that primitive ribosomes, like modern ribosomes, interacted with the *RNA* component of the various aminoacylated tRNAs.

We further suggest that the site of specific base-pairing between the tRNA and the ribosome defined the primitive anticodon. Although such a ribosome could be viewed as template-independent, a better description would be that its template is internal. This *internal template* would then function as a built-in mRNA for protein synthesis.

The precursor of the anticodon loop itself may have served some function independent of protein synthesis—for example, recognition by the replicase, by RNase P, or by another RNA enzyme—that required it to be conserved in all species of the diversifying tRNA population. Initially, the anticodon loop in each species of tRNA may have been free to interact with its cognate peptide-specific ribosome in a different way. Thus, one tRNA and its corresponding peptide-specific ribosome might have employed a provisional genetic code using two contiguous base pairs, whereas other such interactions used three or even four (perhaps noncontiguous) base pairs. As discussed below, the advent of template translocation would have been required to extinguish this polyglot code, and to establish a uniform genetic code consisting of three contiguous bases.

Thermodynamics of the Primitive Codon/Anticodon Interaction

We have argued that the first ribosome consisted of two tRNA-binding sites, and that *additional* interactions between the ribosome and the tRNA determined the specificity of protein synthesis and the sequence of the anticodon. But if the ribosome already had a general affinity for all tRNAs, how could an additional base-pairing interaction with the provisional anticodon allow the ribosome to distinguish between closely related species of tRNA?

The affinity of the tRNA for its binding site(s) on the ribosome may have drawn on both a specific and a nonspecific component. The *non*specific component would represent interactions of the ribosome with many sites on the tRNA other than the future anticodon, and the ribosome/anticodon interaction would represent the specific binding component. For an analogy, consider the interaction between *lac* repressor and *lac* operator. The overall dissociation constant for repressor bound to operator is an impressive 10^{-13} M, but more than half of this (10^{-8} M) can be attributed to nonspecific ionic interactions of repressor with the DNA backbone. The specific component, which primarily reflects hydrogen bonding of the amino acid side chains to the DNA bases, accounts for an increment of only 10^{-5} M (see Ptashne 1986). Thus, despite the high affinity of repressor for nonspecific DNA, the incremental increase in affinity due to specific binding allows repressor to distinguish its own unique site from a million other possible sites on the *Escherichia coli* chromosome. This analogy suggests that the incremental energy of base-pairing between the anticodon loop of each particular tRNA species and a corresponding built-in mRNA segment on the ribosome would have been sufficient to maintain the peptide-specificity of each species of ribosome.

Evolution of the Internal Template

Initially, each tRNA-binding site on the primitive ribosome probably functioned independently, and the first internal template may have consisted of two noncontiguous RNA segments, one for each binding site. What then was the driving force that brought the two anticodon-binding sites together as a continuous inter-

nal template? We suggest that the clues are to be found in the structure of the modern ribosome, where the highly conserved 3' domain of 16S rRNA (for review, see Van Knippenberg 1986) appears to participate in an intricately stacked quaternary complex involving two adjacent bound tRNAs and the mRNA.

Studies of allosteric interactions between aminoacylated tRNAs bound at the A and P sites (Nierhaus et al. 1986), as well as fluorescence transfer measurements between wye base residues located 3' to the anticodon (Fairclough and Cantor 1979), indicate that tRNAs in the A and P sites contact the mRNA simultaneously on the modern ribosome. Simultaneous contact is strictly *unnecessary* for information transfer. Only the incoming aminoacyl-tRNA needs to decode the mRNA; the tRNA bearing the nascent chain has already performed its decoding function. We would therefore interpret these interactions as a molecular fossil, revealing the design of the ancient ribosome rather than the requirements of contemporary protein synthesis.

Not only do both tRNAs appear to contact the mRNA simultaneously, but C_{1400} of 16S rRNA can be photocrosslinked to the wobble base of tRNA bound at the P site (for review, see Ofengand et al. 1986), and the wye base of tRNA at the A site can be photocrosslinked to the 5' base of the corresponding codon in the mRNA (Steiner et al. 1984). In order to accommodate the bulk of two adjacent anticodon stems, the mRNA between the two codons must be kinked (Rich 1974; Sundaralingam et al. 1975). In the modern ribosome, a kinked template would serve to bring the two 3' acceptor ends of the stiff, L-shaped tRNAs into proximity, so that peptide bond formation is rapid, once the four-RNA interaction has occurred.

We therefore suggest that the intricate stacking interactions on the modern ribosome may be a molecular fossil of the primitive ribosome, where such interactions could have promoted *cooperative* binding of tRNAs. The potential for such cooperative binding would favor realignment of the tRNA-binding sites (and perhaps even some reshaping of the tRNAs themselves) to generate adjacent anticodon-binding sites on a continuous internal template.

In principle, each new species of peptide-specific ribosome could have arisen de novo. However, the first ribosome to use stacking interactions between contiguous codon/anticodon triplets to achieve cooperative tRNA binding would have had a powerful selective advantage. We suggest that this particular ribosome was the precursor of the modern ribosome. Natural variation in its internal template would have generated new peptide-specific ribosomes, which in turn recognized new species of tRNA through *specific* base-pairing interactions with the anticodon loop.

Figure 1 diagrams a scheme for the evolution of a peptide-specific ribosome. The scheme begins with an RNA molecule that has a tRNA-binding site. The genomic tag model suggests that such binding sites characterized all early replicases, so a variant replicase may well have been the molecular starting point for the

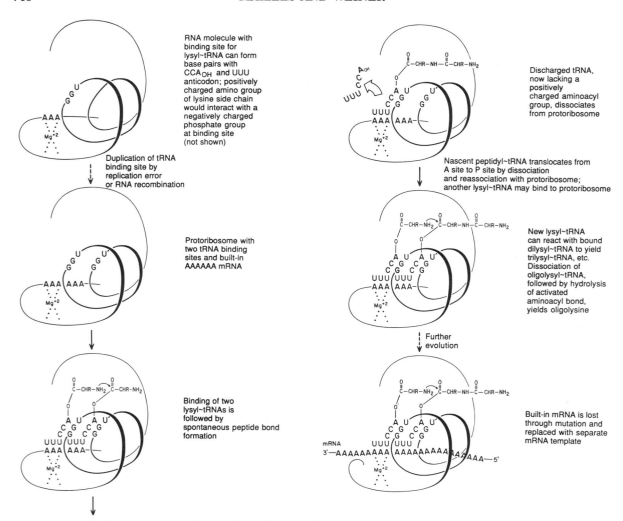

Figure 1. A model for the evolution of a peptide-specific protoribosome into a modern template-dependent ribosome. Since the first tRNA synthetases are likely to have been specific for basic amino acids, a lysine-specific protoribosome is illustrated here. For clarity, the tRNAs are cartooned as hexanucleotides.

evolution of the ribosome. The scheme outlines the development of a relatively sophisticated protoribosome, which carries an internal template and can bind and position two aminoacylated tRNAs for spontaneous peptide bond formation. For simplicity, tRNAs are cartooned as hexanucleotides; all the evidence implies that early tRNAs were in fact much more complex.

tRNA Translocates but the Internal Template Does Not

In the absence of a mechanism for tRNA translocation, a single round of peptide bond formation on the primitive ribosome would usually be followed by release of both the dipeptidyl and the uncharged tRNAs. Synthesis of proteins larger than dipeptides would require successive cycles of association and dissociation, and thus be inefficient.

We suggest that a simple mechanism for tRNA translocation arose early. The two equivalent tRNA-binding

sites on the primitive ribosome might have become nonequivalent, so that the affinity of the peptidyl site (P site) but not the aminoacyl site (A site) was higher for aminoacyl-tRNA than for uncharged tRNA. Following the first round of peptide bond formation, the association constants would favor release of the uncharged tRNA from the P site, and movement of the peptidyl-tRNA from the A site to the P site. Synthesis of longer and longer polypeptides could then occur in this stepwise fashion, as diagrammed in Figure 1.

Previous attempts to imagine the origin of protein synthesis have attributed translocation to conformational changes between the charged and uncharged states of tRNA (Woese 1970, 1979; Crick et al. 1976) or have dispensed with translocation altogether (Crothers 1982). In contrast, we suggest that tRNA is relatively inflexible, and that translocation reflects the differential affinity of the ribosome for the charged and uncharged states of tRNA. For example, the ribosome might discriminate between charged and uncharged tRNA by forming hydrogen bonds to the ester linkage in aminoacyl- or peptidyl-tRNA. Finally, we note that translocation of tRNA without accompanying translocation of the internal template could only occur if the peptide-specific ribosome encoded a homopolymer; otherwise, the *same* tRNA could not bind first to the A site and then to the P site.

tRNA Translocation Preceded External Templates

Following peptide bond formation on the modern ribosome, the peptidyl-tRNA moves from the A to the P site, and the discharged tRNA moves from the P to the E site (Nierhaus et al., this volume). Although translocation was once envisioned as requiring a ratchet or "gating" mechanism to move the mRNA along the ribosome one codon at a time, studies with frameshift suppressor tRNAs demonstrate that a four-base match between the anticodon and the mRNA results in translocation of the mRNA by four rather than three bases during a single round of peptide bond formation (Riddle and Carbon 1973; Atkins et al. 1979; Roth 1981; Bossi and Smith 1984; Weiss et al., this volume). This strongly implies that movement of the tRNA translocates the mRNA. Thus the mRNA is in effect dragged along the ribosome as the tRNA moves from the A site to the P site, and a counting mechanism built into the tRNA anticodon, rather than into the ribosome or the mRNA itself, positions the message in the correct reading frame.

Without a preexisting translocation mechanism, a primitive ribosome could not have translated an external template because random proteins would be synthesized as the mRNA was read in different frames. This problem cannot be overcome by postulating a "code without commas" that only allows the mRNA to be read in one frame (Crick et al. 1957, 1976; Shepard 1983): An mRNA that did not require accurate *unidirectional* translocation could only encode homopolymers.

We therefore suggest that tRNA translocation evolved *before* the advent of external templates, and that the ability of tRNA translocation to drive mRNA translocation on the modern ribosome is a molecular fossil. An important corollary is that prior to the evolution of a template-dependent ribosome, the interaction between the tRNA anticodon and the internal template of the ribosome must have become standardized both in sequence and in codon length. This would not be implausible if all successful ribosomes descended from the first ribosome with two *contiguous* anticodon-binding sites, as described above. Had template-dependent translation preceded a universal code, ribosomes would have synthesized random polypeptides as tRNAs using different genetic codes translated the template.

Was the Three-base Genetic Code Inevitable?

A priori, it is difficult to make an argument against a two-base code encompassing 16 different amino acids, or against a redundant four-base code in which covariance of adjacent nucleotides mitigates the potentially harmful effects of a highly redundant code on the fidelity of translation. However, since a two- or four-base code could not evolve into a three-base code *after* the advent of translocation, it seems likely that the triplet nature of the modern genetic code was established very early, long before the primitive translation apparatus could distinguish 16 or more different amino acids.

We have described a scenario in which an established population of molecules, the early tRNAs, facilitated the evolution of protein synthesis. In this case, demands on tRNA structure predated the development of the code. This leads us to argue that the triplet code may reflect structural *constraints* on variation within the anticodon loop, rather than the necessity of encoding a relatively large number of amino acids.

Charging Specificity Remained Constant during Evolution of the Anticodon

It has always been extremely puzzling that the recognition elements for charging by the tRNA synthetase and for translation are not one and the same. With two exceptions (the glutamine and methionine tRNA synthetases of *E. coli*), mutation of the anticodon does not affect the specificity of charging (see Schimmel 1987 for review of prokaryotes and yeast; Ho and Kan 1987 for recent work on aminoacylation of suppressor tRNAs in vertebrates). The simplest explanation, that structural constraints prevent simultaneous or coordinate recognition of the CCA acceptor and the anticodon loop by a tRNA synthetase, seems unlikely on structural grounds. The distance from the anticodon to the CCA acceptor group at the opposite end of the L-shaped tRNA is a little less than 80 Å (Quigley et al. 1978), a length which could reasonably be spanned by a tRNA synthetase polypeptide (327–937 residues) or an RNA enzyme.

More plausibly, the insensitivity of charging specificity to anticodon sequence is a molecular fossil: It tells us that the anticodon evolved independently of the specificity of charging. In fact, if synthesis of useful polypeptides was the driving force for the evolution of protein synthesis, then the independence of anticodon sequence from charging specificity may have been the *result* of natural selection: only in this way could translational specificity have been maintained while the genetic code underwent fine tuning.

Perpetuation of the Peptide-specific Ribosome

An external template like modern mRNA, entirely separate from the ribosome itself, may well have served to encode the first heteropolymeric peptides. It is, however, an intriguing possibility that the peptide-specific ribosome persisted even as the contemporary translation apparatus emerged. For this to occur, the template for translation would have been an RNA segment that was physically (and thus genetically) a part of the ribosome itself.

Prior to the demonstration of messenger RNA (Volkin and Astrachan 1956; Gros et al. 1961; Hall and Speigelman 1961; Brenner et al. 1962), it was assumed that ribosomes were peptide-specific, and that each ribosome translated part of its own RNA sequence into protein. One great difficulty with such a design, as pointed out by Jacob and Monod (1961), is that unless the ribosomes are unstable, the cell relinquishes vast opportunities for regulation of gene expression. However, a template built into the ribosome itself offers several distinct advantages for the early evolution of protein synthesis. First, the ribosome would gain efficient access to the RNA template. Second, the ribosome would be prevented from translating random RNAs, or RNAs that were already functioning in a nonmessage capacity. Third, early ribosomes would be able to carry internal RNA templates that encoded proteins useful for the replication of the ribosome themselves (a suggestion made to us by L.E. Orgel). In fact, there are many contemporary examples of proteins that function preferentially in *cis*: subunit II of Qβ replicase lies at the 3' end of the single-stranded RNA phage genome, and prefers to replicate the RNA that encoded it (Blumenthal and Carmichael 1979); the high rate of retroposition of mammalian LINE elements (Hattori et al. 1986; Sakaki et al. 1986), as well as insertion elements in lower organisms such as *Drosophila* (Di Nocera and Casari 1987) and *Bombyx* (Burke et al. 1987), may reflect the preference of the reverse transcriptase encoded by the element for copying the mRNA from which it was translated; and the coupling of bacterial translation to transcription enables transposases to act preferentially on the DNA encoding them (Morisato et al. 1983; Derbyshire et al. 1987). Fourth, and most importantly, physical linkage of the ribosome and its RNA template would guarantee genetic linkage, thereby increasing the chances that both be perpetuated.

If ribosomes and their internal templates did remain linked in this way, then detachment of the internal template from the ribosome would be the next landmark in biochemical evolution. This would provide a genetic origin both for the first external template, or mRNA, and for the first gene devoted solely to encoding protein.

REFERENCES

Atkins, J., R. Gesteland, B. Reid, and C. Anderson. 1979. Normal tRNAs promote ribosomal frameshifting. *Cell* **18**: 1119.

Blumenthal, T. and G.C. Carmichael. 1979. RNA replication: Function and structure of Qβ replicase. *Annu. Rev. Biochem.* **48**: 525.

Bossi, L. and D. Smith. 1984. Suppressor *sufj*: A novel type of tRNA mutant that induces translational frameshifting. *Proc. Natl. Acad. Sci.* **81**: 6105.

Brenner, S. 1962. RNA, ribosomes, and protein synthesis. *Cold Spring Harbor Symp. Quant. Biol.* **26**: 101.

Brenner, S., F. Jacob, and M. Meselson. 1961. An unstable intermediate carrying information from genes to ribosomes for protein synthesis. *Nature* **190**: 576.

Burke, W.D., C.C. Calalang, and T.H. Eickbusch. 1987. The site-specific ribosomal insertion element type II of *Bombyx*

mori (R2Bm) contains the coding sequence for a reverse transcriptase-like enzyme. *Mol. Cell. Biol.* **7**: 2221.

Crick, F.H.C. 1957. Discussion. *Biochem. Soc. Symp.* **14**: 25.

———. 1963. The recent excitement in the coding problem. *Prog. Nucleic Acids Res.* **1**: 164.

Crick, F.H.C., J.S. Griffith, and L.E. Orgel. 1957. Codes without commas. *Proc. Natl. Acad. Sci.* **43**: 416.

Crick, F.H.C., S. Brenner, A. Klug, and G. Peiczenik. 1976. A speculation on the origin of protein synthesis. *Origins Life* **7**: 389.

Crothers, D.M. 1982. Nucleic acid aggregation geometry and the possible evolutionary origin of ribosomes and the genetic code. *J. Mol. Biol.* **162**: 379.

Derbyshire, K.M., L. Hwang, and N.D.F. Grindley. 1987. Genetic analysis of the interaction of the IS903 transposase with its terminal inverted repeats. *Proc. Natl. Acad. Sci.* **84**: 8049.

Di Nocera, P.P. and G. Casari. 1987. Related polypeptides are encoded by *Drosophila* F elements, I factors, and mammalian L1 sequences. *Proc. Natl. Acad. Sci.* **84**: 5843.

Fairclough, R.H. and C.R. Cantor. 1979. The distance between the anticodon loops of two tRNAs bound to the 70S *Escherichia coli* ribosome. *J. Mol. Biol.* **132**: 575.

Gros, F., H. Hiatt, W. Gilbert, C.G. Kurland, R.W. Risebrough, and J.D. Watson. 1961. Unstable ribonucleic acid revealed by pulse labelling of *Escherichia coli*. *Nature* **190**: 581.

Hall, B.D. and S. Spiegelman. 1961. Sequence complementarity of T2 DNA and T2-specific RNA. *Proc. Natl. Acad. Sci.* **47**: 137.

Hattori, M., S. Kuhara, O. Takenaka, and Y. Sakaki. 1986. L1 family of repetitive DNA sequences in primates may be derived from a sequence encoding a reverse transcriptase-related protein. *Nature* **321**: 625.

Ho, Y.-S. and Y.W. Kan. 1987. *In vivo* aminoacylation of human and *Xenopus* suppressor tRNAs constructed by site-specific mutagenesis. *Proc. Natl. Acad. Sci.* **84**: 2185.

Hopfield, J.J. 1978. Origin of the genetic code: A testable hypothesis based on tRNA structure, sequence, and kinetic proofreading. *Proc. Natl. Acad. Sci.* **75**: 4334.

Jacob, F. and J. Monod. 1961. Genetic regulatory mechanisms in the synthesis of proteins. *J. Mol. Biol.* **3**: 318.

Jay, D.G. and W. Gilbert. 1987. Basic protein enhances the incorporation of DNA into lipid vesicles: Model for the formation of primordial cells. *Proc. Natl. Acad. Sci.* **84**: 1978.

Lacey, J.C. and D.W. Mullins, Jr. 1983. Experimental studies related to the origin of the genetic code and the process of protein synthesis — A review. *Origins Life* **13**: 3.

Moore, P.B. 1985. Polypeptide polymerase: The structure and function of the ribosome in 1985. In *XXIX Welch Foundation Conference on Chemical Research*, p. 185. R.A. Welch Foundation, Houston, Texas.

Morisato, D., J.C. Way, H.-J. Kim, and N. Kleckner. 1983. Tn10 transposase acts preferentially on nearby transposon ends *in vivo*. *Cell* **32**: 799.

Nierhaus, K.H., H.-J. Rheinberger, U. Geigenmüller, A. Gnirke, H. Saruyama, S. Schilling, and P. Wurmbach. 1986. Three tRNA binding sites involved in the ribosomal elongation cycle. In *Structure, function, and genetics of ribosomes* (ed. B. Hardesty and G. Kramer), p. 454. Springer-Verlag, New York.

Ofengand, J., J. Ciesiolka, R. Denman, and K. Nurse. 1986. Structural and functional interactions of the tRNA-ribosome complex. In *Structure, function, and genetics of ribosomes* (ed. B. Hardesty and G. Kramer), p. 473. Springer-Verlag, New York.

Ptashne, M. 1986. *A genetic switch*. Cell Press and Blackwell Scientific Publications, Cambridge, Massachusetts.

Quigley, G.J., M.M. Teeter, and A. Rich. 1978. Structural analysis of spermine and magnesium ion binding to yeast phenylalanine tRNA. *Proc. Natl. Acad. Sci.* **75**: 64.

Rich, A. 1974. How transfer RNA may move inside the

ribosome. In *Ribosomes* (ed. M. Nomura et al.), p. 871. Cold Spring Harbor Laboratory, Cold Spring Harbor, New York.

Riddle, D.L. and J. Carbon. 1973. Frameshift suppression: A nucleotide addition in the anticodon of a glycine transfer RNA. *Nature New Biol.* **242:** 230.

Roth, J.R. 1981. Frameshift suppression. *Cell* **24:** 601.

Sakaki, Y., M. Hattori, A. Fujita, K. Yoshioka, S. Kuhara, and O. Takenaka. 1986. The LINE-1 family of primates may encode a reverse transcriptase-like protein. *Cold Spring Harbor Symp. Quant. Biol.* **51:** 465.

Schimmel, P. 1987. Aminoacyl tRNA synthetases: General scheme of structure-function relationships in the polypeptides and recognition of transfer RNAs. *Annu. Rev. Biochem.* **56:** 125.

Shepherd, J.C.W. 1983. From primeval message to present-day gene. *Cold Spring Harbor Symp. Quant. Biol.* **47:** 1099.

Spirin, A.S. and V.I. Lim. 1986. Stereochemical analysis of ribosomal transpeptidation: Conformation of nascent peptide. *J. Mol. Biol.* **188:** 565.

Steiner, G., R. Lührmann, and E. Kuechler. 1984. Crosslinking transfer RNA and messenger RNA at the ribosomal decoding region: Identification of the site of reaction on the messenger RNA. *Nucleic Acids Res.* **12:** 8181.

Sundaralingam, M., T. Brennan, N. Yathindra, and T. Ich-ikawa. 1975. Stereochemistry of messenger RNA (codon)-transfer RNA (anticodon) interaction on the ribosome during peptide bond formation. In *Structure and conformation of nucleic acids and protein-nucleic acid interactions* (ed. M. Sundaralingam and M. Rao), p. 101. University Park Press, Baltimore.

Van Knippenberg, P.H. 1986. Structural and functional aspects of the N^6, N^6 dimethyladenosines in 16S ribosomal RNA. In *Structure, function, and genetics of ribosomes* (ed. B. Hardesty and G. Kramer), p. 412. Springer-Verlag, New York.

Volkin, E. and L. Astrachan. 1956. Phosphorus incorporation in *E. coli* ribonucleic acid after infection with bacteriophage T2. *Virology* **2:** 146.

Weiner, A.M. and N. Maizels. 1987. tRNA-like structures tag the 3' ends of genomic RNA molecules for replication: Implications for the origin of protein synthesis. *Proc. Natl. Acad. Sci.* **84:** 7383.

Woese, C.R. 1970. The problem of evolving a genetic code. *Bioscience* **20:** 471.

———. 1979. Just so stories and Rube Goldberg machines: Speculations on the origin of the protein synthetic machinery. In *Structure and conformation of nucleic acids and protein-nucleic acid interactions* (ed. M. Sundaralingam and M. Rao), p. 357. University Park Press, Baltimore.

Genetic Error and Genome Design

D.C. REANNEY*

Department of Microbiology, La Trobe University, Bundoora, Victoria, Australia

According to a fundamental axiom of physics, information cannot be transmitted over long periods of time without experiencing some deterioration in quality due to "noise" (Shannon and Weaver 1949). Nucleic acids obey this general law because, in the absence of selection, the information they encode will be degraded by random errors in the copier process and by environmental damage.

The relationship beween genetic noise and evolution has been systematically explored by Eigen and Schuster (1977), who showed that the information-carrying capacity of any self-reproducing system is inversely proportional to the rate of copy error, according to the equation $\nu_{max} = \ln\sigma/(1-q)$, where ν_{max} represents the upper limit of reproducible information, $1-q$ the error rate per nucleotide, and σ the selective advantage of the wild type over the average of its mutant distribution (Eigen and Schuster 1977).

Some evolutionary consequences of this inverse relationship are set out in Table 1, which compares mutation rates of modern genes with those of very early genes, as measured by the rate of incorporation of noncomplementary nucleotides in template-directed, nonenzymatic oligonucleotide synthesis in simulated pre-life experiments. Table 1 shows that, as one goes back down the path of evolution, the level of error in the mechanism of genetic information transmission rises by a factor of 10^8 or about 100-millionfold (Reanney 1984a, 1986). Reciprocally, the amount of sustainable information contracts from about 10^{10} to about 10^2. It follows that pressures to reduce noise were powerful determinants of genetic structure, especially during early, formative stages of evolution. In this paper, I explore the likely effects of such high noise levels on genome design.

*Present address: Science Focus, 7/497 Burke Road, East Hawthorn, 3123, Victoria, Australia.

Self-replicating RNA Genes

There is now widespread agreement that RNA preceded DNA in evolution (Crick 1968; Reanney 1979; Cech 1985). Although no trace of early RNA genes remains, RNA-based genetic systems still permeate the biosphere in the form of RNA viruses. Throughout this paper, I make frequent reference to RNA viruses as contemporary models of the kinds of problems faced by early RNA genes and the solutions that may have been used to overcome them. In making this statement, I recognize that RNA viruses are subject to selective pressures (to optimize replication rates for host-to-host transmission, for example) that almost certainly did not apply to early RNA genes.

Arguably, the most important difference between naturally occurring DNAs and RNAs lies in the fact that DNA is typically double stranded, whereas RNA is typically single stranded. From a genetic standpoint, double-helical DNA is almost a contradiction in terms because its function is replication, yet the repetitive intertwining of its complementary strands poses an enormous topological barrier to their separation (on which replication depends). In modern DNAs this barrier is overcome by a considerable expenditure of energy (often two ATPs for each base pair melted) and by the concerted action of a variety of sophisticated proteins. The reason selection "pays" this high cost penalty is that the disadvantages of an "unwindable" duplex structure are greatly outweighed by its advantages. Since both "halves" of the internally redundant DNA molecule separate during synthesis, damage to either strand can be repaired using the undamaged partner as a restorative template (Table 2). This has made possible the evolution of a variety of sophisticated mechanisms that detect and repair errors or lesions introduced during synthesis or in the resting state (for review, see Loeb and Kunkel 1982). The result of this error-correcting network is that semi-conservative DNA replication is a "high fidelity" process, with a

Table 1. Error Rates During Evolution

Stage in evolution	Error rate	Strandedness	ν_{max}	Comments
Nonenzymatic synthesis	$10^{-1} \rightarrow 10^{-2}$	single	$\sim 10^2$	first genetic systems
Unrepaired enzyme-catalyzed synthesis	$10^{-3} \rightarrow 10^{-4}$	single	$\sim 10^4$	early cells
Proofreading	10^{-6}	double	$\sim 10^6$	modern genetic systems
Mismatch repair	10^{-10}	double	$\sim 10^{10}$	modern genetic systems

The ν_{max} values are indicative only and assume a constant σ value (see Eigen and Schuster 1977 for details).

Table 2. Strategies Which Minimize the Effects of Error

Redundancy
Internal Redundancy (pairing between complementary strands)
(1) repair processes based on double-helical DNA
Independent Redundancy (multiple copies of [nearly] identical, independent polynucleotides)
(1) genome redundancy
(2) recombination between redundant genomes
(3) sex (regular variations in the level of redundancy)
Subdivision

For explanation see text.

mutation rate generally set at 10^{-9}–10^{-10} substitutions per base per generation (Loeb and Kunkel 1982).

In contrast, single-stranded RNA viruses replicate by mechanisms that avoid the formation of extensive duplex regions. This appears to be because long double-helical RNA molecules cannot be unwound. In the few cases where the viral genomes are double stranded, replication occurs by asymmetric transcription from one strand, and a duplex RNA is regenerated using this newly synthesized strand as template (for discussion, see Reanney 1982, 1984b). These features of RNA synthesis have the fundamental consequence that self-replicating RNA molecules have no (known) capacity to eliminate errors introduced into them by any mechanism. Accordingly, the measured rates of mutation in RNA viral genes fall in the range 10^{-3}–10^{-4} (Eigen and Schuster 1977; Domingo et al. 1978); this is about 100,000 times greater than those in DNA genes (Holland et al. 1982; Reanney 1982, 1984b).

Common examples of RNA mutations are copy errors introduced during RNA synthesis and deaminations brought about by heat from the environment. These are inheritable because they change the nucleotide sequence of an RNA molecule without impairing its capacity to base-pair in the normal fashion. Other classes of damage irreversibly inactivate the molecules: Such damages include cleavages due to (1) the oxidative effects of hydrogen peroxide or superoxide radicals (Fridovich 1978), (2) ribonucleases, or (3) the random hydrolysis of phosphodiester bonds that occurs in RNA molecules at alkaline pH.

Collectively, these observations illustrate the scale of the problem that noise posed to early genetic systems and lead us to look for strategies that would enable RNA genes to overcome the informational "barrier" posed by the Eigen-Schuster relationship. Table 2 sets out the strategies available. Sophisticated repair processes based on the internal redundancy of double-helical polynucleotides were not an option for early single-stranded RNA genes for the reasons just discussed. I will discuss the strategies that were feasible (Table 2) separately, in turn.

Strategy 1—Genome Redundancy

If information is present in multiple copies, then it is statistically highly unlikely that a randomly acting agent will damage all redundant copies at the same sites. This means that redundancy can protect information by

complementation. Some simple mathematical formalism (Reanney et al. 1983) shows that the "selective advantage" of information transfer due to redundancy increases as a function of genome copy number. (Fig. 1). This suggests that small, primitive RNA genomes were "polyploid" (Reanney 1984a).

A contemporary example of a possible cause-and-effect relationship between genetic damage and genome redundancy may be the extremely radiation-resistant bacterium *Dienococcus radiodurans*. Whereas other prokaryotes are traditionally regarded as haploid, *D. radiodurans* has between four and ten whole genomes per cell (Tirgari and Moseley 1980). It is tempting to relate this high genome copy number to this organism's ability to withstand the potential genetic damage that large doses of radiation would be expected to cause.

Redundant genomes were probably an ongoing feature of organisms for long periods of evolution, and, indeed, it is possible to view the diploid genomes of

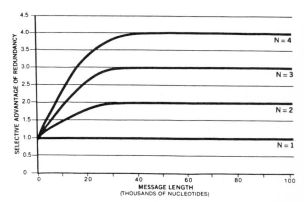

Figure 1. The protective effect of redundancy is plotted by considering four values of N (genome copy number) for an error rate $(1 - q)$ of 10^{-4} substitutions per base per generation. This is within the range of mutation rates measured for modern RNA viruses (see text). The numerical values on the vertical scale indicate the improved fidelity due to redundancy. Attention should be directed to the shapes of the curves as functions of increasing message length. The mathematical relationships on which this graph is based are detailed in Reanney et al. (1983). Note that the graph as given does not take into account the energy cost that increasing levels of redundancy place on the system (Reanney et al. 1983). As the fidelity of replication increases, the advantages of redundancy decrease, and eventually, in high-accuracy systems, redundancy will be selected against. This has evidently happened in the case of prokaryotes (Reanney 1974).

contemporary eukaryotes as lineal descendants of cells with multiple genome copies. This view is consistent with the hypothesis that the eukaryote type of genetic organization preserves more "primitive" features than the prokaryote (Reanney 1974, 1976a). In terms of this argument, the nonredundant, haploid nature of most prokaryote genomes is a derived feature, made possible by the extremely high efficiency of corrective processes in bacterial DNA, under selection to maximize rates of cell division by economizing on genome content (Reanney 1974, 1976a; Doolittle 1978).

Strategy 2—Recombination

The preceding section suggests that genome redundancy was the first error-minimizing strategy in evolution. Redundancy is easily achieved—it merely requires copied RNAs to segregate unevenly after division. However, the presence of multiple copies of essentially the same RNAs in one cell makes possible a variety of RNA/RNA interactions between them (Reanney 1984c, 1986).

Could such RNAs recombine? RNA viruses provide us with a relevant model. Recombination has been demonstrated in three RNA virus families: (1) picornaviruses such as polio (Agol 1984), (2) coronaviruses such as mouse hepatitis virus (Makino et al. 1986), and (3) bromoviruses such as brome mosaic virus (Bujarski and Kaesberg 1986). The process is surprisingly efficient with estimates that 10–20% of picornaviral genomes undergo recombination between homologous RNAs during each infective cycle (King 1987). There is also a high incidence of multiple crossovers in a single growth cycle (King et al. 1985). Using these data, King (1987) suggests that recombination is a common property of RNA viral genomes.

What is the mechanism of RNA recombination? Kirkegaard and Baltimore (1986) addressed this question by crossing a wild-type poliovirus genome with a double mutant under selective conditions that blocked the replication of each parent during mixed infection and made it possible to score for recombinants. The answer was clear cut. When the wild-type parent was allowed to multiply in the presence of a nonreplicating pool of mutant genomes, recombinations were detected. When the roles were reversed, no recombinants were found. This shows that RNA synthesis is needed for RNA recombination and strongly favors a copy choice model in which the viral replicase switches templates while making the anti-sense strand (Kirkegaard and Baltimore 1986).

If this process is widespread, as King infers, what function does it serve? I suggest that generalized RNA recombination, like generalized DNA recombination, functioned from an early stage as a form of "repair," which lowered the "mutational load" due to high noise levels in ancient genes (see Reanney 1977, 1979, 1984c; Maynard-Smith 1978; King 1987). The protective character of such recombination has been examined from a population genetics standpoint by Maynard-

Smith (1978), who noted that if most deleterious mutations are only slightly deleterious, then for a given error rate per site per generation the maximum amount of essential genetic material that can be reproduced without steady deterioration is substantially greater for a population with genetic recombination than for one without it.

Although DNA recombination based on cutting and sealing enzymes is a relatively complex process, RNA recombination based on copy choice is not. It could readily have operated early in evolution.

Strategy 3—Regular Variations in the Level of Redundancy over Time

The previous arguments depend on the assumption that the level of noise in the copier process or the environment is more or less constant or comes and goes at random. What happens, however, when the amount of environmental damage oscillates in a predictable fashion?

I am referring here to the regular changes in the environment that occur as a result of the solar cycle, chiefly the repeating day/night and seasonal cycles. Each year, an average of 260,000 calories reaches each square centimeter of the earth's atmosphere (Orgel 1973). Most of this radiation is mutagenic. The infrared fraction, which constitutes 51% of incident radiation, generates heat, which in turn causes deaminations and depurinations in nucleic acids (Drake 1969). The UV component, although constituting a smaller fraction (9%), is potentially far more damaging, since UV generates cyclobutane pyrimidine dimers in DNA and RNA molecules as well as interchain cross-links and other damages (Drake 1969). The widespread distribution of repair processes, such as the SOS system of E. coli, which erase common photochemical lesions, underscores the reality of the threat posed by UV to genetic structure.

The degree of such genetic damage varies as a function of the seasons (Fig. 2). Seasonal temperature variations of 20°C or more are common in many parts of the world, and such variations may alter the level of heat-induced genetic damage by considerable factors, depending on the effectiveness of repair processes, the pH, and other factors (see Baltz et al. 1976; Reanney and Pressing 1984; L. Loeb, pers. comm.). The effect of UV is arguably much more significant. Each year the UV dosage to which genes are exposed rises from a minimum at the winter solstice to a maximum at the summer solstice, when the length of the exposure period (i.e., the number of daylight hours) is greatest (Fig. 2). Solar radiation is also more intense during summer because of the shorter slant track of its rays through the atmosphere (D.C. Reanney, in prep.).

Paltridge and Barton (1978) have calculated that the amount of physiologically damaging UV in Melbourne, Australia, commonly increases from about 300 dose units in midwinter to about 3,500 dose units in midsummer. I conclude, therefore, that genes in surface-

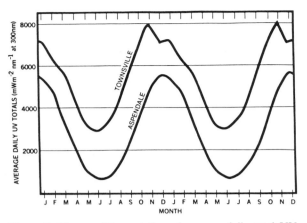

Figure 2. The monthly variation of average daily total UV dose, at two areas in Australia: Aspendale (38° latitude) and Townsville (19° latitude). The values for the first 12 months are measured values taken from Barton (1983). To illustrate the cyclical periodicity of incident UV, the same graph has been duplicated for a second year (D.C. Reanney, in prep.).

dwelling organisms, apart from those near the equator, typically experience a five- to tenfold increase in the amount of potential damage caused by ultraviolet light when winter passes into summer (Fig. 2). When one adds in the effects of heat, which follows the same seasonal periodicity, the degree of potential gene damage rises still further.

Although mutagenic radiation is a significant cause of gene damage today, its effects were probably much greater early in evolution. This is because (1) early RNA genes were probably single stranded and, as we have seen, single-stranded polynucleotides have no capacity to repair genetic lesions, and (2) the early Earth lacked an effective ozone screen (see Orgel 1973), hence the intensity of incident UV was at a maximum at the very time genomes were most vulnerable to its effects (D.C. Reanney, in prep.).

Solar radiation, therefore, constitutes a global selective pressure that has been relentlessly exerted, with characteristic maxima and minima, each year since life began (D.C. Reanney, in prep.). How could selection compensate for the periodicities in the degree of genetic injury that would inevitably ensue? The most readily available form of protection is redundancy, for the reasons already given. However, the protection offered by redundancy during summer (when error rates are high) may be burdensome during winter (when error rates are low). The removal of protection by a primitive form of meiosis would expose defective genes to the full rigor of selection at a time when remaining, faithful copies could reproduce relatively accurately (Reanney and Pressing 1984; Reanney 1986 and in prep.). It is important to remember here that a substantial drop in the density of incident radiation has the same effect on the fidelity of information transfer as the introduction of a repair mechanism—it significantly lowers the frequency of gene damage.

This argument suggests that there was originally

some cause-and-effect relationship between sex and season (Fig. 3) (D.C. Reanney, in prep.). If this concept is correct, then the repetitive alternation of generations between redundant (protected) and nonredundant (unprotected) phases began (at least in part) as an adaptive response to the repetitive alternation of error rates due to seasonal cycles (Reanney and Pressing 1984; Reanney 1986 and in prep.).

Strategy 4—Genome Subdivision

Although genome redundancy is the most widespread of all error-compensating mechanisms developed during evolution, it is not the only one. It is possible to improve the efficiency of information transfer, not by expanding the length of the message, but by dividing it into smaller units (Reanney 1982, 1984b). This is because a small unit of information has a greater chance of passing undamaged through a noisy channel than does a large unit. This strategy of genome segmentation has been followed by many RNA viruses, since RNA viruses as a group retain to this day the high error levels characteristic of unrepaired polynucleotide synthesis (see preceding section and Pressing and Reanney 1984; Reanney 1984b).

The postulate that genome subdivision is an adaptive response to high error rates in RNA virus replication is supported by a well-documented phenomenon called "multiplicity reactivation" (for discussion, see Bernstein et al. 1984). This phenomenon refers to the ability of two viral genomes, each of which has sustained potentially lethal damage, to generate viable progeny if they are allowed to jointly infect a common cell. In the case of divided genomes, the preferred explanation is that undamaged, modular RNAs from each damaged input virus combine to regenerate a complete quota of correct genetic information. Although this phenomenon has also been observed in undivided viral genomes, divided genomes seem better positioned to engage in multiplicity reactivation because the distribu-

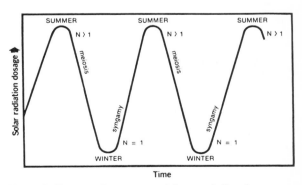

Figure 3. Because the amount of damage inflicted on genes varies with the intensity of solar radiation, a strategy that causes genomes to alternate between redundant (protected) and nonredundant (unprotected) phases should have been selected for during the early period of evolution when repair systems were inefficient or absent (Reanney 1986 and in prep.).

tion of their genetic information among a variety of discrete modular units means that a lethal lesion introduced into any one module does not inactivate the entire chromosome.

The suggested relationship between divided genomes and genetic noise has been explored in detail by Pressing and Reanney (1984). Consider the reovirus group. Reoviruses contain 10–12 separate RNAs in each viral capsid. During the development of this family of viruses, each particle must accumulate the correct combination of 10–12 different modular RNAs, otherwise the viruses are genetically incomplete. Available evidence, summarized by Joklik (1981), suggests that the various RNAs interact selectively during the assembly process by means of specific RNA/RNA or RNA/protein interactions. Lane (1979) has proposed a cooperative process in which the binding of one RNA (A) alters a nucleation complex to create a binding site for a second RNA (B) and so on. A multistep process based on such preferential associations allows for a degree of discrimination against sequences that match imperfectly because they have not bred true (Pressing and Reanney 1984). Mathematical modeling shows that, at equilibrium, a divided genome of this type has a significant selective advantage over its undivided equivalent (D.C. Reanney et al., in prep.).

At first sight it seems that specific RNA/RNA interactions like these would only allow selection to monitor the integrity of the base sequences in the interacting areas of each molecule. However, each "target sequence" in a single-stranded RNA must be unpaired in order to interact with complementary sequences on other RNAs. This means that the target sequence must be stabilized in a "correct" configuration by multiple secondary and tertiary bonds dispersed through the rest of the molecule. In effect, therefore, the target region may serve as a crude form of "quality control" because its availability (i.e., its ability to attract and bind the partner sequence with optimal efficiency) is a function of the correctness of information elsewhere in the molecule (Reanney 1984c). This potential for quality control may be enhanced by chemical kinetics, since interacting sequences synthesized early are probably important for the nucleation of secondary structures that form later.

Such a mechanism seems to make extreme demands on RNA secondary and tertiary structure. However, experimental evidence confirms that mutations that damage RNA topology impair RNA function. Slonimski and his co-workers (Lazowska et al. 1980; Netter et al. 1982) have shown that a variety of cis-acting mutants in group I mitochondrial introns in fungi affect the efficiency of RNA splicing (Davies et al. 1982). These splicing defects can be elegantly explained in terms of the secondary structures of the introns concerned (Davies et al. 1982).

A more important source of error than point mutations arises from large-scale changes in RNA size and structure. In the case of RNA viruses, for example, high multiplicities of infection often cause the forma-tion of defective, interfering RNAs (DI RNAs): these are aberrant versions of the infecting viral RNAs that contain deletions, duplications, or substitutions of the original information. A multistep assembly mechanism based on preferential RNA/RNA interactions seems well suited to preventing such grossly altered molecules from entering the final genome complex. A general screening process like this may well have acted to preserve multicomponent RNA genomes early in evolution, even if experimental evidence eventually shows that it no longer operates in specialized contemporary systems such as segmental RNA viruses.

The dispersion of genetic information among different modular units (chromosomes) is today found in the smallest self-replicating units (RNA viruses) and in the largest (eukaryotic cells). Although most eukaryote chromosomes are physically long elements, they can be functionally subdivided into multiple short modules, each of which corresponds to a unit of replication. This arrangement may preserve a "memory" of their origin (Szybalski and Szybalski 1974; Reanney 1978). The persistence of this modular substructure and the separation of information among separate modules is consistent with the previously mentioned view that "features of very early evolution which have been eliminated from prokaryotes may survive in eukaryotes" (Reanney 1974).

A Refocused Image of Evolutionary Mechanisms

Those of us who studied evolutionary biology in the 1950s accepted on faith the following items of conventional wisdom: (1) The role of sexual recombination is to increase the pool of variation in the population; (2) The role of meiotic recombination is to spread this variation further by exchanging new traits between chromosomes. It is an interesting testimony to the inertia of the educational system that these group selectionist ideas still underpin treatments of evolution in most school and college texts. Nowadays, we know that such ideas are not only suspect, but very likely the wrong way around. Far from being selected for their ability to promote change, sex and recombination may originally have been selected for their ability to reduce it (Reanney 1977, 1986, in prep.; Maynard-Smith 1978; Reanney and Pressing 1984; Bernstein et al. 1985). My thesis in this paper is that key elements of the genetic machinery (i.e., redundancy, segmentation, recombination, and meiosis) represent *protective* strategies that arose in response to the very high levels of noise in the information transmission channels of ancient genes.

This issue cannot be separated from another item of conventional wisdom—the intuitive idea that mutation is somehow a "good thing" because it provides the raw material for evolution. Part of the problem here is semantics. If readers doubt this, they should think of the images called up by the word *mutation* on the one hand and *error* on the other and then remember that, in the context of genetics, both often refer to the same thing.

The point at issue is simple: The word mutation has become a catch-all term, which is often uncritically applied to a spectrum of processes, many of which have little, if anything, in common. Over 12 years ago, I was sufficiently worried by this point to try to construct a "taxonomy" of mutational processes (Reanney 1976b). My primary concern was to differentiate between random copy errors ("point" mutations, etc.) on the one hand and the enormous spectrum of genetic processes that use pre-existing enzymes to translocate, duplicate, and otherwise rearrange polynucleotide sequences on the other (Reanney 1977).

Although the terms I originally coined to describe these processes, "entropic mutation" for the first and "programmed mutation" for the second, may not be suitable, I believe that the distinction between these two categories of genetic variation is fundamental. The first category constitutes "noise" in Shannon's sense (Shannon and Weaver 1949) and should therefore be viewed in the same way as noise in any mechanical system, i.e., as a randomizing agent whose effects on information transfer are almost invariably deleterious. The second category encompasses the array of recombinations brought about by nature's extensive "kit-set" of enzymes tailored to cut and splice polynucleotides. Whereas noise is ultimately a consequence of entropy, enzymes tooled to cleave and reseal phosphodiester bonds are products of natural selection.

If this view is correct, then the positive contribution of noise to adaptive fitness has been rather small·and evolution has been chiefly brought about by processes such as replicative recombination, site-specific recombination, etc., which lead to a plethora of interactions—cointegration, excision, translocation, and so on—among separately evolved DNAs. To appreciate the adaptive power of such processes, one need only look at the molecular genealogy of a genetically engineered DNA construct such as a cosmid and realize that the various steps involved may all occur naturally (for discussion, see Reanney 1976b; Shapiro 1985).

If the idea that noise in genes has only made a minor contribution to evolution seems radical, consider the fact that most mutations with which we are familiar from laboratory studies (auxotrophic mutants, for example) cause loss, not gain, of function. A useful way to think about this is to recognize that no living thing can be uniquely defined by the nucleotide sequence of any of its clonal derivatives, considered in isolation. For large populations of supposedly identical organisms, there is always a statistical spread of sequences, giving a DNA version of the "quasi species" concept that Eigen and Schuster (1977) have advocated for self-replicating RNA genomes. What this means is that the selective protocols developed in the laboratory to isolate mutants often merely trap a variant set of minority sequences and make them the norm until the stress is removed, when the system tends to revert to its original condition. Or to put this another way, most laboratory "mutants" are usually only a few nucleotide substitutions removed from the wild-type genotype and

hence fall within the "normal" range of the consensus sequence that defines and encompasses the identity of the species.

Another difficulty lies in the fact that it is often difficult to distinguish mutations due to noise from those due to the mutagenic effects of transposing elements. A recent study on the adaptation of *Drosophila melanogaster* populations to high mutation pressures is interesting in this regard, since it suggests that transposons act as genetic modifiers that maintain mutagen-mutation equilibria (Nöthel 1987).

Perhaps the most telling evidence for the idea that noise is less important than quantal events comes from what is arguably the best-documented example of evolution in the modern biosphere, namely, the emergence of drug resistance in bacteria. It is easy to construct laboratory mutants that enable bacteria to survive just-lethal concentrations of various antibiotics (see, for example, Nomura 1970). This appears to be a genuine case of adaptation due to genetic noise. As we all know, however, resistance of this type is almost never found in nature. Bacteria become "immune" to antibiotics by acquiring extrachromosomal genetic elements that appear to have collected genes encoding drug-inactivating enzymes from diverse taxonomic sources as a result of transposition and other processes (see Campbell 1972; Reanney 1976b).

Mechanisms discussed in the preceding paragraphs make it possible to see enzyme-based processes that make or break phosphodiester bonds as the principal evolutionary "driving force" in systems based on double-helical DNA. Until recently, however, it was still necessary to assume that noise was the overriding factor in the evolution of self-replicating RNA systems. This has been changed by a growing consensus that RNA "splicing," (which is a bona fide form of RNA recombination [Reanney 1979; Cech 1985]), arose very early in evolution (Darnell 1978; Doolittle 1978), probably before the takeover of genetic function by DNA (Reanney 1979). The discovery of "self-splicing" introns and the recognition that this reaction is potentially reversible (Cech 1985; Sharp 1985) shows how a variety of different RNA phenotypes could have been generated by the programmed insertion/excision of various RNA modules. The importance of these processes for early evolution has been emphasized by Gilbert (1986), who points out that recombination between two common introns in a primitive RNA could excise intervening exons to create an RNA transposon able to migrate from one chromosome to others.

The transposon-like character of self-splicing RNA makes it possible to extend back to the RNA phase of evolution the same enzyme-based, recombinational flexibility that has evidently operated during the DNA phase.

CONCLUSION

To conclude, I believe that noise in genes has not been primarily responsible for evolution. Rather, it has provided an ever-present, remorseless, intrinsic selective pressure (Reanney et al. 1983; Reanney 1986) that has guided the design of protective strategies such as genome redundancy and meiosis. Evolution has been chiefly brought about by quantal recombinations, which have endowed genomes, from early RNAs to modern DNAs, with a quite extraordinary range of genetic options.

REFERENCES

Agol, V.I., V.P. Grachev, S.G. Drozdov, M.S. Kolesnikova, V.G. Kozlov, N. Ralph, L.I. Romanova, E.A. Tolskaya, A.V. Tyufanov, and E.G. Kivtorova. 1984. Construction and properties of intertypic poliovirus recombinants 1st approximation mapping of the major determinants of neuro virulence. *Virology* **136:** 41.

Barton, I.J. 1983. The Australian UV-B monitoring network. In *Division of atmospheric physics technical paper No. 46.* CSIRO, Australia.

Baltz, R.H., P.M. Bingham, and J.W. Drake. 1976. Heat mutagenesis in bacteriophage T4: The transition pathway. *Proc. Natl. Acad. Sci.* **73:** 1269.

Bernstein, H., H.C. Byerly, F.A. Hopf, and R.E. Michod. 1984. Origin of sex. *J. Theor. Biol.* **110:** 323.

———. 1985. Genetic damage, mutation, and the evolution of sex. *Science* **229:** 1277.

Bujarski, J.J. and P. Kaesberg. 1986. Genetic recombination between RNA components of a multipartite plant virus. *Nature* **321:** 528.

Campbell, A. 1972. Episomes in evolution. *Brookhaven Symp. Biol.* **23:** 534.

Cech, T.R. 1985. Self-splicing RNA: Implications for evolution. In *Genome evolution in prokaryotes and eukaryotes* (ed. D.C. Reanney and P. Chambon), p. 3. Academic Press, New York.

Crick, F.H.C. 1968. The origin of the genetic code. *J. Mol. Biol.* **38:** 367.

Darnell, J.E. 1978. Implications of RNA-RNA splicing in evolution of eukaryotic cells. *Science* **202:** 1257.

Davies, R.W., R.B. Waring, J.A. Ray, T.A. Brown, and C. Scazzocchio. 1982. Making ends meet: A model for RNA splicing in fungal mitochondria. *Nature* **300:** 719.

Domingo, E., D. Sabo, T. Taniguchi, and C. Weissman. 1978. Nucleotide sequence heterogeneity of an RNA phage population. *Cell* **13:** 735.

Doolittle, W.F. 1978. Genes-in-pieces: Were they ever together? *Nature* **272:** 581.

Drake, J.W. 1969. Mutagenic mechanisms. *Annu. Rev. Genet.* **3:** 247.

Eigen, M. and P. Schuster. 1977. The hypercycle: A principle of natural self-organization. Part A: Emergence of the hypercycle. *Naturwissenschaften* **64:** 541.

Fridovich, I. 1978. The biology oxygen radicals. *Science* **203:** 875.

Gilbert, W. 1986. The RNA world. *Nature* **319:** 618.

Holland, J., K. Spindler, F. Horodyski, E. Grabau, S. Nichol, and S. Vande Pol. 1982. Rapid evolution of RNA genomes. *Science* **215:** 1577.

Joklik, W. 1981. Structure and function of the reovirus genome. *Microbiol. Rev.* **45:** 483.

King, A.M.Q. 1987. RNA viruses do it. *Trends Genet.* **3:** 60.

King, A.M.Q., D. McCahon, K. Saunders, J.W.I. Newman, and W.R. Slade. 1985. Multiple sites of recombination within the RNA genomes of foot-and-mouth disease virus. *Virus Res.* **3:** 373.

Kirkegaard, K. and J. Baltimore. 1986. The mechanism of RNA recombination in poliovirus. *Cell* **47:** 433.

Lane, L.C. 1979. The RNAs of multipartite and satellite viruses of plants. In *Nucleic acids in plants* (ed. T.C. Hall and J.W. Davies), vol. 2, p. 65. CRC Press, Boca Raton.

Lazowska, J., C. Jacq, and P.P. Slonimski. 1980. Sequence of introns and flanking exons in wild type and box-3 mutants of cytochrome B reveals an interlaced splicing protein coded by an intron. *Cell* **22:** 333.

Loeb, A.A. and T.A. Kunkel. 1982. Fidelity of DNA synthesis. *Annu. Rev. Biochem.* **51:** 429.

Makino, S., J.G. Keck, S.A. Stohlmann, and M.M.C. Lai. 1986. High-frequency RNA recombination of murine coronaviruses. *J. Virol.* **57:** 729.

Maynard-Smith, J. 1978. *The evolution of sex.* Cambridge University Press, Cambridge, England.

Netter, P., C. Jacq, G. Carignani, and P.P. Slominski. 1982. Critical sequences within mitochondrial introns cis dominant mutations of the cytochrome b-like intron of the oxidase gene. *Cell* **23:** 733.

Nomura, M. 1970. Bacterial ribosome. *Bacteriol. Rev.* **34:** 228.

Nöthel, H. 1987. Adaptation of *Drosophila melanogaster* populations to high mutation pressure: Evolutionary adjustment of mutation rates. *Proc. Natl. Acad. Sci.* **84:** 1045.

Orgel, L.E. 1973. *The origins of life. Molecules and natural selection.* Chapman and Hall, London.

Paltridge, G.W. And I.J. Barton. 1978. Erythemal ultraviolet radiation over Australia. *Search* **9:** 372.

Pressing, J. and D.C. Reanney. 1984. Divided genomes and intrinsic noise. *J. Mol. Evol.* **20:** 135.

Reanney, D.C. 1974. On the origin of prokaryotes. *J. Theor. Biol.* **48:** 243.

———. 1976a. Origin of life. In *McGraw-Hill Yearbook of Science and Technology* (ed. D.N. Lapedes), p. 243. McGraw-Hill, New York.

———. 1976b. Extrachromosomal elements as possible agents of adaptation and development. *Bacteriol. Rev.* **40:** 552.

———. 1977. Genetic engineering as an adaptive strategy. *Brookhaven Symp. Biol.* **29:** 248.

———. 1978. Coupled evolution: Adaptive interactions among the genomes of plasmids, viruses and cells. *Int. Rev. Cytol.* (suppl.) **8:** 1.

———. 1979. RNA splicing and polynucleotide evolution. *Nature* **277:** 598.

———. 1982. The evolution of RNA viruses. *Annu. Rev. Microbiol.* **36:** 47.

———. 1984a. Genetic noise in evolution? *Nature* **307:** 318.

———. 1984b. The molecular evolution of RNA viruses. *Symp. Soc. Gen. Microbiol.* **35:** 175.

———. 1984c. RNA splicing as an error-screening mechanism. *J. Theor. Biol.* **110:** 315.

———. 1986. Genetic error and genome design. *Trends Genet.* **2:** 41.

Reanney, D.C. and J. Pressing. 1984. Temperature as a determinative factor in the evolution of genetic systems. *J. Mol. Evol.* **21:** 72.

Reanney, D.C., D.G. MacPhee, and J. Pressing. 1983. Intrinsic noise and the design of the genetic machinery. *Aust. J. Biol. Sci.* **36:** 77.

Shannon, C.E. and W. Weaver, eds. 1949. *The mathematical theory of communication.* University of Illinois Press, Urbana.

Shapiro, J.A. 1985. Mechanisms of DNA reorganisation in bacteria. In *Genome evolution in prokaryotes and eukaryotes* (ed. D.C. Reanney and P. Chambon), p. 25. Academic Press, New York.

Sharp, P.A. 1985. On the origin of RNA splicing and introns. *Cell* **42:** 397.

Szybalski, W. and E.H. Szybalski. 1974. Visualization of the evolution of viral genomes. In *Viruses, evolution and cancer* (ed. E. Kurstak and K. Maramorosch), p. 563. Academic Press, New York.

Tirgari, S. and B.E.B. Moseley. 1980. Transformation in *Micrococcus radiodurans*: Measurement of various parameters and evidence for multiple, independently segregating genomes per cell. *J. Gen. Microbiol.* **119:** 287.

The Phylogeny of tRNA Sequences Provides Evidence for Ambiguity Reduction in the Origin of the Genetic Code

W.M. FITCH* AND K. UPPER[†]

*Department of Biological Sciences, University of Southern California, Los Angeles, California 90089-1481;
[†]Department of Genetics, University of Washington, Seattle, Washington 98195

In 1966, Fitch proposed the ambiguity reduction hypothesis of the origin of the genetic code, based on a view that the origin of life was a process in which local (pre)biological order arose from molecular chaos on the earth, driven by the asymmetric energy budget of the earth's atmosphere, a process in which subsets of random biochemical events gradually became the programmed rule of the system. This in turn led to a view, regarding the origin of the genetic code, that suggests that originally there may have been little specificity regarding which amino acids were charged to the various RNA acceptors that paired to the message. Under such conditions, no messenger RNA is likely to produce exactly the same protein twice. The advantages of obtaining a well-defined protein sequence, however, would have gradually reduced the variability in the assignment of amino acids to codons until the current genetic code emerged. If so, the history of that reduction in ambiguity might be recorded in the phylogenetic history of the tRNAs. This suggests a test of the hypothesis. Does a correspondence exist between the pattern of the genetic code and the inferred phylogeny of the tRNAs? In this paper, we show that, for eight tRNAs, the correspondence is precisely of the type required by the ambiguity reduction hypothesis.

THE HYPOTHESIS

Many of the details of that ambiguity reduction are irrelevant to this study. It does not matter if, at an earlier time, there were more or less than 20 amino acids, nor does it matter to what extent deoxynucleotides might have been involved. Perhaps during this period some of the amino acids that might have been used were gradually excluded. α-Amino butyrate and sarcosine are both common products of attempts to create amino acids abiotically (Miller 1957). If they were common originally, they must have been present in pre-genetic-code proteins and later selected against. The ambiguity reduction hypothesis does require, however, at the time of its occurrence, that the basic method of an acceptor tRNA of about 75 nucleotides, having 3 nucleotides that base-pair with message, had already been reasonably well developed. It further requires that a genetic information-storing system was already present and that the descendant tRNAs are all paralogous, having arisen by gene duplication.

As there are several scenarios that are consistent with the hypothesis, it is useful to elaborate one. The general nature of the reduction can be visualized in the following way. If there were no specificity whatsoever, then any amino acid could be charged to any anticodon acceptor. This could easily be the case since, if the protein sequences were not well specified, the charging enzymes might not be able to distinguish one nucleotide from another. The code would then have been NNN = any amino acid (N = any nucleotide; Fig. 1, top). However, if the system developed a bias that tended to charge hydrophobic amino acids preferentially to tRNAs matching messenger-coding triplets that had a central pyrimidine (Y), and tended to charge hydrophilic amino acids to tRNAs matching messenger-coding triplets that had a central purine (R), then the code would become NYN = hydrophobes, NRN = hydrophiles. Hydrophobes and hydrophiles are broadly descriptive of what the NYN and NRN codons encode today. This is equivalent to separating the codons into two groups, as shown by the column of closed circles in the genetic code (Fig. 1, middle). It is also equivalent to improving the charging enzyme to the point where it can distinguish between the sizes of the two major classes of nucleotides.

It is not important to the test of the hypothesis to know or guess what the first ambiguity reduction step was nor what the selective force furthering that choice was, but it may be useful to suggest how even a first differentiation such as NYN/NRN might have been advantageous. Consider a simple repeat of $(NYNNRN)_n$. Although it does not define a protein, it does define, as suggested by Brack and Orgel (1975), an alternating series of hydrophobic and hydrophilic amino acids, exactly what is required to form β-pleated sheets, one of the two major forms of secondary structure in proteins today. Similarly, α-helical properties would reside in another repeat only slightly more complicated. By so minor a reduction in ambiguity, one may specifically code for the two most important substructures of biologically active proteins.

The second ambiguity reduction step might have been a choice, as shown by the row of filled squares in Figure 1 (bottom), between purines and pyrimidines in the first codon position leading to YYN, RYN, YRN, and RRN, specifying four different groups of amino acids. The cyclic amino acids (tyrosine, histidine, tryp-

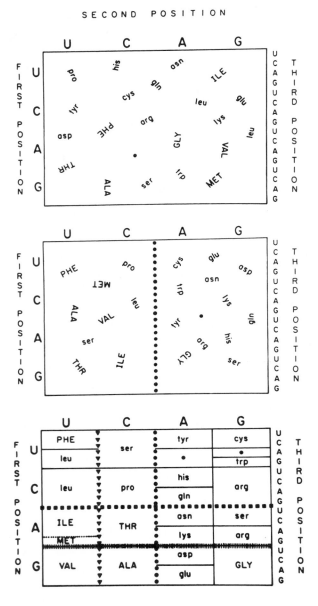

Figure 1. The genetic code. (*Top*) The fully ambiguous "genetic code" as it might have been initially with no particular preference of any amino acid for any particular codon. (*Middle*) The genetic code as it might have been at an early stage if the first reduction in ambiguity had been the institution of a preference for hydrophobic amino acids to be charged to acceptors recognizing a pyrimidine in the middle codon position and for hydrophylic amino acids to be charged to acceptors recognizing a purine in the middle codon position. (*Bottom*) The genetic code as it is today. The various symbols indicate possible evolutionary divergences from an ambiguous ancestral assignment. Squares and circles denote the first differentiation into purine and pyrimidine recognition in the first and second codon positions, respectively; short vertical lines denote the subsequent differentiation into adenine and guanine recognition in the first position purines; triangles denote the subsequent differentiation into cytosine and uracil recognition in the second position pyrimidine; dotted line denotes the differentiation into G and not-G recognition in the third position of the AUN codon. The order of these differentiations is assumed to be independent except that at any one position the purine-pyrimidine differentiation must precede any other differentiation at that position. This restriction was chosen solely on the basis that the purine-pyrimidine differentiation is essentially what is seen in the third position today. Other possible differentiations are omitted because no amino acid reflective of that section of the coding table was used in this study. These differentiation symbols are used to clarify the interpretation of the phylogenies in Fig. 2. All capitalized amino acid abbreviations denote amino acids whose tRNAs are used in this study.

tophan, proline, and phenylalanine) all have codons beginning with a pyrimidine in the first position. In a subsequent step, the pyrimidine might have been separated into the cytidine and uridine specificities that today separate those amino acids with phenyl rings (tyrosine, tryptophan, and phenylalanine) from the heterocyclics histidine and proline (not specifically depicted in Fig. 1).

It is only necessary to continue the process of increasing codon specificity (ambiguity reduction) through additional steps to arrive at a stage where every amino acid has its own set of codons, the ones it uses today (Fig. 1, bottom). This work was started for the purpose of finding evidence that such a process did indeed occur.

The third position of the genetic code is today largely differentiated, if at all, by a purine-pyrimidine division.

Moreover, it could well be that proteins at the earliest stages of evolution were not able to discriminate more finely than between purines and pyrimidines. We have therefore assumed that the purine-pyrimidine division was the first to occur in the first two codon positions as well. There is nothing that forbids, for example, a G-not G(= H) division as in fact is, except for some mitochondria, present today in most methionine-isoleucine codons. These codons must, therefore, either have divided that way initially or else isoleucine later acquired the AUA codon from methionine. Our restriction of the initial division in the first two codon positions into purines and pyrimidines limits the number of possible evolutionary patterns that can be constructed that are consistent with the pattern of the genetic code. This is important to the statistical test to be presented.

METHODS AND RESULTS

General Considerations

Materials. A total of 300 tRNA sequences were examined. For each of the following amino acids there was the accompanying number of tRNAs: Ala, 39; Gly, 43; Ile, 32; Met$_i$, 48; Met$_m$, 20; Phe, 29; Thr, 35; and Val, 54. There may have been inadvertant duplicates in the set in that two sequences obtained from different sources that did not agree completely would both be included, there being no effort to see if the difference might not be a sequencing error as opposed to strain differences. Three fungal met$_m$s are in fact recent duplications of the met$_i$ and are genetically in that category, although they were counted here in the functional met$_m$ category. Sources of sequences were GenBank, EMBO, W. McLain, and H. Nicholas (unpubl.), R. Cedergren (unpubl.), and Sprinzl et al. (1985a,b).

It is important that the sequences be in homologous alignment. The alignment of Sprinzl et al. (1985a,b) is a spatially equivalent alignment because the portions that form the secondary structure are given a dominating preference. In this case the homologous and spatially equivalent alignments are almost always congruent, and we therefore adopted their alignment. In the few cases where it seemed obvious that the spatially equivalent alignment was nonhomologous, we altered the former to the homologous alignment.

Tree construction and ancestral sequence estimation. Given a set of sequences homologously aligned, it is possible, for any particular proposed genealogical (phylogenetic) relationship, to determine the minimum number of nucleotide substitutions necessary to obtain these sequences from their common ancestor by the method of Fitch (1971).

We began by examining the set of tRNAs for each amino acid separately to find the most parsimonious tree for each. We used many different starting trees representing different possible phylogenetic relationships. Each of these trees was subjected to the swapping of its neighboring branches in search of better (more parsimonious) trees until a tree was obtained that could not be improved by swapping neighboring branches. The tree requiring the fewest substitutions, after branch swapping, from among all starting phylogenies was presumed to be the best estimate of the true phylogeny. In these procedures, all positions of the tRNA were treated equally, irrespective of their base pairing and irrespective of any posttranscriptional modifications.

The Test of the Ambiguity Reduction Hypothesis

Imagine that one has a good estimate of the nucleotide sequence for each of eight amino acid tRNAs as they existed in the most recent ancestor common to all the organisms that are alive today, that is, in the cenancestor (cen-, from the Greek kainos, meaning recent, and koinos, meaning common). One can im-agine that the phylogeny of the cenancestral tRNAs for those amino acids might correspond to the pattern of ambiguity reduction shown in the trees of Figure 2. In that case, the tRNA phylogeny and the ambiguity reduction hypothesis would correlate perfectly. One problem is to determine the probability of a favorable outcome.

The test will involve the set of eight tRNAs whose amino acids are shown at the branch tips of Figure 2. The determination of their cenancestral sequences will be the concern in the next section. For now, we need to know how many possible phylogenies there are for eight (cenancestral tRNA) sequences. The number of unrooted trees, t, for n taxa $= (n - 2)!! = \Pi(2i - 1)$ for $i = 1 \rightarrow n - 2$ (Fitch and Margoliash 1968). Thus there are 10,395 unrooted trees. We only count unrooted trees because the procedure we shall use involves a parsimonious estimate of the total number of nucleotide substitutions required for a tree, an estimate that is not affected by the location of the root of the tree.

The next question is, how many of those 10,395 trees are consistent with the genetic code's having a pattern of ambiguity reduction like that in Figure 1? Only the four shown in Figure 2. A favorable outcome for the ambiguity reduction hypothesis would be that at least one of the four ambiguity reduction trees was (among) the most parsimonious of the 10,395 trees.

Constructing the Cenancestral Sequence for Each tRNA

Theory. The test using the eight cenancestral tRNA sequences first requires that we have an estimate of that sequence for each of them. This will require the use of the parsimony method that necessarily has within it, for each node on a tree, an estimate of the ancestral sequence that is consistent with the fewest possible nucleotide substitutions on that tree (Fitch 1971). For that ancestor to be as good an estimate as possible the following must be true. (1) There must be the largest possible number of tRNAs for each amino acid. We used a total of 300 tRNAs. (2) The diversity of the taxa must span the diversity of extant species. If only mammalian species were included, the estimated ancestral tRNA sequence would be only that in the ancestral mammal, not that in the cenancestor. We required that any tRNA have at least one known representative from each of the following five major groups: archaebacteria, eubacteria, eukaryotes (preferably plants, animals, and fungi), chloroplasts, and mitochondria (there is no met$_m$ in mitochondria where one met tRNA serves both purposes and it is of the met$_i$ lineage). (3) The root of the tree of living species must be known. This is not known but is solvable as shown below.

Result. The most parsimonious tree(s) from all starting trees was examined for each amino acid tRNA separately. From these we discovered that each of the five major groups of sequences consistently appeared as a single group on the tree. That is, for any one amino

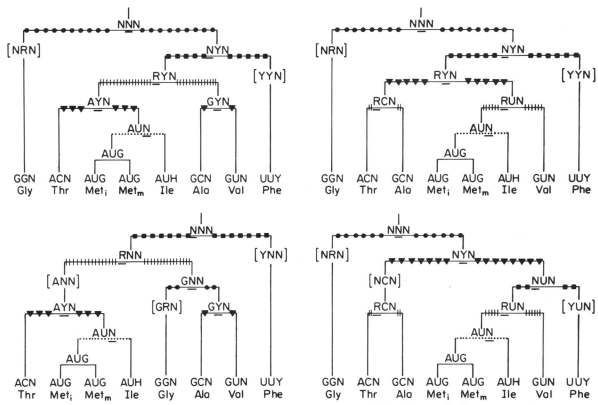

Figure 2. The four possible phylogenies consistent with the codon differentiations of Fig. 1. Each tree starts with an ancestral undifferentiated NNN codon indicating that any amino acid might be incorporated into the polypeptide. Each differentiation divides the set of nucleotides shown by the triplet in the center of a horizontal line into two disjoint subsets shown below the ends of that line. The nucleotide that is differentiated is underlined. The symbols on the lines reflect the divisions seen in Fig. 1. The lengths of the vertical lines carry no meaning in terms of time or amount of change, but the lower divisions should be thought of as temporally occurring after ones above them, with one exception. The upper two trees were rooted on the Gly tRNA lineage, but could equally well have been rooted on the Phe tRNA lineage. Since the length of a parsimonious tree is independent of the location of its root, the rooting of these trees is a consequence solely of requiring the purine-pyrimidine differentiation to precede the differentiation among purines and among pyrimidines. Any intermediate in the tree (e.g., AUN) represents an evolutionary state where any codon, contained in the subset that that ambiguous ancestral triplet represents, would allow any descendant amino acid (e.g., Met, Ile) to be incorporated into a growing polypeptide. A descendant amino acid is one of those at the tips of that subtree that can be reached from the root (NNN) only by passing through that ancestral triplet. Ancestral triplets are shown in brackets whenever a subsequent stage of differentiation not relevant to this study has been omitted. When the tips of the trees are the reconstructed cenancestral tRNAs for these amino acids, the length of these trees is 106 nucleotide substitutions except for the tree in the lower left corner that requires 104 nucleotide substitutions.

acid, the tRNA sequences of all the eukaryotes clustered together, as did all the mitochondria, all the eubacteria, etc. Although there were rare exceptions,[1] the pattern was so consistent that it was clearly reasonable to assume that these five major groups were coherent (monophyletic) and that the tRNAs reflected that fact.

The notable and consistent exception to that coherence was *Anacystis nidulans*. Rather than falling within the eubacteria, it consistently appeared with the chloroplasts. This, however, is not truly a problem. It simply demonstrates that chloroplasts derived from a blue-

green alga-like organism, as suggested some time ago (Margulis 1981) and, since others have added evidence in support of this (e.g., Schwartz and Dayhoff 1978), we thereupon simply made *A. nidulans* a member of the chloroplast group for the purpose of determining the evolutionary relationships of the five major groups.

Within the most parsimonious tree for any one amino acid that utilized tRNAs recognizing different codons (isoacceptors; e.g., valine GUR and GUY codons), one invariably discovered that the pair of tRNAs arose several times in independent lineages. Thus, we are unable to infer separate cenancestral isoacceptor tRNA sequences. This does not mean that separate isoacceptor tRNAs did not exist at the time of the cenancestor, only that, if they did exist, their trace has been lost by competition with a more recently formed paralogous tRNA created by the duplication of the other gene and by the subsequent mutation of its anticodon. Indeed, it

---

[1] Examples of exceptions include the following: *E. coli* met$_m$ tRNA clustered with the chloroplasts rather than the other eubacteria; *Scendesmus obliquus* chloroplast met$_i$ tRNA branched off before *Anacystis nidulans* rather than after; it costs one extra nucleotide substitution to put the *Halobacterium volcanii* Ile tRNA duplication within the archaebacteria.

could well be that there is value in terms of amino-acyl-tRNA-synthetase efficiency if isoacceptor tRNA pairs differ only in their anticodon. If so, and if a pair of isoacceptor tRNAs had drifted genetically apart, there might be positive selection to replace an older form by a newer one created by gene duplication and a G-U interchange in the anticodon of the duplicated gene.

Rooting the Tree

Theory. The characteristics of the most recent ancestor of a group of organisms are potentially inferable from the characteristics of its descendants. One cannot usually infer the characteristics of organisms more ancient than that ancestor due to the absence of other relatives that would provide information. The tRNAs appear to be an exception, however, in that they are presumed to be paralogous, the gene for these various amino acid acceptors having arisen by gene duplications that occurred *prior* to the cenancestor, before the most recent ancestor of all the organisms alive today. That hypothesis of a paralogous relationship will be tested below and found to be statistically supported, but, for the moment, let us consider the consequences if the hypothesis is indeed correct and if all the gene duplications occurred prior to the cenancestor.

Figure 3 illustrates for a group of three taxa and a set of three genes. The question arises, what would happen if a single tree were to be sought using all nine sequences at once? Of the 135,135 possible unrooted trees, three nonrandom examples are shown.

In the second row, the tree has three subtrees, each for a different taxonomic group. This might reflect reality, but it would imply that all the gene duplications occurred subsequent to the divergence of the taxonomic groups being studied.

In the third row is a possible result in which there are again three subtrees, each for a different gene, the divergence of the species having occurred after the gene duplications. Unfortunately, no two of the three subtrees show the same order of taxon divergence.

In the bottom row is the desired result. The three subtrees separate the genes, implying that the genes duplicated prior to the cenancestor and that the order of the taxon divergence within each subtree is the same. This permits us to identify the cenancestral node as the root of those subtrees. This is shown as a closed circle on each of the three subtrees and corresponds to linking the top row trees to each other at their corresponding closed circles. A similar approach to tree rooting using the internal duplication of bacterial ferredoxin was presented by Schwartz and Dayhoff (1978).

In the actual test, there will be sequences for eight genes from each of the major taxonomic groups giving a result rather better than that shown in the third row, but not as perfect as that shown in the bottom row. If, at the level of the major groups of sequences, the tRNAs for each amino acid are orthologous, then one should get the same phylogeny of the groups for each amino acid tRNA. Moreover, if one constructs a large

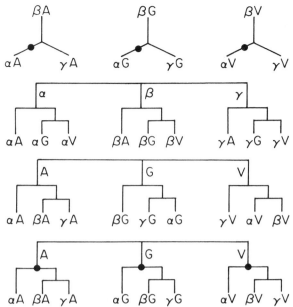

Figure 3. Finding the root of the tree of life, a hypothetical example. The top row shows three trees, each for a separate paralogous gene, A, G, and V. They could be, for example, the tRNAs of alanine, glycine, and valine. For each gene we have a representative from each of three widely divergent taxa, α, β, and γ, that one expects to span the range of all living things. They could be, for example, from archaebacteria, eubacteria, and eukaryotes. The dots represent the roots of that tree. The other three trees show, from the top down, increasing relatedness to their correct phylogeny if all three genes arose via gene duplications prior to the speciation of the organisms in which they reside.

phylogeny that includes simultaneously the five major group ancestral tRNAs (eubacterial, archaebacterial, eukaryotic, chloroplast, and mitochondrial) for all eight amino acid tRNA sets, then one should get a tree with four properties: (1) All the group ancestral tRNAs for any one amino acid set should cluster together; (2) within each such cluster one should observe the same evolutionary relationships among the five major groups; (3) the position possessing the link from any one cluster to the other clusters should locate in the tree where the cenancestral tRNA for that amino acid is to be found; and (4) that position, that amino acid set's root, should be the same for each set. Because the chloroplast and eubacterial sequences always clustered together in the study using all the tRNAs separately, we used the common ancestor of the two, thereby reducing the number of major groups from five to four.

Result. The group ancestors of the tRNA set were examined by the parsimony method with branch swapping with the following results: (1) The four group ancestors in each tRNA set clustered together except for the noninitiating met$_m$ tRNA, which contained the initiating met$_i$ tRNA cluster within it; (2) the tree for each cluster was the same for the seven clustered sets and is shown in Figure 4; (3) the root location for each set (also shown in Fig. 4) is not the same.

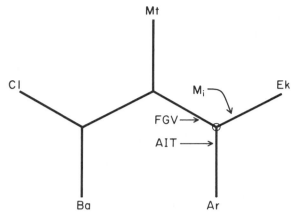

Figure 4. The clustering and rooting of the five major groups for each tRNA. The most parsimonious tree(s) for 31 group ancestral tRNAs was sought. These group ancestral tRNAs were for the eight sets of amino acid tRNAs (the seven shown: A, alanine; F, phenylalanine; G, glycine; I, isoleucine; T, threonine; V, valine; M_i, initiating methionine; plus the not-shown noninitiating methionine) for each of the four groups (Ar, archaebacteria; Ek, eukaryotic; Mt, mitochondrial; and the composite Ba, eubacterial plus Cl, chloroplast). These 32 ($= 8$ sets $\times$ 4 groups) ancestors are reduced to 31 because there are no noninitiating met tRNAs in mitochondria. The tRNAs for any one of the seven amino acids on the figure cluster exclusively among themselves. Moreover, within any one amino acid set, the phylogeny of its four group ancestral tRNAs was, in every case, identical to that shown in the figure. The location of the point in the subtree that connects that subtree to all the others (the root) is shown by the arrows labeled according to the amino acid set whose root is located there. Had all the amino acid tRNA sets rooted at the same location, it would have provided strong evidence that the tree of life was rooted there, that the cenancestor occurs at that point. In the absence of a clear choice, the node with a circle around it was chosen to represent the cenancestor.

From the uniformity of these results, we concluded that the basic arrangement of the five major groups is as shown and supports the earlier suggestion from Woese's laboratory (Fox et al. 1980) of three major kingdoms. Unfortunately, it is not possible to determine from these data where the root lies and hence not possible to determine which was the earliest speciation event, that is, which two of the three kingdoms are the most closely related. Nevertheless, it is clear that the circled node in Figure 4 represents that node closest to the cenancestor, and its sequence was therefore chosen to represent the cenancestor in the final test.

The Tree for Eight Cenancestral tRNAs

None of the species phylogenies for an individual set of tRNAs agreed in detail with any other and we therefore took the preceding results only to indicate the relationships required of the five groups and to determine the node whose sequence would represent the cenancestor. Accordingly, we then constructed, using parsimony, a cenancestral sequence for each set of tRNAs, based upon trees that were consistent among all eight tRNAs and that represented our judgment of what biologists would believe to be the correct tree. Only where we could not discover what that belief

might be did we let the parsimony results from the analyses above influence decisions as to the order of bifurcation within the five major groups. Only in the latter instances did we allow parsimony to influence the nature of the tree.

With the eight cenancestral tRNAs in hand, all possible trees for them were examined by the parsimony procedure. The distribution of the resulting 10,395 tree lengths is shown in Figure 5. The ideal result to support the ambiguity reduction hypothesis would be if one of the four most parsimonious trees (length = 100 nucleotide substitutions) were one of the four trees (Fig. 2) that are consistent with the genetic code. That was not the case. One of the code-consistent trees required 104 nucleotide substitutions, the other three required 106. The details for this tail of the distribution are presented in Table 1. As seen there, all four code-consistent trees reside in the lower 3.5% of the distribution.

An important assumption of this work is that the different tRNA genes are paralogous, that is, homologous by virtue of gene duplications, rather than analogous, that is, similar by virtue of convergence from unrelated ancestral genes. The method of Fitch (1970) permits one to decide between these two choices. This test was applied to each of the interior nodes in the upper left tree of Figure 2. For no node was the probability greater than 10^{-8} that the sequence similarity between its two immediate descendants could, by chance, be as great as that observed. Thus, we have direct evidence that the different tRNA genes arose from a common ancestor as required for the ambiguity reduction hypothesis.

As another by-product of the method, one obtains an estimate of the urancestral tRNA sequence that was the gene that, by gene duplication, gave rise to the various paralogous tRNA genes. This sequence is shown in Figure 6. Immediately below it is the ursequence as proposed by Eigen and Winkler-Oswatitsch (1981), what they called the "master sequence." It was formed from a different, but not disjoint, set of tRNAs by a

Table 1. Distribution of Most Parsimonious Trees in Tail

Substitutions	Trees	Σ Trees	$\Sigma/10{,}395$
100	4	4	0.0004
101	10	14	0.0013
102	21	35	0.0034
103	25	60	0.0058
104	55(1)	115	0.0111
105	89	204	0.0196
106	144(3)	348	0.0335

Column 1 is the number of nucleotide substitutions required to account for the descent of the eight cenancestral tRNAs from their common urancestral sequence. Column 2 is the number of trees that require the number of substitutions shown in column 1. Column 3 is the number of trees that require a number of substitutions equal to or less than the number shown in column 1. Column 4 is the fraction of all trees that require no more than the number of substitutions shown in column 1. (1) and (3) are the number of trees at that number of substitutions that are consistent with the ambiguity reduction hypothesis.

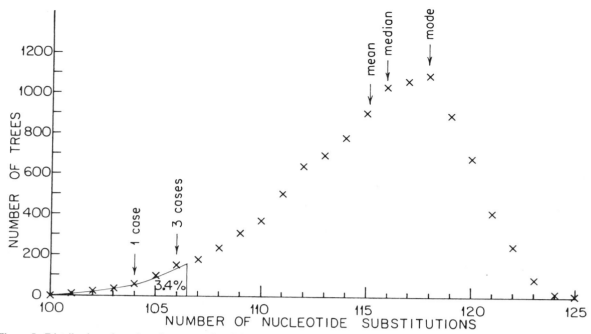

Figure 5. Distribution of tree lengths among the 10,395 possible unrooted trees for the cenancestral tRNAs for eight amino acids. The trees all required between 100 and 125 nucleotide substitutions, inclusive, which number is shown on the abscissa. The number of trees that required any specific number of substitutions is plotted on the ordinate. The locations of the four trees that are consistent with the genetic code as shown in Fig. 2 are indicated at the left of the distribution and they fall, as shown, in the lower 0.0335 of the distribution. That value was found by dividing the number of trees whose length is ≤ 106 substitutions (346) by the total number of trees examined (10,395). The probability that all four trees would fall in the lower 0.0335 of the distribution must be less than 0.0335.

different method. When allowance is made for the four extra positions we have retained from our alignment process, the agreement appears rather good and suggests that the estimates have some validity.

Although the ancestral sequences were reconstructed without regard to whether the secondary structure was retained, as can be seen in Figure 7, the secondary structure has been retained except for the last (fourth)

base pair before the D loop. Only 4 of the 21 base-pairing positions (including the fourth on the D-loop stem) have A or U nucleotides. This is less than the average tRNA but not less than some present-day tRNAs. One should not infer from this that the urancestral sequence was richer in GC pairs to withstand a warmer environment. That might be true but, if the sequences today need a preponderance of GC pairs in

```
GCSSCAGURG  CUCAGUUUGG  UUAGCAGCRY
GGGGGCGUAG  CUCAGUU'GG  'UAG'AGCAC


CAGMCUXYZA  AWCUGGAGGU  CCCSGGUUCG
CGGCCUXYZA  AGCCGGGGGU  CGCGGGUUCG


AUUCCSGGUC  UGSSGCACCA
AUUCCCG'UC  GCCCCCACCA
```

Figure 6. Comparison of our urancestral sequence with the master sequence of Eigen and Winkler-Oswatitsch. The upper sequence is from this work, the lower from Eigen and Winkler-Oswatitsch (1981). The subsequence XYZ represents the anticodon, hyphens are gaps introduced in their sequence to improve the correspondence, and dots between sequences indicate mismatches. The difference in length arises because some tRNAs have extra positions and, since our sequence preserves them all whether they were in fact present in the original ancestral sequence, no disagreement in this respect between the sequences should be inferred. We do, however, believe that an alignment based on homology is preferred to one based on structural equivalence if one is trying to infer ancestral sequences. The single letter IUB code for nucleotides is used, in which Y = C or U, R = A or G, S = C or G, W = A or U, and M = A or C (Nomenclature Committee of the International Union of Biochemistry 1986).

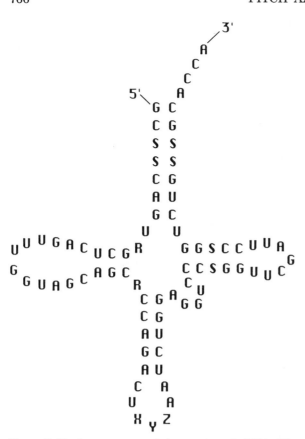

Figure 7. Tertiary structure of the urancestral tRNA. The sequence is the same as the upper sequence of Fig. 6, except that ambiguous nucleotides were made less ambiguous whenever some of the alternative nucleotides were not consistent with normal AU or GC pairing.

their stems but do not care too much where they are, and if through the course of evolution the minority of AU pairs have become distributed across many of the positions, then a simple consensus method must, and a parsimony method is likely to, infer a GC pair to be ancestral in any particular position not functionally required to be an AU pair.

DISCUSSION

Implications of the Result

The shape of the distribution of trees in Figure 5, had it been obtained from random sequences, would have been quite normal looking. Thus its very shape, with its skewed distribution and an extended tail to its lower end, implies the retention of significant biological information in the eight reconstructed cenancestral sequences. This is fortunate since, if the distribution had appeared normal, we would have given less credence to the observation that all four consistent trees were in the lower 3.5% of the distribution.

The probability that any one tree would lie in the lower 3.5% of the distribution is, of course, 0.035. That at least one of the four trees would lie there is consid-

erably greater. That all four would lie there is considerably less than 0.035 but certainly not as low as $(0.035)^4$, since the trees are not independent of each other. It is, nevertheless, a conservative estimate to say that there is less than a 0.035 probability that the null hypothesis is true, that there is no relation between the pattern of the genetic code and the phylogeny of the tRNAs. Said differently, the phylogeny of the tRNAs is consistent with the pattern of the genetic code with better than a 96.5% level of confidence, thus supporting the ambiguity reduction hypothesis.

Limitations to the Significance of the Result

We regard the result as significant in that it rejects the null hypothesis. That is not the same as proving the ambiguity reduction hypothesis that motivated the test in the first instance. Any hypothesis that required this kind of a relationship between the pattern of the genetic code and the phylogeny of the tRNAs is equally supported by our result.

Moreover, the observation of the pattern says nothing about the forces, if any, that might create such a pattern. For example, Woese (1967) has proposed what has been called the *instructive* or *direct recognition* theory (Fitch 1973). In its extreme form, this means that there is a specific interaction between the amino acid and the anticoding triplet so strong that if the evolutionary process were to occur a second time, the identical coding assignments would be made. We are not fond of this version, but in a version closer to Woese's original proposal one can imagine, for example, that there might be preferences or tendencies that made it more likely that hydrophobes would be associated with a second position adenine (A) in the anticodon (that is, with a uracil in the messenger RNA).

Woese (1965) also proposed that his direct recognition process was probably faulty in the early stages of evolution of the translation apparatus. His proposal is not materially different from mine, except that he proposes a mechanism, reduction in the erroneous recognition of the fit between amino acid and adapter.

On the other hand, perhaps the assignment was, as Crick (1968) has suggested, a largely random assignment, a *frozen accident* such that, if that evolutionary process occurred a second time, the coding assignments would have little relation to the present one. Thus, our result may constrain physical theories to forms consistent with an evolutionary development of increasing specificity, but it cannot be in conflict with any physical theory so constrained.

Our results are also not in conflict with special theories such as Jukes's *intruder hypothesis* (1973), which suggests that proteins originally used ornithine and only later was arginine substituted for it. The observation of the pattern does not depend on the presence or absence of subsequent switching of one amino acid for another. Such switching, if it has occurred and is unrecognized, might confound attempts to infer physical bases for the original assignment of amino acids to the tRNAs, but it does not affect the conclusion of a relationship between the genetic code and the history of its tRNAs.

Our results do appear, however, to contradict the proposal of Sheppard (1981) that the primitive code was for only the eight amino acids coded today by the subset of 16 coding triplets defined by RNY. This appears to us an unlikely proposal in that it also requires the recognition system to specifically differentiate all four nucleotides but not use that ability fully in any position.

ACKNOWLEDGMENT

This work was supported by National Science Foundation grant BSR-8796183.

REFERENCES

Brack, A. and L.E. Orgel. 1975. β-Structures of alternating polypeptides and their biological significance. *Nature* **256**: 383.

Crick, F.H.C. 1968. Origin of the genetic code. *J. Mol. Biol.* **38**: 367.

Eigen, M. and R. Winkler-Oswatitsch. 1981. Transfer-RNA: The early adapter. *Naturwissenschaften* **68**: 217.

Fitch, W.M. 1966. Evidence suggesting a partial, internal duplication in the ancestral gene for heme-containing globins. *J. Mol. Biol.* **16**: 1.

———. 1970. Distinguishing homologous from analogous proteins. *Syst. Zool.* **19**: 99.

———. 1971. Toward defining the course of evolution: Minimum change for a specific tree topology. *Syst. Zool.* **20**: 406.

———. 1973. Aspects of molecular evolution. *Annu. Rev. Genet.* **7**: 343.

Fitch, W.M. and E. Margoliash. 1968. The construction of phylogenetic trees. *Brookhaven Symp. Biol.* **21**: 217.

Fox, G.E., E. Stackebrandt, R.B. Hespell, J. Gibson, J. Maniloff, T.A. Dyer, R.S. Wolfe, W.E. Balch, R.S. Tanner, L.J. Magrum, L.B. Zablen, R. Blakemore, R. Gupta, L. Bonene, B.J. Lewis, D.A. Stahl, K.R. Luehrsen, K.N. Chen, and C.R. Woese. 1980. The phylogeny of prokaryotes. *Science* **209**: 457.

Jukes, T.H. 1973. Arginine as an evolutionary intruder into protein synthesis. *Biochem. Biophys. Res. Commun.* **53**: 709.

Margulis, L. 1981. Photosynthesis in plastids (chap. 11). In *Symbiosis in cell evolution*. Freeman Publications, San Francisco.

Miller, S.L. 1957. The mechanism of synthesis of amino acids by electric discharges. *Biochem. Biophys. Acta* **23**: 480.

Nomenclature Committee of the International Union of Biochemistry. 1986. Nomenclature of incompletely specified bases in nucleic acid sequences. *Mol. Biol. Evol.* **3**: 99.

Schwartz, R.M. and M.O. Dayhoff. 1978. Origins of prokaryotes, mitochondria, and chloroplasts. *Science* **199**: 395.

Sheppard, J.C.W. 1981. Periodic correlations in DNA sequences and evidence suggesting their evolutionary origin in a comma-less genetic code. *J. Mol. Evol.* **17**: 94.

Sprinzl, M., T. Voderwulbecke, and T. Hartman. 1985a. Compilation of sequences of tRNA genes. *Nucleic Acids Res.* **13**: r51.

Sprinzl, M., J. Moll, F. Meissner, and T. Hartman. 1985b. Compilation of tRNA sequences. *Nucleic Acids Res.* **13**: r1.

Woese, C. 1965. On the evolution of the genetic code. *Proc. Natl. Acad. Sci.* **54**: 1546.

———. 1967. On the fundamental nature and evolution of the genetic code. *Cold Spring Harbor Symp. Quant. Biol.* **31**: 723.

Evolution of Anticodons: Variations in the Genetic Code

T.H. JUKES,* S. OSAWA,† A. MUTO,† AND N. LEHMAN*

*Space Sciences Laboratory, University of California, Berkeley, California 94720;
†Department of Biology, Nagoya University, Japan

The genetic code consists of the fixed number of 64 three-nucleotide ("triplet") codons and a variable number of complementary anticodons that translate the codons by base-pairing. It was thought until recently that the code was universal with respect to the meaning of the 64 codons, but it is now known that some organisms may have codes that differ slightly from the universal code. For such differences to develop, codons must disappear temporarily from the coding system, and hence from mRNA; otherwise the same codon would have two different meanings, and this would be injurious, probably lethal. The codons that can disappear most readily are the stop codons, provided that any one of the three remains for the function of chain termination. This disappearance is not difficult, because directional mutation pressure (AT pressure) can change UAG and UGA to UAA stop codons and GC pressure can do the reverse.

Because of the wobble rules of codon-anticodon pairing, the 61 codons for amino acids can be translated by as few as 23 or by as many as 53 anticodons (Table 1).

The availability of hundreds of sequences of tRNA molecules has made possible a comparison of anticodons for all the amino acids in many species. The anticodon list varies in different types of organisms and organelles. We have formulated several different codes based on anticodon content; for example, the eukaryotic code differs from the eubacterial code in its anticodon list. We shall describe the following codes: minimal, "early," eubacterial, eukaryotic, halobacterial-methanococcal, chloroplast, and vertebrate mito-chondrial, together with the evolutionary changes linking them.

It has long been known that directional mutational pressure has a pronounced effect on the GC content in bacterial DNA. In some well-known work in 1961 and 1962, Sueoka examined the amino acid content of total protein in many species of bacteria with GC contents ranging from 35% to 73%. He showed that GC content of bacterial DNA influenced the amino acid composition of bacterial protein. In 1965, Jukes pointed out that directional mutation pressure on the silent positions of codons could result in bacterial protein coded by genes containing 73% GC at one extreme, and 40% GC at the other extreme, without any change in its amino acid content. Indeed, the GC content of silent positions in codons of a gene could presumably reach 100% under GC pressure, or 0% under AT pressure. What else could happen?

We have attempted to answer the following questions regarding the evolution of the genetic code. (a) Did an earlier, simpler code give rise to the universal code? (b) Is there a relationship between percentage of GC in the genome and anticodon composition? (c) Why does UGA sometimes code for tryptophan instead of for chain termination? (d) Why is *CAU an isoleucine anticodon in prokaryotes but not in eukaryotes? (e) Why is IGC an arginine anticodon in eubacteria, and why are eight anticodons of this type (INN) found in eukaryotes, with only one, IGC, in eubacteria? (f) How have the mammalian mitochondrial and chloroplast codes evolved from the universal code?

Table 1. Anticodons in the "Universal" Genetic Code

GAA Phe	GGA or IGA Ser	GUA Tyr	GCA Cys
UAA Leu	UGA Ser		
CAA Leu	CGA Ser		CCA Trp
GAG or IAG Leu	GGG or IGG Pro	GUG His	GCG or ICG Arg
UAG Leu	UGG Pro	UUG Gln	UCG Arg
CAG Leu	CGG Pro	CUG Gln	CCG Arg
GAU or IAU Ile	GGU or IGU Thr	GUU Asn	GCU Ser
UAU or *CAU Ile	UGU Thr	UUU Lys	UCU Arg
CAU Met	CGU Thr	CUU Lys	CCU Arg
GAC or IAC Val	GGC or IGC Ala	GUC Asp	GCC Gly
UAC Val	UGC Ala	UUC Glu	UCC Gly
CAC Val	CGC Ala	CUC Glu	CCC Gly

The universal code in eubacteria, halobacteria, and eukaryotes has a maximum of 45 anticodons in any kingdom, not including differences from the universal code found in mitochondria in *Mycoplasma* and ciliated protozoa. *CAU is not present in eukaryotes.

In 1985, one answer to question (c) came when Yamao and co-workers (1985) reported that *Mycoplasma capricolum*, with extremely high AT content, used UGA as a codon for tryptophan. This change in the code was made possible because mutations in the UGA stop codons under AT pressure can change them to UAA, so that codon UGA becomes available for capture by the new tryptophan anticodon UCA that had replaced CCA (Table 2). This finding encouraged us to give thought to other possible effects of directional mutational pressure on evolution of the genetic code, especially in view of the fact that differences from the universal code have also been found in mitochondria and in ciliated protozoa, showing that the code is not as impregnable to change as once was thought. For changes to take place, it is necessary that they be nondeleterious and nondisruptive. The wobble rules of codon-anticodon pairing, first proposed by Crick in 1966, are essential to all considerations of codon-anticodon pairing (Tables 1 and 3). Recently, inosine has been shown to be inserted in anticodons by hypoxanthine-ribosyltransferase (Elliott and Trewyn 1984), rather than being formed by deamination of adenine (Table 3).

What would happen to the UGA codon for tryptophan, found in *Mycoplasma* and mitochondria, if directional mutation was reversed in the direction of GC rather than AT? This possibility is shown in Table 4. UGA tryptophan codons would mutate to UGG, thus rendering possible the acceptance of a mutational change in the tryptophan anticodon from UCA to CCA. As a result, tryptophan would have only one codon, UGG, and UGA would reappear as a stop codon resulting from mutations of UAA, stop, to UGA. None of these changes would be disruptive, and we propose they would have occurred during evolution in the direction of simpler codes (minimal and early codes) proceeding to more complex ones, such as the eukaryotic code.

The simplest code may be defined as the code that has the smallest number of anticodons needed to pair with the 64 possible codons that have always been present in DNA. The simplest code for 20 amino acids (minimal code) is shown in the form of anticodons in Table 5. This is almost identical with the vertebrate mitochondrial code, except that in the vertebrate mitochondrial code there is no UCU anticodon, so that AGA and AGG are stop codons. Also, the mitochondrial code uses CAU instead of UAU as anticodon for methionine codons AUA and AUG.

Table 3. Wobble Rules: Pairing at the Third Position of the Codon

First base on the anticodon	Bases recognized on the codon
U	A, G
C	G
A[†]	U
G	U, C
I	U, C, A

Crick (1966).

[†]It seems likely that inosine will be formed enzymically from an adenine in the nascent tRNA. This may mean that A in this position will be rare or absent.

The other codes now in use contain a considerably larger number of anticodons than does the vertebrate mitochondrial code. The next evolutionary step toward these more complex codes should be to add more GNN anticodons to the minimal code. We propose that this took place as a result of GC pressure, and that the earlier theoretical code shown in Table 6 (Jukes 1983) was the result. All the anticodons shown in Table 6 are also in the present eubacterial code, except for UAU, methionine; UCA, tryptophan; and GCG and UCG, arginine. Anticodon UAU has been found in yeast. UCA is present in *Mycoplasma*; GCG and UCG are present in Halobacteria.

We shall now deal with these exceptions. The conversion of primitive and early codes to the universal code (Table 1) occurred during a period of GC pressure followed by AT pressure. We have given an explanation for tryptophan. A proposal for methionine is shown in Table 7. Methionine lost the AUA codon to isoleucine by the following evolutionary steps: GC pressure converted all methionine codons to AUG, and simultaneously methionine anticodon UAU became CAU, pairing only with AUG. At this point, AUA had disappeared as a codon from coding sequences. tRNA with anticodon CAU duplicated, and one of the duplicate genes changed its recognition site to charging with isoleucine rather than with methionine. Simultaneously, cytidine in the first anticodon nucleotide position of this duplicate became modified. The nature of this modification has recently been identified by S. Yokoyama and co-workers (in prep.) as the addition of a lysine side chain. This modified C in the first anticodon position pairs with A, so that anticodon *CUA will pair with codon AUA. GC pressure then changed to AT pressure, some of the AUC isoleucine codons became changed to AUA, and AUA became re-estab-

Table 2. Stop Codon Capture Following AT Pressure in *Mycoplasma capricolum*

1. UGA stop codons all mutate to UAA.
2. CCA tryptophan anticodon duplicates, and one duplicate mutates to UGA and can pair by wobble with UGG.
3. UGG tryptophan codons mutate to UGA, pairing with UCA. UGA stop codon has been captured by tryptophan.
4. CCA anticodon eventually disappears.

Jukes (1985).

Table 4. UGA Codon for Tryptophan Disappears under GC Pressure and Re-emerges as a Stop Codon

1. UGA tryptophan codons mutate to UGG.
2. UCA tryptophan anticodon mutates to CCA, pairing only with UGG.
3. Some UAA stop codons mutate to UGA stop codons.

UGA tryptophan is captured by UGA stop.

Table 5. Minimal Code and tRNA Anticodons for 20 Amino Acids

First codon base	Second codon base				Third codon base
	U	C	A	G	
U	Phe GAA Leu UAA	Ser UGA	Tyr GUA Stop —	Cys GCA Trp UCA	U, C, A, G
C	Leu UAG	Pro UGG	His GUG Gln UUG	Arg UCG	U, C, A, G
A	Ile GAU Met UAU	Thr UGU	Asn GUU Lys UUU	Ser GCU Arg UCU	U, C, A, G
G	Val UAC	Ala UGC	Asp GUC Glu UUC	Gly UCC	U, C, A, G

The mammalian mitochondrial code is identical except that Met = CAU, and UCU, Arg, is missing.

lished as an isoleucine codon, used rather infrequently. These steps are shown in Table 7.

We turn now to the case of arginine, with its postulated anticodons GCG and UCG in the early code. Under GC pressure, CGU and CGA codons converted to CGC and CGG. Anticodon UCG was then converted to CCG because no CGA codons existed. A new enzyme appeared, tRNA hypoxanthine-ribosyltransferase (HRT) (Elliott and Trewyn 1984), which substitutes A in the first position of anticodons by I, inosine, the nucleoside with the base hypoxanthine, pairing with U, C, and A in the third-codon positions. Under AT pressure, anticodon ACG was produced by mutation from GCG. Anticodon ACG was converted to ICG by HRT, and anticodon ICG paired with arginine codons CGU, CGC, and CGA. The fourth arginine codon, CGG, paired with anticodon CCG. These steps are shown in Table 8.

Not all the 14 CNN anticodons known in eubacteria are found in all eubacteria. Their distribution is related to the GC content of their respective bacterial species. This is discussed by Osawa and co-workers (this volume). For example, anticodons CAC, CUU, and CUC have been found in *Thermus thermophilus* but not in *Escherichia coli*.

The method for establishing the presence of either AT or GC pressure in a gene is as follows. The gene is sequenced and its codons are listed. The content of GC in the silent sites is then calculated. Silent sites are all

sites that can undergo a silent nucleotide substitution (Miyata and Yasunaga 1980; Jukes and Bhushan 1986). The GC content of all the other sites, which are the replacement sites, is then calculated, and the two values for GC content are compared. If the GC content of the silent sites is greater than the GC content of the replacement sites, GC pressure exists, and if the reverse is the case, AT pressure is exerted, as shown in Table 9. The rationale for this is that silent sites respond readily to biased mutational pressure, but replacement sites resist this pressure because of constraints on the amino acid composition of proteins.

We now turn to the eukaryotic code. This is markedly different from the eubacterial code, as a result of AT pressure and the action of tRNA hypoxanthine-ribosyltransferase, which has led to the appearance of INN anticodons in eight family boxes, as shown in Table 10. Therefore, there is a conspicuous difference between the eukaryotic and eubacterial codes in the use of inosine in anticodons, because only one INN anticodon, ICG, is found in bacteria. A possible explanation for this difference is that the HRT enzyme in bacteria may be specific for anticodon ACG, but a second form of the enzyme with a wider range of substrates may exist in eukaryotes. Perhaps it is specific for anticodons with a purine in the second position, except in the case of phenylalanine. There is no way of settling this question without further evidence, because INN anticodons cannot exist complementary to two-

Table 6. Hypothetical Early Code and tRNA Anticodons

First codon base	Second codon base				Third codon base
	U	C	A	G	
U	Phe GAA Leu UAA	Ser GGA Ser UGA	Tyr GUA Stop —	Cys GCA Trp UCA	U, C A, G
C	Leu GAG Leu UAG	Pro GGG Pro UGG	His GUG Gln UUG	Arg GCG Arg UCG	U, C A, G
A	Ile GAU Met UAU	Thr GGU Thr UGU	Asn GUU Lys UUU	Ser GCU Arg UCU	U, C A, G
G	Val GAC Val UAC	Ala GGC Ala UGC	Asp GUC Glu UUC	Gly GCC Gly UCC	U, C A, G

From Jukes (1983).

Table 7. Evolution of Early Methionine Codon AUA into Isoleucine Codon

1. AUA methionine codons change to AUG and UAU anticodon to CAU by GC pressure. AUA codons disappear.
2. Met tRNA with CAU anticodon duplicates. One duplicate mutates to accept isoleucine and anticodon is modified to *CAU.
3. AT pressure changes some AUC isoleucine codons to AUA, isoleucine, pairing with *CAU.

Table 9. Criteria for Presence of AT or GC Pressure in a Gene

1. Calculate GC content of *silent sites* (a). Silent sites are nucleotide sites that can undergo a substitution without causing an amino acid replacement.
2. All other sites are replacement sites, i.e., sites that cannot be substituted without causing an amino acid replacement. Calculate their GC content (b).
If $a < b$, AT pressure exists, e.g., in Trp synthase, *Bacillus subtilis*, $a = 40.5$; $b = 47.3$.
If $b < a$, GC pressure exists, e.g., in Trp synthase, *Pseudomonas aeruginosa*, $a = 92.2$; $b = 55.0$.

Jukes and Bhushan (1986).

codon sets without lethal effects. GNN anticodons, except for GCC, glycine, are not found in family boxes in the eukaryotic code. It may be concluded that INN anticodons were derived from GNN anticodons by AT pressure that produced ANN anticodons.

The presence of anticodon IAU in the eukaryotic code eliminates the need for the special anticodon, *CAU, for isoleucine that is found in bacterial codes. The evolution of IAU is shown in Table 11. Isoleucine anticodon GAU became changed to AAU. This was converted to IAU, which pairs with AUU, AUC, and AUA. *CAU disappeared because its coding function had been assumed by IAU. The eukaryotic code contains a full complement of CNN anticodons, because UNN anticodons are modified in eukaryotes, presumably to pair primarily with NNA, and only weakly or not at all with NNG.

We next examine the case of glutamine codons in ciliated protozoa. The sequence of events is proposed in Table 12 and was discussed by Jukes and co-workers (1987). The first event is the conversion of all stop codons to UGA, so that codons UAA and UAG disappear. Following this, under AT pressure, the stage was now set in ciliated protozoa (GC 20–30%) for the reappearance of UAA and UAG codons as glutamine codons. Anticodon CUG has not been found in *Tetrahymena*, and it may have been converted to UUG by AT pressure. The gene for glutamine tRNA with anticodon UUG duplicated, and one of the duplicates, under AT pressure, acquired anticodon UUA. Later, the tRNA gene with anticodon UUA duplicated again, and, in one of the duplicates, anticodon UUA mutated to CUA, as shown by the close evolutionary relationship of the tRNAs with anticodons UUA and CUA; only four nucleotide differences (Hanyu et al. 1986). Differences in nucleotide sequences between "new" tRNAs, anticodons UUA and CUA, and tRNA

with anticodon UUG are 13 and 11. Meanwhile, some of the glutamine codons CAA and CAG mutated under AT pressure to UAA and UAG. These have been identified as alternate glutamine codons in several ciliated protozoans, including *Tetrahymena*, *Stylonychia*, and *Paramecium* (Caron and Meyer 1985; Helftenbein 1985; Horowitz and Gorovsky 1985; Preer et al. 1985).

The codes for mitochondria and chloroplasts have been derived from a eubacterial code. AT pressure during the evolution of mitochondria was accompanied by the elimination of a number of tRNA genes. AT pressure reduces the number of anticodons by eliminating CNN anticodons. As a result, all CNN anticodons disappeared except for CAU, methionine. Also by AT pressure, GNN anticodons disappeared from family boxes, and the sole anticodons became single UNN anticodons, containing unmodified U, pairing by four-way wobble with sets of four codons ending in U, C, A, and G. In the vertebrate mitochondrial code, anticodon UCU was lost, so that AGA and AGG became stop codons. By these steps, the vertebrate mitochondrial code became closely similar to the minimal code for 20 amino acids, as shown in Table 5.

The mitochondrial code is less stable than the other codes. Mitochondria can apparently tolerate changes in the assignment of codons because mitochondria, especially mammalian mitochondria, have only a small number of protein genes. Evolutionary advantage for

Table 8. Evolution of Codon–Anticodon Pairing in Arginine CGN Codons

1. Arginine anticodon GCG in early code pairs with codons CGU and CGC. Anticodon UCG pairs with CGA and CGG.
2. Under GC pressure, CGA codons disappear. Anticodon UCG is converted to CCG.
3. GC pressure changes to AT pressure. GCG mutates to ACG, which is converted by tRNA-hypoxanthine-ribosyl transferase to ICG, pairing with CGU, CGC, and CGA.
4. CGU and CGA codons reappear by mutation from some CGC and CGG codons. Anticodon CGG remains, pairing with CGG.

Table 10. Anticodons in Eukaryotic Code

GAA Phe	IGA Ser	GUA Tyr	GCA Cys
(UAA Leu)	UGA Ser		
CAA Leu	CGA Ser		CCA Trp
IAG Leu	IGG Pro	GUG His	ICG Arg
UAG Leu	UGG Pro	UGG Gln	UCG Arg
CAG Leu	CGG Pro	CUG Gln	CCG Arg
IAU Ile	IGU Thr	GUU Asn	GCU Ser
UAU Ile		UUU Lys	UCU Arg
CAU Met	(CGU Thr)	CUU Lys	CCU Arg
IAC Val	IGC Ala	GUC Asp	GCC Gly
UAC Val	UGC Ala	UUC Glu	UCC Gly
CAC Val	(CGC Ala)	CUC Glu	CCC Gly

Anticodons in parentheses have not been described but are presumed to exist. UUA and CUA are anticodons for glutamine in ciliated protozoa only. Anticodon UGU may also exist but translation of codon ACA can take place in its absence.

Table 11. Evolution of Isoleucine and Methionine Anticodons in Eukaryotic Code

1. Following changes shown in Table 7, isoleucine anticodon GAU mutates to AAU, and AAU is converted to IAU by hypoxanthine ribosyltransferase. IAU pairs with AUU, AUC, and AUA isoleucine.
2. Anticodon *CAU disappears, its function having been taken over by IAU.

such changes may exist because invading mRNA molecules would be mistranslated (Barrell et al. 1979). Changes in coding assignment in mitochondria also include use of CUN for threonine (yeast) (Li and Tzagoloff 1979), and AGA for serine (*Drosophila*) (de Bruijn 1983).

A second eubacterial family, cyanobacteria, became endosymbiotic in a line of eukaryotes that led to the green plants. Symbiotic residence became accompanied by lowering of DNA content accompanied by AT pressure. The chloroplast code is known completely, as a result of the sequencing of the entire chloroplast genome of *Marchantia* (Ohyama et al. 1986). Anticodons in the chloroplast code are in Table 13. Two, perhaps three, of the family boxes contain a single UNN anticodon with four-way wobbling. Under AT pressure, most of the CNN anticodons have been eliminated from the chloroplast code, with the exception of anticodon CAA pairing with leucine codons UUR, and anticodons *CAU, CAU, and CCA. The last three are needed for pairing with isoleucine (AUA), methionine, and tryptophan codons.

The chloroplast code is in a process of evolution in which it has discarded all but four of the CNN anticodons that are found in the eubacterial code, and has also discarded two GNN anticodons that are present in the eubacterial code. A third GNN anticodon, GGG, is apparently in the process of being discarded (Ohyama et al. 1986), because the tRNA gene containing it has become inactive. Possibly, the chloroplast code may eventually evolve to the code that is found in vertebrate mitochondria.

We do not know the CNN anticodon content of the eubacterial progenitors of mitochondria and chloroplasts.

Halobacterial and methanococcal codes: The remaining group of organisms, named Archaebacteria by Woese (1981), and Metabacteria by Hori and Osawa (1979), contains several families, including the Halobacteria and Methanobacteria. Halobacteria have a high GC content in their DNA, as shown by 68% of

Table 12. Stop Codon "Capture" in Ciliates

1. Stop codons UGA and UAG mutate to UAA (Stop), then UAA mutates to UGA (Stop).
2. *AT pressure:*
Glutamine anticodon UUG duplicates, and one duplicate mutates to UUA. Glutamine codons CAA and CAG mutate to UAA and UAG, pairing with UUA. Later, glutamine anticodon UUA mutates to CUA, pairing strongly with UAG.

GC in the *brp* gene of *H. halobium* (Betlach et al. 1984), and an almost complete set of anticodons for *Halobacterium volcanii* has been discovered by Gupta (1984, 1986). These are shown in Table 14, together with the anticodons so far reported for *Methanococcus*, which has only 31% GC. According to Gupta (1985), INN anticodons, including ICG, are not present in halobacteria. The halobacterial code resembles the eubacterial code except for the absence, as noted, of ICG and the presence of GCG and UCG.

The halobacterial code, as shown in Table 14, may be regarded as complete if the anticodons shown in parentheses are presumed to exist, and if the possible presence of anticodon CCU that is present in the eubacterial code (Table 13) and can be presumed by the presence of an arginine codon AGG in *H. halobium* (Betlach et al. 1984) is included, for a total of 45 anticodons. The halobacterial code is notable for its symmetry of anticodon content, and 25 anticodons, of which 16 are known, can be predicted for the *Methanococcus* code (Table 14). Since no CNN anticodons (except CAU) are included among the 16 known anticodons for *Methanococcus* (Jarsch and Bock 1983; Wich et al. 1984, 1986), it seems likely that *Methanococcus* avoids the use of CNN anticodons, as one would expect from the low GC content of its DNA.

A diagram of the various steps discussed in the text is presented in Figure 1. Downwards, the code is shown as accumulating GNN and CNN anticodons under GC pressure. Loss of codons UGA and AUA takes place. Following this, some UGA stop codons are formed from UAA, and AT pressure then intervenes so that AUA reappears as an isoleucine codon. The enzyme HRT appears, forming anticodon ICG from ACG, which was produced from GCG by mutation, and the progenitor of the eubacterial and eukaryotic codes takes form. Further AT pressure in the eukaryotic line and the action of HRT result in the formation of seven more INN anticodons replacing GNN. Stop codons UAA and UAG are eventually captured by glutamine in ciliated protozoa under strong AT pressure.

The eubacterial code diverges in various directions, depending on GC or AT pressure in bacterial families, leading to codes with varying numbers of CNN anticodons.

A second bacterial "kingdom," including halobacteria and methanogens, has codes resembling a code preceding the introduction of HRT, but this kingdom has similarities to eukaryotes (Hori and Osawa 1979), so its point of divergence is not clear. Anticodons in the halobacterial code are known almost completely, and at least half the anticodons in the methanococcus code have been identified. Methanococci are low in GC (31% of DNA in *M. vannielii*), and are low in content of CNN anticodons, just as in the case of low GC eubacteria.

One of the interesting problems in the code that has been explored only partially is the modification of U in the first anticodon position. Yokoyama and colleagues (1985) reviewed this field. In anticodons for glutamine,

Table 13. Anticodons in Eubacterial Code, Mammalian Mitochondrial Code, and Chloroplast Code

M, C	GAA Phe	C	GGA Ser	M, C	GUA Tyr	M, C	GCA Cys
M, C	UAA Leu	M, C	UGA Ser			C	CCA Trp*
C	CAA Leu		CGA Ser			C	ICG Arg*
	GAG Leu	(C)	GGG Pro	M, C	GUG His		
M, C	UAG Leu	M, C	UGG Pro	M, C	UUG Gln		
	CAG Leu		CGG Pro		CUG Gln	C	CCG Arg
M, C	GAU Ile	C	GGU Thr†	M, C	GUU Asn	M, C	GCU Ser
C	*CAU Ile	M, C	UGU Thr	M, C	UUU Lys	C	UCU Arg
M, C	CAU Met				CUU Lys		CCU Arg
C	GAC Val		GGC Ala	M, C	GUC Asp	C	GCC Gly
M, C	UAC Val	M, C	UGC Ala	M, C	UUC Glu	M, C	UCC Gly
	CAC Val				CUC Glu		CCC Gly

The mitochondrial and chloroplast codes are evidently derived from the eubacterial code; M = mammalian mitochondria; C = chloroplast.

*UCA is the sole mammalian mitochondrial anticodon for tryptophan and UCG for arginine. UCA is the anticodon for tryptophan in *Mycoplasma*.

†AGU is an anticodon for threonine in *Mycoplasma*.

ICG (from ACG) and *CAU (from CAU) are inferred to exist in chloroplasts. (C) The chloroplast gene containing anticodon GGG is apparently inactive. *C = modified C.

lysine, and glutamic acid, U is modified to a 2-thiouridine derivative, which pairs predominantly with A rather than G, and in other cases, U is modified to a derivative of 5-hydroxyuridine, which pairs with A, G, and U in third-codon positions. The latter modification is found in family box anticodons for valine, serine, threonine, and alanine in *E. coli* and *B. subtilis* (Yokoyama et al. 1985; Hara-Yokoyama et al. 1986).

There is very little published information on the nature of a third modification of U occurring in first positions of anticodons pairing with NNR two-codon sets of mitochondria. Such a modification is important in evolution, because it was needed for expansion of the archaetypal code for 14 or 15 amino acids (Fig. 1) to its present complement of 20 amino acids (Jukes 1966, 1983).

When the expansion took place, a crucial change had to take place in the wobble mechanism. When a UNN anticodon pairs with four different codons, it does not need to distinguish between NNY and NNR anticodons. If, however, a distinction must be made between NNY codons pairing with anticodon GNN, and

NNR codons pairing with anticodon UNN, the base U in anticodon UNN must be modified to prevent it from mispairing with NNY codons. In consequence, the U in all UNN anticodons is modified in the eubacterial and eukaryotic codes, except for some UNN anticodons in *Mycoplasma* family boxes as discussed by Osawa and co-workers (this volume). The updated wobble rules are shown in Table 15.

The codons that are most subject to evolutionary reassignments are, obviously, the three stop codons UAA, UAG, and UGA. All three of these have been "captured" by amino acids in some organisms: UGA in *Mycoplasma* and UAA and UAG in ciliated protozoa.

Changes of amino acid assignments of codons and of codon-anticodon pairing during genetic code evolution should have been neutral (Kimura 1983). This could have taken place by various procedures to forestall the appearance of unusable nonsense codons as described above.

The nature of AT/CG pressures has been discussed, but not completely explored. Mutational modifications in DNA-synthesizing systems can bias the mutation

Table 14. Known and Predicted Anticodons in Halobacteria (H) and Methanococcus (M) Codes

H, M	GAA Phe	H	GGA Ser	H, M	GUA Tyr	H(M)	GCA Cys
H(M)	UAA Leu	H(M)	UGA Ser			H(M)	CCA Trp
H	CAA Leu	H	CGA Ser				
H	GAG Leu	H	GGG Pro	H, M	GUG His	H	GCG Arg
H, M	UAG Leu	H, M	UGG Pro	(H)M	UUG Gln	H(M)	UCG Arg
H	CAG Leu	H	CGG Pro	H	CUG Gln	H	CCG Arg
H(M)	GAU Ile	H, M	GGU Thr	H, M	GUU Asn	H(M)	GCU Ser
H, M	*CAU Ile	(H)M	UGU Thr	H, M	UUU Lys	(H)M	UCU Arg
H(M)	CAU Met	H	CGU Pro	H	CUU Lys	(H)	CCU Arg
H	GAC Val	H	GGC Ala	H, M	GUC Asp	H	GCC Gly
H, M	UAC Val	H, M	UGC Ala	H, M	UUC Glu	H(M)	UUC Gly
H	CAC Val	H	CGC Ala	H	CUC Glu	H	CCC Gly

Halobacterial code contains 41 known anticodons and 4 more anticodons can be predicted. Methanococcus code contains 16 known anticodons and nine more anticodons can be predicted. *C = Probably modified C. Predictions for anticodons are in parentheses.

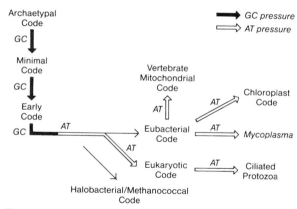

Figure 1. Evolution of genetic codes, showing periods of GC and AT pressure. Details of the codes, shown as anticodons, are in the tables, and are explained in the text.

rate toward either AT pairs or GC pairs (Speyer 1965; Cox and Yanofsky 1967). Methylation and deamination of DNA bases can lead to accumulation of AT pairs in DNA. AT/GC pressure has been exerted on the genome at different rates in various phylogenetic lines, and is always subject to change.

The approach we have used to explore evolution of the code is based on several concepts.

Evolutionary changes or phenomena that have been identified include: neutral evolutionary changes without dislocation of amino acid sequences; gene duplications and mutations that enable new anticodons to appear with change of amino acid assignment (Squires and Carbon 1971; Yamao et al. 1985); disappearance of codons and anticodons resulting from AT/GC pressures; increases in the numbers of CNN anticodons caused by GC pressure; and stop codon capture by amino acids. Changes in the code are adaptive and nondeleterious.

The original minimal code for 20 amino acids contained all 64 three-base codons, and used the minimum number of anticodons (22) needed for codon-anticodon pairing, based on the wobble rules, with four-way wobble in family boxes.

The number of anticodons has increased through various steps. Evolution continued until three existing

Table 15. Anticodon–Codon Pairing

Anticodon first base	Codon third base	Examples
U	U, C, A, G	Mitochondrial code in family boxes
*U	A, G	Mitochondrial code in two-codon sets
†U	A	Eukaryotes
‡U	U, A, G	Eubacteria in family boxes
C	G	All codes
*C	A	Bacteria, isoleucine codon AUA
G	U, C	All codes
A	U	Rare
I	U, C, A	Eukaryotes, ICG in eubacteria

Revised from Crick (1966).

*, †, ‡ = Various modifications of U (Yokoyama et al. 1985),
*C = modified C.

forms of the universal code were produced. These are the eukaryotic code, the eubacterial code, and the code for halobacteria and methanococci. These three codes are distinguished from each other by their anticodon content. No code contains more than 45 anticodons.

Expansion of the code into these three forms was largely influenced by AT/GC pressures in DNA, and evolution of the code has continued within each of the three main groups. In the case of the eubacterial code, evolution has led to differences in the number of CNN anticodons in different bacterial families and higher GC content of DNA is accompanied by larger numbers of CNN anticodons. This is also true of halobacteria as compared with methanococci.

The mitochondrial and chloroplast codes were derived from the eubacterial code through genomic economization and AT pressure, leading to losses of GNN and CNN anticodons. The mitochondrial code has regressed further in this direction than has the chloroplast code. The eukaryotic code is distinctive because it contains eight INN anticodons in family boxes replacing GNN anticodons, except for GCC, glycine. It contains a full complement of CNN anticodons, pairing with NNG codons.

Except for its content of the "magic 20 amino acids" (Crick 1968), the code is not "frozen" (Crick 1968). The use of UGA as a tryptophan codon by *Mycoplasma* and of UAA and UAG as glutamine codons by ciliated protozoa are examples of recent evolutionary changes. Neither *Mycoplasma* nor ciliated protozoans represent "new kingdoms."

Comparisons of the sequences of tRNA molecules should be a fruitful field of study in estimating the recent evolution of the code.

SUMMARY

Clues to evolution of the genetic code can be found by comparing usage of anticodons in various organisms and organelles. GC content of DNA varies, as a result of directional mutation pressure (AT/GC pressure), especially in bacteria. Low GC in *Mycoplasma* is accompanied by use of UGA for tryptophan and, in ciliated protozoa, by use of UAA and UAG for glutamine. These are examples of "stop codon capture," which has been preceded by duplication of tRNA genes followed by nucleotide substitutions in their sequences, including mutational changes in their anticodons. Evolutionary changes in the code may have resulted from disappearance of codons and anticodons resulting from GC pressure and from their reappearance when the direction of the pressure was reversed. In this manner, codon UGA and anticodon UCA for tryptophan could have disappeared under GC pressure and reappeared in *Mycoplasma* under AT pressure. Stop codon UGA may have been the third of the three stop codons to appear, originating from mutations in UAA. Changes in the code are adaptive and nondeleterious.

We propose that the number of anticodons has increased and that evolution continued until three existing forms of the universal code were produced: eukaryotic, eubacterial, and the code for halobacteria and methanococci. These three codes are distinguished from each other by their anticodon pattern. The eukaryotic code contains eight INN (ANN) anticodons that have replaced GNN anticodons as a result of AT pressure. Mitochondrial and chloroplast codes have evolved from the eubacterial code through genomic economization and AT pressure, leading to losses of GNN and CNN anticodons. The mitochondrial code uses "four-way wobble" with UNN anticodons in eight family boxes, and there are three examples of this in the chloroplast code. The code is still evolving except for its content of the present 20 amino acids, from which no exceptions are known. The wobble rules of codon-anticodon pairing were fundamental in the evolution of the code.

ACKNOWLEDGMENTS

T.H. Jukes gratefully acknowledges the support by NASA grant NGR-05 003 460, editing and preparation of the manuscript by Carol Fegte, comments by R. Gupta and R.W. Trewyn, and information from S. Nishimura and Y. Kuchino. S. Osawa and A. Muto were supported by a grant from the Ministry of Education of Japan.

REFERENCES

Barrell, G., A.T. Bankier, and J. Drouin. 1979. A different genetic code in human mitochondria. *Nature* **282:** 189.

Betlach, M., J. Friedman, H.W. Boyer, and F. Pfeifer. 1984. Characterization of a halobacterial gene affecting bacteriorhodopsin gene expression. *Nucleic Acids Res.* **12:** 7949.

Caron, F. and E. Meyer. 1985. Does *Paramecium primaurelia* use a different genetic code in its macronucleus? *Nature* **314:** 185.

Cox, E.C. and C. Yanofsky. 1967. Altered base ratios in the DNA of an *Escherichia coli* mutator strain. *Proc. Natl. Acad. Sci.* **58:** 1895.

Crick, F.H.C. 1966. Codon-anticodon pairing: The wobble hypothesis. *J. Mol. Biol.* **19:** 548.

———. 1968. The origin of the genetic code. *J. Mol. Biol.* **38:** 367.

de Bruijn, M.H.L. 1983. *Drosophila melanogaster* mitochondrial DNA, a novel organization and genetic code. *Nature* **304:** 234.

Elliott, M.S. and R.W. Trewyn. 1984. Inosine biosynthesis in transfer RNA by enzymatic insertion of hypoxanthine. *J. Biol. Chem.* **259:** 2407.

Gupta, R. 1984. *Halobacterium volcanii* tRNAs: Identification of 41 tRNAs covering all amino acids, and the sequences of 33 class I tRNAs. *J. Biol. Chem.* **259:** 9461.

———. 1985. Archaebacteria. In *The bacteria* (ed. C.R. Woese and R.S. Wolfe), vol. 8, p. 311. Academic Press, New York.

———. 1986. Transfer RNAs of *Halobacterium volcanii*: Sequences of five leucine and three serine tRNAs. *Syst. Appl. Microbiol.* **7:** 102.

Hanyu, N., Y. Kuchino, and S. Nishimura. 1986. Dramatic events in ciliate evolution: Alteration of UAA and UAG termination codons to glutamine codons due to anticodon mutations in two *Tetrahymena* tRNAs^Gln. *EMBO J.* **5:** 1307.

Hara-Yokoyama, M., S. Yokoyama, T. Watanabe, K. Watanabe, M. Kitazumi, Y. Mitamura, T. Morii, S.

Takahashi, Y. Kuchino, S. Nishimura, and T. Miyazawa. 1986. Characteristic anticodon sequences of major tRNA species from an extreme thermophile, *Thermus thermophilus* HB8. *FEBS Lett.* **202:** 149.

Helftenbein, E. 1985. Nucleotide sequence of a macronuclear DNA molecule coding for α-tubulin from the ciliate *Stylonychia lemnae*. Special codon usage: TAA is not a translation termination codon. *Nucleic Acids Res.* **13:** 415.

Hori, H. and S. Osawa. 1979. Evolutionary change in 5S RNA secondary structure and a phylogenic tree of 54 5S RNA species. *Proc. Natl. Acad. Sci.* **76:** 381.

Horowitz, S. and M.A. Gorovsky. 1985. An unusual genetic code in nuclear genes of *Tetrahymena*. *Proc. Natl. Acad. Sci.* **82:** 2452.

Jarsch, M. and A. Bock. 1983. DNA sequence of the 16S rRNA/23 rRNA intercistronic spacer of two rDNA operons of the archaebacterium *Methanococcus vannielii*. *Nucleic Acids. Res.* **11:** 7537.

Jukes, T.H. 1966. *Molecules and evolution*. Columbia University Press, New York.

———. 1983. Evolution of the amino acid code: Inferences from mitochondrial codes. *J. Mol. Evol.* **19:** 219.

———. 1985. A change in the genetic code in *Mycoplasma capricolum*. *J. Mol. Evol.* **22:** 361.

Jukes, T.H. and V. Bhushan. 1986. Silent nucleotide substitutions and G + C content of some mitochondrial and bacterial genes. *J. Mol. Evol.* **24:** 39.

Jukes, T.H., S. Osawa, and A. Muto. 1987. Divergence and directional mutation pressures. *Nature* **325:** 668.

Kimura, M. 1983. *The neutral theory of molecular evolution*. Cambridge University Press, Cambridge, England.

Li, M. and A. Tzagoloff. 1979. Assembly of the mitochondrial membrane system: Sequences of yeast mitochondrial valine and an unusual threonine tRNA gene. *Cell* **18:** 47.

Miyata, T. and T. Yasunaga. 1980. Molecular evolution of mRNA: A method for estimating evolutionary rates of synonymous and amino acid substitutions from homologous nucleotide sequences and its application. *J. Mol. Evol.* **16:** 23.

Ohyama, K., H. Fukuzawa, T. Kohchi, H. Shirai, T. Sano, S. Sano, K. Umesono, Y. Shiki, M. Takeuchi, Z. Chang, S.-I. Aota, H. Inokuchi, and H Ozeki. 1986. Chloroplast gene organization deduced from complete sequence of liverwort *Marchantia polymorpha* chloroplast DNA. *Nature* **322:** 572.

Preer, J.R., Jr., L.B. Preer, B.M. Rudman, and A.J. Barnett. 1985. Deviation from the universal code shown by the gene for surface protein 51A in *Paramecium*. *Nature* **314:** 188.

Speyer, J. 1965. Mutagenic DNA polymerase. *Biochem. Biophys. Res. Commun.* **21:** 6.

Squires, C. and J. Carbon. 1971. Normal and mutant glycine transfer RNA. *Nature New Biol.* **233:** 274.

Sueoka, N. 1961. Variation and heterogeneity of base composition of deoxyribonecleic acids: A compilation of old and new data. *J. Mol. Biol.* **3:** 31.

———. 1962. On the genetic basis of variation and heterogeneity of DNA base composition. *Proc. Natl. Acad. Sci.* **48:** 582.

Wich, G., M. Jarsch, and A. Bock. 1984. Apparent operon for a 5S ribosomal RNA gene and for tRNA genes in the archaebacterium *Methanococcus vannielii*. *Mol. Gen. Genet.* **196:** 146.

Wich, G., L. Sibold, and A. Bock. 1986. Genes for tRNA and their putative expression signals in *Methanococcus*. *Syst. Appl. Microbiol.* **7:** 18.

Woese, C.R. 1981. Archaebacteria. *Sci. Am.* **244:** 98.

Yamao, F., A. Muto, Y. Kawauchi, M. Iwami, S. Iwagami, Y. Azumi, and S. Osawa. 1985. UGA is read as tryptophan in *Mycoplasma capricolum*. *Proc. Natl. Acad. Sci.* **82:** 2306.

Yokoyama, S., T. Watanabe, K. Murao, H. Ishikura, Z. Yamaizumi, S. Nishimura, and T. Miyazawa. 1985. Molecular mechanism of codon recognition by tRNAs with modified uridine in the first position of the anticodon. *Proc. Natl. Acad. Sci.* **82:** 4905.

Role of Directional Mutation Pressure in the Evolution of the Eubacterial Genetic Code

S. Osawa,* T.H. Jukes,[†] A. Muto,* F. Yamao,* T. Ohama,* and Y. Andachi*
*Laboratory of Molecular Genetics, Department of Biology, Nagoya University, Nagoya 464, Japan;
[†]Space Sciences Laboratory, University of California, Berkeley, California 94720

GC Contents of Eubacterial Genomes

Among eubacteria, the mean guanine and cytosine (GC) contents of genomic DNA vary approximately from 25% to 75% (Sueoka 1962). The phylogenetic tree to eubacterial 5S rRNA has indicated that bacterial genome GC contents are to some extent related to phylogeny (Hori and Osawa 1986). According to this tree, the gram-negative and the gram-positive bacteria diverged first. Among the gram-positive bacteria, those with low genomic GC content such as *Bacillus subtilis* (genomic GC: 43%), *Lactobacillus viridescens* (40%), *Staphylococcus aureus* (33%), *Clostridium perfringens* (38%), and *Mycoplasma capricolum* (25%) are phylogenetically close, whereas those with high genomic GC, such as *Micrococcus luteus* (74%), *Streptomyces griseus* (73%), and *Mycobacterium tuberculosis* (67%) comprise another phylogenetic group. These two groups separated long ago. The gram-negative bacteria with intermediate GC, such as *Escherichia coli* (50%), *Serratia marcescens* (58%), *Salmonella typhimurium* (51%), and *Pseudomonas fluorescens* (60%) belong to the common gram-negative branch. The differences in the genomic GC contents may have been caused mainly by mutation pressure (Sueoka 1962), the direction and magnitude of this pressure varying among the phylogenetic lines (Muto and Osawa 1987). Such a mutation pressure, which we call GC/AT pressure, is due to biased mutation rates among the four bases and seems to have been exerted on the entire genome during evolution (Jukes and Bhushan 1986; Muto and Osawa 1987). The mutations caused by GC/AT pressure are subject to selective constraints that usually eliminate functionally deleterious changes by negative selection. A certain fraction of nondeleterious mutations are then fixed in the population due to random genetic drift (Kimura 1983). Thus, functionally less important parts in the genome evolve faster than more important parts. For a given species, GC/AT pressure changes the GC content of various parts of the genome in the same direction, but to different extents, depending on their functional importance.

Correlation of GC Contents between the Entire Genome and the Specific Parts of the Genome

The bacterial genome is roughly composed of protein genes (70–80%), spacers, including various signals (20–30%), and stable RNA genes (less than 1%). In Figure 1 are plotted the GC contents of different parts of the genome against the mean GC contents of various bacterial genomes, indicating that all the components positively, but to different extents, correlate with the genomic GC contents (Muto and Osawa 1987). There exists a weak but apparent positive correlation of the GC contents of both rRNA and tRNA with the genomic GC content. In contrast, the GC contents of spacers and protein genes reveal a strong and linear correlation with the genomic GC content. Among various bacteria, the GC content of spacers ranges from

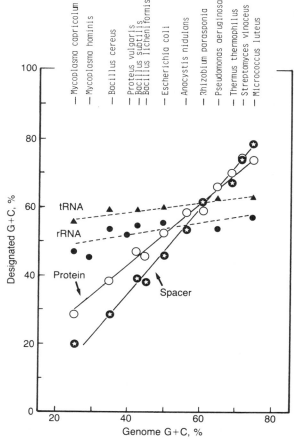

Figure 1. Correlation of GC content between total genomic DNA and designated parts of the genome. (Reprinted, with permission, from Muto and Osawa 1987.)

about 20% to 80%, and that of protein genes from about 30% to 75%, with the variation of genomic DNA GC contents from 25% (*M. capricolum*) to 74% (*M. luteus*). Thus, for a given species, the GC contents of spacers, protein genes, and stable RNA genes are all biased in the same direction as the GC content of the total genome. This bias is stronger for spacers, less so for protein genes, and least for stable RNA genes, although contributions to the average GC content are in the order of protein genes, spacers, and stable RNA genes. These positive colinearities shown in Figure 1 support the idea that GC/AT pressure strongly influences the GC content of entire DNA during evolution. Since spacers are the least functional component of the genome, most mutations in these regions are selectively neutral, and therefore the evolutionary rate is higher than in other parts. The rRNA and tRNA genes are less variable because most of their sequences are important for biological function. Protein genes are more variable than the stable RNA genes because many synonymous codon changes and amino acid replacements occur without deleterious effects.

Codon Usage

A species-specific nonrandom trend in codon usage has been widely recognized (see, e.g., Ikemura and Ozeki 1983). In Figure 2 are plotted the GC contents of the first, second, and third codon positions, respectively, of various bacterial species against the corresponding genome GC contents (Muto and Osawa 1987). The GC contents of all three positions reveal a linear positive relationship with the genome GC content, having different steepness of slope in the rank order of the third, first, and second positions. The most striking observation is that the GC content of the third positions varies linearly from about 10% in *M. capricolum* to more than 90% in *M. luteus*. The strongest correlation in the third position may be largely the result of GC/AT pressure. Note, however, that the slope is steeper in the third nucleotide positions of codons than for spacers. This is due to, in addition to GC/AT pressure, considerable selective constraints by tRNA that are exerted on the third nucleotide positions of codons (see below). In Figure 2, comparisons are made between various protein genes. It is, of course, desirable to use homologous genes for this purpose, but the available data of this kind are limited. Among the most useful genes for such comparisons are those for ribosomal proteins and related proteins, such as elongation factors. The functional structure of ribosomes is well conserved throughout eubacteria, and hence it is expected that most, if not all, of the codon substitutions must be neutral or nearly neutral, because most of the substitutions that can be observed would have no selective advantages for the ribosomal functions.

We compared substitutions of 2769 homologous codon sites in the genes for 20 ribosomal proteins in the S10 and *spc* operon for *M. capricolum* (genome GC: 25%) (Muto et al. 1984; S. Ohkubo et al., unpubl.) and

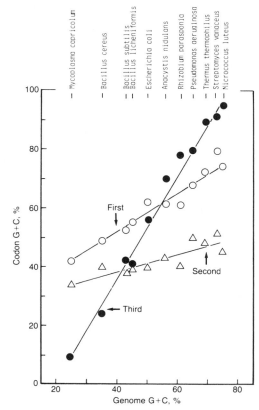

Figure 2. Correlation of GC content between total genomic DNA and the first, second, and third codon positions. (Reprinted, with permission, from Muto and Osawa 1987.)

E. coli (50%) (Cerretti et al. 1983; Zurawski and Zurawski 1985). In the two species, 498 codons (18%) were identical. There were 843 (30%) synonymous (silent) codon substitutions, and 1428 (52%) amino acid replacements. About 98% of the synonymous codon substitutions occurred at the third and/or first positions. In most cases, G or C of codon silent positions in *E. coli* was replaced by A or U(T) in *M. capricolum* (see also Muto et al. 1984; Muto and Osawa 1987). Among 1428 amino acid replacements, 64% of codon changes occurred in the direction of higher AT content in *M. capricolum*, whereas only 11% occurred in the other direction. Altogether, 66% of the substituted codons gained AT, 9% lost AT, and 25% showed no gain or loss of AT. The numbers of total AT gain and loss in the all nucleotide sites (6813) in the substituted codons were 2022 and 229, respectively. All these facts suggest that strong mutation pressure has caused *M. capricolum* to use A and T instead of G and C wherever possible. Several GC-rich codons such as CUC, CUG, UCC, CCC, ACG, CGG, and GGC were absent in sequences studied so far (Table 1), and GUG as initiation codon has never been found.

In contrast, a strongly GC-biased codon usage exists in GC-rich bacteria, such as *Streptomyces* species (Mizusawa et al. 1986; Zalacain et al. 1986) and *M. luteus* (T. Ohama et al., unpubl.). We compared substitutions

Table 1. Codon Usage in S10/*spc* Operon of *M. capricolum* and *E. coli*

	M. cap.[a]	E. coli[b]		M. cap.	E. coli		M. cap.	E. coli		M. cap.	E. coli
Phe (UUU)	112	36	Ser (UCU)	52	58	Tyr (UAU)	69	21	Cys (UGU)	11	6
Phe (UUC)	17	81	Ser (UCC)	0	39	Tyr (UAC)	17	43	Cys (UGC)	4	10
Leu (UUA)	231	13	Ser (UCA)	110	6	Stop (UAA)	15	20	Stop (UGA)	24(Trp)	4
Leu (UUG)	8	23	Ser (UCG)	1	6	Stop (UAG)	7	1	Trp (UGG)	2	22
Leu (CUU)	17	14	Pro (CCU)	42	27	His (CAU)	32	24	Arg (CGU)	50	189
Leu (CUC)	0	15	Pro (CCC)	0	3	His (CAC)	14	39	Arg (CGC)	4	88
Leu (CUA)	26	1	Pro (CCA)	79	17	Gln (CAA)	135	39	Arg (CGA)	2	6
Leu (CUG)	0	206	Pro (CCG)	2	89	Gln (CAG)	2	91	Arg (CGG)	0	1
Ile (AUU)	253	76	Thr (ACU)	131	77	Asn (AAU)	158	24	Ser (AGU)	39	9
Ile (AUC)	33	156	Thr (ACC)	4	88	Asn (AAC)	41	90	Ser (AGC)	9	35
Ile (AUA)	31	1	Thr (ACA)	85	13	Lys (AAA)	415	222	Arg (AGA)	135	3
Met (AUG)	88	98	Thr (ACG)	0	17	Lys (AAG)	35	103	Arg (AGG)	1	0
Val (GUU)	183	164	Ala (GCU)	144	140	Asp (GAU)	118	65	Gly (GGU)	124	197
Val (GUC)	3	48	Ala (GCC)	2	36	Asp (GAC)	13	86	Gly (GGC)	0	106
Val (GUA)	94	85	Ala (GCA)	96	89	Glu (GAA)	204	141	Gly (GGA)	146	7
Val (GUG)	12	50	Ala (GCG)	3	81	Glu (GAG)	12	62	Gly (GGG)	10	16

[a] *M. capricolum.*

[b] *E. coli* (data from Cerretti et al. 1983; Zurawski and Zurawski 1985).

779

at 1291 homologous codon sites in the streptomycin operon genes for two ribosomal proteins (S12 and S7) and elongation factors G and Tu in *M. luteus* versus *E. coli*: 375 (29%) codons were identical. Among 916 (71%) substitutions, there were 468 (36%) synonymous (silent) codon substitutions, and 448 (35%) amino acid replacements. Almost all the synonymous codon substitutions (99%) occurred at the third position, where 82.7% of them resulted in GC increase in *M. luteus*, 15% were without gain or loss of GC, and only 2.3% accompanied a loss of GC. Among amino acid replacements, 55% of codon changes occurred in the direction of higher GC content and 22% of replacements were accompanied by a loss of GC. Among 916 substituted codons out of a total of 1291 codons compared, 66% of the codons gained GC, and 11% of the codons lost GC. The total of the GC gain and loss in all nucleotide sites (2748) in the substituted codons was 670 and 113, respectively. Many codons were completely absent among 1382 codons examined. These were UUU (Phe), UUA (Leu), UUG (Leu), CUA (Leu), AUA (Ile), GUA (Val), UCU (Ser), CCA (Pro), ACA (Thr), UAU (Tyr), CAA (Gln), AAA (Lys), GAA (Glu), UGU (Cys), AGU (Ser), AGA (Arg), and GGA (Gly), all of which have U or A at the third position of codons, with one exception of UUG leucine (Table 2). Codons UUA and UUG were probably converted by GC pressure to CUC or CUG by silent substitutions. The above "nonused" codons are used in high frequencies in *M. capricolum* (GC, 25%; see Table 1).

In *E. coli* or *B. subtilis* (GC, 43%), AUG is the regular initiation codon, although GUG is rarely used. In *M. luteus*, S12, EF-G, and EF-Tu use GUG as initiation codon, although S7 starts with AUG. In contrast, GUG is used only for one EF-Tu in *E. coli* (An and Jriensen 1980), showing that the AUG initiation codons for S12 and EF-G are replaced by GUG in *M. luteus*. In other GC-rich bacteria belonging to *Streptomyces*, three genes start with GUG among seven genes so far analyzed (see Zalacain et al. 1986). Thus, the GC-rich bacteria, including *M. luteus*, seem to use the GUG initiation codon more frequently than *E. coli*, *B. subtilis*, or *Mycoplasma*.

All these facts suggest that strong GC pressure has caused *M. luteus* to discriminate against A and U and to use G and C preferentially, in sharp contrast to the preferential use of A and U in *M. capricolum*.

Since the sequences of the *str* operon in *M. capricolum* and that of the S10/*spc* operon in *M. luteus* are not available, the codon sites in homologous genes of these two bacteria could not be directly compared. Even so, the comparison of the codon usage tables between the two species (Tables 1 and 2) shows a much sharper contrast than the comparison between *M. luteus* and *E. coli*. This is due to intermediary GC content of *E. coli* (50%) between that of *M. luteus* (74%) and *M. capricolum* (25%). For example, in *M. luteus*, 97% of threonine codons are ACC and ACG, whereas in *M. capricolum* 99.5% of threonine codons

are ACA and ACU; all codons for lysine are AAG in *M. luteus*, whereas 90% are AAA in *M. capricolum*; AUA isoleucine codon was not detected in *M. luteus*, although this codon is used considerably in *M. capricolum*. Similar sharp contrasts exist in most other codons in comparisons of these two species.

Amino Acid Composition of Proteins

Constraints that affect the composition of proteins include the relation of amino acid sequence and content to function, the existence of variable and constant regions, the composition of the genetic code, and the presence of GC/AT pressure in the genome. Some proteins, such as histones, change much more slowly in evolution than do others, such as hemoglobins. Near-neutral changes are found in variable regions of proteins and are more common in rapidly evolving proteins. An important constraint is the composition of the genetic code. Amino acids with four codons, such as alanine, valine, and threonine, occur more frequently in proteins than do methionine and tryptophan with only one codon apiece (King and Jukes 1969; Jukes et al. 1975). This constraint is modified, or even magnified, by the fact that the average composition of proteins departs from the proportions of codons in the genetic code. As a result, the percentages of each of the four nucleotides in the first and second codon positions are not uniform. This is shown in Table 3, based on "average" or "consensus" protein Ala-53 Arg-26 Asn-30 Asp-36 Cys-13 Gln-24 Glu-33 Gly-48 His-14 Ile-31 Leu-47 Lys-41 Met-11 Phe-25 Pro-25 Ser-45 Thr-37 Trp-8 Tyr-23 Val-42. In making the calculations, it was assumed that all codon sets were divided equally among synonymous codons. As a result, T, C, A, and G should be approximately equally represented in third positions, except that the exclusion of stop codons will make a slight difference in the percentages.

Percentages of A and G are high in the first position because lysine, aspartic acid, and glutamic acid levels are high in proportion to their representation in the code. A is high in the second position for the same reason, and G is low because arginine is low (Fig. 3).

GC/AT pressure in the genome also affects the amino acid composition of proteins (Sueoka 1962; Jukes and Bhushan 1986). Its effect is exerted on amino acids in near-neutral sites in the protein molecule. Jukes and Bhushan (1986) noted that mitochondrial proteins were higher in phenylalanine, asparagine, and tyrosine in response to AT pressure, and bacterial tryptophan synthase was higher in alanine, arginine (CG codons), and glycine in response to GC pressure.

In response to AT pressure, *M. capricolum* proteins, S10/*spc* operon, were higher in asparagine (AAY), isoleucine (AUY, AUA), and lysine (AAR), and lower in alanine (GCN), glycine (GGN), and valine (GUN) than the corresponding proteins in *E. coli* (Table 1). (Throughout this paper, the following abbreviations are used. N: U,C,A or G; R: A or G; Y: U or C; *U: thiouridine derivatives; **U: 5-hydroxyuridine deriva-

Table 2. Codon Usage in *str* Operon of *M. luteus* and *E. coli*

Codon	M. lut.[a]	E. coli[b]	Codon	M. lut.	E. coli	Codon	M. lut.	E. coli	Codon	M. lut.	E. coli
Phe (UUU)	0	7	Ser (UCU)	0	27	Tyr (UAU)	0	8	Cys (UGU)	0	4
Phe (UUC)	43	37	Ser (UCC)	36	18	Tyr (UAC)	37	28	Cys (UGC)	6	6
Leu (UUA)	0	2	Ser (UCA)	1	3	Stop (UAA)	1	3	Stop (UGA)	3	1
Leu (UUG)	0	2	Ser (UCG)	16	0	Stop (UAG)	0	0	Trp (UGG)	8	8
Leu (CUU)	1	4	Pro (CCU)	5	6	His (CAU)	1	7	Arg (CGU)	23	67
Leu (CUC)	35	5	Pro (CCC)	27	2	His (CAC)	30	24	Arg (CGC)	61	16
Leu (CUA)	0	0	Pro (CCA)	0	5	Gln (CAA)	0	1	Arg (CGA)	1	0
Leu (CUG)	54	78	Pro (CCG)	35	52	Gln (CAG)	47	39	Arg (CGG)	2	1
Ile (AUU)	1	14	Thr (ACU)	3	34	Asn (AAU)	3	2	Ser (AGU)	0	6
Ile (AUC)	73	72	Thr (ACC)	68	40	Asn (AAC)	43	41	Ser (AGC)	1	3
Ile (AUA)	0	0	Thr (ACA)	0	5	Lys (AAA)	0	69	Arg (AGA)	0	0
Met (AUG)	38(1)[c]	36(3)[c]	Thr (ACG)	24	0	Lys (AAG)	89	20	Arg (AGG)	3	0
Val (GUU)	1	70	Ala (GCU)	6	48	Asp (GAU)	5	16	Gly (GGU)	15	76
Val (GUC)	67	1	Ala (GCC)	83	6	Asp (GAC)	71	55	Gly (GGC)	100	38
Val (GUA)	0	39	Ala (GCA)	3	25	Glu (GAA)	0	90	Gly (GGA)	0	2
Val (GUG)	74(3)[c]	12(1)[c]	Ala (GCG)	21	35	Glu (GAG)	113	21	Gly (GGG)	4	2

[a] *M. luteus.*

[b] *E. coli* (data from Yokota et al. 1980; Zalacain et al. 1986; Post and Nomura 1980).

[c] Initiation codons.

Table 3. Nucleotide Percentages in Three Codon Positions

Codon position and protein	Nucleotides (%)			
	U	C	A	G
First position				
consensus protein	18.5	18.2	28.5	34.8
M. luteus, Str	10.7	23.4	25.1	40.9
E. coli, Str	11.2	23.0	25.6	40.2
Second position				
consensus protein	25.3	23.7	33.0	18.0
M. luteus, Str	28.1	23.8	31.9	16.3
E. coli, Str	28.4	22.9	31.5	17.2
Third position				
consensus protein	25.9	25.9	23.3	24.8
M. luteus, Str	4.6	56.7	0.4	38.3
E. coli, Str	29.7	29.4	18.1	22.9

Calculated for a protein of average composition (consensus protein) as compiled by Jukes et al. (1975) and for *str* operons in *M. luteus* and *E. coli* (Table 2).

tives I: inosine.) Also, silent changes from UUA to CUG and from AGA to CGY have evidently taken place during the divergence between *E. coli* and *M. capricolum* (Table 1). In contrast, the amino acid composition coded by the *str* operon in *M. luteus* is almost identical to the corresponding composition in *E. coli* (Table 2). In this case, the difference in GC content between these two species is almost entirely attributable to silent substitutions, except that *M. luteus* has apparently replaced a small number of AUU isoleucine codons in *E. coli* with valine. The protein composition of the *str* gene in *E. coli* is more similar to that in *M. luteus* than it is to the average composition of 199 *E. coli* genes as compiled by Maruyama et al. (1986), despite the great difference in GC content of silent sites

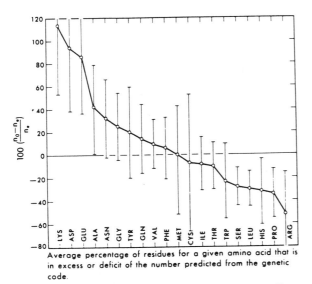

Figure 3. Selection against the genetic code. The ordinate expresses the excess of the observed number n_o of residues of each of the 20 amino acids relative to the expected number n_e in a collection of 189 proteins from 81 families. The vertical bars span one standard deviation. (Reprinted, with permission, from Holmquist 1978.)

between *E. coli* and *M. luteus*, as shown in Table 3. Thus, the *str* operon did not appreciably respond to GC pressure in the replacement of amino acids, probably because it is highly conserved.

The combined effects of GC pressure and compositional nonrandomness are shown in Table 3. In *first codon positions*, all three sequences are high in G as a result of high content of Asp, Glu, Ala, and Gly, also Val in *M. luteus* and *E. coli*. *M. luteus* and *E. coli* are low in T because of low levels of TTR codons, Cys, and Ser. *Second codon positions* are high in A because of high levels of Lys, Asp, and Glu, and low in G because of low levels of Cys, Trp, and Arg. *M. luteus* and *E. coli* show close agreement in nucleotide composition of all first and second positions because of great similarity in amino acid composition of str proteins in these two species. *Third codon positions* are very high in GC in *M. luteus* because of GC pressure and predominance of CNN anticodons.

Anticodons of tRNA

Of the 64 codons in the universal code, 32 are in "family boxes," with four codons for a single amino acid, and most others are in two-codon sets per amino acid. Codon-anticodon pairing involves the wobble rules described by Crick (1966). These state that the second two bases of each anticodon pair with the first two bases of a codon by the usual pairing procedure, A with U, and G with C, but that the first anticodon base pairs with the third codon base by "wobbling" as follows: U in the first position of anticodons pairs with A and G in the third position of codons; C with G; A (very rare) with U; G with U and C; and I (inosine) with U, C, and A. Subsequently, it has been found that unmodified U in the first anticodon position pairs with U, C, A, and G in family boxes in the mitochondrial code (Barrell et al. 1979), but in most other cases, including the universal code, U is modified to restrict its pairing properties (Yokoyama et al. 1985).

Yokoyama et al. (1985) showed that in anticodons for glutamine, lysine, and glutamic acid, U is modified to a 2-thiouridine derivative (*U), which pairs predominantly with A rather than G. Presumably, in anticodons for other two-codon sets, U would also be similarly modified. In family-box anticodons for valine, serine, threonine, and alanine in *E. coli* and *B. subtilis*, U is modified to a derivative of 5-hydroxyuridine, which pairs with A, G, and U in the third-codon positions (Yokoyama et al. 1985). Presumably, in most of the other family-box anticodons, U is modified in a similar way, except for arginine CGN.

When a UNN anticodon pairs with four different codons (such as in family boxes of mitochondria), it does not need to distinguish between NNY and NNR anticodons. If, however, a distinction must be made between NNY codons pairing with anticodon GNN, and NNR codons pairing with anticodon UNN, the base U in anticodon UNN must be modified to prevent it from mispairing with NNY codons. In consequence, the U in all UNN anticodons, especially for two-codon sets, is modified, except for some UNN anticodons in *Mycoplasma* family boxes (see below).

Table 4 includes the anticodons in the eubacterial code as found in *E. coli*. The anticodon list is variable for different classes of eubacteria. As discussed below, this variability is the result of evolution of anticodons from GC/AT pressure in response to the codon choice pattern.

The number of CNN anticodons used in various bacterial species increases with increasing GC content of their DNA, suggesting that the development of the CNN anticodon has been accelerated by GC pressure. The reported number of tRNA having CNN anticodons (not including the obligate CNN anticodons isoleucine [*CAU], methionine [CAU], and tryptophan [CCA]) is seven in *E. coli* (GC, 50%), two in *B. subtilis* (GC, 43%), one in liverwort chloroplasts (GC, 29%) (Ohyama et al. 1986), and none in the *Mycoplasma* group (GC, 25–30%) (see Osawa et al. 1987). Three more CNN anticodons occur, in addition to those found in *E. coli*, in a high GC(69%) bacterium, *Thermus thermophilus* (Hara-Yokoyama et al. 1986).

The low-GC eubacterial families remained low in CNN anticodons, as exemplified by *B. subtilis*, which has only six CNN anticodons as compared with eleven in *E. coli* (Fournier and Ozeki 1985; Sprinzl et al. 1985a,b; Vold 1985).

In extremely AT-rich bacteria, such as *Mycoplasma*, reduction of both CNN and GNN anticodons occurs and an appearance of ANN anticodon (A, unmodified) takes place. In *M. capricolum* (Y. Andachi et al., unpubl.), strong AT pressure accompanies extreme predominance of ACU and ACA threonine codons over ACC and ACG (see Table 1), and tRNA^{Thr} (GGU) disappeared. Replacing it are tRNA^{Thr}(UGU, U unmodified) and tRNA^{Thr}(AGU, A unmodified). tRNA^{Thr}(AGU) was apparently derived by mutation of one of the duplicates of the tRNA^{Thr}(UGU) gene (sequence similarity, 86%). It would appear that codon ACU, which is the most abundantly used threonine

codon (Table 1), is translated by anticodon AGU. Anticodon UGU would mainly be responsible for translating three other threonine codons, ACA, ACG, and ACC. Since unmodified U at the first anticodon position has been reported to be able to pair with A, G, C, and U by four-way wobble in the mitochondrial code (Barrell et al. 1979), tRNA^{Thr}(UGU) could also be used for reading codon ACU as a redundancy of tRNA^{Thr}(AGU).

As postulated previously (Osawa et al. 1987; see also Jukes et al., this volume), the early code would have used the GNN anticodon for translation of codons NNU/C, and anticodon **UNN for codons NNA/G in all the four-codon boxes. This rule can be applied to most of the eubacterial code, except for the arginine four-codon box. Then, two possibilities would exist for the evolution of threonine tRNAs in the *Mycoplasma* line. One is that, first, anticodon UGU became unmodified as a result of partial deprivation of the U-modification enzyme system, so that UGU could translate all the threonine codons by four-way wobble as deduced from the mitochondrial code, and GGU disappeared. An increasing AT pressure led to an extreme predominance of ACU (and ACA) codons over ACC and ACG in the genes. Under these circumstances, one of the genes for tRNA^{Thr} (UGU) mutated to tRNA^{Thr}(AGU). The second possibility is that UGU became unmodified, followed by mutation of one of the genes for UGU to AGU. This would be a transient stage where UGU, AGU, and GGU all existed. GGU then disappeared, for the low demand for translation of codon ACC would be supplied by anticodon UGU, and anticodon GGU would not be needed. In either case, the appearance of tRNA^{Thr}(AGU) is adaptive to fulfill a heavy demand for translation of codon ACU. This may be analogous in the reverse manner to an increase in the content of CNN anticodons in GC-rich bacterial lines, which would have been called for by the predominance of NNG codons in the protein genes (see above).

One significance of the presence of anticodon AGU is that, as mentioned above, it would translate codon

Table 4. Genetic Code and Anticodons of tRNA of *E. coli*

Phe (UUU)	GAA		Ser (UCU)	GGA		Tyr (UAU)	GUA	Cys (UGU)	GCA
Phe (UUC)			Ser (UCC)			Tyr (UAC)		Cys (UGC)	
Leu (UUA)	UAA	CAA	Ser (UCA)	UGA	CGA	Stop (UAA)	—	Stop (UGA)	—
Leu (UUG)			Ser (UCG)			Stop (UAG)	—	Trp (UGG)	CCA
Leu (CUU)	GAG		Pro (CCU)	GGG		His (CAU)	GUG	Arg (CGU)	ICG
Leu (CUC)			Pro (CCC)			His (CAC)		Arg (CGC)	
Leu (CUA)	UAG	CAG	Pro (CCA)	UGG	CGG	Gln (CAA)	UUG	Arg (CGA)	CCG
Leu (CUG)			Pro (CCG)			Gln (CAG)		Arg (CGG) CUG	
Ile (AUU)	GAU		Thr (ACU)	GGU		Asn (AAU)	GUU	Ser (AGU)	GCU
Ile (AUC)			Thr (ACC)			Asn (AAC)		Ser (AGC)	
Ile (AUA)		CAU	Thr (ACA)	UGU		Lys (AAA)	UUU	Arg (AGA)	UCU CCU
Met (AUG)		CAU	Thr (ACG)			Lys (AAG)		Arg (AGG)	
Val (GUU)	GAC		Ala (GCU)	GGC		Asp (GAU)	GUC	Gly (GGU)	GCC
Val (GUC)			Ala (GCC)			Asp (GAC)		Gly (GGC)	
Val (GUA)	UAC		Ala (GCA)	UGC		Glu (GAA)	UUC	Gly (GGA)	UCC CCC
Val (GUG)			Ala (GCG)			Glu (GAG)		Gly (GGG)	

Anticodons were taken from Fournier and Ozeki (1985). Base modifications are not indicated (see text).

ACA more efficiently than anticodon UGU. Moreover, the codon-anticodon pairing 5'ACN3'/3'UGU5' involves only one GC pair, which might cause misreading. Thus, the presence of anticodon AGU would be advantageous in view of both efficiency and correct reading of the most frequently used ACU threonine codon in this organism. In this connection, it is of interest to note that *Mycoplasma mycoides* seems to contain only one species of glycine tRNA having anticodon sequence UCC (Samuelsson et al. 1983). Since codon-anticodon pairing 5'GGN3'/3'CCU5' in the glycine four-codon box involves two GC pairs, all four codons can be translated by four-way wobble more reliably than in the case of the threonine box. The four-codon boxes, where two GC pairs are involved in codon recognition by the second and third anticodon positions, are for proline, alanine, and arginine, in addition to glycine, whereas those containing only one GC pair are for leucine, valine, and serine, in addition to threonine. It is thus possible that codons in the four former boxes could be read by anticodons ANN and UNN (N=C or G, and A or U), whereas in the four latter boxes, four codons could be read only by anticodon UNN (N=G or C), with the exception of the arginine four-codon box. All the eubacterial species so far studied use anticodon IGC for translation of arginine codons CGU, CGC, and CGA, and anticodon CCG for codon CGG. In *M. mycoides*, a gene for tRNA with anticodon ACG has been reported (Samuelsson et al. 1985), although whether A is replaced by I after transcription and whether anticodon CCG exists have not yet been reported.

Change in Amino Acid Assignment of Codons

The codons that are most subject to evolution are, obviously, the three stop codons UAA, UAG, and UGA. All three of these have been "captured" by amino acids in some organisms: UGA in *Mycoplasma* and UAA and UGA in ciliated protozoa (Jukes et al. 1987). This process is made possible by restricting chain termination functions to one or two stop codons, leaving the others available for capture by amino acids (see Jukes et al., this volume). These changes have taken place as a result of AT pressure. High AT pressure in *Mycoplasma* resulted in the appearance of codon UGA for tryptophan (Yamao et al. 1985). A simple conversion of tryptophan codon UGG to UGA by AT pressure could not happen, because UGA was an unusable nonsense codon, resulting from lack of anticodon UCA in the ancestor from which the *Mycoplasma* line branched. The conversion could happen only when tRNA^{Trp}(UCA) appeared. In *M. capricolum*, UGA is predominantly used over UGG as the tryptophan codon (see Table 1). Furthermore, both tRNA^{Trp}(UCA), which can translate both UGA and UGG, and tRNA^{Trp}(CCA) have been found in this bacterium (Yamao et al. 1985). The appearance of the

UGA tryptophan codon took place by the following steps without deleterious or lethal changes (Jukes 1985). AT pressure has led to the replacement of all UGA stop codons by UAA. Then, tryptophan tRNA, with anticodon CAA, duplicated, and one of the duplicates, under AT pressure, mutated to UCA in its anticodon. The new tryptophan anticodon could pair with both UGA and UGG. Since anticodons UCA and CCA both pair with tryptophan codon UGG, this was a neutral change, because it was preceded by the disappearance of UGA stop codons, which had mutated to UAA. Anticodon CCA is no longer needed in *Mycoplasma*, and, although still present, it is apparently disappearing (Yamao et al. 1985; F. Yamao et al., unpubl.).

The UGA tryptophan codon probably appeared fairly recently in the *Mycoplasma* line under strong AT pressure, since UGA codons and UCA anticodons are not used for amino acids in other codes except in mitochondria.

In *M. capricolum*, UGA codons occur preceding termination codons in two ribosomal protein genes, where UGA could very well be read as tryptophan, even though the origin of this UGA could be UAA (Osawa et al. 1987; see also Jukes et al., this volume). On the other hand, in organisms that have only tRNA^{Trp}(CCA), such UGA acts as one of the termination codons. However, it is possible that the UGA termination codon would easily be converted to UGG tryptophan codon, or vice versa. For example, the 3'-codon arrangement of the ribosomal S14 protein gene from liverwort *Marchantia polymorpha* chloroplasts is TGG TAA (Umesono et al. 1985), whereas in *M. capricolum* the corresponding codons are TGA TAA (S. Ohkubo et al., unpubl.). Thus, in both cases the 3'-terminal sense codon before UAA stop is for tryptophan. Since carboxy-terminal tryptophan does not seem to be essential for protein S14 (in *E. coli* S14, no tryptophan exists in the carboxy-terminal region [Yaguchi et al. 1983]), genes for S14 wth UGA (stop) UAA/G (stop) as termination codons could exist in some bacteria. In other words, UGA and UGG would be convertible, when preceding UAA/G and the existence of carboxy-terminal tryptophan would not cause deleterious change for the protein to be synthesized.

No changes in amino acid assignment of the present universal code have been reported to occur from GC pressure, even though almost complete disappearance of NNA and NNU codons takes place in bacteria with DNA high in GC. As mentioned above, in *M. luteus* (74% GC) these include codons UUA and UUG for leucine that were probably converted by GC pressure and silent mutations to CUC and CUG. A complete absence of these two leucine codons suggests the deletion of the corresponding anticodons UAA and CAA. This would leave codons UUA and UUG available for capture by another amino acid. Thus, in this case, GC pressure would produce a condition favorable for changes in codon assignment.

Parts Played by GC/AT Pressure and tRNA in Species-specific Codon Usage

As discussed above and in the previous papers (Jukes and Bhushan 1986; Muto and Osawa 1987), GC/AT pressure may be an important determinant for codon usage in eubacteria. Codon choice pattern is also affected by tRNA. Ikemura and Ozeki (1983) demonstrated a positive correlation between codon usage and tRNA abundance, stressing that tRNA populations may act as selective constraints for determining the codon usage in E. coli, Salmonella, and yeast.

The relation between GC/AT pressure, and tRNA constraints for codon choice has not been studied systematically, and therefore is examined here, partly in collaboration with H. Ozeki and K. Umesono of Kyoto University.

Choice of the third nucleotide of two-codon sets was investigated. Two-codon sets consist of a pair of synonymous codons, NNC and NNU, or NNG and NNA. Synonymous pairs of NNG and NNC or NNA and NNU never exist in two-codon sets. Codons in four-codon boxes, those in the two-codon set plus four-codon box for one amino acid (serine, leucine, and arginine), and codons for isoleucine were not treated, because of the complexity of the codon-anticodon recognition pattern. UGY (cysteine) was also omitted due to the limited number of codons.

We postulate, as the first approximation, that the spacer region is "ideally" free from constraints and its GC content reflects solely GC/AT pressure. If GC/AT pressure is the only factor for determining codon choice, the value of $NNC/(NNC + NNU) \times 100$ in the NNC/U-type two-codon sets or $NNG/(NNG + NNA) \times 100$ in the NNG/A-type two-codon sets (f) is equal to the GC percentage of the "ideal" spacer (s) and will move from $f1$ to $f2$ along with s, when $s1$ changes to $s2$ (Fig. 4a). On the other hand, if tRNA constraints are the only factors, f may be expressed as $50\ (\%) + t\ (\%)$, where t is the fraction of GC percentage of codon third nucleotide deviated from 50 due to tRNA constraints. The f value may change upon change of t (Fig. 4b). Let us then consider the case where both GC/AT pressure and tRNA constraints affect the codon choice. Here, f is expressed as $s + t$. Upon change of GC/AT pressure, $s1$ to $s2$, the GC content of the third nucleotide, $f1$, will shift to $f2$ ($= s2 + t1$) if tRNA constraints, $t1$, do not change (Fig. 4c). When $t1$ changes to $t2$, by, for example, addition of new anticodon, $f1$ will shift to $f3$ even when $s1$ does not change (Fig. 4d). The actual examples shown below clearly indicate that the choice of the third nucleotide of codons is affected by both GC/AT pressure and tRNA constraints in a combination of the schemes shown in Figure 3, a, c, and d.

The two types of codon choice (Table 5; see above)

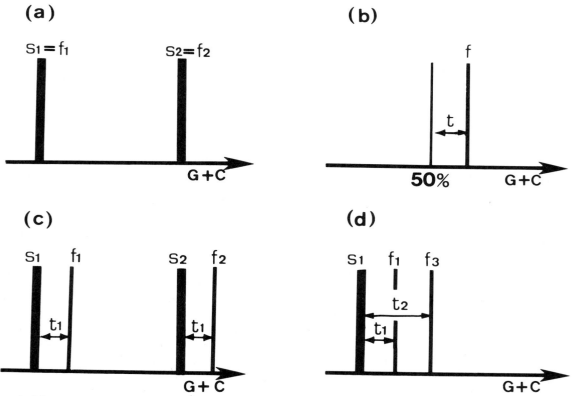

Figure 4. Schematic presentation of the effects of GC/AT pressure and the tRNA constraints on choice of the third nucleotide of two-codon sets (for explanations, see text).

Table 5. Codon Usage in Two-codon sets in Four Species of Eubacteria and Liverwort Chloroplasts

Species[a]			C	M	B	E	L
Spacer G + C(%)[b]			19	20	38	47	80
Amino acid	Codon	Anticodon	Codon usage (%)				
(a) NNU/NNC Type							
Tyr	UAU	GUA	826(90)	69(80)	115(62)	22(24)	0 (0)
	UAC		95(10)	17(20)	96(38)	71(76)	37(100)
His	CAU	GUG	388(85)	32(71)	116(69)	26(26)	1 (4)
	CAC		62(15)	14(29)	53(31)	75(74)	30 (96)
Asn	AAU	GUU	1256(88)	158(79)	179(53)	23(12)	3 (7)
	AAC		175(12)	41(21)	158(47)	166(88)	43 (93)
Asp	GAU	GUC	735(91)	118(90)	266(64)	94(35)	5 (7)
	GAC		72 (9)	13(10)	151(36)	177(65)	71 (93)
Phe	UUU	GAA	1547(94)	112(87)	165(64)	36(21)	0 (0)
	UUC		97 (6)	17(13)	93(36)	133(79)	43(100)
Total	NNU	GNN	4752(90)	490(83)	841(60)	168(26)	9 (4)
	NNC		501(10)	102(17)	551(40)	471(74)	224 (96)
(b) NNA/NNG Type							
Gln	CAA	*UUG	887(94)	135(99)	163(44)	33(20)	0 (0)
	CAG	CUG	53 (6)	2 (1)	138(56)	133(80)	47(100)
Lys	AAA	*UUU	1764(96)	415(92)	395(75)	328(75)	0 (0)
	AAG	CUU	78 (4)	35 (8)	129(25)	109(25)	89(100)
Glu	GAA	*UUC	1133(93)	204(94)	372(70)	304(78)	0 (0)
	GAG	CUC	85 (7)	12 (6)	163(30)	85(22)	113(100)
Total	RNA	*UNY	2897(95)	719(93)	767(73)	632(77)	0 (0)
	RNG	CNY	163 (5)	47 (7)	292(27)	194(23)	202(100)
Total	NNA	*UNN	3784(95)	754(94)	— (–)	— (–)	0 (0)
	NNG	CNN	216 (5)	49 (6)	— (–)	— (–)	451(100)

[a](C) *M. polymorpha* (liverwort) chloroplasts. Taken from all (91) protein genes including open reading frames (Ohyama et al. 1986; K. Ohyama et al., unpubl.). (M) *M. capricolum*. From 20 ribosomal protein genes (S. Ohkubo et al., unpubl.) (B) *B. subtilis*. From 21 protein genes near the replication origin (Ogasawara 1985). (E) *E. coli*. From 30 ribosomal protein genes (Schnier et al. 1986) and elongation factors G and Tu genes (Yokota et al. 1980; Zengel et al. 1984). (L) *M. luteus*. From 2 ribosomal protein genes and elongation factors G and Tu genes (T. Ohama et al., unpubl.).

[b]From K. Ohyama et al. (pers. comm.) for C and Muto and Osawa (1987) for M, B, E, and L.

will be treated using the data of codon usage in the proteins produced at very high rates (Sharp and Li 1986; ribosomal proteins and elongation factors) from *M. capricolum* (genomic GC: 25%; spacer: 20%), *E. coli* (genomic GC: 50%; spacer: 47%), and *M. luteus* (genomic GC: 74%; spacer: 80%), for the codon choice is said to be affected most strongly by the tRNA constraints in these proteins. The codon usage data (Ogasawara 1985) from the genes near the replication origin of *B. subtilis* (genomic GC: 43%; spacer: 38%), which are presumably for "highly produced" and/or "moderately produced" proteins (Sharp and Li 1986) are also included. The actual effect of tRNA constraints for the very highly produced proteins in *B. subtilis* could be a little higher than that used here. In addition to the bacteria, the codon usage data from liverwort chloroplasts (genomic GC: 29%; spacer 19%) are also included, since the genetic system of chloroplasts may be considered as basically prokaryotic and the entire sequence of liverwort chloroplast DNA has been determined (Ohyama et al. 1986 and

unpubl.). The production rate of different proteins in chloroplasts has not been studied. We tentatively assume that nearly all the protein genes are essential and expressed at about the same rate in such an economized system.

Choice of C or U of the third nucleotide of the two-codon sets was first studied for phenylalanine, tyrosine, histidine, asparagine, and aspartic acid, where only one species of tRNA, with anticodon sequence GNN, is involved in the translation, so that the amount of tRNA is not an important factor. In Figure 5a, the $NNC/(NNC + NNU) \times 100$ value ($= f$) of codon two-sets (NNC/U) was plotted against the GC content of the spacer. The f values of chloroplasts, *Mycoplasma*, and *B. subtilis* are, on average, close to the spacer GC content (s), indicating that no appreciable tRNA constraints exist in the range between $s = 20$ and $s = 38$ as in Figure 4a. In *E. coli*, where GC content of spacer (s) is 47%, NNC content (f) shifts to 74% so that the fraction affected by tRNA constraints (t) is 27% ($t = f - s$). The f value reaches the maximum in *Micrococ-*

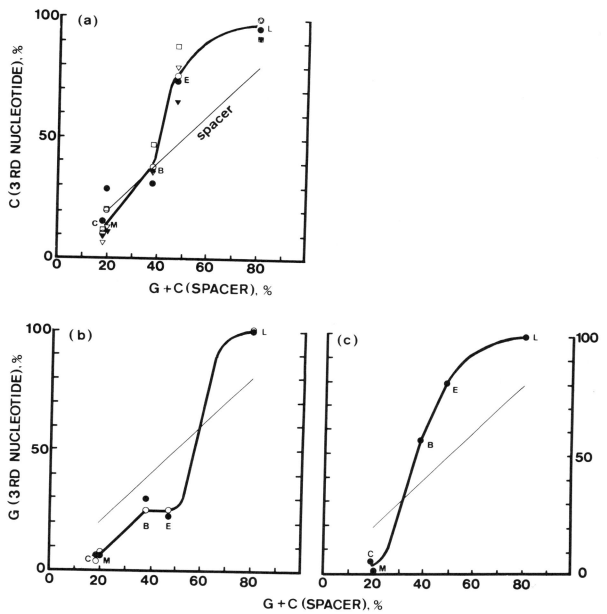

Figure 5. Relation between GC content of spacer and C (*a*) or G (*b* and *c*) content of the third nucleotide of two-codon sets. (*a*) Codons for tyrosine (○), histidine (●), asparagine (□), aspartic acid (▼), and phenylalanine (▽). (*b*) Codons for lysine (○) and glutamic acid (●). (*c*) Codons for glutamine. (C) *Marchantia polymorpha* (liverwort) chloroplasts; (M) *Mycoplasma capricolum*; (B) *Bacillus subtilis*; (E) *Escherichia coli*; (L) *Micrococcus luteus*.

cus ($f = 96$; $t = 16$), indicating that strong tRNA constraints are exerted to choose C rather than U in *E. coli* and *Micrococcus*.

The pairing of the GNN anticodon to the NNC codon is generally stronger than to the NNU codon because of more stable pairing between G (anticodon) and C (codon) than between G and U. However, in a range between $s = 20$ (chloroplasts and *Mycoplasma*) and $s = 38$ (*B. subtilis*), NNU may be nearly as good as NNC, for NNC would not contribute so much to translation efficiency among predominating NNU/A codons in chloroplasts and these high-AT bacteria. This may be

the reason for the lack of tRNA constraints. With increase in s, tRNA constraints appear, for NNU will become less favorable codons than NNC among an increasing amount of NNC/G codons so that the NNU codon acts as a rate-limiting factor in translation.

Next, choice of G or A of the third nucleotide of codons was studied for glutamine (CAR), lysine (AAR), and glutamic acid (GAR), where, depending on the bacterial species, one species (anticodon: *UNN) or two species (anticodons: *UNN and CNN) of tRNA are responsible for translating the codons.

tRNAs with *UNN anticodons have been reported

for glutamic acid, lysine, and glutamine in *E. coli*. It is logical to suppose that *UNN anticodons for these three amino acids are present throughout eubacteria including chloroplasts, for CNN anticodons can read only NNG codons and not NNA codons; NNA codons in two-codon sets must be translated by *UNN anticodons. Yokoyama et al. (1985) showed that *U pairs more readily with A than with G, suggesting that *UNN anticodons are mainly responsible for reading NNA codons.

Genes for tRNA(CUU) for lysine and tRNA(CUC) for glutamic acid are not present in chloroplasts and have not been reported in *E. coli*, *B. subtilis*, and *Mycoplasma* and probably do not exist in these bacteria. On the other hand, tRNAs with anticodons CUC and CUU are members of the major tRNA species in *Thermus*, and therefore presumably exist in *Micrococcus* (GC, 74%). tRNA(CUG) for glutamine has been reported from *E. coli* and *Thermus*, and therefore should exist also in *Micrococcus*. *B. subtilis* may have this tRNA for reasons described below, although its presence has not yet been reported. Chloroplasts lack this tRNA, and there is no sign of its presence in *Mycoplasma*.

In Figure 5, b and c, the NNG/(NNG + NNA) × 100 value (f) of the respective codon two-set (NNG/A) was plotted against the GC content of the spacer (s), as in the case of NNC/U codons. In the cases of AAG/A for lysine and GAG/A for glutamic acid, CNN anticodons are absent in *E. coli*, *B. subtilis*, *Mycoplasma*, and chloroplasts and are presumably present in *Micrococcus*. Only a very small usage (6–8%) of NNG codons is observed in chloroplasts ($f = 5$ as against $s = 19$) and in *Mycoplasma* ($f = 6$ as against $s = 20$), showing considerable constraints against NNG by *UNN anticodons. The percentage of NNG (f) reaches 26% in *B. subtilis*, nearly in parallel with an increase in s (38%), with a similar t value of -11 as in *Mycoplasma* ($t = -14$) (Fig. 4c). The f value does not change in *E. coli* as compared with *B. subtilis*, so that the t value of *E. coli* increases up to -24 as against $t = -11$ of *B. subtilis*, indicating that stronger *UNN constraints are operating here to favor choice of NNA codons. In contrast, the f value of *Micrococcus* reaches nearly 100 with a t value of 20, indicating that strong constraints by CNN anticodons exist to choose NNG codons. In the case of glutamine, CUG anticodon is presumed to exist in *E. coli*, *Micrococcus*, and probably in *B. subtilis*, but is absent in chloroplasts and *Mycoplasma* (see above). CAG usage is almost absent in chloroplasts and in *Mycoplasma* and appears in *B. subtilis* ($f = 56$; $t = 18$). The high value of t is maintained in *E. coli* ($t = 25$) and in *Micrococcus* ($t = 20$).

The above observations suggest that without CNN anticodons, NNG is a very "bad" codon because of poor pairing ability of *UNN anticodons with NNG codons, and the constraints by *UNN are strong so as to keep NNG usage down to around 25%. The appearance of CNN anticodons thus seems to be adaptive, for an increase in s value tends to increase NNG codons, which must be somehow translated. *UNN constraints

cannot accommodate any more of the increasing NNG codons by increasing s value. This is the reason why CNN anticodons need to be generated, presumably by GC pressure, in high-GC bacteria.

The above view is supported by the codon choice pattern for glutamine, lysine, and glutamic acid in *E. coli* (Sharp and Li 1986). Usage of CAG for glutamine is highest in very highly produced proteins (89%) and decreases to 60% with the decreasing production rate of proteins. This pattern can be explained by the constraints of CNN anticodons that are exerted at maximum on very highly produced proteins and decrease in parallel with the decreasing production rate. On the other hand, usage of NNG codons for lysine and glutamic acid is low (about 25%) and nearly unchanged, regardless of the magnitude of the protein production, suggesting that, without CNN anticodons, t value (by *UNN constraints) had been saturated before s had reached 47% ($= s$ of *E. coli*), not only in very highly produced proteins, but also in others, including rarely produced proteins. This suggestion is further strengthened by the fact, as noted above, that usage of NNG codons in *B. subtilis* is almost the same (27%) as that in *E. coli* (23%). In the case of glutamine, the CUG anticodon had developed before the t value reached the maximum (saturation value), whereas for lysine and glutamic acid, CNN anticodons appeared after the t value had been saturated.

From the above discussion, the role of tRNA for choice of the third nucleotide of two-codon sets can be defined as to gain the fraction of GC percentage of the third nucleotide (t) deviated from the GC content of spacer (s) for a given bacterium, which has been determined solely by GC/AT pressure without any constraints. It is noted that, as seen in Figure 5, tRNA constraints observed here generally act additively to GC/AT pressure to produce, in NNA/G-type two-codon sets, more A in the codon third positions by constraints of tRNA(*UNN) in the absence of CNN anticodons, and more G by constraints of tRNA (CNN). In NNC/U-type two-codon sets, third-codon positions gain more C by constraints of tRNA(GNN) only when enough GC pressure is exerted; no appreciable GNN constraints exist when AT pressure predominates.

ACKNOWLEDGMENTS

We thank H. Ozeki, K. Umesono, S. Ohkubo, M. Iwami, and S. Iwagami for supplying published and unpublished data and for helpful discussion. This work was supported by grants from the Ministry of Education, Science and Culture of Japan, by Naito Science Foundation, and by NASA grant NGR-05 003 to the University of California, Berkeley.

REFERENCES

An, G. and F.D. Jriensen. 1980. The nucleotide sequence of *tuf*B and four nearby tRNA structural genes of *Escherichia coli*. Gene **12**: 33.

Barrell, G., A.T. Bankier, and J. Drouin. 1979. A different genetic code in human mitochondria. *Nature* **282**: 189.

Cerretti, D.P., D. Dean, G.R. Davis, D.M. Bedwell, and M. Nomura. 1983. The *spc* ribosomal protein operon of *Escherichia coli*: Sequence and cotranscription of the ribosomal protein genes and a protein export gene. *Nucleic Acids Res.* **11**: 2599.

Crick, F.H.C. 1966. The wobble hypothesis. *J. Mol. Biol.* **19**: 548.

Fournier, M. and H. Ozeki. 1985. Structure and organization of the transfer ribonucleic acid genes of *Escherichia coli*. *Microbiol. Rev.* **49**: 379.

Hara-Yokoyama, M., S. Yokoyama, T. Watanabe, K. Watanabe, M. Kitazume, Y. Mitamura, T. Morii, S. Takahashi, K. Kuchino, S. Nishimura, and T. Miyazawa. 1986. Characteristic anticodon sequences of major tRNA species from an extreme thermophile, *Thermus thermophilus* HB8. *FEBS Lett.* **201**: 149.

Holmquist, W.R. 1978. Evolution of compositional non-randomness in proteins. *J. Mol. Evol.* **11**: 349.

Hori, H. and S. Osawa. 1986. Evolutionary change in 5S rRNA secondary structure and a phylogenic tree of 352 rRNA species. *BioSystems* **19**: 163.

Ikemura, T. and H. Ozeki. 1983. Codon usage and transfer RNA contents: Organism-specific codon-choice patterns in reference to the isoacceptor contents. *Cold Spring Harbor Symp. Quant. Biol.* **47**: 1087.

Jukes, T.H. 1985. A change in the genetic code in *Mycoplasma capricolum*. *J. Mol. Evol.* **22**: 361.

Jukes, T. and V. Bhushan. 1986. Silent nucleotide substitutions and G + C content of some mitochondrial and bacterial genes. *J. Mol. Evol.* **24**: 39.

Jukes, T.H., W.R. Holmquist, and H. Moise. 1975. Amino acid composition of proteins: Selection against the genetic code. *Science* **189**: 50.

Jukes, T.H., S. Osawa, and A. Muto. 1987. Divergence and directional mutation pressures. *Nature* **325**: 668.

Kimura, M. 1983. *The neutral theory of molecular evolution*. Cambridge University Press, England.

King, J.L. and T.H. Jukes. 1969. Non-Darwinian evolution. *Science* **164**: 788.

Maruyama, S., T. Gojobori, S. Aota, and T. Ikemura. 1986. Codon usage tabulated from the GenBank genetic sequence data. *Nucleic Acids Res.* (suppl.) **14**: r151.

Mizusawa, S., S. Nishimura, and F. Seela. 1986. Improvement of the dideoxy chain termination method of DNA sequencing by use of deoxy-7-deazaguanosine triphosphate in place of dGTP. *Nucleic Acids Res.* **14**: 1319.

Muto, A. and S. Osawa. 1987. The guanine and cytosine content of genomic DNA and bacterial evolution. *Proc. Natl. Acad. Sci.* **84**: 166.

Muto, A., Y. Kawauchi, F. Yamao, and S. Osawa. 1984. Preferential use of A- and U-rich codons for *Mycoplasma capricolum* ribosomal proteins S8 and L6. *Nucleic Acids Res.* **12**: 8209.

Ogasawara, N. 1985. Markedly unbiased codon usage in *Bacillus subtilis*. *Gene* **40**: 145.

Ohyama, K., H. Fukuzawa, T. Kohchi, H. Shirai, T. Sano, S. Sano, K. Umesono, Y. Shiki, M. Takeuchi, Z. Chang, S.-I. Aota, H. Inokuchi, and H. Ozeki. 1986. Chloroplast gene organization deduced from complete sequence of liverwort *Marchantia polymorpha* chloroplast DNA. *Nature* **322**: 572.

Osawa, S., A. Muto, T.H. Jukes, T. Ohama, F. Yamao, N. Leheman, and V. Bhushan. 1987. Evolution of anticodons in the genetic code. *Nature* (in press).

Post, L.E. and M. Nomura. 1980. DNA sequence from the *str* operon of *Escherichia coli*. *J. Biol. Chem.* **255**: 4660.

Samuelsson, T., T. Axberg, T. Boren, and U. Lagerkvist. 1983. Unconventional reading of the glycine codons. *J. Biol. Chem.* **258**: 13178.

Samuelsson, T., P. Elias, F. Lusting, and Y.S. Guindy. 1985. Cloning and nucleotide sequence analysis of transfer RNA genes for *Mycoplasma mycoides*. *Biochem. J.* **232**: 223.

Schnier, J., M. Kitakawa, and K. Isono. 1986. The nucleotide sequence of an *Escherichia coli* chromosomal region containing the genes for ribosomal proteins S6, S18, L9 and open reading-frame. *Mol. Gen. Genet.* **204**: 126.

Sharp, P.M. and W.-H. Li. 1986. An evolutionary perspective on synonymous codon usage in unicellular organisms. *J. Mol. Evol.* **24**: 28.

Sprinzl, M., T. Vorderwiibecke, and T. Hartmann. 1985a. Compilation of sequences of tRNA genes. *Nucleic Acids Res.* (suppl.) **13**: r51.

Sprinzl, M., J. Moll, F. Meissner, and T. Hartmann. 1985b. Compilation of tRNA sequences. *Nucleic Acids Res.* (suppl.) **13**: r1.

Sueoka, N. 1962. On the genetic basis of variation and heterogeneity of DNA base composition. *Proc. Natl. Acad. Sci.* **48**: 582.

Umesono, K., H. Inokuchi, K. Ohyama, and H. Ozeki. 1985. Nucleotide sequence of *Marchantia polymorpha* chloroplast DNA: A region possibly encoding three tRNAs and three proteins including a homologue of *E. coli* ribosomal protein S14. *Nucleic Acids Res.* **12**: 9551.

Vold, B.S. 1985. Structure and organization of genes for transfer ribonucleic acid in *Bacillus subtilis*. *Microbiol. Rev.* **49**: 71.

Yaguchi, M., C. Roy, R.A.F. Reithmeier, B. Wittmann-Liebold, and H.G. Wittmann. 1983. The primary structure of protein S14 from the small ribosomal subunit of *Escherichia coli*. *FEBS Lett.* **154**: 21.

Yamao, F., A. Muto, Y. Kawauchi, M. Iwami, S. Iwagami, Y. Azumi, and S. Osawa. 1985. UGA is read as tryptophan in *Mycoplasma capricolum*. *Proc. Natl. Acad. Sci.* **82**: 2306.

Yokota, T., H. Sugisaki, M. Takanami, and Y. Kaziro. 1980. The nucleotide sequence of the cloned *tuf*A gene of *Escherichia coli*. *Gene* **12**: 25.

Yokoyama, S., T. Watanabe, K. Murao, H. Ishikura, Z. Yamaizumi, S. Nishimura, and T. Miyazawa. 1985. Molecular mechanism of codon recognition by tRNA species with modified uridine in the first position of the anticodon. *Proc. Natl. Acad. Sci.* **82**: 4905.

Zalacain, M., A. Gonzarez, M.C. Guerrero, R.J. Mattaliano, F. Malpartida, and A. Jimenz. 1986. Nucleotide sequence of *Escherichia coli fus* gene, coding for elongation factor G. *Nucleic Acids Res.* **14**: 1565.

Zengel, J.M., R.H. Arch, and L. Lindahl. 1984. The nucleotide sequence of *Escherichia coli fus* gene, coding for elongation factor G. *Nucleic Acids Res.* **12**: 2181.

Zurawski, G. and S.M. Zurawski. 1985. Studies of the *Escherichia coli* S10 ribosomal protein operon. *Nucleic Acids Res.* **13**: 4521.

Genetic System of Chloroplasts

H. Ozeki,* K. Ohyama,[†] H. Inokuchi,* H. Fukuzawa,[†‡] T. Kohchi,[†]
T. Sano,[†] K. Nakahigashi,* and K. Umesono*
*Department of Biophysics, Faculty of Science, and [†]Research Center for Cell and Tissue Culture,
Faculty of Agriculture, Kyoto University, Kyoto 606, Japan

Chloroplasts are ubiquitous organelles in green plants and are the sole repositories of photosynthesis. As the abnormalities in phenotype color in plants, such as striped, variegated, pale green, albino, etc., are easily observable, hereditary determinants of green-color characters have been studied in genetics from its beginning, and soon it was found that these abnormalities are often inherited maternally through cytoplasm in a non-Mendelian fashion. Later, it was confirmed that chloroplasts have their own unique DNA. Then, in addition to mutations inherited through the cytoplasm, many cases of Mendelian inheritance due to the mutations in nuclear determinants of the similar green-color characters were also observed.

At present it is well established that chloroplasts are genetically controlled, not only by their own genes but also by numerous nuclear genes. Nuclear-encoded proteins are synthesized in the cytoplasm as precursor molecules and then delivered into chloroplasts, followed by precise processing to mature molecules. The chloroplast genes are expressed within the organelle via chloroplast-specific machinery for protein biogenesis, although the machinery itself is also composed partly of nuclear gene products. In contrast, as no RNA molecules appear to be delivered from the cytoplasm, all the necessary RNAs such as rRNAs or tRNAs ought to be generated within the chloroplasts. To clarify the genetic contribution of the chloroplast genome in plant cells, we have determined the entire nucleotide sequence of chloroplast DNA from a liverwort, *Marchantia polymorpha*, and deduced the genes as far as possible (Ohyama et al. 1986). We chose this organism as a model system of the chloroplast genome because of the shorter size of its chloroplast DNA (~120 kbp) and also because of the availability of a strain of haploid cultured cells in which the chloroplasts are well-developed under laboratory conditions (Ohyama et al. 1983).

Recently, the entire nucleotide sequence of tobacco chloroplast DNA (~150 kbp) has also been determined (Shinozaki et al. 1986). Despite the difference in DNA size, the genetic composition and the genome organization are remarkably similar in the two chloroplasts. Accordingly, in this paper we present mainly the results obtained from liverwort, but these results may

be considered representative for plant chloroplasts. Detailed descriptions of the liverwort chloroplast genes are published elsewhere (H. Fukuzawa et al.; T. Kohchi et al.; K. Ohyama et al.; K. Umesono et al.; all in prep.). Of the many interesting problems in chloroplast study, we chose to focus our discussion here on the genetic system of chloroplasts, on which their functions, maintenance, and genetic continuity are based.

Overall Gene Organization

The liverwort chloroplast genome consists of a double-stranded circular DNA, 121,024 bp in length, containing a pair of inverted repeat sequences, IR_A and IR_B (10,058 bp each), which separate a large single-copy (LSC) region (81,095 bp) and a small single-copy (SSC) region (19,813 bp). Figure 1 presents a new version of the gene map of the liverwort chloroplast genome in which several genes or open reading frames (ORFs) are added to our previous one (Ohyama et al. 1986). The size of liverwort chloroplast DNA is markedly smaller than, for instance, that of tobacco DNA (155,844 bp, Shinozaki et al. 1986). This difference is due mainly to the shorter length in the IR sequences; that is, in tobacco, IR=25,339 bp, LSC=86,684 bp, and SSC=18,482 bp. The shorter DNA does not necessarily mean a reduction in gene composition in the chloroplast genome. Indeed, the counterparts for the genes detected in tobacco IR regions but not in liverwort IR regions are mostly found in the single-copy regions in the liverwort chloroplast genome. Thus, the overall gene composition of both organisms is remarkably similar, if not completely the same. The number of genes in a chloroplast genome has been estimated to be up to 136 (including 9 duplicates in IR regions) in liverwort and about 150 (about 25 duplicates in IR regions) in tobacco.

About half of the genes detected in the liverwort chloroplast genome are involved in the basic transcription and translation machinery, namely, 8 genes for two sets of rRNAs (16S, 23S, 5S, and 4.5S), 36 genes for 31 species of tRNAs, 20 ribosomal protein genes (9 for 50S and 11 for 30S subunits), 4 genes for RNA polymerase subunits, and 1 for initiation factor I (*infA*). Thus, at least 69 out of 136 may be accounted for as the basic genes. These genes are listed in Table 1. Of the rest, about 30 genes have been assigned to photosynthetic or electron transport systems. These are listed in Table 2. At present, 33 possible ORFs still remain to

[‡]Present address: Institute of Applied Microbiology, University of Tokyo, Tokyo 113, Japan.

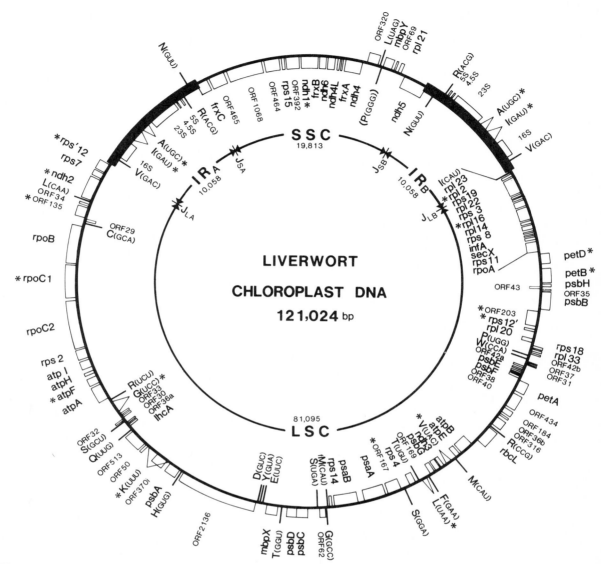

Figure 1. Gene organization of the chloroplast genome of *Marchantia polymorpha*. The inverted repeats (IR_A and IR_B), large single-copy (LSC) and small single-copy (SSC) regions are indicated on the inner circle with their nucleotide numbers (bp). Genes shown outside the map are transcribed anticlockwise, and those inside are transcribed clockwise. Asterisks indicate split genes having introns. Gene symbols refer to Ohyama et al. (1986), although most of them are described in the text. The tRNA genes are indicated by the one-letter amino acid code with their anticodons given in parentheses.

be solved, and are indicated in Figure 1 with numbers of amino acid residues predicted from the coding sequences. Although the products have not been iden-

Table 1. Chloroplast Genes Involved in Protein Biogenesis

tRNA:	31 species
rRNA:	16S, 23S, 4.5S, 5S
RNA polymerase:	*rpoA, rpoB, rpoC1*, rpoC2*
30S r-protein:	*rps2, rps3, rps4, rps7, rps8, rps11, rps12*, rps14, rps15, rps18, rps19*
50S r-protein:	*rpl2*, rpl14, rpl16*, rpl20, rpl21, rpl22, rpl23, rpl33, secX*
Factor:	*infA*
Permease?:	*mbpX, mbpY*

Asterisks indicate split genes. Permease-like genes (*mbp*) are also included.

tified, many of the ORFs in liverwort and tobacco share amino acid sequence homology, suggesting they are likely to be functional. The arrangements of genes in liverwort and tobacco maps are also very similar; an inversion of approximately 30 kbp in the LSC region is the major difference between the two organisms (a region from ORF34 to ORF2136 in Fig. 1). Inversions of this sort have been found frequently in chloroplast genomes (see Palmer 1985).

Genes for Photosynthesis and Electron Transport

Gene-cloning and rapid DNA-sequencing techniques have made possible the identification of chloroplast genes and particularly the accumulation of information for photosynthetic and other related genes. Although

Table 2. Chloroplast Genes for Photosynthesis and Electron Transport

Gene	Product
rbcL	large subunit of ribulose bisphosphate carboxylase
psaA	PSI P_{700} chlorophyll *a* apoprotein A1
psaB	PSI P_{700} chlorophyll *a* apoprotein A2
psbA	PSII 32-kD or D1 protein
psbB	PSII 51-kD P_{680} chlorophyll *a* apoprotein
psbC	PSII 44-kD chlorophyll *a* apoprotein
psbD	PSII D2 protein
psbE	component of cytochrome b_{559}
psbF	component of cytochrome b_{559}
psbG	PSII G protein
psbH	PSII 10-kD phosphoprotein
petA	cytochrome *f*
petB*	cytochrome *b6*
petD*	subunit 4 of cytochrome *b6/f* complex
atpA	F_1-ATPase subunit α
atpB	F_1-ATPase subunit β
atpE	F_1-ATPase subunit ε
atpF*	F_0-ATPase subunit I
atpH	F_0-ATPase subunit III
atpI	F_0-ATPase subunit IV or *a*
frxA	apoprotein of PSI iron-sulfur center
frxB	4Fe-4S type ferredoxin
frxC	*nifH*-like protein
ndh1*	subunit 1 of NADP-PQ oxidoreductase
ndh2*	subunit 2 of NADP-PQ oxidoreductase
ndh3	subunit 3 of NADP-PQ oxidoreductase
ndh4	subunit 4 of NADP-PQ oxidoreductase
ndh4L	subunit 4L of NADP-PQ oxidoreductase
ndh5	subunit 5 of NADP-PQ oxidoreductase
ndh6	subunit 6 of NADP-PQ oxidoreductase
lhcA	bacterial-type light-harvesting polypeptide

Asterisks indicate split genes. Seven *ndh* genes are homologous to human mitochondrial ND genes encoding subunits for respiratory-chain NADH dehydrogenase. PQ: plastoquinone.

the liverwort chloroplast genome is comparatively smaller, as mentioned above, we were able to identify all the counterparts of photosynthetic genes that have been reported previously in a variety of plants (Crouse et al. 1985). This supports the notion that the chloroplast genomes in plants from mosses to higher plants have basically the same gene composition.

Among the genes assigned to photosynthesis and electron transport systems in liverwort chloroplasts

(Table 2), two new groups of genes have been elucidated and designated as *frx* (*A*, *B*, and *C*) and *ndh* (*1*, *2*, *3*, *4*, *4L*, *5*, and *6*) (Ohyama et al. 1986). The *frx* genes were assigned to iron-sulfur proteins based on their characteristic distribution of cysteine residues in the polypeptides deduced from the DNA sequences. A gene product corresponding to *frxA* (for a bacterial-type 4Fe-4S ferredoxin) has been recently identified in spinach chloroplasts; an 8-kD polypeptide has been isolated from the spinach photosystem I complex that has an amino acid sequence highly homologous to that deduced from the *frxA* in liverwort (Oh-oka et al. 1987). Thus the *frxA* may be accounted for as a gene encoding an apoprotein of one of the iron-sulfur centers in photosystem I particles. The *ndh* genes were identified because their deduced amino-acid sequences show significant homology with the components of the NADH dehydrogenase subunits encoded in human and other mitochondrial genomes. Since NADH-plastoquinone (PQ) oxidoreductase activity has been detected in *Chlamydomonas* chloroplasts (Bennoun 1982), these *ndh* genes possibly encode subunits of this enzyme.

Although the photosynthetic genes in liverwort are more or less scattered throughout the chloroplast genome, some functionally related genes tend to form small clusters; e.g., *psaA-psaB*, *psbD-psbC*, *psbE-psbF*, *psbG-ndh3*, *atpB-atpE*, *atpI-atpH-atpF-atpA*, and *psbH-petB-petD* (see Fig. 1). Among them, *psbD* and *psbC* are the overlapping genes sharing 53 bp, and similarly *psbG* and *ndh3* share 10 bp. Each gene cluster may represent a transcription unit. Corresponding gene clusters have also been observed in higher plants (Palmer 1985). As shown in Figure 2, linkage relationships among ATPase subunit genes in prokaryotes and chloroplasts are also comparable to a certain extent (Cozens and Walker 1987).

Genes for Ribosomes

Chloroplast ribosomes are 70S prokaryotic ribosomes sharing the antibiotic sensitivities and im-

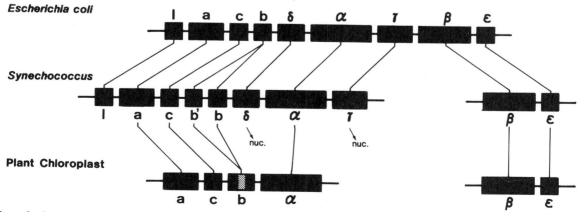

Figure 2. Arrangements of genes for ATPase subunits in prokaryotes and chloroplasts. Thick lines indicate the ATPase genes and the letters show the subunit encoded in the gene. Chloroplast b subunit is also known as I, c as III, and a as IV. Chloroplast b subunit gene (*atpF*) contains an intron (cross-hatched). Chloroplast ATPase subunits II, γ, and δ are nuclear-encoded proteins.

munological similarities with those of *Escherichia coli* (Schmidt et al. 1985). As a specific feature of chloroplast ribosomes, there are four species of rRNAs instead of the usual three species, namely, 16S, 23S, 5S, and 4.5S rRNAs. The additional 4.5S RNA, however, corresponds to the 3′ terminal portion of *E. coli* 23S rRNA, and therefore the RNA components of chloroplast ribosomes are equivalent to those of *E. coli*. Indeed, nearly 70% nucleotide sequence homology has been determined between *E. coli* and liverwort chloroplast rRNA genes (T. Kohchi et al., in prep.). Moreover, the four rRNA genes together with two tRNA genes form a cluster in the order shown in Figure 3a that is quite comparable to the rRNA operons carrying the same species of tRNA genes in *E. coli* or *Bacillus subtilis* (see Ozeki and Inokuchi 1986). In contrast to bacteria, however, both tRNA genes in chloroplast rRNA operons carry an intron (see below). Taking into account this feature, the structure of chloroplast rRNA operons illustrated in Figure 3a may be representative for all plants. In liverwort, there are two sets of rRNA genes or rRNA operons, one in each IR region (Fig. 1).

At present, 20 ribosomal protein genes have been assigned in the liverwort chloroplast genome, all of which have been determined because their amino acid sequences share significant homology with *E. coli* ribosomal proteins. The numbering system has therefore been adopted from *E. coli*; 9 for the 50S large subunit (*rpl*) and 11 for the 30S small subunit (*rps*).

Ten of the genes form a large cluster, whereas the rest are more or less scattered throughout the chloroplast DNA. The gene order in this large cluster is comparable to *E. coli* ribosomal-protein operons as illustrated in Figure 3d (Ohyama et al. 1986). Recently the *X* gene in the *E. coli spc* operon (Fig. 3d) has been identified as encoding a ribosomal protein in the 50S subunit (Wada and Sako 1987), and thus we now assign the *secX* in liverwort chloroplasts to one of the 50S ribosomal protein genes. The linkage of S12-S7 in *E. coli str* operon is also maintained in chloroplasts, although the chloroplast S12 gene (*rps12*) is not only split by two introns but is further separated into two parts (*rps12′* and *rps′12*) that are located far apart, about 60 kbp, on different DNA strands (Fukuzawa et al. 1986) (Fig. 3c). These two parts of *rps12* are transcribed separately and a mature mRNA may be formed after *trans*-splicing (see below).

In spinach chloroplast ribosomes, it has been estimated that about 10 out of 24 ribosomal proteins in the 30S subunit and 6–8 of 33 proteins in the 50S subunit are chloroplast-encoded, whereas the rest are nuclear-encoded proteins (Dorne et al. 1984). These estimated numbers for chloroplast-encoded ribosomal proteins are in good agreement with the numbers of genes assigned *rpl* and *rps* in liverwort chloroplasts. Although a possibility remains that some of the ORFs in chloroplasts may encode ribosomal proteins, there should not be many, judging from their putative amino acid composition. It is very likely that a chloroplast genome carries

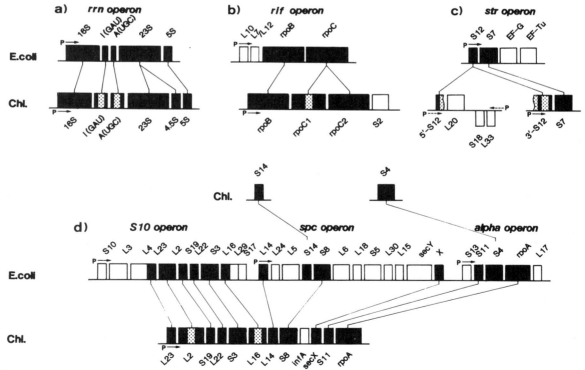

Figure 3. Arrangements of genes, (*a*) for rRNAs, (*b*) for RNA polymerase, and (*c, d*) for ribosomal proteins, in *E. coli* and liverwort chloroplasts. P stands for promoter. Solid arrows indicate the direction of transcription starting from the first gene in each cluster; dotted arrows show the transcription starting farther up. Corresponding genes are connected by thin lines (see text).

only one third of the ribosomal protein genes necessary for the construction of 70S chloroplast ribosomes. This implies that nuclear genomes must contain ribosomal protein genes, not only for eukaryotic 80S ribosomes, but also a considerable number for prokaryotic 70S ribosomes.

Interestingly, all the counterparts for the ribosomal protein genes that have been detected in liverwort chloroplasts have also been detected in tobacco chloroplasts, except *rpl21* (Shinozaki et al. 1986). Similarly, the counterparts of *E. coli* ribosomal protein genes that are not found in liverwort chloroplasts have also not been detected in tobacco, except for *rps16*. It seems, therefore, that the allocation of each gene for ribosomal protein components to either chloroplast or nuclear genome basically follows the same scheme in green plants.

We conclude that the chloroplast ribosomes as well as the ribosomal gene organization are retained as prokaryotic type, but this is so incomplete that without the aid of nuclear genes, chloroplast ribosomes cannot be constructed. We do, however, get a glimpse of the prokaryotic origin of chloroplasts.

Organization of tRNA Genes and Codon Usage

tRNA genes for 31 different tRNA species have been detected throughout the liverwort chloroplast genome. The species of tRNAs are identified by their anticodon triplet sequences in the familiar cloverleaf structure, and the amino acids to be accepted are predicted from their anticodons according to the universal codon table. There are 5 tRNA genes present as duplicates in the IR regions, bringing the total number of tRNA genes to 36. In addition, a possible pseudogene for tRNA^{Pro}(GGG), showing somewhat incomplete cloverleaf structure, was also found. Unmodified cloverleaf structures of all these tRNAs deduced from the DNA sequences, including pseudo-tRNA^{Pro}(GGG), are illustrated in Figure 4. Genes for tRNAs are scattered throughout the genome, and none of them encodes the 3′-CCA sequence. Six tRNA genes are split by an intron at the positions indicated by arrows on the cloverleafs in Figure 4. The structure of introns is described below.

It is generally accepted that no RNA molecules may be transferred from cytoplasm to chloroplasts. If this is the case, all the necessary RNAs such as rRNAs or tRNAs ought to be generated within the chloroplasts. Since all the circumstantial evidence supports the use of the universal codon table in the genetic system of chloroplasts, the 31 species of tRNAs deduced from the DNA analysis must be enough to decode all the universal codons. This number of tRNA species is much smaller than the estimated number of 45–50 in *E. coli* or *B. subtilis* (Fournier and Ozeki 1985; Vold 1985), but higher than the 24 in yeast mitochondria (Bonitz et al. 1980b) or 22 in human mitochondria (Anderson et al. 1981). In these mitochondria, however, the codon table used is not the universal, but a modified version.

It may be said that the complete analysis of chloroplast DNA in liverwort and tobacco has provided the first instances where the entire codon has been correlated with a complete set of tRNAs in one genetic system adopting the universal codon table.

Table 3 summarizes the liverwort case. A distinctive feature in codon usage is that the codons having U or A as the third letter are preferentially used. The liverwort chloroplast DNA is very AT rich (72% AT in total), and about 87% of the third letters of codons in protein-encoding genes are A or T, and spacer regions altogether contain about 80% AT. This problem is discussed in detail by Osawa (this volume), including the present case of liverwort chloroplasts. As is seen in Table 3, all 61 sense codons are used and they must be decoded by the 31 species of tRNAs that are indicated in the table by their unmodified anticodon triplets. In four-codon boxes of CUN-Leu, CCN-Pro, and GCN-Ala, we detected only one species of tRNA gene for each box with T at the wobbling position. Therefore, these codon families may be recognized by expanded U-N wobbling or "two out of three" base interaction that has been proposed in mitochondria (Barrell et al. 1980). In other four-codon boxes of GUN-Val, UCN-Ser, ACN-Thr, and GGN-Gly, two tRNA species are assigned to each box, and thus these codon families as well as the 12 two-codon families may be decoded by allowing ordinary G-U wobbling. In the AUN box, the C residue of the anticodon of tRNA^{Ile}(CAU) is presumably modified to recognize specifically the AUA codon for Ile, preventing the AUG-Met codon being read. In the CGN-Arg box, the anticodon of tRNA^{Arg}(ACG) is usually modified as ICG, and together with tRNA^{Arg}(CCG) this four-codon family may be translated. We conclude that the 31 tRNA species generated in the chloroplasts may be enough to translate all the universal codons properly. To prove this, however, actual production of tRNAs in chloroplasts as well as their modified nucleotides must be worked out. Since we have elucidated all possible tRNA genes in the genome, the hypothesis that no transportation of tRNA from the cytoplasm into the chloroplasts occurs can also be tested by analyzing the tRNA population in chloroplasts.

In tobacco chloroplasts, 30 species of tRNA genes have been reported (Shinozaki et al. 1986). A tRNA gene present in liverwort but not in tobacco is *trnR*(CCG), whereas the rest are the same; a tRNA^{Pro}(GGG) pseudogene was also not detected. It is interesting to see how the tRNA^{Arg}(ACG) alone translates the whole four-codon family of CGN-Arg. In any case, a set of tRNA genes in chloroplasts may not be completely fixed but evolving toward reduction, similar to the case with mitochondria.

It was recently found that a specific glutamyl tRNA with unusual anticodon modification (RNA^{DALA}) is involved in the first step of chlorophyll synthesis in chloroplasts (Schon et al. 1986). The unmodified nucleotide sequence deduced from the *trnQ*(UUC) gene in liverwort chloroplasts shares very high homology

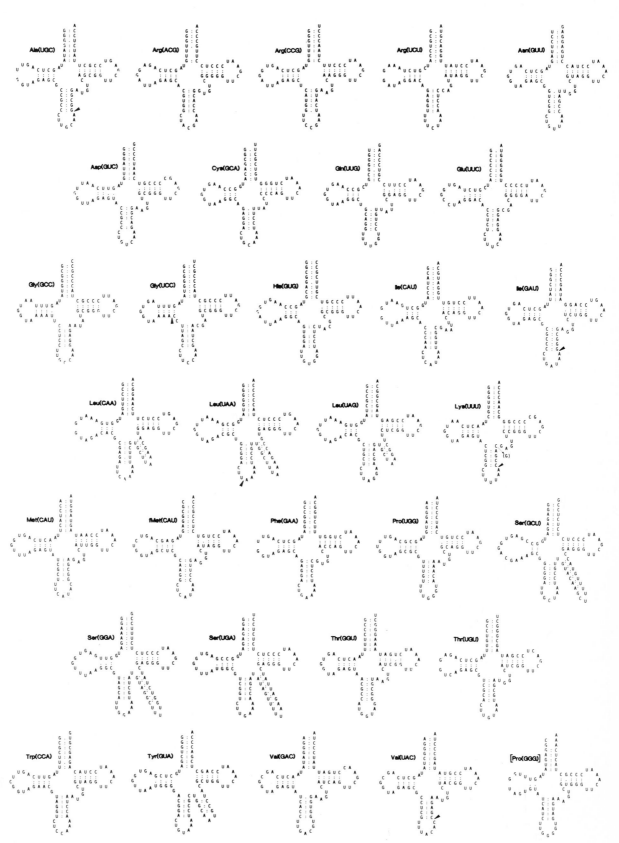

Figure 4. (*See facing page for legend.*)

Table 3. Codon Table and Codon Usage Pattern of Liverwort Chloroplast Protein Genes (91 ORFs)

Codon	tRNA	Usage	Codon	tRNA	Usage	Codon	tRNA	Usage	Codon	tRNA	Usage
UUU	Phe	1547	UCU		628	UAU	Tyr	826	UGU	Cys	219
UUC	GAA	97	UCC	Ser	71	UAC	GUA	95	UGC	GCA	41
UUA	UAA	1867	UCA	GGA	359	UAA	ter	84	UGA	ter	2
UUG	Leu CAA	203	UCG	UGA	48	UAG	ter	5	UGG	Trp CCA	441
CUU		524	CCU		477	CAU	His	388	CGU		357
CUC	Leu	25	CCC	Pro (GGG)	39	CAC	GUG	62	CGC	ACG	47
CUA	UAG	143	CCA	UGG	367	CAA	Gln	887	CGA	Arg	258
CUG		25	CCG		49	CAG	UUG	53	CGG CCG		22
AUU		1519	ACU		616	AAU	Asn	1256	AGU	Ser	414
AUC	Ile GAU	101	ACC	Thr	57	AAC	GUU	175	AGC	GCU	46
AUA	CAU	708	ACA	GGU	499	AAA	Lys	1764	AGA	Arg	382
AUG	Met CAU	430	ACG	UGU	42	AAG	UUU	78	AGG UCU		24
	fMet CAU	91									
GUU		648	GCU		779	GAU	Asp	735	GGU		627
GUC	Val GAC	47	GCC		66	GAC	GUC	72	GGC	Gly	82
GUA	UAC	450	GCA	Ala UGC	452	GAA	Glu	1133	GGA	GCC	678
GUG		48	GCG		50	GAG	UUC	85	GGG UCC		88

tRNA indicates unmodified anticodon sequences of tRNA molecules deduced from the DNA sequence.

with that reported for RNA^{DALA} in higher plants. Since we detected only one gene for tRNA^{Glu} in the chloroplast genome, this gene must have dual functions for both chlorophyll and protein biosynthesis, possibly through differential modification of the primary product.

In the cloverleaf structure of tRNA^{Lys}(UUU), there is a mismatched pair of C-C at the end of the anticodon stem (Fig. 4). Recently we replaced the anticodon region of this tRNA gene with a short synthetic DNA fragment, carrying an amber anticodon (CUA) but not carrying an intron sequence, and then introduced it into *E. coli* amber mutants to test for expression of suppressor activity. No suppressor activity was detected, even at low temperatures. This is presumably due to the aforementioned C-C mismatch, and indeed, it was found that, by a single-base mutation from C to G at that position indicated in Figure 4, the liverwort-derived tRNA gene expressed the suppressor activity in *E. coli* cells (K. Nakahigashi et al., unpubl. results). This result indicates that, at least in *E. coli*, the tRNA^{Lys}(UUU) appears to be defective. Nevertheless, the tRNA carrying the C-C mismatch must be active in protein biogenesis in chloroplasts. Similar mismatching was also found in several other tRNAs in chloroplasts (Fig. 4). Accordingly, these mismatches in chloroplast tRNAs, which may not be permissive in bacteria, may somehow be permissive in the chloroplast machine.

RNA Polymerase Genes

It has been reported that RNA polymerase subunits of spinach chloroplasts are synthesized from poly(A)$^{+}$

RNA, suggesting the possibility of nuclear-encoded proteins (Lerbs et al. 1985). Nevertheless, we could detect the genes presumed to correspond to *E. coli* RNA polymerase subunits in liverwort chloroplast DNA; i.e., *rpoA, B, C1,* and *C2,* following the designation used in *E. coli.* Although in *E. coli* the β′ subunit is encoded by a single gene, *rpoC,* it is separated into two tandemly linked genes, *rpoC1* and *rpoC2,* in the chloroplasts; *rpoC1* and *rpoC2* correspond to the proximal and distal portion of *E. coli rpoC,* respectively. This situation is illustrated in Figure 5, showing the regions for high localized homology. Chloroplast *rpoB* is assigned as the counterpart for *E. coli rpoB* for the β subunit, and as in the *E. coli rif* operon, chloroplast *rpoB* is closely linked to *rpoC1-C2* with a 31-bp spacer (Fig. 3b). Several species of RNA molecules containing these three messages together have been detected, suggesting that this *rpo* gene cluster may be an active transcription unit (K. Nakahigashi and K. Umesono, unpubl. results). Another gene *rpoA* for the α subunit is not linked to *rpoB-C1-C2,* but is found in the cluster of ribosomal protein genes, again like the *rpoA* gene in the *E. coli* α operon (Fig. 3d). Existence of RNA polymerase genes in the chloroplast genome, of course, does not conflict with the presence of a nuclear-encoded RNA polymerase in chloroplasts, because it has been reported that two distinct RNA polymerase activities are detectable in spinach and *Euglena* chloroplasts (Greenberg et al. 1985). It would be interesting to know if they are used for differential expression of chloroplast genes.

Throughout our analysis of liverwort chloroplast DNA, we could not detect an ORF showing significant

Figure 4. Cloverleaf structures of liverwort chloroplast tRNAs. Unmodified nucleotide sequences deduced from tRNA genes are presented in cloverleaf structures. All the species of tRNAs, including an incomplete tRNA^{Pro}(GGG), are presented (see text). Species of tRNAs are indicated by the amino acid with their anticodons in parentheses. Solid triangles indicate the locations of introns. A mutation from C to G in tRNA^{Lys}(UUU) is described in the text.

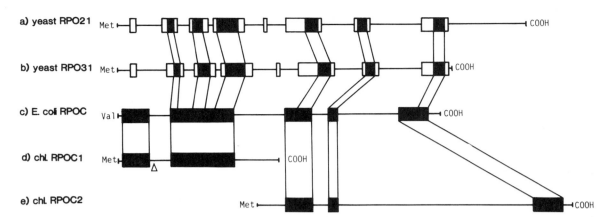

Figure 5. Schematic representation of the location of homologous segments of RNA polymerase β' subunits among yeast, *E. coli*, and chloroplasts. The location of homology segments in *Saccharomyces cerevisiae* and *E. coli* has been worked out by Allison et al. (1985). Closed boxes indicate homologous segments that can be seen in *E. coli* β' polypeptide. Open boxes represent regions of sequence homology between two yeast subunits. An open triangle indicates the location of an intron in the *rpoC1* gene (K. Umesono et al., in prep.).

homology with the σ subunit of RNA polymerase, or even with a common core sequence found in various σ subunits (see Reznikoff et al. 1985). This subunit is known to be essential for accurate promoter recognition of an RNA polymerase. Although it is possible that the chloroplast *rpoD* for the σ subunit was not detected due to the low homology with known prokaryotic σ proteins, we rather suspect that chloroplasts do not carry this gene but depend on the nuclear gene(s) to form an RNA polymerase holoenzyme. In bacteria, a core enzyme, composed of α, β, and β' subunits, can associate with different σ subunits, and then recognize different promoters specifically depending on the σ subunits. Thus, if the chloroplast σ subunit(s) is nuclear-encoded, the nucleus may be capable of controlling the expression of chloroplast genes by σ supply, possibly differentially.

In Figure 1, genes shown inside the circle are transcribed clockwise, and those outside are transcribed anticlockwise, according to the orientation of sense strands of DNA. As the first step of gene expression, recognition by the RNA polymerase holoenzyme of DNA sequences termed promoters results in precise transcription initiation at specific sites with specific orientation. This is presumably accomplished through the sequence-specific binding of a σ subunit. Although the type(s) of chloroplast σ subunit is not known, typical prokaryotic promoter sequences (−35 and −10) can be found at more or less expected positions upstream of genes or gene clusters in liverwort chloroplast DNA. Similarly, prokaryotic terminator sequences in hairpin loops with T-cluster structure are also found downstream. A possible dual terminator structure has been reported in our earlier work (Umesono et al. 1984); that is, within a short spacer region (50 bp) between two end-to-end genes, both DNA strands can be written in similar hairpin loops with T-cluster structures, and they may serve as a dual terminator for both genes, which are transcribed in opposite directions. Rather long-stem loop structures in spacer regions are often

found that may serve to the punctuation of gene clusters in liverwort chloroplast DNA (Umesono et al. 1984). Shine-Dalgarno sequences for ribosome binding in translation initiation are also detected upstream of initiation codons for protein-encoding genes, as the complementary sequences to the 3' terminal part of liverwort 16S rRNA (CCTCCT). Thus, the genetic signals in chloroplasts, such as promoters, terminators, and others, appear to be of a prokaryotic nature.

Experiments to determine the transcription initiation sites as well as the transcription units in liverwort chloroplasts in cultured cells are now under way. Our preliminary results indicate that the primary RNA transcripts are, at least in some cases, rather long, possibly containing two or more messages from the gene clusters described above. These mRNAs may correspond to the polycistronic mRNAs from *E. coli* operons. In contrast to *E. coli*, however, many genes (asterisked in Fig. 1) contain intron sequences that must be spliced out before beginning the translation process. Accordingly, a coupled mechanism of transcription and translation, which is generally observed in *E. coli*, is not likely to occur in chloroplasts, rather the initiation of translation must await completion of intron splicing. For nuclear genes, of course, the two processes of mRNA formation and translation are clearly separated in the nucleus and cytoplasm, respectively. In chloroplasts, no nucleus-like structure is known, but these two processes must somehow be separated in the organelle. A model for built-in structural information contained in the intron sequences to allow precise splicing is presented in the following section.

Split Genes and Their Expression

A split chloroplast gene was first identified in the *Chlamydomonas* 23S rRNA gene (Allet and Rochaix 1979), and the subsequent structural analyses have increased the number of instances in which introns (intervening sequences) in genes encoding tRNAs and proteins have been found. Chloroplast introns can be classified into either group I or group II intron families, as originally proposed in fungal mitochondrial introns (Davies et al. 1982; Michel et al. 1982; Michel and Dujon 1983). Each of the groups contains characteristic sequence elements to be folded into a group-specific secondary structure. Appropriate tertiary folding of the intron portion may confer catalytic activity upon the RNA molecule itself; thus, several instances in both groups have shown an ability to undergo a self-splicing reaction without any protein factors in vitro (Cech and Baas 1986). In the course of self-splicing, group II introns excise lariat intron molecules similar to those of nuclear pre-mRNA splicing (Peebles et al. 1986; Schmelzer and Schweyen 1986; van der Veen et al. 1986).

Taking advantage of the conserved sequences in the group introns, we have postulated 20 introns in 18 different genes (Ohyama et al. 1986; K. Ohyama et al., in prep.). All of the split genes are interrupted only once in their coding messages, except for rps12 and ORF203, which consist of 3 exons. The presumed introns were detected in 6 tRNA genes, such as trnA(UGC) (intron length 768 nucleotides), trnI(GAU) (886), trnG(UCC) (593), trnK(UUU) (2111), trnL(UAA) (315), and trnV(UAC) (530); and in 12 protein genes including atpF (587), ndh1 (712), ndh2 (536), petB (495), petD (493), rps12 (the first intron is split in trans; the second intron, 500, see below), rpl2 (544), rpl16 (535), rpoC1 (596), ORF135 (485), ORF167 (608), and ORF203 (518 and 318). Interestingly, phylogenetic conservation of the split pattern, including the trans-split form of the rps12 gene, can be seen between liverwort and tobacco (no counterpart of ORF135 is found in the tobacco DNA sequence).

The shortest among the liverwort chloroplast introns is an intron found in trnL(UAA) and may be classified as a member of group I, as previously pointed out by Bonnard et al. (1984). The liverwort trnL(UAA) intron contains sequence elements called 9R′ (5′-GUUUUC-3′), A (UCAGGG), B (UCCUGA), 9L (GACUC), 9R (GAAAAC), and 2 (GAGUC), in this order (K. Umesono et al., in prep.), which can apparently form base pairs such as 9R′/9R, A/B, 9L/2 in liverwort as well as in Vicia faba and Zea mays (Bonnard et al. 1984). These interactions play a major role in maintaining a tertiary structure responsible for the splicing reaction in some group I introns (Cech and Baas 1986). Another structural element has been called "IGS" (internal guide sequence), which is located near the 5′ end of the intron and possibly makes base pairs with both 5′ and 3′ exons to keep them in close proximity for splicing (Davies et al. 1982). In fact, this guide sequence has been shown to recognize the 3′ end portion of the 5′ exon, and therefore serves as a sole determinant for 5′ splice-site selection (Been and Cech 1986; Waring et al. 1986). In the liverwort trnL(UAA) intron, however, the interaction between the 5′ exon and presumed IGS is not sufficient, and this may be the

reason why we could not detect self-splicing activity in vitro (K. Umesono, unpubl. results).

The other 19 constituents of the liverwort chloroplast introns can be assigned to group II. According to the proposal of Michel and Dujon (1983), secondary structure models of the trnK(UUU) intron and the second intron of rps12 were constructed (Fig. 6). Although the trnK(UUU) intron is over four times the size of the rps12 intron, it can be folded into a very similar structure; the introns begin at common GUGYG (Y = U or C) pentanucleotides (Table 4) and they are basically composed of six base-paired helices in which the fifth (also called "14bp-hairpin," Keller and Michel 1985) has a highly conserved primary structure (Michel and Dujon 1983; K. Ohyama et al., in prep.). Located on the 3′ side of the sixth helix, a conserved unpaired adenine residue (marked with a circle in the figure) is proposed to be a branch point for lariat formation (van der Veen et al. 1986).

These conserved features may also be applicable to a trans-splicing reaction between the first and second exons of rps12 transcripts (Fig. 7). The model is based on analyses of the liverwort (T. Kohchi and K. Umesono, unpubl. results) and tobacco (Koller et al. 1987) rps12 transcripts and compensatory base changes between them. It is likely that the trans-split form of rps12 genes is initially derived from a nick in the third loop region, indicating that these heterodimer RNA molecules would also undergo normal splicing pathways as seen in nuclear pre-mRNA splicing using artificially separated precursors (Konarska et al. 1985; Solnick 1985). Accordingly, the model also suggests how this bizarre gene is initially formed. The second and third exons of the rps12 gene are tightly linked to the downstream rps7 gene, indicating an evolutionarily conserved arrangement (Fig. 3c). It is therefore likely that the first exon, together with the 5′ half of the intron, could transpose to the 5′ portion of the prerequisite rpl20 gene. The transposition would occur in the early stages of plant chloroplast evolution because the trans-split form of the rps12 gene in chloroplasts can be seen in many plants, but not in Euglena (Palmer 1985; Shinozaki et al. 1986). As an alternative explanation, the exons were usually present separately in primordial organisms, and then came together to form the present style of genes by DNA rearrangements; in this respect, a trans-split gene rps12 may be considered as a "living fossil" of a primitive style.

We have further postulated that there would be some structural requirements responsible for RNA splicing within the first stem loop region because this region always contains 300–400 nucleotides in many group II introns (Figs. 6 and 7, Michel and Dujon 1983). In an attempt to look at this problem, we have compared all of the liverwort group II introns to determine conserved sequence elements in this region. As listed in Table 4, three-sequence stretches such as "AGC," "TATGG," and "CCTAAG" can be observed in nearly all of the introns.

A recent study by Jacquier and Rosbash (1986) has

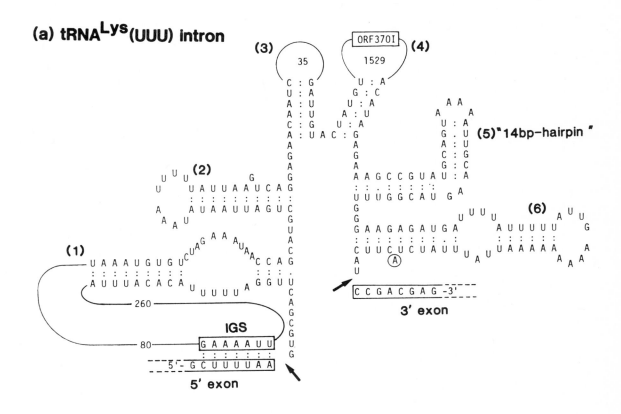

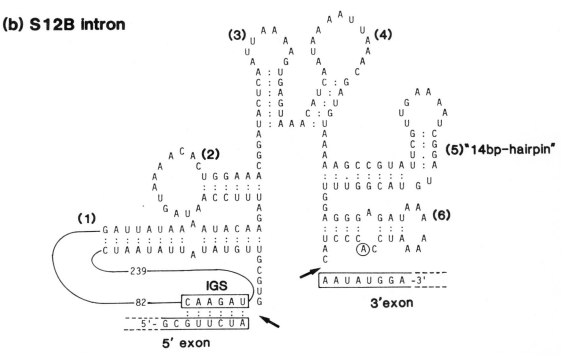

Figure 6. Michel-Dujon models of liverwort chloroplast group II introns. (*a*) An intron found in the *trnK*(UUU) gene contains an ORF, possibly encoding a polypeptide 370 amino acid residues long (ORF370I). Numbers indicate the length of loop regions. (*b*) The second intron of the *rps12* gene. Both introns are composed of six major helices. The fifth hairpin is well conserved in the primary structure. An adenine residue with a circle is a presumed branch point. (IGS) Internal guide sequence that can bind to the 3' end of the 5' exon (see text).

Table 4. Conserved Sequence Elements Found in the First Loop Regions of Group II Introns

Intron	5' Exon/Intron		"AGC"		"TATGG"		IGS		"CCTAAG"
(a) Liverwort chloroplast									
trnA(UGC)	cccTTGCAA/TTGGG-	104	-gAACa-		n.d.	170	-cTTGCGAac-		n.d.
trnI(GAU)	ccCTGATAA/TTGCG-	95	-tAGCa-	45	-tTCAGGt-	97	-cTTATCAGt-	60	-aCCTAATa-
trnK(UUU)	ggCTTTTAA/GTGCG-	103	-tAGCa-	76	-tAATGGa-	89	-gTTAAAAGa-	64	-tCCTAAAc-
trnG(UCC)	gTGGTAAAa/GTGCG-	119	-aAGCg-	38	-cTATGGa-	82	-gTTTGCTAa-	38	-tTCTAAAg-
trnV(UAC)	cgttTACAC/GTGCG-	109	-tAGCc-	47	-aTATGGt-	81	-gGTGTAtaa-	59	-aCCTAAGt-
rps12A	agagTGTAT/GTGCG-		n.d.		n.d.	378	-tATACAaat-	53	-aCCTATTc-
rps12B	ggcGTTCTA/GTGCG-	111	-aAGCa-	57	-cTAGGGt-	73	-tTAGAACaa-	58	-aCCTAAGg-
rpl2	tacCTTTGA/GTGCG-	114	-aGGCa-	51	-aTATGGa-	97	-gTCAAAGac-	34	-tCCTAAGt-
rpl16	atgCTTAGT/GTGTG-	117	-aAGCg-	29	-gTAGGGt-	50	-aACTAAGaa-	38	-aCCTAAAc-
rpoC1	tacTGCGAT/GTGTG-	107	-aAGCt-	51	-cTAGGGt-	88	-cATCGCAaa-	35	-cCCTAAAg-
ndh1	tagCTCTAC/GTGTG-	113	-aAGTc-	145	-aGAAGGt-	76	-aGTAGAGat-	41	-aCCTATCt-
ndh2	taTGAAGGA/GTGCG-	112	-aCGCa-	58	-tTACGGa-	45	-aTTCTTCAa-	51	-tCCTAAAa-
atpF	aggGAGTGT/GTGCG-	113	-tAGCa-	44	-aAATGGt-	89	-aACACTCat-	87	-aCCTATTt-
petB	aatATGGGT/GTGCG-	109	-aAGCa-	21	-cTATGAt-	117	-cACTCATtc-	33	-aTCTACGg-
petD	tatGGGAGT/GTGTG-	103	-aAACt-	36	-cTATGAt-	88	-cATTTCTgt-	37	-aTCTAATg-
ORF135	ttTCTAGAG/GTGTG-		n.d.	111	-cTATGGt-	82	-tCTCTAGAa-	37	-aCCTAAAg-
ORF167	ataGAGATG/GTGTG-	153	-aAACa-	56	-aAAGCCt-	81	-cCATCTCgt-	43	-aGCTAATt-
ORF203A	tgACGTATA/ATGCG-	98	-aAGCg-	33	-cTATGGt-	96	-tTATATGTa-	41	-aCCTAACg-
ORF203B	cctcACGCT/TTGTG-		n.d.		n.d.	109	-tAGCGTtta-		n.d.
(b) Mitochondria									
Sc. aI1	tatTTAATG/GTGCG-	109	-tAGCa-	43	-aCATGGt-	86	-aCGTTGAgg-	57	-aCCTAAAt-
Sc. aI2	tgaTTTTCT/GTGCG-	178	-tAGCa-	49	-cGATGGc-	86	-aAGAAGAgg-	58	-cTGTACGa-
Sc. aI5c	gaCATTTTC/GAGCG-	108	-aAGCt-	77	-aTATGCt-	125	-tGGAAATGa-	41	-aGCTAAGt-
Sc. bI1	atGGACAGA/GTGAG-	125	-aAACt-	40	-aTATAGa-	115	-tTCTGTCTa-	44	-tCCTAAGt-
Sp. cob	ctgATAAAA/TTGCG-	106	-gAGCa-	61	-aTACGGt-	96	-cTTTTATga-	63	-aCCTACGt-
Pa. cox1	ataTTGCAG/GTGCG-	109	-tAGCa-	65	-cTGTGTg-	84	-tCTGCAAgc-	56	-tGCTAAGg-
Zm. cox2	ggTATCGGA/GTGCG-	107	-tAGCa-	62	-cTATGGt-	85	-gTCCGATAa-	53	-aCCTAAGg-

Capitals indicate possible signal sequences. See text. "AGC" sequences have also been pointed out by Lang et al. (1985). Significance of these conserved sequences is evident when a secondary structure model is constructed. "AGC" is always located at the specific bulge, and regions surrounding "TATGG" and "CCTAAG" can form base pairs to loop out "TAT" and "TAAG" sequences, respectively (K. Umesono, in prep.). Each "IGS" is completely conserved in the tobacco counterpart (data are not shown). (Sc) *Saccharomyces cerevisiae.* (Sp) *Schizosaccharomyces pombe.* (Pa) *Podospora anserina.* (Zm) *Zea mays.* Intron sequences were obtained from Bonitz et al. (1980a) (Sc. aI1, aI2, and aI5c), Schmelzer et al. (1983) (Sc. bI1), Lang et al. (1985) (Sp. cob), Osiewacz and Esser (1984) (Pa. cox1), and Fox and Leaver (1981) (Zm. cox2). n.d., not determined.

clearly demonstrated a strong 5' exon-intron interaction using a *trans*-splicing system developed with a short 5' exon transcript and modified group II introns. This study encouraged us to identify the sites of interaction between the 5' exon and the downstream intron, and we have found a penta- or hexanucleotide stretch that is complementary to the 3' end of the upstream 5' exon. All of the sequences are localized between "TATGG" and "CCTAAG" boxes, and their distinctive characteristics would be functionally equivalent to the group I IGS. Therefore, we tentatively propose this sequence motif as group II IGS (Table 4, Figs. 6 and 7). Conservation of these elements is also apparent in mitochondrial (Table 4b) and tobacco chloroplast (data not shown) group II introns. It is also noteworthy that the group II IGSs presented here are present on homologous loops in secondary structure models of *Saccharomyces cerevisiae* aI1 and aI2 (Michel et al. 1982), *Podospora anserina cox1* (Osiewacz and Esser 1984), and *Schizosaccharomyces pombe cob* introns (Lang et al. 1985). Further experimental evidence is needed to confirm this hypothesis, and a more detailed discussion will be published elsewhere (K. Umesono et al., in prep.).

DISCUSSION

In Figure 1, genes and ORFs are drawn more or less to scale, and it can be seen that the map is almost filled up, leaving little room for additional genes. This may allow us to set an upper limit for the genetic capacity of chloroplast genomes in general at 130–140 species of genes.

It becomes evident that the gene organization of chloroplasts is insufficient to support them in cell cytoplasm. It is insufficient because some of the genes for each functional complex or apparatus are absent. For instance: (a) In ribosomes, genes for about two thirds of the ribosomal proteins in 30S and 50S particles are missing, although the genes for other components, including rRNAs, are detected in the chloroplast genome. (b) In the case of the RNA polymerase, a set of genes for the RNA polymerase core enzyme is detected, but a gene for the σ subunit, which is essential to form the RNA polymerase holoenzyme, may be missing. (c) With regard to the translation system, a set of tRNA genes was detected in the chloroplasts that is probably enough to translate all the universal codons. However, many enzymes are needed to make mature

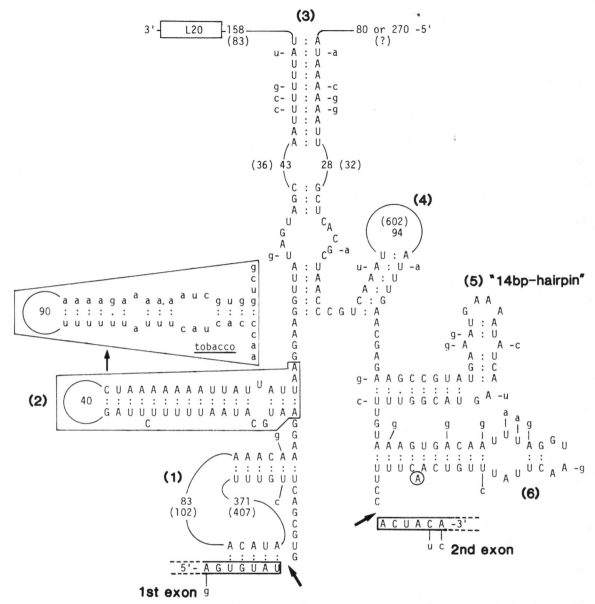

Figure 7. Secondary structure model for *trans*-splicing between the first and second exons of *rps12* gene. Numbers in parentheses and small letters indicate the tobacco sequences (Shinozaki et al. 1986). Note that all of the replacements are compensatory changes and do not affect the structure. The 5′ end of the upstream portion of the liverwort second exon was determined by S1 nuclease mapping (K. Umesono, unpubl.).

tRNAs; for example, those for RNA processing, for various nucleotide modifications, for CCA addition at the 3′ end of tRNAs, etc., and enzymes are required to charge the cognate amino acids to the tRNAs. Many, if not all, of these enzymes may be nuclear-encoded. If an RNase P-type enzyme is involved for tRNA processing in chloroplasts, the RNA component of this enzyme may be coded for in the chloroplast genome if no RNA is introduced from the cytoplasm. Among the factors involved in translation, such as those for initiation (IF) or elongation (EF), a counterpart gene for *E. coli* IF-I has been detected. (d) In the ATPase complex, F_0 subunits of I, III, and IV are chloroplast-encoded, whereas subunit II is nuclear-encoded; and similarly, F_1

subunits of α, β, and ϵ are chloroplast-encoded, whereas γ and δ are nuclear-encoded. (e) A well-known example is that large and small subunits of ribulose bisphosphate carboxylase (RuBisCO) are chloroplast- and nuclear-encoded, respectively. (f) Similarly, the protein components in photosystem I and II complexes are partially encoded by chloroplast genes.

In our analysis, the genes related to DNA replication were not detected. However, chloroplast DNA must be replicated within the organelle, and, consequently, some of the protein components of the DNA replication machinery are likely to be encoded by chloroplast genes. Since the nucleotide sequence of the DNA replication origin is usually specific for each DNA molecule or replicon, it may not be determined directly from DNA sequences. If a factor for replication initiation is also specific for the origin structure, it cannot be determined from a comparison with other data in a bank, either. Accordingly, our failure to assign the genes for DNA replication does not mean that they are absent in the chloroplast genetic system, but rather that some of the unidentified ORFs may code for this machinery. Chloroplasts are well developed in green tissues in plants containing many DNA copies, but not in non-green or etiolated tissues. In these cells, chloroplast DNA must be maintained in proplastids or etioplasts, being replicated and inherited by the progeny cells for their genetic continuity. If a chloroplast gene is essential for DNA replication, other genes basic for the gene expression machinery must be constitutively expressed in proplastids to support the DNA replication, whereas the rest of the genes may be arrested. Since this basic machinery requires many nuclear-encoded proteins, their nuclear genes are also constantly supplying necessary components to proplastids.

As mentioned above, the gene composition worked out for the liverwort chloroplast genome is almost equivalent to that of tobacco, although a few genes are found only in one or the other. In consideration of the data accumulated for a number of other plants, we conclude that the allocation of genes for all chloroplast components to either the chloroplast or nuclear genome is basically the same from liverwort to higher plants. This allocation may have a particular cause, which is not yet evident. However, we prefer to think that it is more likely the result of a "frozen accident." If so, the present genetic system of plant chloroplasts would have to have been established in very early times before the branching of *Bryophytina* and *Tracheophytina*, through the process of prokaryotic endosymbiosis. Then, from this unified single origin, variations, mostly the accumulation of mutations in nucleotide sequences and the rearrangement in genomic DNA, but rarely changes in gene content, in the present chloroplast genome in plants may have evolved.

ACKNOWLEDGMENTS

We thank Yuriko Komine for her excellent help in preparing the illustrations and Karin Knisely for her critical reading of the manuscript. This work was supported by a grant-in-aid for special research projects from the Ministry of Education, Science and Culture of Japan.

REFERENCES

Allet, B. and J.-D. Rochaix. 1979. Structure analysis at the ends of the intervening DNA sequences in the chloroplast 23S ribosomal genes of *C. reinhardii. Cell* **18:** 55.

Allison, L.A., M. Moyle, M. Shales, and C.J. Ingles. 1985. Extensive homology among the largest subunits of eukaryotic and prokaryotic RNA polymerases. *Cell* **42:** 599.

Anderson, S., A.T. Bankier, B.G. Barrell, M.H.L. de Bruijn, A.R. Coulson, J. Drouin, I.C. Eperon, D.P. Nierlich, B.A. Roe, F. Sanger, P.H. Schreier, A.J.H. Smith, R.

Staden, and I.G. Young. 1981. Sequence and organization of human mitochondrial genome. *Nature* **290:** 457.

Barrell, B.G., S. Anderson, A.T. Bankier, M.H.L. de Bruijn, E. Chen, A.R. Coulson, J. Drouin, I.C. Eperon, D.P. Nierlich, B.A. Roe, F. Sanger, P.H. Schreier, A.J.H. Smith, R. Staden, and I.G. Young. 1980. Different pattern of codon recognition by mammalian mitochondrial tRNAs. *Proc. Natl. Acad. Sci.* **77:** 3164.

Been, M.D. and T.R. Cech. 1986. One binding site determines sequence specificity of Tetrahymena pre-rRNA self-splicing, *trans*-splicing, and RNA enzyme activity. *Cell* **47:** 207.

Bennoun, P. 1982. Evidence for a respiratory chain in the chloroplast. *Proc. Natl. Acad. Sci.* **79:** 4352.

Bonitz, S.G., G. Coruzzi, B.E. Thalenfeld, A. Tzagoloff, and G. Macino. 1980a. Assembly of the mitochondrial membrane system. Structure and nucleotide sequence of the gene coding for subunit 1 of yeast cytochrome oxidase. *J. Biol. Chem.* **255:** 11927.

Bonitz, S.G., R. Berlani, G. Coruzzi, M. Li, G. Macino, F.G. Nobrega, M.P. Nobrega, B.E. Thalenfeld, and A. Tzagoloff. 1980b. Codon recognition rules in yeast mitochondria. *Proc. Natl. Acad. Sci.* **77:** 3167.

Bonnard, G., F. Michel, J.H. Weil, and A. Steinmetz. 1984. Nucleotide sequence of the split tRNA$^{Leu}_{UAA}$ gene from *Vicia faba* chloroplasts: Evidence for structural homologies of the chloroplast tRNA^{Leu} intron with the intron from the autosplicable *Tetrahymena* ribosomal RNA precursor. *Mol. Gen. Genet.* **194:** 330.

Cech, T.R. and B.L. Baas. 1986. Biological catalysis by RNA. *Annu. Rev. Biochem.* **55:** 599.

Cozens, A.L. and J.E. Walker. 1987. The organization and sequence of the genes for ATP synthase subunits in the cyanobacterium *Synechococcus* 6301. Support for an endosymbiotic origin of chloroplasts. *J. Mol. Biol.* **194:** 359.

Crouse, E.J., J.M. Schmitt, and H.-J. Bohnert. 1985. Chloroplast and cyanobacterial genomes, genes, and RNAs: A compilation. *Plant Mol. Biol. Rep.* **3:** 43.

Davies, R.W., R.B. Waring, J.A. Ray, T.A. Brown, and C. Scazzocchio. 1982. Making ends meet: A model for RNA splicing in fungal mitochondria. *Nature* **300:** 719.

Dorne, A.-M., A.-M. Lescure, and R. Mache. 1984. Site of synthesis of spinach chloroplast ribosomal proteins and formation of incomplete ribosomal particles in isolated chloroplasts. *Plant Mol. Biol.* **3:** 83.

Fournier, M.J. and H. Ozeki. 1985. Structure and organization of the transfer ribonucleic acid genes of *Escherichia coli* K-12. *Microbiol. Rev.* **49:** 379.

Fox, T.D. and C.J. Leaver. 1981. The *Zea mays* mitochondrial gene coding cytochrome oxidase subunit II has an intervening sequence and does not contain TGA codons. *Cell* **26:** 315.

Fukuzawa, H., T. Kohchi, H. Shirai, K. Ohyama, K. Umesono, H. Inokuchi, and H. Ozeki. 1986. Coding sequences for chloroplast ribosomal protein S12 from liverwort, *Marchantia polymorpha*, are separated far apart on the different DNA strands. *FEBS Lett.* **198:** 11.

Greenberg, B.M., J.O. Narita, C.R. Deluca-Flaherty, and R.B. Hallick. 1985. Properties of chloroplast RNA polymerases. In *Molecular biology of the photosynthetic apparatus* (ed. K.E. Steinback et al.), p. 303. Cold Spring Harbor Laboratory, Cold Spring Harbor, New York.

Jacquier, A. and M. Rosbash. 1986. Efficient trans-splicing of a yeast mitochondrial RNA group II intron implicates a strong 5′ exon-intron interaction. *Science* **234:** 1099.

Keller, M. and F. Michel. 1985. The introns of the *Euglena gracilis* chloroplast gene which codes for the 32-kDa protein of photosystem II. Evidence for structural homologies with class II introns. *FEBS Lett.* **179:** 69.

Koller, B., H. Fromm, E. Galun, and M. Edelman. 1987. Evidence for in vivo *trans*-splicing of pre-mRNAs in tobacco chloroplasts. *Cell* **48:** 111.

Konarska, M.M., R.A. Padgett, and P.A. Sharp. 1985. *Trans* splicing of mRNA precursors in vitro. *Cell* **42:** 165.

Lang, B.F., F. Ahne, and L. Bonen. 1985. The mitochondrial genome of the fission yeast *Schizosaccharomyces pombe*. The cytochrome *b* gene has an intron closely related to the first two introns in the *Saccharomyces cerevisiae cox1* gene. *J. Mol. Biol.* **184:** 353.

Lerbs, S., E. Braurtigam, and B. Parthier. 1985. Polypeptides of DNA-dependent RNA polymerase of spinach chloroplasts: Characterization by antibody-linked polymerase assay and determination of sites of synthesis. *EMBO J.* **4:** 1661.

Michel, F. and B. Dujon. 1983. Conservation of RNA secondary structures in two intron families including mitochondrial-, chloroplast- and nuclear-encoded members. *EMBO J.* **2:** 33.

Michel, F., A. Jacquier, and B. Dujon. 1982. Comparison of fungal mitochondrial introns reveals extensive homologies in RNA secondary structure. *Biochimie* **64:** 867.

Oh-oka, H., Y. Takahashi, K. Wada, H. Matsubara, K. Ohyama, and H. Ozeki. 1987. The 8 kDa polypeptide in photosystem I is a probable candidate of an iron-sulfur center protein coded by the chloroplast gene *frxA*. *FEBS Lett.* **218:** 52.

Ohyama, K., Y. Yamano, H. Fukuzawa, T. Komano, H. Yamagishi, S. Fujimoto, and M. Sugiura. 1983. Physical mappings of chloroplast DNA from liverwort *Marchantia polymorpha* L. cell suspension cultures. *Mol. Gen. Genet.* **189:** 1.

Ohyama, K., H. Fukuzawa, T. Kohchi, H. Shirai, T. Sano, S. Sano, K. Umesono, Y. Shiki, M. Takeuchi, Z. Chang, D. Aota, H. Inokuchi, and H. Ozeki. 1986. Chloroplast gene organization deduced from complete sequence of liverwort *Marchantia polymorpha*. *Nature* **322:** 572.

Osiewacz, H.D. and K. Esser. 1984. The mitochondrial plasmid of *Podospora anserina*: A mobile intron of a mitochondrial gene. *Curr. Genet.* **8:** 299.

Ozeki, H. and H. Inokuchi. 1986. Organization of transfer RNA genes in prokaryotes. *Adv. Biophys.* **21:** 35.

Palmer, J.D. 1985. Comparative organization of chloroplast genomes. *Annu. Rev. Genet.* **19:** 325.

Peebles, C.L., P.S. Perlman, K.L. Mecklenburg, M.L. Petrillo, J.H. Tabor, K.A. Jarrell, and H.-L. Cheng. A self-splicing RNA excises an intron lariat. *Cell* **44:** 213.

Reznikoff, W.S., D.A. Siegele, D.W. Cowing, and C.A. Gross. 1985. The regulation of transcription initiation in bacteria. *Annu. Rev. Genet.* **19:** 355.

Schmelzer, C. and R.J. Schweyen. 1986. Self-splicing of group II in vitro: Mapping of the branch point and mutational inhibition of lariat formation. *Cell* **46:** 557.

Schmelzer, C., C. Schmidt, K. May, and R.J. Schweyen. 1983. Determination of functional domains in intron bI1 of yeast mitochondrial RNA by studies of mitochondrial mutations and a nuclear suppressor. *EMBO J.* **2:** 2047.

Schmidt, R.J., J.P. Hosler, N.W. Gillham, and J.E. Boynton. 1985. Biogenesis and evolution of chloroplast ribosomes: Cooperation of nuclear and chloroplast genes. In *Molecular biology of the photosynthetic apparatus* (ed. K.E. Steinback et al.), p. 417. Cold Spring Harbor Laboratory, Cold Spring Harbor, New York.

Schon, A., G. Krupp, S. Gough, S. Berry-Lowe, C. Gamini Kannangara, and D. Soll. 1986. The RNA required in the first step of chlorophyll biosynthesis is a chloroplast glutamate tRNA. *Nature* **322:** 281.

Shinozaki, K., M. Ohme, M. Tanaka, T. Wakasugi, N. Hayashida, T. Matsubayashi, N. Zaita, J. Chunwongse, J. Obokata, K. Yamaguchi-Shinozaki, C. Ohto, K. Torazawa, B.Y. Meng, M. Sugita, H. Deno, T. Kamogashira, K. Yamada, J. Kusuda, F. Takaiwa, A. Kato, N. Tohdoh, H. Shimada, and M. Sugiura. 1986. The complete nucleotide sequence of the tobacco chloroplast genome: Its gene organization and expression. *EMBO J.* **5:** 2043.

Solnick, D. 1985. *Trans* splicing of mRNA precursors. *Cell* **42:** 157.

Umesono, K., H. Inokuchi, K. Ohyama, and H. Ozeki. 1984. Nucleotide sequence of *Marchantia polymorpha* chloroplast DNA: A region possibly encoding three tRNAs and three proteins including a homologue of *E. coli* ribosomal protein S14. *Nucleic Acids Res.* **12:** 9551.

van der Veen, R., A.C. Arnberg, G. van der Horst, L. Bonen, H.F. Tabak, and L.A. Grivell. 1986. Excised group II introns in yeast mitochondria are lariats and can be formed by self-splicing in vitro. *Cell* **44:** 225.

Vold, B.S. 1985. Structure and organization of genes for transfer RNA in *Bacillus subtilis*. *Microbiol. Rev.* **49:** 71.

Wada, A. and T. Sako. 1987. Primary structures of and genes for new ribosomal proteins A and B in *Escherichia coli*. *J. Biochem.* **101:** 817.

Waring, R.B., P. Towner, S.J. Minter, and R.W. Davies. 1986. Splice-site selection by a self-splicing RNA of *Tetrahymena*. *Nature* **321:** 133.

The Origin of Cells: A Symbiosis between Genes, Catalysts, and Membranes

T. CAVALIER-SMITH

Department of Biophysics, Cell and Molecular Biology, King's College London (KQC), London, WC2B 5RL, United Kingdom

Evolution of catalytic function involves the evolution of the structure of individual catalysts and of their cooperation with other molecules to create an evolving supramolecular community: the living cell. Attempts to understand the origins of cell structure, I think, clarify the origin of enzymes of DNA replication, RNA processing and transcription, active transport, intermediary metabolism, and bioenergetics and shed new light on the crucial relationship between genetics, bioenergetics, and morphology, the fundamental pillars on which biology—and life itself—are built.

Genetic evolution began with the first replication of naked genes (Minchin 1915; Alexander and Bridges 1929; Muller 1929) to form the first living entity: the protobiont. The physical basis for that origin of life—nucleotide pairing and polymerization by prebiotic condensing agents—is now primarily a question of experimental chemistry (Zielinski and Orgel 1987). The next major evolutionary event was the origin of the first true organism: a symbiosis between replicating RNA molecules and primitive ribosomes, making proteins that helped the whole system multiply (Haldane 1965; Crick 1968; Orgel 1968). After much theoretical study (Miller and Orgel 1974; Crick et al. 1976; Eigen and Schuster 1979; Shepherd 1983), a broad outline of how it may have happened is fairly clear, although detailed problems remain (Maizels and Weiner, this volume) and serious experimental study lies in the future.

The gap between such a simple macromolecular system, for which I adopt the term "progenote" (Woese and Fox 1977a), and the simplest cell with a built-in bioenergetic system is immense and largely uncharted. The problem of cellular origins is commonly dismissed in a single sentence, with the assumption that "somehow" primitive ribosomes and chromosomes became enclosed by a lipid membrane to make the first cell, assumed to have been a fermentative heterotroph (Haldane 1929; Oparin 1938). Such ideas ignore the vital role of osmoenzymes, porters, and other catalysts embedded in membranes in chemiosmotic processes essential for all cellular life. Their origin poses major problems for the origin of a cell by simple encapsulation by lipids and for the assumption that fermentation preceded phototrophy (Cavalier-Smith 1985). These problems can be avoided if the first cell was instead a phototrophic heterotroph (Cavalier-Smith 1985) that originated by folding up what Blobel (1980) called an inside-out cell, so as to form a cell bounded, not by a single plasma membrane, but by two distinct membranes, as in gram-negative eubacteria (subkingdom Negibacteria; Cavalier-Smith 1986a, 1987a) such as *Escherichia coli* (Fig. 1). Blobel (1980) and I (Cavalier-Smith 1985) have suggested that many universal features of cells, notably the attachment of chromosomes and ribosomes to membranes and the cotranslational insertion of membrane proteins into membranes by the signal mechanism, first evolved in inside-out cells.

Since the term "inside-out cell" is cumbersome, I propose the term "obcell" instead (the Latin ob- variously means towards, before, and inversely; so it well

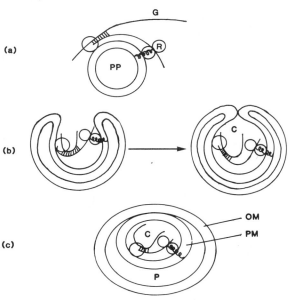

Figure 1. Origin of the first cell: a gram-negative eubacterium. (*a*) Genes (G) and ribosomes (R) associate with the outer surface of prebiotically formed liposome-like membranous vesicles to form an inside-out cell, in which a primitive signal mechanism for the cotranslational insertion of membrane proteins evolved. All early proteins are bound to the genes, ribosomes, or membrane. (*b*) The vesicle folds up to form a protocell bounded by two distinct lipid bilayers; soluble enzymes can evolve for the first time in the newly enclosed cytoplasm (C). (*c*) The outer membrane evolves into the outer membrane (OM) of the gram-negative eubacterium and the inner membrane into its plasma membrane (PM), to the inner surface of which the chromosome, and those ribosomes making membrane proteins, are invariably attached. Both membranes are therefore phylogenetically older than the cytoplasm (C). The periplasmic space (P) is derived from the interior of the inside-out cell, which I therefore call the properiplasm (PP). (After Blobel 1980.)

signifies the inverse relationship between the membrane and ribosomes and chromosome, compared with a true cell, as well as its existence *before* cells and its evolution *into* cells).

I show here that the concept of an obcell enables one to think more concretely about the problems involved in forming the first cell, as well as about the transition from RNA to DNA genomes and the origin of the chromosome. I wrote first "cell" rather than "cells" because I firmly reject the old idea (Minchin 1915), recently surprisingly popular (Woese and Fox 1977b; Woese 1983; Darnell and Doolittle 1986), that bacterial and eukaryotic cells evolved independently from a noncellular progenote. Nor do I accept the recent hypothesis (Woese and Fox 1977b; Woese 1983) that archaebacteria and eubacteria evolved independently from such a progenote. My rejection of these fashionable ideas is based on the immense variety and complexity of the cellular properties shared by the three major lineages (Cavalier-Smith 1987a) and on the fact that I have been able to propose detailed mechanisms for the origin of eukaryote and archaebacterial cells directly from eubacteria (Cavalier-Smith 1987a) and a detailed universal phylogeny (Fig. 2), consistent with both ultrastructural and molecular characters, which places negibacteria at the root of the tree of life. It is useful to group the 20 major steps of evolution summarized in Figure 2 into six phases: (1) chemical evolution; (2) origin and evolution of the protobiont (i.e., origin of replication); (3) origin and evolution of the progenote (origin of the ribosome, genetic code, and protein synthesis); (4) obcellular evolution (origin and improvement of the obcell, i.e., the first symbiosis between genes and membranes); (5) cellular evolution (origin and diversification of cells); and (6) multicellular evolution (origin and diversification of multicells).

The fifth phase, cellular evolution, was responsible for the most fundamental differences within the living world (Table 1; Fig. 2). This structural diversity was caused mainly by changes in membranes and skeletal macromolecules. The same structures, I argue, were equally crucial in the preceding phase of obcellular evolution, which formed the structural framework and raison d'être for the evolution of numerous aspects of catalytic function, notably those involved in the first gene-coded bioenergetic system.

The Minimal Requirements for a Living Cell

In addition to systems for synthesizing nucleic acids and proteins, free-living cells all have six other fundamental features:

1. A lipid-bilayer boundary membrane serves as a permeability barrier to most hydrophilic small molecules and to macromolecules.
2. Active transport enzymes embedded in the plasma membrane are able to pump protons, other ions, and small molecules across the membrane.
3. Intermediary metabolism interconverts low-molecular-weight carbon compounds.
4. Topogenic protein insertion and secretion mechanisms cotranslationally insert proteins into or across a ribosome-bearing membrane (the plasma membrane in prokaryotes; rough endoplasmic reticulum [RER] in eukaryotes).
5. A form of "cell skeleton" provides a rigid framework for the accurate segregation of daughter DNA molecules and the mechanical basis for cell division. In eukaryotes, this cell skeleton is an endoskeleton (the cytoskeleton), and in bacteria, it is an exoskeleton (the cell wall; although apparently absent in mycoplasmas, *Thermoplasma*, and *Planctomyces* and its relatives, they all must have some kind of "envelope skeleton"). The DNA is mechanically attached to the cell skeleton and/or to a

Figure 2. Universal phylogeny and the 20 major steps in evolution. The four steps involving obcells (iv–vii) and the earliest diversification of true cells (viii and ix) are the focus of this paper; for later steps, see Cavalier-Smith 1980 (steps x, xi); 1982 (step xviii); 1986b (step xvii; the symbiotic origin of the kingdom Chromista and the chloroplast endoplasmic reticulum [CER]); 1987a (steps xi, xii, xiii, xiv, xv); 1987b (step xvi); in prep. (step xii, the insertional origin of self-splicing introns from retrotransposons and the origin from them of tRNA and snurp-splicing and pre-RNA introns; step xvi, the invasion of mitochondria and chloroplasts by self-splicing introns); 1987c (step xix, the origin of fungi); in prep. (step xx, the origin of animals from choanomonad protozoa). Note that the origin of eukaryotes, which primitively lack mitochondria (Cavalier-Smith 1987a,d), had nothing to do with symbiosis. Multiple symbiotic events were, however, crucial in the origin of higher eukaryotes (i.e., metakaryotes); the probably simultaneous conversion of three different eubacterial symbionts into chloroplasts, mitochondria, and peroxisomes (Cavalier-Smith 1987b), by greatly diversifying the intracellular membranes, surely stimulated the improvement and diversification of intracellular protein- and vesicle-targeting mechanisms. This, I suggest, was the selective force behind the origin of the stacked Golgi dictyosome and the transition from 70S to 80S ribosomes; it will be important to see if the archezoan cotranslational signal mechanism is closer to that of prokaryotes than metakaryotes. Symbiosis, involving a eukaryotic symbiont, was also involved in the origin of the kingdom Chromista, as confirmed by the presence of nucleomorph DNA in cryptomonads, the only phylum with ribosomes of four kinds in distinct cell compartments (Cavalier-Smith 1986b). There is no fossil evidence for eukaryotes before 1450 million years ago; that between 1450 and 950 million years ago is debatable but plausibly represents a lengthy archezoan phase of evolution. The simplest interpretation of the similarities between eukaryotes and archaebacteria is that their common ancestor evolved nearly 1500 million years ago from a posibacterium (of the actinomycete branch) that lost murein cell walls and evolved introns and glycoprotein. The floppy "L-form" intermediate, osmotically ultrasensitive and incapable of accurately segregating its DNA, was "rescued" in two contrasting ways: (1) by evolution of membrane-rigidifying acid-resistant isoprenoidal ether-linked lipids and an external proteinaceous cell wall to form the first archaebacterium and (2) by the evolution of an internal protein cytoskeleton, which allowed the evolution of cytosis (the controlled budding and fusion of intracellular membrane vesicles), which created the eukaryotic endomembranes and genetic system. The physical segregation of nascent transcripts and ribosomes by the nuclear envelope allowed introns to invade genes for pre-mRNA, and RNA splicing by snurps to evolve (Cavalier-Smith 1987a and in prep.).

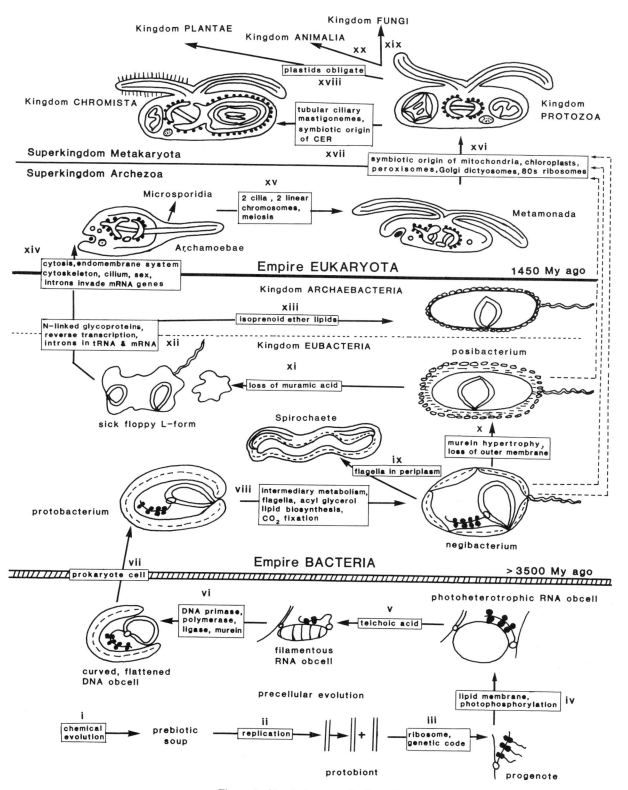

Figure 2. (*See facing page for legend.*)

Table 1. The Eight Kingdoms of Organisms

Empire: BACTERIA[a] (syn. Prokaryota; DNA not separated from ribosomes by an envelope; endomembrane system and
cytoskeleton absent; DNA attached to "envelope skeleton")
   Kingdom 1. Eubacteria (acylglycerol membrane lipids; murein)
   Subkingdom 1. Negibacteria (plasma membrane + outer membrane)
           2. Posibacteria (outer membrane absent)
   Kingdom 2. Archaebacteria (isoprenoid ether lipids; no murein; outer membrane absent)
Empire: EUKARYOTA[a] (nucleated cells; with endomembrane system, cytosis, and internal cytoskeleton; acylglycerol
membrane lipids; no peptidoglycan walls)
   Superkingdom 1. Archezoa[a] (70S ribosomes; Golgi dictyosomes, mitochondria, chloroplasts, and peroxisomes absent)
   Kingdom 1. Archezoa[b]
   Superkingdom 2. Metakaryota[a] (80S ribosomes; Golgi dictyosomes, mitochondria, peroxisomes, and often chloroplasts,
typically present)
   Kingdom 1. Protozoa[c] (chloroplast envelope of three membranes; includes mycetozoa; predominantly phagotrophic)
           2. Chromista (tubular ciliary mastigonemes and/or chloroplast ER present; Cavalier-Smith 1986b)
           3. Plantae (plastids invariably present; chloroplast envelope of two membranes; plastids not in ER)
           4. Fungi (typically with chitinous walls and no chloroplasts or phagocytosis; excludes mycetozoa and pseudo-
fungi; Cavalier-Smith 1987c)
           5. Animalia (triploblastic phagotrophs)

[a]New taxa hereby formally proposed.
[b]Originally a subkingdom of the Protozoa (Cavalier-Smith 1983b); now comprising only the phyla Archamoebae, Metamonada, Microsporidia;
I have removed the Parabasalia (because their hydrogenosome probably evolved from mitochondria – Cavalier-Smith 1987b).
[c]Emended taxon (by removal of the three archezoan phyla to form a separate kingdom – T. Cavalier-Smith, in prep.); includes Parabasalia.

membrane (plasma membrane in bacteria; a specialized part of the ER in eukaryotes, i.e., the nuclear
envelope) throughout the life of the cell. (Note that
I am *not* using cell skeleton as a synonym for cytoskeleton.)

6. There is at least one bioenergetic ATP-generating mechanism.

The last feature is absent in one group of modern
cells, the chlamydias. Chlamydias are prokaryotic intracellular "energy parasites" of eukaryotic cells; since
they almost certainly degenerated from ancestors able
to make ATP (Woese 1987), all six characters were
present in the latest common ancestor of all modern
cells. Thus, the simplest functioning cell comprised four
major systems: (1) the genetic system (replication and
translation), (2) the bioenergetic system (ATP synthesis), (3) the metabolic system (intermediary metabolism), and (4) the structural system (plasma membrane
with active transport molecules and cell skeleton
mediating segregation and division).

The problem of the origin of the cell, therefore, is
how these four systems evolved and came together in a
mutually reinforcing way, allowing the reproducible
growth and division of the whole cell. The structural
system plays a key integrative role, which has been
neglected in most discussions of early life.

Evolution of the plasma membrane, with its active
transport molecules, was a prerequisite for the evolution of a metabolic system composed of soluble substrates and enzymes. It is usually assumed that the first
bioenergetic system was fermentative (Haldane 1929;
Oparin 1938; Raven and Smith 1976, 1982). However,
fermentation depends on intermediary metabolism and
therefore on the prior evolution of a plasma membrane. I argue (see below) that its origin is actually
more complicated than that of photophosphorylation.
In my view, the first bioenergetic system was cyclic
photophosphorylation in an anaerobic heterotroph that

was similar to purple and green sulfur bacteria
(Chromatiaceae and Chlorobiaceae) but much simpler
than either; being necessarily membrane-based, it provided the initial impetus for the association of genes
and ribosomes with membranes and for the extensive
evolution of protein rather than RNA catalysts.

It is also often assumed that the first cell had numerous copies of a much-fragmented genome, and therefore no great need for an accurate division or segregation mechanism (Minchin 1915; Boyden 1953;
Dougherty 1955); however, if division were random,
small cell fragments with unbalanced genetic composition would be liable to be produced (Gabriel 1960).
Moreover, replicative competition between different
nucleic acid molecules in the same cell (Darwin 1868;
Huxley 1873; Dougherty 1955), recently colloquially
dubbed the "selfish DNA" principle (Doolittle and
Sapienza 1980; Orgel and Crick 1980), could be an
additional source of genetic imbalance. Effective controls over replication and segregation, and over cell
growth and division, would therefore almost certainly
have been selected fairly early in evolution, which
would have involved some form of cell skeleton. For
this reason, I believe that DNA replication, circular
chromosomes, and DNA segregation by attachment to
a peptidoglycan skeleton evolved in the obcellular
phase of evolution (Cavalier-Smith 1985) and that a
cell with genes made of RNA (Hartman 1980) probably
never existed.

The RNA World and Metabolism

The idea (Haldane 1965; Lipmann 1965) that early
genomes consisted of RNA rather than DNA has always attracted me for four reasons:

1. DNA is logically superfluous to genetics, since it is
mRNA, rRNA, and tRNA that mediate protein

synthesis, and RNA can be replicated directly by an RNA-directed RNA polymerase as in RNA viruses. Both replication and the genetic code could have evolved with RNA alone but not with DNA alone.

2. RNA replication is simple, often needing only a single enzyme, whereas DNA replication is exceedingly complex, requiring perhaps 30 or more different proteins; the requirement for RNA primers may be a vestige of a time when replication was of RNA rather than DNA. I will argue that DNA primase evolved from an RNA-dependent RNA polymerase, and then DNA-dependent DNA polymerase evolved from DNA primase.

3. In intermediary metabolism, deoxyribonucleotides are synthesized from ribonucleotides and thymine from uracil. Ribose 5′ phosphate and other isomeric phosphorylated pentoses play a central role in intermediary metabolism (i.e., in the pentose phosphate and phospho-gluconate pathways), but deoxyribose does not. Thus, deoxyribose and thymine could easily have been added later by the evolution of a small number of extra enzymes to supplement an established metabolic pattern in which ribose plays the fundamental role.

4. Ribonucleotides play a fundamental role in both bioenergetics and biosynthesis, but deoxyribonucleotides do not. ATP is the most general intermediate energy carrier, being used for many aspects of biosynthesis, for powering active transport and mechanochemical processes involved in DNA replication (e.g., DNA helicases, DNA gyrase, DNA ligase, attachment of primosomes to DNA priming sites), and in transcription (transcriptional termination by the ρ factor RNA helicase), protein synthesis, and recombination (numerous ATP-dependent nucleases as well as DNA ligase). GTP provides energy for protein synthesis, UTP is involved in the biosynthesis of polysaccharides and peptidoglycan, and CTP is involved in the synthesis of phospholipids and teichoic acids. The major carriers of reducing power (NAD and NADP) consist of two ribonucleotides, as does the electron carrier FAD. AMP is also a key constituent of coenzyme A (CoA), which as acetyl CoA, succinyl CoA, and malonyl CoA has a ubiquitous metabolic role. The total absence of comparable roles for deoxynucleotides suggests that the main features of both bioenergetics and macromolecular metabolism became established before the evolution of DNA.

It cannot be concluded that all of the above-mentioned features had necessarily evolved prior to the origin of DNA. It is probable that most of the enzymes that mediate these processes evolved from each other by gene duplication and divergence; thus, they simply inherited the ribonucleotide-binding site from a common ancestor. Even after the evolution of DNA, the same process could continue unchecked if the diverse and well-established ribonucleotide-dependent enzymes were more suitable than DNA ligase and DNA polymerase as ancestors for new metabolic enzymes.

Obcells and the Origin of the Symbiosis between Genes and Membranes

The evolution of RNA well before DNA readily explains why deoxyribonucleotides are not used as coenzymes or energy supplies in metabolism, but it does not solve the long-standing puzzle as to why ribonucleotides themselves should have such an important role (Lipmann 1965). The answer may lie in a very early coupling between bioenergetics and genetics as shown in Figure 3; the reason for the evolution of the membrane-bound proton-motive PPase was to supply nucleoside triphosphate (NTP) for RNA replication and possibly protein synthesis. Thus, the entire raison d'être of this first bioenergetic enzyme was a genetic one: to speed up precellular RNA replication. I suggest that the membrane-bound PPase evolved from the membrane-bound kinase that could have evolved even earlier, possibly from RNA replicase that already would have had an NTP-binding site to use prebiotically synthesized pyrophosphate (Miller and Orgel 1974) to phosphorylate nucleotides and their precursors. Probably the replicase itself had been the first protein to evolve, selected because it increased the efficiency of nucleotide polymerization. If so, its evolution represented the very first effective coupling between replication and translation and so created the first organism by providing a selective advantage for mutations that improved the efficiency of protein synthesis.

The key proteins involved in protein synthesis (aminoacyl-tRNA synthetases and, if it is a protein rather than a rRNA ribozyme, peptidyltransferase) must also have had ribonucleotide-binding sites, and must have catalyzed the joining or cleavage of ribonucleotides (to and from amino acids), and so may also have evolved from the RNA replicase. (The alternative—that the first protein was a single nonspecific enzyme able to act as peptidyltransferase, aminoacyl-tRNA synthetase, and replicase, as suggested by Haldane [1965]—is logically possible only if in at least the earliest stages it was the tRNAs, rather than, as now, the synthetases, that recognized the correct amino acids, as discussed by Crick [1968].) It is conceivable that the PPase evolved during or even before these protein-synthesizing enzymes and thus coupled together the genetic and bioenergetic systems in their very earliest stages. The proton-driven PPase was thus a coupling factor not only in the classical chemiosmotic sense (Mitchell 1961; Harold 1986), but also in the sense that it coupled the proton gradient generated by the photoredox system to the synthesis of RNA.

Since both porphyrins and quinones can be synthesized abiotically, the simple photoredox system of Figure 3 could have originated quite independently of the genetic system. However, as soon as it was coupled to the genetic system by the RNA-coded membrane-bound PPase, it could be improved by the addition of RNA-coded membrane proteins able to bind porphyrins, so as to make distinct chlorophyll-binding pro-

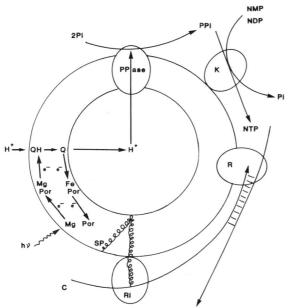

Figure 3. The first photoheterotrophic obcell. An RNA polymerase/replicase (R) is anchored to the outer surface of a lipid bilayer by a hydrophobic signal peptide. Ribosomes (Ri), composed largely, if not entirely, of RNA (possibly a single rRNA molecule; Clark and Gerbi 1982) coded by the coding strand (C) of the RNA genome, translate its protein-coding genes into proteins bearing an amino-terminal signal peptide (SP) that anchors them also to the outer surface of the lipid membrane. The genome codes for at least three proteins: (1) the replicase (R), (2) a pyrophosphate phosphohydrolase (PPase), a membrane protein that makes pyrophosphate from phosphate, and (3) a kinase (K), a membrane protein that uses pyrophosphate to phosphorylate ribose, NMPs, and NDPs to make all four NTPs for polymerization by the replicase (and ATP and GTP for powering protein synthesis). As in purple bacteria (Baltscheffsky 1981), pyrophosphate synthesis is powered by the proton gradient produced by the photoredox system, which "pumps" protons from the environment into the inside-out cell and which consists of metalloporphyrins (MgPor, FePor) and a quinone (Q), all embedded in the membrane. The genome codes also for tRNAs and for an RNase-P-like ribozyme that specifically cleaves the coding strand to make separate tRNA, rRNA, and RNase P ribozyme molecules. It is not essential that aminoacyl-tRNA synthetase or peptidyltransferase enzyme proteins had evolved by this stage, since their functions might have been carried out by the tRNA and rRNAs themselves or by separate ribozyme RNA molecules. Growth was by the thermodynamically spontaneous incorporation of prebiotically synthesized amphipathic lipids (including the porphyrins and quinones) into the membrane, and the polymerization of activated amino acids into the proteins and nucleotides into the RNA. Initially, ribose, bases, and amino acids came from the prebiotic soup, and no enzymes of intermediary metabolism would be essential, although a membrane-bound enzyme able to join purines or pyrimidines to ribose 5′-phosphate might have been the first to evolve. Division was initially caused by random breakage of the membrane by shearing forces in the environment, and the spontaneous resealing of the broken membrane. The initial asymmetry in the arrangement of the MgPor and FePor could have come about by iron-containing liposomes generated on land being washed into Mg-rich seawater.

teins and cytochromes, and of one membrane protein able to bind iron sulfide to make the first ferredoxin. *Chlorobium* ferredoxin is a very simple molecule of 61

amino acids of only 14 different kinds, predominantly those most readily formed in prebiotic experiments. Because of this and because much simpler artificial ferredoxin models made by mixing short oligopeptides with iron sulfide (the most abundant nonsilicate mineral) can act as electron donors and acceptors, Hall et al. (1971) argued that such bacterial (4Fe-4S) ferredoxins were among the very earliest proteins to evolve. These authors based their arguments on the even slightly simpler clostridial ferredoxins rather than the *Chlorobium* ferredoxin because of their acceptance of Oparin's (1938) dogma that the first bioenergetic system was fermentation, rather than anaerobic photophosphorylation as argued here. Oparin's sole reason for preferring fermentation to phototrophy was his belief that it was simpler. This was pure guesswork, since at that time, the molecular basis of neither process was understood. It is now known that all fermentative bacteria have ATP-driven proton pumps in their plasma membrane that are homologous to the F_0F_1 proton-driven ATP synthase of phototrophs and respirers (Harold 1986; Harold and Kanimura 1986). In this respect, therefore, they are no simpler than the others and are equally dependent on sophisticated membranes and chemiosmotic processes. The arguments of Oparin (1938) and Haldane (1929) that the first bioenergetic system was neither autotrophic nor aerobic remain valid. What they did not then appreciate was the fact that anaerobic heterotrophs are not all fermenters: Some (green and purple sulfur bacteria) are photoheterotrophs. The key question is whether fermentation or photoheterotrophy is the primitive condition.

Classic biochemists (Lipmann 1965) regarded substrate-level phosphorylation, on which fermentation depends, as "simpler" than photophosphorylation and oxidative phosphorylation because it could be readily studied in soluble fractions after discarding the membranes. This view, however, predates our present understanding of the universality of chemiosmotic processes (Harold 1986) and is evolutionarily thoroughly misleading. The soluble enzymes and complex metabolic pathways on which fermentation depends could not have evolved until after the origin of the first cell. Glycolysis cannot be regarded as primitive: It depends on ten different enzymes and on the relatively complex coenzyme NAD^+. Moreover, it cannot continuously yield energy in the absence of a separate system for the reoxidation of NADH. Even worse, at two points it requires the input of ATP before energy can be extracted, and thus it is difficult to see how it could have originally evolved except in an organism that made its ATP by photophosphorylation or by oxidative phosphorylation. One cannot take the two ATP-generating steps (catalyzed by phosphoglycerate kinase and pyruvate kinase) out of context and claim that one (or both) of them represents the primitive bioenergetic process; this is because each *starts* with a labile phosphorylated high-energy intermediate that would be most unlikely to have accumulated sufficiently in the prebiotic soup to allow sustained evolution.

In contrast, as Gaffron (1965), Woese (1979), and Baltscheffsky (1981) stressed, light was present in abundance from the very first, and a very early origin for photophosphorylation deserves serious consideration. Moreover, the simple light-driven proton pump shown in Figure 3 places fewer demands on the primitive genetic system than even one single glycolytic enzyme. Even with the addition of a chlorophyll-binding protein and a cytochrome, it involves fewer genes than glycolysis. Above all, the idea of a heterotrophic cyclically phosphorylating obcell (Cavalier-Smith 1985) allows the genetic and bioenergetic systems to be simultaneously evolved to a high level of perfection even before the first cell was formed. The genetic system would have plenty of energy, and both systems could acquire new genes by gene duplication of preexisting ones. Because of the continued loss of pyrophosphates and activated nucleotides and amino acids to the environment, the obcell would have been much less efficient than a true cell, which is why it was eventually superseded. The key point is that it had a distinctly better energy supply than its immediate predecessors; it might have been particularly successful in small rocky seashore crevices periodically fed by spray but not permanently diluted (Cavalier-Smith 1985).

Origin of Facilitated Nutrient Uptake and Storage

One of the key advantages of an obcell phase of evolution is that the obcell would have ready access to amino acids, nucleotides, and lipids from the prebiotic soup and could evolve a high degree of coordination between the genetic, bioenergetic, and structural systems long before the potentially traumatic total encapsulation of genes and ribosomes by a membrane to make a true cell. If such encapsulation had occurred by a crude primitive membrane without a gene-controlled mechanism for growth and division and without gene-encoded facilitated diffusion or active transport enzymes, as traditionally assumed (Harris 1981), it would simply have isolated the genes and ribosomes from their raw materials and caused death by starvation.

Facilitated uptake of sugars, amino acids, bases, phosphates, and cations into the interior of the obcell (the properiplasmic space) would have been advantageous even though RNA and proteins were being made on its outer surface. One reason for this is that if the obcell encountered fluctuations in their supply, such that they were sometimes in excess of its replicative and protein synthetic capacities and sometimes in short supply, they could be sequestered inside when superabundant, stored, and used when supply was suboptimal. Second, iron was specifically needed in the properiplasm, since the Fe porphyrins must be preferentially located on the properiplasmic face of the membrane, and the Mg porphyrins on its outer face, for light-driven proton-translocation to work at all efficiently. Third, at night, the obcell would be starved of energy and unable to grow unless it had an energy store to draw upon. A reversible proton/cation antiporter,

however, could actively accumulate the cation by day, and by night, it could operate in reverse, with the accumulated cation powering proton uptake as it leaked out. Thus, chemiosmotic synthesis of pyrophosphate and therefore synthesis of NTPs, nucleic acids, and proteins could continue.

The main problem for the obcell would have been osmotic swelling and the risk of bursting caused by the internal accumulation of the nutrients. This could have been minimized in two different ways: (1) By polymerizing imported nutrients to minimize their osmotic effects, ribose could be attached to UDP and polymerized to polyribose, amino acids could be polymerized to such polymers as polyaspartate, and phosphate could be polymerized to make polyphosphate. (2) Molecules like iron (needed for Fe porphyrin) that could not be polymerized were bound to iron-binding proteins located in the properiplasm.

Nutrients thus immobilized would not need to be accumulated by active transport but could be taken up by passive facilitated diffusion. Such passive transport molecules are functionally simpler than active transport molecules, and thus probably preceded them. Possibly only one proton/cation antiporter molecule evolved for nocturnal energetics and all other nutrients accumulated passively. If, as proposed in Figure 4, the stored cation was Ca^{++}, it could have formed insoluble calcium polyphosphate in the properiplasm, thus minimizing osmotic effects. Nocturnal hydrolysis of the phosphate would release the Ca^{++} and allow Ca^{++}-driven proton uptake. Thus, I suggest that the Ca^{++}/H^+ antiporter present in all bacteria (de Vrij et al. 1985) first originated in the obcell. A divalent cation would also be better than a monovalent cation, as each ion could pump two protons; Ca^{++} would have been more suitable than Mg^{++} since it is more than 5 times rarer in seawater, so fewer ions would need to be accumulated to establish a given concentration gradient.

Origin of the Obcell Skeleton and the Control of Growth and Division

The properiplasmic storage polymers and binding proteins would nevertheless exert some osmotic effect. A way of totally counteracting this would be for polymer chains to be covalently linked to both internal faces of the membrane, thus causing the obcell to assume either a flattened shape like an ER or Golgi cisterna or a more tubular shape, but supported internally by its polymer skeleton. I originally proposed that the first obcell skeleton consisted of peptidoglycan (Cavalier-Smith 1985); but peptidoglycan biosynthesis is rather complex and might have required too many enzymes to be coded by early RNA genomes. Therefore, I now propose that the obcell skeleton initially consisted of teichoic acids (i.e., [polyol phosphate] copolymers, characteristic of gram-positive bacteria [subkingdom Posibacteria, Cavalier-Smith 1986a, 1987a]).

Teichoic acid polymerizing enzymes might simply have evolved from nucleotide polymerases. The sim-

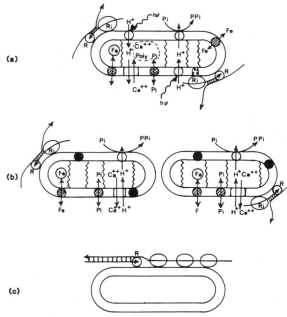

Figure 4. Growth and division of the filamentous DNA obcell. (a) Protection from osmotic bursting is mediated by teichoic acids (zigzag lines) consisting of poly-(glycerol phosphate) covalently bonded to the membrane. Because of their short chain length residues, they would constrain the shape of the obcell into a closed tubule, with a lumen with a radius roughly equal to the thickness of the membrane. The teichoic acids are synthesized by CTP-dependent properiplasmic enzymes, but the lipids, including those of the light-driven proton pump, still insert themselves directly from the prebiotic store; together with the insertion of integral membrane proteins by the ribosomes (Ri), this causes the growth and elongation of the obcell. The integral membrane proteins include the PPase, the iron and phosphate facilitated diffusion proteins (crosshatched circles), and the H^+/Ca^{++} antiporter (square). By day, the latter pumps Ca^{++} into the properiplasm, and by night, as shown in (b), Ca^{++} outflow pumps in protons. The ribosomes also secrete the properiplasmic proteins, which include the teichoic acid synthesizers, Fe-binding protein, and polyphosphate polymerase. (b) Because of the fixed chain length of the teichoic acids, the obcell would grow in length but not in diameter. An approximate equilibrium would be set up between elongation by incorporation of lipid and protein and fragmentation by environmental shearing forces. For a filamentous structure like DNA, shearing tends to break the filament near the middle to produce roughly equal "daughters," so a crude binary fusion would occur. In the dark, the porphyrin/quinone proton pumps (●) would be inactive but protons could still be imported into the properiplasm by the Ca^{++}/H^+ antiporter working in reverse. (c) RNA replication requires not only the synthesis of the coding strand, as shown in the preceding figures, but also of the noncoding strand. This causes conflict between the replicase R, shown here moving to the right along the template, and the ribosomes, shown here moving to the left on the sample template. This conflict was later resolved by the separation of transcription and replication.

plest teichoic acids, substituted polyglycerolphosphates, are covalently attached to membrane lipids, as I suggest was the case in the obcell (Fig. 4). It has been proposed that replication perhaps initially evolved using glycerol nucleotides rather than ribonucleotides (Orgel, this volume). Possibly the first obcells

even had genes of GNA rather than RNA. The fact that CDP-glycerol is involved in the biosynthesis of phospholipids, as well as of glycerol teichoic acid, suggests, however, that enzymes with CTP-binding sites played a key role in the growth of the filamentous obcell (Fig. 4); thus, RNA-specific polymerases had probably already evolved before then.

The usual presence of D-alanine in teichoic acids supports their precellular origin. I earlier argued (Cavalier-Smith 1985) that the composition of the tetrapeptide in the murein peptidoglycan of negibacteria indicates a precellular origin: L-alanine, D-alanine, D-glutamic acid, and diaminopimelic acid (DAP). The presence of D-amino acids suggests that teichoic acids and murein both evolved when obcells were still getting their amino acids from the prebiotic soup: One would not expect D-amino acids if these polymers had evolved after the origin of a complete intermediary metabolism synthesizing L-amino acids. Alanine is much the most abundant amino acid produced by electric discharges in CH_4, N_2, and H_2O mixtures, with only traces of ammonia (Miller and Orgel 1974). Glutamic acid is also produced in reasonable yield, but 100 times less abundantly. It is understandable that the obcell would use D-glutamic acid rather than the L form, since this would not have been depleted by its L-based protein synthesis, and its peptidoglycan synthesis would not compete with its protein synthesis. DAP may also have been favored because it is not used for protein synthesis.

It is interesting that most posibacteria (gram-positive eubacteria; Cavalier-Smith 1986a, 1987a) have replaced DAP by L-lysine, or sometimes L-ornithine: rRNA sequences (Woese 1987) are consistent with the idea that they are derived from negibacteria by peptidoglycan hypertrophy and the loss of the outer membrane (Cavalier-Smith 1980, 1987a). If so, the ancestral posibacterium must already have had a well-developed intermediary metabolism, including the synthesis of L-lysine by the DAP pathway; thus, such substitution would not have harmfully competed with protein synthesis. Replacement of DAP by lysine is associated with the origin of a new bridge peptide to interlink the modified tetrapeptides. The fact that the bridge peptide sometimes contains D-aspartic acid does not mean that the substitution must have occurred very early when D-amino acids were still available, since it could be readily made by modifying the biosynthetic pathway for D-alanine already present in the tetrapeptide.

The pseudomurein peptidoglycan of methanogenic archaebacteria, in contrast, contains only L-amino acids found also in proteins. This is consistent with my thesis that archaebacteria are not an ancient group and evolved only about 1500 million years ago from the actinomycete eubacteria (Cavalier-Smith 1987a), with which they share many metabolic properties (Jones et al. 1987). Although negibacterial murein may be too complex to have formed the first obcell skeleton, one can retain the idea that it evolved during obcellular evolution, and was instrumental in the transition from obcell to eubacterium (Cavalier-Smith 1985), by supposing that it evolved after the origin of DNA replication.

Origin of Chromosomes: Selective Advantages

The increase in the number of different proteins in the filamentous obcell mentioned earlier would probably have occurred mainly by gene duplication and divergence within a single obcell, but possibly also partly by fusion between divergent obcells, especially in the earliest stages. In either case, it seems likely that a large number of different RNA molecules, some coding for single polypeptides and others for several polypeptides, were associated with each obcell. For those RNA molecules coding for single polypeptides, there would have been no distinction between gene duplication and gene replication, and it would be particularly easy for sister genes to diverge and come to code for distinctly different proteins. As it seems unlikely that there would initially have been any synchronization between the replication of the different RNA molecules, they would have been competing with each other for substrates and replicative RNA polymerases. More rapidly replicating RNA molecules, with the least inessential noncoding RNA, would have been favored; direct selection for replicative efficiency could temporarily favor "selfish RNA" molecules that made no contribution to the growth and division of the obcell. Selection, however, would also be acting at the level of obcell multiplication for mutants that made a positive contribution to their growth, survival, and division and for the cooperative interaction of the different gene products with each other and with their parent genes.

Initially, there could have been no distinction between replication and transcription. Although very primitive RNA polymerases might have started at random points, it is likely that selection would be rapid for those starting at the $3'$-OH end of the template so as to make complete complementary transcripts. Both strands would be transcribed and replicated by the same enzyme, as in RNA virus replicases. For protein-coding genes, the RNA polymerase would have a free run along the noncoding strand, but on the coding strand, it would often collide with ribosomes translating it in the opposite direction, and at least one would have to give way (Fig. 4c). This would tend to reduce the rate of synthesis of complementary noncoding strands compared with that of the messenger strands, which would be advantageous for protein synthesis, for which a sufficient number of copies of mRNA would be important. A reduction in the ratio of noncoding to coding strands would be metabolically economical, but it would increase the risk of total loss of a particular gene by random segregation.

It has long been clear (Strasburger et al. 1909; Gabriel 1960) that joining numerous genes together in a large linkage group, coupled with an efficient means of segregation, is how cells have circumvented this difficulty. But the evolution of such a mechanism is by no means simple. In the first place, linkage is useless without a segregation apparatus, and vice versa; so how did things get started? In bacteria, attachment to the rigid peptidoglycan wall plays a key role in DNA segregation (Cavalier-Smith 1987e). I suggest that if obcell growth and division mediated by teichoic acids originated, as suggested above, to ensure osmotic stability, it would have provided a ready-made (although imperfect) segregation mechanism for DNA once DNA chromosomes had evolved, so that one need not postulate the simultaneous origin of chromosomes and a segregation apparatus. All that would be necessary would be the correct temporal and spatial attachment of the chromosomes to a preexisting obcell division mechanism.

Origin of DNA Replication and Transcription: DNA Primase and DNA-dependent RNA Polymerase

The major problem with understanding the origin of DNA chromosomes and the separation of replication and transcription is the immense complexity of DNA replication and the need for it to have evolved in simple stages, each viable and mostly an improvement on preceding stages. The glib assumption that this was achieved by the evolution of reverse transcriptase (Darnell and Doolittle 1986) is inadequate, since it is not explained why reverse transcriptase needs a primer, how all the genes were primed, what its immediate selective advantage was, or how the transition to true DNA replication and transcription was achieved. There is neither evidence nor reason to think that eubacteria ever had reverse transcriptase, and it is also mechanistically implausible to assume that an RNA-directed RNA polymerase, highly specific for polymerizing ribonucleotides and not needing a primer, evolved in a single step into an RNA-directed DNA polymerase, highly specific for deoxyribonucleotides and requiring a specific primer. It is more likely that reverse transcriptase evolved from a DNA-dependent DNA polymerase, to which it is functionally much closer, simply by altering its template requirement.

I suggest that what initiated the evolution of a DNA genome was the origin of DNA primase from a mutant obcellular RNA replicase. Like RNA polymerases, DNA primase requires no primer and can polymerize ribonucleotides. But, uniquely among polymerases, it polymerizes ribonucleotides and deoxyribonucleotides indiscriminately. What it uses depends simply on what is available; this, I suggest, is a frozen relic of its early history, when it mediated a perfectly gradual changeover from RNA to DNA genes.

In the absence of a true DNA polymerase, I suggest that DNA primase would have replicated whole RNA molecules to make mixed ribose/deoxyribose polynucleotides, whose ribose/deoxyribose ratios would depend on that in the local prebiotic soup. If by that time the ribose supply had been much depleted by all of the other RNA-based obcells, the new DNA-rich molecules could have had an immediate replicative advantage, as well as the long-recognized advantage of the greater chemical stability of DNA over RNA. Because this obcell would still have its RNA replicase, it would continue to make some pure RNA molecules as well as the new mixed RNA/DNA molecules. If, however, the ribosomes were less efficient at reading the newer deoxyribose-containing molecules, as is likely, the more they increased relative to pure RNA, the less efficient would be translation. For a given RNA/DNA ratio, it would be advantageous if the RNA polymerase specifically made only mRNA and not the complementary strand: Mutant proteins able to act as primitive σ factors able to confer such specificity, but binding only to the mixed DNA/RNA molecules, would thus be favored, creating a clear separation between replication (by DNA primase to produce mixed DNA/RNA) and transcription by the former RNA polymerase. Their σ binding sites became the first promoters: There must have been a co-evolution of promoters and σ factors to increase strand specificity, which would have been easier the lower the number of different genes at the time of the changeover from RNA to DNA. Without preferential termination also, there would have been no real benefit. As this process proceeded and less and less complementary pure RNA was produced, the RNA polymerase would be increasingly modified to work with a DNA template, thus becoming a DNA-dependent RNA polymerase.

One consequence of the separation of replication and transcription was that there was no longer competition between ribosomes and polymerase on the coding strand, and thus the rate of replication of the two strands would be more nearly equal and they would spend most time in the double-stranded state. With ribosomes no longer able to help separate the complementary strands, single-strand binding proteins and DNA helicase evolved to do this efficiently and speed up replication. Since the mixed DNA/RNA molecules, unlike the original RNA genes, would no longer be attached to the obcell membrane by ribosomes making membrane proteins, specific proteins able to attach them to the membrane would be favored.

Origin of DNA Segregation and Repair: DNA Ligase and Polymerase

If a mutant DNA primase evolved into a DNA ligase by becoming able to join together whole DNA molecules, a very great economy and increase in viability could have resulted: If all the genes were joined into a single molecule, only one copy of each would need to be attached on each side of the division plane to ensure viable offspring. The number of copies of DNA and of DNA-membrane attachment proteins could then be greatly reduced without producing any inviable offspring.

Mutations, rather than segregational mistakes, would become the major source of inviability and more serious as the number of proteins increased. Reduction in gene copy number therefore probably went hand-in-hand with improvements in replication accuracy and the evolution of excision repair. The key step, I suggest, was the evolution from DNA primase of the first true DNA polymerase, i.e., an enzyme that inserted only deoxynucleotides and did so only to a chain already started by DNA primase (the "primer"). By greatly reducing the content of (relatively unstable) ribonucleotides, the frequency of chain breakage would be reduced, much more important for long single-copy chromosomes than for multiple-copy separate genes.

Evolution of 5′ exonuclease activities to remove the RNA-containing primers and of 3′ exonuclease activities specific for terminal unpaired nucleotides (proofreading function) would also greatly reduce mutation rates. Thus, one would have evolved a DNA chromosome replicated in fundamentally the same way as in modern bacteria and segregated by attachment to the obcell membrane. The logical conclusion of the ligation of separate DNA genes would be a single circular chromosome; evolution of DNA topoisomerases and/or endonucleases would have been an essential prerequisite for replication of a circle, and until they evolved, perhaps from mutant polymerases or ligases, the chromosomes must still have been linear. If they evolved before the primer removal mechanism was perfected, there need never have been an end-replication problem (Cavalier-Smith 1983a).

Efficient DNA replication and repair would allow a massive increase in the number of different genes coding for membrane, ribosomal, and properiplasmic proteins and, therefore, a quantum leap in the accuracy and speed of nucleic acid and protein synthesis and membrane growth. Larger and more complex obcells would trap light and nutrients more efficiently but would be more prone to irregular fragmentation to produce pieces lacking a chromosome. As a more highly cross-linked skeleton would prevent this, I suggest that murein evolved at this stage and formed a single covalently bonded two-dimensional sheet inside the properiplasm. Breakage into smaller fragments would now occur only at points where the murein was weakened by murein hydrolases: Spatial control of their position or activity could for the first time give the obcell firm genetic control over its division and allow binary fission to evolve. Possibly the involvement of DNA helicase and DNA gyrase in the segregation of DNA, as postulated for bacterial cells (Cavalier-Smith 1987b), also evolved in obcells (Fig. 5).

Origin of RNA and DNA Viruses

Since during the changeover from RNA to DNA, there would likely be both RNA copies and RNA/DNA copies of the RNA replicase gene, it is possible that some of the RNA copies mutated to make their polymerases even more specific for their own genes and became selfish RNA molecules coding for replicases that did not help in the replication of other obcellular genes. If such a gene happened to be linked to another gene coding for a protein able to bind preferentially to its RNA molecule, then it could readily evolve into a primitive virus. Because there would be no problem in

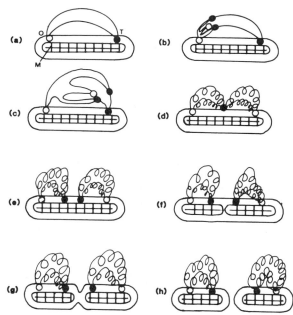

Figure 5. Division and segregation in a flattened DNA obcell. (*a*) The peptidoglycan murein (M) forms a flattened sheet within the properiplasm to which the membrane is covalently attached. The circular DNA molecule is also attached to it at its origin (O) and terminus (T) by integral membrane proteins. (*b*) Elongation of the murein and membrane accompany DNA replication. One sister origin remains attached to the murein and the other attaches to a DNA helicase at one of the replication forks, which pulls it toward the terminus (Cavalier-Smith 1987e). (*c*) At the terminus, the mobile origin becomes attached to the murein instead of the terminus, which is pulled to the center of the obcell by the DNA-gyrase-induced supercoiling of the daughter chromosomes (*d*). (*e*) Two sister termini become attached to the murein on either side of the center line. (*f*) Murein hydrolases cleave the murein specifically between the two terminal attachment sites (*g*). This allows environmental shearing forces to fragment the membrane at this point, which spontaneously reseals to generate two daughter obcells (*h*).

entering or leaving an obcell, it would be much easier for the first RNA virus to evolve on an obcell than in a true cell. I therefore suggest that the basic features of both RNA and DNA viruses first evolved on obcells, rather than in true cells, and were inherited first by bacterial viruses and much later by eukaryote viruses. The phylogenetic distribution of retroviruses suggests that they evolved only after eukaryotes, probably after the evolution of transposons that multiplied by means of reverse transcriptase; such transposons may first have evolved in the immediate common ancestor of eukaryotes and archaebacteria (Cavalier-Smith 1987a).

An Early Origin for DNA Methylation and Restriction Nucleases?

Obcells would be inherently vulnerable to attack by nucleases produced by other obcells, as their chromosomes and RNA were exposed to the environment. Any obcell evolving a nuclease from which it itself was protected could destroy its competitors and greatly increase its food supply. Quite probably soluble nu-

cleases directed at other obcells evolved even in the RNA phase of evolution. They might also have been a major factor in the evolution of thymine, if methylation of uracil protected an obcell's own DNA genome from such attack. Later, with the evolution of DNA endonucleases not inhibited by thymine, postreplication methylation of adenine might have given new protection in the escalating arms race (Dawkins 1982). DNA polymerases would adapt to both thymine and methylated adenine, and both would become integral parts of the control of DNA replication and its distinction from transcription.

Finally, sequence-specific methylation would allow the evolution of restriction nucleases able to attack foreign obcell DNA and also to protect against DNA viruses, which would have been so easily able to infect obcells and, inevitably, would have been a major drain on their resources.

The Origin of the First Cell

It is likely that protection from viruses, and from nucleases and proteases made by other obcells, was a significant factor in the success of the first obcell that managed to fold up and convert itself into a cell. There are three major problems in the origin of a closed cell: (1) the origin of a properly controlled division mechanism, (2) the continued entry of small molecular precursors (if this ceased, the cell would soon die), and (3) the origin of osmotic stability and internal compositional and pH homeostasis. All of these problems are very greatly reduced by the postulate of a preceding phase of obcell evolution.

Eubacterial growth and cell division are integrated and controlled by the spatial control of peptidoglycan synthesis. If this had already evolved in an obcell as discussed above, then it would require only modification, rather than radical innovation, to achieve the same for the first cell. I proposed (Cavalier-Smith 1985) that it was the slightly asymmetric growth of the peptidoglycan that made the obcell curve around to form a closed cell in the first place. Such growth could also force together the lipid membranes of the opposing lip of a semi-open curved obcell (Fig. 6b) to make the first true closed cell. But if the cell simply retained the obcellular division mechanism, a fresh break would tend to occur in the region between the chromosome termini, and the cell would open out again. However, further growth would tend to force the new lipids back again to reclose the cell, which would now have two chromosomes. This process could be repeated over and over again, making a steadily larger and more polyploid cell, which would never be able to divide properly. For this reason, I believe simple lip fusion of an obcell (Fig. 6b) would have been abortive and could not have produced a viable cell. Thus, the transition from a curved obcell to a true eubacterial cell could not have been by random fusion, but must have involved a major gene-controlled innovation. This, I suggested, was the cell septum (Cavalier-Smith 1985).

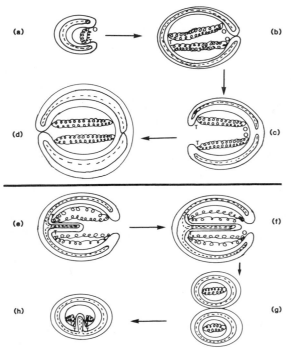

Figure 6. Conversion of an obcell into a protobacterium. Growth of a curved obcell (*a*) would tend to cause its lips to fuse (*b*). Murein hydrolases acting between the chromosome termini (T) would tend to open it out again (*c*); further growth might reseal it (*d*), but this would not yield a viable division mechanism. (*e*) Origin of the septum by the gene-controlled orthogonal outgrowth of two murein sheets (dashed lines) between the two chromosome termini (T) would produce the first reproducible cell-division mechanism (*f*). Fusion of the edge of the growing septum with the obcell lips could close it to produce two topologically closed daughter cells (*g*), each of which would be able to divide by exactly the same septation mechanism that created them in the first place (*h*).

Septum formation depends on the synthesis of two peptidoglycan sheets orthogonally to the preexisting wall. The essential molecular innovation that made this possible, I suggest, was the origin of a protein cofactor for the peptidoglycan polymerizing enzymes that initiated such orthogonal assembly specifically at two adjacent sites, each, in turn, immediately adjacent to the duplicated chromosome termini (Fig. 6e–h). I suggest that from the beginning, these proteins must have specifically bound directly or indirectly to other proteins associated with replication termination, since otherwise septation would not have been properly spatially controlled and thus would have been disadvantageous rather than advantageous. This single extra step could have converted an obcell into a primitive ancestor of the first gram-negative eubacterium, able to grow, divide, and accurately segregate its DNA, which I call the protobacterium.

Differentiation between the Outer Membrane and Plasma Membrane

As both membranes of the newly formed protobacterium would contain facilitated transport proteins, it

would still be able to take up nutrients and grow without immediate interruption. However, those proteins in the outer membrane would no longer be replenished during growth (because ribosomes could only continue to insert them cotranslationally into the inner plasma membrane). Thus, within a dozen generations or so they would be lost, and cell growth would be greatly slowed or would cease altogether unless the outer membrane became more permeable. This, I suggest, happened by the evolution of the first porin proteins able to be cotranslationally inserted through the plasma membrane at points where there were pores in the peptidoglycan, enabling it to adhere to the outer membrane (Fig. 7). These so-called Bayer's patches play a key role in the growth of the negibacterial outer membrane: In modern cells, lipids initially inserted into the plasma membrane must pass outward through them into the outer membrane. In the protobacterium, en-

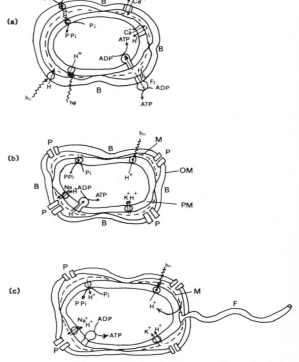

Figure 7. Envelope evolution in the protobacterium. Immediately following obcell closure, the inner and outer membranes would have contained the same proteins (*a*). With the internalization of ribosomes, all existing outer membrane proteins would have soon been lost (*b*); only with the evolution of porins (P), inserted cotranslationally into the outer membranes (OM) via the Bayer's patches (B), where holes in the murein (M) allow adhesion of the outer and plasma membrane, could nutrients continue to be translocated into the cell by the porters in the inner membrane. pH regulation in the newly formed cytoplasm was achieved by the insertion of two new proteins, a K^+/H^+ symporter and a Na^+/H^+ antiporter, into the plasma membrane. (*c*) Evolution of flagella (F), rotated by the periplasmic/cytoplasmic proton gradient, involved the cotranslational insertion and polymerization of proteins into filaments that penetrate the outer membrane as well as the murein.

vironmental, prebiotically made lipids would have inserted into the outer membrane and then passed through the Bayer's patches into the inner membrane, allowing it also to grow. Proteins ensuring the continued existence of the Bayer's patches and proteins catalyzing lipid transfer across them must have evolved during or before the origin of the protobacterium. Phospholipid-synthesizing enzymes using CTP would have been the first to evolve in the protobacterium (or even earlier) and might have evolved from those making glycerol teichoic acid in the obcell.

Since porins allow the entry of all molecules below a molecular weight of about 600, small molecules or ions such as sugars and phosphate could now enter the periplasm by simple diffusion (instead of facilitated diffusion as in the obcell) and interact with periplasmic binding or polymerizing proteins that would continue to be secreted through the plasma membrane. Such ions and small molecules also could cross the plasma membrane by facilitated diffusion, as in the obcell, and thus enter the newly formed cytoplasm. Facilitated uptake of Mg^{++} (essential for polymerases and the Mg porphyrins) and Zn^{++} (essential for replication) would have been vital from the start. Thus, the two most essential steps in the origin of the cell were the evolution of septum-initiating proteins and of porins. As both were needed, the origin of the cell was not highly probable even on the obcell theory. But at least it was possible and reasonably plausible, which is more than one can say for the classic random encapsulation by a liposome-like membrane of naked genes and ribosomes that had not previously co-evolved with membranes; the latter hypothesis implicitly requires the simultaneous sudden origin of numerous different facilitated diffusion proteins and a mechanism for cell division in the absence of any precursors. The obcell theory not only avoids these problems, but also provides the only plausible explanation yet suggested for the origin of the negibacterial outer membrane and for the origin of a complete bioenergetic system.

Origin of Cytoplasmic Ionic Regulation

The PPase and light-harvesting and electron-transport proteins would also inevitably be lost from the outer membrane, but remain in the plasma membrane with the same polarity they have today (Fig. 7b). The proton/Ca^{++} antiporter postulated to maintain the proton gradient at night could function unchanged and be the historical reason why all cells pump calcium outwards across the plasma membrane. By day, however, light-driven proton extrusion would tend to make the cell too alkaline, especially when it was short of internal phosphate and proton-driven PP_i synthesis could not keep up with the light-driven proton pump. I suggest that this problem was solved by the evolution of a K^+/H^+ symporter that allowed proton entry coupled to potassium import (Fig. 7b). This, in turn, could lead under some conditions to excessive internal concentrations of monovalent cations, which might be inhib-

itory to enzymes originally adapted, I assume, to ordinary seawater. Evolution of a Na^+/H^+ antiporter would couple sodium extrusion to H^+ import (Fig. 7b). A proper quantitative balance between the ion carriers would allow the simultaneous regulation of pH and monovalent cation concentration. But the net result would be a low internal Ca^{++} and Na^+ composition and a high internal K^+, quite unlike the ancestral seawater. Newly evolving intracellular enzymes would be adapted to such conditions.

Origin of the Proton-motive F_0F_1 ATP Synthase

A potentially severe problem resulting from the topological closure of the cytoplasm would have been the excessive accumulation of pyrophosphate; produced both by the proton-driven PP synthase and by RNA and DNA polymerases, it would no longer be lost by diffusion and thus would tend to drive the equilibria catalyzed by polymerases toward shortening of nucleic acids, rather than elongation. This problem could have been solved by the replacement of the plasma membrane proton-driven PPase by a proton-driven ATP synthase. It would not even have arisen if the original proton-motive phosphorylation had been of nucleotides to make NTPs, as I originally proposed (Cavalier-Smith 1985). At that time, however, I was not aware of the existence in purple bacteria of proton-driven PPase simpler in structure than the multisubunit ATP synthase. The reason I now suggest that the PPase came first is twofold: (1) Its greater simplicity would make its origin much easier at a time when replication and translation were very primitive and the genome coded for only a handful of polypeptides. (2) As it is likely that prebiotic pyrophosphate rather than ATP served as the energy carrier during preobcellular evolution (Lipmann 1965), kinase(s) able to use it to phosphorylate nucleotides might already have evolved; continuation of this mechanism rather than its immediate replacement by direct phosphorylation of nucleotides makes the origin of obcells a smaller, and therefore more probable, evolutionary step.

As soon as DNA evolved and provided a greater coding capacity, there would have been no obstacle to the evolution of a proton-driven ATP synthase. The evolution of ATPases used in DNA replication would make it relatively easy: A duplicate of one of their genes could have evolved to make the F_1 ATPase, and a duplicate of the PPase (which must have a transmembrane proton channel) could be adapted to make the F_0 proton channel; combination of the two would make the first proton-driven F_0F_1 ATPase, which is present in the plasma membrane of all bacteria, except chlamydias (which make no ATP). I suggest that this happened soon after DNA evolved and that the obcell that underwent closure to form the protobacterium therefore already had two different proton-driven phosphorylating enzymes. Like the PPase, the ATP synthase would simply have been lost from the probacterial outer membrane (Fig. 7b). The pyrophosphate concentration following obcell closure could be reduced to a suitable level by reducing the strength of the PPase promoter; in most cells, the gene was simply lost. ATP synthase would have been useful to the obcell because direct phosphorylation of ATP would be less wasteful than the earlier indirect method using a PP_i/ADP kinase, for much of the PP_i would diffuse away before being used. However, the PPase would still have been retained by the obcell because it would enable the properiplasmic CDP and UDP (used for phospholipid-teichoic acid and peptidoglycan synthesis, respectively) to be rephosphorylated via a transmembrane PP_i/NTP kinase even when starved of extraobcellular adenosine.

Origin of Active Transport of Nutrients

A major consequence of the origin of the protobacterium is that amino acids, bases, phosphate, and sugars could be economically maintained at a higher internal concentration and allow more rapid replication, transcription, and translation. This was probably the primary reason for the success of the first cell, but it would only be possible if the plasma membrane proteins that mediated facilitated diffusion (which simply equalizes internal and external nutrient concentrations) evolved into active transport proteins. This could be done (1) by coupling to inward proton flow and (2) by coupling to ATP hydrolysis on the cytoplasmic face of the plasma membrane. Prior to the folding of the obcell to generate the protobacterium, coupling of endergonic processes to ATP hydrolysis would not have been a favored process because nucleotides and phosphate were continually leaking into the environment, and such coupling would deplete the NTPs needed for nucleic acid and protein synthesis; afterwards, there would be no such competition, and ATP hydrolysis would become very widely used. The fact that import of some amino acids is powered by proton flow and some by ATP hydrolysis suggests that the choice of method used was quite haphazard when the cell first evolved. A third way to power active transport, which also depends on the ready availability of ATP, is to phosphorylate metabolites taken up into the cell by facilitated diffusion, so that they are unable to recross the membrane because of their negative charge. This is the group translocation system used for sugar import by bacteria. But since it depends on phosphoenol-pyruvate, it probably would not have evolved until later, after the origin of intermediary metabolism and substrate level phosphorylation, probably the last major step in the conversion of a protobacterium into a eubacterium.

Origin of Intermediary Metabolism, Autotrophy, and Fermentation

We at last come to Horowitz's (1945) proposal that as the amino acids, sugars, bases, and lipids in the prebiotic soup became depleted, metabolic pathways could evolve backward by a series of single steps. Such a mechanism was probably neither as general nor as simple as commonly supposed. The last enzyme in each pathway could have evolved from the relevant active transport protein, which, as it would already have a binding site for the product, could probably be easily modified to bind its precursor (Holden 1968). However, we would also need a new active transport enzyme for the precursor. Must we postulate a successive backward evolution of active transport proteins as well as enzymes? Is it not easier to imagine an active transport molecule of broad specificity that evolved an enzymatic capacity to catalyze a series of related reactions? More specific enzymes could then evolve by the specialization of such generalist enzymes in different directions following gene duplications. In this way, several steps of a metabolic pathway might be perfected simultaneously. This would avoid the problem of "prescient" forward evolution of pathways without having to make the improbable assumption that every intermediate was already available in the prebiotic soup. Not only biosynthetic pathways, but also catabolic and anaplerotic pathways would evolve to create an interconnecting web of reactions in which no single intermediate was rate-limiting.

Catabolic pathways (such as glycolysis) would not have been metabolically useful in the absence of anaplerotic pathways connecting them to the biosynthetic pathways. The most centrally important, and possibly only truly universal, anaplerotic pathway is the pentose-phosphate pathway. From it lead the biosynthetic pathways to nucleotides, amino acids, lipids, peptidoglycan, and teichoic acids, the key constituents of the obcell. This key role is understandable if it was the first major anaplerotic pathway to evolve. The remarkable fact that pentose phosphates are the immediate substrate not only for nucleotide synthesis, but also for the most widespread method of carbon fixation can readily be understood if, as I suggest, the origin of the pentose-phosphate cycle went hand-in-hand with the origin of autotrophy in the protobacterial cell *before* other intermediary pathways had evolved. The key step was the origin of ribulose-bisphosphate carboxylase, which catalyzed the fixation of CO_2 by reaction with ribulose bisphosphate to form 3-phospho-glycerate. This could be converted to phosphoenol-pyruvate for amino acid and fatty acid synthesis, and reduced to glyceraldehyde-phosphate for making ribose-5'-P for nucleotides and glycerol-phosphate for phospholipids and teichoic acids. Reduction was probably originally by NADPH (Fig. 8) as in the oxidative pentose pathway and in fatty acid synthesis: The use of NADH instead in purple and green bacteria may have arisen later with the evolution of respiration and of NADH-specific dehydrogenases for channeling the hydrogen from catabolites to the respiratory chain. My assumption that glyceraldehyde-3-phosphate dehydrogenase is a particularly primitive enzyme is supported by the fact that it shows more clearly than other proteins the primeval RNY repeat pattern of codons (Shepherd 1983). Interestingly, it lacks introns, contrary to the predictions of Darnell and Doolittle (1986). I suggest

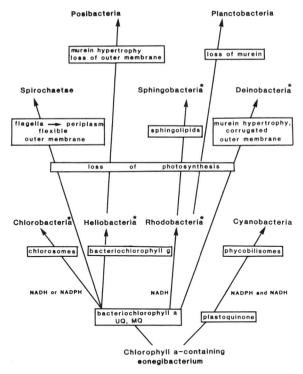

Figure 8. Diversification of eubacteria. With the evolution of intermediary metabolism, the protobacterium became able to make quinones and porphyrins, rather than merely absorb them from the medium. The fundamental bifurcation between cyanobacteria, which use plastoquinone (PQ) and chlorophyll a, and other eubacteria, which use menaquinone (MK) and/or ubiquinone (UQ) and bacteriochlorophyll a, I suggest, dates from the initial origin of quinone and porphyrin biosynthetic pathways. For the reasons given by Olson (1983), the ancestral photosynthetic pigments and reaction centers were probably like those of cyanobacteria; eonegibacterium probably had hydrogenase and used hydrogen as a photoreductant, but it may also have had oxygenic photosynthesis and even phycobilins, and so was actually an early cyanobacterium! The use by cyanobacteria of both NADPH and NADH for photoreduction, I believe, is also primitive and precluded efficient catabolism and heterotrophy because it prevents the occurrence simultaneously of high NAD^+/NADH ratios, which are needed for catabolic pathways such as glycolysis and oxidation of fatty acids, and of high $NADPH/NADP^+$ ratios, which are needed for efficient biosynthesis of lipids and other anabolites. Origin of the ability to use H_2S as photoreductant, as in the cyanobacterium *Oscillatoria limnetica*, the loss of different components of the cyanobacterial photoredox system, and the evolution of different bacteriochlorophylls produced the three phyla of anoxygenic photosynthetic bacteria. The use of NADH alone as photoreductant by purple bacteria (rhodobacteria; new phylum name—asterisks indicate other new phyla) enabled them to evolve glycolysis (absent in cyanobacteria) and efficient photoheterotrophy; this and the origin of a complete Krebs cycle preadapted them for the loss of photosynthesis and the formation of efficiently respiring heterotrophs; it is no coincidence that the vast majority of heterotrophic negibacteria are rhodobacteria. Chlorosomes in the green bacteria (Chlorobacteria including Chlorobiaceae and Chloroflexaceae) are probably an adaptation to very low light intensity (Raven and Beardall 1981). Apart from photosynthetic diversification, the other changes sufficiently important for the results to merit recognition as distinct phyla concern the bacterial envelope: the periplasmic relocation of flagella to make Spirochaetae; hypertrophy of murein causing loss of the outer membrane to make Posibacteria; total loss of peptidoglycan to make Planctobacteria (the *Planctomyces* phylum, in which I include Chlamydiae); evolution of sphingolipids to make Sphingobacteria (the *Bacteroides-Flavobacterium* phylum; Woese 1987); and hypertrophy of murein without loss of the outer membrane to make the radiation-resistant Deinobacteria (e.g., *Deinococcus*). Teichoic acids must have been lost at a very early date from all lines of evolution except heliobacteria/posibacteria, if they were indeed present in the common ancestor.

that it was the evolution of carbon fixation and the consequent superabundant supply of 3-phospho-glycerate that provided the evolutionary stimulus for the evolution of an integrated system of metabolic pathways. The short pathway for making serine, glycine, and cysteine stems directly from 3-phospho-glycerate, and those for other amino acids stem from other constituents of the pentose-phosphate cycle or the side branch leading via PEP and pyruvate to oxaloacetate. Nucleotides are made from pentose phosphates and amino acids. The sudden provision of a newly abundant

internal carbon source would have been a much more potent stimulus for the origin of metabolic pathways than the piecemeal increase in the efficiency of use of prebiotic molecules traditionally assumed (Horowitz 1945). The Krebs cycle probably did not evolve at an early stage, as it is incomplete in most photosynthetic bacteria, from which glycolysis is also typically absent.

Because of the correlations between related codons and the biosynthetic pathways for amino acids (Wong 1975), one might be tempted to suggest that the ambiguity reduction of the genetic code (Fitch and Upper, this volume), which was accompanied by an increase in the number of different amino acids and tRNAs used for making proteins, took place in the protobacterium concomitantly with the evolution of amino acid biosynthesis. If so, then the obcells would have had only a relatively small number of different tRNAs, as well as very few aminoacyl-tRNA synthetase proteins, or even none if the tRNAs were self-charging (Crick 1968) or charged by ribozymal precursors of aminoacyl-tRNA synthetases (Maizels and Weiner, this volume); possibly, therefore, soluble aminoacyl-tRNA synthetase proteins evolved only after the conversion of obcell into protobacterium. However, the preceding suggestions (like the proposal on the same grounds that the biosynthesis of certain amino acids must have evolved at an early stage in evolution of the code; Jurka and Smith 1987) are not the only interpretation of the observed correlation.

One could reasonably argue instead that chemical relatedness of different amino acids *independently* influenced the expansion and ambiguity reduction of a primitive RNY code and the evolution of amino acid biosynthesis. As new tRNAs and their corresponding aminoacyl-tRNA synthetases evolved by gene duplication, it would be almost inevitable that they would be specific for amino acids chemically related to those used by their immediate progenitors, irrespective of whether this happened using amino acids made prebiotically or biosynthetically. Likewise, any biosynthetic pathway necessarily interconverts chemically related amino acids, rather than radically different ones, regardless of whether it evolved early or late. This might be the simplest explanation of the correlations; it allows the genetic code and protein synthesis both to be perfected before the evolution of biosynthetic pathways. Against this, however, is the suggestion that the absence of tryptophan from ribulose-bisphosphate carboxylase might reflect its origin before the full expansion of the code.

As a by-product of the evolution of metabolic pathways, some of the phosphorylated intermediates could be used directly to phosphorylate ATP (substrate-level phosphorylation). When a sufficiently self-sustaining network of pathways evolved that would allow net ATP synthesis by this mechanism, mutations abolishing light-driven proton "pumping" would no longer be lethal and the first fermentative bacterium could evolve. But it would retain the F_0F_1 ATP synthase that evolved in the first photoheterotrophic cell. Instead of providing ATP, it would use it to pump out protons to maintain the cytoplasmic pH regulation mechanism discussed above. The idea that this ATPase evolved originally in a fermentative organism so as to regulate its pH (Raven and Smith 1976, 1982) is unsatisfactory, since it leaves unexplained how any cell without an F_0F_1 ATPase could have evolved intermediary metabolism and substrate level phosphorylation in the first place. Nitrogen fixation in photosynthetic bacteria (Stewart 1983) is the rule rather than the exception, which suggests that it evolved in the earliest photosynthetic eubacteria. It would have given them a huge selective advantage over their progenitors. But once CO_2/N_2 fixation had evolved, it would be less disadvantageous for *some* organisms to lose photosynthesis and N_2 fixation, since they could use their products generated by species that retained them.

Origin of Oxidative Phosphorylation, Respiration, and Methanogenesis

I see no objection to the traditional view that the electron transport molecules and membrane-bound ATP synthase that form the basis for oxidative phosphorylation are derived from those originally evolved for photosynthesis (Broda 1978). This is consistent with both the rRNA phylogeny and my present scenario. In principle, oxidative phosphorylation using H_2 and a membrane-bound hydrogenase might have evolved in an obcell; but in those cases (the vast majority) where the reducing power is provided by soluble dehydrogenases from organic metabolites, it would appear unlikely that it could have evolved prior to the evolution of intermediary metabolism, which would have depended on the prior origin of a cell using photophosphorylation.

This argument applies particularly strongly to methanogenic bioenergetics. Energy production by methanogenesis depends not only on a typical F_1F_0 membrane ATP synthase and a membrane-bound electron transport chain, but also on a very complex metabolic one-carbon cycle of seven enzyme-catalyzed steps; one of these alone requires four different proteins and no less than five different coenzymes including ATP, FAD, the exceedingly complex vitamin B_{12}, and two coenzymes unique to methanogens. For autotrophic methanogenesis, sometimes regarded as a possible "primitive" system, the situation is even worse, since this needs a complete CO_2 fixation system using acetyl CoA and many soluble enzymes essentially similar to those of eubacteria equally able to grow on H_2 and CO_2 alone. The conclusion is inescapable that methanogenesis could only have evolved in an advanced cell already possessing intermediary metabolism and oxidative phosphorylation. This is fully consistent with the rRNA tree which suggests that aerobic oxidatively phosphorylating sulfobacteria (Cavalier-Smith 1986a; Woese 1987), rather than methanogens, were the primitive archaebacterial phenotype.

The only phototrophic archaebacteria, halobacteria, are also not primitive according to the rRNA tree; their light-driven proton pump necessarily depends on a protein-carotenoid covalent complex and is therefore genetically more complex than the original purely "lipid"-based pump postulated for the eubacterial ancestor. The much greater diversity of eubacterial photosynthesizers (and of eubacteria generally; Fig. 8) strongly supports my idea that they were not only the original photosynthesizers, but also the first cells, and that archaebacteria evolved only relatively recently as a result of radical changes in their cell envelope (Cavalier-Smith 1987a), and initially colonized thermal niches for which their tetraether lipids uniquely suit them. Archaebacteria that have colonized mesophilic niches have tended to replace the tetraether lipids by diether lipids that would make their membrane more fluid (Langworthy and Pond 1986). That they have not reacquired acylester lipids is no problem if the enzymes making them, which, I argue, date back at least to the protobacterium, were lost by their thermophilic common ancestor.

Origin of Bacterial Flagella, Spirochetes, and Gliding Motility

As each of the eubacterial phyla (Fig. 8) has flagella, it follows that flagella must also have originated very early, in a common ancestral photosynthetic bacterium (Fig. 7c). I suggest that they evolved by polymerization to form a hollow filament from a mutant outer membrane protein (a porin?), which, like normal outer membrane proteins, would from the start be inserted through the Bayer's patches. Possibly the mutation initially producing such a tubular filament also caused it to stick at the site of a Bayer's patch by adhesion to the outer surface of the plasma membrane.

Berg et al. (1982) proposed that the flagellar motor involves a protein ring embedded in the plasma membrane with a different rotational periodicity to that of the flagellar shaft, such that reversible covalent bonds could be formed between them by oxidation and reduction cycles driven by the proton-motive force in the plasma membrane. If the mutation that produced the flagellar shaft did so by increasing or decreasing the number of subunits per ring by one, and if SH-containing amino acids were appropriately disposed around the base of the ring, then this might have had the correct geometry to form a functional motor by binding to an ancestral single-tiered porin-like ring.

The major difference between spirochetes and other eubacteria is that their flagellar shaft lies in the periplasmic space between the outer membrane and the peptidoglycan layer. This arrangement would automatically result if the flagellar proteins were cotranslationally inserted into modified Bayer's patches that still possessed a hole through the peptidoglycan but no contact with the outer membrane; they would then be forced to grow into the outer compartment of the periplasmic space. The effective mutation might have been one that generally loosened the peptidoglycan/outer membrane connections, which could also allow flagella rotation to make the whole cell rotate in its characteristic corkscrew fashion. Their corkscrewing motility allows them to penetrate semisolid matrices such as sloppy muds rich in organic molecules, a habitat that would have readily allowed the loss of phototrophy. Corkscrewing, however, depends on the spiral shape, controlled by the peptidoglycan. Possibly a single mutation altered the peptidoglycan so as to cause

both spiral growth and less attachment to the outer membrane.

Since some spirochetes glide, rather than spiral, it is also possible that gliding motility preceded corkscrewing. Gliding is almost as widespread as flagellar motility. Since it is present in cyanobacteria, rhodobacteria, and chlorobacteria, it also must have evolved in an early ancestral phototroph. It is driven by the plasma membrane proticity, but its mechanism is unclear. Rotation of proteinaceous filaments visible in the exoperiplasmic space (i.e., between the peptidoglycan and outer membrane, as in spirochete flagella) has been proposed for both cyanobacteria and rhodobacteria (Glagolev 1984). It seems likely that the essential proton-mechanical core of the presumed rotary motor for these filaments and that of flagella had a single common origin. Possibly what differs is mainly the nature and topological location of the shaft attached to the motor. An intriguing possibility is that the topological difference between exoperiplasmic and extracellular rotating filaments may originally have arisen within a single cell; in such a primitive ancestor, insertion might have been poorly controlled—sometimes into the exoperiplasm and sometimes across the outer membrane also. Perhaps an early gene duplication allowed periplasmic and extracellular filaments to be perfected simultaneously, one allowing gliding on surfaces or through viscous media and the other swimming in water.

A possibly more attractive scenario, because of the marked predominance of gliding in the cyanobacteria and the likely primitiveness of chlorophyll a (Fig. 8), is that gliding evolved first and flagella evolved from it. Spirochetes may have arisen as an aberration of the transitional stage between the two. The initial selective advantage of even a poorly controlled filament rotation in the exoperiplasm might have been a stirring effect, increasing the efficacy of nutrient uptake via the newly evolved porins and plasma membrane pumps.

Obviously, the complete evolution of flagella must have been more complicated than outlined here, since their basal region contains about a dozen polypeptides. Most of them may be concerned with perfecting and controlling the basic rotary process or its efficient mechanical coupling to the flagella shaft and anchoring of the flagellum within the envelope, and so might have evolved subsequently, but it seems likely that the original proton-mechanical protein that mediates rotation is one of them.

The original selective advantage of typical flagella would have been to move the bacteria away from regions locally depleted in nutrients. This would occur even with random movement, but as they evolved in a phototroph, it is likely that photokinesis would also soon evolve. Gas vacuoles also probably first evolved in ancestral phototrophic bacteria. Like bacterial flagella, they are homologous structures in both eubacteria and archaebacteria (Jones et al. 1987) and are additional structural evidence that the transition between the two kingdoms occurred in a well-developed flagellated prokaryote cell, and not via a progenote.

Unity of Biochemistry and a Single Origin for All Cells

The great similarity of the metabolic pathways of all organisms was what first led to the general acceptance that all living organisms had a single common ancestor. If, as I argue, metabolic pathways evolved *after* the origin of the first cell, it also shows that all cells evolved from a single common ancestral cell. The similarities in metabolic pathways such as glycolysis, amino acid and nucleotide synthesis, fatty acid synthesis and degradation, squalene synthesis, and pentose-phosphate pathway in the three major lineages can only be explained if all three are descended from a common cellular ancestor possessing all of these. Such a large number of enzymes implies a highly developed DNA replication system with proofreading, as well as very efficient transcription and translation. RNA replication without proofreading could not code for them with sufficient fidelity. The idea that the three major lineages diverged as a crude precellular system with only an RNA genome and an inability to make large proteins (Woese 1983) does not withstand close examination. I have recently tabulated many of the numerous major similarities between the two prokaryotic kingdoms (Cavalier-Smith 1987a) and between them and eukaryotes; in addition, Jones et al. (1987) have stressed the fundamental metabolic similarity between methanogens and eubacteria. More recently, Woese partially retreated from his earlier proposals by suggesting that eukaryotes may have evolved from archaebacteria (Woese and Wolfe 1985) and by recognizing that rRNA sequence data show that there is no unbridgeable gulf between the three groups and cannot tell us the nature of the universal common ancestor. To show that it is not, as Woese (1983) asserted, "impossible" to interconnect the three lineages via cellular intermediates, I have recently shown how all the major features of both archaebacteria and eukaryotes can be explained as logical consequences of the mutational loss of the peptidoglycan murein from a gram-positive eubacterium (Cavalier-Smith 1987a). Anyone who seriously maintains that archaebacteria and eukaryotes originated from a progenote independently of eubacteria should produce a comparably detailed scenario to show that both transitions were possible (and also that they were simpler overall than my scenarios for the origin of the three major lineages) and explain how so many fundamental properties ranging from flagella to metabolic pathways came to be shared by more than one of the three groups.

Likewise, anyone who wishes to maintain the classic idea that the first cell was a clostridial fermenter produced by encapsulation of naked genes and ribosomes should produce a scenario as detailed as the present obcell theory, showing how it might have happened and also how one could evolve a viable and reproducing negibacterial cell with a two-membrane envelope from an ancestral cell with only a single membrane. Unless both are done, the obcell theory will remain the best working hypothesis.

Concluding Remarks: Molecular Co-evolution and Evolutionary Conservatism

The importance of the obcell is that it allowed the close coupling of the primordial genetic system to the solar energy flux on the surface of the earth. This coupling is the keystone of life as we know it. The obcell theory gives a much more fundamental role to membranes than assumed by the classic Oparin-Haldane theory. The origin of a chemiosmotically active coupling membrane was what made cellular life possible. Looking backward, the obcell seems wasteful and inefficient compared with a cell. The system appears too open, with many activated nucleotides and amino acids being lost before they can be polymerized by the particular obcell that made them. However, the obcell would have had a pronounced kinetic advantage over its predecessors, and it is the kinetic advantage of new genotypes over old genotypes that drives evolution, not anthropomorphic concepts of economy. Waste of energy and/or materials is inherent in much progressive genetic evolution (e.g., of homeothermy or deciduousness) just as it is in cultural evolution (compare the modern American economy with that of pre-Columbian Amerindians).

Cells also are fundamentally open systems. The obcell concept allows the gradual evolution not only of their fundamental chemiosmotic properties, but also of the structural system that is the essential link between the genetic and bioenergetic systems, through such processes as membrane growth by lipid and cotranslational protein insertion and the attachment of DNA to membranes and skeletal structures essential for its segregation and cell division. Merely trapping genes and ribosomes inside an inert membrane, as traditionally assumed, would instead have made a closed system, unable to feed and grow, and doomed to an early death. By placing a premium on catalysts able to insert themselves into or onto membranes, the obcell probably played the dominant role in the changeover from primordial ribozymes to protein catalysts. It seems improbable that a ribozyme could act as an osmoenzyme or as a cation porter or to anchor light-harvesting or electron-transport molecules appropriately inside membranes.

Two of the most fascinating features of cell evolution are its extreme conservatism and the intriguing relationships between different molecules and functions. Thus, to understand the evolution of the catalytic functions of human DNA primase, e.g., why it indiscriminately polymerizes ribo- and deoxyribonucleotides, we may have to understand the changeover from RNA to DNA genomes in obcells that lived over 3500 million years ago. Is the fundamental reason that we have D-amino acid oxidases in the peroxisomes in our liver because we have to dispose of useless or potentially harmful products of digested eubacteria, which have D-amino acids in their peptidoglycan primarily because they were abundantly available in the prebiotic soup when obcells first evolved a skeleton? To complicate matters, our peroxisomes themselves, I suggested (Cavalier-Smith 1987b), originated as intracellular posibacterial symbionts..

We must be cautious in assuming that all things that *look* primitive date from the prebiotic soup. Ribozymes, for example, include not only RNase P (which I suggested in Fig. 3 did evolve in the progenote or obcell), but also self-splicing introns, which, as I argue elsewhere in detail (Cavalier-Smith 1987a), go back only about 1500 million years to the common ancestor of eukaryotes and archaebacteria. New things can arise in evolution. Old things can be lost. We cannot assume that widespread properties are necessarily more primitive than restricted ones. Thus, glycolysis enzymes, which figure greatly in speculations about primordial gene assembly (Gilbert et al. 1986), are not among the most ancient proteins, but on my obcell theory represent the very last phase of cellular origins: the evolution of intermediary metabolism. Cytochromes, although not universal, are probably much more ancient.

To decide which molecules actually are ancient and which are recent, and how they evolved, we need, instead of a priori reasoning, detailed *phylogenetic analysis* to reconstruct the complete tree of life using ultrastructural and molecular characters, and also reasoned *integrative scenarios* as to how each of the transitions between the major groups of organisms occurred.

SUMMARY

The gap between early molecular evolution and the origin of the first cell may have been bridged by a photoheterotrophic obcell, consisting of genes and ribosomes attached to the outer surface of a phospholipid vesicle containing a light-driven proton pump and a proton-driven pyrophosphate synthase. I argue that the obcell was the substratum for the origin of DNA replication; DNA segregation by the growth and division of the peptidoglycan murein; periplasmic solute-binding proteins; bioenergetics, including the F_0F_1 proton-driven ATP synthase; active transport of calcium; and facilitated diffusion of nutrients across membranes, and that it played the major role in the replacement of ribozymes by protein catalysts.

Curved growth of the peptidoglycan and a mutation causing septum formation produced the first true cell. Evolution of porins, sodium extrusion and potassium import, conversion of the facilitated diffusion proteins to active pumps, and the evolution of intermediary metabolism, carbon and nitrogen fixation, and of substrate level phosphorylation, completed the origin of the first negibacterial eubacterium, from which all other cells evolved, and from which they have inherited

most of their major catalytic properties—with the notable exceptions of reverse transcriptase, RNA splicing, and methanogenesis, all of which I believe evolved very much later.

ACKNOWLEDGMENTS

I thank Pat Wright for typing and Chris Perera for help with the figures.

REFERENCES

Alexander, J. and C.B. Bridges. 1929. Some physicochemical aspects of life, mutation and evolution. *Colloid Chem.* 1: 9.

Baltscheffsky, H. 1981. Stepwise molecular evolution of bacterial photosynthetic energy conversion. *Biosystems* 14: 49.

Berg, H.C., M.D. Manson, and M.P. Conley. 1982. Dynamics and energetics of flagellar rotation in bacteria. *Symp. Soc. Exp. Biol.* 35: 33.

Blobel, G. 1980. Intracellular membrane topogenesis. *Proc. Natl. Acad. Sci.* 77: 1496.

Boyden, A.A. 1953. Comparative evolution with special reference to primitive mechanisms. *Evolution* 7: 21.

Broda, E. 1978. *The evolution of the bioenergetic process.* Revised reprint. Pergamon Press, Oxford.

Cavalier-Smith, T. 1980. Cell compartmentation and the origin of eukaryote membranous organelles. In *Endocytobiology: Endosymbiosis and cell biology, a synthesis of recent research* (ed. W. Schwemmler and H.E.A. Schenk), p. 893. de Gruyter, Berlin.

———. 1982. The origins of plastids. *Biol. J. Linn. Soc.* 17: 289.

———. 1983a. Cloning chromosome ends. *Nature* 301: 112.

———. 1983b. A 6-kingdom classification and a unified phylogeny. In *Endocytobiology II: Intracellular space as oligogenetic ecosystem* (ed. W. Schwemmler and H.E.A. Schenk), p. 1027. de Gruyter, Berlin.

———. 1985. Genome size during precellular evolution: From RNA to DNA. In *The evolution of genome size* (ed. T. Cavalier-Smith), p. 20. John Wiley, Chichester, England.

———. 1986a. The kingdoms of organisms. *Nature* 324: 416.

———. 1986b. The kingdom Chromista: Origin and systematics. In *Progress in phycological research* (ed. F.E. Round and D.J. Chapman), vol. 4, p. 309. Biopress, Bristol.

———. 1987a. The origin of eukaryote and archaebacterial cells. *Ann. N.Y. Acad. Sci.* 503: 17.

———. 1987b. The simultaneous symbiotic origin of mitochondria, chloroplasts, and microbodies. *Ann. N.Y. Acad. Sci.* 503: 55.

———. 1987c. The origin of fungi and pseudofungi. *Brit. Mycol. Soc. Symp.* 13: 339.

———. 1987d. Eukaryotes without mitochondria. *Nature* 326: 332.

———. 1987e. Bacterial DNA segregation: Its motors and positional control. *J. Theor. Biol.* 127: 361.

Clark, C. and S.A. Gerbi. 1982. Ribosomal RNA evolution by fragmentation of the 23S progenitor: Maturation pathway parallels. *J. Mol. Evol.* 18: 326.

Crick, F.H.C. 1968. The origin of the genetic code. *J. Mol. Biol.* 38: 367.

Crick, F.H.C., S. Brenner, A. Klug, and G. Pieczenik. 1976. A speculation on the origin of protein synthesis. *Origins Life* 7: 389.

Darnell, J.E. and W.F. Doolittle. 1986. Speculations on the early course of evolution. *Proc. Natl. Acad. Sci.* 83: 1271.

Darwin, C. 1868. *The variation of animals and plants under domestication,* vol. 2. Murray, London.

Dawkins, R. 1982. *The extended phenotype.* W.H. Freeman, Oxford.

de Vrij, W.R. Bulthuis, E. Postma, and W.M. Konings. 1985. Calcium transport in membrane vesicles of *Bacillus subtilis*. *J. Bacteriol.* **164**: 1294.

Doolittle, W.F. and C. Sapienza. 1980. Selfish genes, the phenotype paradigm and genome evolution. *Nature* **284**: 617.

Dougherty, E.C. 1955. Comparative evolution and the origin of sexuality. *Syst. Zool.* **4**: 145.

Eigen, M. and P. Schuster. 1979. *The hypercycle*. Springer-Verlag, Berlin.

Gabriel, M.L. 1960. Primitive genetic mechanisms and the origin of chromosomes. *Am. Nat.* **44**: 257.

Gaffron, H. 1965. The role of light in evolution: The transition from a one quantum to a two quanta mechanism. In *The origin of prebiological systems and of their molecular matrices* (ed. S.W. Fox), p. 437. Academic Press, New York.

Gilbert, W., M. Marchionni, and G. McKnight. 1986. On the antiquity of introns. *Cell* **46**:151.

Glagolev, A.N. 1984. *Motility and taxis in prokaryotes*. Soviet Scientific Review, Harwood Academic Publishers, London.

Haldane, J.B.S. 1929. The origin of life. *Rationalist Ann.* **148**: 3.

———. 1965. Data needed for a blueprint of the first organism. In *The origin of prebiological systems and of their molecular matrices* (ed. S.W. Fox), p. 11. Academic Press, New York.

Hall, D.O., R. Cammack, and K.K. Rao. 1971. Role for ferredoxins in the origin of life and biological evolution. *Nature* **233**: 136.

Harold, F.M. 1986. *The vital force. A study of bioenergetics*. W.H. Freeman, New York.

Harold, F.M. and Y. Kanimura. 1986. Primary and secondary transport of cations in bacteria. *Ann. N.Y. Acad. Sci.* **456**: 375.

Harris, D.A. 1981. The coupling ATPase complex: An evolutionary view. *Biosystems* **14**: 113

Hartman, H. 1980. The origin of the eukaryotic cell. *Speculations Sci. Technol.* **3**: 83.

Holden, J.T. 1968. Evolution of transport systems. *J. Theor. Biol.* **21**: 97.

Horowitz, N.H. 1945. On the evolution of biochemical syntheses. *Proc. Natl. Acad. Sci.* **31**: 153.

Huxley, T.H. 1873. *Critiques and addresses*, p. 209. Macmillan, London.

Jones, W.J., D.P. Nagle, and W.B. Whitman. 1987. Methanogens and the diversity of archaebacteria. *Microbiol. Rev.* **51**: 135.

Jurka, J. and T.F. Smith. 1987. β-Turn driven early evolution: The genetic code and biosynthetic pathways. *J. Mol. Evol.* **24**: 15.

Langworthy, T.A. and J.L. Pond. 1986. Archaebacterial ether lipids and chemotaxonomy. *Syst. Appl. Microbiol.* **7**: 253.

Lipmann, F. 1965. Projecting backwards from the present stage of evolution of biosynthesis. In *The origin of prebiological systems and of their molecular matrices* (ed. S.W. Fox), p. 259. Academic Press, New York.

Miller, S.L. and L.E. Orgel. 1974. *The origins of life on the earth*. Prentice-Hall, Englewood Cliffs, New Jersey.

Minchin, E.A. 1915. The evolution of the cell. *Trans. Brit. Assoc. Sect. D* p.437.

Mitchell, P. 1961. Coupling of phosphorylation to electron and hydrogen transfer by a chemi-osmotic type of mechanism. *Nature* **191**: 144.

Muller, H.J. 1929. The gene as the basis of life. *Proc. Int. Congr. Plant Sci.* **1**: 897.

Olson, J.M. 1983. Evolution of two types of photosynthetic reaction centres. In *Endocytobiology II: Intracellular space as oligogenetic ecosystem* (ed. H.E.A. Schenk and W. Schwemmler), p. 913. de Gruyter, Berlin.

Oparin, A.I. 1938. The origin of life. Macmillan, New York.

Orgel, L.E. 1968. Evolution of the genetic apparatus. *J. Mol. Evol.* **38**: 381.

Orgel, L.E. and F.H.C. Crick. 1980. Selfish DNA: The ultimate parasite. *Nature* **284**: 604.

Raven, J.A. and J. Beardall. 1981. The intrinsic permeability of biological membranes to H^+: Significance for the efficiency of low rates of energy transformation. *FEMS Microbiol. Lett.* **10**: 1.

Raven, J.A. and F.A. Smith. 1976. The evolution of chemiosmotic energy coupling. *J. Theor. Biol.* **57**: 301.

———. 1982. Solute transport at the plasmalemma and early evolution of cells. *Biosystems* **15**: 13.

Shepherd, J.C.W. 1983. From primeval message to present-day gene. *Cold Spring Harbor Symp. Quant. Biol.* **47**: 1099.

Stewart, W.D.P. 1983. Natural environments—Challenges to microbial success and survival. *Symp. Soc. Gen. Microbiol.* **34**: 1.

Strasburger, E. 1909. The minute structure of cells in relation to heredity. In *Darwin and modern science*. (ed. A.C. Seward), p. 102. Cambridge University Press, Cambridge, England.

Woese, C.R. 1979. A proposal concerning the origin of life on the planet earth. *J. Mol. Evol.* **13**: 95.

———. 1983. The primary lines of descent and the universal ancestor. In *Evolution from molecules to men* (ed. D.S. Bendall), p. 209. Cambridge University Press, Cambridge, England.

———. 1987. Bacterial evolution. *Microbiol. Rev.* **51**: 221.

Woese, C.R. and G.E. Fox. 1977a. The concept of cellular evolution. *J. Mol. Evol.* **10**: 1.

———. 1977b. Phylogenetic structure of the prokaryotic domain: The primary kingdoms. *Proc. Natl. Acad. Sci.* **74**: 5088.

Woese, C.R. and R.S. Wolfe, eds. 1985. Epilogue. In *The bacteria: Archaebacteria*, vol. 8. Academic Press, New York.

Wong, T.F. 1975. A co-evolution theory of the genetic code. *Proc. Natl. Acad. Sci.* **72**: 1909.

Zielinski, W.S. and L.E. Orgel. 1987. Autocatalytic synthesis of a tetranucleotide analogue. *Nature* **327**: 346.

Earliest Phylogenetic Branchings: Comparing rRNA-based Evolutionary Trees Inferred with Various Techniques

G.J. OLSEN

Department of Biology and Institute for Molecular and Cellular Biology, Indiana University, Bloomington, Indiana 47405

Comparisons of macromolecular sequences offer the greatest potential for inferring phylogenetic relationships spanning the diversity of extant life (Zuckerkandl and Pauling 1965). In addition, molecular comparisons promise to provide insights into the character of the most recent common ancestor of present-day species and the evolution of various metabolic abilities.

There are many methods for inferring evolutionary trees. Each is based on its own assumptions, so it is possible for different methods to yield different results from the same data. This paper demonstrates that when attention is paid to their underlying assumptions, it is possible to infer the same relationships with three diverse techniques: (1) a least-squares, distance matrix method, (2) maximum parsimony, and (3) evolutionary parsimony. A recurring theme is the fact that not all residues in a macromolecule undergo substitution at equal rates; i.e., some sites are more conservative than others.

The analyses presented are limited to 16S rRNA sequences. The molecule is universal, constant in function (at least some functions), readily identified in diverse organisms and organelles, amenable to sequence determination, and sufficiently conservative in primary and secondary structures to permit identification of homologous positions in each sequence. In addition, the molecule is large enough to provide a significant sample of genome evolution.

A 16S rRNA-based View of Evolutionary Relationships

Figure 1 presents a phylogenetic tree based on 16S rRNA sequences from a diverse collection of organisms

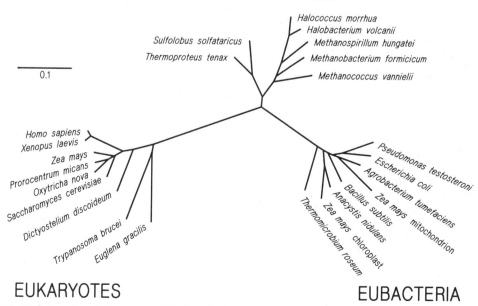

Figure 1. A 16S rRNA-based evolutionary tree. The length of each segment is proportional to the inferred number of fixed point mutations along that segment; the scale bar corresponds to 0.1 nucleotide substitutions per sequence position. The phylogenetic position of the common ancestor to the sequences is not identified; i.e., the tree is unrooted. The least-squares, distance matrix method used to infer the tree is discussed in the text. The sequences are available from Huysmans and De Wachter (1986), Sogin et al. (1986), Herzog and Marteaux (1986), and Oyaizu et al. (1987).

and organelles. This is an "unrooted tree": The lineages diverge from a common ancestral sequence (the location of which is not determined) in the interior of the network, and the contemporary sequences are at the tips of branches. The length of each segment in the tree reflects the inferred amount of sequence change along that segment. The major groups of organisms are identified by the urkingdom designations proposed by Woese and Fox (1977).

The recognition of two fundamentally different groups of prokaryotes, the eubacteria and the archaebacteria, by Woese and Fox (1977) was based on the very different RNase T1 oligonucleotide content of their respective 16S rRNAs. Detailed analyses revealed specific nucleotides that are unique to the eubacterial, eukaryotic, or archaebacterial rRNAs. It was also noted that additional molecular properties, including their membrane lipids and the modified nucleotides of their tRNAs, distinguished the archaebacteria from the eukaryotes and eubacteria (for review, see Woese and Wolfe 1985; Kandler and Zillig 1986).

Analysis of complete 16S rRNA sequences now provides over four times the data per molecule as was available from oligonucleotides. Some of the details of archaebacterial relationships in Figure 1 differ from those originally inferred from the oligonucleotide data, but the archaebacteria remain a coherent group, distinct from the eukaryotes and eubacteria.

The archaebacterial sequences in Figure 1 represent three diverse physiological types: *Sulfolobus solfataricus* and *Thermoproteus tenax* are extreme thermophiles (also referred to as sulfur-dependent archaebacteria or eocytes) and *Halobacterium volcanii* and *Halococcus morrhua* are extreme halophiles; there is also a single representative from each of three major groups of methanogens. Although the thermophilic archaebacteria represented form a single group, other phylogenetically distinct groups of archaebacteria share the thermophilic phenotype (see Klenk et al. 1986; Woese and Olsen 1986; Woese 1987).

Other features in Figure 1 are worth noting. There is relatively little sequence divergence between the animals (*Homo sapiens* [human] and *Xenopus laevis* [frog]), plants (*Zea mays* [corn]), and fungi (*Saccharomyces cerevisiae* [yeast]); the eukaryotic sequence diversity is dominated by the protists, which are represented by *Oxytricha nova* (ciliate), *Prorocentrum micans* (dinoflagellate), *Dictyostelium discoideum* (cellular slime mold), *Trypanosoma brucei* (trypanosoid flagellate), and *Euglena gracilis* (euglenoid flagellate). Among the eubacterial sequences, the green plant (*Z. mays*) chloroplast is specifically related to the cyanobacterium *Anacystis nidulans* (Tomioka and Sugiura 1983). Similarly, the *Z. mays* mitochondrial 16S rRNA is affiliated with the α-group purple bacterium" *Agrobacterium tumefaciens* (Yang et al. 1985), a result consistent with studies of the *c*-type cytochromes (Schwartz and Dayhoff 1978). It will be relevant to later discussions that the β-group purple bacterium (*Pseudomonas testosteroni*) and γ-group purple bac-

terium (*Escherichia coli*) are more closely related to each other than either is to the α-group (nomenclature according to Woese et al. 1985).

Least-squares, Distance Matrix Evolutionary Trees

Sequence alignment: The identification of homologous nucleotides. Before performing any phylogenetic analysis, it is necessary that homologous features be identified. For sequence comparisons, the homologs must be defined for each residue in each sequence. This is critical since subsequent analyses assume that the compared residue from each sequence is derived by nucleotide substitutions from a common ancestral nucleotide. The process of alignment has been discussed elsewhere (Gutell et al. 1985).

The analyses presented in this paper include very diverse rRNA sequences. Because of insertions and deletions in the evolution of the genes, it is not always clear which nucleotide in one sequence corresponds to which nucleotide in another, and sometimes there is no homolog. To satisfy the assumptions of the analyses, it is necessary to omit the regions of sequence that lack a homolog or are of uncertain homology. Consequently, the analyses in this paper are restricted to about 920 sequence positions. In the *E. coli* sequence (Brosius et al. 1981), these are nucleotides 6–38, 49–63, 105–122, 240–393, 499–580, 655–751, 761–825, 875–991, 1047–1115, 1157–1250, 1287–1409, and 1491–1534.

Evolutionary distance and additive trees. Figure 1 is inferred with a least-squares, distance method (Fitch and Margoliash 1967; Olsen 1988). To discuss the method in detail, it is necessary to introduce the concept of "additive trees." A phylogenetic tree is additive if the evolutionary distance separating any two points in the tree is equal to the total of the lengths of the branches that join the two points. Evolutionary distance is the average number of fixed point mutations per sequence position that separate two sequences. Because fixed mutations are events, they can be counted and added. Figure 1 is an example of an additive tree.

To reconstruct the branching order and branch lengths of an additive tree, it is sufficient to know the evolutionary distances between contemporary sequences. For example, Figure 2A presents the evolutionary distances separating pairs of contemporary sequences and Figure 2B is the corresponding unrooted additive tree. For every pair of sequences, the sum of the branch lengths between the two branch tips in Figure 2B equals the corresponding pairwise evolutionary distance in Figure 2A. Panel C presents the same relationships as a "rooted" tree. The location chosen for the root (the common ancestral sequence) is arbitrary in the sense that it cannot be derived from the distance data or the unrooted tree. The tree in panel C is drawn so that three of the four lineages diverge equal amounts from the assumed root; the fourth lineage, that leading to sequence B, diverges significantly more

A.

	A	B	C	D
A	–	0.4	0.4	0.8
B	0.4	–	0.6	1.0
C	0.4	0.6	–	0.8
D	0.8	1.0	0.8	–

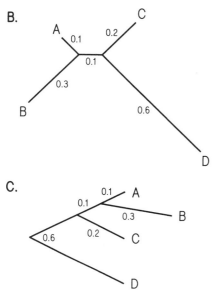

B.

C.

Figure 2. An additive evolutionary tree relating four contemporary sequences. (*A*) Evolutionary distance separating each pair of sequences; (*B*) corresponding unrooted, additive evolutionary tree. The distance between any two sequences is the sum of the lengths of the tree branches joining them. For example, the distance between sequences B and C is 0.3 + 0.1 + 0.2 = 0.6. In an unrooted tree, lineages diverge from an unidentified ancestor in the tree. (*C*) Rooted tree representing the same relationships as those in *B*. The common ancestor is placed at the extreme left, and the rest of the tree is redrawn so that sequence divergence is represented by displacement to the right from the ancestor.

from the presumed root. The evolution of sequence B is reflected in panel A in two specific ways: (1) Because B has diverged more from the common ancestor, it is more distant from D (the most deeply branching sequence) than are either A or C (i.e., BD > AD = CD) and (2) because B is specifically related to A, it is less distant from A than it is from C or D (i.e., AB < BC < BD). Since the contemporary sequences in this illustration have diverged different amounts from their common ancestor, they have changed at different average rates. Additive evolutionary trees are independent of assumptions regarding the rates of change in the lineages; they are based only on the accumulated evolutionary distances.

Estimation of evolutionary distances. Although the evolutionary distances separating contemporary sequences are sufficient for inferring an additive evolutionary tree, we do not have this information directly: we can only observe the number of differences between

contemporary sequences. Because later substitutions at a sequence position can obscure previous events at that position, the observed differences are only a lower limit of the evolutionary distance. In practice, a statistical correction is applied to the observed sequence differences to account for the unobserved substitutions and thereby *estimate* the evolutionary distance. Jukes and Cantor (1969) proposed a correction based on three assumptions: (1) All sequence positions are equally subject to change, (2) when a nucleotide changes, it is equally likely to change to any of the three alternative nucleotides, and (3) there are no insertions or deletions. The first two assumptions result in a conservative correction; deviations from them tend to result in under-estimation of evolutionary distances.

Inference of a tree from evolutionary distance estimates. After converting the number of observed differences between pairs of contemporary sequences into estimated evolutionary distances, the corresponding additive evolutionary tree can be inferred. Although there is an exact relationship between evolutionary distance data and a unique additive tree, mere *estimates* of the evolutionary distances may not precisely fit any additive tree. Given the approximate nature of the data, a least-squares analysis is used here to define the branching order and branch lengths most consistent with the data (Fitch and Margoliash 1967; Olsen 1988). The tree error (the disagreement of the evolutionary distance estimates and a given additive tree) is defined as the weighted squared differences between the distance estimates and the corresponding distances in the additive tree. The weight applied to each squared difference is one over the variance (as a measure of the statistical uncertainty) of the Jukes and Cantor distance estimate (Kimura and Ohta 1972). The tree branching order and branch lengths that minimize the total tree error are the inferred phylogenetic tree.

Effect of Lineage-to-Lineage Differences in the Amount of Nucleotide Substitution

No location in the tree in Figure 1 is equally distant from all of the contemporary sequences, and thus the average rate of sequence change could not have been equal in all lineages. Although additive evolutionary trees do not require that all lineages evolve at equal rates, their accuracy depends on the accuracy of the evolutionary distance estimates. If the amount of sequence change varies from lineage to lineage, then any systematic error in the distance estimates will be lineage-dependent; this can result in systematic errors in the inferred branching order. Because of its assumptions, the Jukes and Cantor treatment tends to underestimate evolutionary distances. Thus, it is important to evaluate the accuracy of the inferred phylogenies.

Mitochondrial evolution as a gauge of systematic errors in tree inference. Mitochondrial rRNA sequences provide dramatic examples of the variation in the amount of sequence divergence: They have undergone much more sequence change than their free-living bacterial relatives (Yang et al. 1985). Although this can be seen for the plant mitochondrial sequence in Figure 1, the differences are greater still when a ciliate (or fungal) sequence is considered. Since the errors in evolutionary distance estimates are expected to increase with the amount of sequence divergence (as the number of un-observed changes increases), the behavior of the mitochondrial lineage in inferred phylogenies will reflect the adequacy of the assumptions used to estimate the distances. Because additional evidence (Gray and Doolittle 1982) supports the origin of the mitochondrial lineage in Figure 1, significant deviations from this result should reflect systematic errors.

Figure 3 tests the effectiveness of the Jukes and Cantor (1969) method of estimating evolutionary distances. Four trees are presented, each of which adds another sequence to the analysis. As the sequence content of the tree is varied, the inferred origin of the ciliate mitochondrial rRNA lineage shifts significantly.

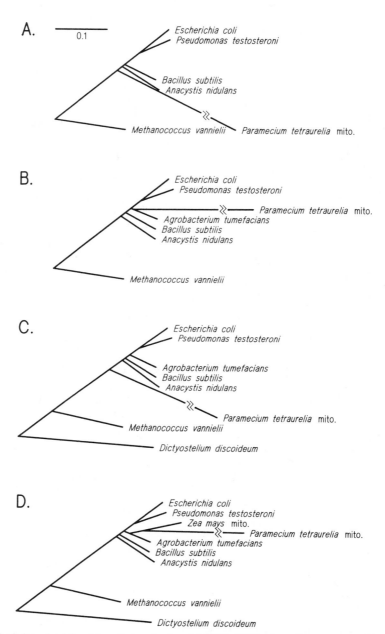

Figure 3. Variation of the inferred origin of the ciliate mitochondrial 16S rRNA when all sequence positions are assumed equally subject to change. The trees were inferred with a least-squares, distance method. Successive panels include one more sequence in the analysis. For compactness, the relationships are presented as rooted trees. Only the horizontal component of the line lengths is significant. The scale bar corresponds to 0.1 substitutions per sequence position. The break in the ciliate mitochondrial lineage is 0.2 substitutions per sequence position. The sequences are available from Huysmans and De Wachter (1986).

The sequences selected for the trees emphasize the perturbations, but the critical elements are (1) a sequence that has changed much more than its specific relatives (the ciliate mitochondrial sequence) and (2) one or more very distant sequences (the archaebacterial and eukaryotic sequences). This combination tends to make the branch point of the mitochondrial sequence leap to a deeper point in the tree (Fig. 3A,C) because the distances from the ciliate mitochondrial sequence to the archaebacterial and eukaryotic sequences are the most underestimated. This effect is countered (Fig. 3B,D) by adding progressively more specific relatives of the mitochondrial sequence (the *A. tumefaciens* and *Z. mays* mitochondrial rRNA sequences) that have diverged from the root of the tree by amounts similar to those of the *A. nidulans*, *E. coli*, and *P. testosteroni* sequences.

Not all sequence positions are equally subject to change. Golding (1983) concluded that significant errors in the estimation of sequence divergence can result from assuming that all sequence positions are equally subject to change. The analysis below investigates the effects of assuming that the 16S rRNA is composed of sequence positions with differing rates of nucleotide substitution, some changing faster than the median rate and others changing more slowly than the median rate. In particular, it is assumed that the rates of change are described by a log-normal distribution.

Estimation of evolutionary distances with site-to-site differences in the substitution rate. When the rate of nucleotide substitution is a function of sequence position, the relationship between sequence similarity, S, and evolutionary distance, x, can be expressed as

$$S(x) = \int_0^\infty f(k) P(kx)\, dk \qquad (1)$$

where $f(k)\,dk$ is the fraction of sequence positions, with nucleotide substitution rates between k and $k + dk$; kx is the average number of substitutions at sequence positions with rate of change k; and $P(kx)$ is the probability of finding identical residues in the two sequences at the sites that have undergone, on average, kx substitutions. If all substitutions are equally likely and if insertions and deletions can be ignored, then

$$P(kx) = \frac{3}{4} \exp\left(-\frac{4}{3} kx\right) + \frac{1}{4} \qquad (2)$$

where exp is the exponentiation operator (Jukes and Cantor 1969). For a log-normal distribution of substitution rates over the positions in the sequences

$$f(k) = \frac{c}{k} \exp\left[-\frac{(\log k)^2}{2\sigma^2}\right] \qquad (3)$$

where σ is the parameter that defines the width of the distribution, log is the natural logarithm operator, and $c = (2\pi\sigma^2)^{-1/2}$. One property of Equation 3 is that

$k = 1$ is the median rate of change, not the average as is commonly employed. Consequently, x is the expected media number of substitutions per sequence position. (It can be shown that the average number of substitutions is $\exp(\sigma^2/2)$ times the median number of substitutions.) To achieve a distribution in which 95% of the sites lie between $1/\alpha$ and α times the median rate of change, $\sigma = (\log \alpha)/2$.

Substituting Equations 2 and 3 into Equation 1 yields

$$S(x) = \int_0^\infty \frac{c}{k} \exp\left[-\frac{(\log k)^2}{2\sigma^2}\right]$$
$$\left[\frac{3}{4} \exp\left(-\frac{4}{3} kx\right) + \frac{1}{4}\right] dk \qquad (4)$$

Letting $\kappa = \log k$, Equation 4 becomes

$$S(x) = \int_{-\infty}^\infty c \exp\left(-\frac{\kappa^2}{2\sigma^2}\right)$$
$$\left\{\frac{3}{4}\exp\left[-\frac{4}{3} \exp(\kappa)x\right] + \frac{1}{4}\right\} d\kappa \qquad (5)$$

or

$$S(x) = \frac{3c}{4} \int_{-\infty}^\infty \exp\left[-\frac{\kappa^2}{2\sigma^2} - \frac{4}{3} \exp(\kappa)x\right] d\kappa + \frac{1}{4} \qquad (6)$$

Equation 6 is easily integrated numerically. However, it is the evolutionary distance, not the similarity, that is desired; consequently, the value of x was found by successive approximation. Given the nth estimate of the evolutionary distance (x_n), the next estimate (x_{n+1}) was determined by

$$x_{n+1} = [S' - S(x_n)]/\left(\frac{dS}{dx}\Big|_{x_n}\right) + x_n \qquad (7)$$

where S' is the observed sequence similarity. The derivative of similarity with respect to evolutionary distance is found by differentiating Equation 5 with respect to x:

$$\frac{dS}{dx} = -\int_{-\infty}^\infty c \exp\left(-\frac{\kappa^2}{2\sigma^2} + \kappa\right) \exp\left[-\frac{4}{3} \exp(\kappa)x\right] d\kappa \qquad (8)$$

Completing the square in the first exponential and taking out the constant factor,

$$\frac{dS}{dx} = -\frac{4}{3} \exp\left(\frac{\sigma^2}{2}\right) \int_{-\infty}^\infty c \exp\left[-\frac{(\kappa - \sigma^2)^2}{2\sigma^2}\right]$$
$$\frac{3}{4} \exp\left[-\frac{4}{3} \exp(\kappa)x\right] d\kappa \qquad (9)$$

Replacing κ with $\lambda = \kappa - \sigma^2$ and rearranging terms,

$$\frac{dS}{dx} = -\frac{4}{3} \exp\left(\frac{\sigma^2}{2}\right)\left(\int_{-\infty}^\infty c \exp\left[-\frac{\lambda^2}{2\sigma^2}\right]\right.$$
$$\left.\left\{\frac{3}{4} \exp\left[-\frac{4}{3} \exp(\sigma^2) \exp(\lambda)x\right] + \frac{1}{4}\right\} d\lambda - \frac{1}{4}\right) \qquad (10)$$

Comparing the integral to that in Equation 5 leads to

$$\frac{dS}{dx} = -\frac{4}{3} \exp\left(\frac{\sigma^2}{2}\right)\left\{S[\exp(\sigma^2)x] - \frac{1}{4}\right\} \quad (11)$$

Thus, Equations 6, 7, and 11 provide an efficient method for estimating evolutionary distances from sequence similarities when the sites in the molecule have a log-normal distribution of substitution rates.

The least-squares evaluation of how well the evolutionary distance estimates fit a given additive tree also requires an estimate of the uncertainties of the distance estimates. The variance in evolutionary distance estimates due to the binomial sampling of sites can be approximated by (1) taking the inferred evolutionary distance to represent the actual value, (2) assuming that all sequence changes are independent, and (3) assuming that the relationship between sequence similarity and evolutionary distance is linear over the relevant range (Kimura and Ohta 1972). Specifically,

$$\text{var}(x) = \text{var}(S)\left(\frac{dS}{dx}\right)^{-2} \quad (12)$$

The variance in sequence similarity is a consequence of the variation in the number of compared residues that happen to be identical. With a homogeneous population, the variance in the number of matching sites is $NP(1 - P)$, where N is the number of sites examined and P is the probability that compared residues are identical. Dividing by N^2 gives the variance of the sequence similarity. Because k, and hence P, varies with position in the molecule, it is necessary to integrate over the distribution. Since a given phylogenetic analysis uses a constant set of sites, the sampling of $f(k)$ can be ignored—the population of sites examined is assumed to be log-normal. Therefore,

$$\text{var}(S) = N^{-2} \int_0^\infty Nf(k)P(kx)[1 - P(kx)]\, dk \quad (13)$$

$$= \frac{1}{N}\int_0^\infty f(k)\left[\frac{3}{4}\exp\left(-\frac{4}{3}kx\right) + \frac{1}{4}\right]$$

$$\left[\frac{3}{4} - \frac{3}{4}\exp\left(-\frac{4}{3}kx\right)\right] dk \quad (14)$$

Rearranging terms,

$$\text{var}(S) = \frac{1}{N}\int_0^\infty f(k)\left\{\frac{1}{2}\left[\frac{3}{4}\exp\left(-\frac{4}{3}kx\right) + \frac{1}{4}\right]\right.$$

$$\left. -\frac{3}{4}\left[\frac{3}{4}\exp\left(-\frac{8}{3}kx\right) + \frac{1}{4}\right] + \frac{1}{4}\right\} dk \quad (15)$$

Comparison with Equations 1 and 2 yields

$$\text{var}(S) = \frac{1}{N}\left[\frac{1}{2}S(x) - \frac{3}{4}S(2x) + \frac{1}{4}\right] \quad (16)$$

Combining Equations 11, 12, and 16 gives

$$\text{var}(x) = \frac{9[2S(x) - 3S(2x) + 1]}{4N\exp(\sigma^2)\{4S[\exp(\sigma^2)x] - 1\}^2} \quad (17)$$

The value of $S(x)$ is the observed sequence similarity. The values of $S(2x)$ and $S[\exp(\sigma^2)x]$ are found using Equation 6, after the evolutionary distance, x, has been estimated as described above. With estimates of the evolutionary distances and their variances, it is possible to infer the corresponding additive tree with the least-squares, distance matrix method.

Effect on the inferred phylogeny of assuming site-to-site differences in the rate of nucleotide substitution. The trees in Figure 3 were based on the assumption that all sequence positions are equally subject to change, and the various inferred trees were inconsistent with one another. The trees in Figure 4, which include the same sequences as those in Figure 3, were inferred with the assumption that 95% of the sequence positions experience between one-eighth and eight times the median rate of nucleotide substitution. These results are self-consistent: Changing the sequence content of the tree has no effect on the inferred branching order and a negligible effect on the inferred branch lengths.

Figure 5 examines the inferred relationships of the urkingdoms for three different compensations for unobserved nucleotide substitutions. The sequence content has been altered from that in Figure 1 so that the placement of the mitochondrial lineage will reflect the adequacy of the distance estimates. In Figure 5A, all the sites are assumed to be equally subject to change. The branching order is the same as that in Figure 1, except for the anomolously deep divergence of the mitochondrial lineage. In Figure 5B, the assumed distribution of rates is the same as that in Figure 4; 95% of the sequence positions analyzed are assumed to experience between one-eighth and eight times the median rate of change. The inferred branching order remains the same, except that the mitochondrial lineage branch point is now in the appropriate place: It branches adjacent to the β and γ purple bacteria, which is the location of the α purple bacterial lineage (see Fig. 1). Figure 5C shows the effect of broadening the assumed distribution of substitution rates still further, such that 95% of the analyzed sequence positions lie between one-eleventh and eleven times the median rate. The ciliate mitochondrial lineage now appears as a specific relative of *P. testosteroni*, to the exclusion of *E. coli*, a branching order inconsistent with the known location of the α purple bacterial (and hence mitochondrial) lineage. Thus, Figure 5C reflects an overcompensation for unobserved substitutions.

Summary. The preceding results show that the inference of reliable phylogenetic trees with a distance method depends on the accurate estimation of evolutionary distances from the sequences differences. However, the only observed errors in branching order invol-

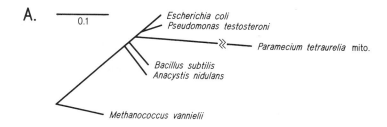

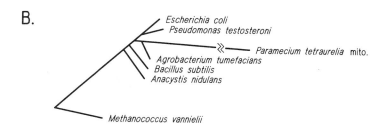

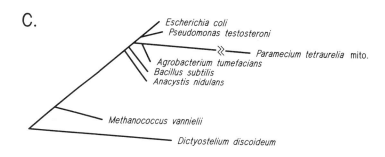

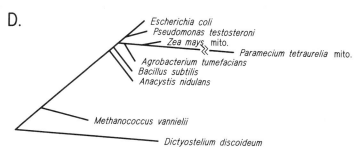

Figure 4. Consistency of the inferred origin of the ciliate mitochondrial 16S rRNA when evolutionary distance estimates acknowledge heterogeneity in the rate of nucleotide change. The rate of change at different sequence positions is assumed to fit a log-normal distribution such that 95% of the sites change at rates between one-eighth and eight times the median rate. The sequences analyzed and the details of the presentation are the same as those in Fig. 3.

ved the very divergent ciliate mitochondrial sequence; other lineages behaved consistently, despite changes in sequence content of the trees and alterations in the method of estimating evolutionary distances. Errors in the distance estimates are most likely to create problems when the tree includes sequences that have diverged varying amounts from their common ancestor and particularly distant outgroups. Such situations should be analyzed with caution. Testing the sensitivity of phylogenetic trees to changes in sequence content provides one simple consistency check. Using a method of estimating evolutionary distances that acknowledges the site-to-site differences in the rate of nucleotide substitution provides more consistent phylogenetic trees than the simpler Jukes and Cantor (1969) method.

A. Undercompensation

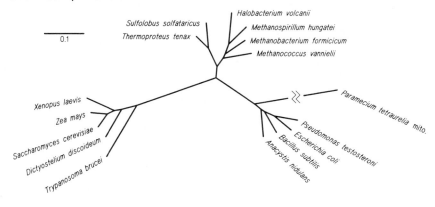

B. Appropriate compensation

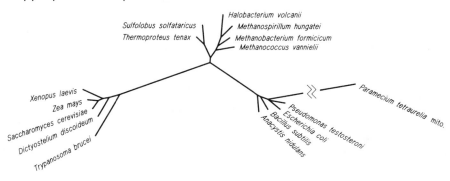

C. Overcompensation

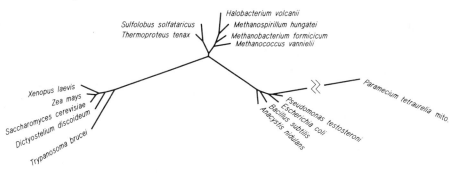

Figure 5. The effect of different amounts of compensation for superimposed substitutions on the inferred urkingdom relationships. Phylogenetic trees that include diverse eukaryotic, eubacterial, and archaebacterial 16S rRNA sequences are presented as a function of the heterogeneity of nucleotide substitution rate assumed in estimating evolutionary distances from observed sequence differences. The behavior of the very divergent ciliate mitochondrial sequence monitors the success of each assumption. (*A*) All sites are assumed to change at the same relative rate; the mitochondrial lineage originates anomolously deeply in the tree, indicating insufficient compensation for superimposed substitutions. (*B*) 95% of the positions are assumed to change at between one-eighth and eight times the median rate; the mitochondrial lineage originates in an appropriate position. (*C*) 95% of the positions are assumed to change at between one-eleventh and eleven times the median rate; the mitochondrial lineage originates as a specific relative of *P. testosteroni*, indicating overcompensation for unobserved nucleotide substitutions in the estimation of evolutionary distances. The sequences are available from Huysmans and De Wachter (1986).

Maximum Parsimony Phylogenetic Trees

Alternative methods of 16S rRNA sequence analysis are discussed with trees relating four taxa, the smallest nontrivial unrooted tree. A tree with four taxa contains five branches: one internal branch and four peripheral branches. The internal branch separates the four peripheral branches into two pairs (sister groups), and, in doing so, it defines the branching pattern of the tree. A specific set of sequence changes occurred in the interval represented by the internal branch; these sequence changes distinguish the ancestors of the two sister groups. Inferring the sequence phylogeny is synonomous with detecting the sequence changes in the internal branch.

Informative sequence positions. Maximum parsimony analysis assumes that the correct phylogenetic tree is consistent with the smallest number of nucleotide substitutions (Fitch 1971). Figure 6A illustrates the evolution of a sequence position that has undergone a substitution in the central branch of the tree. As a consequence of this single change, the two contemporary sequences on one side of the internal branch have one residue (A), and the other two contemporary sequences contain a second residue (C). Whenever a sequence position has one residue shared by two sequences and a second residue shared by the other two sequences, the most parsimonious tree is the one that joins the sequences with identical nucleotides into sister groups, as in Figure 6A; any other branching pattern would require two substitutions to give rise to the observed nucleotides.

Peripheral branch changes can obscure informative events. Figure 6B illustrates a peripheral branch substitution combined with a central branch substitution. Regardless of the assumed branching order, the minimum number of substitutions consistent with the observed nucleotides is two, so a parsimony analysis of this sequence position does not support any particular branching order.

Combinations of peripheral branch changes can be misleading. Figure 6C shows how substitutions in two peripheral branches can mimic a central branch change associated with the wrong branching pattern. On the basis of the observed nucleotides, the sequences containing the A residues appear to be specific relatives, as do the two sequences with G residues. In general, sequence positions at which substitutions have occurred in two or more of the tree branches are problematic.

Slowly changing sequence positions are most reliable. Not all sequence positions accept nucleotide substitutions at the same rate. The rapidly changing sites are most apt to undergo changes in more than one branch. Figure 7A illustrates this point for a tree with peripheral branches six times the length of the internal branch. The curves show the probability that a given sequence position will support the historically correct tree, or one of the two alternative trees, as a function of how rapidly that position is changing. At positions with low substitution rates, the probability of supporting the correct tree is small (because a substitution in the central branch is unlikely), but it is many times greater than the probability of supporting an incorrect tree. Positions with high substitution rates are nearly as apt to support an incorrect branching order as they are the right branching order. Thus, slowly evolving positions provide a small amount of reliable information, whereas rapidly evolving positions superimpose a background of relatively uninformative events.

Felsenstein (1978) pointed out that the nucleotide substitution pattern in Figure 6C is more frequent if two of the peripheral branches, one on either side of

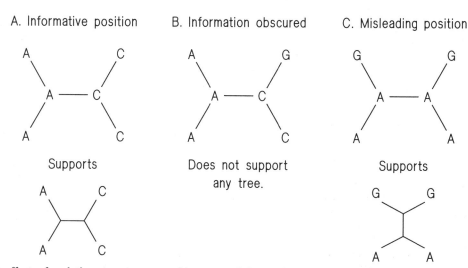

Figure 6. The effects of evolution at a sequence position on tree inference by parsimony. The unrooted trees show the nucleotide found in each of the four contemporary sequences (at the tips) and two ancestral sequences (at the branch points). The identities of the ancestral nucleotides are not available for analysis; they are shown only to clarify the evolutionary events. The branch lengths have no significance. See text for discussion.

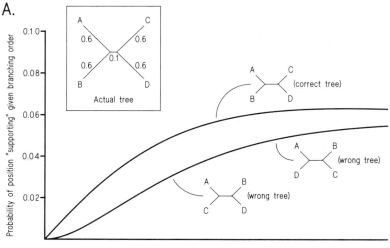

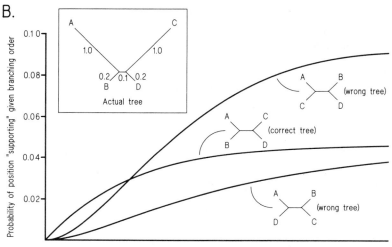

Figure 7. Effect of nucleotide substitution rate on the parsimony information supplied by a sequence position. For each of the three possible branching orders of a four taxa tree, the curves indicate the likelihood that a sequence position will support the given tree branching order (vertical axis) as a function of the relative rate of nucleotide substitution at the position (horizontal axis). (*Insets*) Historically correct trees. The three curves are labeled with their respective branching order and whether or not they represent the historically correct tree. (*A*) All four peripheral tree branches are six times the length of the interior branch. Because the tree is completely symmetrical, the curves indicating the likelihoods of supporting the two incorrect trees are superimposed. (*B*) Two of the peripheral branches are ten times the length of the internal branch, which separates them, and the other two peripheral branches are two times the length of the interior branch. There is a systematic tendency to support the tree that joins the two long branches erroneously.

the internal branch, are particularly long. The tree considered in Figure 7B has two peripheral branches five times the length of the other peripheral branches. Again, the curves give the probability of a sequence position supporting the correct branching order, or one of the incorrect branching orders, as a function of its relative nucleotide substitution rate. As in Figure 7A, positions with low substitution rates preferentially support the correct branching order. However, the more rapidly changing positions in Figure 7B not only increase the noise, but also preferentially support an incorrect branching order (the one that joins the two

longest branches). This is the systematic error described by Felsenstein. These results indicate that the reliability of a parsimony-based analysis is much greater if it is limited to the sequence positions with the lowest nucleotide substitution rates.

Parsimony Analysis of Urkingdom Relationships

Two specific questions are addressed with a parsimony analysis of 16S rRNA data: (1) Are the eubacteria a sister group to the halophiles, to the exclusion of the methanogens, sulfur-dependent archaebacteria, and eukaryotes? (2) Are the eukaryotes a sister group to the sulfur-dependent archaebacteria, to the exclusion of the eubacteria, methanogens, and halophiles?

Limiting the analysis to slowly changing positions. For the purposes of analyzing the relationships of the eukaryotes, eubacteria, and archaebacteria, the slowly changing positions are defined as those with the least intragroup variation. It was required that at least 12 out of 13 eukaryotic (human, rat, frog, brine shrimp, yeast, *Tetrahymena thermophila*, *O. nova*, *P. tetraurelia*, dinoflagellate, *Z. mays*, *D. discoideum*, *T. brucei*, and euglena) sequences contain the same residue and that at least 12 out of 13 eubacterial (*E. coli*, *Myxococcus xanthus*, *Desulfovibrio desulfuricans*, *Thiovulum* sp., *P. testosteroni*, *Rochalimaea quintana*, *A. tumefaciens*, *Flavobacterium heparinum*, *Chlamydiae psittaci*, *Heliobacterium chlorum*, *Bacillus subtilis*, *A. nidulans*, and *Z. mays* chloroplast) sequences share the same residue, although not necessarily the same one as the eukaryotes. Applying a similar stringency (>93% nucleotide conservation) to the available halophile (*Halobacterium volcanii*, *Halobacterium cutirubrum*, *Halobacterium halobium*, and *Halococcus morrhau*), methanogen (*Methanospirilum hungatei*, *Methanobacterium formicicum*, and *Methanococcus vannielii*), and sulfur-dependent archaebacterial (*S. solfataricus* and *T. tenax*) sequences amounts to requiring 100% conservation in these groups. (The sequences are available from Weisburg et al. 1985, 1986; Herzog and Marteaux 1986; Huysmans and De Wachter 1986; Sogin and Elwood 1986; Sogin et al. 1986; Romaniuk et al. 1987.) This criterion for defining slowly changing positions is independent of any assumed intragroup branching order. The rest of this discussion is limited to these sequence positions.

Are the eubacteria specifically related to the halophiles? Lake and co-workers (1985) have proposed that the eubacteria are specifically related to the halophilic archaebacteria. This question can be addressed by a parsimony analysis of four groups: halophiles, eubacteria, methanogens, and sulfur-dependent archaebacteria. In Figure 1, the halophiles and methanogens form a single group, and, without the eukaryotes, the eubacteria are a sister group to the sulfur archaebacteria. Omission of the eukaryotic sequences removes the longest branch from the tree (see Fig. 1), minimizing the potential for systematic error due to long peripheral branches. A parsimony analysis of these four groups indicates that positions (in the *E. coli* numbering system) 34, 289 & 311, 939 & 1344, 982, 1074 & 1083, 1088 & 1097, and 1195 support the tree in Figure 1. Two positions separated by an ampersand (&) are base paired in the 16S rRNA secondary structure (Gutell et al. 1985), and thus are not independently varying traits. The positions supporting an association of the eubacteria with the halophiles (Lake's proposal [Lake et al. 1985]) are 316 & 337 and 940 & 1343. There are no sequence positions supporting the third possible tree, which would associate the eubac-

teria with the methanogens and the sulfur archaebacteria with the halophiles. Thus, in a parsimony analysis that is limited to the most slowly changing sequence positions and that avoids the long branch leading to the eukaryotic sequences, seven positions (or pairs of positions) support the tree in Figure 1, two support Lake's proposal (Lake et al. 1985), and none support the third possible tree.

Are the eukaryotes specifically related to the sulfur-dependent archaebacteria? To address this question, it would be convenient to treat the halophiles and methanogens as a single group (as suggested by Fig. 1). This requires ruling out a relationship of the eukaryotes with the halophiles. By parsimony, positions 245, 283, 284, 503 & 542, 512 & 538, 578, 658, 939 & 1344, 955 & 1255, 1074 & 1083, 1088 & 1097, 1195, 1303 & 1334, 1335, and 1408 support the specific affiliation of the halophiles and methanogens, to the exclusion of the sulfur archaebacteria and the eukaryotes (consistent with Fig. 1). Positions 252 & 274 and 778 suggest an affiliation of the eukaryotes with halophiles, and no positions support an association of the sulfur archaebacteria with the halophiles. Thus, the halophiles and methanogens can be treated as a single group. In keeping with the above criterion of requiring intragroup conservation of the nucleotides analyzed, only those positions in which the halophiles and methanogens share the same nucleotides were utilized in the next analysis.

Figure 1 shows the eukaryotes and eubacteria as sister groups to one another, whereas other proposals (Lake et al. 1984; Wolters and Erdmann 1986) suggest that the eukaryotes are the sister group of the sulfur-dependent archaebacteria, and the eubacteria are the sister group of the halophiles and methanogens. Positions 34, 248 & 276, 338, 339, 549, 923 & 1393, 970, 1202, and 1211 support the unity of the archaebacteria, to the exclusion of the eukaryotes and eubacteria. Positions 955 & 1225, 1303 & 1334, and 1408 unite the eubacteria with the halophiles and methanogens. Positions 34 and 289 & 311 join the eubacteria with the sulfur archaebacteria. Thus, nine positions (or pairs) support the phylogeny in Figure 1, three fit the alternative proposals, and two support the third possible tree.

In summary, the phylogenetic inferences drawn through parsimony analysis are in agreement with those of the distance matrix analysis. I do not wish to argue that these numbers are compelling, that can await additional data.

Evolutionary Parsimony

The method of evolutionary parsimony. Lake (1987) has suggested a new method for inferring the evolutionary relationships between nucleotide sequences. The method, dubbed "evolutionary parsimony," focuses on transversion-type nucleotide substitutions (i.e., the replacement of a purine by a pyrimidine, or vice versa) in the internal segment of a four-organism tree (Fig. 8A).

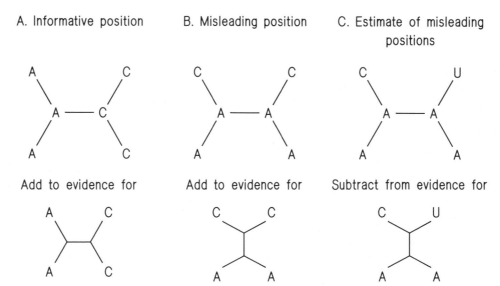

Figure 8. Effects of evolution at a sequence position on tree inference with evolutionary parsimony analysis. The unrooted trees are similar to those in Fig. 6. See text for discussion of the origin and significance of the various possibilities.

The object is to distinguish these central branch transversions from pairs of transversions in peripheral branches that mimic the effects of a central branch transversion (Fig. 8B). The novelty lies in noting that not all pairs of peripheral branch transversions give rise to identical nucleotides; in some sequence positions, they will yield dissimilar nucleotides in the contemporary sequences (Fig. 8C). If transversions are equally likely to give rise to each of the two possible products (e.g., if G is as likely to change to C as it is to U), then the outcomes illustrated in Figure 8B,C will be equally likely (considering only pairs of peripheral branch transversions), and misleading events can be eliminated, on average, by subtracting events of the type in panel C. Accounting for transitions and more complex combinations of transversions yields the following simple rules: (1) Only positions with two purine and two pyrimidine nucleotides are considered; (2) these positions either add or remove support from the phylogeny that unites the two sequences with purines and the two sequences with pyrimidines; (3a) two identical purines and two identical pyrimidines add support; (3b) two different purines and two identical pyrimidines remove support; (3c) two identical purines and two different pyrimidines remove support; and (3d) two different purines and two different pyrimidines add support. The crucial assumption is that transversions are equally likely to yield each of the two possible products (there are also assumptions about the relative likelihood of various types of transitions).

Examining urkingdom relationships with evolutionary parsimony. As in the discussion of parsimony, the rapidly changing sites are most apt to have undergone changes in two or more tree branches; hence, they are more likely to contribute noise than useful information to the inference of the phylogenetic relationships.

Therefore, this analysis is limited to the same "slowly changing" positions as used in the final parsimony analysis (see above). The positions bearing on the unity of the archaebacteria, to the exclusion of the eukaryotes and eubacteria (as in Fig. 1), are +248 & +276, +339, −962 & +973, +1202, and +1211. The sign in front of each position indicates whether it is to be added or subtracted in the evaluation of the branching order. Again, treating each paired position as one-half, the total support for the urkingdom relationships in Figure 1 is four positions. The positions bearing on the possible affiliation of the eubacteria with the methanogens and halophiles, and the eukaryotes with the sulfur archaebacteria, are +1303 & +1334, for a net score of +1. Similarly, the positions bearing on the third possible tree are +289 & +311, for a net score of +1. Thus, an evolutionary parsimony analysis of the most conserved sequence positions in 16S rRNA supports the urkingdom relationships in Figure 1.

CONCLUSIONS

When used with attention to their limitations, three diverse methods of analysis can be used to infer the same phylogenetic relationships of eukaryotes, eubacteria, and archaebacteria. Three points merit emphasis. First, it is possible to infer valid evolutionary relationships in the presence of lineage-to-lineage differences in the average rate of sequence change. Many interesting phylogenetic relationships involve sequences that have diverged to different extents from their common ancestor. However, such studies require an awareness of the assumptions in the method being utilized.

Second, not all sequence positions in a molecule are equally subject to change. In studies of distant phylogenetic relationships, this is particularly significant because the most rapidly changing positions will be completely randomized and hence will have ceased to diverge. This increases both the random errors in tree inferences and the susceptibility to systematic errors.

Finally, there is no substitute for raw data: More information will always yield more reliable phylogenetic inferences. In this regard, the recently published 23S rRNA-based phylogeny of Leffers and coworkers (1987) supports the 16S rRNA-based urkingdom relationships in Figure 1. As other molecules are examined, the clarity with which we can reconstruct early evolutionary events will continue to improve.

ACKNOWLEDGMENTS

I sincerely thank Carl. R. Woese and Norman R. Pace for many discussions about this work, Norman Pace for providing critical comments on the manuscript, and Arthur Koch for commenting on the mathematical section. Much of the work described was supported by Office of Naval Research grant N14-86-K-0268.

REFERENCES

Brosius, J., T.J. Dull, D.D. Sleeter, and H.F. Noller. 1981. Gene organization and primary structure of a ribosomal RNA operon from *Escherichia coli*. *J. Mol. Biol.* **148:** 107.

Felsenstein, J. 1978. Cases in which parsimony or compatibility methods will be positively misleading. *Syst. Zool.* **27:** 401.

Fitch, W.M. 1971. Toward defining the course of evolution: Minimum change for a specific tree topology. *Syst. Zool.* **20:** 400.

Fitch, W.M. and E. Margoliash. 1967. Construction of phylogenetic trees: A method based on mutational distances as estimated from cytochrome *c* sequences is of general applicability. *Science* **155:** 279.

Golding, G.B. 1983. Estimation of DNA and protein sequence divergence: An examination of some assumptions. *Mol. Biol. Evol.* **1:** 125.

Gray, M.W. and W.F. Doolittle. 1982. Has the endosymbiont hypothesis been proven? *Microbiol. Rev.* **46:** 1.

Gutell, R.R., B. Weiser, C.R. Woese, and H.F. Noller. 1985. Comparative anatomy of 16-S-like ribosomal RNA. *Prog. Nucleic Acid Res. Mol. Biol.* **32:** 155.

Herzog, M. and L. Marteaux. 1986. Dinoflagellate 17S rRNA sequence inferred from the gene sequence: Evolutionary implications. *Proc. Natl. Acad. Sci.* **83:** 8644.

Huysmans, E. and R. De Wachter. 1986. Compilation of small ribosomal subunit RNA sequences. *Nucleic Acids Res.* **14:** r73.

Jukes, T.H. and C.R. Cantor. 1969. Evolution of protein molecules. In *Mammalian protein metabolism* (ed. H.N. Munro), p. 21. Academic Press, New York.

Kandler, O. and W. Zillig, eds. 1986. *Archaebacteria '85*. Gustav Fischer Verlag, New York.

Kimura, M. and T. Ohta. 1972. On the stochastic model for estimation of mutational distance between homologous proteins. *J. Mol. Evol.* **2:** 87.

Klenk, H.-P., B. Haas, V. Schwass, and W. Zillig. 1986. Hybridization homology: A new parameter for the analysis of phylogenetic relations, demonstrated with the urkingdom of the archaebacteria. *J. Mol. Evol.* **24:** 167.

Lake, J.A. 1987. A rate-independent technique for analysis of nucleic acid sequences: Evolutionary parsimony. *Mol. Biol. Evol.* **4:** 167.

Lake, J.A., E. Henderson, M. Oakes, and M.W. Clark. 1984. Eocytes: A new ribosome structure indicates a kingdom with a close relationship to eukaryotes. *Proc. Natl. Acad. Sci.* **81:** 3786.

Lake, J.A., M.W. Clark, E. Henderson, S.P. Fay, M. Oakes, A. Scheinman, J.P. Thornber, and R.A. Mah. 1985. Eubacteria, halobacteria, and the origin of photosynthesis: The photocytes. *Proc. Natl. Acad. Sci.* **82:** 3716.

Leffers, H., J. Kjems, L. Østergaard, N. Larsen, and R.A. Garrett. 1987. Evolutionary relationships amongst archaebacteria: A comparative study of 23S ribosomal RNAs of a sulfur-dependent extreme thermophile, an extreme halophile and a thermophilic methanogen. *J. Mol. Biol.* **195:** 43.

Olsen, G.J. 1988. Phylogenetic analysis using ribosomal RNA. *Methods Enzymol.* **164:** (in press).

Oyaizu, H., B. Debrunner-Vossbrink, L. Mandelco, J.A. Studier, and C.R. Woese. 1987. The green non-sulfur bacteria: A deep branching in the eubacterial line of descent. *Syst. Appl. Microbiol.* **9:** 47.

Romaniuk, P.J., B. Zoltowska, T.J. Trust, D.J. Lane, G.J. Olsen, N.R. Pace, and D.A. Stahl. 1987. *Campylobacter pyloridis*: The spiral bacterium associated with human gastritis is not a true *Campylobacter*. *J. Bacteriol.* **169:** 2137.

Schwartz, R.M. and M.O. Dayhoff. 1978. Origins of prokaryotes, eukaryotes, mitochondria, and chloroplasts: A perspective is derived from protein and nucleic acid sequence data. *Science* **199:** 395.

Sogin, M.L. and H.J. Elwood. 1986. Primary structure of the *Paramecium tetraurelia* small-subunit rRNA coding region: Phylogenetic relationships within the ciliophora. *J. Mol. Evol.* **23:** 53.

Sogin, M.L., H.J. Elwood, and J.H. Gunderson. 1986. Evolutionary diversity of eukaryotic small subunit rRNA genes. *Proc. Natl. Acad. Sci.* **83:** 1383.

Tomioka, N. and M. Sugiura. 1983. The complete nucleotide sequence of a 16S ribosomal RNA gene from a blue-green alga, *Anacystis nidulans*. *Mol. Gen. Genet.* **191:** 46.

Weisburg, W.G., T.P. Hatch, and C.R. Woese. 1986. Eubacterial origin of *Chlamydiae*. *J. Bacteriol.* **167:** 570.

Weisburg, W.G., C.R. Woese, M.E. Dobson, and E. Weiss. 1985. A common origin of rickettsiae and certain plant pathogens. *Science* **230:** 556.

Woese, C.R. 1987. Bacterial evolution. *Microbiol. Rev.* **51:** 221.

Woese, C.R. and G.E. Fox. 1977. Phylogenetic structure of the prokaryotic domain: The primary kingdoms. *Proc. Natl. Acad. Sci.* **74:** 5088.

Woese, C.R. and G.J. Olsen. 1986. Archaebacterial phylogeny: Perspectives on the urkingdoms. *Syst. Appl. Microbiol.* **7:** 161.

Woese, C.R. and R.S. Wolfe, eds. 1985. *The Bacteria*, vol. 8: *Archaebacteria*. Academic Press, Orlando, Florida.

Woese, C.R., E. Stackebrandt, T.J. Macke, and G.E. Fox. 1985. A phylogenetic definition of the major eubacterial taxa. *Syst. Appl. Microbiol.* **6:** 143.

Wolters, J. and V.A. Erdmann. 1986. Cladistic analysis of 5S rRNA and 16S rRNA secondary and primary structure— The evolution of eukaryotes and their relation to archaebacteria. *J. Mol. Evol.* **24:** 152.

Yang, D., Y. Oyaizu, H. Oyaizu, G.J. Olsen, and C.R. Woese. 1985. Mitochondrial origins. *Proc. Natl. Acad. Sci.* **82:** 4443.

Zuckerkandl, E. and L. Pauling. 1965. Molecules as documents of evolutionary history. *J. Theor. Biol.* **8:** 357.

Prokaryotes and Archaebacteria Are Not Monophyletic: Rate Invariant Analysis of rRNA Genes Indicates That Eukaryotes and Eocytes Form a Monophyletic Taxon

J.A. LAKE

Molecular Biology Institute and Department of Biology, University of California, Los Angeles, California 90024

Correctly determining the evolutionary origins of extant organisms requires accurate reconstruction of the molecular tree that relates all organisms. Phylogenetic analyses of rRNA to determine the earliest branchings of extant organisms, however, have not properly accounted for the unequal rate paradox and thus have reached erroneous conclusions. This paradox causes even the most robust tree-construction algorithms, such as parsimony, to place organisms from rapidly evolving groups, like eubacteria and eukaryotes, together consistently, even though they may not be phylogenetically related. Recently, a class of rate-invariant treeing algorithms (evolutionary parsimony), not subject to the unequal rate paradox, has been developed to investigate deep evolutionary divergences. Analysis of rRNA sequences by evolutionary parsimony rejects the archaebacterial theory for the origin of eukaryotes and supports the eocyte tree (at the .003% significance level).

The eocyte tree indicates that eukaryotes evolved from the eocytes, a group of extremely thermophilic sulfur-metabolizing prokaryotes. The eocyte tree (shown in Fig. 1) exhibits a fundamental bifurcation into two (not three) taxanomic divisions: a proto-bacterial group (parkaryotes) and a proto-eukaryotic group (karyotes). This bifucation is the deepest division separating extant organisms yet found and renders both the prokaryotic/eukaryotic grouping and the archaebacterial grouping polyphyletic. Hence, both the prokaryotic/eukaryotic and the archaebacterial classifications are improper taxanomic groupings. The tree supports the eocyte classification proposed previously (Lake et al. 1984) and suggests that the ancestor of eukaryotes was an extremely thermophilic and sulfur-metabolizing prokaryote.

METHODS

Sequence alignments. A set of aligned sequences was constructed from 32 small subunit rRNA sequences, representing the eukaryotic (10), eocytic (3), methanogenic (3), halobacterial (4), and eubacterial (12) lineages. Two alignment procedures were followed. In the first, the star alignment, representative members of the four remaining groups were first aligned with the eocyte *Thermoproteus tenax*. These alignments, and all subsequent alignments, were performed using the Align program of the Dayhoff

package. This procedure was chosen because the "star" is not biased toward any particular evolutionary tree. The star alignment is neutral in that it does not favor a particular branching pattern. The second alignment, the archaebacterial alignment, is a reconstruction from the literature of the alignments used to derive the archaebacterial tree. In particular, it uses the eukaryotic-eubacterial alignment of McCarroll et al. (1983). Details will be provided elsewhere (Lake 1987c). Two regions (1–510 and 1431–1469 in the *E. coli* numbering system) could not be aligned consistently among all groups. Hence, these were not included in either alignments.

Tree construction. Trees were constructed using the rate-independent technique of evolutionary parsimony (Lake 1987a), with branch lengths determined by operator metrics (Lake 1987b). Four taxa trees were combined using the neighborliness procedure (Fitch 1981). The tree was rooted using parsimony rooting.

RESULTS

The evolutionary tree that relates all known types of organisms is shown in Figure 1. This tree, derived using evolutionary parsimony analysis, places the eubacteria, halobacteria, and methanogens in the supertaxa consisting of the neighbors on the left side of the tree. They are separated by the deepest phylogenetic division yet known from the supertaxa on the right, consisting of the eocytes and the eukaryotes.

Two features of the tree are unusual. First, the tree contains groups that are characterized by high rates of substitution ("fast-clock" organisms: the eubacteria and the eukaryotes) as well as a group with an intermediate substitution rate, the halobacteria. These fast-clock organisms have substitution rates nearly an order of magnitude greater than the "slow-clock" organisms. Second, the two fast-clock groups, the eubacteria and the nuclear genes of the eukaryotes, are both sister groups of slower-clock organisms. It is this second feature that has made the topology of the tree so difficult to determine (Lake 1986a).

The tree was derived by evolutionary parsimony, using the neighborliness algorithm to extend the individual 4-taxa trees to the complete 32-taxa tree. The deepest branching that is the most susceptible to the unequal rate paradox, and one of the most important

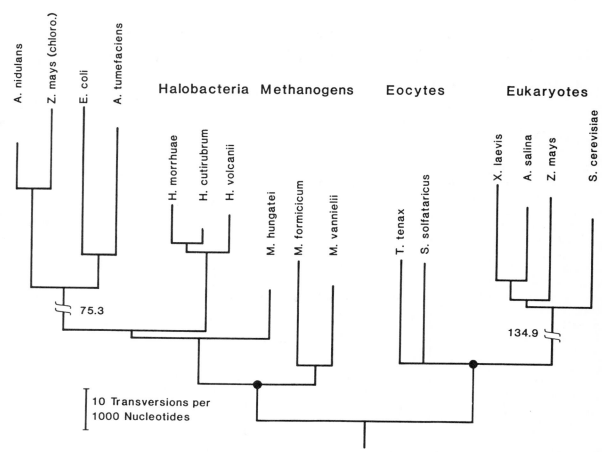

Figure 1. The rooted evolutionary tree that relates all known types of extant organisms. The five groups are (from left to right) eubacteria, halobacteria, methanogens, eocytes, and eukaryotes. Eubacteria and eukaryotes are "fast-clock" organisms; hence, the lengths of the branches leading to each of these groups has been shortened. The true lengths of the branches (75.3 and 134.9 transversion units, respectively) are listed at the sides of the branches.

relationships predicted by the tree, is the 4-taxa subtree that relates the eubacteria, the halobacteria, the eocytes, and the eukaryotes. The significance that can be attached to this topology, in essence, represents the certainty with which the eocyte tree and classification are supported over the archaebacterial tree and classification. Given a tree with the topology of this branch shown in Figure 1, it would be unlikely that parsimony could select the correct tree, since the branch lengths have the pattern for which parsimony is inappropriate. In these cases when the unequal rate paradox (Felsenstein 1978) applies, a rate-invariant algorithm is required. Hence, evolutionary parsimony was employed.

When Can Parsimony Fail?

Two simple examples illustrate when parsimony can fail (Fig. 2). The "true tree" shown in Figure 2a refers to the reference tree topology used to calculate the data, and the "most parsimonious tree" is the tree inferred from analysis of the calculated sequences. In these examples, the probability of substitution is equal for all bases. Thus, for an RNA sequence, an A would

be replaced with equal likelihood by U, C, or G. When there is a high probability of nucleotide substitution in the central branch of the initial tree and low probabilities in the other branches, the pattern xxyy occurs at most positions. This is the informative pattern for parsimony and identifies the tree that positions taxa 1 and 2 together and 3 and 4 together as being the most parsimonious. The absence of other patterns, except for xxxx, indicates that most substitutions are consistent. In this example, parsimony correctly predicts the initial tree.

In the second example (Fig. 2b), the probability of nucleotide substitutions is very high in the peripheral branches leading to taxa 2 and 4 and low in the branches leading to taxa 1 and 3 and in the central branch. Typical sequences are shown in the panel below the true tree, but the expected pattern xxyy that is diagnostic for the true tree is not present. Contrary to expectations, the informative pattern for parsimony that is present is xyxy. (For this example, calculations show that, in the limit of infinite substitution in branches 2 and 4, the xyxy pattern should occur at fully 3 out of every 16 positions.) Hence, the most parsimonious—or

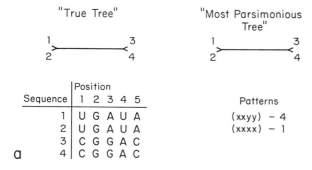

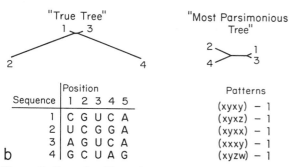

Figure 2. Examples illustrating when parsimony correctly selects a tree and when it fails. Branch lengths (of either 0 or 0.8) represent the relative probabilities of a nucleotide substitution at any one position. The patterns observed in the aligned sequences and the number of their occurrences are shown adjacent to the sequence. (*a*) Parsimony correctly predicts the true tree; (*b*) the tree predicted by parsimony places taxa 1 and 3 and taxa 2 and 4 together in a different topological arrangement from that found in the true tree.

minimum substitution—tree in Figure 2b is not the initial tree but the tree that connects taxa 1 and 3 and connects 2 and 4. In this example, parsimony has picked an incorrect tree because substitutions inserted in peripheral branches of the tree have mimicked the pattern normally produced by substitutions in the central branch of an alternative tree topology. Note that this classic case in which parsimony fails corresponds to the long-short, long-short branch lengths of the motif of the tree illustrated in Figure 1. This explains the need for the rate-invariant method of evolutionary parsimony.

Testing the Critical Central Branch Topology

Testing of the central branch of the eubacterial, halobacterial, eocytic, eukaryotic tree is shown in Figure 3 (Lake 1987c). Using approximately 1.3 million base quartets, calculated from the more than 1000 trees that span these four sets of sequences, the significance of the three alternative trees was calculated using evolutionary parsimony. Calculations were made for two different alignments of the sequences. In the star alignment, rRNA sequences were aligned, using standard computer algorithms, by referencing sequences pairwise with respect to a standard (*T. tenax*) sequence. The archaebacterial alignment is a reconstruction of published alignments using the eubacterial-eukaryotic relationship of C.R. Woese and collaborators as described in Methods. From the significance plot shown in Figure 3, it is apparent that there is highly significant support for the eocyte tree (between .003% and .03%,

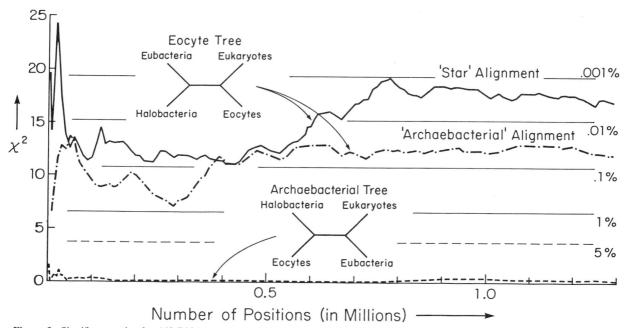

Figure 3. Significance plot for 16S RNA sequences. This plot was derived from sequences from 12 eubacteria, 4 halobacteria, 3 eocytes, and 9 eukaryotes and is based on comparison of approximately 1.3 million sequence quartets. The eocyte tree is selected, at a high significance level, for two sequence alignments. In contrast, there is no support for the archaebacterial tree. The "star" alignment is a global alignment by the Align program of the Dayhoff package. The archaebacterial alignment is a reconstruction from the literature, as described in Methods. (Adapted from Lake 1987c.)

depending on which alignment is used) and no support for the archaebacterial tree. (There is also no support for the third topological alternative; data not shown.) Hence, there is strong and unambiguous support for the early branching orders of this tree. This branching topology is central for understanding the early evolution of organisms and for their proper classification.

The topology and unusual pattern of branch lengths of the tree have obviously contributed to the incorrect view that archaebacteria might be monophylectic, even though they are extremely diverse. In particular, the long length of the peripheral branch leading to the eukaryotes (160 transversion units) and of the peripheral branch leading to the eubacteria (110 transversion units) make these two groups both appear different from all the others. For example, if we compute the distance from the eocytes to the methanogens from the tree in Figure 1 (60 transversion units) and compare it with that from the eocytes to the eukaryotes (180 transversion units), our immediate (and very incorrect) impulse is to say that the eocytes and methanogens are closely related. Reflection and careful analysis show, however, that taxa that are close in distance are not necessarily sister taxa.

DISCUSSION

Importance of the Correct Tree and Classification

The importance of obtaining the correct tree cannot be overemphasized. The tree represents the tangible history of cells and their evolution. Anyone interested in reconstructing the events that led to the development of any enzyme, of a family of enzymes, of the organization of genes and operons, or of mechanisms of RNA processing (to mention a few subjects) must propose and test schemes that are in accord with the evolutionary record. Use of the wrong tree is guaranteed to produce nonsense, or worse, to mislead. The power of a classification based on an incorrect tree to mislead is illustrated by the arginine deiminase pathway found in the photocytes (eubacteria and halobacteria). Because of the high visibility and less than critical acceptance given by many to the archaebacterial tree, this pathway seemed to defy simple (i.e., parsimonious) interpretations since it was found in two "kingdoms." At the time, investigators were misdirected to propose either (1) that the pathway was invented twice or (2) that it was laterally transferred between kingdoms (Stalon 1985). In fact, the arginine deiminase pathway is explained by a single invention when the tree in Figure 1 is used. The incorrect tree and classification had great negative power to obscure and misdirect.

A New Perspective

A new perspective comes with this new tree topology. Most significantly, the eukaryotic cell is seen to be

the topologically nearest neighbor of a thermophilic sulfur-respiring group, the eocytes (and not to the *Escherichia coli*-like eubacteria). Likewise, the bacteria are seen to have arisen from a protobacterial group that used methanogenesis (or possibly even sulfur metabolism; see Stetter and Gaag 1983) as an energy source. This fundamental division into two groups is likewise supported by the distribution of many cellular properties.

Consider the organization of rRNA operons. The operon in eocytes is characterized by the presence of adjacent 16S and 23S genes and the lack of a tRNA spacer between them (see, e.g., Leinfelder et al. 1985). Furthermore, the same rRNA organization is found in eukaryotes. In addition, the 5S rRNA of eocytes is not in the rRNA operon but is found elsewhere on the chromosome, just as the 5S rRNA gene is typically separated from other rRNA genes in eukaryotes. Thus, eocytes and eukaryotes (see, e.g., Gerbi 1985) share a common organization of rRNA genes. rRNA operons of the protobacterial taxon share a different type of organization. Their operons start with the 16S gene; this is followed by a tRNA spacer, by the 23S rRNA, by the 5S rRNA, and then, typically, by another tRNA. This pattern, or minor variations of it, is found in eubacteria (for review, see Gerbi 1985), in halobacteria (Hui and Dennis 1985), and in methanogens (Lechner et al. 1985). Hence, both patterns of rRNA organization are consistent with, and explained by, the dichotomous tree derived here. In contrast, the archaebacterial tree and classification require that both types of operons had to be invented twice. This is an unlikely scenario.

A different type of sequence data, which have recently become available, provides another example of data consistent with this tree. Gas vesicles of halobacteria and eubacteria (and a methanogen) are constructed from a single protein molecule (Walsby 1978). Initially, it was thought that the presence of similar-appearing vesicles, in what were then thought to be unrelated bacterial kingdoms, was an artifact representing either (1) two nonhomologous convergently evolved structures or (2) laterally transferred genes. Protein sequences now available (Walker et al. 1984) from the eubacterial and halobacterial strains indicate that both of these assumptions were false and that the vesicles represent a single evolutionary invention. The sequences show strong homology, at the amino acid level, between halobacterial and eubacterial sequences. Second, the intraeubacterial and intrahalobacterial homologies are even stronger than those of the intergroup (eubacterial and halobacterial). This indicates that lateral transfer of genes between eubacterial and halobacterial species is not likely (unless it occurred at the time one of the groups was forming). Thus, protein sequence data on the gas vesicles support the tree.

Many cellular characteristics support this tree (for a brief compilation, see Lake 1986b). Included among these are the phylogenetic distributions of tetraether lipids, 2Fe-2S ferredoxin, C40 carotenoids, fatty acid esters, C50 carotenoids, ribosomal structures, carotenoid synthesis, and arginine deiminase pathways.

Biological Classification and Polyphyly

Biological thought is profoundly affected by classifications, since they provide the vantage point from which evolutionary relationships of organisms are perceived. For this reason, it is useful to look at the tree presented in this paper and simultaneously to view past and present proposals for the classification of organisms. Three proposals will concern us: the traditional prokaryotic-eukaryotic classification, the more recent archaebacterial classification (Woese and Fox 1977; Woese 1981), and the recently proposed eocyte (Lake et al. 1984) and karyotic classifications (Lake 1987c). Individual ideas on classification are themselves changing. Although some systematists accept the value of paraphyletic groups and some dispute them (for discussions, see Mayr 1969; Wiley 1981), *systematists universally eschew polyphyletic taxa.*

The view that all extant organisms belong to one of two groups defined by the presence of a nucleus or by the lack of a nucleus is the traditional eukaryotic-prokaryotic dichotomy. This classification, illustrated in Figure 4, places those cells with a nuclei into the eukaryotic taxon and places everything else into the prokaryotic taxon. Thus, prokaryote is a description of a group defined in a negative sense; they are organisms that do not have a nucleus (see, e.g., Eldredge 1987). Having the advantage of hindsight, one can recognize that the prokaryotic classification is faulty. The reason is that prokaryotes consist of two groups derived from separate ancestors. Thus, *prokaryotes are a polyphyletic taxon.* One part of the taxon consists of the eubacteria, the halobacteria, and the methanogens and the other part consists of the eocytes. It was a mistake to construct a classification when only one group, the eukaryotes, was known to be monophyletic.

The prokaryotic-eukaryotic concept changed in the late 1970s, when eubacteria were recognized as a monophyletic group (Woese and Fox 1977). Unfortunately, all of the remaining prokaryotic organisms were classified into a separate taxon (the archaebacteria, i.e., the noneubacterial prokaryotes). This grouping is shown in Figure 5. Although this seemed to be an advance at the time, in retrospect, one sees that it did not create a monophyletic grouping. The archaebacteria are a *polyphyletic taxon just as the prokaryotes were.* In this instance, recognition of the eubacteria did not resolve the grouping of the noneubacterial prokaryotes.

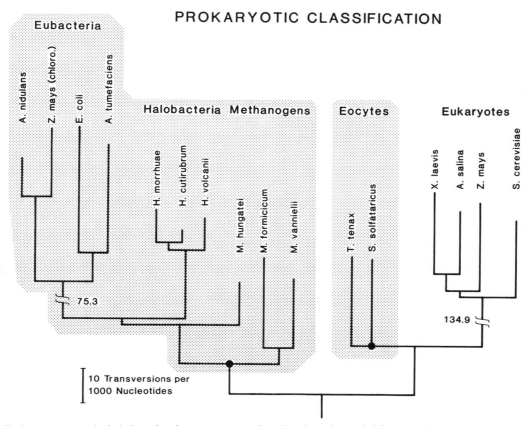

Figure 4. Prokaryotes are polyphyletic and an improper taxon, since they have descended from two last common ancestors. The ancestor on the left gave rise to the eubacteria, halobacteria, and methanogens (including *Thermoplasma*). The remaining prokaryotic group on the right, the eocytes, has a separate origin.

ARCHAEBACTERIAL CLASSIFICATION

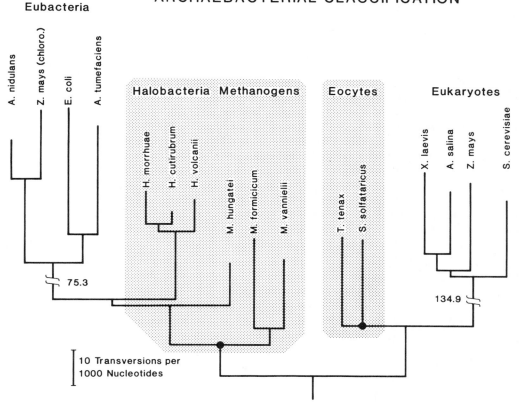

Figure 5. Archaebacteria are polyphyletic and an improper taxon, since they have descended from two last common ancestors. The ancestor on the left gave rise to halobacteria, methanogens, and eubacteria (not in the group). The remaining group on the right, the eocytes, has a separate origin.

To construct a classification that accurately reflects the topology of the tree in Figure 1, one must accommodate the central bifurcation. This is accomplished in the classification shown in Figure 6 by the creation of two superkingdoms (Lake 1987c). The taxon on the right consists of eocytes and eukaryotes. By naming this group karyotes (Karyotae), one removes the redundancy that was previously implied in the name eukaryotes (true + karyotes) and communicates that their common ancestor contributed genes to both eocytes and the nucleus. Karyotes share features of ribosomal operon organization of intron occurrence (Larsen et al. 1986), of ribosome structure (Lake et al. 1984), and of polymerase structure (Zillig et al. 1982) that are eukaryotic. The other branch of the tree, the parkaryotes, has properties much more like those that we expect of bacteria, including ribosomal organization. The name parkaryotes (Parkaryotae) reflects an independent phylogenetic status on a par with that of the karyotes and corrects the antecedent relationship implied by the term *pro*karyotes. This proposal generates monophyletic and balanced superkingdoms. Both taxa are rich in biochemical diversity and both contain large numbers of species. In keeping with standard practice, the common ancestor that gave rise to each of the groups is included in the group, but the ancestor leading to all extant life is not.

The Last Common Ancestor Was Sulfur-metabolizing and Quite Likely Thermophilic

Given the tree that relates all extant organisms, we can ask what the properties of the ancestor that gave rise to this group were. It can be stated with relative confidence that the ancestor was sulfur-metabolizing and quite possibly thermophilic if the distribution of character states is analyzed by parsimony (Fitch 1977). *Thermoproteus tenax* and *S. solfataricus* are both sulfur metabolizers, and it has been reported that sulfur reduction, at low but measurable levels, is a vestigial property of the eukaryotes. Thus, the last common ancestor of the karyotic lineage is most parsimoniously deduced to have been a sulfur-metabolizer. Many methanogens are able to reduce sulfur at low but significant rates in the presence of H_2 (Stetter and Gaag 1983). This ability to reduce sulfur is present in the methanogens *Methanaspirillum hungatei*, *Methanobacterium formicicum*, *Methanococcus vannielii*, and many others. Hence, parsimony predicts that the last common ancestor of the parkaryotes was itself a sulfur-reducer. The most parsimonious interpretation of these data is that the last common ancestor of extant organisms also metabolized sulfur.

This universal ancestor also might have been an extreme thermophile. An analysis, similar to that de-

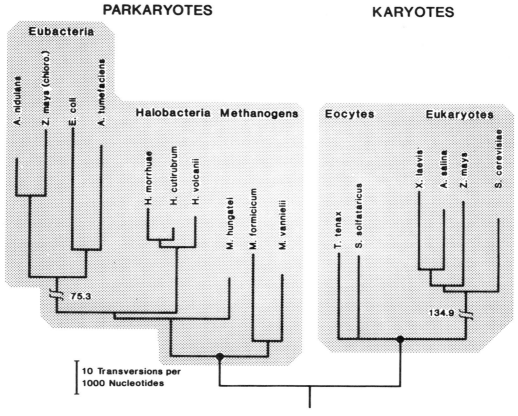

Figure 6. The karyotic-parkaryotic classification defines two useful monophyletic groups. It organizes all taxa into two monophyletic superkingdoms: the karyotes and the parkaryotes. The parkaryotic group contains the eubacteria, halobacteria, and methanogens (including *Thermoplasma*). The karyotic group consists of the eocytes and the eukaryotes. (Adapted from Lake 1987c.) The term paleocyte is suggested for organisms branching before the eubacterial-eukaryotic common ancestor, should any be found subsequently.

scribed above, for the distribution of extreme thermophily indicates that the last common ancestor of all organisms may have been an extreme thermophile. A more complete testing of this conclusion, however, requires more accurately defining the origin of the eukaryotic branch. Until this has been accomplished, parsimony analysis indicates that an extremely thermophilic last common ancestor was likely, but does not entirely exclude a mesophilic one.

Determining the evolutionary tree that relates all organisms has been hampered in the past by a lack of sequence analysis techniques and by a lack of appreciation of the subtleties and pitfalls of the tree-construction process. We are now on the verge of understanding the tree and its earliest branchings. With this knowledge will come, hopefully, a new and deeper comprehension of the origin of extant organisms.

ACKNOWLEDGMENTS

This work was supported by research grants from the National Science Foundation (PCM-83-16926) and the National Institute of General Medical Science (GM-24034).

REFERENCES

Eldredge, N. 1987. *Life pulse*. Facts on File Publishers, New York.

Felsenstein, J. 1978. Cases in which parsimony or compatibility methods will be positively misleading. *Syst. Zool.* **27:** 401.

Fitch, W. 1977. On the problem of generating the most parsimonious tree. *Am. Nat.* **111:** 223.

———. 1981. A non-sequential method for constructing trees and hierarchical classifications. *J. Mol. Evol.* **18:** 30.

Gerbi, S.A. 1985. Evolution of ribosomal DNA. In *Molecular evolutionary genetics* (ed. R.J. MacIntyre), p. 419. Plenum Press, New York.

Hui, I. and P.P. Dennis. 1985. Characterization of the ribosomal RNA gene clusters in *Halobacterium cutirubrum*. *J. Biol. Chem.* **260:** 899.

Lake, J.A. 1986a. An alternative to archaebacterial dogma. *Nature* **319:** 626.

———. 1986b. In defence of bacterial phylogeny. *Nature* **321:** 658.

———. 1987a. A rate-independent technique for analysis of nucleic acid sequences: Evolutionary parsimony. *Mol. Biol. Evol.* **4:** 167.

———. 1987b. Determining evolutionary distances from highly diverged nucleic acid sequences: Operator metrics. *J. Mol. Evol.* (in press).

———. 1987c. Origin of the nucleus: Eukaryotic beginnings deduced by rate-invariant analysis of rRNA sequences. *Nature* (in press).

Lake, J.A., E. Henderson, M. Oakes, and M.W. Clark. 1984. Eocytes: A new ribosome structure indicates a kingdom with a close relationship to eukaryotes. *Proc. Natl. Acad. Sci.* **81**:3786.

Larsen, N., H. Leffers, J. Kjems, and R.. Garrett. 1986. Evolutionary divergence between the ribosomal RNA operons of *Halococcus morrhuae* and *Desulfurococcus mobilis. Syst. App. Microbiol.* **7**: 49.

Lechner, K., G. Wich, and A. Bock. 1985. The nucleotide sequences of the 16S rRNA gene and flanking regions from *Methanobacterium formicicum*: On the phylogenetic relationship between methanogenic and halophilic archaebacteria. *Syst. Appl. Microbiol.* **6**: 157.

Leinfelder, W., M. Jarsch, and A. Bock. 1985. The phylogenetic position of the sulfur-dependent archaebacterium *Thermoproteus tenax*: Sequence of the 16S rRNA gene. *Syst. Appl. Microbiol.* **6**: 164.

Mayr, E. 1969. *Principles of systematic zoology.* McGraw-Hill, New York.

McCarroll, R., G.J. Olsen, Y.D. Stahl, C.R. Woese, and M.L. Sogin. 1983. Nucleotide sequence of the *Dictyostelium discoideum* small-subunit ribosomal ribonucleic acid inferred from the gene sequence: Evolutionary implications. *Biochemistry* **22**: 5858.

Stalon, V. 1985. Evolution of arginine metabolism. In *evolution of prokaryotes* (ed. K.H. Schleifer and E. Stackebrandt), p. 277. Academic Press, New York.

Stetter, K.O. and G. Gaag. 1983. Reduction of molecular sulphur by methanogenic bacteria. *Nature* **305**: 309.

Walker, J.E., P.K. Hayes, and A.E. Walsby. 1984. Homology of gas vesicle proteins in cyanobacteria and halobacteria. *J. Gen. Microbiol.* **130**: 2709.

Walsby, A.E. 1978. The gas vesicles of aquatic prokaryotes. *Symp. Soc. Gen. Microbiol.* **28**: 327.

Wiley, E.O. 1981. *Phylogenetics.* Wiley, New York.

Woese, C.R. 1981. Archaebacteria. *Sci. Am.* **244**: 98.

Woese, C.R. and G.E. Fox. 1977. Phylogenetic structure of the prokaryotic domain: The primary kingdoms. *Proc. Natl. Acad. Sci.* **74**: 5088.

Zillig, W., K.O. Stetter, R. Schnabel, J. Madon, and A. Gierl. 1982. Transcription in archaebacteria. *Zentralbl. Bakteriol. Abt. 1 Orig. Hyg.* **3**: 218.

Reconstruction of Phylogenetic Trees and Estimation of Divergence Times Under Nonconstant Rates of Evolution

W.-H. Li,* K.H. Wolfe,*[†] J. Sourdis,* and P.M. Sharp*[†]
*Center for Demographic and Population Genetics, University of Texas, Houston, Texas 77225;
[†]Department of Genetics, Trinity College, Dublin 2, Ireland

The rate-constancy or "molecular clock" hypothesis has often been taken as a basis for reconstructing phylogenetic relationships among organisms or genes and for dating evolutionary events (see, e.g., Dayhoff 1972; Wilson et al. 1977). However, there is now strong evidence that the rate-constancy assumption is often seriously violated (see, e.g., Britten 1986). For example, among different mammalian orders, the rate of nucleotide substitution may vary by a factor of two or three, and within primates, there is a well-documented slowdown in the lineage leading to man (Wu and Li 1985; Britten 1986; Koop et al. 1986; Li and Tanimura 1987). It is therefore important to take into consideration the possibility of unequal rates among lineages when reconstructing phylogenetic trees and when dating divergence events.

Phylogenetic reconstruction is extremely difficult when the rates of evolution differ greatly among lineages and when the taxa or DNA sequences under study are distantly related. We have studied this problem for the simple case of only four taxa (DNA sequences). We used computer simulation to compare the performance of several methods to see which are most effective against unequal rates of evolution (see also Saitou and Nei 1987).

It is commonly thought that phylogenetic reconstruction becomes much simpler when one or more outgroups are available (Saitou and Nei 1986). However, the usefulness of an outgroup depends on its distance from the taxa under study. We therefore studied how quickly the reliability of an outgroup reference decreases with that distance. We also studied the usefulness of adding a second outgroup. These approaches have been examined by computer simulation.

How to date divergence events is a challenging problem when large differences in rates occur among lineages. We (Li and Tanimura 1987) have recently proposed an approximation method. The method is heuristic and so needs to be examined carefully, using both analytic and simulation approaches.

Finally, we consider the branching order and divergence times among human, chimpanzee, gorilla, and orangutan, using a large amount of DNA sequence data from the four species.

RECONSTRUCTION OF PHYLOGENETIC TREES

Four Taxa with No Outgroup

Three approaches are compared below: maximum parsimony, neighborliness, and evolutionary parsimony. Following Lake (1987), the four DNA sequences under study are labeled 1, 2, 3, and 4. To simplify the representation of data, we work along the sequences from the 5' end to the 3' end and, at each position, recode the nucleotides in all four sequences in terms of their relationship to the nucleotide in sequence 1 at that position. All nucleotides that are the same as the one in sequence 1 are represented by "1"; those related by a transitional mutation are represented by "2," and the two possible transversions are represented by "3" and "4," in the order we come across them, if at all. (Exchanges between A and G [purines] and those between T and C [pyrimidines] are transitions, whereas all other types are transversions.) With this notation, any configuration of four nucleotides can be represented by 1 of 36 four-dimensional vectors (Table 1). For example, the two sets of nucleotides AGCT and GCCA are recoded as vectors 1234 and 1332, respectively.

With four taxa, there are only three possible unrooted trees. In the one shown in Figure 1, taxa 1 and 2 are connected by one node and taxa 3 and 4 are connected by another node. This tree may be represented by the notation ([12] [34]) and will be called tree X. The two other trees are ([13] [24]) and ([14] [23]) and will be called trees Y and Z, respectively.

The maximum parsimony (MP) approach is to find a tree that requires the minimum number of substitutions to explain the nucleotide differences among the sequences under study (Eck and Dayhoff 1966; Fitch 1977). We consider this method because it is one of the most widely used. We also note that in the case of four taxa, the character compatibility method (Le Quesne 1969) is identical to the MP method. In both methods, the configurations (vectors) 1122 and 1133 favor tree X because the number of substitutions required to explain each of the two configurations is only 1 under tree X, but 2 under either Y or Z. For the same reason, the configurations 1212 and 1313 favor tree Y, and the

Table 1. Scores for the X, Y, and Z Trees Under Different Tree-making Methods

	X tree						Y tree						Z tree				
Vector	MP	MPV	NJ	NJV	EP	Vector	MP	MPV	NJ	NJV	EP	Vector	MP	MPV	NJ	NJV	EP
1122	1		2			1212	1		2			1221	1		2		
1133	1	1	2	1	1	1313	1	1	2	1	1	1331	1	1	2	1	1
1233			1	1	−1	1323			1	1	−1	1332			1	1	−1
1322			1			1232			1			1223			1		
1344			1			1343			1			1334			1		
1134			1	1	−1	1314			1	1	−1	1341			1	1	−1
1123			1			1213			1			1231			1		
1132			1			1312			1			1321			1		
1234				1	1	1324				1	1	1342				1	1

The remaining nine vectors (1111, 1222, 1211, 1121, 1112, 1333, 1311, 1131, and 1113) are not utilized by any of the methods. (MP) Maximum parsimony method; (MPV) MP method using transversional differences only; (NJ) neighbor-joining method; (NJV) NJ method using transversional differences only; (EP) evolutionary parsimony method.

configurations 1221 and 1331 favor tree Z. Only these six configurations are informative for inferring the correct tree; all of the others are not informative because, for example, the configurations 1222 and 1233 require at least 1 and 2 substitutions, respectively, under each of the three alternative trees..Thus, a simple procedure for inferring the true tree from sequence data is as follows (Table 1): Give score 1 to each of the six informative configurations and score 0 to each of the other configurations. Let N_{ijmn} be the total score of the configuration $ijmn$ over the length of the sequences and let

$$X = N_{1122} + N_{1133} \tag{1}$$

$$Y = N_{1212} + N_{1313} \tag{2}$$

$$Z = N_{1221} + N_{1331} \tag{3}$$

The tree with the largest score is assumed to be the correct tree. Since transitions usually occur more frequently than transversions (Brown et al. 1982; Li et al. 1984) and since the MP method becomes unreliable when parallel and back mutations occur often (Felsenstein 1978), it may be better to consider only transversional substitutions when dealing with distantly related sequences. We denote this approach as MPV. Under this restriction, $X = N_{1133}$, $Y = N_{1313}$, and $Z = N_{1331}$, and selection of trees is again determined by the relative magnitudes of X, Y, and Z.

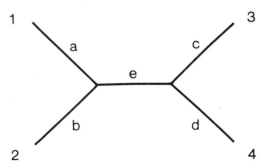

Figure 1. Model tree for four taxa (DNA sequences) labeled *1*, *2*, *3*, and *4*. The tree is unrooted. The branch lengths are denoted by *a*, *b*, *c*, *d*, and *e*.

The neighborliness approach is similar to the MP approach in that it also attempts to find the "minimum evolution" tree, but it makes a further attempt to minimize the distances between neighboring lineages. Three different algorithms for this approach have been proposed (Sattath and Tversky 1977; Fitch 1981; Saitou and Nei 1987), but in the case of four taxa, they all become identical. For ease of discussion, we call this approach the NJ (neighbor-joining) method (Saitou and Nei 1987), because this is also the algorithm used in the next two subsections. In this approach, the X tree is favored if

$$d_{12} + d_{34} < d_{13} + d_{24} \tag{4}$$

$$d_{12} + d_{34} < d_{14} + d_{23} \tag{5}$$

where d_{ij} is the distance between sequences i and j. Here, the distance is taken to be the observed number of nucleotide differences because simulation studies (Saitou and Nei 1987; W.-H. Li et al., unpubl.) suggest that it is usually more advantageous to use this number, rather than a number corrected for multiple hits. This is particularly true for very distantly related sequences because in this case, current methods for estimating the number of substitutions often fail (see, e.g., Li et al. 1985). The essence of conditions 4 and 5 is that taxa 1 and 2 should be joined as neighbors and so should taxa 3 and 4, because this would tend to produce a tree with the minimum total branch length.

There is a simple way to test conditions 4 and 5. We note that for the vector 1122, $d_{12} + d_{34} = 0$, whereas $d_{13} + d_{24} = d_{14} + d_{23} = 2$, and so for this vector, we assign a score of 2 for the X tree (and scores of 0 for the Y and Z trees) (Table 1). For the vector 1233, $d_{12} + d_{34} = 1$ and $d_{13} + d_{24} = d_{14} + d_{23} = 2$, and so we assign a score of 1 to the X tree. In the same manner, we can produce the other scores given in Table 1 in the columns marked NJ. From these scores we define

$$X = 2N_{1122} + 2N_{1133} + N_{1233} + N_{1322} + N_{1344} \\ + N_{1134} + N_{1123} + N_{1132} \tag{6}$$

as the total score for the X tree. Similarly, we define

$$Y = 2N_{1212} + 2N_{1313} + N_{1323} + N_{1232} + N_{1343}$$
$$+ N_{1314} + N_{1213} + N_{1312} \tag{7}$$

$$Z = 2N_{1221} + 2N_{1331} + N_{1332} + N_{1223} + N_{1334}$$
$$+ N_{1341} + N_{1231} + N_{1321} \tag{8}$$

as the total scores for the Y and Z trees, respectively. Then the X, Y, or Z tree is chosen to be the correct tree according to which one has the largest score. If we consider transversional differences only, then the scores become

$$X = N_{1133} + N_{1233} + N_{1134} + N_{1234} \tag{9}$$

$$Y = N_{1313} + N_{1323} + N_{1314} + N_{1324} \tag{10}$$

$$Z = N_{1331} + N_{1332} + N_{1341} + N_{1342} \tag{11}$$

We denote this method as NJV. Note that this is equivalent to classifying nucleotides into R (purines) and Y (pyrimidines) and then applying the maximum parsimony method to the recoded data.

The evolutionary parsimony (EP) method was recently proposed by Lake (1987) for dealing with situations where neighboring lineages differ greatly in substitution rates. In this method, the X, Y, and Z scores are given by

$$X = N_{1133} - N_{1233} - N_{1134} + N_{1234} \tag{12}$$

$$Y = N_{1313} - N_{1323} - N_{1314} + N_{1324} \tag{13}$$

$$Z = N_{1331} - N_{1332} - N_{1341} + N_{1342} \tag{14}$$

The only differences between these equations and Equations 9–11 are the differences in sign in the two middle terms in each equation. In the EP method, the reason for subtracting the two middle terms is that this would make the total score for an erroneous tree statistically zero. Lake (1987) called, for the X tree, $P = N_{1133} + N_{1234}$ the parsimony-like term and $B = N_{1233} + N_{1134}$ the background term and proposed $(P - B)^2/(P + B)$ as a chi-square with 1 degree of freedom for testing the X score to be significantly greater than zero. A tree is considered "proven" if only one of the three chi-squares for the three alternative trees is statistically significant.

Computer simulation was used to test the performance of the above methods. For this purpose, we needed to know how the nucleotides in a DNA sequence change with time. We used Kimura's (1980) two-parameter model, in which the rate of transitional substitution is a and the rate for each of the two types of transversional substitutions is b, both rates being the same for all nucleotides and given in terms of the number of changes per nucleotide site per unit time. The total rate of substitution per nucleotide site is $r = a + 2b$. Under this model, we have

$$p(t) = 1/4 + 1/4 \exp(-4bt) + 1/2 \exp[-2(a + b)t]$$
$$q(t) = 1/4 + 1/4 \exp(-4bt) - 1/2 \exp[-2(a + b)t]$$
$$s(t) = 1/4 - 1/4 \exp(-4bt)$$

where $p(t)$ is the probability that the nucleotide at time t and the initial (time 0) nucleotide are the same, $q(t)$ is the probability that they differ by a transition, and $s(t)$ is the probability that they differ by a particular type of transversion (Li 1986). Using these formulas, one can easily simulate nucleotide changes along an evolutionary lineage.

In our computer simulation, the X tree (Fig. 1) is the true tree. For each of the methods used, the X tree is chosen only if the X score is strictly greater than both the Y and Z scores; ties are neglected. Each of the values shown in Table 2 denotes the proportion of replicates in which the X tree was chosen. In the EP method, we also recorded the number of replicates in which only one of the chi-squares is larger than 3.84 (5% significance level) and also the proportion of X trees among those replicates (values in parentheses). In Table 2, the length of a branch denotes the expected number of substitutions per nucleotide site on the branch, i.e., the rt value. The "proportion of transitions" denotes the proportion of substitutions that are transitions. When this proportion is 33%, substitution occurs randomly among the four types of nucleotides, i.e., $a = b$. The other value (66%) used is close to that observed in nuclear pseudogenes (Li et al. 1984).

In Table 2, the first two cases (lines 1 and 2 and 3 and 4) were intended to show the effect of the length of the central branch (e). In the first case, e is fairly long (15%), and both the MP and NJ methods perform well, even though the substitution rates in neighboring lineages differ by a factor of 2. In the second case, e is reduced to 10% and the probability (P) of obtaining the correct tree is considerably reduced for both the MP and NJ methods. The second, third (lines 5 and 6), and fourth (lines 7 and 8) cases were intended to show the effect of increasing the difference in rates between neighboring lineages. It is seen that the P values for the MP and NJ methods become very low and approach zero as the difference increases from twofold (case 2) to fourfold (case 3), and then to tenfold (case 4). Note that in cases 3 and 4, the P value decreases as the length of the sequences (L) increases. Thus, under such extreme conditions, the performance of the MP and NJ methods cannot be improved by increasing L. Remarkably, the performance of the EP method improves with the difference in substitution rates between neighboring lineages. For example, if the proportion of transitions is 66% and if L is 4000, P is only 37% when the difference in rates between neighboring lineages is twofold (case 2) but is 64% when the difference becomes tenfold (case 4). Furthermore, for this method, P increases with L, and so if L is increased, P will eventually become very high. The fifth case (lines 9 and 10) shows that by excluding transitional differences from comparison, the MP and NJ methods (i.e., MPV

Table 2. Probability (%) of Obtaining the Correct (Unrooted) Tree with Four Taxa

Branch lengths (%)[a]					L[b]	Prob. of transitions = 33%						Prop. of transitions = 66%					
a	b	c	d	e		MP	MPV	NJ	NJV	EP		MP	MPV	NJ	NJV	EP	
40	80	40	80	15	1000	78	68	81	67	46	(58, 17)[c]	77	79	80	91	35	(37, 13)
					4000	95	92	94	84	60	(72, 29)	93	99	96	100	43	(44, 18)
40	80	40	80	10	1000	53	50	52	48	41	(48, 17)	58	62	55	76	32	(38, 15)
					4000	69	68	51	51	52	(84, 19)	72	83	57	96	37	(29, 17)
20	80	20	80	10	1000	7	9	3	4	52	(70, 16)	8	35	0	35	42	(42, 16)
					4000	0	0	0	0	73	(90, 29)	0	23	0	25	52	(56, 18)
8	80	8	80	10	1000	0	0	0	0	59	(78, 21)	0	11	0	6	45	(49, 17)
					4000	0	0	0	0	85	(94, 53)	0	0	0	0	64	(83, 18)
8	80	8	80	20	1000	19	23	0	4	79	(93, 31)	18	67	1	74	55	(74, 19)
					4000	4	3	0	0	97	(100, 79)	2	89	0	89	77	(91, 23)
6	60	6	60	6	1000	0	1	0	0	68	(85, 30)	0	18	0	10	47	(57, 14)
					4000	0	0	0	0	93	(99, 67)	0	7	0	1	61	(75, 32)
40	40	40	80	5	1000	68	62	81	68	40	(46, 13)	68	65	77	79	34	(45, 16)
					4000	89	83	97	83	48	(50, 18)	92	90	94	98	39	(53, 17)
20	60	40	80	5	1000	40	39	28	35	43	(50, 14)	35	49	29	57	33	(30, 16)
					4000	35	37	12	21	53	(71, 17)	27	63	18	71	33	(33, 15)

(MP) Maximum parsimony method; (MPV) MP method using transversional differences only; (NJ) neighbor-joining method; (NJV) NJ method using transversional differences only; (EP) evolutionary parsimony method.

[a] Branch lengths are in terms of the number of nucleotide substitutions per site.

[b] L indicates number of nucleotides in each sequence. The number of replicates conducted is 400 for L = 1000 and 100 for L = 4000.

[c] The first value in parentheses is the probability of obtaining the correct tree among the replicates in which one and only one of the three chi-squares is greater than 3.841 (5% significance level), and the second value denotes the percentage of such replicates among all replicates.

and NJV) also work under extreme conditions if the central branch is very long ($e = 20\%$) and if the proportion of transitions is 66% or higher. In the sixth case (lines 11 and 12), e is only 6% but the EP method performs somewhat better than in case 4 ($e = 10\%$) because the lengths of the peripheral branches are shorter in case 6 than in case 4. The seventh case (lines 13 and 14) shows that if only one of the four lineages has evolved faster than the others, then the MP and NJ methods work well, even though e is only 5%. In the last case (lines 15 and 16), where the rates differ in all lineages, the EP method performs better than the other methods when the proportion of transitions is 33%; the MPV and NJV methods perform better than the EP method when the proportion of transitions is 66%.

The results in Table 2 suggest that the MP and NJ methods work with very similar limitations and that, in general, the NJ method is somewhat better than the MP method. The results also suggest that when considering distantly related sequences, it is better to use transversional differences only, i.e., to use MPV and NJV because, in general, the proportion of transitions is higher than 33% (Brown et al. 1982; Li et al. 1984). The EP method was proposed to complement the MP method under conditions where the latter performs poorly. Our simulation results suggest that the method indeed performs well under extreme conditions, although poorly under moderate conditions (e.g., case 1). However, it may not work well when the proportion of transitions is high, in contrast to the MPV and NJV methods; furthermore, it often requires a large L value.

Three Taxa with One or Two Outgroups

In the case of three taxa, our purpose is to infer which two of the three taxa are more closely related or,

in other words, have split more recently. This is equivalent to determining the root of the tree. In the absence of outgroups, the only way to infer the root is to assume that the two taxa with the shortest distance are more closely related and that the root of the tree is somewhere between the ancestral node of these two taxa and the third taxon. This approach is the unweighted pair group (UPG) method (Sokal and Sneath 1963). In the presence of one or more outgroups, many other methods can be used (see, e.g., Nei 1987). We use the NJ method and the transformed distance (TD) method (Farris 1977; Klotz and Blanken 1981; Li 1981). In the TD method, the known outgroup (or outgroups) is used as a reference for making corrections for unequal rates among the ingroups and then the ingroups are clustered according to the new distances.

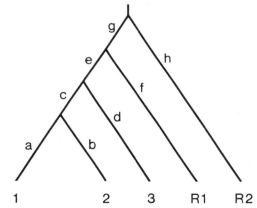

Figure 2. Model tree for three taxa with one or two outgroups. The three ingroup taxa are denoted *1*, *2*, and *3*, and the two outgroups are denoted R1 and R2. The branch lengths are denoted by *a*, *b*, *c*, etc.

To treat the problem, we follow Saitou and Nei (1986) but remove the assumption of rate constancy. We use the model tree shown in Figure 2, in which taxa 1 and 2 are more closely related to each other than either is to the third taxon, and R1 and R2 denote the two outgroup references. If only one outgroup (R1) is available, then the conditions for obtaining the correct branching order are the same as conditions 4 and 5, with taxon 4 replaced by R1 (Saitou and Nei 1986). Thus, in this case, the TD and NJ methods (and also the methods of Sattath and Tversky [1977] and Fitch [1981]) are identical. When two outgroups are available, we combine them as a single (composite) outgroup and infer the branching order as in the case of one outgroup. Conditions 4 and 5 then become

$$d_{12} + (d_{34} + d_{35})/2 < d_{13} + (d_{24} + d_{25})/2$$
$$d_{12} + (d_{34} + d_{35})/2 < d_{23} + (d_{14} + d_{15})/2$$

in which taxa 4 and 5 refer to R1 and R2 (Saitou and Nei 1986).

Table 3 shows our simulation results. We first consider the situation where the rate of nucleotide substitution has become progressively faster toward more recent lineages. In this situation, the UPG method has a very low probability of obtaining the correct branching order (Table 3), and it should be useful to have an outgroup. In Table 3, the proportion of transitions is

Table 3. Probability (%) of Obtaining the Correct Branching Order for Three Ingroup Taxa with One or Two Outgroup References

		Branch lengths (%)[a]						Prop. of transitions = 1/3			Prop. of transitions = 10/11		
									TD			TD	
a	b	c	d	e	f	g+h	L[b]	UPG	1 ref.	2 refs.	UPG	1 ref.	2 refs.
A. Acceleration toward more recent lineages													
4	3	0.5	2	0.5	3	6	500	6	83	85	6	73	78
							1500	1	99	100	1	98	97
				10	15	16	500	6	49	53	6	40	44
							1500	1	64	67	1	49	51
							3000	0	76	80	0	54	57
				40	40	45	500	6	18	19	6	16	16
							3000	0	7	5	0	3	2
								(0)[c]	(16)	(13)	(9)	(43)	(53)
30	25	2	25	2	26	28	500	22	63	69	24	49	54
							1500	16	84	87	17	64	70
							3000	7	92	94	11	76	86
				15	40	45	500	22	49	53	24	42	45
							1500	16	60	65	17	46	49
							3000	7	72	78	11	59	61
								(13)	(60)	(54)	(21)	(76)	(81)
50	40	5	40	5	40	42	500	26	72	75	29	56	60
							1500	17	91	95	27	74	79
							3000	7	99	99	19	91	92
				15	55	55	500	22	56	63	29	49	51
							1500	17	72	80	27	62	64
							3000	9	83	89	19	72	74
								(17)	(70)	(72)	(16)	(96)	(99)
				50	100	100	1500	16	41	37	27	41	43
							3000	10	35	33	19	48	39
								(17)	(42)	(36)	(16)	(89)	(88)
B. Deceleration toward more recent lineages													
2.5	3	0.5	4	10	14	16	500	84	76	83	84	69	77
							1500	98	95	99	98	93	96
				35	40	45	500	84	73	80	84	70	76
							1500	98	94	98	98	92	94
23	25	2	28	2	30	35	1500	93	87	92	85	70	78
							3000	100	92	99	95	83	86
				12	40	44	1500	93	85	90	85	74	81
							3000	100	91	98	95	82	92
35	40	5	45	15	60	60	1500	98	94	94	90	81	83
							3000	100	99	99	97	90	94
				50	120	120	1500	97	91	95	90	78	85
							3000	100	99	100	97	92	94

The methods used are the unweighted paired group method (UPG) and the transformed distance method (TD).

[a]Branch lengths are in terms of the number of nucleotide substitutions per site. See Fig. 2 for the branch notations a, b, c, etc.

[b]L indicates the number of nucleotides in each sequence. The number of replicates conducted is 100 for L = 3000, 200 for L = 1500, and 600 for L = 500.

[c]The value in parentheses was obtained using transversional differences only.

1/3 or 10/11, the latter being the value observed in mitochondrial DNA (Brown et al. 1982). In case 1 (lines 1–7), the three ingroup sequences are closely related and the distances among them ($a + b$, $a + c + d$, $b + c + d$) are 7% or smaller. When the outgroup used (R1) is also closely related to the ingroups, the probability (P) of obtaining the correct branching order is high even if L is only 500 nucleotides. When the distance between R1 and the ingroups (e.g., $f + e + d$) becomes about 30%, P is at most 76% if $L \leq 3000$ and if the proportion of transitions is 1/3 or higher. When the distances between R1 and the ingroups become 80% or larger, P becomes low and decreases with increasing L. Therefore, such an outgroup is not useful for inferring the branching order. In case 2 (lines 8–13), the distances among the ingroups are 50% or larger. It is seen that if $L = 3000$, P is still high even if the distances between R1 and the ingroups are 80% or larger. These results may seem contradictory to those for case 1. However, in case 1, the length of branch c is only 0.5%, whereas in case 2 it is 2%; thus, an outgroup is still useful even when its distance to the ingroups is 80%. In case 3 (lines 14–21), the ingroups are distantly related, but c is fairly large (5%). In this case, if $L \geq 1500$, P is high even if the distances between R1 and the ingroups are about 120%. However, P becomes low when the distances between R1 and the ingroups become larger than 190%. We note that adding a second outgroup reference (R2), in general, increases P but usually only to a small extent. Furthermore, if R2 is very distantly related to the ingroups, then adding R2 may reduce the P value. We also note that if the outgroups are distantly related to the ingroups and if the proportion of transitions is higher than 1/3, then it is better to exclude transitional differences from comparison (see the P values in parentheses).

We next consider the situation in which the substitution rate has become progressively slower toward more recent lineages. We impose the condition that d_{12} is substantially smaller than both d_{13} and d_{23} so that the UPG method performs well. It is clear from Table 3B that the P value often becomes smaller when an outgroup is used. Fortunately, in all cases with $L = 3000$, the P value is high even when an outgroup is used. Since in practice, if no outgroup is available, we cannot distinguish between the two situations (acceleration or deceleration), we may conclude from the results in Table 3 that a suitable outgroup is quite useful for inferring the branching order among three taxa.

Six Taxa with One Outgroup

The TD and NJ methods are considered here. For each method, we compare the performance with an outgroup against the performance with no outgroup. We consider obtaining the correct *unrooted* tree because the NJ method does not give the tree root. In the NJ method, when an outgroup is used, we assume that it is the last taxon to be joined to the other taxa. In the absence of outgroups, the TD method employed an

algorithm (Li 1981) in which the UPG method is first applied to determine the tree root, then the taxa on one side of the root are used as references for making corrections for unequal rates of evolution among the taxa on the other side of the root, and finally, the taxa on each side of the root are clustered according to the new distances.

Figure 3 shows the model tree used in our simulation, and Table 4 shows the simulation result. Note that in all but the last case, the NJ method performs better without an outgroup. This is surprising. Apparently, if the number of taxa is four or larger, the NJ algorithm is effective in detecting unequal rates even with no known outgroup. However, it should be pointed out that if the outgroup is not distantly related to the ingroups and if the internal branches (i.e., the h values) are not short, then the availability of an outgroup will eventually improve the performance of the NJ method as L increases. This can be seen from the rapid increase in the P value, with increasing L in all cases in Table 4. The availability of an outgroup improves the performance of the TD method when the ingroups are not very closely related; when they are closely related, the TD method performs well without outgroups. In summary, an outgroup is needed only when fairly distantly related sequences are being considered.

ESTIMATION OF DIVERGENCE TIMES

The model tree in Figure 4 was used to illustrate a method (proposed by Li and Tanimura 1987) for estimating the divergence time between two sequences. Suppose that we know T_2 and want to estimate T_1. The standard approach under the assumption of rate constancy is

$$T_1 = 2d_{12}T_2/(d_{13} + d_{23}) \qquad (15)$$

If the rate-constancy assumption does not seem to hold and if an outgroup (R) is available, the following

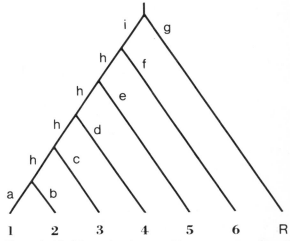

Figure 3. Model tree for six taxa with one outgroup. The six taxa are denoted *1–6*, the outgroup by R, and the branch lengths of the tree by a, b, c, etc.

Table 4. Probability (%) of Obtaining the Correct Unrooted Tree for Six Taxa with One Outgroup Reference or None

| | | | | | | | | | | Prop. of transitions = 1/3 | | | | | Prop. of transitions = 10/11 | | | | |
| | | | | | | | | | | | NJ | | TD | | | NJ | | TD | |
a	b	c	d	e	f	h	i+g	L[b]	UPG	no ref.	1 ref.	no ref.	1 ref.	UPG	no ref.	1 ref.	no ref.	1 ref.
4	3	2	3	3.5	4	0.5	5	1500	1	97	94	94	95	1	91	90	85	90
								3000	0	100	100	100	100	0	100	98	99	100
30	25	25	30	25	25	2	30	1500	9	77	70	66	60	7	42	32	36	29
								3000	2	95	94	89	82	2	65	63	58	52
35	25	25	40	25	25	2	30	1500	0	64	54	52	53	1	33	24	21	27
								3000	0	85	77	72	80	0	58	50	42	43
45	40	40	50	40	40	3	45	1500	17	52	43	48	41	11	54	43	47	52
								3000	19	74	78	73	77	18	80	71	69	74

(UPG) Unweighted pair-group method; (NJ) neighbor-joining method; (TD) transformed distance method.
[a]Branch lengths are in terms of the number of nucleotide substitutions per site. For the branch notation, see Fig. 3.
[b]L indicates the number of nucleotides in each sequence. The number of replicates conducted is 200 for L = 1500 and 100 for L = 3000.

method (proposed by Li and Tanimura 1987) may be used. Suppose the difference between d_{1R} and d_{3R} is smaller than that between d_{2R} and d_{3R}. This indicates that the rate-constancy assumption holds better in lineage 1 and so we estimate T_1 by

$$T_1 = aT_2/(a + c) \qquad (16)$$

where a and $a + c$ are estimated by

$$a + c = (d_{1R} + d_{13} - d_{3R})/2 \qquad (17)$$

$$a = (d_{13} + d_{12} - d_{23})/2 \qquad (18)$$

If the difference between d_{1R} and d_{3R} is larger than that between d_{2R} and d_{3R}, then T_1 should be estimated by b $T_2/(b + c)$. If we know T_1 and want to estimate T_2, then Equation 16 becomes $T_2 = (a + c) T_1/a$.

Table 5 shows our simulation results. In all cases, the true value of T_1 is 1. In cases 1 and 2 (lines 1 and 2), the rate-constancy assumption holds and Equations 15 and 16 both give, on average, an estimate of 1.01 or 1.00 for $T_1 = 1$. In case 3 (lines 3 and 4), a rate slowdown occurs in both lineages 1 and 2, with a stronger tendency in lineage 2, and the average estimates of T_1 obtained from the formulas in Equations 15 and 16 are 0.77 and

0.89, respectively, the latter being closer to 1. In case 4 (lines 5 and 6), the rate slowdowns in lineages 1 and 2 are stronger than in case 2, and the average estimate obtained under the rate-constancy assumption, i.e., from Equation 15, is only 0.56, whereas that obtained from Equation 16 is 0.87. In the last case (line 8), an acceleration in rate occurs in lineages 1 and 2 and the average estimates obtained from Equations 15 and 16 are 1.36 and 1.05, respectively, the latter being considerably more accurate than the former. These examples show that if the substitution rates differ greatly among lineages, Equation 16 gives considerably better estimates than does Equation 15.

Actually, once the expected branch lengths a, b, c, and d are specified, the average estimates based on Equations 15 and 16 can be calculated readily. For example, in case 5 (line 7), $a = 4.5\%$, $b = 3.0\%$, $c = 3.0\%$, and $d = 10.0\%$, and thus the expected values of d_{12}, d_{13}, and d_{23} are 7.5%, 17.5%, and 16.0%. Putting these values and $T_2 = 1.5$ into Equations 15 and 16, we obtain 0.67 and 0.90. These theoretical values and the average estimates based on simulation (0.68 and 0.91) are almost identical. The same comment applies to the other cases in Table 5. Note that in case 5, the outgroup is not closely related to the ingroups because $e + f = 50\%$. Thus, as long as an outgroup is fairly closely related to the ingroups, it can serve as a good reference.

DISCUSSION

The simulation results in Table 2 suggest that as long as the central branch is fairly long, it is not very difficult to determine the phylogenetic relationships among four distantly related taxa, even if the substitution rates are quite different among different lineages. However, the problem becomes extremely difficult when the central branch is short and thus requires further investigation.

Our simulation study shows that the availability of an outgroup can greatly facilitate the determination of branching order among three taxa. However, adding a second outgroup is of limited value. Furthermore, if there are four or more ingroup taxa, having an outgroup does not facilitate the determination of the

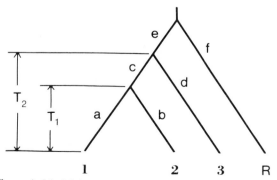

Figure 4. Model for estimating divergence times. The three ingroup taxa are denoted by *1*, *2*, and *3* and the outgroup by R. T_1 and T_2 denote the divergence times; one is known, but the other is unknown and to be estimated. The branch lengths are denoted by a, b, c, etc.

Table 5. Estimation of Divergence Time (T_1) with and without the Assumption of Rate Constancy

Branch lengths (%)[a]					T_2	L[b]	Estimates of T_1	
a	b	c	d	e + f			constancy assumption	no constancy assumption
1.7	1.7	1.7	3.4	6.0	2.0	1000	1.01 (0.17)[c]	1.01 (0.18)
4.0	4.0	2.0	6.0	10.0	1.5	1000	1.00 (0.11)	1.00 (0.11)
1.4	1.0	1.7	3.4	6.0	2.0	1000	0.77 (0.15)	0.89 (0.20)
						3000	0.76 (0.08)	0.89 (0.11)
2.0	1.4	1.5	6.0	10.0	1.5	1000	0.56 (0.09)	0.87 (0.14)
						3000	0.56 (0.05)	0.87 (0.07)
4.5	3.0	3.0	10.0	50.0	1.5	3000	0.68 (0.04)	0.91 (0.08)
3.5	4.0	1.5	3.0	10.0	1.5	3000	1.36 (0.08)	1.05 (0.07)

The true value of T_1 is 1 time unit in all cases. In the simulation, nucleotide substitutions were assumed to be random and the distances between sequences were estimated according to the formulae of Jukes and Cantor (1967).

[a]Branch lengths are in terms of the number of nucleotide substitutions per site. See Fig. 4 for the branch notations a, b, c, etc.

[b]L indicates the number of nucleotides in each sequence. The number of replicates conducted is 300 for $L = 1000$ and 100 for $L = 3000$.

[c]Values in parentheses are the standard deviations estimated from the replicates. This value indicates the variability of the estimate among different replicates.

phylogenetic relationships among the ingroups, except when the ingroups are relatively distantly related and when the DNA sequences under study are fairly long. Of course, having an outgroup should be of help in the determination of the ancestral root of the ingroups.

Estimation of divergence times is difficult when substitution rates differ greatly among lineages. The method (proposed by Li and Tanimura 1987) gives only approximate estimates but is preferable to the assumption of rate constancy. To obtain more accurate estimates, a more rigorous treatment of the problem is needed.

Branching Order among Apes and Humans

To illustrate the methods described in this paper, we considered the branching order and divergence times among apes and humans. These are controversial subjects in evolution. We used 10.2 kb of noncoding DNA sequence data from the η-globin pseudogene region of human (H), chimpanzee (C), gorilla (G), and orangutan (O), of which two parts totaling 5.3 kb have also been sequenced in rhesus (Rh) and New World monkeys (NWM) (Koop et al. 1986; Miyamoto et al. 1987; Maeda et al. 1988). We applied the MP and NJ (or TD) methods to the 10.2-kb sequences to determine the branching order of H, C, G, and O (a known outgroup). For the MP method, there are only 14 informative configurations (see Table 1 for definition), of which 7 favor the topology ([HC] [GO]) (i.e., the X score is 7), 4 favor ([HG] [CO]) (i.e., $Y = 4$), and 3 favor ([HP] [CG]) (i.e., $Z = 3$). Since the X score is the largest, the topology ([HO] [GO]) is chosen. This topology is also favored by five "gaps" (insertion or deletion events) shared by H and C but by neither G nor O; ([HO] [CG]) is favored by one difference of this type, and ([HO] [CO]) is favored by none. Thus, both the substitutions and the gap events indicate that H and C are the closest relatives. For the NJ method, the terms in conditions 4 and 5 are $d_{HC} + d_{GO} = 428$ substitutions, $d_{HG} + d_{CO} = 429$, and $d_{HO} + d_{CG} = 432$. Since the first number is the smallest, this method also favors the

topology ([HC] [GO]). However, the three numbers are so similar that we cannot be certain of the branching order. In view of this uncertainty, despite the large amount of sequence data used, we wonder if the branching order for H, C, and G is very close to a trichotomy.

The pairwise distances between H, C, G, O, Rh, and NWM for the 5.3-kb sequences mentioned above are given in Table 6. We have used these distances to calculate the branch lengths in Figure 5 as follows. Using NWM as a reference, we find from Table 6 that the Rh and the H lineages, particularly the former, have evolved faster than the other lineages. Therefore, we take Rh and H as taxa 1 and 2 and NWM as taxon 3. From Table 6, we have $d_{12} = 7.51$, $d_{13} = 12.86$, and $d_{23} = 11.28$, and from Equation 18, we obtain $a = 4.54$ as the branch length from K to Rh (Fig. 5). Further-

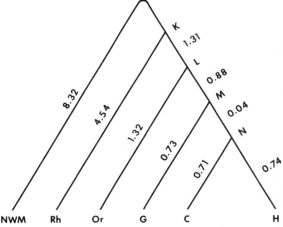

Figure 5. A phylogenetic tree for higher primates. (H) Human; (C) chimpanzee; (G) gorilla; (Or) orangutan; (Rh) rhesus monkey; (NWM) New World monkeys. The branching order for H, C, G, and Or were determined by the MP and NJ methods, using a 10.2-kb DNA region from the four species (see text). The branch lengths are in terms of the number of substitutions per 100 sites and are determined as described in the text.

Table 6. Mean (Below Diagonal) and Standard Error (Above Diagonal) of the Number of Nucleotide Substitutions per 100 Sites between Species

Species	Human	Chimpanzee	Gorilla	Orangutan	Rhesus	New World monkey
Human		0.17	0.18	0.25	0.41	0.53
Chimpanzee	1.45		0.18	0.25	0.42	0.52
Gorilla	1.51	1.57		0.26	0.41	0.52
Orangutan	2.98	2.94	3.04		0.40	0.52
Rhesus	7.51	7.55	7.39	7.10		0.56
New World monkey	11.28	11.16	11.20	11.02	12.86	

The mean and standard error were calculated according to the method of Kimura (1980). The sequence data used are 5.3 kb of noncoding DNA, which is made up of two separate regions: (1) the η-globin locus (2.2 kb) described by Koop et al. (1986), for which the New World monkey species is owl monkey, and (2) 3.1 kb of the η-δ globin intergenic region sequenced by Maeda et al. (1983 and unpubl.), for which the New World monkey species is spider monkey. The human allele used in the latter region is the T allele. The two regions are about 3.3 kb apart, and both form part of the 10.2-kb continuous sequence available for human, chimpanzee, gorilla, and orangutan. We have excluded a number of anomalous regions (poly[A] tails of Alu elements, a polypyrimidine tract, and some regions in which the correct alignment was not apparent) from the analysis.

more, we obtain $d_{12} - 4.54 = 2.97$ as the branch length from K to H and $d_{13} - 4.54 = 8.32$ as the branch length from K to NWM. Next, we use NWM and Rh as a composite reference, i.e., taxon 3, and take O and H as taxa 1 and 2. We then have $d_{13} = (11.02 + 7.10)/2 = 9.06$, $d_{23} = 9.40$, and $d_{12} = 2.98$. Putting these values into Equation 18, we obtain 1.32 as the branch length from L to O. Moreover, we obtain $d_{12} - 1.32 = 1.66$ as the branch length from L to H and $2.97 - 1.66 = 1.31$ as the branch length from K to L, because the branch length from K to H is 2.97 (see above). Finally, using NWM, Rh, and O as a composite reference, we obtain the other branch lengths in Figure 5.

Using Equation 16 and assuming that the branching date for Rh is $T_2 = 25 \pm 5$ million years (Myr) (Pilbeam 1984), we estimate that the branching date for O is $T_1 = T_2 \, d_{LH}/d_{KH} = 14.0 \pm 2.8$ Myr, where d_{KH} and d_{LH} are the branch lengths from K and L to H, respectively. This estimate is somewhat older than Pilbeam's (1986) estimate of 12 Myr from fossil records. Note that in the estimation, we have used the H lineage, rather than the O lineage, because the latter seems to have evolved more slowly than the other lineages. Similarly, taking the branching date for O as estimated above, we estimate the branching date for G to be 6.6 ± 1.3 Myr and that for C to be 6.3 ± 1.2 Myr.

ACKNOWLEDGMENTS

We thank Drs. M. Miyamoto and N. Maeda for allowing us to use their unpublished sequence data. This study was supported by National Institutes of Health grant GM-30998.

REFERENCES

Britten, R.J. 1986. Rates of DNA sequence evolution differ between taxonomic groups. *Science* **231:** 1393.

Brown, W.M., E.M. Prager, A. Wang, and A.C. Wilson. 1982. Mitochondrial DNA sequences of primates: Tempo and mode of evolution. *J. Mol. Evol.* **18:** 225.

Dayhoff, M.O. 1972. *Atlas of protein sequence and structure*, vol. 5. National Biomedical Research Foundation, Silver Spring, Maryland.

Eck, R.V. and M.O. Dayhoff. 1966. *Atlas of protein sequence and structure*. National Biomedical Research Foundation, Silver Spring, Maryland.

Farris, J.S. 1977. On the phenetic approach to vertebrate classification. In *Major patterns in vertebrate evolution* (ed. M.K. Hecht et al.), p. 823. Plenum Press, New York.

Felsenstein, J. 1978. Cases in which parsimony or compatibility methods will be positively misleading. *Syst. Zool.* **27:** 401.

Fitch, W.M. 1977. On the problem of discovering the most parsimonious tree. *Am. Nat.* **111:** 223.

———. 1981. A non-sequential method for constructing trees and hierarchical classifications. *J. Mol. Evol.* **18:** 30.

Jukes, T.H. and C.R. Cantor. 1967. Evolution of protein molecules. In *Mammalian protein metabolism* (ed. H.N. Munro), p. 21. Academic Press, New York.

Kimura, M. 1980. A simple method for estimating evolutionary rates of base substitutions through comparative studies of nucleotide sequences. *J. Mol. Evol.* **16:** 111.

Klotz, L.C. and R.L. Blanken. 1981. A practical method for calculating evolutionary trees from sequence data. *J. Theor. Biol.* **91:** 261.

Koop, B.F., M. Goodman, P. Xu, K. Chan, and J.L. Slightom. 1986. Primate η-globin DNA sequences and man's place among the great apes. *Nature* **319:** 234.

Lake, J.A. 1987. A rate-independent technique for analysis of nucleic acid sequences: Evolutionary parsimony. *Mol. Biol. Evol.* **4:** 167.

Le Quesne, W.J. 1969. A method of selection of characters in numerical taxonomy. *Syst. Zool.* **18:** 201.

Li, W.-H. 1981. Simple method for reconstructing phylogenetic trees from distance matrices. *Proc. Natl. Acad. Sci.* **78:** 1085.

———. 1986. Evolutionary change of restriction cleavage sites and phylogenetic inference. *Genetics* **113:** 187.

Li, W.-H. and M. Tanimura. 1987. The molecular clock runs more slowly in man than in apes and monkeys. *Nature* **326:** 93.

Li, W.-H., C.-C. Luo, and C.-I. Wu. 1985. Evolution of DNA sequences. In *Molecular evolutionary genetics* (ed. R.J. MacIntyre), p.1. Plenum Press, New York.

Li, W.-H., C.-I. Wu, and C.-C. Luo. 1984. Nonrandomness of point mutation as reflected in nucleotide substitutions in pseudogenes and its evolutionary implications. *J. Mol. Evol.* **21:** 58.

Maeda, N., J.B. Bliska, and O. Smithies. 1983. Recombination and balanced chromosome polymorphism suggested by DNA sequence 5′ to the human delta-globin gene. *Proc. Natl. Acad. Sci.* **80:** 5012.

Maeda, N., C.-I. Wu, J. Bliska, and J. Reneke. 1988. Molecular evolution of higher primates: Intergenic structure, rate and pattern of DNA changes and origin of simple sequences. *Mol. Biol. Evol.* (in press).

Miyamoto, M.M., J.L. Slightom, and M. Goodman. 1987. Phylogenetic relationships of humans and African apes from DNA sequences of the $\psi\eta$-globin region. *Science* **238:** 369.

Nei, M. 1987. *Molecular evolutionary genetics.* Columbia University Press, New York.

Pilbeam, D. 1984. The descent of hominoids and hominids. *Sci. Am.* **252:** 84.

———. 1986. Hominoid evolution and hominoid origins. *Am. Anthropol.* **88:** 295.

Saitou, N. and M. Nei. 1986. The number of nucleotides required to determine the branching order of three species with special reference to the human-chimpanzee-gorilla divergence. *J. Mol. Evol.* **24:** 189.

———. 1987. The neighbor-joining method: A new method for reconstructing phylogenetic trees. *Mol. Biol. Evol.* **4:** 406.

Sattath, S. and A. Tversky. 1977. Additive similarity trees. *Psychometrika* **42:** 319.

Sokal, R.R. and P.H.A. Sneath. 1963. *Principles of numerical taxonomy.* W.H. Freeman, San Francisco.

Wilson, A.C., S.S. Carlson, and T.J. White. 1977. Biochemical evolution. *Annu. Rev. Biochem.* **46:** 573.

Wu, C.-I. and W.-H. Li. 1985. Evidence for higher rates of nucleotide substitution in rodents than in man. *Proc. Natl. Acad. Sci.* **82:** 1741.

Reliability of Evolutionary Trees

D. PENNY,* M.D. HENDY,[†] AND I.M. HENDERSON*
*Departments of *Botany and Zoology, and* [†]*Mathematics and Statistics,*
Massey University, Palmerston North, New Zealand

Previous work (Penny and Hendy 1985, 1986) has shown that evolutionary trees reconstructed from sequence data converge to a consistent answer as longer sequences become available. The rate of convergence can be used to test hypotheses concerning both the results and methods. However, conditions are known where convergence to an incorrect tree can occur (Felsenstein 1978; Lake 1986). Maximum likelihood calculations have a theoretical advantage (Felsenstein 1982), but there has been no simple method for their calculation and a priori assumptions about the rates of evolution were required.

In this paper, we describe a simple method for maximum likelihood for 2-state characters, using Hadamard matrices. Because these matrices are easily inverted, we can, for a given tree, calculate rates of evolution directly from the data. The method has allowed us to compare maximum likelihood, minimal length, and distance methods for reconstructing evolutionary trees.

When the molecular clock hypothesis applies, then the minimal length method will converge on the correct tree for four taxa, but with five or more taxa, errors are possible. In general, "long edges attract." Methods for overcoming this include adding new taxa that intersect long unbranched edges, giving a higher weight to nucleotide positions that change more slowly, and testing closely related trees by maximum likelihood calculations. These methods are discussed here using biological examples.

Evolutionary theory has in the past been criticized on the grounds that it did not make "falsifiable predictions" and therefore was not fully scientific (Popper 1972; but see also Popper 1978). Much of our earlier work was carried out to show that this criticism is invalid and that indeed both qualitative and quantitative predictions from evolutionary theory are possible.

Our approach has been to show that evolutionary trees from different protein sequences (but from the same set of species) are very similar, as predicted by the theory of evolution with a stochastic mechanism. This work involved the development of (1) methods that were guaranteed to have found all optimal trees, (2) a tree comparison metric that was calculable, and (3) the expected distribution of this tree composition method. These three developments made it possible to show that minimal trees from five different protein sequences were extremely similar (Penny et al. 1982). Since then, two additional approaches have been used. The first approach shows that a shorter tree is a good predictor (Penny and Hendy 1985), and the second approach

shows that, as more sequences became available, the results converge toward a single tree (Penny and Hendy 1986).

It has been known for some time (Felsenstein 1978), however, that some evolutionary models, even with only four taxa, would converge to an incorrect tree. In such cases, the more data that are available, the more certain it is that the shortest tree will be incorrect. Likelihood methods have a theoretical advantage in handling these difficult cases, but they lack an efficient implementation that guarantees to have found the optimal rates for a given tree and that handles more than about five taxa. On the other hand, distance methods (see Sneath and Sokal 1973), and to a lesser extent parsimony (Hendy and Penny 1982), can handle more taxa and so have had a practical advantage.

We have recently described (M.D. Hendy; M.D. Hendy and D. Penny; both in prep.) a new likelihood method that seems to be particularly suitable for the long sequences of ribosomes. These sequences are sufficiently long to test for convergence to a single tree and to allow estimates of deviations from a simple model.

DATA

The data we have used in our main example are eight ribosomal sequences from the EMBL DNA database (Hamm and Cameron 1986). The sequences are from soybean *Glycine max*, yeast *Saccharomyces cerevisiae*, a nematode *Caenorhabditis elegans*, brine shrimp *Artemia salina*, toad *Xenopus laevis*, human *Homo sapiens*, mouse *Mus musculus,* and rat *Rattus norvegicus*. The entries in EMBL are GMRN18S, SCRNA5, CERDNA, ASRRNA18S, XLRGEO14, HSRGE, MMRNA18, and RNRGEA.

METHOD

The method can start either with a model (a tree with expected rates of change along each edge) or from a set of sequences. In the first case, the method predicts the expected partition frequencies in the sequences, and in the second case, it gives the expected rates on each edge of the specified tree. The basic theorem will be described by M.D. Hendy (in prep.).

Two-state characters: The forward calculation.

$$q = -\ln(1 - 2\rho)/2 \qquad (1)$$

$$\rho = Kq \qquad (2)$$

$$r = \exp(-2\rho) \qquad (3)$$

$$s = 2^{1-n}Hr \qquad (4)$$

The entries of p are the probabilities that the vertices at the two ends of an edge on a tree T will have different codes (see Fig. 1): i.e., the number of changes on the edge is an odd number. Values of p range from 0 (no change) to 0.5 (complete randomization). q contains the expected (average) number of changes along an edge; i.e., it allows for multiple changes along the edge. Entries in q can vary from zero to infinity. Both p and q have $2n - 3$ entries.

Matrix K ($2^{n-1} \times 2n - 3$) records the edges linking all even-sized subsets of n taxa, and there are 2^{n-1} such subsets. A value of 1 indicates that the edge is on the minimal set of paths linking pairs of taxa in the subset; otherwise the entry is 0. The first row is for the null set, the second row is for the subset of taxa [1,2], the third row is for the subset [1,3], and so forth. Subsets of four or more taxa are joined in pairs so that paths linking these pairs in the tree T are nonintersecting; this is unique for each subset. The matrix can be generated recursively (M.D. Hendy, in prep.), with a row of zeros as the first row. The construction uses a $(2n - 3)$-tuple (Π $(1,m)$, whose jth entry is 1 if the edge e_j is on the path from taxon 1 to taxon m; otherwise the entry is 0. K is then generated row by row with $K_1 = 0$ and $K_{i+g} = K_i + \Pi(1,m)$ (mod 2), $1 \le i \le g = 2^{m-2}$, for $2 \le m \le n$.

ρ is the product Kq. Entries in ρ can also vary from zero to infinity and are the expected number of changes along a path (or set of paths), summing those on the individual edges of the paths. The paths connect all even-sized subsets of the n taxa. δ is derived from ρ (see Fig. 2), and the entries are the probability that an even number of vertices in a subset of taxa have the same character state. This gives distance values directly, where a subset has only two taxa (Fig. 2). We call r parity values, and it is also derived from ρ. Entries are related to the probability that an even number of vertices in a subset of taxa have the same character state.

H is a Hadamard matrix that depends only on the number of taxa n. A Hadamard matrix is any square matrix H whose entries are ± 1 and with orthogonal rows. This property makes inversion particularly simple; it is easy to see that $H^{-1} = H^t/h$, where h is the number of rows of H and H^t is the transpose of H. In Equation 4, $h = 2^{n-1}$. The matrix can be generated recursively as follows:

$$\text{Let} \quad H^{(1)} = [1] \text{ and } H^{(m+1)} = \begin{vmatrix} H^{(m)} & -H^{(m)} \\ H^{(m)} & H^{(m)} \end{vmatrix}$$

$$\text{for} \quad 1 \le m \le n-2 \quad \text{and} \quad H = H^{(n)}$$

The output s is the frequency of each of the 2^{n-1} partitions of the taxa. A partition is a subset of taxa having the same code at the binding site being considered. The order of partitions is [1], [1,2], [1,3], [1,2,3], [1,4], ..., [1,2,3, ..., n]. This order is calculated recursively by adding each new taxon in turn to all previous partitions. Initially, $P_1 = [1]$; thereafter, $P_{i+g} = P_i U[m]$ for $1 \le i \le g = 2^{m-2}$, $2 \le m \le n$.

Two-state characters: The inverse calculation.

K is a $2^{n-1} \times (2n - 3)$-order matrix of full rank, and hence there exists a left-handed inverse K^* (known as a generalized inverse) such that $K^*K = I$, the identity matrix of order $(2n - 3)$ (sect 5.6; Noble 1969). An infinite number of such generalized inverses exist; however, $K^* = (K^tK)^{-1}K^t$ is the inverse that minimizes the Euclidean distance between ρ and $\rho^* = K.K^*\rho$. Consequently, it is possible, for a given tree, to calculate the rates of change that would best fit the observed data. It is shown (M.D. Hendy, in prep.) that $K^tK = 2^{n-3}(I + J)$, where J is the square matrix of order $(2n - 3)$ whose entries are all 1s. It is easily seen that $(K^tK)^{-1} = (I - (2n - 2)^{-1}J)/2^{(n-3)}$; so $K^* = (I - (2n - 2)^{-1}J) K^t/2^{n-3}$.

A worked example with $n = 4$ taxa is given in Figure 3. In this case, the fit is precise because we are dealing with limiting values for infinitely long sequences. Sampling errors, selecting the wrong tree, and trees being an inappropriate model can all lead to a lack of agreement between the initial values and the final calculated values of s.

Other calculations are possible on the basis of the values generated (see Fig. 2). For example, the expected distance matrix D can be calculated from ρ. There will be a loss of information in converting to D because it goes from $2^{n-1} - 1$ independent values (in ρ) to $n(n - 1)/2$ values in D. q can also be estimated from D with an appropriate matrix.

The method described here is for two-state characters, but it can be made more general. We have shown that with four codes, it is possible to allow three different rates for changes between codes, and the results will still be related by a Hadamard matrix (and consequently invertible). However, this results in large numbers of partitions, most of which will not occur in a given set of sequences. An alternative is to consider all pairs of "codes": A/~A(not A); C/~C, purines/

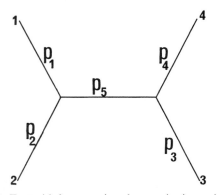

Figure 1. Tree with four taxa (pendant vertices), one internal edge, and two internal vertices (ancestors). The probability that the adjacent vertices have different codes is shown on each edge; these values form p.

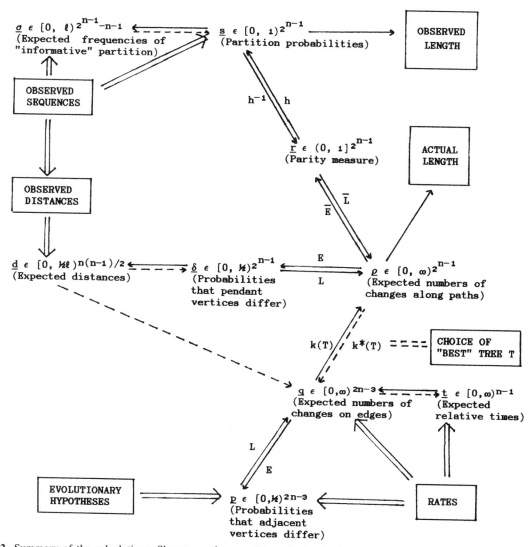

Figure 2. Summary of the calculations. Shown are the quantities calculated, their interrelationships, and their relation to the observed data.

$$
\underline{p} = \begin{bmatrix} 0.10 \\ 0.08 \\ 0.09 \\ 0.11 \\ 0.05 \end{bmatrix}, \quad \underline{q} = -\ln(1-2\underline{p})/2, \quad \underline{\rho} = K\underline{q} = \begin{bmatrix} 00000 \\ 11000 \\ 10101 \\ 01101 \\ 10011 \\ 01011 \\ 00110 \\ 11110 \end{bmatrix} \begin{bmatrix} 0.11157 \\ 0.08718 \\ 0.09923 \\ 0.12423 \\ 0.05268 \end{bmatrix} = \begin{bmatrix} 0.00000 \\ 0.19875 \\ 0.26384 \\ 0.23908 \\ 0.28848 \\ 0.26409 \\ 0.22346 \\ 0.42221 \end{bmatrix}, \quad \underline{r} = e^{-2\underline{\rho}}
$$

$$
\underline{s} = \frac{H \cdot \underline{r}}{8} = \frac{1}{8}
\begin{bmatrix}
1 & -1 & -1 & 1 & -1 & 1 & 1 & -1 \\
1 & 1 & -1 & -1 & -1 & -1 & 1 & 1 \\
1 & -1 & 1 & -1 & -1 & 1 & -1 & 1 \\
1 & 1 & 1 & 1 & -1 & -1 & -1 & -1 \\
1 & -1 & -1 & 1 & 1 & -1 & -1 & 1 \\
1 & 1 & -1 & 1 & 1 & -1 & 1 & -1 \\
1 & -1 & 1 & -1 & 1 & -1 & 1 & 1 \\
1 & 1 & 1 & 1 & 1 & 1 & 1 & 1
\end{bmatrix}
\begin{bmatrix}
1.00000 \\
0.67200 \\
0.59400 \\
0.61992 \\
0.56160 \\
0.58968 \\
0.63960 \\
0.42981
\end{bmatrix}
=
\begin{bmatrix}
0.07442 \\
0.04748 \\
0.01460 \\
0.08270 \\
0.01496 \\
0.06794 \\
0.06002 \\
0.63788
\end{bmatrix}
\begin{array}{l}
\{1\} \\
\{1,2\} \\
\{1,3\} \\
\{1,2,3\} \\
\{1,4\} \\
\{1,2,4\} \\
\{1,3,4\} \\
\{1,2,3,4\}
\end{array}
$$

Figure 3. Worked example of the calculation of partition frequencies s with four taxa as described in Fig. 1. $p_1 = 0.1$, $p_2 = 0.08$, $p_3 = 0.09$, $p_4 = 0.11$, $p_5 = 0.05$.

pyrimidines, and so forth. This avoids the problem of large numbers of partitions and allows several estimates of both trees and rates to be compared. Consequently, this approach has been developed first and some applications will be discussed below.

RESULTS

Several applications have been described recently (M.D. Hendy and D. Penny, in prep.). For example, it can be shown that when the molecular clock hypothesis is valid, and when only four taxa are being considered, then the minimal length tree will always be correct when the sequences are long enough to overcome sampling effects. However, this is the only value of n for which this will always be true.

With five or more taxa, the minimal tree may be not the shortest when long and short edges are interspersed throughout the tree. Indeed, in one example with five taxa with short internal edges and with equal rates of change, the correct tree was the thirteenth shortest (third longest) of the 15 possible unrooted trees. This demonstrates that parsimony cannot guarantee a correct result even with equal rates of change. In another example with four taxa but with unequal rates, the correct tree was the longest of the three trees. With these examples, it was possible to get the correct tree by parsimony when additional taxa were available that intersected long edges. We paraphrase this contradiction with parsimony by long edges attract. However, we should note that current parsimony methods underestimate the actual number of changes on the tree. The parsimony model should be based on the actual, rather than the observed, number of changes on T.

Similar tests have been made with UPGMA, a method of building trees from distance matrices. We have found examples (M.D. Hendy and D. Penny, in prep.) where UPGMA works and parsimony fails; one example is the five taxa with equal rates but with short internal edges. Conversely, there are many cases where parsimony finds the correct tree and UPGMA fails; cases with unequal rates and additional taxa intersecting long edges are examples. So far, we have found a method of overcoming the cases where UPGMA fails. However, there are many other methods that use distance matrices and each needs to be studied. From Figure 2, it is clear that there is a loss of information in going from sequences to distances. With sequences, there are $2^{n-1} - 1$ independent values, but with distances, there are only $n(n - 1)/2$ independent values.

Quartets and Distance from a Tree

With four taxa, there are only three unrooted binary trees, and all trees can be tested to find the tree that gives the frequencies of partitions that are in closest agreement with the data. Starting with s, the vectors r, ρ, and q can be calculated for each of the three trees. The generalized inverse K^* gives entries in q that minimize the sums of squares of the deviations. These

values of q can then be used to calculate the predicted probabilities of the partitions, $s' \cdot s$ and s' (for each of the three trees) can then be tested by standard goodness-of-fit tests.

ρ' are the predicted values Kq' and so $\rho' = KK^* \rho$. If we let

$$\varepsilon(1) = \rho'(2) + \rho'(7) - \rho'(8)$$
$$\varepsilon(2) = \rho'(3) + \rho'(6) - \rho'(8)$$
$$\varepsilon(3) = \rho'(4) + \rho'(5) - \rho'(8)$$

then the distances from ρ' to ρ^* for each tree can be calculated as follows:

$$\Delta^2(1) = \varepsilon(1)^2/3 + (\varepsilon[2] - \varepsilon[3])^2/4$$
$$\Delta^2(2) = \varepsilon(2)^2/3 + (\varepsilon[1] - \varepsilon[3])^2/4$$
$$\Delta^2(3) = \varepsilon(3)^2/3 + (\varepsilon[1] - \varepsilon[2])^2/4$$

An example using purines/pyrimidines with four ribosomal sequences (nematode, brine shrimp, *Xenopus*, and mouse) is given in Table 1. In these sequences, taxon 1 (nematode) has a different code from the other taxa 189 times; taxa 1 and 2 share the same code, which differs from the code of taxa 3 and 4, 58 times; and so on (see Table 1, column 1). Column 2 shows the values of the corresponding r; these are independent of the tree chosen.

The values in r are converted to q for each of the three unrooted trees spanning four taxa, using the appropriate K^* for each tree. q is converted back to r' using the K matrix for each of three trees (each tree will give a different r'). The r' values are then used to calculate the expected frequencies for the partitions s' ($s' = Hr'$). These are shown in the next three columns in Table 1 and are the best fit that can be obtained for each of the three trees to the original sequences.

Tree 1 links nematode with brine shrimp and mouse with *Xenopus*; this gives the best fit to the original data. The distance between the observed and predicted ρ values are 14 times greater in trees 2 and 3 than in tree 1 (Table 1). In addition, the agreement between the observed and predicted s values is good for tree 1, in contrast to those for the other two trees. The only value not in close agreement is that for partition [1,4]/[2,3], where the branches to the nematode and mouse appear to share two more coincident changes than expected. This could be an illustration of the covarion hypothesis (Fitch and Markowitz 1970).

The fit is not exact for several reasons; there is "sampling" error, and of course the model may be too simple (it assumes that each nucleotide position has equal for change). Another reason for not fitting exactly is the reduction in the number of independent variables in going from the level of r or s ($2^{n-1} - 1$) to the level of p and q ($2n - 3$), the number of edges on the tree. It is usually not possible to do this exactly; K^* is chosen to minimize the sums of squares of differences (distance squared) between ρ and ρ^*.

Table 1. Observed and Predicted Partition Frequencies

s (observed)	r	$T_1 \to s'$ (predicted)	$T_2 \to s'$ (predicted)	$T_3 \to s'$ (predicted)	Partitions
189	1.0000	189.69	198.26	197.51	{1}/{2, 3, 4}
58	0.7207	58.72	7.18	7.05	{1, 2}/{3, 4}
1	0.7005	1.24	12.04	2.78	{1, 3}/{2, 4}
8	0.8659	8.12	17.16	17.89	{1, 2, 3}/{4}
5	0.6999	1.30	2.96	15.41	{1, 4}/{2, 3}
7	0.8652	7.53	17.51	15.96	{1, 2, 4}/{3}
47	0.9788	47.70	49.84	49.15	{1, 3, 4}/{2}
1403	0.7054	1403.71	1413.04	1412.25	{1, 2, 3, 4}
Δ_i		0.00825	0.11614	0.11457	

s is the observed frequency of partitions derived from transversions between four taxa (nematode, brine shrimp, *Xenopus*, and mouse). r is calculated from s ($r = H's$). q is calculated for each tree (T_1–T_3), and these are then used to calculate the predicted values r' and s'. The distances from the observed to predicted ρ values are shown as Δ_1, Δ_2, and Δ_3 are about 14 times larger. T_1 (joining *Xenopus* and nematode) gives the best fit to the observed data. The last column gives the taxa in each partition.

Quartets with Eight Eukaryotes

The number of unrooted binary trees for n taxa is $(2n - 5)!!$, where the double factorial notation (!!) for odd numbers represents $1.3.5. \ldots (2n - 5)$. With values of $n \geq 9$, it becomes impractical to test every tree. Several branch-and-bound methods are available when selecting minimal length trees (Penny and Hendy 1987), and this allows large numbers of trees to be searched efficiently. However, a branch-and-bound approach has not yet been developed for the present calculations.

As an alternative, we have tried testing all quartets of taxa and selecting the tree that the data fit most closely, as described above. We have tried this approach with the eight sequences described earlier. In two cases, the internal edge had zero length, and thus these quartets did not distinguish between the three possibilities. The other 68 quartets (giving 70 combinations of 4 taxa from 8) gave a consistent tree (see Fig. 4). Thus, none of the quartets contradicts the present tree, but any other tree will be contradicted by at least some quartets. Until additional examples are tried, it is premature to conclude whether this method will be generally useful.

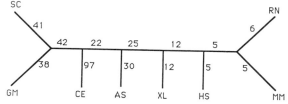

Figure 4. Tree for the eight species calculated according to the method of quartets from the data in Table 2. (GM) Soybean *Glycine max*; (SC) yeast *Saccharomyces cerevisiae*; (CE) nematode *Caenorhabditis elegans*; (AS) brine shrimp *Artemia salina*; (XL) *Xenopus laevis*; (HS) human *Homo sapiens*; (MM) mouse *Mus musculus*; (RN) rat *Rattus norvegicus*. Numbers associated with each edge are the quantities q_i, which represent the expected number of nucleotide changes on that edge. If we assume the molecular clock, these are proportional to time, and we would place the root on the edge to nematode.

It is simple to apply the inverse calculation to this tree with the observed frequencies of the partitions (Table 2). The values of p from this calculation are also shown in Figure 4. The root of the tree is not given directly, but the assumption of equal rates of change (the molecular clock) is best satisfied by placing the root on the edge leading to nematode.

DISCUSSION

Figure 2 gives a framework for many calculations and tests on evolutionary trees, only a few of which have been discussed here. Examples discussed above include evaluating methods of tree construction; we have found many realistic examples where choosing the apparent shortest tree, or using a simple distance matrix, will lead to the selection of an incorrect tree, even when sequences are sufficiently long to overcome sampling errors. We have shown that adding additional taxa that intersect long edges will increase the reliability of the parsimony method, but apparently not that of UPGMA.

Calculating the q values (the expected number of changes on each edge) for any tree allows a simple test for deviations from the molecular clock. Underlying assumptions of the model can also be examined. For instance, finding that the changes on the nematode and mouse lineages were more similar than expected (Table 1) could be an example of the covarion hypothesis (Fitch and Makowitz 1970). This hypothesis predicts that some sites change more rapidly than others and that these sites may vary on different lineages.

It is possible with quartets of taxa to measure the distance from the observed to predicted data for any tree. This gives an objective measure of how well the data fit a specific tree.

An additional advantage is being able to calculate directly the optimal q values for a tree. This avoids the use of a heuristic "hill-climbing" algorithm whose properties are unknown. The functional relationship between the q and s values will allow additional calculations. It provides the potential for an efficient and objective tree-building method for distance data.

Table 2. Frequency of Partitions for Eight Eukaryotyes

Pn	Freq	Pn	Freq	Pn	Freq	Pn	Freq
1	158	29	3	123	0	231	4
3	166	31	33	125	4	233	3
5	35	33	0	·		235	6
7	83	35	0	·		237	2
9	18	37	0	143	3	239	30
11	38	39	0	·		241	32
13	23	41	2	·		243	52
15	91	·		167	1	245	21
17	7	·		·		247	112
19	4	91	1	·		249	67
21	4	·		225	6	251	405
23	8	·		227	5	253	146
25	1	121	1	229	2	255	7430
27	10						9017

Frequency of partitions for the eight ribosome sequences. Pn is the taxa in the partition when taxa are numbered in binary (1, 2, 4, 8, . . .). Pn = 7 is the case where the first three taxa share the same code (1 + 2 + 4 = 7). Freq indicates the number of times each partition occurs, summed over all five comparisons (A, ~ A; C, ~ C; . . . ; purines, pyrimidines). Partitions not shown do not occur.

It is anticipated that more objective analyses of evolutionary tree construction will be generally useful and that the study of evolutionary trees will become more scientific.

REFERENCES

Felsenstein, J. 1978. Cases in which parsimony or compatibility methods will be positively misleading. *Syst. Zool.* **27:** 401.

———. 1982. Evolutionary trees from DNA sequences: A maximum likelihood approach. *J. Mol. Evol.* **17:** 368.

Fitch, W.M. and E. Markowitz. 1970. An improved method for determining codon variability in a gene and its application to the rate of fixation of mutations in evolution. *Biochem. Genet.* **4:** 579.

Hamm, G.H. and G.N. Cameron. 1986. The EMBL data library. *Nucleic Acids Res.* **14:** 5.

Hendy, M.D. and D. Penny. 1982. Branch and bound algorithms to determine minimal evolutionary trees. *Math. Biosci.* **59:** 277.

Lake, J. 1986. In defence of bacterial phylogeny. *Nature* **321:** 658.

Noble, B. 1969. *Applied linear algebra.* Prentice-Hall, Englewood Cliffs, New Jersey.

Penny, D. and M.D. Hendy. 1985. Testing methods of evolutionary tree construction. *Cladistics* **1:** 266.

———. 1986 Estimating the reliability of evolutionary trees. *Mol. Biol. Evol.* **3:** 403.

———. 1987. TurboTree: A fast algorithm for minimal trees. *CABIOS* **3:** 183.

Penny, D., L.R. Foulds, and M.D. Hendy. 1982. Testing the theory of evolution by comparing phylogenetic trees constructed from five different protein sequences. *Nature* **297:** 197.

Popper, K.K. 1972. *Objective knowledge: An evolutionary approach.* Oxford University Press, Oxford, England.

———. 1978. Natural selection and the evolution of mind. *Dialectica* **32:** 339.

Sneath, P.H.A. and R.R. Sokal. 1973. *Numerical taxonomy.* W.H. Freeman, San Francisco.

Male-driven Molecular Evolution: A Model and Nucleotide Sequence Analysis

T. Miyata, H. Hayashida,[†] K. Kuma,[*] K. Mitsuyasu,[*] and T. Yasunaga[‡]

*Department of Biology, Faculty of Science, Kyushu University, Fukuoka 812, Japan;
†National Institute of Genetics, Mishima 411, Japan; ‡ The Institute of Physical and
Chemical Research, Wako, Saitama, 351-01, Japan

Mutation rates and functional constraints against mutational variations are known to be the major factors that determine the rate of molecular evolution (Wilson et al. 1977; Kimura 1983). Although much effort has been made to understand the evolutionary properties of genes and proteins on the basis of functional constraints (Wilson et al. 1977; Kimura 1983), little is known about the mutational factor. Knowing the source of mutations might be essential for a comprehensive understanding of the mechanisms underlying molecular evolution. Among several known mechanisms by which mutations are generated (Watson et al. 1987), DNA replication and repair are probably the major source of mutations that contribute to molecular evolution (Wilson et al. 1977; Britten 1986). Rapid rates of evolution of virus-coded genes (Palese and Young 1982; Hayashida et al. 1985) and mammalian mitochondrial genes (Brown et al. 1982; Miyata et al. 1982), as compared with those of cellular genes, may support this idea.

It is generally thought that the number of cell divisions in sperm cells differs greatly from that in eggs (Alberts et al. 1983; Winter et al. 1983). Coupled with replication errors, this factor was shown to generate a marked difference between autosomes and sex chromosomes in mutation frequency, which is consistent with the observed pattern of evolutionary rate in highly divergent portions of genes (Miyata et al. 1987). We describe below the important influence this factor has had on mutation frequencies and evolutionary rates, and we suggest that males serve as mutation generators, at least in mammalian evolution.

Differences in Mutation Frequency between Autosomes and Sex Chromosomes

We have considered (Miyata et al. 1987) a simple model of mutation frequency based on the assumptions that (1) errors in DNA replication during germ-cell division are the major source of mutations that contribute to molecular evolution and (2) the number of germ-cell divisions differ between males and females. This simple model predicts that the asymmetry in the number of germ-cell divisions between male and female results in differences in mutation frequency between autosomes and sex chromosomes.

In the XX female/XY male system of diploid animals, the autosomes generally occur in duplicate, with one copy from each parent. Since the probability that a certain set of autosomes carried by the male is 1/2 and that by the female is 1/2, the mutation frequency per generation for autosomes is expected to be proportional to $(\alpha + 1)/2$, if a long evolutionary time span is considered, where α represents the male-to-female ratio of the number of germ-cell divisions. On the other hand, the expected mutation frequency per generation for the Y chromosome is α, because the Y chromosome is always carried by the male. The female carries two X chromosomes, whereas the male carries only one. Thus, the expected mutation frequency per generation for the X chromosome is given as $(\alpha + 2)/3$.

The expected mutation frequencies of the X chromosome relative to that of autosomes ($R_{X/A}$) is $R_{X/A} = (2/3)(2 + \alpha)/(1 + \alpha)$. Similarly, the relative mutation frequency for the Y chromosome is $R_{Y/A} = 2\alpha/(1 + \alpha)$. It is generally believed that the number of cell divisions in sperm is extremely large compared with that in egg (i.e., $\alpha \gg 1$). In such an extreme case, we have $R_{X/A} = 2/3$ and $R_{Y/A} = 2$, the maximum difference in mutation frequency between autosomes and sex chromosomes. This implies that the contribution of the female to mutation is negligibly small, whereas the male serves as a major generator of mutations that contribute to molecular evolution.

The ZW female/ZZ male system shows a distinct pattern of mutation frequency: This system differs from the XX/XY system only in a reversal of sex. Thus, the expected relative mutation frequencies could be obtained from the same expression for the XX/XY system by replacing α with $1/\alpha$; $R_{Z/A} = (2/3)(2\alpha + 1)/(1 + \alpha)$ and $R_{W/A} = 2/(1 + \alpha)$ (Fig. 1). Table 1 summarizes the mutation frequencies and relative mutation frequencies between the XX/XY system and ZW/ZZ system. Figure 1 demonstrates interesting differences in mutation frequency between the two systems: The degree of relative mutation frequencies of the ZW/ZZ system is in the reverse order to those of the XX/XY system in the case of $\alpha > 1$, and $R_{W/A}$ of the W chromosome is strikingly small if the male-to-female ratio α of germ-cell division is very large. Note that the difference in mutation frequency between autosomes and sex chromosomes is derived from the presence of asymmetry in the number of germ-cell divisions.

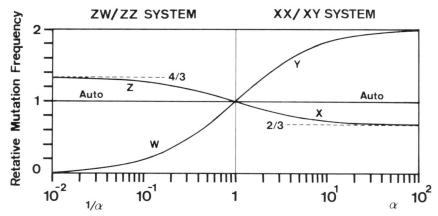

Figure 1. Dependence of the relative mutation frequency on male-to-female ratio α of the number of germ-cell divisions. For the ZW/ZZ system, the relative mutation frequencies were plotted against the inverse of α. For both systems, the relative mutation frequencies were shown for $\alpha > 1$.

Evolutionary Properties of Silent Positions

Comparisons of the evolutionary rates at highly divergent portions of autosome-linked genes with those of X- and Y-linked genes provide useful information for testing the model described above. These gene regions are known to be constrained very weakly, if at all, against base alternations (Kimura 1977, 1983; Miyata et al. 1980, 1982, 1985; Miyata and Hayashida 1981; Miyata and Yasunaga 1981; Hayashida and Miyata 1983) and thus are expected to reflect mutational properties almost directly. Among the highly divergent regions, synonymous codon alternating (silent) positions of protein-encoding regions might be best for our present purpose: First, many gene sequences are available for comparison between different species. Second, the nucleotide sequences of protein-encoding regions could be aligned easily without introducing many gaps. Third, the rates of evolution at silent positions are similar for different genes, which is in contrast to the rates at amino-acid-changing (replacement) positions, which differ greatly for different genes (Miyata et al. 1980, 1982, 1985; Hayashida and Miyata 1983) and are therefore possible to compare between different genes.

Recently, we found an additional characteristic of the evolution of silent substitutions (Miyata et al. 1987). We compared 35 autosome-linked gene sequences between human and mouse (or rat) and calculated the number of nucleotide substitutions per site (K_S^c) at the silent positions as well as that (K_A^c) at the replacement positions (Miyata and Yasunaga 1980). Figure 2 shows a plot of K_S^c against K_A^c for the autosome-linked genes. The K_S^c values appear to be divided into two distinct groups, depending on the K_A^c values. A statistical analysis of the 35 genes showed that a group of genes (divergent type or d-type) with high K_A^c values (≥ 0.08) is slightly higher in K_S^c value than another group of genes (conservative type or c-type) with low K_A^c values (< 0.088) (Miyata et al. 1987). The average value of K_S^c is 0.76 ± 0.10 for the d-type genes and 0.55 ± 0.07 for the c-type genes.

Most of the d-type genes correspond to a gene group (specific or s-type) that occurs mostly in vertebrates or expresses only in specific cells, whereas most of the c-type genes correspond to a gene group (general or g-type) that might be vital for most organisms and cells (Fig. 2). This indicates that the nucleotide sequences of important genes are conserved not only at the replacement positions, but also at the silent positions, although slightly.

Table 1. Comparison of the Expected Mutation Frequencies between the XX Female/XY Male System and ZW Female/ZZ Male System

	Autosome	X(Z) chromosome	Y(W) chromosome
Mutation frequency			
XX/XY system	$(1 + \alpha)/2$	$(2 + \alpha)/3$	α
ZW/ZZ system	$(1 + \alpha)/2$	$(1 + 2\alpha)/3$	1
Relative mutation frequency			
XX/XY system	1	$(2/3)(2 + \alpha)/(1 + \alpha)$	$2\alpha/(1 + \alpha)$
ZW/ZZ system	1	$(2/3)(1 + 2\alpha)/(1 + \alpha)$	$2/(1 + \alpha)$
For $\alpha \geqslant 1$			
XX/XY system	1	$2/3$	2
ZW/ZZ system	1	$4/3$	$0(1/\alpha)$

α, male-to-female ratio of the number of germ-cell divisions; $0(1/\alpha)$, order of $1/\alpha$.

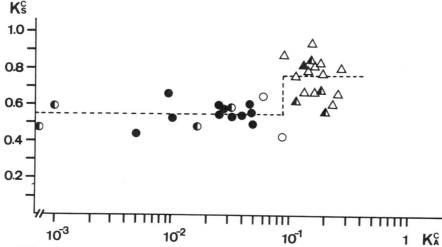

Figure 2. K_S^c versus K_A^c plot for autosome-linked genes. Each of 35 autosome-linked gene sequences was compared between human and mouse (or rat), and the K_S^c value was plotted against the K_A^c value. Circles and triangles indicate genes belonging to the conservative group (c-type) with K_A^c less than 0.088 (vertical dashed line) and divergent group (d-type) with K_A^c greater than 0.088, respectively. (●▲) Genes classified as general type (g-type); (○△) genes classified as specific type (s-type) (ambivalent genes were indicated by half-filled circles or triangles). Horizontal dashed lines represent the average value ($= 0.55 \pm 0.07$) of K_S^c of the c-type genes and the average value ($= 0.76 \pm 0.10$) of K_S^c of the d-type genes. (For the values of K_S^c and K_A^c and the classification of genes, see Miyata et al. 1987.)

X-linked and Y-linked Gene Evolution

At present, four X-linked genes are available for nucleotide sequence comparison between human and mouse or rat. Figure 3 shows their K_S^c values, together with the corresponding values of autosome-linked genes for comparison. Even at weakly constrained silent positions, the X-linked genes are apparently conserved much more strongly than autosome-linked c-type genes. To facilitate comparison with the relative mutation frequency described above, we introduced an index $R'_{X/A}$ representing the relative evolutionary rate of silent substitution: $R'_{X/A} = K_S^c$ (X-linked gene)/K_S^c(autosome-linked gene). The relative evolutionary rate could be compared directly with the relative mutation frequency of the X chromosome ($R_{X/A}$).

Since the K_S^c differs in value between d- and c-type genes and all four X-linked genes appear to belong to the conservative group, the c-type genes should be used for estimates of relative evolutionary rate. Interestingly, the $R'_{X/A}$ value ($= 0.60$) is close to the expected value (2/3) of the relative mutation frequency corresponding to the case where $\alpha \gg 1$. We have also analyzed (Miyata et al. 1987) the relative evolutionary rate for genes involved in the general-type genes, and a similar result was obtained.

At present, no Y-linked gene sequence is available for comparison between human and mouse (or rat). However, comparison of evolutionary rates between Y-linked and autosome-linked genes is possible for human argininosuccinate synthetase (AS) pseudogenes ψAS-7 and ψAS-Y, which are mapped to chromosome 7 and the Y chromosome, respectively. Their phylogenetic relationship is interesting in that ψAS-7 was copied from ψAS-Y or vice versa, but not directly from

the functional gene (Nomiyama et al. 1986). Using the AS functional gene as a reference, we (Miyata et al. 1987) estimated the evolutionary distance K^c(ψAS-a/ψAS-Y) between the ancestral pseudogene ψAS-a and ψAS-Y as well as the evolutionary distance K^c(ψAS-a/ψAS-7) between ψAS-a and ψAS-7 as described previously (Miyata and Hayashida 1982). By introducing the relative evolutionary rate of the Y-linked gene, defined as $R'_{Y/A} = K^c(\psi AS\text{-}a/\psi AS\text{-}Y)/K^c(\psi AS\text{-}a/\psi AS\text{-}7)$, the $R'_{Y/A}$ was estimated to be 2.2 on average for the silent position and the 3′-noncoding region. This figure is close to the expected value ($= 2$) of relative mutation frequency of the Y chromosome for the case where $\alpha \gg 1$.

In summary, the silent positions of the X-linked genes are conserved much more strongly than the corresponding positions of autosome-linked genes encoding conservative types of proteins. In contrast, the Y-linked AS pseudogene evolved much more rapidly than the homologous autosome-linked pseudogene. The relative evolutionary rates were on average $R'_{X/A} = 0.60$ and $R'_{Y/A} = 2.2$. These observations are obviously parallel with the prediction of the present model based on the assumptions that the male-to-female ratio of the number of germ-cell divisions is extremely large and that DNA replication errors are the major source of mutations.

An alternative intepretation may be posssible for the observed rates of silent substitutions. The limited rate of silent substitutions in X-linked genes is due to functional reasons but not to different numbers of germ-cell divisions between male and female. Because many vital genes exist on the X chromosome, mutation frequency is limited to a lesser extent for the X chromosome than for the autosomes and the Y chromosome by efficient

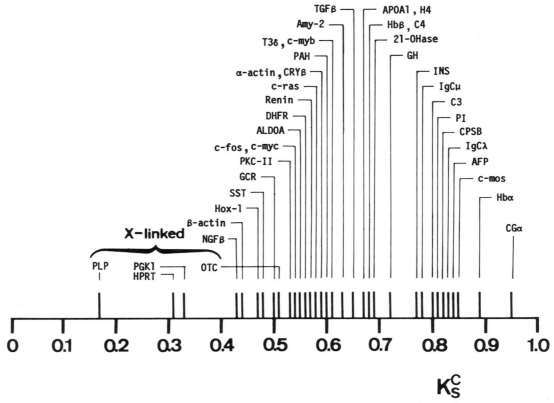

Figure 3. Comparison of the K_s^c values between autosome-linked genes and X-linked genes. (The K_s^c values and the abbreviations of genes were taken from Miyata et al. 1987.)

DNA repair or other unknown mechanisms. Although we do not exclude the possibility that these factors may be involved in part, the present model might be more plausible. Indirect evidence indicates that, at the individual level, the mutation frequency of the male is about ten times as high as that of the female (Winter et al. 1983); furthermore, our model explains the observed pattern of silent substitutions quantitatively.

Analyses of the avian ZW female/ZZ male system would provide clear-cut proof. If the alternative interpretation is true, the R' values are expected to be of the order $R'_{W/A} > 1 > R'_{Z/A}$. In contrast, our model predicts a reverse order $R'_{Z/A} > 1 > R'_{W/A}$ and the $R'_{W/A}$ value is very much lower than unity. Since the K_s^c value of α- and β-globin genes was estimated to be about 0.37 between chicken and duck, the corresponding value of W-linked genes is expected to be much lower when the same species are compared.

The most remarkable conclusion from the present analysis is that males serve as a major source of mutations that contribute to molecular evolution. This may provide insight into the mechanisms underlying molecular evolution. It remains to be solved why the rate of molecular evolution is constant with respect to absolute time, but not to generation time (Wilson et al. 1977). In addition, recent nucleotide sequence analyses revealed that, in some lineages, the rate of molecular evolution is not constant (Kikuno et al. 1985; Wu and

Li 1985; Britten 1986). The present result suggests that the constancy and nonconstancy of the molecular clock should be reexamined on the basis of the number of germ-cell divisions of males.

Since evolutionary rates of silent substitutions differ between autosome-linked genes and sex chromosome-linked genes, the molecular clock could not be applied directly to certain cases. For example, in estimating dates of divergence of X-linked duplicated genes by applying the molecular clock calibrated by autosome-linked genes, the observed number of nucleotide substitutions between the genes in question should be corrected by multiplying by a factor of 3/2 (Kuma and Miyata 1987).

As shown above, the relative mutation frequency R correlates well with the relative evolutionary rate R'. This result is consistent with the neutral theory which predicts that the rate of molecular evolution increases linearly with increasing mutation rate (Kimura 1968, 1977, 1983).

ACKNOWLEDGMENTS

We thank Drs. M. Sekigutchi, Y. Iwasa, and N. Yamamura for valuable comments and discussion. This work was supported in part by grants from the Ministry of Education, Science, and Culture of Japan.

REFERENCES

Alberts, B., D. Bray, J. Lewis, M. Raff, K. Roberts, and J.D. Watson. 1983. *Molecular biology of the cell*. Garland Publishing, New York.

Britten, R.J. 1986. Rates of DNA sequence evolution differ between taxonomic groups. *Science* **231:** 1393.

Brown, W.M., E.M. Prager, A. Wang, and A.C. Wilson. 1982. Mitochondrial DNA sequences of primates: Tempo and mode of evolution. *J. Mol. Evol.* **18:** 225.

Hayashida, H. and T. Miyata. 1983. Unusual evolutionary conservation and frequent DNA segment exchange in class I genes of the major histocompatibility complex. *Proc. Natl. Acad. Sci.* **80:** 2671.

Hayashida, H., H. Toh, R. Kikuno, and T. Miyata. 1985. Evolution of influenza virus genes. *Mol. Biol. Evol.* **2:** 289.

Kikuno, R., H. Hayashida, and T. Miyata. 1985. Rapid rate of rodent evolution. *Proc. Jpn. Acad.* **61(B):** 153.

Kimura, M. 1968. Evolutionary rate at molecular level. *Nature* **217:** 624.

———. 1977. Preponderance of synonymous changes as evidence for the neutral theory of molecular evolution. *Nature* **267:** 275.

———. 1983. *The neutral theory of molecular evolution*. Cambridge University Press, Cambridge, England.

Kuma, K. and T. Miyata. 1987. Limited divergence of X-linked gene: Further supporting evidence for male-driven molecular evolution. *Proc. Jpn. Acad.* **63(B):** 332.

Miyata, T. and H. Hayashida. 1981. Extraordinarily high evolutionary rate of pseudogenes: Evidence for the presence of selective pressure against changes between synonymous codons. *Proc. Natl. Acad. Sci.* **78:** 5739.

———. 1982. Recent divergence from a common ancestor of human IFN-α genes. *Nature* **295:** 165.

Miyata, T. and T. Yasunaga. 1980. Molecular evolution of mRNA: A method for estimating evolutionary rates of synonymous and amino acid substitutions from homolo-gous nucleotide sequences and its application. *J. Mol. Evol.* **16:** 23.

———. 1981. Rapidly evolving mouse α-globin-related pseudo gene and its evolutionary history. *Proc. Natl. Acad. Sci.* **78:** 450.

Miyata, T., T. Yasunaga, and T. Nishida. 1980. Nucleotide sequence divergence and functional constraint in mRNA. *Proc. Natl. Acad. Sci.* **77:** 7328.

Miyata, T., H. Hayashida, K. Kuma, and T. Yasunaga. 1987. Male-driven molecular evolution demonstrated by different rates of silent substitutions between autosome- and sex chromosome-linked genes. *Proc. Jpn. Acad.* **63(B):** 327.

Miyata, T., H. Hayashida, R. Kikuno, H. Toh, and Y. Kawada. 1985. Evolution of interferon genes. *Interferon* **6:** 1.

Miyata, T., H. Hayashida, R. Kikuno, M. Hasegawa, M. Kobayashi, and K. Koike. 1982. Molecular clock of silent substitution: At least six-fold preponderance of silent changes in mitochondrial genes over those in nuclear genes. *J. Mol. Evol.* **19:** 28.

Nomiyama, H., K. Obaru, Y. Jinno, I. Matsuda, K. Shimada, and T. Miyata. 1986. Amplification of human argininosuccinate synthetase pseudogenes. *J. Mol. Biol.* **192:** 221.

Palese, P. and J.F. Young. 1982. Variation of influenza A, B, and C viruses. *Science* **215:** 1468.

Watson, J.D., N.H. Hopkins, J.W. Roberts, J.A. Steitz, and A.M. Weiner. 1987. *Molecular biology of the gene*, volume 1. Benjamin Cummings, Menlo Park, California.

Wilson, A.C., S.S. Carlson, and T.J. White. 1977. Biochemical evolution. *Annu. Rev. Biochem.* **46:** 573.

Winter, R.M., E.G.D. Tuddenham, E. Goldman, and K.B. Matthews. 1983. A maximum likelihood estimate of the sex ratio of mutation rates in haemophilia A. *Hum. Genet.* **64:** 156.

Wu, C.-I. and W.-H. Li. 1985. Evidence for higher rates of nucleotide substitution in rodents than in man. *Proc. Natl. Acad. Sci.* **82:** 1741.

Reconstructing the Evolution of Vertebrate Blood Coagulation from a Consideration of the Amino Acid Sequences of Clotting Proteins

R.F. DOOLITTLE AND D.F. FENG
Department of Chemistry, University of California, San Diego,
La Jolla, California 92093

Vertebrate blood coagulation is a delicately balanced phenomenon whose central feature is the thrombin-catalyzed conversion of fibrinogen to fibrin. A large number of accessory proteins are involved, both in the generation of thrombin and in the mobilization, degradation, or neutralization of other components. The general theme of events embodies restrained and highly selective proteolysis. To this end, there are two main routes for the production of thrombin, denoted the extrinsic and intrinsic systems, respectively.

The extrinsic system begins with the release or exposure of the membrane-associated tissue factor (TF) that activates the protease precursor denoted factor VII. Activated factor VII, in turn, attacks factor X, which, in league with the accessory protein factor V and calcium ions, converts prothrombin to thrombin (Fig. 1). The intrinsic system runs a roughly parallel course, beginning with a plasma-based contact factor, XII, which itself may be activated by "foreign" substances or by a plasma protein prekallikrein. Activated factor XII converts factor XI to an activated form, which in turn attacks factor IX. Factor IX, in concert with the accessory protein factor VII, and in an analogous fashion to the (extrinsic) factor VII, activates factor X. Prothrombin, factor VII, factor X, and factor IX, are typified by having unique calcium-binding domains near their amino termini, the characteristic feature of

which is the unusual amino acid γ-carboxyglutamic acid ("Gla").

The evolution of these parallel proteolytic amplification systems has long been a subject of interest, since at first glance, it is difficult to imagine how any part of the scheme could function without the whole ensemble (Doolittle 1961). One of our longstanding goals has been to derive a logical step-by-step scenario depicting the evolution of the process. In this regard, we long ago undertook comparative studies aimed at finding creatures with simpler clotting systems that might provide clues to the relative appearance of some of the clotting factors (Doolittle and Surgenor 1962).

Since then, the amino acid sequences of many mammalian clotting proteins have been determined, including all of the factors mentioned above, as well as a number of others involved in fibrinolysis and the inactivation of various factors. Largely as a result of the efforts of Davie et al. (1986), the sequences of most of the serine proteases involved have been reported. As anticipated, these sequences are all homologous, and as a result, it should be possible to reconstruct their evolutionary appearance merely by sequence comparison. The situation is complicated, to a degree, in that "exon shuffling" has played a significant role in their invention. Thus, an assortment of identifiable modules occurs in their amino-terminal "halves," including struc-

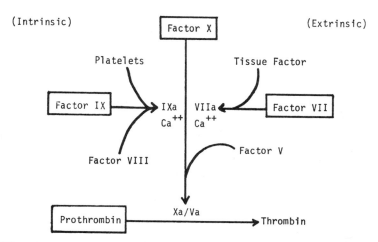

Figure 1. Outline of reactions involved in intrinsic and extrinsic clotting schemes in mammals. Thrombin generated by either course leads to the transformation of fibrinogen into fibrin.

Table 1. Shuffled Exonic Structures in the Amino-terminal Regions of Clotting and Lysis Proteins

	Gla	Finger	EGF	Kringle	CF
Factor X	+		2		
Factor IX	+		2		
Factor VII	+		2		
Prothrombin	+			2	
Factor XII		1 + 1	1 + 1	1	
Plasminogen				5	
Plasminogen activator		1	1	2	
Urokinase			1	1	
Factor XI					4
Prekallikrein					4

(Gla) γ-Carboxyglutamic acid region; (Finger) fibronectin fingers I or II; (EGF) epidermal growth factor domain; (Kringle) pretzel-like structure first identified in prothrombin; (CF) contact factor domain.

tural domains referred to as kringles, EGF domains, fibronectin fingers, and gla domains. At the same time, these characters can themselves be used as pointers to the order of appearance of the various factors (Table 1).

In the present study, we attempt to reconstruct events surrounding the appearance of the principal proteases involved in vertebrate blood clotting by comparing the sequences of their carboxy-terminal halves. These regions have not been subject to exon exchange, so far as we can tell, and have the further advantage that they can be compared with other serine proteases not involved in blood clotting. In this regard, we have aligned the sequences of 13–15 proteases and constructed phylogenetic trees by a progressive alignment scheme designed to reflect as accurately as possible the evolutionary process (Feng and Doolittle 1987). We have compared the results with both early conclusions based on comparative studies, on the one hand, and inferences made on the basis of characteristic amino-terminal domains, on the other.

MATERIALS AND METHODS

Progressive alignment. The computer-based progressive alignment scheme employed makes the alignment strictly by objective criteria (no "eyeball shifting"). The tree-building program used was based on principles first described by Fitch and Margoliash (1967) and includes various modifications subsequently introduced by other investigators (Klotz and Blanken 1980). The novel feature of the procedure is that it builds the alignment progressively, beginning with the most similar sequences, and employs the rule "once a gap, always a gap." The premise is that the most reliable data are those involving the most recently diverged sequences. A full description of the procedure appears elsewhere (Feng and Doolittle 1987).

Protease sequences. The 15 sequences used in the study were taken from the published literature: human prothrombin (Friezner-Degen et al. 1983), human factor IX (Kurachi and Davie 1982), bovine factor X (Enfield et al. 1980), human factor XII (McMullen and Fujikawa 1985), human factor XI (Fujikawa et al. 1986), human factor VII (Hagen et al. 1986), bovine

protein C (Long et al. 1984), human prekallikrein (Chung et al. 1986), human plasminogen (Wiman 1977), human plasminogen activator (Pennica et al. 1983), human urokinase (Steffens et al. 1982), human complement factor B (Woods et al. 1982), human complement factor C1r (Arlaud and Gagnon 1983), bovine trypsinogen (Walsh and Neurath 1964), bovine chymotrypsinogen B (Smillie et al. 1968), and porcine elastase (Shotton and Hartley 1970). Various subsets of the sequences were aligned during the course of the study, the most important of which is shown in Figure 2.

RESULTS

Several different aspects are considered in the interpretation of evolutionary trees derived from sequence alignments. First, an examination is made to determine whether there is a clustering by function. Second, a search is made for independent origins for agents involved in similar interactions. In our case, the sequences fell into two main groups (Fig. 3). Not unexpectedly, those proteases whose amino-terminal segments have gla-containing sequences form a discrete cluster. The deepest division in the cluster is between prothrombin and the others, implying that a prothrombin-like protein was the first of these agents on the scene. Although not shown in Figure 3, in other trees, we found that the next most closely related sequence, surprisingly, was C1r, the first protease in the complement system.

A separate subcluster exists also for tissue plasminogen activator, urokinase, and factor XII. Plasminogen seems to have emerged on an independent line direct from a "root stock." Factor XI and prekallikrein constitute a somewhat remotely situated pair that appears to have budded off from the pancreatic zymogen group. These two proteins have distinctive amino-terminal halves (not used in the comparisons here) and are known to be closely related (Chung et al. 1986). In some of our trees, we included the more distantly related complement B, and it consistently assumed the "outlier" position.

Even with a casual inspection of the tree shown in Figure 3, it is clear that the branching order is only partly consistent with a wholly parsimonious treatment

```
f11hu    IVGGTASVRGEWPWQVTL  HTTSPTQR  HLCGGSIIGNQWILTAAHCF    YGVESPKILRVYSGILNQSEIKEDTSFFGVQEIII  HDQYKMAES
prek     IVGGTNSSWGEWPWQVSL  QVKLTAQR  HLCGGSLIGHQWVLTAAHCF    DGLPLQDVWRIYSGILNLSDITKDTPFSQIKEIII  HQNYKVSEG
chyb     IVNGEDAVPGSWPWQVSL    QD  STGF HFCGGSLISEDWVVTAAHC     GVTTSDV  VVAGEFDQGLETEDTQVLKIGKVFK  NPKFSILTV
elap     VVGGTEAQRNSWPSQISL  QYRSGSSWAHTCGGTLIRQNWVMTAAHC      VDRELTFRVVVGEHNLNQNNGTEQVVGVQKIVV  HPYWNTDDVAA
tryb     IVGGYTCGANTVPYQVSL    N    SGY HFCGGSLINSQWVVSAAHCY    KSGIQVRL    GQDNINVVEGNQQFISASKSIV  HPSYNSNTL
plsh     VVGGCVAHPHSWPWQVSL    RT  RFGM HFCGGTLISPEWVLTAAHCL    EKSPRPSSYKVILGAHQEVNLEPHVQEIEVSRLFL  EP        T
paht     IKGGLFADIASHPWQAAIFAKHRRSPGERFLCGGILISSCWILSAAHCF    QERFPPHHLTVILGRTYRVVPGEEEQKFEVEKYIV  HKEFDDDT  Y
f12hu    VVGGLVALRGAHPYIAALY    WGHS  FCAGSLIAPCWVLTAAHCL      QDRPAPEDLTVVLGQERRNHSCEPCQTLAVRSYRL  HEAFSPVS  Y
lmuh     IIGGEFTTIENQPWFAAIY  RRHRGGSVTYVCGGSLISPCWVISATHCF    IDYPKKEDYIVYLGRSRLNSNTQGEMKFEVENLIL  HKDYSADTLAH
f7hu     IVGGKVCPKGECPWQ  VL    L  LVNGAQLCGGTLINTIWVVSAAHCF    DKIKNWRNLIAVLGEHDLSEHDGDEQSRRVAQVIIP  STYVPGTT
f9hu     VVGGEDAKPGQFPWQVVL      NGKVDAFCGGSIVNEKWIVTAAHC      ETG   VKITVVAGEHNIEETEHTEQKRNVIRAIIPHHNYNAAINKY
f10b     IVGGRDCAEGECPWQALL     V  NEENEGFCGGTILNEFYVLTAAHCL    HQA   KRFTVRVGDRN  TQEGDEEMAHEVEMTVKHSRFVKET  Y
proc     IVDGQEAGWGESPWQAVL     L  DSKKKLVCGAVLIHVSWVLTVAHCL    DSR   KKLIVRLGEYDMRRWESWEVDLDIKEVII  HPNYTKSTS
prot     IVEGSDAEIGMSPWQVML   FRKSPQELLCGASLISDRWVLTAAHCLLYPPWDKNFTENDLLVRIGKHSRTRYERNIEKISMLEKIYIHPRYNWREN  L
```

```
f11hu    GYDIALLKL  ETT    VNYTDSQRPICLPSKG  DRNV  I YTDCWVTGWGYRKLR   D KIQNTLQKAKIPLVTNEECQK  RYR    GHKITHKMI
prek     NHDIALIKL  QAP    LNYTEFQKPICLPSKG  DTST  I YTNCWVTGWGFSKEK   G EIQNILQKVNIPLVTNEECQK  RYQ    DYKITQRMV
chyb     RNDITLLKL  ATP    AQFSETVSAVCLPSAD  EDFP  A GMLCATTGWGKTKYN   ALKTPDKLQQATLPIVSNTDC R KYW     GSRVTDVMI
elap     GYDIALLRL  AQS    VTLNSYVQLGVLPRAG  TILA  N NSPCYITGWGLTRTN   G QLAQTLQQAYLPTVDYAICSSSSYW     GSTVKNSMV
tryb     NNDIMLIKL  KSA    ASLNSRVASISLPTSC  A  S  A GTQCLISGWGNTKSS   GTSYPDVLKCLKAPILSNSSCKS  AYP    G QITSNMF
plsh     RKDIALLKL  SSP    AVITDKVIPACLPSPN  YVVA  D RTECFITGWGETQ     GTFGAGLLKEAQLPVIENKVCNRYEFL     NGRVQSTEL
paht     DNDIALLQL  KSDSSRCAQESSVVRTVCLPPAD  LQLP  D WTECELSGYGKHEAL   SPFYSERLKEAHVRLYPSSRCTSQHLL     NRTVTDNML
f12hu    QHDLALLRLQEDADGSCALLSPYVQPVCLPSG  AARP  SETTLCQVAGWGHQFEG     AEEYASFLQEAQVPFLSLERCSAPDVH     GSSILPGML
lmuh     HNDIALLKIRSK EGRCAQPSRTIQTICLPSM  YNDP  QFGTSCEITGFGKENST    DYLYPEQLKMTVVKLISHRECQQPHYY     GSEVTTKML
f7hu     NHDIALLRLHQP    VVLTDHVVPLCLPERTFSERTL AFVRFSLVSGWG QLLD      RGATALELMVLNVPRLMTQDCLQQSRKVGDSPNITEYMF
f9hu     NHDIALLEL  DEP    LVLNSYVTPICIADKE  YTNIFLKFGS GYVSGWG RVFH    KGRSALVLQYLRVPLVDRATCLRSTK     FTIYNNMF
f10b     DFDIAVLRLKTP     IRFRN VAPACLPEKDWAAETL  QTKTGIVSGFG RTHE     KGRLSSTLKMLEVPYVDRSTCKLSSS     FTITPNMF
proc     DNDIALLRLAKP    ATLSQTIVPICLPDSGLSERKLTQVGQETVVTGWGYRDET     KRNRTFVLSFIKVPVVPYNACVHAME     NKISENML
prot     DRDIALMKLKKP    VAFSDYIHPVCLPDRETAASLL QAGYKGRVTGWGNLKETWTANVGKGQPSVLQVVNLPIVERPVCKDSTR     IRITDNMF
```

```
f11hu    CAGYREGG      KDACKGDSGGPLSCKHNE    VWHLVGITSWGE  GCAQRERPGVYTNVVEYVDWILE  KTQAV
prek     CAGYKEGG      KDACKGDSGGPLVCKHNG    MWRLVGITSWGE  GCARREQPGVYTKVAEYMDWILE  KTQSSDGKAQMQSPA
chyb     CAG  ASG      VSSCMGDSGGPLVCQKNG    AWTLAGIVSWGS  STCSTSTPAVYARVTALMPWVQE  TLAAN
elap     CAG GNVG      RSGCQGDSGGPLHCLVNG    QYAVHGVTSFVSRLGCNVTRKPTVFTRVSAYISWINN  VIASN
tryb     CAGYLEGG      KDSCQGDSGGPVVCSG      KLQGIVSWGS  GCAQKNKPGVTKVCNYVSWIKQ  TIASN
plsh     CAGHLAGG      TDSCQGDSGGPLVCFEKD    KYILQGVTSWGL  GCARPNKPGVYVRVSRFVTWIEG  VMRNN
paht     CAGDTRSGGPQANLHDACQGDSGGPLVCLNDG    RMTLVGIISWGL  GCGQKDVPGVYTKVTNYLDWIRD  NMRP
f12hu    CAGFLEGGT      DACQGDSGGPLVCEDQAAERRLTLQGIISWGS  GCGDRNKPGVYTDVAYYLAWIRE  HTVS
lmuh     CAADPQWKT      DSCQGDSGGPLVCSLQG    RMTLTGIVSWG  GCALKDKPGVYTRVSHFLPWIRS  HTKEENGLAL
f7hu     CAGYSDGSK      DSCKGDSGGPHATHYRG    TWYLTGIVSWGQ  GCATVGHFGVYTRVSQYIEWLQKLMRSEPRPGVLLRAPFP
f9hu     CAGFHEGGR      DSCQGDSGGPHVTEVEG    TSFLTGIISWGE  ECAMKGKYGIYTKVSRYVNWIKE  KTKLT
f10b     CAGYDTQPE      DACQDSGGPHVTRFKD    TYFVTGIVSWGE  GCARKGKFGVYTKVSNFLKWIDKIMKARAGAAGSRGHSEAPATWTVPPPLPL
proc     CAGILGDPR      DACEGDSGGPMVTFFRG    TWFLVGLVSWGE  GCGRLYNYGVYTKVSRYLDWIYGHIKAQEAP   LESQVP
prot     CAGYKPDEGKR   GDACEGDSGGPFV  MKSPFNNRWYQMGIVSWGE  GCDRDGKYGFYTHVFRLKKWIQKVIDQFGE
```

Figure 2. Alignment of sequences from 11 serine proteases involved in blood clotting and fibrinolysis and three pancreatic digestive enzymes. (elap) Porcine elastase; (tryb) bovine trypsin; (chyb) bovine chymotrypsin; (prek) prekallikrein; (plsh) human plasminogen; (paht) human plasminogen activator; (lmuh) human urokinase; (proc) bovine protein C; (prot) human prothrombin; (f11hu) human factor XI; (f12hu) human factor XII; (f9hu) human factor IX; (f7hu) human factor VII; (f10b) bovine factor X.

of the "shuffled exons" found in the regions of the proteins that were not used in the alignments. Thus, single events can account for the introduction of the gla domain, on the one hand, and the two EGF domains in factor IX, factor X, and protein C, on the other. Similarly, the occurrence of four "contact factor" domains in factor XI and prekallikrein can also be explained by a single happening. On separate occasions, however, single EGF domains must have been added to a common ancestor of factor XII, plasminogen activator, and urokinase. Moreover, kringles have been added or deleted to or from prothrombin and the factors involved in fibrinolysis on several occasions. So far as we know, the sequence of the amino-terminal half of Clr has not yet been reported, and it will be of great interest to determine whether it contains a kringle structure of the sort found in prothrombin, given the similarity of their protease sections.

The quantitative features of the tree in Figure 3 are also revealing. For example, it is obvious that the di-

versification of the gla-containing proteins took place in parallel with that of the plasminogen-activator family. In contrast, the divergence of factor XI and prekallikrein was a relatively recent event that took place well after all the other factors were in place (Fig. 3). Indeed, we can make some estimates about when all of these gene duplications took place by availing ourselves of sequence data from various species. For example, human and bovine sequences have both been reported for prothrombin, plasminogen, protein C, and factor IX, inter alia, and each of the pairs is 85–86% identical over the regions used in our alignment. Knowing that artiodactyls and primates diverged about 80 million years ago, we can extrapolate the observed differences between various factors and gauge the times of duplication. Thus, prekallikrein and factor XI are 68% identical, and, allowing for the exponential course of sequence divergence, we can estimate they must have begun their separate existences about 200 million years ago. By this same kind of reckoning, the major diver-

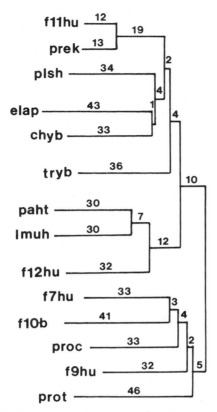

Figure 3. Phylogenetic tree showing relationship of sequences from 14 serine proteases aligned in Fig. 2. Sequence lengths compared ranged from 223 to 259 residues.

Table 2. An Inferred Order of Appearance for Some Blood-clotting and Fibrinolytic Proteins

Factor	MYA[a]
Fibrinogen	600
Prothrombin	
Tissue factor	
Plasminogen	
Factor XII	500
Factor X	
Factor VII	
Factor V	
Urokinase	450
Factor IX	
Factor VIII	
Factor XI	
Prekallikrein	200

[a]MYA indicates millions of years ago.

gence of gla-containing factors began about 600 million years ago, a time that corresponds to the divergence of the fibrinogen γ and β chains (Doolittle 1984).

DISCUSSION

Extrapolations based on sequence comparisons, if they are valid, should be in accord with the actual distribution of the proteins among existing creatures. For example, if prekallikrein and factor XI are the result of a gene duplication that took place only 200 million years ago, then all those vertebrates that di-

verged prior to that time should have only a single preduplication representative. This suggests that fish and amphibians only have a single factor of this sort. The divergence of reptiles and birds from the mammalian line is usually put at about 250 million years, and it will be interesting to determine whether either or both of these classes have both proteins.

With regard to more ancient happenings, it is known that lampreys, which along with hagfish diverged from vertebrate lines about 450 million years ago, definitely have fibrinogen, prothrombin, tissue factor, XIII, and plasminogen (Doolittle et al. 1962; Doolittle 1984); there is circumstantial evidence that these creatures also have factors VII, V, and X, a surmise based on the observation that lampreys have a well-developed extrinsic system that responds to exogenous (human) factor V (Doolittle and Surgenor 1962). The intrinsic clotting system in lampreys is largely confined to factors associated with thrombocytes, the nucleated equivalent of the mammalian blood platelet, and it will be of more than passing interest to determine if lampreys have factors IX and VIII. In the event they do not, it should be possible to pinpoint the invention of these proteins

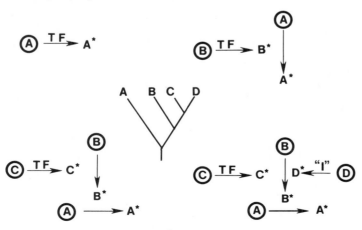

Figure 4. Four hypothetical stages of blood clotting showing how alternate pathways may have appeared during evolution. (TF) Tissue factor; (I) intrinsic stimulus. The tree in the center shows how three gene duplications would lead to genes for four precursor enzymes (circled). Asterisk designates the activated proteases. According to this scheme, a direct TF-activated path existed first. The way events are shown here, A corresponds to prothrombin, B is factor X, C is factor VII, and D is factor IX.

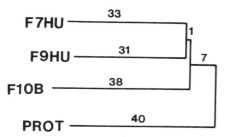

Figure 5. Computer-plotted cladogram based on sequences of four gla-containing factors listed in Table 3.

by finding those lower organisms in which these two important factors do occur.

In the meantime, we can pose a scenario of how and when the various clotting and lysis proteins made their appearance by combining the results of the sequence comparisons with observations as to which factors occur in the lamprey (Table 2). The scheme logically begins with the thrombin-fibrinogen reaction that may have come into being as long ago as 600 million years. With the evolution of the blood clot came the need to remove it, and the equivalent of plasminogen must have appeared soon thereafter. The progenitor factor XII, according to our tree, should have been involved with plasminogen activation.

Four hypothetical early stages in the evolution of parallel intrinsic and extrinsic schemes are depicted in

Figure 4, and, by way of comparison, a computer-derived tree based on the actual sequences of prothrombin and factors X, VII, and IX is shown in Figure 5. The eventual incorporation of factor XII, factor XI, and prekallikrein is predicted in Figure 6. In contemporary mammals, this group of proteins may be involved in coupling, clotting, and lysis, consistent with the presumed role for a factor XII ancestor in ancient creatures. (The depictions in Figs. 4 through 6 only include the serine protease factors and do not show non-protease factors such as fibrinogen and factors V and VIII.)

In conclusion, the elucidation of the sequences of many of the mammalian blood-clotting factors allows inferences to be made about the time and order in which these proteins were introduced during evolution. In some cases, the validity of the extrapolations can be checked by comparative studies on lower vertebrates like the lamprey. In other cases, it will be necessary to explore even more rudimentary systems in protochordates and appropriate invertebrates.

REFERENCES

Arlaud, G.J. and J. Gagnon. 1983. Complete amino acid sequence of the catalytic chain of human complement subcomponent Clr. *Biochemistry* **22**: 1758.

Chung, D.W., K. Fujikawa, B.A. McMullen, and E.W. Davie. 1986. Human plasma prekallikrein, a zymogen to a serine

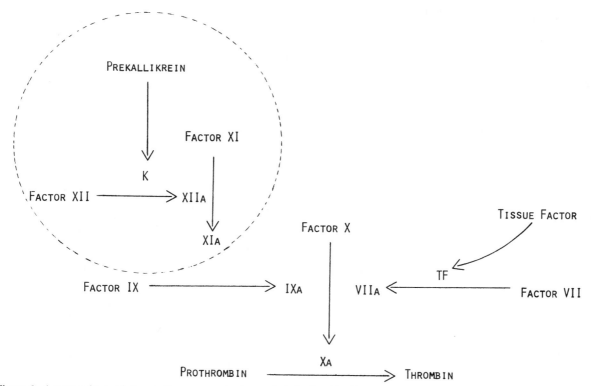

Figure 6. A more advanced stage in the procoagulant cascade is depicted in this rendition, which shows the incorporation of three more reactions in the "front end." None of the three newly added proteins are of the gla type; it is likely that all or some of these reactions do not exist in the clotting schemes of primitive vertebrates like the lamprey.

protease that contains four tandem repeats. *Biochemistry* **25:** 2410.

Davie, E.W., A. Ichinose, and S.P. Leytus. 1986. Structural features of the proteins participating in blood coagulation and fibrinolysis. *Cold Spring Harbor Symp. Quant. Biol.* **51:** 509.

Doolittle, R.F. 1961. "The comparative biochemistry of blood coagulation." Ph.D. thesis, Harvard University, Cambridge, Massachusetts.

———. 1984. Evolution of the vertebrate plasma proteins. In *The plasma proteins* (ed. F. Putnam), p. 317. Academic Press, New York.

Doolittle, R.F. and D.M. Surgenor. 1962. Blood coagulation in fish. *Am. J. Physiol.* **203:** 964.

Doolittle, R.F., J.L. Oncley, and D.M. Surgenor. 1962. Species differences in the interaction of thrombin and fibrinogen. *J. Biol. Chem.* **237:** 3123.

Enfield, D.L., L.H. Ericsson, K. Fujikawa, K.A. Walsh, H. Neurath, and K. Titani. 1980. Amino acid sequence of the light chain of bovine factor X$_1$ (Stuart factor). *Biochemistry* **19:** 659.

Feng, D.-F. and R.F. Doolittle. 1987. Progressive sequence alignment as a prerequisite to correct phylogenetic trees. *J. Mol. Evol.* **25:** 351.

Fitch, W.M. and E. Margoliash. 1967. Construction of phylogenetic trees. *Science* **15:** 279.

Friezner-Degen, S.J., R..A. MacGillivray, and E.W. Davie. 1983. Characterization of the complementary deoxyribonucleic acid and gene coding for human prothrombin. *Biochemistry* **22:** 2087.

Fujikawa, K., D.W. Chung, L.E. Hendrickson, and E.W. Davie. 1986. Amino acid sequence of human factor XI, a blood coagulation factor with four repeats that are highly homologous with plasma prekallikrein. *Biochemistry* **25:** 2417.

Hagen, F.S., C.L. Gray, P. O'Hara, F.J. Grant, G.C. Saari, R.G. Woodbury, C.E. Hart, M. Insley, W. Kisiel, K. Kurachi, and E.W. Davie. 1986. Characterization of a cDNA coding for a human factor VII. *Proc. Natl. Acad. Sci.* **82:** 2412.

Klotz, L.C. and R.L. Blanken. 1980. A practical method for calculating evolutionary trees from sequence data. *J. Theor. Biol.* **91:** 261.

Kurachi, K. and E.W. Davie. 1982. Isolation and characterization of a cDNA coding for human factor IX. *Proc. Natl. Acad. Sci.* **79:** 6461.

Long, G.L., R.M. Belagaje, and R.T.A. MacGillivray. 1984. Cloning and sequencing of liver cDNA coding for bovine protein C. *Proc. Natl. Acad. Sci.* **81:**5653.

McMullen, B.A. and K. Fujikawa. 1985. Amino acid sequence of the heavy chain of human factor XIIa (activated Hageman factor). *J. Biol. Chem.* **260:** 5328.

Pennica, D., W.E. Holmes, W.J. Kohr, R.N. Harkins, G.A. Vehar, C.A. Ward, W.F. Bennett, E. Yelverton, P.H. Seeburg, H.L. Heyneker, D.V. Goeddel, and D. Collen. 1983. Cloning and expression of human tissue-type plasminogen activator cDNA in *E. coli. Nature* **301:** 214.

Shotton, D.M. and B.S. Hartley. 1970. Amino-acid sequence of porcine pancreatic elastase and its homologies with other serine proteinases. *Nature* **225:** 802.

Smillie, L.B., A. Furka, N. Nagabhushan, D.J. Stevenson, and C.O. Parks. 1968. Structure of chymotrypsinogen *B* compared with chymotrypsinogen *A* and trypsinogen. *Nature* **218:** 343.

Steffens, G.J. W.A. Günzler, F. Otting, E. Frankus, and L. Flohé. 1982. The complete amino acid sequence of low molecular mass urokinase from human urine. Hoppe-Seyler's Z. Physiol. Chem. 363:1043.

Walsh, K. and H. Neurath. 1964. Trypsinogen and chymotrpysinogen as homologous proteins. *Proc. Natl. Acad. Sci.* **52:** 884.

Wiman, B. 1977. Primary structure of the B-chain of human plasmin. *Eur. J. Biochem.* **76:** 129.

Woods, D.E., A.F. Markham, A.T. Ricker, G. Goldberger, and H.R. Colten. 1982. Isolation of cDNA clones for the human complement protein factor B, a class III major histocompatibility complex gene product. *Proc. Natl. Acad. Sci.* **79:** 5661.

Globins: A Case Study in Molecular Phylogeny

M. Goodman,[*][†] J. Czelusniak,[*] B.F. Koop,[*][†] D.A. Tagle,[*] AND J.L. Slightom[*][‡]

*Departments of *Anatomy and Cell Biology and †Molecular Biology and Genetics, Wayne State
University School of Medicine, Detroit, Michigan 48201; ‡Division of Molecular Biology,
The Upjohn Company, Kalamazoo, Michigan 49001*

Amino acid sequences are now known for several hundred globin chains, and nucleotide sequences are now known for over 100 globin genes. The sequenced globin chains and genes represent a wide range of eukaryotes, including some plants, some invertebrates, and a large number of vertebrates. The best represented mammalian order is Primates. Nucleotide sequences on extensive flanking DNA regions in the case of ϵ-, γ-, and $\psi\eta$-globin genes for humans and other primates also exist. These comparative sequence data are a rich repository of information on the evolutionary history of both the genes and the species represented by the sequences. In the present study, as in previous ones (Goodman 1981; Goodman et al. 1984), we use the maximum parsimony algorithm to extract this evolutionary information.

The maximum parsimony algorithm constructs genealogical trees of species lineages and also of gene lineages. For the species trees, only sequences supposed to be orthologous are aligned against one another. For the gene trees, the aligned homologous sequences consist not only of orthologues, but also of paralogues (sequences encoded by duplicated genes). The largest portion of amino acid sequence data that elucidate the phylogenetic relationships of vertebrates comes from globins, but αA lens crystallins, cytochrome c, fibrinopeptides A and B, and ribonucleases also contribute useful data. A species tree constructed from these different protein sequences combined in an extended alignment agreed closely with the morphological picture of vertebrate phylogeny; this congruence helped identify the genealogical arrangement for orthologous sequences within paralogous branches of the gene tree of globins. Then, in light of knowledge on the three-dimensional structure and functional residues of vertebrate hemoglobin (Perutz and Fermi 1981; Dickerson and Geis 1983), we examined tempos and modes of amino acid sequence evolution in the globin tree. The results call into question the molecular clock hypothesis and are consistent with Darwinian concepts on natural selection.

Among the more significant episodes in the later history of the globins was a series of gene duplications that occurred in the early mammals and gave rise to a cluster of five linked β-related hemoglobin loci ($5'$-ϵ-γ-η-δ-β-$3'$) (Hardison 1984; Harris et al. 1984; Goodman et al. 1984). Evolutionary reconstructions indicate that only two progenitors of the five genes existed in the

last common ancestor of Eutheria (placental mammals) and Metatheria (marsupials) but that these two genes already differed with respect to times of developmental expression (Koop and Goodman 1988). One locus was the progenitor of δ and β genes; its expression became developmentally delayed and its coding sequence evolved at a threefold faster rate than the embryonically expressed locus, the latter being the progenitor of ϵ, γ, and η genes. This pattern continued in marsupials and also in placentals, where embryonic ϵ genes evolved at the slowest rate. A detailed analysis of the fate of the γ-hemoglobin locus in primates shows that gene duplication per se does not initiate faster rates of coding sequence evolution. This locus duplicated in the catarrhine stem, and the catarrhine γ-coding sequences evolved, after the duplication, at much slower rates than in preceding evolutionary periods. The fastest rate of nonsynonymous substitutions occurred in the single γ locus of earlier primates, when the embryonic hemoglobin that the γ gene encoded was redesigned to be the fetal hemoglobin of simian primates. We suggest that selected substitutions brought about adaptive changes in the allosteric properties of embryonic, fetal, and adult hemoglobins and that the patterns of sequence changes in these hemoglobins exemplify Darwinian evolution.

MATERIALS AND METHODS

Genomic DNA isolation and cloning of primate globin genes. Genomic DNAs were isolated from primate liver or blood samples (Blin and Stafford 1976; Kan and Dozy 1978), followed by a CsCl-ethidium bromide gradient banding. Specifically, DNA was isolated from blood samples of gorilla (Tomoka, National Zoo, Washington, D.C.), chimpanzee-1 (Yerkes Primate Center, Atlanta, Georgia), and rhesus monkey-1 (California Primate Center); from liver samples of orangutan, YO-1 (Yerkes Primate Center), and orangutan, NZO-1 (National Zoo, Washington, D.C.); and from fibroblast tissue-culture cells of spider monkey-1 (H. Villas Zoo, Madison, Wisconsin).

Purified primate DNAs were cloned into λ replacement vectors (either Charon 4A, 30, 32, 35, or 40) after the primate DNAs were partially digested with either *Eco*RI, *Mbo*I, or *Sau*3AI. From these partial digests, DNA fragments of 15–20 kb were size-selected by sedimentation velocity centrifugation on a 5–20% NaCl gradient, as described by Slightom et al. (1980). These size-selected primate DNA fragments were cloned into the appropriate λ replacement vector arms.

Each primate recombinant phage library (at least 1×10^6 pfu) was screened in situ using the nitrocellulose filter contact developed by Benton and Davis (1977), and the filters were hybridized against the nick-translated ^{32}P-labeled *Ava*II to *Eco*RI fragment (245 bp) isolated from the human γ cDNA clone pJW151 (Wilson et al. 1978). This probe is specific for exon 2 of the fetal globin genes; γ genes were thus isolated from each of the above-mentioned libraries, along with clones that contained additional regions of the β-globin gene clusters of these primate species (Giebel et al. 1983; Slightom et al. 1985, 1987, and in prep.; Koop et al. 1986). The nucleotide sequences of the primate fetal globin genes were then obtained by sequencing from the λ clones and from the plasmid subclones.

Nucleotide sequencing of primate globin gene regions. Nucleotide sequences were obtained using the chemical sequencing method developed by Maxam and Gilbert (1980). Isolation of the end-labeled DNA fragments and DNA sequencing reactions were done as described by Maxam and Gilbert (1980) and Chang and Slightom (1984). After the chemical reactions, DNA fragments were subjected to electrophoresis on 16% (40 cm) and 4% (104 cm) acrylamide–7 M urea gels. Pouring of these gels was simplified by using a 1/8-inch hole drilled into the face plate, as described by Slightom et al. (1987). Efficiency of the DNA sequencing gels was increased by using wedge-shaped spacers (Olsson et al. 1984) obtained from CBS Scientific. The wedge spacers measured 60 cm long and their thickness ranged from 0.2 mm (top) to 0.4 or 0.6 mm (bottom); on the longer gels, a 0.2-mm spacer was used for the remaining 44 cm. Hence, these longer gels are referred to as "bell-bottom" gels. A typical 4% acrylamide bell-bottom gel is run until the xylene cyanol dye is about 65 cm from the top; in general, nucleotide sequence reads start about 50 bp from the end-labeled site and read out to about 550 bp. Nucleotide sequence reads greater than 600 bp can be obtained using a 4% gel fitted with a uniform 0.2-mm spacer. The capacity of these gels can be increased by using a comb with 3-mm slots (from International Biotechnologies, Inc.) that allows 32 loads to be made across a 20-cm wide gel. This gel system has been used to obtain as much as 4000 bp of readable nucleotide sequence from a single gel.

Maximum parsimony programs. The minimum number of nucleotide replacements needed to account for a phylogeny, the maximum parsimony score, was determined by two programs (mpalmx and mpafep) that use an algorithm that accurately takes into account the genetic code. These procedures allow subtrees to be fixed: The set of codons corresponding to the parsimony solution for the ancestor of each subtree is computed and is used as a terminal taxon. The program mpalmx computes the scores of all possible trees with eight terminal taxa, and the program mpafep iteratively tries to lower the score of an input tree by branch swapping.

Ancestral codons and branch lengths were calculated by the program tpab, which determines these sequences and lengths by the parsimony method. Ambiguities in parsimony assignments of codons, different ancestral codons each giving the same NR score, were resolved by choosing codons that would minimize the sum of the distances on the tree for every pair of terminal taxa. The distance between terminal taxa on the tree was the sum of lengths of the branches connecting the two taxa. Numbers of nucleotide replacements on each link were corrected for superimposed mutations by the program tava, which propagates mutational information from pairs of nodes more populated by intervening links to those less populated.

All of these programs were run on a Cray-2 computer at the University of Minnesota. Time on this computer was obtained through the NSF supercomputer access program. These four programs are written in Fortran and are available from the authors.

RESULTS AND DISCUSSION

History of Earlier Globins

Figure 1 shows representative lineages from a genealogical tree describing the descent of 245 eukaryotic globins. The maximum parsimony method used to find this tree divided the 245 amino acid sequences into five major phylogenetic clades (Fig. 1). All plant globins (6) group in the first clade, all annelid globins (7) in the second, all arthropod globins (13) in the third, all mollusc globins (6) in the fourth, and all vertebrate globins (213) in the fifth. The extracellular multisubunit hemoglobins of annelids and arthropods group more closely to monomeric hemoglobins of their respective Metazoa phyla than to each other. Within the phylum Annelida, the extracellular hemoglobin sequences of the earthworm and *Tylorrhynchus* form a monophyletic branch that joins the lineage, leading to the intracellular monomeric hemoglobin of the bloodworm *Glycera*. Similarly within Arthropoda, one branch leads to the extracellular multisubunit hemoglobin of *Artemia* (a branchiopod crustacean) and the other branch leads to the monomeric and dimeric forms of the insect *Chironomus*.

The primitive hemoglobin of metazoans was probably monomeric. If so, the multisubunit hemoglobins represent independently derived states in Annelida and Arthropoda. Lending support to this hypothesis, the ancestral sequence that the parsimony method found for annelid globins diverges much less from the single-chain hemoglobin of *Glycera* than from any domain of extracellular annelid hemoglobins (see Fig. 1). Similarly, the ancestral sequence found for arthropod globins diverges less from certain of the monomeric hemoglobins of *Chironomus* than from the multisubunit hemoglobin of *Artemia*.

The lineages of the globin tree shown in Figure 1 illustrate another noteworthy finding, namely, that separate hemoglobin and myoglobin branches emerged more than once from generalized ancestors. The mol-

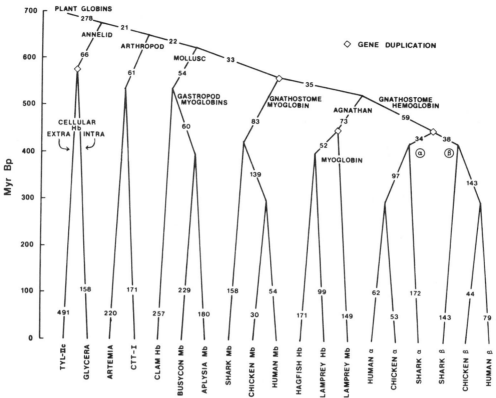

Figure 1. Representative lineages from the genealogical tree for 245 globin amino acid sequences. The branching arrangement for this tree was found using parsimony programs mpalmx and mpafep. The number of nucleotide replacements shown on the lines of descent have been corrected for superimposed mutations by the augmentation algorithm, tava, described in Baba et al. (1981) and based on a procedure that propagates mutational information from pairs of nodes more populated by intervening links to those less populated (Moore 1977). The ordinate scale Myr BP (millions of years before the present) is based on paleontological views, as previously used (Goodman 1981), concerning the ancestral separations of the organisms from which the 245 globins came. In the full tree, extracellular multisubunit hemoglobin sequences of the earthworm *Lumbricus* (an oligochaete) join those of *Tylorrhynchus* (a polychaete); then this extracellular branch joins the lineage to the intracellular monomeric hemoglobin of *Glycera* (a polychaete). Thus, the separation between annelid intracellular and extracellular globins is attributed to a gene duplication that preceded the ancestral separation of annelid subphyla Polychaeta and Oligochaeta. Of the 245 sequences, 219 were previously cataloged (Goodman et al. 1987). New sequences in the present study include *Tylorrhynchus* chain IIc (Suzuji and Gotoh 1986), a domain of the extracellular hemoglobin of *Artemia salina* (Moens et al. 1986), a chain from the tetrameric hemoglobin of the clam *Anadara trapezia* (Como and Thompson 1980), and lamprey myoglobin (A.E. Romero-Herrera and M. Goodman, in prep.).

lusc myoglobins group with clam hemoglobin rather than with vertebrate myoglobins, and the myoglobin of lamprey (an agnathan or jawless vertebrate) groups with lamprey and hagfish hemoglobins rather than with gnathostome (i.e., jawed vertebrate) myoglobins. Of the two types of mollusc myoglobins, the monomeric type found in *Aplysia* (an opisthobranch gastropod) accumulated fewer sequence changes than the dimeric type found in such prosobranch gastropods as *Busycon*, again supporting the idea that the primitive globin of metazoans was a single-chain protein.

The clustering of lamprey myoglobin with lamprey and hagfish hemoglobins is well supported by the parsimony criterion. At least 11 NRs (nucleotide replacements) must be added to the parsimony length to find a tree that breaks up this clade of jawless vertebrate globins. The best genealogical arrangement for the jawed vertebrate myoglobin and hemoglobin branches with respect to the jawless vertebrate globins, however, is not so clear. In previous studies (Goodman et al.

1975, 1987; Goodman 1981), the maximum parsimony results placed the paralogous separation of gnathostome myoglobin and hemoglobin branches in the early gnathostomes not long after the orthologous separation of the lineage to agnathan globins and not long before the paralogous separation of gnathostome α and β hemoglobin branches. In the present reconstruction on the enlarged body of globin amino acid sequences, it is slightly more parsimonious to switch the positions to agnathan globin and gnathostome myoglobin branches or, alternatively, to first group agnathan globin and gnathostome myoglobin branches. The former arrangement (agnathan globin grouping with gnathostome hemoglobin) saves three NRs, and the latter alternative saves four NRs. If we add up the lengths at only those sequence positions where residues in heterotetrameric vertebrate hemoglobins are either heme contacts or intersubunit contacts, then the lowest length (by a savings of just one NR) favors grouping agnathan globin and gnathostome hemoglobin branches first (the arrangement depicted in Fig. 1). In each of these three alternatives, the maximum parsimony reconstruction places the origin of the gnathostome myoglobin branch at a time that is much later than the billion-year-old dates found in molecular clock calculations (Dickerson 1971; Dayhoff 1972). By placing all vertebrate globins together in a monophyletic group apart from other metazoan globins, the parsimony reconstruction allows fossil evidence on the first appearances of vertebrates and metazoans to place limits on how far back to go to date paralogous separations within the vertebrate globin clade. The earliest remains indicative of vertebrate life are from sediments of the mid-Ordovician period about 475 Myr BP (millions of years before the present) (Romer 1966; Janvier 1985), and unequivocal evidence of metazoan life does not appear until about 680 Myr BP (Cloud and Glaessner 1982). Thus, in Figure 1, the gene duplication that separated gnathostome myoglobin and hemoglobin branches falls in between the node for the orthologous separation of molluscs and vertebrates and the later node for the orthologous separation of agnathans and gnathostomes, i.e., at about 575 Myr BP. Inasmuch as this date is only one-half as old as the molecular clock date, it calls into question the molecular clock hypothesis.

A Period of Fast Rates

As in previous studies (Goodman et al. 1975, 1987; Goodman 1981), the present analysis provides evidence that rates of globin evolution were much faster in the early jawed vertebrates and tetrapods than in the amniotes descending to mammals and birds. Rates in the earlier period averaged at about 69 NR% (nucleotide replacements per 100 codons per 10^8 years), whereas rates in the later period averaged about 16 NR%. This marked slowdown in rates depends, however, on the time scale provided by fossil evidence, a scale that places (Fig. 1) the orthologous separation of sharks from birds and mammals at about 425 Myr BP and, in turn, the later orthologous separation of birds and mammals at about 300 Myr BP. The latter date presupposes that birds are more closely related to extant reptiles than to mammals. If birds were more closely related to mammals, then the "molecular clock" date for the bird-mammal divergence node (about 170 Myr BP) would be acceptable, and the evidence for faster rates in the early vertebrates would be much weaker. It is in the context of this issue that the cladistic relationships depicted in the species tree (Fig. 2) for combined protein sequence data are important. As

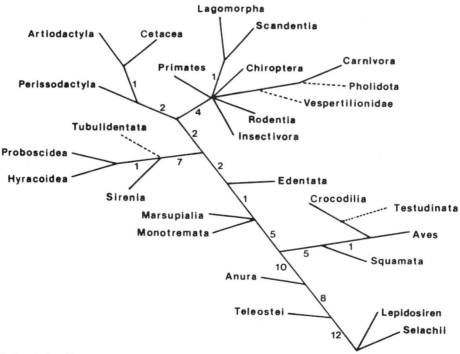

Figure 2. Cladistic relationships among mammalian orders and nonmammalian vertebrate clades from the most parsimonious species tree constructed for 107 taxa using combined protein sequence data (J. Czelusniak et al., in prep.). The amino acid sequences represent 93 β-hemoglobin, 92 α-hemoglobin, 53 myoglobin, 52 αA lens crystallin, 41 fibrinopeptide, 33 cytochrome c, 23 ribonuclease, and 10 embryonic α-hemoglobin chains. The eight types of amino acid sequences were arranged in an extended alignment, with each of the eight segments of the alignment consisting of putative orthologues aligned against one another. Numbers on the stems (links between internodes) are in each case the minimum number of nucleotide replacements required above the maximum parsimony score to find a tree that breaks up the group defined by that stem in the maximum parsimony tree. For example, to break up Tetrapoda requires addition of eight nucleotide replacements, to break up Amniota requires ten replacements, and to break up Mammalia requires five replacements. The taxa represented by dashed lines are poorly represented by sequences (e.g., the aardvark or Tubulidentata only by αA lens crystallin); therefore, these taxa are not included in the calculations of "strength of grouping."

shown in Figure 2, Aves and reptilian taxa still share a common ancestor after the separation of the lineage to Mammalia; at least 5 NRs must be added to the parsimony length to have birds closest to mammals. With cladistic protein evidence placing birds in the reptilian clade of crocodilians, turtles, and squamates, rather than in the clade of mammals, the finding that rates of globin evolution were four to five times faster in earlier vertebrates than in the last 300 million years gains credibility.

Selection of Heterotetrameric Hemoglobin

The fast rates occurred as the primitive monomeric hemoglobin of the early vertebrates evolved into an allosteric tetramer whose subunits interacted cooperatively. During this same time, the vertebrates were evolving into larger more active animals and thus needed an allosteric hemoglobin that could efficiently deliver oxygen to respiring tissues. As illustrated in Figure 3, results from the maximum parsimony recon-

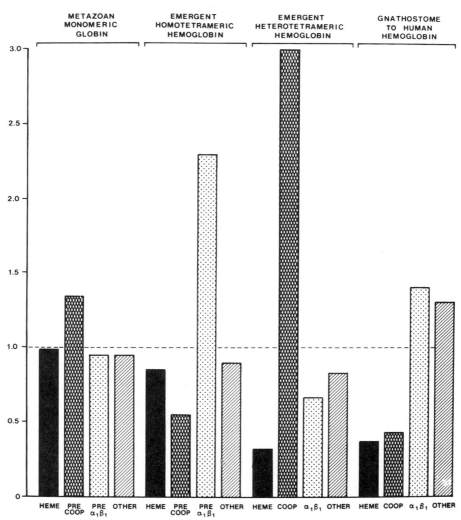

Figure 3. Relative rates of amino acid replacements in different functional groups of hemoglobin sites as deduced from ancestral amino acid sequences found by the parsimony method. The relative rate of a functional group is its percentage of NRs (number of NRs at positions in the functional group to total numbers of NRs) divided by its percentage of positions (number of positions in the functional group to total number of positions). The relative rate of amino acid replacements for all positions is 1.0. During the first (metazoan to vertebrate ancestor) and second (vertebrate to α-β ancestor) periods of descent, HEME designates the functional group consisting of heme contacts; PRE COOP (precursors of cooperative sites) designates those positions that became $\alpha_1\beta_2$ contacts in both α and β chains and those that became associated with either the Bohr effect or DPG binding; PRE $\alpha_1\beta_1$ (precursors of $\alpha_1\beta_1$ contacts) designates those positions that became $\alpha_1\beta_1$ contacts in both α and β chains; OTHER designates the remaining interior and exterior positions. The elevated rate of substitutions in the precursors of $\alpha_1\beta_1$ contacts during the second period of descent plus the fact that almost all subunit contact sites in α chains and almost all in β chains occur in both α and β chains at the same helical positions (see Table 12 in Goodman 1981) supports the idea that a homotetramer had emerged by the time of the α-β duplication. During the third ($\alpha\beta$ to gnathostome α ancestor plus $\alpha\beta$ to gnathostome β ancestor) period of descent, a markedly elevated rate of substitutions at cooperative positions in nascent α and β chains supports the idea that positive selection brought about the emergence of a heterotetrameric hemoglobin with allosteric properties. This idea is further supported by the markedly reduced rate of substitutions at cooperative sites in the subsequent descent of α and β chains. The grouping of residue positions according to function follows the scheme presented in Table 12 in Goodman (1981).

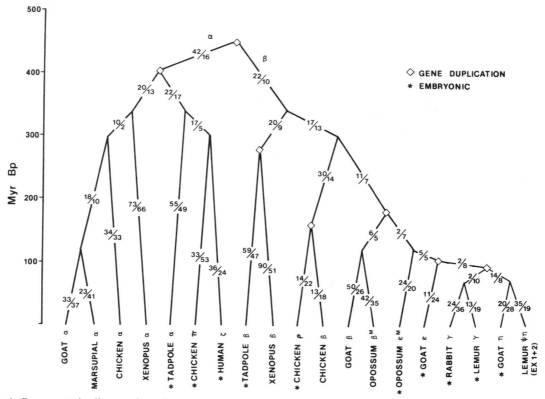

Figure 4. Representative lineages from the most parsimonious genealogical tree for the coding sequences from 112 globin genes. Branch lengths, calculated by the method described by Czelusniak et al. (1982), are presented as fractions, with the numerator giving the number of amino-acid-changing substitutions and the denominator giving the number of silent substitutions. Since these numbers have not been augmented to correct for hidden (back) substitutions, in contrast to the link lengths in Fig. 1, these branch lengths are likely to be underestimated on lines of descent with few internodes relative to those with many internodes.

struction of ancestral globin sequences indicate that the evolutionary transition of monomeric hemoglobin to a tetramer with allosteric properties occurred in two stages. In the first stage, an elevated rate of amino acid replacements at prospective $\alpha_1\beta_1$ contact sites accompanied the emergence of a homotetramer. The second stage began with the gene duplication that produced separate α and β genes. The fastest evolving sequence positions in the nascent α and β chains of the emerging tetramer were the $\alpha_1\beta_2$ contact sites, the salt-bridge-forming sites associated with the Bohr effect, and the 2,3-diphosphoglycerate (DPG)-binding sites. These are sites responsible for the subunit cooperativity that permits efficient unloading of oxygen in respiring tissues. Natural selection first perfected these important functional sites and then preserved them, as evident from the fact that later—from the amniote ancestor to present—they along with heme contacts were the slowest-evolving positions.

Divergence of Embryonic and Adult Hemoglobin Genes

The origin of α- and β-hemoglobin branches (~ 450 Myr BP) and the subsequent rapid evolution of coopera-

tivity in the nascent heterotetrameric hemoglobin of jawed vertebrates preceded the ancestral separation of cartilaginous and bony fishes. Not long afterwards in the primitive bony fishes, about 400 Myr BP, an α-locus duplication was the source of two diverging paralogous gene lines. One line led, presumably through regulatory changes, to α genes expressed in embryonic life, whereas the other line led to α genes expressed from fetal through adult life. In contrast to this monophyletic origin of avian and mammalian embryonic α genes (π and ζ, respectively), independent β gene duplications, much later in phylogeny, were the source of the embryonic ρ locus in birds and embryonic ϵ, γ, and η loci of mammals (Czelusniak et al. 1982; Goodman et al. 1984).

Whereas eutherians (placental mammals) have five types of β-hemoglobin loci (ϵ, γ, η, δ, and β), the opossum (a marsupial) has only two β-hemoglobin genes: one gene ϵ^M has coding and promoter sequences much like those of eutherian prenatally expressed ϵ, γ, and η genes; the other gene β^M codes for adult opossum hemoglobin β chains and has eutherian adult β-type promoters (Koop and Goodman 1988). Apparently, only two progenitors of the five types of eutherian β-hemoglobin genes existed in the last common ancestor of Metatheria (marsupials) and Eutheria, but these two ancestral genes were already differentiated with respect to their times of developmental expression. The two paralogous gene lines (represented by ϵ^M and β^M in opossum) trace back to a single gene duplication that occurred after the ancestral separation of Aves and Mammalia but before the separation of Metatheria and Eutheria. Later in the early eutherians, two further gene duplications separated ϵ, γ, and η loci. Only ϵ, of the three loci, served as an indispensable eutherian gene. The η locus became a pseudogene in the basal primates and was deleted in the stem of rodents and lagomorphs. In turn, artiodactyls lost the γ locus.

The evidence for these deduced historical features of mammalian adult-type and embryonic-type β-hemoglobin genes comes from a genealogical reconstruction carried out by the maximum parsimony method on nucleotide sequence data representing the exons of over 100 globin genes (Koop and Goodman 1988). Figure 4 illustrates the paralogous relationships found in this genealogical reconstruction, and Figure 5 illustrates the orthologous relationships of those mammals that are best represented by sequenced α, β, ϵ, and γ genes. The numbers shown as a fraction on each branch in these figures are, in the numerator, the number of amino-acid-changing base replacements and, in the denominator, the number of silent base replacements.

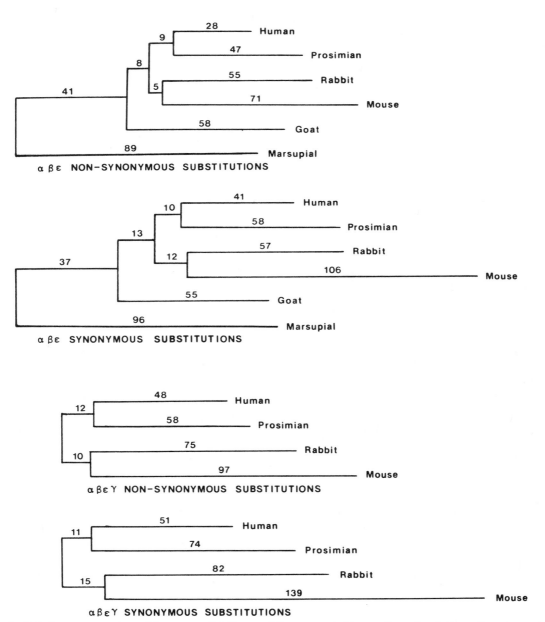

Figure 5. Orthologous separations of the mammalian lineages fully represented by α-, β-, and ϵ-globin coding sequences (*top*) and by α-, β-, ϵ-, and γ-globin sequences (*bottom*). The number of nonsynonymous and synonymous base substitutions along the orthologous lines of descent was obtained from the most parsimonious tree for the coding sequences from 112 globin genes.

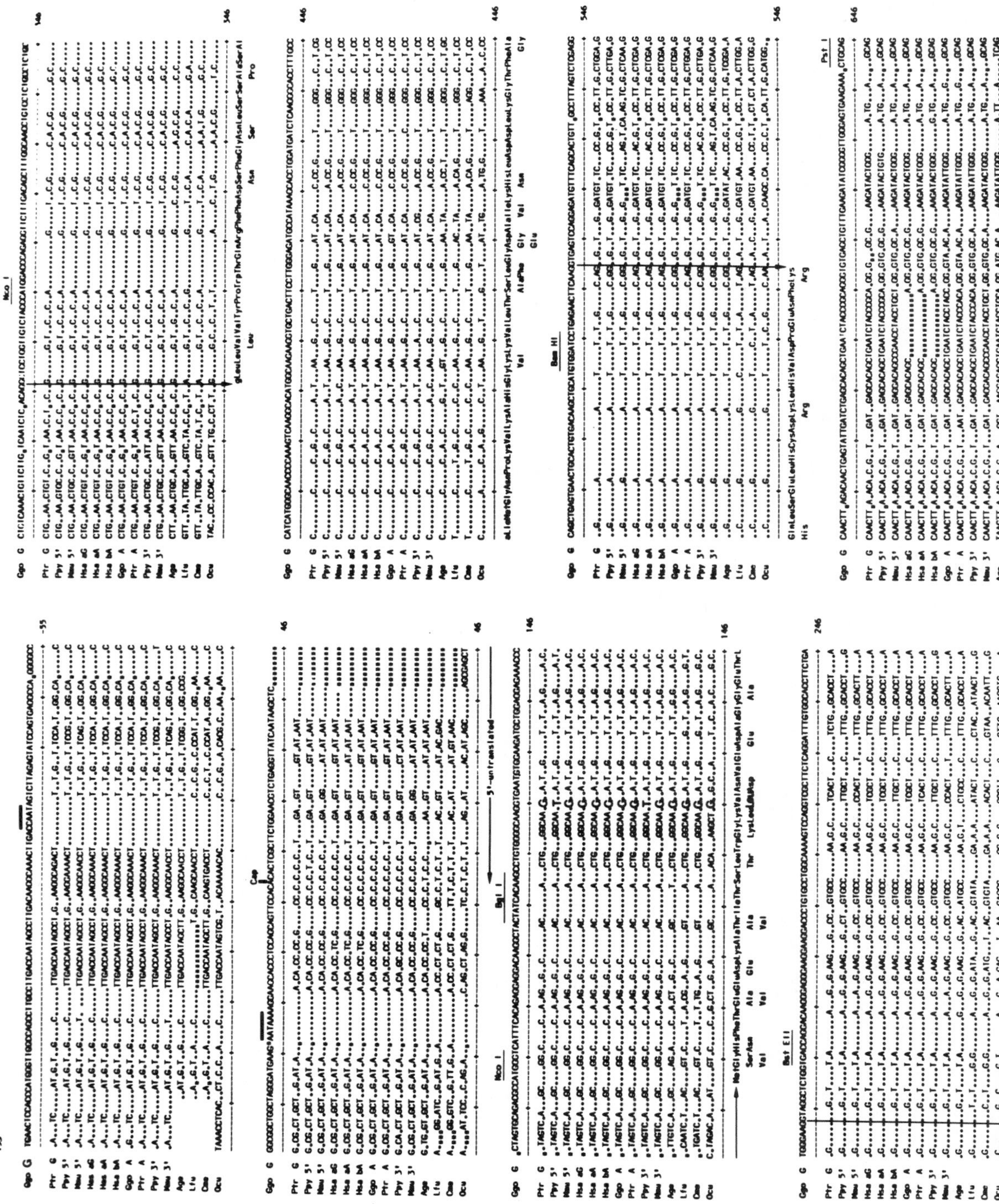

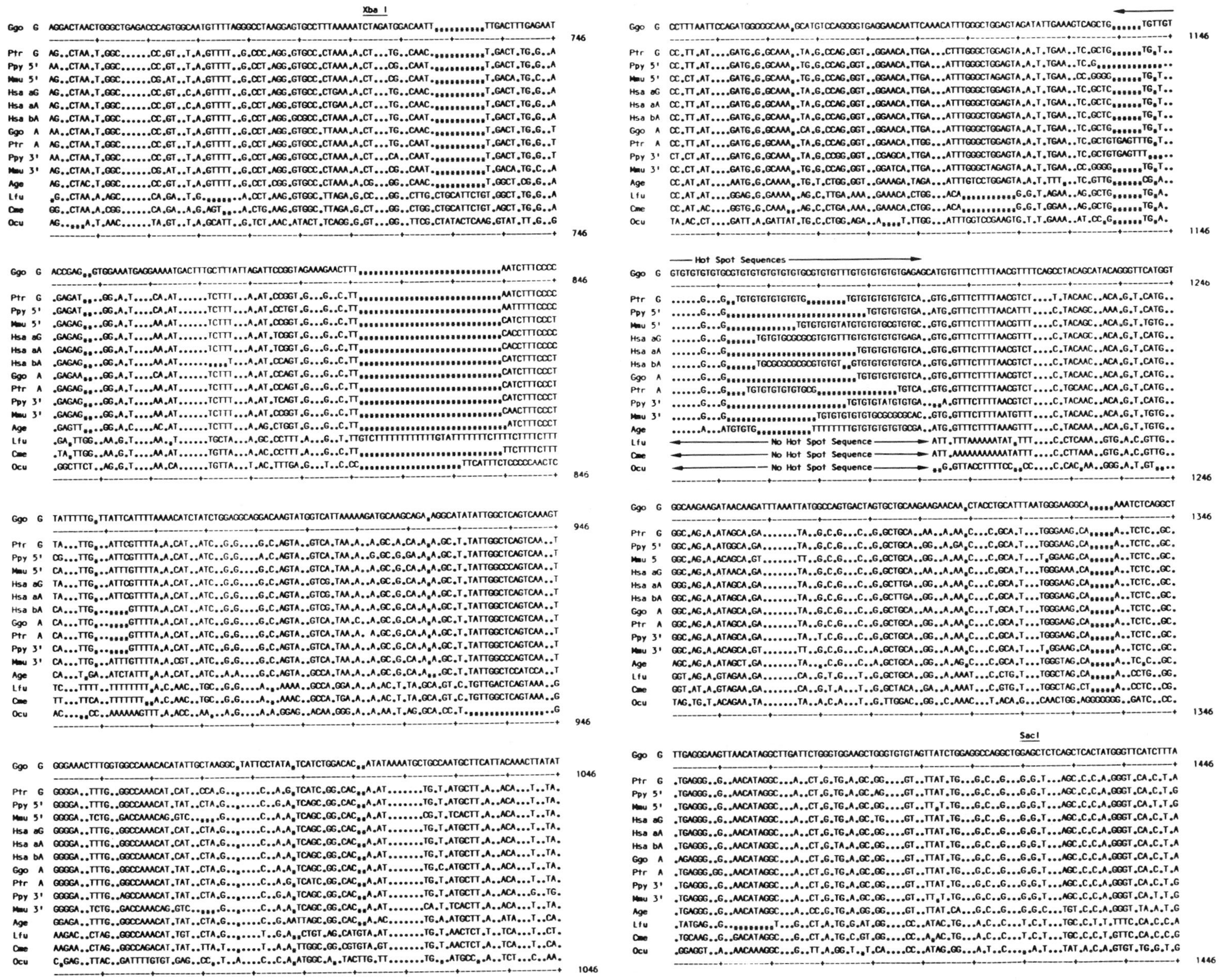

Figure 6. (Continued on following page.)

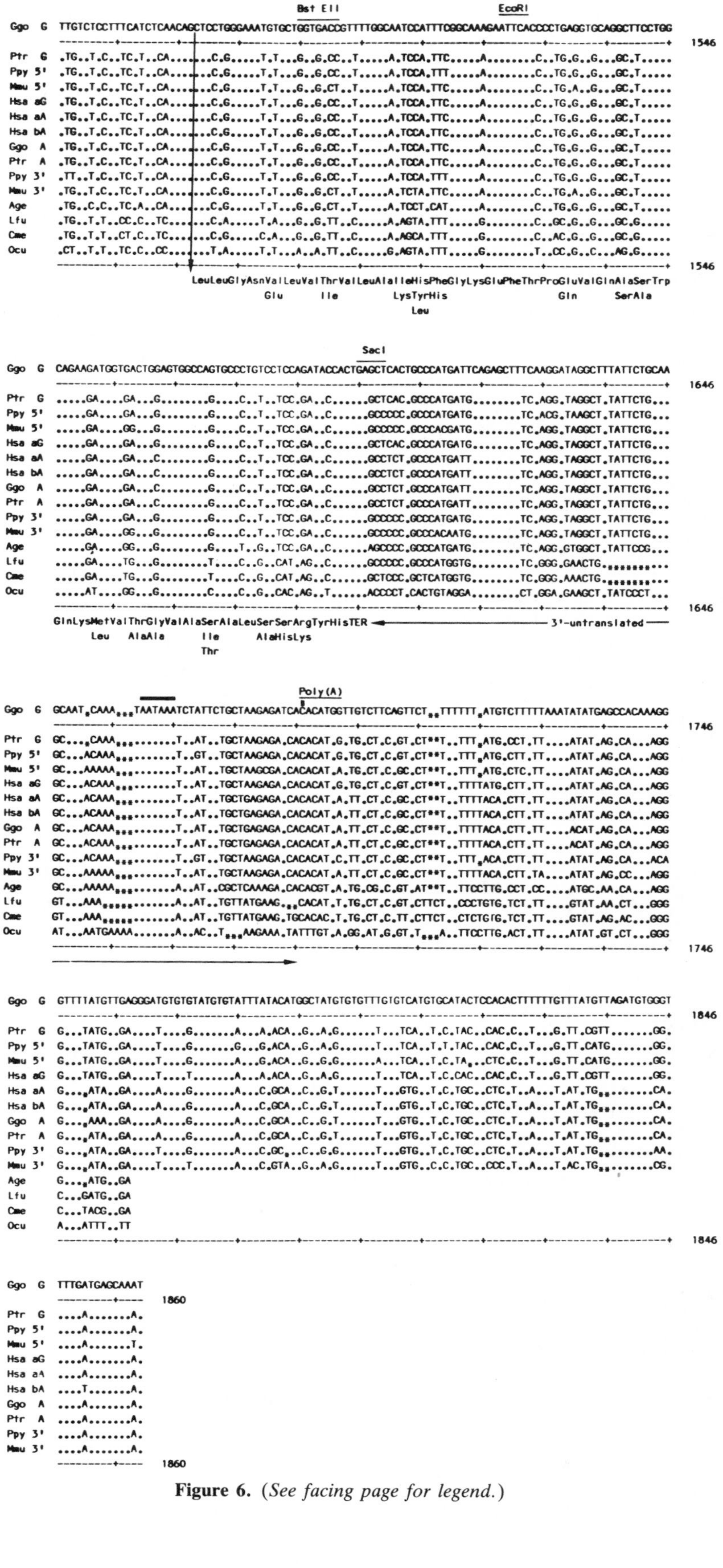

Figure 6. (*See facing page for legend.*)

The quotient of these two magnitudes, i.e., ratio of amino acid changing to silent substitutions or R_{cs} value, serves as a guide as to whether the gene lineage in question evolved under the surveillance of stabilizing selection, R_{cs} values of 1 or less indicating that such surveillance was indeed in force (Czelusniak et al. 1982). The proportion of nonsynonymous substitutions rises when a redundant copy of a functional gene becomes a pseudogene ($R_{cs} = 3$ in randomly mutating codons), but also tends to rise when adaptive amino acid replacements are positively selected. In the latter case, a shift back in a later evolutionary period from higher to lower R_{cs} value is a sure indication that adaptive substitutions were selected. Thus, in addition to rates of amino acid replacements and distributions of replacements in functionally different parts of the hemoglobin molecule, R_{cs} values provide a third parameter for evaluating the role of natural selection in the evolution of hemoglobin genes.

On comparing different mammalian species lineages, we find that both nonsynonymous and synonymous substitutions show the same pattern of nonuniform rates. Among eutherian mammals, rates are fastest in the lineage to mouse and slowest in the human lineage (Fig. 5). As the synonymous or silent substitutions that elude selection show this pattern, the nonuniform rates probably do not involve differences in the intensity of stabilizing selection. Rather, differences in mutation pressure may be the cause. Possibly, the de novo occurrence of mutations is higher in rodents with their short generation times than in primates with their long generation times (Goodman 1985; Wu and Li 1985; Britten 1986). However, on comparing substitution rates in different paralogous gene lineages, we find that the nonsynonymous or amino-acid-changing rate was much slower in embryonic ϵ genes than in the developmentally later expressed β genes, both in opossum and eutherians (see examples in Fig. 4). It would seem that stabilizing selection acted more pervasively on embryonic ϵ genes than on adult β genes. It may well be that less room exists for variation of internal conditions in the embryonic stage of life than in later stages.

After the initial β gene duplication in the stem therian mammals that existed before the metatherian-eutherian split, the nascent ϵ locus became restricted in its expression to embryonic life and the nascent adult-type β locus became developmentally delayed in its expression. During this evolutionary period in which the two genes (nascent ϵ and nascent β) came under different regulatory controls, there was only one-third the number of nonsynonymous substitutions in the emerging embryonic gene as in the emerging adult gene (Fig. 4). Of the reconstructed amino acid changes (in embryonic ϵ: L → F and A → S at positions 3 and 52; in adult β: D → E, N → D, I → V, M → L, I → V, and A → D at positions 43, 47, 54, 78, 111, and 116), perhaps the most significant was the replacement of leucine by phenylalanine at position 3 of the embryonic chain. As position 3 (NA3 in the helical notation) borders NA2, a position involved in DPG binding, it is possible that the R group of phenylalanine—which is larger than the R group of leucine (a phenyl ring compared to an isopropyl moiety)—distorted the space where DPG fits and thus reduced the affinity of the binding site for its ligand. Reduced DPG binding would increase the oxygen affinity of embryonic hemoglobin over that of maternal hemoglobin, thereby favoring the transport of oxygen from mother to embryo. That the replacement of leucine by phenylalanine at NA3 in the progenitor of marsupial and placental ϵ chains had adaptive significance is suggested by this phenylalanine persisting in opossum ϵ^{M} and eutherian ϵ, γ, and η chains.

With respect to the six hypothesized amino acid changes in the nascent adult-type β-chain, three occurred at known functional sites: $\beta43$ is an $\alpha_1\beta_2$ contact site, $\beta54$ an interior position, and $\beta116$ an $\alpha_1\beta_1$ contact site. Moreover, not only was the replacement at $\beta116$ from a neutral to an acidic residue, but the replacement at $\beta47$ (an exterior position) was also charge changing. Thus, it seems reasonable to suggest that the emerging adult hemoglobin had different functional properties from its predecessor. If so, some of the amino acid changes might have led to an adult hemoglobin that was better adapted to external environmental conditions.

Figure 6. Aligned nucleotide sequences of primate γ globin genes along with the orthologous rabbit $\beta3$-globin gene. The nucleotide sequences of the primate γ-globin genes are from the following publications: human $^{A}\gamma$- and $^{G}\gamma$-globin genes are denoted as Hsa aG and Hsa aA ($^{G}\gamma$- and $^{A}\gamma$-genes, respectively) from chromosome a and Hsa bA ($^{A}\gamma$-gene) from chromosome b of a single individual (Slightom et al. 1980; Shen et al. 1981). Gorilla (Ggo), chimpanzee (Ptr), orangutan (Ppy), and rhesus monkey (Mmu) from 5' and 3' γ-gene sequences (equivalent to $^{G}\gamma$ and $^{A}\gamma$ in the case of Ggo and Ptr) are from Scott et al. (1984), Slightom et al. (1987), and J.L. Slightom et al. (in prep.), respectively. The nucleotide sequences of the single fetal-globin gene from spider monkey (Age), brown lemur (Lfu), and dwarf lemur (Cme) are from Giebel et al. (1985) and Harris et al. (1986), respectively. The orthologous rabbit (Ocu) $\beta3$ globin gene sequence is from Hardison (1981). The numbering system used was set by the overall alignment of the 15 γ-gene sequences: asterisks indicate gaps that were used to increase sequence identities among these genes. The complete nucleotide sequence of the gorilla $^{G}\gamma$ gene (which is the longest gene) is presented on the top line (above the first counting line). For any position where one sequence differs from another, the nucleotide or asterisk(s) for that position in each gene is shown. Nucleotide sequence elements that may have biological importance are noted: promoter sequences CCAAT and AATAAA and poly(A)-addition signals are overlined. The γ-chain amino acid sequences are shown below the bottom counting line, and amino acid differences are printed below the appropriate codon. The translation initiator codon is the first Met and the terminator codon is designated TER. Vertical arrows show the location of exon-intron boundaries, which all conform to the GT/AG rule (Breathnach et al. 1978). Horizontal arrows indicate the size expected for the 5'- and 3'-untranslated regions; however, it should be noted that these regions have only been substantiated for the human and for the 3' region of the spider monkey γ-globin genes (Slightom et al. 1980; Giebel et al. 1985; respectively).

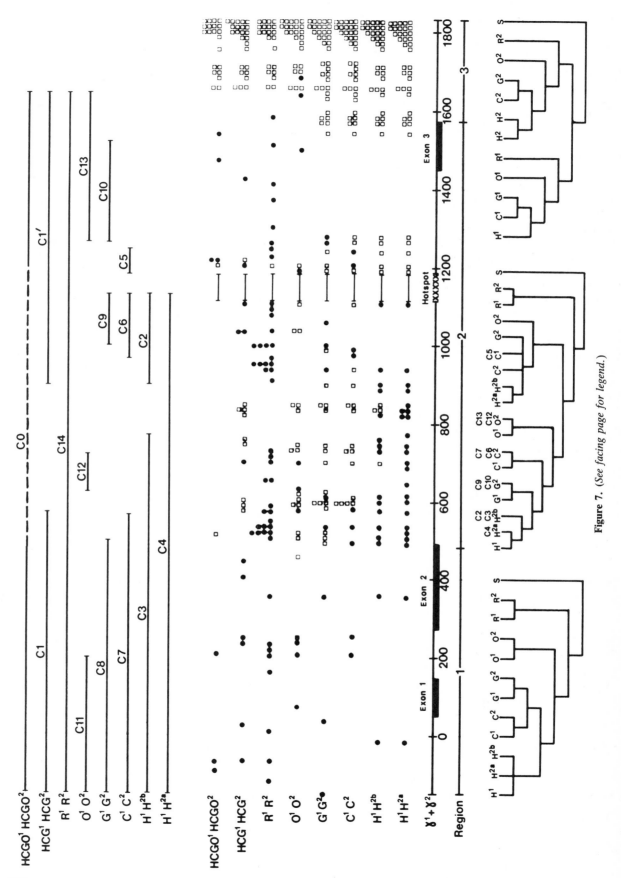

Figure 7. (*See facing page for legend.*)

886

Certainly, after the metatherian-eutherian split, as the descendant marsupials and placentals radiated, their new ecological environments could serve as a selective agency for further sequence changes in adult hemoglobins. Clear evidence that positive natural selection was a force directing the evolution of mammalian hemoglobins comes from examining the fate of the γ locus in primates (see below).

Emergence of Primate Fetal Hemoglobin

A detailed analysis of the genealogical history of primate γ-hemoglobin genes is now possible, because the nucleotide sequences are known for γ genes from a wide range of primates: five catarrhines (human, chimpanzee, gorilla, orangutan, and rhesus monkey), a platyrrhine (spider monkey), and two lemuroid prosimians (brown lemur and dwarf lemur). These gene sequences (aligned in Fig. 6 against the orthologous sequence of the rabbit's single γ locus) represent the duplicated γ loci of catarrhines and single γ locus of the other primates. In addition, the tentative nucleotide sequence of the single γ gene in galago (a lorisoid prosimian) and the partial amino acid sequences of ϵ and γ chains isolated from galago embryonic hemoglobins (R.T. Jones, unpubl.) help elucidate the history of the γ locus in primates (D. Tagle et al., in prep.).

The γ gene in galago, like γ in mouse and rabbit, is turned on in embryonic life and turned off at the beginning of fetal life, at which time β is turned on. In contrast, γ genes in simian primates (catarrhines and platyrrhines) are turned on in fetal life and turned off in postnatal life. Lemur and galago γ gene sequences diverge less from each other than from simian γ sequences; also, the amino acid sequences encoded by prosimian γ-hemoglobin genes diverge less from ϵ-hemoglobin amino acid sequences than have simian γ amino acid sequences (D. Tagle et al., in prep.). These developmental and genealogical facts led to the conclusion that in the first primates, the γ locus, like the ϵ locus, encoded an embryonic hemoglobin chain, but later in primate phylogeny in the lineage to Anthropoidea, γ evolved into a fetally expressed gene.

In the most parsimonious genealogy, low ratios of amino acid changing to silent substitutions (R_{cs} values of only 0.2 to 0.8) occur on the ancestral eutherian γ line and then on the lineages leading to extant lagomorph, rodent, and prosimian γ genes, as illustrated

for rabbit and lemur in Figure 4. These are the lineages where γ genes, behaving as ϵ genes, encoded embryonic hemoglobin chains and were therefore under surveillance of strong stabilizing selection.

On the γ branch leading from the early primates to extant platyrrhine and catarrhine γ genes, the single γ locus duplicated in the early catarrhines, after which (as revealed by the parsimony analysis presented in Fig. 7) the two catarrhine loci experienced gene conversions of varying extents in each catarrhine species lineage. Figure 8 shows those branches of the genealogical reconstruction that describe the descent of the coding sequences in the primate γ genes. In contrast to the low ratios of amino acid changing to silent substitutions in the ancestral eutherian γ line, there is a markedly elevated ratio ($R_{cs} = 3.25$) on the presimian lineage leading to the common ancestor of platyrrhine and catarrhine γ genes. This higher rate of nonsynonymous substitutions coincides with regulatory changes that caused the γ locus to encode a fetal hemoglobin chain rather than an embryonic one.

Of the 13 nonsynonymous substitutions detected on the presimian γ lineage, three occurred at DPG-binding sites: valine at NA1 mutated to glycine and histidine at H21 mutated through two amino-acid-changing base replacements to serine. These mutations must have markedly reduced the DPG-binding capacity of fetal hemoglobin, ensuring a favorable balance in the transport of oxygen from mother to fetus, and thereby helped make possible the extended intrauterine fetal life and extensive prenatal brain development of simian primates. Four other amino acid replacements were also at known functional sites: A→T at interior position $\beta 9$ and I→T, N→I, and Q→E at $\alpha_1\beta_1$ contact positions G14, G18, and H3. A fifth amino acid replacement K→R, at HC1, which borders the DPG-binding position H21, might have also influenced the degree of DPG binding.

In contrast to the high ratio of amino acid changing to silent substitutions and the fast rate of amino acid replacements in the presimian γ lineage, there is a low ratio (average R_{cs} value of 0.75) and a much reduced replacement rate in the catarrhine γ lineages. This pattern of results supports the inference (Goodman 1981; Czelusniak et al. 1982) that positive selection acted at the DPG-binding sites and many other moderating amino acid positions of the precatarrhine γ chains to fix adaptive amino acid replacements. The

Figure 7. A parsimony analysis of aligned γ^1 and γ^2 (or 5' and 3') genes of human (H), chimpanzee (C), gorilla (G), and rhesus monkey (R), plus the hypothetical ancestor of human, chimpanzee, and gorilla (HCG) and the hypothetical ancestor of human, chimpanzee, gorilla, and orangutan (HCGO). Directly above the map of the duplicated γ^1 and γ^2 genes are the results of a position by position parsimony analysis using the single γ gene of spider monkey, brown lemur, dwarf lemur, and rabbit to indicate where intraspecific similarity of γ^1 and γ^2 genes (paralogous positions) is greater than the interspecific similarity of γ^1 or γ^2 (orthologous positions). Open boxes indicate positions where interspecific similarity between γ^1 (or γ^2) genes is greater than intraspecific similarity between γ^1 and γ^2 genes. Two consecutive dots indicate greater intraspecific similarity and suggest a conversion event (labeled C0-C14). Below the map of γ^1 and γ^2 genes, we have indicated three regions, and using regional parsimony analysis, we have estimated the overall phylogenetic order for these three distinct γ gene regions. The complex nature of region 2 necessitated breaking up sequences into small subsequences that reflect patchy conversion regions (for discussion, see Slightom et al. 1987).

natural selection that was positive in the precatarrhines continued to act in the catarrhines, but now in its purifying or stabilizing form.

Darwinian Interpretation

The evolution of globin genes should not be viewed in isolation from the evolution of the organisms in which the genes occur. That a correlation exists between the fate of the genes and the fate of the organisms is obvious when viewed on a macroevolutionary time scale, but it is not so apparent on the short time scale of microevolution. The difference between marsupials and placentals in the number of their β-related hemoglobin genes illustrates the point. As judged from our opossum findings (Koop and Goodman 1988), marsupials have only two developmentally regulated β genes, embryonic ϵ^M and adult β^M. Placentals, on the other hand, have β clusters of up to five or more developmentally regulated genes. In correlation, intrauterine embryonic and fetal life is very brief in marsupials but considerably extended in placentals. Nevertheless, the expansion of a two-gene cluster to a five-gene cluster may not have given the early placental mammals any initial advantage over marsupials. At the time the two-gene cluster expanded, the additional loci may have been redundant. The long-term significance of the expansion is that the additional loci contributed to the success of later evolutionary experiments such as at the γ locus, where an embryonic hemoglobin was redesigned to be the fetal hemoglobin of simian primates.

Just because a gene is redundant, it does not necessarily accumulate mutations freely. It has to become a pseudogene (silenced and nonfunctional) to do so. The duplicate γ locus in catarrhines might be redundant and catarrhines could get along with only one γ locus, as the early catarrhines must have before the duplication occurred. Yet the coding sequences in both loci (the $5'\gamma^1$ and the $3'\gamma^2$) are clearly not able to accumulate nonsynonymous mutations freely. The encoded amino acid sequences of both loci are closely scrutinized by purifying selection, as evident from the low ratios of amino acid changing to silent substitutions in the catarrhine γ^1 and γ^2 genes (Fig. 8). For nonsynonymous mutations to accumulate freely in a catarrhine γ gene, that gene would have to be repressed in its expression. But selection would not tolerate mutations in the two presently expressed catarrhine γ genes when such mutations harm the functioning of fetal hemoglobin.

Although extra loci encoding embryonic hemoglobin chains might well have been redundant in the early placental mammals in the sense that one ϵ locus would have sufficed, the extra loci (γ and η) when expressed did not escape purifying selection. This is especially evident in the gene line of the pre-γ and nascent γ locus, where very low ratios of amino acid changing to silent substitutions (R_{cs} values of 0.25 and 0.20) are found in the genealogical reconstruction (Fig. 4). As many as 30–40 million years had elapsed from the time

of the duplication that separated ϵ, γ, and η genes in a stem lineage of Eutheria (a lineage that existed about 110–90 Myr BP) to the time in the presimians (~ 60–40 Myr BP) when the burst of nonsynonymous substitutions occurred at the γ locus.

Two different explanations have been offered for the elevated rate of nonsynonymous substitutions in the presimian γ locus. The Darwinian explanation, detailed above, implicates positive selection of advantageous mutations. Selected mutations at the γ locus shaped a fetal hemoglobin that served the needs of those evolving primates with extended prenatal brain development. By having the presimian and nascent simian γ locus experience a significant number of selected nonsynonymous substitutions, the Darwinian model explains why a slow replacement rate ensued in catarrhine γ genes. In the second explanation for the presimian burst of replacements, the proportion of acceptable neutral replacements increases during a period of reduced selective constraint, indeed during a period when the γ gene may have been completely silenced prior to reactivation and adoption as a fetal hemoglobin gene (Harris et al. 1986). The trouble with such a neutralist model is that it is incomplete. It does not account for substitutions fixed during the transition from reduced selective constraint to intensified selective constraint.

Kimura (1983) deduces that "when an exceptionally high rate is encountered in molecular evolution, we should suspect the loss of constraint rather than acquirement of new function" and that "the high rate is usually caused by removal of preexisting functional constraint, allowing a large fraction of previously harmful mutations to become selectively neutral so that they become fixed by random drift." If this happened in the evolution of the primate fetal hemoglobin locus, as would be expected if the presimian γ locus had been silenced, we are still left with harmful amino acid replacements in the fetal hemoglobin chain encoded by the reactivated γ locus. The Darwinian model readily allows such a silenced and reactivated gene as long as one or more mutations resulted in an advantageous function (e.g., loss of DPG-binding capacity in fetal hemoglobin). However, in the Darwinian model, selection not only preserves those mutations that previously had been spread by random drift and proved to be adaptive in the reactivated gene, but also spreads any new mutations that reverse the damage from harmful amino acid replacements due to prior mutations that had previously—in the silenced gene—escaped selection. Positive selection must also spread mutations that improve newly arisen functions. The Darwinian model explains how new useful adaptations emerge in molecules and in the organisms that synthesize the molecules.

ACKNOWLEDGMENTS

We thank Serge Vinogradov, Jack Farmer, Bill Schopf, Richard Jones, and David Hess for useful discussions. We also thank Janet Pedwaydon for able

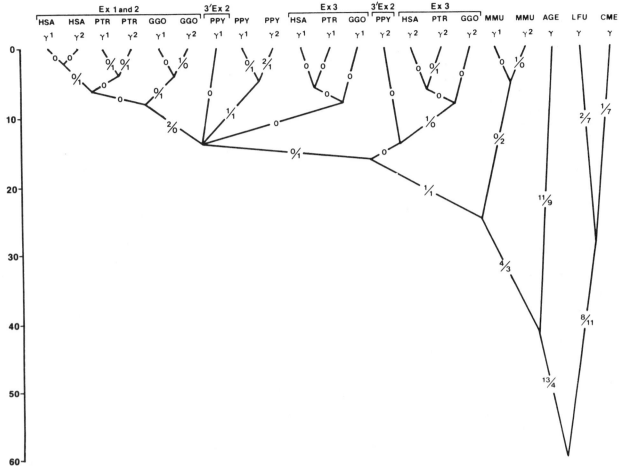

Figure 8. Detailed view of the primate γ gene branches from the genealogical reconstruction carried out by the parsimony method of coding sequences of 112 globin genes. The primates from which the genes come are designated by the three-letter convention for species names employed in Fig. 6. As in Fig. 4, link lengths are shown as fractions, the quotients of these fractions are R_{cs} values (ratios of amino acid changing to silent substitutions). The ordinate scale indicates the time level in Myr BP for each branching node. Different homology regions in the coding sequences show different evolutionary histories due to the varying extents of gene conversion regions in each pair of catarrhine γ¹ and γ² genes (see Fig. 7). For example, one of the features of the composite of the different regional histories presented is that the 3′ part of exon 2 of orangutan (Ppy) and γ¹ and γ² genes has not been involved in conversions from the time that the orangutan lineage separated from the African apes and humans, whereas the remaining exon regions (exon 1, most of exon 2, and exon 3) all were involved in conversions during descent of the orangutan lineage.

assistance in the computer processing of the data. This work was supported by grants from the National Institutes of Health (HL-33940), the National Science Foundation (BSF-86-07202), and the Alfred P. Sloan Foundation.

REFERENCES

Baba, M.L., L.L. Darga, M. Goodman, and J. Czelusniak. 1981. Evolution of cytochrome *c* investigated by the maximum parsimony method. *J. Mol. Evol.* **17:** 197.

Benton, W.D. and R.W. Davis. 1977. Screening λgt recombinant clones by hybridization to single plaques *in situ. Science* **196:** 180.

Blin, N. and D.W. Stafford. 1976. A general method for isolation of high molecular weight DNA from eukaryotes. *Nucleic Acids Res.* **3:** 303.

Breathnach, R.C., C. Benoist, K. O'Hare, F. Ganow, and P. Chambon. 1978. Ovalbumin gene: Evidence for a leader sequence in mRNA and DNA sequences at the exon-intron boundaries. *Proc. Natl. Acad. Sci.* **75:** 4853.

Britten, R.J. 1986. Rates of DNA sequence evolution differ between taxonomic groups. *Science* **231:** 1393.

Chang, L.-Y.E. and J.L. Slightom. 1984. Isolation and nucleotide sequence analysis of the β-type globin pseudogene from human, gorilla, and chimpanzee. *J. Mol. Biol.* **180:** 767.

Cloud, P. and M.F. Glaessner. 1982. The Ediacaran period and system: Metazoa inherit the earth. *Science* **217:** 783.

Como, P.F. and E.O.P. Thompson. 1980. Amino acid sequence of the α-chain of the tetrameric hemoglobin of the bivalve mollusc *Anadara trapezia. Aust. J. Biol. Sci.* **33:** 653.

Czelusniak, J., M. Goodman, D. Hewett-Emmett, M.L. Weiss, P.J. Venta, and R.E. Tashian. 1982. Phylogenetic origins and adaptive evolution of avian and mammalian hemoglobin genes. *Nature* **298:** 297.

Dayhoff, M.O., ed. 1972. *Atlas of protein sequence and structure,* volume 5. National Biomedical Research Foundation, Washington, D.C.

Dickerson, R.E. 1971. The structure of cytochrome *c* and the rates of molecular evolution. *J. Mol. Evol.* **1:** 26.

Dickerson, R.E. and I. Geis. 1983. *Hemoglobin: Structure, function, evolution, and pathology.* Benjamin-Cummings, Menlo Park, California.

Giebel, L.B., V.L. van Santen, J.L. Slightom, and R.A. Spritz. 1985. Nucleotide sequence, evolution, and expression of the fetal globin gene of the spider monkey *Ateles geoffroyi. Proc. Natl. Acad. Sci.* **82:** 6985.

Goodman, M. 1981. Decoding the pattern of protein evolution. *Prog. Biophys. Mol. Biol.* **38:** 105.

———. 1985. Rates of molecular evolution: The hominoid slowdown. *Bioessays* **3:** 9.

Goodman, M., M.M. Miyamoto, and J. Czelusniak. 1987. Pattern and process in vertebrate phylogeny revealed by coevolution of molecules and morphology. In *Molecules and morphology in evolution: Conflict or compromise* (ed. C. Patterson), p. 141. Cambridge University Press, Cambridge, England.

Goodman, M., G.W. Moore, and G. Matsuda. 1975. Darwinian evolution in the genealogy of haemoglobin. *Nature* **253:** 603.

Goodman, M., B.F. Koop, J. Czelusniak, M.L. Weiss, and J.L. Slightom. 1984. The η-globin gene: Its long evolutionary history in the β-globin gene family of mammals. *J. Mol. Biol.* **180:** 803.

Hardison, R.C. 1981. The nucleotide sequences of rabbit embryonic globin gene β3. *J. Biol. Chem.* **256:** 11780.

———. 1984. Comparison of the β-globin gene families of rabbits and humans indicates that the gene cluster 5'-ε-γ-δ-β-3' predates the mammalian radiation. *Mol. Biol. Evol.* **1:** 390.

Harris, S., P. Barrie, M. Weiss, and A. Jeffries. 1984. The primate ψβ1 gene: An ancient β-globin pseudogene. *J. Mol. Biol.* **180:** 785.

Harris, S., J.R. Thackeray, A.J. Jeffries, and M.L. Weiss. 1986. Nucleotide sequence analysis of the lemur β-globin gene family: Evidence for major rate fluctuations in globin polypeptide evolution. *Mol. Biol. Evol.* **3:** 465.

Janvier, P. 1985. Environmental framework of the diversification of the Osteostraci during the Silurian and Devonian. *Philos. Trans. R. Soc. Lond. B* **309:** 259.

Kan, Y.W. and A.M. Dozy. 1978. Polymorphisms of DNA sequence adjacent to minor β-globin structural gene: Relationship to sickle mutation. *Proc. Natl. Acad. Sci.* **75:** 5631.

Kimura, M. 1983. *The neutral theory of molecular evolution,* p. 89. Cambridge University Press, Cambridge, England.

Koop, B.F. and M. Goodman. 1988. Evolutionary and developmental aspects of two β-hemoglobin genes ($ε^M$ and $β^M$) of opossum. *Proc. Natl. Acad. Sci.* (in press).

Koop, B.F., M.M. Miyamoto, J.E. Embury, M. Goodman, J. Czelusniak, and J.L. Slightom. 1986. Nucleotide sequence and evolution of the orangutan ε globin gene region and surrounding *Alu* repeats. *J. Mol. Evol.* **24:** 94.

Maxam, A. and W. Gilbert. 1980. Sequencing end-labelled DNA with base-specific chemical changes. *Methods Enzymol.* **65:** 499.

Moens, L., M.L. Van Houwaert, D. Geelen, G. Verproten, and J. Van Beeumen. 1986. The amino acid sequence of the structural unit isolated from the higher molecular weight globin chains of *Artemia* sp. In *Invertebrate oxygen carriers* (ed. B. Linzen), p. 81. Springer-Verlag, Berlin.

Moore, G.W. 1977. Proof of the populous path algorithm for missing mutations in parsimony trees. *J. Theor. Biol.* **66:** 95.

Olsson, A., T. Moks, M. Uhlén, and A.B. Gaal. 1984. Uniformly spaced banding pattern in DNA sequencing gels by use of field-strength gradient. *J. Biochem. Biophys. Methods* **10:** 83.

Perutz, M.F. and G. Fermi. 1981. *Hemoglobin and myoglobin: Atlas of molecular structures in biology,* volume 2. Oxford University Press, New York.

Romer, A.S. 1966. *Vertebrate paleontology.* University of Chicago Press, Chicago, Illinois.

Scott, A.F., P. Health, S. Trusko, S.H. Boyer, W. Prass, M. Goodman, J. Czelusniak, L.-Y.E. Chang, and J.L. Slightom. 1984. The sequence of the gorilla fetal globin genes: Evidence for multiple gene conversions in human evolution. *Mol. Biol. Evol.* **1:** 371.

Shen, S., J.L. Slightom, and O. Smithies. 1981. A history of the human fetal gene duplication. *Cell* **26:** 191.

Slightom, J.L., A.E. Blechl, and O. Smithies. 1980. Human $^Gγ$ and $^Aγ$-globin genes: Complete nucleotide sequences suggest that the DNA can be exchanged between these duplicated genes. *Cell* **21:** 627.

Slightom, J.L., L.-Y.E. Chang, B.F. Koop, and M. Goodman. 1985. Chimpanzee fetal $^Gγ$ and $^Aγ$ globin gene nucleotide sequences provide further evidence of gene conversions in hominine evolution. *Mol. Biol. Evol.* **2:** 370.

Slightom, J.L., T.W. Theisen, B.F. Koop, and M. Goodman. 1987. Orangutan fetal globin genes: Nucleotide sequences reveal multiple gene conversions during hominid phylogeny. *J. Biol. Chem.* **262:** 7472.

Suzuki, T. and T. Gotoh. 1986. The complete amino acid sequence of giant multisubunit hemoglobin from the polychaete *Tylorrhynchus heterochaetus. J. Biol. Chem.* **261:** 9257.

Wilson, A.T., L.B. Wilson, J.K. de Riel, L. Villa-Komaroff, A. Efstratiadis, B.G. Forget, and S.M. Weissman. 1978. Insertion of synthetic copies of human globin genes into bacterial plasmids. *Nucleic Acids Res.* **5:** 563.

Wu, C.-I. and W.-H. Li. 1985. Evidence for higher rates of nucleotide substitutions in rodents than in man. *Proc. Natl. Acad. Sci.* **82:** 1741.

Sequence Convergence and Functional Adaptation of Stomach Lysozymes from Foregut Fermenters

C.-B. Stewart* and A.C. Wilson
Department of Biochemistry, University of California, Berkeley, California 94720

Until about 1974, a basic assumption guiding investigations on the molecular basis of adaptive evolution was that amino acid replacements in proteins are the basis for the observed differences among individuals, populations, and species. However, quantitative studies of protein evolution, considered in relation to knowledge of taxonomic distance, led Wilson and co-workers (1977) to question this assumption. They hypothesized that regulatory mutations were responsible for most observed variations in anatomy, physiology, and lifestyle of organisms. There is considerable evidence that the concentrations of well-known proteins vary greatly from one species to another, but the adaptive significance of these differences is often unclear.

Lysozyme and Digestion in Foregut Fermenters

Lysozyme provides plausible cases of an association between a major regulatory shift and species adaptation (Dobson et al. 1984). Twice during the evolution of placental mammals, once in the ruminants (e.g., cow) and later in the colobine monkeys (e.g., langur; see Bauchop and Martucci 1968), foregut fermentation has independently evolved (Fig. 1) as a means of utilizing otherwise indigestible plant parts. In both cases, lysozyme *c* has been recruited to function as an enzyme in the true stomach, where it probably degrades the cell walls of bacteria coming from the foregut (see Fig. 2; Dobson et al. 1984) so that their contents can then be hydrolyzed by the conventional digestive enzymes (Beintema et al. 1977; Vonk and Western 1984).

Our approach to studying the molecular basis of adaptive evolution has been to compare the events concerning lysozyme that occurred on these two lineages of mammals and to contrast them with those occurring on lineages leading to organisms with simple stomachs. This bacteriolytic enzyme is expressed at high levels (~1–2 mg/g tissue) in the anterior region of the true stomachs of ruminants and langur (Pahud and Widmer 1982; Pahud et al. 1988; Dobson et al. 1984; Stewart 1986) and at much lower levels in most nonstomach tissues and secretions (Padgett and Hirsch 1967; Dobson et al. 1984; Stewart 1986). In contrast (Fig. 3), most other mammals examined express lower

levels of lysozyme in the stomach, and the chief location where expression occurs is the posterior (pyloric) region (Florey 1930; Dobson et al. 1984; Stewart 1986). Consistent with the regulatory hypothesis, altered patterns of lysozyme gene regulation appear to be involved in these and other (McHenery et al. 1979; Cámara and Prieur 1984; Hammer and Wilson 1987; Hammer et al. 1987) cases of dietary adaptation.

Functional Changes in Ruminant Lysozymes

In addition to these regulatory changes, ruminant stomach lysozymes have functional and structural characteristics that are consistent with action in the stomach, which is acidic and contains pepsin. At physiological ionic strengths, the ruminant lysozymes tested all have narrow ranges of activity, with their optima centered near pH 5, whereas the "conventional" lysozymes have optimum activities that extend to about pH 8 (Pahud and Widmer 1982; Dobson et al. 1984). Ruminant and Old World monkey lysozymes are also unusually resistant to digestion by pepsin (Dobson et al. 1984). In addition, the amino acid sequence of cow stomach lysozyme has some unusual features that may reflect adaptation to stomach conditions. For example, cow stomach lysozyme has lost an acid labile aspartyl-prolyl bond (Jauregui-Adell and Marti 1975) between residues 102 and 103,[1] which is found in other mammalian lysozymes, and also has fewer amides than other lysozymes (Jollès et al. 1984). However, it was not

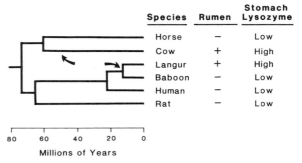

Species	Rumen	Stomach Lysozyme
Horse	−	Low
Cow	+	High
Langur	+	High
Baboon	−	Low
Human	−	Low
Rat	−	Low

80 60 40 20 0
Millions of Years

Figure 1. Independent evolution of foregut fermentation in mammals for which lysozyme sequences are known. Arrows point to the approximate times when the rumen or foregut arose, i.e., about 50 million years ago on the lineage leading to ruminants and about 15 million years ago on the lineage leading to leaf-eating (colobine) monkeys. These are probably also the times at which lysozyme was recruited as a major enzyme in the stomachs of these foregut fermenters.

---

*Present address: Hormone Research Institute, University of California, San Francisco, California 94143.

[1] Throughout this paper, we use the numbering system for human lysozyme (see Stewart et al. 1987).

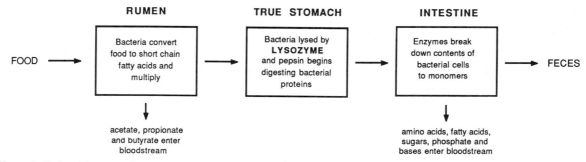

Figure 2. Role of lysozyme in ruminant and colobine digestive physiology, as proposed by Dobson (1981).

clear if these features were the result of neutral drift (King and Jukes 1969; Kimura 1983) or if they were selected for because they are critical to function. To test which of these features might be critical for stomach function, we have studied the structural and functional characteristics of langur lysozyme and compared them with those of cow stomach lysozyme.

Convergent Evolution of Lysozyme Sequences

The amino acid sequence of langur stomach lysozyme was determined and compared with cow and other lysozymes of known sequence (Stewart et al. 1987). This protein is similar in size (130 amino acids) and overall sequence to baboon (14 differences) and human (18 differences) lysozymes, yet shares several residues with cow stomach lysozyme that are not found in most other lysozymes of known sequence. The lysozyme sequences were analyzed by methods (referred to as parsimony methods) that use the characters in the sequences (i.e., the amino acids) to build trees that require the fewest amino acid replacements and thereby provide the assignment of specific amino acid replacements along specific lineages (Stewart et al. 1987). Parsimony trees can be powerful tools for analyzing sequences regarding adaptive evolution and

structure/function relationships, since correlations between given amino acid replacements and functional changes can sometimes be made.

Tree analysis of the lysozyme sequences indicated that, after foregut fermentation arose along the lineage leading to langur, its lysozyme converged in sequence upon cow stomach lysozyme; i.e., it gained sequence similarity to cow stomach lysozyme. As illustrated in Figure 4, about half of the replacements along the langur lysozyme lineage were in parallel or were convergent (Fig. 5) with those along the cow stomach lysozyme lineage (Stewart et al. 1987). The langur lysozyme lineage also appears to be evolving about twice as fast as the other primate lineages (Fig. 4; C.-B. Stewart et al., in prep.). This was an unexpected result because the usual direction of evolution is divergent (Fig. 5); i.e., after speciation or gene duplication, differences steadily accumulate in the separate lineages until the descendants are both different from each other and different from their common ancestor (Dawkins 1986). Furthermore, functional convergence, whether in evolutionarily unrelated (i.e., analogous) proteins or related (i.e., homologous) proteins, is usually achieved by divergent mechanisms (Garavito et al. 1977; Creighton 1983; Gurnett et al. 1984).

Parallelism and convergence are sometimes referred to as homoplastic evolution (Fig. 5) and are often cited as evidence for positive selection on the assumption that similar selection pressures produced similar adaptive responses, but a certain amount can occur by chance or coincidence (Zuckerkandl and Pauling 1965; Peacock and Boulter 1975). For langur and cow stomach lysozymes, the number of homoplastic replacements is higher than can be explained by chance alone (Stewart et al. 1987). Therefore, adaptive explanations for these replacements are in order.

Lysozyme *c* is an ideal enzyme for such a study because it is exceptionally well-characterized (for reviews, see Imoto et al. 1972; Osserman et al. 1974; Jollès and Jollès 1984). Thus, specific amino acid replacements can be examined in light of the enzyme's three-dimensional structure and catalytic mechanism. In this paper, we compare the kinetic behaviors of langur and cow stomach lysozymes on bacterial cells and attempt to correlate the functional and sequence convergence of these two enzymes.

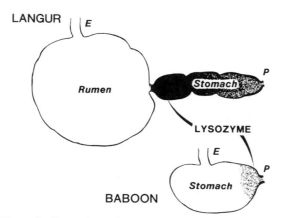

Figure 3. Comparison of lysozyme expression in langur and baboon stomachs. Stippled areas indicate relative levels of lysozyme activity in the stomach mucosa (Stewart 1986). The esophagus (E) and pyloric sphincter (P) are indicated.

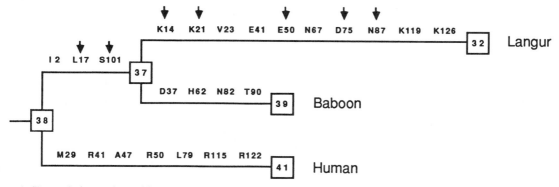

Figure 4. Tree relating amino acid sequences of three primate lysozymes (based on Stewart et al. 1987). The lengths of the lineages are proportional to the number of amino acid replacements along them. Arrows point to seven replacements that occurred in parallel or convergently to those on the cow lineage. The numbers of amino acid differences from cow stomach lysozyme 2 (Jollès et al. 1984) are in boxes.

METHODS

Assays. Lysozyme assays were performed in a 3-ml volume using a concentration of *Micrococcus lysodeikticus* cells (NCTC 2665; Sigma) that produced an absorbance at 450 nm of 0.50 ± 0.01. Sodium acetate (from pH 3.65 to 5.2) and 2(*N*-morpholino)ethanesulfonic acid (from pH 5.2 to 7.2) buffers were mixed to constant molarity (0.05) and ionic strength (0.10) according to the method of Perrin and Dempsey (1974). Initial rates of cell lysis were monitored at 450 nm (Maurel and Douzou 1976), with a Linear chart recorder attached to a Zeiss spectrophotometer (Stewart 1986).

Langur stomach lysozyme was purified by a combination of ion-exchange and sizing column chromatography (Stewart 1986). Purified cow stomach lysozyme 2, human lysozyme, and baboon lysozyme were those described previously (Dobson et al. 1984). Chicken lysozyme was purchased from Sigma.

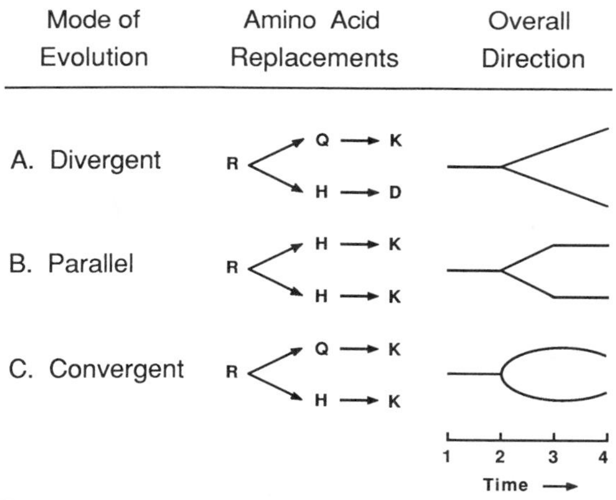

Molecular modeling. Modeling was performed with the program INSIGHT (Dayringer et al. 1986) on an Evans and Sutherland molecular graphics system at the University of California at San Francisco. The human lysozyme coordinates (data set 1LZ1 in the Brookhaven Data Bank) were used, and the amino acid differences between langur and human lysozymes were made by "replacing" the given human residue with the one found in langur lysozyme.

Mode of Evolution	Amino Acid Replacements	Overall Direction
A. Divergent	R → Q → K, R → H → D	
B. Parallel	R → H → K, R → H → K	
C. Convergent	R → Q → K, R → H → K	

Time → 1 2 3 4

Figure 5. Three modes of amino acid sequence evolution. (*A*) Divergence is the usual direction of evolution. In the upper lineage, the ancestral arginine (R) is replaced by a glutamine (Q) and then by a lysine (K). In the lower lineage, R is first replaced by a histidine (H) and then by an aspartic acid (D). Thus, both lineages continually diverge over time. (*B*) Parallelism is independent evolution of similar characters (amino acids or nucleotides) from the same ancestral state. (*C*) Convergence is the evolution of similar characters from different initial states (Haas and Simpson 1946; Sneath and Sokal 1973; Wiley 1981). Convergence can occur in related (homologous) or unrelated proteins. (Parallel and convergent events in homologous sequences are detected by assigning replacements in the most parsimonious manner along a known genealogical tree and looking for independently acquired amino acids in two lineages [Sneath and Sokal 1973]. Parallelism and convergence are subsets of *homoplasy*; convergence is also used as the general term [rather than homoplasy] to express the concept of independent evolution of similar or identical functional and/or structural characteristics [see, e.g., Dawkins 1986].)

RESULTS

pH Dependence

Under the condition of ionic strength used here, which was chosen to mimic the average of that found in the ruminant stomach contents, the langur and cow stomach lysozymes produced nearly superimposable pH-dependence curves. Both are relatively more active at lower pH (~ 4) and less active at higher pH (~ 6–7) than is human lysozyme (Fig. 6). Baboon lysozyme produces a curve similar to that of cow and langur lysozymes (Dobson et al. 1984; Stewart et al. 1984; Stewart 1986). Like the cow and langur enzymes, chicken lysozyme has relatively high bacteriolytic activity at pH 4; yet it also has high activity at neutral pH, similar to the human enzyme (Dobson et al. 1984; Stewart 1986).

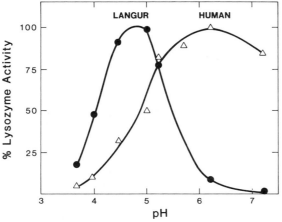

Figure 6. Dependence of catalytic activity on pH for purified lysozymes from langur and human. The activities are expressed as a percentage of the activity at the pH optimum (Stewart 1986).

The "lag" in the progress curves of ruminant and langur lysozymes at neutral pH and above (Dobson 1981; Dobson et al. 1984) was not found under the more carefully defined conditions used in the present study (not shown). The known kinetic similarities between langur and cow stomach lysozymes appear to be reconciled with their pH and ionic strength dependencies (for details, see Stewart 1986).

Molecular Modeling

The two parallel replacements along the lineage leading to baboon and langur lysozymes (producing Leu-17 and Ser-101) and the five homoplastic replacements along the langur lysozyme lineage (producing Lys-14, Lys-21, Glu-50, Asp-75, and Asn-87) that are depicted in Figure 4 were modeled onto the three-dimensional structure of human lysozyme.

None of these replacements caused obvious steric hindrance (not shown). As shown in Figure 7 (top), residue 101 lies near the substrate-binding cleft. In human lysozyme, Arg-101 and Met-17 are involved in a hydrogen bond network with Tyr-20; this network appears to be disrupted when Arg-101 is replaced by a serine. (Most vertebrate lysozymes of known sequence [see Jollès and Jollès 1984; McKenzie and Shaw 1985; Rodríguez et al. 1985; Stewart et al. 1987] have either Arg-101 and Met-17 or Ser-101 and Leu-17. Tree analysis shows that these two replacements must have occurred independently at least twice during evolution [C.-B. Stewart, unpublished analysis]. Thus, they may be coupled or compensatory changes [Kimura 1986].)

The five homoplastic replacements along the langur lysozyme lineage involve amino acid residues whose side chains appear to be external. As shown in Figure 7 (bottom), these residues are on the backside (relative to the substrate-binding cleft) of the molecule. Residue 21 lies near residue 101, but it is not known to be a contact residue for the polysaccharide substrate (Imoto

et al. 1972; Sarma and Bott 1977; Artymiuk and Blake 1981; Smith-Gill et al. 1984; Veerapandian et al. 1985).

DISCUSSION

Classically, homoplasy has been interpreted as resulting from adaptation to similar environments (Zuckerkandl and Pauling 1965; Dawkins 1986), in this case, the true stomachs of foregut fermenting mammals. Can these parallel and convergent replacements account for the observed functional similarity between ruminant and Old World monkey lysozymes? What can these replacements further tell us about the selection pressures on stomach enzymes?

Dependence on pH

Since the catalytic activity of baboon lysozyme has a pH dependence similar to that of langur and cow stomach lysozymes (Fig. 6), the five homoplastic replacements along the langur lineage are probably not responsible for this particular shift in function. The basis for the shift must lie in features shared by these three enzymes and not by the human enzyme. One of the replacements that made baboon and langur lysozymes more similar to cow stomach lysozyme (see Fig. 4) was that of an arginine by a serine at position 101. This residue is at subsite F in the polysaccharide-binding cleft of chicken lysozyme (Imoto et al. 1972) and is therefore a likely candidate for conferring a functional difference. Langur, baboon, cow, and chicken lysozymes, which all exhibit relatively high activity at pH 4, have serine at residue 101, whereas human lysozyme has arginine at this position. Thus, this replacement may be at least partly responsible for the increased activity at lower pH values. The effect of this residue on lytic activity can now be directly tested through site-specific mutagenesis.

The loss of activity at neutral pH shown by cow stomach, langur, and baboon lysozymes may primarily be accounted for by their lower isoelectric points (~7–9), compared to chicken and human lysozymes (~11–12) (Pahud et al. 1983; Dobson et al. 1984; Stewart 1986). This interpretation is consistent with the standard electrostatic explanation for the dependence of lysozyme's bacteriolytic activity on pH (Davies et al. 1969; Maurel and Douzou 1976; Dobson et al. 1984; Price and Pethig 1986).

The five parallel and convergent replacements along the langur lineage are scattered over the exons of the lysozyme gene (Jung et al. 1980) and structural units of the protein (Gō 1983). These replacements involve external, charged side chains (Fig. 7b). None are in the active cleft or in known binding sites for the peptidoglycan substrate (Imoto et al. 1972; Sarma and Bott 1977; Artymiuk and Blake 1981; Smith-Gill et al. 1984; Veerapandian et al. 1985); thus, they are unlikely to alter the basic catalytic mechanism. Such external residues are often assumed to be of little adaptive significance and are often cited as evidence of neutral re-

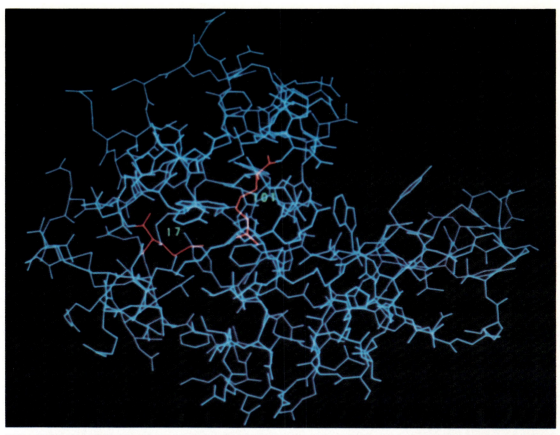

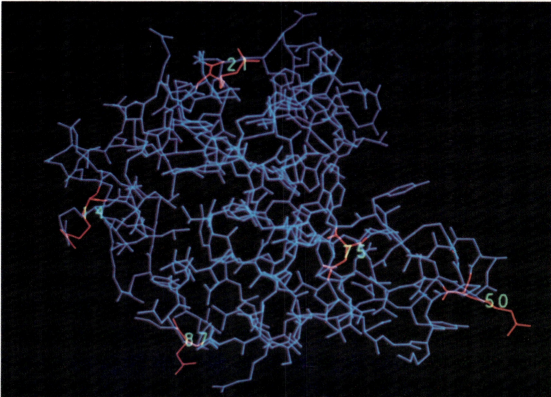

Figure 7. Molecular models showing (in red) the positions of seven convergent or parallel replacements in lysozyme (based on the three-dimensional structure of human lysozyme). (*Top*) The positions of the two replacements (producing Leu-17 and Ser-101) along the lineage leading to baboon and langur. (*Bottom*) Five replacements (producing Lys-14, Lys-21, Glu-50, Asp-75, and Asn-87) along the langur lineage.

placements (Doolittle 1979). Yet, because the number of convergent and parallel replacements between langur and cow stomach lysozymes is greater than can be explained by chance alone (Stewart et al. 1987), adaptive explanations for these surface replacements are in order. What can these replacements tell us about the adaptive evolution of stomach lysozymes?

Positively Charged Residues and Arginine Deficiency

Two of the putatively adaptive events (at positions 14 and 21) involve the replacement of an arginine by a lysine in langur and cow stomach lysozymes. This observation highlights the inference (Fig. 4) that, after their divergence, the langur lysozyme lineage gained four lysines (at positions 14, 21, 119, and 126), whereas the human lysozyme lineage gained four arginines (at positions 41, 50, 115, and 122). As shown in Table 1, the result is that langur lysozyme now has 9 lysines and 6 arginines, whereas human lysozyme has 5 lysines and 14 arginines. The cow lineage also appears to have lost arginines in favor of lysines (Stewart 1986), with a final result of 3 arginines and 12 lysines (Jollès et al. 1984). (Although horse milk lysozyme [McKenzie and Shaw 1985] has a low arginine content [four], it also has an overall higher number of positively charged residues than cow or langur lysozymes.)

Lysine and arginine are often considered to be the epitome of conservative, neutral replacements (Zuckerkandl and Pauling 1965; Doolittle 1979, 1986). The present study suggests, however, that arginine has been actively selected *against* and/or lysine has been actively selected *for* during the relatively recent evolutionary history of the langur stomach lysozyme lineage. What might the selection pressure(s) be upon lysozymes found in the guts of foregut fermenters that would cause them to lose arginines in favor of lysines? One possibility is that lysyl bonds are less sensitive to hydrolysis by pancreatic trypsin than are arginyl bonds (Vonk and Western 1984; Craik et al. 1985). Another selection pressure could be irreversible modification of arginine by bacterial fermentation products such as diacetyl (Yankeelov 1972); this reaction is illustrated in its simplest form in Figure 8. Modification of arginine residues by diacetyl is known to decrease the bacteriolytic activity of lysozyme (Davies and Neuberger 1969; Kaiser et al. 1985). A lysozyme with fewer arginines might survive and function longer in the intes-

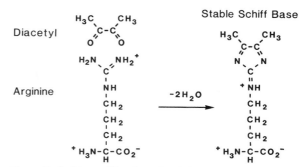

Figure 8. Stable modification of arginine by diacetyl, a product of fermentation in the rumen.

tine, thus providing the host animal with greater nutritional benefits. Whatever the driving force, the replacements of arginines by lysines would maintain positive charges on the surface of the molecule that appear to facilitate binding to bacterial cells, which bear a negative surface charge (Price and Pethig 1986).

Another possible source of bias against arginine was postulated by King and Jukes (1969), who noted that, unlike other amino acids, arginine is underrepresented in most proteins compared to expectation from the number of arginine codons, which is six (AGR and CGX). Lysine, on the other hand, has only two codons (AAR). Thus, all other things being equal, one would expect arginine to be present in proteins three times as often as lysine, which is rarely the case (Jukes 1973). Part of this general bias away from arginine may be explained by an underrepresentation in the genome of the CG dinucleotide (King and Jukes 1969). However, avoidance of this dinucleotide cannot totally explain arginine deficiency in ruminant stomach lysozymes for two reasons. First, complete avoidance of the CGX codons would result in an expected ratio of arginine to lysine of 1.0; as shown in Table 1, the ratio in cow stomach lysozyme (0.25) is significantly less. Second, cow stomach lysozyme is known to use a CGX codon for arginine (R.T. White and D. Irwin, pers. comm.). Therefore, additional factors must be selecting against arginine in stomach lysozymes of foregut fermenters, as well as in many other proteins (Jukes 1973, 1974; Wallis 1974).

Joysey and co-workers (Gurnett et al. 1984) have proposed that arginine appears to be selected for in myoglobins of diving and burrowing animals. Thus, in two cases where adaptive evolution in protein molecules has been proposed, namely, in lysozyme and myoglobin, arginine and lysine replacements appear not to be neutral. Although these amino acids may at first glance appear to be "functionally conservative" to the protein chemist, they may not always be so to the selection process (Wallis 1974).

Other Potentially Adaptive Features

Jollès et al. (1984) postulated that there was a gain in stability to acid along the lineage leading to cow stomach lysozyme. This stabilization was inferred from

Table 1. Numbers of Basic Amino Acids in Some Lysozymes c

Species	Arg	Lys	Arg/Lys ratio
Cow	3	12	0.25
Langur	6	9	0.67
Baboon	8	5	1.6
Human	14	5	2.8
Rat	12	6	2.0
Horse	4	15	0.27
Chicken	11	6	1.8

the low content of amides and the absence of an aspartyl-prolyl bond in this enzyme. In contrast, conventional mammalian lysozymes possess this most acid-
labile of all peptide bonds and, in addition, have a high
amide content. Yet, langur lysozyme does not have
fewer amides and has not lost the aspartyl-prolyl bond
between residues 102 and 103. It might therefore appear that these features are not important for survival
in the acidic stomach of foregut fermenting animals.

Such a conclusion might, however, be premature.
Since Pro-103 is at a bend in the human lysozyme
molecule, this residue may be hard to lose by a simple
one-step process without causing problems in folding.
Most primates appear to express only one lysozyme
gene (Stewart 1986; D. Irwin, pers. comm.), whereas
lysozyme is a multigene family in ruminants (Dobson et
al. 1984; Stewart 1986; E.M. Prager and D. Irwin,
unpubl.). Multiple copies of a gene may provide adaptive flexibility by allowing intermediate evolutionary
states to occur that might be deleterious to the organism if in a single-gene copy. Primates may thus have
been less able genetically than the ruminants to carry
out the process of losing Pro-103 while maintaining a
functional lysozyme.

Adaptation and Positive Selection in Proteins

Accelerated evolution has accompanied the convergence upon cow stomach lysozyme displayed by the
langur enzyme (Stewart et al. 1987). This suggests that
some changes in primary sequence are necessary for
functioning in the stomach of foregut fermenters. So, at
least in this case, some changes in protein structure and
function (see Table 2 for a summary) appear to be
necessary for adaptive evolution at the organismal
level. Whether these replacements were the primary
adaptive events or were of secondary importance to the
regulatory changes is a question that may be answered
by comparative studies of other ruminants and leaf-
eating monkeys.

Table 2. Potentially Adaptive Features of Mammalian
Stomach Lysozymes of Known Sequence

	Anterior stomach level[a]	Lower pH optimum[b]	Asp-Pro bond[c]	Arg/Lys ratio
Cow	high	+	−	<1
Langur	high	+	+	<1
Baboon	low	+	+	>1
Human	low	−	+	>1
Rat	low	−	+	>1

[a]Data from Dobson et al. (1984) and Stewart (1986).

[b]Data from Dobson et al. (1984) and Stewart (1986). + refers to
those lysozymes with sharp, acidic pH profiles similar to those of
langur stomach lysozyme (Fig. 6); − refers to lysozymes with broader,
more basic curves.

[c] + means there is an aspartyl-prolyl bond in the lysozyme between
residues 102 and 103 (primate lysozyme numbering system).

ACKNOWLEDGMENTS

We thank Jack Kirsch and the members of the Wilson lab for many helpful discussions and Robert Fletterick for the access to the computer modeling system.
This work received support from the National Institutes
of Health.

REFERENCES

Artymiuk, P.J. and C.C.F. Blake. 1981. Refinement of human
lysozyme at 1.5 Å resolution: Analysis of non-bonded and
hydrogen-bond interactions. *J. Mol. Biol.* **152:** 737.

Bauchop, T. and R.W. Martucci. 1968. Ruminant-like digestion of the langur monkey. *Science* **161:**698.

Beintema, J.J., W. Gaastra, J.A. Lenstra, G.W. Welling, and
W.M. Fitch. 1977. The molecular evolution of pancreatic
ribonuclease. *J. Mol. Evol.* **10:** 49.

Cámara, V.M. and D.J. Prieur. 1984. Secretion of colonic
isozyme of lysozyme in association with cecotrophy in
rabbits. *Am. J. Physiol.* **247:** G19.

Craik, C.S., C. Largman, T. Fletcher, S. Roczniak, P.J. Barr,
R. Fletterick, and W.J. Rutter. 1985. Redesigning trypsin:
Alteration of substrate specificity. *Science* **228:** 291.

Creighton, T.E. 1983. *Proteins: Structures and molecular
properties.* W.H. Freeman, New York.

Davies, R.C. and A. Neuberger. 1969. Modification of lysine
and arginine residues of lysozyme and the effect on enzymatic activity. *Biochim. Biophys. Acta* **178:** 306.

Davies, R.C., A. Neuberger, and B.M. Wilson. 1969. The
dependence of lysozyme activity on pH and ionic strength.
Biochim. Biophys. Acta **178:** 294.

Dawkins, R. 1986. *The blind watchmaker.* W.W. Norton,
London.

Dayringer, H.E., A. Tramontano, S.R. Sprang, and R.J.
Fletterick. 1986. Interactive program for visualization and
modelling of proteins, nucleic acids and small molecules. *J.
Mol. Graphics* **4:** 82.

Dobson, D.E. 1981. "Evolution of ruminant lysozymes."
Ph.D. thesis, University of California, Berkeley.

Dobson, D.E., E.M. Prager, and A.C. Wilson. 1984. Stomach
lysozymes of ruminants. I. Distribution and catalytic properties. *J. Biol. Chem.* **259:** 11607.

Doolittle, R.F. 1979. Protein evolution. *The proteins* (3rd
edition) **4:** 1.

———. 1986. *Of URFs and ORFs: A primer on how to
analyze derived amino acid sequences.* University Science
Books, Mill Valley, California.

Florey, H. 1930. The relative amounts of lysozyme present in
the tissues of some mammals. *Br. J. Exp. Pathol.* **11:** 251.

Garavito, R.M., M.G. Rossmann, P. Argos, and W. Eventoff.
1977. Convergence of active center geometries. *Biochemistry* **16:** 5065.

Gō, M. 1983. Molecular structural units, exons, and function
in chicken lysozyme. *Proc. Natl. Acad. Sci.* **80:** 1964.

Gurnett, A.M., J.P. O'Connell, D.E. Harris, H. Lehmann,
K.A. Joysey, and E. Nevo. 1984. The myoglobin of rodents: *Lagostomus maximus* (viscacha) and *Spalax ehren-
bergi* (mole rat). *J. Protein Chem.* **3:** 319.

Haas, O. and G.G. Simpson. 1946. Analysis of some phylogenetic terms, with attempts at redefinition. *Proc. Am.
Philos. Soc.* **90:** 445.

Hammer, M.F. and A.C. Wilson. 1987. Regulatory and structural genes for lysozymes of mice. *Genetics* **115:** 521.

Hammer, M.F., J.W. Schilling, E.M. Prager, and A.C. Wilson. 1987. Recruitment of lysozyme as a major enzyme in
the mouse gut: Duplication, divergence, and regulatory
evolution. *J. Mol. Evol.* **24:** 272.

Imoto, T., L.N. Johnson, A.C.T. North, D.C. Phillips, and
J.A. Rupley. 1972. Vertebrate lysozymes. In *The enzymes*
(ed. P.D. Boyer), vol. 7, p. 665. Academic Press, New
York.

Jauregui-Adell, J. and J. Marti. 1975. Acidic cleavage of the aspartyl-proline bond and the limitations of the reaction. *Anal. Biochem.* **69:** 468.

Jollès, P. and J. Jollès. 1984. What's new in lysozyme research? *Mol. Cell. Biochem.* **63:** 165.

Jollès, P., F. Schoentgen, J. Jollès, D.E. Dobson, E.M. Prager, and A.C. Wilson. 1984. Stomach lysozymes of ruminants. II. Amino acid sequence of cow lysozyme 2 and immunological comparisons with other lysozymes. *J. Biol. Chem.* **259:** 11617.

Jukes, T.H. 1973. Arginine as an evolutionary intruder into protein synthesis. *Biochem. Biophys. Res. Commun.* **53:** 709.

———. 1974. The "intruder" hypothesis and selection against arginine. *Biochem. Biophys. Res. Commun.* **58:** 80.

Jung, A., A.E. Sippel, M. Grez, and G. Schütz. 1980. Exons encode functional and structural units of chicken lysozyme. *Proc. Natl. Acad. Sci.* **77:** 5759.

Kaiser, E.T., D.S. Lawrence, and S.E. Rokita. 1985. The chemical modification of enzymatic specificity. *Annu. Rev. Biochem.* **54:** 565.

Kimura, M. 1983. *The neutral theory of molecular evolution.* Cambridge University Press, Cambridge, England.

———. 1986. The role of compensatory neutral mutations in molecular evolution. *J. Genet.* **64:**7.

King, J.L. and T.H. Jukes. 1969. Non-darwinian evolution. *Science* **164:** 788.

Maurel, P. and P. Douzou. 1976. Catalytic implications of electrostatic potentials: The lytic activity of lysozyme as a model. *J. Mol. Biol.* **102:** 253.

McHenery, J.G., T.H. Birkbeck, and J.A. Allen. 1979. The occurrence of lysozyme in marine bivalves. *Comp. Biochem. Physiol.* **63B:** 25.

McKenzie, H.A. and D.C. Shaw. 1985. The amino acid sequence of equine milk lysozyme. *Biochem. Int.* **10:** 23.

Osserman, E.F., R.E. Canfield, and S. Beychok, eds. 1974. *Lysozyme.* Academic Press, New York.

Padgett, G.A. and J.G. Hirsch. 1967. Lysozyme: Its absence in tears and leukocytes of cattle. *Aust. J. Exp. Biol. Med. Sci.* **45:** 569.

Pahud, J.-J. and F. Widmer. 1982. Calf rennet lysozyme. *Biochem. J.* **201:** 661.

Pahud, J.-J., D. Schellenberg, J.C. Monti, and J.C. Scherz. 1983. Lysozyme, an abomasal enzyme in the ruminants. *Ann. Rech. Vét.* **14:** 493.

Peacock, D. and D. Boulter. 1975. Use of amino acid sequence data in phylogeny and evaluation of methods using computer simulation. *J. Mol. Biol.* **95:** 513.

Perrin, D.D. and B. Dempsey. 1974. *Buffers for pH and metal ion control.* Chapman and Hall, London.

Price, J.A.R. and R. Pethig. 1986. Surface charge measurements on *Micrococcus lysodeikticus* and the catalytic implications for lysozyme. *Biochim. Biophys. Acta* **889:** 128.

Rodríguez, R., L. Menéndez-Arias, G. González de Buitrago, and J.G. Gavilanes. 1985. Amino acid sequence of pigeon egg-white lysozyme. *Biochem. Int.* **11:** 841.

Sarma, R. and R. Bott. 1977. Crystallographic study of turkey egg-white lysozyme and its complex with a disaccharide. *J. Mol. Biol.* **113:** 555.

Smith-Gill, S.J., J.A. Rupley, M.R. Pincus, R.P. Carty, and H.A. Scheraga. 1984. Experimental identification of a theoretically predicted "left-sided" binding mode of (GlcNac)$_6$ in the active site of lysozyme. *Biochemistry* **23:** 993.

Sneath, P.H.A. and R.R. Sokal. 1973. *Numerical taxonomy: The principles and practice of numerical classification.* W.H. Freeman, San Francisco.

Stewart, C.-B.R. 1986. "Lysozyme evolution in Old World monkeys." Ph.D. thesis, University of California, Berkeley.

Stewart, C.-B., D.E. Dobson, and A.C. Wilson. 1984. Lysozyme as a major digestive enzyme in a colobine monkey. *Am. J. Phys. Anthropol.* **63:** 222.

Stewart, C.-B., J.W. Schilling, and A.C. Wilson. 1987. Adaptive evolution in the stomach lysozymes of foregut fermenters. *Nature* **330:** 401.

Veerapandian, B., D.M. Salunke, and M. Vijayan. 1985. X-ray characterisation of an additional binding site in lysozyme. *Fed. Eur. Biochem. Soc. Lett.* **186:** 163.

Vonk, H.J. and J.R.H. Western. 1984. *Comparative biochemistry and physiology of enzymatic digestion.* Academic Press, London.

Wallis, M. 1974. On the frequency of arginine in proteins and its implications for molecular evolution. *Biochem. Biophys. Res. Commun.* **56:** 711.

Wiley, E.O. 1981. *Phylogenetics.* John Wiley, New York.

Wilson, A.C., S.S. Carlson, and T.J. White. 1977. Biochemical evolution. *Annu. Rev. Biochem.* **46:** 573.

Yankeelov, J.A., Jr. 1972. Modification of arginine by diketones. *Methods Enzymol.* **25B:** 566.

Zuckerkandl, E. and L. Pauling. 1965. Evolutionary divergence and convergence in proteins. In *Evolving genes and proteins* (ed. V. Bryson and H.J. Vogel), p. 97. Academic Press, New York.

The Exon Theory of Genes

W. GILBERT

The Biological Laboratories, Harvard University, Cambridge, Massachusetts 02138

Since the intron/exon structure of genes was discovered 10 years ago (Berget et al. 1977; Broker et al. 1977), only a few generalities about the properties of introns have emerged. Most vertebrate genes, but not all, have an intron/exon structure. The length distribution of exons is rather narrow, peaking at about 40 or 50 amino acids. However, introns are an order of magnitude longer than the exons; their length distribution is very broad, the shortest introns being only 50 bases long, the longest extending out to some 50,000 bp. No essential function has been found that requires the presence of all the introns in a gene. If one compares genes from different species, separated by a sufficient evolutionary distance, the exon sequences of homologous genes drift slowly, the positions coding for amino acids being conserved, whereas the intron sequences drift as rapidly as third-base positions, indicating that they are evolutionarily silent. Nonetheless, there is a general role that introns might play, solely because of their length and position, by participating in genetic recombination and hence increasing the rate at which the exons reassort as independent elements. This is the concept of exon shuffling (Blake 1978, 1979, 1983; Gilbert 1978).

The argument that introns increase the rate of recombination is straightforward. We know that there exist recombinational processes that can create interchanges between contiguous parts of a gene. Such recombinational processes, often called illegitimate recombination, would involve the recombination between DNA sequences at a few matched bases. A single such recombination could be used to make a double-length gene out of a simple structure; a double recombination might be used to insert a fragment of one gene into another. Such recombinations are observed in microorganisms. An example in humans is hemoglobin Lepore. However, if the two regions to be recombined were to be separated by a 10,000-base intron in the finished gene, the illegitimate recombination that combines them need not take place exactly at the end of one exon or exactly at the beginning of a second, but anywhere within 10,000 bases after the end of one exon or within 10,000 bases before the beginning of the second. On a combinatorial basis alone, this recombination process is 10^8 times more rapid than that involving exact recombination. Thus, the introns represent hot spots for recombination; by their mere presence and length they increase the rate of recombination, and hence shuffling of the exons, by factors of the order of 10^6 or 10^8. Under this model, the presence of an intron/exon structure in recent genes reflects the most probable way for new genes to arise: through the coupling of exons by intron-mediated recombination.

This picture provides a way of creating new genes from the combination of exons, in a way more in keeping with the requirements of natural selection than that of the classic model for domain doubling. For example, the classic model suggests that the putting together of domains to make a protein with a repeated domain structure will involve an extremely rare recombination event that would produce a large amount of a correct gene product. The intron/exon model suggests that a frequent recombination event creates a long intron separating the exons of the two domains. This new gene need not produce, at least initially, a large amount of product, but is instead a trial gene that produces only a small amount of product. Natural selection will then work on variations of this gene selecting for splicing mutants that make splicing more effective and accurate, and thus increase the yield of the gene product. The traditional hypothesis involves a rare event leading to an immediately useful product. In contrast, the shuffling hypothesis involves a common event that occurs as the first of a series of small steps leading to a new, complex gene product.

There are now many examples of the shuffling of exons in the genes that have arisen throughout Metazoan evolution. The most striking of these is the LDL receptor, EGF precursor, and blood factors IX and X story (Südhof et al. 1985a,b). But where did this intron/exon structure originate?

The Exon Theory of Genes

We suggest that the first genes were assembled by recombination within introns linking exons serving as minigenes (Doolittle 1978; Gilbert 1979). The complete form of this hypothesis is that the first exons encoded very short polypeptide fragments, essentially statistically occurring open reading frames, ranging in length from 15 to 20 amino acids. The very first genes might simply have made such polypeptide products, which then assembled into multimeric structures with enzymatic activity. The splicing mechanism would also have permitted the assemblage, using *trans*-splicing, of multiexon protein chains, through the intermediate existence of multimeric RNA complexes. However, it is only recombination between introns that creates at the DNA level, at the genetic level, a single heritable gene, made up of exons, that will dictate a single, complex protein subunit. This picture asserts that the small peptides used in that original set of exons probably had structure in solution, or structure in an appropriate hydrophobic environment, that gave them the ability to serve as elements of form and function. The structures need not be as three-dimensionally stable as those of today's proteins, because we are looking at the slow biochemical processes occurring at the beginning of evolution.

The polypeptides encoded by the first exons would be small and compact and represent elements that fold up in space (modules in Mitiko Gō's sense, circumscribed by a sphere 28 Å in diameter [Gō 1981]).

Over the sweep of evolutionary time, introns are lost and more complicated exons are formed. The exon theory of genes hypothesizes that the only processes with appreciable rates are those of intron loss. Although the probability of intron loss by exact deletion is very rare, and the probability of intron loss by an approximate deletion that removes the intron and some of the surrounding material is rather rare, there is one process known that over evolutionary time removes introns—retroposition: A mature message is copied back into DNA and then part of all of that DNA is recombined into the chromosome. This process will remove introns singly and, as in pseudogene formation, will take an entire complex structure, remove all of its introns, and reinsert it into DNA. In general, this does not lead to a functional gene because the reinsertion is in some region of DNA that is not transcribed. However, if the reinsertion is into an intron within a previously existing gene, the reinserted element will serve as a complex exon, often carboxy-terminal, in the new gene. This process, slow over evolutionary time, combines the elementary exons into more complicated structures, which will be shuffled in their turn. The immunoglobulin fold, a preeminent example of a single exon used throughout an entire gene family, is a complex exon of this kind, since its length, at 120 amino acids, would be that of some 5–6 minimal exons. This offers an explanation for the additional introns found in CD4 and in N-CAM: They are remnants of the original immunoglobulin structure.

An extensive piece of evidence for this general exon theory is the gene structure of triosephosphate isomerase (TIM) (Straus and Gilbert 1985; Marchionni and Gilbert 1986). TIM, an enzyme of glycolytic metabolism, is an extremely ancient protein, which evolved completely before the divergence of the Eukaryotes from the Eubacteria and the Archaebacteria. This gene has six introns in animals and eight introns in plants. Five of these introns are in identical positions, and one is a closely matched position. This high identity argues that the gene was split before the divergence of plants and animals, approximately a billion years ago. This gene has also been sequenced in *Aspergillus* (McKnight et al. 1986), where it has five introns, and *Saccharomyces* and *Escherichia coli*, where it has none. Three of the five introns in *Aspergillus* agree in their positions with those of the plant gene, but two are at

novel positions. Superficially, these numbers might suggest that the gene evolved from one of no introns in bacteria to added introns as one moved up through the fungi, alternative ones in alternative lines, to a set of eight introns in the lineage that led to the plants and animals. However, a more subtle interpretation of the positions of the introns (Gilbert et al. 1986) shows that all of the introns, including the ones in *Aspergillus* that are not represented in the plant/animal line, fall upon divisions of the protein that break the protein into modules, as defined by Mitiko Gō (1979): The exons represent compact elements of polypeptide structure, each lying within a sphere about 28 Å in diameter. If we assume that all ten of the TIM introns that have thus far been found in corn, chicken, and *Aspergillus* were already present in some ancestral TIM gene, then 10 of the 11 exons of that gene are modules in this sense, and one is not. That peculiar exon, we hypothesize, will turn out to be divided by an intron in the ancestral gene.

The exon theory suggests that the first genes had an intron/exon structure. The intron's role was to assemble and reassort the exons as individual elements during the formation of those genes. Over evolutionary time, simple exons are fused to make complicated ones. Can we push this model back before the origin of DNA?

The force of the intron/exon idea is that it is efficient to make genes out of building blocks that can be rearranged by the evolutionary process. Of course, this is true on a larger scale when one makes an entire organism out of smaller elements, or one makes complex proteins out of dissimilar subunits encoded by genes on different chromosomes. The assortment of elements onto different chromosomes, or even into separate genes, provides the ability to reassort those elements in each generation to provide for the variation that drives evolution. The intron structure permits the assortment of elements *within* genes over a much longer time span; still by a process rapid compared to the full sweep of geological history. This ability to reassort the genetic elements of the biological molecules might have been the role of the intron/exon structure at the very beginning of evolution.

The RNA World

Our view of the origin of life has been drastically changed in the last few years by the discovery of several enzymatic activities in RNA molecules, notably those involved in the making and breaking of phosphodiester bonds (the work of Cech, Altman, and their colleagues described in papers in this volume [Been et al.; Lawrence et al.]). This raises the possibility that RNA might show a wide variety of other enzymatic activities. Ulenbeck (Sampson et al., this volume) has given a simple demonstration that there can be metallo-RNA enzymes. White (1976) suggested several years ago that many of the enzymatic cofactors used to carry out chemical reactions might be the remnants of RNA molecules.

Thus, one might imagine a purely RNA-catalyzed

world in which RNA enzymes, ribozymes, using their own functionalities as well as cofactors (metals, NAD, FMN, etc.), carry out all of the enzymatic reactions needed for primitive life (Gilbert 1986). Here RNA would serve as the holder of genetic information, copied by ribozymes. The intron/exon hypothesis distinguishes between the genetic material and the ribozyme gene products. The genetic material would have an intron/exon structure, initially involving self-splicing introns. The base-pairing and secondary structure features of this molecule can be specialized as a substrate for replication. Then, when the genetic material with its complete intron/exon structure is copied by the ribozymes, many copies are made: Some of the daughter copies splice out their introns and combine their exons, thus producing functional ribozymes. Those ribozyme RNAs are specialized for enzymatic activity. They are three-dimensional structures that are not constrained by the need to be copied by an RNA-replicating mechanism.

How might such structures arise? The self-splicing intron, which can splice itself out of an RNA molecule, will presumably, at some rate, be able to splice itself back into an RNA molecule and serve as an insertion sequence. (This has not yet been demonstrated experimentally.) Thus, insertion sequences are implicit in the RNA enzymology that we already know. However, two insertion sequences around an intervening region of RNA serve to construct a transposon and will be able to carry that intervening region around from one RNA molecule to another. In this way, a structure with self-splicing introns can also be viewed, over a much longer time scale, as a pattern of transposons that permit the shuffling of exons. In addition, RNA recombination, once an intron/exon structure arises, will permit the shuffling of exons for the same reasons that it does at the DNA level.

This picture of the RNA world is one in which the intron/exon structure is used to make ribozymes, the ribozymes provide the full enzymology of an RNA cell, and short, presumably 1,000–10,000 long RNA molecules serve as genetic material. We hypothesize that this RNA state had a long history and existed all the way through the period of the first isolation of RNA molecules within membranes. If among the molecules made by the RNA are basic molecules for charge neutralization, a requirement for many of the RNA-RNA interactions, then the RNA molecules may be wrapped up within membranes, which would serve to isolate the genetic structures from the outside world and permit them to compete with each other so that natural selection could be effective.

The first proteins would be simple homopolymer chains or simple dipeptide/tripeptide structures involving very few amino acids. The first oligopeptides involved basic amino acids whose properties would enhance the likelihood of RNA being wrapped in membranes (Jay and Gilbert 1987) and thus improve the ability of cells to function. A second role of such early polypeptides would be to serve as pores through membranes. A third role would be to support the three-dimensional structure of ribozymes.

The transition to an RNA-protein world could be quite gradual. The ability to activate amino acids and insert them into oligopeptide chains can emerge slowly, a few amino acids at a time, because the first role of the oligopeptides is supportive rather than enzymatic. In this picture of the sweep of evolution, the role of protein enzymes is not required by some unusual chemical feature of enzymology. Rather, the hypothesis is that RNA molecules and cofactors are a sufficient set of enzymes to carry out all the chemical reactions necessary for the first cellular structures. Protein enzymes offer improvements in the rate of catalysis rather than in the types of reactions catalyzed. One can imagine a gradual supplanting of many of the ribozyme functions, first by protein-RNA combinations and later by complete protein structures. Because the oligopeptides will be coded by RNA messages that have undergone splicing, like the ribozymes, and that are derived from an underlying genetic material with an intron/exon structure, the proteins, too, are assembled from exons from the very beginning. Of course, the protein exons and the enzymes that they finally create are unrelated in an evolutionary sense to the ribozyme functions they replace. Many enzymatic activities will represent novel combinations of polypeptide exons that solve an underlying enzymological problem differently than does a ribozyme.

After the emergence of proteins, one would have a world of cells containing RNA as the genetic material, ribozymes involved in protein synthesis (rRNA and tRNAs, and possibly activating enzymes), ribozymes involved in RNA splicing, or a group II self-splicing pattern, as well as having protein enzymes and structural elements. In addition, lipid membranes would permit the separation of inside from outside and provide the boundaries between independent replicating entities. The genetic material would be rather small RNA molecules, with an intron/exon structure, with each cell having many copies of each gene. Such genetic molecules are small, because their effective size is determined roughly by the inverse of mutation rate.

DNA would arise as a genetic material after the introduction of the enzymatic process of reverse transcription and the other enzymatic processes needed to convert the ribonucleotide precursors into the deoxyribonucleotide precursors. DNA as a genetic material offers a double-strand structure whose error correction mechanisms permit the creation of very long genomes and hence a simpler transmission of information to the progeny. On this view, the DNA has a very late-developed, protein-based enzymology. This is consistent with the fast conversions of nucleotides into deoxynucleotides and the ultrafast synthesis rate of DNA. Because the genetic RNA molecules that were copied into DNA had an intron/exon structure, the DNA itself preserves that intron/exon structure.

The progenote cell's DNA more closely resembled that of the modern eukaryotic cell than that of a current prokaryote. Over evolutionary time the descendants of this original cell have diversified, branched, and specialized. One line gave rise to the Eubacteria, simplifying ribosomal structures and specializing its DNA and its cell structure for rapid multiplication, consequently losing the intron structure. Another line gave rise to the Archaebacteria, also losing the intron/exon structure. A third line maintained the intron/exon structure and introduced effective splicing mechanisms, probably making a transition from group II splicing, where the guide sequences are internal in the intron, to a development of a *trans*-splicing mechanism involving a fully developed splicesome. The cell line that makes this transition is the ancestor of the eukaryotes. It eventually develops a nuclear membrane, maintains a complex ribosomal structure, and picks up prokaryotic symbiotes to create mitochondria and chloroplasts. This line leads to the multicellular organisms. But the genomes of modern metazoa still have retained an intron/exon structure that resembles and has arisen from that in the very first DNA-containing organism.

The Numerology of Evolution

The intron/exon hypothesis, the notion that genes are assembled from small modules, provides a clear resolution of the numerical paradox that is often seen as circumscribing the possibilities of evolution. How is it possible to find a protein structure consisting of 200 amino acids by some random walk through evolution? This question reflects the fact that a 200-amino-acid-long structure is one out of some 20^{200} possible structures, and there is neither time nor carbon in the universe to explore all those possible structures and find the relevant one. How then is it possible for natural selection to create the protein enzymes that we see around us? The exon theory provides a simple explanation. It suggests that the first genes are selected out of a group of 20^{20} possibilities, a far smaller universe of possibilities (15 kg of random proteinaceous material contains all possible 20-long sequences). In fact, it may be the case that only a small fraction of the 20^{20} possible 20-long sequences actually have relevant three-dimensional shapes. For example, suppose that only 10^6 such different shapes exist in the space of exons. Then the evolutionary path leading to a 200-amino-acid-long protein would be the selection of a first exon out of the space of 10^6 possibilities, followed by the subsequent choice of a second exon again as one of 10^6 shapes, then the choice of a third, and so forth. If done in order, the ten choices required to produce a 200-amino-acid-long final protein explore only 10^7 possibilities (rather than the 10^{60} possibilities if a simultaneous choice were being made), far less than the 10^{260} possibilities we contemplated originally. This argument shows that the numerology of evolution is not an insurmountable problem, and it implies further that evolution could have examined only an extremely tiny fraction of the possible structures of proteins. There may be very, very many different three-dimensional con-figurations that can solve a given enzymatic problem with the same efficiency.

What is the total number of shapes available in the world of exons? (Above, we hypothesized there to be only 10^6.) One can try to estimate that from our current knowledge by assuming that one can assemble from the gene products that have been studied so far, a group that represents random draws from an underlying world of exon shapes. If this were the case, one could compare the total number of exons studied with the number of repeats of exon structures to get some idea of the full universe of exon shapes represented in all proteins. If the sampling were random, then we would expect the number of repeats to be approximately $n^2/2N$, where N is the total number of exons, and n is the number of exons that have been observed. (This is essentially the birthday problem. $1/N$ is the probability one exon drawn from the pool will match a specified earlier one, and $n^2/2$ is the number of pairs of possible matches of n objects.) These numbers are difficult to determine, in part because we do not know how to compare shapes rather than amino acid sequence. But one can make very rough guesses. If one has observed about 3000 exons and has seen about 100 repeats, then the total universe of exons would be 10^5. These estimates are very crude but do suggest that there is a very small world of shapes from which all gene products were formed.

REFERENCES

Berget, S.M., A.J. Berk, T. Harrison, and P.A. Sharp. 1978. Spliced segments at the 5′ termini of adenovirus-2 late mRNA: A role for heterogeneous nuclear RNA in mammalian cells. *Cold Spring Harbor Symp. Quant. Biol.* **42:** 523.

Blake, C.C.F. 1978. Do genes-in-pieces imply proteins-in-pieces? *Nature* **273:** 267.

———. 1979. Exons encode protein functional units. *Nature* **277:** 598.

———. 1983. Exons—Present from the beginning? *Nature* **306:** 535.

Broker, T.R., L.T. Chow, A.R. Dunn, R.E. Gelinas, J.A. Hassell, D.F. Klessig, J.B. Lewis, R.J. Roberts, and B.S. Zain. 1978. Adenovirus-2 messengers—An example of baroque molecular architecture. *Cold Spring Harbor Symp. Quant. Biol.* **42:** 531.

Doolittle, W.F. 1978. Genes in pieces: Were they ever together? *Nature* **272:** 581.

Gilbert, W. 1978. Why genes in pieces? *Nature* **271:** 501.

———. 1979. Introns and exons: Playgrounds of evolution. *ICN-UCLA Symp. Mol. Cell. Biol.* **14:** 1.

———. 1986. Origin of life, the RNA world. *Nature* **319:** 618.

Gilbert, W., M. Marchionni, and G. McKnight. 1986. On the antiquity of introns. *Cell* **46:** 151.

Gō, M. 1979. Eucaryotic gene regulation. *ICN-UCLA Symp. Mol. Cell. Biol.* **14:** 1.

———. 1981. Correlation of DNA exonic regions with protein structural units in haemoglobin. *Nature* **291:** 90.

Jay, D. and W. Gilbert. 1987. Basic protein enhances the incorporation of DNA into lipid vesicles: Model for the formation of primordial cells. *Proc. Natl. Acad. Sci.* **84:** 1978.

Marchionni, M. and W. Gilbert. 1986. The triosephosphate isomerase gene from maize: Introns antedate the plant-animal divergence. *Cell* **46:** 133.

McKnight, G.L., P.J. O'Hara, and M.L. Parker. 1986. Nucleotide sequence of the triosephosphate isomerase gene from *Aspergillus nidulans:* Implication for a differential loss of introns. *Cell* **46:** 143.

Straus, D. and W. Gilbert. 1985. Genetic engineering in the precambrian: Structure of the chicken triosephosphate isomerase gene. *Mol. Cell. Biol.* **5:** 3497.

Südhof, T.C., J.L. Goldstein, M.S. Brown, and D.W. Russell.

1985a. The LDL receptor gene: A mosaic of exons shared with different proteins. *Science* **228:** 815.

Südhof, T.C., D.W. Russell, J.L. Goldstein, M.S. Brown, R. Sanchez-Pescador, and G.I. Bell. 1985b. Cassette of eight exons shared by genes for LDL receptor and EGF precursor. *Science* **228:** 893.

White, H.B., III. 1976. Coenzymes as fossils of an earlier metabolic state. *J. Mol. Evol.* **7:** 101.

What Introns Have to Tell Us: Hierarchy in Genome Evolution

W.F. DOOLITTLE

Department of Biochemistry, Dalhousie University, Halifax, Nova Scotia B3H 4H7, Canada

I argue here that (1) although as molecular biologists we often assign "evolutionary functions" to parts of genomes, most such functions cannot be understood within the tenets of the modern (neo-Darwinian) synthesis; (2) that neo-Darwinian synthesis is the only theoretical framework within which the facts of molecular biology have been addressed to date; and (3) it is only when we affirm the reality of a biological hierarchy—a hierarchy in which entities at different organizational levels (genes, organisms, populations, or species) independently experience evolutionary sorting processes such as selection—that such evolutionary functions make sense.

Confusion about such issues has, I believe, cropped up over and over in evolutionary speculations stemming from molecular data, the debates over the meaning of repetitive DNAs and the origins of introns being two recent examples. I will review these debates at some length, in an effort to convince the reader that this confusion is a general one. I will then attempt to show how this confusion can be relieved if we accept hierarchical views.

"SELFISH," "POLITE," AND "JUNK" DNA

Two Traditions of Argument

During the 1960s and 1970s, experimental developments in three areas led to our current understanding of genomes as evolutionarily plastic structures. First, plant genomes were shown to harbor mobile "controlling elements," whose coming and going did not fit with notions of the stability of genomic structure and function. Second, animal genomes were shown to be composed in large part of evolutionarily unstable repetitive sequences, clustered or dispersed throughout unique sequence DNA (Britten and Davidson 1971). Third, a large fraction of spontaneous mutations in bacteria was shown to be due to the insertion of copies of elements already present at other locations (Nevers and Saedler 1977). The kinds of arguments we used then in dealing with the question of the function of repetitive and/or transposable elements have recently been summarized by the evolutionary biologists Gould and Vrba (1982):

"A survey of previous literature reveals two emerging traditions of argument, both based on the selectionist assumption that repetitive DNA must be good for something if so much of it exists. One tradition holds that repeated copies are conventional adapta-

tions, selected for an immediate role in regulation... We do not doubt that conventional adaptation explains the preservation of much repeated DNA in this manner.

"But many molecular evolutionists now strongly suspect that direct adaptation cannot explain the existence of all repetitive DNA: there is simply too much of it. The second tradition therefore holds that repetitive DNA must exist because evolution needs it so badly for a flexible future—as in the favored argument that 'unemployed,' redundant copies are free to alter because their necessary product is still being generated by the original copy. While we do not doubt that such future uses are vitally important *consequences* of repeated DNA, they simply cannot be the *cause* of its existence, unless we return to certain theistic views that permit the control of present events by future needs." (Gould and Vrba 1982; emphasis mine).

The first tradition of argument, that of "current adaptation," was most thoroughly elaborated, for repeated elements in animal DNA, by Britten and Davidson (1971). Their model, in which the majority of repetitive sequences have a role in the regulation of gene expression, has, in various forms (e.g., Davidson and Britten 1979), survived into the mid-1980s, although most writers now take an agnostic position. Recognizing the constraint that whatever function repetitive DNAs may have, that function cannot depend on sequence, position, or amount—because these are so variable even between closely related species—Cavalier-Smith, for instance, has constructed a variety of arguments around the notion that extra DNA plays a structural role for chromosomes or for the nucleus (Cavalier-Smith 1985). Zuckerkandl (1986) has argued that, however useless such "junk" DNA may be, it must at least be "polite," conforming to overall constraints of chromosome size and structure.

The second, or "future utility" tradition of argument was already accommodated in the Britten-Davidson model in its earliest (1971) form. That is, the genomic flexibility potentiated by recombination between (or mobility of) repetitive sequences could allow dramatic alterations in regulatory networks, with consequent neo-Goldschmidtian alterations in organismal form and function (see Doolittle 1982). The existence of transposable elements in bacteria was rationalized in a similar way—they were there to allow genomes to change quickly and in a modular manner; evolution was their function. Strobel et al. (1979), for instance, suggested that "it is possible that the sole function of these elements is to promote genetic variability...." Campbell (1985) has recently carried such reasoning further still, suggesting that genomes contain "evolutionary drivers" of a variety of sorts. Some, like Tn917 or the SOS system, are responsible for "inducible evolution" (as Echols [1981] had pointed out before). They disrupt genomes under environmental conditions where new mutants would be a good thing to have around ("sensory evolution"). Some, of which Campbell admits there are no documented examples, might give organisms "the capacity to evolve according to what will occur in the future instead of what the environment is like at present" ("projective evolution").

What Is Wrong Here

Selectively advantageous traits are fixed within populations of organisms because their bearers leave more progeny, in the short run. The long-run advantage of evolutionary flexibility will not directly lead to fixation of a trait, and most transposable and repetitive elements, unless they bear "useful" genes (like IS50; Hartl et al. 1985), should confer disadvantage in the short run. Traits conferring greater evolutionary flexibility can be fixed indirectly, by "hitchhiking"—in asexual species because of favorable mutations they can cause in clones bearing them, and in sexual species because of favorable mutations that they cause and to which they are physically linked (Maynard Smith 1985). Bacterial transposable elements might be maintained through hitchhiking, although they are unlikely to have originated in this way (Brookfield 1985; Hartl et al. 1985). The thousands of copies of repetitive sequences riddling most eukaryotic genomes can neither have originated nor be maintained through hitchhiking. To repeat the words of Gould and Vrba (1982), "although evolutionary flexibility may be an important *consequence* of repeated DNA, it simply cannot be the *cause* of its existence."

These kinds of problems are not new to evolutionary biology: they appear again and again in discussions of the selection pressures responsible for the origins and maintenance of mutation, recombination, and sex, which also serve evolutionary flexibility. These now are most often dealt with by arguing that, although flexibility may provide advantages at the group or population level, such advantages are usually too weak to account for the maintenance of these genetic mechanisms within populations, and almost always too weak to be responsible for their origins within species (Maynard Smith et al. 1985). Some short-term advantage must be sought, either in contemporary populations or in ancestral populations, in those cases where the genetic mechanism is now so developmentally wired in that it cannot be eliminated, no matter what the immediate selective effect. (It might be advantageous for me as an individual to reproduce clonally, but too many mutations are required for me to acquire that competence.)

Thus, explanations for the origin of recombination and sex now address the current or earlier short-term advantages of these processes to individual organisms within populations. These advantages are seen to be, for example, repair of mutation, competition between siblings (which are more likely all to survive if they are not identical), or the avoidance of parasites (for review, see Stearns 1985). Such individual level effects must be the cause of recombination and sex, even though recombination and sex undoubtedly do have important evolutionary consequences at the level of species. Maynard Smith's (1982) analogy to horses' backs illustrates very well what we as biologists *should* mean by "function" (that property of a trait that is the cause of its existence) and "effect" (other consequences of its existence). He writes, "horses have very stiff backbones, and a consequence of this is that people can ride them. However, we would not say that the function of a horse's backbone is to enable people to ride horses, because we do not think that horses' backbones evolved as they did so as to enable people, in the future, to ride."

SELFISH DNA AND SELECTION
AT THE LEVEL OF THE GENOME

For transposable elements, short-term advantage is best sought at the level of the elements themselves. Most transposable elements have, by definition, the ability to replicate within genomes. They will thus, for instance, come to "contaminate" element-free chromosomes in hybrids between element-bearing and element-free individuals, and for that reason will spread through sexually reproducing populations even if they reduce organismal fitness—by 50% in the most extreme example (Hickey 1982). Their ability to spread in this way will be increased by selection operating among variant elements. No other explanation for the origin or maintenance of transposable elements is required (Orgel and Crick 1980; Sapienza and Doolittle 1980). To the extent that repetitive sequences in general are more or less well transposable and their ability to be transposed (now or in the recent past) depends on element sequence, the existence of repetitive DNAs in eukaryotic genomes is thereby rationalized. The conferral of evolutionary flexibility is a consequence, not a cause—and it need not even be an advantageous consequence. The evidence suggests, for instance, that P elements are, on balance, a bad thing for *Drosophila melanogaster* to have, either as individual flies, or as populations of flies, or as a species of insect (Engels 1986).

HIERARCHY

Natural Selection

This line of reasoning initially encountered opposition within the molecular biological community, in part because, as practitioners of the "new synthesis," we are used to seeing selection as something that affects only the differential reproductive success of individual organisms within populations. That differential success is, of course, due to differences between genes, so that we can model evolution in terms of the frequencies of genes in populations, but the "benchmark" (Sober 1985) against which success is measured still remains the individual organism, even in such extremely gene-centered discussions as Dawkin's (1976). Molecular biology is part of the neo-Darwinian "modern synthesis," of which Hull (1981) is right, I think, in saying that "the current view is that *genes mutate, organisms are selected, and species evolve*" (emphasis mine). That is, the level of genes is seen only as that at which variation is generated; this variation is only sorted by selection at the level of organisms (through expressions in phenotype), whereas events at the level of species (e.g., speciation and extinction, evolutionary "trends") follow passively, as a consequence of what happens to individual organisms.

Nevertheless, we are aware that Darwin's theory of natural selection is generalizable. Business firms, for instance, reproduce (from year to year, or by starting new branches) and have phenotypes (business practices) that determine how well they survive and reproduce in their environment (the "free" market), and we are used to thinking of economics in Darwinian terms. In principle, any entities which, like organisms or business firms, reproduce and show *heritable variation in fitness,* such that variation that affects survival and reproduction is passed on, will evolve by natural selection.

Levels of Selection

Eldredge, Gould, Vrba, Salthe, and others have recently elaborated on the implications of the notion that the biological world is hierarchically constructed, and that at each level of the hierarchy legitimate evolutionary processes can be seen (Gould 1982; Vrba and Eldredge 1984; Eldredge 1985; Salthe 1985). They mean us to take such hierarchy seriously, not just in the metaphorical way in which even the most thorough-going reductionist will admit that genes fit into organisms and organisms into species, in the manner of Chinese boxes. Rather, these evolutionary theorists argue, entities at levels below and above that of organisms are every bit as *real* as organisms are, and experience real selection, so that biological evolution is to be seen as a much more complex process than it is in the modern synthesis.

With transposable elements, such arguments are quite easy to construct and difficult to counter. Stretches of DNA show heritable variation in fitness, heredity being mediated by transposition, variation being effected by mutation, and fitness being defined in terms of the ability to transpose and the ways in which this process interacts with cellular replication machinery and regulatory mechanisms. The genome is the environment, and other nonselective processes, analo-

gous to genetic drift in populations of organisms, affect events at this level. Gene conversion, unequal crossing-over, and "molecular drive" phenomena (Dover 1982) all influence the composition of the population of nongenic sequences in genomes—contributing to sorting (selection and drift). Arguably, most of what we will see when we sequence the human genome will be the products of such genome-level sorting, not of selection in the usual neo-Darwinian sense. Although the stretches of DNA that are the analogs of individual organisms at this level are usually all strung together on chromosomes, it is not difficult to see them as discrete evolutionary entities (individuals in the ontological sense [Ghiselin 1974; Hull 1981]) bounded by the nucleotides that mark their ends as transposable elements of conversion patches or the like.

Species Selection

Ghiselin (1974), Hull (1981), Eldredge (1985), and others would also have us see species as *individuals* in the ontological sense. They have births (speciation), deaths (extinction), and a cohesiveness defined by their shared gene pools (at least in sexually reproducing organisms). They have ontogeny (phyletic evolution). They also have proper names. If we discovered creatures on Mars identical to ourselves, we would still not call these creatures *Homo sapiens* unless we knew them to be related to us biologically, by descent. However, if we found lakes or trees we would call them lakes or trees. "Lakes" and "trees" designate classes; *H. sapiens* designates an individual.

Philosophers disagree as to how necessary this ontological argument is to the further notion that species can undergo selection in a way analogous to, but not reducible to, selection at the level of organisms in a population (Kitcher 1986). The process of species selection is, however, easy to imagine, as in the following passage from Sober's (1985) book, *The Nature of Selection.*

"We might visualize how this process works by a simple hypothetical example. Let's begin with two species, one winged and the other nonwinged, which initially have the same census sizes. Suppose that winged organisms survive and reproduce exactly as well as their wingless counterparts. But there is a difference: small colonies of wingless individuals become separated from the main population rather frequently; winged organisms, on the other hand, in virtue of their greater mobility, very rarely form isolated subpopulations. If this system is allowed to evolve, we may later find a large number of rather small wingless species and a small number of rather large winged species. Wingless species speciate, whereas winged species grow. Notice that although wingless *species* have had more daughter species, wingless *organisms* are no more reproductively successful than winged ones."

In pointing out that this kind of selection is truly not reducible to the level of the individual organism, and thus that species-level selection (a "macroevolutionary" process) is truly uncoupled from individual-level selection (a "microevolutionary" process), Sober (1985) says further that "this point goes beyond the fairly obvious idea that macro-phenomena may be studied 'at their own level,' rather than from a micro point of view. That is a relatively uncontroversial epistemological or methodological thesis. Rather, we have here an ontological claim to the effect that an item at the macro-level is not identical with anything at the micro-level. It is not to be doubted that species are *composed* of organisms. Rather, the idea is that a certain causal mechanism—species selection—is distinct from the array of mechanisms acknowledged by the individual-level science."

Equivocations

Perhaps in an attempt to avoid charges of gratuitous holism, Vrba and Eldredge (1984) and Vrba (1984) have defined, rather rigorously, conditions under which species selection can be said to have occurred. First, to be the product of species selection, a trait must exist because it affects what species do: give rise to new species, persist in geological time, and go extinct. Winglessness is such a trait in Sober's example. Second, the trait must be "emergent" at the level of species—not simply something that all organisms within the species have as a result of individual-level selection operating on them. Third, although he by no means sees it as a requirement, Gould (1982) points out that species-level selection is easiest to demonstrate when it runs counter to organism-level selection, just as the "selfishness" of transposable elements is easiest to see when they reduce organismal fitness.

I find these constraints unnecessarily rigid. If Sober is right about the validity of the uncoupling of macro- and micro-evolution, then it seems reasonable to say that any trait that is more prevalent among *species* than it would otherwise have been, because of its effects on *species* reproduction (speciation) or survival, is to that extent maintained by *species* selection. Fully analogous definitions for the organismic or genomic levels can be formulated, with "organism" or "pieces of DNA" substituted for species.

Importance

Many logically possible evolutionary processes do not actually often occur, and it was important to the selfish DNA argument (not in terms of the logic but in terms of the biology) to show that some real DNAs actually are selfish. Mainstream neo-Darwinists have argued against group selection processes (of which species selection can be seen as an example) by showing that the conditions under which these processes are likely to be important (compared to the overwhelming power of organismal selection) are severely limited (Maynard Smith 1978). In a recent summary of arguments for the group-selective advantages of sex and recombination, Maynard Smith et al. (1985) conclude: "A major difficulty stands in the way of this approach to the plasticity and directive power of the genome. It stems from the fact that selection between populations or species is likely to be a weak force compared to selection between individuals or genes. If genetic structures are to evolve because they promote evolution, this "weakness" of selection between populations and species must be compensated by the cumulative advantageous effect of the operation of those structures over long spans of evolutionary time." I will return to this argument, as it affects our understanding of introns.

THE EVOLUTION OF INTRONS

In 1978, Gilbert suggested that introns could be understood as serving an evolutionary function by allowing for the rapid modular construction of genes with novel and interesting complex activities through any of several processes, including "exon shuffling" (Gilbert 1978). This view was combined, although not specifically by Gilbert, with the then prevalent assumption that eukaryotes evolved relatively recently (1.4 billion years ago) from prokaryotes not altogether unlike *Escherichia coli*. Since prokaryotes like *E. coli* seem to lack introns in their protein-coding genes, one could only logically conclude that introns were inserted into genes during or after the prokaryote-to-eukaryote transition. Given that most introns appear to play no essential role in gene expression, the only imaginable type of selection that could have favored their insertion was the long-term one of speeding the evolutionary process.

Darnell (1978) and I (Doolittle 1978) could not see the long-term evolutionary payoffs as sufficiently strong or persistent to outweigh the obvious short-term disadvantage involved in massively disrupting the structures of thousands of already functioning intact genes (even if precise splicing mechanisms were already, for some other reason, in place). Instead, we suggested, the last common ancestor of eukaryotes and prokaryotes must have had introns in its genes, with prokaryotes having subsequently lost them through selection for reduction in genome size and for increased efficiency of gene expression, expected to be more severe in such small, rapidly growing (k-selected) cells (for review, see Darnell and Doolittle 1986). We noted that such a suggestion also implied that there was no prokaryote-eukaryote transition 1.4 billion years ago, and that this view was consistent with data then emerging from Woese's laboratory (Woese 1987). These showed that eukaryotes and prokaryotes (eubacteria, at least) have comprised separate evolutionary lineages since before the evolutionary divergences that gave rise to all modern groups of eubacteria, some 3.5–4.0 billion years ago, and suggested that their last common ancestor was a primitive cell (the "progenote") in which genes were inefficiently organized and expressed. Finally, we proposed that introns might have had some (difficult to specify) role in the initial, precellular assembly of genomes.

Blake (1978) suggested that if exon shuffling were to be of any real evolutionary use, introns would have to break up genes in a specific way. Each exon (or collection of exons) would have to encode modules of structure and/or function at the protein level ("domains") or elements of "supersecondary structure"), so that new genes assembled by shuffling would have some hope of producing proteins of stable and potentially functional sorts.

Exons actually often do encode bits of protein that seem to be structural and/or functional modules (Lonberg and Gilbert 1985; Duester et al. 1986; Marchionni and Gilbert 1986). If this correlation is assumed to be statistically meaningful, then the whole subsequent debate about whether introns were introduced recently or were always there hinges on how the coincidence is to be explained. There seem to be only two possibilities. First, introns were inserted by some kind of transposition process that targeted itself in such a way as to divide genes in places corresponding to linkers between domains or elements of supersecondary structure. Several suggestions along these lines have been made (Craik et al. 1983; Hickey and Benkel 1985), but they seem (to me) contrived. The other possibility is that exons that encode modules at the level of protein structure and/or function are themselves the product of some prolonged period of selection. L. Altenberg and D. Brutlag (in prep.) call this "constructional selection," arguing that, among exons that code randomly for bits of protein, those that by chance encode shuffle-able modules would be selected by shuffling itself, since they would come to be used again and again in the construction of new genes (and thus, in passing, new organisms or species). This seems intrinsically reasonable, and one then needs only ask when such shuffling started, and how long it has been going on.

At least in some cases, one can show that it has been going on since before the separation of eukaryotes and prokaryotes. As Gilbert (1985) pointed out, the observation that the exons of a given gene encode modules of protein structure is prima facie evidence that that gene was assembled by shuffling, and that the introns were therefore there before the gene was assembled. There are, Gilbert reasoned, a number of proteins produced by both prokaryotes and eukaryotes for which structural and functional homology, down to the level of domains and supersecondary structure, can be demonstrated. Unquestionably, such genes were assembled prior to the eukaryote-prokaryote divergence. If their eukaryotic versions contain introns that delimit module-encoding exons, then shuffling must have created them, and those introns must have been present before the eukaryote-prokaryote divergence. There are now perhaps half a dozen instances in which such analyses have been made and confirm the early presence of introns (see Marchionni and Gilbert 1986; Duester et al. 1986).

We can also now envision, at least in a rough way, how introns might have played a role in precellular genome assembly (Cech 1986; Darnell and Doolittle 1986). Cech (1986) has presented a scheme by which RNAs with a structure related to that of the *Tetrahymena* 28S rRNA intron might replicate themselves, in the absence of any other macromolecule. Such self-replicating molecules, at first randomly assembled, would experience Darwinian selection for improved replicability. When self-replicating RNAs came to encode polypeptides, the phenotype-genotype coupling would have been established. Whatever structural or catalytic role these first polypeptides might have served, they were likely to have experienced selection for stability, and hence come to resemble domains or elements of supersecondary structure—first establishing the correlation between exon structure and protein structure. This correlation would have been further refined when polypeptide-encoding self-replicating RNAs were spliced together to produce unstable RNA genomes with multiple coding regions (for which we can easily imagine advantages) by the kind of selection for shuffle-ability discussed above. Darnell and I (1986) imagined then a stage in which primitive (cellular) "organisms" had RNA genomes (with introns) but produced at least occasionally spliced mRNAs. Conversion of the RNA genome to DNA would have "frozen" introns in place (DNA introns cannot self-excise), producing a primitive eukaryote-like genome. Darnell and I suggested also that the progenote had such a genome, so that prokaryotes (or at least eubacteria) have since slowly lost introns. It is worth noting here that, alternatively, conversion to DNA of the spliced mRNA products of intron-containing RNA genomes might give rise to prokaryote-like primitive genomes.

THE ROLE OF INTRONS IN EVOLUTION

Exon Shuffling in Vertebrate Evolution

Gilbert's (1978) contention that exon shuffling should be important in eukaryote evolution and allow a kind of flexibility and innovativeness in the development of novel, complex function that has been denied to prokaryotes has been amply supported by the data. There are now examples of eukaryotic genes that clearly have been assembled from pieces of other genes, those pieces being exons. The low-density-lipoprotein receptor gene (Sudhoff et al. 1985) is perhaps still the best instance. Proteins of the vertebrate blood system in general offer a wealth of instances of shuffling (Doolittle 1985) and one could sensibly argue that this and many other complex vertebrate systems, involving proteins that recognize several ligands and cell surface components, simply could not have come into existence if there had not been introns.

Although it is inappropriate to think of introns as having "driven" eukaryotic evolution, it is reasonable to describe them as important genetic "constraints" (Maynard Smith et al. 1985). That is, the range of variants presented to selection by members of a species will be strongly constrained, both quantitatively and qualitatively, by the species' repertory of shuffle-able exons. Two otherwise similar species should respond to environmental challenges in different ways if their introns are differently disposed, ways that would in principle be partly predictable, given complete knowledge of genome structure. It is difficult to think of any other process for generating variants (simple mutations, transpositions, gene conversions, chromosomal rearrangements) that could constrain evolution so strongly or in such an interesting fashion.

Cause and Consequence at the Level of Organisms

Nevertheless, it is neither necessary nor appropriate to think of introns as serving an evolutionary function, at the level of individual organisms. In the words of a previous section, we could not argue that introns are more prevalent among organisms within a species than they would otherwise have been, because of their effects on organism reproduction or survival. An intron that participates in a beneficial exon shuffle does indeed "hitchhike" on the selective advantage of the new gene, but probably most introns have never participated in a shuffle, and yet there they are. The larger character of "intron-ness" need not be seen as favored by hitchhiking. In a sense, we have explained introns away as a relic of a prebiotic era, during which selection at the genomic level (or the organismal level, if we define self-replicating RNAs as organisms) did pay attention to them. Currently, their activities at the level of organisms are, like the straightness of the horse's back, an effect or consequence.

Introns and Species Selection

We could, on the other hand, quite easily argue that introns are, because of their effects on species reproduction and survival, more prevalent among species than they would otherwise have been, and thus are to that extent maintained by species selection. Species differ in their repertories of introns. Species that have more introns, or more advantageously placed introns, will be able to come up with evolutionary solutions that less well-endowed species cannot attain. (Organisms within favored species will of course also benefit in this way, but all organisms within a species are likely to be the same with respect to intron disposition—there will be no selection *between* them.) There will be selection between species—species favored by well-placed introns will more likely successfully reproduce (speciate), if adaptation plays any role whatsoever in the process of speciation (Rose and Doolittle 1983). In this context, it makes sense to say that introns have an evolutionary function, and Gilbert's (1978) initial claim for the importance of introns *can* be understood as a statement about selection.

The argument here is not that introns arose through species-level selection. Nor have they been particularly well maintained by such selection; their overall evolutionary history seems to be one of random loss (Blake

1985). Rather, the claim is that species that have lost relatively less of their ancestral complement of introns—for whatever reason (weak selection for efficiency in genomic organization, relative infrequency of germ-line processes that might eliminate introns)—have done relatively better (given rise to more new species). And because they have done better, introns are more prevalent among species (and for that reason, but only that reason, more prevalent among organisms at large) than they would otherwise have been.

Introns are apparently quite difficult to lose: Losses can be shown, but they occur over times that are long compared to events of speciation and extinction (Blake 1985). Thus, the usual sorts of objections to group-level selective processes that maintain elements of genomic plasticity—that these forces are weak compared to forces operating on individuals within populations (Maynard Smith 1978; Maynard Smith et al. 1985)—do not stand. Species-level selection of the sort argued for here will not override selection at the level of organisms, but when genomic plasticity is maintained *within* species for other reasons (genome level processes for selfish DNAs, sluggishness of loss for introns), then it should operate on differences *between* species.

ACKNOWLEDGMENTS

Research in this laboratory is supported by grants from The Medical Research Council and Natural Sciences and Engineering Research Council of Canada. I wish to thank the Canadian Institute for Advanced Research for fellowship support.

REFERENCES

Blake, C.C.F. 1978. Do genes-in-pieces imply proteins-in-pieces? *Nature* **273:** 267.
———. 1985. Exons and the evolution of proteins. *Int. Rev. Cytol.* **93:** 149.
Britten, R.J. and E.H. Davidson. 1971. Repetitive and non-repetitive DNA sequences and a speculation on the origins of evolutionary novelty. *Q. Rev. Biol.* **46:** 111.
Brookfield, J.F.Y. 1985. The population biology of transposable elements. *Philos. Trans. R. Soc. Lond. B Biol. Sci.* **312:** 27.
Campbell, J.H. 1985. An organizational interpretation of evolution. In *Evolution at a crossroads* (eds. D.J. Depew and B.H. Weber), p. 133, MIT Press, Cambridge.
Cavalier-Smith, T. 1985. *The evolution of genome size.* John Wiley and Sons, New York.
Cech, T.R. 1986. A model for the RNA-catalyzed replication of RNA. *Proc. Natl. Acad. Sci.* **83:** 4360.
Craik, C.S., W.J. Rutter, and R. Fletterick. 1983. Splice junctions: Associations with variation in protein structure. *Science* **220:** 1125.
Darnell, J.E. 1978. Implications of RNA:RNA splicing in evolution of eukaryotic cells. *Science* **202:** 1257.
Darnell, J.E. and W.F. Doolittle. 1986. Speculations on the early course of evolution. *Proc. Natl. Acad. Sci.* **83:** 1271.
Davidson, E.H. and R.J. Britton. 1979. Regulation of gene expression: Possible role of repetitive sequences. *Science* **202:** 1257.
Dawkins, R. 1976. *The selfish gene.* Oxford University Press, New York.
Doolittle, R.F. 1985. The genealogy of some recently evolved vertebrate proteins. *Trends Biochem. Sci.* **10:** 233.

Doolittle, W.F. 1978. Genes in pieces: Were they ever together? *Nature* 272: 581.

———. 1982. Selfish DNA after fourteen months. In *Genome evolution* (ed. G.A. Dover and R.B. Flavell), vol. 20, p. 3. Academic Press, New York.

Dover, G.A. 1982. Molecular drive: Cohesive mode of species evolution. *Nature* 299: 111.

Duester, G., H. Jornvall, and G.W. Hatfield. 1986. Intron-dependent evolution of nucleotide-binding domains within alcohol dehydrogenase and related enzymes. *Nucleic Acids Res.* 14: 1931.

Echols, H. 1981. SOS functions, cancer and inducible evolution. *Cell* 25: 1.

Eldredge, N. 1985. Unfinished synthesis: Biological hierarchies and modern evolutionary thought. Oxford University Press, New York.

Engels, W.R. 1986. On the evolution and population genetics of hybrid-dysgenesis-causing transposable elements in *Drosophila*. *Philos. Trans. R. Soc. Lond. B Biol. Sci.* 312: 205.

Ghiselin, M.T. 1974. A radical solution to the species problem. *Syst. Zool.* 25: 536.

Gilbert, W. 1978. Why genes-in-pieces? *Nature* 271: 501.

———. 1985. Genes-in-pieces revisited. *Science* 228: 823.

Gould, S.J. 1982. Darwinism and the expansion of evolutionary theory. *Science* 216: 380.

Gould, S.J. and E.S. Vrba. 1982. Exaptation—A missing term in the science of form. *Paleobiology* 3: 115.

Hartl, D.L., M. Medhorn, L. Green, and D.E. Dykhuizen. 1985. The evolution of DNA-sequences in *Escherichia coli*. *Philos. Trans. R. Soc. Lond. B Biol. Sci.* 312: 191.

Hickey, D.A. 1982. Selfish DNA: A sexually-transmitted nuclear parasite. *Genetics* 101: 519.

Hickey, D.A. and B.F. Benkel. 1985. Splicing and the evolution of introns. *Nature* 316: 582.

Hull, D.L. 1981. Units of evolution: A metaphysical essay. In *The philosophy of evolution* (eds. U.L. Jensen and R. Harré), p. 23. Harvester Press, Brighton, England.

Kitcher, P. 1986. Bewitchment of the biologist. *Nature* 320: 649.

Lonberg, N. and W. Gilbert. 1985. Intron/exon structure of the chicken pyruvate kinase gene. *Cell* 40: 81.

Marchionni, M. and W. Gilbert. 1986. The triosephosphate isomerase gene from maize: Introns antedate the plant-animal divergence. *Cell* 46: 133.

Maynard Smith, J. 1978. *The evolution of sex*. Cambridge University Press, Cambridge, England.

———. 1982. Overview—Unsolved evolutionary problems. In *Genome evolution* (ed. G.A. Dover and R.B. Flavell), vol. 20, p. 375. Academic Press, New York.

———. 1985. The evolution of recombination. *J. Genet.* 64: 159.

Maynard Smith, J., R. Burian, S. Kauffman, P. Alberch, J. Campbell, B. Goodwin, R. Lande, D. Raup, and L. Wolpert. 1985. Developmental constraints and evolution. *Q. Rev. Biol.* 60: 265.

Nevers, P. and H. Saedler. 1977. Transposable genetic elements as agents of gene instability and chromosomal rearrangements. *Nature* 268: 109.

Orgel, L.E. and F.H.C. Crick. 1980. Selfish DNA: The ultimate parasite. *Nature* 284: 604.

Rose, M.R. and W.F. Doolittle. 1983. Molecular biological mechanisms of speciation. *Science* 220: 157.

Salthe, S.N. 1985. *Evolving hierarchical systems: Their structure and representation*. Columbia University Press, New York.

Sapienza, C. and W.F. Doolittle. 1980. Genes are things you have whether you want them or not. *Cold Spring Harbor Symp. Quant. Biol.* 45: 177.

Sober, E. 1985. *The nature of selection*. MIT Press, Cambridge.

Stearns, S.C. 1985. The evolution of sex and the role of sex in evolution. *Experientia* 41: 1231.

Strobel, E., P. Dunsmuir, and G.M. Rubin. 1979. Polymorphisms in the chromosomal locations of elements of the 412, copia, and 297 dispersed repeated gene families in *Drosophila*. *Cell* 17: 429.

Sudhoff, J.C., L.J. Goldstein, M.S. Brown, and D.W. Russell. 1985. The LDL receptor gene: A mosaic of exons shared with different proteins. *Science* 228: 815.

Vrba, E.S. 1984. What is species selection? *Syst. Zool.* 33: 318.

Vrba, E.S. and N. Eldredge. 1984. Individuals, hierarchies and processes: Towards a more complete evolutionary theory. *Paleobiology* 10: 146.

Woese, C.R. 1987. Bacterial evolution. *Microbiol. Rev.* 51: 221.

Zuckerkandl, E. 1986. Polite DNA: Functional density and functional compatibility in genomes. *J. Mol. Evol.* 24: 2.

Protein Architecture and the Origin of Introns

M. Gō AND M. NOSAKA

Department of Biology, Faculty of Science, Kyushu University 33, Fukuoka, 812, Japan

Two possibilities have been proposed for the origin of split structures observed in protein-coding eukaryotic genes. One is that most of the introns were positioned in their present locations in primordial genes and have served during evolution as mediators of exon shuffling to yield new functional proteins by allowing different combinations of functional units (Gilbert 1978). The other is that the origin is rather new and introns were created by insertion of such DNA sequences as retroposons into eukaryotic genes (Cavalier-Smith 1985; Sharp 1985).

A clue to the relative plausibilities of the two hypotheses can be obtained by studying the conformational characteristics of polypeptide segments encoded by exons. In some cases they code segments, which are recognized as structural domains. Because domains behave as more or less independent folding units, an assembly of such segments is likely to yield a new functional and stable protein (Blake 1978).

However, introns are not always located at the domain boundaries. Sometimes they are found within domains (Dennis et al. 1984; Chang and Meyerowitz 1986; Duester et al. 1986). For example, the maize alcohol dehydrogenase (ADH) gene has one intron at the boundary of domains 1 and 2, but it has eight more introns within the domains (Dennis et al. 1984). There are many cases where introns split genes encoding mono-domain proteins.

In hemoglobin α and β chains (Gō 1981) and lysozyme (Gō 1983), positions of introns in the genes are closely correlated with compact structural units, called modules by one of the authors (Gō 1983). Modules are defined as compact, or least-extended, substructures within a globular domain. One intron whose presence was predicted by assigning one-to-one correspondence between exons and modules has been found in the leghemoglobin gene of soybean (Blake 1981; Jensen et al. 1981). Leghemoglobin consists of four modules, and each module is encoded by an exon; this split gene is probably the ancestral form of the globin family which originated more than a billion years ago (Gō 1985).

Hemoglobin and lysozyme consist of a single domain, and the identification of modules was based on a visually oriented algorithm utilizing distance maps (Gō 1981, 1983). This algorithm was applied to triosephosphate isomerase (TIM) (Straus and Gilbert 1985) and a different version to ADH (Brändén et al. 1984). The intron positions in TIM genes of chicken, maize, and *Aspergillus nidulans* appear closely correlated with

module junctions recognized in the distance map (Gilbert et al. 1986).

In an earlier paper (Gō 1981), it was made clear that this algorithm is applicable only for monolayer proteins. In these proteins each domain is composed of only such modules, one surface of which is exposed to the solvent and the other surface of which faces the interior of the domain. Large proteins or domains sometimes contain core modules that are entirely buried in their interior. In such cases the distance plot is not directly applicable.

Intron-exon structures of many genes encoding large proteins are now known. We wished to investigate whether the intron positions are correlated with module junctions even in large proteins. For this purpose we extended the algorithm originally developed for identification of modules in small monolayer proteins to be widely applicable for larger proteins or domains. The boundaries of modules and those of domains can be detected simultaneously using an extended algorithm given in two versions.

METHOD

Modules introduced originally are segments defined by partitioning a globular domain into relatively compact regions consisting of about 20–40 contiguous amino acid residues (Gō 1981). The algorithm was applied to a small protein such as lysozyme (Gō 1983) and cytochrome *c* (Gō 1985), a small domain such as ovomucoid third domain (Gō 1985), and a small subunit, hemoglobin α and β chains (Gō 1981). In these monolayer domains or subunits having no core modules buried inside, the joints of the modules are characterized by their locations not being close to the surface of the domains or subunits (Gō 1981). Utilization of this characteristic as well as the compactness itself makes easier the identification of modules in a small domain or subunit consisting of monolayer modules; the modules can be identified by the fact that their joints are located not far from all the other residues. Search for such joints was carried out by using a distance map on which amino acid residues separated from each other by more than a certain distance were marked.

The spatial relationships between modules are more complicated in multilayer domains or subunits than in small monolayer domains or subunits, thus the visually oriented method by distance map used in monolayer domains or subunits must be modified for application to larger proteins. Carboxypeptidase A is one protein having a core module; it consists of 307 amino acid residues and contains one core module that is encoded by one exon in rat gene of preprocarboxypeptidase A. Residues within this module have little or no relative accessible surface area as shown in Figure 1. Such proteins, where not all of the modules face onto the surface, are called multilayer. The limitation in application of the previous method to multilayer proteins was noted in the first stage of its introduction (Gō 1981). A less clear correlation between intron positions and module junctions in carboxypeptidase A (Blake 1983) was caused by this limitation.

Module Joints Recognized by Centripetal Profile

In a large protein, junctions of modules are not necessarily located close to its center. Even in such a case, they are located close to local centers, i.e., to centers of long contiguous segments. This property allows detection of module junctions by considering not a whole protein molecule, but only contiguous segments of a certain length and by locating their center. In practice we do so by locating minima of F_i; mean-square distance between C^α atom of ith residue and C^α atoms of the residues, which are within k residues along the polypeptide chain from ith residue, i.e.,

$$F_i = \sum_{j_1 \leq j \leq j_2} r_{ij}^2 / (j_2 - j_1) \qquad (1)$$

where $j_1 = \max(1, i - k)$, $j_2 = \min(n, i + k)$, and n is the number of residues in the protein. F_i is an index of centripetal character of the ith residue within a window length of $(2k + 1)$ residues. F_i was calculated for various k between 40 and 90; it was found that most of the local minima of F_i depend little on the value of k in this range (Fig. 2a). This makes the local minimum of F_i easy to detect. Those minima are candidates for the junctions of modules. The compactness of modules should be confirmed by another profile described below.

Modules as Compact Units within Domains

The candidates of module junctions by centripetal profile (Fig. 2a) were confirmed by an alternative algorithm called an extensity profile, in which relative compactness of a local segment along the backbone was employed to apportion a globular domain into compact units. This algorithm is based on an observation of protein conformation that atomic density or relative accessibility of a residue has an autocorrelation of 8–10 residues (Gō and Gō 1980). When the backbone is followed in one direction along the residue number, it comes out onto the surface of the protein, then turns on the surface and goes into the interior, then again comes out onto the surface and so on. In the interior of proteins the backbone has a tendency to have extended conformations, and it often makes β sheets. Thus, straight interior parts and curved surface regions appear alternatively along the backbone. From the autocorrelation length of 8–10 residues, the average length of this repeat is suggested to be about 16–20 residues. This value is expected to be the average length of modules for proteins whose three-dimensional structure was analyzed by X-ray crystallographic study.

Extensity Profile

Extensity of a backbone segment having a certain length of backbone (e.g., 21 residues) was formulated and calculated as in the following. Each pairwise distance between two α carbons was calculated within a window composed of $2k + 1$ residues centered at the ith residue; then the average of $k(2k + 1)$ pairwise distances was calculated. This quantity plotted for each residue in a subunit is hereafter referred to as the extensity profile of the subunit. Local maxima of the extensity profile were identified (Fig. 2b) and modules were defined as the segments bordered by two consecutive local maxima of the profile. Modules identified in such a way are the contiguous portions having least extended local structures in protein tertiary structures. In evaluating the extensity profile, less weight was given to the residue pairs that are separated by more

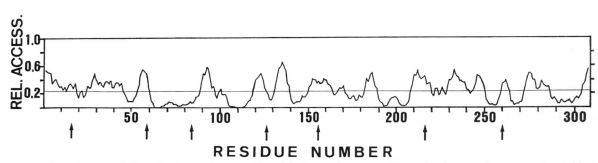

Figure 1. Relative accessibility of bovine carboxypeptidase A is shown after a smoothing operation over five consecutive residues. The arrows indicate intron positions in rat gene of preprocarboxypeptidase A (Quinto et al. 1982). Relative accessibility of a residue is defined as the ratio of its accessible surface area to solvent in a native protein conformation to that in the denatured state (Gō and Miyazawa 1980).

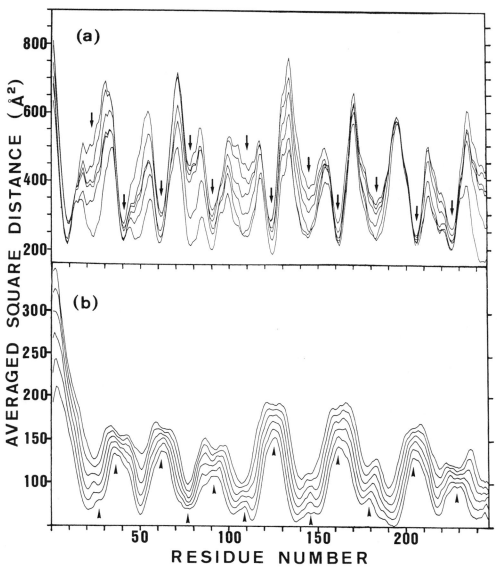

Figure 2. (*a*) Centripetal profile of chicken TIM. Curves of F_i with the windows of 81, 101, 121, 141, 161, and 181 residues, corresponding to $k = 40, 50, 60, 70, 80,$ and 90 in Eq. 1, respectively, are drawn from the bottom to the top. F_i is smoothed over five residues to facilitate the detection of their local minima. The common local minima among the curves marked by the arrows are employed as module junctions; at least 12 junctions are identified. To confirm the compactness of the segments apportioned by these minima, it was searched as to whether correspondents are present in the maxima of extensity curve E_i. (*b*) Extensity profiles E_i of chicken TIM with window length ($= 2k + 1$) of 21, 23, 25, 27, 29, and 31 residues, from the bottom to the top, respectively. The local maxima marked by arrows were employed as module junctions; at least 13 modules were identified. Local maxima within $2k + 1$ residues from the amino- or carboxy-terminal residues are less reliable, because the window of full length ($2k + 1$ residues) cannot be taken centering at these residues. The X-ray coordinates of chicken TIM used in the calculation of F_i and E_i were supplied by the Protein Data Bank of Brookhaven National Laboratory (Bernstein et al. 1977).

than k residues sequence-wise. This weighting operation was applied to take into account the interactions primarily between the residue pairs located closely rather than of those separated from each other sequence-wise. This was found to be useful in avoiding noise brought into the extensity profile by the residues located a short distance space-wise but a long distance sequence-wise from the residue under consideration. The weighted extensity of ith residue E_i is given by

$$E_i = \frac{1}{(j_2 - j_1)(j_2 - j_1 + 1)} \sum_{j_1 \leq m < j \leq j_2} G_{mj} \quad (2)$$

and

$$G_{mj} = \begin{cases} r_{mj}^2 & \text{for } j - m \leq k \\ r_{mj}^2/(j - m) & \text{for } j - m > k \end{cases} \quad (3)$$

where r_{mj} is the distance between the jth and the mth α

carbons. Theoretically speaking, the length of window should be chosen in a self-consistent way; it is thus best to use the length of modules identified. Since this is difficult to realize because the size of modules is not unique, we changed the length of the window empirically and obtained satisfactory results with a k value between 10 and 20 in various proteins.

RESULTS

Modules of TIM

Triosephosphate isomerase (TIM; EC 5.3.1.1) is a good subject for the study of protein evolution, since it is an enzyme in the glycolytic pathway, is distributed widely from bacteria to mammals, and is also a slowly evolving protein (Forthergill-Gilmore 1986). Chicken TIM functions as a dimer of identical subunits, each of which is composed of 247 amino acid residues. The structure of the subunit of chicken TIM is known by X-ray crystallographic studies (Banner et al. 1975) to consist of a single domain having a typical barrel structure where (α/β) repeats eight times.

Modules identified by the centripetal profile and those identified by the extensity profile correspond to each other (Table 1), except that one minimum at residue 10 in the centripetal profile (Fig. 2a) has no correspondent in the extensity profile (Fig. 2b). Junctions of modules identified by the two profiles are not exactly the same. This means that the boundaries of the identified modules have inevitable deviations of several residues, depending on the profile employed. Despite the deviation between the two profiles, the module junctions they identify are essentially very similar. In the regions near the amino and carboxyl termini, the identified minima and maxima in the profiles inevitably

contain some artificial effect from the short window length. This is why deviation occurs between the two profiles and the identification of modules is less certain at the amino- and carboxy-terminal regions.

An extensity profile was drawn for k in the range of 10–15 (Fig. 2b). It was found that the residue numbers at the local maxima of extensity profiles for the different k values are essentially similar, although they shift occasionally by several residues. The local maxima of the extensity profile for $k = 10$ were employed in the final identification of modules (Table 1). Thus, at least 13 and possibly 14 modules were identified in TIM. Since identification of short modules consisting of ten or so residues is beyond the sensitivity of the present method, there remains the possibility that the modules can be decomposed into two. Thus, we have identified the minimum number of modules.

Modules as Building Blocks

The spatial arrangement of the modules of TIM is shown in stereo pictures of the space-filling model (Fig. 3,a–c). Each module is positioned in a localized way. Modules making the carboxyl ends of β strands, i.e., M1, M3, M4, M6, M8, M10, M12, and M13 are seen with different colors in Figure 3a, and those making the other ends, i.e., M2, M5, M7, M9, and M11 are seen in Figure 3b.

The modules are also shown in a smoothed wire model (Feldmann et al. 1986) in blue and yellow alternatively (Fig. 4,a–c). The locations of the junctions between modules are seen clearly in the figure; many of them are located in the interior of the subunit but a few are positioned close to the surface. Most of the module junctions are found on the secondary structures, on α helices or on β strands. Interactions between the side

Table 1. Modules of TIM and Introns of Its Genes

Module boundary	Residue number[a]		Corresponding intron[b]		
	A	B	chicken[c]	maize[d]	A. nidulans[e]
	10 (β)		—	12–13	12
M1–M2	23 (α)	28 (α)	—	—	—
M2–M3	42 (β)	37 (β)	37	37	—
M3–M4	63 (β)	63 (β)	—	—	—
M4–M5	79 (α)	78	78	78	—
M5–M6	92 (β)	93 (β)	—	—	—
M6–M7	111 (α)	109 (α)	106–107	106–107	106–107
M7–M8	125 (β)	127 (β)	—	—	131–132
M8–M9	146 (α)	147 (α)	151	151	—
M9–M10	162 (β)	162 (β)	—	—	168
M10–M11	185 (α)	179 (α)	179–180	182–183	—
M11–M12	207 (β)	204 (β)	209	209	—
M12–M13	227 (β)	230 (β)	—	236–237	239

[a]Local minima in the centripetal profile are shown as A and local maxima in the extensity profile are shown as B. Secondary structures at these minima and maxima are shown in parentheses.

[b]Numbers show the intron positions aligned to the amino acid sequence of chicken TIM.

[c]From Straus and Gilbert (1985).

[d]From Marchionni and Gilbert (1986).

[e]From McKnight et al. (1986).

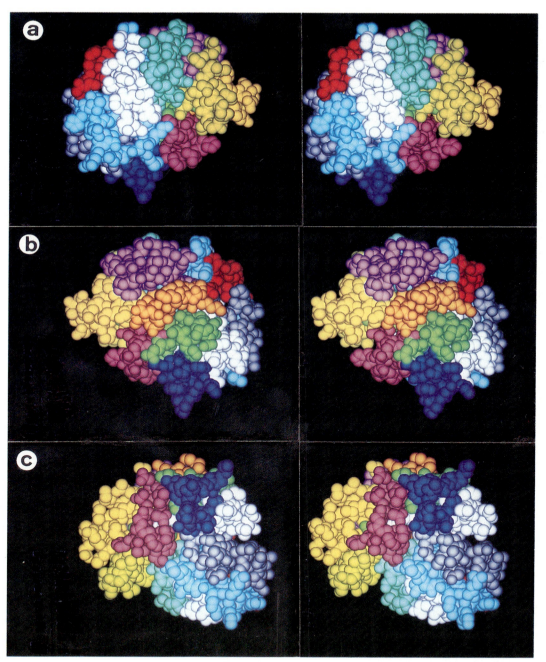

Figure 3. Spatial arrangements of modules in a TIM subunit are shown in space-filling model in stereo (crossed-eye) pairs (*a*) from the direction of the carboxyl termini of β strands; (*b*) from that of the amino termini of β strands; and (*c*) from that of one side of the barrel. The modules are colored light blue (M1), red (M2), grey (M3), dark blue (M4), white (M5), red violet (M6), yellow green (M7), yellow (M8), orange (M9), green yellow (M10), purple (M11), blue-green (M12), and white (M13). Both M5 and M13 are colored white, but only M13 is seen in *a* and M5 in *b*. M5 and M13 are seen in *c* at the upper and lower parts, respectively. See a guide by Young (1987) for a technique telling how to focus on the stereo drawings if necessary.

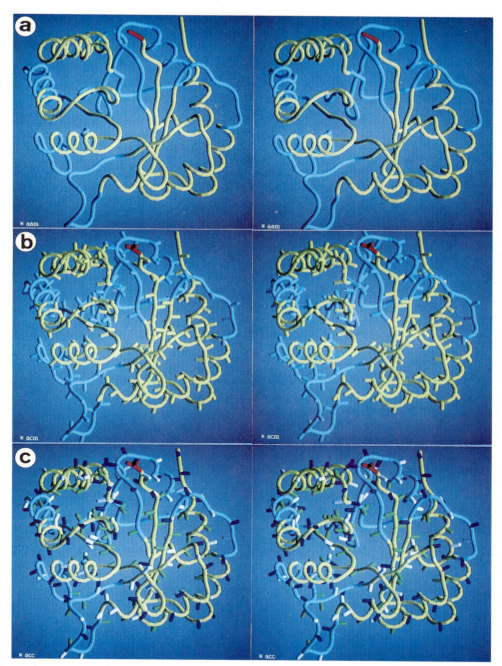

Figure 4. Stereo (not crossed-eye) drawings of a subunit of TIM are shown in smoothed wire model (Feldmann et al. 1986) from the direction of the amino termini of β strands. Modules of TIM with odd numbers are colored yellow and those with even numbers blue. Amino terminal of the chain is shown in red. Only the backbone is drawn in *a*, the backbone with shortened branches of the side chains in *b*, and the same as that in *b*, except that hydrophilic, hydrophobic, and ambivalent side chains are colored in blue, green, and white, respectively, in *c*.

chains within the modules are recognized as well as those between the side chains belonging to different modules (Fig. 4,b and c). Hydrophilic side chains are localized on each module on the surface exposed to solvent. A part of the hydrophobic side chains contributes to stabilize the modules themselves, and the left part is involved in making contacts between the modules. The latter yields a stable globular subunit by making an assembly of 13 modules (Fig. 4c).

Modules and Function of TIM

The exon shuffling hypothesis (Gilbert 1978) is based on the assumption that an exon is a functional or structural unit of proteins. What is the function of each module, and how are functionally important residues distributed on modules in TIM? Possible catalytic site Glu-164 and phosphate-binding site Gly-232 are located on modules M10 and M13, respectively. It is noted that the modules having even numbers (except M2) are involved in TIM function (Table 2), i.e., the active sites (Banner et al. 1975) are distributed mainly on M4, M6, M8, M10, and M12, and on the terminal modules M1 and M13. These are the modules building the carboxyl ends of the eight β strands, i.e., the top of the β barrel structure (Figs. 3a and 4). Module M2 and those of odd numbers M5, M7, M9, and M11 make up the bottom of the β barrel of TIM (Fig. 4b). Intersubunit contact sites (Banner et al. 1975) are located on M1 and M3–M7 (Table 2), which are localized on one side of the β barrel (Fig. 3c).

Correlation of Module Junctions with Intron Positions in TIM

Split gene structures of TIM have been reported for several species. Human (Brown et al. 1985) and chicken (Straus and Gilbert 1985) genes of TIM were sequenced and were revealed to be split into seven exons;

the six introns are located at exactly the same positions in the genes. The maize gene of TIM, being interrupted by eight introns (Marchionni and Gilbert 1986), has the largest number of introns among the genes of TIM whose structures were analyzed so far. The *Saccharomyces cerevisiae* gene of TIM is not interrupted by introns (Alber and Kawasaki 1982); however, the TIM gene of *A. nidulans* is split by five introns (McKnight et al. 1986). The amino acid sequence of TIM of chicken has approximately 50% identity to that of *S. cerevisiae* (Alber and Kawasaki 1982). Based on the fact that the tertiary structure is conserved better than the primary structure, the three-dimensional structures of human, maize, and *A. nidulans* TIMs are thought to be similar to that of chicken analyzed by X-ray crystallographic study.

All positions of the six introns in TIM genes of chicken and human correspond to the module junctions identified in the present analysis within the deviation of five residues, no matter which profile is used, i.e., to the junctions between modules M2 and M3, M4 and M5, M6 and M7, M8 and M9, M10 and M11, and M11 and M12, respectively (Table 1). It should be noted that these six introns are also conserved in the gene of maize, but only one intron corresponding to the junction of M6–M7 is conserved in the *A. nidulans* gene.

The position of intron 8 in the maize TIM gene corresponds to the junction of M12–M13. Introns 1 of maize and *A. nidulans* TIM genes correspond closely to the amino-terminal minima at residue 10 in the centripetal profile; however, no maximum is observed in the extensity profile (Fig. 2b). The positions of introns 1, 2, and 5 in the gene of *A. nidulans* are either exactly the same as or very similar to those in the gene of maize. Introns 3 and 4 of the gene of *A. nidulans* correspond to the junctions M7–M8 and M9–M10, respectively, although they do not have correspondents in the genes of chicken, human, or maize. Intron positions except those in the amino- and carboxy-terminal

Table 2. Modules of TIM, Their Secondary Structure and Function

Module	Residue number	Secondary structure[a,b]	Active sites[b]	Subunit contact sites[b]
M1	1–28	[β][α	10–12	13, 14
M2	29–37	α][β		
M3	38–63	β][α][β]		44, 45, 47, 52, 63
M4	64–78	none	71–74	64, 66, 68, 71–77
M5	79–93	[β][α		79, 81, 82, 84, 85, 91
M6	94–109	[α][α	94–96, 99, 100	96, 97, 103
M7	110–127	α][β	125, 127	111
M8	128–147	β][α	128, 129	
M9	148–162	α][β		
M10	163–179	β][α	162–166, 169 (Glu-164)	
M11	180–204	α]		
M12	205–230	[β][α][β	208, 209, 211, 229, 230	
M13	231–247	β][α]	231–234 (Gly-232)	

[a] α helix and β strand are shown by [α] and [β], respectively. When a boundary of the modules falls on a stretch of the secondary structures, amino-terminal parts of them are denoted by [α or [β, carboxy-terminal parts by α] or β].
[b] From Banner et al. (1975).

regions correspond to the module junctions within the deviation of zero to six residues.

Module Length

Chicken TIM consisting of 247 amino acid residues is decomposed into at least 13 modules by the compactness observed in the extensity profile. The mean length of TIM modules is 18 residues; it seems shorter than those in hemoglobin and lysozyme. We identified modules in subunits composed of less than 200 amino acid residues using the original version of the algorithm (Fig. 5,a–c). The reason only small subunits were considered in the analysis is that small subunits contain almost no core modules and the simple visually oriented method is still effective for them. The mean length of the modules in 29 subunits is approximately 18 residues, and they are distributed mostly within the range of 10–40 residues. The average length of modules, 18 residues, satisfies the expected value by the autocorrelation length observed in protein folding (Gō and Gō 1980). When the subunits are grouped into 'two categories depending on their sources, i.e., whether they are derived from eukaryotes or prokaryotes, each group shows a similar distribution of module length (Fig. 5,b and c). We see no difference in the protein architecture built from modules whether it is encoded by prokaryotic or eukaryotic genes. This implies that there is no reason to suppose that only the genes of eukaryotes have been split for a long time and that prokaryote genes have never been split. An intron in the thymidilate synthase gene of T4 phage (Chu et al. 1984) might be such a remnant in contemporary prokaryotic genes.

DISCUSSION

It is easier to build a complex protein when its construction is modular—that is, when it is built from smaller units of standard size and shape. The secondary structure of the modules in TIM is of three types: The first type consists of α helix and β strand in the order of chain direction from amino to carboxyl termini or consists of only α helices (M2, M6, M7, M9, and M11); the second type consists of β strand and α helix or consists of β strand, α helix, and β strand (M1, M3, M5, M8, M10, M12, and M13); the third type has no secondary structure (M4) (Table 2).

Most of the module junctions are located on the secondary structures (Table 1); this implies that proteins are designed in nature by making module joints rigid utilizing the secondary structures as the joints of modules. This character of the module junctions is also observed in alcohol dehydrogenase (M. Gō and M. Nosaka, in prep.) Secondary structures seem to hold flexible loops, on which active sites are often located, facilitating foundations of protein architecture. This phenomenon is noted to be a principal part of the design of artificial proteins in which short segments are joined to yield stable globular proteins.

All of the introns in chicken and human TIM genes correspond to the boundaries of the identified modules within a deviation of zero to five residues, and most of the introns, except those close to the terminals in maize and *A. nidulans* genes, also correspond to these boundaries within a deviation of zero to six residues. Could such close correlation of module boundaries with intron positions happen only by chance? Given the maize TIM gene, the probability of eight introns falling by chance within seven residues from the module joints is extremely small. A small probability is retained also for the other TIM genes, thus the correlation is scarcely expected from random process.

The most probable explanation for the correspondence of the intron positions to the module boundaries is that an ancestral gene of TIM was interrupted by at least 12 introns corresponding to the module junctions identified in the present paper; some of these, however, have been lost. According to this hypothesis at least six, five, and seven introns have been lost from chicken, maize, and *A. nidulans* TIM genes, respectively, during the course of evolution. Introns are located close to 10

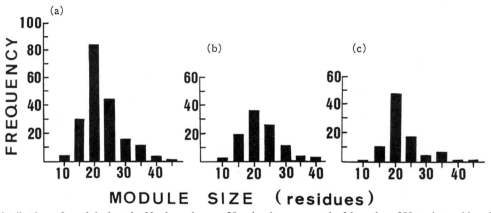

Figure 5. Distribution of module length. Nonhomologous 29 subunits composed of less than 200 amino acid residues were decomposed into modules using their three-dimensional structure by X-ray crystallography. The module size and its frequency are shown (*a*) for all the subunits, (*b*) for the subunits of proteins from eukaryotes, and (*c*) for those from prokaryotes, respectively.

out of 12 junctions of modules when the TIM genes of four species are aligned and at least two more introns are thought to be or have been present close to the junctions of M3–M4 and M5–M6 (Table 1).

Given modules encoded by mini-genes, is such a short segment of about 20 or less amino acid residues stable in aqueous solution? There is some evidence that the length of 20–40 amino acid residues might be the minimum requirement for a segment to be stable in aqueous solution (Wetlaufer 1981). S-peptide obtained by limited proteolysis of ribonuclease A consists of 20 amino acid residues. α helix in isolated S-peptide has been demonstrated to have significant stability in water (Kim and Baldwin 1984). Even isolated C-peptide, which corresponds to residues 1–13 of ribonuclease A, shows α helix formation, and charged groups play a critical role in the helix stability (Shoemaker et al. 1987). This fact shows that even such a short segment can have a stable conformation depending on its amino acid sequence.

Primitive enzymes might be assemblies of such short segments that are supposed to be more or less stable themselves but can be more stabilized by making spatial interactions with each other in the assemblies. Strong selection might have worked on conformations of such segments through a period of trial and error. The split genes might be the remnants of recruitment of useful modules into functional proteins in prebiological evolution.

Introns presumably existed in ancient genes (Darnell 1978; Doolittle 1978) and the RNA-catalyzed process (Cech 1986) possibly facilitated the splicing of the introns (Gilbert 1986; Darnell and Doolittle 1986). At some point in prebiological evolution, RNA and protein are supposed to have begun interacting with each other. It is noted that the average length of a module is ~ 20 amino acid residues, which is consistent with the length of polymerized RNA using a template in simulation of prebiological conditions (Acevedo and Orgel 1986).

ACKNOWLEDGMENTS

We thank Richard Feldmann for his drawings of smoothed wire models of TIM, Haruki Nakamura for computer software of 3-D graphics, Tomoo Monji and Junji Matsuguma for taking photographs of CPK models, Nobuhiro Gō for suggestive discussions, and Professor Hirotsugu Matsuda for continuous encouragement on this work. Recognition is made of the Centre Européen de Calcul Atomique et Moléculaire (CECAM) workshop held in 1979 in Orsay where a part of this work was initiated. Computation was done by FACOM M380S at the computer center in Kyushu University. A part of this work was supported by the Kurata Research Grant and by Grants-in-Aid for Special Project Research and for Scientific Research from the Ministry of Education, Science and Culture of Japan.

REFERENCES

Acevedo, O.L. and L.E. Orgel. 1986. Template-directed oligonucleotide ligation on hydroxylapatite. *Nature* **321:** 790.

Alber, T. and G. Kawasaki. 1982. Nucleotide sequence of the triose phosphate isomerase gene of *Saccharomyces cerevisiae. J. Mol. Appl. Genet.* **1:** 419.

Banner, D.W., A.C. Bloomer, G.A. Petsko, D.C. Phillips, C.I. Pogson, and I.A. Wilson. 1975. Structure of chicken muscle triose phosphate isomerase determined crystallographically at 2.5 Å resolution. *Nature* **255:** 609.

Bernstein, F.C., T.F. Koetzle, G.J.B. Williams, E.F. Meyer, Jr., M.D. Brice, J.R. Rodgers, O. Kennard, T. Shimanouchi, and M. Tasumi. 1977. The protein data bank: A computer-based archival file for macromolecular structures. *J. Mol. Biol.* **112:** 535.

Blake, C.C.F. 1978. Do genes-in-pieces imply proteins-in-pieces? *Nature* **273:** 267.

———. 1981. Exons and the structure, function and evolution of haemoglobin. *Nature* **291:** 616.

———. 1983. Exons–present from the beginning? *Nature* **306:** 535.

Bränden, C.-I., H. Eklund, C. Cambillau, and A.J. Pryor. 1984. Correlation of exons with structural domains in alcohol dehydrogenase. *EMBO J.* **3:** 1307.

Brown, J.R., I.O. Daar, J.S. Krug, and L.E. Maguart. 1985. Characterization of the functional gene and several processed pseudogenes in the human triosephosphate isomerase gene family. *Mol. Cell. Biol.* **5:** 1694.

Cavalier-Smith, T. 1985. Selfish DNA and the origin of introns. *Nature* **315:** 283.

Cech, T. 1986. The generality of self-splicing RNA: Relationship to nuclear mRNA splicing. *Cell* **44:** 207.

Chang, C. and E.M. Meyerowitz. 1986. Molecular cloning and DNA sequence of the Arabidopsis thathiana alcohol dehydrogenase gene. *Proc. Natl. Acad. Sci.* **83:** 1408.

Chu, F.K., G.F. Maley, F. Maley, and M. Belfort. 1984. Intervening sequence in the thymidylate synthase gene of bacteriophage T4. *Proc. Natl. Acad. Sci.* **81:** 3049.

Darnell, Jr., J.E. 1978. Implications of RNA · RNA splicing in evolution of eukaryotic cells. *Science* **202:** 1257.

Darnell, J.E. and W.F. Doolittle. 1986. Speculations on the early course of evolution. *Proc. Natl. Acad. Sci.* **83:** 1271.

Dennis, E.S., W.L. Gerlach, A.J. Pryor, J.L. Bennetzen, A. Inglis, D. Llewellyn, M.M. Sachs, R.J. Ferl, and W.J. Peacock. 1984. Molecular analysis of the alcohol dehydrogenase (*Adh1*) gene of maize. *Nucleic Acids Res.* **12:** 3983.

Doolittle, W.F. 1978. Genes in pieces: Were they ever together? *Nature* **272:** 581.

Duester, G., H. Jornvall, and G.W. Hatfield. 1986. Intron-dependent evolution of the nucleotide-binding domains within alcohol dehydrogenase and related enzymes. *Nucleic Acids Res.* **14:** 1931.

Feldmann, R.J., B.R. Brooks, and B. Lee. 1986. *Understanding protein architecture through stimulated unfolding.* Division of Computer Research and Technology, National Institutes of Health, Bethesda, Maryland.

Forthergill-Gilmore, L.A. 1986. The evolution of the glycolytic pathway. *Trends Biochem. Sci.* **11:** 47.

Gilbert, W. 1978. Why genes in pieces? *Nature* **271:** 501.

———. 1986. The RNA world. *Nature* **319:** 618.

Gilbert, W., M. Marchionni, and G. McKnight. 1986. On the antiquity of introns. *Cell* **46:** 151.

Gō, M. 1981. Correlation of DNA exonic regions with protein structural units in haemoglobin. *Nature* **291:** 90.

———. 1983. Modular structural units, exons, and function in chicken lysozyme. *Proc. Natl. Acad. Sci.* **80:** 1964.

———. 1985. Protein structures and split genes. *Adv. Biophys.* **19:** 91.

Gō, M. and N. Gō. 1980. Comparison of method to define the surface of protein. In *Rapport d'activite scientifique du*

CECAM (ed. C. Mosaer), p. 135. Centre Européen de Calcul Atomique et Moléculaire, Orsay.

Gō, M. and S. Miyazawa. 1980. Relationship between mutability, polarity and exteriority of amino acid residues in protein evolution. *Int. J. Pept. Protein Res.* **15**: 211.

Jensen, E.O., J.K. Pauldan, J.J. Hyldig-Nielsen, P. Jorgensen, and K.A. Marcker. 1981. The structure of a chromosomal leghaemoglobin gene from soybean. *Nature* **291**: 677.

Kim, P.S. and R.L. Baldwin. 1984. A helix stop signal in the isolated S-peptide of ribonuclease A. *Nature* **306**: 329.

Marchionni, M. and W. Gilbert. 1986. The triosephosphate isomerase gene from maize: Introns antedate the plant-animal divergence. *Cell* **46**: 133.

McKnight, G.L., P.J. O'Hara, and M.L. Parker. 1986. Nucleotide sequence of the triosephosphate isomerase gene from *Aspergillus nidulans:* Implications for a differential loss of introns. *Cell* **46**: 143.

Quinto, C., M. Quiroga, W.F. Swain, W.C. Nikovits, Jr., D.N. Stadring, R.L. Pictet, P. Valenzuela, and W.J. Rutter. 1982. Rat preprocarboxypeptidase A: cDNA sequence and preliminary characterization of the gene. *Proc. Natl. Acad. Sci.* **79**: 31.

Sharp, P.A. 1985. On the origin of RNA splicing and introns. *Cell* **42**: 397.

Shoemaker, K.R., P.S. Kim, E.J. York, J.M. Stewart, and R.L. Baldwin. 1987. Tests of the helix dipole model for stabilization of α-helices. *Nature* **326**: 563.

Straus, D. and W. Gilbert. 1985. Genetic engineering in the precambrian: Structure of chicken triosephosphate isomerase gene. *Mol. Cell. Biol.* **5**: 3497.

Wetlaufer, D.B. 1981. Folding of protein fragments. *Adv. Protein Chem.* **34**: 61.

Young, D.C. 1987. Viewing stereo drawings. *Science* **235**: 623.

Exon and Domain Evolution in the Proenzymes of Blood Coagulation and Fibrinolysis

C.C.F. Blake, K. Harlos, and S.K. Holland
Laboratory of Molecular Biophysics, University of Oxford, Oxford, OX1 3QU, England

Gilbert's explanation (1978) of the mosaic structure of eukaryotic genes in terms of its ability to promote exon-encoded protein functions being reassorted in novel protein molecules, a process subsequently referred to as exon shuffling, represents a potentially major new mechanism for molecular evolution. It was immediately obvious to some of us (Blake 1978) that exon shuffling might be an explanation of the common occurrence of domain enzymes, and particularly of those that seem to use a domain of the same structure for the same function in combination with other different domains, such as the NAD-binding unit of the dehydrogenases (Rossmann et al. 1974). This proposal seemed to identify exon-encoded fragments with structural domains, and also to imply that exon-mediated evolution was an early mechanism (Blake 1983), which had already been proposed on other grounds (Darnell 1978; Doolittle 1978; Reanney 1979). Both these ideas have proved contentious; and although further analysis (Blake 1985; Holland and Blake 1987) has suggested that exons can be more readily correlated with supersecondary structures that could represent the primordial building blocks of proteins, those who believe that introns and exons are early or late aspects of gene structure have developed into two opposing schools (see Orgel and Crick 1980; Cavalier-Smith 1985).

Until recently, direct evidence of exon shuffling was not available, but now a number of apparent examples of evolution by exon shuffling have appeared. On the basis of Gilbert's original suggestion (Gilbert 1978), the validation of exon shuffling could be argued to involve the identification of two or more structural genes, each of which contains an exon or exon cluster, that encodes a similar protein structural unit with a similar function, but that are otherwise distinct. The supposition of the discovery of such genes is that a common exon or exon cluster has been shuffled into the genes to incorporate a common function into the expressed proteins. A good example of this type of behavior seems to be offered by the blood coagulation and fibrinolytic system whose proenzymes have related structure and functions that appear to be the result of exon shuffling events.

Proteins of Blood Coagulation and Fibrinolysis

The proteins of the blood coagulation system and of fibrinolysis are shown in Figure 1. Many of the proteins are involved in the cascade of sequential conversion of zymogens into active enzymes through proteolytic cleavage of their polypeptide chains. Studies on the primary structures have now been completed for nearly all these proteins, either through chemical determination of amino acid sequence or through gene or cDNA sequencing. These studies have shown that the zymogens all have pancreatic serine proteinase units at the carboxyl termini of their polypeptide chains, and amino-terminal extensions containing between three and six copies of small homology units. The homology units are composed of between 40 and 85 amino acid residues linked by one to three disulfide bridges. Among the coagulation and fibrinolytic zymogens, the number of distinct types of homology unit is very limited. As shown in Figure 2, Kringle units of 85 amino acid residues linked by three disulfide bridges (Magnusson et al. 1975) occur in prothrombin and blood coagulation factor XII, and in plasminogen and its two activators, urokinase (uPA) and tissue plasminogen activator (tPA). Calcium-binding units of about 47 amino acid residues, with one disulfide bridge (Di Scipio et al. 1977) and containing between 10 and 12 γ-carboxyglutamic acid residues, formed in a vitamin-K-dependent posttranslational modification (Nelsestuen et al. 1974), are present in the amino termini of prothrombin, factors VII, IX, X, and some inhibitors of coagulation, such as proteins C and S. Epidermal growth factor (EGF)-like units, containing about 40 amino acid residues linked by three disulfide bridges (Doolittle et al. 1984) occur in factors VII, IX, X, proteins C and S, and uPA and tPA. The final types of homology unit, the fibronectin type I and type II units, originally defined in the fibronectin molecule, have been shown to be related to the EGF (Doolittle 1985) and the Kringle (Patthy et al. 1984; Holland et al. 1987) units, respectively. The ten coagulation and fibrinolytic proteins shown in Figure 2 contain 36 small homology units of three different types in patterns that cannot be easily derived from any potential ancestral protein.

The Exon Pattern

Gene structures are known for bovine and human prothrombin (Degen et al. 1983; Irwin et al. 1985), factor IX (Anson et al. 1984), factor X (Leytus et al. 1986), protein C (Plutzky et al. 1986), tPA (Ny et al. 1984), and uPA (Verde et al. 1984). The relation between gene structure and homology pattern can therefore be established for five copies of the Kringle, four

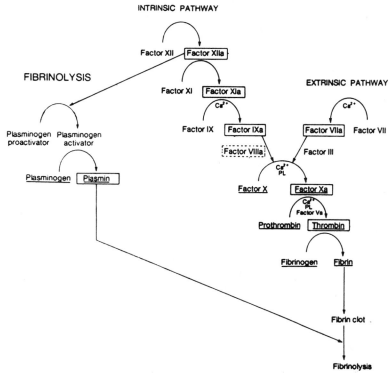

Figure 1. A schematic diagram of the blood coagulation and fibrinolytic systems. Proenzymes are shown unboxed; active forms are boxed. PL signifies phospholipid.

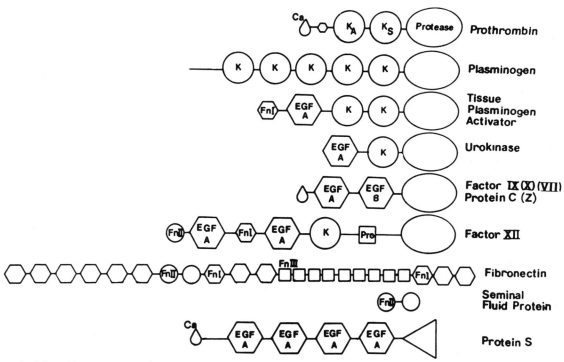

Figure 2. Schematic representation of the arrangement of homology units in the coagulation and fibrinolytic proenzymes. Fibronectin is also shown. The calcium-binding unit is marked Ca, the Kringle is marked K, and the epidermal growth factor-like unit is labeled EGF. The shapes; teardrop, circle, hexagon, and ellipse, are intended to signify units of homologous structures, but squares represent other units.

copies of the calcium-binding unit, and eight copies of the EGF-like unit. Those relationships are demonstrated in Figures 3–5, which show the exon-encoded patterns for the three types of unit. The correlation between gene structure and protein structure is least good for the Kringle units (Fig. 3). Here four of the five examples are encoded by two exons, with a similar intron location for three but quite a different location for the fourth. In addition, the termini of the chains,

and particularly the carboxyl terminus, are somewhat variable in length, although the sliding junction hypothesis of Craik et al. (1983) may be relevant here. It should be noted that the amino acid homology in the Kringles (20% identity over 11 copies) is sufficiently high for derivation from a common ancestor to be certain. The correlation of gene structure and protein structure for the calcium-binding unit, which is encoded on two exons with a common intron location in all our

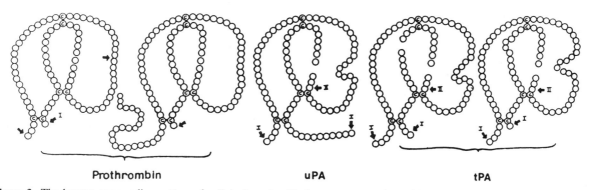

Figure 3. The known exon-coding patterns for Kringle units. Circles represent amino acid residues; those with an inscribed C represent cysteine residues. Arrows indicate the location of introns. The phase of the exon/intron junction is indicated by 0 where the junction is between coding triplets, I where it occurs after the first base of the triplet, and II where it occurs after the second base of the triplet.

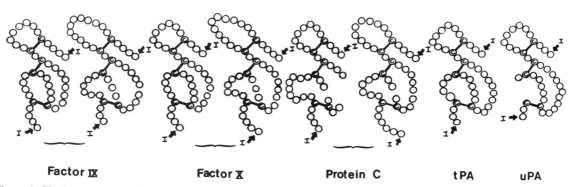

Factor IX **Factor X** **Protein C** **tPA** **uPA**

Figure 4. The known exon-coding patterns for epidermal growth factor-like units. Circles and arrows have the same significance as in Fig. 3.

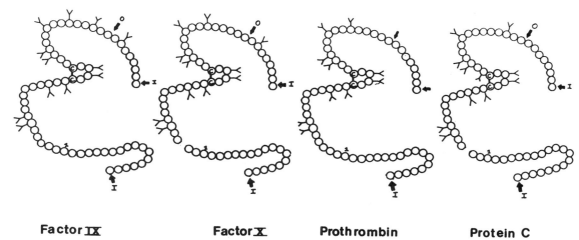

Factor IX **Factor X** **Prothrombin** **Protein C**

Figure 5. The known exon-coding patterns for calcium-binding unit. Circles and arrows have the same significance as in Fig. 3.

examples, and the EGF-like unit, which is always encoded by a single exon in these examples, is remarkably clear.

Despite the less than perfect result for the Kringle it seems reasonable to conclude that these small homology units are discretely encoded on exons, and that those proteins that have been discussed in which they occur have obtained the units through an exon-shuffling mechanism.

Structural Analysis

X-ray structural analysis of proteins in the coagulation and fibrinolytic systems would clarify the true relationship between gene and protein structure, but unfortunately none of the complete proteins appears to crystallize. The only usable crystals that have been reported are of fragment 1 of bovine prothrombin (Aschaffenburg et al. 1977; Hu Kung and Tulinsky 1980;

Olsson et al. 1982), which consist of the calcium-binding unit and the first Kringle unit. The structure of fragment 1 has been carried out independently by Park and Tulinsky (1986) and ourselves (Harlos et al. 1987). The division of the fragment into structural domains is very revealing in relation to the exon pattern of prothrombin, as shown in Figure 6. The Kringle unit, represented by residues 64–156, is a very compact structure with a clearly defined hydrophobic core and is demonstrably a single structural domain encoded precisely by exons 4 and 5. The calcium-binding unit is more complex than had been thought previously and appears to consist of two parts. Residues 1–36, which contain all nine invariant γ-carboxyglutamic acid residues that bind calcium, appear to be totally disordered in the crystal. Residues 36–63, in contrast, are well ordered, organized in a compact structure consisting of two α helices linked by a disulfide bridge. There is a good correlation between the disordered unit and exon 1,

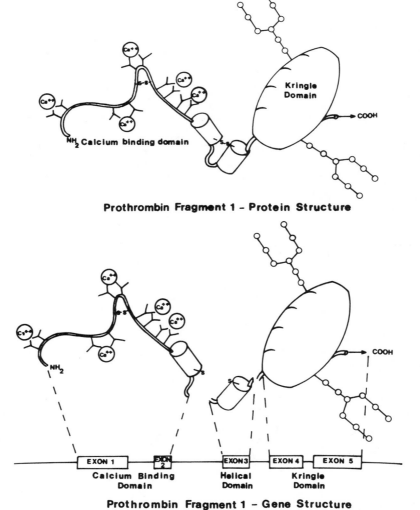

Prothrombin Fragment 1 – Protein Structure

Prothrombin Fragment 1 – Gene Structure

Figure 6. A schematic drawing of the relationship between the three-dimensional structure of fragment 1 of bovine prothrombin and the fine structure of its gene.

and exons 2 and 3 correspond very closely to the two helices in the ordered unit. It is interesting to note that the calcium-binding unit in factors IX, X, and protein C is composed of the products of exons 1 and 2 only, and the chain then immediately enters the EGF-like unit. The second helix, therefore, seems unique to prothrombin, where it perhaps acts as a "spacer" between the calcium-binding unit and the Kringle, and exon 3 of the prothrombin gene appears to have no equivalent in the genes of factors IX, X, and protein C. The calcium-binding unit in prothrombin may therefore be considered to be made up of three parts, each encoded by a single exon, but only two of these parts are present in other proteins containing the calcium-binding unit.

Functions of the Homology Units

The final aspect to consider is whether these small homology units have discrete functions, whose incorporation in the novel protein molecules provides the driving force for the proposed exon shuffling. These functional aspects are not particularly easy to study, and the picture is far from complete. The general nature of the functions of the small homology units can be understood by considering the current view of the complexes that are required for zymogen activation in the later stages of the blood coagulation cascade. As Figure 7 shows, the converting complex for prothrombin is a multiprotein assembly located on a membrane surface. Converting complexes for factor X and perhaps for factors VII and IX are similar. Plasminogen and its activators may also form multiprotein converting complexes involving interactions between themselves and fibrin.

The common factor in considering the function of the Kringle and EGF-like units, and the related type I and type II fibronectin domains, is protein binding. Table 1

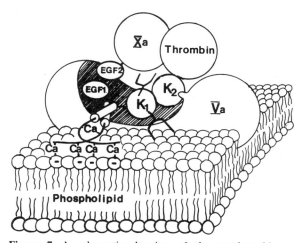

Figure 7. A schematic drawing of the prothrombinase-converting complex, showing the possible interactions of prothrombin, factor X_a and factor V_a on a phospholipid surface. Cylinders represent the helices of the calcium-binding unit, and the calcium ions shown are proposed to be bound by γ-carboxyglutamic acid residues.

shows what is known about the particular protein that interacts with individual units. The only specific binding site known is located on the Kringle units, where in plasminogen it interacts with arginine or lysine amino acids. This binding site is located in a cleft in the Kringle structure, with a bipolar charge pattern due to the presence of aspartic acid and arginine side chains.

Our X-ray studies on fragment 1 indicate that the calcium-binding unit also functions as a protein-binding unit, in addition to its phospholipid-binding ability, the function in each case being mediated by calcium ions. The protein-binding aspect can be more narrowly defined as a dimerization of the calcium-binding units. The interface includes not only the γ-carboxyglutamic acid region, which dimerizes through shared calcium ions, but also the exon-2-encoded helix, which makes a hydrophobic dimer interface through invariant aromatic amino acid residues. This reinforces the proposal that the calcium-binding unit is composed of two parts by allocating to the two structural parts two distinct functional roles. It is important to realize that dimerization of the calcium-binding units could link any two proteins containing the unit such as prothrombin and factor X (see Fig. 7) or factors IX and X, which must interact in the converting complex. No interaction between such pairs of protein has been described previously.

CONCLUSION

This analysis of the gene structure/protein structure relationships in the proenzymes of blood coagulation and fibrinolysis indicates that small-exon-encoded protein units of three specific types make up the non-catalytic amino-terminal extensions of the proteins. The observed patterns in which the small protein units occur in the different proenzymes are such that no simple derivation from a single ancestral protein seems possible. It is more reasonable to see the one or two exons that encode each small unit acting as autonomous genetic elements to be recruited into specific genes as required. The small protein units appear to carry particular binding functions, usually for other proteins in the coagulation or fibrinolytic systems, which enable the particular roles of the zymogens in the system to be specified. This set of proteins seems to fulfill in all respects the exon-mediated functional reassortment type of evolution first proposed by Gilbert (1978).

Through the EGF-like units, the evolutionary history of the coagulation and fibrinolytic zymogens is linked to that of the low-density lipoprotein receptor (LDLR) and the epidermal growth factor precursor (EGFP) proteins (Südhoff et al. 1985). A region encoding 400 amino acids containing three copies of the EGF-like unit is equivalent in the LDLR and EGFP genes, and as in the coagulation and fibrinolytic system, the EGF units are encoded by single exons. The LDLR protein also contains seven tandem repeats of a 40-residue unit otherwise found in the complement 9 protein (Di Scipio et al. 1984). In all, the LDLR gene contains 18

Table 1. Binding Function of Protease Domains

Domain	Source		Function
Kringle	prothrombin	K_A	?
		K_S	factor V binding
	plasminogen	K_1	Lys binding
		K_4	fibrin binding
		K_2	
		K_5	
	tissue plasminogen activator	(2)	fibrin binding
	urokinase	(1)	?
Fibronectin type II	fibronectin	(2)	collagen binding
	factor XII		collagen binding?
	bovine seminal fluid protein BSFP	(2)	?
EGF A	EGF	(8)	transmembrane receptor binding
	TPA, UK, FACXII		?
A/B	factor IX	(2)	
	factor X	(2)	factor V binding
	protein C	(2)	
Fibronectin type I	fibronectin	(5)	fibrin binding
			actin binding
			heparin binding
		(3)	fibrin binding
		(3)	collagen binding
	factor XII	(1)	fibrin binding ?
	tissue plasminogen activator	(1)	fibrin binding

exons, of which 13 encode segments homologous to those found in other proteins and which are also often encoded by separate exons. This is major evidence of exon shuffling (Gilbert 1985).

ACKNOWLEDGMENTS

We are grateful to the Medical Research Council for financial support. We also acknowledge the financial support of the Medical Research Council, the Deutsche Forschungsgemeinshaft (grant Ha-1291/1-2) and the Environmental Protection Agency Cephalosporin Fund to K.H. C.C.F.B. is a member of the Oxford Enzyme Group, which is supported by the Science and Engineering Research Council.

REFERENCES

Anson, D.S., K.H. Choo, D.J.G. Rees, F. Gianelli, K. Gould, J.A. Huddleston, and G.G. Brownlee. 1984. The gene structure of human anti-haemophilic factor IX. *EMBO J.* **3:** 1053.

Aschaffenburg, R., C.C.F. Blake, J.M. Burridge, and M.P. Esnouf. 1977. Preliminary X-ray investigation of fragment 1 of bovine prothrombin. *J. Mol. Biol.* **114:** 575.

Blake, C.C.F. 1978. Do genes-in-pieces imply proteins-in-pieces? *Nature* **273:** 267.

———. 1983. Exons—Present from the beginning? *Nature* **306:** 535.

———. 1985. Exons and the evolution of proteins. *Int. Rev. Cytol.* **93:** 149.

Cavalier-Smith, T. 1985. Selfish DNA and the origin of introns. *Nature* **315:** 283.

Craik, C.S., W.J. Rutter, and R. Fletterick. 1983. Splice junctions: Association with variation in protein structure. *Science* **220:** 1125.

Darnell, J.E. 1978. Implications of RNA. RNA splicing in evolution of eukaryotic cells. *Science* **202:** 1257.

Degen, S.J.F., R.T.A. MacGillivray, and E.W. Davie. 1983. Characterization of the cDNA and gene coding for human prothrombin. *Biochemistry* **22:** 2087.

Di Scipio, R.G., M.A. Hermodson, S.G. Yates, and E.W. Davie. 1977. A comparison of human prothrombin, factor IX, factor X and protein S. *Biochemistry* **16:** 698.

Di Scipio, R.G., M.R. Gehring, E.R. Podack, C.C. Kan, T.E. Hugli, and G.H. Fey. 1984. Nucleotide sequence of cDNA and derived amino acid sequence of human complement component C9. *Proc. Natl. Acad. Sci.* **81:** 7298.

Doolittle, R.F. 1985. The genealogy of some recently evolved vertebrate proteins. *Trends Biochem. Sci.* **10:** 233.

Doolittle, R.F., D.F. Feng, and M.S. Johnson. 1984. Computer-based characterization of epidermal growth factor precursor. *Nature* **307:** 558.

Doolittle, W.F. 1978. Genes in pieces: Were they ever together? *Nature* **272:** 581.

Gilbert, W. 1978. Why genes in pieces? *Nature* **271:** 501.

———. 1985. Genes in pieces revisited. *Science* **228:** 823.

Harlos, L., C.W.G. Boys, S.K. Holland, M.P. Esnouf, and C.C.F. Blake. 1987. Structure and order of the protein and carbohydrate domains of prothrombin fragment 1. *FEBS. Lett.* (in press).

Holland, S.K. and C.C.F. Blake. 1987. Proteins, exons and molecular evolution. *Biosystems* **20:** 181.

Holland, S.K., K. Harlos, and C.C.F. Blake. 1987. Deriving the generic structure of the fibronectin type II domain from the prothrombin Kringle I crystal structure. *EMBO J.* **6:** 1875.

Hu Kung, W.J. and A. Tulinsky. 1980. X-ray crystallographic structure determination of proteins involved in the onset of blood coagulation. *Dev. Biochem.* **8:** 81.

Irwin, D.M., K.G. Ahern, G.D. Pearson, and R.T.A. Mac-Gillivray. 1985. Characterization of the bovine prothrombin gene. *Biochemistry* **24:** 6854.

Leytus, S.P., D.C. Foster, K. Kurachi, and E.W. Davie. 1986. Gene for human factor X; a blood coagulation factor whose gene organisation is essentially identical with that of factor IX, and protein C. *Biochemistry* **25:** 5098.

Magnusson, S., T.-E. Petersen, L. Sottrup-Jensen, and H. Claeys. 1975. Complete primary structure of prothrombin: Isolation, structure and reactivity of ten carboxylated glutamic acid residues and regulation of prothrombin activation by thrombin. *Cold Spring Harbor Conf. Cell Proliferation* **2:** 123.

Nelsestuen, G.L., T.H. Zytovicz, and B.J. Howard. 1974. The mode of action of vitamin K. *J. Biol. Chem.* **249:** 6347.

Ny, T., F. Elgh, and B. Lund. 1984. The structure of the human tissue type plasminogen activator gene: Correlation of intron and exon structure to functional and structural domains. *Proc. Natl. Acad. Sci.* **81:** 5355.

Olsson, G., L. Andersen, O. Lindquist, L. Sjölin, S. Magnusson, T.E. Petersen, and L. Sottrup-Jensen. 1982. A low resolution model of fragment 1 from bovine prothrombin. *FEBS Lett.* **145:** 317.

Orgel, L. and F.H.C. Crick. 1980. Selfish DNA: The ultimate parasite. *Nature* **284:** 604.

Park, C. and A. Tulinsky. 1986. Three-dimensional structure of the Kringle sequence: Structure of prothrombin fragment 1. *Biochemistry* **25:** 3977.

Patthy, L., M. Trexler, Z. Vali, L. Banyai, and A. Varadi. 1984. Kringles: Modules specialised for protein binding. *FEBS Lett.* **171:** 131.

Plutzky, J., J.A. Hoskins, G.L. Long, and G.R. Crabtree. 1986. Evolution and organization of the human protein C gene. *Proc. Natl. Acad. Sci.* **83:** 546.

Reanney, D.C. 1979. RNA splicing and polynucleotide evolution. *Nature* **277:** 598.

Rossmann, M.G., D. Moras, and K.W. Olsen. 1974. Chemical and biological evolution of a nucleotide binding protein. *Nature* **250:** 194.

Südhoff, T.C., J.L. Goldstein, M.S. Brown, and D.W. Russell. 1985. The LDL receptor gene: A mosaic of exons shared with different proteins. *Science* **228:** 815.

Verde, P., M.P. Stopelli, P. Galeffi, P.D. Nocera, and F. Blas. 1984. Identification and primary sequence of an unspliced human urokinase poly (A)$^+$ RNA. *Proc. Natl. Acad. Sci.* **81:** 4727.

Summary

A.M. WEINER

*Department of Molecular Biophysics and Biochemistry, Yale University School of Medicine,
New Haven, Connecticut 06510*

Few meetings have been as intellectually challenging or as physically exhausting as the 1987 Symposium. The talks we heard were incredibly diverse, and so were the scientists who presented them: biophysical chemists, organic chemists, evolutionary biologists, molecular biologists, virologists, and enzymologists. However useless such professional labels may be, they serve to remind us that we attended this Symposium because we hoped to broaden our perspectives and to bring new ideas into our own research.

This Symposium on "The Evolution of Catalytic Function" was itself intended to be catalytic—and we the participants, like self-cleaving RNAs, were both catalysts and substrates. The catalytic effect was further augmented by the rather devilish (some might say diabolical) organization of the Symposium. Sessions on RNA catalysis were interspersed with molecular dynamics, and phylogenetic trees were sandwiched between protein structure and function. This interdigitation of subjects and techniques made it very difficult to *avoid* being educated—even for the more experienced *avoiders* among us.

The Bible tells us it took 6 days to create the world and that the seventh day was a day of rest. We covered 4.6 billion years of evolution in 8 days and that averages out to just about 400,000 years per minute of meeting time. We touched on almost every major topic in molecular evolution, ranging from the prebiotic synthesis of the building blocks of life in the primordial soup about 4.6 billion years ago to the recent emergence of our own species, *Homo sapiens*, less than 100,000 years ago.

No summary could possibly do justice to all of the papers, and I apologize in advance to those who may feel neglected. Instead, I will attempt to review the proceedings of this Symposium from a larger perspective. There is no better place to start than to remember the Dorcas Cummings lecture of Ernest Mayr, whose wit, energy, and wisdom at age 83 are an inspiration to us all. Mayr recalled the words of Dobzhansky that "nothing in biology makes sense except in light of evolution"—a point that is illustrated repeatedly in this volume. Whether we seek to understand the mechanism of RNA catalysis or the pathway of protein folding, an evolutionary perspective can make our experiments more powerful and can save us from the silliest of mistakes.

All references cited without a date refer to papers in this volume.

This volume begins with the prebiotic soup—as is only proper from the chemical, biological, and *culinary* point of view. Ever since Oparin's revolutionary suggestion in 1936 that the most primitive life forms would have had to be built from preexisting, prebiotically synthesized molecules, organic chemists have sought to simulate in the modern laboratory the very same conditions that are thought to have prevailed on the primitive earth. The first experiments were truly exhilarating—yields of glycine exceeding 2% were achieved simply by passing a spark discharge through a refluxing aqueous mixture of N_2, NH_3, and CH_4 (Miller). Such early success generated great optimism, and for some time, a host of prebiotic chemists (by which I mean *contemporary* chemists working on prebiotic problems) sought to extend these experiments. Plausible prebiotic pathways were soon described for a number of other amino acids, as well as for purines and pyrimidines, but then the serious problems began (Orgel; Ferris et al.). Ribose was an extremely minor condensation product of formaldehyde, and even if such sugars could be made, ribose would only condense with the nucleic acid bases to form mononucleosides under the harshest of conditions. Equally harsh conditions were required to condense the mononucleotides into typical polynucleotides or to condense the amino acids into peptides. Finally, lipids—those long aliphatic chains that were almost certainly required to form some kind of primitive membrane—never appeared in the simulated prebiotic brew. Such failures were difficult to bear, and it required courage to continue in the field.

In considering the primordial soup, perhaps the only conclusion universally agreed upon was made by Westheimer (1987) in his recent article entitled "Why Nature Chose Phosphates." Phosphate chemistry offers the best of all possible worlds for life: (1) Trivalency allows linear polymers linked by phosphodiester bonds to retain a negative charge, thereby trapping nucleic acids, mononucleotides, and many metabolites within the negatively charged phospholipid membranes, a point first made by Davis (1958) in his article "The Importance of Being Ionized." (2) Phosphoester bonds uniquely combine thermodynamic instability with kinetic stability, thereby allowing enzymes to carry out downhill reactions while preventing spontaneous hydrolysis, a point first made by F. Lipmann (1951). (3) The reversibility of phosphoester bond transfers allows phosphodiester bonds to be rearranged without additional energy input—a critical requirement for early evolution of the RNA world.

The discovery of catalytic RNA by Cech in 1981 gave the prebiotic chemists a temporary reprieve from the merciless complexity of prebiotic synthesis (for review, see Cech and Bass 1986). Now at least the chemists could concentrate on making RNA precursors and short oligoribonucleotides; the amino acids and peptides—once potentates of the prebiotic world—were dethroned. But the reprieve did not last long, because even catalytic RNA posed a terribly serious problem, and that is the danger of enantiomeric cross-inhibition (Joyce; Orgel; Schwartz et al.). Simulated prebiotic synthesis of mononucleosides (and most other biologically interesting compounds) inevitably yields equal amounts of the D and L forms, since chiral templates do not generally exist in the nonliving world. These mononucleosides would have had to condense to generate a population (or library) of oligonucleotides, before any catalytic RNA could arise. The details of such a condensation are speculative at best, but one particularly attractive scenario is that template-directed polymerization of activated mononucleotides played a critical role in building up the size and variety of the prebiotic oligonucleotide library (Orgel). An especially dramatic example of template-directed prebiotic polymerization is the ability of poly(D-C), in the presence of divalent magnesium, to direct polymerization of the D enantiomer of guanosine 5'-phospho-2-methylimidazole (D-2-MeImpG) into polymers as long as G_{50} having almost exclusively 3'-5' phosphodiester bonds (Joyce). Unfortunately, the new snag is that such prebiotic polymerizations are poisoned by precursors of the opposite handedness. This makes it exceedingly difficult to imagine how oligonucleotides large enough to be catalytically active could have arisen prebiotically. In fact, if we did not know better, we might even be forced to conclude from these results that life as we know it is impossible. Our presence here today is compelling evidence against this hypothesis.

The prebiotic chemists now agree (in the words of Orgel) that RNA is "an evolutionarily advanced molecule" and must have been preceded by "something like RNA, but simpler." The leading candidate today is a prochiral nucleic acid analog based on a glycerol-pyrophosphate backbone instead of a ribose-phosphate backbone, and having the ability (at least according to molecular dynamics calculations performed by Levitt) to form a stable base-paired duplex (Joyce et al. 1987). Now for those of us who have not attempted an organic synthesis since college or university, this is very disconcerting. How could life have gotten started on the wrong foot, with a compound so different from RNA? This line of reasoning makes it very tempting to dismiss the current state of affairs in prebiotic chemistry and to go back to the comfortable assumption that RNA as we now know it *did* arise prebiotically, one way or the other. One of these random RNA molecules would then function miraculously as a crude RNA replicase, and the purely prebiotic era would come to an end. The trouble with this assumption is that we are almost certainly assuming too much. Quarrel as we will with

the details of any particular prebiotic simulation, the general point remains that RNA is exquisitely difficult to make. And even if we assume the existence of a modern ribose-phosphate backbone in primitive RNA, we still have no good reason for supposing that the modern four bases existed at the time. More likely there were two bases, or ten, and since all modern nucleic acids use only the canonical four bases (thymine is uracil in disguise), the evidence appears to be lost forever.

My point is that we must take each other seriously. We simply cannot skip the soup and start with the main course. To put the matter differently, what is dessert for the prebiotic chemist is merely an appetizer for the molecular biologist. And herein lies the problem that this Symposium was meant to address. We are all specialists, and we naturally tend to assume (or even in weak moments to *hope*) that events outside our field will prove irrelevant to our experiments and interests. Such assumptions should be avoided, since they could be dangerous to our scientific health.

Molecular Phylogeny

The construction of evolutionary trees provides a particularly vivid example of the dangers involved in casually assuming that evolutionary issues are trivial or uncomplicated. In the section devoted to the construction of evolutionary trees, Doolittle and Feng noted that the alignment of distantly related (and especially *un*related!) sequences is not simple and can strongly bias the resulting tree. In addition, evolutionary trees can be "steered to the left" by addition of a distant relative to the dataset and "steered to the right" by addition of a close relative. These somewhat light-hearted words seemed especially poignant, given the serious dispute between those who follow Woese (Pace et al. 1986) in using 16S ribosomal RNA sequences to divide all life into the three kingdoms of eubacteria, archaebacteria, and eukaryotes (Olsen) and those who advocate an alternative formulation based on rRNA gene organization which results in five kingdoms not including archaebacteria (Lake).

Further complications in the construction of trees arise because rates of sequence evolution are clearly nonconstant (Li et al.; Penny et al.), and because the evolution of certain gene families cannot be reconstructed without a major experimental commitment to characterizing gene organization in nonstandard (some would say obscure) organisms that are not usually subjected to experimental investigation. For example, the evolution of vertebrate blood coagulation can only be reconstructed by analyzing the proteins present in cyclostomes such as the lamprey, and the analysis might benefit by examining the even more primitive protochordates (Doolittle and Feng). Likewise, the evolutionary history of the mammalian fetal globin genes has benefitted from the compilation of sequences for over 400 globin chains and 100 globin genes, ranging as far back as elasmobranches like the shark (Goodman et al.). Finally, striking evidence for convergent evolution can make the construction of trees even more perilous (Stewart and Wilson). Lysozyme *c*, a bacteriolytic enzyme present in many tissues as well as in tears and milk, has twice been recruited as a digestive enzyme (once in the cow, and once in the colobine monkeys). The newly recruited lysozymes exhibit convergent evolution driven by positive Darwinian selection for adaptation to the acidic, pepsin-containing environment of the stomach.

Intriguing experimental evidence has also been accumulating for a "male-driven" view of mammalian evolution (Miyata et al.). The idea here is that mutations resulting from errors in DNA replication would accumulate more rapidly in sperm than in eggs, since sperm are the product of a far greater number of cell divisions. If true, male animals would supply a greater fraction of natural variation than females—a dubious distinction if most mutations are neutral or harmful.

Since phylogenetic comparisons have become the stock in trade for many of us—regardless of field—I suspect that nonphylogeneticists were somewhat disturbed to discover that the construction of a tree not only involves a lot of judgment and some art, but is also exquisitely sensitive to the quality and variety of the available data. Gilbert went so far as to suggest that "evolutionary trees reflect the will of the person who constructed them"—strong language indeed, but perhaps more realistic than many of us would like to admit.

Catalytic RNA

The discovery of catalytic RNA has of course transformed much of molecular biology, as well as the ways we think about the origins of life, and four different kinds of catalytic RNAs were examined: self-splicing group I and group II introns, RNase P, self-cleaving "hammerhead" structures, and the splicing of mRNA precursors. The group I and group II self-splicing introns are found in such diverse locations as the genes for ribosomal RNA in the ciliate *Tetrahymena* and many genes within fungal mitochondria (Been et al.; Kay and Inoue; Davis et al.; Michel and Jacquier, Doudna et al.; Tabak et al.; Peebles et al.). Cech (Been et al.) reviewed his earlier experiments showing that the excised linear intron could function as a poly(C) polymerase, and we were alerted to the fact that two laboratories (Been et al.; Doudna et al.) are hard at work trying to transform the *Tetrahymena* intron by sophisticated genetic engineering into a template-dependent RNA polymerase. These polymerases would use random oligonucleotides as a source of activated nucleotides to faithfully copy an RNA template. The motivation for these experiments is to show that it is *not utterly inconceivable* for prebiotically synthesized oligonucleotides to have functioned as an enzyme capable of assembling other shorter oligonucleotides into faithful copies of a template. Supposing these efforts

are successful—and at least in my mind there is little doubt that they will be—what will the rest of us make out of these experiments in *de*evolution? For the skeptics, little will have been accomplished, but for those who are wise (or foolish) enough to adopt a more flexible standard of evidence, it will be clear that these experiments bring us closer to understanding the origins of life.

Now lest the idea of an RNA molecule copying itself strike anyone as a stylish fantasy devised by those who are inebriated with the potential of catalytic RNA, I wish to quote from a 1968 paper by Francis Crick (1968). In considering how sufficiently large RNA molecules could have arisen to carry out primitive protein synthesis, Crick wrote:

> For all we know, the structure of the large rRNA molecules may have been partly repetitive. These repetitions might have been produced rather easily if there were an RNA replicase available. Possibly the first "enzyme" was an RNA molecule with replicase properties. Thus a system based mainly on RNA is not impossible. Such a system could then start to synthesize protein and thus could evolve very rapidly by natural selection.

RNase P was the second catalytic RNA to be discovered. A provisional tertiary structure for this large, phylogenetically variable RNA was described, and evidence was presented suggesting that the main role of the RNase P C5 protein is to function as a "salt puddle" to neutralize the negative charge of the RNA backbone of both enzyme and substrate, thereby enabling the substrate to approach the enzyme even in low salt (Pace et al.). This is such a simple role that even a crude positively charged protein, made by a very unsophisticated translation apparatus, might have played the part (Maizels and Weiner). Thus, the role of the C5 protein in RNase P may be a paradigm for how the RNA world (Gilbert; Benner et al.) began to make the transition to the ribonucleoprotein or RNP world. Evidence was also presented showing that the minimal substrate for RNase P may be as simple as a stem-and-loop structure with a 3′-terminal CCA sequence (Lawrence et al.). If RNase P is in fact an ancient enzyme, such substrate specificity suggests that the first tRNA-like structures were very much simpler than those we know today.

The self-cleaving "hammerhead" structures first discovered in plant viroids (Forster et al.) have now been found more recently and mysteriously in Satellite 2 of the newt *Notopthalmus viridescens* (Epstein and Gall). A mere 13 positions within the hammerhead structure must be conserved for self-cleavage; when the hammerhead is reconstituted in vitro from two separate oligonucleotides (a 19-mer and a 24-mer), the 24-mer is cleaved and the 19-mer is released unchanged (Samson et al.). The existence of this—"the world's smallest ribozyme" consisting of only 19 nucleotides—makes the first template-dependent RNA polymerase a good deal less *im*plausible. Perhaps we are not merely lucky to be alive, but likely to be so. It is even possible that life on this planet was *inevitable*.

Nuclear mRNA splicing was likely to have evolved from group II self-splicing introns (Sharp et al.; Frendewey et al.). Both kinds of introns are excised by a lariat mechanism, the splice junction sequences are vaguely similar, and in each case the lariat is formed when the 5′ splice site is attacked by the 2′-OH of a bulged A (A*) residing within a sequence resembling UACUA*AC (Peebles et al.). Seen in this light, splicing functions that were originally performed by the group II intron itself in *cis* might now be performed by the snRNAs in *trans*. Perhaps the snRNAs can be thought of as a group II intron in pieces, and the mRNA spliceosome as Nature's way of reassembling the intron from its parts. In this extreme view, the proteins that complex with snRNAs to form the small nuclear ribonucleoprotein particles (snRNPs) function to fine tune yet another instance of RNA catalysis.

Our understanding of how RNA can do what it does depends on a detailed knowledge of RNA anatomy. The most commonly used rules for RNA base pairing have been carefully refined for maximum predictive power (Turner et al.) and intricate RNA structural motifs like pseudoknots are being subjected to physical analysis (Tinoco et al.). An impromptu talk by Klug reminded us that even yeast phenylalanine tRNA can specifically cleave itself in the presence of divalent lead cations (Brown et al. 1985). Here, the known crystal structure of the tRNA makes it possible in this *solitary* case to propose a specific mechanism for the self-cleavage reaction. A lead hydroxide ion nestled in the metal binding pocket of the tRNA serves as a general base to deprotonate the 2′-OH adjacent to the scissile bond. This mechanism also explains why divalent zinc, manganese, and magnesium are all bound, but lead alone allows catalysis: The pK_a of divalent lead falls in the neutral range (7.2), whereas the pK_a values of the other divalent metals exceed 9. (Without betraying a smile, Klug concluded his talk with these words: "Of course, as they say, 'it did not escape our notice' that RNA could function as a metalloenzyme." Only a few are entitled to invoke these famous words, and in this case, it was entirely appropriate.)

Protein Synthesis

The section devoted to ribosomes—the most sophisticated RNA machine within the cell—is particularly inspiring. Protein synthesis was very stylish in the 1960s and early 1970s, but then fell out of favor as the scope of molecular biology expanded at a breakneck pace. There were simply more interesting subjects than there were molecular biologists to study them. Fortunately, the 15-year loneliness of the ribosomologists is now over. In the words of Moore, "the discovery of catalytic RNA has made the ribosome respectable again." Noller noted drily that before this "post-ribozyme era," the idea that rRNA might be anything more than a passive

scaffold for intelligent proteins was "condemned to play to an empty house." Nomura built a careful case for catalytic RNA within the ribosome. In particular, many mutations conferring antibiotic resistance map within the rRNA itself, and deletion of many of the ribosomal proteins genes, although harmful, is not necessarily fatal.

All 21 proteins in the 30S subunit of the *E. coli* ribosome have now been localized by neutron scattering techniques (Moore). The resulting three-dimensional map is fully consistent with the immunoelectron microscopic map (Oakes et al.), as well as with the assembly pathway established earlier for ordered addition of ribosomal proteins onto rRNA (Nomura/Nomura et al.). The detailed secondary (and some tertiary) structures of 16S and 23S rRNAs have also been firmly established by phylogenetic and physical techniques, and the precise binding sites of the ribosomal proteins on the rRNA are being mapped (Noller et al; Gerbi et al.). Equally exciting, the 50S subunits of *Halobacterium halobium* have been crystallized and diffract to 5.5 Å (Yonath et al.).

Given the pace of the structural studies, it is only a matter of time before the ribosome begins to yield some of its secrets. But these studies will not reveal the detailed mechanism of protein synthesis unless we know how tRNA and mRNA bind and move during peptide bond formation and translocation. An allosteric three-site model of the ribosome was presented, strongly suggesting that the ribosome has, in addition to the P and A sites, an E or exit site for the discharged tRNA (Nierhaus et al.). The order of these three sites on the ribosome, reading 5′ to 3′ along the mRNA, would be E, P, A. The allosteric three-site model, together with the studies of "shifty" codons that cause abnormal translocation (Weiss et al.), suggests that translocation of mRNA may be a passive process: The mRNA would remain *bound* to the discharged tRNA, as well as to the peptidyl-tRNA, and would simply be dragged along when the *pair* of tRNAs moved *as a unit* from the P and A sites to the E and P sites.

Understanding the mechanism by which the largest and most complex of ribozymes is able to catalyze protein synthesis should help us to make better guesses than are currently possible about the origin of translation. In fact, the idea that the ribosome may be a ribozyme predates the discovery of catalytic RNA by over 20 years. In that same 1968 article from which I quoted earlier, Crick also wrote:

> In looking at the present-day components of the mechanism of protein synthesis, one is struck by the considerable involvement of non-informational nucleic acid. The ribosomes are mainly made from RNA and the adaptor molecules (tRNA) are exclusively RNA, although modified to contain many unusual bases. Why is this? One plausible explanation, especially for rRNA, is that RNA is "cheaper" to make than protein. If a ribosome were made exclusively of protein the cell would need *more*

ribosomes (to make the extra proteins, which would not be a negligible fraction of all the proteins in the cell) and thus could only replicate more slowly. Even though this may be true, we cannot help feeling that the more significant reason for rRNA and tRNA is that *they were part of the primitive machinery* for protein synthesis. Granted this, one could explain why their job was not taken over by protein, since (i) for rRNA, it would be too expensive, (ii) for tRNA, protein may not be able to do such a neat job in such a a small space. In fact, as has been remarked elsewhere, tRNA looks like Nature's attempt to make RNA do the job of a protein (Crick 1967).

If indeed rRNA and tRNA were essential parts of the primitive machinery, one naturally asks how much protein, if any, was then needed. It is tempting to wonder if the primitive ribosome could have been made *entirely* of RNA. Some parts of the structure, for example the presumed polymerase, may now be protein, having been replaced because a protein could do the job with greater precision. Other parts may not have been necessary then, since primitive protein synthesis may have been rather inefficient and inaccurate. Without a more detailed knowledge of the structure of present-day ribosomes it is difficult to make an informed guess.

These words are as appropriate in 1987 as in 1968. Perhaps Crick was right to go off and contemplate the human brain, while the rest of us are left behind to fill in the molecular biological details.

The section on protein synthesis and the genetic code is filled with controversial ideas. The complexity of every biological system is limited by the prevailing level of replication error and irreversible environmental damage. Such errors and damage are generally fatal for single-stranded RNA genomes, but they can be repaired in DNA genomes because the intrinsic redundancy of the duplex allows one strand to serve as template for repair of the other (Reanney). Cavalier-Smith alerted us to the unseemly preoccupation of molecular biologists with the role of information transfer in evolution (DNA makes RNA makes protein) while the role of membranes in metabolism and bioenergetics is woefully neglected. Without membranes, there would be no metabolism, no energy, and no cells. Maizels and Weiner presented a novel scheme for the origin of protein synthesis. The key idea in this "genomic tag model" was that 3'-terminal tRNA-like structures, much like those found today in RNA bacteriophage (Biebricher; Priano et al.) and plant viruses (Marsh and Hall), may have tagged primordial genomes for replication in the RNA world. Charging of these tRNA-like structures by an aberrant activity of the RNA replicase would then have provided a facile pathway for the evolution of protein synthesis. The design of the genetic code was also discussed. Ambiguity reduction clearly played a role in the evolution of the code (Fitch and Upper). The point was also made that codons generally cannot change meaning without enormous risk to the organism, although instances of "stop codon capture" show that termination codons are an exception to this rule (Jukes et al.). In addition, GC and AT pressure can strongly bias evolution of the code (Osawa et al.).

Finally, Ozeki et al. presented (fortunately in schematic form) all 121,024 nucleotides of the liverwort chloroplast genome. The lowly liverwort was chosen for this honor because it is the only plant for which *green* cell lines have been obtained, and thus the only chloroplast genome that can currently be subjected to straightforward genetic analysis in the laboratory. The organization of the chloroplast operons encoding ribosomal proteins, ribosomal RNA, RNA polymerase subunits, and ATPase left no doubt that the chloroplast is a eubacterial endosymbiont. This poses an interesting evolutionary problem, since certain chloroplast tRNA genes are split by group II self-splicing introns, whereas modern eubacteria appear to lack self-splicing introns. How then did chloroplasts acquire group II introns? One possibility is that modern eubacteria have purged themselves of the burden of introns in order to survive in a hostile world, while their endosymbiotic eubacterial relatives have had the luxury of retaining the introns because survival in the protected environment of a eukaryotic host cell presents a very different kind of challenge. Another possibility is that chloroplasts and mitochondria have acquired self-splicing introns by *horizontal* gene transfer from another phylum, mediated perhaps by a viral vector such as T4 bacteriophage, whose host range may have been broader in the past than it is now (Belfort et al.; Shub et al.).

Viruses

Although most of the material in this volume is obviously relevant to the theme of molecular evolution, the papers devoted to the replication and transcription of RNA viruses might benefit from a few words of explanation. These viruses exhibit extraordinary diversity and (at least to the nonvirologist) a baffling array of genomic structures, replication schemes, and transcriptional mechanisms. For example, $Q\beta$ is a simple plus-strand bacteriophage (Biebricher; Priano et al.); poliovirus and corona virus are plus-strand animal viruses (Paul et al.; Lai et al.); brome mosaic virus (BMV) is a segmented plus-strand plant virus (Marsh and Hall); vesicular stomatitis virus is a minus-strand animal virus (Wertz et al.); influenza is a segmented minus-strand animal virus (Krug et al.); and bunyaviruses are segmented minus-strand viruses infecting both the insect vector that transmits them as well as the mammalian host cell (Kolakofsky et al.).

Is there any method in this viral madness? Despite such very different life styles, each of these viruses shares the same preoccupation with achieving a functional separation of replication and transcription. Replication must copy the entire viral genome without loss of terminal sequences, whereas transcription must regulate expression of the viral genes. This is true even when the same polymerase carries out both replication and transcription.

What we make of the universal imperative of viral life to separate replication and transcription depends on how we view viruses. If we think of viruses as evolutionary latecomers that have somehow assembled an infectious unit from off-the-shelf parts in a highly evolved host, then we have only to marvel at how cleverly the parts of the cell can be rearranged to usurp the cell itself. Seen in this way, BMV with its 3′-terminal tRNA structures could be thought of as representing, in Hall's words, "the evolution of a timid tRNA into an RNA virus." But another more exciting view of viruses (and the RNA viruses in particular) is that they might be molecular fossils of earlier stages in cellular or even precellular evolution that have managed to *coevolve* with their ever more sophisticated hosts. Thus, the diversity of viral replicative and transcriptional strategies may be showing us the molecular biology of the gene as it existed a billion or more years ago. Supposing, then, that viruses are a valuable repository of outmoded life forms, we might (in the extreme case) think of positive single-stranded RNA viruses as fossils of the most ancient RNA world (Maizels and Weiner), negative single- and double-stranded RNA viruses as fossils of a more advanced RNP world after the primitive ribosome came into existence, retroviruses as fossils of a world in transition from RNA to DNA genomes, and double-stranded DNA viruses like SV40 as pieces of nearly contemporary chromosomes that have escaped to build a life of their own.

Protein Structure and Function

I now turn to proteins. In an evolutionary context, it is only proper to discuss RNA before proteins, but I apologize to those who still insist on thinking the old-fashioned way. The sections on protein structure and function address three main questions: (1) What do proteins look like at atomic resolution and what structural motifs are used to construct them? (2) How does the polypeptide chain fold uniquely into its lowest energy conformation? (3) How do proteins catalyze chemical reactions? These questions have obvious evolutionary interest, since evolution is simply Nature's way of groping through amino acid "sequence space" in search of stable units of protein folding and useful enzymatic activities. (The notion of amino acid sequence space was originally invented by Maynard Smith in 1961 [see Ninio 1983], and Eigen introduced sequence space early in the Symposium by discussing a mathematically tractable way of representing all possible RNA sequences as points in multidimensional space.) In fact, it becomes apparent that there is sometimes little difference between Nature's groping through sequence space and the use of site-directed mutagenesis to explore enzyme structure and function. Perhaps the major difference is that Nature can afford to be patient, whereas

useful mutations in the laboratory must be fixed and tested within the typical 5-year granting period.

Two basic philosophies have guided the experimentalists who are exploring amino acid space. In the *analytical* approach—exemplified by the studies of Hermes et al. and Alber et al. on triose phosphate isomerase, and Higaki et al. on trypsin—a nearly perfect catalyst is injured by site-directed mutagenesis, the effects are assessed, and then an attempt is made to repair the damage either by further site-directed mutagenesis or by biological selection for pseudorevertants (i.e., intragenic second site revertants). The strength of this approach is that it starts with an interesting and exceedingly well-characterized enzyme, so that interpretation of the data can be spectacularly detailed and complex. The potential disadvantage is that triose phosphate isomerase is so nearly perfect already that almost all mutations are likely to be deleterious. Because of this, the region of sequence space that can be explored is generally very limited.

In the *synthetic* approach to the exploration of amino acid sequence space—exemplified by efforts to transmute antibodies into enzymes (Tramontano et al.; Pollack and Schultz) or synthetic peptides into transmembrane ion channels (DeGrado et al.)—site-directed mutagenesis is used in an effort to transform a noncatalytic molecule (an "almost-catalyst" in Plückthun's words) into the real thing. This approach to understanding enzymatic function has the advantage that the amino acid sequence space to be explored is relatively unconstrained by preexisting structures and thus that many mutations may be advantageous for function. However, such freedom is also a potential limitation, since the experiments may have little to say about the obvious fine tuning of enzymes.

Exon Shuffling

Gilbert, W.F. Doolittle, Go and Nosaka, and Blake et al. suggest a way to reconcile the synthetic and analytic approaches to the experimental investigation of protein structure and function. To evolve a 20,000-dalton protein, Nature cannot search through all of sequence space (20^{200} possible sequences). Suppose, however, that proteins are constructed from compact domains of 15–20 amino acids roughly 30 Å in diameter. (These domains would correspond in size to the primordial exons of triose phosphate isomerase as deduced by phylogenetic comparisons of intron positions in the genes of maize, chicken, and *Aspergillus*.) Suppose further, for the sake of argument, that 20 different primordial exons were assorted and reassorted to produce a variety of proteins. Then, 20^{20} alternative sequences (or perhaps 10^6 shapes) might be a manageable number for an evolutionary search pattern. These compact domains of protein structure could have been as simple as an α-helix (Shoemaker et al.) or a calcium-binding "EF hand" (Kretsinger), or as advanced as the nucleic acid binding "zinc fingers" (Klug; Berg). In this *synthetic* phase of the evolution of a new protein, Nature would be putting together compact units of protein structure into new combinations, and asking whether any hopeful monster had emerged. Once synthetic evolution had produced a crude but marginally useful polypeptide, the *analytic* phase of evolution would take over and make smaller changes (analogous to site-directed mutagenesis) that might help to accommodate the compact domains of protein structure to each other and to fashion a more efficient active site.

In this context, it would probably be useful to make a distinction between the hypothetical primordial exons encoding compact domains of protein structure (let us call these *micro*exons) and certain contemporary exons (*macro*exons) encoding clearly defined and autonomous units of structure such as an immunoglobulin fold, an EGF-type segment (first identified in epidermal growth factor), or a proprotease "kringle" (Doolittle and Feng). The microexons, selected primarily for the ability to encode stable, compact domains of protein *structure*, would initially have been assembled by random recombination (exon shuffling) into larger genetic units encoding domains of protein *function*. Loss of introns from such genetic units would then yield macroexons, which could serve as the raw material for additional rounds of exon shuffling, ultimately yielding complex proteins with multiple domains. Further rounds of duplication and divergence could then yield even more complex structures, as exemplified by ferredoxin, soybean trypsin inhibitor, and perhaps pepsin (McLachlan).

Thus, exon shuffling really describes two simultaneous but very different kinds of genetic assembly: the de novo assembly of substantial protein domains from microexons and the subsequent reassortment of macroexons constructed from fused microexons. In both cases, exon shuffling speeds evolution by assembling preexisting units of structure and/or function. This (admittedly artificial) distinction between microexons and macroexons provides a way out of much current confusion surrounding the question of whether we should expect intron positions to coincide with the boundaries of proteins domains. The idea of exon shuffling was *originally* developed for the shuffling of macroexons, and in these instances, the introns usually do define the boundaries of recognizable proteins domains. But for the de novo assembly of new protein domains, it is quite possible that the introns will oftentimes appear *not* to fall at the boundaries of protein domains simply because we do not yet understand the rules for protein folding well enough.

Model Enzymes

Taken together, the studies of protein structure and evolution suggested that the protein chemists and the enzymologists often mimic Nature. Perhaps we would even be justified in saying that the ontogeny of experimental science recapitulates natural phylogeny. But as Mayr pointed out, we humans alone have the ability to use our minds to escape from at least some of the constraints of evolution. And indeed, at least one chemist frankly advocated the virtues of *retrograde* evolution from biotic to prebiotic metabolism. Breslow described his efforts to scan biochemistry for ways to strengthen chemistry. If methods can be found to replace the protein framework of an enzyme, but to preserve the catalytic strategy, the repertoire of useful chemical reactions might be expanded. In fact, this is the highest compliment a chemist can pay to biologists: Imitation, they say, is the sincerest form of flattery. An utterly novel variation on this theme was a successful effort to relocate the histidine of subtilisin's "catalytic triad" onto the peptide substrate itself. The resulting mutant subtilisin, with an alanine replacing the histidine at position 64, provides the first example of "substrate-assisted" catalysis: The enzyme specifically cleaves substrates at histidine, albeit inefficiently (Wells et al.).

Other enzymologists (Bruice; Frey and Moss; Jencks; Lin et al.) described model reactions designed to better understand enzyme mechanisms. In one particularly interesting case, a lysine 2,3-aminomutase from *Clostridium* was shown to use *S*-adenosylmethionine (SAM) as a primitive form of cobalamin (Moss and Frey). The ability of this especially simple modified nucleotide to serve as a cofactor in a sophisticated metabolic reaction reinforces the view originally proposed by H.B. White that cofactors, most of which are chemically related to nucleotides, are molecular fossils of primitive metabolic pathways. In fact, the "null" hypothesis (i.e., the simplest, but not necessarily the correct interpretation) would be that all cofactors resembling nucleotides are fossils of metabolic pathways that existed in the primordial world when precellular (or cellular) organisms were made also exclusively of RNA (Gilbert; Benner et al.). Now of course it could be argued that the ring structure of nucleotide cofactors so greatly extends the catalytic range of proteins that proteins would inevitably have adopted or even modified nucleotide metabolites to serve as cofactors. However, it should be remembered that in addition to having a nucleotide-related "business end," many cofactors also have an AMP "handle" (NAD and FAD, for example). Although the business end may be explained away as a recent invention, the AMP handle still smacks of an ancient RNA past.

Many participants in the Symposium were uncomfortable with even entertaining the notion that metabolism in the RNA world could have been very sophisticated. Future historians of science may be amused to note that 6 years after the discovery of catalytic RNA had pushed proteins off center stage, students of molecular evolution were still hesitant to accept the ultimate implications of this change in the prevailing paradigm. Unfortunately, the Symposium did not have the opportunity to hear experimental evidence supporting the Abstract of Shvedova et al. that a 2.5S RNA is the catalytic component of the 1,4-α-glucan branching enzyme from rabbit muscle. If substantiated, this would be the first *direct* evidence for the involvement of RNA in intermediary metabolism, and as such it would be strong evidence in favor of significant metabolism in the RNA world.

Protein Folding

A solution to "the protein-folding problem," i.e., a theoretical determination of the three-dimensional structure of a protein given only the primary sequence of the polypeptide chain, remains the Holy Grail of biophysical chemistry. Despite rapid advances in molecular dynamics, it is likely to be some time before these difficult and computationally intensive techniques can be used to determine the structure of a protein of modest size de novo (Karplus et al.). An additional problem is that most molecular biologists would not know where to find (let alone *afford*) the many hours of supercomputer time required for even the most streamlined of these programs.

Supercomputers are smart, but not superhuman, so it was encouraging to learn that the protein-folding problem, although difficult, was not infinitely complex (Ponder and Richards). Since the main chain of a polypeptide accounts for over 60% of the atoms in a protein, the individuality of each protein structure must be due entirely to the remaining 30–40% of the atoms in amino acid side chains. Most protein-folding programs start with a defined primary sequence and allow that chain to fold using empirical rules. An alternative, and very informative approach, is to turn this classical approach around. Instead of asking "What structures are compatible with a given sequence?", Ponder and Richards suggest that we try asking "What sequences are compatible with a given structure?" If the coordinates of a known crystal structure are used to fix the polypeptide backbone in space, it is possible to ask (using accepted parameters for tight packing of the amino acid side chains) how many different primary sequences could fill (i.e., be compatible with) the available internal space within the protein. Fortunately, the answer is *not many*; only 18 different amino acid sequences could substitute for the 5 amino acids at the core of crambin. Consideration of packing rules also led Ponder and Richards to the intriguing speculation that methionine might be rare because it is the most flexible of all the amino acids. Perhaps a protein containing too much methionine would be unable to fold uniquely.

Despite progress in molecular dynamics and other direct assaults on the protein folding problem, X-ray crystallography remains the best and most satisfying way to determine protein structure. A picture is really still worth 10^3 words (or perhaps 10^5 words, at current rates of exchange). Perutz et al. treated us to the most recent efforts to understand the origin of cooperativity in hemoglobin. (In the meeting, the X-ray structures of oxy- and deoxyhemoglobin came to life with the help of molecular graphics in the form of a movie that gave those present an opportunity to experience life as it must appear to Maxwell's demon.)

Conformational Change

The role of protein conformational changes in catalytic and regulatory functions received considerable emphasis. Crystallographic evidence was presented for huge movements within adenylate kinase upon substrate binding (Schulz) and for the activation of phospholipase A_2 (perhaps resulting from a conformation change) which can be induced by lipid bilayers but not by single lipid molecules below the critical micellar concentration (Achari et al.). This could be seen as a warning to those who work on catalytic RNAs that proteins (or at least individual polypeptide chains) are potentially just as flexible as the "softer" RNA structures.

The active sites of bacterial glutamine synthetase have been localized by crystallography to the *interface* between the 12 identical subunits (Eisenberg et al.). This important result has the potential to explain why many oligomeric enzymes are functional in the assembled form but not as monomers. In the particular case of glutamine synthetase, the result also suggests that the greatest possible allosteric control may be achieved by using subtle conformational changes *within* the subunits to induce much larger relative motions *between* the subunits. Movements of one subunit relative to another may also regulate ribulose bisphosphate carboxylase/oxygenase in both tobacco (Eisenberg et al.) and spinach (Branden et al.). Perhaps it is worth noting here that there is no obvious reason a priori why we should expect evolution to produce active sites that lie *within* rather than *between* the subunits of an oligomer. The greater mystery, surely, is why certain proteins oligomerize specifically in the first place (McLachlan).

A very different kind of conformational change must occur in the 23-amino-acid transmembrane domain of the aspartate receptor (*tar* protein), which is responsible for transmitting sensory information across the bacterial membrane bilayer to the flagellar motor (Thorsness et al.). Conformational changes in the *tar* protein appear to be especially subtle, since both aspartate and the maltose-binding protein can bind to the *tar* product, and the bacterium can adapt to either attractant *independently* by progressive methylation of glutamic acids within the intracellular domain of the *tar* protein. Spectacular progress in molecular neurobiology, molecular endocrinology, and the derangement of cell-growth control in neoplasias has focused attention on the molecular mechanisms of transmembrane signaling. Many of the proteins responsible for such transmembrane signaling have been (or soon will be) cloned, expressed, and subjected to site-directed in vitro mutagenesis. However, few if any of these proteins can be analyzed using the full power of genetics in vivo, where it is possible to select, rather than to screen for, interesting or rare phenotypes. For this reason, work on the genetically accessible *tar* protein is likely to be one of our best hopes for understanding the basic mechanisms of transmembrane signaling in the near future.

Protein Crystallography

Quiocho et al. presented stunning crystallographic results showing that the sulfate-binding protein of gram-negative bacteria holds the charged sulfate group using seven hydrogen bonds but not one single ionic pair. Thus, arrays of hydrogen bonds can hold charged groups with great specificity, while ultimately dispersing the charge to solvent by polarization of the protein itself. This is clearly a discovery of profound importance for understanding how proteins achieve their extraordinary specificity.

Aided and inspired by the crystal structure of DNA polymerase I (Steitz et al.) as well as by extensive site-directed mutagenesis of the enzyme (A. Polesky et al., unpubl.), Fierke et al. showed us how DNA polymerase I—which makes an error in only 1 out of every 10^8 nucleotides added—uses kinetic proofreading to balance catalytic efficiency with enzymatic selectivity. The tradeoff between speed and accuracy in enzymatic systems was also addressed from a theoretical point of view (Ninio).

Positive Selection

Finally, powerful evidence was provided for positive Darwinian selection of protease inhibitors (Creighton and Charles; Carrell et al.; Laskowski et al.) and lysozymes (Stewart and Wilson). This is potentially irritating to neutralists, who have long labored to convince the rest of us that most mutations are neutral, and thus that these mutations must be randomly fixed in the population before natural selection can work upon them. However, given a clear and pressing threat to the organism (such as microbial infection of a seed or egg) or a clear and pressing advantage (such as the ability to digest bacteria in a protorumen), advantageous mutations may be directly selected without prior fixation in the population.

Here again, experimental ontogeny appears to recapitulate natural phylogeny. Interesting mutations that confer a positive advantage on a particular research group can be directly selected by preferential funding and international attention. These mutations subsequently spread to other laboratories, and eventually become fixed in the scientific population.

This concludes my summary of the unsummarizable. I apologize once again for not having all of evolution in the proper perspective, but evolution is not yet over, and thus the papers in this volume represent only a beginning.

I would also like to thank Jim Watson on behalf of all of us for having both the foresight and courage to conceive of this Symposium and to risk bringing such disparate company together. Jim has always had a prophetic view of science—he can tell not just where science is going, but also where it *ought* to go.

REFERENCES

Brown, R.S., J.C. Dewan, and A. Klug. 1985. Crystallographic and biochemical investigation of the lead (2)-catalyzed hydrolysis of yeast phenylalanine tRNA. *Biochemistry* **24**: 4785.

Cech, T.R. and B.L. Bass. 1986. Biological catalysis by RNA. *Annu. Rev. Biochem.* **55**: 599.

Crick, F.H.C. 1967. The genetic code—yesterday, today and tomorrow. *Cold Spring Harbor Symp. Quant. Biol.* **31**: 3.
———. 1968. The origin of the genetic code. *J. Mol. Biol.* **38**: 367.

Davis, B.D. 1958. On the importance of being ionized. *Arch. Biochem. Biophys.* **78**: 497.

Joyce, G.F., A.W. Schwartz, S.L. Miller, and L.E. Orgel. 1987. The case for an ancestral genetic system involving simple analogues of the nucleotides. *Proc. Natl. Acad. Sci.* **84**: 4398.

Lippmann, F. 1951. In *Phosphorus metabolism* (ed. W.D. McElroy and H.B. Glass), vol. 1, p. 521. Johns Hopkins Press, Baltimore, Maryland.

Ninio, J. 1983. Sequence space. In *Molecular approaches to evolution*, p. 92. Princeton University Press, Princeton, New Jersey.

Pace, N.R., G.J. Olsen, and C.R. Woese. 1986. Ribosomal RNA phylogeny and the primary lines of evolutionary descent. *Cell* **45**: 325.

Westheimer, F.H. 1987. Why nature chose phosphates. *Science* **235**: 1173.

Author Index

A

Achari, A., 441
Ahmed, S.A., 537
Alber, T.C., 603
Allemann, R.K., 53
Almassy, R.J., 483
Altman, S., 233
Andachi, Y., 777
Andersson, I., 491
Ares, Jr., M., 709
Arnberg, A.C., 213
Ashley, G.W., 587
Atkins, J.F., 687

B

Bakker, C.G., 37
Baldwin, R.L., 391
Barfod, E.T., 147
Barlow, P., 441
Bartkiewicz, M., 233
Bartlett, P.A., 83
Been, M.D., 147
Beese, L., 465
Behlen, L.S., 267
Belfort, M., 181
Bellocq, C., 373
Benatan, E.J., 223
Benkovic, S.J., 91, 631
Benner, S.A., 53
Berg, J.M., 579
Biebricher, C.K., 299
Blacklow, S.C., 597
Blake, C.C.F., 925
Boswell, D.R., 527
Brändén, C.-I., 491
Breslow, R., 75
Brimacombe, R., 665
Broni, B., 353
Bruice, T.C., 567
Brünger, A.T., 381
Brunie, S., 441
Burke, J.M., 147

C

Carrell, R.W. 527
Carter, P., 647
Cascio, D., 483
Cavalier-Smith, T., 805
Cech, T.R., 147
Chandry, P.S., 181
Changchien, L.-M., 695
Chapman, M.S., 483
Charles, I.G., 511
Cherry, J.M., 173
Chothia, C., 399
Craik, C.S., 615
Creighton, T.E., 511
Cunningham, B.C., 647
Czelusniak, J., 875

D

Davenport, Jr., R.C., 603
Davies, R.W., 165
Davis, N., 367
Davis, P.W., 135
DeGrado, W.F., 521
DiRenzo, A.B., 267
Dock-Bregeon, A.C., 113
Doolittle, R.F., 869
Doolittle, W.F., 907
Doudna, J.A., 173
Dunn, D.M., 687

E

Eigen, M., 307
Eisenberg, D., 483
Elber, R., 381
Ellington, A.D., 53
Epstein, L.M., 261
Estell, D.A., 647

F

Fairman, R., 391
Feng, D.F., 869
Fermi, G., 555
Ferris, J.P., 29
Fierke, C.A., 631
Fitch, W.M., 759
Fleming, J.O., 359
Forster, A.C., 249
Freemont, P.S., 465
Freier, S.M., 123
Frendewey, D., 287
Frey, P.A., 571
Friedman, J.M., 465
Fukuzawa, H., 791

G

Gall, J.G., 261
Ge, L., 53
Gerber, A.S., 173
Gerbi, S.A., 709
Gesteland, R.F., 687
Giammona, D.A., 603
Giannousis, P.P., 83
Gibson, B.W., 615
Gilbert, W., 901
Glasfeld, A., 53
Glockshuber, R., 105
Gō, M., 915
Gold, H., 233
Goodman, M., 875
Gott, J.M., 193
Grabowski, P.J., 277
Graycar, T.P., 647
Grivell, L.A., 213
Guerrier-Takada, C., 233

H

Hall, T.C., 331
Hanson, J.E., 83
Hardin, C.C., 135
Harlos, K., 925
Hayashida, H., 863
Henderson, I.M., 857
Hendy, M.D., 857
Hermes, J.D., 597
Higaki, J.N., 615
Ho, S.P., 521
Holland, S.K., 925
Howard, M.B., 367

I

Inokuchi, H., 791
Inoue, T., 159

J

Jacquier, A., 201
Jaeger, J.A., 123
James, B.D., 239
Janda, K., 91
Jang, S.-K., 343
Janson, C.A., 483
Jarrell, K.A., 223
Jeffries, A.C., 249
Jencks, W.P., 65
Jeppesen, C., 709
Johnson, K.A., 631
Joyce, G.F., 41
Jukes, T.H., 769, 777
Jurka, J., 407

K

Karplus, M., 381
Kato, I., 545
Kay, P.S., 159
Keck, J.G., 359
Keller, W., 287
Kierzek, R., 123
Kim, P.S., 391
Klug, A., 473
Knight, S., 491
Knowles, J.R., 597
Kohchi, T., 791
Kohr, W.J., 545
Kolakofsky, D., 373
Konarksa, M.M., 277
Koop, B.F., 875
Koshland, Jr., D.E., 1, 623
Krämer, A., 287
Kramer, F.R., 321
Krauch, T., 53
Kräusslich, H.-G., 343
Kretsinger, R.H., 499
Krug, R.M., 353
Kuchta, R.D., 631

Kuhn, R.J., 343
Kuma, K., 863
Kuriyan, J., 381
Kwakman, J.H.J.M., 213

L

Lai, M.M.C., 359
Lake, J.A., 675, 839
Lamond, A.I., 277
Laskowski, Jr., M., 545
Lawrence, N., 233
Leanz, G.F., 53
Lee, C.-K., 343
Lehman, N., 769
Leonard, K.R., 729
Lerner, R.A., 91
Lesk, A.M., 399
Li, W.-H., 847
Liddington, R.C., 555
Lin, A.I., 587
Lindqvist, Y., 491
Lolis, E., 603
Longfellow, C.E., 123
Lorimer, G., 491
Luisi, B., 555

M

MacPherson, L.J., 53
Maizels, N., 743
Makino, S., 359
Marciniak, R., 277
Marlowe, C.K., 83
Marsh, L.E., 331
Matthews, C.R., 537
McClain, W.H., 233
McLachlan, A.D., 411
Michel, F., 201
Miles, E.W., 537
Miller, S.L., 17
Mills, D.R., 321
Mitsuyasu, K., 863
Miyata, T., 863
Moazed, D., 695
Moore, P.B., 721
Moras, D., 113
Moroney, S., 53
Moss, M.L., 571
Mowbray, S.L., 623
Muto, A., 769, 777

N

Nakahigashi, K., 791
Napper, A.D., 91
Nicklin, M., 343
Nierhaus, K.H., 665
Ninio, J., 639
Noller, H.F., 695

943

Subject Index

A

Accessible surfaces of proteins, 400
Acetamidophenyl ester
  in catalytic hydrolysis, 94
  as transition-state analog, 94
Active site, 1–7
  of adenylate kinase, 432
  of bovine trypsin inhibitor, 515
  conservation of during evolution, 403
  of DNA polymerase, 465
  of glutamine synthetase, 483–489
  location of, 72
  of RuBisCO, 483
  of serine proteases, 615–620, 647–652
  of TIM, 607
    location of, 605
    mutations in, 609–612
Active transport, 453
  origins of, 811, 817–818
Actomyosin
  catalytic efficiency of, 637
  free energy profile of, 637
Adaptation of stomach enzymes, 891–899
Adaptive evolution, of lysozyme, 891–899
Adenine nucleotides, 429
S-Adenosylcobalamin
  in lysine-2′3′-aminomutase, 571–577
  in ribonucleotide reductase, 587–596
Adenovirus
  E1A proteins, 581
  pre-mRNA splicing substrates, 288
Adenylate kinase, 429–435
  similarity plot of structures, 432
  variants of, 432
Alignment
  of adenylate kinase structures, 430–435
  of globin nucleotide sequences, 882–885
  progressive, 870
  of protease inhibitors, 530–531
  of serpin sequences, 530–531
Allosteric control, 450, 555
Allosteric theory in hemoglobin, 563
Amino acid
  biosynthesis, 408
  composition
    of β-turns, 407
    constraints due to genomic composition, 780
    extensions in trypsin and spleen inhibitor, 511–512
  prebiotic synthesis of, 18–20
  replacements, 879, 891–899
  sequence homology
    of adenylate kinases, 429–433
    of antitrypsin and antithrombin, 528

in blood-clotting proteins, 871
to bovine trypsin inhibitor, 516
divergence in, 399
of globins, 875–889
of glutamine synthetases, 484–486
of ovomucoid, 547
in serpins, 530–531
sequence of tryptophan synthase α subunit, 538
Aminoglycosides, 706
Anacystis nidulans, 762
  relationship to green plant chloroplast, 826
Angiotensin, 528–532
Antibodies, 4
  as catalysts, 91–97
  design of, 105
  as enzyme mimics, 77
  expression of, 106
  in stabilization of transition state, 97
Antibody-catalyzed reactions
  kinetics of, 99–102
  rates of, 99–102
  specificity of, 101
Anticodon
  CNN and GNN, 783
  codon interactions
    effects on genomic composition, 782
    evolution of arginine CGN codon, 772
    in frame shifting, 687
    phylogenetic differences, 775
    primitive thermodynamics, 745
    in rRNA 1400 site, 679
    wobble rules, 769–770, 782
  evolution, 759–775
  inosine in, 771
  loop
    cleavage, 115, 120
    conformation, 113
    dimerization, 113, 118
    flexibility, 117
    methylation, 115
Antigens, design of, 96
Antiplasmin, 530–531
Antithrombin, 530–532
α1-antitrypsin, 527–535
Anion hole, of adenylate kinase, 438
Anion protein interactions, 438
Arabinose, complex with binding protein, 454
L-Arabinose-binding protein, 453–456
Archaebacteria, 234, 825–845
  in cellular origin, 904
  in evolution, 806, 812–815
Architectural motifs. *See* Helix; Loop; Protein structure; Secondary structure
Arginine, in lysozyme adaptation, 897
Artificial enzymes, 75–80
Aspartate transcarbamylase, 582

Aspartyl-proline bond, in lysozyme adaptation, 891–894
Autonomous folding units, 391. *See also* Domains; Protein folding

B

Bacillus stearothermophilus, 729
Bacillus subtilis, ribonuclease P, 239
Bacterial genome
  codon usage, 778, 785
  composition, 777
  constraints on amino acid composition, 780
  GC-rich species, 778
Barley Z protein, 530–531
Bacteriophage Qβ
  genome evolution, 316, 329
  mechanism of RNA synthesis, 321
  mutant production equation, 303
  quasi-species distribution, 299, 303
  sequence heterogeneity, 302
Bacteriophage T4 introns, 187
  evolutionary origin, 187
  in thymidylate synthase gene, 181–197
Baculoviruses, 354
α/β Barrel structure
  in glycolate oxidase, 492
  in other enzymes, 605
  in RuBisCO, 487, 494–496
  in TIM, 604
Basic genes, of chloroplast, 791
Bestatin, 88
β-Sheets, conformational flexibility of, 401
β-Turns, as structural elements, 407–410
Binding energy
  in catalysis, 67
  in phosphonate ester inhibitors, 84
Binding functions of protein domains, 930
Binding pocket of antibodies, 95
Binding proteins
  arabinose-, 453
  calcium-, 459–462. *See also* Calcium-binding proteins
  galactose-, 453, 461
  interactions with ionic substrates and ligands, 453–462
  maltose, 627–629
  mononucleotide-, 429–437
  sulfate-, 453, 456–458
Binding specificity in immune system, 91–95
Bioenergetics, evolution of, 805–824
Biological classifications, 843
  karyotes and parkaryotes, 844–845
Biological information, 307
Biomimetic chemistry. *See* Artificial enzymes

945

DATE DUE

DEMCO 38-297